HOLISTIC MIDWIFERY

A COMPREHENSIVE TEXTBOOK FOR MIDWIVES IN HOMEBIRTH PRACTICE

VOLUME II

CARE OF THE MOTHER AND BABY FROM THE ONSET OF LABOR THROUGH THE FIRST HOURS AFTER BIRTH

SECOND EDITION

ANNE FRYE, CPM
BA HOLISTIC MIDWIFERY

ILLUSTRATED BY RHONDA BAKER
WITH OVER ONE-THOUSAND, SIX-HUNDRED DRAWINGS

FOREWORD TO THE FIRST EDITION BY ELIZABETH DAVIS, CPM
INTRODUCTION TO THE FIRST EDITION BY ROBBIE DAVIS-FLOYD, PHD

LABRYS PRESS, PUBLISHER
A DIVISION OF MATRIX MIDWIFERY ENTERPRISES, LTD.
PORTLAND, OREGON

First edition, 5,408 copies
Second edition, 4,000 copies
Printed in the United States of America by Sheridan Books, Inc., Chelsea, MI

ISBN (paperback): 978-1-891145-67-4

Library of Congress Control Number: 98-104092

Cover photography: Joy Jech, CPM, LDM, Birth Photographer, www.blossommidwifery.com

Other publications by Anne Frye and Labrys Press:

HOLISTIC MIDWIFERY, A COMPREHENSIVE TEXTBOOK FOR MIDWIVES IN HOMEBIRTH PRACTICE:
VOL. I: CARE DURING PREGNANCY
UNDERSTANDING DIAGNOSTIC TESTS IN THE CHILDBEARING YEAR
HEALING PASSAGE: A MIDWIFE'S GUIDE TO THE CARE AND REPAIR OF THE TISSUES INVOLVED IN BIRTH
UNDERSTANDING FEMALE PELVIC ANATOMY IN 3D DVD, program and 5 short vignettes describing selected soft tissue regions of the female pelvis.

For more information or customer service please contact:
Labrys Press, 7528 NE Oregon St., Portland, OR 97213 USA
(503) 255-3378, FAX (503) 255-1474, www.midwiferybooks.com, midwiferybooks@gmail.com

Errata: Errata can be posted to the website using the contact form provided there. Noted errors, omissions and corrections can be found there as well.

This edition is a high quality paperback. It is constructed of archival quality acid-free paper. It has a sew-wrap binding, the finest binding money can buy. To open it for the first time: lay the book on a table. Lift the entire book, leaving the spine flat on the table. Gently open it in the center, laying each side on the table. Close the book. Pick it up as before and divide the first half of the pages in half and open them completely, then do the same on the other side. Do this in several places throughout the book. This gently breaks in the binding. Should you discover any defects in materials or workmanship please report them as soon as they are noted.

COPYRIGHT INFORMATION AND HISTORY OF PUBLICATION

In researching copyright information for my own writing, I have become acutely aware of the need for a clear and accurate history of copyright in every text, although this is rarely done. The only person who can provide that is the author. Therefore, to make it easier for future generations to reuse and republish this work, should they deem it worthy of such attention, I offer this history of copyright for their benefit.

The conception of this textbook began in late 1979 as a handout in workbook form that was used as the primary workbook for a five-day midwifery skills workshop sponsored by Informed Homebirth, then headquartered in Boulder, Colorado. Accompanying it were manuals entitled "Lab Work for Midwives" and "Suturing for Midwives," both written by Anne Frye and "Complications of Labor and Delivery" and "Herbs for Midwives," both written by Valerie Hobbs. Beginning in 1980, these workshops were co-taught by these midwives across the United States. During this period, the lab work, herbal suturing manuals were enthusiastically received by those attending the workshops, so much so that requests for copies came in from the midwifery community at large. In response, overruns were printed and sold through Moonflower Birthing Supply in Boulder, Colorado. However, only these three manuals made it to the general midwifery public, the main manual, consisting of a master workbook, being less complete, was never published for circulation outside the participants in the workshops. By 1984, times had changed, Informed Homebirth had changed, Anne and Valerie's lives had changed and the call for these workshops had diminished as more formal educational settings began to be established for independent midwifery. The workshop manuals sold out. Since the workshops were no longer being offered, the manuals were not reprinted, but the demand for them steadily increased, leading to the revision, expansion and evolution of Anne's written work. The comprehensive textbook has waited all these years to come into being.

Manuscript and copyright history

"Informed Homebirth Midwifery Skills Workshop Manual, Days 1, 2, 3, 5," unregistered copyright 1980, by Informed Homebirth, never available to the public, with contributions by Anne Frye and Valerie Hobbs. This manual was the original seed of HOLISTIC MIDWIFERY. However, the book you hold in your hands, as well as Volume I, differ so much from these original manuals that I considered the difference too great to count the first printing of HOLISTIC MIDWIFERY as a second edition. Therefore, the copyright on HOLISTIC MIDWIFERY does not start with this manual.

At the termination of my formal relationship with Informed Homebirth, ownership of the workshop manuscripts was turned over to Anne. In 1996, Anne incorporated Matrix Midwifery Enterprises, Ltd, and started doing business as Labrys Press. The corporation became active on January 1, 1997. At that time, the copyright was transferred to the business, and copyright registrations for all subsequent publications began to be filed with the US Copyright Office in Washington DC in the name of Labrys Press.

HOLISTIC MIDWIFERY, VOLUME I: CARE DURING PREGNANCY, was first published September 1, 1995, under an unregistered copyright. Copyright for this title was registered September 16, 1997, reg. no. TX-4-636-668. This copyright covers the entire textbook, including all illustrations (although the illustrations are not specifically mentioned in the copyright registration information).

HOLISTIC MIDWIFERY, VOL. I was revised and reprinted in 1998 under an unregistered copyright. Revisions were primarily typographical, with a few technical corrections and minor content expansion. They were not deemed substantial enough to warrant reregistration of copyright.

HOLISTIC MIDWIFERY, VOLUME II: CARE OF THE MOTHER AND BABY DURING LABOR THROUGH THE FIRST HOURS AFTER BIRTH, went to press in October of 2004. Copyright for this title was registered as soon a copies of the book were available to send in with the application.

To all my teachers and friends in the childbirth community, without whom I would be at a great loss

Thank you.

TABLE OF CONTENTS

FOREWORD

While hard at work on the fourth edition of HEART & HANDS: A MIDWIFE'S GUIDE TO PREGNANCY AND BIRTH, I was thrilled that Anne agreed to let me see and utilize information from the manuscript pages of this text. We have been friends for many years–we met in 1978, when she was my student at the now defunct Holistic Childbirth Institute in San Francisco, CA–and have enjoyed working together on many occasions for the preservation and advancement of midwifery. I particularly recall working on a revision of the MANA Core Competencies document with her and being struck by the depth of her integrity and compassion for birthing women.

As I read deeper and deeper into this manuscript, my overwhelming reaction was that, if awards were given for texts such as these, Anne surely deserved one. Her thorough and innovative research has led her to core information on the physiology of birth–for example, on the cardinal movements of the baby and mechanisms of newborn stabilization–that I have not seen in any other contemporary textbook. At all times, she has been exhaustively inclusive and yet discriminating in suggesting appropriate responses to labor and birth complications. In fact, here is where I see the greatest evolution in her work since Volume I: in the maturation of both her understanding and her ability to articulate complex concepts incisively.

A stellar example is Anne's chapter on shoulder dystocia. She first clarifies the problem with relevant anatomy and physiology, and then elucidates a variety of treatments and their respective efficacy according to the situation. Other texts merely give a list of possibilities that leaves the reader wondering where to begin–and anyone who has handled this complication knows that time is of the essence!

For this and many other reasons, I consider this an excellent text for student midwives. Throughout, students are given concrete ways to interact with the information; for example, directions for finding the biparietal dimension on their own head, or for holding a doll and pelvis against their own body to better understand the left and right of fetal position. Terms are vividly described; for example, the meninges are characterized as fitting against brain tissue like a glove, with fingers encapsulating sections of gray matter. And the text is well organized, laying a solid foundation in all mechanisms of cephalic descent before treating the complexities of the breech. Her outstanding chapter on breech birth features tables the like of which I have never seen, showing what is happening with each part of the baby's body at every stage of descent.

Above all else, Anne's book heralds a return to what is truly natural in birth, what is physiologic. It represents the appreciation that, to some extent, midwifery has failed its mission by becoming increasingly, and sometimes carelessly, interventive. Anne teaches us to look deeper, and to understand that all we do–no matter how well intentioned or holistic–must be considered an intervention. She reminds us in her very style of presenting information that our primary charge is to do no harm. She encourages us to use our intuition, our gut, our compassion. She cautions us to be constantly aware of personal issues, shortcomings or shortsightedness that can influence how we do our work.

In short, this treasure trove of information is unmatched for breadth and depth by any other midwifery or obstetrical text. It is essential reading for every student and every practitioner, no matter how seasoned.

Any midwifery program worth its salt must midwife the midwife, and any decent midwifery text must do the same. To my dear friend and beloved sister in midwifery, I have but two last words to say: mission accomplished!

Elizabeth Davis, BA, CPM
Co-director, National Midwifery Institute, Inc.
Author, HEART & HANDS: A MIDWIFE'S GUIDE TO PREGNANCY AND BIRTH

PREFACE

In this new edition, many technical errors and typos have been corrected and some new and updated information has been added, however the main content remains largely unchanged. This book has been widely successful in its first edition and I trust will continue to serve as a resource to the community for years to come. The balance of this preface appeared in the first edition.

This book continues the three-volume series begun with HOLISTIC MIDWIFERY, VOL. I. In writing Volume I, I knew I was doing something unique and that made it relatively easy, as most texts devote but few pages to prenatal care. In writing this volume, I was well aware of the trend in obstetrics to devote more pages to the process of labor than any other aspect of pregnancy. I therefore felt much more internal pressure to create something that would really fill a gap in the existing literature. In doing so, I have endeavored to reinvent the modern textbook; to articulate a model of care that is truly foreign to those outside of homebirth; to show the world how midwives think, how we process at a birth and what leads us to respond the way we do. It is my hope that by writing these things down that our standard of care will be better understood and respected. In addition, I wanted to remind us all of our roots and what can be accomplished without the use of machines and other technologies that separate us from the organic process of birth. The result is several books in one: labor handbook, skills handbook, newborn handbook, plus a wealth of information on complex birthing and neonatal situations. It includes all this because midwives working at home must be well-versed in many more aspects of care than is the case for any one hospital practitioner.

I have tried to incorporate the wisdom of the many midwives who shared their insights and personal techniques with me, although this is just a smattering of the broad range of midwifery wisdom that exists. I have also relied on a variety of historical sources, because that is where the rich clinical detail that is the mainstay of the physical aspects of midwifery care is found. This may aggravate educators who want references to be "current" but the fact is, the most basic aspects of care have not changed for millennia, making much of the older material just as relevant today as it was when it was first published. Very often, these sources describe the rationale for or history of a technique or include vivid discussion of basic anatomy or physiology that is too often missing in today's texts.

Most people unfamiliar with midwifery wonder what it is that we do when birth does not go entirely smoothly. They will find plenty of answers here. Although I have been discriminating in the options I present, note that this, like the rest of my texts, is not a cookbook. I expect the reader to study and compare various options and then use those approaches and procedures that make the most sense to her and for her, considering her personal practice style and setting; her experience and training; the mother with whom she is working, and the individual birthing situation. Choices can vary widely, as can the circumstances at births. I also know that the complication that has never happened in the practice of any midwife you know can happen the very next day in your own, so I have tried to address every conceivable possibility and offer at least some information on how to handle any problem that may arise. Whenever possible, I have explained why a particular technique is or is not recommended so that midwives are well prepared to make intelligent decisions when faced with a birth that does not match any written description.

Some of the things I have included in this book will, no doubt, spark controversy. I have tried to include what might be done if the midwife is the only care provider available, with no prospects for transport. Thus I present some historical techniques that have been abandoned in favor of surgical delivery. In some cases, placenta previa comes to mind, the choices outside the hospital are all pretty grizzly. In those few cases, I have tried hard to find what appeared to be the (relatively) least harmful way of dealing with the problem under discussion and have done my best to include the risks of those interventions proposed as they were described in the historical literature. These authors had extensive experience with the hands-on techniques they discuss, and thus much wisdom was gleaned from texts for situations with which I have thankfully, never been confronted myself.

In looking over decades of English-language writings on midwifery and obstetrics, I believe I have achieved my goal of making a unique contribution to the field. I hope that you find it useful and that it helps you better serve the women and babies in your care.

September 30, 2013
Portland, OR

ACKNOWLEDGMENTS

Special thanks to the following people who helped make this book possible. Because each one made an important and unique contribution, they are listed in alphabetical order.

Ruth Ancheta for permission to adapt her drawings of women in various positions and activities during labor.
Rhonda Baker, independent midwife and artist extraordinaire, for her time, incredible talent and wholehearted commitment to getting the drawings just right
Randy Baker for formatting the dilation chart on the computer
Maggie Banks for granting permission to use her breech photos, for reviewing the chapter on breech births and for sharing her considerable wisdom and expertise with me
Diane Barnes, CNM, for loaning me her copy of THE PRINCIPLES AND PRACTICE OF OBSTETRICS by Greenhill, 1951, which was such a help in writing certain portions of the text
Cecily Bartlett for her help with German translation
Birthingway College of Midwifery students for reviewing portions of early versions of the draft
Beth Cachat for reviewing the chapters covering skull anatomy and moulding
Jill Cohen, independent midwife, for reviewing portions of the section on the cardinal movements of birth. Her recommendations prompted a major overhaul of the content resulting in a vast improvement in the text
Mary Cronk for granting permission to use her breech photos and for freely offering her wisdom in helping refine the sections on the cardinal movements of birth in breech presentations and on assisting at breech births
Elizabeth Davis, CPM, for her support, her valuable editing comments, her permission to publish her technique for turning a posterior baby and her willingness to endorse this text with her lovely foreword
Robbie Davis-Floyd, PhD, for her general support and encouragement and her eloquent introduction
Peter Dunn, MD, for sending me copies of many of his articles on physiologic neonatal transition
Doug Ehrmantraut for scanning and labeling the drawings
William Emerson, PhD, for reviewing the chapters covering skull anatomy and moulding
Karen Erlich, CPM, for reviewing the section on the cardinal movements of birth
Jane Evans for collaborating with Mary Cronk on editing the breech sections and offering her own experienced insights and wisdom on the process of breech birth
Linda Garcia, RN, for reviewing and editing the chapter on IV use
K Hindall for copyediting with great care
Abby Hoffer, CPM, for reviewing portions of the section on the cardinal movements of birth
Ed Hoffman-Smith, ND, for helping with the math to figure out the proportionate sizes of the drawings representing newborn sizes at different weights and gestational ages
Pamela Hunt, CPM, for reviewing the chapter on assisting breech births
Mary Jean Kidd for finding the perfect astrological time to send the manuscript to the printer
Shari McBride, for doing a final review and proofread of the summaries of breech descent
Judy Mercer, CNM, for reviewing the chapters on newborn anatomy and physiology and the cord chapter
Martha Morgan, for helping with German translation
George Morley, MD, for reviewing the chapters on placental transfusion and resuscitation and other portions of the text as they relate to physiologic newborn transition
Sales representatives at Orion Medical Supply, Vancouver, WA for reviewing current medical devices with me
Kathy Pollock, for her proofreading skills
Jane Poznar, RPh, for reviewing and editing the sections on allopathic pharmaceuticals
Jean Robinson for photocopying an otherwise unobtainable book for me from a UK library
Carrie Rothburd for plowing through the tough first copy editing of the first two-thirds of the text
John Schleiff, EMT, for reviewing the material on shock, IV use and oxygen equipment
Hilary Schlinger, CPM, for her content editing skills, midwifery expertise and revision suggestions
Holly Scholles, CPM, for reviewing numerous portions of the manuscript and her invaluable support
Penny Simkin for allowing me access to her files of articles and for her support
Karen Strange, CPM, for extensive review of the entire section on the cardinal movements of birth and selected chapters on anatomy and resuscitation skills and for her help and support
Last but not least, to my family and friends, for their incredible support throughout this long process

THE POSTMODERN MIDWIFE AS A SOURCE OF AUTHORITATIVE KNOWLEDGE[1]

This second volume in Anne Frye's HOLISTIC MIDWIFERY series has been long-awaited and will be widely welcomed and eagerly received by the national and international midwifery communities. Since the publication of the first volume in the series, HOLISTIC MIDWIFERY: VOLUME I: CARE DURING PREGNANCY, I have been fascinated to note that in the home-, birth-center, or hospital office of almost every midwife I have visited, three textbooks sit prominently juxtaposed on the bookshelf. On the left is WILLIAMS OBSTETRICS, the classic ob/gyn text; in the middle is VARNEY'S MIDWIFERY, the classic midwifery text for hospital-based practice; and on the right is Anne Frye's HOLISTIC MIDWIFERY Volume 1. (Perhaps the left-to-right positioning of these books is unintentional, or perhaps it represents midwives' sense of the spectrum these books encompass, from left-brained separation-based values to right-brained gestaltic and inclusive ways of thinking.) The presence of these three volumes together on one shelf clearly illustrates the broad-based and eclectic approach of what I call **the postmodern midwife**–one who balances knowledge systems, weighing each in a relative sense and choosing what works in her experience. In what follows, I will explain this concept in relation to Frye's books, because almost all midwives who read them will exemplify my definition of the postmodern midwife.

For past millennia, midwives have served women in childbirth. In premodern times, midwives were usually the only birth attendants. With the Industrial Revolution and the arrival of modernism, male physicians either replaced midwives or superceded them in the modernist medical hierarchy, leaving them with plenty of women to attend but with relatively little autonomy. "Modernism" arrived in various parts of the world at various times; first in the industrializing countries of the North, and more slowly in the colonized and exploited countries of the South. So anthropologists consider "modernism" not to be a particular point in time but rather a singular orientation toward "progress," defined in terms of Westernized forms of education, technologization, infrastructural development (highway, rail, water, and air systems etc.), factory production, economic growth, and the development of the global marketplace. This singular orientation identifies a single point in a given area toward which development should be progressing: in economics, that single point is capitalism; in health care, it is Western biomedicine. Thus in modernizing societies traditional systems of healing, including traditional and homebirth midwifery, have become increasingly regarded by members of the growing middle and upper classes as "premodern vestiges" of a more backward time that must necessarily vanish as modernization/ biomedicalization progresses. Modernist midwives, for example, tend to practice only in hospitals or clinics, to accept biomedical hierarchies of knowledge and status, to reject alternative knowledge systems, and to avoid political involvement in efforts to effect humanistic change (for examples, see Kirkham & Perkins, 1997).

Yet around the world, the singular orientations of modernization are increasingly contested in the new "postmodern" era. Postmodern thinking moves beyond uncritical acceptance of modernization as good, noting the enormous environmental, social, and cultural damage modernization entails, and seeking to generate more polymorphous societies in which multiple knowledge and belief systems can coexist and complement each other. In postmodern societies, conservation and preservation of the environment and of indigenous or traditional languages, cosmologies, health care, and economic systems take on particular urgency and importance, and such endeavors are sometimes considered to be more important than expanding the reach of industrialization, capitalism, and biomedicine.

These postmodern efforts at conservation are fueled both by global organizations and by myriad local grass-roots social movements. In the cultural arena of childbirth, for example, as governments and development planners urge the elimination of traditional birthways, some international workers seek to conserve them in various countries, and many indigenous women who have tried out government-funded hospitals and clinics reject the impersonal care they receive there, and deliberately return to traditional midwives and out-of-hospital birth (Barnes-Josiah et al.,1998; Kolenda 1998; Davis-Floyd 2000). And while in some regions, professional midwives trained in a modernist ideology of biomedical superiority act, in fact, superior, in others both professional and traditional midwives are displaying a variety of creative and highly relativistic responses to biomedical encroachment and constraints (for examples, see Kroeger 1996; Davis-Floyd 2003; Davis-Floyd, Cosminsky, & Pigg 2001; Dieteker 2005).

Informed relativism: the characteristics of the postmodern midwife

Around the world we are witnessing the emergence of a phenomenon that I call "postmodern midwifery"–a term aimed at capturing precisely those aspects of contemporary midwifery practice that fall outside the easy distinctions between traditional birthways, professional midwifery, and modern biomedicine. With this term, I am trying to make salient the qualities emergent in the practice, the discourse, and the political engagement of a certain kind of contemporary midwife–one who often constructs a "radical critique" (Marcus, 1993) of unexamined conventions and narrow assumptions. Postmodern midwives as I define them are educated, articulate, organized, political, and highly conscious of both their cultural uniqueness and their global importance. In other words, by "postmodern midwife" I specifically do not mean midwives who uncritically accept either their own ethno-obstetric system or that of biomedicine, but rather midwives who fully understand these in a relative way, as different ways of knowing about birth, discrepant systems that often conflict but can be complementary.

The postmodern midwife is scientifically informed: she knows the limitations and strengths of the biomedical system and of her own, and moves fluidly between them to serve the women she attends. She plays with the paradigms, working to ensure that the uniquely woman-centered dimensions of midwifery are not subsumed by biomedicine. She is a shape-shifter–she knows how to subvert the medical system while appearing to comply with it, a bridge-builder, creating collaborations with biomedicine where possible, and a networker.

Lacking or actively rejecting a sense of structural inferiority to biomedicine, she is free to observe the benefits of traditional midwifery practices common in many cultures such as massage, external version, eating and drinking during labor, birthing in upright positions, birthing at home, and uninterrupted contact between mother and baby, all of which have been scientifically validated. She compares these with what she sees in the hospital and what she learns of the scientific evidence presented here and elsewhere, concludes that there is value in the midwifery approach that biomedicine does not recognize, and develops both a vision and a sense of mission around preserving that approach in the face of biomedical encroachment. She works with the resources at hand, such as this book, to accomplish this mission. When she can, she travels to attend regional, national, and international conferences on childbirth and midwifery; at such conferences she increases her ability to translate between systems and makes connections with midwives in other parts of the world, learning the meaning of midwifery as a social movement and how to create networks of communication to unite midwives in her region and beyond. Through such transnational interlinkages, she works to create a global culture of midwifery as well as to preserve, carry forward, and teach to others the best of her own cultural traditions around birth.

The postmodern midwife often feels spiritually "called" to midwifery, and regards this calling as an additional impetus to the sense of vision and mission she develops. She understands the worldwide role of obstetricians in eliminating or subordinating midwives and discounting their knowledge, and has a sense of relationship to midwifery history and her personal role in continuing it. The postmodern midwife desires and values many forms of education, constantly seeking to learn more in order to better serve the women she attends. She works to assure that the education she receives will serve not to further coopt midwifery into medicine, but to add to midwifery's knowledge base and to improve and publicize its intrinsic worth. She constructs her own midwifery knowledge and that of her community as a primary and valuable source of authoritative knowledge (Jordan 1993, Part 2) in ways that make it available to others, through writing pamphlets, articles, and books (as Frye has done), and by offering seminars to local, regional, or transnational midwives through which she can share this knowledge by speech and bodily demonstration. In so doing, she invents ways to make discrepant knowledge systems complementary. She is proud of her strength in organization, which her ancestor midwives were often unable to achieve. She understands that ***for a midwife, the professional is always political***, and that she and her colleagues must have an organized political voice if they are to survive. So she works to build midwifery organizations in her community, to join national and international midwifery organizations, and to work with them for policies and legislation that support midwives and the mothers they attend.

It would be easy to conclude that only professional midwives, with their greater access to high technologies and international networking systems can achieve the **informed relativism** I am highlighting as the primary characteristic of the postmodern midwife. But traditional midwives in many countries are undergoing radical changes, and an emergent postmodern consciousness sometimes characterizes their responses. Such traditional midwives, who are literate, politically savvy, and eager to absorb new knowledge, would benefit tremendously from access to this volume and its predecessor; therefore I issue a call to postmodern midwives in multiple countries to translate this book in order to make it accessible to both the professional and the traditional midwives in their regions who desire access to the knowledge this volume contains.

In 1978 with the first publication of BIRTH IN FOUR CULTURES, Brigitte Jordan issued a call for the replacement of top-down, culturally inappropriate, biomedically oriented systems with models of mutual accommodation between Western and indigenous systems. But the worldwide hegemony of Western biomedicine has made this kind of mutual accommodation an elusive goal. Why bother to accommodate to a system you regard as inferior? Why not, as has so often been done, demand instead that the midwifery system change to accept biomedical ways of knowing and managing birth? The answer is quite clear of course: *biomedicine is an inappropriate model for birth in any culture. It is too costly, too interventive, too drug- and technology-oriented, and does too much harm to mothers and babies*. Nevertheless, because of the general global dominance of the West, the legacy of colonialism, and the various dramatic successes of biomedicine, almost all developing countries do aspire to meet the standards set by Western medicine, despite the fact that these standards have been scientifically demonstrated to be inappropriate for normal birth and indeed for many of the world's health needs. And all midwives in developed countries must continually challenge biomedical standards with whatever resources they can muster to preserve the knowledge and ideology midwives have developed: this book, which encodes so much midwifery knowledge about labor and birth, is an essential element in midwives' ability to sustain that challenge. The nature and the quality of the knowledge provided its pages are essential for all midwives practicing everywhere. It is significant that Frye incorporates into this volume much of the knowledge early obstetricians, like midwives, obtained from direct experience with birth. As medical traditions crystallized around higher technology, much of this earlier knowledge was lost to or discounted by modern obstetrics, and is re-encountered and renewed here within a holistic midwifery context.

Postmodern midwives, for all their value, often find themselves living in a constant state of stress, lobbying legislatures for the right to exist, struggling to balance conflicting ideologies and knowledge systems (for examples, see Davis-Floyd 1998), and arguing with each other about appropriate standards for education and practice. In developed and developing countries alike, the tensions between biomedical, traditional, and alternative knowledge systems permeate professional midwifery training and practice and generate conflicts between midwifery educators, between educators and students, and among practicing midwives and those who regulate them. The professional midwives of the industrialized North are accelerating their long struggle for autonomy even as traditional midwives in the less affluent countries of the South continue to lose the autonomy they formerly held. In short, today nothing is easy about being a midwife of any type. Yet motivated by a shared desire to offer viable long-term options to biomedical birth, these daughters of time*[1] and tradition continue their struggle, with varying degrees of success, but always with the necessary determination to make sure that midwives, with all their limitations *and* all their power, remain available to serve the mothers and babies of the postmodern world. Frye's work is one of the keys that can unlock the doors that hold them back, enabling midwives of all types to study and then to build on the knowledge base that Frye presents in these richly detailed pages.

I suggest that the primary challenge for postmodern midwives is to realize the promises of science and technology while removing their threat to normal birth, and to create and practice a more fluid, holistic, and globally inclusive ideology of birth. Today we have the great advantage that we can perceive the full spectrum of birth knowledge and ideology. With this broad and inclusive perspective, midwives can create a **knowledge spiral** that combines the best of technocratic medicine, professional midwifery, and the birth wisdom of ancient and indigenous cultures, much of which is encoded in these pages, to create the most comprehensive and effective knowledge system about birth that the world has ever known. The future of midwifery is entirely in the hands of postmodern midwives–in other words, it's up to you! This book will help you to create that future in a viable, authoritative, and sustainable form.

Robbie Davis-Floyd, PhD
Cleveland, Ohio, 2004

Acknowledgments

My deepest thanks to Anne Frye for the honor of writing this Foreword, for her years of midwifery apprenticeship and practice, and for her enormous and rewarding efforts to encode, for the first time in the history of English language texts, an out-of-hospital midwifery knowledge base in a three-volume series that will benefit midwives around the world.

Endnotes

1. I have adapted much of the material in this Foreword from the following sources, which I have either authored or co-authored: Davis-Floyd & Davis 1997; Davis-Floyd 2000, 2001, 2003, nd; Davis-Floyd, Cosminsky & Pigg, 2001a.

2. The phrase "daughters of time" in relation to midwives springs from a formative moment in the history of the new midwifery in the United States. Santa Cruz midwife Karen Erlich described that moment to me as follows (personal communication 2000):

The First International Conference of Practicing Midwives was held in El Paso in January of 1977. It was an amazing, emotional gathering, the first ever, of homebirth midwives who had sprung up all over the continent, thinking they were the only ones who existed. Among the concerns expressed was whether we wanted to stay as iconoclastic, outside-the-system lay care givers, or allow a process of professionalization . . . During the open mike, women spoke passionately, eloquently, angrily, tactfully and not tactfully, about this calling and the political issues already confronting us. In the midst of this hot, compelling, fascinating, provocative session, Mary Offermann got up and, instead of politicizing, sang this song. It was fantastic! The conference ended awash in the true emotions of birth and womankind.

Daughters of Time

I am a daughter of time, My mother walked these hills in years gone by.
Her mother too once watched these trees, in blossom, bearing fruit and losing leaves.

> We are the daughters, the daughters of time . . .
> Last night I held a woman who was giving birth, She brought another daughter here to earth.
> I feel happy with my man and with our son, but I wonder if a little girl will ever come to me
> To join the daughters, the daughters of time. (Copyright1975 Mary Offermann.)

For these midwives, the poetic sense of "daughters of time," with its image of birth as the moment that embodies the continuity of generations of women, helped solidify a sense of what their project was about. The image expresses a hope that women today will be empowered to recuperate knowledge and skills maintained by women in the past, revitalize them for the present, and preserve them for the future. The phrase was further cemented in American midwifery lore in the early 1980s through a film about nurse-midwives called "Daughters of Time" (Durrin 1982), and by an article by Barbara Katz Rothman with that title (1998).

A brief biography of the author:

Robbie Davis-Floyd, Ph.D., is a Senior Research Fellow in the Department of Anthropology at the University of Texas, Austin and Adjunct Associate Professor at Case Western Reserve University in Cleveland, Ohio. She lectures nationally and internationally, and is author of over 80 academic articles, and of BIRTH AS AN AMERICAN RITE OF PASSAGE (1992), co-author of FROM DOCTOR TO HEALER: THE TRANSFORMATIVE JOURNEY (1998) and THE ANATOMY OF RITUAL (forthcoming), and co-editor of eight collections, including CHILDBIRTH AND AUTHORITATIVE KNOWLEDGE: CROSS-CULTURAL PERSPECTIVES, CYBORG BABIES: FROM TECHNO-SEX TO TECHNO-TOTS, DAUGHTERS OF TIME: THE SHIFTING IDENTITIES OF CONTEMPORARY MIDWIVES (a special triple issue of MEDICAL ANTHROPOLOGY 20:2/3-4), and MAINSTREAMING MIDWIVES: THE POLITICS OF PROFESSIONALIZATION (2005).

References and Further Reading

Barnes-Josiah D, Myntti C, Augustin, A. "The 'three delays' as a framework for examining maternal mortality in Haiti," SOC SCI MED, 46(8);981-993, Apr 1998.

Davis-Floyd.R."The ups, downs, and interlinkages of nurse- and direct-entry midwifery: status, practice, and education," 67-118, in Tritten J, Southern J, eds. GETTING AN EDUCATION: PATHS TO BECOMING A MIDWIFE, 4th ed. Midwifery Today, Eugene OR, 1998.*

Davis-Floyd R. " Global issues in midwifery: Mutual accommodation or biomedical hegemony?" MIDWIFERY TODAY (53);12-16, 68-69, Spring, 2000.*

Davis-Floyd, R "La partera profesional: articulating identity and cultural space for a new kind of midwife in Mexico," MED ANTHROPOL, 20(2-3, special triple issue "Daughters of Time: the shifting identities of contemporary midwives");185-243, 2001.*

Davis-Floyd R. "Home birth emergencies in the U.S. and Mexico: The trouble with transport," SOC SCI MED, 56(9, special issue: "Reproduction Gone Awry");1911-1931, May 2003.

Davis-Floyd R "Daughter of time: The postmodern midwife." Unpublished ms, nd.

Davis-Floyd, R, Davis E. "Intuition as authoritative knowledge in midwifery and homebirth," 315-349, in Davis-Floyd R, Sargent C, eds. CHILDBIRTH AND AUTHORITATIVE KNOWLEDGE: CROSS-CULTURAL PERSPECTIVES, Berkeley: U California Press, 1997.

Davis-Floyd R, Cosminsky S, Pigg SL. "Introduction: Daughters of Time: the shifting identities of contemporary midwives" in MED ANTHROPOL, 20(2-3, special triple issue "Daughters of Time: the shifting identities of contemporary midwives");105-139, 2001a.

Davis-Floyd R, Cosminsky S, Pigg SL, eds. "Daughters of Time: The Shifting Identities of Contemporary Midwives," a special triple issue of MED ANTHROPOL, 20(2-3), 2001b.

Dieteker, M. "The construction of urban midwife identities in popular neighborhoods in Mexico City," in Good Maust M, Guëmez Piñeda M, Davis-Floyd R, eds. MIDWIVES IN MEXICO: CONTINUITY, CONTROVERSY, AND CHANGE. Austin, University of Texas Press, 2005.

Durrin, G. DAUGHTERS OF TIME: THE CLASSIC FILM ON NURSE-MIDWIVES TODAY. Durrin, Washington, DC, 1982. (1-800-536-6843 durrinprod@aol.com)

Jordan B. BIRTH IN FOUR CULTURES: A CROSS-CULTURAL INVESTIGATION OF CHILDBIRTH IN YUCATAN, HOLLAND, SWEDEN AND THE UNITED STATES, 4th ed. Waveland, Prospect Heights, IL, 1993.

Katz-Rothman B, "Daughters of Time," in Tritten J, Southern J, eds. GETTING AN EDUCATION: PATHS TO BECOMING A MIDWIFE, 4th ed. Midwifery Today, Eugene OR, 1998.

Kirkham M J, Perkins ER. REFLECTIONS ON MIDWIFERY. Balliere Tindall, London England, 1997.

Kolenda P. "Fewer deaths, fewer births: decline of child mortality in a UP village," MANUSHI, 105;5-13, Mar-Apr 1998.

Kroeger M. Final consultant report. CHN 3 Project, Provincial Department of Health Central Java, Indonesia, 1996.

Marcus GE. What comes just after "post"? the case of ethnography," 95-115, in N. Denzin N, Lincoln Y, eds. THE HANDBOOK OF QUALITATIVE SOCIAL SCIENCE. Sage, Beverly Hills CA, 1993.

*This article is also available for viewing and downloading at www.davis-floyd.com.

BECOMING FAMILIAR WITH VOLUME II

NOTE: Further details regarding using this three volume text can be found in Volume I in the chapter entitled "An Overview of the Text." There you will find information on conventions of vocabulary such as the use of the word yoni instead of vagina and clitorotomy instead of episiotomy. Here, you will find information that is particular to this volume concerning changes I have incorporated since the first volume was published.

The organization of the text

Most students hardly look at a table of contents and this is often a mistake. However, the table of contents is the outline of a book and you are referred to it for an overview. The text follows the format of Volume I, beginning with anatomical and physiological information that forms a foundation for what follows. It then discusses uncomplicated labor, birth, neonatal care and the hours following birth, followed by a discussion of situations that demand additional or more specific skills, ending an extensive section amounting to a crash course in bedside high risk neonatal triage for the midwife. As with Volume I, information builds from chapter to chapter. If referring to a single chapter, at least read through it in its entirety to avoid missing basic information that may be vital to your understanding.

Midwifery skills and equipment

There are many skills that pertain to the period spanning labor, birth and the hours immediately following. While some of these skills are used at every, or nearly every, birth, many are just as important but pertain only to certain circumstances or may be used only rarely. It has been difficult to decide which to describe as general skills and which to link to specific circumstances that may arise during labor. The section entitled "Supplies and Equipment for Labor and Birth." The first chapter in this section mentions every piece of equipment you might want or need to carry, from the most basic to the most rarely needed tools and supplies. In some cases, notably IV equipment, injection equipment, and oxygen and resuscitation equipment, the use of the equipment is intimately interwoven with an understanding of the equipment itself, in part because this equipment is often foreign to students and midwives who do not have hospital training. Therefore, these tools are mentioned in the main chapter, but detailed lists and descriptions are found in the chapters that cover those skills, which are also found in this section. Suturing skills and equipment are covered in my text HEALING PASSAGE.

Numerous skills are described throughout the text, which may, at times, be essential to the midwife's art. Those that seemed suitable for description separate from their specific clinical application are described in their own chapters. Criteria for assigning a separate chapter to a skill included the complexity of the skill and the depth of detail required, whether the skill might be useful for both the baby and mother (such as the skill of giving an injection or the use of oxygen) and whether the skill might come in handy in various circumstances throughout the labor, birth and immediate postpartum period. Many of these are located in the part entitled "Remedies, Skills and Equipment for Complex Labor Situations" under the major topic heading entitled "When Labor and Birth Demand Specific Midwifery Skills." For example, the use of intravenous therapy is sufficiently complex that it has been assigned its own chapter, although it is certainly not needed at most births. It is therefore allocated to the section covering complex labors. When a skill is described in its own chapter, how it is done and when it is used will be discussed there. The skill will be mentioned again in appropriate locations throughout the text when the need for it is likely to arise.

However, there are many essential skills that are only used in very specific circumstances; these seemed most appropriately described in the context of when they would be used. For example, skills pertaining to the birth of the placenta, such as fundal checks, cord traction and manual removal of the placenta (to name a few) seemed best discussed in the context of the process of the birth of the placenta in its totality, so they are not included as general skills. Likewise, those skills that are only used during newborn care and assessment are included in separate sections and are usually discussed in the context in which they are used.

Finding specific skills: Some skills have an entire chapter devoted to them such as "Manual Removal of the Placenta." These can easily be picked out by scanning the table of contents. Most, however, are interwoven in numerous chapters throughout the text. I have made every effort to index and cross-reference skills so that they are easy to find. Therefore, the best way to locate a specific skill is to use the index. See the entries under "skills" (where nearly all the skills in the book should be found), also see "abdominal examination," "labor positions & activities," "newborn examination," "placental detachment and birth," "placental examination," "rebozo techniques," "reflexes in the newborn," "resuscitation, newborn," "version in labor," "vital signs, maternal," "yoni exams, internal." This is not a complete list.

You can also look up the specific skill (such as "transillumination,") depending upon what type of skill you are trying to find.

Using the index

Finding specific information: The index is designed to help you find specific information as quickly as possible. Look for the most specific topic first. For example, if you want information on how to perform a specific type of examination on the newborn arm, see "Arm, newborn." If you go to the entry on "Newborn examination" you will find the page which begins the discussion of examining the newborn arms, but no detailed entries. The Skills entry lists rebozo relaxation techniques, but if you want a listing of specific types of rebozo techniques, you're better off going straight to "Rebozo techniques." Nearly every topic heading in each chapter is indexed somewhere.

Note that indexing topics are given by subject and may not always match the exact wording as found on the page being referenced. This was necessary because the indexing feature in Wordperfect had limited capabilities as far as how many words could be used in a header or subheader.

In most cases, substantial information can be found on the topic for each page given. If the word was mentioned incidental to other subject matter, I refrained from indexing it; in other words, not every instance of every word is indexed. I did, however, endeavor to give separate entries for proper names, methods, techniques and maneuvers as well as anatomical parts, specific findings (such as each individual reflex), etc.

Page numbers given: The page numbers generally indicate where the discussion of the topic you are looking up begins. A notation such as 93-97 required imbedding index codes on every consecutive page and I was worried about moving text around and messing up the sequence, so I abandoned this convention. Therefore, in many cases, the discussion may continue for several consecutive pages. When this isn't the case, the next page where the discussion of the same topic picks up is also given. If only one page is mentioned, that is either the only place the topic is discussed or where the most information about it can be found.

Cross-referencing: Many topics are cross-referenced, some with complete listings under both headings. For example the header, "pendulous abdomen" is completely cross-referenced with the header "abdomen, pendulous." Some topics only have one complete listing. For instance the header "Reflexes in the newborn" contains a complete listing of every reflex mentioned in the text, the cross-reference "newborn reflexes," contains only a general and very short list of where groups of reflexes are discussed. For some major topics, I have also referred you to other headers for additional information.

WHAT IS LABOR?

Labor is much more than the physical process by which women give birth and by which babies are born, awesome as those experiences appear in and of themselves. Labor is also the transformational opening of a woman's entire being. Women who give birth unhindered are open to the elemental forces of nature that bring the baby forth. Heart, mind, spirit, emotions and sexual self, as well as the woman's physical body, open to allow another life to begin an independent existence on this planet. Thus, labor is a spiritual experience of enormous importance to both the woman and her baby. While women experience various life-changing events during pregnancy, the experience of giving birth is so significant that most women in old age continue to remember their birth experiences as though they had happened yesterday. This makes the totality of the birth experience one of the most pivotal in a woman's life.

The transition from intrauterine life to life outside the womb has tremendous impact upon the infant as well, in ways that will influence a person for their entire life. Unless unusual circumstances have created a challenging situation during gestation, the processes of labor and birth represent the new child's first challenging physical accomplishment. A baby's own experience of gestation and birth and his or her mother's responses to those experiences form an imprint on the baby's psyche that will influence the person's own attitudes, feelings and beliefs about childbirth. The incredible sensitivity of the baby during the process of birth should never be underestimated. The comments and attitudes of care providers, parents and others present during this important transition shape the ways in which the baby interprets her birth experience, frequently reinforcing experiences and decisions the baby has already begun to formulate in the womb.

Birth attendants who respect labor as a life-changing, empowering and spiritually expansive event strive to hold open the environment as a sacred container in which birth can unfold. The entire birth process then takes place in an arena of expanded consciousness. The multifaceted nature of this process also demands an environment of minimal stress so that the woman can feel safe and let go. The optimal environment is usually the mother's home, although it may be any physical setting in which the mother feels safe and comfortable. Western society, with its focus on the dangers of birth, often overlooks that institutional settings typically provide none of these vital criteria for keeping birth normal.

Many of the problems that arise from the medicalization of childbirth occur because hospital staff see labor as something that happens to a woman; not as something a woman does (Rothman, 1982). The medical model focuses on ways to manage labor and any accompanying pain, ways to make the uterus function according to hospital schedules and protocols and ways to make each woman's labor conform to artificially formulated averages, rather than on how to assist each individual woman as she gives birth. Medical texts often discuss how to involve the woman in her care or how to help her participate in her birth, as though the birth of her child were something external to her. Labor is, to a certain extent, involuntary, but this does not mean that the woman herself does not actively give birth. Breaking with this tendency, this book honors and recognizes the uniqueness of each woman, each labor, each baby. With that in mind, we proceed.

Katz-Rothman B. In Labor: Women and Power in the Birthplace. WW Norton & Co, New York NY, 1982.

NOTES:

ANATOMY AND PHYSIOLOGY OF THE MOTHER AND BABY RELEVANT TO LABOR AND BIRTH

The Evolution of Our Understanding of Fetal Descent

This portion of the book covers the anatomy and physiology of the baby's adaptation and movement through the mother's pelvis during the birth process. Each chapter builds on the next; therefore new students should read each chapter sequentially. Birth with the baby in cephalic presentations is covered first, followed by all other presentations. The material in this section builds on information covered in detail in Volume I of HOLISTIC MIDWIFERY. The chapter entitled "Discussing How the Baby Is Situated in the Uterus" covers fetal position, lie, variety, attitude, denominator, presentation and presenting part prior to the onset of labor. The chapter's entitled "The Fine Art of Palpation," "The Skeletal System" and "Pelvimetry" explain the anatomical features of the female pelvis. Review these topics in Volume I thoroughly before studying this part of the book.

Understanding the cardinal movements of birth

In 1752 William Smellie, the "father" of British midwifery, was the first to publish a textbook more or less accurately describing the cardinal movements of birth. No doubt, many midwives before him had also scrutinized the process; however, since many were not literate and men generally wrote the textbooks, it was a man who first put these observations into print.

Throughout the ages, the study of the process of labor has presented numerous difficulties. Observation of the process as a woman gives birth, of course, is the most available and least invasive method used by midwives and doctors alike. Additionally, internal exams offer information about the lowermost portion of the presenting part. However, what the examiner can see and feel is limited and offers little definitive information about how the rest of the baby's body is navigating the birth canal during labor. External abdominal palpation is informative but only offers a snapshot of the process between contractions. Aside from these methods, for centuries men have had the distinct advantage of having access to "study material" in the form of the cadavers of women who had died at various stages of childbirth. Dissection of fresh or frozen cadavers revealed more complete information about the process of labor, and our current understanding of the cardinal movements is still based on observations made during these antique studies. There are problems with this approach, however. Labor is a fluid, organic process that takes place in living women. Cadaver material is inevitably going to be somewhat distorted and nuances of the natural process missed. In addition, each cadaver can only offer information about a moment in the process.

The baby can also be observed during Cesarean surgery prior to removal from the uterus. This offers information about the natural process in a living woman. However, prior to the advent of antibiotics in the mid-1940s, surgical births were only performed in situations in which labor had taken a decidedly pathological turn, because the risk of surgery was so great. This makes findings gathered during emergency surgery somewhat unreliable when applied to normal labors. In addition, women receiving surgery are drugged and supine before the baby's position in utero can be seen.

Realizing these problems, some researchers pushed stillborn babies through the pelvises of their deceased and dissected mothers to glean more information about the dynamics of descent. Of course, the woman's body was supine, and having students push the baby through a cadaver is not the same as natural labor (to say the least). Nevertheless, internal rotation often occurs with such experiments, and many other details can be observed with this method of study.

Wilhelm Roentgen introduced a new arena of study when he discovered X-rays in the late nineteenth century. By 1897, Eduard Albert, a physician in Dresden, Austria, as well as Doctors Pierre Budin of France and H Varnier were all experimenting with X-rays to study pelvic architecture, and a whole new world of study opened up. Over the next 25 years, methods were refined and by the 1930s X-rays were being widely used in pregnancy (Jarcho, 1933). X-rays allow the internal process to be observed in living women during labor. A few studies were done that confirmed many of the details already outlined in previous work, although most studies focused on the nuances of descent and rotation of the head.

However, X-ray investigations are fraught with problems as well. For research purposes, each woman must be positioned in exactly the same manner as the films are shot or the angle will be off, rendering the films almost useless for this type of study. Varying thicknesses of tissue layers can affect the quality of the image. Asking women to stay stone still during a portion of their labor is not only difficult and cruel, it is hardly representative of the natural process. Because of all such difficulties, study populations have usually been small. Many studies focus on only a single detail of the birth process; other information that could have been gleaned from the same X-ray films was often not collected. Each X-ray image is only a moment in a continuous process. Furthermore, the exact circumstances under which the films were obtained is often not discussed; for example, was the woman drugged? The position she was required to maintain is usually mentioned (it was often some sort of semi-seated, supine or lateral position), but its effect on the results is usually not taken into consideration. Sometimes the parity of the mothers is not given, leaving one wondering if the same ratio of results would occur in nulliparas. While "normal births" were usually the only ones included in studies intended to research normal labor, the limitations of the technique present numerous confounding factors.

Researching the movements (mechanisms) of labor: I have done an exhaustive (and exhausting) study of the cardinal movements of birth (aka the mechanisms of labor). I have looked at nearly all the most current editions of modern textbooks. I have studied numerous textbooks from 1752 to the present as well. I have tracked down the few articles that I could find in English that review aspects of the cardinal movements of birth using serial X-ray studies in living women. My studies have been hindered by some articles with promising titles being in languages that I do not speak and many of them being published prior to 1953, which means the articles cannot be located on Medline searches (which, as of this printing, only catalogue articles from 1953 to the present). I had to pick through old bibliographies, find the most promising titles and look them up one by one.

As far as I have been able to determine, hardly any research has been done on the cardinal movements of birth since the late sixties. Studies falling in this category include those looking at how the baby moves through the pelvis and characteristics of the passageway, notably those by Borell and Fernström in the late 1950s and early 1960s and studies focusing upon the timing and rate of descent in relationship to contraction patterns, cervical dilation and the like, notably those by Emanuel Friedman (1950s-1960s). So the material in this part is based on the best research I have been able to dig up. What this means is that I have rewritten portions of this part as many as five times. New material would often come to light as I researched other topics seemingly not directly related.

The movements the baby makes during labor were given quite a bit of detailed attention in the old textbooks. At the turn of the century, many doctors seeking to provide midwifery services had never seen a birth because women distrusted men in their labor rooms. Books were written to try and fill this gap by doctors who had had the opportunity to attend births in or out of hospitals (notable authors include William Smellie [1752], William Dewees [1824], Hugh Hodge [1864], J. Whitridge Williams [1903] and Joseph De Lee [1913] [dates indicate first editions of their texts]). Much of what is accepted today about fetal movements and pelvic characteristics was laid down in such writings. As the practice of midwifery evolved more and more into the surgical specialty of obstetrics, the profession lost interest in the process of normal labor and today devotes many more textbook and journal article pages on technological and surgical solutions to problems in labor and the minutia of the biochemical aspects of labor in the hope of one day attaining complete control over the process. For example, MANAGEMENT OF LABOR AND DELIVERY by Robert Creasy (1996), which has 570 pages of text, dedicates 37 of these to a chapter entitled "Normal Labor and Delivery." This chapter covers uterine activity and pelvic architecture with only 12 pages devoted to the fetus and the way he passes through the birth canal. By comparison, the sixth edition of De Lee's PRINCIPLES AND PRACTICE OF OBSTETRICS (1934) has 18 pages on the actual process of occiput anterior descent alone, plus additional whole chapters covering fetal adaptation and other topics directly relevant to the processes of birth. The most extensive treatment of the subject seems to be by Alfred C. Beck in his text OBSTETRICAL PRACTICE, first published in 1935. He devotes some 200 pages and hundreds of drawings to the mechanism of labor. Happily, this text has fallen into the public domain, and most of the illustrations in this part of the book have been adapted from it.

As always, I evaluated what I found with what I know from my own experience. I found studies that have heretofore been largely ignored, but whose findings matched my own observations of the process. I believe these studies have been ignored for three reasons. One, they found details of the process differ from what is taught and therefore were rejected by authors who were set in their beliefs. In some cases, looking at the process with fresh eyes has been difficult for me as well, as my understanding from studying current literature differed from what the research showed. Two, there is much less interest in the normal process today; either the baby falls out or physicians rush to intervene with drugs, instruments or surgery. The in-depth understanding of the process has given way to laboring by the clock, with the result being far less appreciation of the totality of labor by the average medical practitioner. Finally, some of the best, most enlightened research was done by non-American doctors and therefore has not been incorporated into the literature in the way it might have been if a US team had done the work.

To an extent, understanding how it all works is academic as long as labor is progressing and the baby comes out easily. However, I believe it is important for birth practitioners of all kinds to be able to visualize the unseen process of descent. We should know the natural process intimately. This way, they will know better what might be happening and how they might help. I believe it is important for texts to validate what can be observed and to state, as accurately as possible, what cannot be observed directly. Such knowledge helps to confirm the practitioner's impressions that things are going smoothly and helps to troubleshoot what the problem might be when they are not. Finally, as the process of labor is in many ways the core of what birth attendants are there to assist on the physical level, students should not feel they must hunt through the literature to find a decent, in-depth discussion of these basic concepts. Every textbook on midwifery or obstetrics that presents itself as "comprehensive" should cover the process of birth in all its variations as thoroughly as did the writers of the past.

The following chapters represent my best research to date. They offer a fresh look at the process. As far as I have been able to determine, it is one of the most thorough, if not the most thorough, review of the process of birth that has ever been published. Future editions may be modified as more is uncovered about the fascinating, complex and sometimes controversial details of this process.

Do not skip this part

You will miss a great deal if you skip over this part. Do not think because you have been practicing many years, or because you have studied the material that is presented in a more succinct manner in another contemporary text, that you already know this stuff. I have been practicing many years, and much of the material presented here was no less than illuminating to me. A thorough knowledge of this part of the text will provide a foundation for understanding the recommendations that follow regarding supporting women in labor. It will also assist you in evaluating new ideas about what might help and what won't as you experiment with new maternal positions and activities in your own practice. It will help you immensely as you watch women labor because it will offer better insight into what their responses might mean in terms of fetal position. In short, this is foundation information that is vital to your practice. Not scrutinizing these basic details has led to obstetrical and, sadly, midwifery practices that arise out of an unfamiliarity with the very things that help the baby be born most easily, particularly regarding how maternal posture facilitates or impairs descent.

Studying this material: Understanding and visualizing the descriptions and illustrations in this section will be greatly facilitated by obtaining a doll with moveable limbs, a cloth body and a plastic head with moulded sutures or on which sutures have been drawn and a model of the female pelvis (ideally, one with flexible joints that will allow the doll to pass through the cavity). Do not think this is a waste of money. Having models will make this material so much easier to study and you will grasp it so much faster. These models will serve you throughout your career as a midwife. Label the models to assist in identifying landmarks. Rubber bands can be used to hold the doll's limbs and head in different positions as you move through the following chapters. If you have trouble with remembering right or left orientations on your body as opposed to someone else's, it may help to position the sacrum of the pelvic model toward you as you study the summaries. That way, the left and right for the pelvis will be the same as your own. After some practice, you will be able to visualize the pelvis so well that you will only need to hold the doll up against your torso to review the movements of fetal descent. Arrange the doll, hold it in place against your body, then look in a mirror. From here, you will be well on your way to visualizing what is happening in the mother's body during labor. Your goal is to become fluent in the nuances of fetal descent.

Note to international students: In North America, the word "transverse" is used when the baby's denominator is positioned directly to one side of the mother. In other countries, the term "lateral" is used instead. Thus, the designation LOT (Left Occiput Transverse) becomes LOL (Left Occiput Lateral). I have chosen to retain the North American terminology in my texts; however, I realize that the use of the word "transverse" can be confusing because the side-to-side diameter that runs across the maternal pelvis is referred to as the transverse diameter. Thus the baby's denominator is referred to as being transverse when it is positioned to the mother's side, and the long axis of the baby's shoulders or pelvis is said to be transverse when either are aligned with the transverse diameter of the pelvic brim (i.e., straight across the width of the mother's pelvis).

Basic Physical Principles of Birth

Features of Fetal Anatomy Pertinent to the Birth Process

We begin with a discussion of features of fetal anatomy that help the baby's body pass through the mother's pelvis during labor. The following chapters explain more about how the baby's and the mother's bodies work together during labor and birth.

The Head and Neck

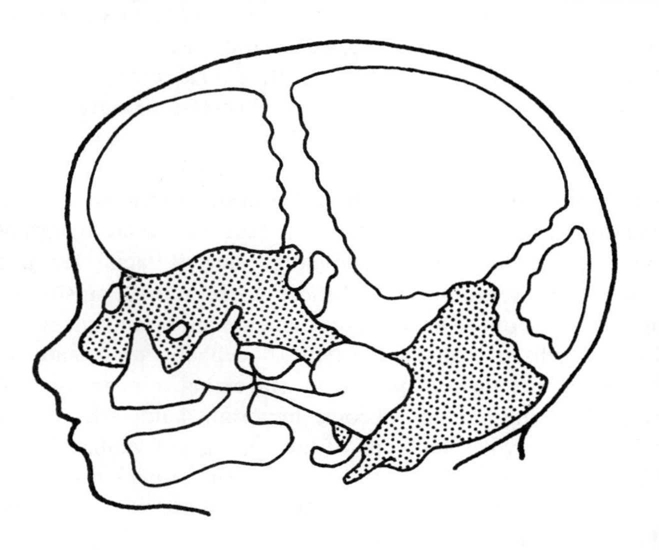

Fetal skull at 16 weeks gestation. The unshaded areas ossify intramembranously. The shaded areas ossify endochondrally.

The skull is, by far, the most important part of the fetal anatomy as far as the birth process is concerned. It is the largest, most ossified and least compressible region of the term baby's skeletal structure, making the size and position of the head the most critical factor regarding the relative ease or difficulty the baby will encounter as he moves through the birth canal, whether in a breech or cephalic presentation.

The skull is the most complex bony structure in the body. Its parts fit together like an intricate three-dimensional jigsaw puzzle to create the face, jaws, eye sockets, nasal passages, sinuses and ear canals as well as to protect the brain. Many of the skull bones have intricate, irregular, three-dimensional shapes. Some that are harder to visualize are illustrated separately. Any anatomy book will give you information on the features of the adult skull. Descriptions of the newborn skull are harder to come by, yet there are many features of the newborn skull that differ dramatically from the adult. For example, the face is smaller because the jaw and nasal sinuses are less developed and the teeth have not erupted, resulting in the cranial dome appearing comparatively large. The focus of this discussion will be on features unique to the term fetus and newborn that have to do primarily with birth. The depth of detail given here will help you understand how the head moulds during labor and the importance of treating the head gently both during and after birth and lays the foundation for the discussion of osteopathic treatment that is found in Volume III of this text.

An overview of skull development

The newborn skull consists of 51 bony elements separated by either cartilage or connective tissue. The skull bones are only partially ossified at birth. They develop by way of two ossification processes: intramembranous or endochondral. **Membranous bones** form by hardening or ossifying outward from a central region called the growth center. Numerous thin spikes of bone fan out from this region, denser at their growth center and more fragile and flexible near their edges.

In the newborn, the edges of membranous bones are smooth and slightly separated from each other by a gap spanned by a flexible bridge of fibrous membranous tissue. These gaps are called **sutures**. The width of each suture varies depending upon the bones in question.

The ossification of **endochondral (en-de-KON-drel) bones** is somewhat more complex. A cartilaginous template in the shape of the eventual bone forms first. This cartilage is gradually reabsorbed and replaced by hard, calcium-filled bone as the baby matures. During ossification, which occurs uniformly throughout the cartilaginous template, regions of uniform thickness become consistently firm throughout, making them much less flexible than membranous bones at the same stage of development.

Endochondral bones are separated by hyaline cartilage or fibrocartilage and meet at **synchondrodial (syn-kon-DRO-de-al) joints**. At birth, these joints are much less flexible than sutures but do allow some movement of the surrounding more ossified regions of bone. At some point after birth, the timing of which varies with the individual bone, some synchondrodial joints become far less mobile. Others fuse completely, joining ossified regions into one solid bone. The most important synchondrodial joints related to birth join the occipital and sphenoid bones and are described in detail in this chapter.

While the term fetal skull is more ossified than a preterm skull, the newborn's skull bones are still not nearly as dense as they will be at maturity. At the time of birth, the skull bones are more flexible and even more mobile than is generally taught. Movement of the skull bones will be discussed in the next chapter.

Regions of the skull

The skull is divided into three regions: the face, the vault, and the base. Some of the skull bones extend into two or more of these regions. For example, the occiput makes up part of the vault and part of the base of the skull. Therefore, each bone is listed according to its primary location in each regional category below.

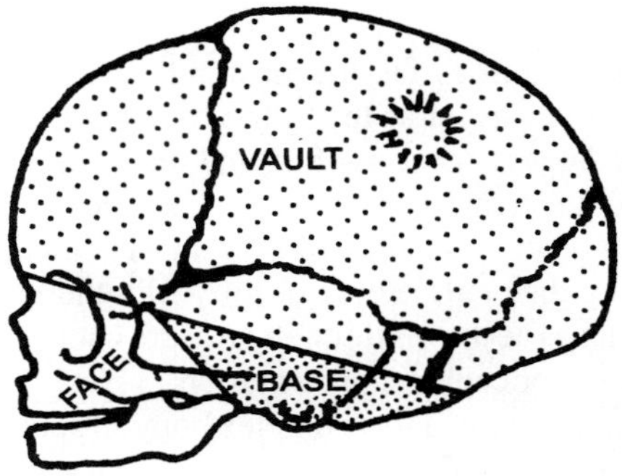

Regions of the skull

The face: The face extends from the bridge of the nose to the junction of the chin and neck. The face can be an important landmark during labor. Clinically relevant facial features include the **mentum** or chin, the **mouth**, and the **nasion** or **bridge (root) of the nose**. All of these are important landmarks during births of babies in extended cephalic presentations. Together, the **lower jaw line (inferior border of the mandible)** and mentum become important landmarks during breech births when the nape of the neck is not visible due to maternal positioning during pushing. The **superior border of the maxilla** consists of the bony ridge that extends horizontally to either side of the nostrils. It provides a safe location to place fingertips during certain manipulations of the head during breech births.

All of the facial bones are intramembranous in origin except for the inferior nasal conchae, which ossify endochondrally. Immature development of the jaws, sinuses and nasal cavities account for the small size of the newborn face. (One-eighth of the newborn skull makes up the face, compared to one-third of the skull in the adult.) The chart below outlines the names and locations of the facial bones; however, they are not illustrated separately in this volume.

BONE NAME AND NUMBER	LOCATION AND FUNCTION
Lacrimal bones (2)	Medial walls of orbits
Mandible bones (2)	Lower jaw bones
Maxillary bones (2)	Upper jaw & central facial bone
Inferior nasal conchae (2)	Part of lateral walls of nasal cavity
Nasal bones (2)	Bridge of nose
Palatine bones (2)	L-shaped. Posterior hard palate, lateral wall of nose
Vomer bone (1)	Part of nasal septum
Zygomatic (malar) bones (2)	Cheekbones

The shape of the newborn mandibles (which fuse into one in adults and function as one in infants) differ significantly from the adult's, making it ideally suited for nursing. The teeth have not yet erupted, the paranasal sinuses are tiny, and the maxilla and mandible are small. The angle of the mandible is slight and the arms or rami connecting it to the head on either side are very short. Its lower border is level with the foramen magnum. The mandible bones meet at the intermandibular suture at the center of the chin, where they later fuse.

The facial bones are relatively stable during birth but can become misaligned due to pressure from other bones that receive direct stress during descent. The face may also receive direct pressure when the head is deflexed.

Ethmoid: Sometimes classified as a facial bone, the ethmoid resembles a rough, rectangular natural sponge. It lies between the sphenoid and the nasal bones and is the most deeply situated bone of the skull. It forms the bony walls of the upper nasal cavity and a portion of the medial wall of the orbital cavity, and its lowermost border forms part of the skull base. It is only partially ossified at birth.

The vault of the skull (cranium): In the newborn, the sides of the cranium are made up of the two parietal bones, the two temporal bones, the pterygoid processes of the temporal bones and the lateral extremities of the greater wings of the sphenoid. Anteriorly, the two frontal bones make up the forehead. The back of the vault is comprised of the interparietal region of the occiput. Most of these unfused bones are thin and incompletely ossified, making them easily bendable as well as compressible. Sutures also permit these bones to move and, in some cases, overlap under pressure so that the shape of the head can adapt or mould to the shape of the pelvis.

Parietal bones: The two parietal bones extend from the center of the top of the head down to the ears on either side of the skull to form most of the sides of the skull vault. (See the drawing of the lateral view of the skull on page 13 for an illustration of the parietal bone.) Each parietal bone has four blunt corners and is shaped like a shallow bowl. Each is bordered by the opposite parietal bone superiorly, the frontal bones anteriorly, the occipital bone posteriorly, and the temporal and sphenoid bones inferiorly. The parietal bones form intramembranously and make up the bulk of the sides of the skull vault. These bones are thin and can become "dented" during a difficult birth involving excessive pressure, much like a ping-pong ball or an empty aluminum drink can when pressed with your thumbpad. The parietal bones have three clinically important landmarks:

Parietal eminence (boss, protuberance or prominence) (2): The eminence is the hardest part of the parietal bone and is the highest point on either side. It is located in the upper posterior center of each bone (see illustration). The distance between the two parietal eminences marks the widest transverse diameter of the fetal skull.

Vertex: The vertex is bounded in front by the anterior fontanelle, in back by the posterior fontanelle, and on each side by the parietal eminences and is divided down the center by the sagittal suture. The term "vertex" is also used in a descriptive sense when referring to any more-or-less flexed cephalic presentation in which the vertex region of the head is presenting.

Crown of the head (or of the vertex): The most protuberant region of the vertex anterior to the posterior fontanelle. It is included in the presenting circumference of the head when the head is well flexed.

Parietal foramina: These openings in the parietal bones are found bilaterally to either side of the sagittal suture about two-thirds of the way posterior to the anterior fontanelle. They each admit an emissary vein to the superior sagittal sinus. These are usually clinically insignificant, tiny openings 1 mm in diameter or less and may be absent or closed at birth.

As parietal ossification progresses during fetal development, it radiates in such a way as to leave a cleft at the upper part of the bone in front of the posterior fontanelle, the cleft on the two sides forming a round space across the sagittal suture known as the **sagittal fontanelle**, which has usually closed by the 5th month. The parietal foramina can be regarded as the remains of this fontanelle. In about 5% of all babies, impaired ossification results in parietal foramina that are large enough to be clinically evident. This presents either as a persistent sagittal fontanelle (discussed in more detail under "Fontanelles" on page 17) or, much less commonly, an irregular opening in the parietal bone on one or both sides which can, very rarely, be as large as 3 cm in diameter. These holes present more like fontanelles than anything else and may be large enough to allow bulging or pulsation of the overlying scalp. Large parietal foramina represent a lack of mineralization, but may appear in otherwise normal infants (Chasler, 1972; Jackson, 1933; Rudolph, 1997, Vol. 3).

Frontal bones: The vertical portion of each of the two frontal bones consists of a slightly curved plate of bone that forms half of the forehead. These bones meet in the center of the forehead at the **frontal** or **meiotic suture** (see the suture section on page 16 for more details). The lower portion of each frontal bone is shaped like bilateral partial cups with a notch between them for the nose. The cups form the roof of the orbital and nasal cavities, thus contributing to the floor of the anterior portion of the cranium. (For a drawing of the frontal bones, see page 14.)

Within each frontal bone is a cavity, the frontal air sinus, which is present but undeveloped in the newborn. The upper border of each plate-shaped portion of the frontal bones meets a parietal bone on either side of the skull. The lower borders form the orbital ridge at the eyebrow line. The frontal bones develop intramembranously. Together, they articulate with twelve other bones: the sphenoid, ethmoid, two parietals, two nasals, two maxillae, two lacrimals and two zygomatics. In addition to the frontal suture, the clinically significant landmarks of the frontal bones are:

Frontal eminence (boss, protuberance or prominence): This is the highest point on each frontal bone on either side. They are roughly centered on the anterior surface of each frontal bone, above each eyebrow. This is the hardest region of these bones.

Glabella: The elevated area between the eyebrows, above the root of the nose.

Orbital ridge: The portion of the frontal bones underlying the eyebrows.

Sinciput (brow or forehead): The major anterior portion of the frontal bones, which is bounded superiorly by the anterior fontanelle, laterally by the coronal sutures and inferiorly by the glabella and the orbital ridges.

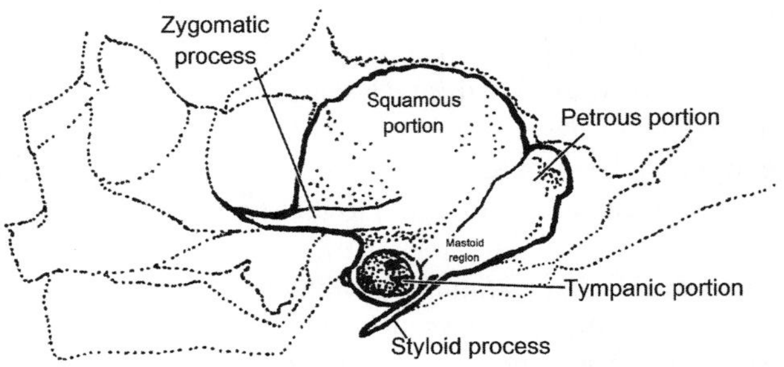

Newborn temporal bone, exterior view

Temporal bones: The two temporal bones contribute to the lower lateral surface of the vault as well as the central portion of the cranial base. The temporal bones provide many passageways for cerebral nerves and blood vessels. The various parts are connected by sutures and fissures, which render these bones quite flexible. The temporal bone has a complex shape. In the newborn, each bone is divided by sutures into three main parts, in addition to the styloid process:

Squamous portion: This part is a rough-edged, oval, relatively flat plate of bone. Its upper border meets the parietal bones on either side along the squamous sutures. It has a horizontal bar of bone (the zygomatic process) that projects forward to meet the tip of the zygomatic bone of the face, where they form the lateral parts of the cheekbone (this can be felt as the elevation that extends from in front of your ears toward your cheeks on either side). Below the origin of the zygomatic process is the mandibular fossa, which is the attachment point for the condyle of the mandible, forming the temporomandibular or jaw joint.

Tympanic portion: A semicircular plate surrounds the opening for the ear canal. It is located below the origin of the zygomatic process. Below that is a needle-like projection called the **styloid process**, which serves as an attachment point for connective tissues of the tongue, neck and hyoid bone.

Petrous portion: The petrous part projects from the inside lower surface of the temporal bone and contributes to the cranial base. It looks like a slightly posteriorly curved, wedge-shaped, mountain ridge that is largest where it meets the squamous portion and tapers toward the center of the skull on either side. It meets the occiput posteriorly and the edges of the sphenoid bone anteriorly. The posterior slope of this ridge forms a depressed part (fossa) of the posterior cranial floor, which can be seen when you look down inside the skull from above. The anterior slope of this ridge, together with the sphenoid bone, forms the midcranial fossa, which provides cup-like supports for the temporal lobes of the brain. The large base of mountain ridge proper houses the middle and inner ear cavities behind the tympanic portion.

The mastoid portion lies behind the ear and serves as an attachment point for some of the muscles of the neck, notably the sternomastoid muscle, and is full of air cavities or sinuses. Nipple-shaped mastoid processes are virtually absent at birth, leaving the facial nerves close to the surface where they are vulnerable to damage, especially from forceps.

The petrous part and the styloid process develop endochondrally, while the squamous and tympanic parts develop intramembranously. Union of the three parts of the temporal bone begins at birth and is complete by the first year, with the exception of the styloid process, which does not fuse until puberty.

Occiput: The occiput is located at the back of the skull. Parts of the occiput contribute to both the vault and the base of the skull. The newborn occiput is commonly described as a solid bone. It is actually comprised of four regions of ossification: the squamous part, the two condylar (lateral or exoccipital) parts and the basilar part. The illustration on page 15 shows the occiput in relationship to the other bones of the skull. The occiput is not completely fused at term. Synchondrodial joints separate these regions, facilitating mobility of adjacent bones. These regions are described below.

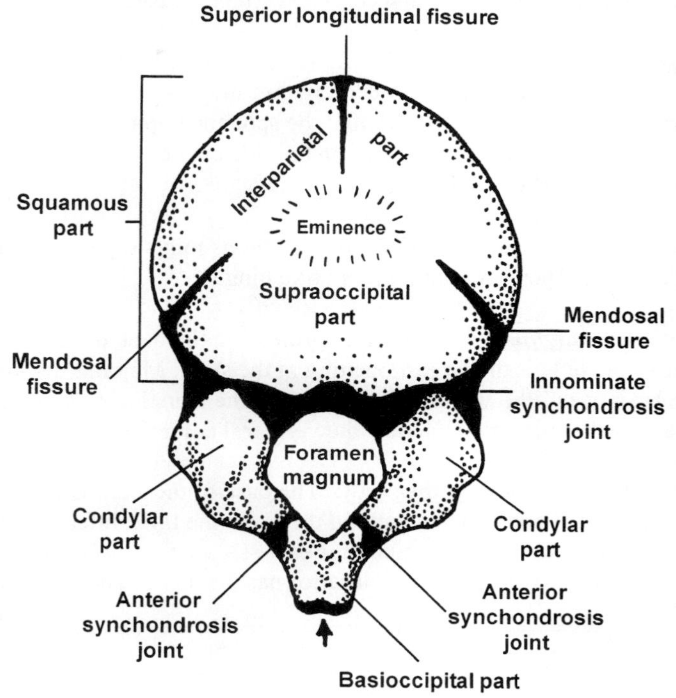

Newborn occiput, viewed from below
(arrow indicates basioccipital side of the sphenooccipital joint)

Squamous part: The squamous part of the occiput consists of a convex protective plate extending upward from the nape of the neck, across the back of the head in a broad, blunt-tipped triangle. This is the part generally referred to when the occiput is discussed in most midwifery and obstetric textbooks. It consists of a single structure divided into two regions or parts, as follows:

Interparietal (upper) part: This forms the upper portion of the vault of the occiput and is the only part which contributes to the vault of the skull. It is a relatively smooth, gently curved, flat plate of bone lying between the two parietal bones, bordered by the lambdoid suture above and the mendosal suture-fissures below. This is the only portion of the occiput that ossifies intramembranously.

The newborn has three cartilaginous fissures which allow slight flexibility of this otherwise solid bone, contributing to the mobility of the interparietal part during moulding, as follows:

Superior longitudinal (medial) fissure: This consists of a partially fused split extending from the center of the upper border of the interparietal part downward, terminating roughly where the elevation of the occipital eminence begins.

Mendosal suture-fissures (2): These splits begin at the edge of the bone on either side and proceed at a slightly upward slant, following the angle up from each lower corner of the occiput. These fissures serve as a partial line of demarcation separating the interparietal (upper) part from the supraoccipital (lower) part. They terminate on either side approximately where the elevation of the occipital eminence begins.

Supraoccipital (lower) part: This is the lower region of the squamous part of the occiput. Its upper border is located along the angles of the mendosal suture-fissures. The lower border meets the condylar parts on either side and the foramen magnum in the center. Its shape is an extension of the interparietal plate. The surface is roughened due to the attachment of many muscles. The supraoccipital region is bounded from below by the **innominate synchondrodial joints.** These cartilaginous joints separate the supraoccipital region from the condylar parts of the occiput on either side. They contribute to the slight mobility of the occiput during birth, and have been called the obstetric joints.

The most clinically relevant landmark of the squamous part is the **external occipital eminence (protuberance, prominence or boss).** This is the most elevated region on the vault of the occiput at the back of the head. This landmark is located roughly in the center of the squamous part, bounded from below by the points of the Mendosal suture-fissures and above by the point of the medial fissure. The eminence is an important landmark when measuring certain skull diameters.

Condylar (exoccipital or lateral) parts of the occiput: At birth, the condyles are two elongated oval facets of bone that lie horizontal to the top of the head, deep within the upper neck, where they contribute to the base of the skull. The condylar parts border the lower edge of the temporal bone at the petrooccipital suture. The inside edges of these bones form the sides of the foramen magnum in a flattened, widened, short, fat, rounded "V"; they rest upon (articulate with) the atlas, which forms the first cervical vertebra. Posteriorly, they meet the edge of the supraoccipital part on either side.

Basioccipital part of occiput: The lowermost, central, portion of the occiput forms the anterior border of the foramen magnum (closest to the chin) deep within the base of the skull. It is shaped like a short, fat "Y." The tail of the "Y" meets the sphenoid bone in front at the sphenooccipital synchondrodial joint. The tip of each arm of the "Y" meets the anterior border of a condylar part on the sides. The outside edges of the basioccipital part are bordered on either side by the petrous portion of the temporal bone.

***Anterior synchondroses*:** These cartilaginous joints separate the condylar and the basioccipital parts of the occiput on either side. They act as slightly mobile hinges.

Foramen magnum: In addition to protecting the back of the brain, the occiput also forms the foramen magnum. This four-sided hole is the largest opening in the skull. Major structures passing through it include the medulla oblongata of the brain stem, the vertebral arteries, and the spinal accessory nerves. Ligaments around the margins of the foramen attach to the joints that connect the vertebral column to the base of the skull.

Cranial base (floor) of the skull: The base of the skull is formed by portions of several bones: the central portion of the sphenoid bone which is behind the eyes; the thick inferior petrous portion of the temporal bones; the basioccipital and condylar parts of the occiput; the ear ossicles; the lowermost border of the frontal and ethmoid bones; and the inferior parts of the maxillae, palatine, inferior nasal conchae and vomer bones of the face.

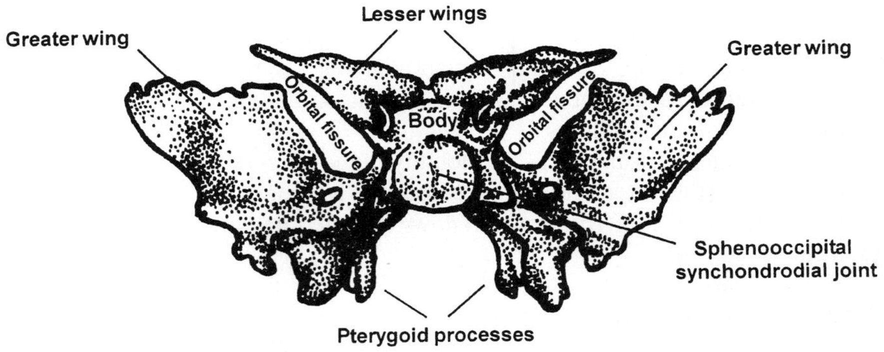

Newborn sphenoid bone (posterior view)

Sphenoid (SFEE-noid) bone: This intricate bone, shaped roughly like a bat in flight, consists of a central body and three pairs of processes or projections (the greater wings, the lesser wings and the pterygoid [TER-ih-goid] processes). It is wedged between the frontal, temporal and basilar part of the occipital bones and spans the width of the midcranial cavity. Its central body is more or less a cube and lies behind the bridge of the nose. The central body is hollow, containing a pair of air sinuses, separated by a septum. The tops of these sinuses meet on top of the bone to form an enclosure for the pituitary gland. The greater wings project laterally from the central body, forming the posterior walls of the eye sockets and part of the sidewalls of the skull (flag-shaped bony areas on the sides of the skull in front of each ear). The horn-like lesser wings form part of the floor of the anterior cranial cavity and part of the side walls of the orbits. The trough-shaped pterygoid processes project inferiorly from the central body, anchoring the pterygoid muscles, which are used in chewing.

The sphenoid bone is called the keystone of the cranium because it articulates with all the other cranial bones. Major points of contact include articulation with the frontal and ethmoid bones above and the vomer and palatine bones (small facial bones) below. On the sides it meets the zygomatic (cheek), parietal and temporal bones. The central posterior border of the sphenoid bone and the central anterior border of the basioccipital bone meet to form the **sphenooccipital synchondrodial joint**. This joint acts as a hinge that allows the entire occipital region slight mobility during moulding in labor and during respiration after birth.

The body of the sphenoid, its lesser wings and the roots of the greater wings ossify endochondrally. The pterygoid processes and the bulk of the greater wings ossify intramembranously. These parts unite by the end of the first year.

Auditory ossicles: The three tiny bones of each ear are the **malleus**, **incus**, and **stapes**. They develop intramembranously and have nearly reached adult size by term.

Intercalary (Wormian, sutural, intrasutural, fontanelle or intrafontanelle) bones

These tiny, irregularly shaped bones or bony clusters are extra bones not present in all individuals that may develop within the borders of a suture. They are often found along the lambdoidal sutures and much more rarely in the anterior fontanelle. They are structurally insignificant and represent additional ossification centers that appear during fetal development. The bones themselves pose no problem but are sometimes associated with cretinism, cleidocranial dysostosis and osteogenesis imperfecta.

Openings in and attachments to the skull

There are a total of 85 openings for the passage of nerves, organs and blood vessels to and from the head. Many muscles and ligaments attach to the skull as well. Misalignment of the bones can affect any of these structures.

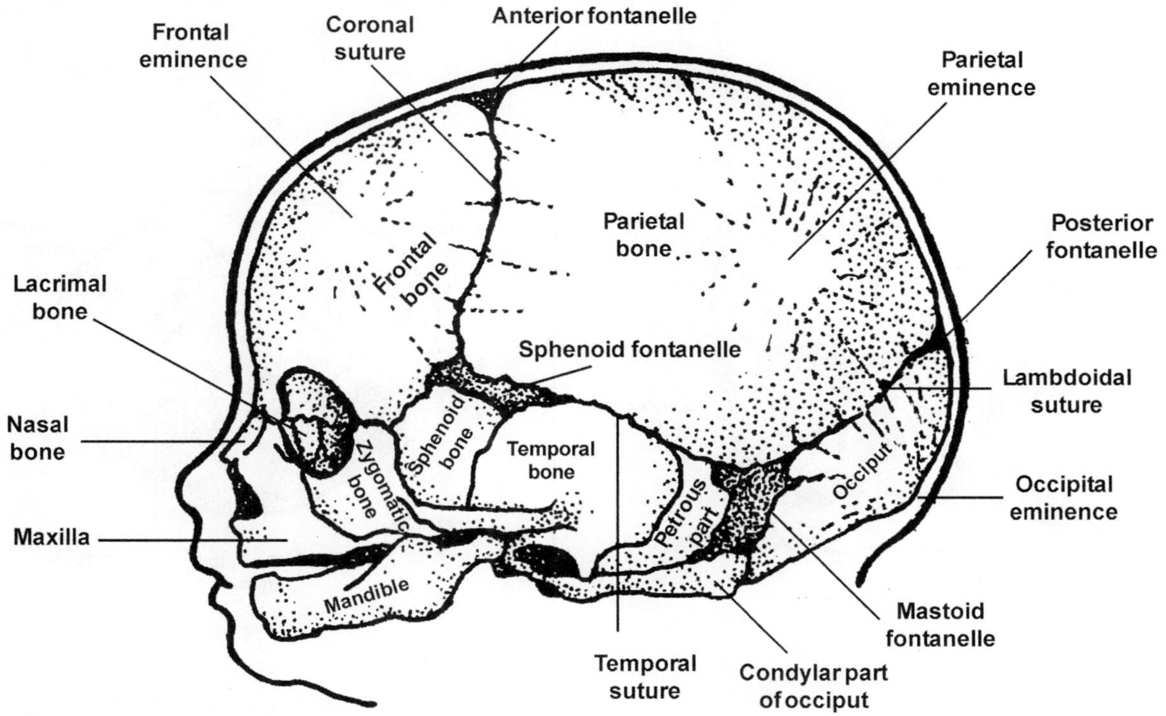

Newborn skull: external side view showing lateral sutures, fontanelles and other features

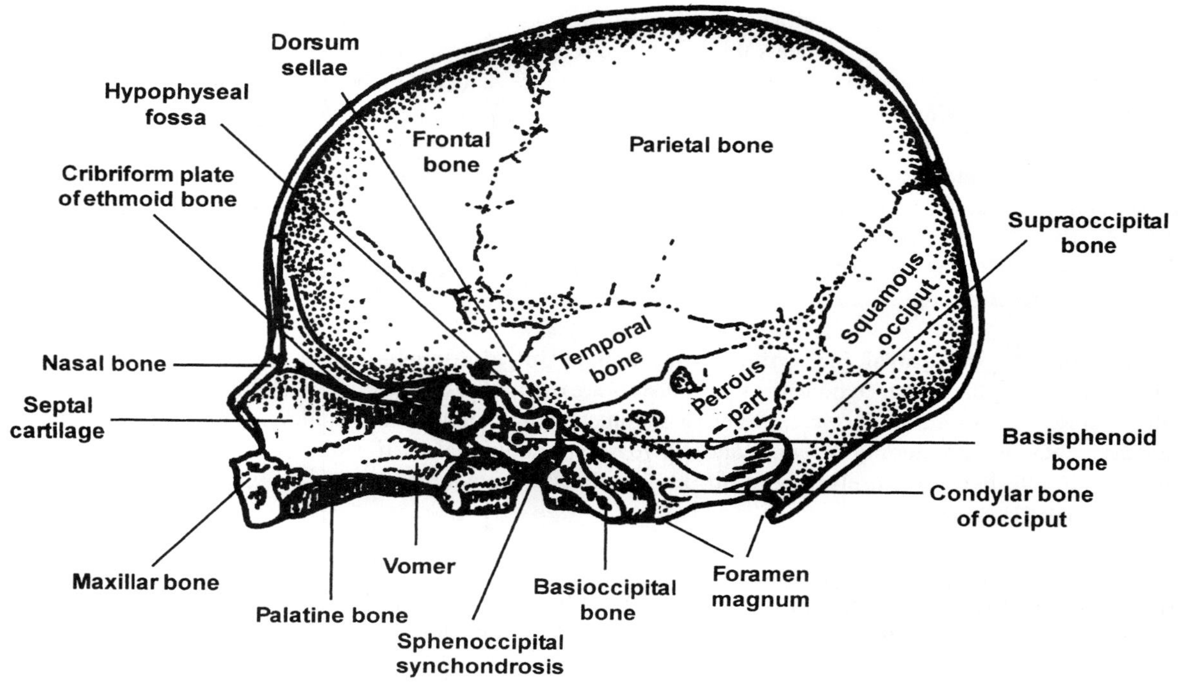

Newborn skull: viewed from inside (sagittal section)

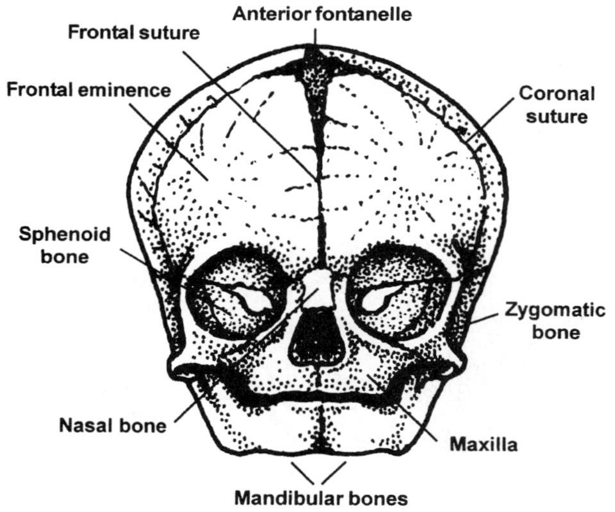

Newborn skull: anterior view

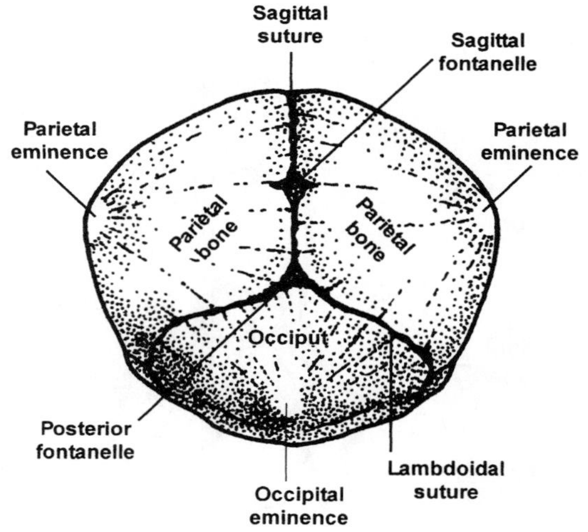

Newborn skull: posterior view

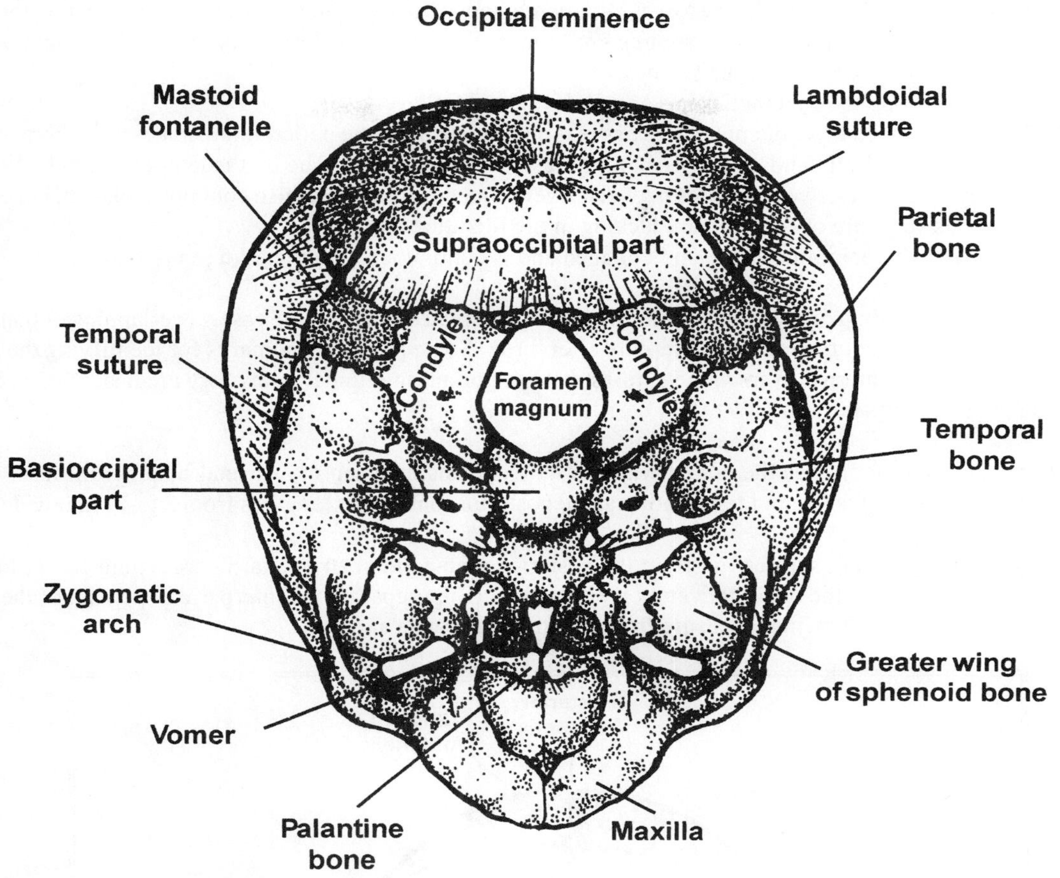

Newborn skull viewed from below (showing typical asymmetrical moulding)

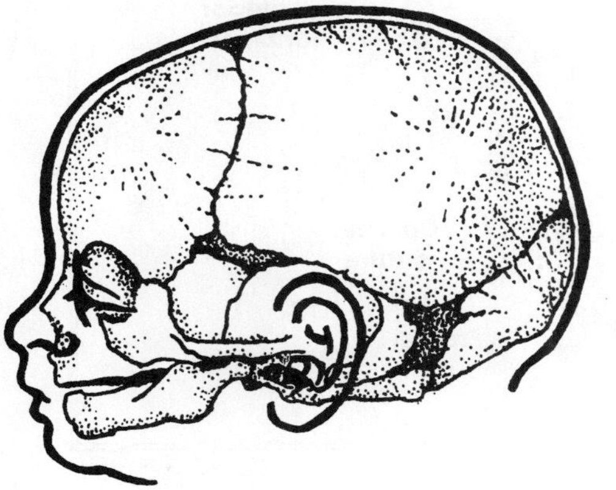

Relationship of external anatomy to skull bones: lateral view

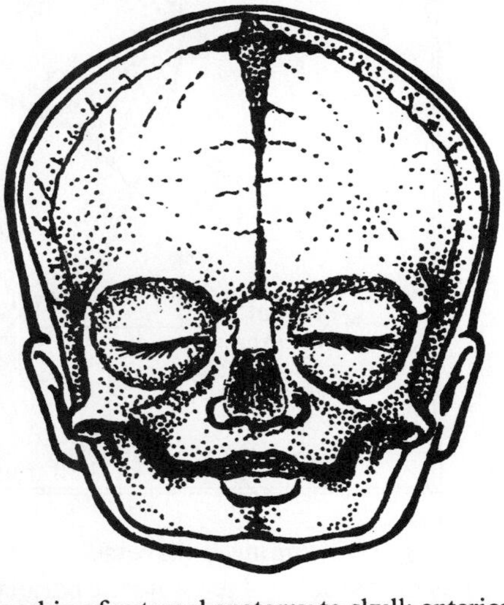

Relationship of external anatomy to skull: anterior view

Sutures of the skull of primary clinical significance

Anatomy: Sutures are the meeting points between intramembranous bones. Fontanelles are located where the sutures intersect. By term, the tissues spanning the sutures and fontanelles consist of four primary layers (Scammon, 1923; Sundaresan, 1990). These are, from the surface down:

Skin: The skin overlying the fontanelles has a well-developed fat layer.

Level 2: This well-defined layer of connective tissue is continuous with the pericranium contains the bony skull plates. It is rich in elastin and consists of highly vascular connective tissue that is later replaced by bone.

Level 3: This layer of connective tissue lies between level 2 and the dura which also contains collagen, but other details as to its structure or function are lacking in the literature.

Level 4: This layer also contains elastin and collagen and is continuous with the dura (endocranium).

The sutures allow moulding or movement of the adjacent bony plates and, in some cases, overlapping of bony edges. They also allow the brain to continue growing rapidly after birth. Some provide landmarks for identifying the position of the fetal skull during an internal exam. The sutures most important in clinical midwifery are described below (see illustrations on pages 13, 14 and 16):

Sagittal suture: This suture divides the cranial vault in half. It runs between the parietal bones from front to back, originating at the anterior fontanelle and terminating at the posterior fontanelle. It ranges from 3 to 17 mm wide at term.

Lambdoidal sutures (2): These sutures run from the posterior fontanelle in an outwardly sweeping curve, following down and around the border of the occipital vault on either side. They separate the interparietal portion of the occiput from the two parietal bones. They may measure from 1.5 to 11 mm wide at term.

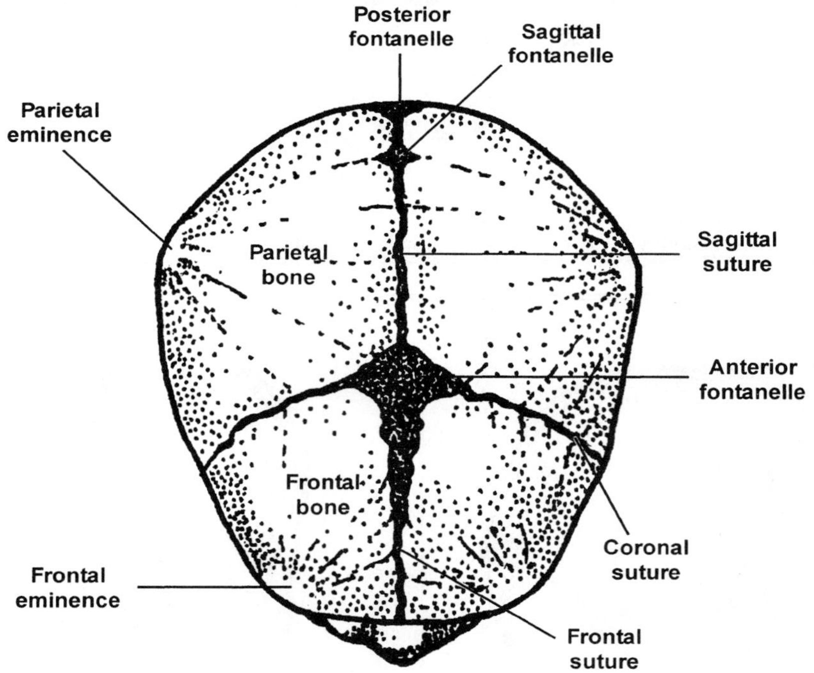

View of skull from above, showing sutures and fontanelles

Coronal sutures (2): Running transversely and downward from the anterior fontanelle to the sphenoid fontanelle on either side, the coronal sutures separate the parietal bones from the frontal bones. They measure 1 to 11 mm wide at term.

Frontal (metopic) suture: Located between the two frontal bones, the frontal suture is an anterior continuation of the sagittal suture. It extends from the central, anterior point of the anterior fontanelle to the glabella (down the center of the forehead to the area between the eyebrows above the bridge of the nose). It may be mistaken for the sagittal suture in deflexed presentations during internal exams and can help to distinguish a face presentation.

Temporal (lateral or squamous) sutures (2): The temporal sutures separate the temporal bone from the parietal bone on either side of the head. Each extends from the temporal fontanelle in front, forming a gentle arch, dipping down near the uppermost tip of the pinna and running almost straight to the posterolateral fontanelle in back. During birth, the temporal suture allows some upward and downward mobility of the parietal bones. It also allows the temporal bone to move upward and forward toward the sphenoidal fontanelle.

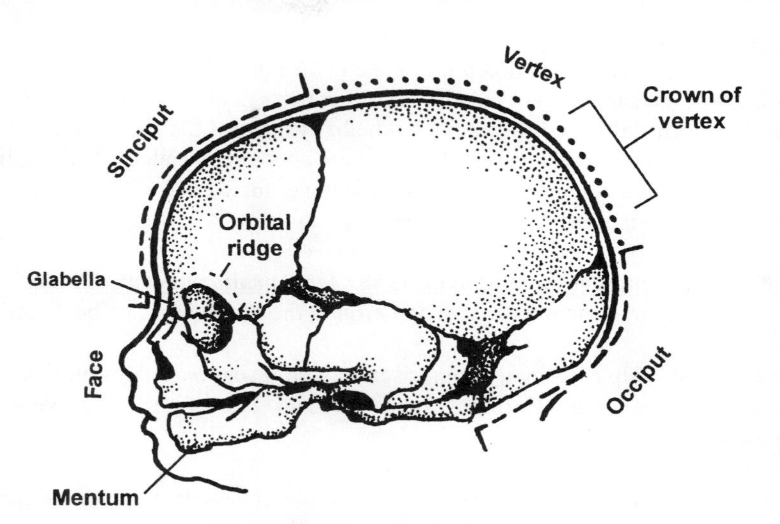

Other clinically relevant external landmarks of the fetal skull

Fontanelles of primary clinical significance

Membrane and skin-covered openings or spaces known as "fontanelles" are located at the intersection of each suture line. The anterior and the posterior fontanelles are the most clinically important of these landmarks. Their position and shape help identify the position of the vertex of the fetal skull in the mother's pelvis during labor. Other fontanelles are clinically relevant primarily because they allow movement of the adjacent bones.

Anterior fontanelle (bregma): This fontanelle is located at the junction of the sagittal, frontal, and coronal sutures. It is a diamond-shaped opening bordered by the two frontal and two parietal bones. It is the largest fontanelle, averaging about 3 cm in width by 2 cm in length at term. The bregma refers to both the fontanelle and the region immediately surrounding it.

Posterior fontanelle (lambda): This fontanelle is located where the sagittal suture meets the two lambdoidal sutures. Bordered by the interparietal occiput posteriorly and the parietal bones anteriorly, it forms an inverted "Y." The tail of the "Y" becomes the sagittal suture and the arms of the "Y" begin the lambdoidal sutures on either side. The posterior fontanelle is much smaller than the anterior fontanelle and is more a meeting point for the bones than a fontanelle in the strictest definition of an open space.

Sagittal or interparietal fontanelle (false, Gerdy's): This is a developmental fontanelle that usually continues to ossify so that by the fifth month of gestation, the tiny parietal foramina in each parietal bone are all that remain. However, in 5% of babies, a well-developed sagittal fontanelle is present at birth. It consists of a small, diamond-shaped space, usually located one-quarter of the distance anterior to the posterior fontanelle in the sagittal suture. If found during an internal exam, it is most likely to be mistaken for the anterior fontanelle because it is similarly diamond-shaped. This feature is often benign but may be associated with certain fetal anomalies. The parietal foramina may also fail to ossify by term, leaving openings in this area on one or both sides of the sagittal suture, which also may resemble fontanelles. These are described in more detail under "Parietal bones" on page9.

Anterolateral (sphenoidal) fontanelles (2): Formed at the junction of the parietal, frontal, sphenoid and temporal bones on either side of the skull, the sphenoidal fontanelles allow the temporal bone to move upward and forward. They cannot be palpated during a normal labor and therefore do not serve as important directional landmarks.

Posterolateral (mastoid) fontanelles (2): These roughly rectangular membranous openings are located laterally and posteriorly (well behind the ears) at the junction of the parietal, temporal and occipital bones. They allow the temporal and the occipital bones to move during labor, but cannot normally be palpated. They are not relevant directional landmarks.

Newborn-to-adult changes in the skull

After skeletal ossification is complete in the adult, the number of skull bones is reduced from 51 to 29 (including the ossicles of the ear and the hyoid bone). There are 15 bones in the face, 8 in the cranium and 6 located in the inner ears. The newborn skull has 34 sutures. As the baby matures the edges of membranous bones gradually become serrated and finally interlock. However, the edges of these bones are beveled allowing slight movement during respiration throughout most of the life span. Depending upon the bone, fusion takes place at various times during the maturation process. By adulthood, the number of sutures is reduced to 25.

Soft tissue structures in and around the fetal brain relevant to birth

A variety of structures within and around the brain may also be directly impacted by the birth process, as follows:

Scalp: The scalp is formally comprised of skin layers only; however, the tissue layers between the skull bone and the skin surface are commonly referred to as the scalp. It consists of five layers of tissue, listed here from the most superficial to the deepest layer:

Epidermis: Tough, elastic skin surface.

Dermis: Subcutaneous layer containing blood vessels, lymphatics, hair follicles and dense connective tissue.

Epicranial aponeurosis (galea): A thin layer of tendon that covers the vertex, connecting the frontal and occipital portions of the occipitofrontalis muscle. Laterally, it is attached to the zygomatic arch, the auricular muscles and the tissues of the posterior triangle (the region of the neck bounded by the sternocleidomastoid muscle, the trapezius muscle, and the upper border of the clavicle, including the omoclavicular triangle, which is bounded by the clavicle, the omohyoid muscle, and the sternocleidomastoid muscle and contains the subclavian artery and vein. This tendon forms a large potential space with poorly defined margins, allowing any subgaleal bleeding to cross suture lines and travel into the region of the ear, forehead or neck.

Loose connective tissue: A loose, irregularly arranged layer of connective tissues permits limited movement of the scalp muscles and the three superficial layers above it.

Pericranium: The pericranium is the periosteum of the skull. It covers the outer surfaces of the cranial bones, firmly adhering at their edges. It forms a protective covering that contains any bleeding that may occur beneath it.

Meninges: There are three primary protective membranous layers that surround the brain: the dura mater, the arachnoid mater and the pia mater. To fully appreciate the following description, it will be most helpful to review the material on the shape and lobes of the brain in the part of the text covering anatomy in the chapter entitled "The Nervous System" of Volume I before studying this section.

Dura mater (tough mother): The dura mater has two layers that cover the brain like a glove. The outer endosteal layer is a strong, thick, inelastic fibrous membrane that forms the endocranium (periosteum of the skull cavity). Its inner meningeal layer forms a thin, exceptionally smooth membrane next to the brain. These layers are fused, but are separated more easily in children than in adults. The dura mater extends downward through the foramen magnum to enrobe the entire spinal cord. In the skull, it is especially adherent to the cranial base, along the edges of sutures and around the foramen magnum. These attachments help to limit the motion of the skull bones. In the spaces between membranous bones (at the sutures and fontanelles), the dura mater fuses with the pericranium (the periosteum of the skull surface). The dura also forms protective channels for the major venous sinuses that drain the head. Several of these channels are formed in special grooves on the interior of the skull at the margins of the dura mater and where the partitions meet.

In the same way that the material of a glove is a continuous covering that encases the body of the hand and forms folds between the fingers in communicating compartments to simultaneously separate, enclose and protect the fingers, the dura mater consists of a continuous sheet of tissue that covers the brain and has several folds that extend between various regions of the brain. These folds form two primary and two smaller partitions, dividing the brain into communicating compartments. These partitions stabilize and support the brain within the skull and provide conduits for some of the cranial blood vessels. In order to visualize the three-dimensional structure of these partitions, the brain and the outer covering of the dura must be removed, leaving these internal folds intact. The primary extensions of the dura are the **falx cerebri** and the **tentorium cerebelli**. The smaller extension of the dura mater are the **falx cerebelli** and the **diaphragma sellae**. These extensions function like ligaments for the skull.

Falx cerebri: This sickle-shaped, double-layered fold of dura mater extends downward from the sagittal suture as a tough vertical membrane between the hemispheres of the brain, dividing the cranial cavity into right and left hemispheres. Its lower border lies just above the corpus callosum. The upper border of the falx cerebri forms a continuous attachment to the inside of the skull beginning just beneath the occipital eminence, following the sagittal and frontal sutures, continuing along the midline and ending at the crista galli on the ethmoid bone at the interior root of the nose. Below the occipital eminence, the lowermost posterior edge of the falx cerebri forms an inverted, wide-armed "Y" with the tentorium cerebelli. The arms of the inverted "Y" have an anteriorly oriented slant and are not attached to bone.

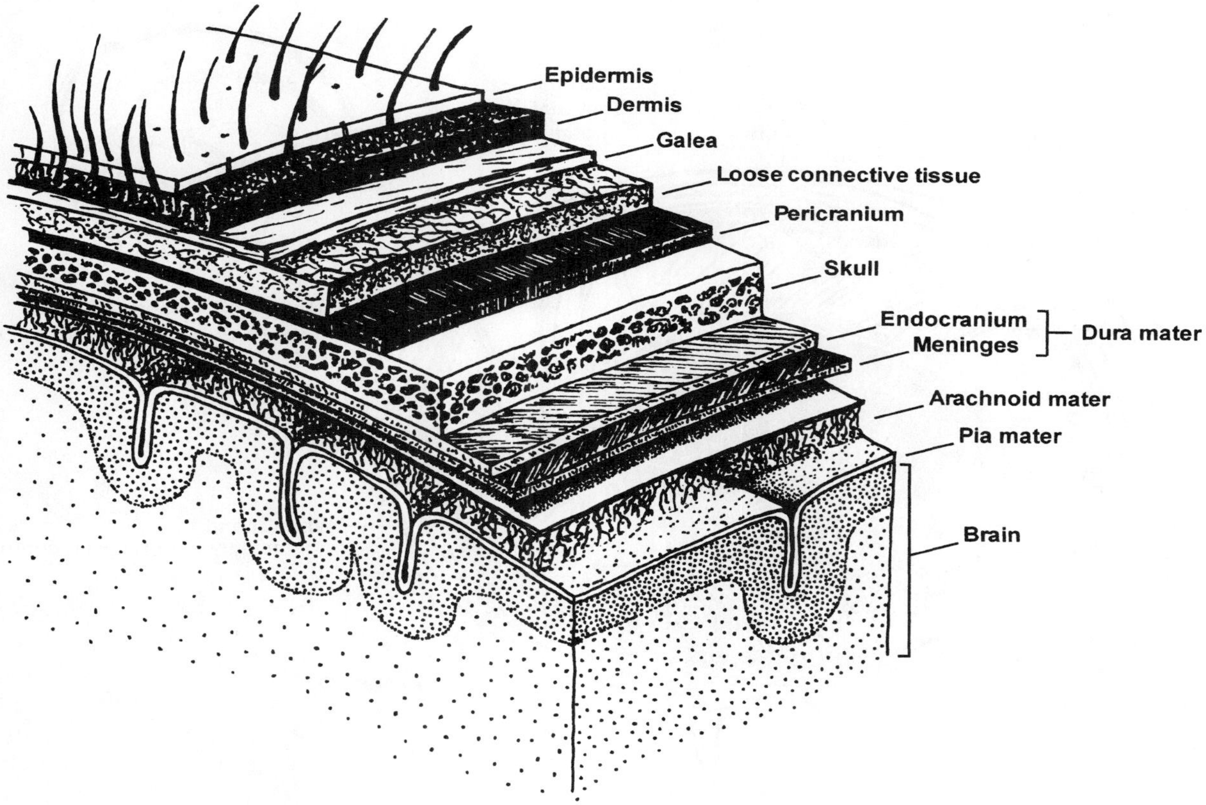

Layers of the scalp and dura mater

Tentorium cerebelli: The posterior center of this fold of dura is located at the level of the occipital eminence. Here the widest portion of the tentorium is attached to the posterior free edge of the falx cerebri in an inverted "Y," which forms a peak, like an A-frame tent, over the cerebellum. On either side, the walls of the tent flair sideways and around the border of the skull at a slight downward angle and then curve forward on each side to form a broad, horizontal crescent-shaped membranous "shelf" under the occipital lobe of the brain.

The outer edge of the shelf extends along the grooves of the transverse venous sinuses of the occipital bone, where it forms a canal for the transverse sinus. It continues along the posteroinferior angle of the parietals to the upper borders of the petrous portion of the temporal bone on each side (at about the level of the tragus of the newborn ear).

From the anterior border of the petrous part of the temporal bone (at the about the level of the posterior corner of the baby's lower jaw), the outer edge is unattached and continues anteriorly. This suspended portion narrows sharply as it extends into the anterior midcranium. The anterior tips of the unattached border are connected on either side to the two anterior and two posterior clinoid processes on the upper posterior surface of the lesser wing of the sphenoid bone, in the center of the anterior third of the skull. At the point where the tentorial shelf leaves its peripheral attachment, the outer edge of the lower layer of the tentorium continues down on either side, forming two teardrop-shaped cups with the wide end of the tear toward the front of the skull. These cups cradle the temporal lobes on either side of the brain behind the eyes. The outer wall of each cup sweeps up and is continuous with the dura mater which overlies the outer surface of the brain.

The inside horizontal free edge of the tentorium forms a U-shaped opening called the **incisura** or **tentorial notch**. The brain stem passes to the spinal cord through this opening. This notch is somewhat larger than the structures that must pass through it, allowing some downward displacement of the brain stem when sufficient pressure is applied to the head.

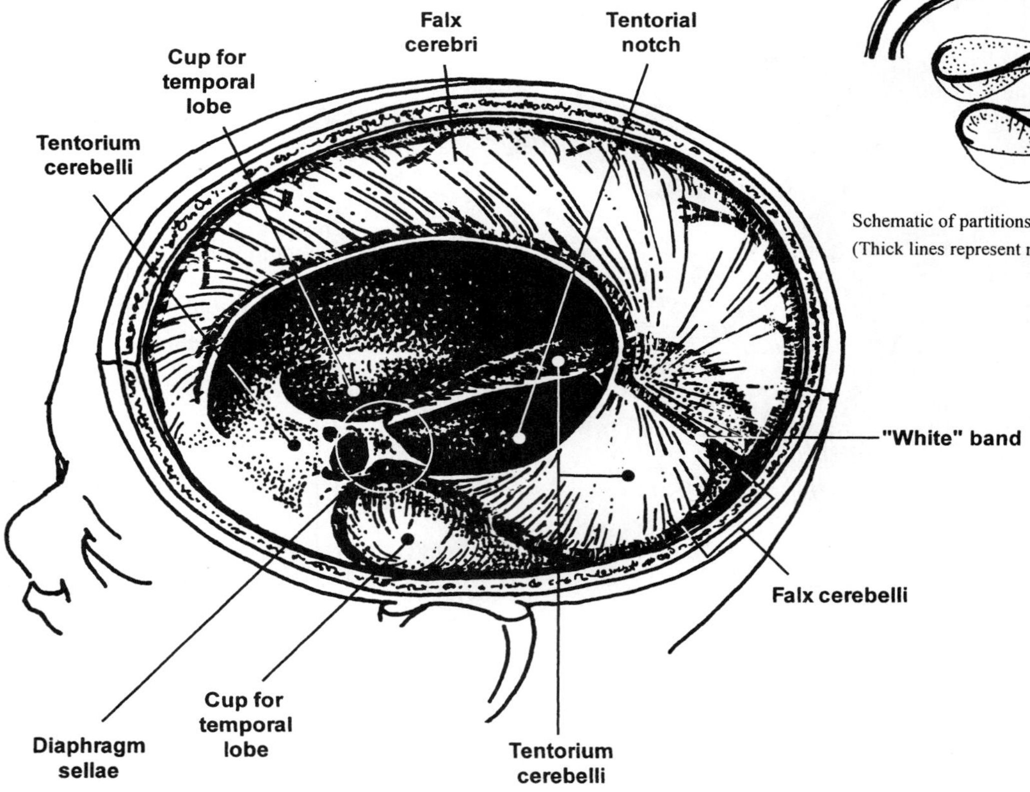

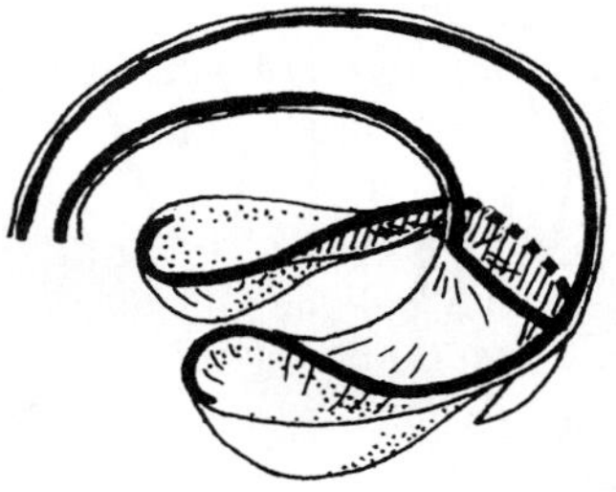

Schematic of partitions showing their shape (Thick lines represent major blood vessels)

Cut away view with brain removed showing partitions of the dura mater

Falx cerebelli: The falx cerebelli is a small, crescent-shaped fold of dura. Its upper border is attached to the posterior third or so of the inferior border of the tentorium cerebelli. Its posterior edge is attached vertically to the internal occipital crest (a ridge which extends downward from the occipital eminence). Its anterior, vertical free edge curves downward in an anteroposterior orientation and projects into the notch between the two cerebellar hemispheres. Its inferior end is often divided into two small folds which terminate at the edge of the foramen magnum.

Diaphragma sellae: This is a small, horizontal layer of dura mater overlying the posterior, superior surface of the sphenoid bone. It nearly covers the cavity where the pituitary gland is situated.

Fibrous structure of the dura: The fibers of the tentorium and falx cerebri blend to form a strong thin band (white line) beneath the straight sinus (a blood vessel described below). The fibers of the tentorium fan out from the broad posterior edges of the white line and again converge as they pass forward to their anterior attachment. These horizontal bands resist excessive cranial stress. Vertical fibers from the middle two-thirds of the falx cerebri and the lateral tentorium converge in the anterior fifth of the white line, forming a vertical band of strong fibers. These fibers are also arranged to withstand the normal stresses of moulding.

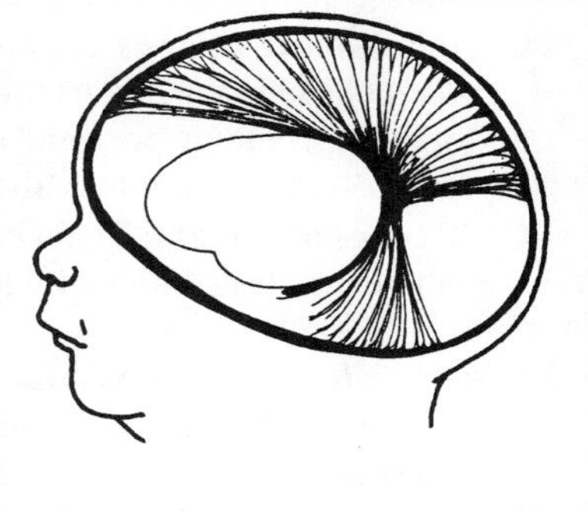

Fibrous structure of dura ("white" line is the deep black region)

Beneath the dura mater are two additional membranes which, when considered together, are sometimes referred to as the leptomeninges or piarachnoid. These membranes line the dura mater and also extend into the folded partitions described above.

Arachnoid (spider-like) mater (parietal layer of leptomeninges): This thin membrane is tenuously attached to the dura and is loosely applied to the pia mater. It is separated from the pia mater by the subarachnoid space, which is filled with cerebrospinal fluid and contains the largest blood vessels which supply the brain. A gauzy web of fine strands form connections which span this space and anchor the arachnoid mater to the pia mater.

Pia (tender) mater: A delicately thin, highly vascular membrane which is closely applied to the surface of the brain, following its every convolution. The leptomeningeal space is that which lies between the arachnoid and pia maters.

The cerebral vascular system: The brain and its vascular system undergo rapid growth and remodeling throughout gestation. Between ten weeks gestation and term, the entire development of the cerebral hemispheres takes place and the weight of the brain increases by about 100-fold. By term, the brain's arterial system is more mature than the venous system. Certain cerebral veins are more susceptible to birth-related strains and injury because they are attached to the dura mater. In addition these venous sinuses are devoid of the elastic muscle tissue found in all other veins, making them more vulnerable to trauma.

The superficial cerebral veins consist of three main groups: the **ascending veins** pass up and over the outer hemisphere of the brain on either side to join the veins of the medial surface and drain into the superior sagittal sinus via a series of **superior cerebral bridging veins**. A descending group of veins drain partly down and forward to enter the sphenoparietal or cavernous sinus and partly down and backward to the transverse sinus. The **inferior (basal) veins** drain mainly into the sphenoparietal and cavernous sinus, into the basal vein, then into the **great cerebral vein (great vein of Galen)**, and finally into the superior and transverse sinuses. Venous drainage of the cerebellum occurs via a surface network that empties into the adjacent venous sinuses in the dura mater.

There are several medium to large midline venous sinuses which drain blood from the brain.

Superior sagittal (longitudinal) sinus: This large vessel runs along the inside of the skull from front to back along the upper border of the falx cerebri, extending from the level of the bridge of the nose, up the frontal suture, along the sagittal suture and down to the occipital eminence. It receives the superior cerebral veins and veins from the pericranium. This vessel is often incompletely formed at term.

Inferior sagittal (longitudinal) sinus: This large vessel runs along the lower border of the falx cerebri to its junction with the tentorium cerebelli. It receives veins from the falx cerebri and some drainage from the medial aspects of the brain. This sinus is fully developed at birth.

Straight sinus: This large vessel is a continuation of the inferior longitudinal sinus. It extends from front to back along the junction of the falx cerebri and tentorium cerebelli until it joins the superior longitudinal sinus. It drains the inferior longitudinal sinus and the great cerebral vein.

Great cerebral vein (great vein of Galen): This vessel receives blood returning from many vessels of the brain, including the basal vein, the thalamostriate (terminal) vein and other internal cerebral veins. These vessels unite to form the great cerebral vein which joins the straight sinus at its junction with the inferior longitudinal sinus.

Occipital sinus: This vessel runs from the occipital eminence, through the posteriorly attached border of the falx cerebelli and then down to the foramen magnum. It receives blood from small vessels of the inferior surface of the cerebellum, pons and medulla and empties into the confluence of sinuses. This vessel is quite variable in size and is sometimes absent.

Confluence of sinuses: The meeting point of the superior sagittal, straight and occipital sinuses at the occipital eminence. It is drained by the two transverse sinuses of the dura mater.

There are also four bilateral venous sinuses:

Transverse sinuses (2): Beginning at the confluence of sinuses, these vessels run around the outer edge of the tentorium. They continue as the sigmoid sinuses and empty into the internal jugular vein.

Superior petrosal sinuses (2): These run from the cavernous to the transverse sinus, within the attached margin of the tentorium along the petrous ridge of the temporal bone.

Inferior petrosal sinuses (2): These run from the cavernous sinus along the groove between the petrous portion of the temporal bone and the occiput to the jugular foramen and the internal jugular vein.

Cavernous sinuses (2): These run on each side of the body of the sphenoid bone between the superior orbital fissure and the highest point of the petrous portion of the temporal bone. Each receives blood from the ophthalmic vein and empties into the petrosal sinuses posteriorly.

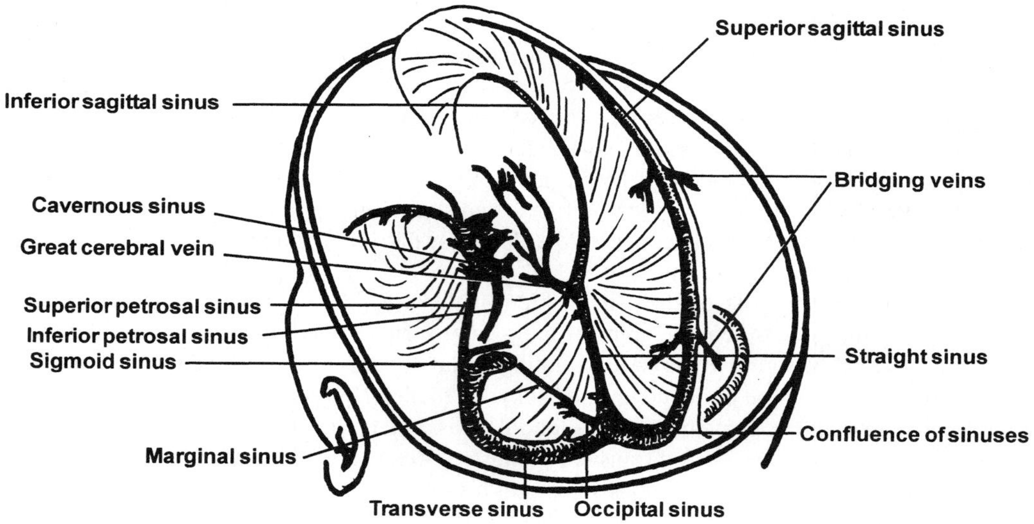

Major venous sinuses within the fetal skull near term

As the baby descends through the pelvis, these intracranial vessels are all subjected to tension and pressure as the head changes shape during labor. The fetal head can withstand considerable compression when pressure is evenly applied. The skull bones are designed so that even pronounced moulding occurs in a way that minimizes strain on these structures. Thus, the brain is protected during the normal stresses of birth. Injury is more likely to occur in very difficult or obstructed labors, when instruments or strong fundal pressure are used to extract the head or if the baby is premature. Excessive occipitofrontal or oblique distortion can cause tearing of veins which bridge the dura or the dural folds themselves. Damage can result in intercranial hemorrhage, which, when severe, leads to brain damage or death. For more details about these types of damage, see the subchapter entitled "Cranial Injuries."

Germinal matrix: The germinal matrix is a developmental feature of the fetal brain that plays a central role in brain growth and maturation. It consists of a layer of specialized tissue located in the brain's subependymal layer. The **ependyma** consists of a cellular membrane that lines the ventricles of the brain as well as the central canal of the spinal cord. This vascular structure is covered with cilia that secrete spinal fluid, thus contributing to the regulation of interventricular pressure. The germinal matrix lies adjacent to this lining at the external angle of the ventricles on either side over the head and body of the caudate nucleus. The **caudate nucleus**, when fully developed, is an elongated curved mass of gray matter with a thick anterior portion called the caput or head, which protrudes into the anterior horn of the lateral ventricle; the corpus or body, which extends along the floor of the body of the lateral ventricle; and the cauda or tail, a thin, elongated, curved portion which curves downward, backward, and forward into the dorsolateral wall of the lateral ventricle.

Having a gelatinous texture, the structure of the germinal matrix is extremely fragile. It serves as a highly active nursery for neurological stem cells. At predetermined times, a wave of rapidly multiplying stem cells will stop dividing and differentiate (early in development they become neuronal cells; later on in development they become glial cells). These cells move outward from the matrix to the developing basal ganglia, cerebral cortex and other forebrain regions.

Within the germinal matrix, amid dense islands of cells, lies a large, complex network of very fragile immature blood vessels and capillaries that are almost devoid of supportive connective tissue. The vessels have extensive connections between them during most of midgestation. The venous drainage system for the germinal matrix forms a "U" before it merges with the great cerebral vein. Prior to 32 weeks, most of the cerebral blood flow occurs in this central brain region. The U-shaped drainage vessels can easily become overloaded, which causes the area to be very intolerant of pressure changes. If venous pressure rises, as it can in the presence of hypoxic-ischemic events or even postural changes after birth (such as holding the baby head-down), delicate vascular walls can be damaged, resulting in bleeding into the adjacent tissue and sometimes into the ventricle cavities, where blood mixes with cerebral spinal fluid. Extensive destruction of the subependymal capillary bed can occur without arterial or venous rupture. (Please note that this is a very simplified explanation of an extremely complex and as-yet incompletely understood process.)

The germinal matrix is meant to develop and then disappear in the gravity-free environment of the uterus, where its fragility is not an issue. It reaches maximal size around 23 weeks gestation with an average diameter of 2.3 mm. As the brain matures, the size of the germinal matrix gradually diminishes as cells in this area migrate away. It decreases to half its maximum size by 32 weeks, is even smaller by 36 weeks and usually involutes entirely by 39 weeks. Injury is most likely to occur around the 23rd week of gestation and is much less frequent after 28 weeks. As gestation proceeds, blood vessels branch out toward the brain's periphery, which reduces the concentration of blood flow in the center of the brain. By term, most of the brain's circulation takes place in the cerebral cortex. Therefore, bleeding tends to occur closer to the surface of the brain, in the cortical region, in near-term infants who suffer cerebral trauma.

The neck

The neck is a specialized region of the spinal column that connects the thoracic spine to the skull at the occipital condyles. It allows the skull to rotate in either direction as much as 110°, and sometimes more, in preterm infants and about 80° by term. It makes it possible for the skull to flex forward or laterally as well as extend backward. Its mobility makes it prone to injury. The clinical landmark of the neck most relevant during breech birth is the **nape of the neck.** This is the region of the scalp just below the occipital eminence. It is demarcated by the posterior hairline.

Atlas: While not a part of the skull per se, the atlas is integral to the consideration of the impact of birth on the baby. The atlas is the first cervical vertebra and serves as the seat for the base of the skull. From above, it resembles the pelvis. The atlas is small and relatively flat at birth, consisting of a ring of bone with an anterior and posterior arch and two lateral masses. The rounded anterior arch forms one-fifth of the ring, and the posterior arch forms two-fifths of the ring. The atlas forms endochondrally and ossifies from three centers, with the entire anterior arch being cartilaginous at birth, as is the symphysis of the posterior arch, which consists of a thin plate at term.

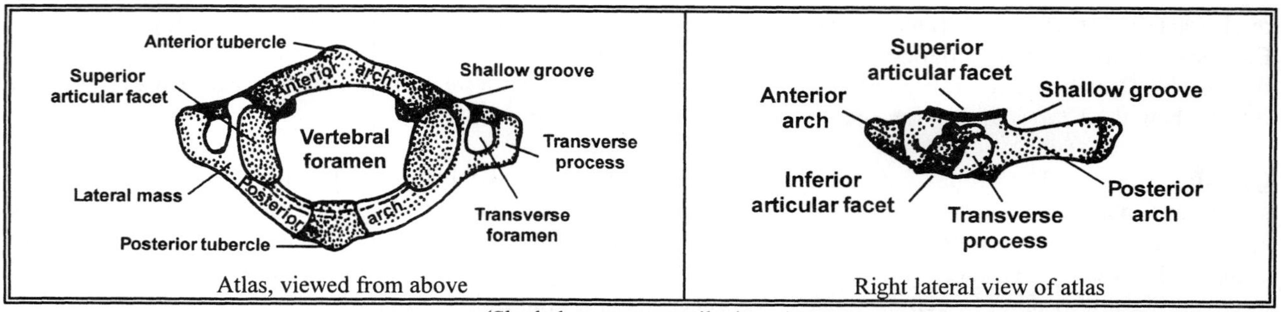

Atlas, viewed from above

Right lateral view of atlas

(Shaded areas are cartilaginous)

The posterolateral portions of the upper surface form concave oval facets to either side of the arches. These facets are angled at an upward, backward slant and are tipped toward the midline, although this angulation is slight in the newborn. They serve as cups into which the occipital condyles fit. Behind each of these depressions is a groove through which the first spinal nerve and the vertebral artery pass to the head. Because the articular facets are incompletely developed at birth, this groove is very shallow in the newborn. On the underside, two circular cups, angled downward and toward the midline, serve as articulations for the axis, the second cervical vertebra, immediately below the atlas.

Two transverse processes project like knob-ended little handles from either side of the outer border of the ring, at the level of the superior facets. The hole in the center of each provides a passageway for the vertebral artery before it enters the groove. The central foramen of the atlas is generously large and has nearly achieved its adult size at term. There is much more room in the opening than is required to allow passage of the spinal cord, thus, the atlas can be considerably out of alignment without resulting in life-threatening spinal compression. (Gilles et al., 1979; Goss, 1973; Williams, 1995).

Atlantooccipital (atloid) joint: The occiput articulates with the spinal column where the condyles rest on the superior facets of the atlas at the base of the skull. This articulation is nearest the posterolateral border of the foramen magnum. This joint is supported by a variety of ligaments and membranes which render it quite mobile.

Spine

The newborn spine forms the long axis of the body. It consists of a series of elastic, cartilaginous vertebrae surrounded by less-elastic connective tissue; otherwise its general anatomy resembles the adult spine except that the infant spine has a convex curve throughout its length. The vertebral column can be stretched about 2 inches (5 cm). When the spine is dissected from the surrounding tissue, it is highly flexible and can be twisted and bent in a half circle forward and backward (Crelin, 1973). However, the spinal cord and meninges are far less elastic, meaning that injudicious traction can cause significant spinal cord damage while leaving no obvious bony injury (Yashon, 1986).

The ability of the fetal spine to flex forward, extend backward, straighten, flex laterally and stretch are important factors in how the baby's body rotates as it descends through the birth canal. In both cephalic and breech labors, the requirement of the spine to flex laterally allows the body to accommodate the shape of the chest as it descends. These are the determining factors in rotation of the upper torso during descent in cephalic presentations. Likewise, the shape of the lower torso and breech, as well as the lateral flexibility of the spine, influence the descent and rotation of the lower torso in breech births. The upper and lower torsos can move independently of each other to a limited extent by virtue of spinal flexibility as well as the rotational mobility at the waist. The fetal spine does not serve as a clinical landmark in most labors. The student is referred to the description of basic adult spinal anatomy found in the chapter entitled "The Skeletal System" in Volume I and to the subchapter entitled "Examining the Back, Spine, Scapulae and Buttocks."

The Upper Torso and Arms

Shoulder girdle

The shoulder girdle is the second most clinically important anatomical feature of the fetus during the birth process.

They must rotate within and beneath the pelvic bones without difficulty. The shoulders also act as the denominator for the chest as it moves through the pelvis. In contrast to the oval shape of the head, the shoulders form a longer, more narrow axis consisting of a clavicle in front and a scapula in back on either side. The shoulder girdle consists of endochondral bones that are not densely ossified and still have cartilaginous ends at the time of birth. The important landmarks of the shoulder are the clavicles, scapulae and acromion.

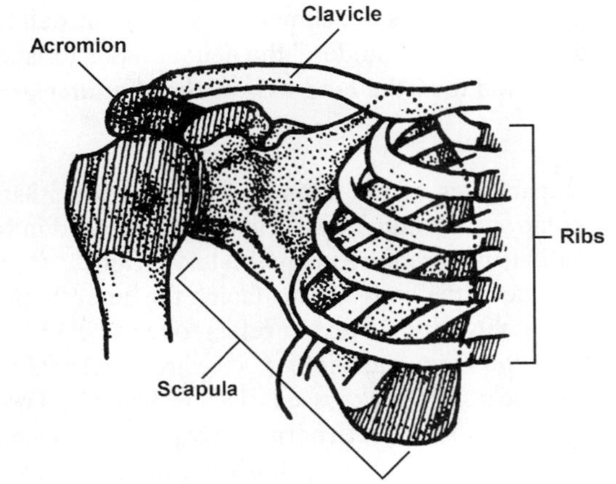

Anatomy of the right shoulder: anterior view

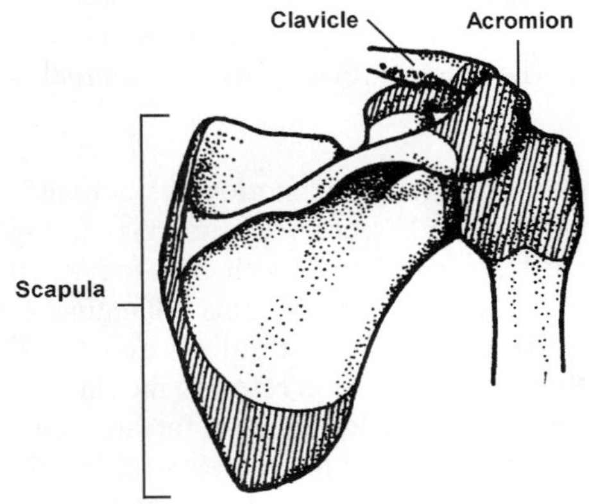

Anatomy of the right shoulder: posterior view

(Cartilaginous areas of the shoulder bones are indicated with thin-line shading.)

The anterior shoulder and armpit provide a passageway for the **brachial plexus of nerves**, which extends from the ventral divisions of spinal nerve roots C4 to T1 under the clavicles on either side to the armpit to the first rib where they divide into anterior and posterior branches to supply the arms on either side. (Note that the nerve roots are numbered according to the cervical vertebra immediately *below* them.) The shoulders are designed for mobility rather than stability, and the soft tissues in this region can be easily damaged with inappropriate handling. (This possibility is covered in depth in the chapters entitled "Assisting at the Birth of a Breech Baby" and "Shoulder Dystocia.") While not part of the brachial plexus proper, the phrenic nerves, which run from the brachial plexus to the diaphragm on either side, are attached to this plexus, primarily as a branch of C4, and it therefore is vulnerable to injury when the brachial plexus injured. The brachial plexus also receives small branches from C3 and C5.

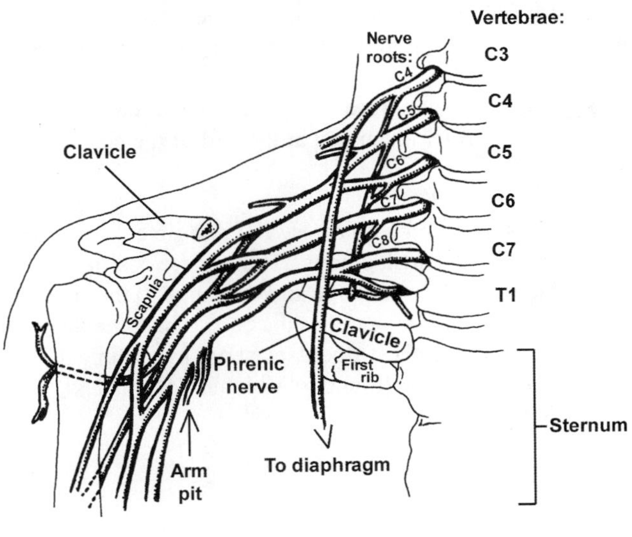

Brachial plexus and phrenic nerve (right anterior view)

Clavicles (collar bones): These long bones extend horizontally from the sternum to the scapula in the uppermost anterior region of the thorax. Each clavicle is curved at both ends. Each is cone-shaped at its sternal end and flattened at its outer end, where it articulates with a scapula. The middle two-thirds of the bone is gracefully curved, convex anteriorly while its lateral third is concave anteriorly. The clavicles transmit pressure from the upper limbs to the axial skeleton.

Scapulae (shoulder blades): These large, thin, flat, triangular bony plates are located to the side of the upper spine, where they overlay the posterior rib cage between ribs two and seven on either side. The anterior surface articulates laterally with the clavicle on either side and with the humerus at the shoulder joint.

Acromion (ah-KRO-me-on): The acromion is the lateral end or process of the scapula that projects as a broad, flattened structure overhanging the shoulder joint. It articulates with the clavicle and gives attachment to parts of the deltoid and trapezius muscles. Its lateral border is a palpable landmark– "the point of the shoulder," the denominator for shoulder presentations. The diameter that spans the acromial processes is referred to as the **long axis of the shoulder girdle**.

Arms

Understanding the range of motion, flexion and extension capabilities of the arms is important when assisting complicated cephalic and breech presentations. In cephalic presentations, shoulder dystocia may occur, and in breech presentations, extension of one or both arms may occur; both situations may require manual intervention.

The anatomical position for the arms is hanging relaxed, by the side of the body, palms facing the outer thighs. The arms flex and extend at the shoulder, elbow and, to a limited extent, at the wrist. Flexion refers to moving a body part closer to another, while extension refers to moving the same parts farther from one another. The arms can fold in over the chest, elbows against the lower chest, forearms and hands toward the midline or crossed. This is the normal position in breech descent. This positioning or arms stretched downward along the torso are both normal in cephalic presentations.

If an arm is stretched across the chest (hand over opposite shoulder) in a breech baby, the arm can safely be brought down by hooking a finger over the elbow and sweeping the arm across the chest; this naturally draws the forearm and hand down. When the arms are extended over the head, the elbow bends either directly forward or laterally, away from the midline of the chest, in order to flex the arm and bring it downward. If the forearm is positioned behind the head, the elbow must be directed laterally or downward in an anterior oblique arc to restore it to an anatomical position. While babies are generally more flexible than adults, their basic range and limits of motion are similar. Practice placing your arms in different positions and then moving them to other positions, being very aware of the ways in which the arms move most easily. This will help bring to consciousness how the upper limbs can be safely manipulated. Practice manipulating the arms of babies (explain to them what you are doing) to become proficient in the event of an emergency at a birth.

Hands and wrists: On very rare occasions a hand may present and you will need to distinguish it from a foot. These considerations are further discussed at the end of the chapter under the heading "Feet and ankles."

Chest

The fetal chest is round with a very flexible rib cage made more mobile by the thoracic spine. At birth the sternum and xiphoid process are cartilaginous. The ribs are ossified. While the chest is usually not considered in discussions of the process of labor, in fact its shape and the range of thoracic spinal flexibility dictate how the upper torso rotates (and therefore how the shoulders rotate) as the baby's body navigates the curve of the birth canal in both cephalic and breech presentations. The fetal chest does not serve as a clinical landmark in most labors. The student is referred to the description of chest anatomy found in Volume I of this text.

The Lower Torso and Legs

The lower torso

The lower pole of the fetal torso is known as the breech or region of the buttocks. It is the third largest region of the fetus after the head and upper torso. However, in a term breech baby, the rump closely approximates the size of the head, especially when the buttocks are presenting with the legs extended up along the torso. The bones of the pelvis are endochondral in origin, and are only partially ossified at birth. The thinner regions near the edges are somewhat flexible. The cartilaginous joints between the bones are wide, and the vertebrae of the sacrum are not yet fused. The unfused innominate bones are made up of three separate bones on each side (the ilium, the ischium and the pubis), which are united by a Y-shaped cartilage, with the three bones meeting in the acetabulum. The bones of the iliac crests and the acetabula, as well as most of the ischiopubic rami, are cartilaginous at birth and can be compacted together to a limited extent. Ossification occurs gradually, with the acetabula usually fusing during puberty and the innominate bones fusing between the 20th and 25th year. Important landmarks of and terms pertaining to the pelvic bones and soft structures include the following:

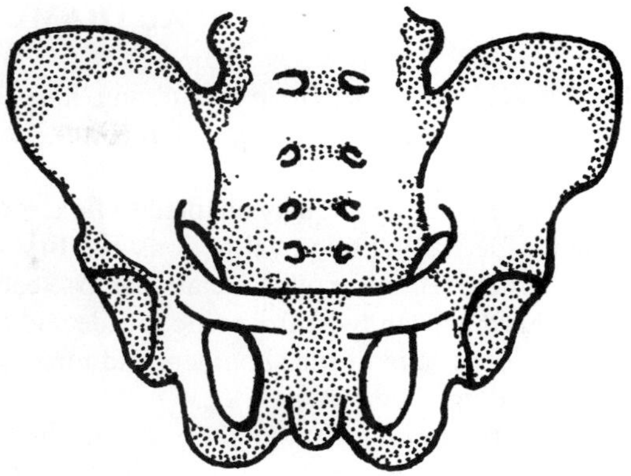

Fetal pelvis anterior view
(shaded areas are cartilaginous)

Anus: Opening of the rectum, found centered between the buttocks in a straight line with the tuberosities.

Breech (rump): Region of the buttocks.

External genitalia: The vulva, labia, clitoris and yoni orifice in girls; the scrotum and penis in boys. The groove that is formed between the legs from the pubic bone to the coccyx is sometimes referred to as the **genital crease**.

Gluteal cleft: Groove of the buttocks.

Iliac crests: The upper borders of the wings of the ilia on either side, commonly referred to as the hip bones. The bisiliac diameter between the top of the crests is sometimes used to designate the **long axis of the pelvis**.

Podalic pole: This is the lower (foot) end of the baby's torso.

Greater trochanters of the femurs: The large bony prominences distally adjacent to the ball joint of each of the femurs. The bitrochanteric diameter runs between the greater trochanters. This diameter is most often referred to as the presenting diameter in a breech and as the long axis of the pelvis. The bisiliac diameter and the bitrochanteric diameter are usually identical.

Tuberosities: Terminating ends of the ischia, also known as the "sit bones." The tuberosities are clinical landmarks used during internal exams to distinguish the breech from the face.

Spines of the sacrum: Small, bony projections that run the length of the exterior surface of the sacrum. These landmarks are unique features of the breech and help distinguish it from the face on internal exam.

Legs

Manipulation of the fetal legs in a breech may be necessary on rare occasions. The need to manipulate the fetal legs during a cephalic birth almost never presents itself, except perhaps in the very rare event that a fetal limb is involved in a compound presentation.

The anatomical position for the legs is standing, toes and knees forward. When the legs are flexed, they may bend at the hip, the knee or, to a limited extent, at the ankle. The knees have limited lateral flexibility when the legs are straight as well, especially when normal fetal outbowing is straightened by splinting of the legs in a frank breech presentation.

Extended legs in a frank breech presents the most likely scenario in which assistance may be needed. To disengage the legs when they are extended upward against the anterior torso, the knee must be flexed toward the side and slightly posteriorly, away from the midline of the body. This moves the lower leg and foot across the anterior torso and downward. A leg that is flexed against the lower torso can be brought down by grasping the ankle and moving it away toward the opposite side of the body (away from the hip joint of the leg being manipulated). This will sweep the knee across the midline and downward. The flexed leg can also unfold by extending the upper leg forward, away from the torso, although this movement is not usually possible if the legs are still in the birth canal.

Practice these maneuvers on yourself, although your limbs will generally be far less flexible that those of a newborn. Also practice with cooperative, informed babies when you get a chance.

Feet and ankles: There will be times that the feet, heels and ankles must be distinguished from a hand. This is pertinent to breech presentations and whenever a small part presents. The heel of the foot will not disappear, regardless of the relationship of the foot with the lower leg. However, the "heel" of the hand will vanish when the hand and wrist are taken out of a right-angle relationship. Examine your own foot and hand to see how this works. The toes and fingers also have distinct differences which allow them to be differentiated on internal exam. These differences are further discussed in the chapter entitled "Performing Internal Exams during Labor."

Ways in Which the Baby's Body Adapts during Descent: Anatomical Diameters, Attitude and Moulding

NOTE: Visual aids will help in studying this chapter. A doll can be used; alternatively, use a jumbo hen's egg. This approximates the shape of the skull, with the occiput at the widest end and the chin at the narrowest end.

The baby's body is uniquely adapted to flex, rotate and reshape itself to fit through the pelvis. The baby's body can be thought of as having two oval regions–the first is the head, and the second is the chest and shoulders (considered together). These regions move in relationship to each other at the neck, which acts as a hinge, and throughout the length of the spine, which can twist from side to side and flex forward, backward and laterally. Note that the long axis of the head and the long axis of the shoulders and torso are at right angles to each other when the body is in the anatomical position (standing, face forward).

The term **fetal pole** refers to either end of the longitudinal axis of the baby's body. The term cephalic (cephalad) refers to the cranium and refers to the head; the term podalic (literally, the foot) refers to the breech.

Flexion, Extension and Rotation of the Head and Understanding the Cephalic Diameters

Knowledge of the way birth works is enhanced by an intimate understanding regarding the shape and movement of the fetal head. The head is the most commonly presenting part of the baby. It is normally slightly larger than the shoulders at term. Viewed from above, the top of the head is oval, with the larger end toward the back and the slightly narrower end toward the face.

The head is freely mobile from back to front and side to side on the neck, allowing it to be positioned in a wide variety of ways. The flexible cervical spine of the term infant allows the head to turn to either side at least 80° easily. The baby will position her head to take the path of least resistance as she passes through the birth canal.

Each attitude of the head presents a more or less favorable set of diameters for birthing. A **diameter** is defined as a straight line connecting two opposite points across a plane of a spherical or cylindrical body–in other words, the distance from side to side across a circle. A **plane** is an imaginary flat surface that spans the object at the level of the diameter. (When an apple is sliced from any angle, the resulting flat surface represents a plane. Measuring straight across this surface between the farthest points gives the diameter of the apple at that plane.)

The diameters of the skull are relevant in relationship to the attitude of the fetal head as it descends. The medical literature describes a number of diameters of the fetal skull, some of which are more clinically useful than others simply because they are associated with more common attitudes of the head. A diameter is designated by naming the location of two anatomical features (landmarks) on the anatomical part that mark the beginning and ending points for the measurement. The designation of specific landmarks is necessary to denote the level of the imaginary plane through which the diameter passes because no part of the fetus is perfectly round. These landmarks are found at the two most distant points, either from side to side or from the most anterior point to the most posterior point, straight over the plane in question. These principles can be applied to all anatomical planes. For example, the biparietal diameter, which marks the widest transverse plane of the skull, is measured from the highest lateral point of one parietal eminence through the skull to the highest point of the other parietal eminence. Thus, the plane of the biparietal diameter passes transversely through the skull at the level of the parietal eminences. (Refer to the charts beginning on page 33 to find each diameter as it is mentioned throughout this chapter.)

The various diameters of the skull are considered more or less favorable in relationship to the diameters of the pelvis through which it must pass. The presenting diameter of the skull must be small enough to fit through the available space in the pelvis at all levels. A diameter that fits through the pelvic brim may be too large to fit through a lower plane in the same pelvis as descent proceeds. The presenting diameter usually changes (for better or worse) as descent advances.

Flexion describes how near the baby's chin is to his chest. When the head is ideally flexed, the chin is on or nearly on the chest, making the crown of the vertex the part of the head that leads the way through the pelvis. In this attitude the suboccipitobregmatic diameter and the biparietal diameters intersect. The suboccipitobregmatic diameter extends from the junction of the scalp and the back of the neck below the occipital protuberance to the center of the anterior fontanelle and is the smallest, most circular anteroposterior diameter of the baby's head. The biparietal forms the transverse diameter (at right angles to the suboccipitobregmatic) at the same plane. These and other cephalic diameters are illustrated in the charts starting on page 33.

The longest diameter of a given part may also be referred to as an axis. The longest axis of the skull will always be an anteroposterior diameter (because the skull's anteroposterior length encompasses all its longest diameters) and the longest axis of the shoulders and pelvis are always transverse diameters (because the longest span of those parts is always from side to side).

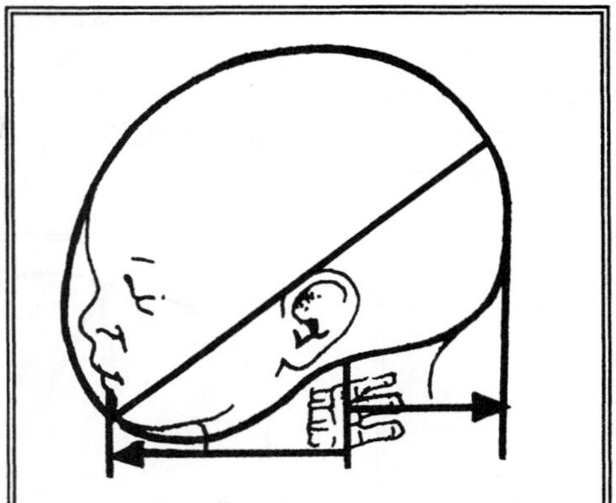
Lima-bean shape of the head. Atlas as fulcrum between two unequal halves divided by the verticomental diameter.

How head flexion occurs

Viewed from the side, the fetal head is a bent, oval body shaped like a lima bean, with the indentation located where the head joins the neck. When the skull is divided vertically from the junction of the spine and the occipital condyles upward, it has a characteristic asymmetry. The bulk of its volume is on the facial or sincipital side, with the smaller "half" made up of the occipital area in the back. These two unequally sized regions of the skull cause the head to behave like a two-armed lever, with the fulcrum (pivot point) located where the occipital condyles contact the atlas (the atlantooccipital joint).

The longest diameter of the skull is the verticomental, which divides the length of the skull starting at the tip of the chin and extending upward to the crown of the vertex. This division also places the larger "half" of the skull on the sincipital side.

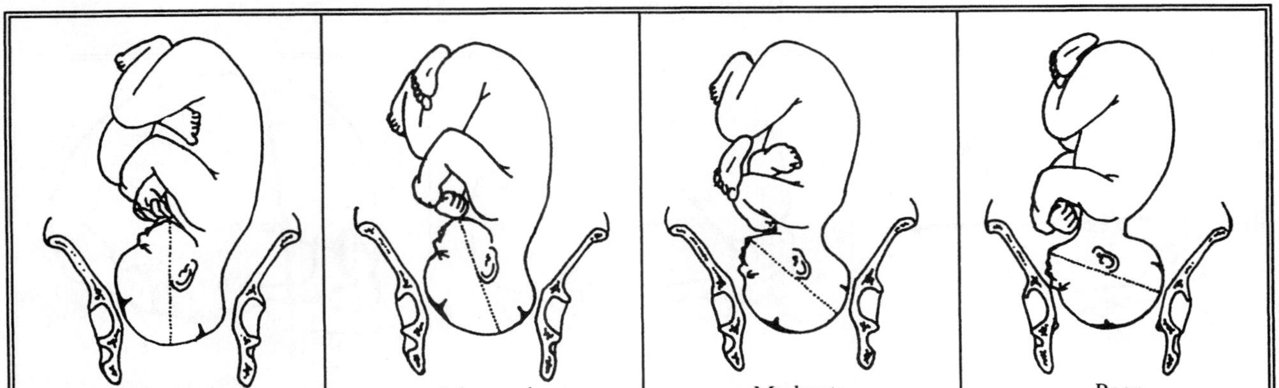

(Degrees of flexion in vertex presentations: the dotted line indicates the verticomental diameter)

Adequate flexion is encouraged by the shape and elasticity of the soft and, to a lesser extent, the bony tissues of the pelvis working in concert with the shape of the baby's head. An elliptical body (the head) passing through a round canal avoids resistance by adapting its long axis to the long axis of the canal. In late pregnancy, as the uterus becomes more active and toning contractions become stronger, the baby's head is pressed down into the lower uterine segment. The sinciput and occiput usually meet equal resistance in the birth canal of a normal pelvis; however, the sincipital end of the head lever is longer and the anterior region in front of the verticomental diameter is larger than the occipital end. This causes this larger region to catch when it meets the resistance of the pelvic walls, directing the baby's chin toward her chest and causing the larger, more rounded crown of the vertex to tip downward. Thus the elliptical shape of the head accommodates itself to the relatively round birth canal.

As the occiput is forced downward, the crown of the vertex leads the way, causing the axis of the verticomental diameter to be directed straight downward in line with the axis of the pelvic cavity. This shift results in a favorable presenting diameter. Flexion of the spine also tends to encourage head flexion. Flexion of head and spine usually commence and are often complete prior to the onset of labor, especially in first-time mothers (Rydberg, 1954).

The posterior fontanelle is more or less centered in the birth canal when the head is completely flexed, presenting the 9.5 cm suboccipitobregmatic diameter, with a circumference of 29 cm. When the head is not so well flexed, it may be because the pelvis is large and does not require more flexion for the head to pass, or that the pressure from contractions is insufficient to encourage better flexion, or that other factors are interfering. In any event, larger (i.e., longer), anteroposterior diameters of the head must negotiate the pelvis. For example, with the baby in a median vertex attitude, the wide biparietal diameter and the long occipitofrontal diameter present a longer shape with a larger circumference than the suboccipitobregmatic diameter. This is increasingly true as the head tilts backward into a brow presentation.

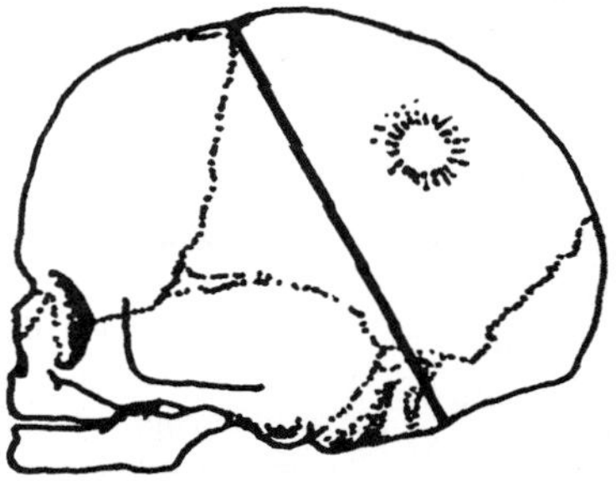

Lateral view of the presenting diameter in a well-flexed vertex presentation

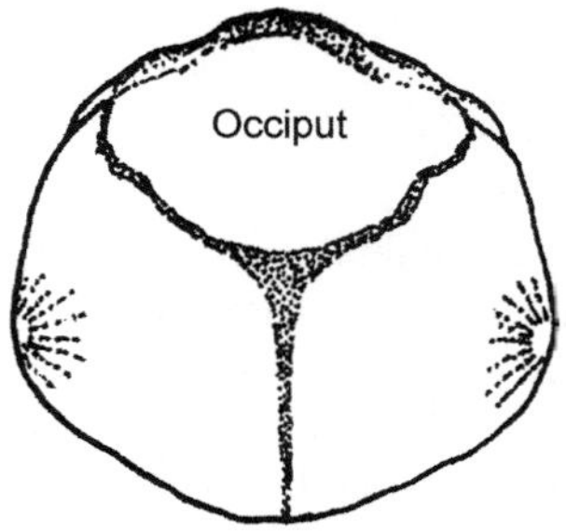

Looking directly down on the well-flexed head

When the baby's head reaches full extension and the face presents with the chin near the pubic bone, the diameter of the face is roughly the same as that of the well-flexed vertex. In the face presentation below, the suboccipitobregmatic diameter is comparable to the submentobregmatic diameter, both of which are 9.5 cm.

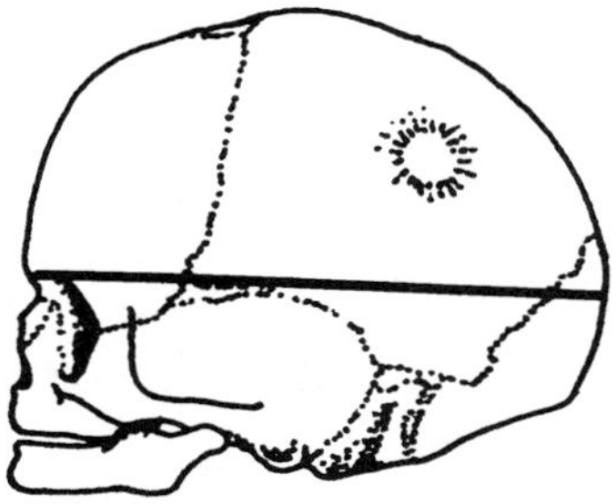

Median vertex

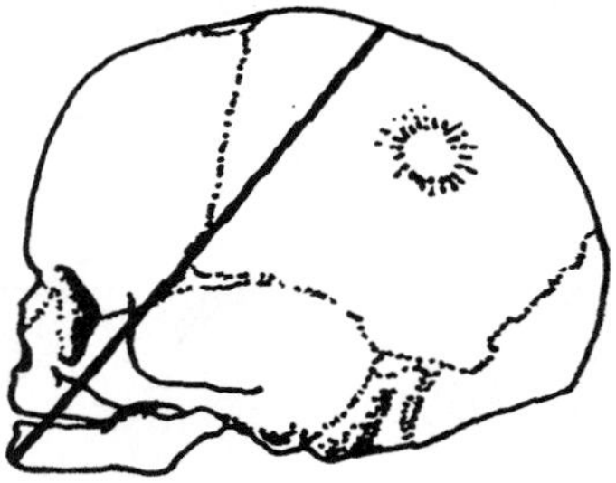

Brow

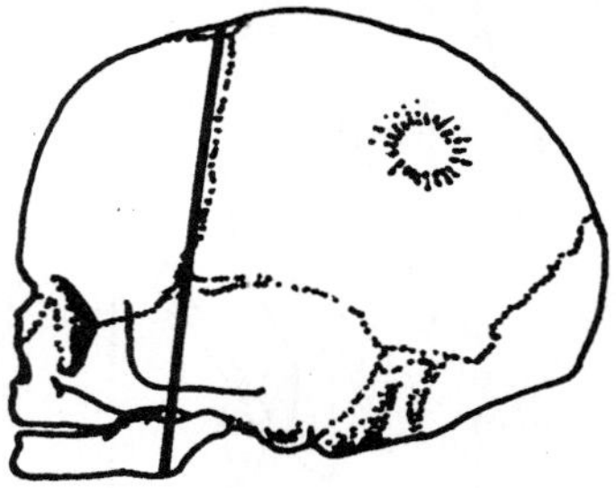

Face

Flexion and extension of the fetal spine and torso

By virtue of spinal mobility, the head can tilt to the side (bringing the shoulder closer to the hip) and can twist at the neck. The torso can flex in a forward direction and extend, to a lesser degree, in a backward direction. The torso can also twist at the waist, temporarily taking the pelvic girdle out of anatomical alignment with the shoulder girdle. Flexion of the fetal spine prior to labor encourages the head to bend forward. This produces a favorable angle in relation to the atlantooccipital articulation, causing the larger bulk on the facial side of the verticomental diameter (toward the forehead) to dip downward when the head meets the resistance of the maternal soft tissues.

A spine that is not well flexed at the onset of labor tends to be accompanied by a deflexed head. The pressure from contractions can produce either flexion or extension of the head, depending upon the other factors in play. Extension is especially encouraged when the baby is occiput posterior. Should the large occiput start to tip back, flexion becomes even more difficult. If the force of contractions and the maternal pelvic structures cannot overcome this tendency toward extension, maternal postural changes can help promote flexion. (See details in the chapter entitled "The Process of Birth in Mentum Anterior Face Presentations.") Extension of the upper spine and neck normally occur as the flexed head passes beneath the pubic arch and through the soft tissues of the birth canal during pushing.

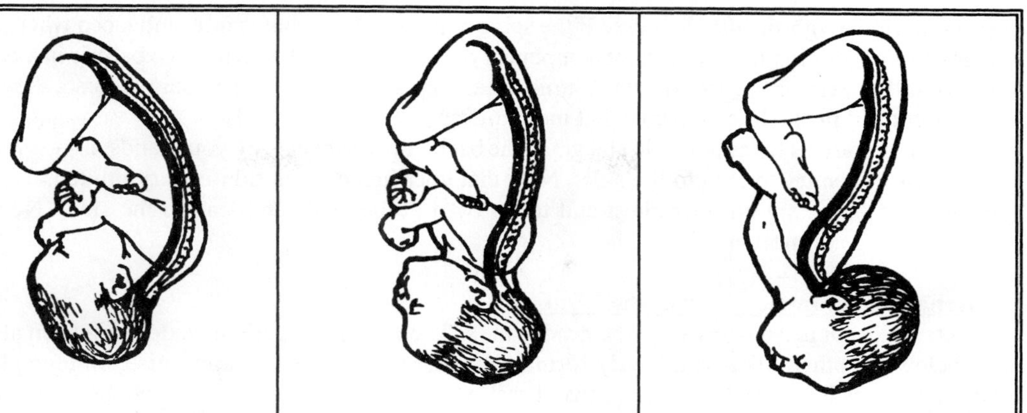

Curved spine in early labor | Straighter spine with head slightly extended in early labor | When the head is extended, pressure from contractions, pelvic structure or the tilt of the uterus may encourage further extension.

The posture of the baby's spine changes as labor progresses. The baby usually starts out with the head and spine well flexed. Contractions from above and a closed cervix below cause the baby's body to become compacted in this flexed posture in early labor. Stronger contractions narrow the uterine walls, resulting in intermittent straightening of the spine.

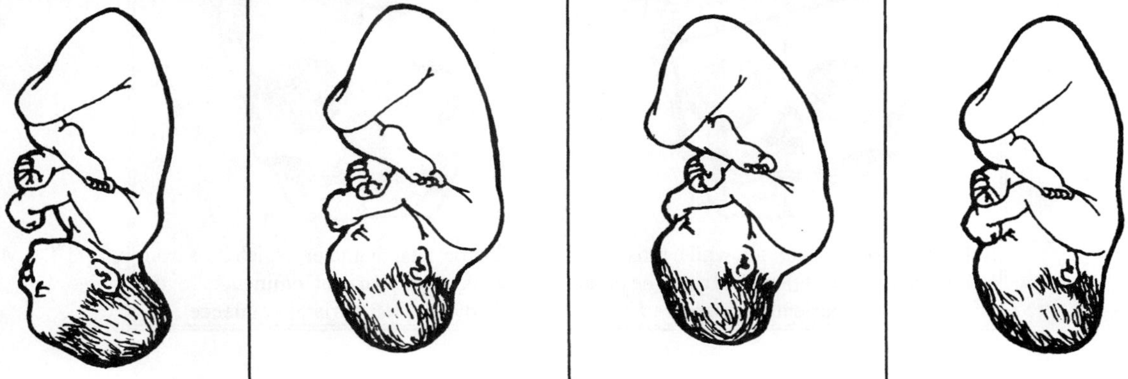

1. 2. 3. 4.

1. The axes of the head and spine prior to flexion
2. Flexion of the head and body into the ideal position is encouraged by toning or labor contractions, the shape of the head and the soft and bony pelvic structures.
3. Compaction of the baby's body as labor commences because the soft tissues of the pelvis are not yet dilated.
4. Straightening of the back occurs during late labor and pushing as the soft pelvic tissues make room for and simultaneously help maintain flexion of the head.

As the pelvic soft tissues dilate to admit the head during active labor, the back begins to remain straightened as the head finds more space in the pelvis. This reduces the angle between the cervical spine and the base of the skull. As descent proceeds, in most cases, the baby's cervical and upper thoracic spine straighten, becoming lordotic in some. In spite of this straightening, the head is maintained in a posture of flexion by virtue of being held firmly during descent through the pelvic cavity. Moulding also helps to maintain the head in a flexed posture. Although the angle between the long axis of the head and the axis of the spine can vary greatly, forward bending of the spine is rare in late labor.

Straightening of the spine enhances axial pressure, which facilitates passage of the torso through the cervix and later through lower birth canal. As the baby's torso approaches the curve of the birth canal, it rotates so the spine occupies an anterior oblique or transverse position, allowing it to take full advantage of its ability to flex laterally and twist.

Lateral flexion would be significantly impaired if the spine remained flexed but is fully enhanced when it is straightened. The full range of spinal motion is an important component of normal descent, whether the baby is in a cephalic or breech presentation (Borell & Fernström, 1958). If the arms or legs are straight against the baby's torso, they can limit lateral flexion to an extent and make descent somewhat more difficult.

Try this: bend forward as far as possible and grasp the back of your knees with your hands; now try to twist from side to side at the waist. Then try to lean to the side. Note that your range of motion is very limited. Next, stand up in a relaxed posture, put your chin on your chest and try to twist at the waist and lean to the side. Notice the dramatic difference in your range of motion.

The subsuperparietal diameters and asynclitism

The diameter relevant to asynclitism of the head is the 8.25 cm subsuperparietal, extending from above one parietal eminence to below the other. This is the only formal diameter that transects a transverse, oblique plane of the skull. While not designated as left or right, there are two directions from which this diameter can be measured, as illustrated below. Presentation of this oblique diameter is made possible by the lateral flexibility of the fetal neck, allowing a larger head to descend through the brim more easily. There are two attitudes of asynclitic vertex descent: anterior and posterior. (This attitude, unique to flexed vertex descent, is covered in the chapter entitled "Synclitism and Asynclitism.") In a breech presentation, the aftercoming head may also descend at an oblique angle.

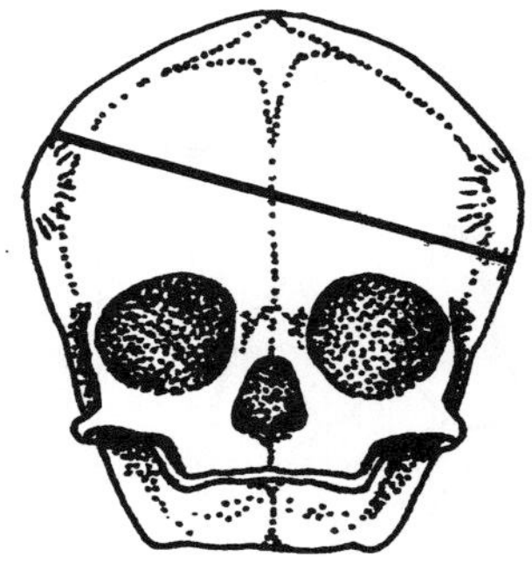

Subsuperparietal diameter, which runs from below the left parietal eminence to the point above the right parietal eminence.

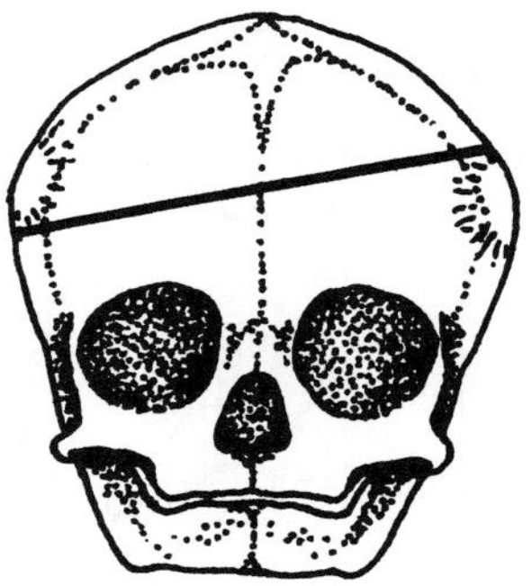

Subsuperparietal diameter, which runs from below the right parietal eminence to the point above the left parietal eminence.

Diameters of the Fetal Body

The following tables describe the most clinically significant fetal diameters. Those of the head, pelvis and shoulder girdle are included for easy reference and comparison. Many diameters are mentioned in the literature. While some older books describe most of these, others only include the few most relevant. No authorities agree entirely upon the length of each diameter, primarily because the populations from which the measurements have been derived varied. Measurements are averages only, although statements as to which are relatively "longest" or "shortest" are correct.

There is some debate regarding the landmarks for some measurements: when sources differed, those differences are included, with the most accepted description given first. Some diameters have rather vague landmarks at one end; these have been described as precisely as possible. In a few cases, the clinical relevance of a particular diameter given in one source did not match what was stated elsewhere. In such cases, I either left out the stray description if it just seemed incorrect (mistakes do creep into textbooks), or I included it beneath the primary indication as given in most sources. In several cases, different names were used to describe the same diameter (based upon a description or an illustration or both). When this is the case, the multiple names are given under the one most commonly mentioned.

Diameters of the Fetal Skull, Shoulders and Torso

(•Most clinically significant diameters.   Measurements key: AP: anteroposterior diameter; Trans: transverse diameter; Circ: circumference)

Diameter	Description	Location	Relationship to Other Diameters	Presentation	Measurement	
					Centimeters	Inches
The most important transverse diameters of the fetal skull						
•Biparietal (Parietal)	Located at the level of the parietal eminences	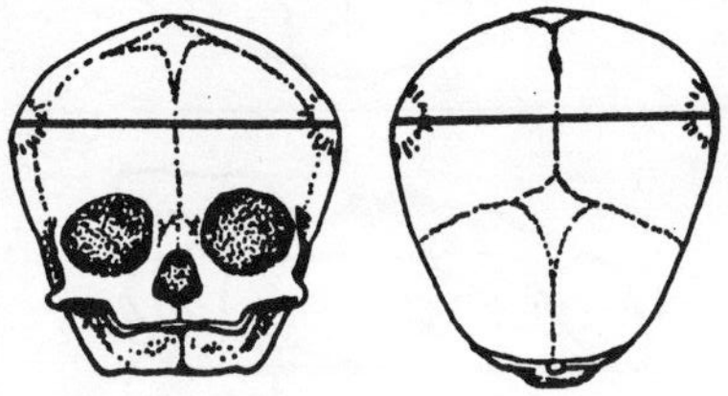	Longest transverse diameter of the head, regardless of presentation	Cephalic	Trans: 9.5	3.75
•Subsuper-parietal (superparietal subparietal)	Extends diagonally from side to side through the skull from above one parietal eminence to below the other	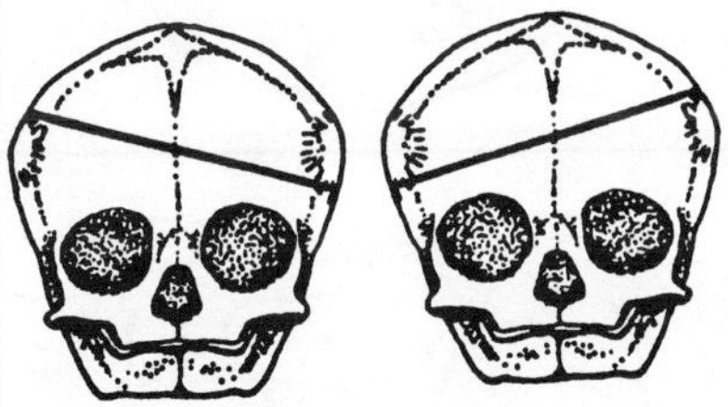	Smallest transverse diameter in flexed vertex when the occiput is transverse and the head is tilted to one side, causing the parietal eminence to present	Asynclitic, flexed vertex as it passes through the brim	Trans: 8.25 (moulded)	3.25
•Bitemporal	Between the extremities of the coronal sutures	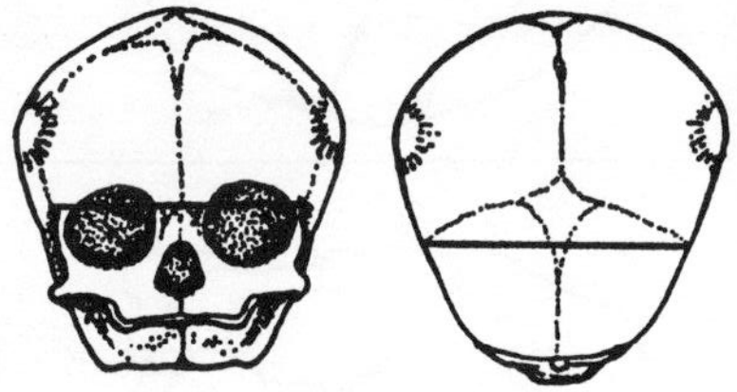	Shortest transverse diameter of the skull; bisects the submento-bregmatic diameter (the first AP diameter to engage in a face presentation).	The bitemporal diameter is the first transverse diameter to engage in a face or a brow presentation.	Trans: 8.25	3.25
Bimastoid	Between the nipplelike projections on the posterior tip of the petrous part of the temporal bone (behind ear and level with upper gum line)	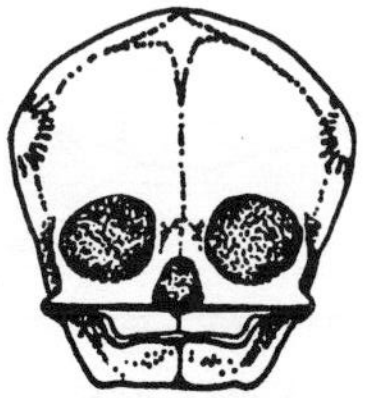	Next largest transverse diameter after the neck when moving up toward the vertex	Flexed aftercoming head in a breech	Trans: 7.5	3

Diameter	Description	Location	Relationship to Other Diameters	Presentation	Measurement	
					Centimeters	Inches
Anteroposterior diameters of the skull in different presentations						
Suboccipito-frontal	Extends from junction of scalp and back of neck below occipital protuberance to the prominence of the forehead (some say to root of nose)	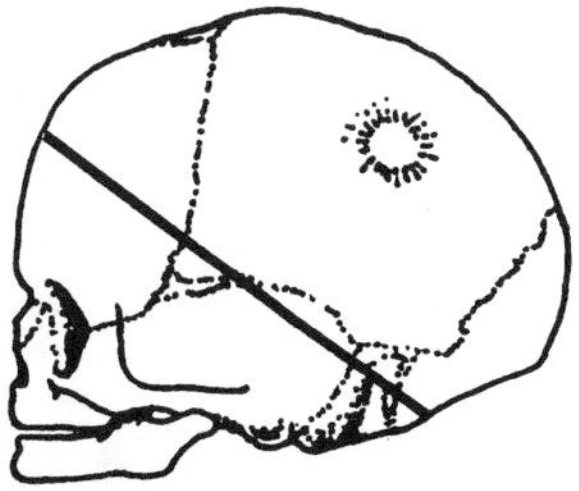	Normal engaging diameter in vertex or well-flexed breech presentations; second-longest diameter of the skull in vertex presentations	Partially flexed occiput anterior vertex as head enters brim; good flexion in a persistently occiput posterior baby or in a well-flexed aftercoming head in a breech presentation	AP: 10.5+ Trans. 9+ Circ: 30	4 ⅛ 3.5 12
•Suboccipito-bregmatic	Extends from junction of scalp and back of neck below the occipital protuberance to the center of the anterior fontanelle	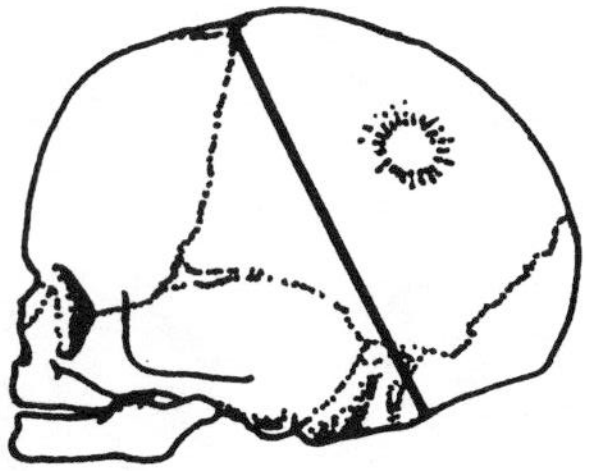	Anteroposterior diameter in well-flexed vertex presentation	Crown of the vertex; fully flexed anterior vertex	AP: 9.5 Trans: 9+ Circ: 29 (28 after moulding)	3.75 3.5+ 11.5
•Occipitofrontal	Extends from the root of the nose (between the brows) to just below the lower border of the posterior fontanelle (some sources say to the occipital eminence)	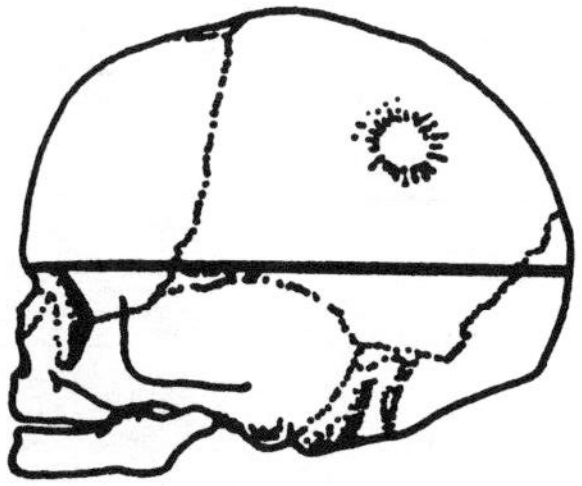	Anteroposterior diameter in deflexed vertex presentations	Median vertex; persistently posterior vertex when the head is not well flexed	AP: 11 Trans: 9+ Circ: 35	4.5 3.5+ 13.75
Suboccipito-mental	Extends from the junction of the scalp and back of neck to the tip of the chin	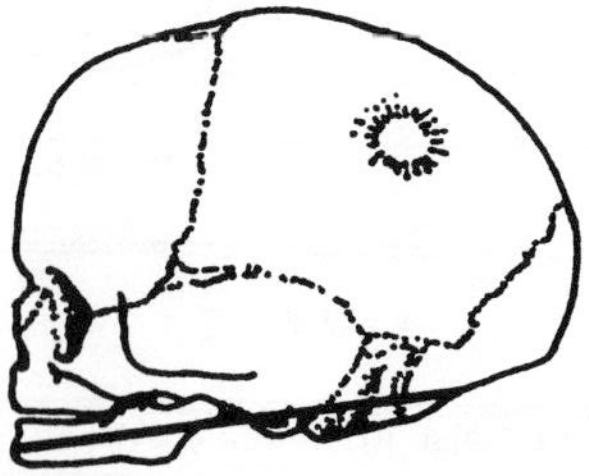	First anteroposterior diameter of aftercoming head	Well-flexed aftercoming head in a breech baby as he starts to emerge	AP: 9.5	3.75

Diameter	Description	Location	Relationship to Other Diameters	Presentation	Measurement	
					Centimeters	Inches
Occipitomental (Mentoccipital)	Extends from the tip of the chin to the occipital eminence (some sources say to the posterior fontanelle, which is also known as the occipital fontanelle)	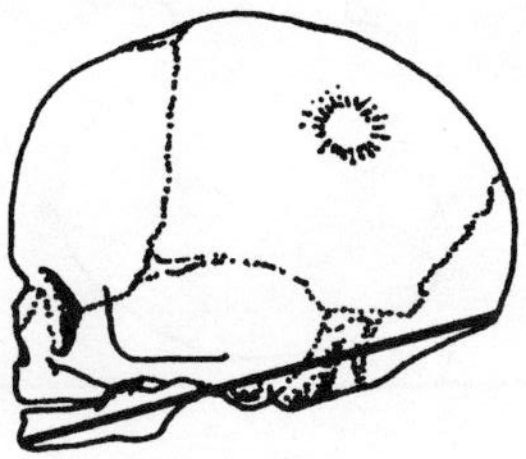	Longest anteroposterior diameter of the most posterior portion of the head	Presenting diameter of extended aftercoming head in a breech	AP: 13 Trans: 9+	5.12 3.5+
•Submento-bregmatic (Trachelobregmatic; Cervicobregmatic; Tracheloparietal)	Extends from the junction of neck and chin to the center of the anterior fontanelle	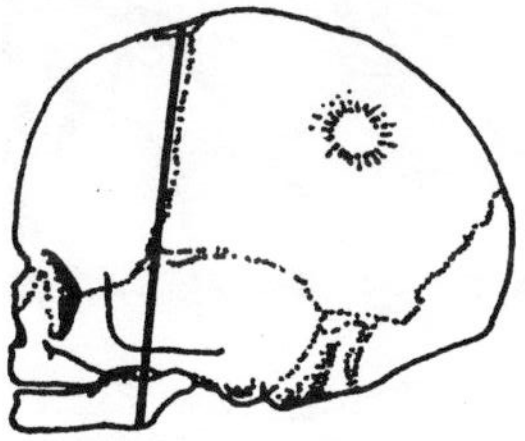	Anteroposterior diameter when the head is fully extended	Face, mentum anterior	AP: 9.25	3.75
Frontomental	From the center of the forehead to the center of the lower margin of the chin	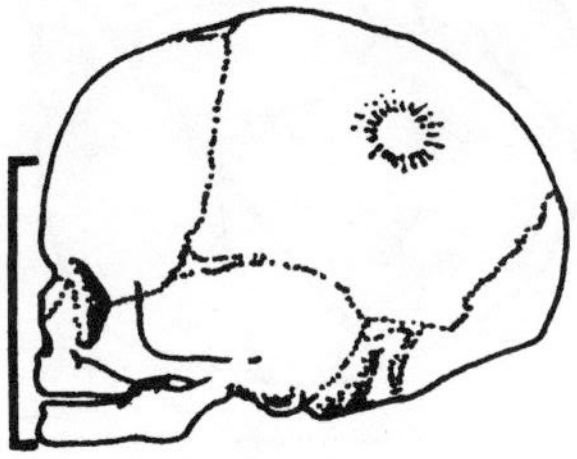	Diameter of face proper	Face as it begins to crown	AP: 8.25	3.25
Sterno-bregmatic	Extends from the center of the anterior fontanelle to the top of the sternum	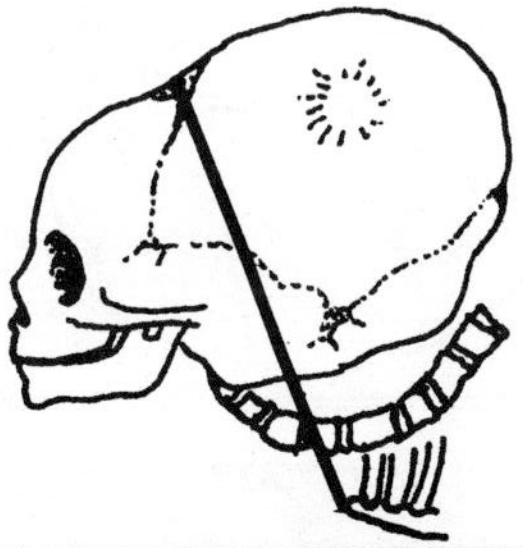	Longest possible presenting diameter in a longitudinal lie	Face, mentum posterior	AP: 18	7

Diameter	Description	Location	Relationship to Other Diameters	Presentation	Measurement	
					Centimeters	Inches
•Verticomental (Mentovertical; some sources call this occipitomental)	Extends from the point of chin to the highest point of the vertex (some sources say a point anterior to the posterior fontanelle)	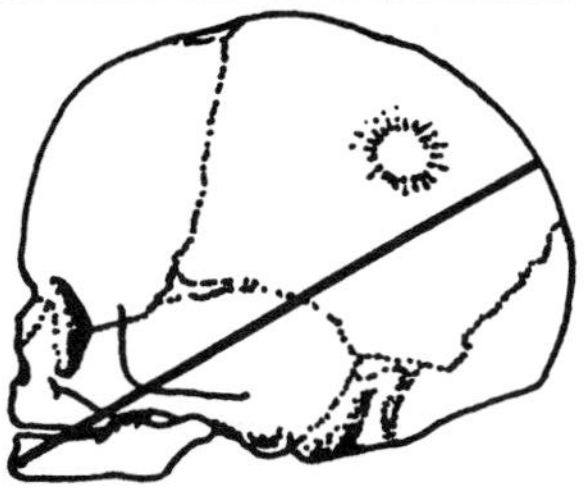	Longest diameter of the fetal skull. Many sources say this diameter is horizontal to the path of descent in a brow.	Longitudinal to path of descent in a well-flexed vertex. Many sources say this is the presenting diameter in an unmoulded brow presentation.	AP: 13.3	5.25
•Mentobregmatic (Mentoparietal)	Extends from the tip of the chin to the posterior angle of the anterior fontanelle. (Some sources say through the biparietal diameter to the vertex; defined this way it is similar to the verticomental)	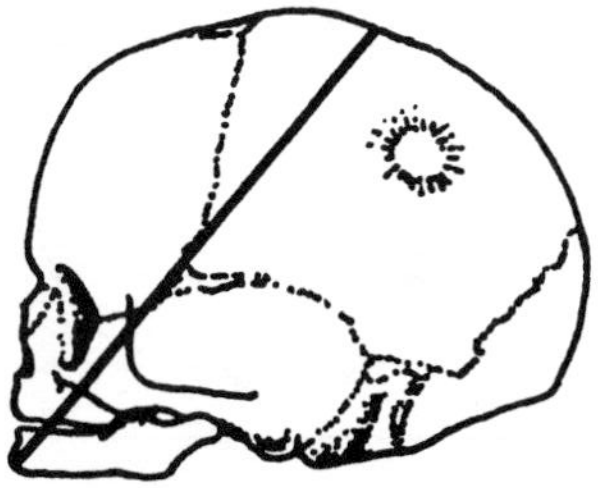	Deflexed cephalic	Presenting diameter of brow (Borell & Fernström, 1960)	AP: 12.2	4.8
Submento-vertical	Extends from the junction of the head and neck in front to the furthest part of the crown of the vertex	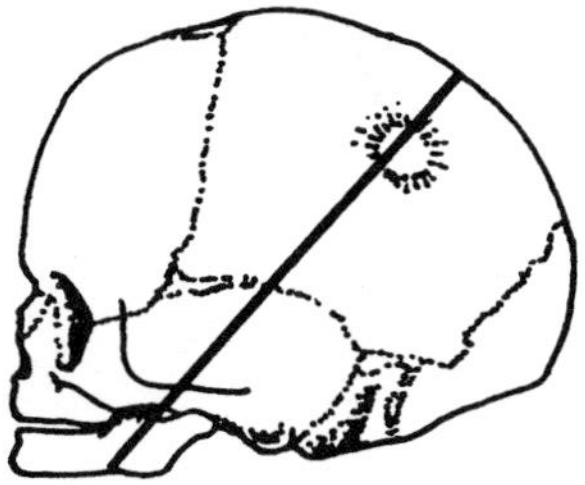	One of the three longest AP diameters of the skull	Brow-face	AP: 11	4.5
Other clinically relevant diameters						
Bisacromial	Between the acromial processes of the scapulae	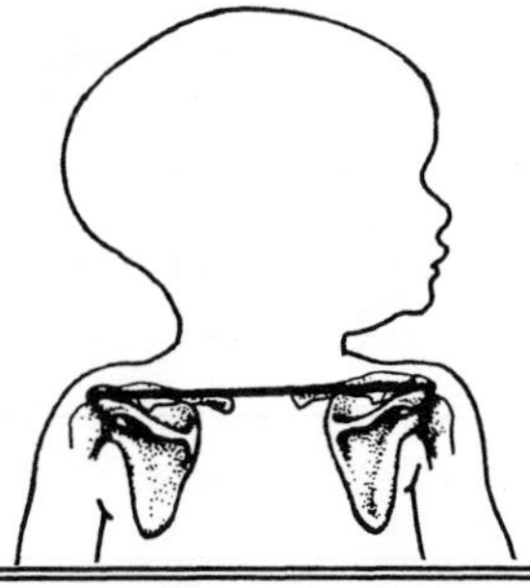	Widest transverse diameter of unflexed shoulder girdle. Passage of this diameter through the brim marks engagement of the chest.	Presenting shoulder diameter in longitudinal lie; compresses by at least 1 in.	Trans: 12 Circ: 32-34	4.75

Diameter	Description	Location	Relationship to Other Diameters	Presentation	Measurement	
					Centimeters	Inches
Other clinically relevant diameters (cont.)						
Bitrochanteric	Between greater trochanters of femurs	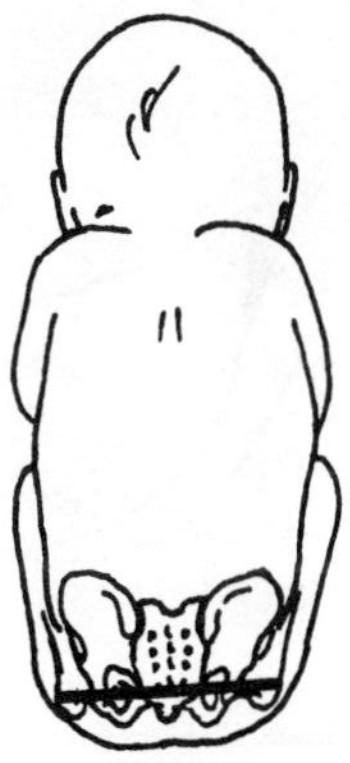	Third widest anatomical diameter of fetus after the head and shoulders; usually matches the bisiliac. Passage of this diameter through the brim marks engagement of the pelvis in a breech presentation.	Breech	Trans: 9-10.1	3.5-4
Bisiliac	Widest diameter between the iliac crests.	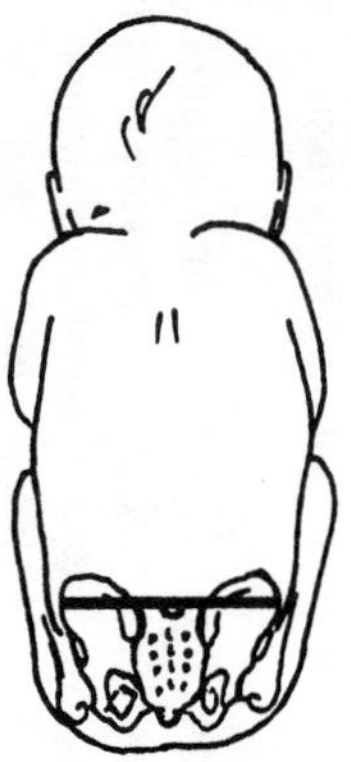	Passage of this diameter through the brim marks engagement of the pelvis in a cephalic presentation. In a breech baby, this diameter sweeps perineum after the bitrochanteric diameter has done so.	Breech	Trans: 9-10.1	3.5-4

The following chart summarizes the most clinically significant circumferences of the newborn skull. The first column gives the longest anteroposterior (AP) and widest transverse (T) diameters that transect each other (AP X T) at the same level or plane of the fetal skull. The distance around these diameters is the circumference of the skull at this plane. Each presentation presents a different circumference. The chart also notes the largest diameter over which the perineum will retract as the spine extends during birth. The "sweeping" diameter is larger than the presenting diameters; however, because there is more space at the outlet, this diameter is born without difficulty.

Largest Engaging Cephalic Diameters in the Same Plane (AP × T)	These Diameters Present in These Presentations	Widest Diameter That the Perineum Sweeps over as Head Is Born	Average Circumference of Engaging Diameters
Suboccipitobregmatic X biparietal	Well-flexed vertex	Suboccipitofrontal, head born by spinal extension	29 cm 11.5 in
Occipitofrontal X bitemporal & biparietal	Deflexed vertex, military position, especially in OP position	Occipitofrontal, head born by spinal extension	35 cm 13.75 in
Mentobregmatic X bitemporal, followed by the biparietal on engagement	Brow presentation	Mentovertical, head born by flexion of the neck and upper spine	35.5 cm 14 in
Submentobregmatic X bitemporal, followed by the biparietal on engagement	Anterior face presentation	Submentovertical, head born by flexion of the neck and upper spine	29 cm 11.5 in

Moulding and Compression of the Fetal Skull

"Moulding" refers to the influence of the external pressures and forces of labor on the fetal parts. The shape and structure of the baby's head and spine, shoulder girdle, chest and pelvis may be altered by these pressures as well as by contact with the soft and bony tissues of the pelvis.

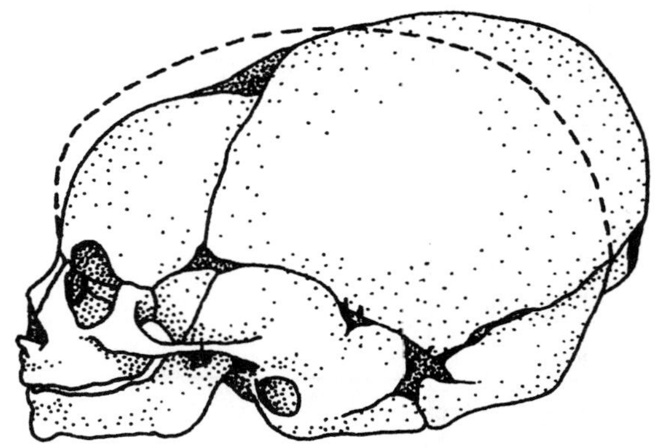

Basic principle of moulding: one diameter is compressed while the diameter at a right angle bulges.

The term "moulding" is most commonly applied to the skull. The skull is designed to provide maximum accommodation to the forces of labor, minimum trauma to the delicate nervous system within and complete restoration to free mobility of all its parts once the stress of labor is over (Frymann, 1998b). The membranous bones in the vault of the fetal skull are flexible and unfused in most term newborns, allowing the head to change shape. The skull bones that undergo the most obvious repositioning include the parietal, temporal and occipital bones and the upper portion of the frontal bones. These bones can adapt themselves in various ways; they can flex, flatten, compress or bend, as well as separate, move together and pivot along suture lines and joints. Moulding temporarily changes the shape of the head and sometimes its size, especially its circumference. The overall volume of the skull is not reduced by normal moulding; as the presenting diameter of the skull becomes compressed, the areas at right angles begin to bulge.

Movement of the bones in the vault

The bones in the vault can move in a variety of complex ways. In most labors, moulding is produced by direct contact between the soft tissues of the mother's lower uterine segment and pelvis and is usually minimal. Uniform pressure applied over each parietal eminence bends the bones inward slightly, reducing all transverse skull diameters as the bones accommodate to the shape of the pelvis. More pronounced moulding causes the bones to straighten (flatten slightly) and the upper borders to rise upward. Extreme rising can only occur by separation at the temporal suture line on either side of the skull. Unequal separation occurs along this suture if the parietal bones become pushed forward or backward by unequal pressure from either the frontal or occipital bones. The lower borders of the parietal bones may also slide under the squamous portions of the temporal bones and the greater wings of the sphenoid.

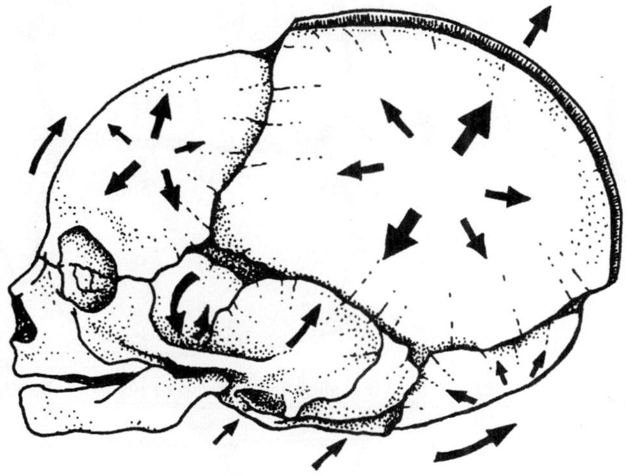

Side view: movement of bones in the vault (the edges of the sagittal suture become staggered like this when pressure is extreme)

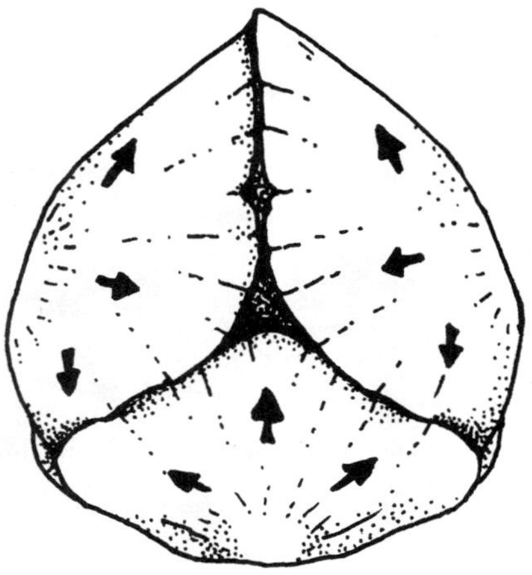

Movement of bones in the vault: posterior view showing flattening of the parietal bones and staggering of the edges of the sagittal suture

The frontal bones tend to move slightly backward and upward and may also be flattened if not too ossified. The edges of the frontal suture may become staggered or actually overlap slightly, especially during difficult labors.

The tip of the interparietal portion of the occiput becomes elevated and displaced slightly forward, a result of corresponding changes in the base of the skull. The occiput can also flex slightly at the junction of the squamous and the interparietal parts along the Mendosal suture-fissures (Moloy, 1942). The temporal bones move like wobbling wheels when responding to compression (Frymann, 1998a). How the head actually changes shape has to do with the complex, changing pressures and forces it receives during labor.

Sutton (2001) states that a wide bitemporal diameter (giving the head a roundness) or a shortened occipitofrontal diameter (giving the head a squareness) makes entering the pelvis and moulding more difficult at term.

Staggering and locking at suture lines: While it has been widely taught for decades that the edges of the parietal bones normally overlap along the sagittal suture, in fact, this is a relatively rare and often pathological occurrence at term. The attachments of the bony plates to the underlying connective tissues and the narrow fibrous connections at the sagittal suture prevent any significant overlap without first tearing loose those attachments. The thickness of the bony edges is also a limiting factor. Physiological overlap is impossible when the width of the membranes spanning a suture is less than the thickness of the adjacent bony plates. Other limitations include each parietal bone being relatively fixed at its base (preventing a true sliding motion at the sagittal suture), as well as the manner in which the dura and underlying venous sinuses are attached at the sagittal suture. When a baby has a wide sagittal suture and parietal overlap is induced by excessive pressure, it rarely exceeds 3 mm (⅛ inch) at term (Baxter, 1946; Carlan et al., 1991). More overlap is possible in preterm babies whose sutures are spaced more widely apart and whose skull bones are less ossified.

In most labors, external pressure from the birth canal causes the parietal bones to mould by bending inward and flattening. This deflects the entire vault of the skull upward and forward approximately 0.5 cm. Flattening elevates both edges of the sagittal sutures to an almost identical degree. More pronounced moulding may cause the edge of one parietal bone to be elevated slightly above the edge of the other along the sagittal suture. During descent, the posterior parietal bone is the one closest to the mother's sacrum. It is usually subjected to more pressure than the anterior parietal bone, which is nearest the mother's pubic bone. Therefore, the edge of the posterior parietal bone tends to be depressed slightly below the edge of the anterior parietal bone. However, the reverse can occur as well, with the posterior parietal bone becoming more flattened as the result of pressure and its edge rising above that of the anterior parietal bone.

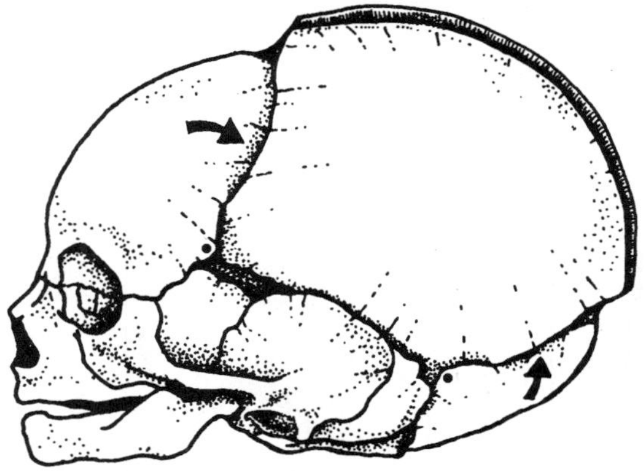

Sites of locking (dots indicate where the bone overlaps; arrows show where the bone goes under the adjacent bone)

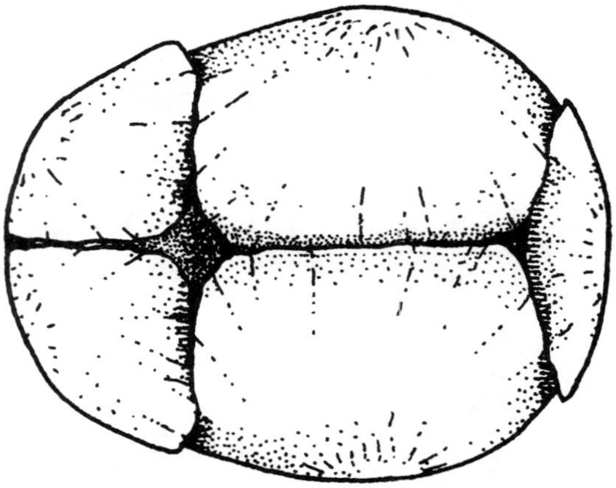

Overhead view showing overlap of bones at the dots

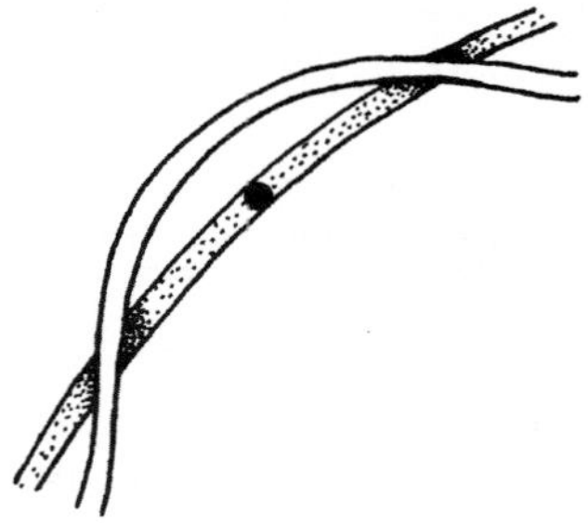

Closeup of overlapping at the dot at the base of the left lambdoidal suture (occiput unshaded, parietal bone shaded)

Overlap is also prevented by a unique locking feature of the parietal, occipital and frontal bones, which comes into play when the parietal bones are compressed. In the unmoulded head, the edges of each frontal bone are flush with the edges of each parietal bone along the full length of the coronal suture. Slight pressure causes the parietal bones to bend inward and flatten. At the same time, the edge's of the frontal bones may be pressed inward slightly beneath the edges of the parietal bones, down the length of the coronal suture to the point just above the sphenoid fontanelle. Below this level, the edges of the frontal bones slightly overlap the edges of the compressed parietal bones. This unequal matching at the edges of the bones, as well as the strong membranes spanning the sutures, causes the edges of the frontal bones to catch (become braced) against the edges of the parietal bones at the level of the sphenoid fontanelles, preventing the frontal bones from collapsing under the edges of the parietal bones. This locking effect along the coronal suture also limits forward displacement of the parietal bones. Because these relationships resolve as soon as pressure on the parietal bones is released, it is unusual to find any overlapping along the coronal suture after birth. Apparent overlapping near the anterior fontanelle is really due to elevation of the edges of the parietal bones above the edges of the frontal bones, which also lifts the posterior boundary of the anterior fontanelle, causing the membrane in the fontanelle to slant upward at a more vertical angle.

Simultaneously, a similar but less effective locking or bracing occurs at the edges of the occipital and posterior parietal borders along the lambdoidal suture. In the uncompressed head, the bony edges of the lambdoidal suture are flush. The newborn occipital plate has quite a lot of forward and backward mobility when the parietal bones are not compressed, which allows it to be pushed under the free posterior edges of the parietal bones. However, when pressure is applied to the parietal bones, the upper portion of the occiput rises upward and is normally prevented from moving inward because the lower third of the occipital bone extends slightly beyond the edge of the parietal bones, beginning just above the mastoid fontanelles at the level of the Mendosal suture-fissures. This severely restricts the range of motion of the occipital plate, and in most cases, overlapping of the interparietal portion of the occiput is arrested as well. This locking between the parietal and occipital bones along the mismatched edges of the lambdoidal suture prevents the occipital bone from being pushed deeply into the cranial cavity. It is less effective than the locking that occurs along the coronal suture, probably due to the wide mastoid fontanelle.

During labor, the occipital plate may tend to slip under the parietal bones at the lambdoidal suture, and the frontal bones may slide under the parietal bones slightly between contractions. However, during contractions, additional compression of the biparietal diameter causes the frontal, parietal and occipital bones to lock into place as described above, which reduces and may even prevent overlapping, thus protecting the cranial contents from injury. Locking still allows bending and upward displacement of the vault because the parietal bones flatten, and there are compensating changes in the base of the skull (details below) (Moloy, 1942).

Variations in moulding during labor: Dr. William Emerson (2002) points out that moulding is a dynamic, adaptive process that varies as the baby descends through the birth canal, irrespective of the degree to which the head is flexed. Slight moulding occurs at the inlet. During the dilation phase of labor and prior to pushing, the sides of the fetal skull are subjected to bilateral pressures that flatten and lift the top edges of the parietal bones upward and compress the temporal bones inward and slightly downward, narrowing the head from side to side and resulting in the locking described above.

Some torsional (twisting) action happens as the head undergoes internal rotation. This torsional force increases as the occiput rotates left or right. In the early second phase of labor, after full dilation has occurred and the mother is beginning to push, the pressure shifts and torsional forces increase. The vertical axis of the head and spine is twisted because when the chest and shoulders reach the curve of the birth canal, they usually rotate 45° out of anatomical alignment with the head. This occurs by turning at the neck, a twisting motion that extends to the skull bones, skewing the bones of the vault slightly out of alignment with the base of the skull. If you imagine a thread running down through the top, at the center of a baby's head and into the neck, that thread is the vertical axis around which torsional forces occur. The greatest degree of moulding typically occurs when the head is at about +3 station, as it begins to round the bend of the birth canal.

As descent progresses to crowning, the pressure on the cranium is primarily anteroposterior. That is, the head becomes compressed from front to the back and vice versa, with a pronounced downward thrust, reforming the cranium into a very round shape. After the head exits the bony pelvis but is still in the soft birth canal, the degree of moulding decreases and often disappears (Borell & Fernström, 1967).

As soon as the head is born and the pressure is released, the parietal, occipital and frontal bones spring outward, increasing the head circumference by up to one-half cm. As the baby begins to breathe, the cranium responds by expanding more and returning all the bones to their anatomic relationship. Crying assists in this process. However, if the baby has undergone undue, unusual or prolonged stress during labor, resolution of all the moulding may not resolve at the time of birth and can persist much longer (Emerson, 2002; Moloy, 1942).

Abnormal moulding of the vault: Emery (1972) and de la Fuente (1991) reported a small number of fetal fatalities involving a variety of rare and unusual forms of moulding. Among these findings, they noted cases where the edges of the sagittal suture became pushed against each other forming a firm, apparently fused ridge, accompanied by a variety of other unusual displacements of adjacent skull bones that were still present at the time of autopsy. They postulated that this fusion at the sagittal suture caused the parietal bones to lift upward along the sagittal suture during descent, transmitting the force of moulding downward. At autopsy, they found that the lower borders of the parietal bones were displaced inward on either side resulting in inward pinching along the lateral suture. Numerous intracranial lesions such as hemorrhages were associated with these findings. Both authors believed that normal moulding consists of overlapping at the sagittal suture. In any event, in all of Emery's cases and several of de la Fuente's, it was felt that this unusual moulding alone caused the baby to die. In some of de la Fuente's cases, it was hard to assign the cause of death when this moulding was considered along with other associated damage.

Landmarks commonly displaced by moulding: In summary, the following bones are affected by normal to moderate moulding:

Parietal bones: Most notably, with the pressure of descent, the parietal bones become elevated above their unmoulded position by a process of bilateral elongation or flattening as the parietal eminences are pressed inward. This raises their upper borders at the highest point of the vault. This process, along with corresponding movement of the occipital and frontal bones, typically reduces the occipitofrontal diameter by as much as 1 cm at the point of maximal anterior vertex moulding (Borell & Fernström, 1967).

Frontal bones: The frontal eminences are pressed backward, moving the posterior, superior angle of the frontal bones either upward or downward slightly.

Occipital bones: The posterior tips of the condyles and the entire occipital plate are pushed forward and upward 0.5 to 1 cm.

Temporal bones: When compressed laterally, the posterior, uppermost tips of the petrous portion of the temporal bones become elevated, moving the sphenoid and temporal bones closer together. This change occurs as the sphenooccipital synchondrosis bends to allow elevation of the occiput. The squamous portion of the temporal bone and the greater wing of the sphenoid are also displaced inward slightly, a type of moulding made possible by the movement of the unfused parts of these bones. These changes decrease the transverse diameter of the skull bones in the region of the lateral sutures. These shifts are facilitated by accompanying changes in the base of the skull.

Movement in the base of the skull

It is widely acknowledged that the bones of the cranial vault move during moulding. It is much less well known how responsive the other skull bones are to the forces of birth, with the face and base of the skull typically described as solid and immobile. However, there is a great deal of mobility in these regions as well.

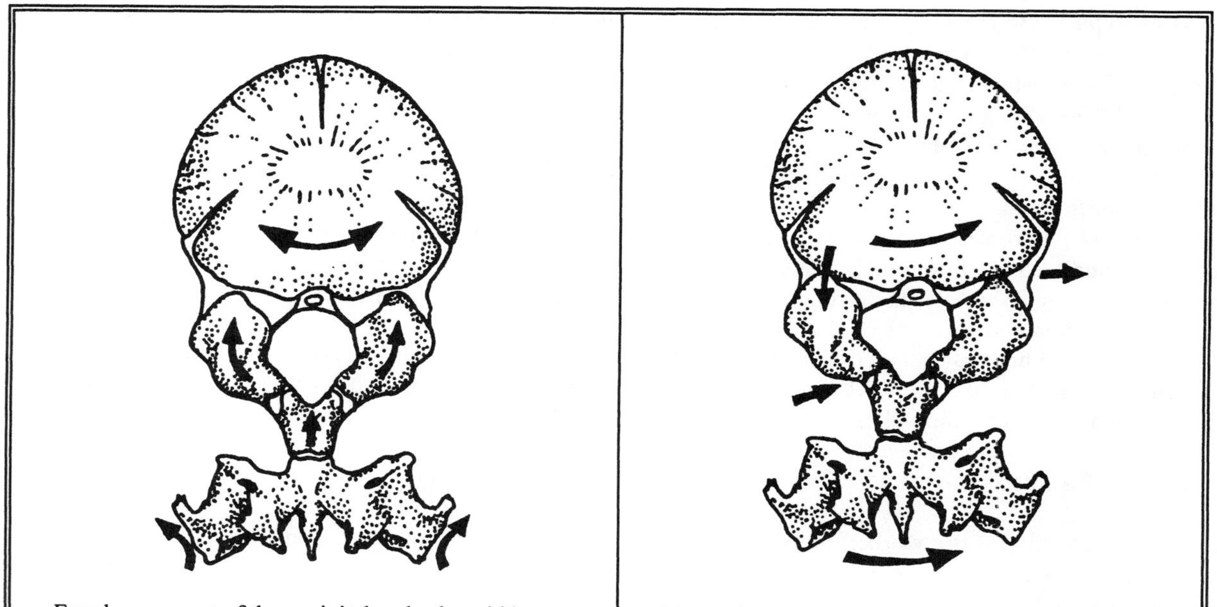

Equal movement of the occipital and sphenoid bones during compression

Unequal displacement of the occipital and sphenoid bones producing a domino effect with adjacent bones

The interparietal and squamous occipital bones pivot at their base, rising upward slightly during compression in most normal births. The joints at the sphenooccipital and sphenopetrosal synchondroses and at the occipitomastoid and petrooccipital sutures allow the bones that make up the occipital region to rise upward together at an angle in response to the normal compression that occurs when the head is flexed. The posterior portion of the temporal bone is elevated as well, causing the petrous portions to protrude into the posterior-inferior region of the cranial cavity slightly. The slope of the squamous portion of the temporal bone and the greater wing of the sphenoid bone become more vertical during moulding. The most obvious moulding of the base of the skull usually resolves immediately after most births, which is why it is not noted on newborn examination and why it is so hard to research (Moloy, 1942).

If the baby's head is in a less-than-ideal position during labor, it can get jammed down onto the neck, resulting in exaggerated occipital rotation. The occiput has limited movement left and right, moving much like the dial on a rotary telephone. When it rotates out of alignment to either the right or left, the resulting imbalance of pressure causes the condyle on that side to be displaced forward. Unequal displacement of the condyles presses the basiocciput forward at an angle, which misaligns the sphenoid bone. The condyles rest on the atlas, which is also affected. Therefore, movement of the bones in the base of the skull can result in a domino effect, with slight shifts in adjacent bones in the face, cranium and spinal column. When the skull bones are misaligned, corresponding asymmetries can be noted in the contour of the skull vault and the child's facial features.

If the mother gives birth on her back on a hard surface with her legs supported wide apart in stirrups (lithotomy position), the sacrum is held firmly in place with its tip in the way of descent and the woman's coccyx is rendered less mobile as well. Even when her baby's head is in an ideal position, the posterior cheekbone (the one closest to the coccyx) will scrape over the coccyx as the head passes through the outlet, dragging that cheekbone backward as it descends and resulting in a downward facial slant, depressed cheekbone and droopy upper lip on that side. This, in turn, lifts the eye socket on the opposite side of the face (Dobson, 1994).

Nerve networks and circulatory vessels traverse numerous passages in the skull. The skull is also the locus of four of the five physical senses. Even slight misalignments of the bones can lead to constriction of nerve and circulatory pathways resulting in muscle and ligament tension and other sequelae such as digestive and respiratory problems. The best time to treat such misalignments is in early infancy, before ossification is complete (Dobson, 1994). (Craniosacral assessment and adjustment for newborns is covered in Volume III of this text.) (Thanks to Dr. William Emerson of California for his review and contributions to this section.)

Abnormal moulding of the base of the skull

Occipital osteodiastasis: This rare and usually fatal accident of moulding results from excessive pressure on the suboccipital region resulting in traumatic separation of the innominate synchondrodial joint on one or both sides. The lower edge of the supraoccipital portion of the squamous occipital bone is torn free of its attachment and becomes displaced forward and inward, compressing the brain stem. In its most serious form, this causes injury to the attached dura and occipital vascular sinuses, resulting in severe subdural bleeding into the posterior skull. The edge of the displaced bone may also lacerate the cerebellum. On rare occasions, it has been known to occur during normal vertex births and after difficult instrumental delivery. However, it happens most often during breech births, when the fetal neck has been forcibly hyperextended while the occipital eminence is still trapped beneath the symphysis pubis (Pape & Wigglesworth, 1979).

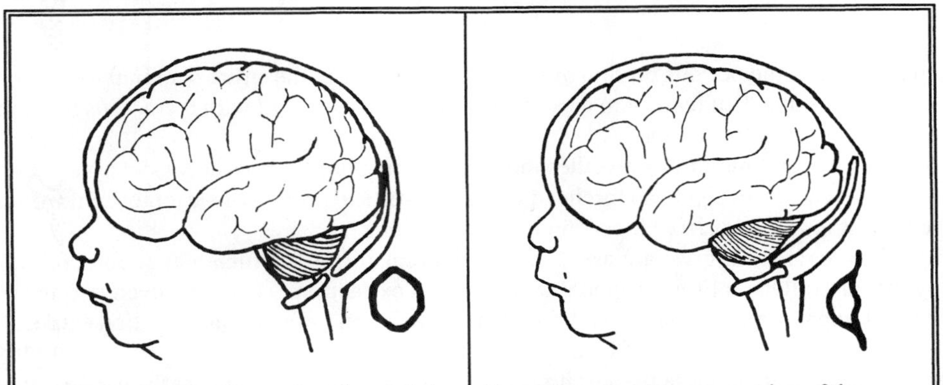

Normal alignment of bones in suboccipital region. Inset shows normal shape of foramen magnum viewed from above.

Osteodiastasis with compression of the cerebellum. Inset shows posterior distortion of the foramen magnum viewed from above.

Atlantooccipital inversion: The atlas has a great deal of anteroposterior and lateral mobility where it joins the occiput. The foramen magnum is an ellipse with its long axis in the anteroposterior diameter, while the atlantal foramen is closer to a circle in newborns, which enhances the mobility of this joint. In ten newborn autopsy examinations performed in 1979, Gilles and coauthors noted that extension of the head resulted in inversion (protrusion) of the posterior arch of the atlas up through the foramen magnum, producing bilateral compression of the vertebral arteries as they traverse this area to enter the foramen magnum. In addition, when the head of some of these babies were flexed, a portion of the axis (the second cervical vertebra) protruded a short distance into the anterior foramen magnum. Neither of these are usual findings and they postulated that this could be one mechanism of death for neonates, infants with disease or unanticipated death. It is not clear whether this had anything to do with the deaths of the infants they autopsied. Fortunately, most infants are well equipped to tolerate vertebral artery compression because blood flow is easily rerouted through the circle of Willis from the carotid arteries, which makes up for any deficiency. In addition, the ability to do something with force on a cadaver does not easily translate into a subtle mechanism of death. Extension of the head has not been found in association with the discovery of dead babies in their cribs (Guntheroth, 1995). However, one-fifth of the population has abnormally small, string-like posterior communicating arteries on both sides. Gilles postulates that those with small vessels may not be able to compensate for sudden bilateral occlusion of the vertebral arteries. In short, this type of vertebral artery occlusion may be a rare, little-recognized reason for some otherwise unexplainable fetal distress in babies in extended cephalic presentations or in some fetal or newborn deaths.

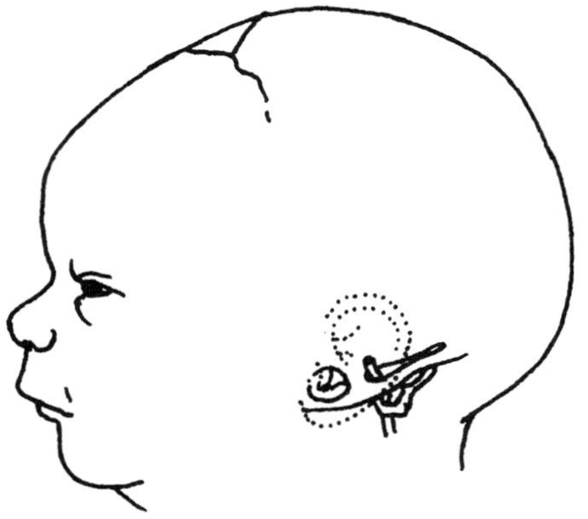

Anatomical alignment of atlantooccipital joint

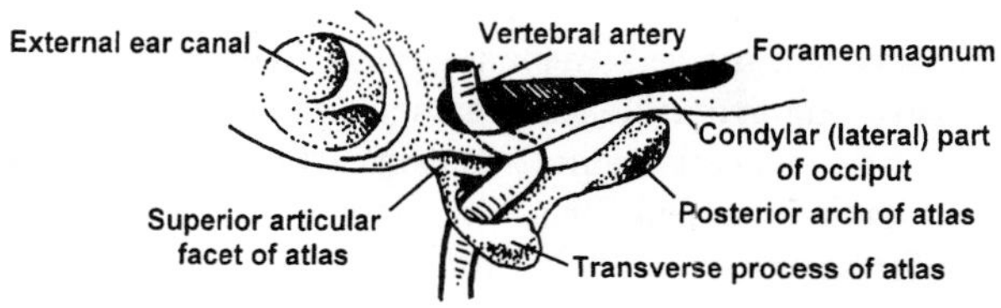

Close-up of normal anatomical alignment

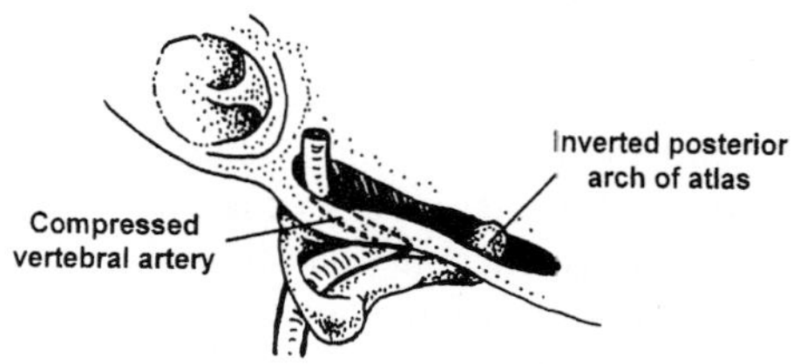

Partial extension of the head producing atlantooccipital inversion with compression of the vertebral artery.

Cerebral soft tissues and moulding

Normal moulding causes the petrous portion of the temporal bone and the entire occipital base to rise along with the parietal bones, carrying the attached tentorium cerebri and falx cerebri upward with them, thus minimizing tension and protecting these internal tissues from injury.

Excessive compression and moulding stretches the cerebral membranes and the vascular sinuses contained within them. Compression between the occiput and forehead strains the vertical portion of the tentorium. Compression between the vault and the base strains the horizontal portion of the tentorium.

The majority of intracranial injuries are associated with prematurity, instrumental or forceful delivery or manual manipulations by the birth attendant such as podalic version and extraction. However, even during spontaneous labor, abrupt or severe moulding or any excessive moulding that occurs in an unfavorable direction (especially upward), can result in these membranes and blood vessels becoming severely stretched or torn.

Damage can occur anywhere in these tissues; however, it most commonly occurs at the point of attachment between the tentorium cerebri and falx cerebri. When the mobility of the parietal, temporal and basioccipital bones reaches its limit, they cannot rise up any further. As a result, the temporal and occipital bones and the attached tentorium become relatively fixed. In order for more extreme moulding to occur, the lateral sutures must stretch (widen) to allow the parietal bones to continue to rise. The falx cerebri is dragged upward along with the parietal bones, first becoming tense and finally tearing away from its attachment to the tentorium cerebri. The weakest point in this area is located where the great vein of Galen joins the straight sinus. Any tearing of the dura or blood vessels results in intracranial hemorrhage. Resulting complications include brain damage and death, depending on the severity of bleeding and the location of injury (Moloy, 1942).

Overlapping of the occipital and parietal bones may compress the superior sagittal sinus and slow cerebral circulation, leading to increased cerebral venous pressure. This may precipitate intracerebral hemorrhage with associated respiratory distress. Problematic overlap occurs most frequently during anteroposterior compression in preterm babies with soft skulls and wide sutures, when the normal locking which occurs at the lambdoidal suture may not be sufficient to protect against venous compression. After birth, overlap may occur in these babies when they are placed supine and is particularly dangerous because protective locking cannot occur if the parietal bones are not also compressed. Turning the head to one side or laying the baby on her side promptly resolves the overlap. Excessive rotation of the head may compress the ipsilateral internal jugular vein and should be avoided (Newton & Gooding, 1975).

Moulding and head position

Visible moulding that is unresolved at birth varies depending upon the baby's presentation. For example, if the baby is well flexed and LOT or LOA, the suboccipitobregmatic diameter presents. Moulding causes the head to elongate in the verticomental diameter, with bulging centered near the posterior fontanelle. The occiput is pressed upward, the base of the skull rises slightly, and the face and forehead are flattened. The following chart describes typical moulding for various cephalic presentations.

Moulding can either help or hinder fetal descent. If the head becomes moulded while in a deflexed or asynclitic position, subsequent repositioning of the head becomes more difficult. This is even more exaggerated when a caput develops (see details below). Although the term "moulding" is formally applied to the skull, other parts of the baby's body, especially the shoulder girdle, may be said to mould as well. Note that moulding shortens the presenting anteroposterior diameter of the head.

Position of the Head	Presenting Diameter Shortened by Moulding	Presenting Diameter Lengthened by Moulding
1. Flexed vertex, occiput anterior	Suboccipitobregmatic	Verticomental
2. Flexed vertex, occiput posterior	Suboccipitofrontal	Submentovertical
3. Median or deflexed posterior vertex	Occipitofrontal	Submentovertical
4. Breech (flexed aftercoming head)	Suboccipitofrontal	Submentovertical
5. Anterior face	Submentobregmatic	Occipitofrontal
6. Anterior brow	Mentobregmatic	Suboccipitofrontal

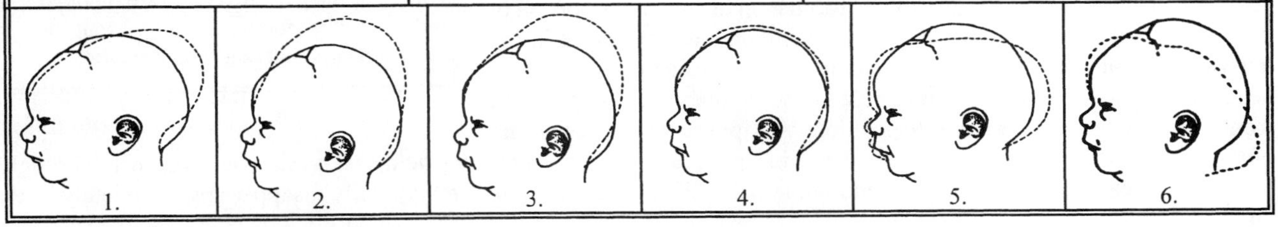

Moulding and gestational age

Preterm babies are especially prone to intracranial damage because their skeletons are less ossified and their intracranial structures are more immature and fragile. The normal pressure of birth can produce excessive moulding due to the extreme malleability and wider suture lines that characterize the soft preterm skull. Conversely, if the baby is postmature, the skull is more ossified and the bones not as compressible, possibly leading to difficulty with descent.

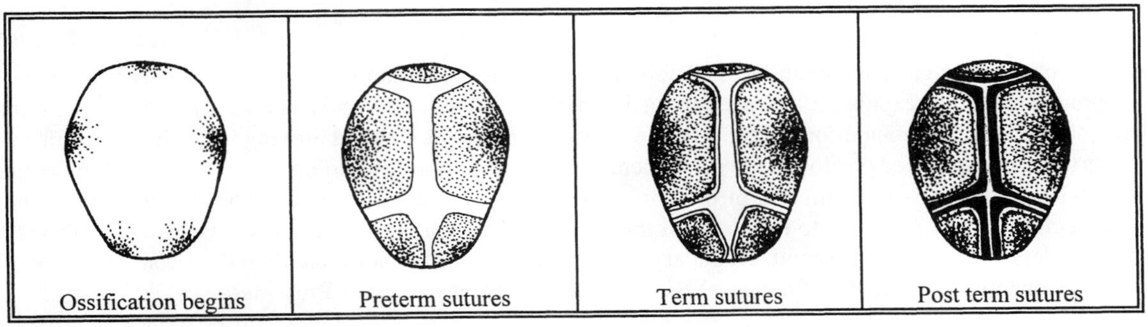

Caput succedaneum

In contemporary obstetrics, a caput is defined as a localized swelling of the scalp which occurs during some labors as a result of direct pressure on the head. Caputs may contain serum with or without some blood mixed in. A caput by itself is, in most cases, a benign by-product of birth. It presents as a soft, diffuse edematous swelling that pits on finger-pressure and that usually overlies suture lines. The fluid collects between the subcutaneous scalp tissue and the pericranium as a result of impaired venous return. This typically occurs prior to full dilation, when the cervical ring becomes closely and directly applied to the lowermost region of the presenting part. Once the cervix is fully dilated, a caput can form as the result of obstructed descent when the birth canal is tight all around. The more direct and sustained the circumferential pressure on the presenting part, the more likely it is that a caput or similar swelling will form. Thus, the size and depth of a caput is an indication of how much pressure the presenting part sustained during descent. A large caput suggests strong pressure from above and resistance from below. A small one suggests a short period of impaired descent, little resistance from the soft tissues of the birth canal or weak contractions, even if impairment of descent was prolonged.

The development of a caput is encouraged by early rupture of membranes, which removes the cushion of forewaters and allows the scalp to come in direct contact with the cervix. Even with ruptured membranes, a caput usually will not form unless a woman is in good labor with the fetal head well applied to her cervix. Caputs also do not form in babies that have died. Caput formation is minimized or entirely absent when the mother labors in warm salt water (see the chapter entitled "Hydrotherapy and Waterbirth" for additional information). Similar-appearing localized regions of edema may develop on any dependent part of the fetus that receives sufficient localized pressure for an extended period of time during labor.

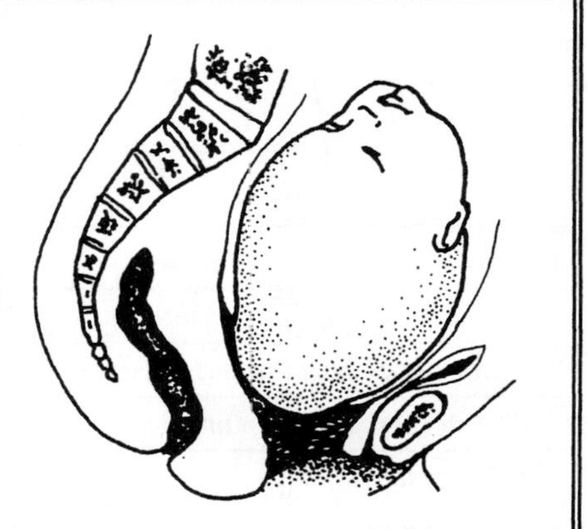
This LOA baby's membranes are ruptured and a caput has formed. A large caput can act as a plug, hindering further rotation.

The location of a caput depends upon the position of the head. In an LOA position, a caput may be formed on the posterior region of the right parietal bone near the sagittal suture, because that is the area closest to the cervix. In an ROA position, the caput is formed on the posterior portion of the left parietal bone. A caput may be palpable on internal exams during labor and can interfere with efforts to determine the exact position of the head. It can also act as a plug that impedes or sometimes prevents the head from changing to a more favorable position. A caput that enlarges during labor indicates that the baby is probably stuck in a particular position or is being held back as she tries to descend through the pelvis. A caput is largest at birth and immediately begins to reduce in size, typically disappearing completely after 24 to 36 hours.

As distinct from a caput, a cephalohematoma occurs when bleeding becomes trapped beneath the pericranium of one or more skull bones. It is uncommon for a cephalohematoma to be obvious at the time of birth; it usually takes several hours for it to develop. (More details are found in the subchapter entitled "Examining the Head and Neck.")

Moulding and Adaptations of Other Parts of the Fetal Body

Adaptations of the shoulder girdle

The most clinically significant diameter of the shoulder girdle is the bisacromial, which runs between the tips of the acromial processes of the scapula. It averages about 12 cm (4.75 in) in length and has a circumference of 34 cm (13.5 in). The shoulders tend to become compacted by either being depressed downward, flexing forward or hunching upward as they pass through the curved portion of the pelvis beneath the pubic bone. Moulding can reduce the shoulder diameter by 25% to 33% or more, thus facilitating birth. They may also descend on an angle. The shoulders may alter their position several times as they adapt to the shape of the birth canal during descent (Borell & Fernström, 1958).

The shoulders move as they descend, secondary to the movement of the head and then the chest. This is explained in detail in the chapter entitled "The Process of Birth in Occiput Anterior Vertex Presentations."

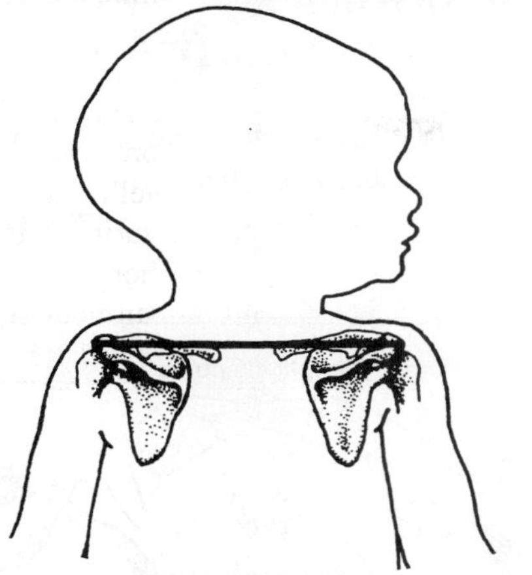

Bisacromial diameter

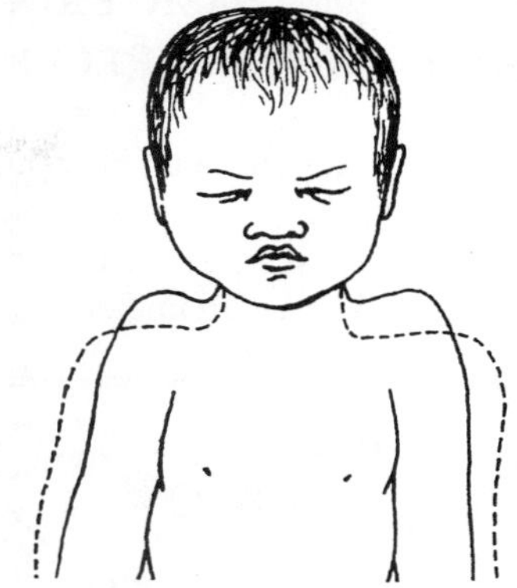

Shoulders may flex forward, hunch upward (as shown) or descend at a slant as they accommodate their shape to that of the birth canal.

Adaptations of the fetal pelvis

Like the shoulder girdle, the fetal pelvis consists of a bony structure that is wider from side to side than it is deep in its anteroposterior dimension. The bisiliac diameter is the widest diameter between the iliac crests. The bitrochanteric diameter, which runs between the greater trochanters of the femurs, is usually the same length as the bisiliac. In vertex presentations, the long axis of the fetal pelvis follows the movements of the torso as the spine changes position to negotiate the birth canal.

Once the head and the shoulders of a baby in a cephalic presentation are born, the rest of the body slides out or can be guided out safely with slight traction. The exception to this generalization occurs when there is a mechanical problem, such as a short or entangled cord, or some rare fetal anomaly that causes the baby's abdomen or thorax to be unduly large and rigid. In a breech presentation, the malleability of the fetal pelvis allows it to compact to a limited extent. While this may facilitate the birth of the breech, it poses a potential danger because the head may still be too large to pass through, especially if the baby is preterm (when the head is even more disproportionately large, than the trunk than at term).

How the head, neck and torso move in relationship to each other

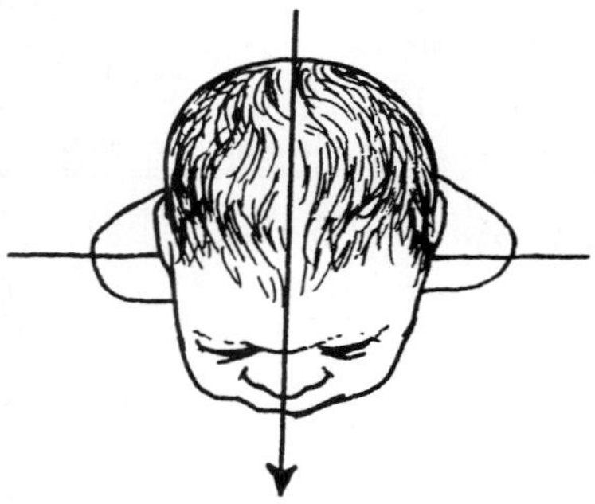

Viewed from above, the long axis of the head runs from the center of the forehead to the posterior fontanelle. The long axis of the shoulders is their transverse diameter, a narrow, elongated axis with rounded ends.

The natural tendency is for the cervical vertebrae to remain in a straight line with the thoracic spine, causing the head to face forward. Thus, the long axes of the head and shoulders are at right angles to each other in their normal anatomical relationship. During descent, the baby's body rotates, turning the head, or the baby himself may consciously or unconsciously turn his head to navigate the birth canal. The head returns to its natural anatomical relationship at right angles to the axis of the shoulders as soon as it has an opportunity to do so. This tendency is reflected in the cardinal movements of birth during internal rotation, restitution and external rotation. These movements are explained in detail in the chapters entitled "The Process of Birth in Occiput Anterior Vertex Presentations," "The Process of Birth in Mentum Anterior Face Presentations," "The Process of Birth in Frontum Anterior Brow Presentations," and "The Process of Birth in Sacrum Anterior Breech Presentations."

Basic Principles of How the Mother's Soft and Bony Pelvic Structures Influence Fetal Descent

In Volume I, the chapter entitled "Pelvimetry" focused on describing pelvic architecture and on the clinical aspects of assessing pelvic dimensions. Review that chapter before studying this one. This chapter goes into more detail regarding the specifics of pelvic structure as related to fetal descent during the birth process. For easy reference, the most important landmarks and pelvic diameters are repeated below.

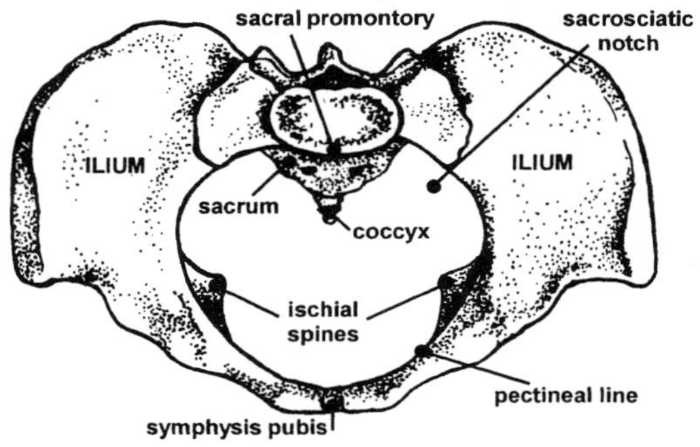

Pelvis: superior view, looking straight down

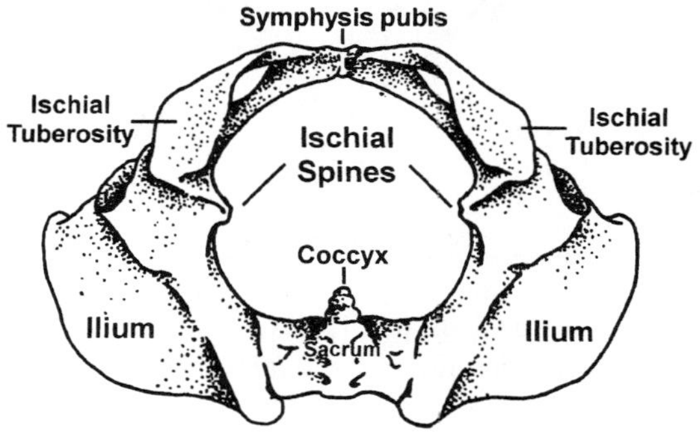

Pelvis: inferior view, looking straight up

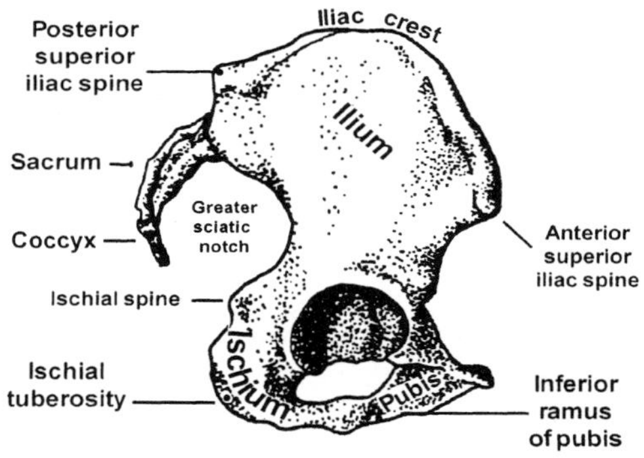

Pelvis: lateral view, standing position

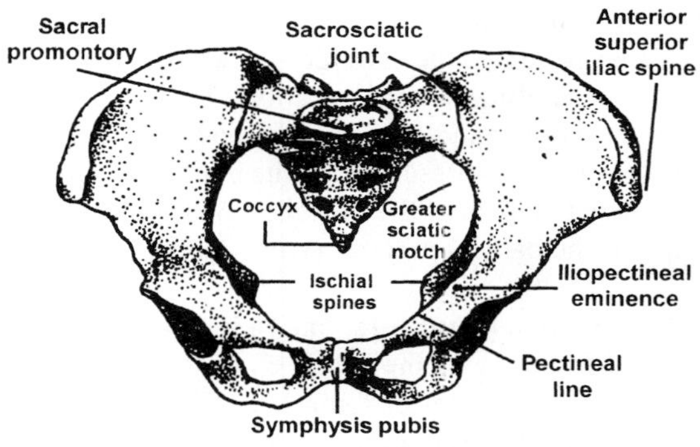

Pelvis: anterior view, standing position

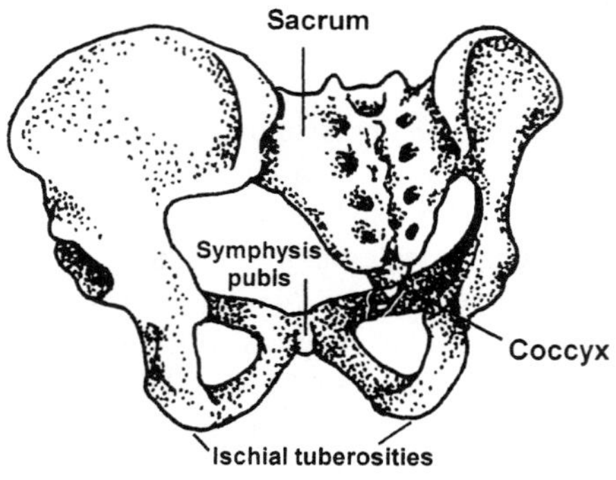

Pelvis: posterior-oblique view, standing position

Examine the drawings above. Note the level of the sacrum and coccyx in relationship to the upper border of the pubic bone; when the woman is standing, the distance between the sacral promontory and the upper border of the pubic bone is usually 6.5 cm. This will be important as we discuss how the pelvis and baby work together during labor and birth.

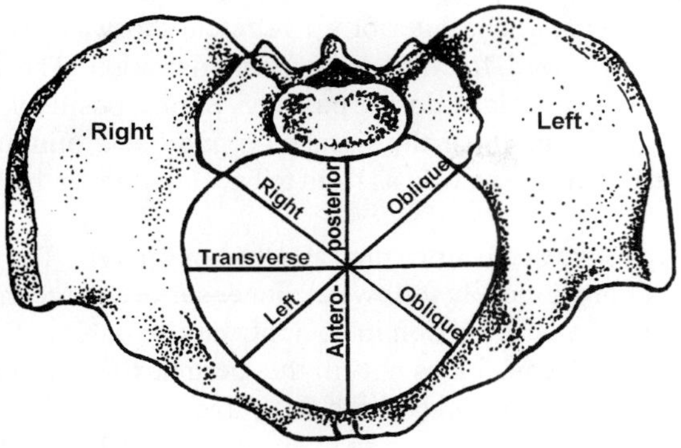

Pelvic diameters viewed from above the brim

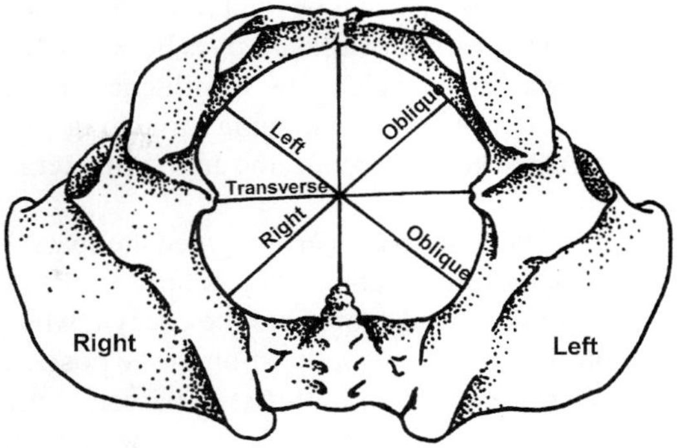

Pelvic diameters viewed from below

Directional locators and references to degrees of rotation given for the pelvis in this text will be from the perspective of looking up into the pelvis from between the mother's legs (inferior view). Time references put the 6 o'clock point in the center of the sacrum, 12 o'clock in the center of the pubic arch, the 3 o'clock point, to the *mother's* left (your right) and the 9 o'clock point to the *mother's* right (your left). The oblique diameters extend across the pelvis, creating an "X." The right oblique diameter originates from the *mother's* right sacroiliac joint and the left oblique diameter originates from the *mother's* left the sacroiliac joint. Each extends diagonally across the brim to the point just anterior to the opposite iliopectineal eminence.

Pelvic diameters are useful when studying how the baby shifts position as she descends through the pelvis. I strongly encourage you to obtain a pelvic model and label it with the diameters described above. If you don't have access to a pelvic model, make an enlarged copy of these pictures to refer to when studying with a doll.

The Soft Birth Canal

The course of the dilated birth canal

The soft birth canal consists of the lower uterine segment, the cervix, the yoni and the surrounding muscles and other soft tissues framed by the bony pelvis. The birth canal is a passageway that enlarges dynamically as the descending presenting part fills it during labor.

Most texts state that the curve of Carus follows the curve of the dilated birth canal, i.e., straight to the level of the ischial spines and lower border of the pubic arch, at which point it curves sharply forward. The course of the dilated birth canal was investigated by Borell and Fernström (1957c), who studied 21 laboring women (16 nulliparas, 5 multiparas) and found that it differs considerably from what is usually taught.

Their research showed that the upper portion of the dilated birth canal curves slightly. The middle part of the birth canal, in the region of the ischial spines, begins to curve forward. The lower part, in the region of the tuberosities, forms an angle of about 90° with the upper part. This angle was less acute in multiparas. The more pronounced curve begins about 1 cm below the level of the ischial spines and reaches its deepest curve either at or just above the level of the tuberosities. In no case was the

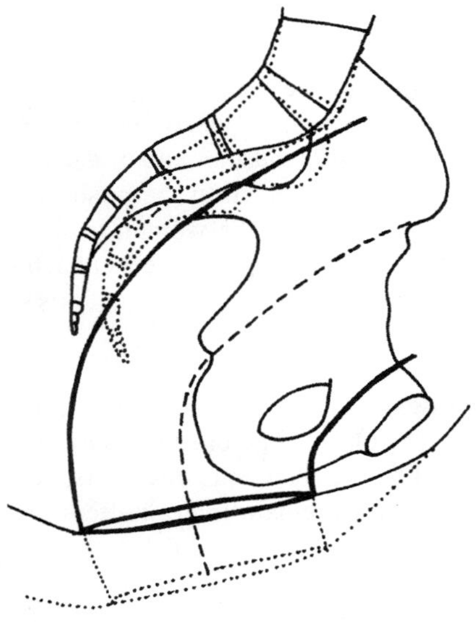

Shape and course of the birth canal: Solid lines show the sacral mobility and lesser perineal stretching that tends to occur when the mother is upright. Dotted lines show sacral immobility and excessive perineal stretching that can occur when the mother is supine.

deepest curve found to be beneath the pubic arch. Stretching and thinning of the periurethral and perineal tissues results in extension of the birth canal beyond the bony outlet as the head emerges. The anterior wall stretches forward between 3 to 6 cm and the posterior wall stretches between 4 and 8 cm in a downward, forward and outward direction. The actual degree to which the canal elongates is influenced by maternal position, especially during pushing. Supine positions pivot the soft tissues forward, maximizing stretching, while upright positions pivot the tissues up and back, minimizing stretching. As the head descends, the anal sphincter is stretched to either side as well as front to back, flattening the lower rectal canal.

Borell and Fernström also investigated the spacial relationship between the birth canal and the bony pelvis. The canal is generally of uniform width when it is fully formed. Its posterior border closely follows the inner surface of the sacrum near the promontory and again near the coccyx, which helps to enhance head flexion in occiput anterior babies. During occiput anterior labors, the midportion of the posterior wall of the birth canal does not fill the sacrum, which is usually more deeply curved than the soft tissue passage. Anteriorly, the soft birth canal (behind the pubic bone) begins at the anterior fornix of the yoni. At the level of the upper border of the pubic bone, there is an average depth of 1 cm of tissue between the inner wall of the birth canal and the inner surface of the pubic bone. Between the midportion and the lower border of the pubic bone, there is a thickness of soft tissue ranging from a minimum of 1 cm and up to 3 cm in depth between the baby's head and the inner surface of the bone.

The pelvic gates

(It will be most helpful for you to study the chapter entitled "Pelvic Anatomy" in HEALING PASSAGE and construct the model of the pelvic muscles found in the back of that text before studying this section.) Before the baby can be born she must pass through three muscular gates: the cervix, the muscles of the levator ani sling and the genital opening consisting of the urogenital diaphragm, perineum and vulva.

When the pelvis is normally shaped, the soft tissues of the pelvis and perineum form the primary passageway during descent and have the most direct influence over flexion and rotation. The walls of this passageway are firm and resistant to stretching, especially in first-time mothers. The presenting part is first pressed like a broad-tipped wedge against the cervix as the os gradually thins and dilates. (For centuries, the term "wedge" has been used to describe the leading portion of the presenting part because of the way it divides or "wedges" itself between the soft pelvic tissues.) Uterine retraction draws the lower segment (and along with it the surrounding attached structures) up and over the fetal presenting part. Labor contractions also apply pressure from above to the advancing head or breech. Together, these forces result in the stretching and dilating of the lower segment of the uterus and cervix, as well as of the pelvic soft tissues.

Internal rotation of the presenting part: In most cases, the presenting part passes through the cervix before it reaches the pelvic floor, where it begins to dilate the levator ani muscles radially. The pubococcygeus portion of the levator ani is the strongest of these muscles and is usually the first pelvic floor muscle that the presenting part encounters. The tips of the pubococcygeus attach to the posterior surface of the pubic bones, forming a teardrop-shaped opening that is directed downward when the woman is standing and leaning forward. From here, the sling angles posteriorly and inferiorly to where the deeper muscles attach to the coccyx. As the most anterior portion of the presenting part meets the resistance of the anterior sidewalls of this sling-shaped opening, it is assisted to rotate anteriorly (see the next section for more details).

Pelvic ligaments: The pelvic ligaments allow the bones to move and provide support for the pelvic floor muscles as stretching takes place. The ones that have the most direct influence over how the fetus rotates are the sacrotuberous ligaments and the sacrospinous ligaments, both of which take up space in the back and sides of the pelvis. They assist the presenting part to remain anterior after internal rotation has occurred and may help flex the shoulders when they have descended to this level (Tully, 2003).

Observations regarding the influence of the pelvic soft tissues on the birth process are highly relevant to the midwifery model of care. The soft tissues, and therefore the flexibility of the pelvic joints, are more easily influenced by maternal distress or relaxation, leading to correspondingly more difficult or easy labors. That the pelvic soft tissues (rather than the bones) are the primary influence over the movements of the presenting part in the average pelvis underscores the relationship between the maternal emotional state and the physical aspects of labor and explains the ability of maternal activities and position changes to dramatically alter the course of labor for the better. More details regarding the influence of the soft tissues will be found in the chapter entitled "The Process of Birth in Occiput Anterior

Vertex Presentations."

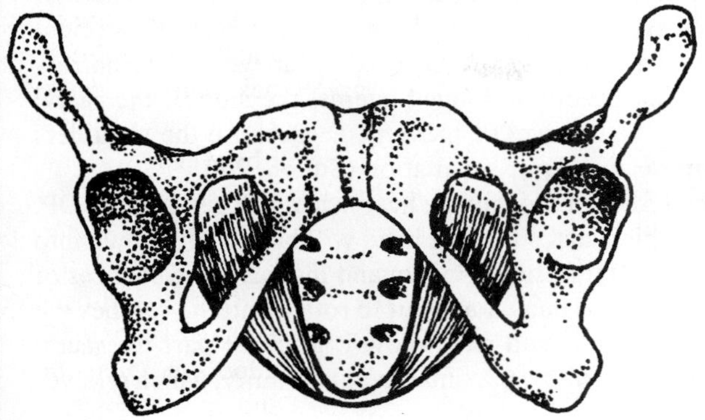

Levator ani muscles being converted to a sling by the pressure of the presenting part (not shown); anteroinferior view.

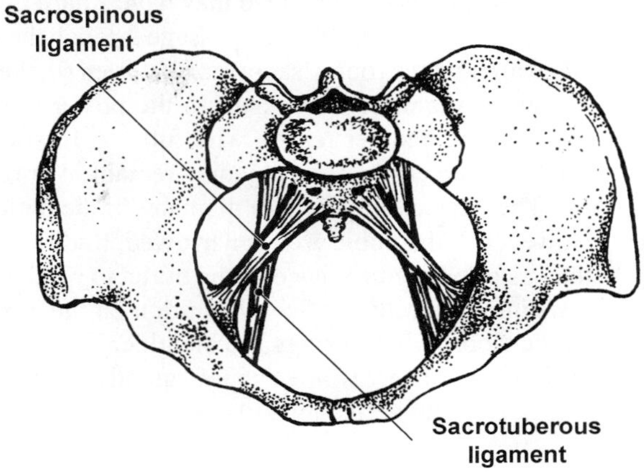

Pelvic ligaments

Engagement Through the Anterior or Posterior Pelvis

Steer (1975) discusses the head engaging through the posterior or anterior region of the pelvic cavity. Although there isn't enough space in most pelvises for this tendency to be dramatic, the head may navigate the inlet closer to the sacrum or closer to the pubic bone or centrally, according to the shape of the pelvis. The head then adapts itself to the shape of the segment through which it is descending. (More details will be found in the chapter entitled "Synclitism and Asynclitism.")

How Variations in Pelvic Bone Structure Might Affect Labor

While there is compelling evidence regarding the ability of the soft passages to affect birth, the shape of the pelvic bone structure can also have an impact upon the position in which the baby chooses to descend as well as the progress of labor. According to the Caldwell-Moloy system of pelvic classification (1933), none of the four basic pelvic types described below is considered abnormal, although each variation can influence the ease with which birth takes place, especially when the shape is extreme and the pelvis small. It must be kept in mind that the soft tissues are the main influence over fetal descent in the vast majority of labors, but that the bones create the surrounding structure for the soft tissues and thus influence their shape as well. Even given the various problems described for each of these pelvic types, they will be minimized when the woman's posture keeps the brim wide open and allows maximal pelvic mobility.

Gynecoid

The gynecoid, or "female" type of pelvis, is the most nearly round at all levels (brim, cavity and outlet). It is spacious posteriorly, with a relatively short, moderately curved sacrum, straight sidewalls and wide interspinous and intertuberous diameters. It is the ideal childbearing pelvis and, as, such, offers no peculiarities that may adversely affect the course of labor.

Anthropoid

This pelvis has an egg-shaped brim, with the larger part of the "egg" in back, giving it a long anteroposterior diameter and a reduced transverse diameter. Otherwise, the measurements are roughly equivalent to a gynecoid pelvis. This shape impacts birth in the following ways:

Brim: The long anteroposterior diameter of the brim encourages the baby to assume an occiput posterior position, since the larger portion of the oval, which best accommodates the biparietal diameter, is nearest the mother's sacrum.

Cavity: Once engagement has occurred, the rest of the birth usually proceeds without problems. If the baby enters the pelvis OP, the head may have a hard time rotating to an OA position because of the more narrow transverse diameter, although passage through the spines often occurs easily because of the relatively straight sidewalls and the roomy sacral curve. Even so, the chances of a persistent OP position are good. The narrow transverse diameter may result in the posterior shoulder becoming lodged against the side of the sacral promontory, another reason why full OA rotation may be delayed or prevented. Because the shoulders cannot rotate easily, the baby may remain in or return to a posterior orientation (Sutton, 2001).

Outlet: The long anteroposterior diameter of the outlet helps accommodate the head when it is persistently OP. However, if the pubic arch is narrowed, traditional teaching states that the head will have to dip down into the posterior sagittal space of the outlet to be born. This strains the perineum and increases the chances of tears into the rectum. (See illustration on the next page.) The baby may wait to rotate until he reaches the pelvic floor, which brings the shoulder deeper into the pelvis and may allow it to move past the sacral promontory. These women benefit greatly from positions that allow maximal sacral mobility, which relieves pressure on the perineum and creates more room in the posterior pelvis.

<u>Android</u>

The male-type pelvis has a heart-shaped brim, with the narrow portion toward the symphysis. The pelvic cavity is funnel-shaped as the sidewalls descend toward the outlet. This results in a labor with the following characteristics at different planes:

Brim: The more triangular or heart-shaped inlet may predispose the baby to assume an occiput posterior position, although many of these babies engage easily in an anterior position (Sutton, 2001). The large sacral promontory and the narrow sacrocotyloid diameter can cause the biparietal diameter to become hung up at the brim when the android shape is extreme, thus increasing the incidence of occiput posterior position as well as sometimes encouraging deflexion.

In many android pelvises, the sacrum is longer than average and the promontory more prominent. These factors together can delay engagement and make it more difficult. The long sacrum makes the pelvis deeper so that the head has further to travel in the confines of the cavity. If the shoulder axis is oblique, the posterior shoulder may become lodged against the side of the sacral promontory, encouraging rotation to the posterior.

Cavity: The sidewalls of the android pelvis converge, encroaching on the space; the spines are prominent and protruding, and the sacrum is relatively flat. This funneling may make descent impossible unless the overall pelvic dimensions are large. Arrest usually occurs in the pelvic cavity with the head in either an OP or OT position because the prominent ischial spines prevent the occiput from rotating. Changing positions from upright to side-lying and sometimes even flat on the back for a few contractions can help move the pelvic bones and work the baby down. Stair-climbing is ideal for this purpose.

Outlet: The narrow subpubic arch forces the head backward to take up the posterior sagittal space of the outlet. There can be a delay during late descent and pushing because of the tight space in the lower pelvic cavity and at the outlet. The baby may move up and down several times as she moulds and works her head through the tight fit. Whenever the posterior sagittal space of the outlet must stretch to accommodate more than half of the circumference of the head, the mother is at greater risk for large perineal lacerations. The narrow pubic arch makes it difficult for the shoulders to emerge and increases the risk for shoulder dystocia at the outlet. Full sacral mobility is very important for this mother and baby.

<u>Notes on the role of the pubic arch during labor</u>: In studying anterior vertex positions, Borell and Fernström (1957c) found that the distance between the anterior boundaries of the soft birth canal and the pubic bone was typically greater than has been widely taught. As traditionally presented, the presenting part fills the anterior pelvis to capacity during descent, with only the thinnest depth of tissue between the baby and the inner surface of the pubic bone. In their studies, Borell and Fernström found that in no case was the birth canal flush with the lower border of the symphysis, regardless of the width or angle of the pubic arch. They concluded that, in any case, the uppermost pubic arch occupies only a small segment of the birth canal and that the part it plays in the descent of the head has probably been overrated. These interesting findings suggest that the types of dystocia illustrated in figures 2 and 3 on the next page are most likely to occur when the pelvic architecture is extreme and especially in women who are kept supine, thus limiting sacral mobility. How the birth canal is altered by the passage of a somewhat deflexed occiput posterior infant was not studied, but such a position may diminish the space in the anterior pelvis.

It is generally taught that, when the angle of the pubic arch is less than 80° degrees, the anterior sagittal diameter of the outlet (that is, the space immediately below the pubic arch) is rendered impassable by the fetal head. The research described above suggests that the angle may need to be even more extreme than this to actually reduce the usable space in the anterior outlet. However, if the arch is narrow enough, some or all of the space from the symphysis to the tuberosities will be unusable because the available space cannot accommodate the skull. Instead, as the baby rocks under the pubic bone, the head is displaced posteriorly. The size of the posterior sagittal diameter, the concavity of the sacrum, and the level of the ischial spines in relationship to the sacral tip and the amount of space that can be created by optimal maternal postures are critical in determining whether this woman can have her baby normally.

Likewise, the anterior shoulder, which normally rotates beneath the symphysis pubis or one of the pubic rami, may become lodged above (inlet shoulder dystocia) or against (outlet shoulder dystocia) a low, thick or steeply angled pubic bone, creating difficulty with the birth.

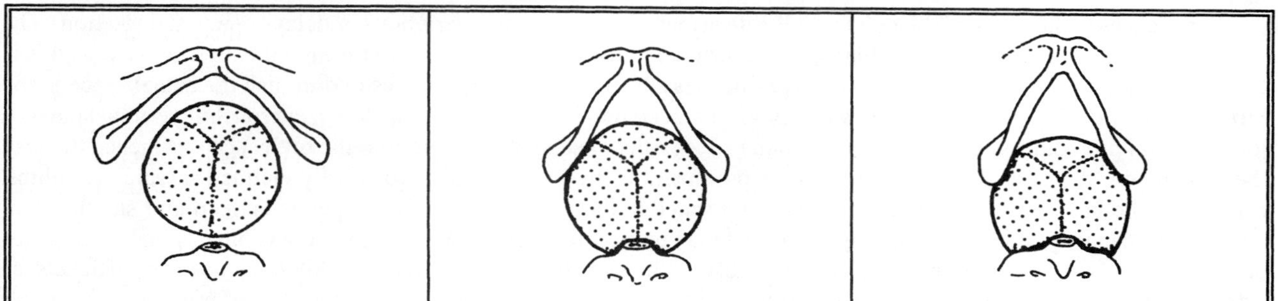

1. 2. 3.

1. The head passes easily through the rounded pubic arch and roomy, shallow sacrum of a gynecoid pelvis, as well as all other pelvises of adequate size.
2. A very narrow arch displaces the head into the posterior segment of the outlet. In this case the posterior sagittal diameter is large enough to allow birth. Displacement backward stresses the perineum and may lead to unusual or extensive tears. Sacral mobility becomes critical to allow the baby to pass without problems.
3. Here the posterior sagittal diameter is too short to accommodate the head, making birth via the yoni more difficult. The best chance for a normal birth lies in allowing full sacral mobility; however, if the passage is too narrow, the bones will not be able to move sufficiently to overcome the restriction.

Platypelloid

This pelvis has a long transverse diameter and a narrow anteroposterior diameter. This impacts labor as follows:

Brim: The wide, shallow brim often results in the baby entering the pelvis with her occiput transverse. Getting through the brim, which is narrowed in the anteroposterior diameter, is difficult and painful for the mother who may experience long, erratic early labor contractions as the baby works to get her head in a transverse position so she can engage. Deflexion may occur, leading to a brow presentation.

Cavity: Once past the brim, the head may also have trouble negotiating the midcavity because the antero-posterior diameter can prevent normal rotation and the sacral curve is flattened. However, once the head is through the brim, descent very often proceeds without further problems (Sutton, 2001).

Outlet: Once the head is past the midcavity, the birth should proceed smoothly, although a low pubic arch can lead to shoulder dystocia at the inlet.

Assimilation pelvis

"Assimilation" is a term applied to the most common structural variation in the pelvis, with every fifth or sixth pelvis displaying one of the following characteristics:

High-assimilation pelvis: The sacrum of a high-assimilation pelvis is longer than usual, with six segments instead of five and five foramina instead of four. This deepens the posterior segment of the pelvis, and in some cases causes the sacral promontory to be higher than usual, where it may impair transverse rotation of the shoulder axis because the posterior shoulder becomes lodged against the side of the promontory. The long sacrum may also result in some funneling in the lower pelvic cavity. It favors engagement of the occiput directly OA or OP and is a feature common to android pelvises.

Low-assimilation pelvis: In a low-assimilation pelvis the union of the ilia with the spinal column is lower than usual. Six lumbar vertebrae instead of five are present, and the sacrum has three or four foramina, making it shorter than average. This causes the posterior pelvis to be very shallow and has no special influence on the course of labor.

Mixed pelvic types and individual variations

Each woman's pelvis is unique and may have multiple minor variations. A significant percentage of women, if not most, have a pelvis that is a mixture of these pure types.

The pelvic examination described in Volume I gives an idea of the shape, contours and rough dimensions of the pelvis. A woman with narrow diameters in any plane of her pelvis will need expert guidance from her midwife to maximize her chances of a successful birth.

Differences in the shape of the pelvic cavity at various planes can cause variations or delays in internal rotation. The available space at the level of the ischial spines is critical to the passage of the head through the lower cavity, as this is the plane of least pelvic dimension. Excessive thickness of the bones (which serves to diminish the actual space in the birth canal), inwardly inclining pelvic walls, or pronounced pelvic features (such as large, encroaching ischial spines, a jutting sacral promontory, or a previously broken coccyx that healed sticking up into the outlet) can influence the way the baby enters or passes through the pelvis. A prominent, convexly curved, or forwardly inclined sacrum can inhibit rotation of the baby in the midpelvis by taking up space in the pelvic cavity. If the pelvis is deep and smaller than average, the capacity of the lower cavity and outlet may be significantly reduced. Women who have spinal deformities or previous pelvic fractures are particularly likely to have pelvic features that inhibit fetal descent. Rickets or osteoporosis will permanently deform the pelvis in a variety of ways. (See a recent edition of Volume I for a full discussion of how pelvic deformities may impact the progress of labor.)

Taking into account all the above, remember that just about any kind of pelvis can birth a baby, as long as it is large enough to accommodate that particular baby. Given a well-fitting presenting part, good strong contractions, postures that maximize pelvic dimensions as the baby descends and a positive mental and emotional attitude on the part of the mother and birth attendants, babies can and do get born even when the pelvic contours and dimensions are seemingly far from ideal.

Pelvic Mobility and Labor

Opening the angle of the superior strait (spinopubic or inlet angle)

The spinopubic angle extends from the uppermost border of the sacral promontory to the top of the pubic bone. Fetal descent is facilitated when the mother's lower spine and pubic bone are kept at a wide angle (120° is optimal), allowing maximum room for the contractions to center the baby's presenting part over the pelvic cavity so that it can descend through the brim. This angle remains open as long as the mother's knees are kept lower than her tuberosities (or as long as her weight is centered in front of or directly over her tuberosities). Note that, while I am calling this the spinopubic angle, in reality the space immediately above the bony landmarks is equally important because, practically speaking, it must also remain open for the baby to have room to fit his presenting part and move in order to navigate the inlet.

The more the brim tips forward, the more the sacrum, coccyx and pelvic floor are pivoted up and out of the way posteriorly (causing the genitals to "face" the floor). Jean Sutton (2002) points out that only minor changes in posture can produce dramatic differences in the angle of the brim and the degree to which the pelvic passageway is curved. If the woman stands or kneels with her butt sticking out in back, she will automatically tip her pubic bone down and forward so that the circular pelvic inlet is also tipped forward or outward, away from the spine (Sutton & Scott, 1996). The natural lordosis of late pregnancy facilitates this wide angle, especially when the woman leans forward (Sutton, 2002). Any position that does not involve direct pressure against the sacrum will assist in keeping this angle wide; however, take note that leaning back (arching the back) before the baby's head is well down in the pelvis may lock the lowest lumbar vertebra against the upper sacrum, thus preventing the upper sacrum from rocking backward. However, as descent progresses and the baby fills the pelvis, thrusting the pelvis forward (if the mother is upright) or swaying the back (if she is leaning forward) usually occur naturally as the entire sacrum glides backward to facilitate descent.

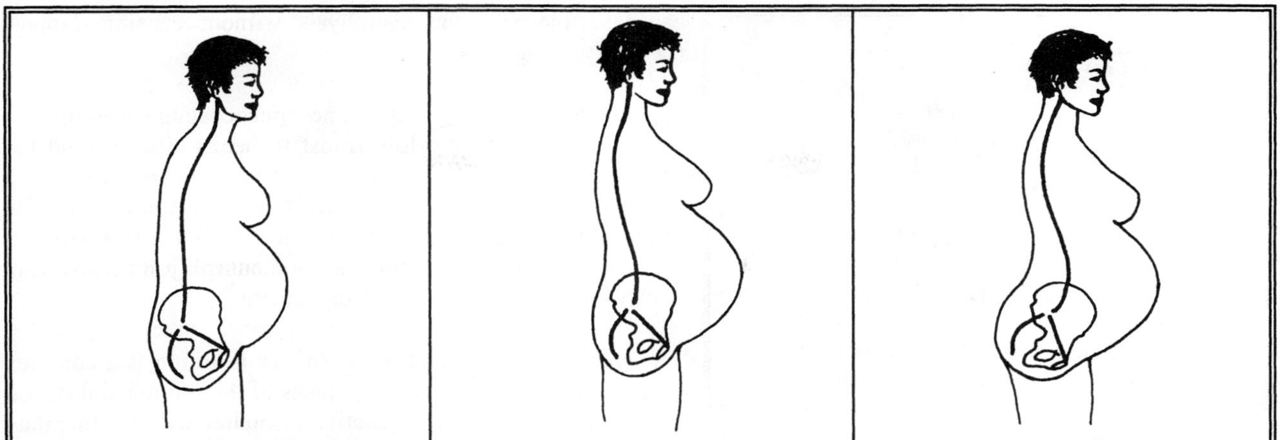

1. Spine curled forward | 2. Standing straight | 3. Brim tipped forward

1. Curving the spine forward lifts the pubic bone and levels the brim. It simulates semi-sitting, lithotomy and other supine positions with the knees up. This positioning moves the upper border of the pubic bone closer to the lower spine as well as maximizing the curve of the birth canal. Instead of the sacral promontory being 6.5 cm higher than the top of the symphysis, it is only 1 to 2 cm higher thus the brim is level rather than tilted. This narrows the brim and pivots the sacrum, coccyx and levator ani sling forward into the pelvic cavity, increasing the curve through which the baby must navigate. Deep squatting only closes these diameters even more.
2. Standing increases the angle between the pubic bone and spine, opening both the inlet and outlet; it moves the levator ani sling back and causes the genitals to face the floor at an angle.
3. When the brim is tipped forward, the lordosis of late pregnancy is exaggerated, the brim maximally opens and the sacrum, coccyx and levator ani sling pivot back and out of the way, creating the most room for the baby. The sacral promontory is now 6.5 cm above the upper border of the symphysis.

(Sutton, 2001)

Opening the midpelvis and outlet

Once the widest part of the head has passed through the brim, it is beneficial for the mother to assume positions that open the midpelvis and outlet. Positions that place the knees below the hips, such as forward-leaning postures with the knees spread, maximize pelvic mobility and fetal descent through the lower pelvis as well.

Movement of the pelvic bones in labor

(It will be helpful to review the basic information the chapters entitled "The Skeletal System" in HOLISTIC MIDWIFERY, Vol. I, before studying this section.) During labor, the pelvis goes through dramatic changes that facilitate the birth. While Hippocrates believed that the transverse diameter widened during labor, pelvic mobility is by and large ignored or outright denied throughout much of obstetrical history and still is in much of contemporary obstetrics. The pelvis is made up of four bones: the two ilia, the sacrum and the coccyx. The meeting points between each of these bones forms a joint. These joints are supported and held in place by muscles, tendons and ligaments. The placement of these supporting tissues is such that each joint is allowed to move in various anatomical directions that minimize stress and injury. Pregnancy hormones relax all the connective tissues in the body, which results in increased flexibility of the pelvic joints in late pregnancy and during labor.

The symphysis pubis: The joining point or symphysis of the pubic bones is a **cartilaginous synarthrosis (sin-are-THROW-sis) joint**. This joint consists of a slightly movable articulation made up of fibrocartilaginous tissue without a synovium or synovial fluid. The bony surface on each side is firmly attached to a thin layer of hyaline cartilage, which blends with the surface of a thick, strong but malleable disc of fibrocartilage. Collagenous ligaments extend from the periostea (lining tissues) of the rami, across the symphysis and blend with the hyaline and fibrocartilaginous tissues. They do not form a complete capsule, but do contain plexuses of afferent nerve terminals. The combined strength of these connective tissues exceeds that of the adjacent bones, allowing them to tolerate a wide range of stresses. The primary way this joint moves is by separating laterally as well as allowing the adjacent bones to move up or down slightly when in motion or when the legs are positioned asymmetrically. In pregnancy, separation of up to 1.25 cm and sometimes more

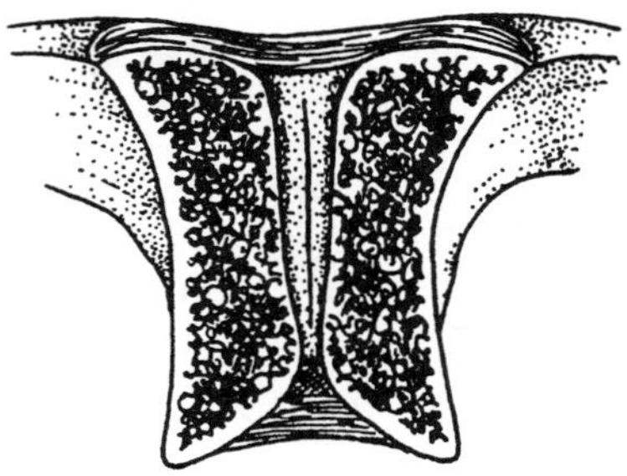

A cutaway of the symphysis and surrounding bone, revealing the tissues in the joint

can take place at the symphysis without causing damage (O'Grady, 1998).

The sacrococcygeal joint: The **sacrococcygeal joint** is a symphysis between the lowermost tip of the sacrum and the uppermost coccygeal base. These bony ends are united by a fibrocartilaginous disk that is covered with a hyaline membrane of varying thickness. Normally this joint has limited forward and backward mobility, but in some individuals this joint is synovial, which would allow even more movement.

The sacroiliac joints: The **sacroiliac junction** is a complex joint formed by the articular surfaces of the sacrum and ilia on either side. In women, this junction is smaller and smoother than in men and remains mobile throughout the childbearing years. The joint has two components. The posterior two-thirds of the space between the sacrum and ilia on either side consists of a fibrous articulation called a **syndesmodial (sin-dis-MOW-de-al) joint**. In this region, the bony surfaces are bound together by fibrous bands referred to as the **interosseous sacroiliac ligament**. This ligament allows stretching and rotational movement between the sacrum and ilia. Anterior to these ligaments are synovial joints proper, which allow the sacrum to slide up and down. The illustration shows a coronal section through the midportion of the sacroiliac joints, with the pelvis in the standing position, reveal these two types of articulation.

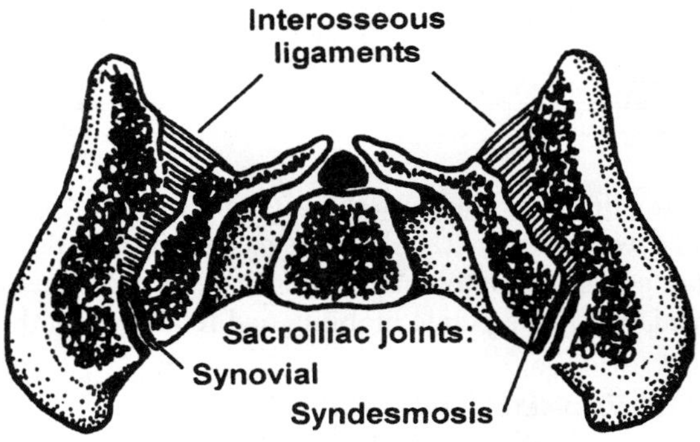

Sacroiliac joints

Studies done on nonpregnant individuals and cadavers confirm that the sacrum does move; however, they differ somewhat as to the types and extent of the motion observed, as natural movement in this part of the body is very difficult to study with X-rays. Investigators have described sacral joint motion characterized as flexion (moving forward), extension (moving backward), rotation (anteroposterior nodding or rotation around a transverse axis [called **nutation**]) and latero-flexion (turning slightly toward one side) as well as upward and downward gliding.

The motion of the sacrum during labor has been studied by Borell and Fernström (1957b). Upon examining a total of 191 women of reproductive age, they found the pelvis to be highly mouldable during late pregnancy and labor. Women were X-rayed using three variations of supine positioning and standing. Movements in the sacroiliac joint occurred around a transverse axis as well as by gliding were noted. Joint motion resulted in both upward and downward displacement of the symphysis, by as much as 2 to 3 cm in some women. Movements seemed to occur, regardless of the woman's posture; from this, they concluded that further changes would result if the woman assumed other positions. Displacement of the symphysis often resulted in a greater increase in the sagittal diameter of the outlet than in the sagittal diameter of the true conjugate. During labor, pelvic joint movement was even more dynamic and showed great variation among the women studied. They found the true conjugate of the inlet increased as the head passes through the inlet and the sagittal diameter of the outlet increased as the head leaves the pelvis.

With all the ways the sacrum, as well as the other pelvic joints, can move in the nonpregnant individual, it is obvious that all ranges of motion would be enhanced by pregnancy. Certainly, passage of a baby through the pelvis is a unique circumstance that presents the opportunity for the sacrum to be maximally displaced backward and the ilia to move sideways during birth. Spreading the legs can separate the ischial tuberosities and spines, widening both the midpelvis and the outlet (Beal, 1982; Williams, 1995).

<u>"Opening the back"</u>: Jean Sutton (2001) states that, once the presenting part descends enough to apply pressure to the nerve plexus at the junction of the bladder and the urethra, a neurohormonal response is triggered, which results in the sacrum moving backward as the body of the baby passes through the pelvis. Jamaican midwives refer to this as "opening the back," a phenomenon rendered invisible if the woman is clothed and which is hindered by modern hospital-based obstetrics where women give birth lying down. Other midwives have reported a "flattening" of the sacral area, which they first notice as the biparietal diameter passes the sacral promontory, prior to pushing. The region that visibly changes is the rhombus of Venus (Michaelis), which includes the last (fifth) lumbar vertebra and the sacrum and coccyx. During a true fetal ejection reflex, the entire sacrum moves backward 1 to 2 cm, pushing the wings of the ilia outward at the sacroiliac joints, which widens the pelvis, increasing its measurements in all dimensions as well as straightening the posterior pelvic wall. This can result in a widening of the inlet as much as 2 to 3 cm; the midpelvis (at the level of the ischial spines), some 1 to 3 cm; the outlet as much as 2 to 3 cm (Corkill, unpublished lecture, quoted by Sutton, 2001).

Pelvic Measurements Before and After the Sacrum Moves Backward During Pushing			
Before the sacrum moves backward			
Diameters	**Transverse**	**Oblique**	**Anteroposterior**
Inlet (brim)	13 cm	12 cm	11 cm
Midpelvis	12 cm	12 cm	12 cm
Outlet	11 cm	12 cm	13 cm
After the sacrum moves backward			
Inlet (brim)	15 cm	14 cm	13 cm
Midpelvis	14 cm	14 cm	14 cm
Outlet	13 cm	14 cm	15 cm

(Sutton, 2001)

Women move intuitively during labor. During a spontaneous birth, a woman works with the changes that occur within her body to facilitate an easy birth. When labor is difficult or the woman loses her ability to tell what to do (because of fear, excessive pain, etc.), the midwife can suggest various techniques, such as maternal position changes and activities to expand and rearrange the dimensions of the pelvis in various ways, to help labor move forward (Balaskas, 1992; Williams, 1995).

For more details on how the mother's body and the baby's body work together to accomplish birth, see the chapter entitled "Other Considerations Regarding the Mother's Body, the Baby's Body and the Process of Labor."

PURE PELVIC TYPES	GYNECOID	ANDROID	ANTHROPOID	PLATYPELLOID
Entering the brim	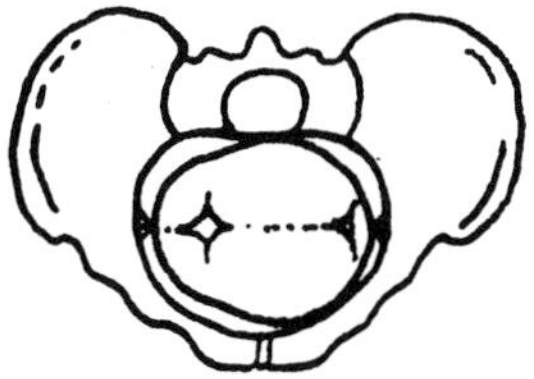	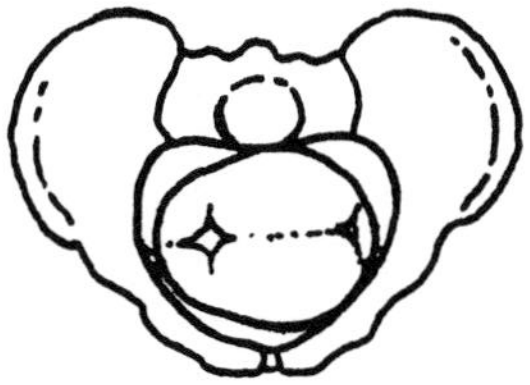	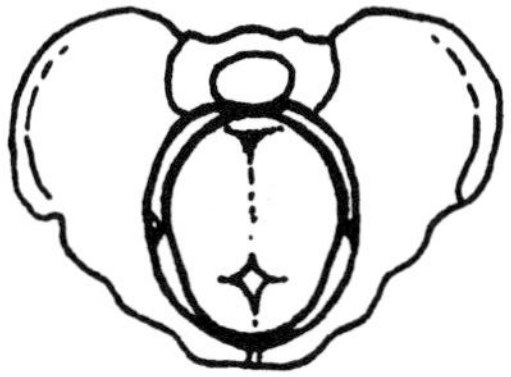	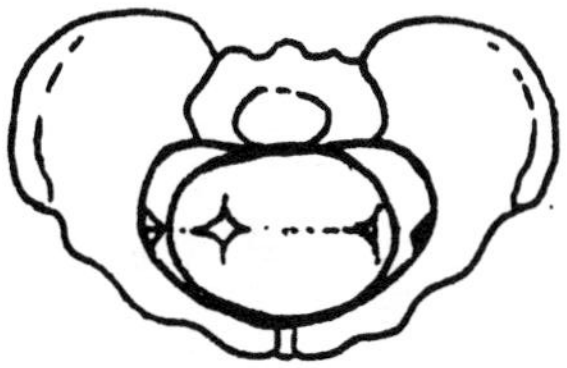
Fetal head **Position at engagement** **Attitude** **Asynclitism** **Moulding**	OT or LOA Flexion Slight to moderate Minimal	OT or OP Partial deflexion Marked Marked	OA or OP or ROP Variable Variable Variable	OT Variable Marked Marked
Engagement	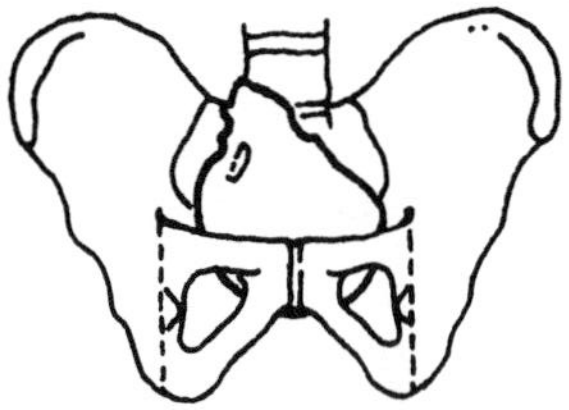	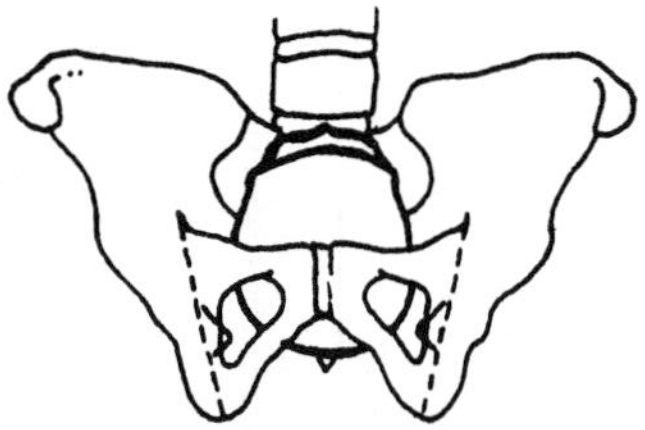	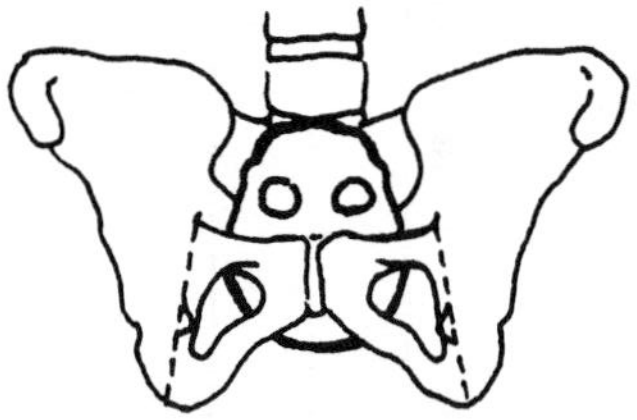	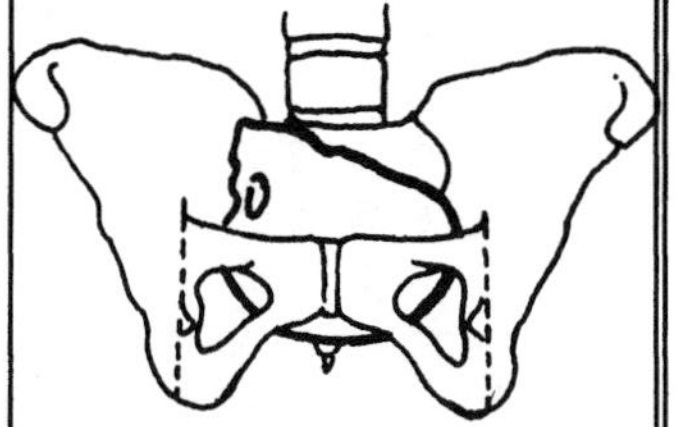
Descent through the cavity	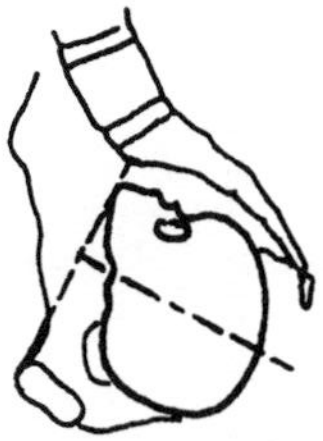	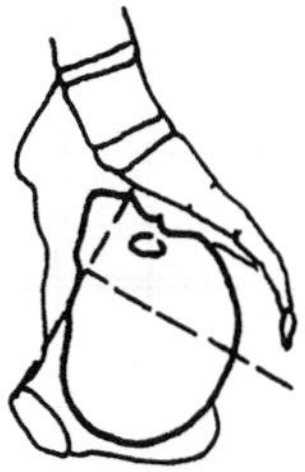	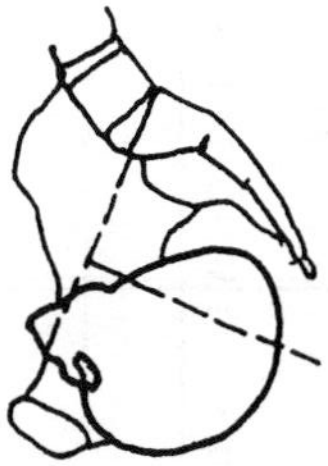	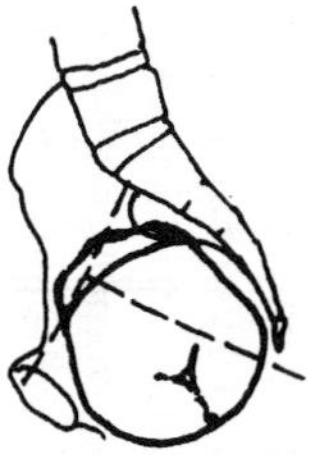

PURE PELVIC TYPES	GYNECOID	ANDROID	ANTHROPOID	PLATYPELLOID
Usual course of labor	Good with early, complete internal rotation	Delayed, especially at the end of first phase, possible persistent OP or deep transverse arrest	Good; possible persistent posterior	Delayed at beginning of labor with possible arrest at the inlet; deep transverse arrest may also occur prior to engagement
Prognosis for normal vertex birth	Excellent	Expect delays, unless overall dimensions are large	Good; prone to persistent OP births	Good once the biparietal diameter is past the narrowest AP diameter of the brim
Prognosis for normal breech birth	Favorable	Entrapment of aftercoming head is likely	Favorable	Deflexion and entrapment of aftercoming head is likely
Prognosis for deflexed cephalic birth	Most favorable	Least favorable, expect delays, poor prognosis for brow	Favorable	Delay at beginning with possible arrest at inlet
Risk of shoulder dystocia•	Minimal	Outlet dystocia increased due to narrow pubic arch with accompanying impingement of anterior shoulder on the rami.	Minimal	Inlet dystocia increased due to low pubic arch
Chances of perineal tears	Not increased	Increased due to narrowed pubic arch, which, when extreme, leads to increased pressure into perineal body	Increased if baby is OP due to perineum retracting over the partially flexed occiput	Not increased

•For a full discussion, see the chapter entitled "Shoulder Dystocia."

THE STATION OF THE PRESENTING PART

The term **station** describes the relationship between the lowest bony portion of the presenting part of the fetus and various bony pelvic landmarks of the mother. Station provides a way of communicating the location and progressive descent of the presenting part in the bony portion of the birth canal. To determine station, an imaginary line is drawn down through the pelvic cavity, centered between the sacrum and the pubic bone, following the path the presenting part must take as it descends through the bony pelvis. The ischial spines mark the midpoint in this pathway, halfway between the inlet and the outlet. The ischial tuberosities mark the outlet of the bony pelvis.

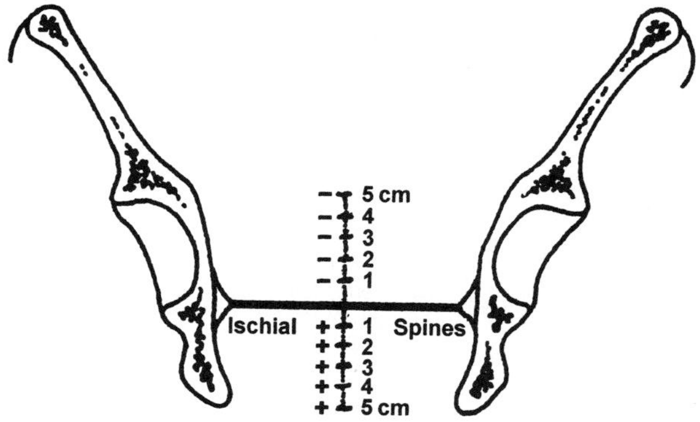

Stations of the pelvis viewed anteriorly with the mother seated.

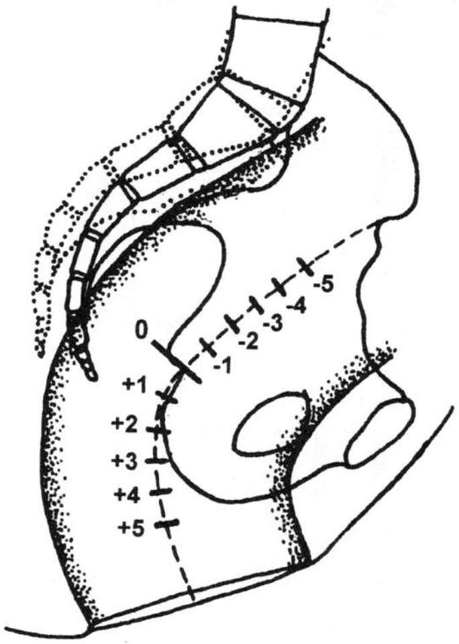

Lateral, standing view with the perineum maximally stretched showing how the stations follow the slight curve of the bony birth canal within the pelvic cavity.

The level of the ischial spines is designated as **zero (0) station**. From this point, there are five stations above the spines and five stations below the spines. They are spaced one centimeter apart; thus there are 11 stations in all (–5, –4, –3, –2, –1, zero, +1, +2, +3, +4, + 5), each representing one centimeter of descent. Those stations above the spines are expressed as negative numbers and designated as **minus** stations. The physical landmark for -5 is located just below the anatomical plane of the brim, at the level of the obstetric conjugate, and represents the uppermost boundary of the birth canal. Each minus station represents the number of centimeters the presenting part is *above the ischial spines* (i.e., at -4 the leading edge of the presenting part is 4 cm above the spines). At zero station, the leading edge of the presenting part is *level with the ischial spines*, marking 5 cm of depth and the midpoint of the bony passage as well as the narrowest transverse diameter of the bony pelvic cavity. Those stations below the spines are expressed as positive numbers and designated as **plus** stations. The plus stations represent the number of centimeters the leading edge of the presenting part is *below the ischial spines*. Plus stations increase numerically as the outlet is approached. The conjugate of the outlet at the level of the ischial tuberosities is designated as +5 and is the lowermost boundary of the bony birth canal. At this point, the presenting part is usually visible at the introitus, at least during pushing contractions. From +5, the presenting part advances out of the pelvic outlet and into the soft birth canal until it has fully emerged.

These landmarks correlate with adequately sized gynecoid pelvises. As with all anatomical measurements, they represent an average. For a woman with a large, deep pelvis, the distance from the brim to the outlet may span more than 11 centimeters; for women with shallow pelvises, the distance will be less. Even so, the level of the ischial spines is always used to indicate the midpelvis and is always designated as "zero station." If the woman's spines are not directly parallel to each other, station is best assessed by using the lowermost spine as the zero point. This will help compensate for any corresponding asymmetry higher in the pelvis.

Prior to 1988, the concept of station was less standardized than it is today. One very old system started at -3 through zero and ended at + 4 or +5. The most widely used older system, popularized by De Lee, divided the regions above and below the spines into thirds (-3, -2, -1, zero, +1, +2, +3). The 11 station system described here has long since replaced these older formats, but other systems should be kept in mind when studying older textbooks.

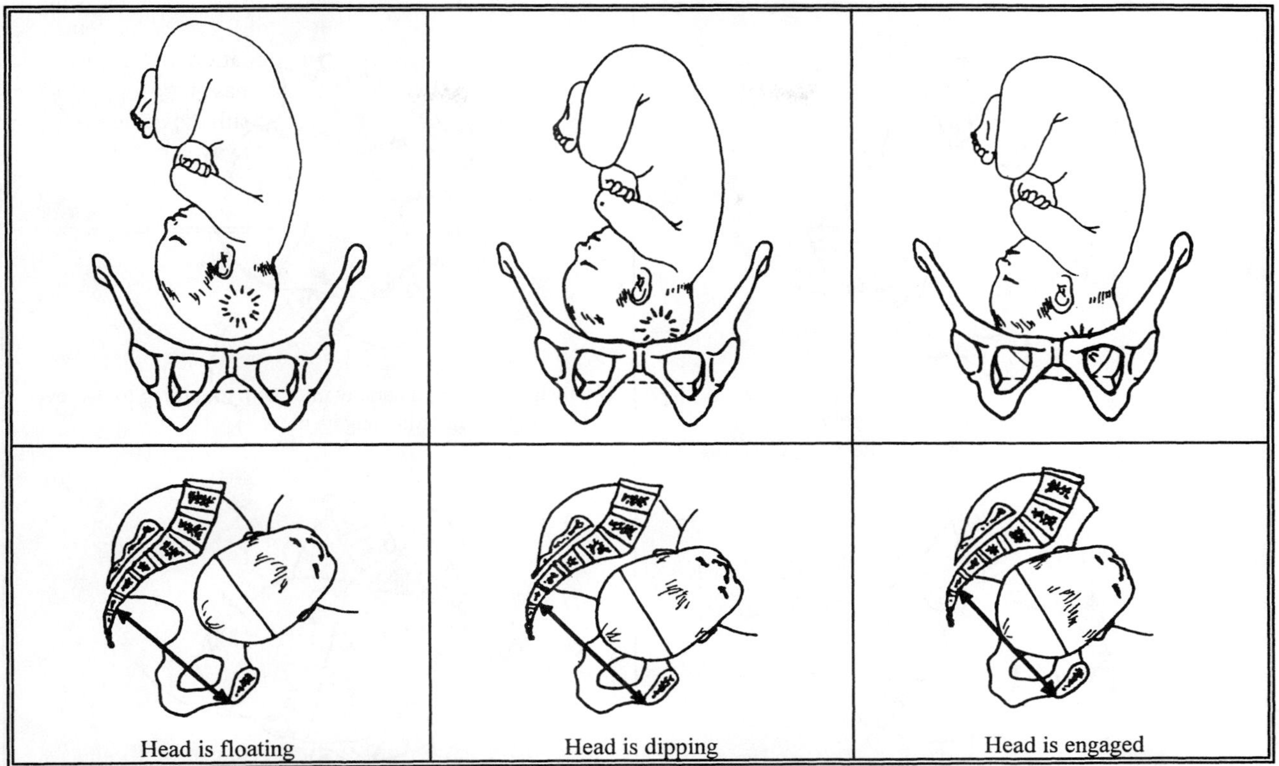

(Upright views show mother supine; side views show mother standing)

Descent to Engagement

The presenting part is said to be **floating** when it is entirely above the pelvic brim and is freely mobile on palpation. It is said to be **dipping** and is typically much less freely mobile on palpation when it has passed through the pelvic brim but engagement has not yet occurred. The presenting part is **fixed** when it becomes immobile in the pelvis. The level of descent at which fixation occurs varies depending upon the size of the presenting part and the pelvis.

Engagement occurs when the widest diameter of the presenting part has passed through the pelvic brim. In cephalic presentations, the parietal eminences are the anatomical landmarks of this diameter. When the top of the skull reaches or nearly reaches the level of the ischial spines in a flexed vertex presentation of an average sized (7.5 to 8.5 lbs) term fetus, engagement has usually occurred. The distance between the crown of the head and the biparietal eminence in the average-sized fetal head is usually no less than 3.5 cm and averages about 4.5 cm (1 3/8 to 1 6/8 in). The distance between the pelvic brim and the ischial spines in the average-sized maternal pelvis is about 5 cm. This means most heads are engaged when the lowermost portion of the vertex has descended to between −2 and −1. Thus, in most flexed vertex presentations, you can be certain that the biparietal diameter has passed through the brim when the top of the head reaches or nearly reaches the spines (zero station). This is considered a landmark in labor because the widest part of the head has passed through the narrowest diameter of the inlet. In cephalic presentations, engagement indicates that the pelvic inlet is large enough to allow for birth, but it gives no indication of the size of the midpelvis or the outlet.

A variety of factors can alter these typical findings, however. For example, if the baby's head is large, the vertex may be at the level of the spines, but the biparietal diameter may still not have descended fully through the brim. If the pelvis is shallow, the vertex must be at a plus station before the head has engaged. If the mother's pelvis is deep, the head could be engaged well before the vertex is level with the spines.

It is important to distinguish the *bony* portion of the presenting part when judging station; otherwise, an enlarging caput may be mistaken for descent in station. (An enlarging caput sometimes develops precisely because the presenting part is *not* advancing.) Conversely, the bones can fool you as well, because a head that is quite moulded through a narrow brim may descend to zero station before engagement has occurred.

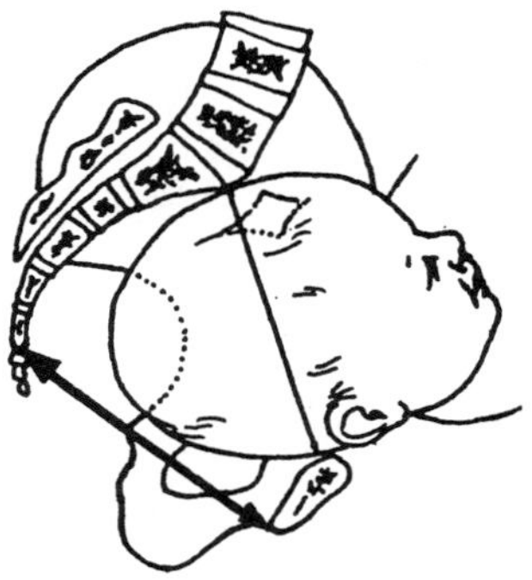

Head engaged in a deep pelvis

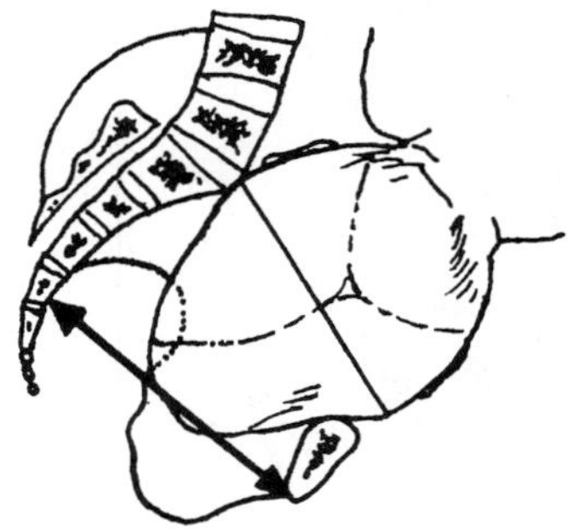

Unengaged head in a narrow inlet with moulding to the level of the spines, simulating engagement

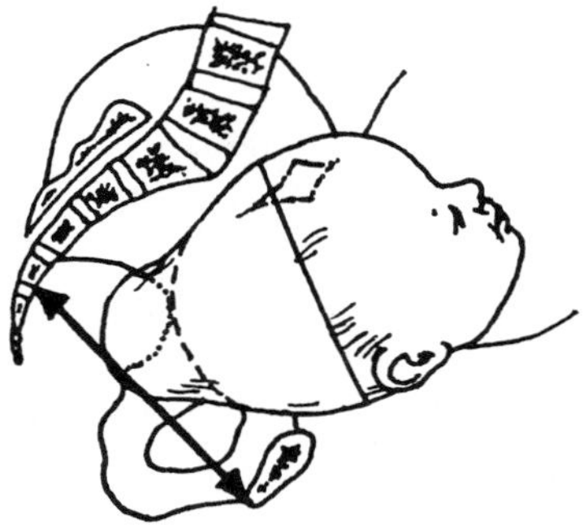

A large caput mimicking engagement

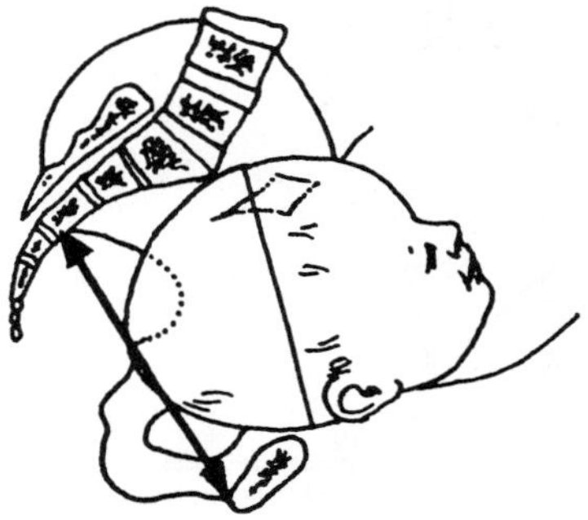

Unengaged head with vertex below spines in a very shallow pelvis

Timing of engagement

Engagement of the vertex may occur as early as 2 to 3 weeks prior to the onset of labor or before the clinical recognition of labor in some first-time mothers (this is accompanied by "lightening"). A tendency to early engagement is attributed to strong muscles and a firm pelvic floor. It was once thought that engagement in a primigravida was strongly indicative of a normally sized pelvis. In fact, the normal level to which the baby descends prior to labor varies widely among all mothers, and lack of engagement is not, in itself, a sign of a problem. In a review of 462 first-time mothers, Weekes and Flynn (1975) found only 50% to be engaged at term. However, it is true that, regardless of parity, descent to engagement or below prior to labor bodes well for efficient dilation when labor contractions begin because the presenting part will be more firmly applied to the cervix.

In multiparous mothers, whose musculature has already stretched to accommodate one or more babies, engagement of the vertex may also occur in late pregnancy but is most often delayed until labor is well underway. Juntunen and Kirkinen (1994) looked at descent in a group of grand multiparas and found that the baby stays higher throughout labor, with 7% still unengaged at 7 cm of dilation; all had normal births. Engagement frequently does not occur in deflexed cephalic presentations or in breech presentations until labor is well underway, regardless of the mother's parity.

Engagement of the deflexed head

The attitude of the head has everything to do with when and at what level engagement occurs. For example, when the head is deflexed, the biparietal diameter must descend further before it passes through the brim. The more deflexed the head, the further the biparietal diameter will be from the lowermost portion of the presenting part. In a face presentation, the face can be at the level of the spines while the biparietal diameter is still well above the brim. In most cases, the face must be at +2 before the biparietal diameter passes through the brim. Engagement of the face and brow will be discussed in more detail in the chapters entitled "The Process of Birth in Mentum Anterior Face Presentations," and "The Process of Birth in Frontum Anterior Brow Presentations."

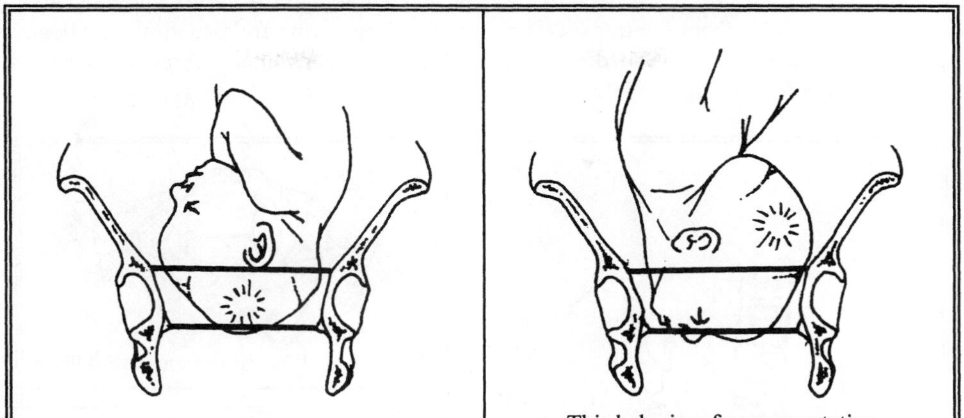

Engagement in a vertex presentation

This baby in a face presentation is not yet engaged.

(The mother is supine.)

Visualizing cephalic engagement

The following exercise can be performed on your own head, or with the use of a doll and pelvis, to help you better understand engagement. Tip your chin to your chest and place your index finger on the highest point at the top of the head (the crown of the vertex). Now place your thumb on the widest point of your skull directly above the ear (the parietal eminence on one side). If you were a well-flexed engaged baby, the place where your index finger rests would be at the level of the spines; where your thumb rests would be just below the pelvic inlet. Note the distance between your fingers.

Keeping your thumb in place, straighten your neck and move your index finger about halfway toward the front of the head, between the crown of the vertex and the brow. This is the bregmatic region, and is the lowest part of the head that presents in a deflexed posterior baby. Notice the distance between your thumb and forefinger. It may be as much as one-third longer than when the head is well flexed!

Next, still keeping your thumb in place, stretch your index or ring finger to the center of your forehead and note the distance; this is the distance for engagement in a brow presentation. Again keeping your thumb in place, stretch your little finger as far as you can to reach for the tip of your nose. See how far that is? This distance is why a baby presenting by his face does not engage until the face is well advanced into the pelvic cavity (adapted from Gentlebirth Midwifery archives, 1999).

Breech engagement is covered in the chapter entitled "The Process of Birth in Sacrum Anterior Breech Presentations."

Synclitism and Asynclitism

"Synclitism" and "asynclitism" are terms used to describe ways in which the vertex baby's head commonly enters and moves through the pelvic brim from the transverse position. These terms are also applied whenever the centering of the presenting part within the birth canal is discussed. Material in this chapter references Greenhill, 1951; Oxorn, 1986; Simkin & Ancheta, 2000 and Varney, 1997.

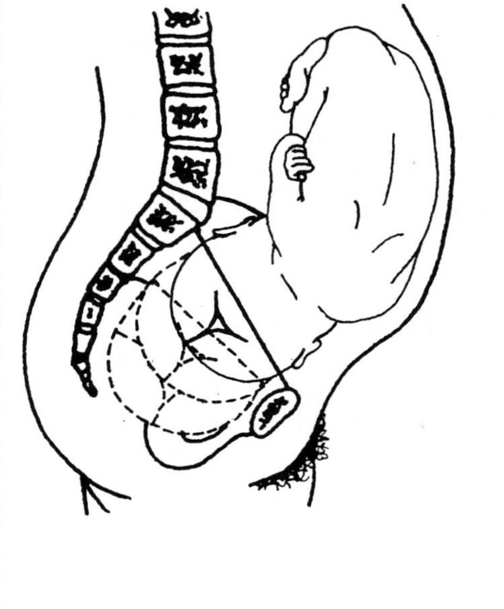
Synclitic descent

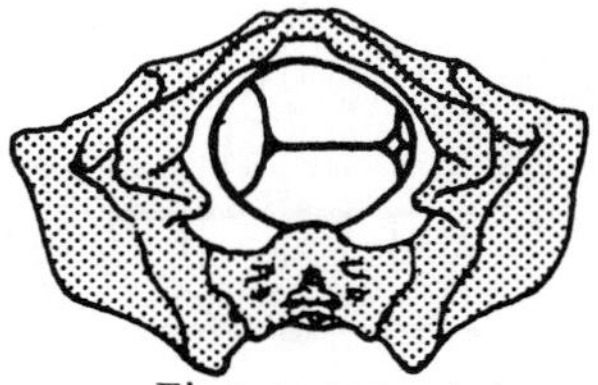
First movement

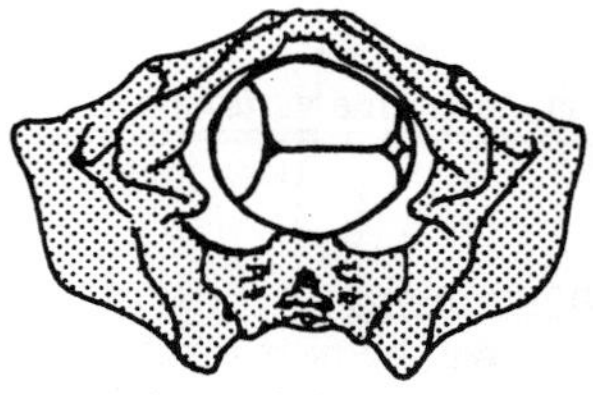
Second movement

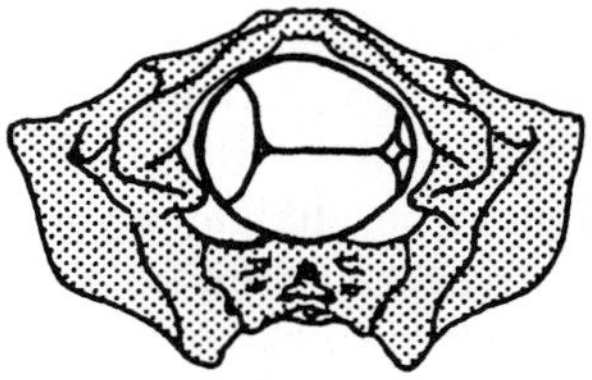
Third movement

Synclitism (SIN-kli-tism)

Synclitism exists when the biparietal diameter of the fetal head or the bitrochanteric diameter of the breech is parallel with the planes of the pelvis. The sagittal suture or genital crease is centered in the birth canal. In vertex presentations, synclitism allows the parietal eminences to descend through the pelvis simultaneously. Synclitic engagement occurs when the uterus is directly above the inlet (tilted forward slightly) and the pelvis is roomy, affording the head plenty of room to descend with the biparietal diameter parallel with the plane of the inlet. When the two parietal eminences enter the pelvis simultaneously, the presenting transverse (biparietal) diameter is 9.5 cm.

Asynclitism

The presenting part is said to be "asynclitic" (a-sin-KLI-tick) whenever the sagittal suture (or the genital crease) is cocked off center as it passes through the pelvis. This often occurs as the head enters the transverse diameter of the pelvis, either LOT or ROT (occiput at 3 or 9 o'clock).

In asynclitism, the parietal eminences enter the pelvis one after the other. The presenting diameter is the subsuperparietal of 8.13 to 8.75 cm, a half-inch (.75 cm) or so smaller than the biparietal diameter. Asynclitic descent through the brim to engagement allows a larger head to descend into the pelvis than is possible when the biparietal diameter descends parallel with the plane of the pelvic brim. There are two types of asynclitic descent.

Posterior asynclitism (Litzmann's obliquity): Posterior asynclitism is the most common way for a flexed head to enter the pelvic brim. Posterior asynclitism is associated with well-toned abdominal muscles that support the uterus tightly within the maternal torso. The baby's head is occiput transverse with the sagittal suture running across the pelvic cavity.

As toning or labor contractions begin, pressure from the fundus causes the fetal neck to bend sideways to a varying degree, tipping the baby's anterior ear toward her anterior shoulder. This moves the sagittal suture anteriorly, toward the pubic arch, which centers the posterior parietal eminence over the brim as the head approaches the inlet (and places the biparietal diameter at an oblique angle to the plane of the brim).

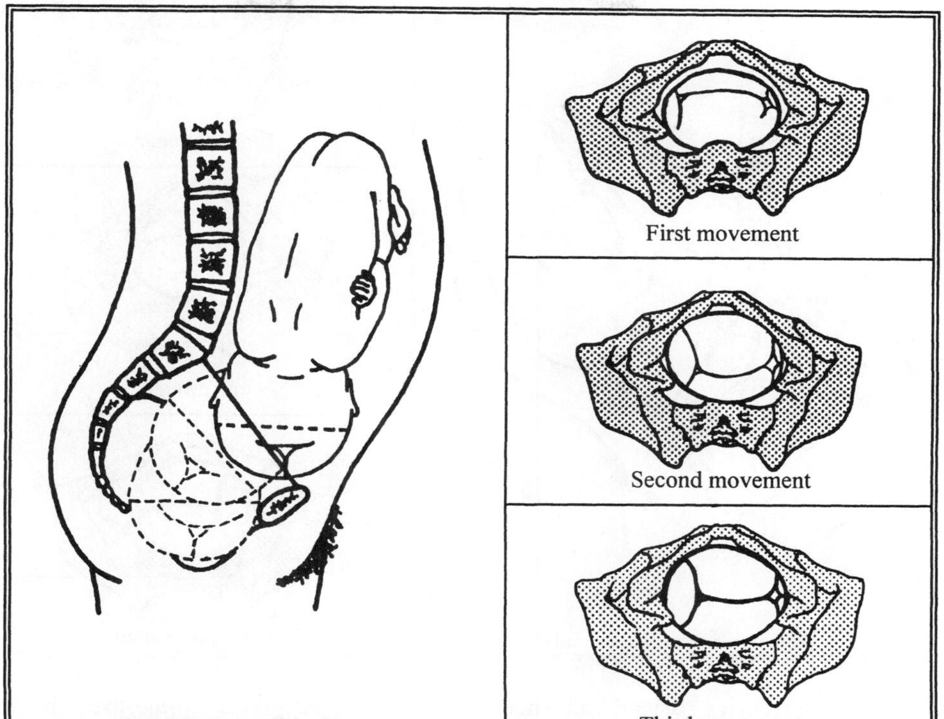

Posterior asynclitic descent

(Maternal abdominal muscle tone is exaggerated to clearly show how good tone encourages posterior asynclitism.)

This results in the posterior parietal eminence leading the way into the posterior pelvis. Strengthening contractions apply downward pressure, causing the baby to maintain the tilt of her head. The posterior parietal eminence enters the brim as the region between the posterior parietal eminence and the baby's posterior ear pivots around the sacral promontory. As this occurs, the posterior parietal eminence drops below the promontory and the baby takes advantage of the concavity of the upper sacral curve by tilting the posterior parietal bone backward into this space. The sagittal suture swings through the midpelvis toward the posterior pelvis as the anterior parietal bone descends past the pubic bone in front. This causes the head to temporarily assume an attitude of anterior asynclitism (head tipped laterally with posterior ear toward posterior shoulder). Both parietal bones have now passed through the pelvic brim. The head may level at this point (see below) or it may continue to descend in an attitude of anterior asynclitism with the posterior parietal bone tilted toward the sacrum to a varying degree, causing the anterior parietal bone to be lowermost in the pelvis until the end of the dilation phase of labor or until internal rotation is complete. When this occurs, the sagittal suture will be tipped posteriorly on internal exam (Javert & Steele, 1942).

As the head dips back into the hollow of the sacrum, the cervical os tends to be pulled backward as well. When a posterior cervix is discovered during an internal exam, this is an indirect indication that the head is descending in the roomiest portion of the pelvic cavity.

Anterior asynclitism (Näegele's obliquity): This occurs when the anterior parietal eminence leads descent. Here, the abdominal muscles are typically lax, allowing the uterus and baby to lean further away from the mother's spine. Anterior asynclitism may also occur if the pelvic brim is contracted or otherwise abnormal or if the inclination of the brim is marked, thus preventing the more common posterior asynclitism. As contractions begin, pressure from the fundus causes the fetal neck to bend sideways to a varying degree, tipping the baby's posterior ear toward his posterior shoulder. This moves the sagittal suture toward the mother's spine and centers the anterior parietal eminence over the brim as the head approaches the inlet (and places the biparietal diameter at an oblique angle to the plane of the brim).

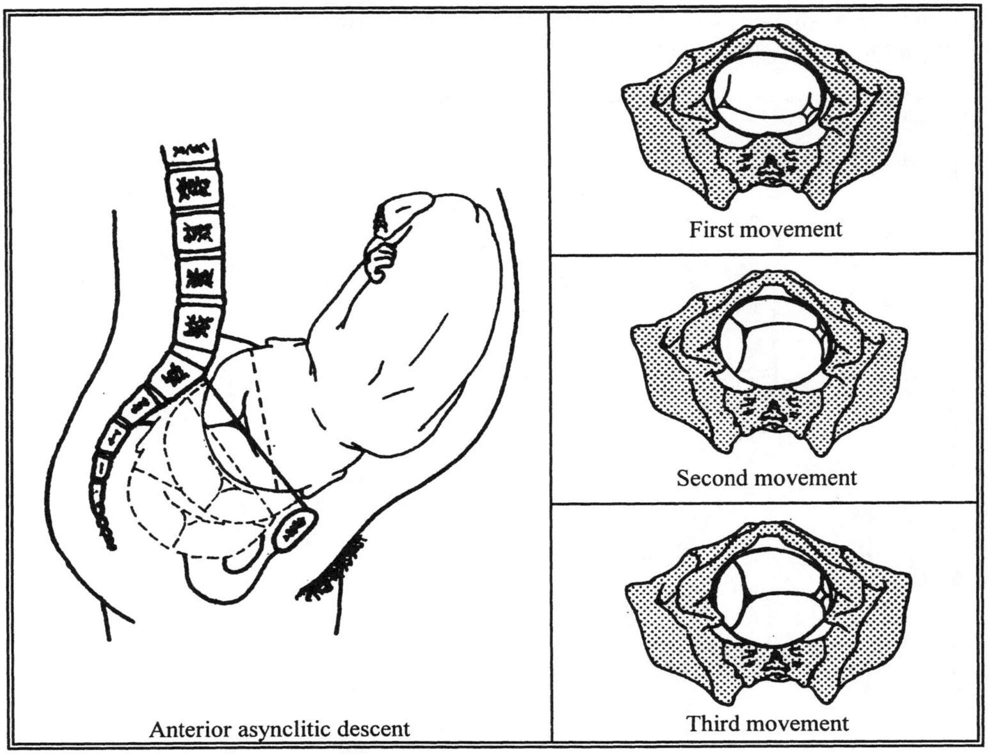

Anterior asynclitic descent

The region between the anterior parietal eminence and the baby's ear pivots around the pubic bone causing the anterior parietal eminence to descend into the pelvis. Once the anterior parietal bone is below the obstetric conjugate, the baby pivots the anterior parietal eminence into the limited space beneath the pubic bone. The sagittal suture swings forward toward the pubic bone as the posterior parietal bone descends past the sacral promontory in back. This causes the head to temporarily assume an attitude of posterior asynclitism (head tipped laterally with anterior ear nearer the anterior shoulder). Both parietal bones are now through the brim. The head may level at this point (as below) or it may continue to descend with the anterior parietal bone tilted toward the pubic rami to a varying degree, causing the posterior parietal bone to be lowermost in the pelvis until the end of the dilation phase of labor or until internal rotation is complete. When this occurs, the sagittal suture will be tipped toward the pubic bone on internal exam. Depending upon the reason the baby entered the pelvis via anterior asynclitism, he could continue to wiggle the head through the pelvis alternating anterior and posterior inclinations until undergoing internal rotation.

When the anterior parietal eminence descends into the pelvis first, the cervical os may be pulled forward, nearer to the pubic bone, indicating that the head is coming through the less roomy anterior pelvis.

Leveling

Leveling occurs as the head gradually resumes a centered orientation, with the sagittal suture more or less midway between the front and back of the pelvis; resulting in the head assuming an attitude of synclitism (as illustrated above). This may occur before or after internal rotation.

Other types of asynclitic positioning

Before or after the head is engaged, the sagittal suture may remain off center until internal rotation is complete, or it may be restored to a nearly centered position within the pelvis. However, the sagittal suture usually becomes asynclitic while internal rotation is occurring, until the head undergoes internal rotation and settles into its new position resting in the trough of the pelvic floor.

Asynclitic positioning also occurs whenever the head is laterally flexed, presenting in any off-center or cocked position as it passes through the pelvic cavity. Persistent asynclitism commonly occurs when the baby has her fist tucked up under her chin or near her neck but may also be present if there is a tight cord around the neck pulling the head to one side, if there is a large caput preventing the head from repositioning itself, if the baby has congenital deformities of the neck or shoulder, or if true cephalopelvic disproportion exists. If extreme asynclitism persists until the head has descended deeply into the pelvis, it may slow or even prevent descent of the baby through the birth canal and delay or prevent internal rotation. If a caput forms, asynclitism may not be correctable as the caput tends to act as a plug in the cervix, fixing the head in place.

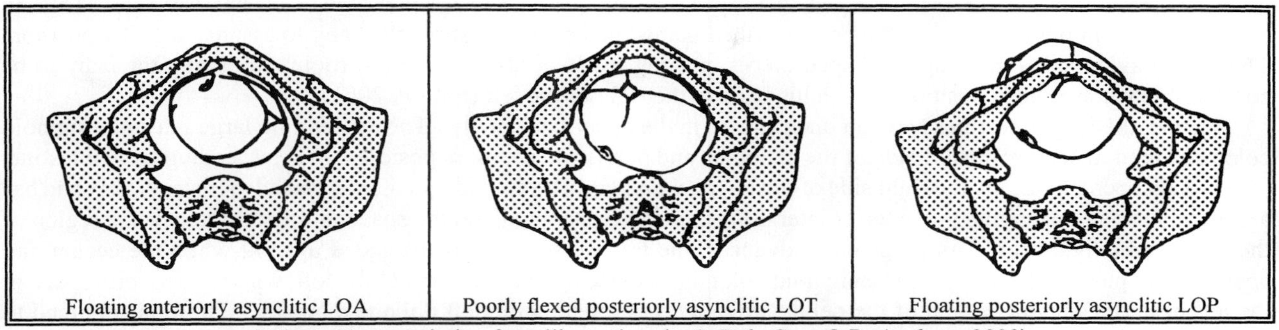

(Adapted by permission from illustrations by S. Dela Cruz © R. Ancheta, 2000)

Anterior or posterior?
The labeling of one variety of asynclitism as "posterior' and the other "anterior" can be confusing. Remember that in posterior asynclitism the *posterior* parietal bone is lowermost in the pelvis while in anterior asynclitism, the *anterior* parietal bone is lowermost in the pelvis.

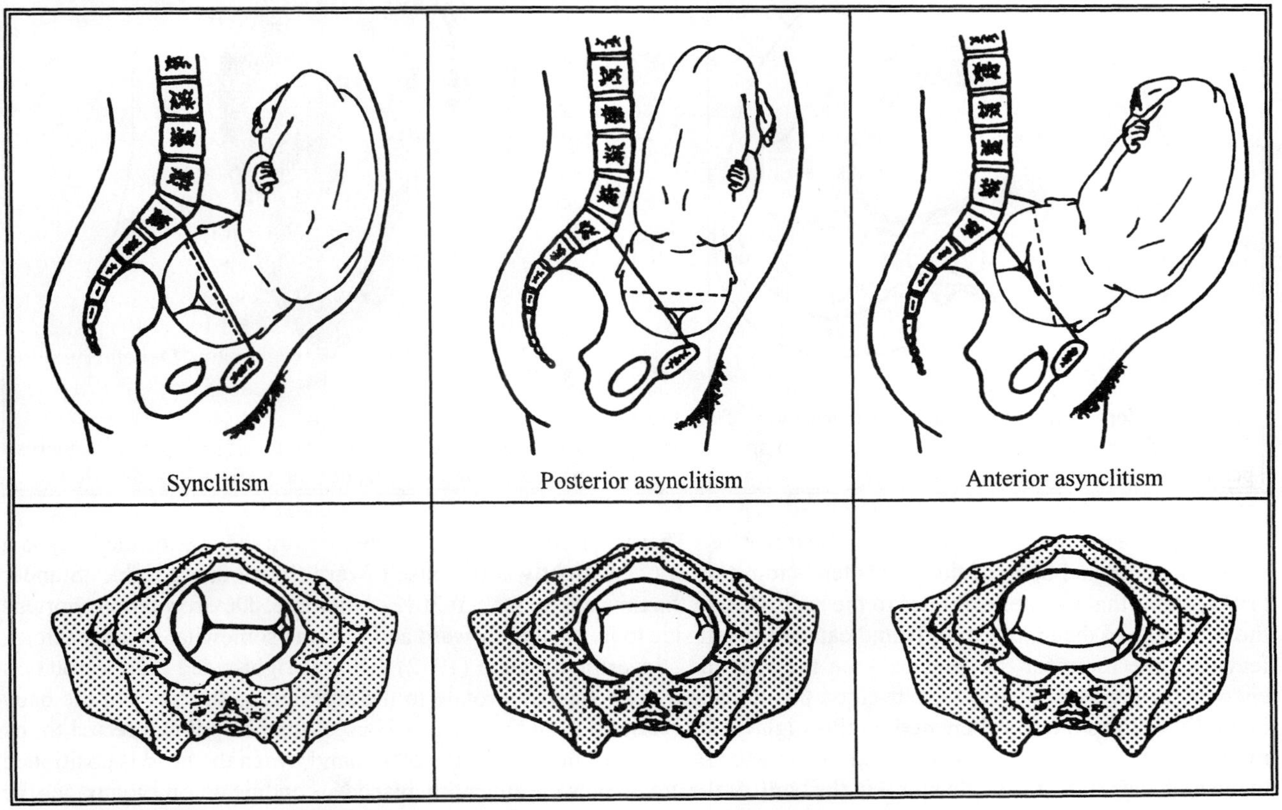

OTHER CONSIDERATIONS REGARDING THE MOTHER'S BODY, THE BABY'S BODY AND THE PROCESS OF LABOR

Why does the baby favor the left side of the mother's body for positioning and descent?

This question was hotly debated for many decades among doctors. As a result, several theories were presented. Of course, all these factors can vary from woman to woman, which is why babies do not all descend in the same position.

First, the nulliparous uterus is shaped like a pear, resulting in a less spacious lower uterine segment. This, in combination with the anatomical changes described below, makes it easiest for the baby to assume an LOA position. The multigravida has a more apple-shaped uterus, making the lower segment more roomy, allowing the baby to be comfortable whether he is positioned with his back to the right or the left (Sutton, 2001).

Second, the large intestines form an open square in the abdominal cavity. The descending large intestine, sigmoid colon and rectum occupy the left side of the abdomen and pelvis and are more posterior. The ascending large intestine, cecum and appendix occupy the right side of the lower abdomen. The ascending colon is placed more anteriorly and has a larger diameter, occupying the anterior lateral torso and encroaching upon the space in the right transverse region of the torso and pelvic brim. As pregnancy advances, the transverse colon is displaced upward while the cecum and appendix are pushed to the right. The sigmoid colon is displaced posteriorly and to the left, where it occupies space in the left posterior oblique region of the pelvis, effectively shortening the left oblique diameter. These factors tend to encourage left-sided engagement and the LOT or LOA baby to rotate in an anterior direction and to encourage the posterior rotation of the ROT, ROA or ROP baby, especially if the ascending bowel is full.

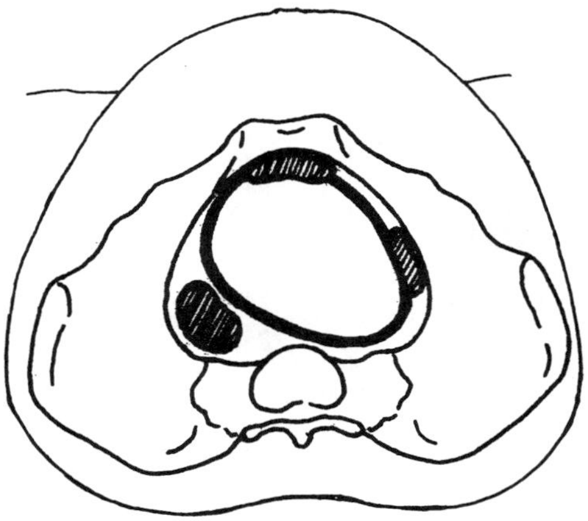

Sagittal section of maternal abdomen superior view from the supine position showing other parts that take up space in the pelvis.

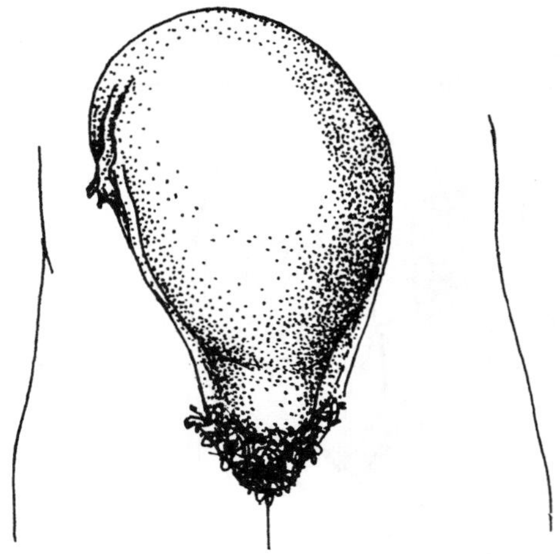

Dextrorotation and right obliquity of the pregnant uterus favoring anterior rotation when the fetal back is to the left

Third, the pregnant uterus tends to dextrorotate. That is, at about 20 weeks, well before the size of the baby is a factor, the enlarged body of the uterus tends to rotate or twist slightly at the base toward the mother's right. Stander (1945) states that the uterus rotates to the right 80% of the time and to the left 20% of the time. Dextrorotation shortens the right side of the uterus slightly and causes the left side to be pushed forward and become somewhat more spacious, leaving more room for the fetal back on the left side. Javert and Steele (1942) felt that right-sided uterine rotation encourages the baby to assume left-sided positions and helps the baby rotate to the anterior, as the body of the baby naturally follows the spiral created by the slightly clockwise twist in the uterus. Thus, if the occiput is directed to the mother's left, it is naturally encouraged to move to her anterior midline. On the other hand, when the head is positioned to the mother's right, the slight spiral in the body of the uterus plus the anteriorly placed ascending colon encourages the head to move in the direction of the uterine rotation, that is, toward her spine to a posterior position. As a result of dextrorotation, the uterine fundus also tilts to the right slightly. This is referred to as right-sided obliquity. These changes assist in flexion of the cephalic baby whose back is to the mother's left (explained in detail in the chapter entitled

"The Process of Birth in Occiput Anterior Vertex Presentations").

Finally, Calkins (1939) found that the full maternal bladder tends to swell more on the right side. Although he realized that the bladder is considerably flattened by the term uterus, he nevertheless conjectured that the full bladder may take up slightly more space on the mother's right and thus may make a minor contribution to the fetal propensity for left-sided anterior positions.

The angle of descent

The angle of the pelvic brim is oblique to the vertical axis of the maternal spine. The brim tips forward at about a 120° angle in most women (this angle is figured by placing the zero line of a protractor on a vertical line through the maternal spine with the curve toward her anterior torso). The anterior inclination of the brim is exaggerated by the lordosis that is natural to late pregnancy. Obviously the angle of the pelvic brim will influence the angle of fetal descent. This angle facilitates fetal flexion and rotation when the baby's back is anterior because, with the curve of the back pushed forward to rest in the curve of the anterior uterine wall, the contractions push down on the baby and the back and neck tend to curl forward. Conversely, when the baby is posterior, deflexion and spinal extension are more likely because the pressure from contractions and the lordosis of the mother's lower spine next to the fetal back tend to encourage the fetal spine to straighten. The angle of descent is also an important consideration when looking at illustrations and forming realistic mental images about the process of labor. In addition, taking the angle into consideration helps make sense of what you are feeling when you perform an internal exam, because when the woman lies down for the exam, the baby moves toward her spine; when she stands, the baby is once again tilted forward.

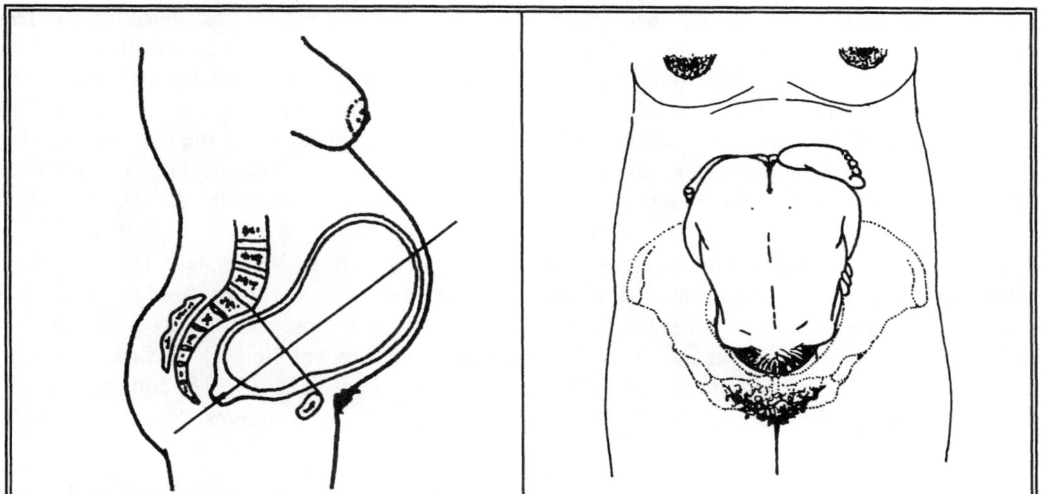

Especially during contractions, the uterus tips forward, exaggerating the angle of descent, which is usually depicted accurately from the side.

The woman on the left: anatomical directly anterior view.

Beginning at about 12 weeks gestation, the uterus starts to rise out of the pelvis. As it enlarges, the lordosis of the mother's lower back as well as the abdominal organs above and around the uterus cause the uterus to tip forward with the lower segment resting largely at the level of the iliac crests, placing the cervix roughly at the level of the pelvic brim. When the mother has good abdominal muscle tone, the baby and uterus are firmly supported at a forward-leaning angle in relation to her spine when she stands. During contractions, the uterus tips forward, which increases this angle even more. This forward-leaning angle is easy to see when looking at a cross section of the baby in the uterus, but largely ignored in drawings that show a frontal view of the mother's torso. There are several reasons for this. First of all, most of the early drawings of babies in utero were done from dissected cadavers, not from living, standing women. These images have been copied over and over while a discussion of the angle of descent quietly dropped out of the textbooks. Secondly, the forward-leaning angle of the fetus makes the details that the artist is trying to illustrate (such as head flexion, rotation, shoulder girdle angle, etc.) hard to see when the frontal view is a completely accurate anatomical representation, with the observer standing directly in front of the standing mother. Therefore, the artist and the student must reach a compromise. Keep in mind that the angle of uterus is tipped forward about 30° at all times and a little more during contractions, placing the presenting part directly over the brim (Sutton, 2002).

The frontal views in this text are drawn of a first-time mother with firm abdominal muscles in a standing position who is between contractions. Imagine that you are lying on the floor in front of the mother with your feet between the mother's feet and your head propped looking up at her belly. This brings your view of the baby into a more vertical plane, even though the uterus and baby are tilted forward.

The process of dilation

For labor to progress, the cervix must ripen (a change that, in most cases, happens in the days or weeks before birth), efface and dilate. In a first-time mother, ripening and thinning of the cervix, descent to engagement and dilation happen more or less sequentially, while in a multiparous mother, all except descent occur more or less simultaneously. When a woman has had a few babies, descent occurs later in labor and then takes place more rapidly because her muscle tone is less firm.

At the onset of most labors, the uterus is directed at an angle into the pelvic brim with the cervical os pointing toward the junction of the sacrum and coccyx. Contrary to the images presented in many texts, which show the cervix pointing straight down in line with the birth canal and dilating in perfectly centered, round circles, during most labors the os actually dilates in an elliptical shape starting from behind and expanding forward. This is because the rim of the normally posteriorly placed cervix has a relatively shorter distance to open toward the back of the pelvis than the wide anterior rim does in the front, where it must stretch over the largest part of the baby's head.

The first 3 cm or so of dilation are only slightly elliptical; then the cervix begins to form a more pronounced ellipse until dilation is complete. This elliptical shape is more exaggerated the more posteriorly the cervix is placed. An equally influential factor is the shape of the fetal head. When the flexed occiput anterior head is positioned more or less centrally in the pelvis, the wide biparietal diameter and overall contour of the head tends to encourage the elliptical shape because the edges of the os are held back by the biparietal diameter. When the head is well flexed, the last parts of the cervix to disappear are often the sides and finally the anterior rim as it recedes from over the crown of the vertex. Thus cervical opening follows the shape of the head, with the last portion of cervix to disappear being the anterior edge that overlies the widest and lowermost portion of the vertex (Sutton, 2002). This is why posterior cervical lips are so rare and usually seen only with posterior babies, when the widest part of the head is toward the back of the pelvis.

Vectors and labor: A "vector" is a quantity possessing both force and direction. Vectors are represented by arrows to indicate that they can move in only one direction at a time. In labor, the baby's body forms a vector in relationship to the pelvic cavity. During a contraction, the entire uterus tilts forward. If the presenting part is optimally positioned (which is the case when the baby is occiput anterior and the head and spine are well flexed), the force of the contractions is transmitted through the posteriorly situated os toward the roomy posterior pelvic cavity. The contractions are effective, the baby moves down through the brim, the head dilates the soft tissues, and labor moves along rapidly (King, 1993).

Compound Presentation

A compound presentation occurs when two or more fetal parts (usually an extremity and the presenting pole of the baby) present simultaneously at the inlet. Typically, a hand, arm, foot or leg presents alongside the head or the breech and both parts enter the pelvis at the same time. A hand beside the head is, by far, the most common. In transverse lie, a hand and a foot occasionally present together. Other far less common combinations include one or two feet with the head (very rare), two hands or arms with the head or breech, the head and three or four extremities, and a complete prolapse of the arm past the head in a longitudinal vertex lie. Footling or kneeling breeches and shoulder presentations with a single extended arm are not classified as compound presentations. Always keep in mind that multiple presenting limbs could belong to different babies. Most of the time, compound presentations are purely positional, but on rare occasions they may be secondary to cord entanglement, which means they will be difficult or impossible to reduce.

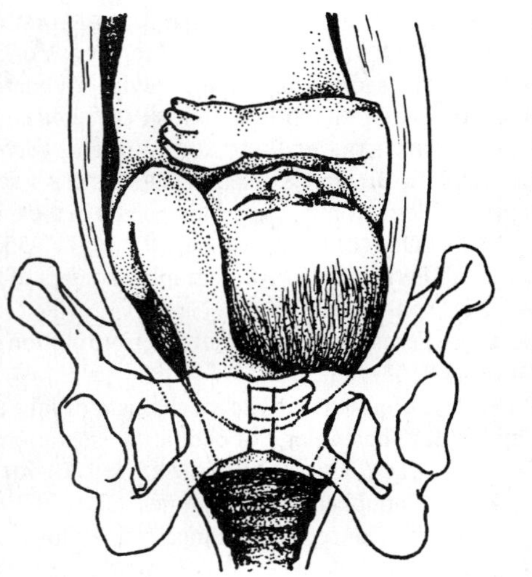
Compound presentation with hand over head (mother supine)

In an unusual case reported by Hahl (1901), a breech baby was positioned so that his head was between his legs, resulting in the vertex and the scrotum being simultaneously palpable on internal exam. These complex compound presentations are much more likely when the baby is premature or muscle tone is weak or absent, as would be the case if the baby had a congenital muscular defect or were dead.

Easily detected compound presentations occur roughly once in every 500 to 1000 births; however, minor degrees of compound presentation probably occur much more frequently, with the baby retracting her limb up inside the uterus before the problem is detected. The most commonly associated factor is prematurity, since compound presentation is facilitated when the presenting part does not fill the pelvic inlet. Other factors include contracted pelvis, pendulous abdomen, multiple gestation (including conjoined twins), anomalous extra limbs, large head, nonvertex presentation, and polyhydramnios.

Nuchal extremities

An extremity or small part extended around the back of the neck is said to be **nuchally placed**. One or both arms extended behind the neck can arrest labor. (See the chapter entitled "Assisting a Woman Whose Baby Is in a Compound Presentation" for more details.)

References and Further Reading on the Basic Physical Principles of Birth

References used in multiple chapters

Balaskas J. ACTIVE BIRTH: THE NEW APPROACH TO GIVING BIRTH NATURALLY, rev ed. Harvard Common Press, Harvard MA, 1992.

Baudelocque J. PRINCIPES SUR L'ART DES ACCOUCHEMENTS. Méquignon, Paris France, 1775. Cited in Jarcho J. THE PELVIS IN OBSTETRICS. Paul B Hoeber Inc, New York NY, 1933.

Beal M."The sacroiliac problem: review of anatomy, mechanics, and diagnosis," JAOA, 81(10);667-679, June, 1982.

Beard R. THE OCCIPITO-POSTERIOR POSITION: ITS MECHANISM AND TREATMENT, 2nd ed. FW Preece & Sons, Adelaide Australia, 1937.

Beck A. OBSTETRICAL PRACTICE. Williams & Wilkins Co., Baltimore MD, 1935.

Bennett VR, Brown LK, eds. MYLES TEXTBOOK FOR MIDWIVES, 13th ed. Churchill Livingstone, Edinburgh UK, 1999.

Borell U, Fernström I. "The movements in the mechanism of disengagement with special reference to the attitude of the foetal head." ACTA OBSTET GYNECOL SCAND, 36;347-355, 1957a.

Borell U, Fernström I. "Radiographic studies of the rotation of the foetal shoulders during labour." ACTA OBSTET GYNECOL SCAND, 37(1);54-61, 1958.

Borell U, Fernström I. "Internal anterior rotation of the fetal head: a contribution to its explanation," ACTA OBSTET GYNECOL SCAND, 38(1);103-108, 1959a.

Borell U, Fernström I. "The mechanism of labour," RADIOL CLIN N AM, 5(1);73-85, Apr, 1967.

Calkins L. "The etiology of occiput presentations," AM J OBSTET GYNECOL, 74(4);618-623, 1939.

Corkill T. LECTURES ON MIDWIFERY AND INFANT CARE, 6th ed. Whitcombe and Tombs Ltd, Christchurch New Zealand, 1958.

Corkill T. Unpublished lecture notes. Cited in Sutton J, Scott P. UNDERSTANDING AND TEACHING OPTIMAL FOETAL POSITIONING, 2nd ed. Birth Concepts, Tauranga NZ, 1996.

De Lee J. THE PRINCIPLES AND PRACTICE OF OBSTETRICS, 6th ed. WB Saunders Co, Philadelphia PA, 1934.

De Lee J. THE PRINCIPLES AND PRACTICE OF OBSTETRICS, 7th ed. WB Saunders Co, Philadelphia PA, 1938.

Dobson J. BABY BEAUTIFUL: A HANDBOOK OF BABY HEAD SHAPING. Heirs Press, Carson City NV, 1994.

Edgar J. THE PRACTICE OF OBSTETRICS: DESIGNED FOR THE USE OF STUDENTS AND PRACTITIONERS OF MEDICINE, 5th rev. ed. P Balkiston's Son & Co, Philadelphia PA, 1916.

Gilles F. "Infantile atlantooccipital instability: the potential danger of extreme extension," AM J DIS CHILD, 133(1);30-37, Jan, 1979.

Greenhill JP. PRINCIPLES AND PRACTICE OF OBSTETRICS, 10th ed. WB Saunders Co, Philadelphia PA, 1951.

Hahl. "Stricture des os internum als Geurtshinderniss," AARCHI F GYNECOL, Ixiii;684-694, 1901. Cited in Williams JW. OBSTETRICS: A TEXTBOOK FOR THE USE OF STUDENTS AND PRACTITIONERS, 4th ed. D Appleton & Co., New York NY, 1919.

Hirst B. A TEXT-BOOK OF OBSTETRICS, 5th ed. WB Saunders Co, Philadelphia PA, 1906.

Hughes E, ed. OBSTETRIC–GYNECOLOGIC TERMINOLOGY. FA Davis Co, Philadelphia PA, 1972.

Jarcho J. THE PELVIS IN OBSTETRICS. Paul B Hoeber Inc, New York NY, 1933.

Javert C, Steele KB. "The transverse position and the mechanism of labor. A historical collective review," INTERNAT ABSTR SURG, 75;507, 1942.

King J. BACK LABOR NO MORE!, WHAT EVERY WOMAN SHOULD KNOW BEFORE LABOR. Plenary Systems, Inc, Dallas TX, 1993.

O'Grady J. Section III: "Pelvic conditions," Chapter 29: "Pelvic relaxation syndrome," in O'Grady J, Buckman R, eds. OBSTETRIC SYNDROMES AND CONDITIONS. Parthenon Pub Group, New York NY, 1998.

Oxorn H. OXORN–FOOTE HUMAN LABOR AND BIRTH, 5th ed. Appleton-Century-Crofts, Norwalk CT, 1986.

Rydberg E. THE MECHANISM OF LABOUR. Charles C Thomas, Springfield IL, 1954.

Scott P. SIT UP AND TAKE NOTICE: POSITIONING YOURSELF FOR A BETTER BIRTH. Great Scott, Tauranga NZ, 2003.

Simkin P, Ancheta R. THE LABOR PROGRESS HANDBOOK. Blackwell Science, Oxford UK, 2000.

Stander H, ed. TEXTBOOK OF OBSTETRICS, 3rd ed. (9th ed. WILLIAMS OBSTETRICS). D Appleton-Century Co, New York NY, 1945.

Steer C. MOLOY'S EVALUATION OF THE PELVIS IN OBSTETRICS, 3rd ed. Plenum Medical Books Co, New York NY, 1975.

Stern D. COMYNS BERKELEY'S PICTORIAL MIDWIFERY: AN ATLAS OF MIDWIFERY FOR PUPIL MIDWIVES, 5th ed. Baillière, Tindall & Cox, London UK, 1956.

Sutton J. LET BIRTH BE BORN AGAIN! REDISCOVERING AND RECLAIMING OUR MIDWIFERY HERITAGE. Birth Concepts, Bedfont UK, 2001.

Sutton J. "Optimal fetal positioning," REACHE workshop, Seattle WA, May 15, 2002.

Sutton J, Scott P. UNDERSTANDING AND TEACHING OPTIMAL FOETAL POSITIONING, 2nd ed. Birth Concepts, Tauranga NZ, 1996.

Varney H. VARNEY'S MIDWIFERY, 3rd ed. Jones & Bartlett, Sudbury MA, 1997.

Williams JW. OBSTETRICS: A TEXT-BOOK FOR THE USE OF STUDENTS AND PRACTITIONERS, 6th ed. D Appleton & Co., New York NY, 1930.

Williams P, ed. GRAY'S ANATOMY: THE ANATOMICAL BASIS OF MEDICINE AND SURGERY, 38th American ed. Churchill Livingstone, New York NY, 1995.

The Evolution of Our Understanding of Fetal Descent

Creasy R. MANAGEMENT OF LABOR AND DELIVERY. Blackwell Science, Boston MA, 1996.

De Lee J. THE PRINCIPLES AND PRACTICE OF OBSTETRICS, WB Saunders Co, Philadelphia PA, 1913.

Dewees W. A COMPENDIOUS SYSTEM OF MIDWIFERY CHIEFLY DESIGNED TO FACILITATE THE INQUIRIES OF THOSE WHO MAY BE PURSUING THIS BRANCH OF STUDY. HC Carey & L Lea, Philadelphia PA, 1824.

Hodge H. THE PRINCIPLES AND PRACTICE OF OBSTETRICS. Blanchard and Lea, Philadelphia PA, 1864.

Smellie W. A TREATISE ON THE THEORY AND PRACTICE OF MIDWIFERY, VOL 1. D Wilson, London, 1752. Reprint ed. in Classics in Obstetrics and Gynecology Library, Gryphon Editions, New York NY, 1990.

Williams JW. OBSTETRICS: A TEXTBOOK FOR THE USE OF STUDENTS AND PRACTITIONERS. D Appleton & Co, New York NY, 1903.

FEATURES OF FETAL ANATOMY PERTINENT TO THE BIRTH PROCESS

Berkovitz B, Moxham B. A TEXTBOOK OF HEAD AND NECK ANATOMY. Year Book Medical, Chicago IL, 1988.

Bosma J. ANATOMY OF THE INFANT HEAD. Johns Hopkins U P, Baltimore MD, 1986.

Chasler C. ATLAS OF ROENTGEN ANATOMY OF THE NEWBORN AND INFANT SKULL. Warren H Green, St. Louis MO, 1972.

Crelin e. FUNCTIONAL ANATOMY OF THE NEWBORN. Yale U Press, New Haven ST, 1973.

Gilles F. Chapter 9: "Perinatal neuropathology," in Davis R, Robertson D, eds. TEXTBOOK OF NEUROPATHOLOGY, 3rd 3ed. Williams and Wilkins, Baltimore MD, 1997.

Goss CM, ed. ANATOMY OF THE HUMAN BODY BY HENRY GRAY, 29th American ed. Lea & Febiger, Philadelphia PA, 1973.

Guntheroth W. Chapter II: "Pathology of SIDS," in HIS CRIB DEATH: THE SUDDEN INFANT DEATH SYNDROME, 3rd ed. Futura Co, Armonk NY, 1995.

Jackson C, ed. MORRIS' HUMAN ANATOMY: A COMPLETE SYSTEMATIC TREATISE, 9th ed. P Blakiston's Sons Inc, 1933.

Kapit W, Elson L. THE ANATOMY COLORING BOOK, 3rd ed. Benjamin Cummings, San Francisco CA, 2002.

Lewis W, ed. ANATOMY OF THE HUMAN BODY BY HENRY GRAY, 20th American ed. Lea & Febiger, Philadelphia PA, 1918.

Magoun H, ed. OSTEOPATHY IN THE CRANIAL FIELD, 2nd ed. Journal Printing Co, Kirksville MO, 1966.

Marieb E. HUMAN ANATOMY AND PHYSIOLOGY, 4th ed. Benjamin/Cummings, Menlo Park CA, 1998.

McMinn M, et al. COLOR ATLAS OF HEAD AND NECK ANATOMY. Year Book Medical, Chicago IL, 1981.

Netter F, au, Colacino S, ed. ATLAS OF HUMAN ANATOMY. CIBA-Geigy, Summit NJ, 1989.

Rudolph A. ATLAS OF THE NEWBORN: VOL. 3: HEAD AND NECK, EYE, CENTRAL NERVOUS SYSTEM. BC Decker, London UK, 1997.

Scammon R. Chapter 3: "A summary of the anatomy of the infant and child," in Abt I, ed. PEDIATRICS, VOL. 1. WB Saunders Co, Philadelphia PA, 1923.

Sundaresan M, et al. "Anatomy and development of the fontanelle," ARCH DIS CHILD, 65(4);386-387, Apr, 1990.

Tortora G, Anagnostakos N. PRINCIPLES OF ANATOMY AND PHYSIOLOGY, 6th ed. Harper & Row, New York NY, 1990.

Yashon D. SPINAL INJURY, 2nd ed. Appleton-Century-Crofts, Norwalk CT, 1986.

WAYS IN WHICH THE BABY'S BODY ADAPTS DURING DESCENT: ANATOMICAL DIAMETERS, ATTITUDE AND MOULDING

Baxter J. "Moulding of the foetal head," J OBSTET GYNECOL BRIT EMP, 53(3);212-218, 1946.

Borell U, Fernström I. "X-ray diagnosis of muscular spasm in the lower part of the uterus from the degree of moulding of the foetal head," ACTA OBSTET GYNECOL SCAND, 38;181-189, 1959b.

Borell U, Fernström I. "The mechanism of labour in face and brow presentation," ACTA OBSTET GYNECOL SCAND, 39;626-644, 1960.

Carlan S, et al. "Fetal head molding : diagnosis by ultrasound and a review of the literature," J PERINATOL, 11(2); 105-111, June, 1991.

de la Fuente A. "Locking and reverse molding of the fetal skull," PEDIATR PATHOL, 11(2):271-280, Mar-Apr, 1991.

Dobson J. "Birthing choices," MIDWIFERY TODAY, (33);17-18, Spring, 1995.

Emerson W, perinatal psychologist. Personal communications, Winter/Spring, 2002.

Emery JL. "Locking and reverse moulding of the foetal skull related to cerebral birth trauma," Daamen nummer; VROEGER NE TIJDSCHR VERLOSK GYNACC, pp. 13-23, Dec, 1972.

Frymann V. "Relation of disturbances of craniosacral mechanism to symptomatology of the newborn: study of 1,250 infants," J AM OSTEOPATH ASSOC, 65(10):1059-1075, June, 1966, in King H, ed. THE COLLECTED PAPERS OF VIOLA M. FRYMANN: LEGACY OF OSTEOPATHY TO CHILDREN. American Academy of Osteopathy, Indianapolis IN, 1998a.

Frymann V. "The trauma of birth," OSTEOPATHIC ANNALS (5):197-205, May, 1976, in King H, ed. THE COLLECTED PAPERS OF VIOLA M. FRYMANN: LEGACY OF OSTEOPATHY TO CHILDREN. American Academy of Osteopathy, Indianapolis IN, 1998b.

Frymann V. "Birth trauma: the most common cause of developmental delays," NEW DEVELOPMENTS, 1(4), in King, H, ed. THE COLLECTED PAPERS OF VIOLA M. FRYMANN: LEGACY OF OSTEOPATHY TO CHILDREN, American Academy of Osteopathy, Indianapolis IN, 1998c.

Frymann V. "Lateral strains of the sphenobasilar synchondrosis (symphysis)," CRANIAL LETTER, 41(2):4-5, in King, H, ed. THE COLLECTED PAPERS OF VIOLA M. FRYMANN: LEGACY OF OSTEOPATHY TO CHILDREN. American Academy of Osteopathy, Indianapolis IN, 1998d.

Guntheroth W. CRIB DEATH–THE SUDDEN INFANT DEATH SYNDROME, 3rd ed. Futura Pub Co Inc, Armonk NY, 1995.

Hellman L, Pritchard J. WILLIAMS OBSTETRICS, 14th ed. Appleton-Century-Crofts, New York NY, 1971.

Hemsath F. "Birth injury of the occipital bone with a report of thirty-two cases," AMER J OBSTET GYNECOL, 27(2);194-203, 1934.

Holland E. "Cranial stress in the foetus during labour and on the effects of excessive stress on the intracranial contents; with an analysis of 81 cases of torn tentorium cerebelli and subdural cerebral hemorrhage," J Obstet Gynaecol Br Emp, 29(4, new series);549-571, 1922.

Lapeer R, Prager R. "Fetal head moulding: finite element analysis of a fetal skull subjected to uterine pressures during the first stage of labour," J Biomech, 34(9);1125-1133, Sept. 2001.

Moloy H. "Studies on head molding during labor," Amer J Obstet Gynecol, 44:762-781, 1942.

Newton T, Gooding C. "Compression of superior sagittal sinus by neonatal calvarial molding," Radiology, 115(3);635-640, June, 1975.

Pape K, Wigglesworth J. Haemorrhage, Ischaemia and the Perinatal Brain, Spastics International Medical Pub, London UK, 1979.

Sorbe B, Dahlgren S. "Some important factors in the molding of the fetal head during vaginal delivery–a photographic study," Int J Obstet Gynaecol, 21(3);205-212, June, 1983.

Basic Principles of How the Mother's Soft and Bony Pelvic Structures Influence Fetal Descent

Abramson D, et al. "Relaxation of the pelvic joint in pregnancy," Surg Gynecol Obstet, 58;595-613, 1934.

Borell U, Fernström I. "The movements at the sacro-iliac joints and their importance to changes in the pelvic dimensions during parturition," Acta Obstet Gynecol Scand, 36(1);42-57, 1957b.

Borell U, Fernström I. "The shape and course of the birth canal; a radiographic study in the human," Acta Obstet Gynecol Scand, 36(2);166-178, 1957c.

Caldwell W, Moloy H. "Anatomical variations in the female pelvis and their effect in labor with a suggested classification," Am J Obstet Gynecol, 26:479, 1933.

Duncan M. "The behavior of the pelvic articulations in the mechanism of parturition," Dublin Qtrly J Med Sci, 18;60-69, Aug, 1854.

Heyman J, Lundqvist A. "The symphysis pubis in pregnancy and parturition," Acta Obstet Gynaecol Scand, 12(2);191-226, 1932.

Kotarions R. "Pelvic articulations during parturition, part one: the obstetric pelvis," J Obstet gynaecol Physical Therapy, pp 6-8, Mar, 1988.

Moloy H. Clinical and Roentgenologic Evaluation of the Pelvis in Obstetrics. WB Saunders Co, Philadelphia PA, 1951.

O'Conner L. "The female pelvis: part one," Bull Section Obstet Gynaecol APTA, 10(1);6-7, Mar, 1986.

Russell J. "Moulding of the pelvic outlet," Obstet Gynaecol Br Cwlth, 76(9);817-820, Sept, 1969.

Tully G. Resolving Shoulder Dystocia: the Three R's. Spinning Babies Workshops, 10545 Humboldt Ave. So., Minneapolis MN, 2003.

The Station of the Presenting Part

Gentlebirth midwifery archives, http://www.gentlebirth.com, accessed 1999.

Juntunen K, Kirkinen P. "Partogram of a grand multipara: different descent slope compared with an ordinary parturient," J of Perinatal Medicine, 22(3);213-218, 1994.

Weekes A, Flynn M. "Engagement of the fetal head in primigravidae and its relationship to duration of gestation and time of onset of labor," Brit J Obstet Gynaecol, 82(1); 7-11, Jan, 1975.

The Birth Process When the Baby Is in a Flexed Cephalic Presentation

The Frequency of Different Vertex Positions

Vertex presentations occur in about 95% of all labors. In over 60% of these, the head enters the pelvis with the sagittal suture in the transverse diameter of the pelvic brim (LOT). The following table is based on 1,040 X-ray studies of women at the onset of labor without regard to pelvic type (Javert & Steele, 1942).

PERCENTAGE OF VARIOUS TYPES OF VERTEX POSITIONS AT DIFFERENT STATIONS								
Station at the onset of labor	**LOT**	**ROT**	**LOA**	**ROA**	**ROP**	**LOP**	**OA**	**OP**
Above or at the brim (≥ -5)	39.9	23.5	13.2	9.6	7.3	3.0	1.8	0.6
At, just above or just below the spines	33.7	28.8	11.9	5.7	11.5	3.2	2.8	1.8

From a midwifery point of view, the "ideal" fetal position has the back directed to the mother's left side or anterior left, with the head LOT or LOA. This positioning offers the best insurance that the baby will rotate anteriorly and will descend with the greatest ease for both the mother and baby. The LOA baby will often turn at the neck to assume a transverse position (LOT) which allows the head to descend most easily through the brim.

The Process of Birth in Occiput Anterior Vertex Presentations

Introducing the Cardinal Spiraling Movements of Birth

The principal movements of the baby through the pelvis are known as the "cardinal movements of birth." This process is also referred to by the medical model as the "mechanisms of labor," in keeping with the tendency of the technocratic mentality to reduce the mysteries of birth to the workings of a machine.

At conception, the chromosomes organize and assemble themselves into the miraculous spiral of life: a DNA molecule. Development ensues with a continuing duplication of these spirals as each cell is born. Likewise, the birth process consists of spiraling movements of the baby's head and torso as she enters and moves through the pelvis. This chapter focuses on the spiraling movements of the baby through the pelvis in vertex presentations. The differences encountered with extended cephalic and breech presentations will be covered at the beginning of their respective sections.

It is important to remember that each mother's body and each baby combine to create unique circumstances that influence the way that the baby will actually move during descent. Therefore, take these descriptions as a useful guide, knowing that the more you understand the ways in which a baby *can* move through the pelvis, the more accurately you will be able to assess how each individual labor is unfolding.

In a cephalic presentation, the process of birth involves moving the baby's body, consisting of two ovoid regions (the head and chest) connected by a hinge (the neck) joined to a flexible spine, through the three primary regions of the mother's birth canal: the inlet, the midpelvis and the outlet. The cephalic baby's lower torso and pelvis follow the lead of the upper torso as it navigates the birth canal and therefore require no particular movements to be born. The bony portion of the birth canal presents a slightly curved passage that bends somewhat more just below the level of the ischial spines and even more at the level of the tuberosities and through the soft birth canal beyond the bony outlet. It is also wider transversely at the inlet and anteroposteriorly at the outlet. These features require the fetal head and body to move in various ways as they pass through the pelvis to best accommodate their shape to the shape of the soft birth canal and the bony pelvic cavity. The head, the torso and shoulders usually make three movements:

Engagement occurs as the widest diameter of a fetal part passes through the pelvic brim
Rotation or positional adaption of a fetal part to the shape and resistance of the birth canal
Disengagement or emergence of a fetal part from the outlet of the birth canal

The way these processes occur varies, depending upon the lie, position and attitude of the baby as well as the shape of the mother's pelvis. When the pelvis is roomy, the canal formed by the soft tissues exerts the primary influence over flexion, rotation and other movements as the baby's head and body descend through the pelvis (Borell & Fernström, 1967; Rydberg, 1954a). However, when fetal parts do come into contact with the bony pelvis due either to positioning or a snug bony passage, this also influences how the baby descends and rotates. Therefore, the ways in which both the soft and bony pelvic structures accommodate fetal descent are described here.

There are universally applicable terms used to designate the characteristic movements the baby makes as he comes through the pelvis. Seven mechanisms of labor are discussed in virtually every modern obstetrical textbook. These steps focus on the movements of the head and leave out many important nuances of the process. Some of the accepted descriptions of the mechanisms are anatomically incorrect. This chapter presents a new paradigm for understanding the birth process and includes much more detail than other modern textbooks. This expanded understanding will be officially called the "cardinal spiraling movements of birth" but may also be abbreviated to the "cardinal movements of birth" in the text. This information has been gleaned from studying older research and textbooks (asterisks throughout this part of the text indicate the contemporary "mechanisms" of labor). The following chart offers a comparative overview of these two approaches. Numbered movements on the right correspond to details in the following explanations and accompanying illustrations. The movements are described here as they relate to descent of a baby in a vertex presentation through a normal pelvis. Since more babies engage in a left occiput transverse or anterior oblique position, illustrations in this chapter demonstrate the movements from this perspective. However, most of these details can be applied to the cardinal spiraling movements in other vertex positions as well.

Obstetrical Mechanisms of Labor (Cardinal movements of birth)	Cardinal Spiraling Movements of Birth (movements are numbered, those marked with an * match the obstetrical mechanisms; associated changes are marked with a •)
1. Flexion of the head	*1. Flexion of the head and spine (and later the shoulders)
2. Descent	*2. Descent
	-Angle of descent
	• Dilating the soft birth canal
3. Engagement of the head	*3. Engagement of the head
	-Transverse descent to engagement
	-Asynclitic descent to engagement
4. Internal rotation of the head	*4. Internal rotation of the head
	5. First internal rotation of the chest and shoulders
	6. Engagement of the shoulders
	• Flexion/extension of the shoulders and arms
	7. Spinal extension occurs as the head descends into the birth canal
	• Dilating the perineum
	8-1. Second internal rotation of the chest and shoulders begins
	• Crowning of the head
5. Extension of the neck just below the occiput	*9. Birth of the flexed head by extension of the lower neck and upper spine
6. Restitution of the head	*10. Restitution of the head
	8-2. Second internal rotation of the chest and shoulders is completed
7. External rotation of the head	*11. External rotation of the head
	12. Birth of the posterior and anterior shoulders
	13. Birth of the arms, torso and legs with a spiraling motion

Studying this material

This material is detailed and complex. Be sure you throughly understand the material in all the preceding chapters before you begin. Have a doll and a pelvis on hand as you move through each description. Even those adept with spacial relationships may find it challenging to grasp the interaction between two three-dimensional objects with complicated shapes which are constantly in motion. Label the various diameters, right and left sides and anatomical features on your models; this is especially helpful for students or dyslexics. Be sure you understand each movement before proceeding to the next. While the basic principles of the obstetric mechanisms of labor are incorporated into the expanded understanding presented here, you will notice that the explanation of the way certain movements (mechanisms) occur differ dramatically from other texts. Each discrepancy is noted. To maintain the flow of this material, the background information that supports these changes is included at the end of this chapter under the heading "Notes on Changes Incorporated into the Cardinal Spiraling Movements of Birth." The numbers in the drawings throughout this section correspond to the numbered cardinal movements in the above table.

Understanding Each Cardinal Spiraling Movement of Birth

*1. Flexion of the head

Flexion describes the degree to which the baby's chin is tucked against her chest. In contemporary obstetrics, the cardinal movement of "flexion" refers exclusively to the baby's head. Flexion will tend to occur only to the degree necessary to allow the baby's head to pass through the pelvis. Therefore, complete flexion does not occur in every labor or may be delayed until the head has descended to a point where smaller cephalic diameters are required for further descent to take place. When the head is completely flexed, the presenting diameter changes from the occipitofrontal of 11.0 cm (the typical diameter of engagement), to the smaller and rounder suboccipitobregmatic diameter (9.5 cm), which reduces the presenting diameter by 1.5 cm or more. This shift causes the axis of the verticomental diameter to be directed straight down, parallel with the pelvic passage.

The head is typically not well flexed when it rests above the brim during late pregnancy. As it enters the brim, it is often, but not invariably, fairly well flexed (note that optimal diameters are not required for passage through the brim in most pelvises). When a substantial degree of flexion is present at the onset of labor, in most cases it remains unchanged until internal rotation begins or until the head reaches the sacral tip (Rydberg, 1954b).

If the head is not well flexed before entering the brim, some flexion usually occurs prior to or early in labor. If descent past the spines occurs prior to complete dilation, flexion can be encouraged by the resistance of a firm cervical os, which mimics the resistance of the pelvic floor. In some cases, the baby's head is in more of a sinciput than a vertex presentation as the head enters the brim. When this happens, the forehead tends to remain stationary until the back of the vertex is pushed downward by contractions and the head tips forward at the neck.

In some labors, optimal flexion does not take place until the head has reached the pelvic floor, where flexion and rotation can occur almost simultaneously. When flexion is delayed, it tends to occur toward the end of dilation in first-time mothers and in all labors as the head passes through the cervix. Flexion becomes exaggerated as the occiput contacts the anterior pelvic floor and again when it passes through the deepest curve of the birth canal.

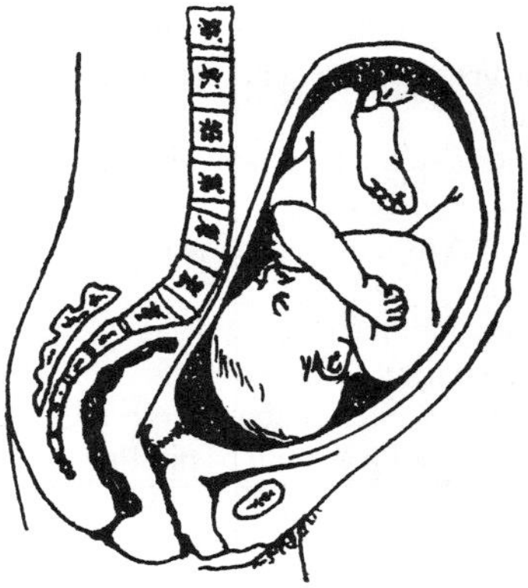

(1) Lateral view of a LOA baby prior to labor showing flexion of the fetal spine into the hammock of the abdomen.

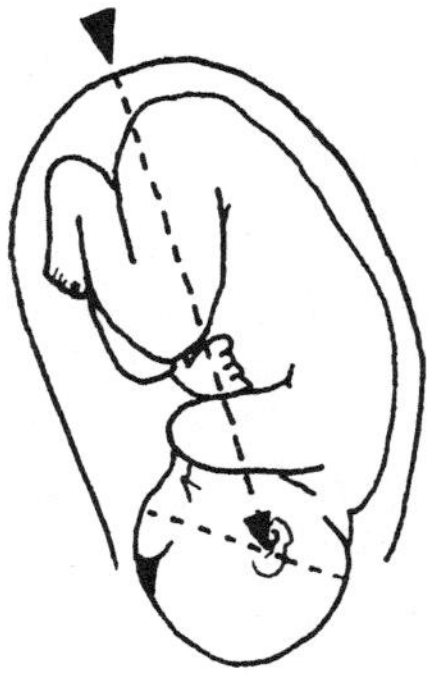

Anterior view showing how slight right-sided obliquity of the uterine fundus also encourages flexion when the fetal back is to the mother's left (this baby is LOT)

<u>Flexion of the fetal spine</u>: The baby's head, neck and spine work together, tending to curl forward as labor draws near, especially in first-time mothers. The exaggerated lordosis of the mother's lower spine tends to push her anterior torso forward, causing the baby to be most comfortable with his back nestled into the "hammock" created by the mother's abdominal wall. If spinal flexion has not occurred before labor, early labor contractions encourage both the head and spine to curl forward, especially when the fundus is leaning slightly to the mother's right, and the baby's back is to her left. The baby whose occiput is anterior is also ideally positioned to receive the force of the uterine contractions and transmit them directly to the dilating os.

<u>*2. Descent</u>

Descent is the process, continuing throughout normal labor, by which the presenting part moves through the mother's pelvis, from the brim to the outlet and then through the portion of the birth canal extending beyond the bony pelvis to birth. The other cardinal spiraling movements occur simultaneously during descent of the baby. Descent is considered a separate process only insofar as it is a necessary prerequisite to internal rotation of the presenting part.

In some women, considerable descent takes place in the last days or weeks prior to the onset of labor. In other mothers, descent to engagement often does not begin until labor is well underway. In labor, descent occurs due to the combination of downward pressure from uterine contractions, the cervical os opening and finally retracting over the presenting part, the stretching and relaxation of the pelvic soft tissues, maternal pushing efforts and, to a lesser extent, gravity. While gravity can significantly facilitate descent and the mother's pushing efforts during labor, its influence does not supersede that of the uterine muscle and active bearing down in cephalic presentations. If the full influence of gravity were essential, women could not give birth spontaneously in the lithotomy position.

The rate of descent varies widely during normal labor. Following engagement, descent tends to be minimal and slow in some women until the cervix is nearing full dilation. In others, continual descent occurs throughout dilation. More rarely but just as normally, the baby may remain high after dilation is complete and descend only when the resting phase is over and the uterus begins to press the baby downward. A strong bag of waters can inhibit descent. The most dramatic and rapid descent often occurs after full dilation when the uterus starts actively bearing down and maternal pushing efforts assist the process, especially in women who have given birth before. All the other cardinal movements of birth optimize continued descent.

Angle of descent: The baby enters the pelvis at a 30° anteriorly slanting angle in relation to the mother's spine. This places the longitudinal axis of the anterior vertex baby directly over the center of the pelvic brim. This angle is exaggerated when the mother's abdominal muscles are lax and is always slightly increased during contractions.

Dilation of the soft birth canal: A major result of descent is the dilation of the soft tissues as the presenting part makes its way through the pelvis. While this is not considered a cardinal movement, it is a vital part of normal labor.

***3. Engagement of the head**

This describes the descent of the biparietal diameter, the widest portion of the fetal skull, through the pelvic inlet. Although engagement is considered one of the cardinal movements of birth, it actually occurs prior to labor in some mothers. (Engagement is described in more detail in the chapter entitled "The Station of the Presenting Part.")

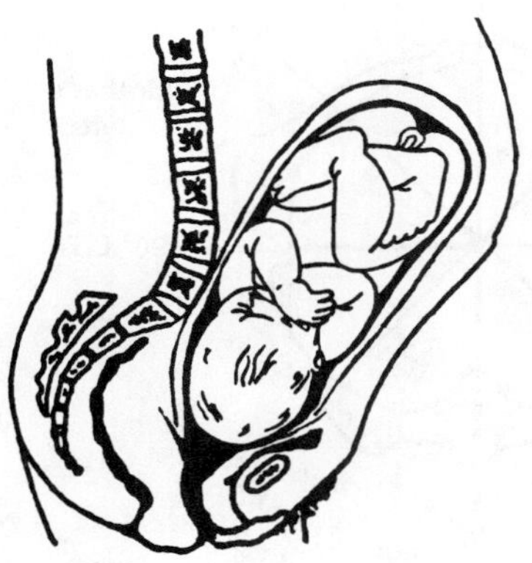

(3) LOT baby undergoing posterior asynclitic descent to engagement: first movement past promontory

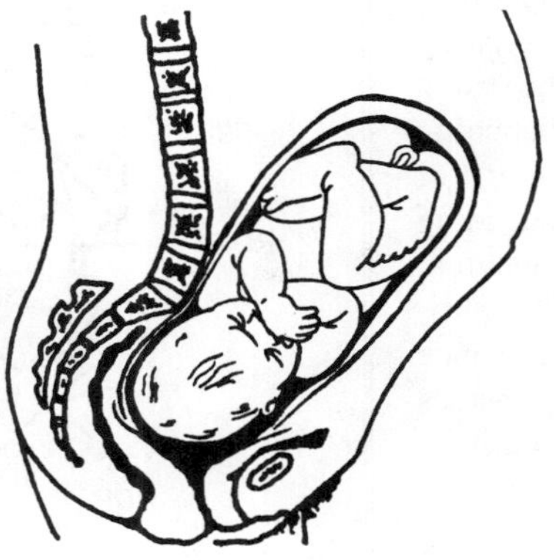

(3) Asynclitic descent switches to anterior as the head swings down past the promontory

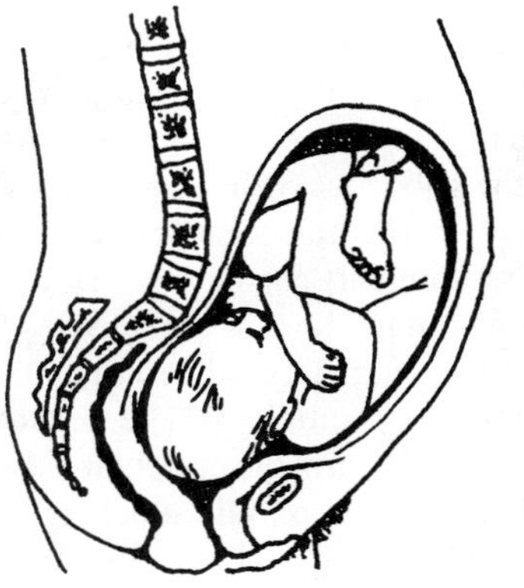

(3) Alternatively, the head may engage through the oblique diameter

Transverse descent to engagement: Regardless of the position of the body, the head will often enter the brim with the occiput transverse. If the baby does not begin labor with her occiput transverse, she will tend to turn her head at the neck so that the occiput is moved to a transverse orientation before the head enters the brim. This occurs for two reasons:

The long axis of the head seeks the long axis of the brim: Babies often choose to enter the brim with their head transverse because the long axis of the vertex best accommodates itself to the long axis of the brim. In addition, occiput transverse descent places the biparietal diameter in the anteroposterior diameter of the pelvis, to the side of the sacral promontory, where there is more room for it to descend.

Asynclitic descent to engagement: In addition, babies favor an occiput transverse position because it allows them to take advantage of asynclitic engagement, entering the brim via slight to moderate posterior asynclitism, which is maintained until the posterior parietal eminence becomes relatively fixed beneath the sacral promontory. The anterior parietal bone then slips downward behind the symphysis, as the head assumes an attitude of anterior asynclitism. The head often remains somewhat anteriorly asynclitic until internal rotation is complete. (Synclitic and asynclitic descent are covered in detail in the chapter entitled "Synclitism and Asynclitism.") If the head is sufficiently flexed, the baby rotates her head to OT to take advantage of asynclitic engagement even if she is in an oblique orientation prior to the onset of descent

(LOA, ROA, LOP or ROP). The torso may or may not move along with the head as this occurs; if it does not, the head rotates by turning at the neck.

If the head does not engage transverse, the baby will usually enter the pelvis and engage with her head aligned with one of the oblique diameters of the pelvis.

***4. Internal rotation of the head**

Internal rotation occurs as the baby's head moves to accommodate itself to the shape of the birth canal as it descends.

The extent of internal rotation: The distance the head usually rotates is determined by how far the denominator must travel to reach a more or less directly anterior (or directly posterior) position in the pelvis. This distance is expressed in degrees of arc, as it is a portion of a 360° circle that is being traversed. For ease of discussion, the movement of the head is usually broken down into eighths of a circle (or 45° increments). When labor begins with the baby's head in a transverse orientation, the occiput moves a total of 90° to OA, which is expressed in short arcs of movement consisting of 45° each (for example from LOT to LOA to OA). When labor begins with the head in an anterior oblique orientation and engages oblique–for example, LOA–internal rotation moves the occiput only 45°, from LOA to OA.

Why rotation occurs: The best research indicates that internal rotation is brought about primarily by the shape of the head as it descends and adapts to the resistance offered by the walls of the dilating soft tissues of the birth canal, especially the strong and resistant sidewalls of the loop-shaped opening of the pubococcygeus muscle, which is the first of the levator ani muscles that the descending presenting part encounters. Beyond this opening, the rest of the levator ani muscles form a forward-slanting sling that cradles and guides the head once rotation is complete. The levator ani muscles collectively form the muscular pelvic floor with the pubococcygeus muscle attaching superiorly behind the pubic arch. Typically, the region of the presenting part that reaches the pelvic floor first, which is usually the portion closest to the pubic bone, leads the rotation. (See the notes at the end of this chapter for a discussion of this rationale.)

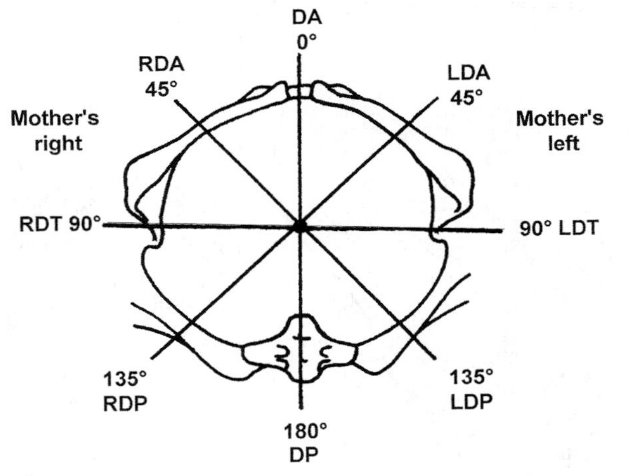

Degrees of rotation from different locations. The same principles apply to all types of fetal presentations, therefore "D" is used here generically to indicate the denominator.

When internal rotation occurs: The point at which internal rotation of the head takes place is highly variable. In a study of thirty women with occiput anterior babies and normal labors in the hospital, first-time mothers usually experienced internal rotation as the occiput met the resistance of the most anterior portion of the levator ani near the pubic bone, above the bend in the birth canal (−3 to 0 station) or as the head entered the upper third of the more curved portion of the birth canal (just below the level of the spines, about +1 station) (Borell & Fernström, 1959). Most of the time, full dilation precedes internal rotation. Prior to full dilation, rotation may be encouraged by the resistance of a partially dilated cervix, which mimics the resistance of the pelvic floor. In multiparas, the occurrence of internal rotation is even more variable and tends to occur at a lower level in the pelvis because the levator ani has been stretched, offering less counterpressure.

Calkins (1955) performed an extensive X-ray study on 5,400 women laboring (and probably drugged, which relaxes the pelvic tissues) in the hospital. He discovered that internal rotation takes place during descent to the pelvic floor or was completed at least by the time the head reached the pelvic floor in roughly 75% of multiparas and 60% of nulliparas. He called this "early internal rotation." This was commonly seen in women who had previously given birth and in those who had very efficient uterine contractions. Even so, 58% of the early group were primigravidas with poor contractions. When early rotation failed to occur, he felt this was probably the result of a lack of necessity at that point in descent more than anything else.

In the remaining women, "late" internal rotation occurred during distension of the pelvic floor (between +2 and +4 station) or even as late as crowning. If the head waits to rotate until it reaches the pelvic floor, rotation typically takes place during the next one or two contractions in multiparas and during the next three to five contractions in first-time mothers. Rotation may also occur during the resting phase of labor. About 5% of the time, internal rotation to the anterior does not occur. Some of these babies rotate to the posterior. A total of 1.6% primigravidas and 1.4% multigravidas had no internal rotation, with their babies heads born in the same position that they assumed during descent.

Level of Internal Rotation among 30 Women with Normal Labors		
Level in the birth canal	**Nulliparas**	**Multiparas**
1. Above the curve	9	1
2. Upper third of curve	11	3
3. Middle third of curve	0	5
4. Lower third of curve	0	1
5. Below the curve	0	0

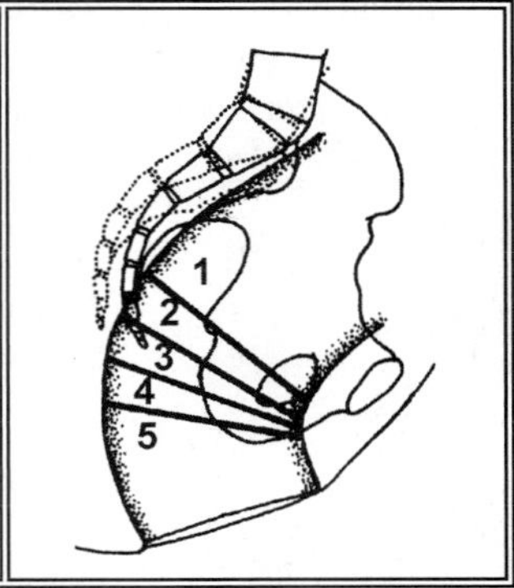

(Borell & Fernström, 1959)

How internal rotation occurs: The crown of the vertex leads the way through the midpelvis followed by the posterior fontanelle, the occiput, the parietal bones, the anterior fontanelle (bregma) and finally the sinciput. The levator ani forms a muscular funnel, which, with pressure, is converted to a sling. When the vertex contacts its upper, anterior band (part of the iliococcygeus muscle), the downward pressure from uterine contractions, the shape and resistance of these soft tissues, and the shape of the head encourages the occiput to rotate forward 90°, toward the mother's symphysis pubis.

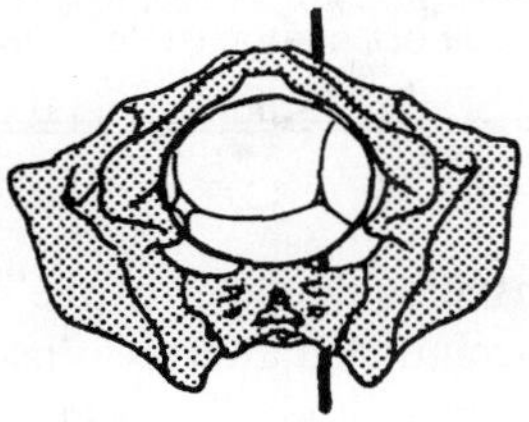

This LOT baby has already engaged via posterior asynclitism.

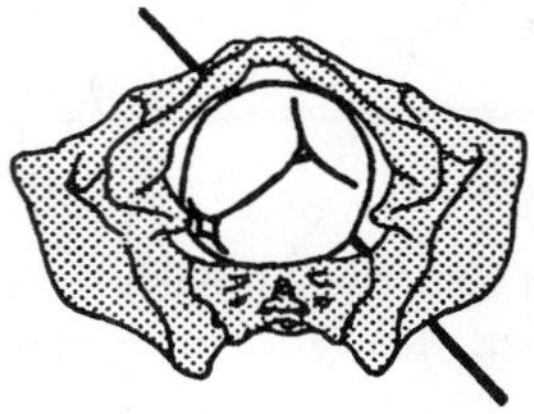

Internal rotation begins as the head rotates 45° to LOA

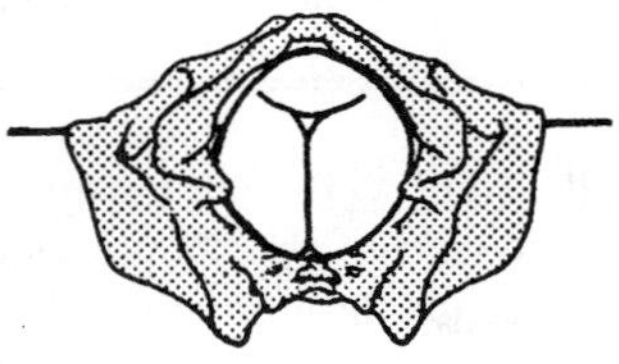

Internal rotation is complete as the head rotates another 45° to OA

(Black line denotes the angle of the shoulders)

The well-flexed head rotates around the axis formed by the verticomental diameter. Rotation occurs in a downwardly spiraling motion, thus furthering descent. Rotation results in the sagittal suture (long axis of the skull) and occiput rotating from the transverse or oblique diameter through which they entered the brim to the anteroposterior diameter of the pelvis (for example, LOT to LOA to OA). During internal rotation, it is not unusual for the sagittal suture to remain (or become) asynclitic until the head is cradled in the levator ani muscles. After internal rotation has occurred, the baby's face is to the mother's back with the sinciput near the sacrum and the occiput behind the symphysis. The head presses down, converting the levator ani into a sling, and is ready to begin descent through the curve of the birth canal. Often, perfect rotation with the posterior fontanelle precisely in the midline does not occur, and the baby's head is born slightly oblique. To descend further, the head may not need to rotate at all if the baby is small or if the mother's pelvis is large.

5. First internal rotation of the body and shoulders

As the head undergoes internal rotation to a directly occiput anterior position, the baby's body and shoulders usually follow the motion of the head by rotating from the diameter occupied by the long axis of the shoulders (anteroposterior or oblique) into the transverse diameter of the brim. Full rotation of the body bringing the shoulder axis to transverse is especially likely when the mother is upright, mobile and leaning forward and the fetal spine is well flexed.

Other possibilities for shoulder rotation: Less commonly, the fetal body and shoulders may undergo a partial first internal rotation, following the head for the first 45° of movement. For example, as the head rotates from occiput transverse to occiput anterior oblique, the shoulders rotate internally 45°, into the adjacent oblique diameter of the pelvis. Here the shoulders remain as the head continues to rotate another 45°, to OA, by turning at the neck. This temporarily takes the long axis of the vertex and the long axis of the shoulders out of their normal anatomical alignment.

Finally, the shoulders may remain aligned with the diameter they originally occupy as the head turns, either 45° or 90°, to become occiput anterior. (The concepts presented here regarding shoulder rotation differ somewhat from those found in other texts. They are further discussed at the end of this chapter.)

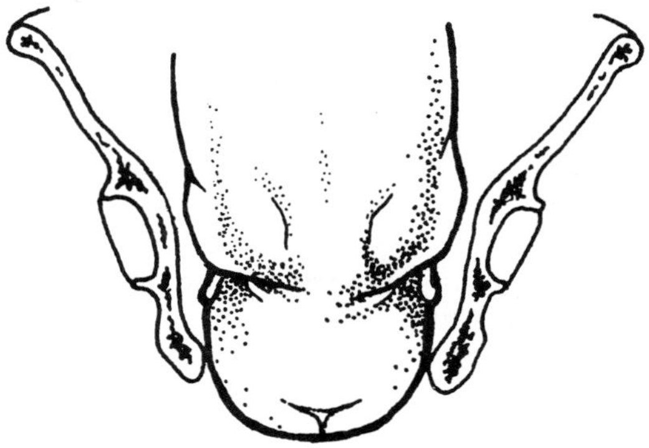

(5) Full internal rotation of the shoulders to the transverse diameter.

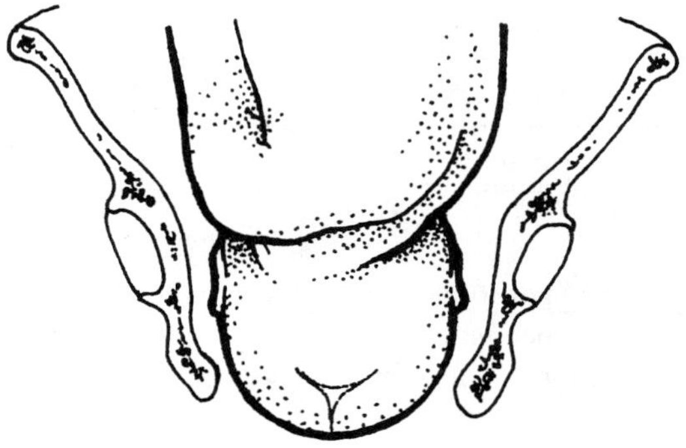

(5) Partial internal rotation; the twisting of the neck allows the shoulders to remain in an oblique orientation (note moulding as they enter the brim)

6. Engagement of the shoulders

Engagement of the shoulders occurs as the bisacromial diameter, the widest transverse diameter of the shoulder girdle, descends through the brim. It usually takes place after internal rotation of the occiput and after the first internal rotation of the shoulders (when it takes place), as the head continues to descend to or past the ischial tuberosities. Exactly when it occurs varies, depending upon the size of the baby and the depth of the pelvis. If the shoulder girdle has followed the head completely during internal rotation, they will enter the transverse diameter of the brim. Less commonly, they may descend through an oblique or the anteroposterior diameter of the pelvis.

• The attitude of the shoulders and arms (a component of skeletal adaptation as described in 1)

Adaptation continues when the shoulders change their attitude by flexing or extending in relation to the chest several times as they adapt to the changing shape of the birth canal during descent, particularly as they pass through the lower half of the birth canal. They may mould as engagement occurs. Most commonly, they become pressed in a downward slope along the torso. Alternatively, the scapulae can move together with the shoulders hunching toward the ears (see top right illustration on page 82). Or one shoulder may be hunched while the other is pressed down. The arms are typically crossed over the chest, which allows maximal spinal flexibility. They may also be extended along one or both sides of the body, where they may impair lateral spinal flexion to a certain extent (Borell & Fernström, 1958).

7. Spinal extension begins

As the head moves deeper into the pelvis, more room is created for the baby to stretch out her body somewhat. The spine becomes less flexed, and spinal extension begins as the tucked head fits nicely into the curve of the birth canal.

• Dilating the perineum

As the head becomes firmly pressed against the pelvic floor near the level of the tuberosities (+4 to +5), it is poised to begin rocking back and forth as the mother bears down and pushes. With each push, the head rocks forward, then recedes as the mother relaxes and the force of pushing subsides. This process massages the pelvic floor, naturally dilating it to minimize trauma, making more and more room for the sinciput in the hollow of the sacrum so that the occiput and then the neck can pass beneath the pubic bone. This causes the perineum to form a resistant channel for the head to pass through, which encourages continued flexion. How long a channel is formed depends upon the mother's position. When she is upright, the levator ani sling is rotated up and back, and the stretching is less extreme. When she is supine, the levator ani sling is maximally elongated, especially when her legs are flexed toward her abdomen. When the pelvic floor has sufficiently stretched, the biparietal diameter is positioned under the lower border of the pubic arch, which usually corresponds with the onset of crowning. Soon, the biparietal diameter moves past the pubic bone to the level of the conjugate of the outlet. At this point, the head has mostly left the confines of the bony pelvis and is now almost entirely contained within the soft birth canal.

8-1. Second internal rotation of the chest begins

As the vertex distends the perineum, the midchest enters the curve of the birth canal near the level of the ischial spines. Here, it usually begins to rotate from the transverse or anteroposterior diameter it occupies to an oblique diameter to allow the spine to flex laterally. The shoulders move in concert with the chest. Where they go depends upon the diameter through which they entered the brim: if they entered the brim transverse, they rotate 45° to an oblique diameter. If they entered the anteroposterior diameter of the brim, they may remain there, or they can rotate 45° into the right or left oblique diameter of the pelvis. If the shoulders entered an oblique diameter of the brim, they usually do not begin further rotation at this point. (The concepts presented here regarding chest rotation and spinal flexion differ from those found in other texts. They are further discussed in the notes found at the end of this chapter.)

• Crowning of the head

"Crowning" is sometimes defined as visualization of the presenting part at the introitus. However, in this text (and in most others), it is defined as the point during pushing when the presenting part no longer recedes between contractions. This usually corresponds with the point at which the biparietal diameter reaches the level of the pubic arch, although exactly when crowning begins varies among individual women.

A full crown may be defined as the point at which the widest diameter of the presenting part is encircled by the introitus. In vertex presentations, this is usually when the suboccipitobregmatic and biparietal diameters of the head are distending the vulvar ring. Although crowning is a significant landmark during pushing because it indicates that the widest diameter of the head is past the bony outlet, it is not considered one of the cardinal movements of birth.

***9. Birth of the flexed head by extension of the lower neck and upper spine**

The flexed head continues descent and dilates the lower birth canal. Flexion may be further exaggerated as the head meets the pelvic floor and again as the forehead meets the resistance of the sacrosciatic ligaments and the posterior levator ani sling. At this point, the head is about to leave the bony outlet and enter the outermost portion of the curved birth canal created by the perineal tissues.

A combination of downward pressure from contractions, further descent of the fetal head, maintenance of flexion and the resistance afforded by the pelvic floor cause the crown of the baby's head to show as the head glides continuously downward under the arch of the pubic rami, past the bony outlet and through the dilated soft tissues. This moves the lower part of the baby's cervical spine and the upper part of the thoracic spine into the deepest bend of the birth canal. As the head continues to distend the perineum, the upper thoracic spine undergoes marked extension (curving backward), allowing the head to remain almost completely flexed. The baby's nose stays in contact with the posterior wall of the birth canal until the head emerges.

Visible crowning at the introitus toward the end of pushing is evidence that the forehead has passed the bony outlet and that spinal extension has begun. As spinal extension continues, the head remains flexed against the stretched perineum until it begins to disengage. Once the biparietal diameter (the widest part) passes through the mouth of the yoni, the soft parts around the head retract, the fetal neck lengthens, and the head is born. As the perineum retracts, it sweeps posteriorly over the baby's vertex, bregma, forehead, brows, nose, mouth and chin and anteriorly over the occiput. Note that the head will tend to flex only to the extent necessary to traverse the passageway it must navigate, but it need not and *usually does not* deflex to any significant degree in order to be born. (The concepts presented here regarding how extension occurs differ from those presented in other texts. They are further discussed in notes at the end of this chapter.)

Maintenance of head flexion is facilitated by passage through the resistance birth canal. Intrauterine pressure, combined with the pressure from the mother's pushing efforts, forces the baby's head more deeply into the pelvic soft tissues. The brow is held back by the sling-shaped floor of the levator ani. This causes the sincipital portion of the head to flex further forward, since the occipital portion is still beneath the pubic arch. The parietal eminences impinge on the sides of the levator ani as the head passes under the pubic bone. This holds the head in a flexed posture while the crown of the vertex is pressed through the opening of the perineum. The perineum gradually stretches as the occiput and vertex pass through the bony outlet, leaving the lower neck under the pubic arch. In order for the head to continue advancing, the upper thoracic and lower cervical spine arch upward. The crown of the vertex emerges as the perineum is stretched and thinned downward and outward (if long enough or the mother is supine) or backward (if the perineum is quite short or the mother is upright).

***10. Restitution of the head**

"Restitution" refers to the unique tendency of the head to reposition its long axis to its original anatomical orientation at a right angle with the long axis of the shoulders once the head is born and is free of counterpressure. If the long axes of the shoulders and head are out of alignment, the neck untwists, causing the head to return or restitute 45° to an oblique angle (OA to LOA for example) to restore its right-angle relationship with the shoulders and normal alignment with the spine. In contemporary obstetrics, the term "restitution" is used exclusively for discussing cephalic presentations.

8-2. Second internal rotation of the chest and shoulders is completed

After the head is born, the pause before the next contraction relieves downward pressure on the baby's chest and shoulders slightly. This, coupled with the need for the spine to flex laterally due to the shape of the soft tissues at the outlet, causes the chest to finish rotating to the side 45°, moving the shoulders into the anteroposterior diameter of the pelvis. Rotation may occur before the next contraction or as it is building and causes the posterior shoulder to move into the hollow of the sacrum, where it presses against the pelvic floor. This positions the long axis of the shoulders in the longest diameter of the pelvic outlet.

The second rotation of the shoulder axis does not always take place as described above. Less commonly, the shoulders may emerge through the oblique or transverse diameter of the outlet. These variations are discussed in more detail in the chapter entitled "Variations in Vertex Descent and Rotation."

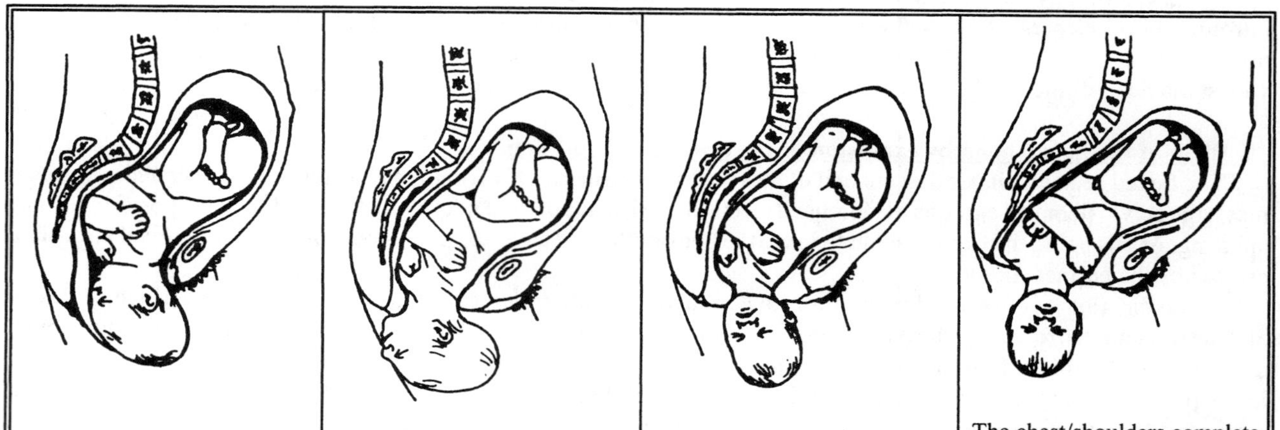

The chest/shoulders begin their 2nd internal rotation to oblique (8-2) as head crowns	The head is born face down.	The head restitutes (10) restoring the anatomical alignment with the shoulders.	The chest/shoulders complete their 2nd internal rotation to AP (8-2); the head followss, rotating externally (11)

(The mother is in an upright, kneeling position.)

***11. External rotation of the head**

The head rotates externally in concert with the movements of the chest and shoulders as they move into the anteroposterior diameter of the outlet.

12. Birth (disengagement) of the shoulders

Once the head is out, the shoulders are born as the torso flexes laterally. The shoulder girdle descends at a slightly sloping angle, with the anterior shoulder usually leading the way. If the birth occurs spontaneously, especially if the mother is in an upright, forward-leaning position, the anterior shoulder may be seen first, but the posterior shoulder will usually be born first.

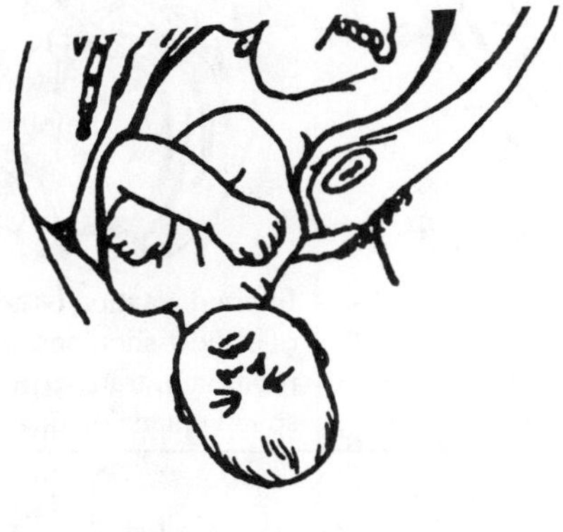

Birth of the posterior shoulder

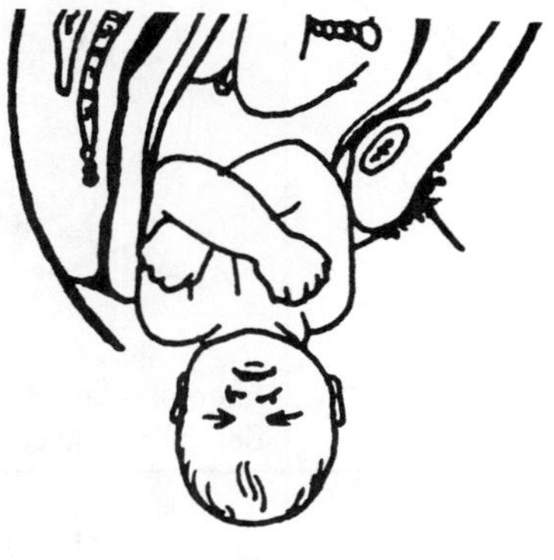

Birth of the anterior shoulder

Birth of the posterior shoulder: The anterior shoulder reaches the level of the pubic bone. A combination of lateral trunk flexion and the weight of the head as it swings forward causes the anterior shoulder to pivot against the pubic arch or ramus, especially when the infant's head is not manipulated. At this point, the anterior shoulder is often visible. With the force of the next contraction, the anterior shoulder braces beneath the pubic bone, the posterior shoulder moves forward, the perineum bulges, and the posterior shoulder flexes slightly toward the baby's chest and slides out first.

Birth of the anterior shoulder: The birth of the posterior shoulder reduces the diameter of the upper torso as well as allowing it to drop back into the posterior outlet. Both of these changes free the anterior shoulder, allowing it to slip past the pubic bone and emerge (Sutton & Scott, 1996). (The concepts presented here regarding the birth of the shoulders differ from those presented in other texts. They are further discussed in the notes at the end of this chapter.)

13. Birth of the arms, torso and legs

The arms, torso and the legs generally slide out easily in a subtle spiraling motion once the shoulders have been born. This spiraling motion is most obvious when the baby emerges with no assistance during a vertical birth or during birth into warm water. Warm water allows the baby to participate in his birth more actively with the triggering of several primitive reflexes resulting in the baby himself actively making a spiraling exit. This is further explained in the chapter entitled "Hydrotherapy and Waterbirth."

Moulding

Moulding in anterior vertex presentations reduces the suboccipitobregmatic diameter and elongates the verticomental diameter. A caput would develop over the posterior parietal bone in the region of the crown of the vertex near the sagittal suture on the side that was directly over the os during descent.

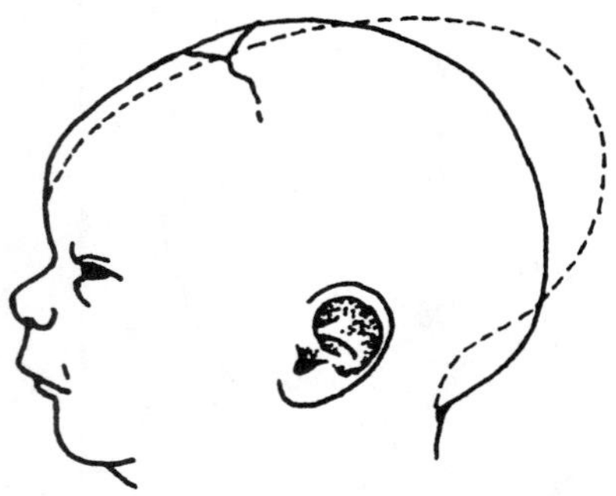

Typical moulding in occiput anterior vertex presentations

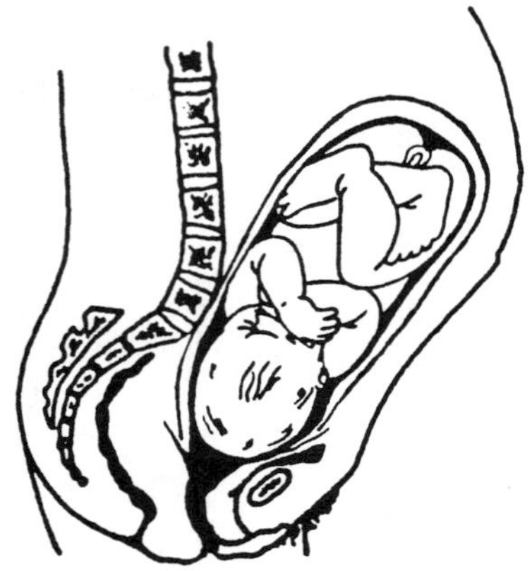

Baby LOT; dilation well underway, posterior asynclitic descent (2) to engagement (3)

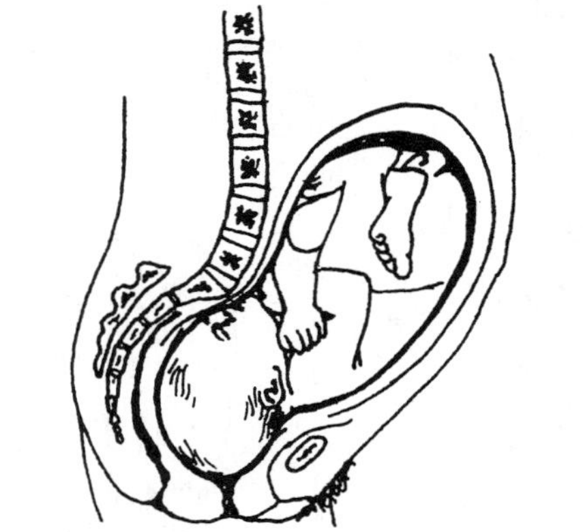

Internal rotation (4) begins to LOA; spinal flexion enhanced (1)

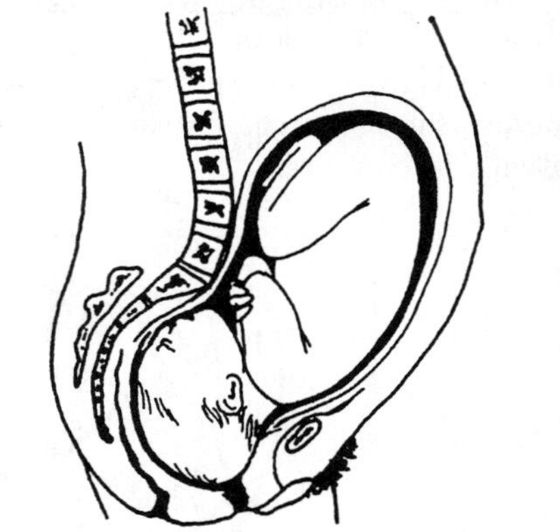

Internal rotation of head to OA complete (4); chest-shoulders undergo 1st internal rotation to transverse (5) and engage (6); spinal extension begins (7)

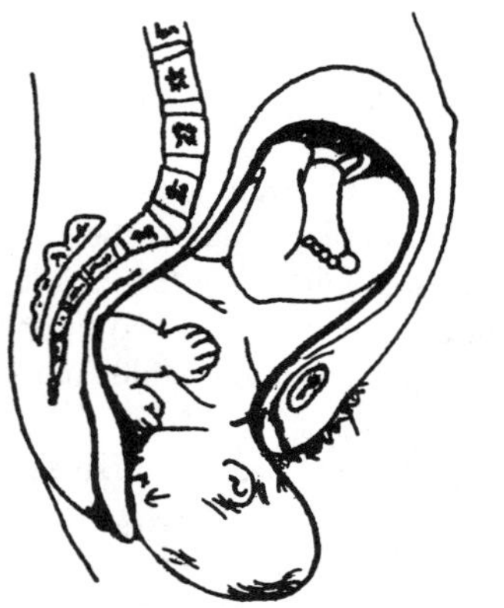

Chest-shoulders begin 2nd internal rotation to oblique (8-1); upper spine extends (9) as flexed head crowns

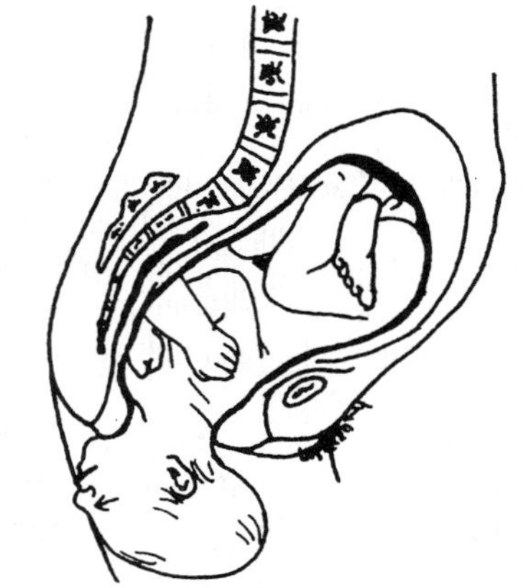

Chest-shoulders are now oblique (8-1); head is born OA by spinal extension (9)

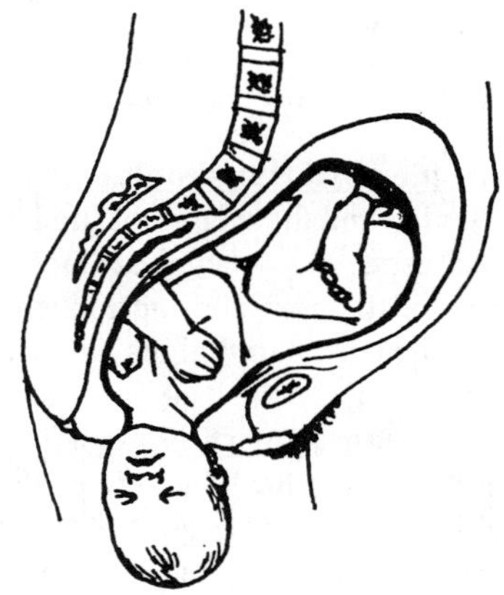

Head restitutes to LOA (10)

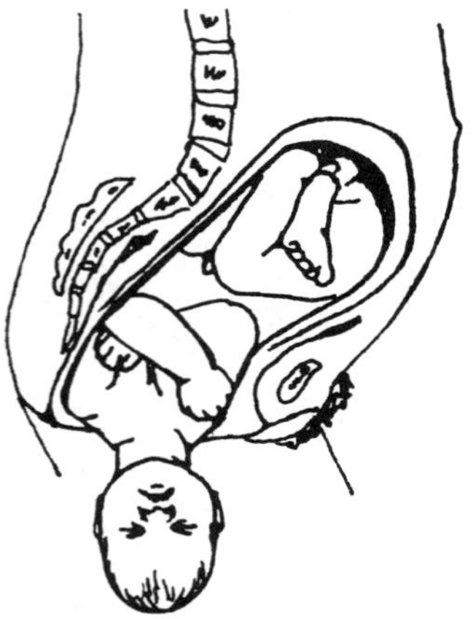

Chest/shoulders finish 2nd internal rotation to AP (8-2); head follows, rotating externally to LOT (11)

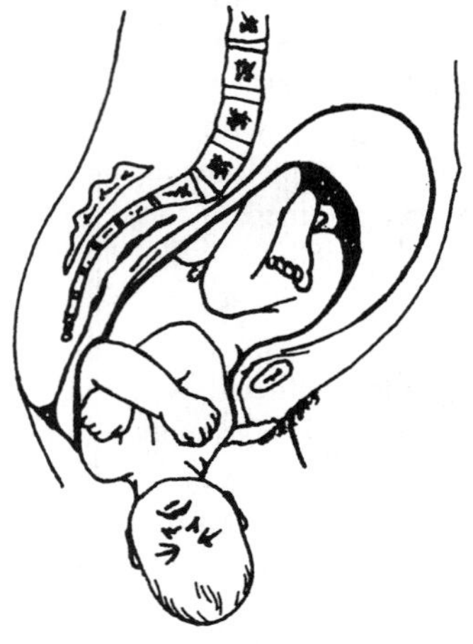

Posterior shoulder born (12)

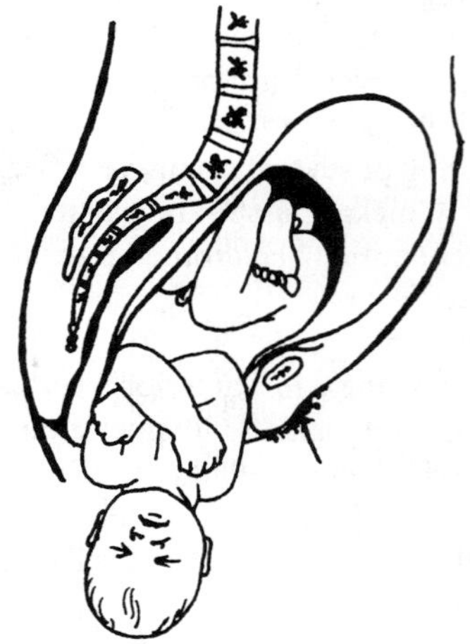

Anterior shoulder is born (12); body follows with a spiraling motion (13)

(Numbers in the drawings match the explanatory notes in this chapter associated with each cardinal spiraling movement.)

Notes on the Changes Incorporated into the Cardinal Spiraling Movements of Birth

This chapter contains several radical departures from the standard teaching regarding the obstetric mechanisms of labor. These notes provide the background research for these changes.

Why internal rotation occurs (movement 4)

Why internal rotation occurs has been hotly debated for centuries. It has often been stated that the lowermost portion of the presenting part reaches the pelvic floor first and therefore leads rotation. However, Beard (1937) offers a compelling rationale to explain his view that the most anterior portion leads rotation. He studied the specific muscles of the pelvic floor and felt that the pubococcygeus muscle was the strongest of all the levator ani muscles and thus must have the most influence over internal rotation. Since the most anterior portion of the presenting part meets the upper end of the pubococcygeus first (in the anterior pelvis between the pubic bone and the spines), he felt this was what triggers rotation. The iliococcygeus and ischiococcygeus muscles are more inferiorly and posteriorly placed in relation to the brim as well as weaker than the pubococcygeus. Because of the placement of these muscles, he reasoned that the anterior, rather than the lowermost, portion of the presenting part would reach the pelvic floor first and be triggered to rotate forward. Borell and Fernström (1967) confirm Beard's impressions and add that the loop-shaped opening of the pelvic floor best accommodates the head in either an OA or OP orientation. If the muscles are lax or if the largest part of the head is posterior, the counterpressure afforded by the entire sling of muscles surrounding the presenting part is probably required to prompt rotation, because in some cases the head must descend further before rotation begins.

Shoulder descent and rotation (movements 5, 8-1 and 8-2)

Only one in vivo English-language research project has specifically looked at the process of shoulder engagement and rotation. Borell and Fernström (1958) did a small study of 40 laboring women to determine if, when, where, why and to what extent shoulder rotation occurred. They do not mention parity, but these were totally spontaneous births with no interventions other than the X-rays themselves. Thirty-eight of the 40 babies were born OA and two were born OP.

They found that the conventional teaching that internal rotation of the shoulders occurs for the same reasons as does internal rotation of the head–that is, that the shape of the shoulder girdle initiates rotation to align itself with the shape of the passageway–is not correct. The way the shoulders come through the birth canal is more complex. As a result of their careful observations using serial X-rays, they found that the shoulders usually undergo two internal rotations:

First internal rotation of the body and shoulders: The shoulders start out aligned in one of the oblique diameters or in the anteroposterior diameter of the brim. As the head rotates internally to a directly OA or OP position, the body and shoulders usually lag behind only slightly, following the movement of the head as they rotate to become aligned with the transverse diameter of the brim in the majority of labors. *At this point, shoulder rotation is prompted by internal rotation of the head.* When the shoulders undergo full rotation, the normal right-angle alignment of the shoulder axis to the long axis of the head is maintained as the shoulders rotate into the transverse diameter and then engage. Since the head has just dilated the birth canal, the shape of the soft tissues is not a critical factor in determining the diameter through which the shoulders engage.

Second internal rotation of the chest and shoulders: Lateral flexibility of the spine has long been recognized as an important component of breech descent and rotation. Borell and Fernström's research emphasizes the importance of spinal flexibility during descent in cephalic presentations as well and concludes that the shape of the shoulders is not the primary determinant of their rotation. This is a major departure from what is generally taught, which is that the first internal rotation generally does not occur and that the second internal rotation is prompted entirely by the shape of the shoulders adapting to the shape of the outlet.

They observed that, as the vertex passes the tuberosities, the midchest and spine enter the curve of the birth canal near the level of the ischial spines with the shoulders aligned in the transverse diameter. The midchest rotates, moving the shoulders into an oblique diameter, which allows the spine to take advantage of lateral flexion. (Because the occiput is directly anterior and the shoulders usually are transverse, the chest could rotate to the right or to the left. To avoid confusion, the descriptions of each movement will assume that the chest rotates to occupy the oblique diameter that correlates with the original position of the head, which is usually how it occurs.) After the head is born, the midchest usually finishes its second internal rotation by moving into the anteroposterior diameter, allowing the spine maximum lateral flexibility through the deepest curve in the birth canal. *The second internal rotation of the shoulders occurs in concert with movement of the upper torso and is prompted by the need for the chest and spine to flex laterally as they navigate the curve of the birth canal.* Thus, the shoulders become the denominator for the chest and spine, indicating their movement.

Most observations of shoulder position in labor have been incidental to the study of diagnostic images obtained for some other purpose. It is obvious from these findings that if a researcher weren't specifically studying the movement of the shoulders with a series of images, a lot of these nuances would be missed. The following charts show the positions of the fetal shoulders as they rotate during different points in descent.

Position of Bisacromial Diameter	**Station of Shoulders (bisacromial diameter)**					
	2-3 cm above brim	**Brim (-5)**	**Ischial spines (0)**	**Tuberosities (+5)**	**3-4 cm below tuberosities**	**After birth of shoulders**
AP	60%	21%	5%	0%	50%	60%
Oblique	23%	24%	50%	58%	40%	35%
Transverse	17%	55%	45%	42%	10%	5%

To read this chart fill in this sentence: "When the shoulders are (at one of the stations in the top row), they are in the ____ position ___% of the time." For example, "When the shoulders are 2-3 cm above the brim they are in the AP position 60% of the time." In 55% of the cases studied, the shoulders were transverse at the brim, placing their long axis at right angles with the long axis of the head. It is very likely that the shoulders and torso move to the transverse diameter much more often in women who are upright and mobile in labor and who favor forward-leaning positions. The women in these studies were constrained to specific postures during X-ray.

Borell and Fernström also studied the level of the shoulder axis as the head progresses through the birth canal. The following chart may help you visualize where the shoulders are while the head is descending.

Position of Shoulders	**Depth of Descent of the Vertex**		
	At ischial tuberosities (+5)	**Maximally distending perineum**	**Head just born**
Shoulders 3 cm above brim	5%		
Shoulders 2 cm above brim	5%		
Shoulders 1 cm above brim	55%		
Shoulders at the brim (–5)	35%	4%	
Shoulders between brim & ischial spines (–5 to 0)		40%	
Shoulders level with ischial spines (0)		41%	18%
Shoulders between spines & tuberosities (0 to +5)		6.5%	28%
Shoulders at ischial tuberosities (+5)		6.5%	32%
Shoulders 2 to 3 cm below tuberosities			22%

To read this chart, fill in the blanks as follows: In (the given percentage) of all labors, the shoulders are (at a station listed in the left column) when the head has descended to the level of (a point listed in the top row)." For example: "In 5% of all labors, the shoulders are 3 cm above the brim when the vertex has descended to the pelvic floor at the level of the tuberosities (+5)."

The basic principle of internal rotation is universal, regardless of the longitudinal polarity or variety of the baby. The shoulders may not always be able to follow the head. For example, deflexion of the baby's spine prior to engagement of the head would tend to cause the shoulders (and head) to assume a more military attitude. In these cases (such as occiput posterior positions), the spine will flex less, possibly resulting in the posterior shoulder becoming lodged beside the sacral promontory, which may impair rotation. In these cases, it is more likely that the shoulders will not rotate to the transverse before entering the brim (Sutton, 2001). (Internal rotation of the head is further explained in chapters covering descent with the head in other attitudes.) The next table describes what happens when the fetal body and shoulders do and do not follow the head around completely.

Internal Rotation of the Denominator and First Internal Rotation of Shoulder Axis in Cephalic Presentations

Position of denominator in mother's pelvis	Distance denominator must rotate	Destination of denominator	Possible ways the body will respond to internal rotation of the head (using the anterior shoulder as the denominator)*
Transverse	90°	Directly anterior	Start AP**, rotate 45° to an oblique diameter, then 45° to transverse to enter brim
			Start AP, rotate 45° to an oblique diameter, as head turns at the neck
			Remain AP as head turns at the neck
Anterior oblique	45°	Directly anterior	Start oblique, rotate 45° to enter brim transverse
Posterior oblique		Short-arc rotation to direct posterior	Remain oblique as head turns at the neck
Directly anterior	0°	No rotation	Remain transverse to enter brim
Posterior oblique	135°	Long-arc rotation to direct anterior	Start oblique, rotate 45° to AP, 45° to opposite oblique, then 45° to transverse as head turns at the neck (135° in all)
			Start oblique, rotate 45° to AP then rotate 45° to opposite oblique diameter as head turns at the neck
			Start oblique, rotate only 45° to AP as neck turns the last 90° to bring denominator anterior
Directly posterior	0°	No rotation	Remain transverse to enter brim
	180°	Long-arc rotation to direct anterior	Start transverse, rotate 45° to oblique, then 45° to AP, then 45° to opposite oblique, then 45° to engage transverse (180° in all)
			Start transverse, rotate 45° to oblique, then rotate 45° to AP, then 45° to opposite oblique diameter (135° in all). The head turns at the neck during its last 45° of rotation to allow the shoulders to enter the oblique diameter of the brim.
			Start transverse, rotate 45° oblique then 45° to AP. Neck twists to achieve its last 90° of rotation, allowing shoulders to engage AP.***

*Listed in probable order of frequency **AP=anteroposterior ***Possible but unlikely because of the distance the neck must twist

To read the preceding chart, fill in the blanks: "When labor begins with the (cephalic denominator [occiput, mentum or frontum]) in the (given position), it must rotate a total of (distance denominator must rotate in degrees) to become (destination of denominator). As this occurs, the shoulders, which started out (original orientation of shoulders) will (respond to internal rotation of the head in this way) before entering the brim." For example, with vertex babies: "When labor begins with the occiput in the transverse position, it must rotate a total of 90° to become directly anterior. As this occurs, the shoulders, which started out AP, rotate 45° to an oblique diameter, then 45° to transverse before entering the brim."

Notes on the birth of the head by extension (movement 9)

It has been widely taught that birth of the head takes place during a process of extension that occurs at the atlantooccipital joint, where the neck meets the occiput. It is said that once the lower margin of the occiput has cleared the pubic bone, the head, which is still in the birth canal, begins to extend from the base of the occiput as the chin lifts off the chest, causing the baby's face to sweep over the perineum as the head emerges, then the head is said to tip posteriorly and the occiput is said to escape. Several routine obstetrical interventions have worked to keep this myth alive: the long-standing practice of cutting the perineum and the use of heavy anesthetics that profoundly relax the pelvic floor to an abnormal degree. Both interventions lessen the normal resistance of the perineum and favor early extension; the historical use of the Ritgen maneuver, (a technique used to compensate for the lack of voluntary pushing when women are under general anesthesia) to manually produce deflexion as the head emerges; and the use of forceps, during which early extension can be produced by artificially deflexing the head after the occiput clears the pubic bone. Being able to effect extension in these ways has fostered the idea that this is the way spontaneous birth occurs as well.

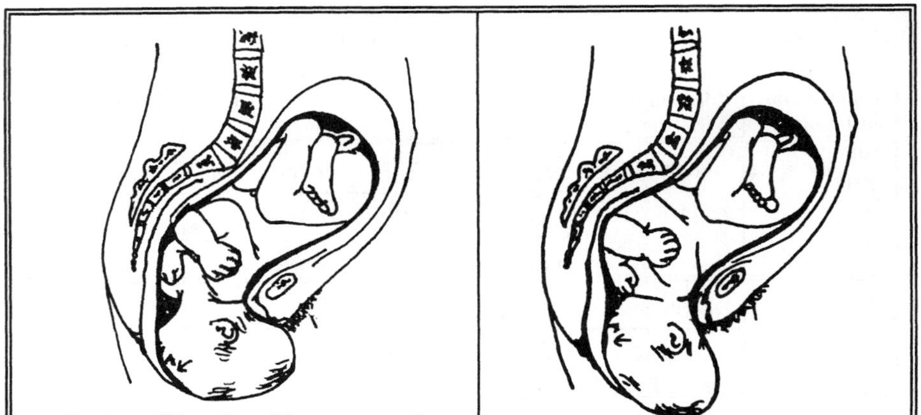

What is traditionally said to occur as the head is born | What really occurs

Anyone who has attended spontaneous births over intact perineums knows that the top of the flexed head presents and the perineum retracts around it, leaving the flexed head exposed at the introitus. A few older texts have stated that the head remains flexed until emergence. Borell and Fernström (1959) did detailed X-ray studies that showed that what appears to occur matches what is going on internally. Once the head is past the tuberosities, it is surrounded by the soft birth canal, leaving the upper spine and lower neck under the pubic arch where they do most of the extending, allowing the head to remain mostly flexed with optimal cephalic diameters emerging as the perineum retracts.

Notes on the birth of the shoulders (movement 12)

Many older midwifery and obstetrical textbooks, such as Greenhill's PRINCIPLES AND PRACTICE OF OBSTETRICS (1951, p. 205)–and even some newer textbooks such as Varney's MIDWIFERY (1997, p. 437)–teach that the posterior shoulder is usually born first when the shoulders are born spontaneously. However, it is standard practice to teach that the anterior shoulder is normally born prior to the posterior shoulder. For decades, this outcome has been fostered by having the mother in a supine position. This unanatomical position, coupled with decades of drugged mothers having their perineums cut followed by instrumental deliveries, has fostered a fear regarding shoulder dystocia. To counter this, the anterior shoulder, which is the one most likely to become impacted behind the pubic bone, is encouraged to come first. When the mother is flat on her back, the weight of the head as it hangs toward the floor favors the presentation of the anterior shoulder and most certainly impairs the ability of the posterior shoulder to birth first. The attendant grasps the head and exaggerates the downward angle of the neck, thus forcing the anterior shoulder to emerge first. If the process was designed to work like this, manipulation to birth the anterior shoulder would be unnecessary most of the time.

In fact, as soon as the head is born, most doctors manipulate it without regard for the timing of contractions, showing little patience in waiting for the uterus to do the work of shoulder rotation. Sutton and Scott point out that if the mother is upright in a forward-leaning position and the shoulders are allowed to be born spontaneously, the need to cut the perineum is rare and the incidence of shoulder dystocia is, in their experience, almost nonexistent (Sutton & Scott, 1996).

Applying These Basic Concepts to All Vertex Presentations

The chapters that follow discuss the variety of ways the vertex baby can be born (LOT, ROT, LOA, etc.). The basic cardinal spiraling movements must always be taken into account, regardless of the baby's position. Keeping all this straight can be difficult, and there is no substitute for studying each movement in detail.

The Cardinal Spiraling Movements: Left Occiput Transverse (LOT)

This chapter will describe the birth of the baby in the left occiput transverse position (LOT), the most common fetal position at the onset of labor. It is essential to have a solid understanding of the material presented in the chapters entitled "Features of Fetal Anatomy Pertinent to the Birth Process," "Synclitism and Asynclitism" and "The Process of Birth in Occiput Anterior Vertex Presentations" prior to studying this chapter, since they contain more detailed explanations of the basic concepts that are applied to LOT descent here.

The manner in which LOT descent proceeds is explained here in great detail, elaborating upon variations in the process of normal shoulder rotation and other movements that may occur in the majority of all births. LOT birth is employed here as the template for understanding all other types of descent, The variations in LOT descent and rotation may also be applied to all other cephalic presentations.

Study and understand this chapter *thoroughly* (including relevant maternal anatomy), both on paper and in three dimensions using a doll and pelvic model, prior to studying the other presentations. This material can be very confusing because it describes the movement of two three-dimensional objects from a variety of angles. Once descent in the LOT position is fully understood, use the models to visualize birth in the other positions. Remember that left and right maternal landmarks refer to the mother's left and right, regardless of the angle of view.

Historical Highlights

In the first printed descriptions of the cardinal movements of birth as generally understood today, William Smellie (1752) stated that the baby most commonly assumes a transverse position of the occiput as she enters the brim, although he mentions that descent through an oblique pelvic diameter also occurs occasionally (Rydberg, 1954a). Those following Smellie studied and refined his explanations of labor and pelvic architecture, but the concept of the transverse orientation of the occiput fell out of obstetrical textbooks for nearly two centuries. This was because John Louis Baudelocque (1775) put forth the notion that the oblique diameter of the brim was longer than the transverse diameter. This idea was furthered when Bard (1807) presented the first drawing of the pelvis in an American textbook, stating that the transverse diameter was longer in the skeleton but that the oblique diameter was longer in living women due to the presence of soft tissues, which shortened the transverse diameter. This turned out to be an error, but it went uncorrected for quite a long time (as so many errors in obstetrics tend to do). Throughout those many years, the position of the denominator was described as either directly anterior or posterior; right or left anterior oblique; or right or left posterior oblique, with no consideration of a transverse orientation. Babies who were occiput transverse were usually designated as posterior. Thus, many illustrations in older texts show a vertex baby that is clearly in an occiput transverse orientation by today's definition with a caption indicating that the baby is posterior oblique.

In 1942, Javert and Steele revived the concept of the occiput transverse position and engagement via posterior asynclitism in their landmark paper, which articulated LOT descent and made clear that it is the most common way for the vertex baby to descend through the brim. In spite of this, many modern textbooks persist in presenting the LOA position as the most common. Logically, the anterior abdomen offers the baby the most room to expand at he grows in late pregnancy. The bony ridge of the mother's spine causes the baby to place his back as far away from it as possible. Right up to term, the baby's back can frequently be felt to be anterior oblique. However, we must remember that the "O" in "LOT" refers to nothing other than the occiput. As the baby's *head* descends near term or during early labor, it tends to seek the transverse diameter to engage. The back may follow so that the entire baby is transverse or the head can turn 45° at the neck, leaving the baby's back in an anterior oblique orientation while the head assumes an occiput transverse position (Morison, 1971).

The Cardinal Movements of Birth When Labor Starts with the Baby in the LOT Position

This summary describes the three possibilities for chest and shoulder rotation. Follow each lettered description through to the end of the summary (i.e., 5-A, 6-A, 9-A and 12-A follow the same pattern of descent). Subsequent summaries will only describe "A," which is the most common of these three. Asterisks refer to the cardinal movements as recognized by contemporary obstetrics. You will note that the numbered steps correspond to the steps first outlined in the table describing the cardinal movements of birth found at the beginning of the chapter entitled "The Process of

Birth in Occiput Anterior Vertex Presentations."

The orientation of the baby to the mother's pelvis

Prior to labor, the baby's occiput is in the left transverse region of the mother's pelvis, directed toward her left hip, with the sagittal suture aligned with the transverse diameter of the brim. The shoulders are aligned with the anteroposterior diameter of the brim, at right angles with the long axis of the head, or the shoulders and back may be somewhat more anterior oblique. The head and spine are flexed forward, the natural position of the fetus. The head may not be completely flexed, as optimal diameters may not be required for some babies to enter the pelvis. Fetal small parts are on the mother's right side.

Birth of the LOT baby

Babies tend to favor a transverse position because it places the wide biparietal diameter to the side of the promontory and affords the advantage of asynclitic engagement, as detailed in the chapter entitled "Synclitism and Asynclitism."

***1.** The degree of head and spinal flexion varies; however, many babies are fairly well flexed prior to the onset of labor. After complete dilation, flexion of the head is often enhanced as it contacts the pelvic floor.

***2.** The baby descends throughout labor. Prior to engagement, the head is in an attitude of posterior asynclitism, with the sagittal suture above or slightly behind the symphysis.

***3.** The head engages as the biparietal diameter passes through the anteroposterior diameter of the brim. Posterior asynclitism allows the posterior parietal bone (the baby's left) to descend into the roomy sacral curve. The process of engagement converts the attitude to one of anterior asynclitism, which may persist until internal rotation is complete.

***4.** The head rotates internally a total of 90°, from LOT to OA, as it adapts to the loop-shaped opening of the levator ani sling. Rotation consists of a downwardly spiraling movement, which facilitates descent. Internal rotation usually occurs after dilation is complete and the vertex has passed the ischial spines. It begins as the head rotates 45° from the LOT position to LOA. Then the head rotates another 45° to OA.

5. The baby's body moves with the shoulders if they undergo their first internal rotation.

5-A. Following the rotation of the occiput from LOT to LOA, the shoulders rotate 45° from the anteroposterior diameter, to align with the left oblique diameter. As the occiput rotates from LOA to OA, the shoulders rotate another 45° to align with the transverse diameter of the brim, 90° in all. (See illustrations at the end of this chapter. Follow "A" entries below.)

5-B. Following the rotation of the occiput from LOT to LOA, the shoulders rotate 45° from the antero-posterior diameter to align with the left oblique diameter. As the head rotates 45° from LOA to OA, the neck twists, allowing the body and shoulders to remain aligned with the left oblique diameter until the head is born. (Not illustrated. Follow "B" entries below.)

5-C. The baby's body remains aligned with the anteroposterior diameter of the brim as the head rotates internally 90° by turning at the neck. (Not illustrated. Follow "C" entries below.)

6. The shoulders engage though the diameter into which they rotated. As the head passes through the ischial tuberosities, the bisacromial diameter enters:

6-A. the transverse diameter of the brim.

6-B. the left oblique diameter of the brim.

6-C. the anteroposterior diameter of the brim.

The attitude of the shoulders shifts during descent as the torso accommodates to the shape of the birth canal.

7. The spine begins to extend as the head enters the pelvis more deeply.

8-1. Internal rotation of the chest may occur between the time the head distends the perineum and is born. As the midchest and spine enter the curve of the birth canal near the level of the ischial spines, they may rotate 45°:

8-1-A. moving the shoulders from the transverse into the left oblique diameter as they undergo their second internal rotation. This adjustment allows the spine to flex laterally. The neck twists as this occurs, allowing the head to remain OA.

8-1-B. but as the chest and shoulders are already oblique, the internal shoulder rotation does not begin now.

8-1-C. moving the shoulders from the anteroposterior to the left oblique diameter as they undergo their first internal rotation. The neck partially untwists as this occurs, allowing the head to remain OA.

Rotation of the chest and spine to an oblique orientation allows the spine to flex laterally.

***9.** The head glides down past the pubic arch and begins to crown as the lower neck and upper spine extend under the pubic arch, allowing the head to remain flexed as it emerges. The perineum retracts and the head is born.

***10.** Restitution occurs as the neck untwists to allow the occiput to rotate 45°, from OA back to the LOA position, restoring the long axis of the vertex to a 90° angle with the long axis of the shoulders.

8-2. The chest and shoulders rotate internally according to their position.

8-2-A. The chest and shoulders complete their second internal rotation, moving 45° from the left oblique into the anteroposterior diameter before or during the next contraction.

8-2-B. The chest and shoulders complete their first internal rotation, moving 45° from the left oblique diameter into the anteroposterior diameter before or during the next contraction.

8-2-C. The chest and shoulders complete their second internal rotation, moving 45° from the left oblique diameter into the anteroposterior diameter before or during the next contraction.

This movement brings the anterior shoulder under the pubic arch.

***11.** Concurrent with the internal rotation of the chest, the head rotates externally 45° from LOA to LOT.

12. The anterior shoulder braces against the pubic bone as the posterior shoulder is born by a process of lateral spinal flexion. Birth of the posterior shoulder reduces the diameter of the upper torso, allowing the anterior shoulder to slip past the pubic bone and emerge.

13. The torso and legs are born by a process of lateral flexion and a spiraling motion.

Moulding is similar in all anterior vertex positions. Any caput that forms in an LOT baby will appear over the posterior portion of the left parietal bone near the crown of the vertex and may overlie suture lines.

LOT orientation, head partially flexed	Posterior asynclitic descent to engagement	Anterior asynclitism after engagement.	Internal rotation of head begins: LOT to LOA.
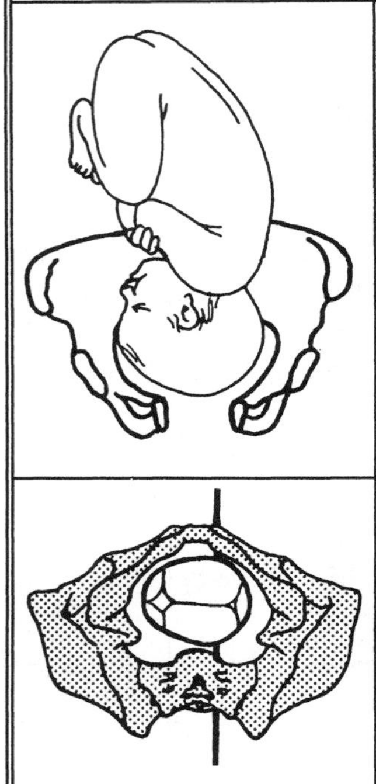	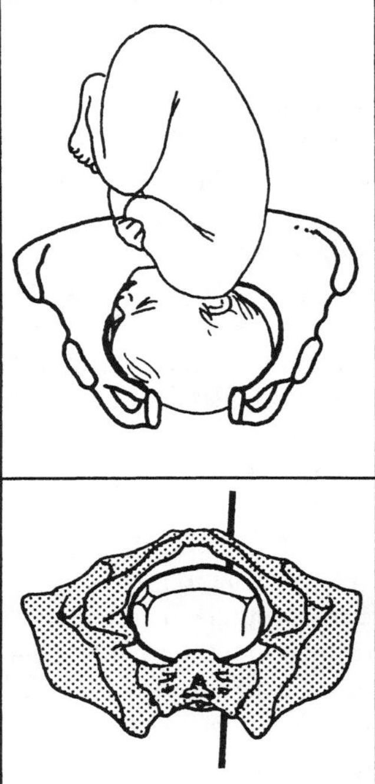	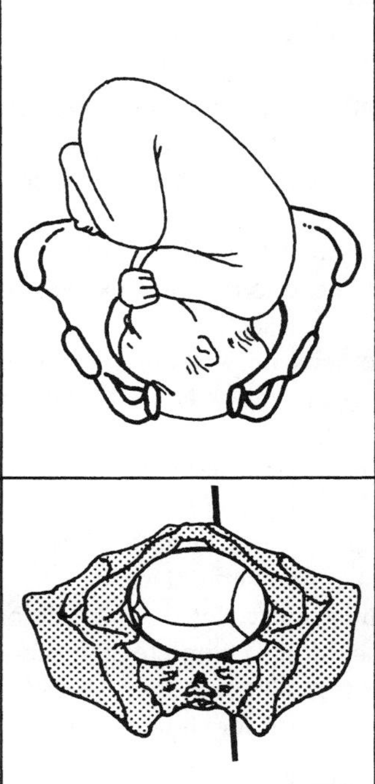	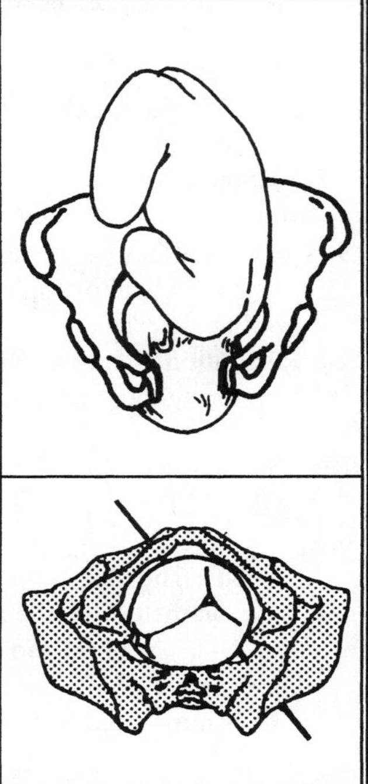
Internal rotation from LOA to OA; shoulders follow the head and engage transverse.	Midchest descends, rotates to oblique. Upper spine extends as head is born.	The head restitutes 45° from OA to LOA.	Chest rotates AP; head follows, rotating externally LOA to LOT. Shoulders are born.
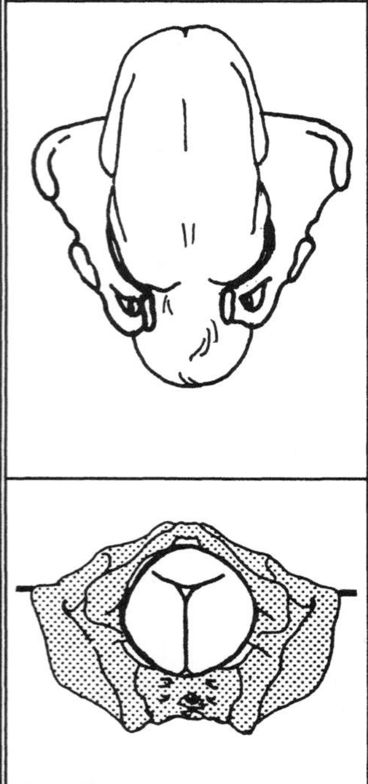	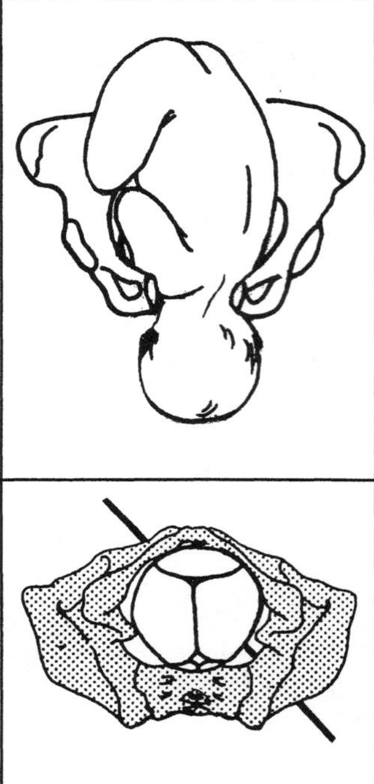	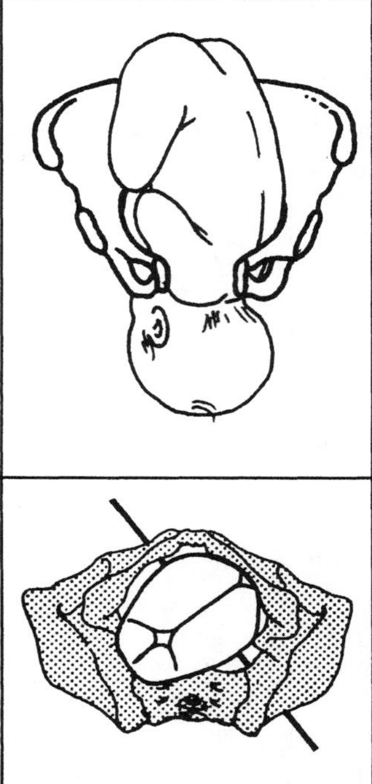	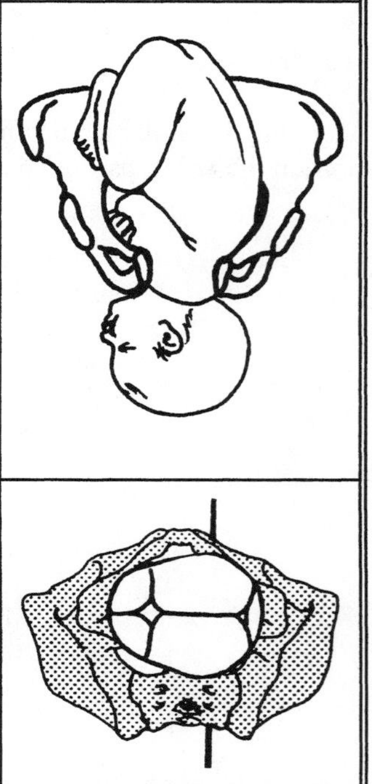

Summary of the Cardinal Spiraling Movements: Right Occiput Transverse (ROT)

Birth from the ROT position is the mirror opposite of birth from the LOT position. Most of the details given for LOT descent in the previous chapter, such as variations in the way the shoulders rotate and are born, apply to all vertex presentations. This chapter and most that follow will summarize the cardinal movements unique to each anterior vertex position. For more details regarding why things occur as well as possible variations, reread the chapter entitled "The Process of Birth in Occiput Anterior Vertex Presentations" and the subchapter entitled "The Cardinal Spiraling Movements: Left Occiput Transverse."

Orientation of the baby to the mother's pelvis

The sagittal suture is aligned with the transverse diameter of the brim, while the occiput is to the mother's right. The shoulder axis is aligned with the anteroposterior diameter.

Birth of the ROT baby

***1.** The degree of head and spinal flexion varies; however, many babies are fairly well flexed prior to the onset of labor. After complete dilation, flexion of the head is often enhanced as it contacts the pelvic floor.

***2.** The baby descends throughout labor. Prior to engagement, the head is in an attitude of posterior asynclitism, with the sagittal suture above or slightly behind the symphysis.

***3.** The head engages as the biparietal diameter passes through the anteroposterior diameter of the brim. Posterior asynclitism allows the posterior parietal bone (the baby's right) to descend into the roomy sacral curve. The process of engagement converts the attitude to one of anterior asynclitism, which may persist until internal rotation is complete.

***4.** The head rotates internally a total of 90° from ROT to OA, as it adapts to the loop-shaped opening of the levator ani sling. Rotation consists of a downwardly spiraling movement, which facilitates descent. Internal rotation usually occurs after dilation is complete and the vertex has passed the ischial spines. It begins as the head rotates 45° from the ROT position to ROA. Then the head rotates another 45° to OA.

5. The baby's body moves with the shoulders as they undergo their first internal rotation. Following the rotation of the occiput from ROT to ROA, the shoulders rotate 45° from the anteroposterior diameter to align with the right oblique diameter. As the occiput rotates from ROA to OA, the shoulders rotate another 45° to align with the transverse diameter of the brim, 90° in all.

6. The shoulders engage when the bisacromial diameter enters the transverse diameter of the brim, as the head passes through the ischial tuberosities. The attitude of the shoulders shifts during descent as the torso accommodates to the shape of the birth canal.

7. The spine begins to extend as the head enters the pelvis more deeply.

8-1. The second internal rotation of the shoulders begins between the time the head distends the perineum and is born. As the midchest and spine enter the curve of the birth canal near the level of the ischial spines, they rotate 45°, moving the shoulders from the transverse into the right oblique diameter. This adjustment allows the spine to flex laterally. The neck twists as this occurs, allowing the head to remain OA.

***9.** The head glides down past the pubic arch and begins to crown as the lower neck and upper spine extend under the pubic arch, allowing the head to remain flexed as it emerges. The perineum retracts and the head is born.

***10.** Restitution occurs as the neck untwists to allow the occiput to rotate 45°, from OA back to the ROA position, restoring the long axis of the vertex to a 90° angle with the long axis of the shoulders.

8-2. The chest and shoulders complete their second internal rotation, moving 45° from the right oblique into the anteroposterior diameter before or during the next contraction. This brings the anterior shoulder under the pubic arch.

***11.** Concurrent with the internal rotation of the chest, the head rotates externally 45° from ROA to ROT.

12. The anterior shoulder braces against the pubic bone as the posterior shoulder is born first by a process of lateral spinal flexion, after which the anterior shoulder slips past the pubic bone and emerges.

13. The torso and legs are born by a process of lateral flexion and a spiraling motion.

Moulding is similar in all occiput anterior positions. Any caput that forms in an ROT baby will appear over the posterior portion of the right parietal bone near the crown of the vertex and may overlie suture lines.

ROT orientation, head partially flexed	Posterior asynclitic descent to engagement	Anterior asynclitism after engagement.	Internal rotation of head begins: ROT to ROA.
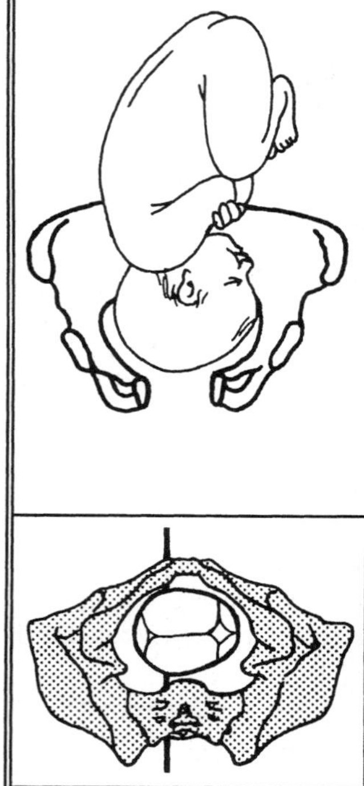	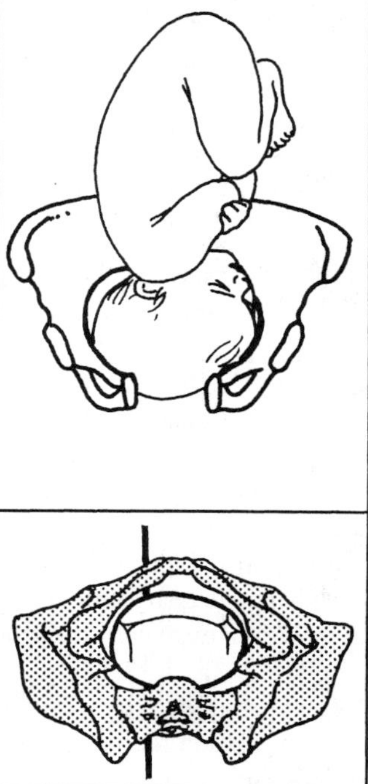	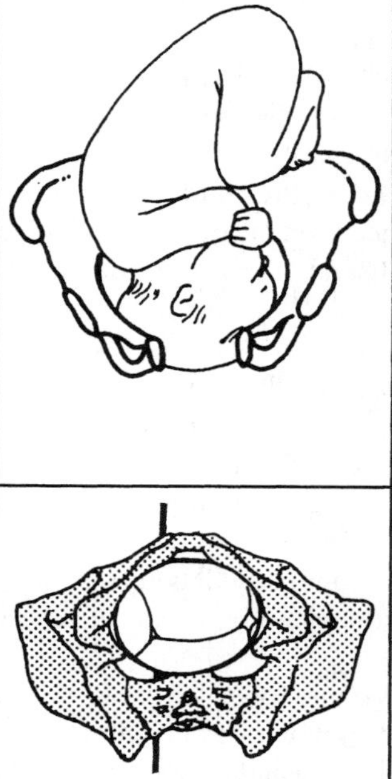	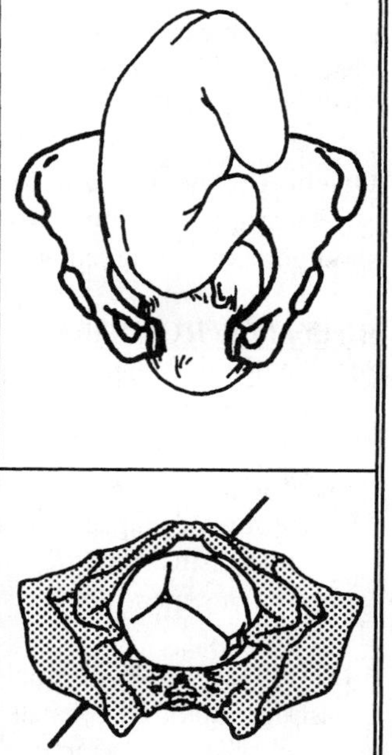
Internal rotation from ROA to OA; shoulders follow the head and engage transverse.	Midchest descends, rotates to oblique. Upper spine extends flexed head is born.	The head restitutes 45° from OA to ROA.	Chest rotates AP; head follows, rotating externally: ROA to ROT. Shoulders are born.
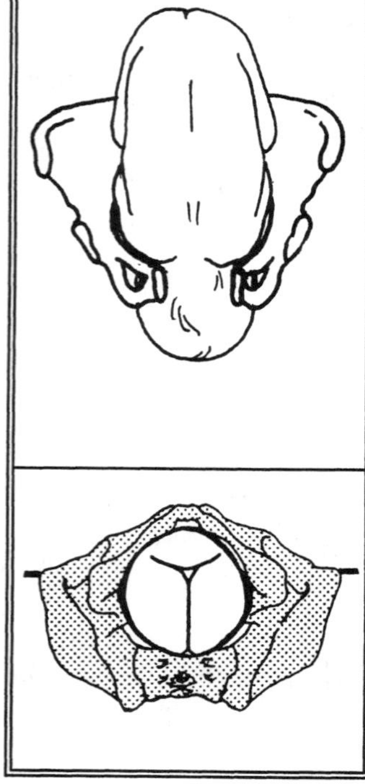	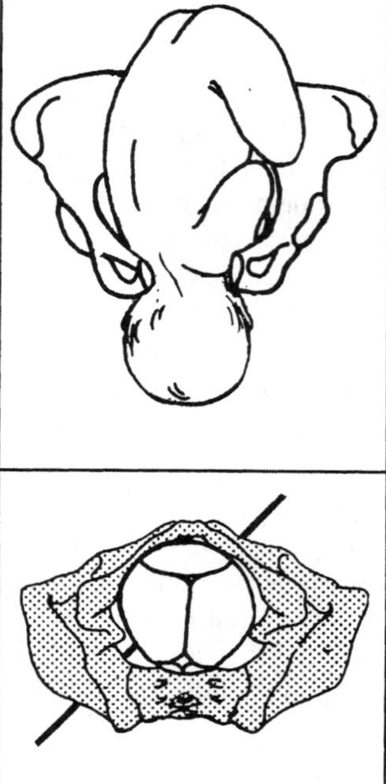	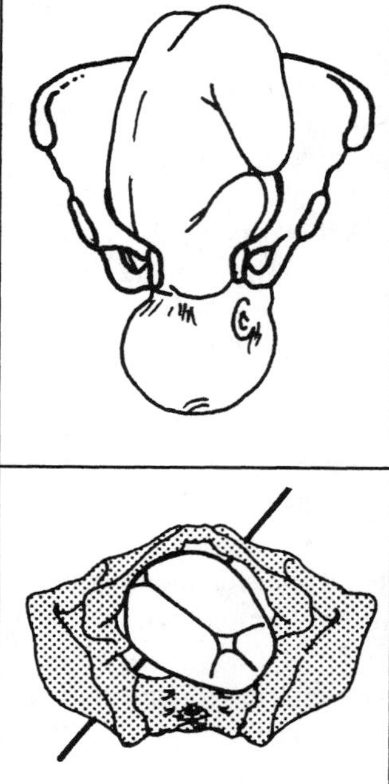	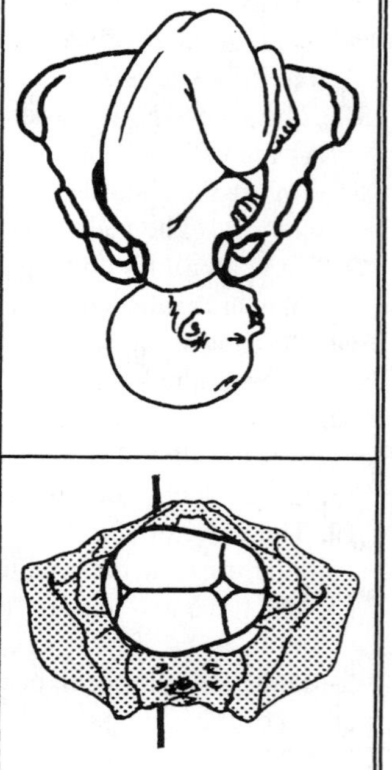

Summary of the Cardinal Spiraling Movements: Left Occiput Anterior (LOA)

The process of birth when the baby is in the left occiput anterior position (LOA) is similar in most respects to birth in the LOT position; the primary difference is that the head only rotates internally 45° to reach the OA position.

Orientation of the baby to the mother's pelvis

The sagittal suture is aligned with the right oblique diameter while the occiput occupies the left anterior corner of the pelvis. The shoulder axis is aligned with the left oblique diameter.

Birth of the LOA baby

***1.** The degree of head and spinal flexion varies; however, many babies are fairly well flexed prior to the onset of labor. After complete dilation, flexion of the head is often enhanced as it contacts the pelvic floor.

***2.** The baby descends throughout labor.

***3.** The head engages as the biparietal diameter passes through the brim. The head often rotates 45° from LOA to LOT by turning at the neck so that the baby can take advantage of posterior asynclitic descent. Once engaged, the head restitutes to an LOA orientation.

***4.** The head rotates internally a total of 45° from LOA to OA, as it adapts to the loop-shaped opening of the levator ani sling. Rotation consists of a downwardly spiraling movement, which facilitates descent. Internal rotation usually occurs after dilation is complete and the vertex has passed the ischial spines. Pressure from the pelvic soft tissues often results in slight asynclitism until rotation is complete.

5. The baby's body moves with the shoulders as they undergo their first internal rotation. Following the rotation of the occiput from LOA to OA, the shoulders rotate 45° from the left oblique diameter to align with the transverse diameter of the brim.

6. The shoulders engage when the bisacromial diameter enters the transverse diameter of the brim, as the head passes through the ischial tuberosities. The attitude of the shoulders shifts during descent as the torso accommodates to the shape of the birth canal.

7. The spine begins to extend as the head enters the pelvis more deeply.

8-1. The second internal rotation of the shoulders begins between the time the head distends the perineum and is born. As the midchest and spine enter the curve of the birth canal near the level of the ischial spines, they rotate 45°, moving the shoulders from the transverse into the left oblique diameter. This adjustment allows the spine to flex laterally. The neck twists as this occurs, allowing the head to remain OA.

***9.** The head glides down past the pubic arch and begins to crown as the lower neck and upper spine extend under the pubic arch, allowing the head to remain flexed as it emerges. The perineum retracts and the head is born.

***10.** Restitution occurs as the neck untwists to allow the occiput to rotate 45°, from OA back to the LOA position, restoring the long axis of the vertex to a 90° angle with the long axis of the shoulders.

8-2. The chest and shoulders complete their second internal rotation, moving 45° from the left oblique into the antero-posterior diameter before or during the next contraction. This brings the anterior shoulder under the pubic arch.

***11.** Concurrent with the internal rotation of the chest, the head rotates externally 45° from LOA to LOT.

12. The anterior shoulder braces against the pubic bone as the posterior shoulder is born first by a process of lateral spinal flexion, after which the anterior shoulder slips past the pubic bone and emerges.

13. The torso and legs are born by a process of lateral flexion and a spiraling motion.

Moulding is essentially the same for all anterior vertex positions. Any caput that forms in an LOA baby will appear on the posterior portion of the left parietal bone near the crown of the vertex and may overlie suture lines.

LOA orientation, head partially flexed	Descent to engagement, flexion enhanced	Internal rotation of head: LOA to OA. Shoulders follow to engage transverse.
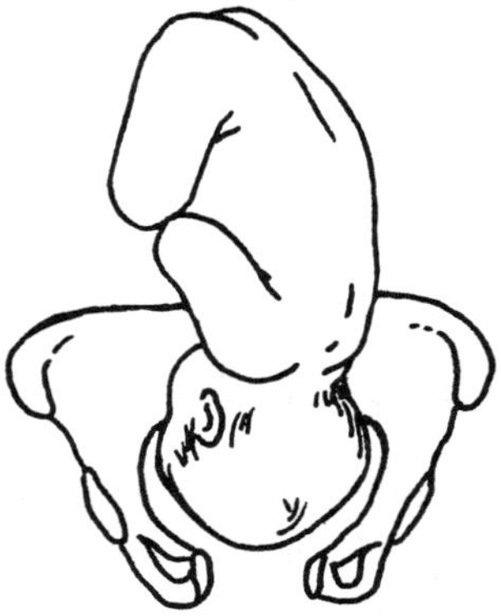	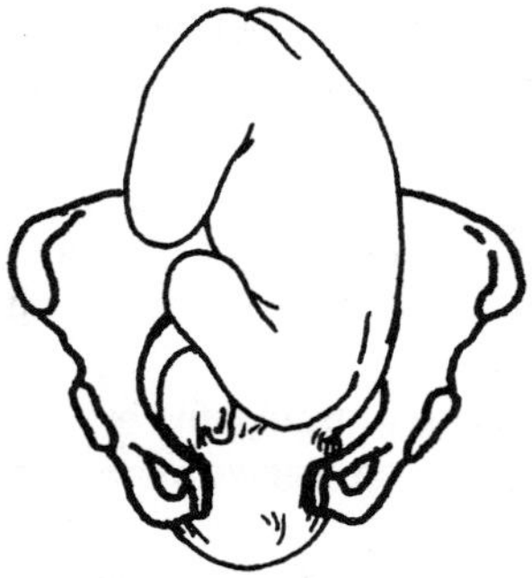	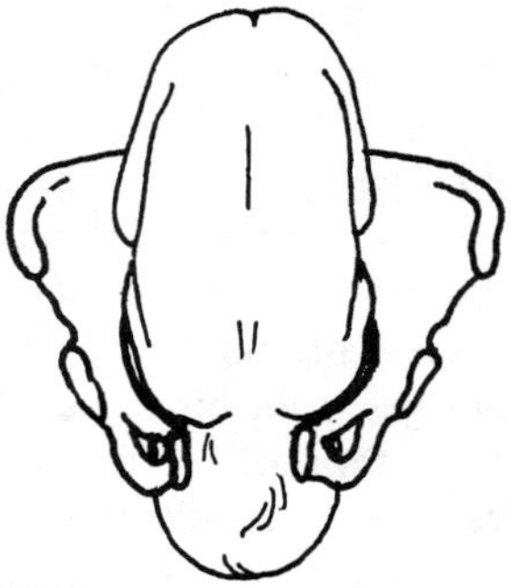
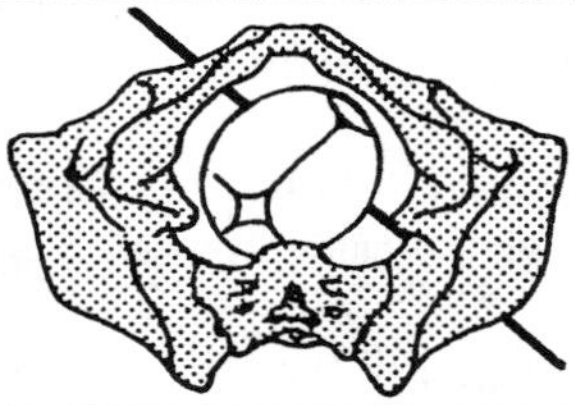	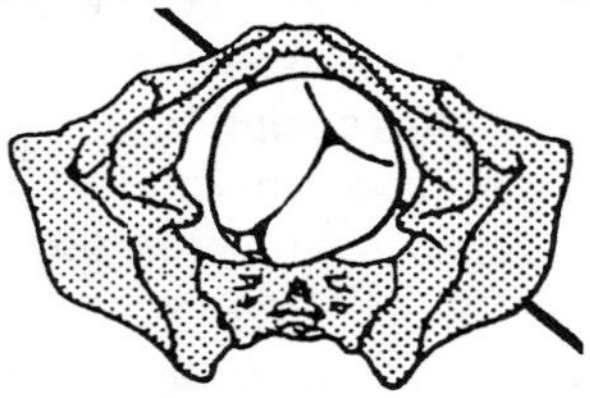	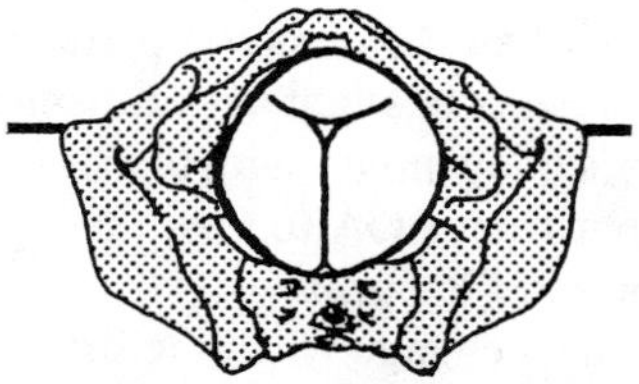

Midchest descends, rotates to oblique. Upper spine extends as head is born.	The head restitutes 45° from OA to LOA.	Chest rotates AP; head follows, rotating externally: LOA to LOT. Shoulders are born.
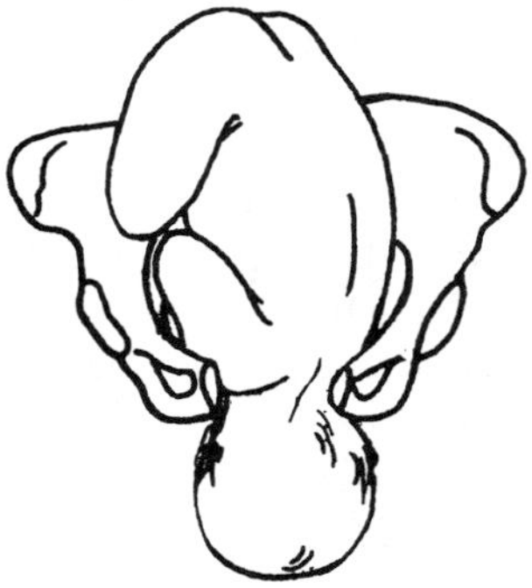	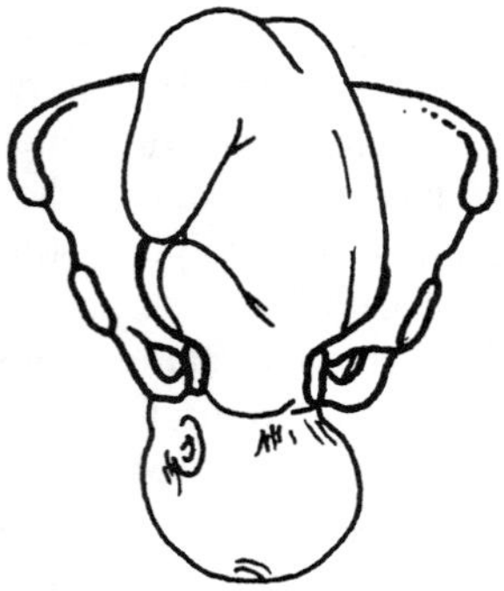	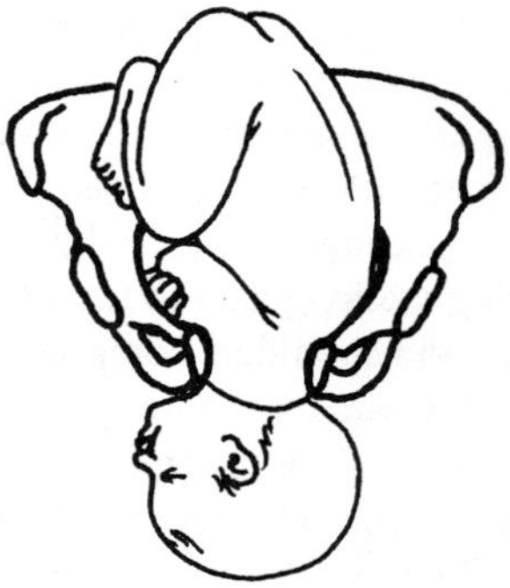
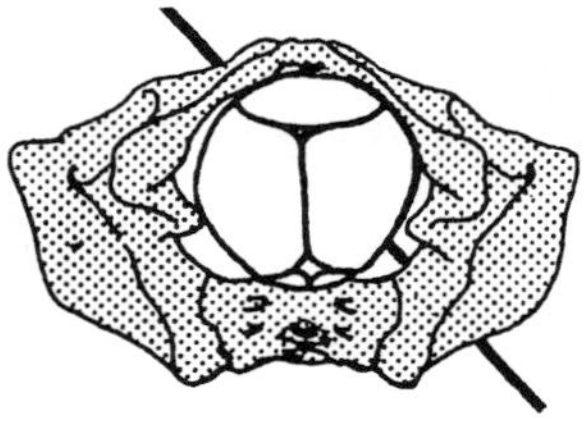	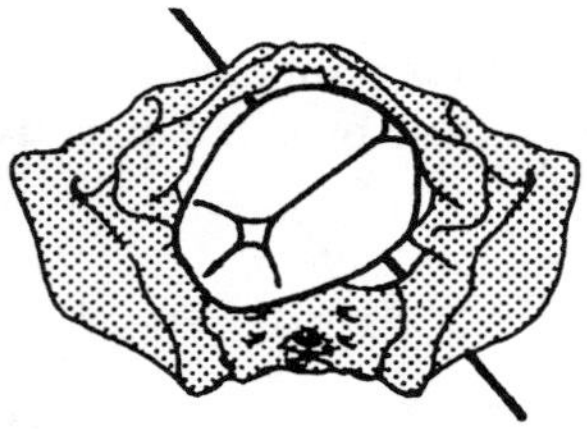	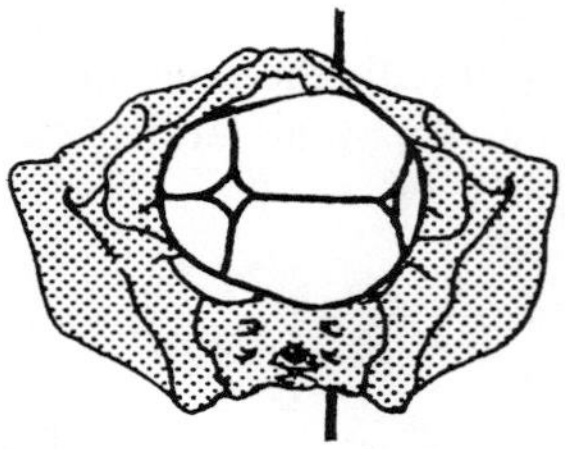

Summary of the Cardinal Spiraling Movements: Right Occiput Anterior (ROA)

The process of birth when the baby is in the right occiput anterior position (ROA) is a mirror image of birth in the LOA position.

Orientation of the baby to the mother's pelvis

The sagittal suture is aligned with the left oblique diameter while the occiput occupies the right anterior corner of the pelvis. The shoulder axis is aligned with the right oblique diameter.

Birth of the ROA baby:

***1.** The degree of head and spinal flexion varies; however, many babies are fairly well flexed prior to the onset of labor. After complete dilation, flexion of the head is often enhanced as it contacts the pelvic floor.

***2.** The baby descends throughout labor.

***3.** The head engages as the biparietal diameter passes through the brim. The head often rotates 45° from ROA to ROT by turning at the neck so that the baby can take advantage of posterior asynclitic descent. Once engaged, the head restitutes to an ROA orientation.

***4.** The head rotates internally a total of 45° from ROA to OA, as it adapts to the loop-shaped opening of the levator ani sling. Rotation consists of a downwardly spiraling movement, which facilitates descent. Internal rotation usually occurs after dilation is complete and the vertex has passed the ischial spines. Pressure from the pelvic soft tissues often results in slight asynclitism until rotation is complete.

5. The baby's body moves with the shoulders as they undergo their first internal rotation. Following the rotation of the occiput from ROA to OA, the shoulders rotate 45° from the right oblique diameter to align with the transverse diameter of the brim.

6. The shoulders engage when the bisacromial diameter enters the transverse diameter of the brim, as the head passes through the ischial tuberosities. The attitude of the shoulders shifts during descent as the torso accommodates to the shape of the birth canal.

7. The spine begins to extend as the head enters the pelvis more deeply.

8-1. The second internal rotation of the shoulders begins between the time the head distends the perineum and is born. As the midchest and spine enter the curve of the birth canal near the level of the ischial spines, they rotate 45°, moving the shoulders from the transverse into the right oblique diameter. This adjustment allows the spine to flex laterally. The neck twists as this occurs, allowing the head to remain OA.

***9.** The head glides down past the pubic arch and begins to crown as the lower neck and upper spine extend under the pubic arch, allowing the head to remain flexed as it emerges. The perineum retracts and the head is born.

***10.** Restitution occurs as the neck untwists to allow the occiput to rotate 45°, from OA back to the ROA position, restoring the long axis of the vertex to a 90° angle with the long axis of the shoulders.

8-2. The chest completes its second internal rotation, moving the shoulders 45° from the right oblique into the antero-posterior diameter before or during the next contraction. This brings the anterior shoulder under the pubic arch.

***11.** Concurrent with the internal rotation of the chest, the head rotates externally 45° from ROA to ROT.

12. The anterior shoulder braces against the pubic bone as the posterior shoulder is born first by a process of lateral spinal flexion, after which the anterior shoulder slips past the pubic bone and emerges.

13. The torso and legs are born by a process of lateral flexion and a spiraling motion.

Moulding is essentially the same for all anterior vertex positions. Any caput that forms in an ROA baby will appear on the posterior portion of the right parietal bone near the crown of the vertex and may overlie suture lines.

ROA orientation, head partially flexed	Descent to engagement, flexion enhanced	Internal rotation of head: ROA to OA. Shoulders follow to engage transverse.
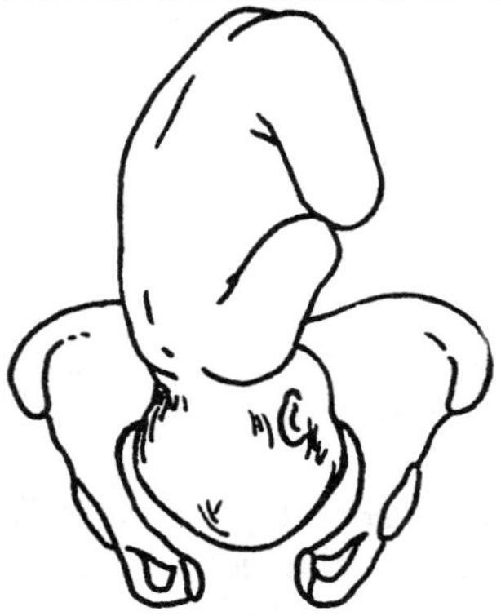	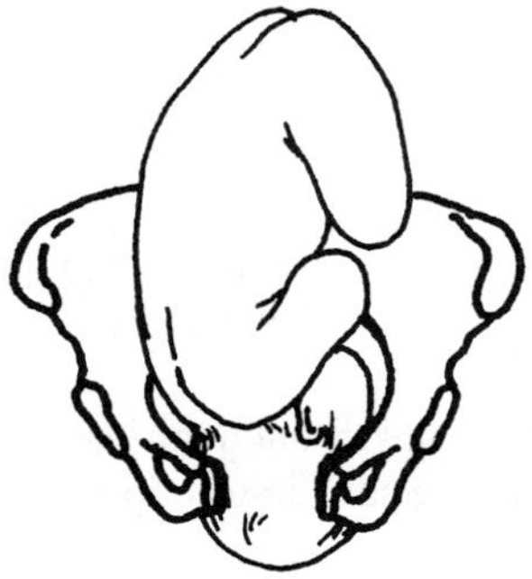	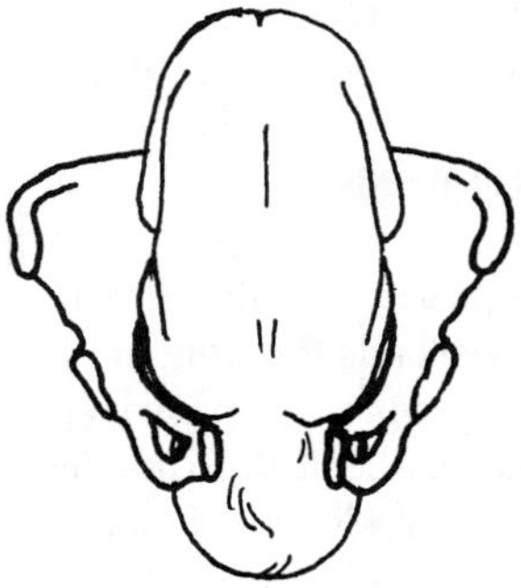
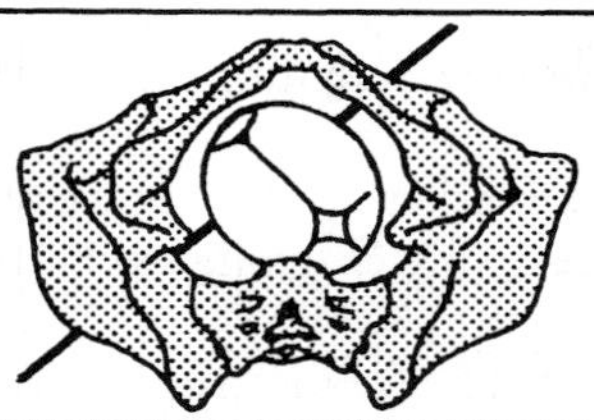	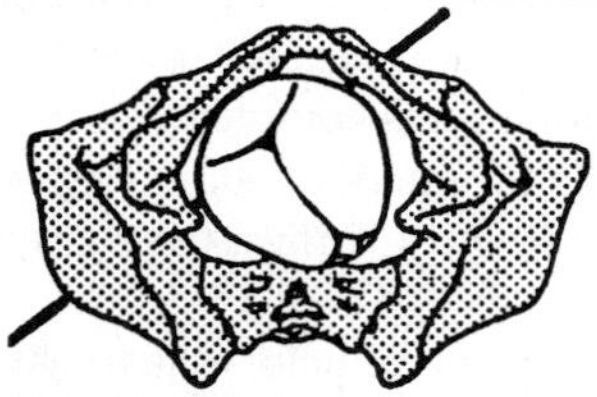	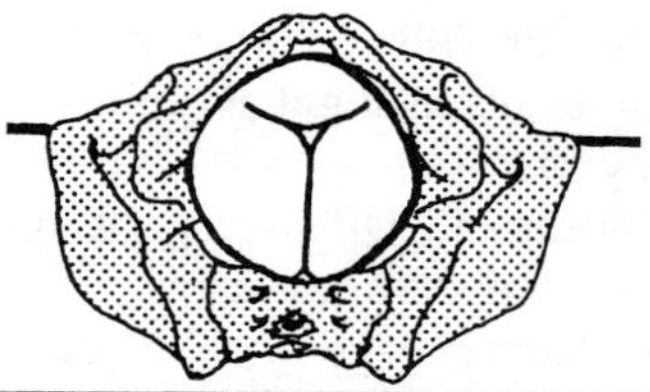
Midchest descends, rotates to oblique. Upper spine extends as head is born.	The head restitutes 45° from OA to ROA.	Chest rotates AP; head follows, rotating externally: ROA to ROT. Shoulders are born.
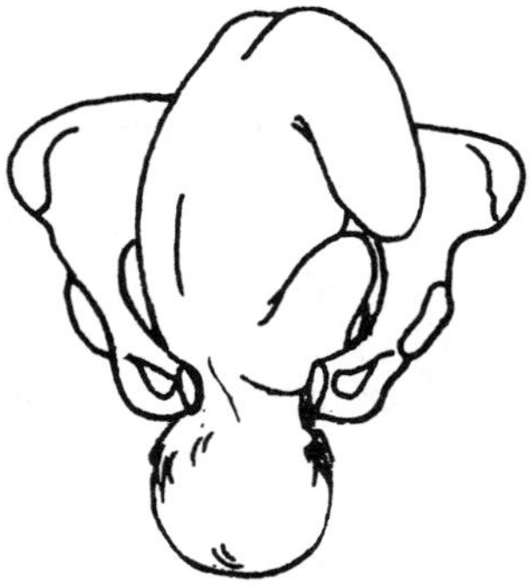	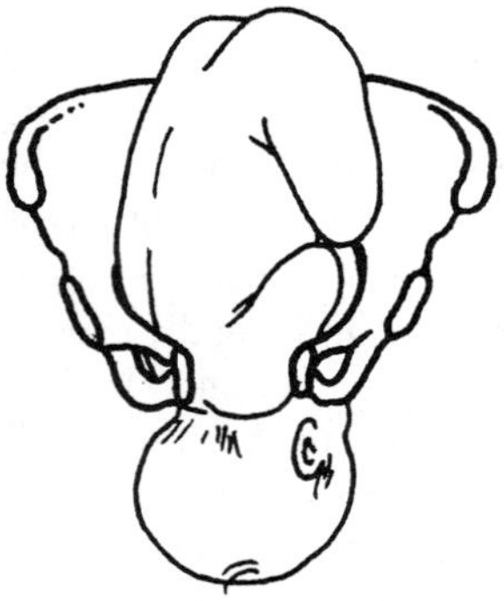	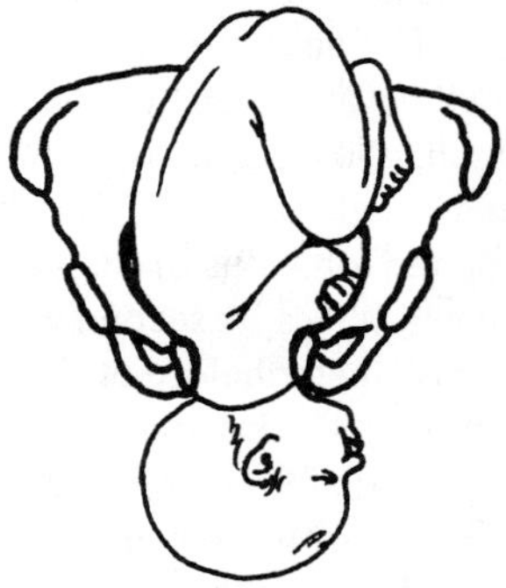
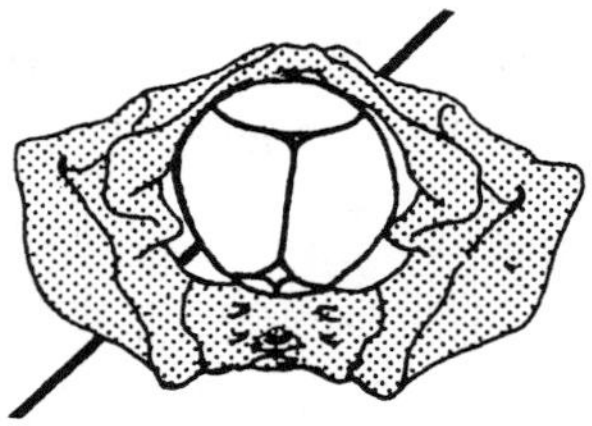	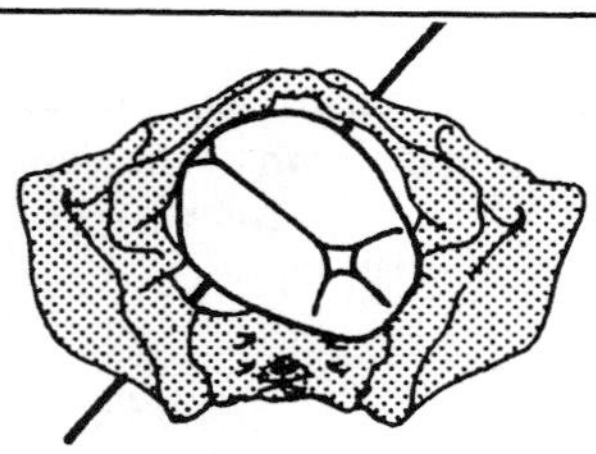	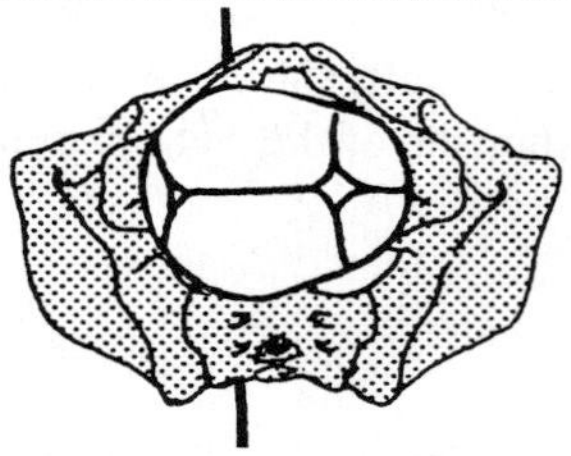

SUMMARY OF THE CARDINAL SPIRALING MOVEMENTS: OCCIPUT ANTERIOR (OA)

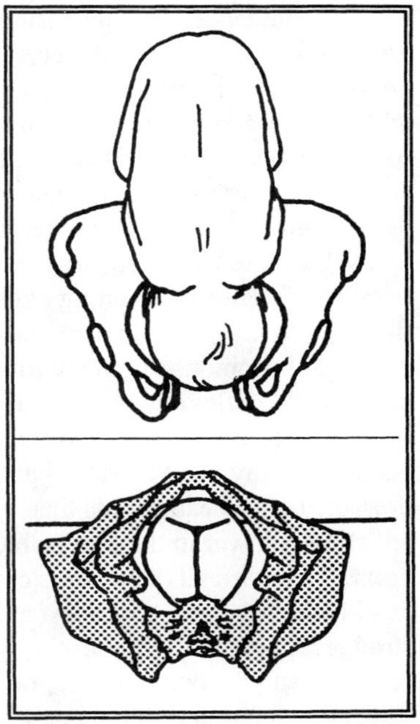

The baby may occasionally assume a direct OA position when the head is still well above the brim, although rotation usually occurs before labor unless the maternal pelvis is unusually large or the baby unusually small, because the long axis of the vertex best accommodates to a transverse or oblique diameter of the brim. Shoulder rotation may occur in either a left or a right direction. Subsequent movements of the occiput will follow accordingly.

Orientation of the baby to the mother's pelvis

The sagittal suture is aligned with the anteroposterior diameter and the occiput is directly anterior, behind the symphysis pubis. The shoulders are aligned with the transverse diameter.

Birth of the directly OA baby (movements not illustrated)

***1.** The degree of head and spinal flexion varies; however, many babies are fairly well flexed prior to the onset of labor. Head flexion is often enhanced after complete dilation, as the head contacts the pelvic floor.

***2.** The baby descends throughout labor.

***3.** The head engages as the biparietal diameter passes through the brim.

***4.** Internal rotation of the head does not occur.

5. The shoulder axis remains aligned with the transverse diameter of the brim.

6. The shoulders engage when the bisacromial diameter enters the transverse diameter of the brim, as the head passes through the ischial tuberosities. The attitude of the shoulders shifts during descent as the torso accommodates to the shape of the birth canal.

7. The spine begins to extend as the head enters the pelvis more deeply.

8-1. Internal rotation of the shoulders begins between the time the head distends the perineum and is born. As the midchest and spine enter the curve of the birth canal near the level of the ischial spines, they rotate 45°, moving the shoulders from the transverse into:

- **8-1-A.** the left oblique diameter (Follow "A" entries below.)
- **8-1-B.** the right oblique diameter (Follow "B" entries below.)

This allows the spine to flex laterally. The neck twists as the torso moves, allowing the head to remain OA.

*** 9.** The head glides down past the pubic arch and begins to crown as the lower neck and upper spine extend under the pubic arch, allowing the head to remain flexed as it emerges. The perineum retracts and the head is born.

***10.** Restitution occurs as the neck untwists to allow the occiput to rotate 45° from OA back to:

- **10-A.** the LOA position.
- **10-B.** the ROA position.

The movement restores the long axis of the vertex to a 90° angle with the long axis of the shoulders.

8-2. The chest completes its second internal rotation, moving the shoulders 45° from:

- **8-2-A.** the left oblique diameter
- **8-2-B.** the right oblique diameter

into the anteroposterior diameter before or during the next contraction. This brings the anterior shoulder under the pubic arch.

***11.** Concurrent with the internal rotation of the chest, the head rotates externally 45°:

- **11-A.** from LOA to LOT.
- **11-B.** from ROA to ROT.

12. The anterior shoulder braces against the pubic bone as the posterior shoulder is born first by a process of lateral spinal flexion, after which the anterior shoulder slips past the pubic bone and emerges.

13. The torso and legs are born by a process of lateral flexion and a spiraling motion.

Moulding is essentially the same for all anterior vertex positions. Any caput that forms will appear on the posterior portion of the posterior parietal bone near the crown of the vertex and may overlie suture lines.

THE PROCESS OF BIRTH IN OCCIPUT POSTERIOR VERTEX PRESENTATIONS

The incidence of babies assuming a posterior (face up or "sunny-side up") position during late pregnancy ranges from 15 to 30%. There are a variety of reasons why babies assume posterior positions prenatally, including an anthropoid pelvis, an anterior placenta, cold maternal abdomen (according to Native Alaskans), and any habitual maternal posture that keeps the knees higher than the tuberosities during pregnancy (Sutton & Scott, 1996) Most of these babies rotate to an occiput anterior position before they are born, although a few are born OP. Right occiput posterior positioning is five times more common than left occiput posterior positioning. One reason for this may be the presence of the descending colon on the mother's right, which may impede the ROP baby from rotating forward to an ROA position.

Why some babies rotate backward rather than forward has been hotly debated for centuries. Beard (1937) studied occiput posterior positioning extensively from a clinical point of view and felt that the posterior shoulder and flank of the persistently posterior baby become jammed against the adjacent lateral aspects of the mother's lower lumbar vertebrae and sacral promontory, preventing rotation. He also felt that the proximity of the lordotic lower spine of the mother encouraged deflexion of the fetal spine and head as the baby tried to get comfortable beside this bony ridge.

He theorized that, once dilation is complete, the fetal head is born into the upper yoni. No internal rotation has yet occurred. Any head flexion that was produced by the tightly applied cervix during dilation is now lessened, releasing pressure on the head, which then becomes somewhat extended. This happens because the posterior portion of the levator ani sling is lower in the pelvis than the anterior end; thus the occiput is not yet in contact with the pelvic floor. At this point, the biparietal diameter is cramped into the space between the sacrum and the ischial spines. The widest part of the head is thus above the weakest and most distant part of the pelvic floor. The forehead contacts the pubococcygeus, the strongest portion of the muscle, which is nearest the anterior pelvic brim. This contact prompts the forehead to rotate forward (and the occiput to rotate backward). (This view is supported by the work of Borell and Fernström [1959] who found that internal rotation begins when the most anterior portion of the presenting part contacts the mouth of levator ani behind the pubic bone.) Beard felt that, by the time the back of the head reaches the pelvic floor (at a lower level in the rear of the pelvis than would be the case if the occiput were anterior), the shoulders will have just entered the brim. At this point, further descent of the head must occur so it can clear the sacrosciatic notch and rotate to the posterior. The shoulders being wedged into the space beside the promontory and the ascending colon probably encourages the shoulders and chest to maintain their oblique orientation as they engage and descend. However, not every persistently posterior labor follows this pattern, and the etiology of persistent posterior positioning and rotation remains not fully understood.

Sutton (2001) believes that maternal postures that close the spinopubic angle impede rotation to the anterior both during late pregnancy and during labor. Conversely, opening the spinopubic angle maximizes space for the baby to turn.

Long-Arc Rotation of the OP Baby

The head may rotate a long way around, so that when the occiput starts out in a posterior oblique orientation, the baby is born OA. This is termed "long-arc rotation" because the baby rotates 135°. The head starts out in the posterior oblique position. If all goes well, descent continues throughout labor and pushing. However, because OP babies tend to have trouble flexing their heads and spines, engagement and descent may be delayed.

Full flexion may not occur until the head reaches the pelvic floor, where the soft and bony tissues encourage better flexion as well as internal rotation. The occiput will eventually rotate 135°, winding up beneath the pubic bone. First, the occiput moves 45° from an oblique posterior position to OT. At the same time, the baby's body and shoulders begin their first internal rotation, rotating 45° to arrive in the anteroposterior pelvic diameter. The occiput continues to rotate another 45° from OT to oblique anterior. The shoulder axis moves into the adjacent oblique pelvic diameter as this occurs. Internal rotation is complete when the occiput rotates an additional 45° to arrive directly beneath the pubic bone (OA). As this occurs, the head usually spirals deeper into the pelvis.

In many cases, the shoulders continue to follow the head, rotating 45° into the transverse diameter of the pelvis. When this occurs, they typically return to the oblique diameter that they passed through most recently during their second internal rotation. The shoulders may also lag behind to remain in the oblique diameter as the occiput rotates its last 45° from oblique anterior to OA. Now birth proceeds, depending upon the position of the torso, as for an LOT or ROT position. Moulding may present as a combination of that typically seen with OA and OP positions. Due to the changes in position during descent, the baby's head may also appear to have typical OA moulding.

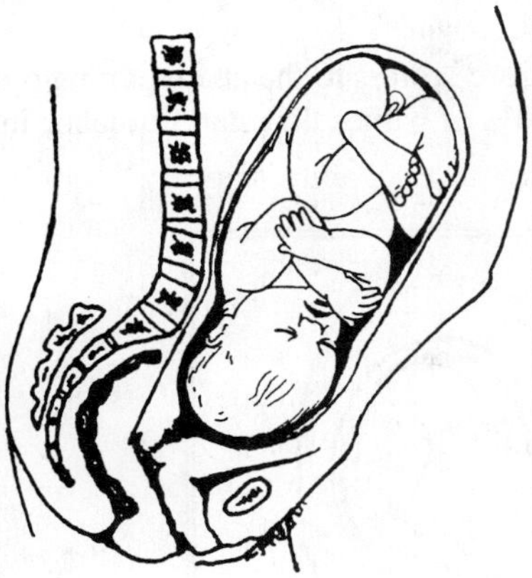

Baby LOP at onset of labor

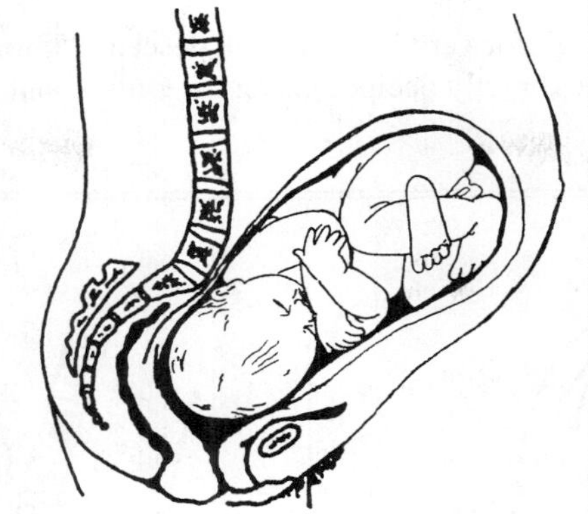

Dilation underway, descent (2) to engagement (3), spinal flexion enhanced (1)

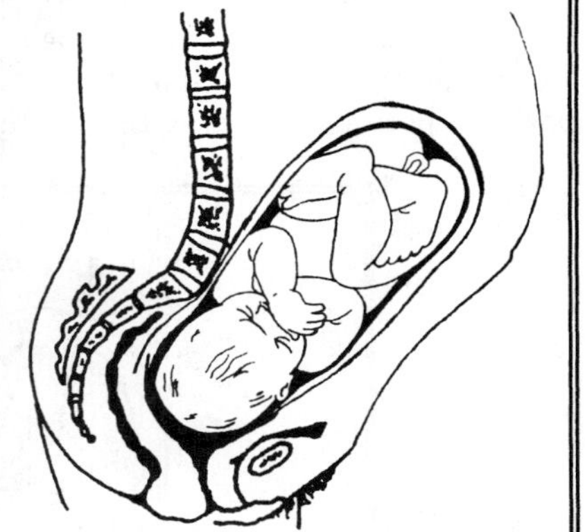

Internal rotation of head begins (4): LOP to LOT. Chest moves to AP (5).

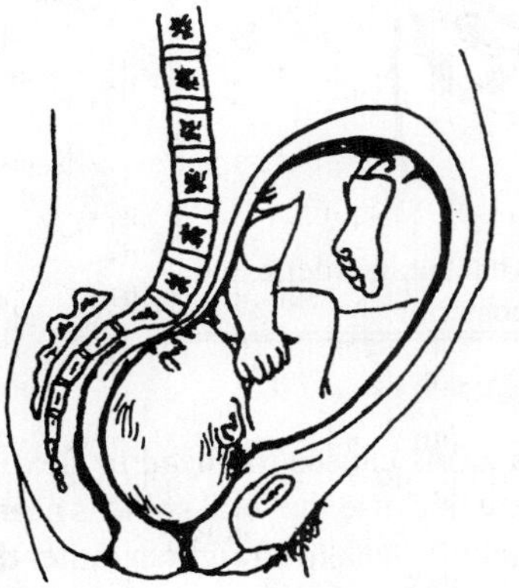

Internal rotation of head: LOT to LOA (4). Chest follows, rotating internally to oblique (5)

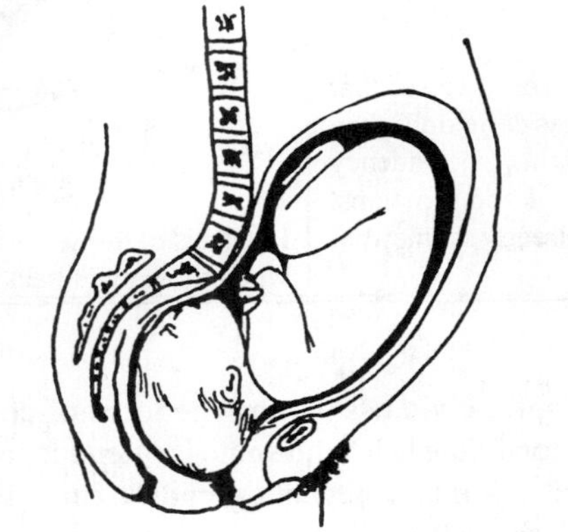

Internal rotation of head: LOA to OA (4). Chest follows to transverse and engages(6)

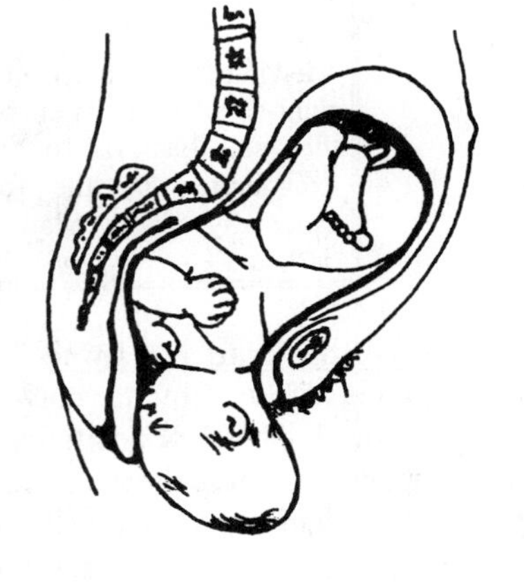

Shoulders rotate to oblique (8-1), spine extends (7, 9) as head is born

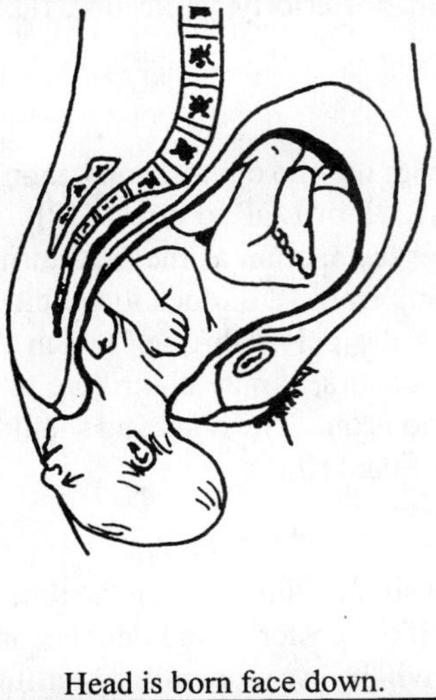

Head is born face down.

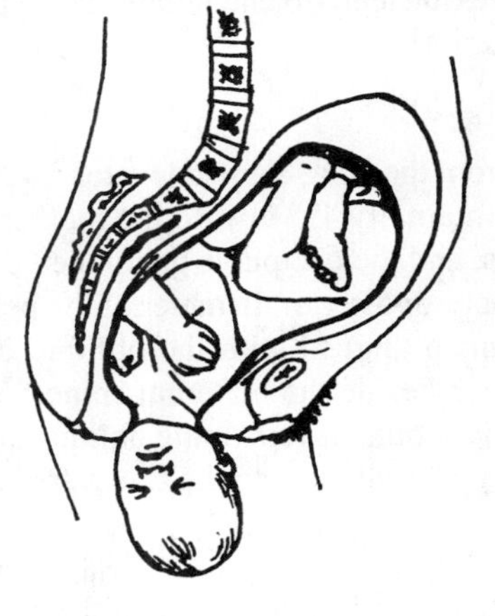

Restitution of head (10)

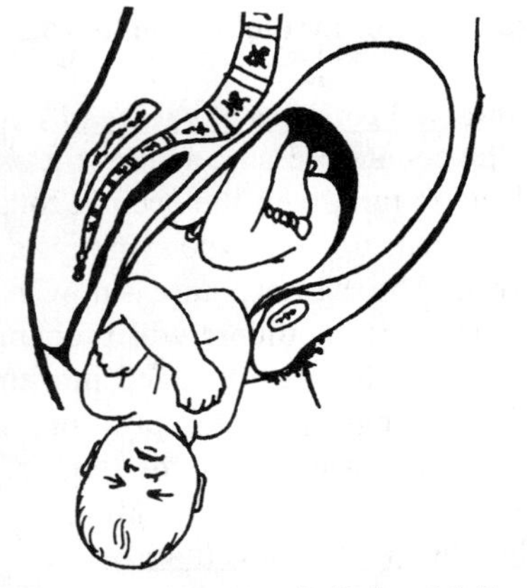

Chest rotates to AP (8-2), head follows, rotating externally to LOT (11), shoulders and body are born (12, 13)

(Numbers in the drawings match the explanatory notes in this chapter associated with each cardinal spiraling movement.)

Short-Arc Rotation of the OP Baby

Short-arc rotation occurs during straightforward LOP or ROP descent. "Short-arc" refers to the head rotating only 45° toward the mother's spine to become directly occiput posterior. Only about 10% of babies that start out labor in a posterior position remain so until birth.

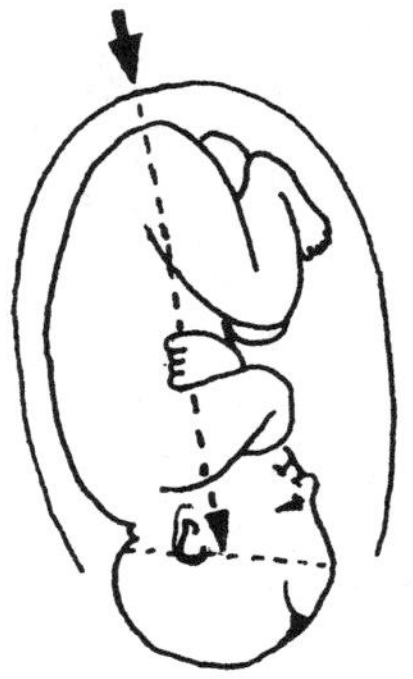

Viewing the mother from the front, we see that right-sided obliquity encourages deflexion when the fetal back is to the right., a tendency exaggerated by the force of contractions, especially if the head is already somewhat deflexed.

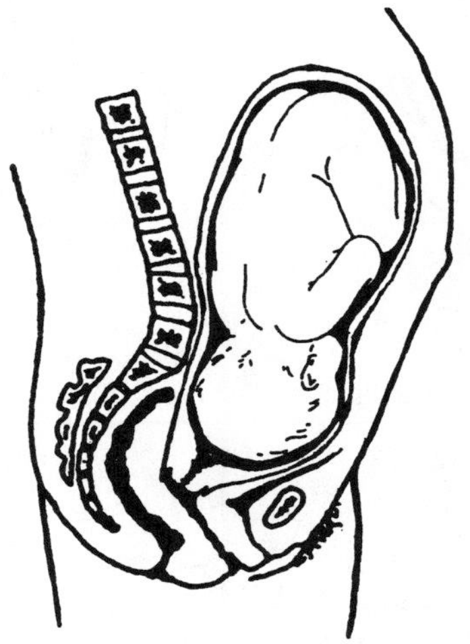

Lordosis of the spine also encourages deflexion when the baby's back is posterior.

***1. Flexion of the head and spine**

Resistance afforded by the bony and soft pelvic tissues and the force of contractions causes the head to flex to a varying degree. In posterior positions, flexion of the head and spine is often incomplete because the fetal spine is nearest the mother's spine, where the increased lordosis of late pregnancy tends to cause the baby's back to straighten rather than curl forward, a tendency enhanced once contractions begin. Furthermore, in those women who have a right-sided obliquity (tilt) of the uterine fundus, the fetal back being to the right causes uterine activity to encourage deflexion; when the pressure is applied directly over the back, the back tends to extend.

As a result, the larger occipitofrontal diameter of the skull may present, often delaying descent and dilation, and prolonging the pushing phase of labor. Deflexion tends to encourage the occiput to rotate posteriorly, while more flexion makes it easier for the occiput to rotate anteriorly.

***4. Internal rotation of the head**

The counterpressure against the skull from the sling-shaped levator ani, coupled with uterine contractions, prompts the head to turn, with the occiput rotating internally 45° toward the mother's spine (ROP or LOP to direct OP). The sinciput ends up under the symphysis pubis, and the occiput is positioned directly over the sacrum as the head turns at the neck. The sagittal suture is now in the anteroposterior diameter of the pelvis (running from 12 o'clock to 6 o'clock). The chest and shoulders will probably remain aligned with the oblique diameter of the pelvis through which they descended if they are wedged into the space beside the maternal spine. When this occurs, it may contribute to the persistent occiput posterior position, with the shoulders remaining oblique until the head is out. The body and shoulders may also follow the head, rotating 45° from the oblique into the transverse diameter of the brim.

5. Engagement of the shoulders

The shoulders begin their descent through an oblique diameter of the pelvic inlet at some point between the time the head reaches the pelvic floor and crowning. Rotation to the transverse may be impaired if the posterior shoulder becomes lodged against the sacral promontory. If the baby's spine is extended, the shoulder axis will be in a more military attitude, which may also result in the anterior shoulder becoming impinged on the pubic bone, impairing rotation to the transverse diameter and making engagement of the shoulders more difficult (Sutton, 2001).

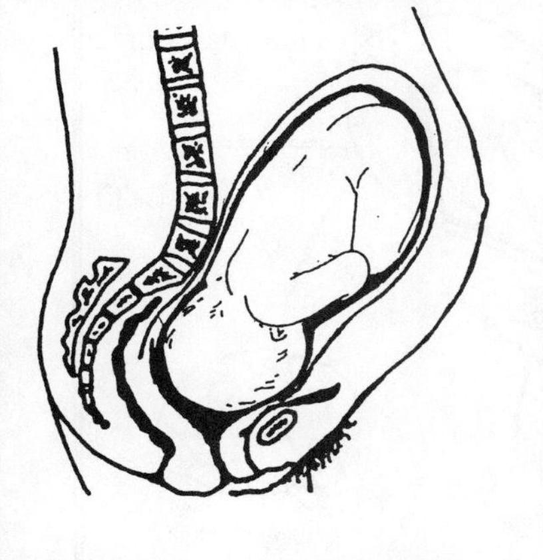

Baby ROP, descent well underway (2), dilation complete; engagement (3) has occurred; spine is somewhat deflexed (1)

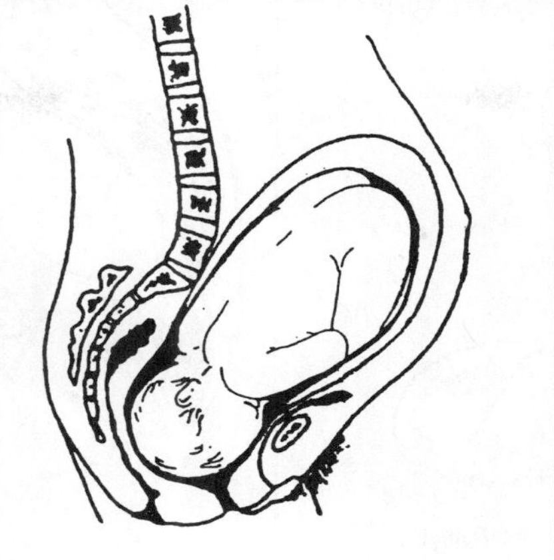

Flexion (1) is enhanced; internal rotation (4) ROP to OP

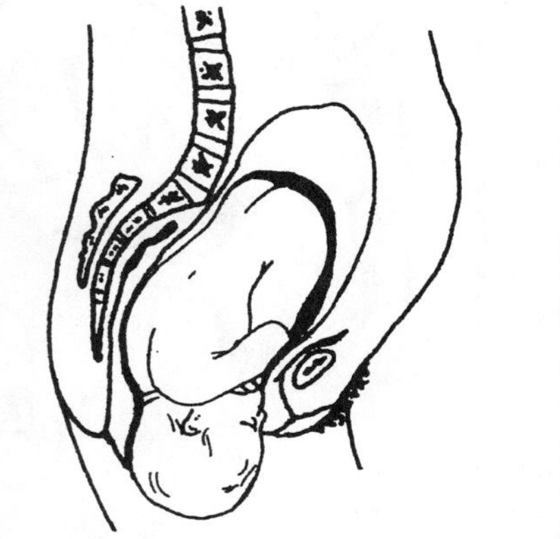

Shoulders remain oblique (5) and engage (6) as head passes ischial tuberosities

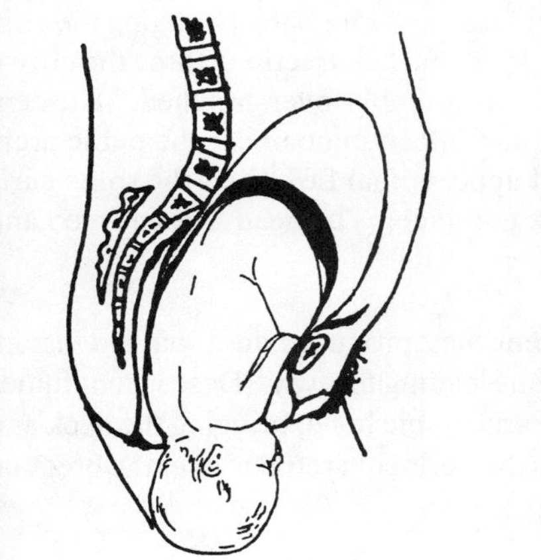

The head is born "sunny side up" by spinal flexion and extension (9)

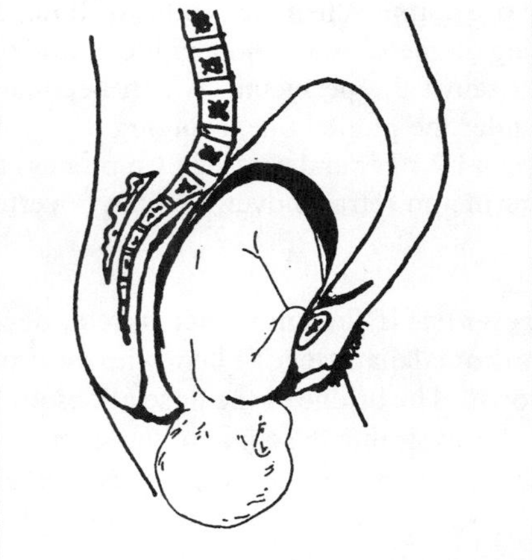

Head restitutes 45° from OP to ROP (10)

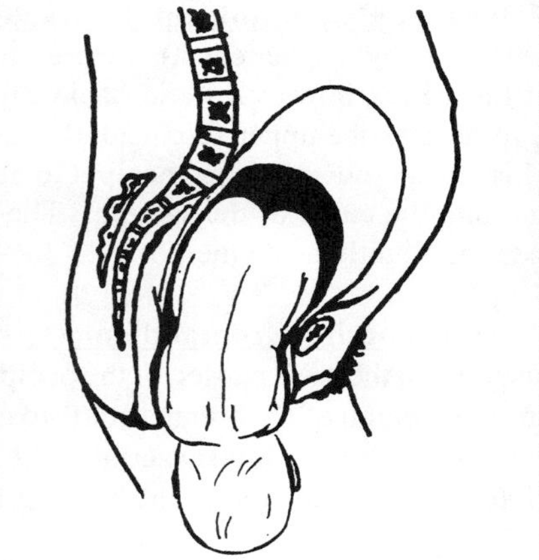

Shoulders rotate AP (8-2) as head rotates externally 45°: ROP to ROT (11); shoulders (12) and body (13) are born

• Dilating the perineum

The head is pressed firmly against the pelvic floor, poised to begin rocking back and forth as the mother pushes. The head rocks forward with each push and then recedes between contractions. This process presses the occiput into the perineal floor, massaging the soft tissues, making more and more room for the occiput in the hollow of the sacrum. Once the pelvic floor is sufficiently softened, the biparietal diameter will stay beneath the pubic bone, and crowning begins.

***9. Birth of the head by a process of spinal flexion and extension**

In light of the work of Borell and Fernström (1957b), as well as what can be observed during birth itself, the way the posterior head emerges from the lower birth canal is not described accurately in most texts. There are two ways the birth of the head can occur in a direct OP birth. Which of these occurs depends upon the degree to which the head is flexed. These descriptions apply to all posterior births, regardless of the position the baby assumes prior to labor (ROP, LOP or direct OP).

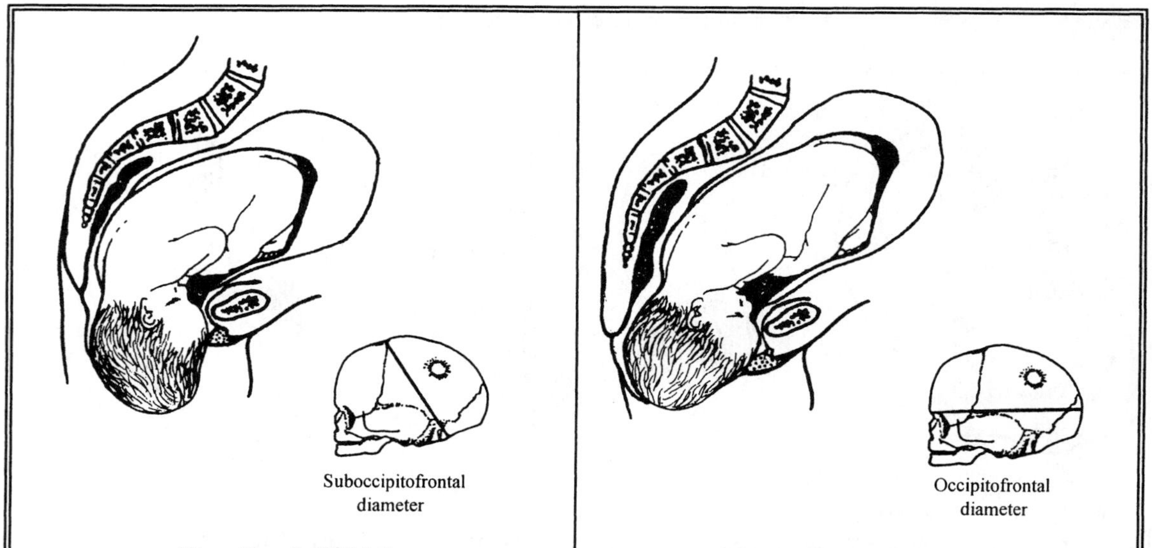

Flexed head: OP birth

Incompletely flexed head: OP birth

When the suboccipitofrontal diameter presents: When the head is well flexed for a posterior baby (bringing the chin near the baby's upper chest), the presenting diameter is the suboccipitofrontal of 10.5 cm. Contractions force the crown of the vertex downward and backward against the perineum, which becomes considerably overstretched. Descent continues as the upper forehead glides under the pubic bone, bringing the neck and upper spine under the pubic arch. This allows the vertex and occiput to descend further and emerge by a process of upper spinal flexion as the spine curls and into the curve of the sacrum. The perineum retracts over the baby's vertex and face. The head is then freed and extends slightly as it emerges.

When the occipitofrontal diameter presents: If flexion is incomplete, descent may produce additional extension, resulting in the presentation of the occipitofrontal diameter of 11 cm with the bregma leading the way. Descent continues until the region of the bregma starts to crown. The bridge of the nose glides under the pubic bone, bringing the neck and upper spine into the lower sacrum. The spine curls into the curve of the sacrum as the perineum retracts over the bregma, vertex, face and occiput. The head is then freed and extends slightly as it emerges.

***10. Restitution**

Restitution occurs after the head is out. The neck untwists, and the occiput returns 45° to a posterior oblique orientation (OP to ROP or LOP), realigning the long axis of the head to a 90° relationship with the long axis of the shoulders, which are still in an oblique diameter of the pelvis.

8-2. Internal rotation of the chest and shoulders

Once the head is born, the upper torso and shoulders have descended further and are now more free to move. The chest now rotates internally 45° with the next contraction, moving the anterior shoulder from an oblique orientation toward the mother's symphysis, bringing the bisacromial diameter into the anteroposterior diameter of the outlet.

***11. External rotation of the head**

The head follows the shoulders, and the occiput rotates externally another 45° toward the mother's side (ROP to ROT or LOP to LOT).

The process of shoulder emergence and the birth of the body is the same for all cephalic presentations.

Moulding

In persistent occiput posterior descent, moulding of the head varies with the degree of flexion. Flexed moulding causes the bones to rise steeply in front and back, lengthening the verticomental diameter and shortening the suboccipitobregmatic diameter. The caput, if one develops, is located over the sagittal suture just in front of the posterior fontanelle (or the portion that was encircled by the cervical os). The caput is most often centered in posterior babies, but may also be off to one side. An indentation overlies the bregma, which is produced by pressure when this region is pressed against the pubic arch.

If the head was extended, the skull is shortened in the occipitofrontal diameter and lengthened in the suboccipitobregmatic and submentovertical diameters. This was first described as "sugar loaf" moulding by William Smellie because the shape resembles the solid loaves of sugar which were sold in England in the 1700s. The caput is centered more anteriorly and may overlie the bregma. This type of moulding, along with the centering of any caput over the anterior fontanelle, makes it more difficult to detect a deflexed OP attitude during an internal exam.

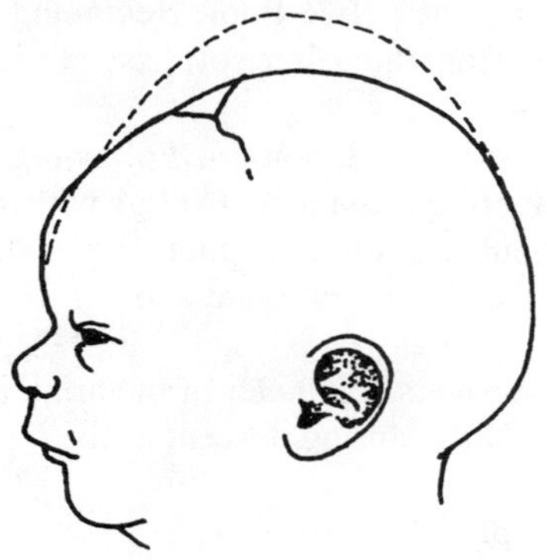

Flexed OP moulding

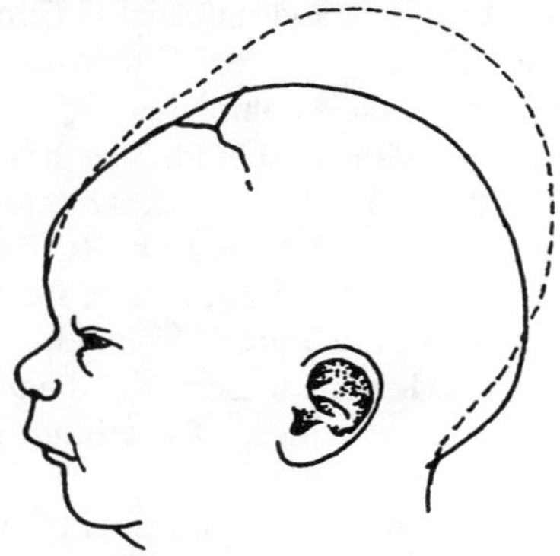

Extended "sugarloaf" OP moulding

SUMMARY OF THE CARDINAL SPIRALING MOVEMENTS: RIGHT OCCIPUT POSTERIOR (ROP)

Orientation of the baby to the mother's pelvis

The sagittal suture is aligned with the right oblique diameter, while the occiput is in front of the sacroiliac joint in the right posterior corner of the pelvis. The shoulders are aligned with the left oblique diameter.

Long-arc rotation of the ROP baby

***1.** The degree of spinal flexion varies; however, most babies are only partly flexed prior to labor because the baby's back is adjacent to his mother's. Flexion may be enhanced after full dilation once the head is firmly pressed against the pelvic floor, but often remains incomplete until anterior rotation occurs.

***2.** The baby descends throughout labor.

***3.** The head engages as the biparietal diameter passes through the brim.

***4.** The head rotates internally a total of 135°, from ROP to OA, as it adapts to the shape of the levator ani sling. Rotation consists of a downwardly spiraling movement, which facilitates descent. Internal rotation usually occurs after dilation is complete and the head is firmly pressed against the pelvic floor. Beginning at ROP, the head rotates 45° to ROT, then 45° to ROA, then 45° to OA. Pressure from the pelvic soft tissues often results in slight asynclitism until rotation is complete.

5. The baby's body moves with the shoulders as they undergo their first internal rotation. Following the rotation of the occiput from ROP to ROT, the shoulders rotate 45° from the left oblique diameter to align with the anteroposterior diameter. As the occiput rotates from ROT to ROA, the shoulders rotate another 45° to align with the right oblique diameter. As the occiput rotates from ROA to OA, the shoulders rotate another 45° to align with the transverse diameter of the brim, 135° in all.

6. The shoulders engage when the bisacromial diameter enters the transverse diameter of the brim, as the head passes through the ischial tuberosities. The attitude of the shoulders shifts during descent as the torso accommodates to the shape of the birth canal.

7. The spine begins to extend as the head enters the pelvis more deeply.

8-1. The second internal rotation of the shoulders begins between the time the head distends the perineum and is born. As the midchest and spine enter the curve of the birth canal near the level of the ischial spines, they rotate 45°, moving the shoulders from the transverse into the right oblique diameter. This adjustment allows the spine to flex laterally. The neck twists as this occurs, allowing the head to remain OA.

***9.** The head glides down past the pubic arch and begins to crown as the lower neck and upper spine extend under the pubic arch, allowing the head to remain flexed as it emerges. The perineum retracts and the head is born.

***10.** Restitution occurs as the neck untwists to allow the occiput to rotate 45°, from OA back to the ROA position, restoring the long axis of the vertex to a 90° angle with the long axis of the shoulders.

8-2. The chest completes its second internal rotation, moving the shoulders 45° from the right oblique to the antero-posterior diameter before or during the next contraction. This brings the anterior shoulder under the pubic arch.

***11.** Concurrent with the internal rotation of the chest, the head rotates externally 45° from ROA to ROT.

12. The anterior shoulder braces against the pubic bone as the posterior shoulder is born first by a process of lateral spinal flexion, after which the anterior shoulder slips past the pubic bone and emerges.

13. The torso and legs are born by a process of lateral flexion and a spiraling motion.

Moulding may be similar to that of an ROA baby if descent was not obstructed for a time. If it was, moulding may present a combination of posterior and anterior features. Any caput formation occurs over the mid to posterior right parietal bone, beside or overlying the sagittal suture. Exactly where it develops will depend upon the degree of flexion.

ROP orientation, head partially flexed	Descent to engagement	Internal rotation begins: ROP to ROT	Internal rotation of head continues: ROT to ROA.

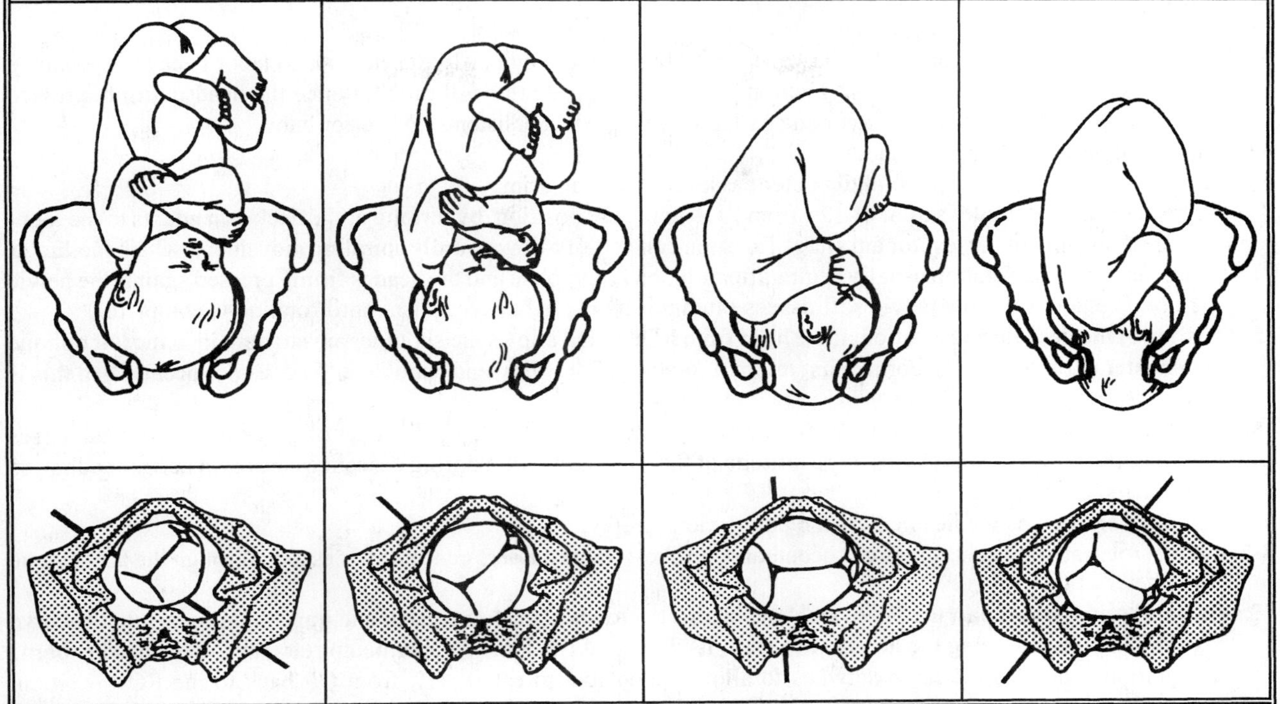

Internal rotation: ROA to OA; shoulders follow the head and engage transverse.	Midchest descends, rotates to oblique. Upper spine extends, flexed head is born.	The head restitutes 45° from OA to ROA.	Chest rotates AP; head follows, rotating externally: ROA to ROT. Shoulders and body are born.

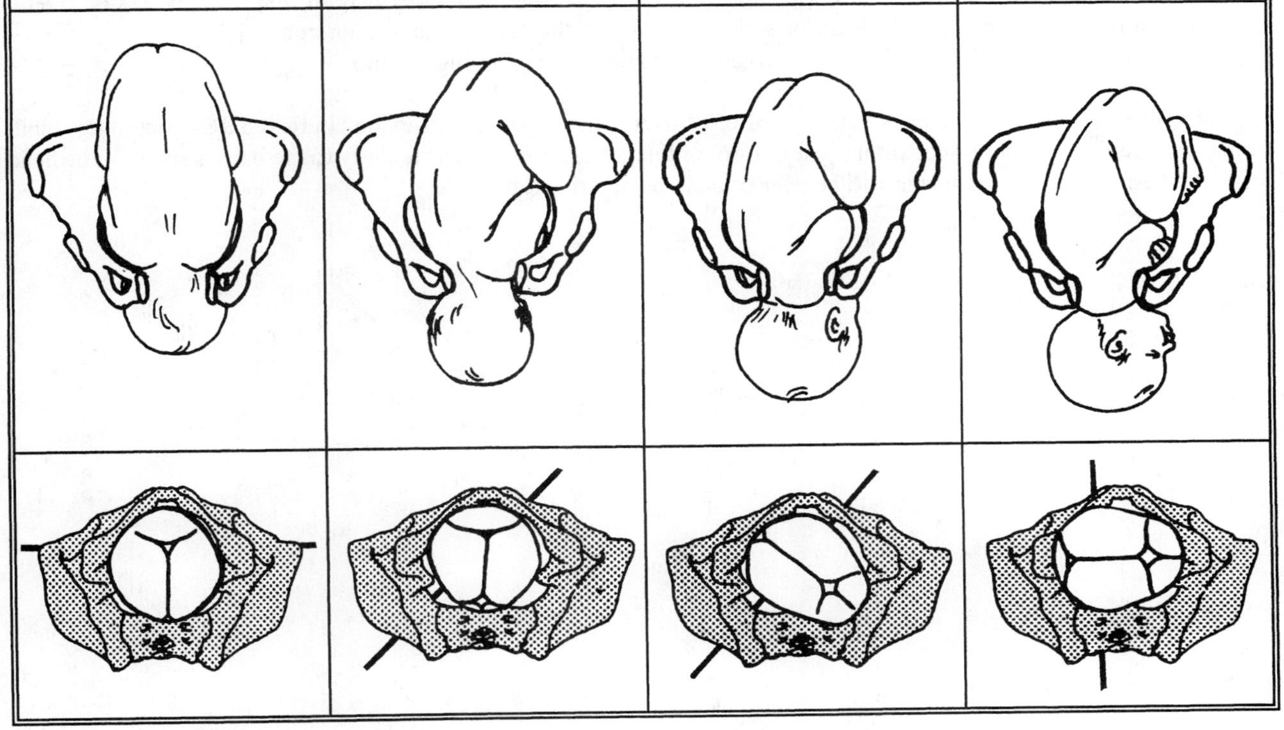

Short-arc rotation of the ROP baby

The movements are slightly different than for occiput anterior descent: numbered movements have been changed to reflect these differences.

***1.** The degree of spinal flexion varies; however, most babies are only partly flexed prior to labor because the baby's back is adjacent to his mother's. Flexion may be enhanced after full dilation once the head is firmly pressed against the pelvic floor, but often remains incomplete in the persistently posterior baby.
***2.** The baby descends throughout labor.
***3.** The head engages as the biparietal diameter passes through the brim.
***4.** The head rotates internally a total of 45°, from ROP to the OP position, by turning at the neck as it adapts to the loop-shaped opening in the levator ani sling. Rotation consists of a downwardly spiraling movement, which facilitates descent. Internal rotation usually begins after dilation is complete and the head is firmly pressed against the pelvic floor. Pressure from the pelvic soft tissues often results in slight asynclitism until rotation is complete.
5. Twisting of the neck during rotation of the head from ROP to OP allows the shoulder axis to remain in the left oblique diameter until the head is born. (First internal rotation of the body and shoulders (5) does not occur when this is the case.)
6. The shoulders engage when the bisacromial diameter enters the left oblique diameter of the brim, as the head passes through the ischial tuberosities. The attitude of the shoulders shifts during descent as the torso accommodates to the shape of the birth canal.
7. The spine extends as the head enters the pelvis more deeply.
8-1. Internal rotation of the chest may not occur, and the chest and shoulders continue to descend through the left oblique diameter of the pelvis.
***9.** The head glides down past the pubic arch and begins to crown as the lower neck and upper spine curl into the curve of the sacrum, allowing the head to maintain its degree of flexion. The perineum retracts and the head is born.
***10.** Restitution occurs as the neck untwists to allow the occiput to rotate 45°, from OP back to the ROP position, restoring the long axis of the vertex to a 90° angle with the long axis of the shoulders.
8-2. The chest rotates internally, moving the shoulders 45° from the left oblique into the anteroposterior diameter before or during the next contraction. This brings the anterior shoulder under the pubic arch.
***11.** Concurrent with the internal rotation of the shoulders, the head rotates externally 45° from ROP to ROT.
12. The anterior shoulder braces against the pubic bone as the posterior shoulder is born first by a process of lateral spinal flexion, after which the anterior shoulder slips past the pubic bone and emerges.
13. The torso and legs are born by a process of lateral flexion and a spiraling motion.

Moulding in all persistently posterior vertex positions varies with the degree of flexion. In flexed ROP moulding, caput formation occurs over the sagittal suture just in front of the posterior fontanelle slightly to the baby's right. If the head was extended, any caput that forms will be over or near the anterior fontanelle.

ROP orientation, head partially flexed	Descent to engagement, flexion is enhanced	Internal rotation of head: ROP to OP. Neck twists, leaving shoulders oblique.
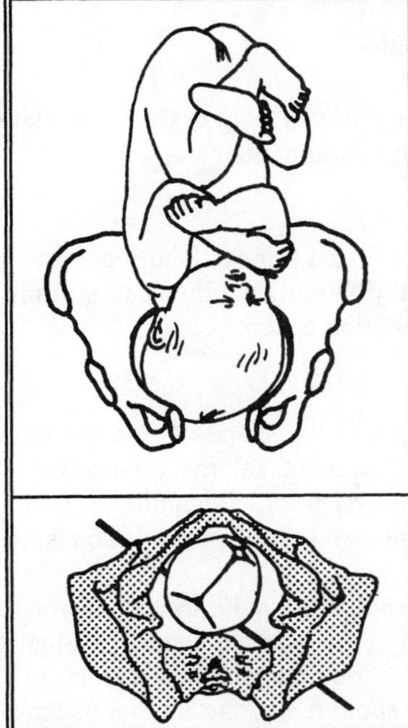	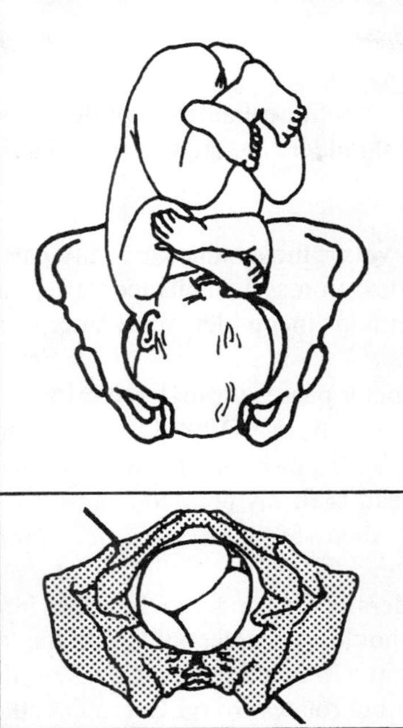	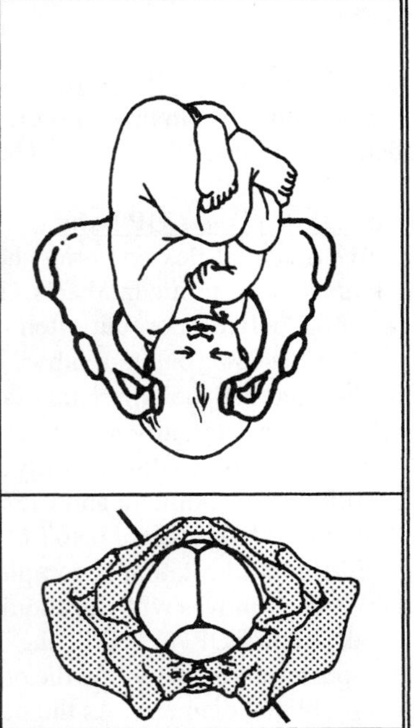
Birth of head face up as spine flexes and extends; chest descends oblique	Head restitutes: OP to ROP	Chest rotates internally to AP; head follows rotating externally ROP to ROT, shoulders are born.
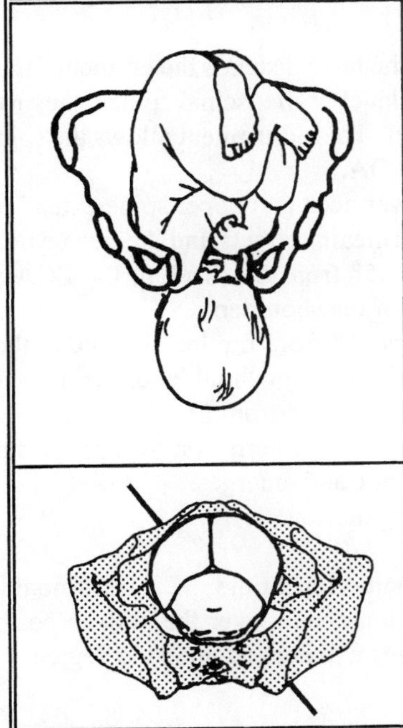	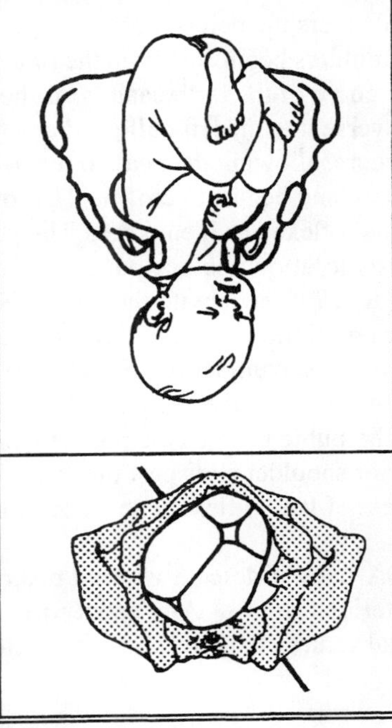	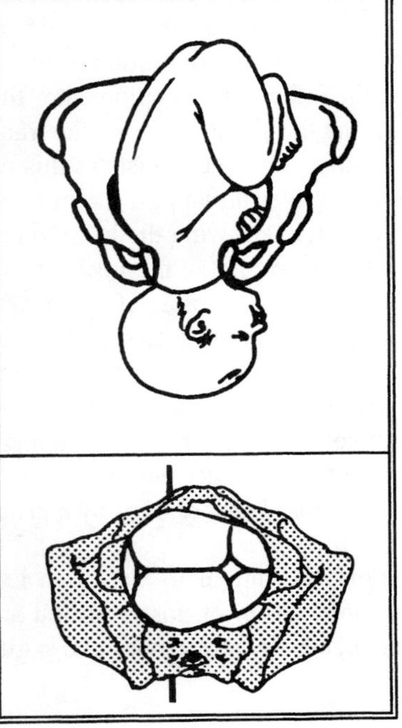

SUMMARY OF THE CARDINAL SPIRALING MOVEMENTS: LEFT OCCIPUT POSTERIOR (LOP)

Left occiput posterior positioning is much less common than right occiput posterior. LOP descent is a mirror image of ROP descent.

Orientation of the baby to the mother's pelvis

The sagittal suture is aligned with the left oblique diameter, while the occiput is in front of the sacrosciatic joint in the left posterior corner of the pelvis. The shoulders are aligned with the right oblique diameter.

Long-arc rotation of the LOP baby

***1.** The degree of spinal flexion varies; however, most babies are only partly flexed prior to labor because the baby's back is adjacent to his mother's. Flexion may be enhanced after full dilation once the head is firmly pressed against the pelvic floor, but often remains incomplete until anterior rotation occurs.

***2.** The baby descends throughout labor.

***3.** The head engages as the biparietal diameter passes through the brim.

***4.** The head rotates internally a total of 135°, from LOP to OA, as it adapts to the shape of the levator ani sling. Rotation consists of a downwardly spiraling movement, which facilitates descent. Internal rotation usually begins after dilation is complete and the head is firmly pressed against the pelvic floor. Beginning at LOP, the head rotates 45° to LOT, then 45° to LOA, then 45° to OA. Pressure from the pelvic soft tissues often results in slight asynclitism until rotation is complete.

5. The baby's body moves with the shoulders as they undergo their first internal rotation. Following the rotation of the occiput from LOP to LOT, the shoulders rotate 45° from the right oblique diameter, to align with the anteroposterior diameter. As the occiput rotates from LOT to LOA, the shoulders rotate another 45° to align with the left oblique diameter. As the occiput rotates from LOA to OA, the shoulders rotate another 45° to align with the transverse diameter of the brim, 135° in all.

6. The shoulders engage when the bisacromial diameter enters the transverse diameter of the brim, as the head passes through the ischial tuberosities. The attitude of the shoulders shifts during descent as the torso accommodates to the shape of the birth canal.

7. The spine begins to extend as the head enters the pelvis more deeply.

8-1. The second internal rotation of the shoulders begins between the time the head distends the perineum and is born. As the midchest and spine enter the curve of the birth canal near the level of the ischial spines, they rotate 45°, moving the shoulders from the transverse into the left oblique diameter. This adjustment allows the spine to flex laterally. The neck twists as this occurs, allowing the head to remain OA.

***9.** The head glides down past the pubic arch and begins to crown. The lower neck and upper spine extend under the pubic arch, allowing the head to remain flexed as it emerges. The perineum retracts and the head emerges.

***10.** Restitution occurs as the neck untwists to allow the occiput to rotate 45° from OA back to the LOA position, restoring the long axis of the vertex to a 90° angle with the long axis of the shoulders.

8-2. The chest completes its second internal rotation, moving the shoulders 45° from the left oblique to the antero-posterior diameter before or during the next contraction. This brings the anterior shoulder under the pubic arch.

***11.** Concurrent with the internal rotation of the chest, the head rotates externally 45° from LOA to LOT.

12. The anterior shoulder braces against the pubic bone as the posterior shoulder is born first by a process of lateral spinal flexion, after which the anterior shoulder slips past the pubic bone and emerges.

13. The torso and legs are born by a process of lateral flexion and a spiraling motion.

Moulding may be similar to that of an LOA baby if descent was not obstructed for a time. If it was, moulding may present a combination of posterior and anterior features. Any caput formation occurs over the mid- to posterior left parietal bone, beside or overlying the sagittal suture. Exactly where it develops will depend upon the degree of flexion.

LOP orientation, head partially flexed	Descent to engagement	Internal rotation begins: LOP to LOT	Internal rotation of head continues: LOT to LOA.
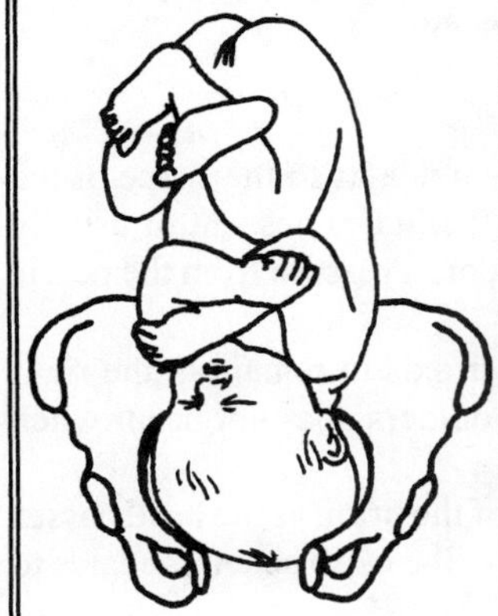	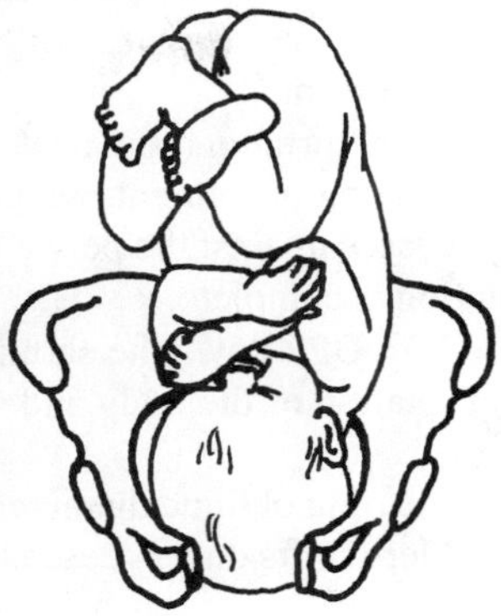	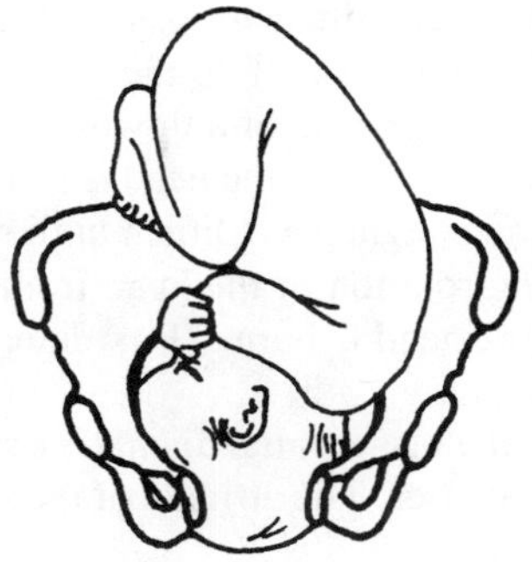	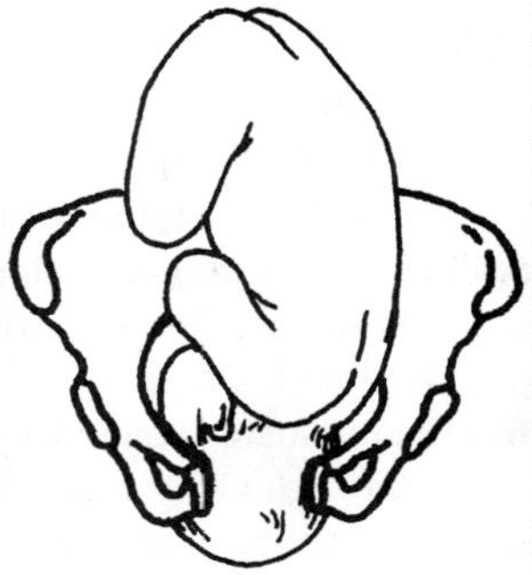
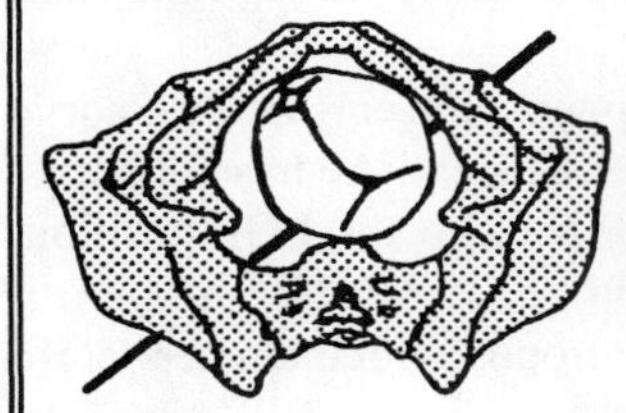	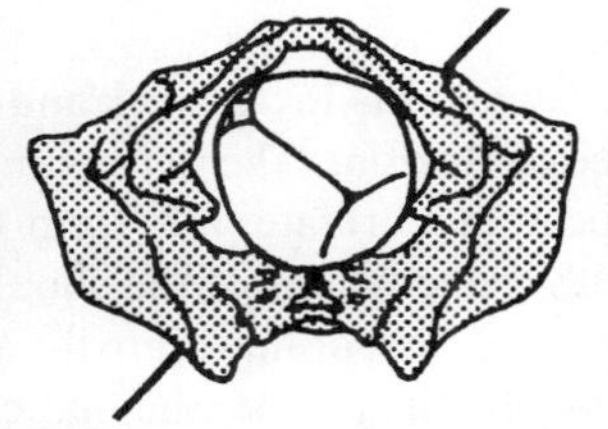	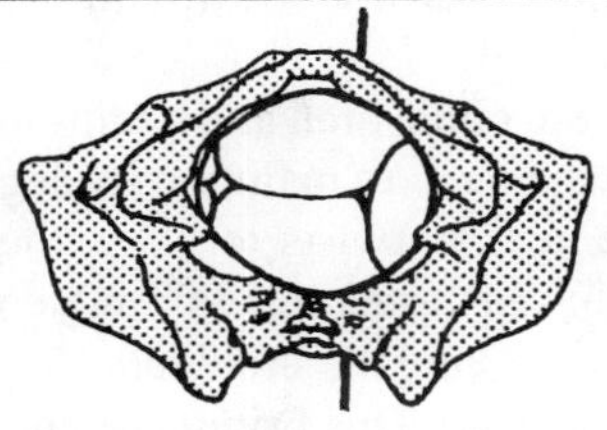	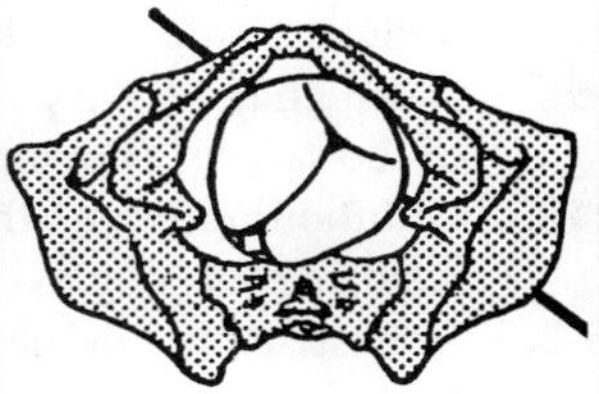

Internal rotation: LOA to OA; shoulders follow the head and engage transverse,.	Midchest descends, rotates to oblique. Upper spine extends; flexed head is born.	The head restitutes 45° from OA to LOA.	Chest rotates AP; head follows, rotating externally: LOA to LOT. Shoulders and body are born.
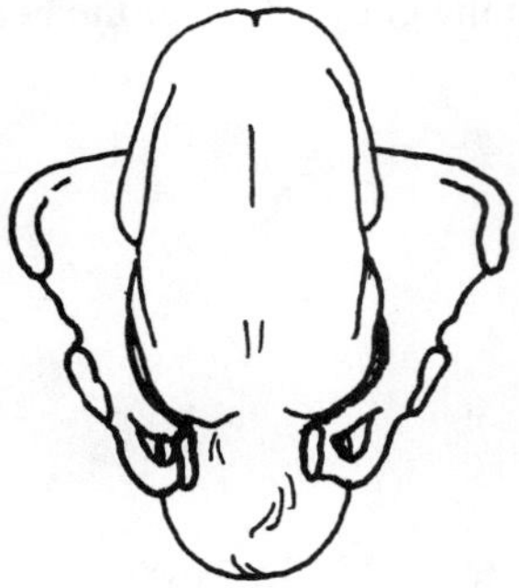	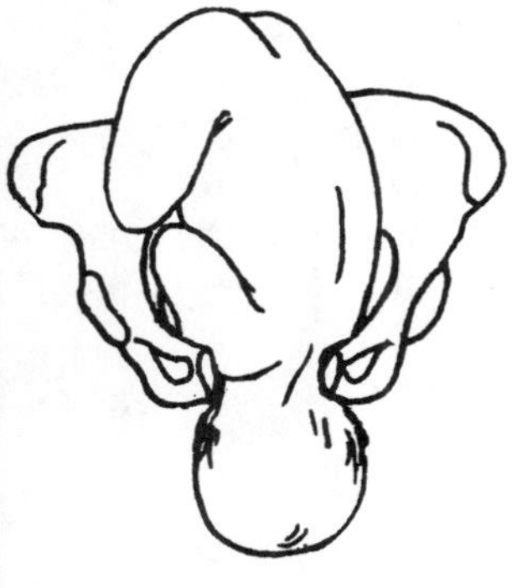	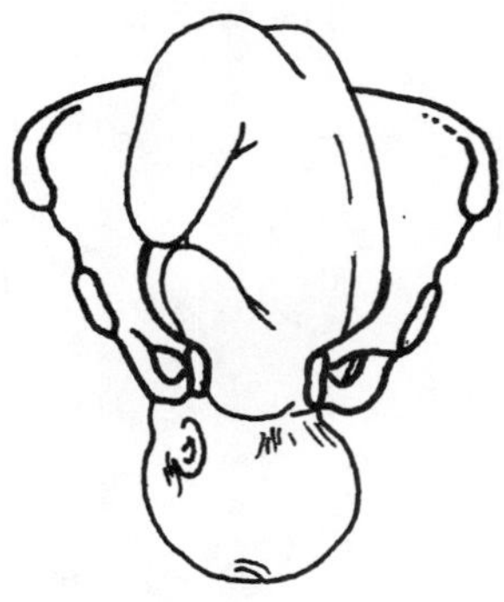	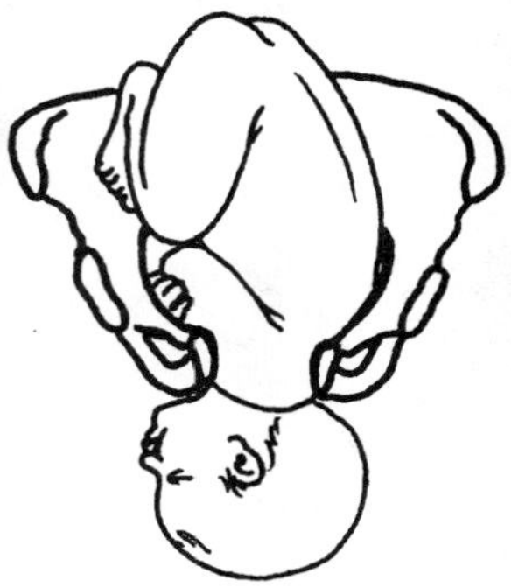
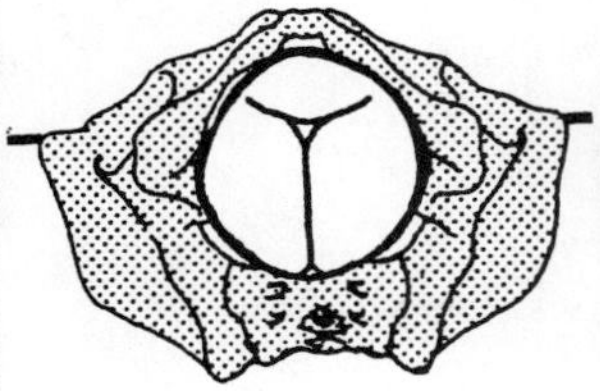	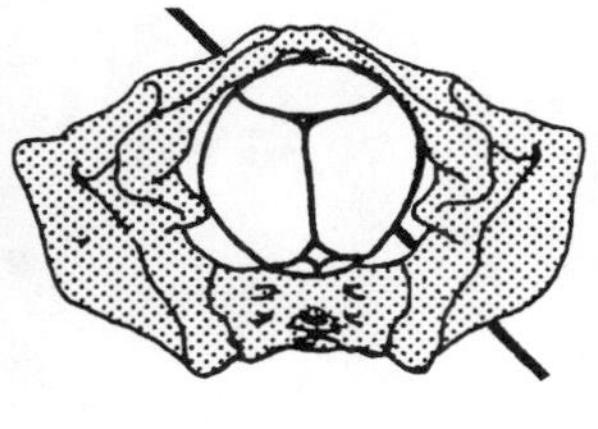	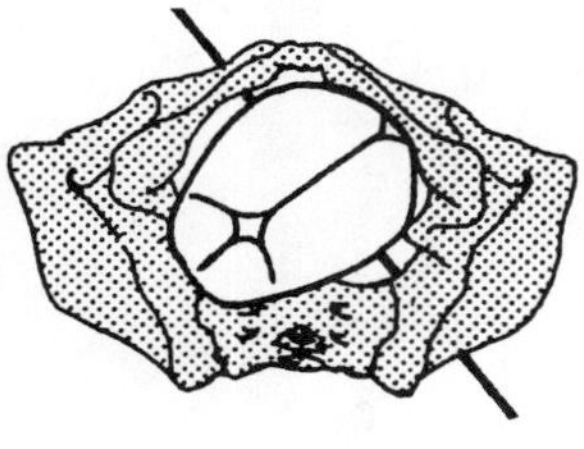	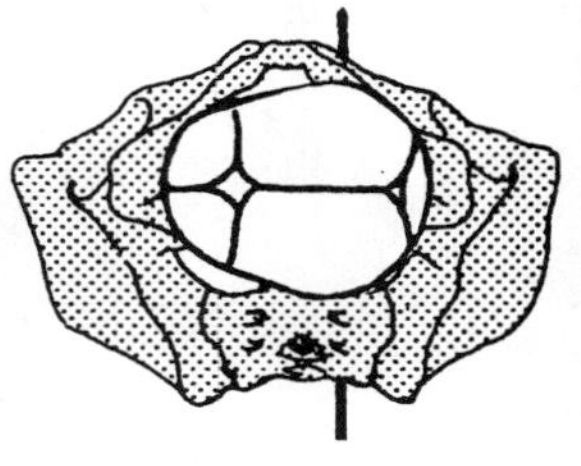

Short-arc rotation of the LOP baby

***1.** The degree of spinal flexion varies; however, most babies are only partly flexed prior to labor because the baby's back is adjacent to his mother's. Flexion may be enhanced after full dilation once the head is firmly pressed against the pelvic floor, but often remains incomplete in the persistently posterior baby.

***2.** The baby descends throughout labor.

***3.** The head engages as the biparietal diameter passes through the brim.

***4.** The head rotates internally 45° from LOP to the OP position by turning at the neck as it adapts to the shape of the levator ani sling. Rotation consists of a downwardly spiraling movement, which facilitates descent. It usually begins after dilation is complete and the head is firmly pressed against the pelvic floor. Pressure from the pelvic soft tissues often results in slight asynclitism until rotation is complete.

5. Twisting of the neck during rotation of the head from LOP to OP allows the shoulder axis to remain in the right oblique diameter until the head is born. (First internal rotation of the body and shoulders does not occur when this is the case.)

6. The shoulders engage when the bisacromial diameter enters the right oblique diameter of the brim, as the head passes through the ischial tuberosities. The attitude of the shoulders shifts during descent as the torso accommodates to the shape of the birth canal.

7. The spine extends as the head enters the pelvis more deeply.

8-1. Internal rotation of the chest may not occur, and the chest and shoulders continue to descend through the right oblique diameter of the pelvis.

***9.** The head glides down past the pubic arch and begins to crown as the lower neck and upper spine curl into the curve of the sacrum allowing the head to maintain its degree of flexion. The perineum retracts and the head is born.

***10.** Restitution occurs as the neck untwists to allow the occiput to rotate 45°, from OP back to the LOP position, restoring the long axis of the vertex to a 90° angle with the long axis of the shoulders.

8-2. The chest rotates internally, moving the shoulders 45° from the right oblique into the anteroposterior diameter before or during the next contraction. This brings the anterior shoulder under the pubic arch.

***11.** Concurrent with the internal rotation of the shoulders, the head rotates externally 45° from LOP to LOT.

12. The anterior shoulder braces against the pubic bone as the posterior shoulder is born first by a process of lateral spinal flexion, after which the anterior shoulder slips past the pubic bone and emerges.

13. The torso and legs are born by a process of lateral flexion and a spiraling motion.

Moulding in all persistently posterior vertex positions varies with the degree of flexion. In flexed moulding, caput formation occurs over the sagittal suture just in front of the posterior fontanelle slightly to the baby's left. If the head was extended, any caput that forms will be over or near the anterior fontanelle.

LOP orientation, head partially flexed	Descent to engagement, flexed enhanced	Internal rotation of head: LOP to OP. Neck twists, leaving shoulders oblique.
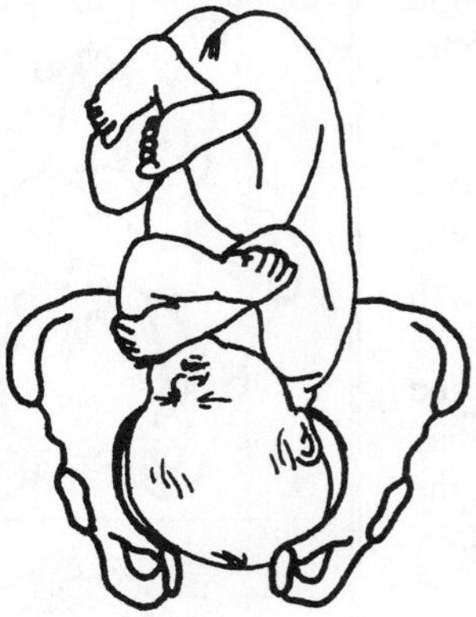	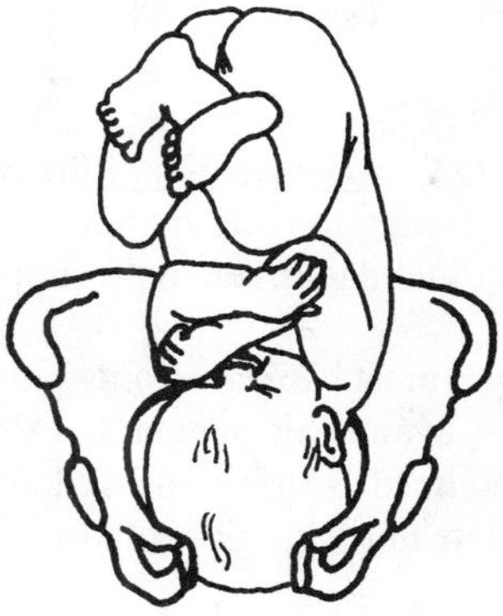	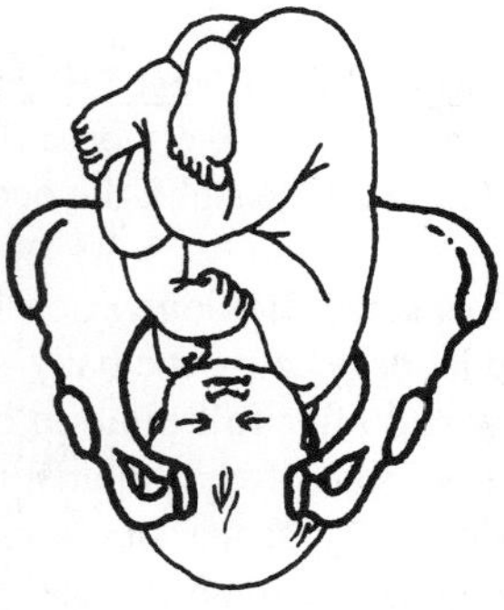
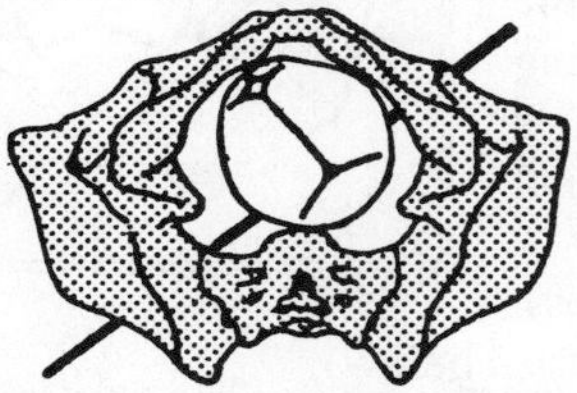	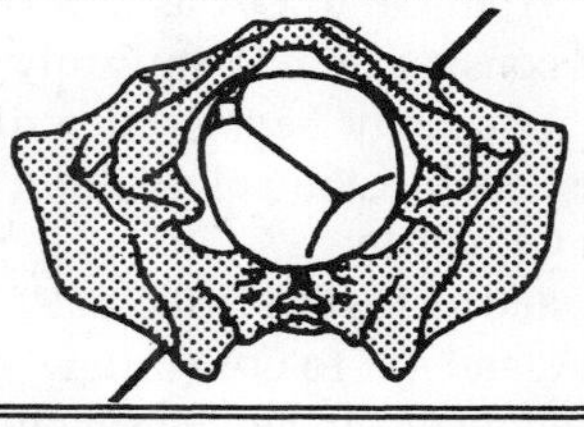	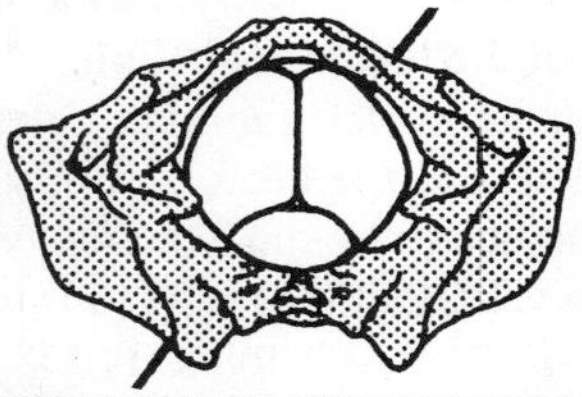
Birth of head face up as spine flexes and extends; chest descends oblique	Head restitutes: OP to LOP	Chest rotates internally to AP; head follows rotating externally LOP to LOT, shoulders are born.
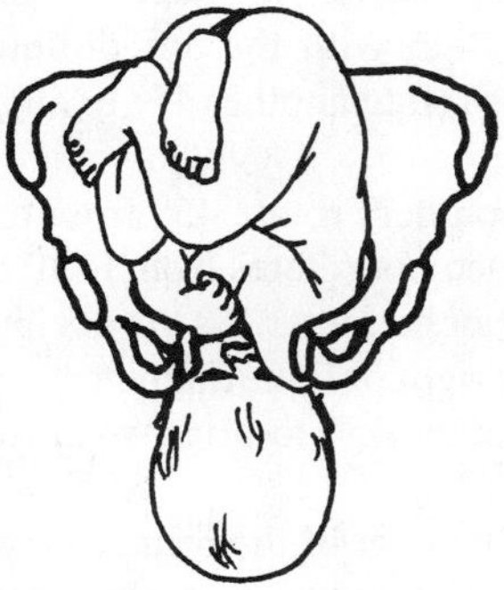	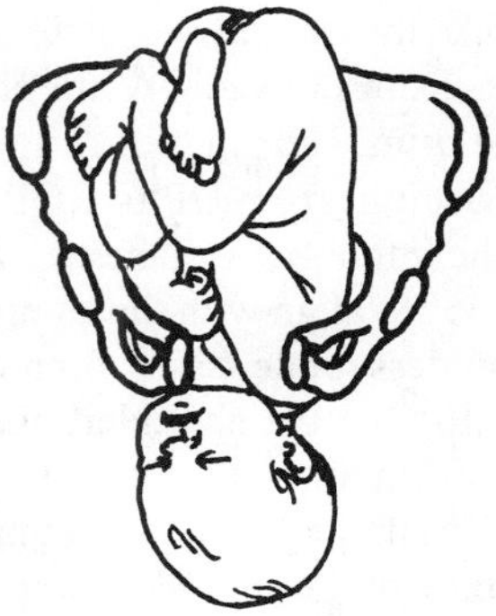	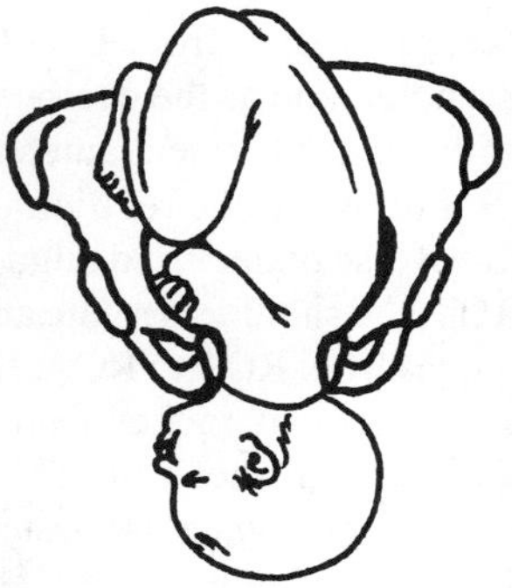
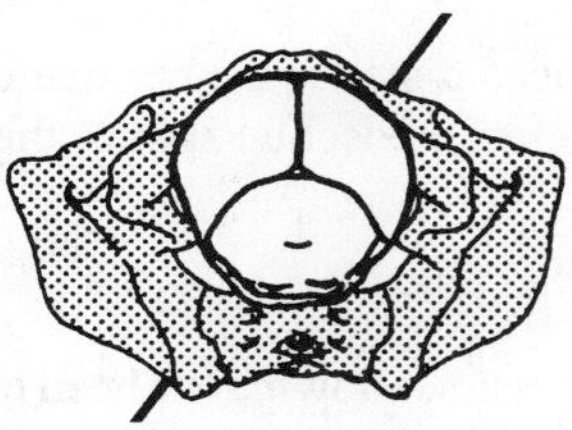	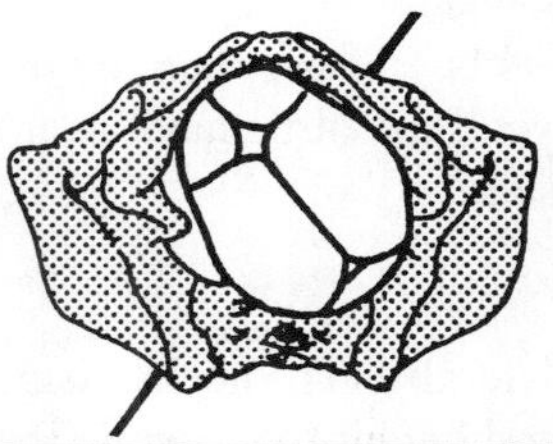	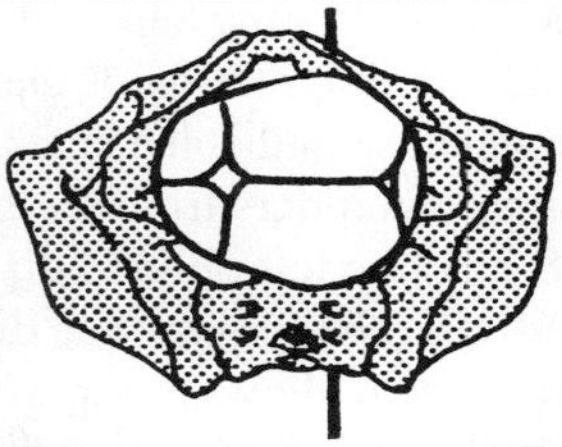

SUMMARY OF THE CARDINAL SPIRALING MOVEMENTS: OCCIPUT POSTERIOR (OP)

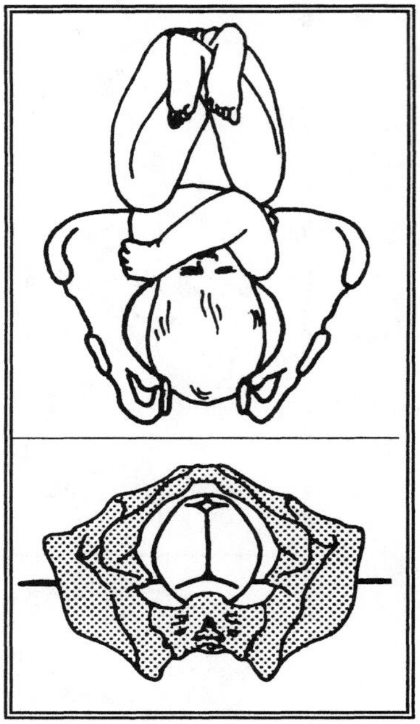

Orientation of the baby to the mother's pelvis

The sagittal suture is aligned with the anteroposterior diameter of the brim, while the occiput is directly posterior, in front of the lower spine. The shoulders are aligned with the transverse diameter.

Long-arc rotation of the direct OP baby to OA (movements not illustrated)

Rotation may occur in either a left or a right direction, but because the descending colon is on the right, the occiput will tend to rotate to the mother's left.

***1.** The degree of spinal flexion varies; however, most babies are only partly flexed prior to labor because the baby's back is against his mother's. Flexion may be enhanced after full dilation once the head is firmly pressed against the pelvic floor, but often remains incomplete until anterior rotation occurs.

***2.** The baby descends throughout labor.

***3.** The head engages as the biparietal diameter passes through the brim.

***4.** The head rotates internally a total of 180° from OP to OA as it adapts to the shape of the levator ani sling. Rotation consists of a downwardly spiraling movement, which facilitates descent. It usually begins after dilation is complete and the head is firmly pressed against the pelvic floor. Internal rotation occurs as the head moves from OP 45° to:

4-A. LOP, 45° to LOT, 45° to LOA, and 45° to OA (follow "A" entries).

4-B. ROP, 45° to ROT, 45° to ROA, and 45° to OA (follow "B" entries below).

Pressure from the pelvic soft tissues often results in slight asynclitism until rotation is complete.

5. The baby's body moves with the shoulders as they undergo their first internal rotation.

5-A. Following the rotation of the occiput from OP to LOP, the shoulders rotate 45° from the transverse diameter to align with the right oblique diameter. As the occiput rotates from LOP to LOT, the shoulders rotate another 45° to align with the anteroposterior diameter. As the occiput rotates from LOT to LOA, the shoulders rotate 45° to align with the left oblique diameter, and as the occiput rotates from LOA to OA, the shoulders rotate another 45° to align with the transverse diameter of the brim, 180° in all.

5-B. Following the rotation of the occiput from OP to ROP, the shoulders rotate 45° from the transverse diameter to align with the left oblique diameter. As the occiput rotates from ROP to ROT, the shoulders rotate another 45° to align with the anteroposterior diameter. As the occiput rotates from ROT to ROA, the shoulders rotate 45° to align with the right oblique diameter, and as the occiput rotates from ROA to OA, the shoulders rotate another 45° to align with the transverse diameter of the brim, 180° in all.

6. The shoulders engage when the bisacromial diameter enters the transverse diameter of the brim, as the head passes through the ischial tuberosities. The attitude of the shoulders shifts during descent as the torso accommodates to the shape of the birth canal.

7. The spine extends as the head enters the pelvis more deeply.

8-1. The second internal rotation of the shoulders begins between the time the head distends the perineum and is born. As the midchest and spine enter the curve of the birth canal near the level of the ischial spines, they rotate 45°, moving the shoulders from the transverse into:

8-1-A. the left oblique diameter.

8-1-B. the right oblique diameter.

This adjustment allows the spine to flex laterally. The neck twists as this occurs, allowing the head to remain OA.

*** 9.** The head glides down past the pubic arch and begins to crown as the lower neck and upper spine extend, allowing the head to remain flexed as it emerges. The perineum retracts and the head is born.

***10.** Restitution occurs as the neck untwists to allow the occiput to rotate 45° from OA to:

10-A. the LOA position.

10-B. the ROA position.

The movement restores the long axis of the vertex to a 90° angle with the long axis of the shoulders.

8-2. The chest completes its internal rotation, moving the shoulders 45° from:

8-2-A. the left oblique diameter

8-2-B. the right oblique diameter

into the anteroposterior diameter before or during the next contraction. This brings the anterior shoulder under the pubic arch.

***11.** Concurrent with the internal rotation of the chest, the head rotates externally 45°:

11-A. from LOA to LOT.

11-B. from ROA to ROT.

12. The anterior shoulder braces against the pubic bone as the posterior shoulder is born first by a process of lateral spinal flexion, after which the anterior shoulder slips past the pubic bone and emerges.

13. The torso and legs are born by a process of lateral flexion and a spiraling motion.

Birth of the directly OP baby (movements not illustrated)

The first rotational direction is to the right, because babies that remain posterior tend to stay to the mother's right.

***1.** The degree of spinal flexion varies; however, most babies are only partly flexed prior to labor because the baby's back is adjacent to his mother's. Flexion may be enhanced after full dilation once the head is firmly pressed against the pelvic floor, but often remains incomplete in the persistently posterior baby.

***2.** The head descends throughout labor.

***3.** The head engages as the biparietal diameter passes through the brim.

***4.** Internal rotation of the head does not occur.

5. The shoulder axis remains aligned with the transverse diameter of the brim.

6. The shoulders engage when the bisacromial diameter enters the transverse diameter of the brim as the head passes through the ischial tuberosities. The attitude of the shoulders shifts during descent as the torso accommodates to the shape of the birth canal.

7. The spine extends as the head enters the pelvis more deeply.

8-1. Internal rotation of the shoulders begins between the time the head distends the perineum and is born. As the midchest and spine enter the curve of the birth canal near the level of the ischial spines, they rotate 45°, moving the shoulders from the transverse into:

8-1-A. the left oblique diameter. (Follow "A" entries below.)

8-1-B. the right oblique diameter. (Follow "B" entries below.)

This adjustment allows the spine to flex laterally. The neck twists as this occurs, allowing the head to remain OA.

***9.** The head glides down past the pubic arch and begins to crown as the lower neck and upper spine mould into the curve of the sacrum and extend along it, allowing the head to maintain its degree of flexion. The perineum retracts and the head is born.

***10.** Restitution occurs as the neck untwists to allow the occiput to rotate 45° from OP back to the:

10-A. the ROP position.

10-B. the LOP position.

The movement restores the long axis of the vertex to a 90° angle with the long axis of the shoulders.

8-2. The chest completes its second internal rotation, moving the shoulders 45° from:

8-2-A. the left oblique diameter

8-2-B. the right oblique diameter

into the anteroposterior diameter with the next contraction. This brings the anterior shoulder under the pubic arch.

***11.** Concurrent with the internal rotation of the chest, the head rotates externally 45°:

11-A. from ROP to ROT.

11-B. from LOP to LOT.

12. The anterior shoulder braces against the pubic bone as the posterior shoulder is born first by a process of lateral spinal flexion, after which the anterior shoulder slips past the pubic bone and emerges.

13. The torso and legs are born by a process of lateral flexion and a spiraling motion.

Moulding will be consistent with the way the baby descended.

MEDIAN VERTEX POSITIONING (MILITARY ATTITUDE)

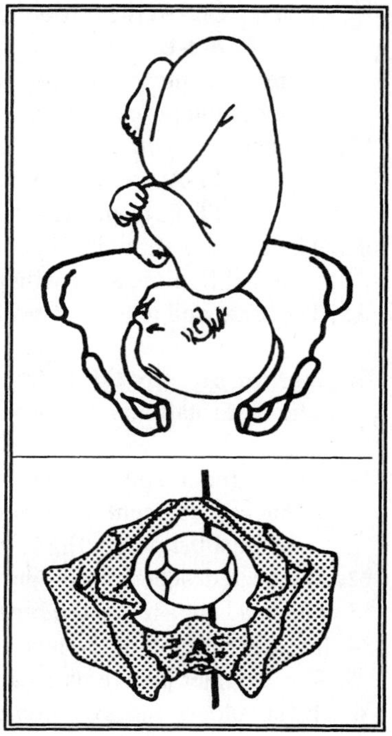

In this case, the baby's head is neither fully flexed nor extended. The brow and the occiput are at the same level in the pelvis, as though the baby is facing straight ahead in an attitude variously referred to as a military, sinciput, bregma or median vertex attitude it has also been called "commonly deflexed." The presenting diameter is the occipitofrontal of 11 cm rather than the more favorable suboccipitobregmatic diameter of 9.5 cm. Along with deflexion of the head, the spine and the shoulders are usually straighter than they would otherwise be as well. The baby may assume a median attitude in any vertex position: i.e., LOA, LOT, LOP, ROA, ROT, ROP, OA or OP.

Engagement usually occurs with the occiput in the transverse region of the maternal pelvis (the sagittal suture running side to side). Because the head and spine are deflexed, the baby may descend more slowly than it would otherwise, usually with the head asynclitic until the center of the vertex is pressed against the pelvic floor. Poor and sometimes infrequent uterine contractions are more common, and pushing may be considerably prolonged. As labor progresses, several things can happen:

- Many babies start labor in a median vertex attitude. In the majority of cases, the head and spine flex more, the occiput rotates and birth proceeds as for an occipitoanterior position. Flexion is facilitated by maternal positions that open the spinopubic angle.
- The head can remain deflexed and rotate to an occiput anterior position as birth proceeds. The most common reason for persistent deflexion is the presence of a fist under the chin or in the groove of the baby's neck. Other, less common reasons include tight multiple loops of cord around the neck or a tumor of the neck.
- The head can descend as far as the ischial spines and become stuck, unable to descend or rotate beyond this level, which is the narrowest plane of the bony pelvis. The medical model refers to this as "deep transverse arrest". It is more likely to occur when women are kept on their back, not allowed to move or are given drugs that decrease pelvic muscle tone. In fact, maternal position changes often prompt internal rotation.
- Even if the head remains transverse for a time, it may simply require additional moulding before it can descend further. The midwife must assess the well-being of mother and baby and have patience, which will sometimes be rewarded with the transformation of the medical model's deep transverse arrest into the midwifery model's deep pelvic moulding (Lemay, 2001). Once sufficient moulding has occurred, the baby may then rotate to an OA or OP position or may continue descent in the transverse position. On rare occasions, the head may even emerge with its long axis in the transverse diameter of the outlet.
- The head can rotate to an occiput posterior position. Further flexion may or may not occur. The occiput is in the hollow of the sacrum, and the forehead is against the pubic bone. The birth proceeds the same as for a persistent occipitoposterior position.
- The head can continue to extend, and the birth proceed as a brow or face presentation.

VARIATIONS IN VERTEX DESCENT AND ROTATION

The following variations are set forth as examples of the ways in which labor can take an unexpected turn (so to speak). They generally apply to cephalic presentations and illustrate that just about anything can and does happen from time to time during labor.

Variations in chest rotation and birth

The rotation of the chest and shoulder axis can vary widely. The shoulders should birth without difficulty as long as they rotate beneath, rather than above, the upper border of the pubic bone and don't get hung up behind one of the pubic rami. Wherever the shoulder diameter winds up, the long axis of the head will usually resume its right-angle relationship to the long axis of the shoulders once it is free to do so. Thus, as a rule, the position of the long axis of the head is a reliable indicator of the location of the long axis of the shoulders, which should be perpendicular. Occasionally, however, factors such as a tight perineum, a tight cord around the neck, the proximity of a fetal extremity or the presence of an anatomical abnormality may prevent the head from realigning normally with the shoulder axis. Many of the ways the shoulders can rotate are summarized below.

ROTATIONAL ACTIVITIES OF THE CHEST AND SHOULDERS DURING DESCENT (IN APPROXIMATE ORDER OF FREQUENCY)

Shoulders start*	First internal rotation of shoulders (as head rotates internally)	Shoulders engage	Second internal rotation begins (as chest enters pelvic curve)	Second internal rotation of shoulders completes (after birth of head)
AP**	AP to oblique to transverse	Transverse	Oblique	AP
AP	AP to oblique to transverse	Transverse	Oblique	No rotation, emerge oblique
Oblique	Oblique to transverse	Transverse	Oblique	AP
Oblique	No rotation	Oblique	Stays oblique	No rotation, emerge oblique
Transverse	No rotation	Transverse	Shoulders remain transverse	No rotation, emerge transverse
Oblique	No rotation	Oblique	Shoulders remain oblique	AP to opposite oblique
AP	AP to oblique to transverse	Transverse	Shoulders remain transverse	No rotation, emerge transverse
AP	No rotation	AP	Oblique	AP
AP	No rotation	AP	Transverse	AP

*The original position of the shoulders depends on the orientation of the entire fetal body and head **Anteroposterior

Overrotation (internal superrotation) during vertex descent: Anterior rotation of the occiput can be exaggerated in either a left or right direction especially in a mother with a roomy pelvis, a small baby or both. For instance, occasionally a baby starting labor LOA converts to ROA during internal rotation. The occiput rotates 90° across the anterior pelvis, past the symphysis to the opposite anterior oblique position (e.g., LOA to OA to ROA). The back and shoulders may superrotate along with the occiput to the opposite oblique diameter (i.e., left oblique to anteroposterior to right oblique); this maintains a relatively normal alignment. On rare occasions, the shoulders and torso may remain in their original position, which in this example would be an LOA orientation (the left oblique diameter). When this occurs, the baby's spine is twisted considerably out of its usual alignment, which is made possible by the uniquely flexible fetal body. If the shoulders do remain in the left oblique diameter, the occiput restitutes 90° from ROA to OA to LOA once the head is born. If the shoulders have rotated to match the head, the occiput should restitute from OA to LOA. No restitution will occur if the sagittal suture is aligned in one oblique pelvic diameter with shoulders occupying the opposite oblique diameter. The reverse can happen as well (ROA to OA to LOA).

Sometimes, in a posterior position, the occiput will rotate 90° across the posterior pelvis past the hollow of the sacrum. (For example, it may move LOP to OP to ROP.) If the torso follows, the baby's back, which at first was on the mother's posterior left, now lies on her posterior right side. Another form of internal superrotation occurs when the head rotates normally and then reverses its internal rotation during birth (as in LOA to OA to LOA). The shoulders and back may lag behind the head as the baby twists at the neck once again, creating a markedly twisted posture, or they may superrotate to the same side as the occiput, which maintains them in more typical alignment.

<u>Other rotational variations in occiput posterior births</u>: While 90% of all posterior babies rotate to a directly anterior position, variations in rotation of the posterior occiput can occur:

- The occiput may rotate 90° from an oblique posterior position, through the transverse, to an oblique anterior position. For example, the head might go from ROP to ROT to ROA and be born from an oblique angle. See the table at the beginning of the chapter regarding options for shoulder rotation.
- The head may rotate only 45° to a transverse diameter. Here it is likely to delay labor while it moulds to fit through the pelvic cavity. If this cannot be accomplished, or anterior rotation does not occur, the head may become stuck or it may be born transverse.
- The head may not undergo rotation at all, remaining in its original posterior oblique location. This may prevent further progress, or the head may emerge oblique (Oxorn, 1986).

THE BIRTH PROCESS WHEN THE BABY IS IN AN EXTENDED CEPHALIC PRESENTATION

NOTE: Even though breech presentations are far more common than either face or brow presentations, these are presented first so that the student will be thoroughly versed in cephalic descent before tackling the even more complex process of breech descent.

FACE PRESENTATIONS: GENERAL PRINCIPLES

A face presentation occurs when the baby's head is fully extended, causing the face to be the presenting part. The incidence of face presentation ranges between 1 in 380 to 1 out of every 800 births, with an average of 1 in every 545 births. While considered unusual, labor generally progresses, and birth occurs naturally when the chin rotates anteriorly because the presenting diameter is not much different than that of a flexed vertex baby.

Presenting diameter

Face presentation can be defined as a fully deflexed head, with the region of the face between the glabella and the chin presenting. The denominator for face presentations is the **mentum** or chin, which leads descent. Borell and Fernström (1960) confirmed what most textbooks state, which is that the submentobregmatic (also called the trachelobregmatic, the cervicobregmatic or the tracheloparietal) diameter most often presents, which ranges from 9.5 to 10.2 cm in length, almost the same as for the suboccipitobregmatic diameter of 9.5 cm in a fully flexed vertex presentation.

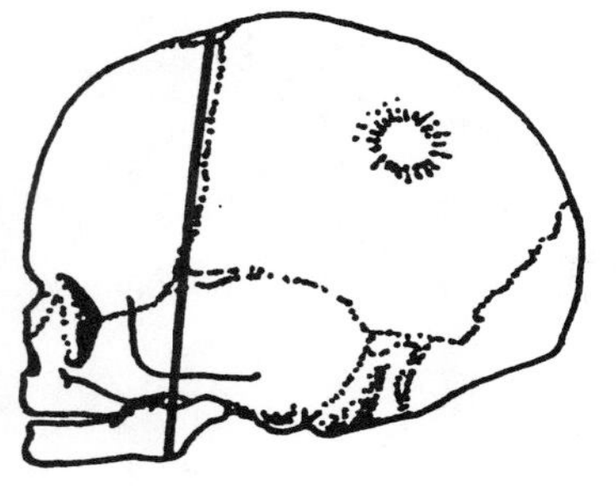

Submentobregmatic diameter

Associated factors

A long list of "associated factors" has accumulated over the years in an attempt to explain why some babies fully extend their heads. Hyperextension is thought to be related to maternal conditions that may interfere with the normal positioning of the uterus, such as pendulous abdomen, polyhydramnios, pelvic disproportion, multiple pregnancy, high parity, obliquity of the uterus (sideways tilting of the entire uterus) and certain uterine anomalies. Presumed fetal associations have included placenta previa, polyhydramnios, a small or premature baby, and a nuchal or short cord, as well as certain abnormalities that could interfere with proper flexion, such as enlargement of the thyroid, tumors of the neck, anencephaly, spasm of the muscles in the back of the neck, intrauterine death and dolichocephaly (a defect where the breadth of the fetal skull is less than four-fifths of its length). Large fetuses are often mentioned in reports, but the definition of "large" varies, with weights ranging from over 8 lb (3,629 grams) to over 8 lb 13.5 oz (over 4000 grams). External version to turn a breech is believed to contribute to some cases of extension, especially if version is performed close to term. Rupture of membranes prior to engagement has been thought to trap the head in an attitude of extension. However, even with all these proffered "reasons," the majority of face presentations have no discernable etiology.

After doing an extensive review of the literature between 1940 and 1981, Cruikshank and Cruikshank (1981) found that there was no unanimity of opinion on these proposed associations and that none could stand up to close statistical scrutiny with the exception of anencephaly and, to a lesser extent, high parity. They concluded that it is most likely that almost all face presentations occur primarily due to conditions related to the fetus rather than conditions related to the mother. In most babies, the flexor muscles of the upper body predominate. In the occasional situation where the extensors predominate, the thrust of contractions through the fetal spine may support the maintenance of an extended cephalic presentation in these babies. Tension in the spine and fetal neck for other reasons can also cause the baby to resist flexion. Anencephaly is strongly associated with face presentation because the vault of the skull is missing.

Primary or secondary?

A primary presentation is one that the fetus assumes prior to the onset of labor. A secondary presentation is one that develops during labor as a result of fetal or maternal factors and usually there is an interplay between the two. It has long been taught that the vast majority of face and brow presentations are secondary and develop as a partially deflexed head descends into the pelvis. In fact, in reviewing reports of X-rays taken of 1762 women prior to the onset of labor, Cruikshank and Cruikshank (1981) found that 1 out of every 251 fetuses was presenting his face before labor began, over twice the reported incidence of babies who remained in a face presentation by the time they were born. This means that something caused the majority of these babies to flex their heads as labor progressed, with the remaining babies maintaining full extension throughout labor.

These data, coupled with the conflicting reports concerning etiologic factors, support the conclusion that there are no particular predisposing maternal etiologic factors. The apparent association of multiparity with deflexed presentations is compatible with this observation. For example, let's say an intrinsic fetal factor, such as dominant extensor muscles, causes the baby to hold her head in a slightly deflexed attitude. If the mother were a primigravida and the baby's head were engaged prior to labor, the fixation of engagement would prevent the head from extending more. If the mother were a multipara and therefore carrying the baby unengaged at term, the baby is more likely to remain deflexed as labor begins.

The Process of Birth in Mentum Anterior Face Presentations

In cephalic presentations, the head and shoulders almost always make three movements, regardless of the degree of flexion: engagement or entry of the part into the pelvis, rotation or positional adaption of the part to the shape of the birth canal and disengagement or emergence of the part from the pelvis. While the movements of birth in flexed and extended cephalic presentations are similar, the way the head negotiates the pelvis and the way it is born differ in several important respects, which are noted. Asterisks next to a number indicate the movements mentioned in modern textbooks.

Descent of the Baby in an Anterior Face Presentation

***1. Full extension of the head**

"Extension" describes the degree to which the baby's chin is lifted away from his chest. Most face babies enter the pelvis fully extended or nearly so. If the baby is only in a partially extended face presentation, the pelvic tissues and contractions produce counterpressure on the head, increasing extension until the baby's chin (mentum) leads the way as descent proceeds. Note that the soft, probably edematous face would be felt at this point during an internal exam because the bony vertex is completely out of reach.

***2. Descent**

Descent is likely to take place in a manner similar to the fully flexed head because the presenting diameters are almost the same as in flexed anterior vertex presentations.

Asynclitic descent to engagement: At any given station, the biparietal diameter is much higher in the pelvis in face presentations than it is in a vertex presentation. Because the bulk of the head precedes the biparietal diameter, asynclitic descent would not offer any advantage and is therefore an ineffective adaptation for engagement of the face. As the biparietal diameter descends to the level of the brim, the baby may be able to wiggle his head through at somewhat of an angle, but this would be most likely to occur if the baby were small in comparison to the pelvis.

***3. Engagement of the head**

Descent of the biparietal diameter–the widest transverse diameter of the fetal skull– through the pelvic inlet happens late in labor. A face presentation is unique in that considerable descent of the head is required before engagement can occur. The first plane of the head to engage is the face. The face can be at the level of the ischial spines (indicated in the chart below by the dotted lines) while the biparietal diameter is still well above the brim.

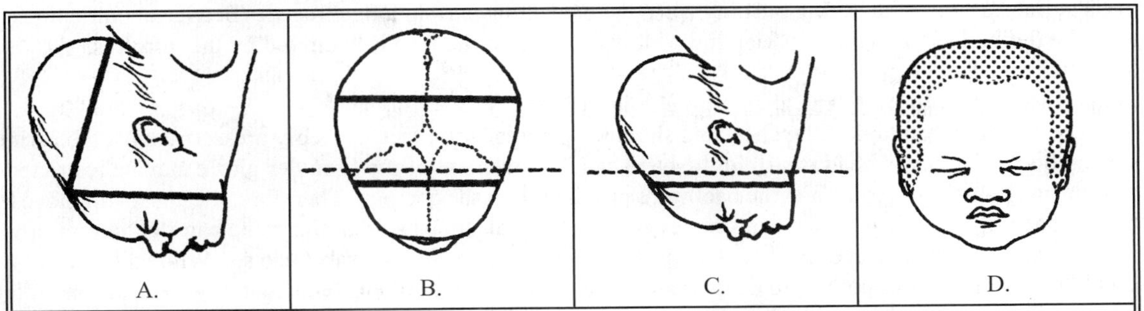

A. The suboccipitobregmatic diameter compared to the submentobregmatic diameter
B. The bitemporal diameter bisects the submentobregmatic in the same plane. These engage together. Note that the biparietal diameter is still well above the brim.
C. Side view showing the engagement of the submentobregmatic diameter
D. The pale areas engage first, followed by the shaded areas.

The longest anteroposterior diameter of the face is the submentobregmatic (which is about the same size as the suboccipitobregmatic diameter of the well-flexed vertex presentation). The transverse diameter of the face is the bitemporal. In vertex presentations, the suboccipitobregmatic and biparietal diameters, which are at 90° angles to each other, are in the same plane when the head is flexed and engage together. In a face presentation, the submentobregmatic diameter and the biparietal diameter are in different planes. First, the submentobregmatic and bitemporal diameters pass through the brim. After further descent the biparietal diameter passes through the brim, marking the actual engagement of the head. In most cases, the face must be at +2 station before engagement occurs.

***4. Internal rotation of the head**

The baby's head accommodates itself to the shape of the mother's levator ani in extended cephalic presentations just as it does in flexed attitudes. This usually occurs between the ischial spines and the tuberosities. The mentum rotates to a directly anterior position. This allows the bulky and less compressible posterior portion of the head to occupy the roomier sacral curve and places the upper spine in position to flex under the pubic bone as the head is born.

5. First internal rotation of the body and shoulders

As the face undergoes internal rotation to bring the chin directly anterior, the shoulders and body are likely to follow completely, moving to align with the transverse diameter of the brim. Full extension of the head as it passes under the pubic arch presses the occiput backward against the upper spine, causing the back to arch. This results in the shoulders usually assuming a transverse orientation, which maintains them in a 90° angle with the long axis of the head.

6. Engagement of the shoulders

The shoulders enter the transverse diameter of the inlet between the time the face reaches the pelvic floor and when it distends the perineum as it passes through the ischial tuberosities.

• Flexion of the shoulder and arms

As in vertex presentations, the attitude of the shoulders can shift as necessary to facilitate descent.

7. Spinal straightening begins

As the head passes deeply into the pelvic cavity, space is created in the uterus for the baby's body to stretch out, and the spine begins to straighten. This prepares the baby's body to flex laterally when the spine reaches the deepest curve of the birth canal.

• Dilating the perineum

As the face descends, it becomes firmly pressed against the pelvic floor.

• Crowning of the face

This is defined as the point during pushing when the presenting part no longer recedes between contractions. A full crown may be defined as the point at which the widest diameter of the face is encircled by the introitus.

8-1. Second internal rotation of the chest and shoulders begins

The second internal rotation of the chest and shoulders begins as the face is deeply pressed against the perineum or as it is being born. While the head is still in the birth canal, movement of the shoulder girdle may be restricted by the posture of the neck and upper spine and the backward pressure from the occiput. Therefore, the chest will move to adapt itself to the shape of the pelvic cavity near the level of the ischial spines so that the spine can flex laterally, with the shoulders following to assume an oblique orientation to the extent that they are able to do so. While this type of twisting may sound impossible, it is important to keep in mind the extreme flexibility of fetal anatomy. The second rotation of the chest and shoulders is accomplished as the baby turns his head, allowing the chin to remain directly anterior.

***9. Birth of the head by flexion of the upper spine and lower neck**

Traditionally, the head is said to deflex at the atlantooccipital joint as the chin pivots under the pubic arch, allowing the face to emerge as the head tips forward and the large posterior portion of the vertex sweeps the perineum. In fact, this would cause increasingly wider diameters to traverse the outlet as the head emerges, making birth more difficult. Borell and Fernström (1960) did X-ray studies of face and brow presentations and found that the head more or less maintains its degree of full extension throughout its birth. If full cervical extension has been maintained during labor, the head will be born by a process of spinal flexion that occurs in the lower cervical to upper thoracic areas as the head emerges from the birth canal.

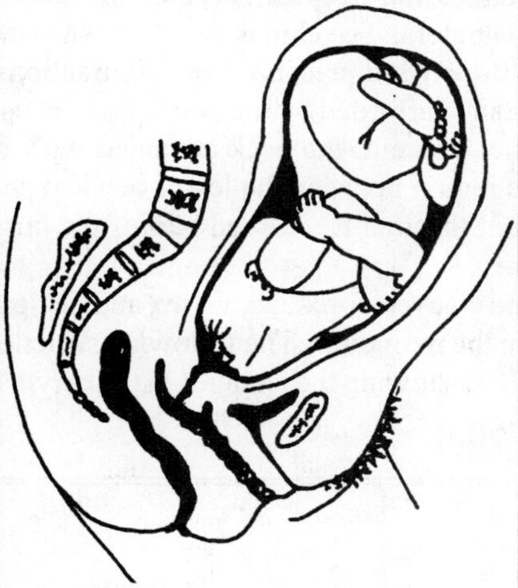

Head floating RMA and spine extended

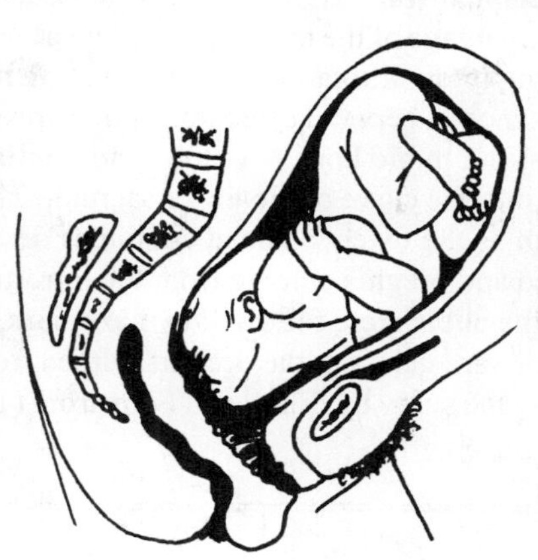

Descent (2) to engagement (3), spinal extension enhanced (1)

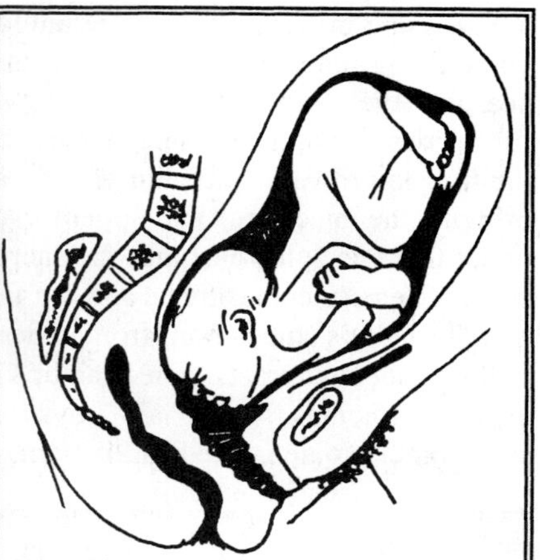

Internal rotation of head to MA (4) and 1st internal rotation of chest/shoulders to transverse (5)

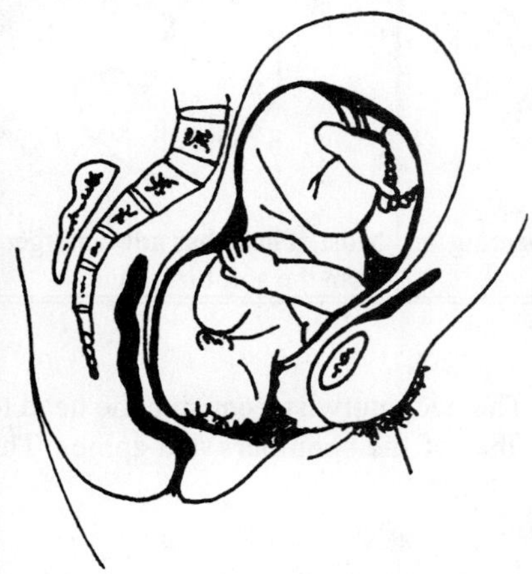

Shoulders engage transverse (6)

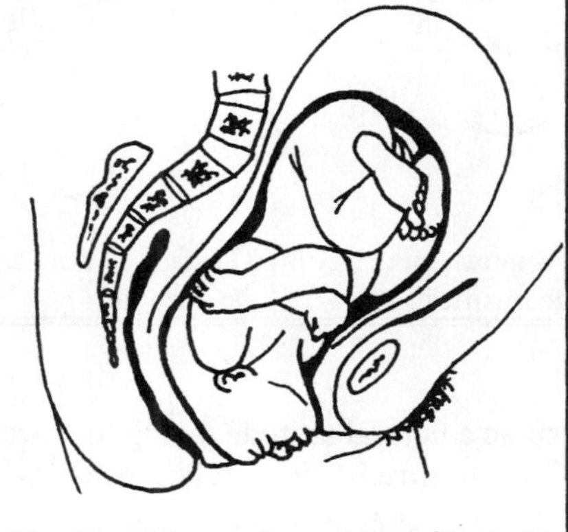

Shoulders/chest undergo their 2nd internal rotation to oblique (8-1); spinal flexion (7) allows head to remain extended (9); face is born MA and perineum retracts

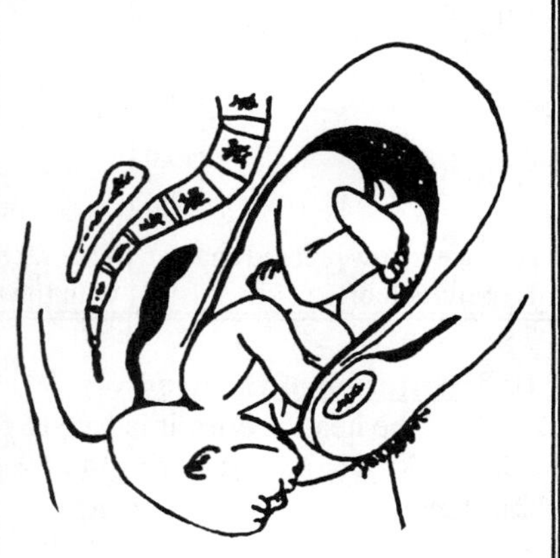

Shoulders/chest are now oblique (8-1); Head is born facing up OP (MA)

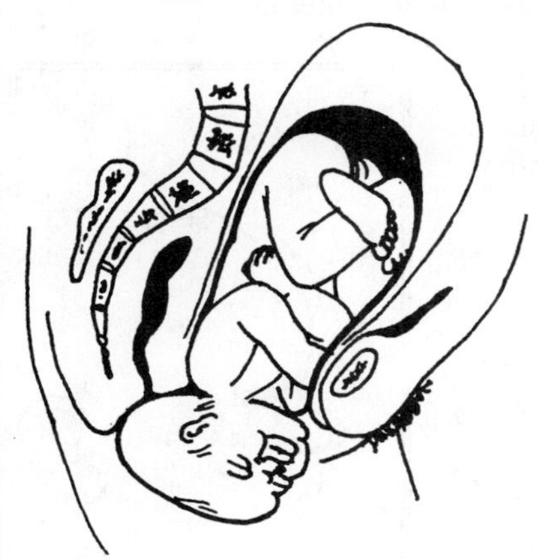

Head restitutes to LOP (RMA) (10)

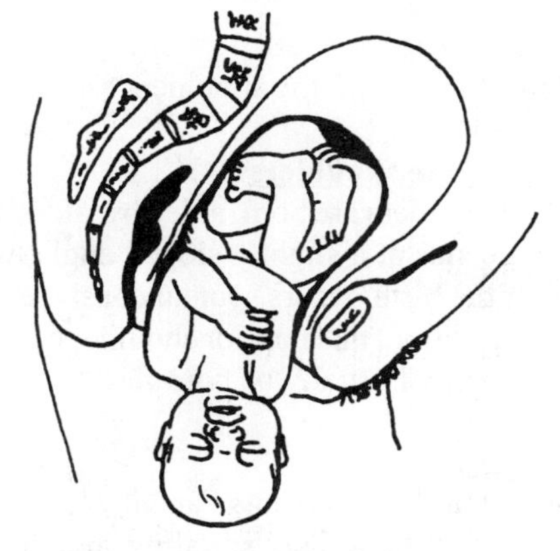

Shoulders/chest complete 2nd internal rotation to transverse (8-2); the head rotates externally to LOT (RMA) (11); the posterior and anterior shoulders are then born (12)

While some movement at the atlantooccipital joint does occur as the head rounds the deepest curve of the outlet, maintaining almost full extension takes advantage of the most optimal cephalic diameters. The chin is usually positioned near the level of the tuberosities following internal rotation. A combination of downward pressure from contractions, further descent of the fetal head, maintenance of cervical extension and the resistance afforded by the pelvic floor cause the face to crown as the chin glides past the pubic bone. As the head continues descent, the neck advances with it, bringing the lower neck and upper torso into the curve of the lower sacrum. The region between the lower cervical and upper thoracic spine curl into the sacrum as the extended head continues descent through the curved part of the birth canal. The perineum retracts and the face and bregma emerge from the introitus.

The baby's chin is born from under the pubic arch, followed by the mouth, nose, eyes, forehead, vertex and occiput as the perineum retracts. The head tips forward gently as the occiput is freed from the perineum. The following sketches are direct tracings from serial X-rays from the study by Borell and Fernström (1960) showing the changes in the cervical and thoracic spine as the head is born.

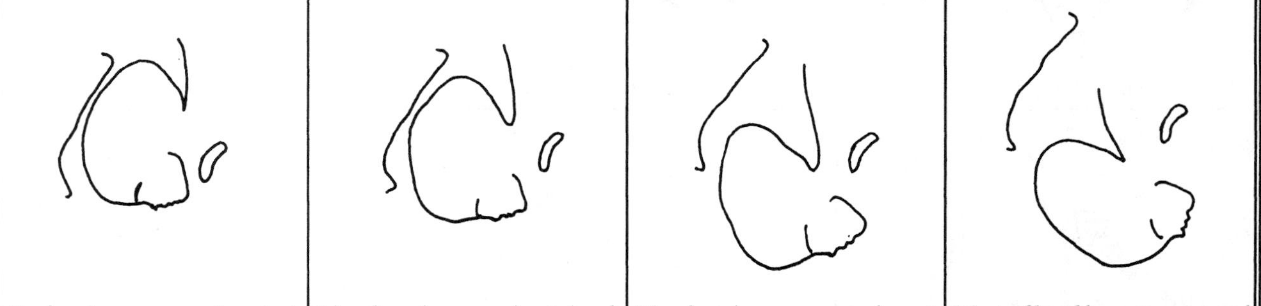

The face is now pressed against the pelvic floor.	The face is now about level with the tuberosities.	The face is now appearing at the introitus.	Most of head has now emerged from the soft birth canal.

***10. Restitution of the head**

Once the head is born it is free to resume a natural attitude facing forward. The neck untwists, causing the head to rotate back 45°, thus restoring its long axis to a right-angle relationship with that of the shoulders and spine. The shoulders remain at an oblique angle.

8-2. Second internal rotation of the chest and shoulders is completed

The upper spine will straighten out as soon as the head is born. The chest will rotate 45° moving the shoulders into an anteroposterior position.

***11. External rotation of the head**

The head rotates 45° in concert with the shoulders as they move into the anteroposterior diameter of the outlet.

12. Birth (disengagement) of the shoulders

Once the head is out, the shoulders are born, aided by lateral flexion. The long shoulder girdle descends at a slightly sloped angle, with one shoulder leading the way. If the birth occurs spontaneously, especially if the mother is in an upright position, the anterior shoulder may be seen first, but the posterior shoulder will usually be born first.

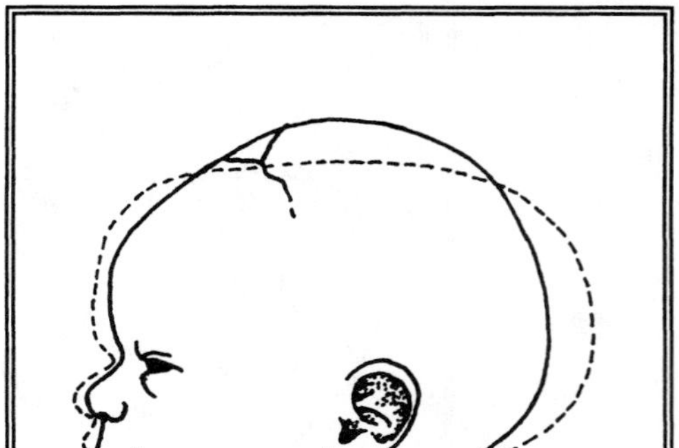

13. Birth of the torso and legs

Once the shoulders have been born, the torso and the legs generally slide out easily in a spiraling motion. This spiraling motion is most obvious when the baby is allowed to emerge with no assistance during a waterbirth (Greenhill, 1951; Sutton & Scott, 1996).

Moulding

Moulding in an anterior face presentation results in the head becoming elongated in its anteroposterior diameter. The parietal bones are flattened along the sagittal suture which flattens the vertex. There is no misalignment along the sagittal suture. Depression of the parietal bones increases the occipitofrontal diameter and decreases the submentobregmatic diameter, a desirable occurrence in face presentations. This causes the occiput to protrude and the forehead to be displaced forward slightly. The face is bruised and swollen from the pressure of birth. Caput formation can be expected, with the caput forming over the anterior cheek and eye.

Applying These Basic Concepts to all Face Presentations

The next chapters discuss the various ways the face baby can be born (LMA, RMA, LMT, etc.). Keep in mind that the basic movements must always be taken into account, regardless of the baby's position.

Summary of the Cardinal Spiraling Movements: Left Mentum Anterior (LMA)

The frequency of the different positions for face presentations is not discussed in great detail in the obstetric literature, although it is mentioned that LMA is the most frequent. An LMA position is a fully extended ROP.

Orientation of the baby to the mother's pelvis

The long axis of the face is aligned with the right oblique diameter, while the chin (mentum) occupies the left anterior corner of the brim. The shoulders are aligned with the left oblique diameter.

Birth of the LMA baby

***1.** The head is often fully extended prior to labor and the upper spine is arched. If not, extension becomes complete as the face encounters the resistance afforded by the soft tissues of the pelvic cavity.

***2.** The baby descends throughout labor.

***3.** The head engages as the biparietal diameter passes through the brim, which has usually occurred by the time the face reaches +2 station, late in labor.

***4.** The face rotates internally a total of 45°, from LMA to MA, as it adapts to the loop-shaped opening of the levator ani sling. Rotation consists of a downwardly spiraling movement, which facilitates descent. It usually occurs after dilation is complete and the face has passed the ischial spines.

5. The baby's body moves with the shoulders as they undergo their first internal rotation. Following the rotation of the mentum from LMA to MA, the shoulders rotate 45° from the left oblique diameter to align with the transverse diameter of the brim.

6. The shoulders engage when the bisacromial diameter enters the transverse diameter of the brim, as the face passes through the ischial tuberosities. The attitude of the shoulders shifts during descent as the torso accommodates to the shape of the birth canal.

7. The spine begins to straighten as the head enters the pelvis more deeply.

8-1. The second internal rotation of the shoulders begins between the time the face distends the perineum and is born. As the midchest and spine enter the curve of the birth canal near the level of the ischial spines, they rotate 45°, moving the shoulders from the transverse into the left oblique diameter. This adjustment allows the spine to flex laterally. The neck twists as this occurs, allowing the face to remain MA. Internal rotation of the shoulders may be hampered by the proximity of the occiput.

***9.** The chin glides down past the pubic arch, and the face begins to crown. The anterior neck is now under the pubic arch and the head is in the soft birth canal. The lower neck and upper spine begin to flex into the curve of the sacrum, allowing the head to remain almost fully extended as it advances. The perineum retracts and the head is born. The head is no longer held back in an attitude of extension, and the vertex now leads the way.

***10.** Restitution occurs as the neck untwists, allowing the occiput to rotate 45° from OP (MA) back to the ROP (LMA) position, restoring the long axis of the vertex to a 90° angle with the long axis of the shoulders.

8-2. The chest completes its second internal rotation, moving the shoulders 45° from the left oblique into the antero-posterior diameter before or during the next contraction. This brings the anterior shoulder under the pubic arch.

***11.** Concurrent with the internal rotation of the chest, the head rotates externally 45° from ROP (LMA) to ROT (LMT).

12. The anterior shoulder braces against the pubic bone as the posterior shoulder is born first by a process of lateral spinal flexion, after which the anterior shoulder slips past the pubic bone and emerges.

13. The torso and legs are born by a process of lateral flexion and a spiraling motion.

Moulding is similar in all anterior face positions. Caput formation will occur over the left cheek and eye.

LMA: head extended before labor	Descent to engagement	Internal rotation: LMA to MA	Chest-shoulders rotate internally following the head and engage transverse.

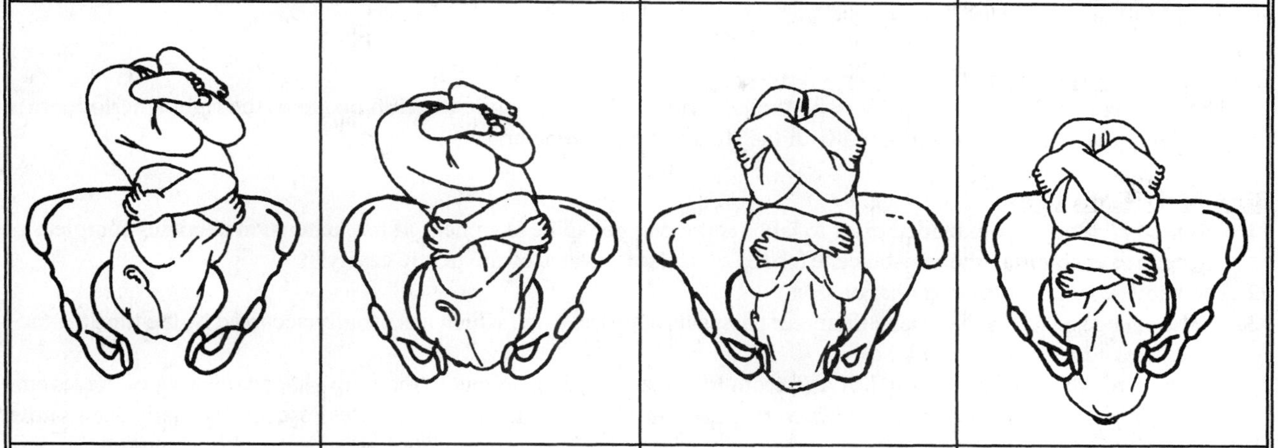

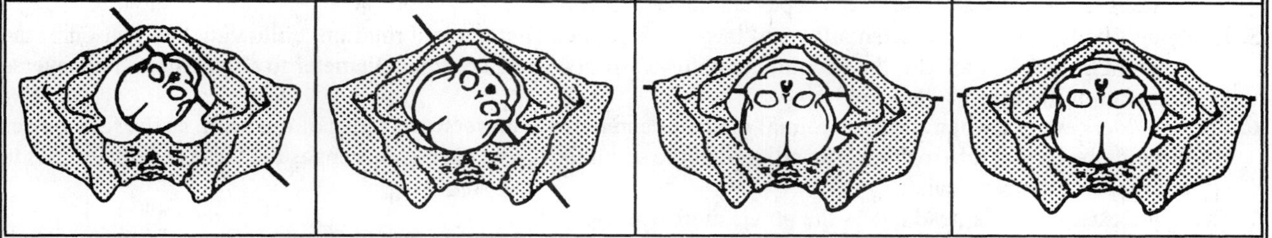

Chest-shoulders rotate to left oblique as descent proceeds. Upper spine flexes as head is born.	Head restitutes 45° from OP to ROP (MA to LMA)	Chest-shoulders rotate to transverse; head rotates externally 45°: ROP to ROT (LMA to LMT)

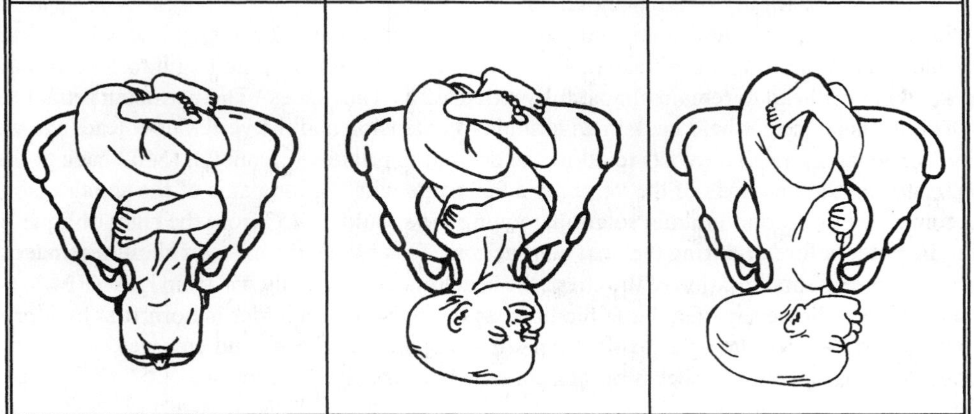

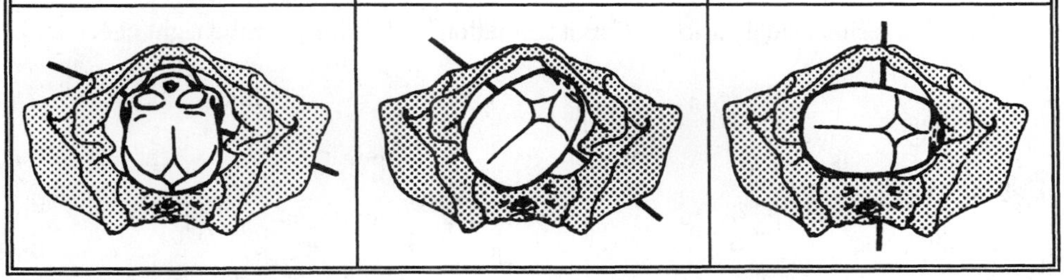

SUMMARY OF THE CARDINAL SPIRALING MOVEMENTS: RIGHT MENTUM ANTERIOR (RMA)

Birth with the baby in an RMA position is the mirror image of birth with the baby LMA. An RMA position is a fully extended LOP.

Orientation of the baby to the mother's pelvis

The long axis of the face is aligned with the left oblique diameter while the chin occupies the right anterior corner of the pelvis. The shoulders are aligned with the right oblique diameter.

Birth of the RMA baby

***1.** The head is often fully extended prior to labor and the upper spine is arched. If not, extension becomes complete as the face encounters the resistance afforded by the soft tissues of the pelvic cavity.

***2.** The baby descends throughout labor.

***3.** The head engages as the biparietal diameter passes through the brim, which has usually occurred by the time the face reaches +2 station, late in labor.

***4.** The face rotates internally a total of 45°, from RMA to MA, as it adapts to the loop-shaped opening of the levator ani sling. Rotation consists of a downwardly spiraling movement, which facilitates descent. It usually occurs after dilation is complete and the face has passed the ischial spines.

5. The baby's body moves with the shoulders as they undergo their first internal rotation. Following the rotation of the mentum from RMA to MA, the shoulders rotate 45° from the right oblique diameter to align with the transverse diameter of the brim.

6. The shoulders engage when the bisacromial diameter enters the transverse diameter of the brim, as the face passes through the ischial tuberosities. The attitude of the shoulders shifts during descent as the torso accommodates to the shape of the birth canal.

7. The spine extends as the head enters the pelvis more deeply.

8. The second internal rotation of the shoulders begins between the time the face distends the perineum and is born. As the midchest and spine enter the curve of the birth canal near the level of the ischial spines, they rotate 45°, moving the shoulders from the transverse into the right oblique diameter. This adjustment allows the spine to flex laterally. The neck twists as this occurs, allowing the face to remain MA. Internal rotation of the shoulders may be hampered by the proximity of the occiput.

***9.** The chin glides down past the pubic arch, and the face begins to crown. The anterior neck is now under the pubic arch and the head is in the soft birth canal. The lower neck and upper spine begin to flex into the curve of the sacrum, allowing the head to remain almost fully extended as it advances. The perineum retracts and the head is born. The head is no longer held back in an attitude of extension and the vertex now leads the way.

***10.** Restitution occurs as the neck untwists to allow the occiput to rotate 45° from OP (MA) back to the LOP (RMA) position, restoring the long axis of the vertex to a 90° angle with the long axis of the shoulders.

11. The chest completes its second internal rotation, moving the shoulders 45° from the right oblique into the antero-posterior diameter before or during the next contraction. This brings the anterior shoulder under the pubic arch.

***12.** Concurrent with the internal rotation of the chest, the head rotates externally 45° from LOP (RMA) to LOT (RMT).

13. The anterior shoulder braces against the pubic bone as the posterior shoulder is born first by a process of lateral spinal flexion, after which the anterior shoulder slips past the pubic bone and emerges.

14. The torso and legs are born by a process of lateral flexion and a spiraling motion.

Moulding is similar in all anterior face positions. Caput formation will occur over the right cheek and eye.

RMA: head extended before labor	Descent to engagement	Internal rotation: RMA to MA	Chest-shoulders rotate internally following the head and engage transverse.
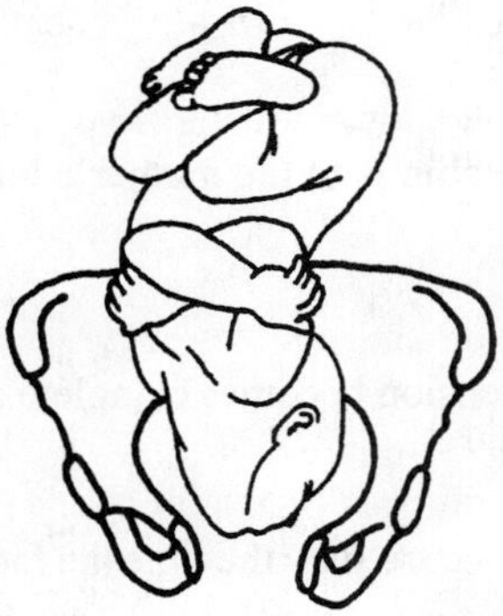	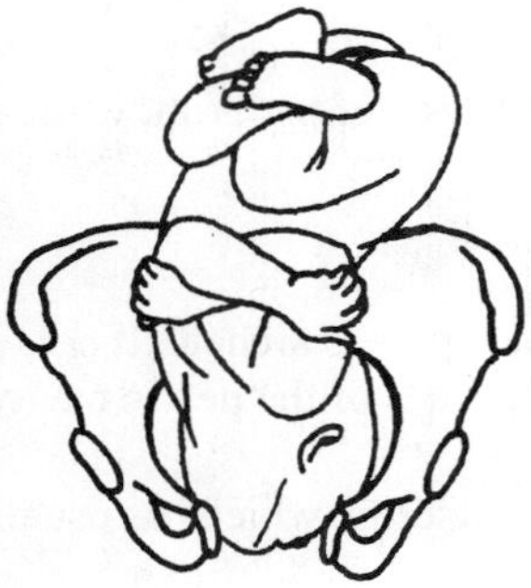	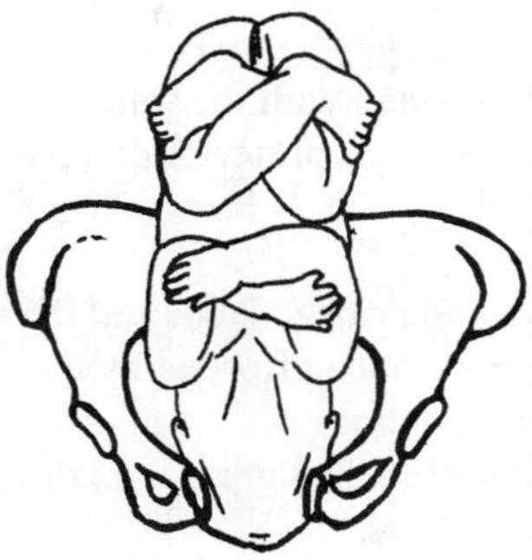	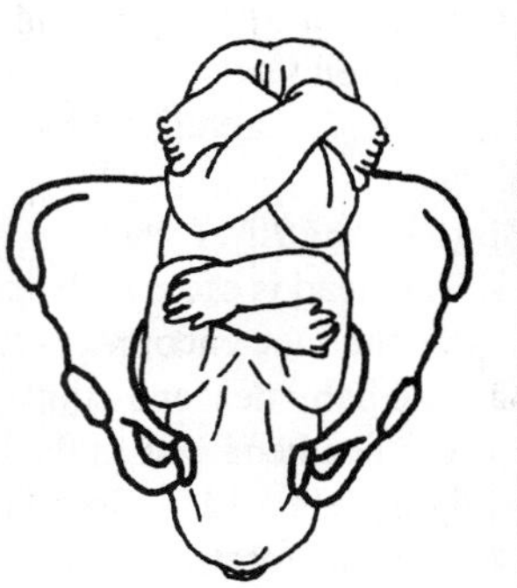
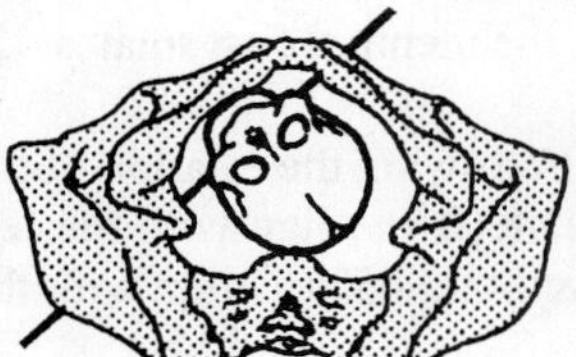	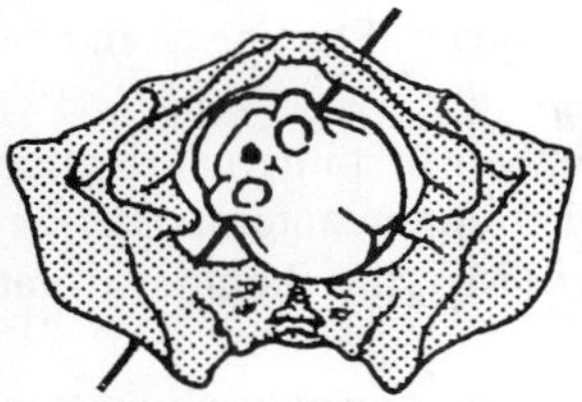	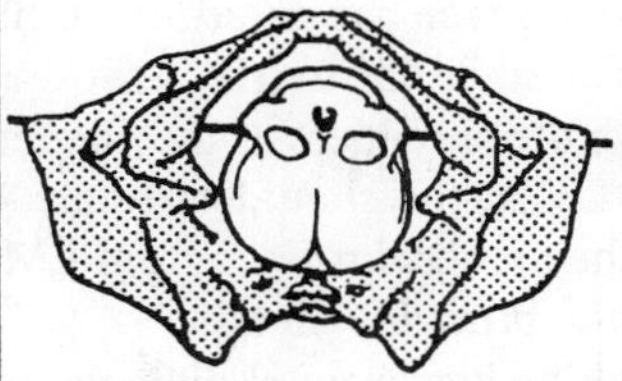	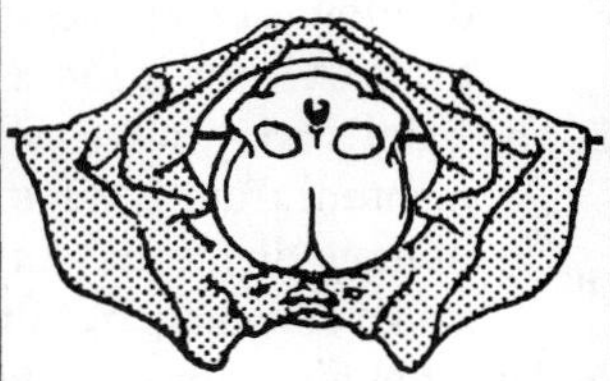

Chest-shoulders rotate to right oblique as descent proceeds. Upper spine flexes as head is born.	Head restitutes 45° from OP to LOP (MA to RMA)	Chest-shoulders rotate to transverse; head rotates externally 45°: LOP to LOT (RMA to RMT)
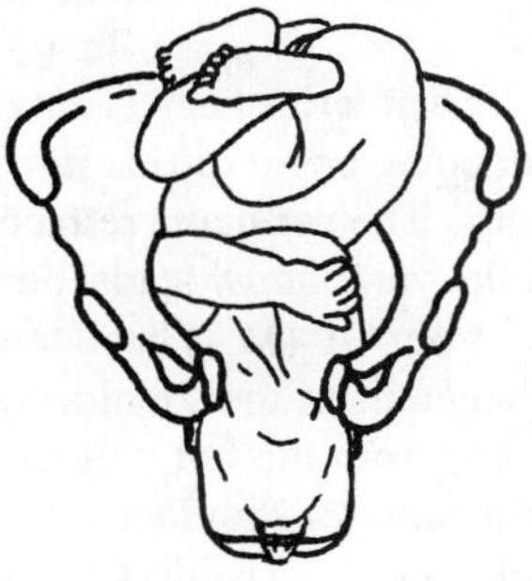	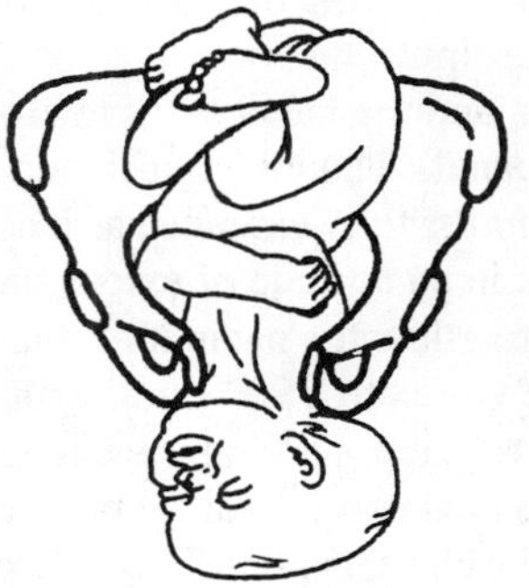	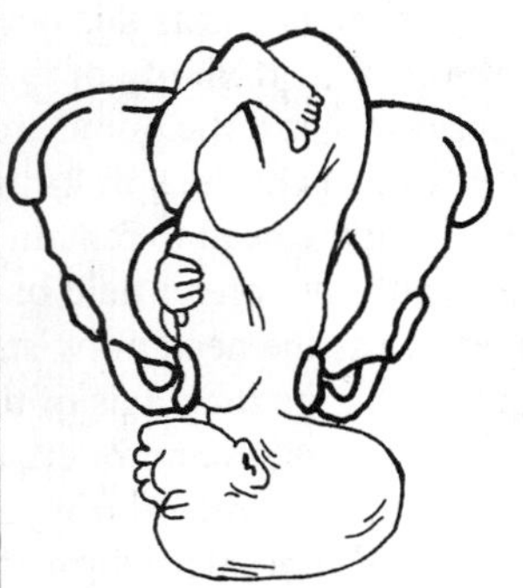
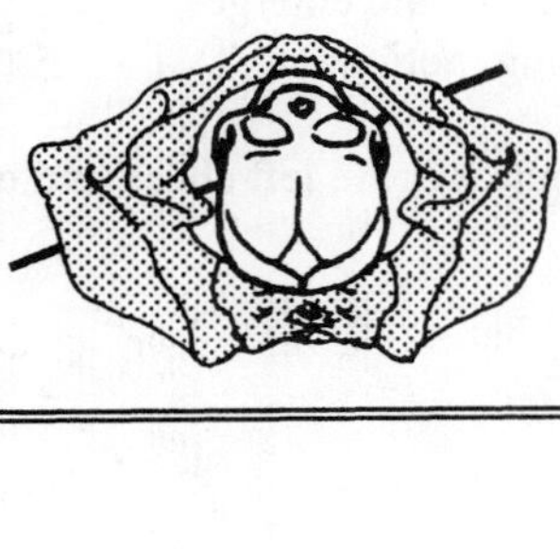	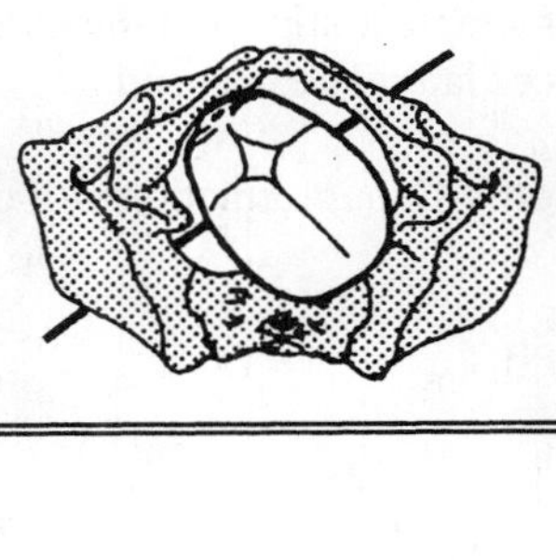	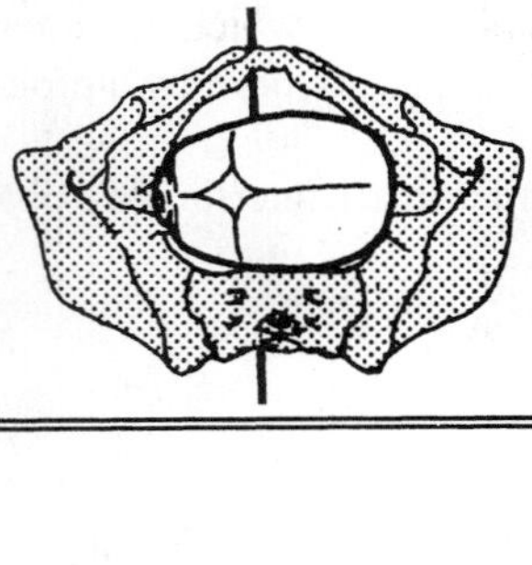

SUMMARY OF THE CARDINAL SPIRALING MOVEMENTS: LEFT MENTUM TRANSVERSE (LMT)

LMT positioning represents a fully extended ROT position. When the transverse face has descended into the pelvis, spontaneous rotation to anterior almost always occurs.

Orientation of the baby to the mother's pelvis

The long axis of the face is aligned with the transverse diameter of the brim, while the chin is to the mother's left. The shoulder are aligned with the anteroposterior diameter.

Birth of the LMT baby

***1.** The head is often fully extended prior to labor and the upper spine is arched. If not, extension becomes complete as the face encounters the resistance afforded by the soft tissues of the pelvic cavity.

***2.** The baby descends throughout labor.

***3.** The head engages as the biparietal diameter passes through the brim, which has usually occurred by the time the face reaches +2 station, late in labor.

***4.** The face rotates internally a total of 90°, from LMT to MA, as it adapts to the loop-shaped opening of the levator ani sling. Rotation consists of a downwardly spiraling movement, which facilitates descent. It usually occurs after dilation is complete and the face has passed the ischial spines. Starting from LMT, the mentum first rotates 45° to LMA, then it rotates another 45° to MA.

5. The baby's body moves with the shoulders as they undergo their first internal rotation. Following the rotation of the mentum from LMT to LMA, the shoulders rotate 45° from the anteroposterior diameter to align with the left oblique diameter. As the mentum rotates from LMA to MA, the shoulders rotate another 45° to align with the transverse diameter of the brim, 90° in all.

6. The shoulders engage when the bisacromial diameter enters the transverse diameter of the brim, as the face passes through the ischial tuberosities. The attitude of the shoulders shifts during descent as the torso accommodates to the shape of the birth canal.

7. The spine extends as the head enters the pelvis more deeply.

8-1. The second internal rotation of the shoulders begins between the time the face distends the perineum and is born. As the midchest and spine enter the curve of the birth canal near the level of the ischial spines, they rotate 45°, moving the shoulders from the transverse into the left oblique diameter. This adjustment allows the spine to flex laterally. The neck twists as this occurs, allowing the face to remain MA. Internal rotation of the shoulders may be hampered by the proximity of the occiput.

***9.** The chin glides down past the pubic arch, and the face begins to crown. The anterior neck is now under the pubic arch and the head is in the soft birth canal. The lower neck and upper spine begin to flex into the curve of the sacrum, allowing the head to remain almost fully extended as it advances. The perineum retracts and the head is born. The head is no longer held back in an attitude of extension and the vertex now leads the way.

***10.** Restitution occurs as the neck untwists to allow the occiput to rotate 45° from OP (MA) back to the ROP (LMA) position, restoring the long axis of the vertex to a 90° angle with the long axis of the shoulders.

8-2. The chest completes its second internal rotation, moving the shoulders 45° from the left oblique into the antero-posterior diameter before or during the next contraction. This brings the anterior shoulder under the pubic arch.

***11.** Concurrent with the internal rotation of the chest, the head rotates externally 45° from ROP (LMA) to ROT (LMT).

12. The anterior shoulder braces against the pubic bone as the posterior shoulder is born first by a process of lateral spinal flexion, after which the anterior shoulder slips past the pubic bone and emerges.

13. The torso and legs are born by a process of lateral flexion and a spiraling motion.

Moulding is similar in all anterior face positions. Caput formation will occur over the left cheek and eye.

LMT: head extended	Descent to engagement	Internal rotation of head and shoulders: LMT to LMA	Internal rotation of head continues: LMA to MA
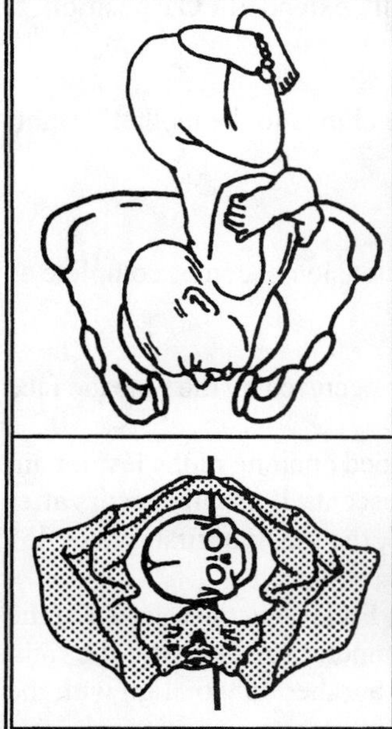	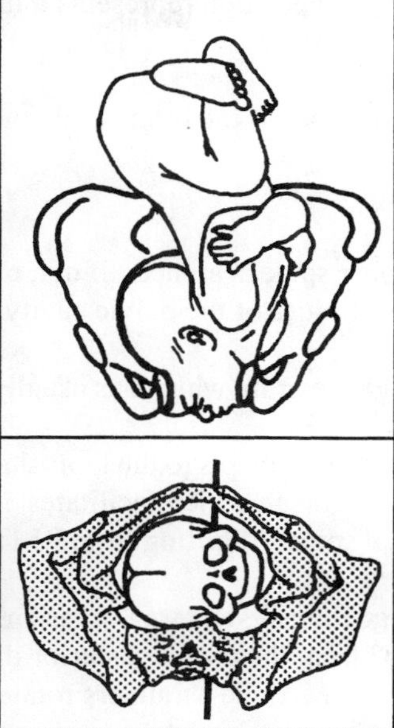	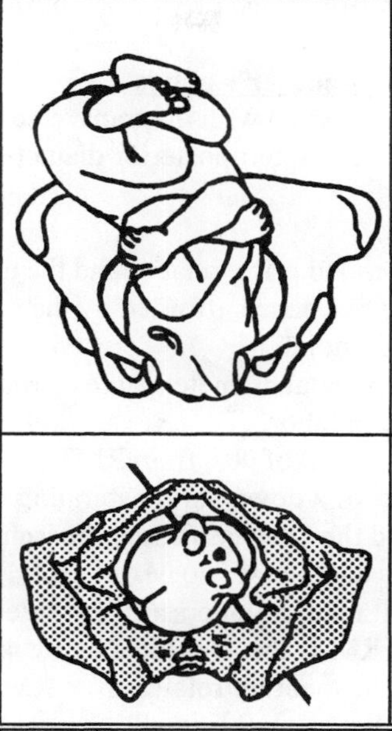	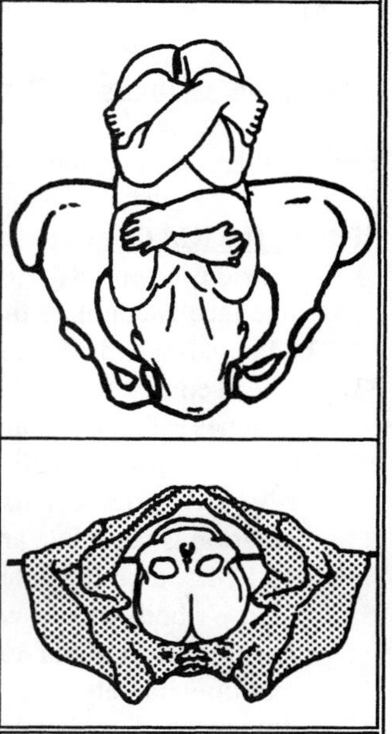
The shoulders follow the head and engage transverse.	Chest rotates as descent proceeds, bringing shoulders left oblique. Upper spine flexes as head is born.	The head restitutes: 45° from OP to ROP (MA to LMA)	Shoulders rotate to AP as head rotates externally: ROP to ROT (LMA to LMT)
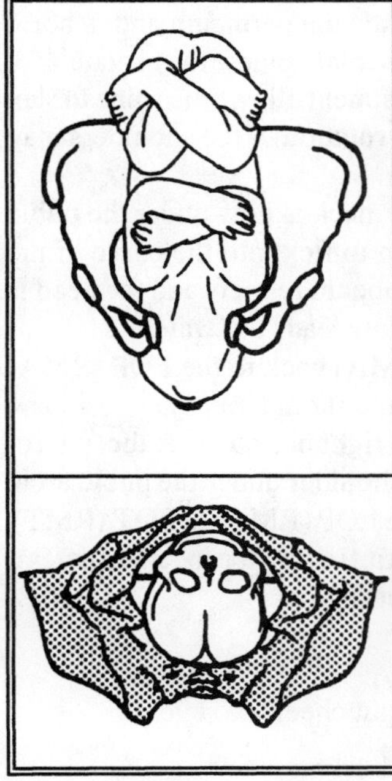	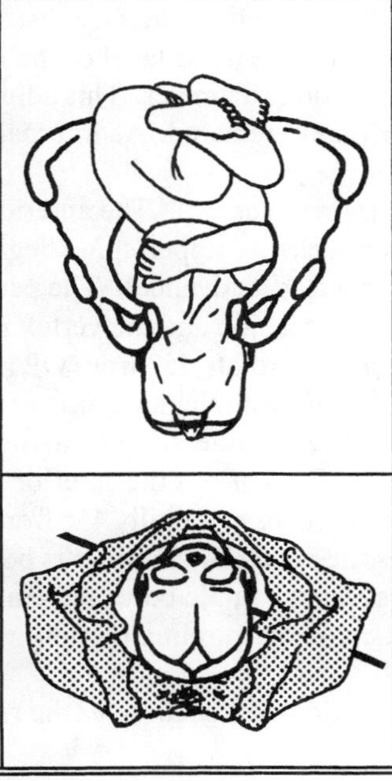	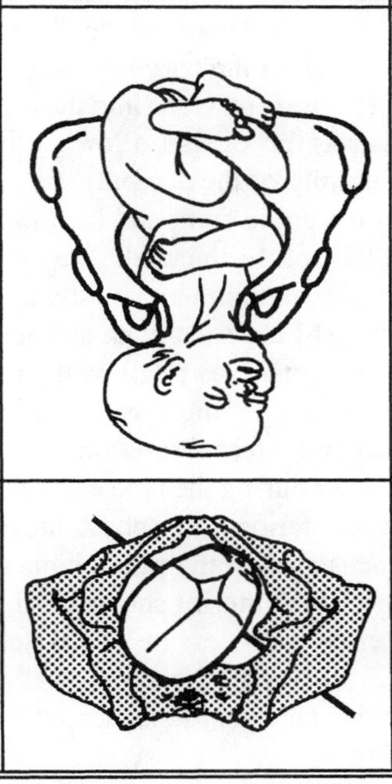	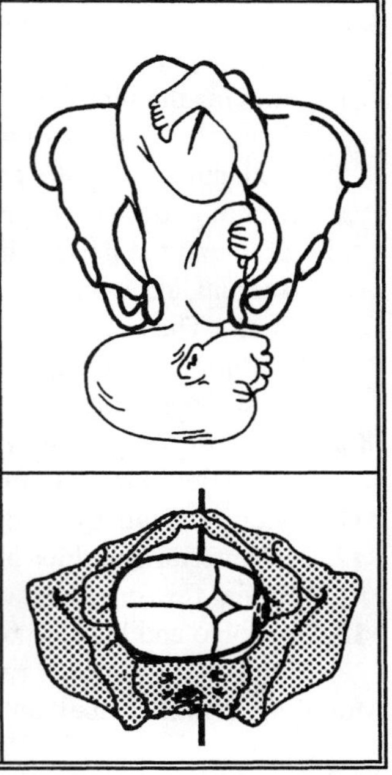

SUMMARY OF THE CARDINAL SPIRALING MOVEMENTS: RIGHT MENTUM TRANSVERSE (RMT)

An RMT position is the mirror image of an LMT birth. This position represents a fully extended LOT position.

Orientation of the baby to the mother's pelvis

The long axis of the face is aligned with the transverse diameter of the brim, while the chin is to the mother's right. The shoulders are aligned with the anteroposterior diameter.

Birth of the RMT baby:

***1.** The head is often fully extended prior to labor and the upper spine is arched. If not, extension becomes complete as the face encounters the resistance afforded by the soft tissues of the pelvic cavity.

***2.** The baby descends throughout labor.

***3.** The head engages as the biparietal diameter passes through the brim, which has usually occurred by the time the face reaches +2 station, late in labor.

***4.** The face rotates internally a total of 90°, from RMT to MA, as it adapts to the loop-shaped opening of the levator ani sling. Rotation consists of a downwardly spiraling movement, which facilitates descent. It usually occurs after dilation is complete and the face has passed the ischial spines. Starting from RMT, the mentum first rotates 45° to RMA, then it rotates another 45° to MA.

5. The baby's body moves with the shoulders as they undergo their first internal rotation. Following the rotation of the mentum from RMT to RMA, the shoulders rotate 45° from the anteroposterior diameter to align with the right oblique diameter. As the mentum rotates from RMA to MA, the shoulders rotate another 45° to align with the transverse diameter of the brim, 90° in all.

6. The shoulders engage when the bisacromial diameter enters the transverse diameter of the brim, as the face passes through the ischial tuberosities. The attitude of the shoulders shifts during descent as the torso accommodates to the shape of the birth canal.

7. The spine extends as the head enters the pelvis more deeply.

8-1. The second internal rotation of the shoulders begins between the time the face distends the perineum and is born. As the midchest and spine enter the curve of the birth canal near the level of the ischial spines, they rotate 45°, moving the shoulders from the transverse into the right oblique diameter. This adjustment allows the spine to flex laterally. The neck twists as this occurs, allowing the face to remain MA. Internal rotation of the shoulders may be hampered by the proximity of the occiput.

***9.** The chin glides down past the pubic arch, and the face begins to crown. The anterior neck is now under the pubic arch and the head is in the soft birth canal. The lower neck and upper spine begin to flex into the curve of the sacrum, allowing the head to remain almost fully extended as it advances. The perineum retracts and the head is born. The head is no longer held back in an attitude of extension and the vertex now leads the way.

***10.** Restitution occurs as the neck untwists to allow the occiput to rotate 45° from OP (MA) back to the LOP (RMA) position, restoring the long axis of the vertex to a 90° angle with the long axis of the shoulders.

8-2. The chest completes its second internal rotation, moving the shoulders 45° from the right oblique into the anteroposterior diameter before or during the next contraction. This brings the anterior shoulder under the pubic arch.

***11.** Concurrent with the internal rotation of the chest, the head rotates externally 45° from LOP (RMA) to LOT (RMT).

12. The anterior shoulder braces against the pubic bone as the posterior shoulder is born first by a process of lateral spinal flexion, after which the anterior shoulder slips past the pubic bone and emerges.

13. The torso and legs are born by a process of lateral flexion and a spiraling motion.

Moulding is similar in all anterior face positions. Caput formation will occur over the right cheek and eye.

RMT: head extended	Descent to engagement	Internal rotation of head and shoulders: RMT to RMA	Internal rotation of head continues: RMA to MA.
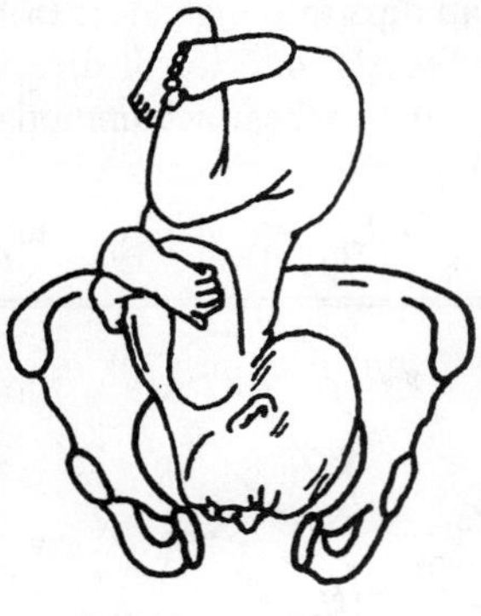	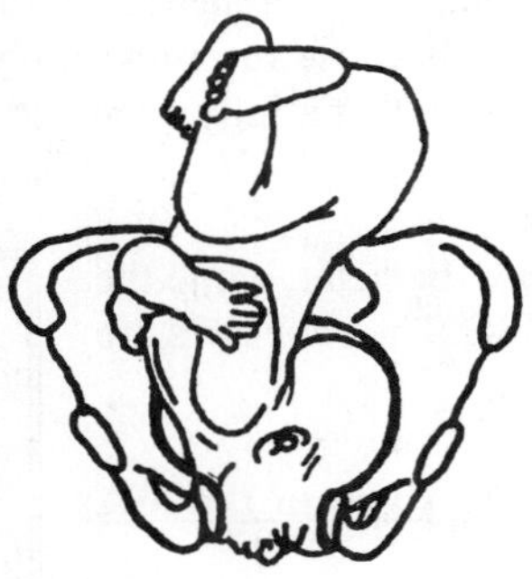	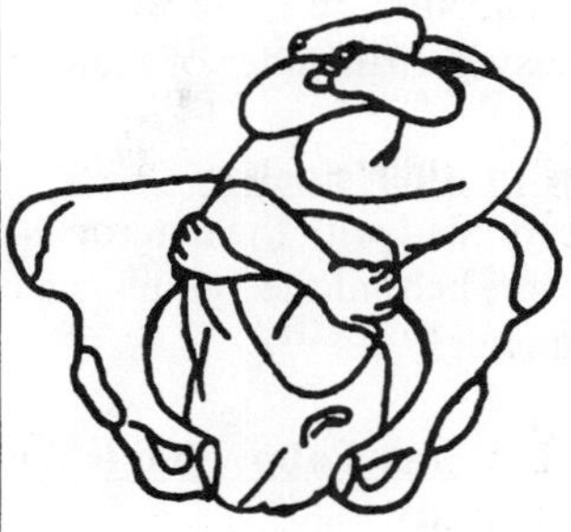	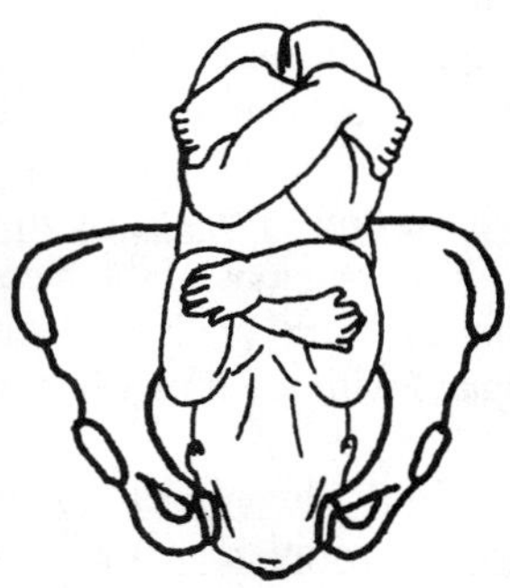
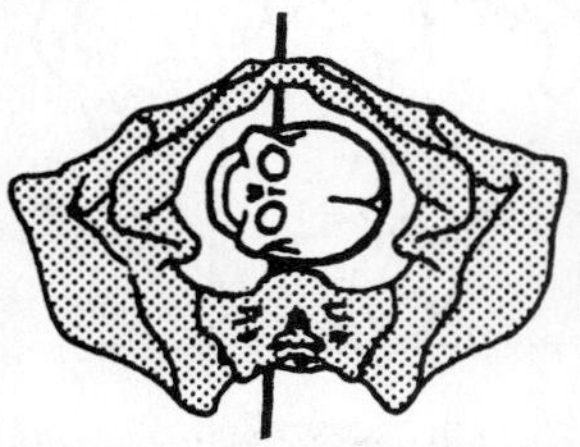	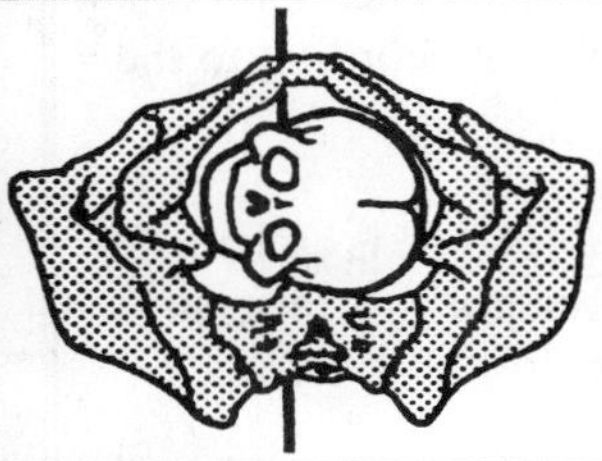	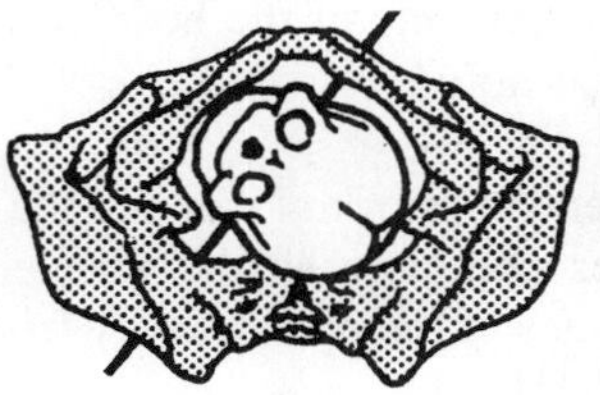	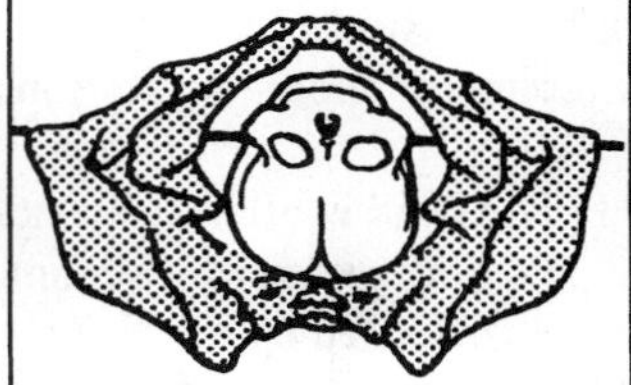

The shoulders follow the head and engage transverse.	Descent rotates chest, bringing shoulders to right oblique. Upper spine flexes as head is born.	The head restitutes: 45° from OP to LOP (MA to RMA)	Shoulders rotate to AP as head rotates externally 45°: LOP to LOT (RMA to RMT)
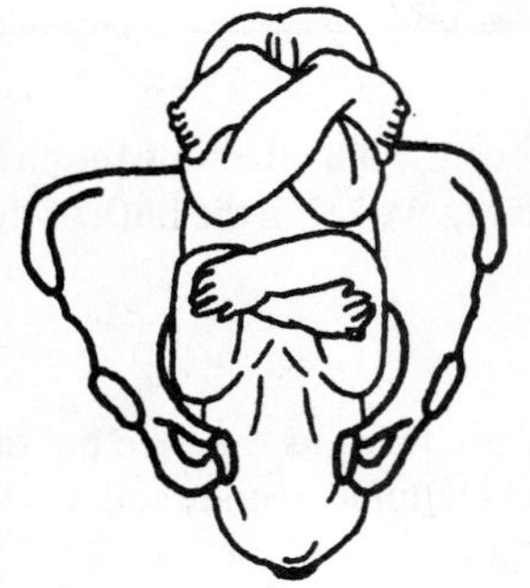	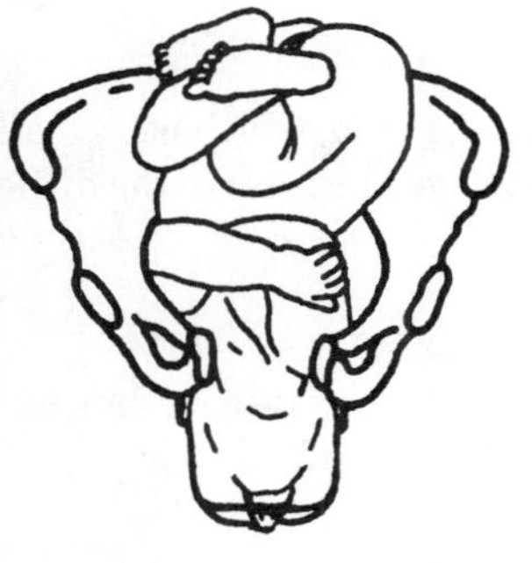	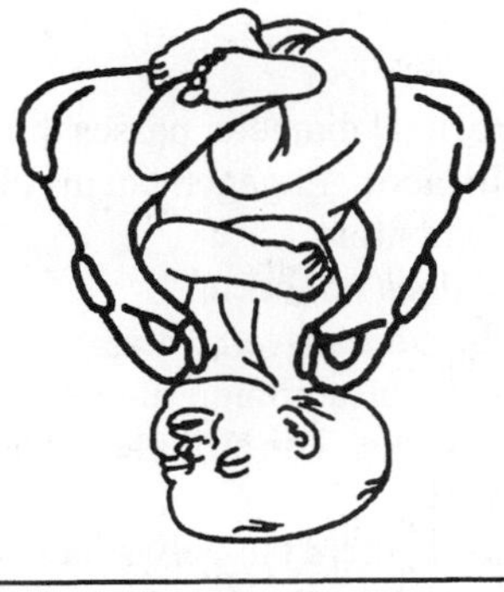	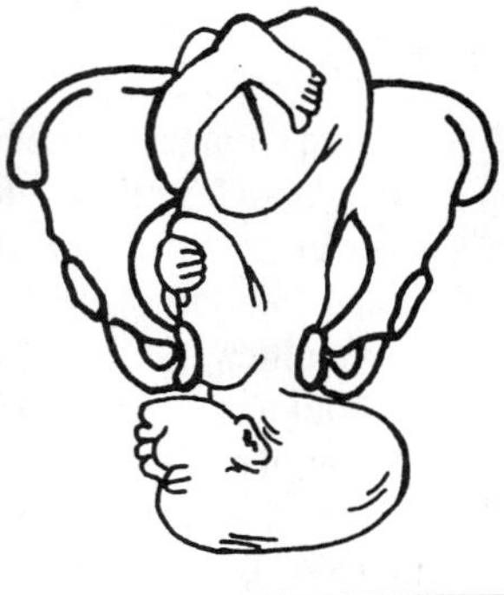
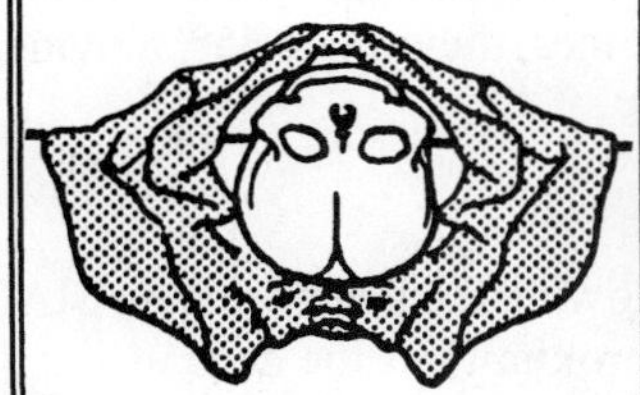	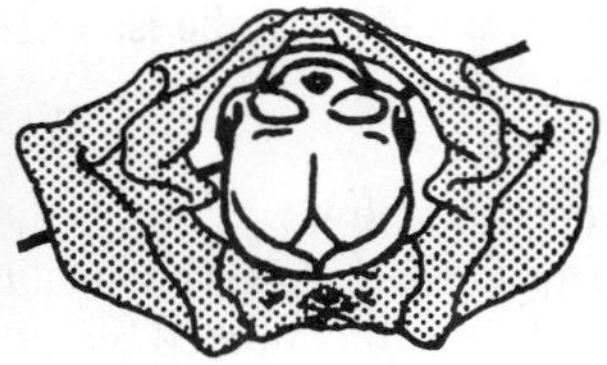	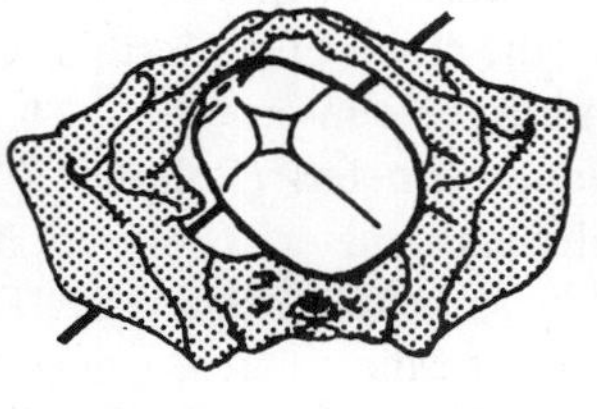	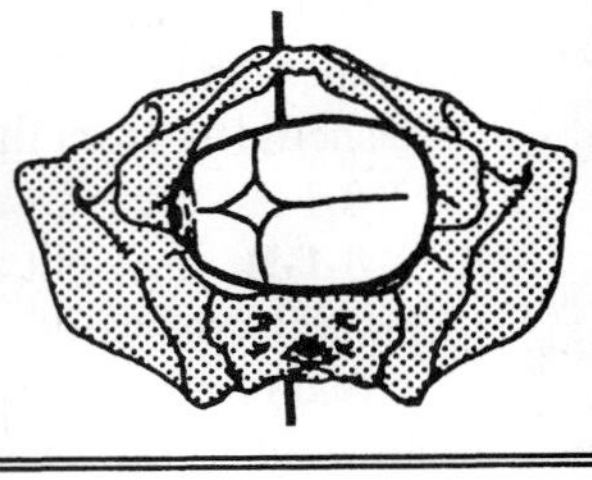

Summary of the Cardinal Spiraling Movements: Mentum Anterior (MA)

Theoretically, the baby may assume a direct MA position prior to labor, before the head dips into the pelvic brim. While it may be possible for a tiny baby to present and descend with the mentum either directly anterior or directly posterior, in reality these mechanisms are quite rare. This is because the presenting diameters best accommodate themselves to an oblique or transverse diameter of the brim. Note that a fully extended OP position becomes MA.

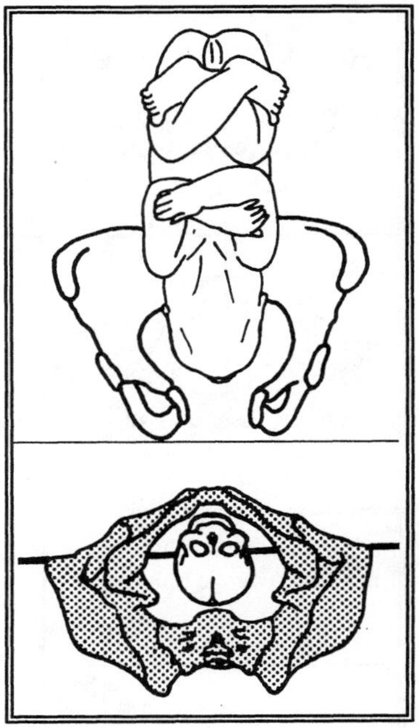

Orientation of the baby to the mother's pelvis

The long axis of the face is aligned with the anteroposterior diameter, while the chin (mentum) is directly anterior, behind the symphysis pubis. The shoulders are aligned with the transverse diameter.

Cardinal Movements of Birth When Labor Starts with the Baby in the MA Position (movements not illustrated)

When the baby is directly MA, shoulder rotation may occur in either a left or a right direction. Subsequent movements of the head will follow according to the direction of shoulder rotation, as noted.

***1.** The head is often fully extended prior to labor and the upper spine is arched. If not, extension becomes complete as the face encounters the resistance afforded by the soft tissues of the pelvic cavity from below.

***2.** The baby descends throughout labor.

The entire body of the baby may assume an LMA or RMA position to enter the brim. When this occurs, the birth proceeds as for an LMA or RMA position. The head may temporarily rotate to an LMA or RMA orientation prior to entering the brim, to facilitate descent. If this occurs, the neck may twist, allowing the shoulders to remain transverse. The following description assumes that the head enters the pelvis directly MA.

***3.** The head engages as the biparietal diameter passes through the brim, which has usually occurred by the time the face reaches +2 station, late in labor. Engagement may be delayed because of the difficulty in wedging the bulk of the vertex past the sacral promontory.

***4.** Internal rotation of the head does not occur.

5. The shoulder axis remains in the transverse diameter of the brim.

6. The shoulders engage when the bisacromial diameter enters the transverse diameter of the brim as the face passes through the ischial tuberosities. The attitude of the shoulders shifts during descent as the torso accommodates to the shape of the birth canal.

7. The spine extends as the head enters the pelvis more deeply.

8-1. Internal rotation of the shoulders begins between the time the face distends the perineum and is born. As the midchest and spine enter the curve of the birth canal near the level of the ischial spines, they rotate 45°, moving the shoulders from the transverse into:

8-1-A. the left oblique diameter. (Follow "A" entries below.)

8-1-B. the right oblique diameter. (Follow "B" entries below.)

This adjustment allows the spine to flex laterally. The neck twists as this occurs, allowing the face to remain MA. Internal rotation at the level of the shoulders may be somewhat hampered by the proximity of the occiput.

***9.** The chin glides down past the pubic arch and the face begins to crown. The anterior neck is now under the pubic arch and the head is in the soft birth canal. The lower neck and upper spine begin to flex into the curve of the sacrum, allowing the head to remain almost fully extended as the perineum retracts and the head is born. The head is no longer held back in an attitude of extension, and the vertex now leads the way.

***10.** Restitution occurs as the neck untwists to allow the occiput to rotate 45° from OP (MA) back to:

10-A. the ROP (LMA) position.

10-B. the LOP (RMA) position.

Restitution restores the long axis of the vertex to a 90° angle with the long axis of the shoulders.

8-2. The chest completes its second internal rotation, moving the shoulders 45° from:

8-2-A. the left oblique diameter

8-2-B. the right oblique diameter

into the anteroposterior diameter before or during the next contraction. This brings the anterior shoulder under the pubic arch.

***11.** Concurrent with the internal rotation of the chest, the head rotates externally 45°:

11-A. from ROP (LMA) to ROT (LMT).

11-B. from LOP (RMA) to LOT (RMT).

12. The anterior shoulder braces against the pubic bone as the posterior shoulder is born first by a process of lateral spinal flexion, after which the anterior shoulder slips past the pubic bone and emerges.

13. The torso and legs are born by a process of lateral flexion and a spiraling motion.

Moulding is similar for all anterior face positions. The caput will form over the anterior cheek and eye.

THE PROCESS OF BIRTH IN MENTUM POSTERIOR FACE PRESENTATIONS

In a persistently posterior face presentation, the baby typically starts out either LMP or RMP, and the chin rotates to a posterior position. *As a rule, the birth of a normal term baby in a face presentation requires that the chin rotate anteriorly to arrive beneath the pubic bone.* However, studies confirm that many mentum posterior babies will rotate spontaneously to a mentum anterior position from which they can be born more safely. Rotation usually occurs very late in labor, after the face is well applied to the pelvic floor. Three studies report a rate of spontaneous rotation of 50 to 63% (Cruikshank & White, 1973; Cucco, 1966; Tucker et al., 1957).

Why posterior face presentations become arrested

The anterior pelvis is short and shallow compared to the posterior pelvis. When the chin is posterior, the anterior neck must traverse both the posterior pelvic wall from the center of the sacral promontory to the tip of the coccyx, a distance of about 12.5 to 15 cm, as well as the distance from the tip of the coccyx to the edge of the fully distended perineum, which is another 3 to 8 cm. The anterior neck, which averages 5 cm in length in a term infant, becomes maximally stretched during full extension but is still much too short to span the length of the posterior birth canal.

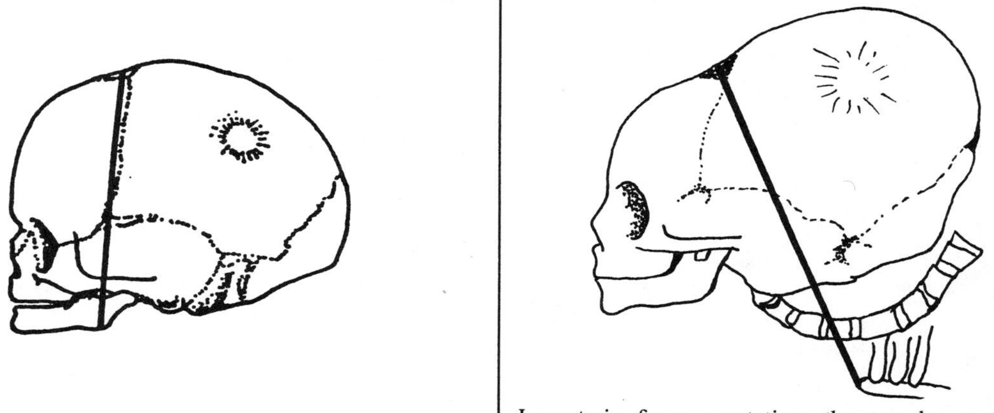

The submentobregmatic diameter presents in anterior face presentations.

In posterior face presentations, the sternobregmatic diameter presents. Here it is shown with the profound moulding of the posterior skull which makes this posture possible.

In addition, the inflexible dome of the vertex becomes maximally moulded in a posterior direction and then gets stuck above and behind the pubic bone, which prevents descent. The large posterior skull gets pressed against the pubic bone at the bregma; as this occurs, the dome of the head pushes against the anterior shoulder, forcing it backward. The dome of the head wedges between the scapulae, locking the shoulder axis into a transverse orientation. The upper spine is maximally arched and the lower spine is equally lordotic, causing the entire spine to form a rigid "S" curve. With the neck already stretched to its limit, the biparietal diameter, shoulders and the upper chest try to descend and engage together, compounding the improbability of advancement. The locking of the shoulders also limits or prevents upper spinal mobility. This combination of factors render further descent with the head fully extended impossible. After posterior rotation of the chin takes place, the sternum impinges upon the promontory of the sacrum or slightly below this point. The presenting anteroposterior diameter thus becomes the sternobregmatic, which is 18 or 19 cm in length in the average term fetus, far too long for all but the largest pelvis combined with a very small, preterm or dead (and therefore very malleable) baby.

When labor progresses

Only rarely is a persistently MP baby born with minimal trauma; in such cases the baby is usually small and the pelvis huge. Most commonly, labor progresses only because long-arc rotation to MA takes place, starting as the chest begins its second internal rotation, moving the shoulders 45° into the oblique diameter through which they most recently passed.

Should a persistently posterior labor progress, birth is usually accomplished by a difficult and often damaging process of maximum extension as the anterior chest and neck is stretched along the sacrum and as the bregma and vertex are squeezed under the pubic arch. At this point, the face, bregma, vertex and occiput are born by a difficult process of being squeezed through the outlet. The head is then freed to resume an OA orientation and the shoulders are released. The shoulders will then undergo internal rotation of 45° to an oblique angle, or they move on to rotate another 45° into the anteroposterior diameter. The head will follow them, externally rotating to match their motion. The shoulders and body are then born as for all other cephalic presentations.

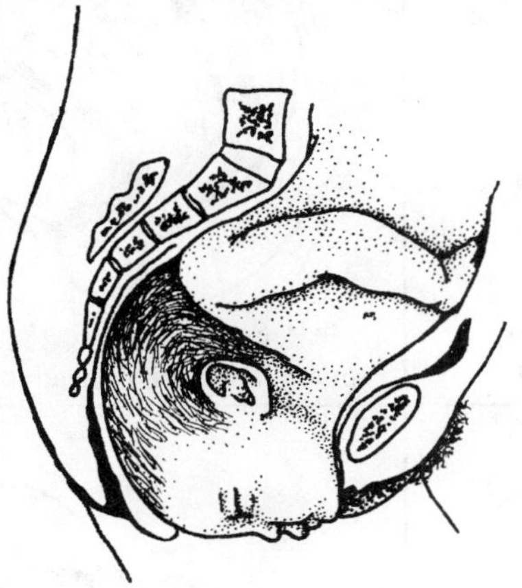

When the chin is anterior, there is room in the sacral curve for the upper spine to flex, allowing the head to pass beneath the pubic arch while maintaining full extension.

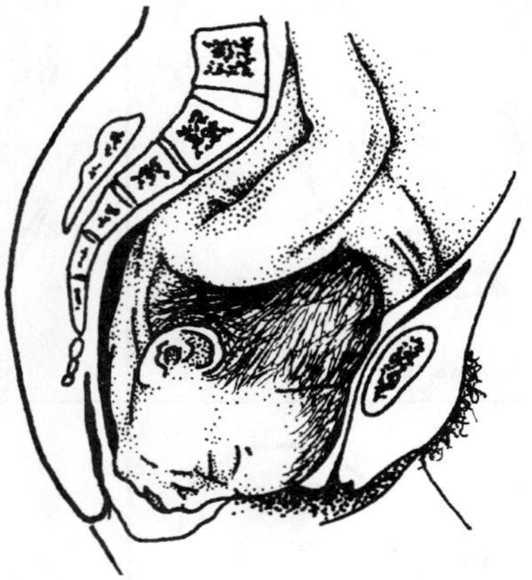

The crown of the vertex is trying to mould under the pubic arch. Head, chest and shoulders are attempting to enter the pelvis together. There is no room for any part of the spine to extend further; with descent, crushing of the vault and occiput is likely unless anterior rotation of the mentum occurs or the pelvis is quite large.

Moulding in the persistently posterior face presentation

The head is extremely distorted, with a deep horizontal depression across the skull at the level of the anterior fontanelle. The posterior vertex is much elongated, and the top of the head is flattened along the sagittal suture. The basiocciput is displaced downward. The membranes and venous sinuses in the skull have undergone an undue amount of stress, and intracranial hemorrhaging is a likely result. Caput formation occurs over the anterior cheek and eye.

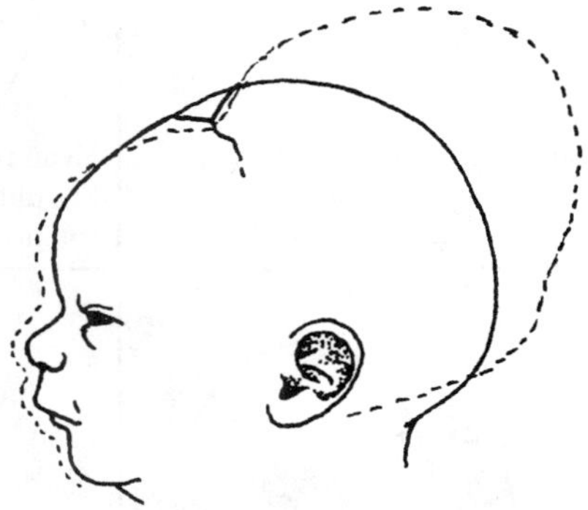

Risks to the baby

The baby born persistently mentum posterior is at great risk of brain and spinal trauma from the extreme distortion required for the dome of the cranium to navigate underneath the pubic arch. In preterm babies, this is dangerous because the skull is less ossified and the brain more fragile. In term babies, the skull is less compressible, and the danger of damage is just as great.

Risks to the mother

It is to be expected that the mentum posterior labor will not progress. Any type of obstructed labor that continues unresolved places the mother at grave risk of infection, uterine rupture, hemorrhage and death. For a full description of the course and sequelae of obstructed labor, see the chapter entitled "Transverse Lie." If labor does progress, extensive perineal and periurethral tearing may occur.

Happily, most babies who start out in a posterior face presentation rotate to anterior and are born normally.

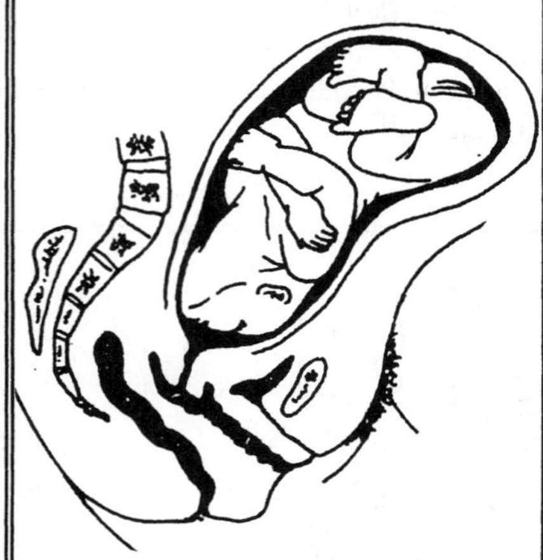

RMP, head floating, spine extended (1)

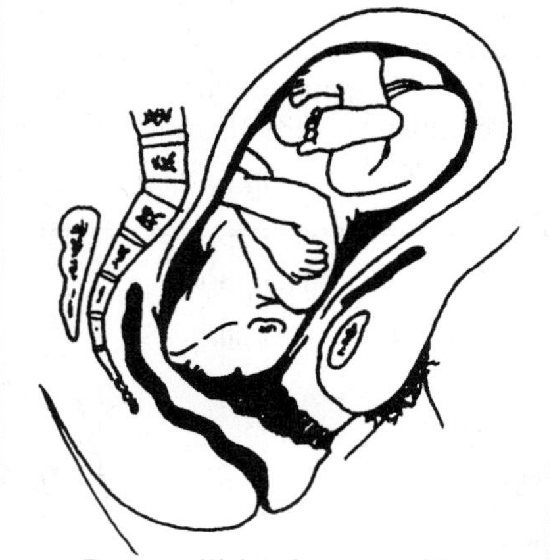

Descent (2) head engages (3), spinal flexion is enhanced (1)

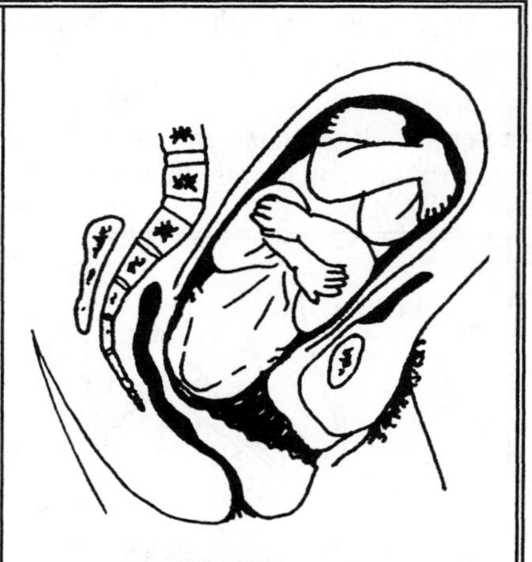

Internal rotation of head to RMT (4)

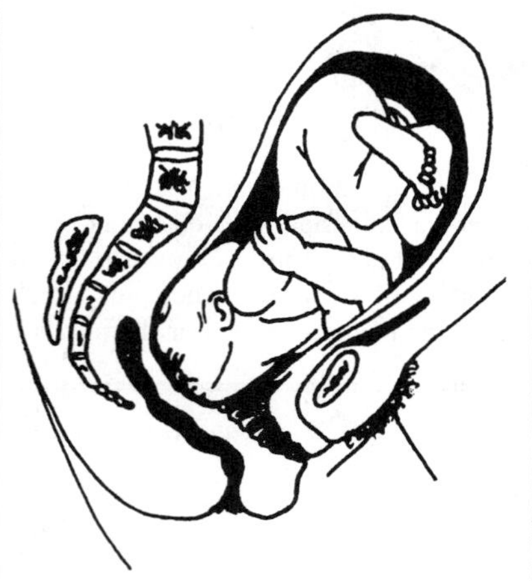

Internal rotation of head to RMA (4); chest/shoulders begin 1st internal rotation (5)

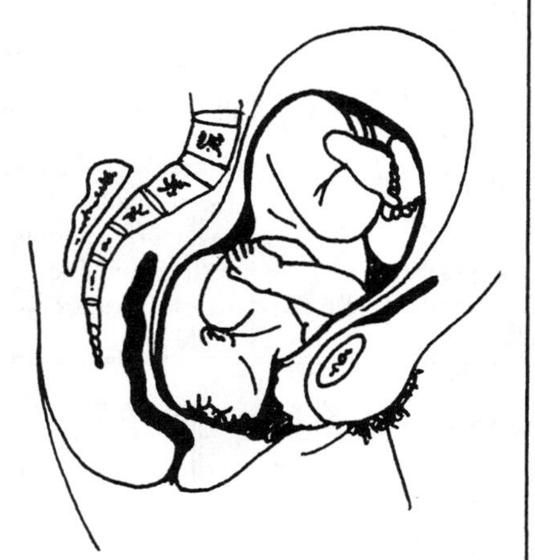

Head rotates internally to MA (4); Shoulders/chest complete 1st internal rotation to transverse (5) and engage (6)

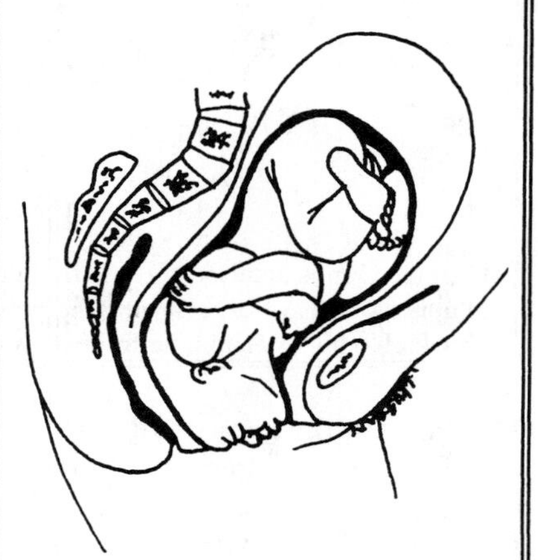

Chest/shoulders begin 2nd internal rotation to oblique (8-2); head crowns and is born by cervical flexion (9)

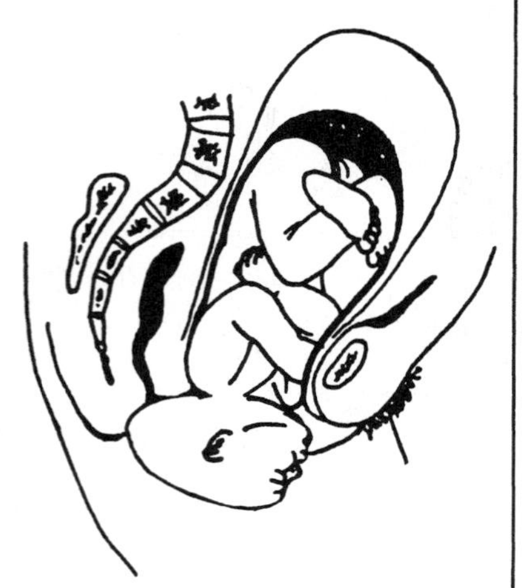

Head is born MA

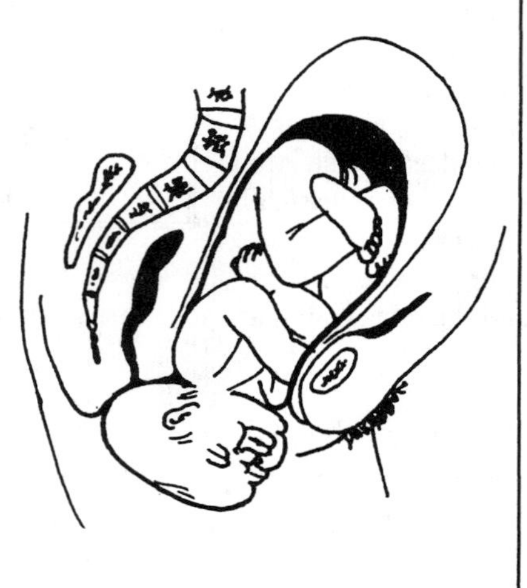

Head restitutes to LOP (RMA) (10)

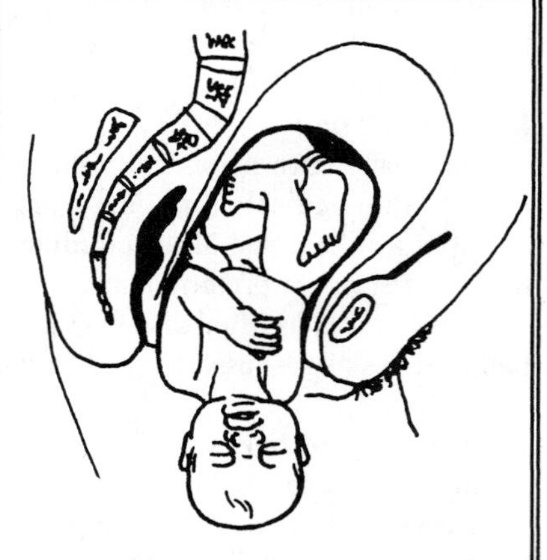

Shoulders finish 2nd internal rotation to AP (8-2); head follows with external rotation to LOT (RMT) (11); posterior shoulder born (12)

Summary of the Cardinal Spiraling Movements: Left Mentum Posterior (LMP)

Posterior face presentations typically start out either LMP or RMP. As is the case in occiput posterior positions, the baby may travel 135° via a long-arc rotation to an MA position or 45° via short-arc rotation to direct MP. This chapter reviews both movements for an LMP baby. LMP positioning occurs when an ROA baby's head becomes fully extended.

Orientation of the baby to the mother's pelvis

The long axis of the face is aligned with the left oblique diameter, while the chin occupies the left posterior corner of the pelvis. The shoulders are aligned with the right oblique diameter.

Long-arc rotation of the LMP baby

***1.** The head is often fully extended prior to labor and the upper spine is arched. If not, extension becomes complete as the face encounters the resistance afforded by the soft tissues of the pelvic cavity from below and as the bregma impinges on the superior ramus of the pubic bone anteriorly.

***2.** The baby descends throughout labor.

***3.** The head engages as the biparietal diameter passes through the brim, which has usually occurred by the time the face reaches +2 station, late in labor.

***4.** The face rotates internally a total of 135°, from LMP to MA, as it adapts to the loop-shaped opening of the levator ani sling. Rotation consists of a downwardly spiraling movement, which facilitates descent. It usually occurs after dilation is complete and the face is firmly pressed against the pelvic floor. Starting from LMP, the chin rotates 45° to LMT, then 45° to LMA and 45° to MA.

5. The baby's body moves with the shoulders as they undergo their first internal rotation. Following the rotation of the mentum from LMP to LMT, the shoulders rotate 45° from the right oblique diameter to align with the anteroposterior diameter. As the mentum rotates from LMT to LMA, the shoulders rotate 45° to align with the left oblique diameter. As the mentum rotates from LMA to MA, the shoulders rotate another 45° to align with the transverse diameter of the brim, 135° in all.

6. The shoulders engage when the bisacromial diameter enters the transverse diameter of the brim, as the face passes through the ischial tuberosities. The attitude of the shoulders shifts during descent as the torso accommodates to the shape of the birth canal.

7. The spine extends as the head enters the pelvis more deeply.

8-1. The second internal rotation of the shoulders begins between the time the face distends the perineum and is born. As the midchest and spine enter the curve of the birth canal near the level of the ischial spines, they rotate 45°, moving the shoulders from the transverse into the left oblique diameter. This adjustment allows the spine to flex laterally. The neck twists as this occurs, allowing the face to remain MA. Internal rotation of the shoulders may be hampered by the proximity of the occiput.

*** 9.** The chin glides down past the pubic arch and the face begins to crown. The anterior neck is now under the pubic arch and the head is in the soft birth canal. The lower neck and upper spine begin to flex forward, allowing the head to remain almost fully extended as it advances. The perineum retracts and the head is born. The head is no longer held back in an attitude of extension, and the vertex now leads the way.

***10.** Restitution occurs as the neck untwists to allow the occiput to rotate 45° from OP (MA) back to the ROP (LMA) position, restoring the long axis of the vertex to a 90° angle with the long axis of the shoulders.

8-2. The chest completes its second internal rotation, moving the shoulders 45° from the left oblique into the anteroposterior diameter before or during the next contraction. This brings the anterior shoulder under the pubic arch.

***11.** Concurrent with the internal rotation of the chest, the head rotates externally 45° from ROP (LMA) to ROT (LMT).

12. The anterior shoulder braces against the pubic bone as the posterior shoulder is born first by a process of lateral spinal flexion, after which the anterior shoulder slips past the pubic bone and emerges.

13. The torso and legs are born by a process of lateral flexion and a spiraling motion.

Moulding is similar in all face positions that rotate to anterior. Caput formation occurs over the left cheek and eye.

LMP orientation, head almost completely extended	Descent to engagement, extension complete	Internal rotation begins: LMP to LMT	Internal rotation of head continues: LMT to LMA.
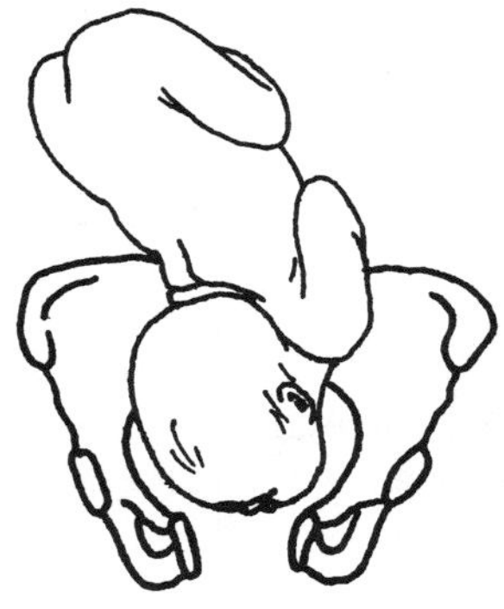	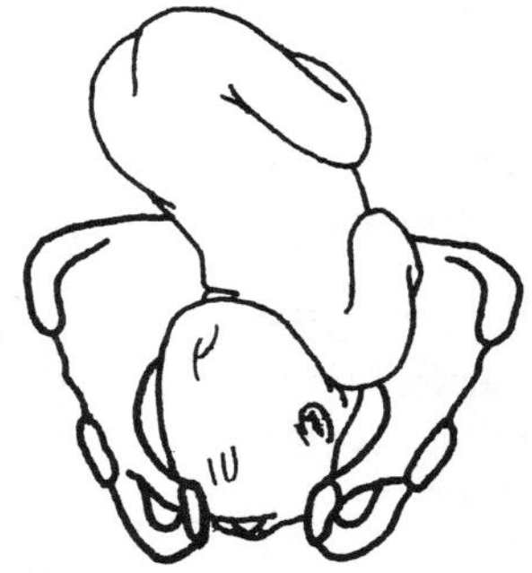	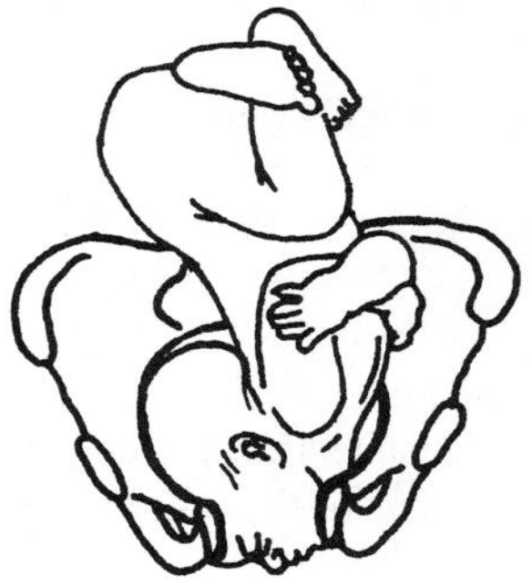	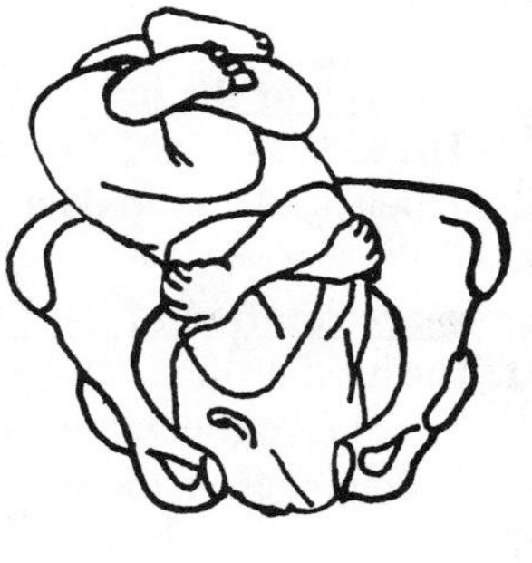
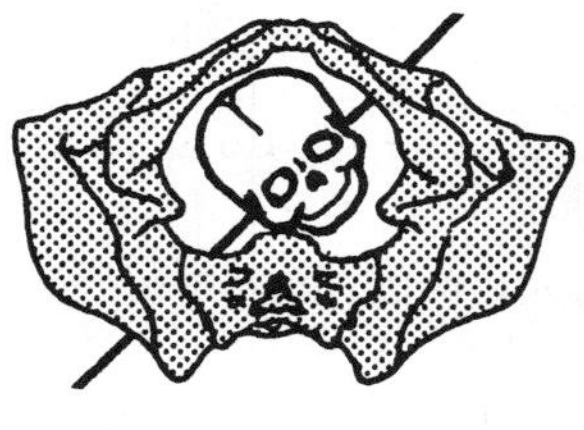	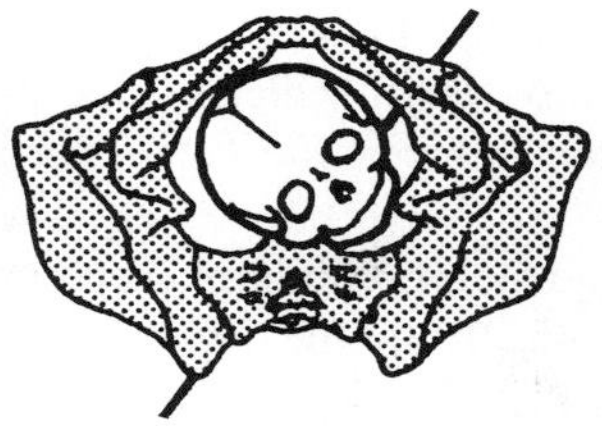	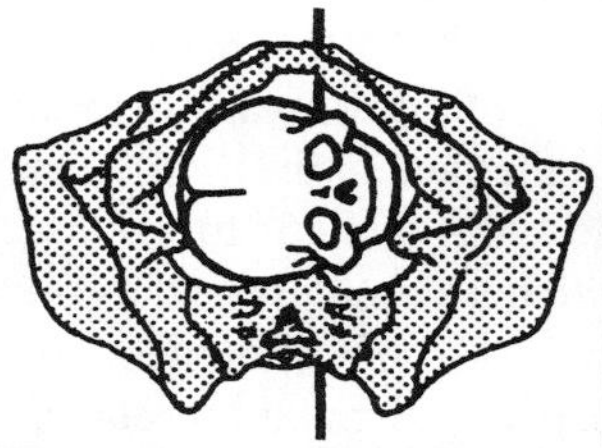	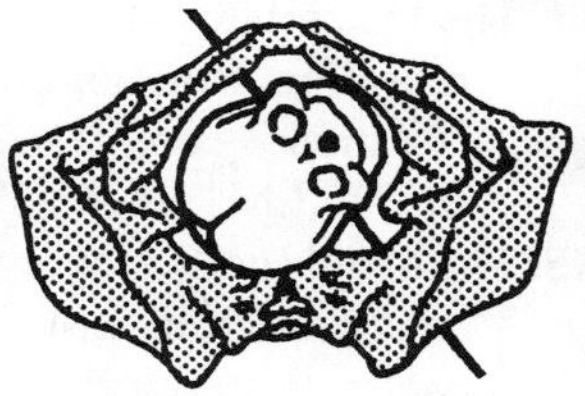
Internal rotation: LMA to MA; shoulders follow the head and engage transverse.	Midchest descends, rotates to oblique. Upper spine extends; flexed head is born OP (MA).	The head restitutes 45° from OP to ROP (MA to LMA).	Chest rotates AP; head follows, rotating externally: ROP to ROT (LMA to LMT). Shoulders and body are born.
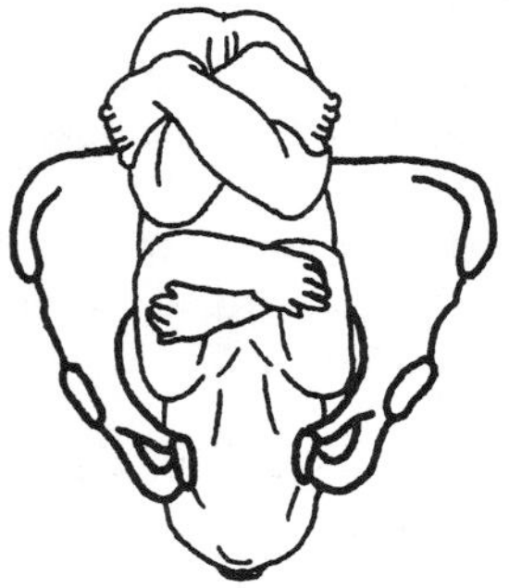	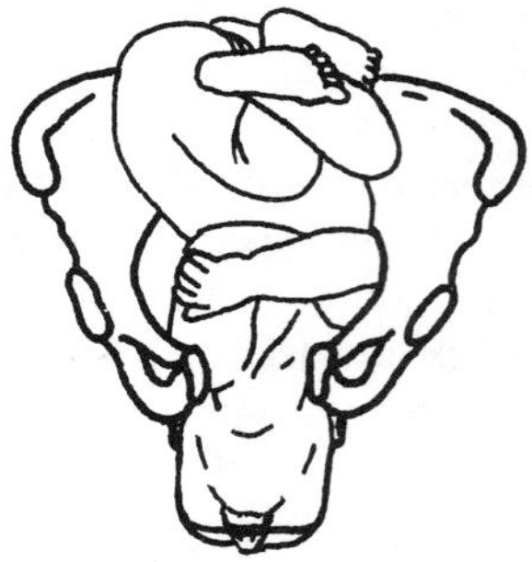	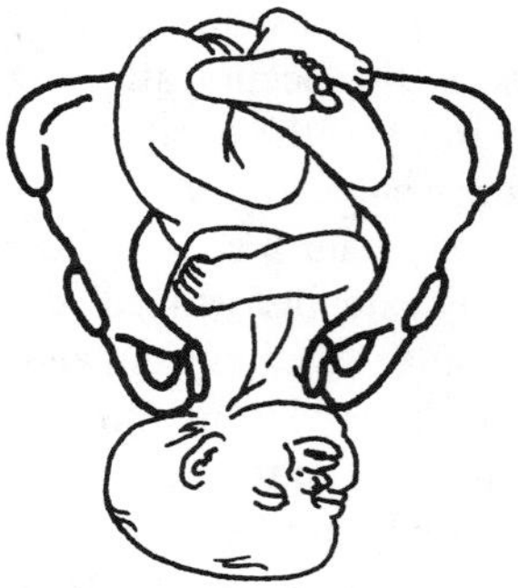	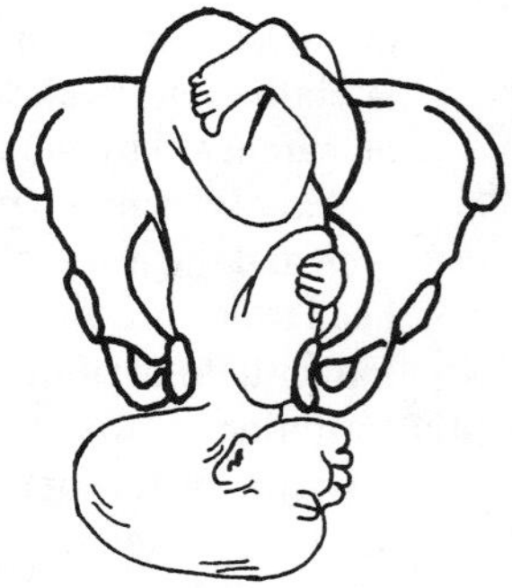
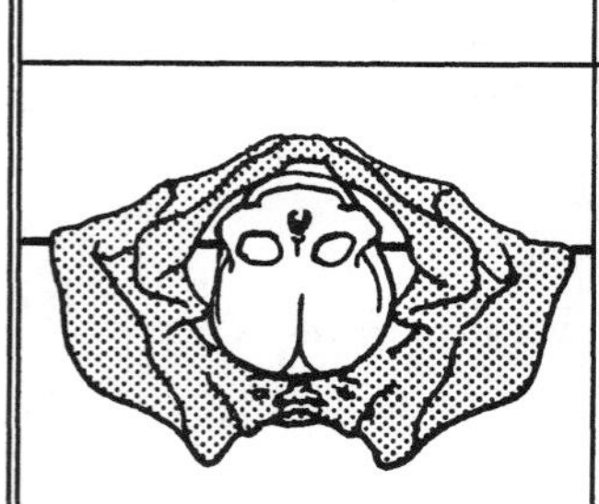	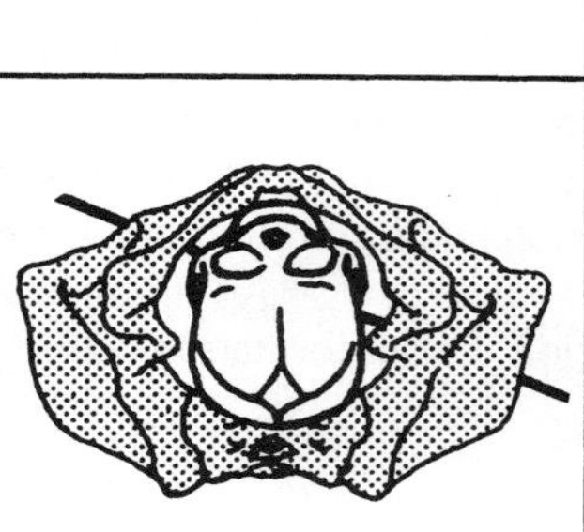	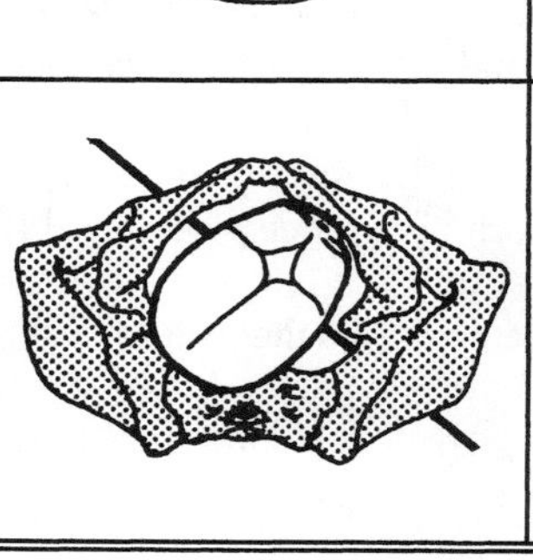	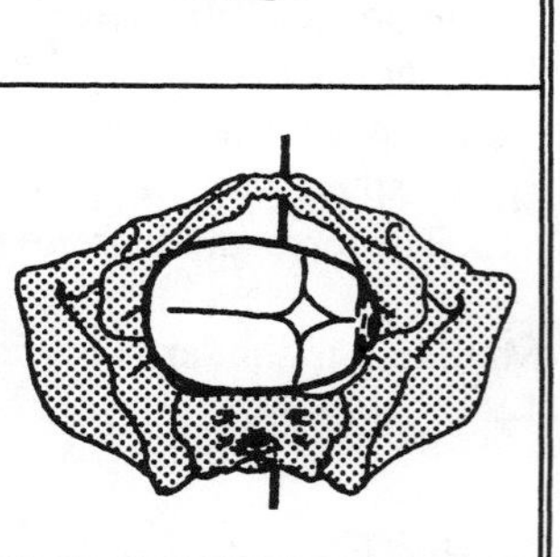

Short-arc rotation of the LMP baby (movements not illustrated)

Direct MP birth is virtually impossible for a full-term, living baby. You will note that the cardinal movements occur out of their usual sequence and that some of the steps are missing.

***1.** The head is often fully extended prior to labor and the upper spine is arched. If not, extension becomes complete as the face encounters the resistance afforded by the soft tissues of the pelvic cavity from below and as the bregma impinges on the symphysis anteriorly.

***2.** The baby attempts to descend throughout labor, although in most cases this becomes increasingly difficult as labor advances.

***3.** The face rotates internally from LMP 45° to MP.

4. The baby's body moves with the shoulders as they undergo their first internal rotation. Concurrent with the rotation of the mentum from LMP to MP, the shoulders rotate 45° from the right oblique diameter to align with the transverse diameter. This occurs as the bregma becomes pressed against the pubic bone, which pushes the occiput backward, where it becomes jammed between the scapulae. This fixes the shoulders in a transverse position and results in the head and shoulders attempting to descend together. The dome of the skull resists further moulding, and further descent is usually impossible. The bulk of the head becomes arrested above the brim.

Further descent will proceed, with great difficulty, only if the baby is quite small and the mother's pelvis quite large.

***5.** The head engages as the biparietal diameter, shoulders and upper sternum squeeze through the brim together.

6. The attitude of the shoulders remains fixed as long as the head is jammed between the scapulae.

7. The spine is fixed in an "S" curve with the upper spine maximally arched and the lower spine lordotic.
The face crowns.

***8.** The face is born by a difficult process of compression as the large dome of the vertex is squeezed from beneath the pubic arch. The face eventually moves beyond the pelvic outlet as the upper neck remains maximally extended and the lower neck and upper spine remain maximally arched. The perineum retracts and the head is born. The head is no longer held back in an attitude of extension, and the vertex now leads the way. The shoulders are free to move once the head emerges.

***9.** Because the shoulders have descended transverse, the neck is not twisted; restitution of the head does not occur.

10. The second internal rotation of the chest and shoulders begins after the head is born, to allow the spine to flex laterally. Beginning from the transverse, the shoulders rotate 45° to right oblique diameter and may rotate another 45° to the anteroposterior diameter.

***11.** Concurrent with the internal rotation of the chest, the head rotates externally 45° from OA (MP) to ROA (LMP). If the chest rotated a full 90°, the head will rotate externally another 45° to ROT (LMT).

12. The anterior shoulder braces against the pubic bone as the posterior shoulder is born first by a process of lateral spinal flexion, after which the anterior shoulder slips past the pubic bone and emerges.

13. The torso and legs are born by a process of lateral flexion and a spiraling motion.

Moulding is similar in all posterior face positions. The caput will appear over the left cheek and eye.

SUMMARY OF THE CARDINAL SPIRALING MOVEMENTS: RIGHT MENTUM POSTERIOR (RMP)

Labor with the baby in an RMP position is the mirror opposite of labor with an LMP position. Full deflexion from an LOA position results in an RMP baby.

Orientation of the baby to the mother's pelvis

The long axis of the face is aligned with the right oblique diameter, while the chin (mentum) occupies the right posterior corner of the pelvis. The shoulders are aligned with the left oblique diameter.

Long-arc rotation of the RMP baby

***1.** The head is often fully extended prior to labor and the upper spine is arched. If not, extension becomes complete as the face encounters the resistance afforded by the soft tissues of the pelvic cavity from below and as the bregma impinges on the superior ramus of the pubic bone anteriorly.

***2.** The baby descends throughout labor.

***3.** The head engages as the biparietal diameter passes through the brim, which has usually occurred by the time the face reaches +2 station, late in labor.

***4.** The face rotates internally a total of 135°, from RMP to MA, as it adapts to the loop-shaped opening of the levator ani sling. Rotation consists of a downwardly spiraling movement, which facilitates descent. It usually occurs after dilation is complete and the face is firmly pressed against the pelvic floor. Starting from RMP, the chin rotates 45° to RMT, then 45° to RMA and 45° to MA.

5. The baby's body moves with the shoulders as they undergo their first internal rotation. Following the rotation of the mentum from RMP to RMT, the shoulders rotate 45° from the left oblique diameter to align with the anteroposterior diameter. As the mentum rotates from RMT to RMA, the shoulders rotate 45° to align with the right oblique diameter. As the mentum rotates from RMA to MA, the shoulders rotate another 45° to align with the transverse diameter of the brim, 135° in all.

6. The shoulders engage when the bisacromial diameter enters the transverse diameter of the brim, as the face passes through the ischial tuberosities. The attitude of the shoulders shifts during descent as the torso accommodates to the shape of the birth canal.

7. The spine extends as the head enters the pelvis more deeply.

8-1. The second internal rotation of the shoulders begins between the time the face distends the perineum and is born. As the midchest and spine enter the curve of the birth canal near the level of the ischial spines, they rotate 45°, moving the shoulders from the transverse into the right oblique diameter. This adjustment allows the spine to flex laterally. The neck twists as this occurs, allowing the face to remain MA. Internal rotation of the shoulders may be hampered by the proximity of the occiput.

*** 9.** The chin glides down past the pubic arch and the face begins to crown. The anterior neck is now under the pubic arch and the head is in the soft birth canal. The lower neck and upper spine begin to flex into the curve of the sacrum, allowing the head to remain almost fully extended as it advances. The perineum retracts and the head is born. The head is no longer held back in an attitude of extension, and the vertex now leads the way.

***10.** Restitution occurs as the neck untwists to allow the occiput to rotate 45° from OP (MA) back to the LOP (RMA) position, restoring the long axis of the vertex to a 90° angle with the long axis of the shoulders.

8-2. The chest completes its second internal rotation, moving the shoulders 45° from the right oblique into the antero-posterior diameter before or during the next contraction. This brings the anterior shoulder under the pubic arch.

***11.** Concurrent with the internal rotation of the chest, the head rotates externally 45° from LOP (RMA) to LOT (RMT).

12. The anterior shoulder braces against the pubic bone as the posterior shoulder is born first by a process of lateral spinal flexion, after which the anterior shoulder slips past the pubic bone and emerges.

13. The torso and legs are born by a process of lateral flexion and a spiraling motion.

Moulding is similar in all face positions that rotate to anterior, with caput formation over the right cheek and eye.

RMP orientation, head almost completely extended	Descent to engagement, extension complete	Internal rotation begins: RMP to RMT	Internal rotation of head continues: RMT to RMA.
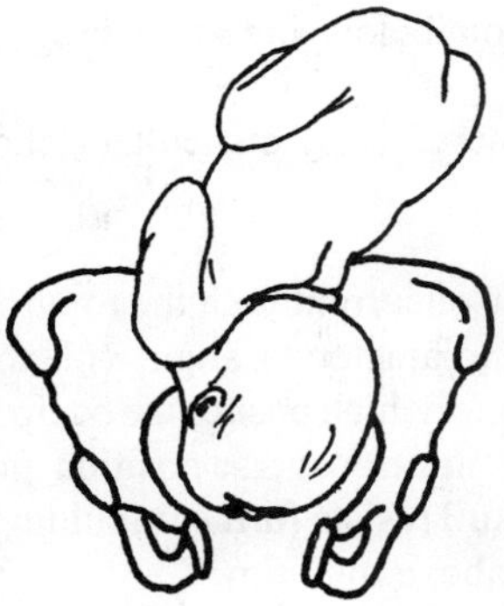	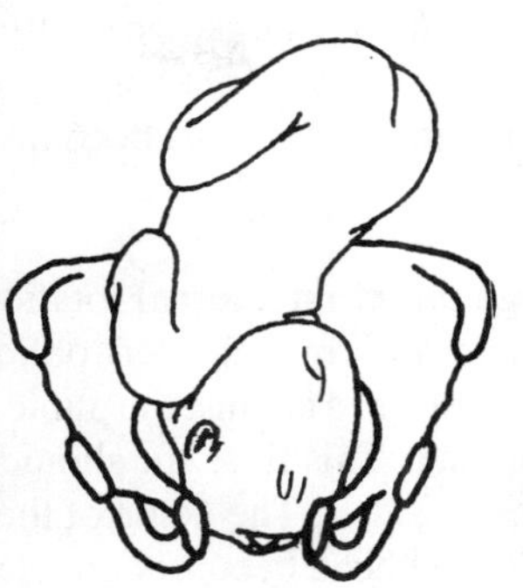	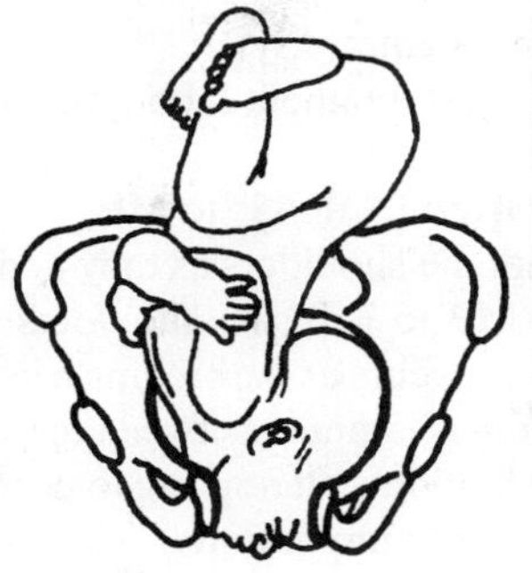	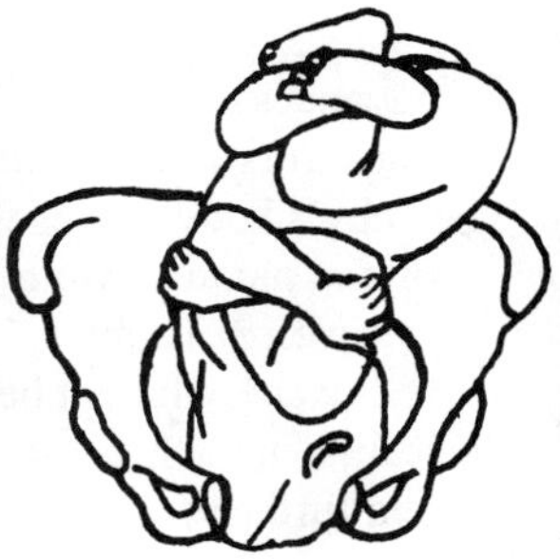
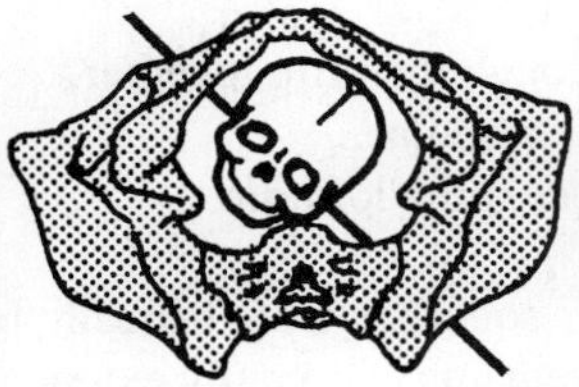	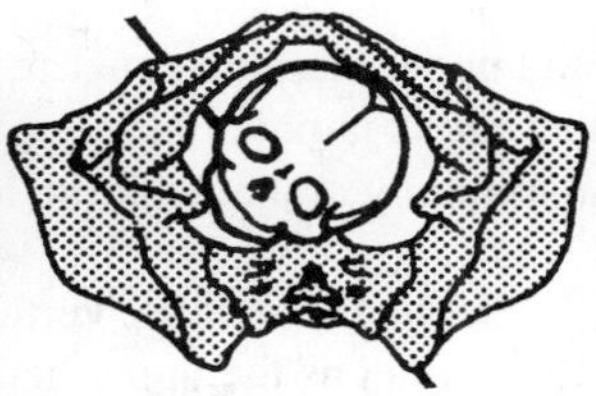	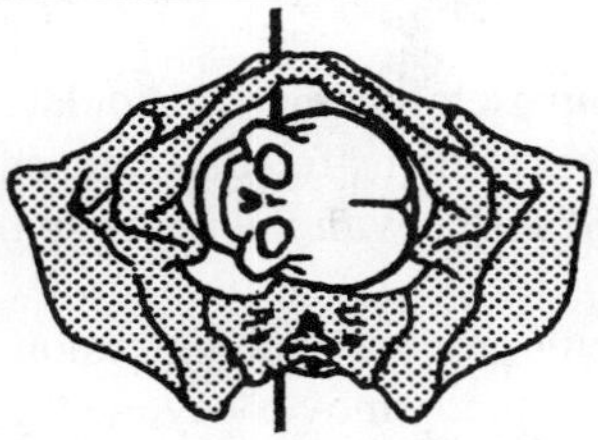	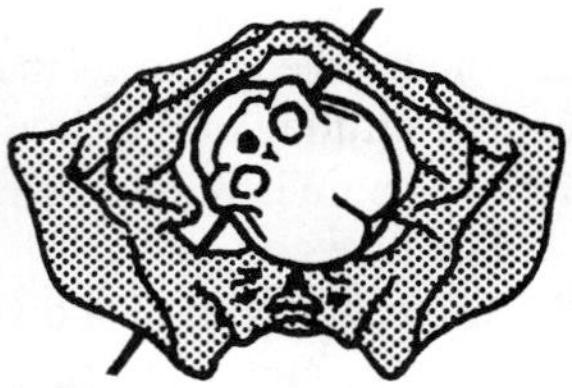

Internal rotation: RMA to MA; shoulders follow the head and engage transverse,	Midchest descends, rotates to oblique. Upper spine extends flexed head is born OP (MA).	The head restitutes 45° from OP to LOP (MA to RMA).	Chest rotates AP; head follows, rotating externally: LOP to LOT (RMA to RMT). Shoulders are and body are born.
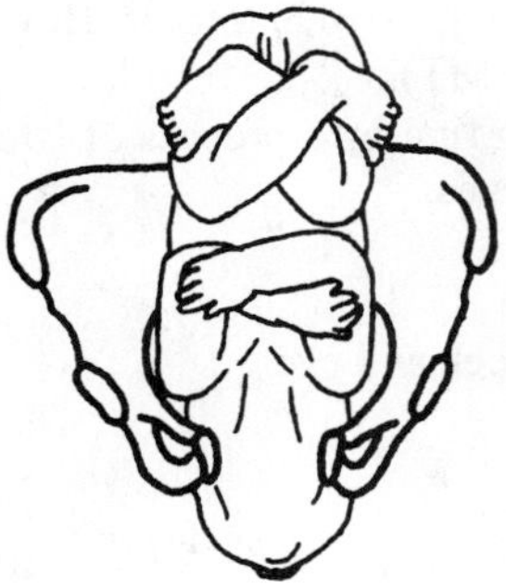	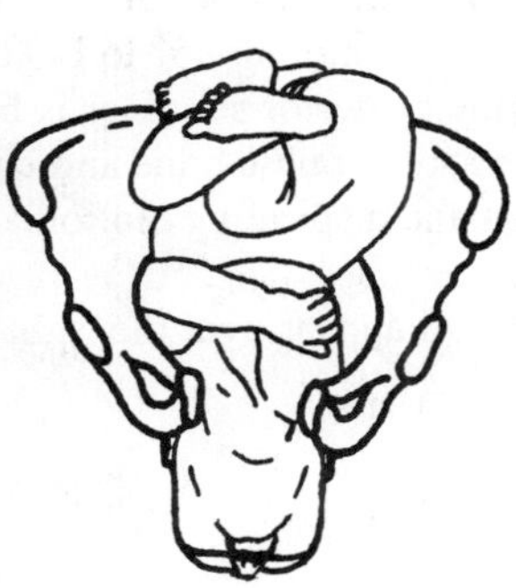	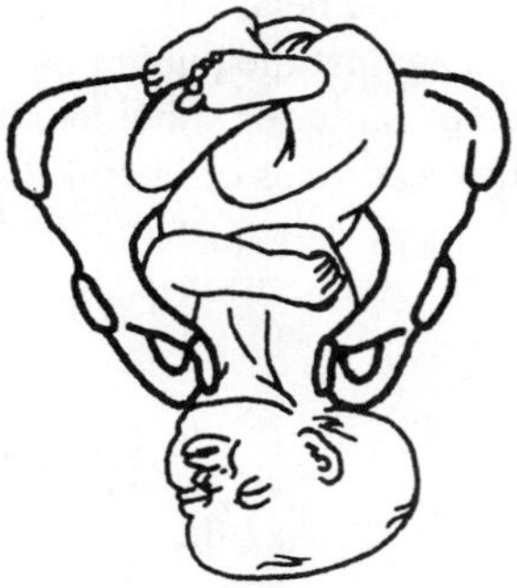	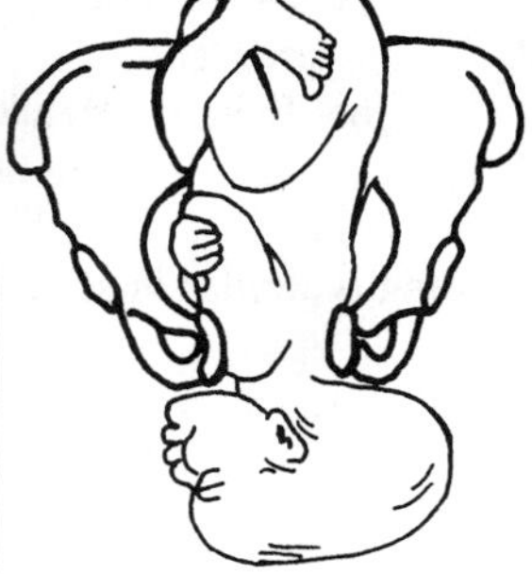
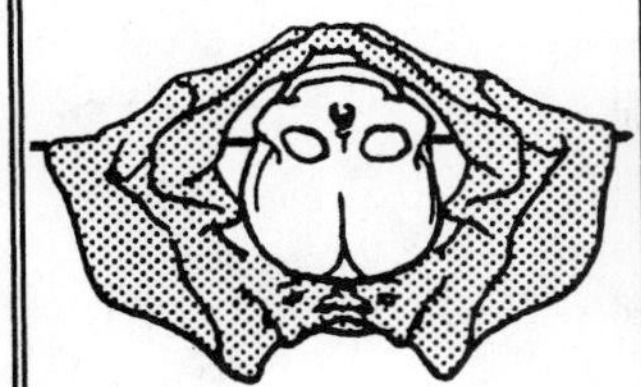	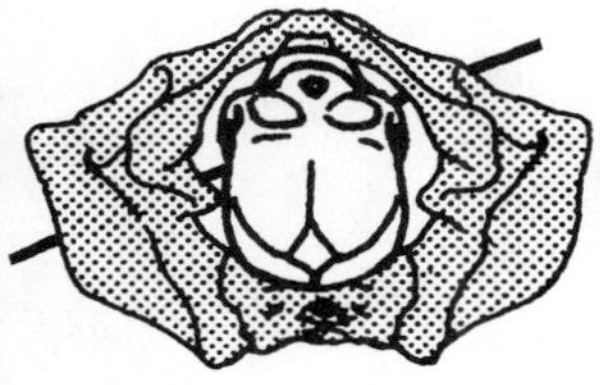	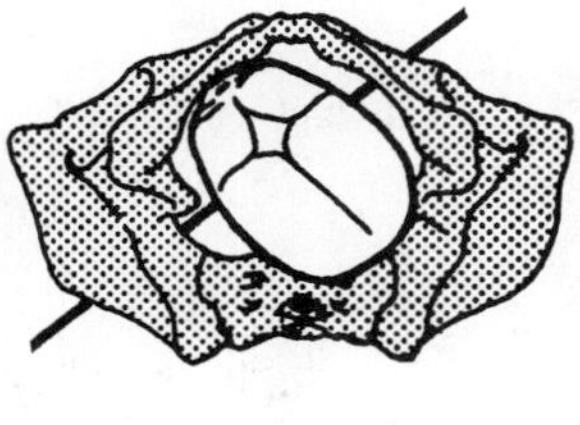	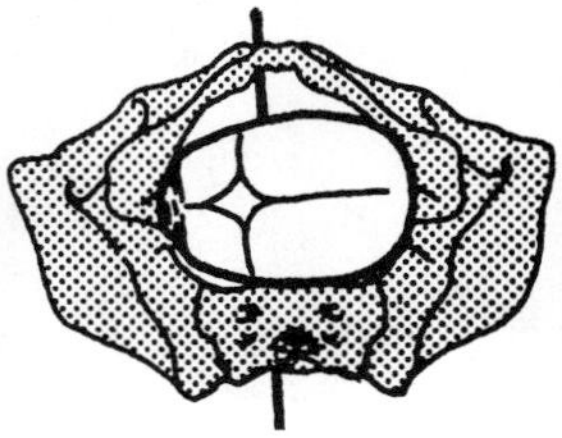

Short-arc rotation of the RMP baby (movements not illustrated)

Direct MP birth is virtually impossible for a full-term, living baby.

***1.** The head is often fully extended prior to labor and the upper spine is arched. If not, extension becomes complete as the face encounters the resistance afforded by the soft tissues of the pelvic cavity from below and as the bregma impinges on the symphysis anteriorly.

***2.** The baby attempts to descend throughout labor, although in most cases this becomes increasingly difficult as labor advances.

***3.** The face rotates internally from RMP 45° to MP.

4. The baby's body moves with the shoulders as they undergo their first internal rotation. Concurrent with the rotation of the mentum from RMP to MP, the shoulders rotate 45° from the left oblique diameter to align with the transverse diameter. This occurs as the bregma becomes pressed against the pubic bone, which pushes the occiput backward, where it becomes jammed between the scapulae. This fixes the shoulders in a transverse position and results in the head and shoulders attempting to descend together. The dome of the skull resists further moulding, and further descent is usually impossible. The bulk of the head becomes arrested above the brim.

Further descent will proceed, with great difficulty, only if the baby is quite small and the mother's pelvis quite large.

***5.** The head engages as the biparietal diameter, shoulders and upper sternum squeeze through the brim together.

6. The attitude of the shoulders remains fixed as long as the head is jammed between the scapulae.

7. The spine is fixed in an "S" curve with the upper spine maximally arched and the lower spine lordotic.
The face crowns.

***8.** The face is born by a difficult process of compression as the large dome of the vertex is squeezed from beneath the pubic arch. The face eventually moves beyond the pelvic outlet as the upper neck remains maximally extended and the lower neck and upper spine remain maximally arched. The perineum retracts and the head is born. The head is no longer held back in an attitude of extension, and the vertex now leads the way. The shoulders are free to move once the head emerges.

***9.** Because the shoulders have descended transverse, the neck is not twisted; restitution of the head does not occur.

10. The second internal rotation of the chest and shoulders begins after the head is born, to allow the spine to flex laterally. Beginning from the transverse, the shoulders rotate 45° to left oblique diameter and may rotate another 45° to the anteroposterior diameter.

***11.** Concurrent with the internal rotation of the chest, the head rotates externally 45° from OA (MP) to LOA (RMP). If the chest rotated a full 90°, the head will rotate externally another 45° to LOT (RMT).

12. The anterior shoulder braces against the pubic bone as the posterior shoulder is born first by a process of lateral spinal flexion, after which the anterior shoulder slips past the pubic bone and emerges.

13. The torso and legs are born by a process of lateral flexion and a spiraling motion.

Moulding is similar in all posterior face positions. The caput will appear over the right cheek and eye.

SUMMARY OF THE CARDINAL SPIRALING MOVEMENTS: MENTUM POSTERIOR (MP)

Theoretically, the baby may assume a direct MP position prior to labor, before the head dips into the pelvic brim. While it may be possible for a tiny baby to present and descend with the mentum either directly anterior or directly posterior, in reality these mechanisms are quite rare. This is because the presenting diameters best accommodate themselves to an oblique or transverse diameter of the brim. Note that a fully extended OA position becomes MP.

Orientation of the baby to the mother's pelvis

The long axis of the face is aligned with the anteroposterior diameter, while the chin (mentum) occupies the directly posterior space in front of the sacrum. The shoulder axis is aligned with the transverse diameter.

When the baby is directly mentum posterior, the shoulders, once they are free to move, may rotate internally in either a left or a right direction. Subsequent movements of the head will follow according to the direction of shoulder rotation, as noted.

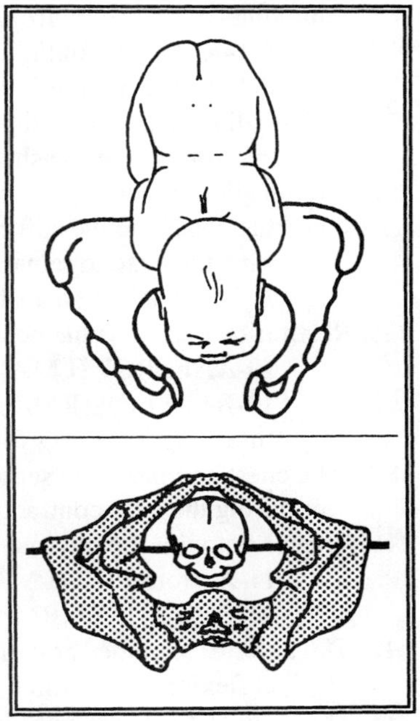

Long-arc rotation when the baby is MP (movements not illustrated)

***1.** The head is often fully extended prior to labor and the upper spine is arched. If not, extension becomes complete as the face encounters the resistance afforded by the soft tissues of the pelvic cavity from below and as the bregma impinges on the anterior brim. At this point, descent usually becomes arrested.

***2.** The head attempts to descend throughout labor, although this becomes increasingly difficult as labor advances.

The entire body of the baby may assume an LMP or an RMP position to enter the brim. When this occurs, labor may proceed as for an LMP or RMP baby undergoing long-arc or short-arc rotation, the head may temporarily rotate to an LMP or RMP orientation prior to entering the brim to facilitate descent. If this occurs, the neck may twist 45°, allowing the shoulders to remain transverse. The following description assumes that the head enters the pelvis directly MP.

***3.** The head engages as the biparietal diameter passes through the brim, which has usually occurred by the time the face reaches +2 station, late in labor. Engagement may be delayed because of the difficulty in wedging the bulk of the vertex under the pubic bone.

***4.** Because the head is directly MP, internal rotation can proceed in either a left or right direction, a total of 180°. Rotation consists of a downwardly spiraling movement, which facilitates descent. It usually occurs after dilation is complete and the face is firmly pressed against the pelvic floor. Starting from MP, the mentum rotates:

- **4-A.** 45° to LMP, 45° to LMT, 45° to LMA, 45° to MA. (Follow "A" entries below.)
- **4-B.** 45° to RMP, 45° to RMT, 45° to RMA, 45° to MA. (Follow "B" entries below.)

5. The baby's body moves with the shoulders as they undergo their first internal rotation.

- **5-A.** Following with the rotation of the mentum from MP to LMP, the shoulders rotate from the transverse diameter to align with the right oblique diameter. As the mentum rotates from LMP to LMT, the shoulders rotate 45° to align with the anteroposterior diameter. As the mentum rotates from LMT to LMA, the shoulders rotate 45° to align with the left oblique diameter, and as the mentum rotates from LMA to MA, the shoulders rotate another 45° to align with the transverse diameter of the brim, 180° in all.
- **5-B.** Following with the rotation of the mentum from MP to RMP, the shoulders rotate 45° from the transverse diameter to align with the left oblique diameter. As the mentum rotates from RMP to RMT, the shoulders rotate 45° to align with the anteroposterior diameter. As the mentum rotates from RMT to RMA, the shoulders rotate 45° to align with the right oblique diameter, and as the mentum rotates from RMA to MA, the shoulders rotate another 45° to align

with the transverse diameter of the brim, 180° in all.

6. The shoulders engage when the bisacromial diameter enters the transverse diameter of the brim, as the face passes through the ischial tuberosities. The attitude of the shoulders shifts during descent as the torso accommodates to the shape of the birth canal.

7. The spine extends as the head enters the pelvis more deeply.

8-1. The second internal rotation of the shoulders begins between the time the face distends the perineum and is born. As the midchest and spine enter the curve of the birth canal near the level of the ischial spines, they rotate 45°, moving the shoulders from the transverse into:

8-1-A. the left oblique diameter.

8-1-B. the right oblique diameter.

This adjustment allows the spine to flex laterally. The neck twists as this occurs, allowing the face to remain MA. Internal rotation of the shoulders may be hampered by the proximity of the occiput.

***9.** The chin glides down past the pubic arch and the face begins to crown. The anterior neck is now under the pubic arch and the head is in the soft birth canal. The lower neck and upper spine begin to flex into the curve of the sacrum, allowing the head to remain almost fully extended as the perineum retracts and the head is born. The head is no longer held back in an attitude of extension, and the vertex now leads the way.

***10.** Restitution occurs as the neck untwists to allow the occiput to rotate 45° from OP (MA) back to:

10-A. the ROP (LMA) position.

10-B. the LOP (RMA) position.

This movement restores the long axis of the vertex to a 90° angle with the long axis of the shoulders.

8-2. The chest completes its second internal rotation, moving the shoulders 45° to the anteroposterior diameter before or during the next contraction. This brings the anterior shoulder under the pubic arch.

***11.** Concurrent with the internal rotation of the chest, the head rotates externally 45°:

11-A. from ROP (LMA) to ROT (LMT).

11-B. from LOP (RMA) to LOT (RMT).

12. The anterior shoulder braces against the pubic bone as the posterior shoulder is born first by a process of lateral spinal flexion, after which the anterior shoulder slips past the pubic bone and emerges.

13. The torso and legs are born by a process of lateral flexion and a spiraling motion.

Moulding is similar in all face positions that rotate anteriorly; any caput forms over the anterior cheek and eye.

<u>Direct MP descent and birth (movements not illustrated)</u>

***1.** The head is often fully extended prior to labor and the upper spine is arched. If not, extension becomes complete as the face encounters the resistance afforded by the soft tissues of the pelvic cavity from below and as the bregma impinges on the brim anteriorly.

***2.** The baby attempts to descend throughout labor, although, in most cases, this becomes increasingly difficult as labor advances.

***3.** Internal rotation of the face does not occur. The shoulders remain transverse.

4. The bregma becomes pressed against the pubic bone, which pushes the occiput backward, where it becomes jammed between the shoulder blades. This fixes the shoulders in a transverse position and results in the head, shoulders and upper chest attempting to descend together. The dome of the skull resists further moulding and descent is usually impossible. The bulk of the head becomes arrested above the brim.

Further descent will proceed, with great difficulty, only if the baby is quite small and the mother's pelvis quite large.

***5.** The head engages as the biparietal diameter, shoulders and upper sternum squeeze through the brim together.

6. The attitude of the shoulders remains fixed as long as the head is jammed between the scapulae.

7. The spine is fixed in an "S" curve with the upper spine maximally arched and the lower spine lordotic. The face crowns.

***8.** The face is born by a difficult process of compression as the large dome of the vertex is squeezed from beneath the pubic arch. The face eventually moves beyond the pelvic outlet as the upper neck remains maximally extended and the lower neck and upper spine remain maximally arched. The perineum retracts and the head is born. The head is no longer held back in an attitude of extension, and the vertex now leads the way. The shoulders are free to move once the head emerges.

***9.** Because the chest and shoulders have descended transverse, the neck is not twisted; restitution of the head does not occur.

10. Internal rotation of the chest and spine occurs after the head is born, to allow the spine to flex laterally. Beginning from the transverse, the shoulders rotate 45° into:

10-A. the left oblique diameter. (Follow "A" entries below.)

10-B. the right oblique diameter. (Follow "B" entries below.)

They may rotate another 45° into the anteroposterior diameter before or during the next contraction. This brings the anterior shoulder under the pubic arch.

***11.** Concurrent with the internal rotation of the chest, the head rotates externally 45°:

11-A. from OA (MP) to LOA (RMP). If the shoulders rotated a full 90°, the head will rotate externally another 45° to the LOT (RMT) position.

11-B. from OA (MP) to ROA (LMP). If the shoulders rotated a full 90°, the head will rotate another 45° to the ROT (LMT) position.

12. The anterior shoulder braces against the pubic bone as the posterior shoulder is born first by a process of lateral spinal flexion, after which the anterior shoulder slips past the pubic bone and emerges.

13. The torso and legs are born by a process of lateral flexion and a spiraling motion.

Moulding is similar in all persistently posterior face positions. Any caput forms over the anterior cheek and eye.

BROW PRESENTATION: GENERAL PRINCIPLES

Brow presentation occurs when the baby's head is tipped back about three-quarters of the way in an attitude of partial extension. The presenting part is bordered by the glabella, the temples on either side and the anterior fontanelle (bregma); the denominator is the forehead, which is also called the **sinciput** or **frontum**. Brow presentations are the rarest of all fetal attitudes, with the reported incidence ranging between 1 in every 468 births to 1 in every 3543 births, depending on the study. The average incidence is 1 in every 1444 births (Cruikshank & Cruikshank, 1981).

Presenting diameters

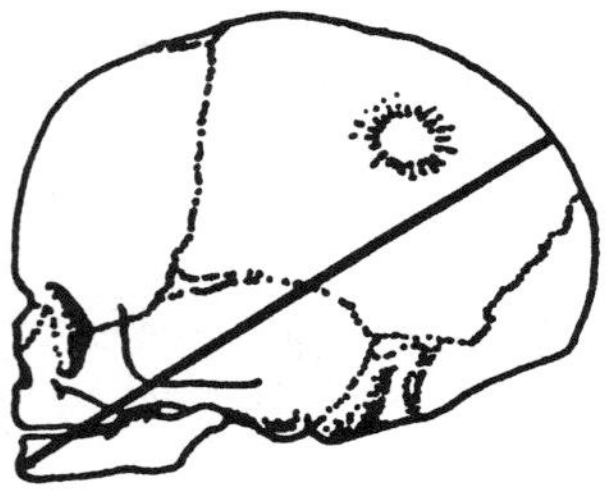

Verticomental diameter

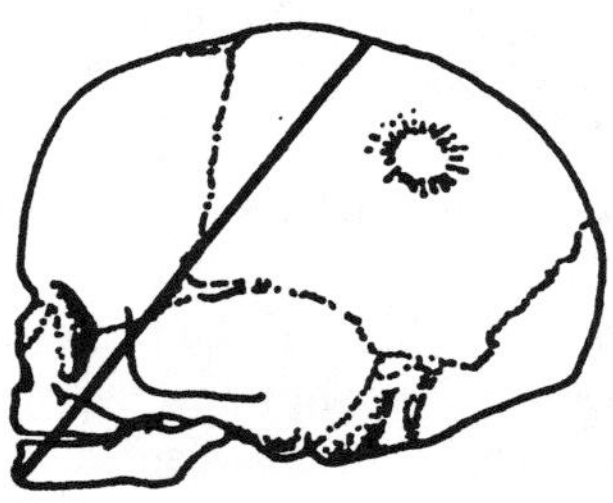

Mentobregmatic diameter

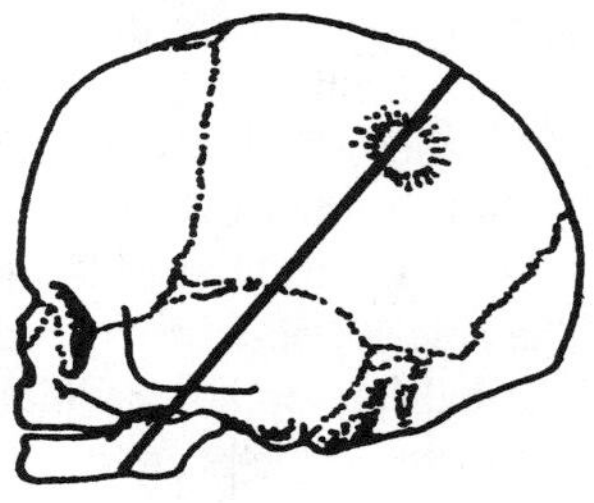

Submentovertical diameter

There is some debate regarding the diameter that presents in a brow. Traditionally, the verticomental (in some sources called the occipitomental) of 14 cm is said to present, which is the longest anteroposterior diameter of the head. However, Borell and Fernström (1960) did X-ray studies of 16 face, brow and brow-face presentations and noted that the mentobregmatic (mentoparietal) diameter of 12.2 cm more frequently presents. The difference is significant. The mentobregmatic diameter is 1.8 cm shorter and therefore much more favorable to progressive labor. Since the diameter of the mother's bony pelvic brim is usually no larger than 12.5 cm, passage of the verticomental diameter would be difficult if not impossible except in a large pelvis. The mother's sacrum cannot move back and out of the way until the baby fills the pelvis; with such a large presenting diameter, the baby might never descend to this point. Thus, brow presentation with the verticomental diameter presenting may be a physical impossibility unless the baby is small, the pelvis quite large and mobile, or moulding excessive. Conversely, the mentobregmatic diameter is a bit smaller than the transverse diameter of most pelvic brims. Considering that pelvic soft tissues fill some of the space within this diameter, the fit is still tight, but some heads could fit through if sufficient time and patience are brought to bear during labor to give the head a chance to mould.

Brow-face presentation

A well-extended brow presentation is the same as a partially extended face presentation (and vice versa). Any presentation that is midway between a face and a brow is likely to either extend more to become a face, become slightly more flexed to become a brow or flex more deeply to become a vertex. The head may also remain in a brow-face attitude as labor progresses, although this is less likely, as the pressure of the soft tissues will usually encourage further extension or flexion unless something interferes (Borell & Fernström, 1960). Stern (1956) states that the submentovertical diameter of 11 cm presents when the face is incompletely extended.

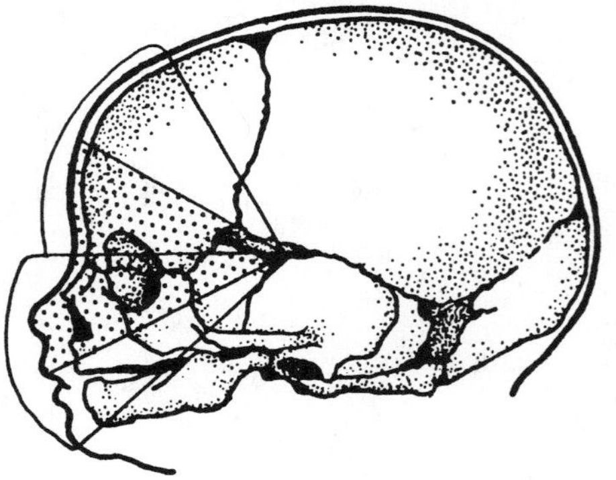

Boundaries of face (lower division), Brow (upper division), Brow-face (shaded portion)

Associated factors

As with face presentation, a number of factors have been offered as explanations regarding why brow presentations occur. The three most serious contenders for "associated factor" are high parity, low birthweight and cephalopelvic disproportion, none of which hold up to close scrutiny.

In spite of this general statement, Cruikshank and Cruikshank (1981) did find an association between brow presentation and the size of the maternal pelvis. Pelvic size issues are thought to involve relative cephalopelvic disproportion with a suggestion in the literature that the baby's size is the problem, since these researchers believed that the verticomental diameter is presenting. However, the data are contradictory because the definition of a "large" infant varies among studies. Some quote weight ranges over 7 lb (3175 grams), while others use weights over 8 lb 13.5 oz (over 4000 grams) as the cutoff for "large" babies. The thinking is that brow presentation probably persists more frequently in larger babies, even if the pelvis is normal, as well as in women who have smaller pelvises. If the pelvis were larger or the baby were smaller, the baby would have more room to flex to vertex or fully extend into a face. However, even if one accepts that all cases in which "small" pelvis and "large" infant are causative, this still leaves 70.4% of all brow presentations without specific etiology. If factors intrinsic to the baby are causative, then excessive muscle tone in the extensor muscles of the neck may play a part (Donald, 1979). The bottom line is that nothing is known for certain about the cause of brow presentations.

Primary or secondary?

While it has been taught that brow presentation is invariably a secondary presentation (i.e., it is most likely a step in the process of conversion to either a face or a vertex attitude), in fact, not all the data support this view. Cruikshank and Cruikshank (1981) point out that, if nearly all face presentations are primary, then nearly all brow presentations must also be primary, with fetal factors being the main reason for brow presentation in the majority of cases. It is hard to gauge exactly what percentage of brow presentations are primary, however, because most are detected only after labor has been underway for a while. Ingolfsson (1969) found that 78% of brow babies that emerged spontaneously were not diagnosed until the time of birth.

Unstable presentation

Many babies presenting their brow at the onset of labor do convert to more favorable diameters once labor is underway. Even if the brow presentation is primary to begin with, that it is an unstable presentation seems well supported by the high ratio of conversions to either face or vertex prior to birth.

THE PROCESS OF BIRTH IN FRONTUM ANTERIOR BROW PRESENTATIONS

Even if most babies who present their brow do so prior to the onset of labor, the course of labor is very variable. When labor does progress with a brow presentation, the head and shoulders almost always make three movements, as is true with all presentations. These are engagement or entry of the part into the pelvis, rotation or adaption of the part to the shape of the birth canal and disengagement or emergence of the part from the pelvis. Because brow presentations are so rare, because many will convert to another presentation prior to birth, because progress to birth as a brow in a term baby is not anticipated by most authors and because many, if not most, brow presentations are only recognized late in labor, descriptions of the cardinal movements for different positions are essentially nonexistent in medical textbooks, both old and new, with the notable exception of the description found in OXORN-FOOTE HUMAN LABOR AND BIRTH (Oxorn, 1986). While the process of birth in face and brow presentations is similar, the way the head negotiates the pelvis and the way it is born differ in some respects. (Asterisks next to a number indicate the cardinal movements mentioned in contemporary textbooks.)

The Frequency of Different Brow Positions

Eight formal positions are theoretically possible for brow presentation, as for all presentations. There is some debate about which occur most frequently. Many authors state that, in most cases, the head enters the transverse diameter of the pelvis. This makes sense, as the long presenting diameter is accommodating itself to the longest pelvic diameter. McCormick (1944) states that LFA and RFP occur most frequently. Oxorn (1986) makes no mention of the frequency of each variety, although the only variety he describes is LFA. We will go with common sense, as well as the observation of many researchers, and assume that most brow babies start labor transverse.

Persistent Brow Presentation

While it is generally stated that there is no process of descent for a term baby presenting by the brow, progressive labors and births do occur. This is most likely if the baby is of small or average size, the pelvis is normal to large, contractions are of excellent quality and the mother has given birth before. In most of these cases, the head engages in the transverse diameter and the brow rotates anteriorly. The birth will be greatly facilitated if the mother is upright during descent and pushing. Progress in labor is the key to safety for the mother and baby. Both face grave risks from nonprogressive labor, with excessive moulding leading to intracranial injury, fetal distress or death and uterine rupture being likely if obstructed labor is neglected. For a full description of the course and sequelae of obstructed labor, see the chapter entitled "Transverse Lie."

Open fetal mouth

Since so many brow babies convert their positions so that more desirable diameters present, it is interesting to note that a fairly frequent cause of persistent, nonprogressive brow presentation occurs when the fetal mouth is open and the lower jaw becomes lodged against the pelvis, either on the sacral promontory, elsewhere around the perimeter of the brim or even at the level of the ischial spines. It is easy to see how this occurs, as the mouth is perfectly positioned for such an accident of labor to occur. This splints the head at that level, preventing both further flexion and further extension. The open jaw increases the presenting mentobregmatic diameter as well as locking the mouth against the pelvis, thus compounding the problem because the baby has no room to maneuver out of this position unaided.

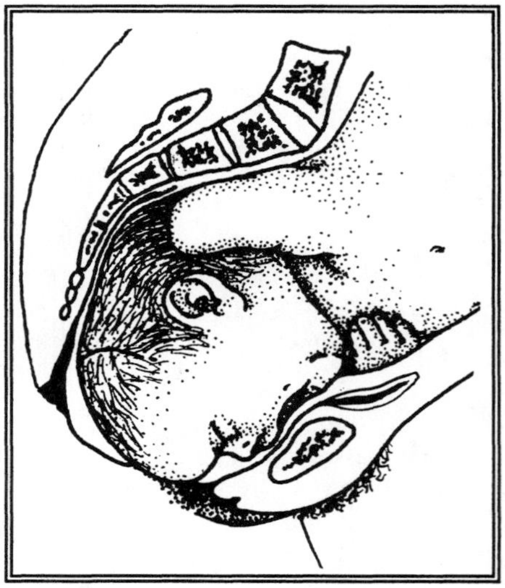

Full bladder

Ian Donald (1979) points out that a very full bladder can keep a baby in a persistent brow presentation with no descent below the brim. This is particularly true in multiparous women.

Labor in a Brow Presentation

1. Conversion to another attitude (further flexion or complete extension)

As labor attempts to advance, there are three possibilities: the attitude of the baby may convert to face, it may convert to vertex, or it may persist as a brow. Spontaneous conversion to a face or a vertex presentation occurs, on the average, 50% of the time, with about 30% converting to face and 20% to vertex.

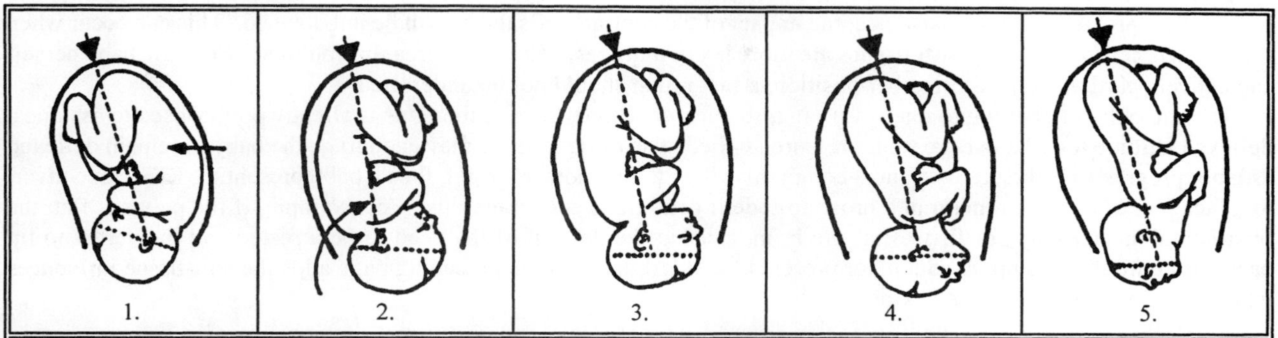

1. Right-tilted obliquity of the uterus, LOT baby, with contractive force encouraging flexion
2. Right obliquity of the fundus with an ROT baby, contractive force encouraging deflexion
3. If the fetus is already deflexed, contractive force will encourage the fetal back to remain straightened rather than flex.
4. Straightening of the spine puts pressure on the back of the fetal head, encouraging the bulk of the head to tip back. If the process arrests here, brow presentation will result.
5. Further extension of the neck and spine result in a face presentation.

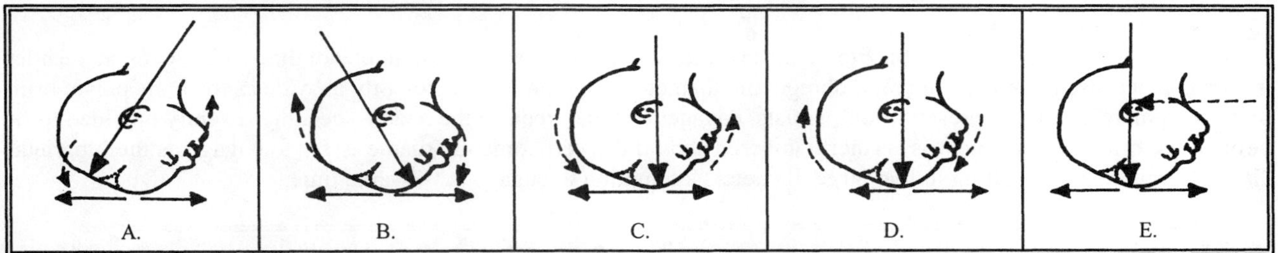

A. If downward force from contractions originates on the side the baby is facing, and the force is directed obliquely through the baby's buttocks toward his vertex, and if the mother's pelvic tissues offer equal resistance from below, flexion will be encouraged. The vertex is pressed down into the pelvis, while the anterior bulk of the head is directed toward the chest.

B. If downward force from contractions originates on the side of the baby's back and is directed obliquely through the buttocks toward the brow, and if the pelvic tissues offer equal resistance from below, head and spinal extension will tend to be exaggerated. The face is pressed down into the pelvis, with the posterior bulk of the head directed toward the back.

C. If pressure from contractions is directed straight down and the maternal pelvic tissues are tense and unyielding on the side nearest the baby's face, the brow will be held back, causing the vertex to descend, resulting in more flexion.

D. If pressure from contractions is directed straight down and the maternal pelvic tissues are tense and unyielding on the side nearest the back of the head, the vertex will be held back on that side, encouraging further extension of the spine and neck.

E. If the head is partly deflexed and the application of force is balanced (direct downward force from contractions above and equal resistance around the circumference of the inlet below), the head will tend to stay partially extended at the brim; encouraging the baby to remain in a brow presentation.

NOTE: Oblique thrust from the force of the contractions and unequal resistance from the pelvic tissues may augment or neutralize each other. (adapted from Miller & Callander, 1989)

However, in study populations where brow presentation was detected in early labor, spontaneous conversion rates of 67 to 75% have been reported. In fact, some researchers believe that the conversion rate to vertex is probably much higher than this because it is theorized that many occiput posterior babies may enter the pelvis in an undetected brow or brow-face attitude with the baby flexing further during labor. The process of each type of conversion is described below. Conversion to a face or vertex presentation may also occur before the head enters the brim and is often required before descent can occur, therefore conversion is described as part of the cardinal movement of extension in these descriptions.

There are several theories regarding how conversion may occur. If the spine is not well flexed when labor starts, the head is likely to be deflexed as well. The positioning of the head in a brow presentation causes the bulk of the head in front of and behind the pivot point of the atlantooccipital joint to be roughly equal; thus the leverage to encourage flexion or extension is about the same. Which occurs may depend upon the direction of force from the fundus above and the resistance from the soft and bony pelvic structures below. Downward thrust from toning contractions push down on the head and spine, which tends to assist the baby in bending her spine one way or the other. If the soft or bony structures of the pelvis provide unequal resistance, the impact of the contraction's thrust will be imbalanced. This can occur when the pelvis is contracted or the soft tissues are more lax or more resistant in one area than another. Plus, the baby herself can actively participate in altering her position, a factor that should not be underrated.

Uterine obliquity (tilting to one side) can also encourage extension. If the fetus is already predisposed to assume a deflexed attitude for whatever reason, pressure applied at an oblique angle may encourage the baby to remain deflexed as labor progresses. The uterus is most commonly tilted to the mother's right, thus a baby presenting RFT can convert to a face presentation or remain in a brow attitude if conditions encourage this. For example, if the pelvis is flat, the biparietal diameter may not fit well at the brim, causing the descent of the head to be arrested and the vertex to tip backward until the bitemporal diameter presents. The last chart on the preceding page adds the soft-tissue influences which may foster extension or flexion.

<u>*2. Descent</u>

Regardless of the eventual outcome, most brow presentations enter the pelvis transverse. The baby would naturally seek the longest pelvic diameter to engage a long cephalic diameter. This can occur even if the baby is in an oblique position prior to the onset of labor, as the head turns at the neck. The baby may then resume her frontum oblique orientation after engagement and proceed with internal rotation. Descent occurs, or attempts to take place, throughout labor and is a necessary prerequisite to all the other cardinal movements.

<u>*3. Engagement of the brow</u>

Engagement usually occurs as the biparietal descends through the transverse diameter of the pelvis. Arrest at the inlet is common because the presenting mentobregmatic diameter in a term baby is roughly as wide as the bony pelvic brim of most women. If a brow presentation persists, engagement may require the head to become severely moulded to fit through the brim. Engagement is further hampered should the verticomental diameter try to engage as the biparietal diameter transects it, resulting in two large diameters attempting to engage at the same time.

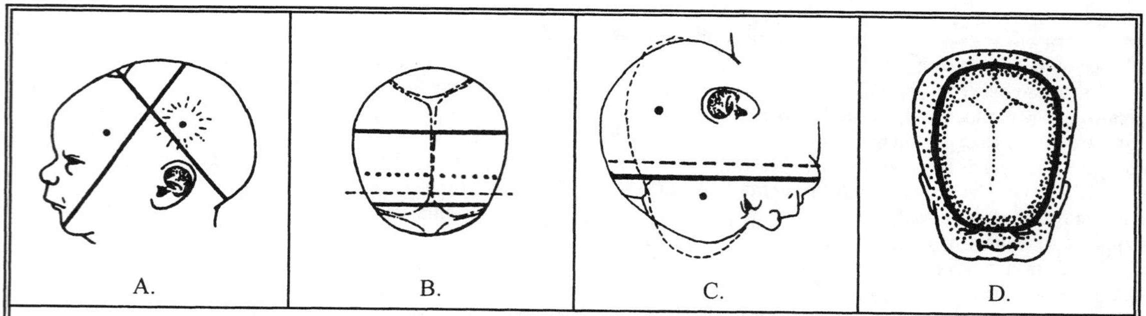

A. The suboccipitobregmatic diameter compared to the mentobregmatic diameter. Dots show locations of the bitemporal and biparietal diameters.
B. The solid lines show the levels of the bitemporal and biparietal diameters. The dotted line shows the level of the mentobregmatic diameter. The bitemporal diameter enters the brim (dashed line) first. Note that the mento-bregmatic and biparietal diameters are still well above the brim.
C. Moulding of the mentobregmatic diameter which must occur before the bulkiest anteroposterior diameter can engage; even more moulding is necessary before the biparietal diameter can fit through the brim.
D. The pale areas engage first, followed successively by the variously shaded areas.

In vertex presentations, the suboccipitobregmatic and biparietal diameters, which are at 90° angles to each other and are in the same plane, engage together. As is true for face presentations, in a brow presentation the mentobregmatic (mentoparietal) diameter and the biparietal diameter are in different planes (although the distance from the brow to the parietal eminences is not as far as the distance from the face to the eminences). First, the mentobregmatic and bitemporal diameters pass through the brim. After further descent, the widest transverse diameter, the biparietal, passes slowly through the brim, marking the actual engagement of the head. In most cases, the brow must have descended to at least +1 before engagement occurs.

Asynclitic engagement? As is true for face presentations, the biparietal diameter is farther from the inlet in brow presentations than in vertex presentations. Because the bulk of the head precedes the biparietal diameter through the brim, asynclitic descent does not facilitate engagement.

***4. Internal rotation of the head**

Once the baby has maneuvered her head through the brim, the brow typically rotates anteriorly as it contacts the uppermost edge of the levator ani sling. The large posterior portion of the head needs all the room to be found in the sacral curve in order to descend further. There must be sufficient room in the pelvic cavity to allow the extended head to rotate and the lower face and chin to lodge behind and partly under the pubic arch.

5. First internal rotation of the body and shoulders

The shoulders rotate with the head as it rotates internally, moving from the anteroposterior diameter to an oblique and then to the transverse diameter of the pelvis.

Conversion possibilities after further descent: Once internal rotation has occurred, one of the following conversion mechanisms may still come into play at any point between now and crowning.

Brow-to-face conversion: After anterior rotation, the vertex becomes lodged in the maternal sacrum. Force from contractions presses the face downward, extending the head into a mentum anterior face presentation. This may not occur until the head is deep in the pelvis.

Brow-to-vertex conversion: After engagement and anterior rotation of the brow, the force of contractions causes the spine to flex, and the head converts to an occiput posterior position. When this occurs is debated among researchers. While it can occur as late as after descent to the pelvic floor (Arthure, 1957; Jennings, 1968), this is extremely rare. Most authors state that brow-to-vertex conversion will occur at the brim, prior to engagement, or not at all.

Conversion usually requires good contractions and is more likely in women who have given birth before. Whether a brow will be able to convert to a vertex presentation or even a face is also very dependent upon the degree of moulding the head has undergone. If moulding is already pronounced, the head will become locked into a brow presentation and be prevented from moving one way or the other. This is especially true if a caput has formed. If conversion does not occur, labor may or may not become arrested, depending upon the overall situation.

6. Engagement of the shoulders

The shoulders descend through the brim as the brow passes the ischial tuberosities.

• **Flexion of the shoulders:** The attitude of the shoulders adjusts as the torso moves down, moulding and compacting as necessary to negotiate the curve of the birth canal.

7. Spinal extension increases

The spine is already somewhat extended in a brow presentation. As the head moves deeply into the pelvis, it leaves space in the uterus and the baby naturally takes advantage of this space by stretching out.

8-1. Second internal rotation of the chest and shoulders

As the shoulders and chest descend, they encounter the curve of the pelvic cavity near the level of the ischial spines. To negotiate the birth canal, the upper torso rotates, moving the chest and shoulders into an oblique diameter. This movement allows the spine to flex laterally. As this occurs, the head turns at the neck, allowing the head to remain in an FA orientation.

***9. Birth of the head**

The upper torso moves into the sacrum as the bulk of the very moulded head moves past the ischial tuberosities into the soft birth canal. A combination of downward pressure from contractions and the resistance afforded by the pelvic floor result in the upper spine and lower cervical vertebrae curling into the curve of the lower sacrum, causing the chin to tip toward the chest slightly. The perineum retracts as the vertex and upper occiput emerge posteriorly and most of the face emerges anteriorly. When the vault of the head is almost free from the birth canal, the neck extends slightly and the rest of the face is born. After its birth, the head is no longer held back in an attitude of extension, and the vertex now leads the way.

Notes on the birth of the head: While Borell and Fernström (1960) studied labors in both brow and face presentations, they give no details regarding the disengagement of the brow baby's head from the birth canal, and there are no other similar studies to which we can refer. Williams (1903), states that the birth of the head in anterior brow presentation occurs as the superior maxillae impinge on the lower border of the pubic bone, after which ". . . the rest of the head is born by extreme flexion, the brow, bregma, and occiput appearing in succession over the anterior margin of the perineum." This observation is noteworthy because Williams did not favor the use of clitorotomy, so the birth canal was in a more natural state, even if the women under his care were flat on their backs. Greenhill (1951) states that sometimes the head is born to the mouth before the occiput is born. In general, birth of the head is said to take place by a process of flexion at the atlantooccipital joint as a part of the face presses against the pubic bone anteriorly, allowing the head to pivot forward as it flexes and the brow, vault and occiput are born. After that, the nape of the neck is said to rest on the edge of the perineum, the head tips backward, and the face is born.

This teaching ignores the possible role of the upper thoracic and lower cervical spine. Nor does it take into account the considerable moulding that must take place before most babies' heads will descend to the point that emergence is even a possibility. Extreme moulding flattens the vertex and elongates the cranial vault, making the proposed movements, as described, less likely. Borell and Fernström do state that the spine, rather than the atlantooccipital joint, is where the movement occurs, as is true for all other cephalic presentations. In the case of a brow, the spine flexes as the head emerges. My description extrapolates from that assumption, with reference to those found in the older literature.

***10. Restitution of the head**

The neck untwists as the head restitutes to realign its long axis at a right angle with the long axis of the shoulders.

8-2. Second internal rotation of the chest is completed

The chest rotates 45°, moving the shoulders into the anteroposterior diameter of the pelvis, before or during the next contraction, bringing the anterior shoulder under the pubic arch.

***11. External rotation of the head**

The head rotates externally to 45° to arrive at a frontum transverse position, thus maintaining its long axis at a right-angle with the shoulders.

The shoulders and torso emerge as for any cephalic presentation.

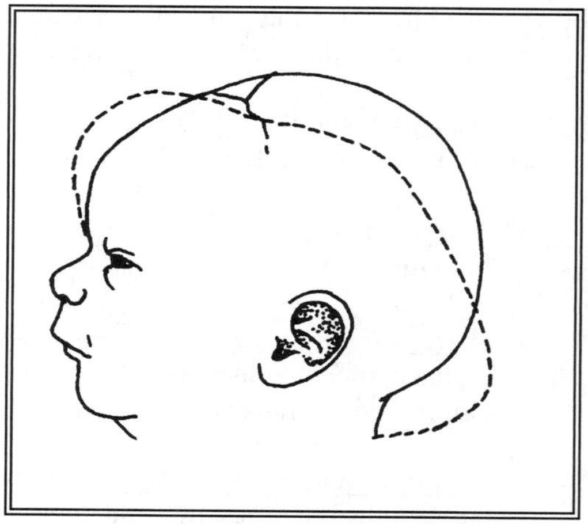

Moulding

Moulding in an anterior brow presentation results in elongation of the anteroposterior diameter and flattening of the vertex. The parietal bones are depressed an identical distance in relation to the frontal and occipital bones; this increases the occipitofrontal diameter and decreases the mentobregmatic diameter, a desirable feature in brow presentation. This causes the forehead to protrude. The forehead is bruised and swollen from the pressure of birth and may sport a large caput between the upper forehead and the bregma, slightly off center to the side that was most anterior during descent. There is no misalignment along the sagittal suture.

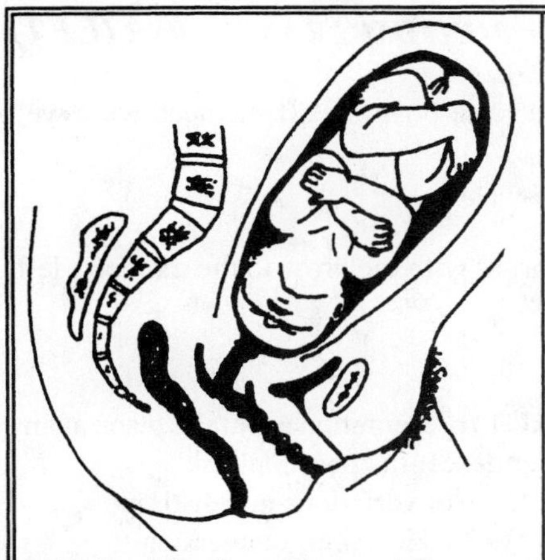

RFT, head floating, spine partially extended (1)

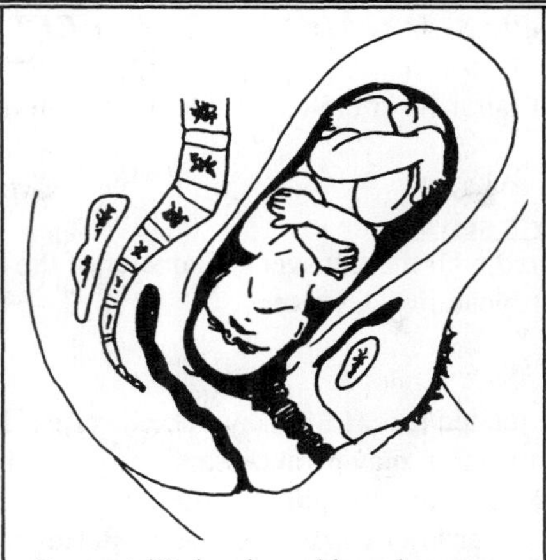

Descent (2); head moulds and engages (3), spinal extension is maintained (1)

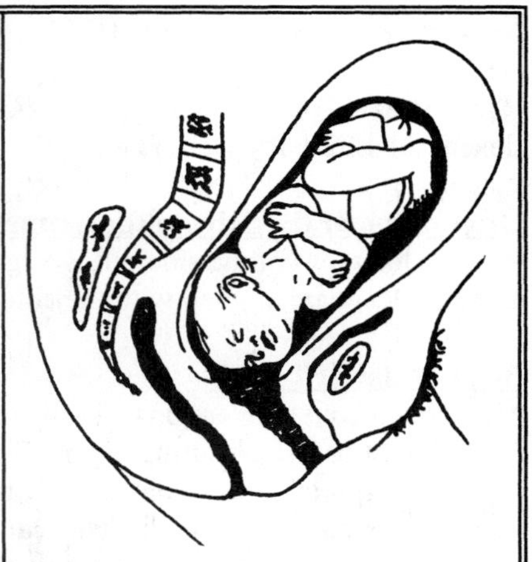

Internal rotation of head to RFT (4)

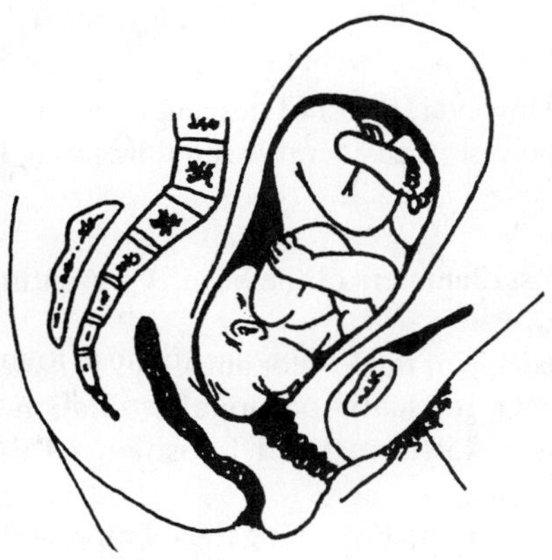

Internal rotation of head to RFA (4); chest/shoulders begin 1st internal rotation (5)

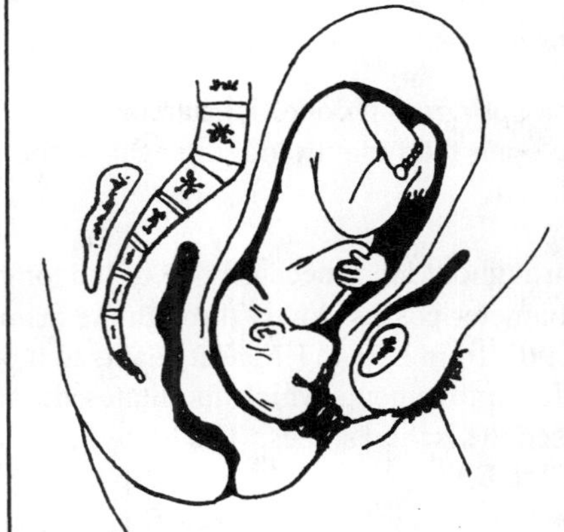

Head rotates internally to FA (4); Shoulders/chest complete 1st internal rotation to transverse (5) and engage (6)

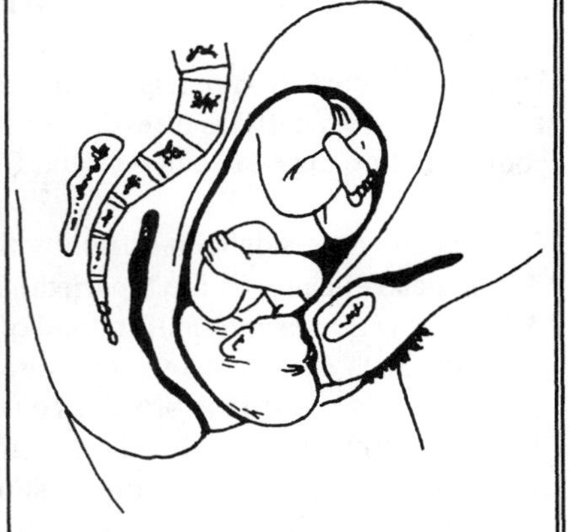

Chest/shoulders begin 2nd internal rotation to oblique (8-2); head crowns and is born by cervical flexion (9)

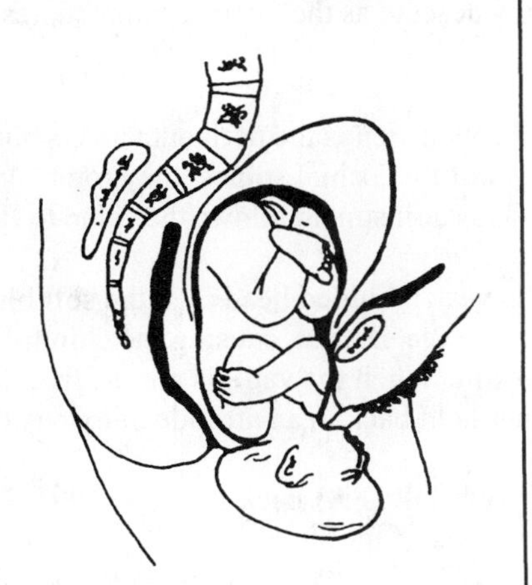

Head is born FA

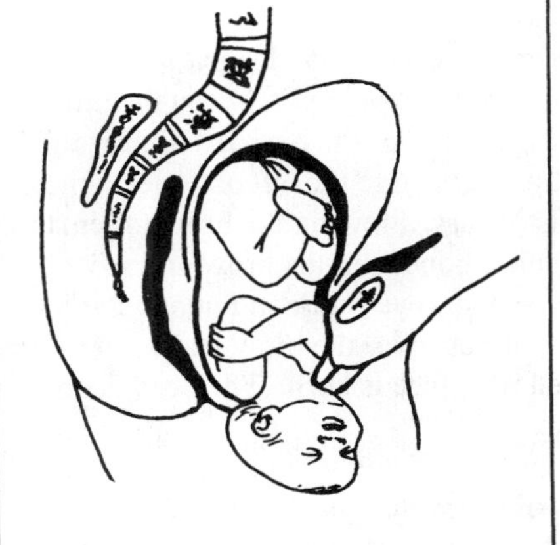

Head restitutes to LOP (RFA) (10)

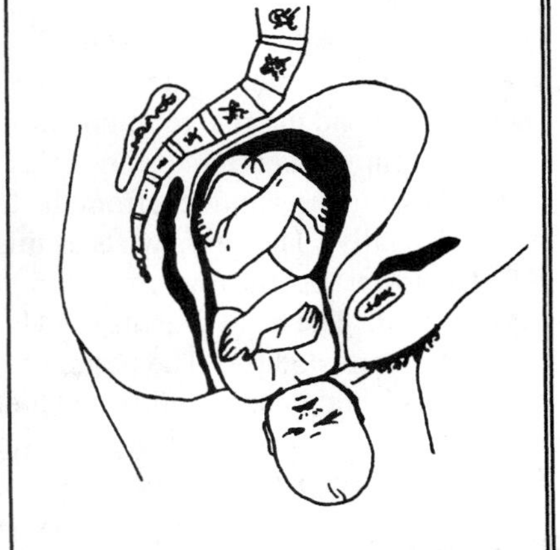

Shoulders finish 2nd internal rotation to AP (8-2); head follows with external rotation to LOT (RFT) (11); posterior shoulder born (12)

SUMMARY OF THE CARDINAL SPIRALING MOVEMENTS: LEFT FRONTUM TRANSVERSE (LFT)

We shall first review the process of labor for a baby in a left frontum transverse position. If the head were well flexed, the LFT baby would be ROT.

Orientation of the baby to the mother's pelvis

The long axis of the sinciput is aligned with the transverse diameter of the brim, with the brow to the mother's left. The shoulders are aligned with the anteroposterior diameter.

Birth of the LFT baby

***1.** Spontaneous conversion to a fully extended face (LMT) or a flexed vertex (ROT) presentation may take place at any point before or during labor. Conversion may be necessary before further descent is possible.

Unequal forces: Conversion can occur due to obliquely directed uterine force or variations in soft-tissue resistance or both. This can occur after engagement and anterior rotation. However, conversion to vertex usually occurs at or above the brim, with descent proceeding as an ROT position.

Impaction of the vertex: After anterior rotation, when the head is deeply descended, the vertex can become lodged against the maternal sacrum. Force from contractions presses the face downward, converting the baby to LMT.

When partial extension persists, labor may progress if conditions are optimal. However, arrest of descent could occur at any time, frequently as a result of the open fetal mouth lodging against the pelvis. Considerable moulding may be required before the head can descend further.

***2.** The baby descends with difficulty throughout labor because one of the longest diameters of the head is presenting.

***3.** The head engages as the biparietal diameter passes slowly through the brim.

***4.** The brow rotates internally a total of 90°, from LFT to FA, as it adapts to the shape of the levator ani sling. Rotation consists of a downwardly spiraling movement, which facilitates descent. It usually occurs after dilation is complete, when the brow has passed the ischial spines. The brow first rotates 45° from the LFT position to LFA. Then the brow rotates another 45° to FA.

5. The baby's body moves with the shoulders as they undergo their first internal rotation. Following the rotation of the head from LFT to LFA, the shoulders rotate 45° from the anteroposterior diameter to align with the left oblique diameter. As the brow rotates from LFA to FA, the shoulders rotate 45° to align with the transverse diameter of the brim, 90° in all.

6. The shoulders engage when the bisacromial diameter enters the transverse diameter of the brim, as the brow passes through the ischial tuberosities. The attitude of the shoulders shifts during descent as the torso accommodates to the shape of the birth canal.

7. The spine extends as the head enters the pelvis more deeply.

8-1. The second internal rotation of the shoulders begins between the time the brow distends the perineum and is born. As the midchest and spine enter the curve of the birth canal near the level of the ischial spines, they rotate 45°, moving the shoulders from the transverse into the left oblique diameter. This adjustment allows the spine to flex laterally. The neck twists as this occurs, allowing the brow to remain FA.

*** 9.** The lower face is now under the pubic bone, and the brow and most of the very moulded head is in the soft birth canal. The head crowns slowly as the lower neck and upper spine flex into the sacrum, causing the chin to tip forward slightly. The perineum retracts over the brow and vault of the skull. When the vault is almost free, the head straightens slightly and the lower face is born. The head is no longer held back in an attitude of extension, and the vertex now leads the way.

***10.** Restitution occurs as the neck untwists, allowing the head to rotate 45° from OP (FA) back to the ROP (LFA) position, restoring the long axis of the vertex to a 90° angle with the long axis of the shoulders.

8-2. The chest completes its second internal rotation, moving the shoulders 45° from the left oblique into the anteroposterior diameter before or during the next contraction. This brings the anterior shoulder under the pubic arch.

***11.** The head follows the internal rotation of the shoulders by rotating externally 45° from ROP (LFA) to ROT (LFT).

12. The anterior shoulder braces against the pubic bone as the posterior shoulder is born first by a process of lateral spinal flexion, after which the anterior shoulder slips past the pubic bone and emerges.
13. The torso and legs are born by a process of lateral flexion and a spiraling motion.

Moulding is similar in all brow presentations, with any caput forming over the upper left forehead and bregma.

LFT: unmoulded head before labor	Descent to arrest or engagement, moulding begins	Internal rotation begins: LFT to LFA, body follows to oblique	Internal rotation of head LFA to FA, chest/shoulders rotate transverse and engage
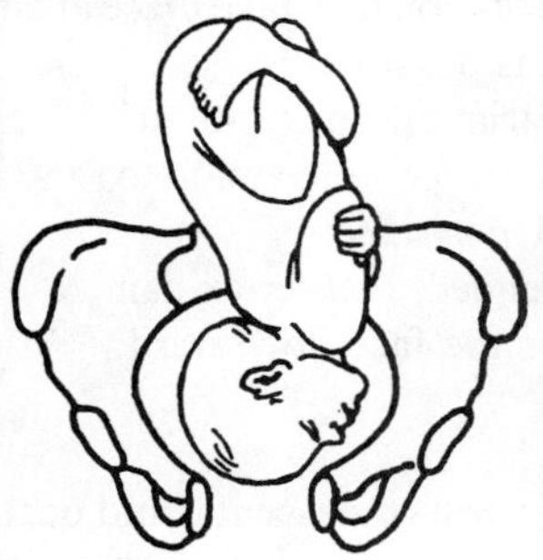	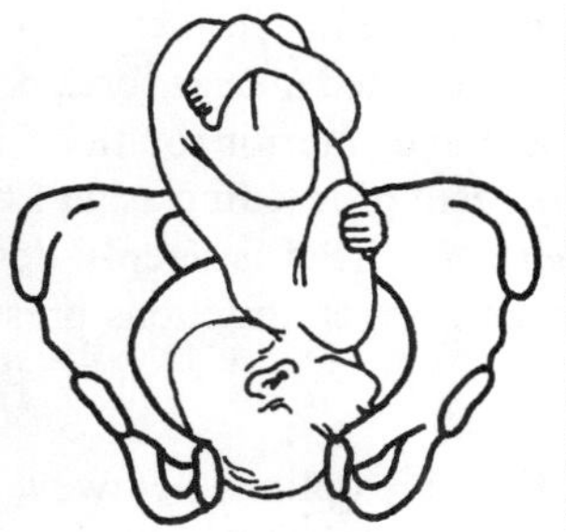	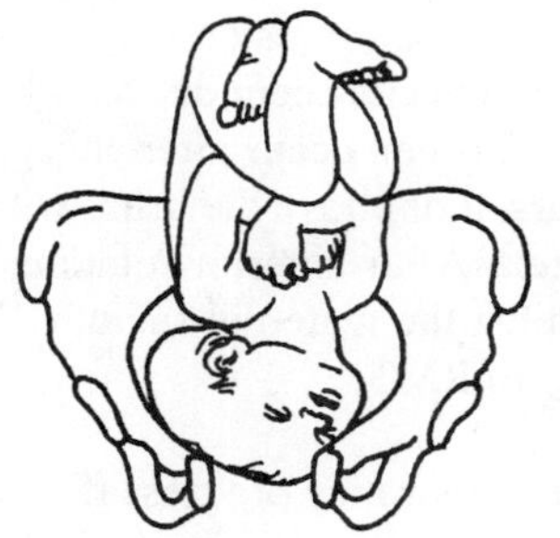	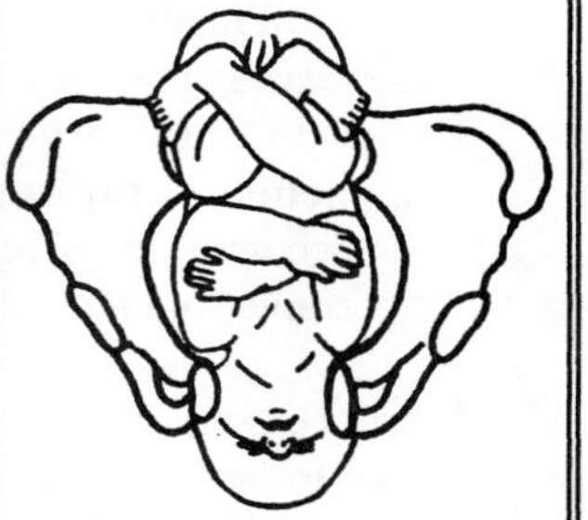
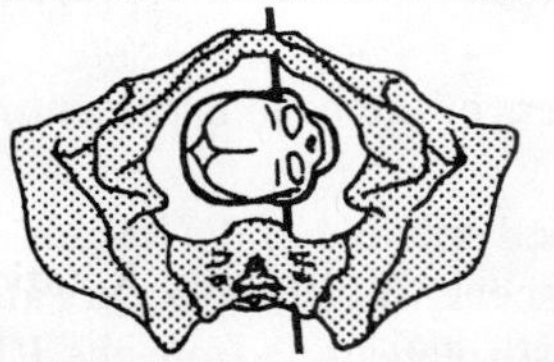	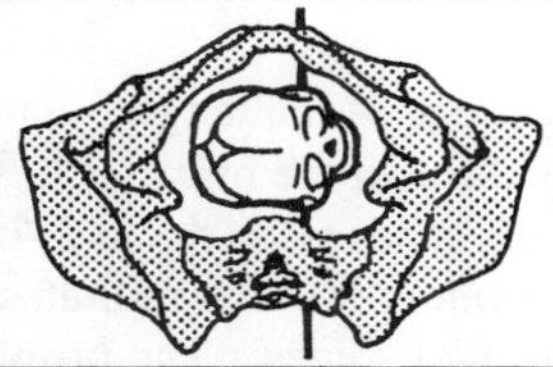	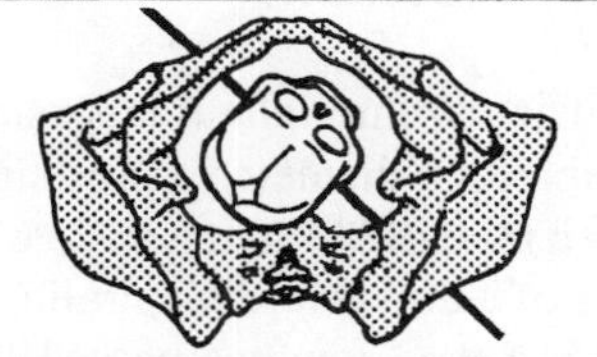	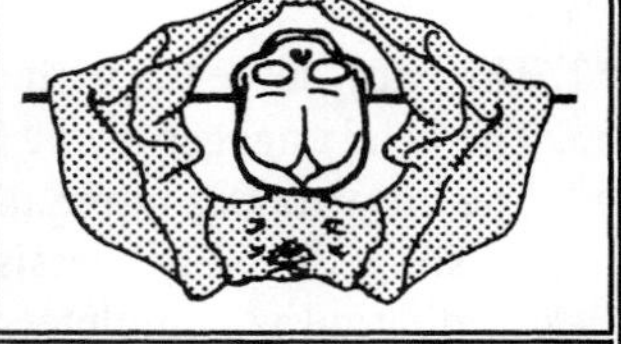
2nd internal rotation of chest/shoulders to oblique. Head born by combination of spinal flexion and cephalic extension	Head is born directly OP (FA)	Restitution : OP to ROP (FA to LFA).	Chest-shoulders complete 2nd internal rotation, head rotates externally to ROT (LFT), posterior and anterior shoulders emerge
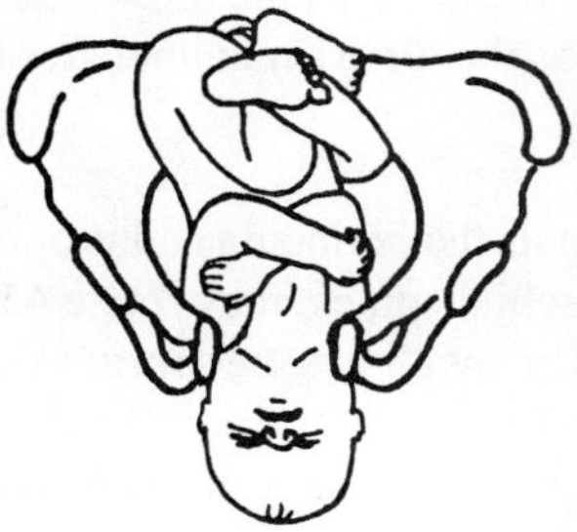	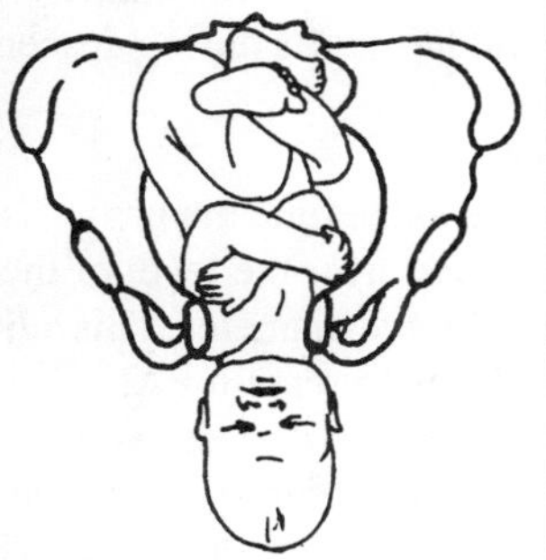	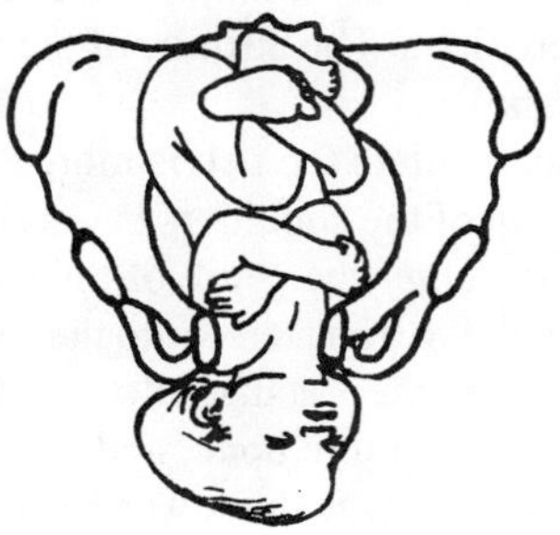	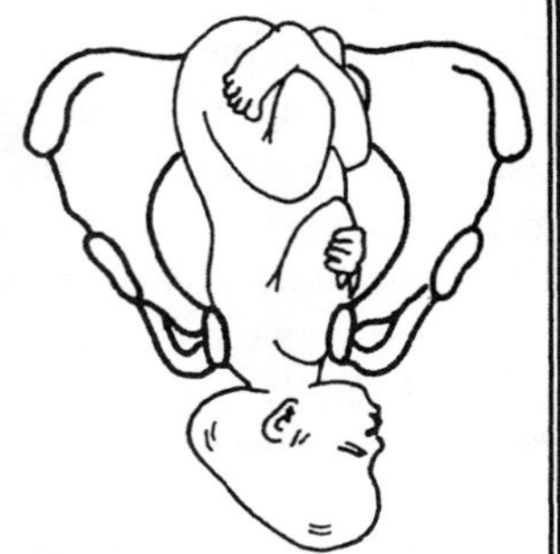
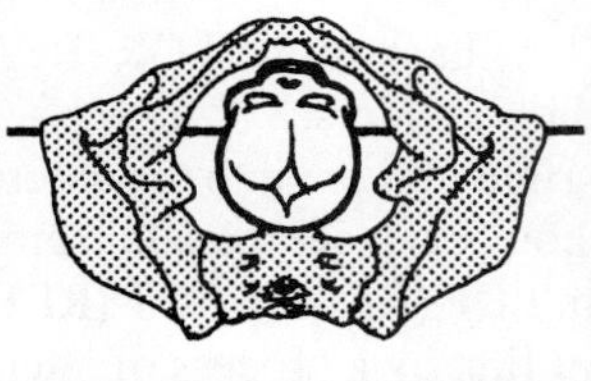	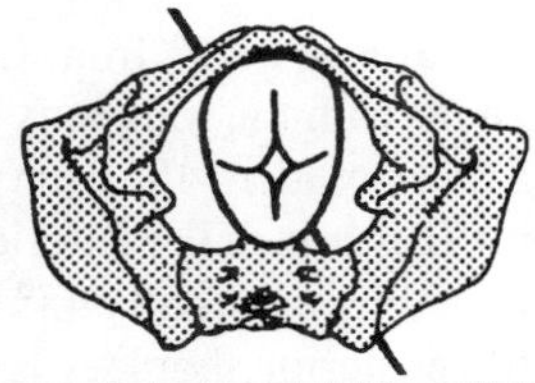	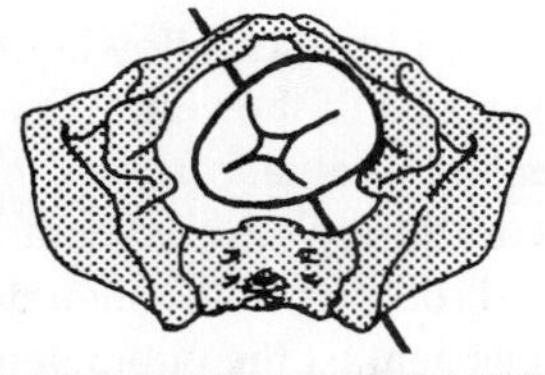	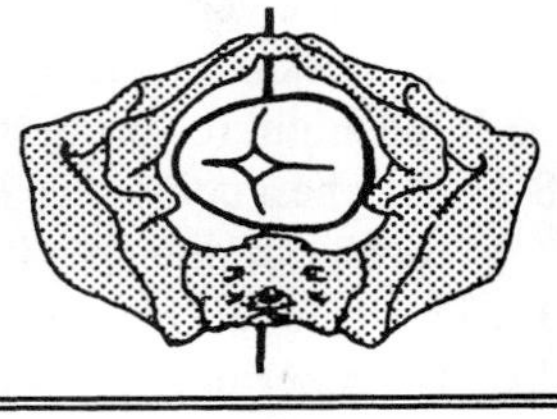

Summary of the Cardinal Spiraling Movements: Right Frontum Transverse (RFT)

The flexed RFT baby converts to an LOT position and is the mirror image of LFT descent.

Orientation of the baby to the mother's pelvis

The sinciput is aligned with the transverse diameter of the brim, with the brow to the mother's right. The shoulders are aligned with the anteroposterior diameter.

Birth of the RFT baby

***1.** Spontaneous conversion to a fully extended face (RMT) or a flexed vertex (LOT) presentation may take place at any point before or during labor. Conversion may be necessary before further descent is possible.

Unequal forces: Conversion can occur due to obliquely directed uterine force or variations in soft-tissue resistance or both. This can occur after engagement and anterior rotation. However, conversion to vertex usually occurs at or above the brim, with descent proceeding as an LOT position.

Impaction of the vertex: After anterior rotation, when the head is deeply descended, the vertex can become lodged against the maternal sacrum. Force from contractions presses the face downward, converting the baby to RMT.

When partial extension persists, labor may progress if conditions are optimal. However, arrest of descent could occur at any time, frequently as a result of the open fetal mouth lodging against the pelvis. Considerable moulding may be required before the head can descend further.

***2.** The baby descends with difficulty throughout labor because one of the longest diameters of the head is presenting.

***3.** The head engages as the biparietal diameter passes slowly through the brim.

***4.** The brow rotates internally a total of 90°, from RFT to FA , as it adapts to the loop-shaped opening of the levator ani sling. Rotation consists of a downwardly spiraling movement, which facilitates descent. It usually occurs after dilation is complete, when the brow has passed the ischial spines. The brow first rotates 45° from the RFT position to RFA. Then the brow rotates another 45° to FA.

5. The baby's body moves with the shoulders as they undergo their first internal rotation. Following the rotation of the head from RFT to RFA, the shoulders rotate 45° from the anteroposterior diameter to align with the right oblique diameter. As the brow rotates from RFA to FA, the shoulders rotate another 45° to align with the transverse diameter of the brim, 90° in all.

6. The shoulders engage when the bisacromial diameter enters the transverse diameter of the brim, as the brow passes through the ischial tuberosities. The attitude of the shoulders shifts during descent as the torso accommodates to the shape of the birth canal.

7. The spine extends as the head enters the pelvis more deeply.

8-1. The second internal rotation of the shoulders begins between the time the brow distends the perineum and is born. As the midchest and spine enter the curve of the birth canal near the level of the ischial spines, they rotate 45°, moving the shoulders from the transverse into the right oblique diameter. This adjustment allows the spine to flex laterally. The neck twists as this occurs, allowing the brow to remain FA.

***9.** The lower face is now under the pubic bone, and the brow and most of the very moulded head is in the soft birth canal. The head crowns slowly as the lower neck and upper spine flex into the sacrum, causing the chin to tip forward slightly. The perineum retracts over the brow and vault of the skull. When the vault is almost free, the head straightens slightly and the lower face is born. The head is no longer held back in an attitude of extension, and the vertex now leads the way.

***10.** Restitution occurs as the neck untwists, allowing the head to rotate 45° from OP (FA) back to the LOP (RFA) position, restoring the long axis of the vertex to a 90° angle with the long axis of the shoulders.

8-2. The chest completes its second internal rotation, moving the shoulders 45° from the right oblique into the anteroposterior diameter before or during the next contraction. This brings the anterior shoulder under the pubic arch.

***11.** The head follows the internal rotation of the shoulders by rotating externally 45° from LOP (RFA) to LOT (RFT).

12. The anterior shoulder braces against the pubic bone as the posterior shoulder is born first by a process of lateral spinal flexion, after which the anterior shoulder slips past the pubic bone and emerges.

13. The torso and legs are born by a process of lateral flexion and a spiraling motion.

Moulding is similar in all brow presentations, with any caput forming between the upper right forehead and bregma.

RFT: unmoulded head before labor	Descent to arrest or engagement, moulding begins	Internal rotation: RFT to RFA	Internal rotation of head & 1st of body: RFA to FA, chest-shoulders engage
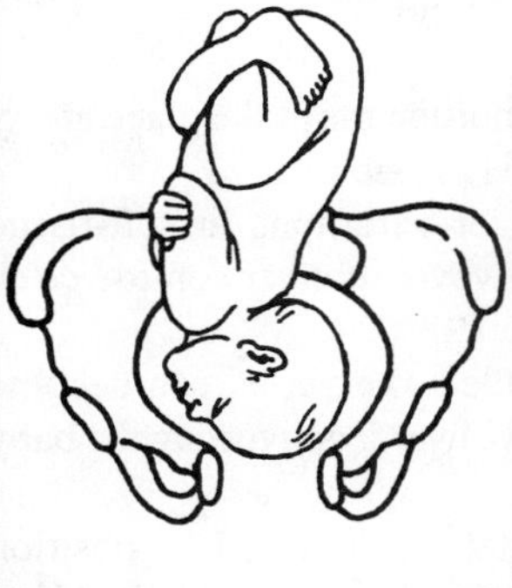	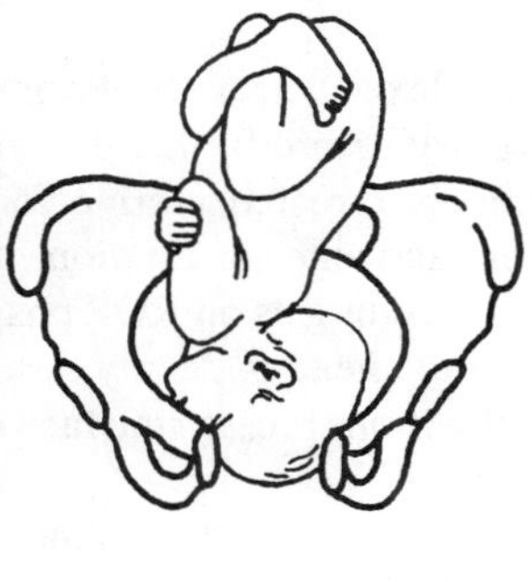	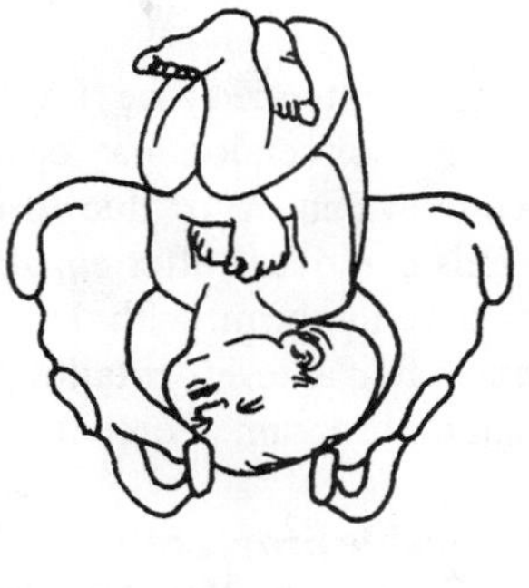	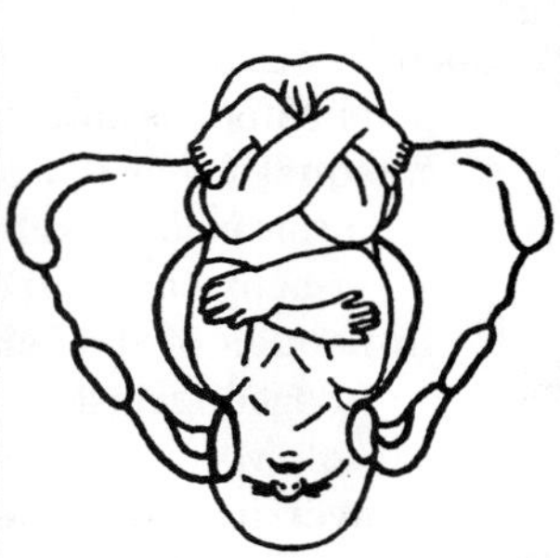
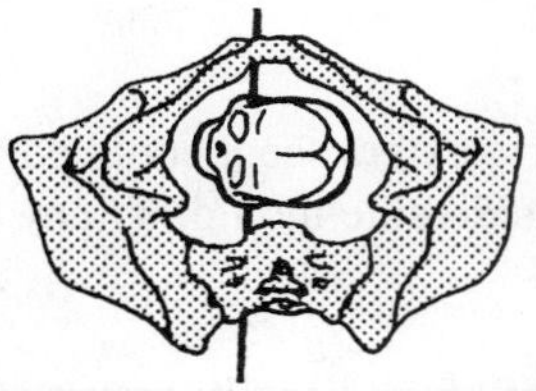	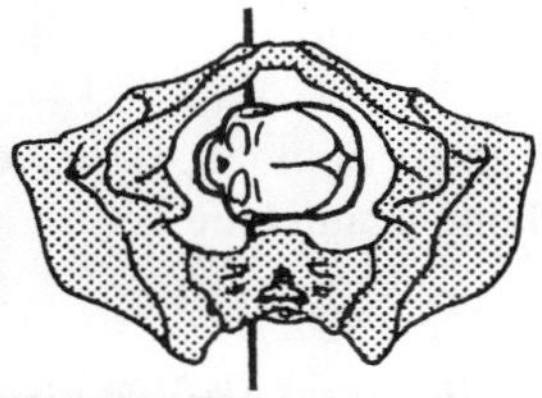	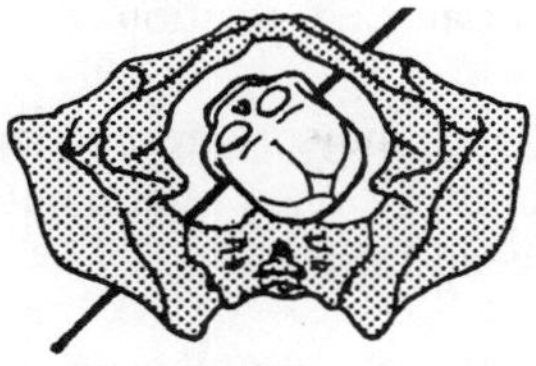	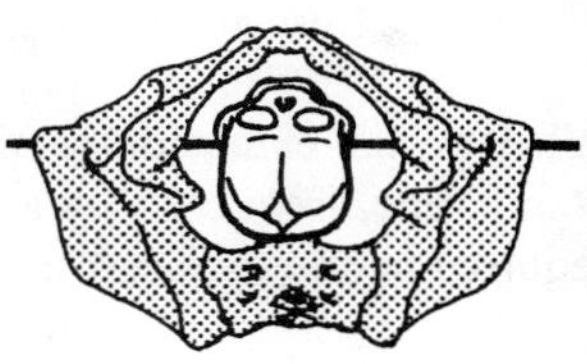
2nd internal rotation of chest/shoulders to oblique. Head born by combination of spinal flexion and cephalic extension	Head is born directly OP (FA) to LOP (FA to RFA)	Restitution : OP to LOP (FA to RFA)	Chest/shoulders complete 2nd internal rotation, head rotates externally to LOT (RFT), posterior and anterior shoulders emerge
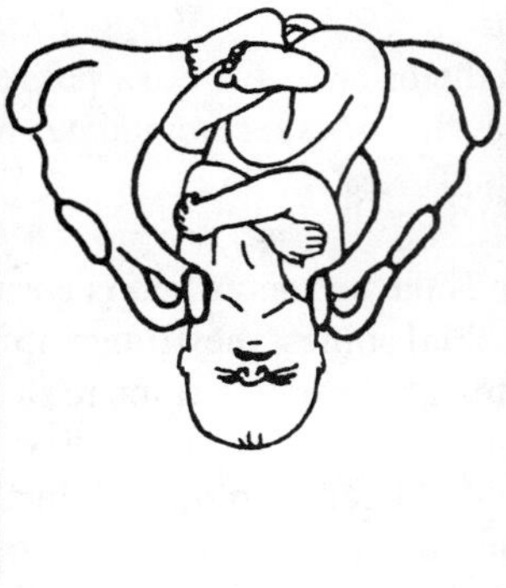	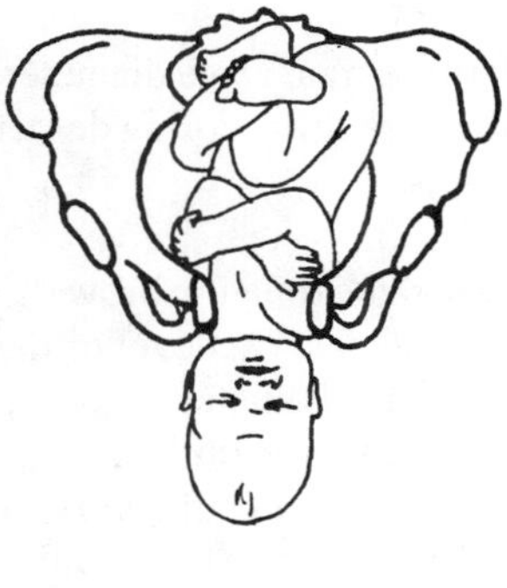	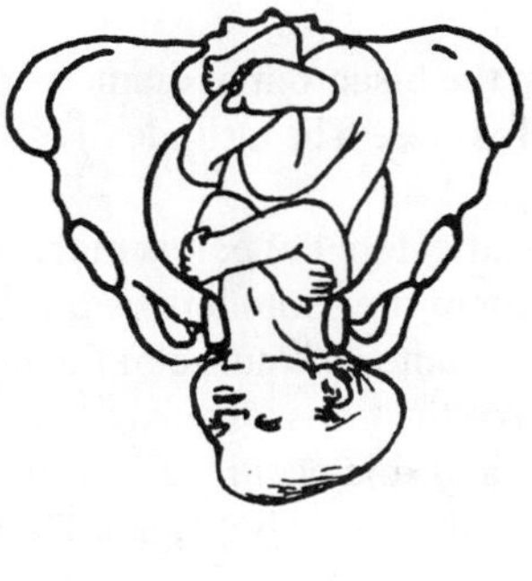	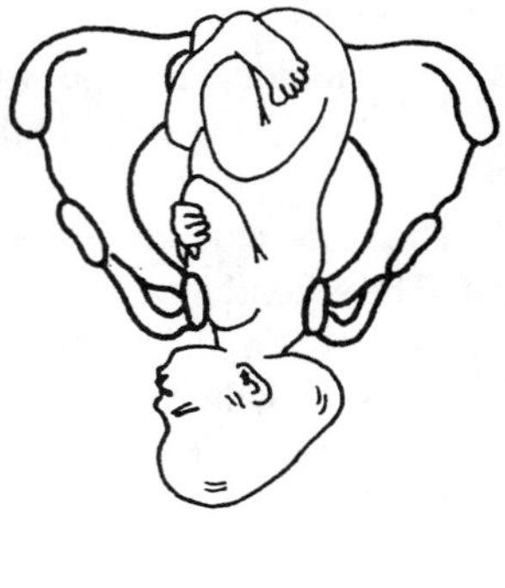
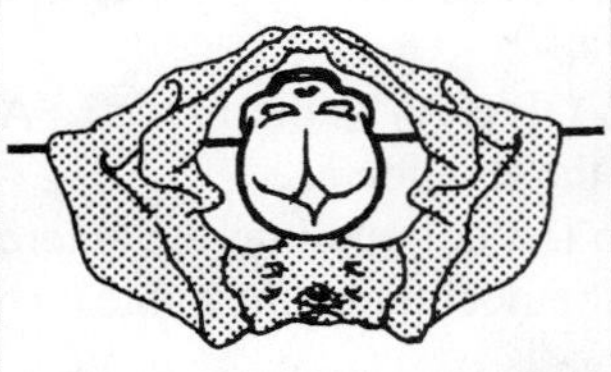	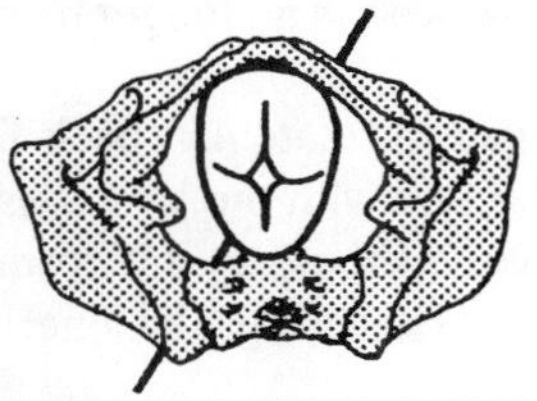	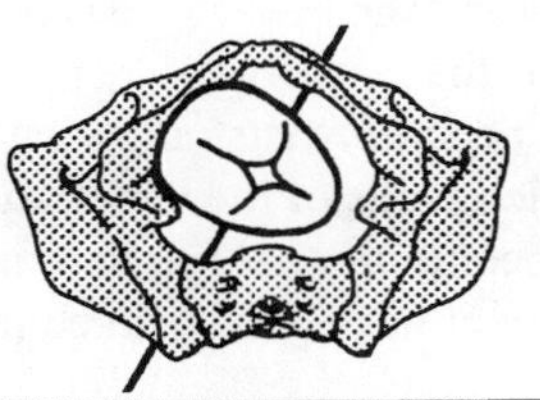	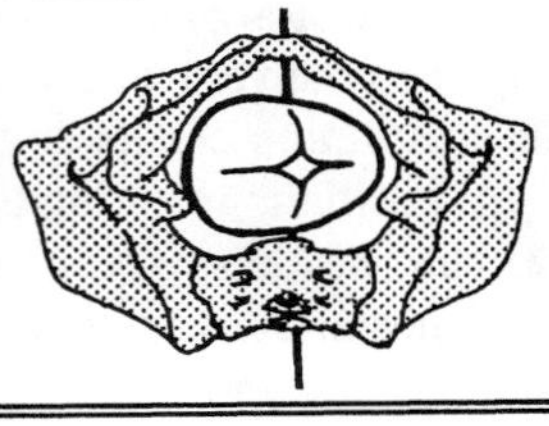

Summary of the Cardinal Spiraling Movements: Left Frontum Anterior (LFA)

The flexed LFA baby presents as an ROP.

Orientation of the baby to the mother's pelvis

The long axis of the sinciput is aligned with the right oblique diameter, while the brow occupies the left anterior corner of the brim. The shoulders are aligned with the left oblique diameter.

Birth of the LFA baby

***1.** Spontaneous conversion to a fully extended face (LMA) or a flexed vertex (ROP) presentation may take place at any point before or during labor. Conversion may be necessary before further descent is possible.

Unequal forces: Conversion can occur due to obliquely directed uterine force or variations in soft-tissue resistance or both. This can occur after engagement and anterior rotation. However, conversion to vertex usually occurs at or above the brim, with descent proceeding as an ROP position.

Impaction of the vertex: After anterior rotation, when the head is deeply descended, the vertex can become lodged against the maternal sacrum. Force from contractions presses the face downward, converting the baby to LMA.

Conversion to a more favorable brow position: The baby's head and body may rotate 45° into an LFT position before entering the brim, which allows the long axis of the head to enter a longer diameter of the brim. Descent proceeds as for an LFT position.

When partial extension persists, labor may progress if conditions are optimal. However, arrest of descent could occur at any time, frequently as a result of the open fetal mouth lodging against the pelvis. Considerable moulding may be required before the head can descend further.

***2.** The baby descends with difficulty throughout labor because one of the longest diameters of the head is presenting.

***3.** The head engages as the biparietal diameter passes slowly through the brim.

***4.** The brow rotates internally a total of 45°, from LFA to FA , as it adapts to the loop-shaped opening of the levator ani sling. Rotation consists of a downwardly spiraling movement, which facilitates descent. It usually occurs after dilation is complete and the brow has passed the ischial spines.

5. The baby's body moves with the shoulders as they undergo their first internal rotation. Following the rotation of the head from LFA to FA, the shoulders rotate 45°, from the left oblique diameter to align with the transverse diameter of the brim.

6. The shoulders engage when the bisacromial diameter enters the transverse diameter of the brim, as the brow passes through the ischial tuberosities. The attitude of the shoulders shifts during descent as the torso accommodates to the shape of the birth canal.

7. The spine extends as the head enters the pelvis more deeply.

8-1. The second internal rotation of the shoulders begins between the time the brow distends the perineum and is born. As the midchest and spine enter the curve of the birth canal near the level of the ischial spines, they rotate 45°, moving the shoulders from the transverse into the left oblique diameter. This adjustment allows the spine to flex laterally. The neck twists as this occurs, allowing the brow to remain FA.

***9.** The lower face is now under the pubic bone, and the brow and most of the very moulded head is in the soft birth canal. The head crowns slowly as the lower neck and upper spine flex into the sacrum, causing the chin to tip forward slightly. The perineum retracts over the brow and vault of the skull. When the vault is almost free, the head straightens slightly and the lower face is born. The head is no longer held back in an attitude of extension, and the vertex now leads the way.

***10.** Restitution occurs as the neck untwists, allowing the head to rotate 45° back from OP (FA) to the ROP (LFA) position, restoring the long axis of the vertex to a 90° angle with the long axis of the shoulders.

8-2. The chest completes its second internal rotation, moving the shoulders 45° from the left oblique into the antero-posterior diameter before or during the next contraction. This brings the anterior shoulder under the pubic arch.

*11. The head follows the internal rotation of the shoulders by rotating externally 45° from ROP (LFA) to ROT (LFT).

12. The anterior shoulder braces against the pubic bone as the posterior shoulder is born first by a process of lateral spinal flexion, after which the anterior shoulder slips past the pubic bone and emerges.

13. The torso and legs are born by a process of lateral flexion and a spiraling motion.

Moulding is similar in all brow presentations, with any caput forming between the upper left forehead and bregma.

LFA orientation, head partially flexed	Descent to engagement	Internal rotation of head and shoulders: LFA to FA	The shoulders follow the head and engage transverse.

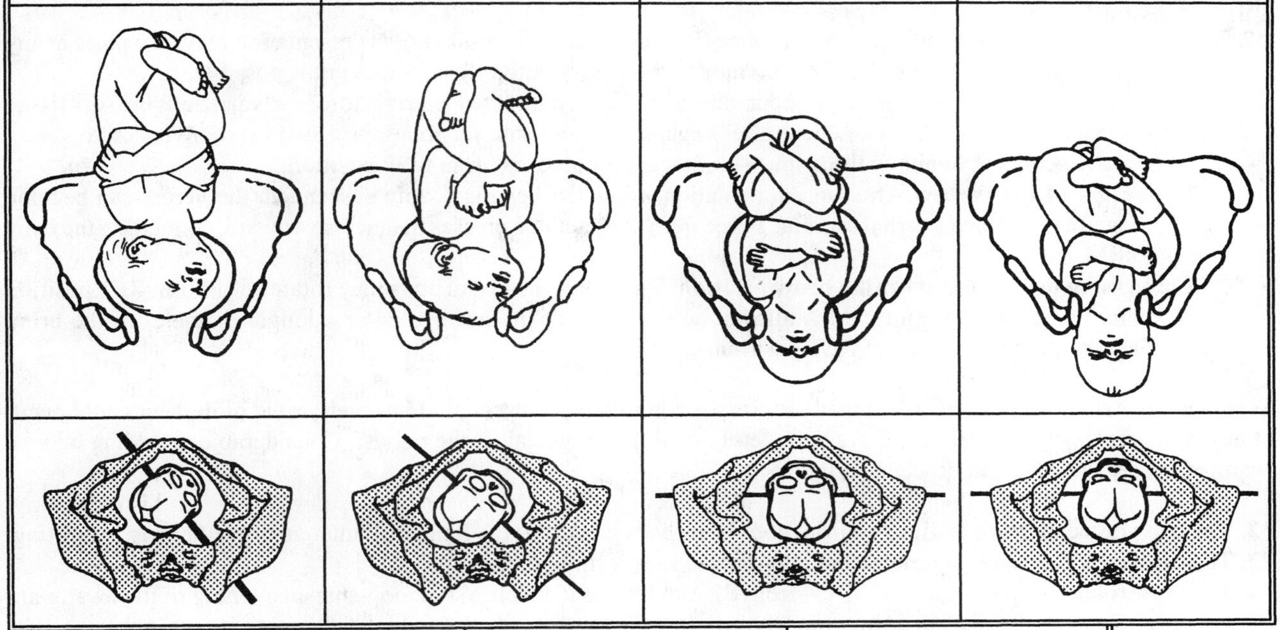

Descent rotates chest, bringing shoulders oblique. The upper spine extends as head is born.	The head restitutes 45° from OP to ROP (FA to LFA)	Shoulders rotate to AP diameter as head rotates externally 45°: ROP to ROT (LFA to LFT)

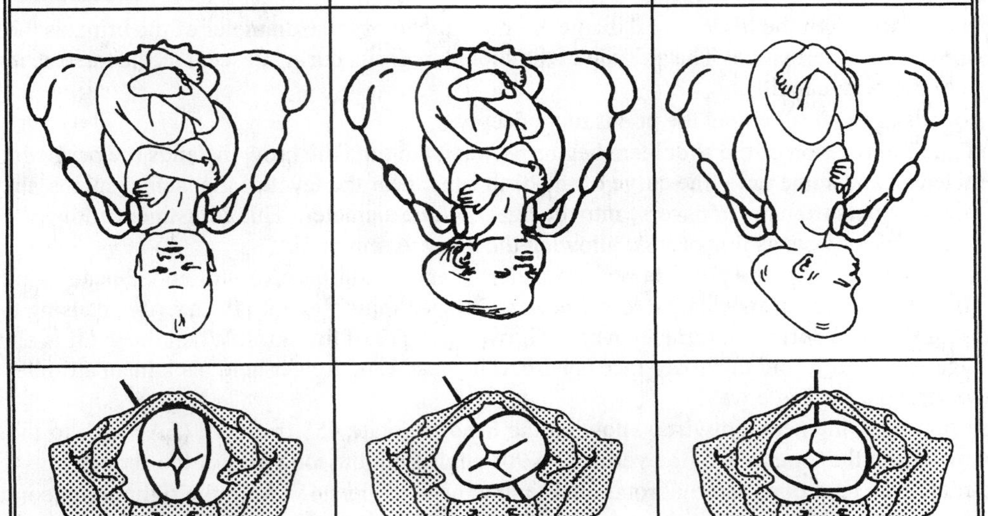

SUMMARY OF THE CARDINAL SPIRALING MOVEMENTS: RIGHT FRONTUM ANTERIOR (RFA)

Birth in the RFA position is the mirror image of birth in the LFA position. If the head were well flexed, the RFA baby's would be LOP.

Orientation of the baby to the mother's pelvis

The long axis of the sinciput is aligned with the left oblique diameter, while the brow occupies the right anterior corner of the brim. The shoulders are aligned in the right oblique diameter.

Birth of the RFA baby

***1.** Spontaneous conversion to a fully extended face (RMA) or a flexed vertex (LOP) presentation may take place at any point before or during labor. Conversion may be necessary before further descent is possible.

Unequal forces: Conversion can occur due to obliquely directed uterine force or variations in soft-tissue resistance or both. This can occur after engagement and anterior rotation. However, conversion to vertex usually occurs at or above the brim, with descent proceeding as an LOP position.

Impaction of the vertex: After anterior rotation, when the head is deeply descended, the vertex can become lodged against the maternal sacrum. Force from contractions presses the face downward, converting the baby to RMA.

Conversion to a more favorable brow position: The baby's head and body may rotate 45° into an RFT position before entering the brim, which allows the long axis of the head to enter a longer diameter of the brim. Descent proceeds as for an RFT position.

When partial extension persists, labor may progress if conditions are optimal. However, arrest of descent could occur at any time, frequently as a result of the open fetal mouth lodging against the pelvis. Considerable moulding may be required before the head can descend further.

***2.** The baby descends with difficulty throughout labor because one of the longest diameters of the head is presenting.

***3.** The head engages as the biparietal diameter passes slowly through the brim.

***4.** The brow rotates internally a total of 45° from RFA to FA , as it adapts to the loop-shaped opening of the levator ani sling. Rotation consists of a downwardly spiraling movement, which facilitates descent. It usually occurs after dilation is complete and the brow has passed the ischial spines.

5. The baby's body moves with the shoulders as they undergo their first internal rotation. Following the rotation of the head from RFA to FA, the shoulders rotate 45°, from the right oblique diameter to align with the transverse diameter of the brim.

6. The shoulders engage when the bisacromial diameter enters the transverse diameter of the brim, as the brow passes through the ischial tuberosities. The attitude of the shoulders shifts during descent as the torso accommodates to the shape of the birth canal.

7. The spine extends as the head enters the pelvis more deeply.

8-1. The second internal rotation of the shoulders begins between the time the brow distends the perineum and is born. As the midchest and spine enter the curve of the birth canal near the level of the ischial spines, they rotate 45°, moving the shoulders from the transverse into the right oblique diameter. This adjustment allows the spine to flex laterally. The neck twists as this occurs, allowing the brow to remain FA.

***9.** The lower face is now under the pubic bone, and the brow and most of the very moulded head is in the soft birth canal. The head crowns slowly as the lower neck and upper spine flex into the sacrum, causing the chin to tip forward slightly. The perineum retracts over the brow and vault of the skull. When the vault is almost free, the head straightens slightly and the lower face is born. The head is no longer held back in an attitude of extension, and the vertex now leads the way.

***10.** Restitution occurs as the neck untwists, allowing the head to rotate 45° from OP (FA) back to the LOP (RFA) position, restoring the long axis of the vertex to a 90° angle with the long axis of the shoulders.

8-2. The chest completes its second internal rotation, moving the shoulders 45° from the right oblique into the antero-posterior diameter before or during the next contraction. This brings the anterior shoulder under the pubic arch.

*11. The head follows the internal rotation of the shoulders by rotating externally 45° from LOP (RFA) to LOT (RFT).
12. The anterior shoulder braces against the pubic bone as the posterior shoulder is born first by a process of lateral spinal flexion, after which the anterior shoulder slips past the pubic bone and emerges.
13. The torso and legs are born by a process of lateral flexion and a spiraling motion.

Moulding is similar in all brow presentations, with any caput forming between the upper right forehead and bregma.

RFA orientation, head partially flexed	Descent to engagement	Internal rotation of head and shoulders: RFA to FA	The shoulders follow the head and engage transverse.
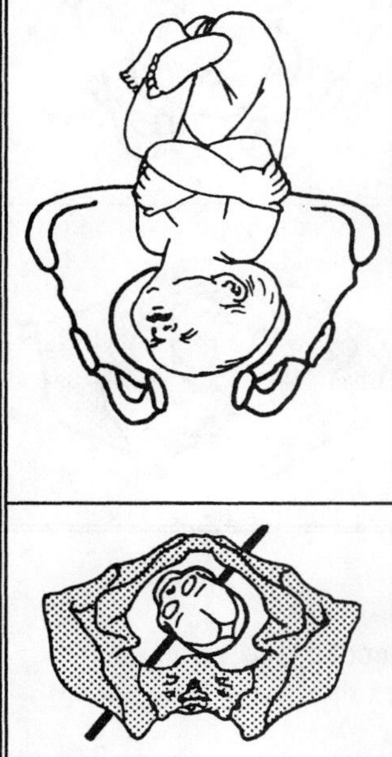	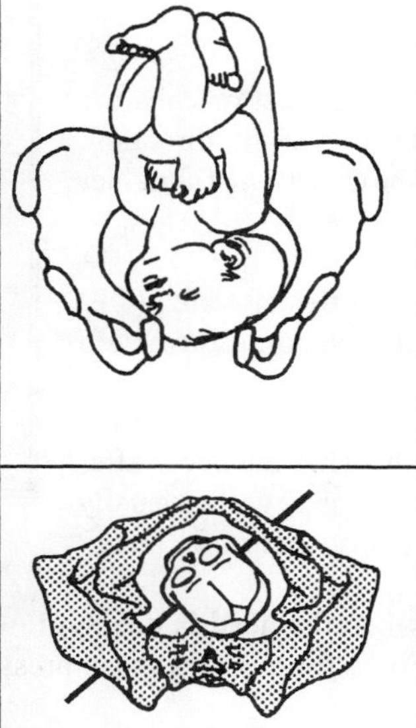	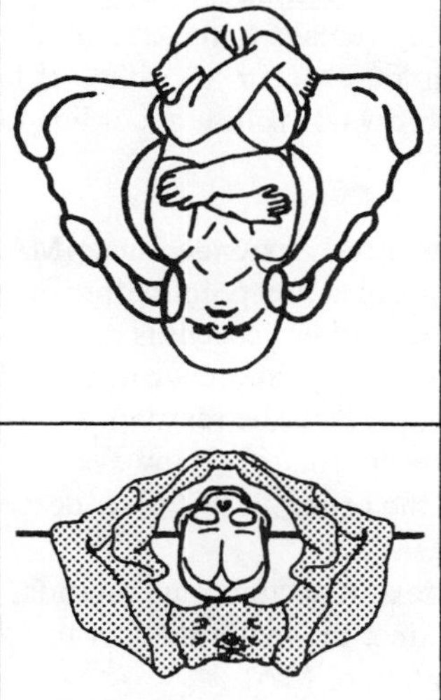	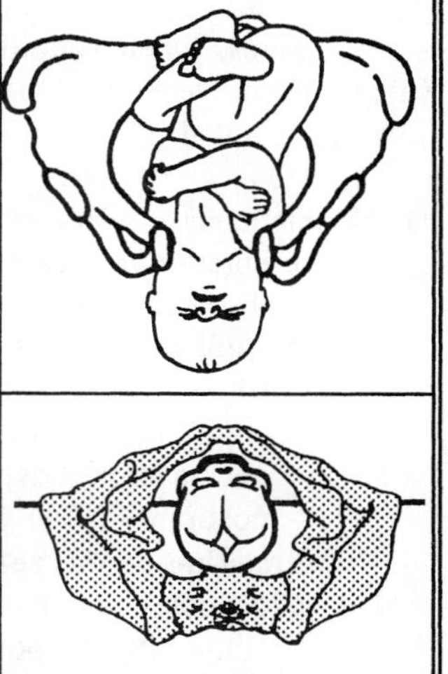

Descent rotates chest, bringing shoulders oblique. The upper spine extends as head is born.	The head restitutes 45° from OP to LOP (FA to RFA)	Shoulders rotate to AP diameter as head rotates externally 45°: LOP to LOT (RFA to RFT)
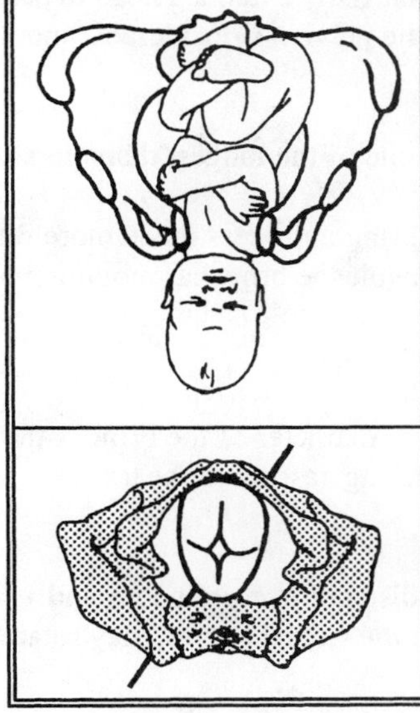	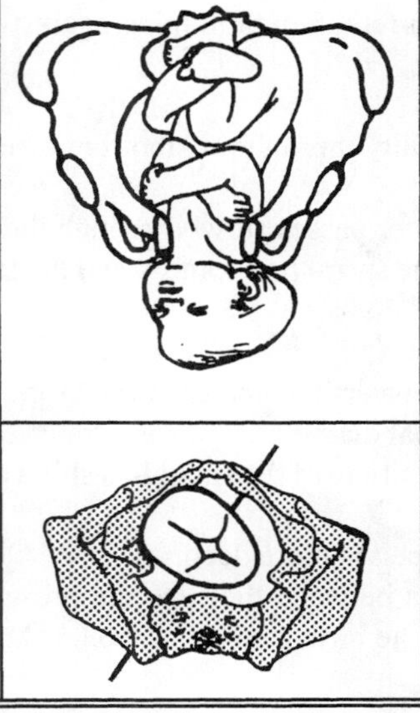	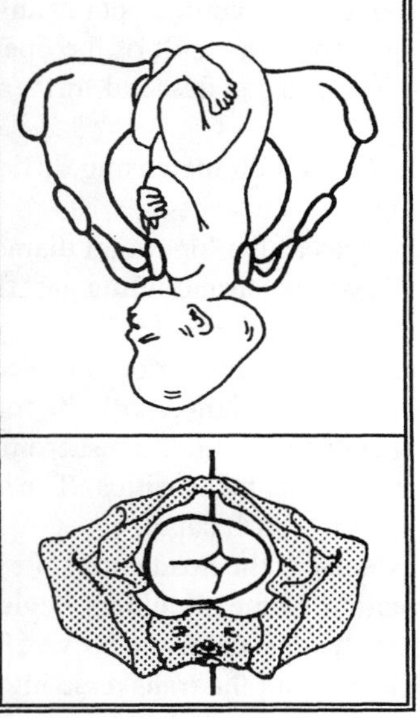

SUMMARY OF THE CARDINAL SPIRALING MOVEMENTS: FRONTUM ANTERIOR (FA)

Theoretically, it is possible for a brow baby to present and descend with the sinciput directly anterior, however, this mode of descent is even more improbable than the positions already contemplated because the long presenting diameter accommodates best to an oblique or transverse diameter of the brim.

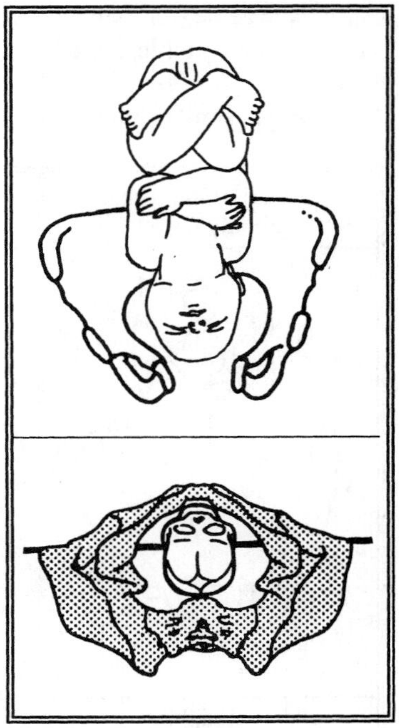

Orientation of the baby to the mother's pelvis

The long axis of the sinciput is aligned with the anteroposterior diameter, with the brow directly anterior, behind the symphysis. The shoulders are aligned with the transverse diameter.

Birth of the directly FA baby (movements not illustrated)

The shoulders will probably remain transverse until the midchest reaches the ischial spines, when rotation may occur in either a left or a right direction. Subsequent movements of the brow will follow according to the direction of shoulder rotation, as noted.

***1.** Spontaneous conversion to a fully extended face (MA) or a flexed vertex (OP) presentation may take place at any point before or during labor. Conversion may be necessary before further descent is possible.

Unequal forces: Conversion can occur due to obliquely directed uterine force or variations in soft-tissue resistance or both. This can occur after engagement and anterior rotation. However, conversion to vertex usually occurs at or above the brim. In this case, descent proceeds as for an OP position.

Impaction of the vertex: After anterior rotation, when the head is deeply descended, the vertex can become lodged against the maternal sacrum. Force from contractions presses the face downward, converting the position to MA.

Conversion to a more favorable brow position: The baby's head and body may rotate 45° into an RFA or LFA position before entering the brim, which allows the long axis of the head to enter a longer diameter of the brim. Descent proceeds as for an RFA or LFA position.

When partial extension persists, progressive labor usually requires an unusually small baby, a large pelvis or both. However, arrest of descent could occur at any time due to an inability of the partially extended head to pass through the birth canal, frequently as a result of the open fetal mouth lodging against the pelvis. Considerable moulding may be required before the head can descend further.

***2.** The baby descends with increasing difficulty throughout labor because one of the longest diameters of the head is presenting.

***3.** The head engages as the biparietal diameter passes slowly through the brim, a process made more difficult by the trouble the vertex has moulding past the sacral promontory and the trouble the brow has moulding past the pubic bone.

***4.** Internal rotation of the brow does not occur.

5. The shoulders remain aligned with the transverse diameter of the brim.

6. The shoulders engage when the bisacromial diameter enters the transverse diameter of the brim as the brow passes through the ischial tuberosities. The attitude of the shoulders shifts during descent as the torso accommodates to the shape of the birth canal.

7. The spine extends as the head enters the pelvis more deeply.

8-1. Internal rotation of the shoulders begins between the time the brow distends the perineum and is born. As the midchest and spine enter the curve of the birth canal near the level of the ischial spines, they rotate 45°, moving the shoulders from the transverse into:

8-1-A. the left oblique diameter. (Follow "A" entries below.)

8-1-B. the right oblique diameter. (Follow "B" entries below.)

This adjustment allows the spine to flex laterally. The neck twists as this occurs, allowing the brow to remain FA.

***9.** The lower face is now under the pubic bone, and the brow and most of the very moulded head is in the soft birth canal. The head crowns slowly as the lower neck and upper spine flex into the sacrum, causing the chin to tip forward slightly. The perineum retracts over the brow and vault of the skull. When the vault is almost free, the head straightens slightly and the lower face is born. The head is no longer held back in an attitude of extension, and the vertex now leads the way.

***10.** Restitution occurs as the neck untwists, allowing the head to rotate 45° from OP (FA) back to:

10-A. the ROP (LFA) position.

10-B. the LOP (RFA) position.

This movement restores the long axis of the vertex to a 90° angle with the long axis of the shoulders.

8-2. The chest completes its internal rotation, moving the shoulders 45° from:

8-2-A. the left oblique diameter

8-2-B. the right oblique diameter

into the anteroposterior diameter before or during the next contraction. This brings the anterior shoulder under the pubic arch.

***11.** The head follows the internal rotation of the shoulders by rotating externally 45°:

11-A. from ROP (LFA) to ROT (LFT).

11-B. from LOP (RFA) to LOT (RFT).

12. The anterior shoulder braces against the pubic bone as the posterior shoulder is born first by a process of lateral spinal flexion, after which the anterior shoulder slips past the pubic bone and emerges.

13. The torso and legs are born by a process of lateral flexion and a spiraling motion.

Moulding is similar in all brow positions. Any caput will form between the anterior upper forehead and bregma.

The Process of Birth in Frontum Posterior Brow Presentations

The baby starts out either LFP or RFP in posterior brow presentations, and the forehead persists in a posterior position. Birth is almost always impossible when the baby is presenting in this position, unless the baby is very premature or stillborn, because the long presenting diameters are the least compressible of all the cephalic diameters, making it extremely unlikely that the vertex of a full term baby can mould beneath the pubic bone to allow for descent. As with any posterior presentation, the baby may rotate 135° from the posterior via a long-arc rotation to an FA position or via short-arc rotation to a directly frontum posterior position. As with anterior brow presentations, spontaneous conversion to a fully extended face or a flexed vertex position may occur at any time, provided that moulding or the formation of a caput do not prevent this from occurring.

Long-arc rotation of the posterior brow baby

Descent proceeds very slowly if partial extension is maintained. The presenting part remains high until sufficient moulding occurs to allow the vertex to pass through the shallow anterior portion of the pelvic inlet.

From the posterior oblique position, the brow rotates 45° to FT, then 45° to anterior oblique and then another 45° to directly FA. The shoulders may follow the head, rotating 90° to align with the transverse diameter, or they may lag behind by 45°, so that when the head is FA, the shoulders are still aligned with an oblique diameter of the pelvis. It is unlikely that birth will occur naturally, even if the baby manages to rotate to FA and pushing begins.

As the midchest and shoulders enter the curve of the pelvic cavity near the spines, they undergo internal rotation into the oblique diameter through which they most recently passed. If progress continues and partial extension has been maintained during labor, the head will be born by a process of spinal flexion as it emerges from the birth canal. The bridge of the nose is usually positioned near the level of the tuberosities following internal rotation. A combination of downward pressure from contractions, further descent of the fetal head, maintenance of extension, and the resistance afforded by the pelvic floor cause the brow to crown as the bridge of the nose squeezes past the pubic bone. As the head continues to advance, the neck advances with it, bringing the upper torso deeper into the curve of the birth canal. The upper spine and lower cervical vertebrae curl into the curve of the sacrum as the head flexes toward the chest. The perineum retracts, and the brow and bregma emerge from the introitus. In a brow presentation, the vertex emerges as the perineum retracts, followed by the face as the head tips backward slightly.

The head is then freed to resume a vertex orientation. The head restitutes 45° as the neck untwists to resume an anatomical relationship with the shoulders. The force of the next contraction and the mother's pushing efforts rotate the upper chest and shoulders from an oblique diameter to the anteroposterior diameter of the pelvis, with the head rotating externally to become OT (FT). The birth of the shoulders and body is the same as for any cephalic presentation.

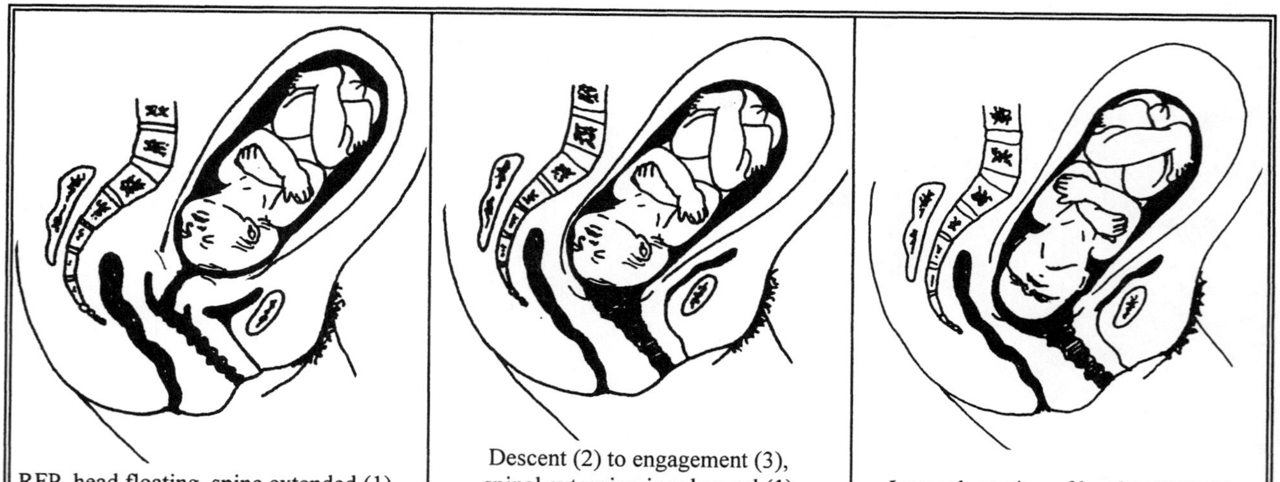

RFP, head floating, spine extended (1) | Descent (2) to engagement (3), spinal extension is enhanced (1) | Internal rotation of head to RFT (4)

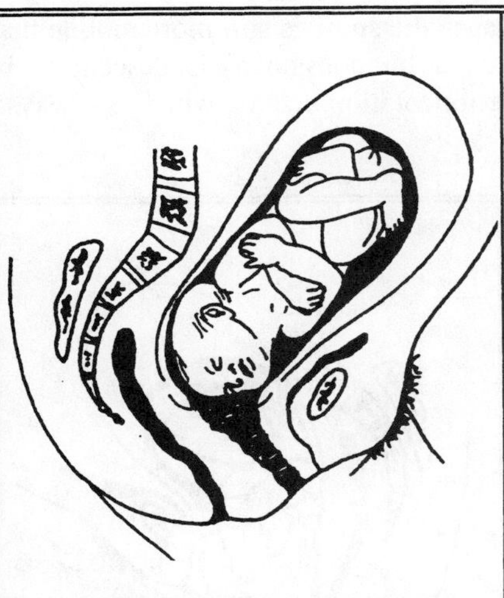

Internal rotation of head to RFA (4); chest/shoulders begin 1st internal rotation (5)

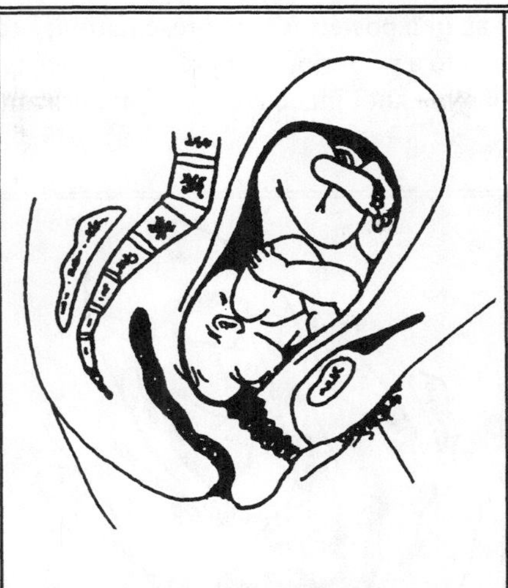

Head rotates internally to FA (4); Shoulders/chest complete 1st internal rotation to transverse (5) and engage (6)

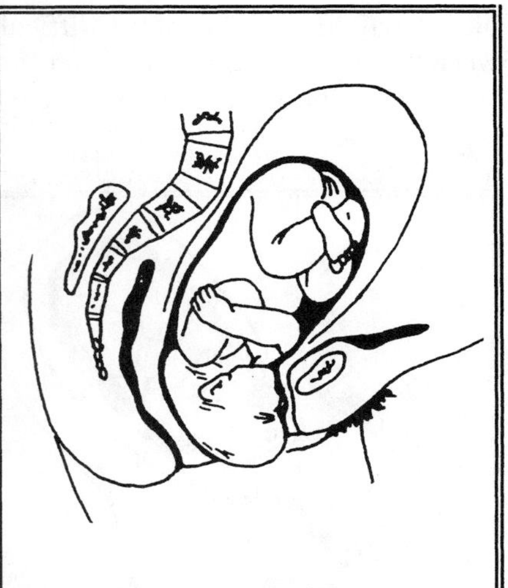

Chest/shoulders begin 2nd internal rotation to oblique (8-1); head crowns and is born by cervical flexion (9)

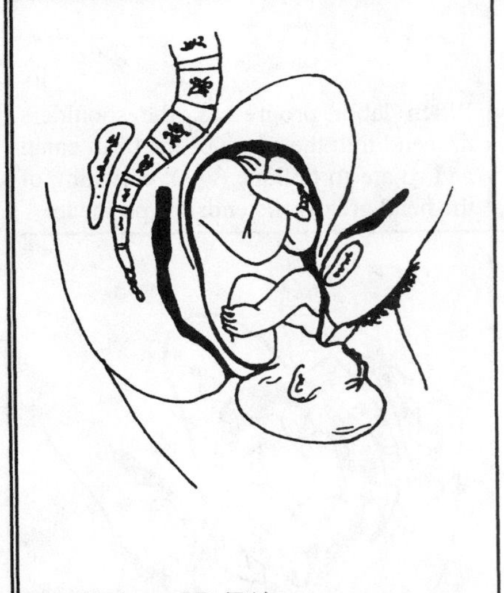

Head is born OP (FA)

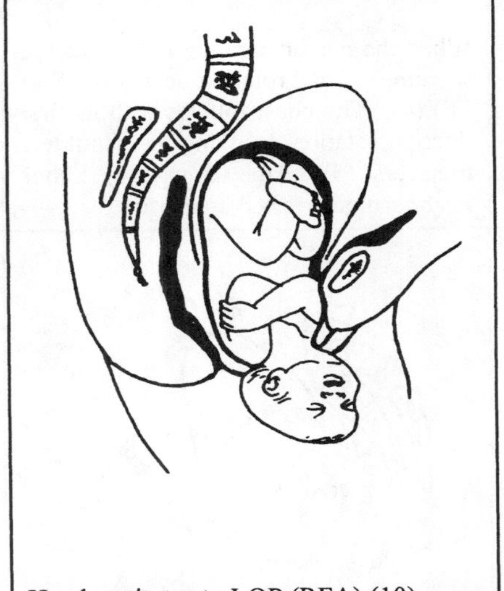

Head restitutes to LOP (RFA) (10)

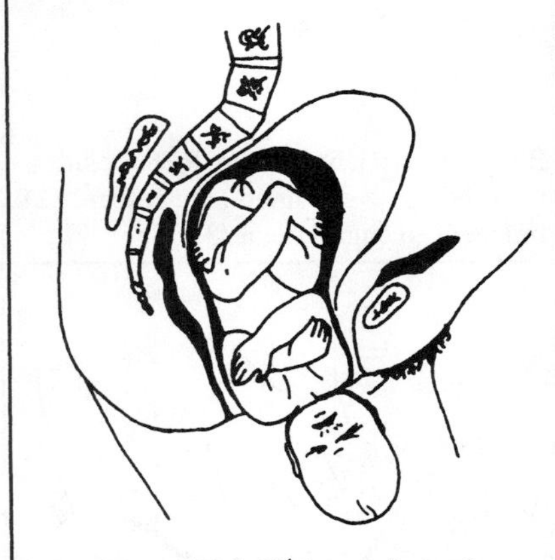

Shoulders finish 2nd internal rotation to AP (8-2); head follows with external rotation to LOT (RFT) (11); posterior shoulder born (12)

Short-arc rotation of the posterior brow baby

Upon reaching the pelvic floor, the head turns as the forehead rotates 45° posteriorly into the hollow of the sacrum. This usually brings the labor to a standstill. The shoulder axis may remain in an oblique diameter of the pelvis, at a 45° angle to the axis of the head, or as the bulk of the cranial dome presses backward, the occiput may become impinged in the space between the scapulae, encouraging the shoulder axis to move into the transverse diameter of the pelvis.

Conversion to a more favorable presentation is unlikely if the head becomes extremely moulded, impacted deep in the pelvis or if a caput forms. If the baby does not flex into a vertex presentation or fully extend his head into a face presentation and rotate to mentum anterior, a surgical birth may be necessary at this point. Any attempt to force the cranial vault beneath the pubic arch is likely to result in brain injury. Birth by yoni may be possible if the baby is early, very small or dead (with a softer skull than in a live baby), if the mother has an exceptionally large pelvis or a combination of these factors is present. Labor should be allowed to proceed only if there is steady, spontaneous progress and the baby is doing well.

While rare, birth of babies in the frontum posterior position does infrequently occur. However, because of its rarity, there are no descriptions of the movements of the emerging head in posterior brow presentations. This position presents specific problems. Cervical and thoracic flexion or extension are impaired, rendering descent through the curve of the birth canal difficult, but not as difficult as in a posterior face presentation, because the spine is still more mobile than when the mentum is posterior. Conversion to a posterior face presentation may occur but does not assist descent, as the head is then locked into place and the baby cannot maneuver at all, unless anterior rotation occurs, which is always a possibility.

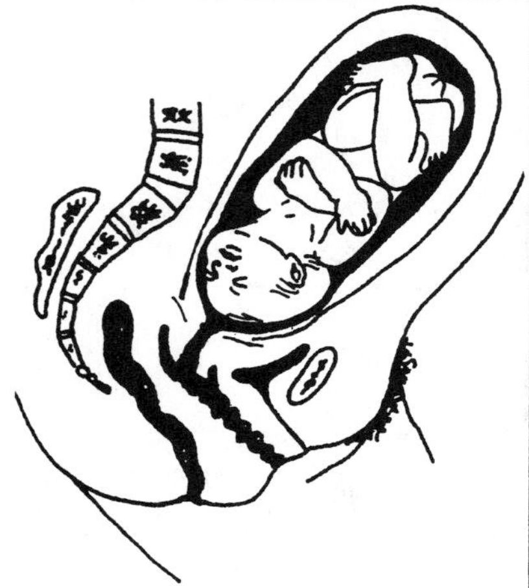

Baby begins labor in an RFP position with the spine extended (1); descent (2) proceeds to engagement (3).

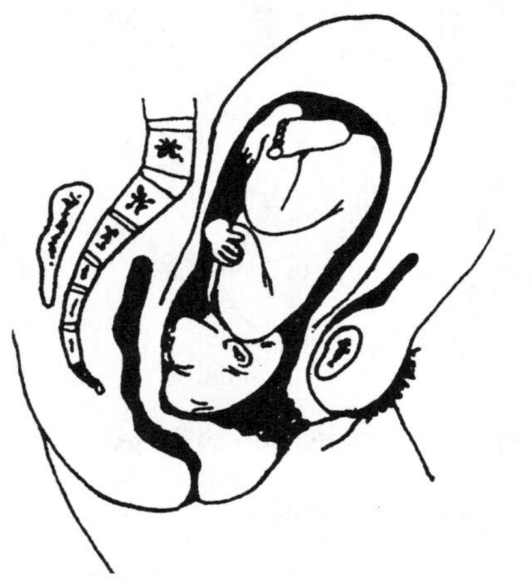

When the head enters the hollow of the sacrum, internal rotation occurs (RFP to FP) (4). The chest follows with its first internal rotation, bringing the shoulders transverse (5) and they engage (6). Labor may become arrested at any time.

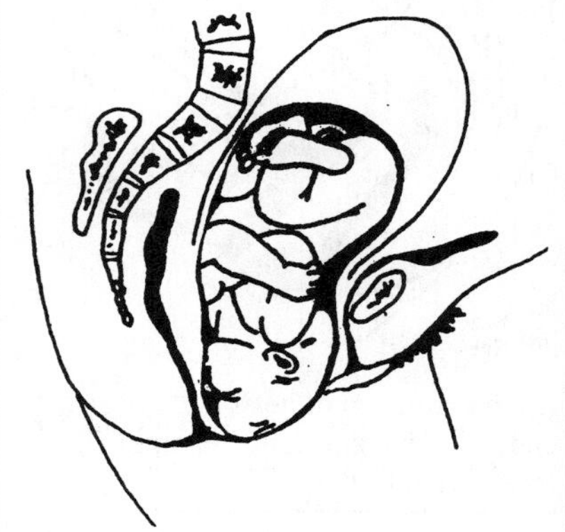

When labor progresses, the shoulders descend into the curve of the birth canal and rotate to oblique (8-1); crowning of the head greatly distends the perineum.

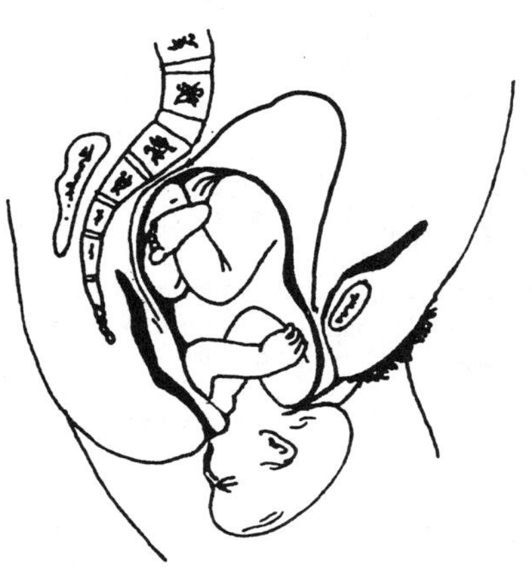

The head is born by a combined process of extension and flexion (9) and the vertex now leads the way.

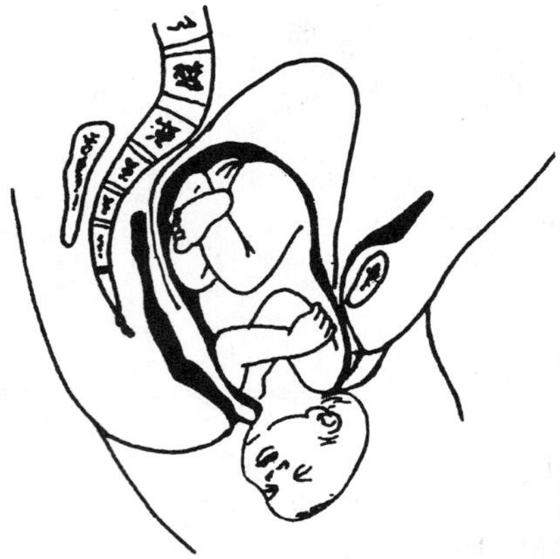

The head restitutes from OA to LOA (FP to RFP) (10).

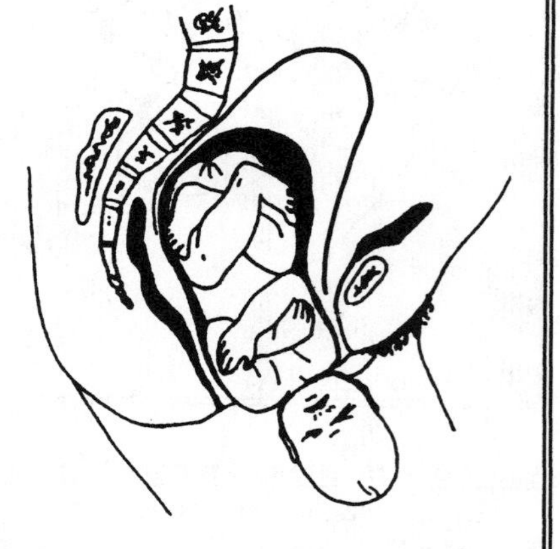

The shoulders complete their 2nd internal rotation (8-2) to AP; the head follows, rotating externally to LOT (RFT) (11). The posterior shoulders is born first (12).

If the baby remains in a brow presentation and descent proceeds, it is likely that the lower neck and upper thoracic spine will become pushed into the mother's lower sacrum, where they will probably undergo extreme extension as the upper spine arches. The large cranial vault is lodged under the pubic arch. The brow and upper face are squeezed forward, the vertex becomes flattened and the perineum is excessively stretched and is likely to tear. The head is extruded slowly from the introitus. Once the head is born, the rotation and birth of the shoulders, torso and legs proceed as for any posterior cephalic presentation.

Summary of the Cardinal Spiraling Movements: Right Frontum Posterior (RFP)

Labor with the baby in an RFP position is the mirror opposite of an LFP position. Flexion produces an LOA position.

Orientation of the baby to the mother's pelvis

The long axis of the sinciput is aligned with the right oblique diameter, while the brow occupies the right posterior corner of the brim. The shoulders are aligned with the left oblique diameter.

Long-arc rotation of the RFP baby

***1.** Spontaneous conversion to a fully extended face (RMP) or a flexed vertex (LOA) presentation may take place at any point before or during labor. Conversion may be necessary before further descent is possible.

Unequal forces: Conversion can occur due to obliquely directed uterine force or variations in soft-tissue resistance or both. This can occur after engagement and anterior rotation. However, conversion to vertex usually occurs at or above the brim, with descent proceeding as an LOA position.

Impaction of the vertex: After anterior rotation, when the head is deeply descended, the vertex can become lodged against the maternal sacrum. Force from contractions presses the face downward, converting it into an RMP position, which may undergo long-arc-rotation to MA.

Conversion to a more favorable brow position: The baby's head and body may rotate 45° into an RFT position before entering the brim, which allows the long axis of the head to enter a longer diameter of the brim. Descent proceeds as for an RFT position.

When partial extension persists, progressive labor usually requires a small baby, a large pelvis or both. Labor may progress if conditions are optimal. However, arrest of descent could occur at any time due to an inability of the partially extended head to pass through the birth canal, frequently as a result of the open fetal mouth lodging against the pelvis. Considerable moulding may be required before the head can descend further.

***2.** The baby descends with difficulty throughout labor because one of the longest diameters of the head is presenting.

***3.** The head engages as the biparietal diameter passes slowly through the brim, a process made more difficult by the trouble the vertex has moulding past the pubic bone.

***4.** The brow rotates internally a total of 135°, from RFP to FA, as it adapts to the loop-shaped opening of the levator ani sling. Rotation consists of a downwardly spiraling movement, which facilitates descent. It usually occurs after dilation is complete and the brow is firmly pressed against the pelvic floor. The brow rotates 45° from the RFP position to RFT, then 45° to RFA, and finally 45° to FA.

5. The baby's body moves with the shoulders as they undergo their first internal rotation. Following the rotation of the brow from RFP to RFT, the shoulders rotate 45° from the left oblique diameter to align with the anteroposterior diameter. As the brow rotates from RFT to RFA, the shoulders rotate 45° to align with the right oblique diameter. As the brow rotates from RFA to FA, they rotate another 45° to align with the transverse diameter of the brim, 135° in all.

6. The shoulders engage when the bisacromial diameter enters the transverse diameter of the brim, as the brow passes through the ischial tuberosities. The attitude of the shoulders shifts during descent as the torso accommodates to the shape of the birth canal.

7. The spine extends as the head enters the pelvis more deeply.

8-1. The second internal rotation of the shoulders begins between the time the brow distends the perineum and is born. As the midchest and spine enter the curve of the birth canal near the level of the ischial spines, they rotate 45°, moving the shoulders from the transverse into the right oblique diameter. This adjustment allows the spine to flex laterally. The neck twists as this occurs, allowing the brow to remain FA.

***9.** The lower face is now under the pubic bone, and the brow and most of the very moulded head is in the soft birth canal. The head crowns slowly as the lower neck and upper spine flex into the sacrum, causing the chin to tip forward slightly. The perineum retracts over the brow and vault of the skull. When the vault is almost free, the head straightens slightly and the lower face is born. The head is no longer held back in an attitude of extension, and the vertex now leads the way.

***10.** Restitution occurs as the neck untwists, allowing the head to rotate 45° from OP (FA) back to the LOP (RFA) position, restoring the long axis of the vertex to a 90° angle with the long axis of the shoulders.

8-2. The chest completes its second internal rotation, moving the shoulders 45° from the right oblique into the antero-posterior diameter, before or during the next contraction. This brings the anterior shoulder under the pubic arch.

***11.** The head follows the internal rotation of the shoulders by rotating externally 45° from LOP (RFA) to LOT (RFT).

12. The anterior shoulder braces against the pubic bone as the posterior shoulder is born first by a process of lateral spinal flexion, after which the anterior shoulder slips past the pubic bone and emerges.

13. The torso and legs are born by a process of lateral flexion and a spiraling motion.

Moulding is similar in all brow positions, with any caput forming over the upper right forehead and bregma.

RFP orientation, head partially flexed	Internal rotation to RFT; descent to engagement	Internal rotation of head and shoulders: RFT to RFA	Internal rotation: RFA to FA; chest rotates to transverse and engages

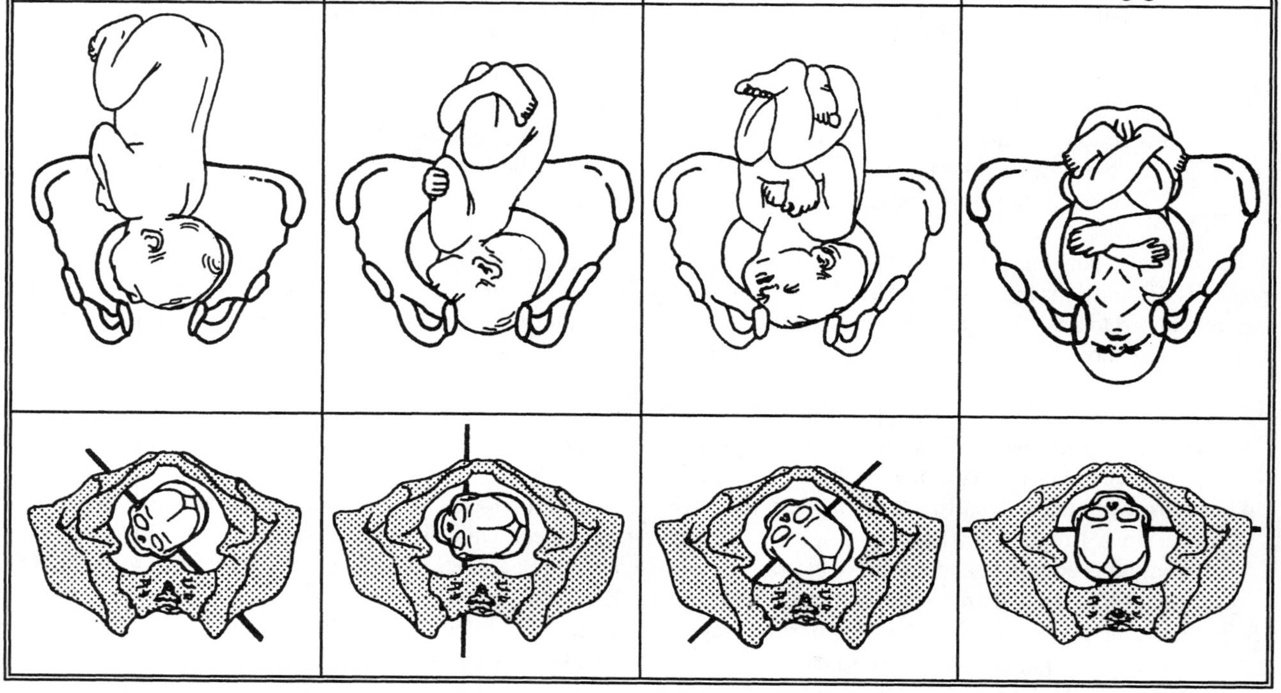

Midchest rotates as descent proceeds; bringing shoulders oblique. Upper spine extends as head is born.	The head is born FA (OP).	The head restitutes 45° from OP to LOP (FA to RFA) as the spine realigns.	Shoulders rotate to AP diameter as head rotates externally 45°: LOP to LOT (RFA to RFT)

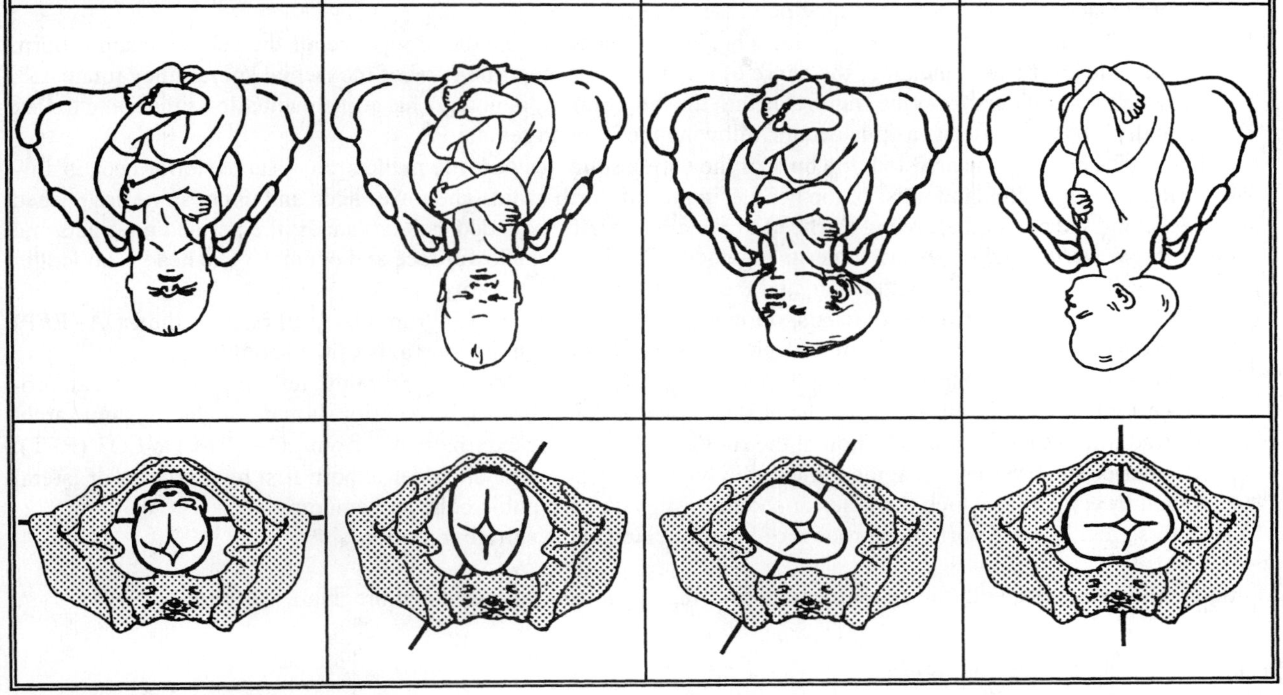

Short-arc rotation of the RFP baby (movements not illustrated)

***1.** Spontaneous conversion to a fully extended face (RMP) or a flexed vertex (LOA) presentation may take place at any point before or during labor. Conversion may be necessary before further descent is possible.

Unequal forces: Conversion can occur due to obliquely directed uterine force or variations in soft-tissue resistance or both. This can occur after engagement and anterior rotation. However, conversion to vertex usually occurs at or above the brim, with descent proceeding as an LOA position.

Impaction of the vertex: After anterior rotation, when the head is deeply descended, the vertex can become lodged against the maternal sacrum. Force from contractions presses the face downward, converting it into an RMP position, which may undergo long-arc-rotation to MA.

Conversion to a more favorable brow position: The baby's head and body may rotate 45° into an RFT position before entering the brim, which allows the long axis of the head to enter a longer diameter of the brim. Descent proceeds as for an RFT position.

When partial extension persists, progressive labor requires an unusually small baby, a very large pelvis or both. Arrest of descent could occur at any time because of the difficulties of posterior descent, as a result of the open fetal mouth lodging against the pelvis or other reasons. Considerable moulding may be required before the head can descend further.

***2.** The baby descends with difficulty throughout labor because one of the longest diameters of the head is presenting.

***3.** The head engages as the biparietal diameter passes slowly through the brim, a process made more difficult by the trouble the vertex has moulding past the pubic bone.

***4.** The brow rotates internally 45°, from RFP position to FP, as it adapts to the shape of the levator ani sling. Rotation consists of a downwardly spiraling movement, which facilitates descent. It usually occurs after dilation is complete and the brow is firmly pressed against the pelvic floor.

5. The baby's body moves with the shoulders as they undergo their first internal rotation. Following the rotation of the brow from RFP to FP, the shoulders rotate 45° from the left oblique diameter to align with the transverse diameter of the brim.

6. The shoulders engage when the bisacromial diameter enters the transverse diameter of the brim, as the brow passes through the ischial tuberosities. The attitude of the shoulders shifts during descent as the torso accommodates to the shape of the birth canal.

7. The spine extends as the head enters the pelvis more deeply.

8-1. The second internal rotation of the shoulders begins between the time the brow distends the perineum and is born. As the midchest and spine enter the curve of the birth canal near the level of the ischial spines, they rotate 45°, moving the shoulders from the transverse into the left oblique diameter. This adjustment allows the spine to flex laterally. The neck twists as this occurs, allowing the brow to remain FP.

***9.** If labor does not become arrested, the bulk of the vertex squeezes past the pubic arch. The posterior neck is now under the pubic arch and most of the head is in the soft birth canal. The lower neck and upper spine are pushed up behind the occiput, allowing the head to remain partially extended as it advances; the perineum retracts and the brow, vertex and upper face emerge together followed by the lower face and occiput. The head is no longer held back in an attitude of extension, and the vertex now leads the way.

***10.** Restitution occurs as the neck untwists, allowing the head to rotate 45° from OA (FP) back to the LOA (RFP) position, restoring the long axis of the vertex to a 90° angle with the long axis of the shoulders.

8-2. The chest completes its second internal rotation, moving the shoulders 45° from the left oblique into the antero-posterior diameter before or during the next contraction. This brings the anterior shoulder under the pubic arch.

***11.** The head follows the internal rotation of the shoulders by rotating externally 45° from LOA (RFP) to LOT (RFT).

12. The anterior shoulder braces against the pubic bone as the posterior shoulder is born first by a process of lateral spinal flexion, after which the anterior shoulder slips past the pubic bone and emerges.

13. The torso and legs are born by a process of lateral flexion and a spiraling motion.

Moulding will be severe, with the caput forming over the upper right forehead and bregma.

Summary of the Cardinal Spiraling Movements: Left Frontum Posterior (LFP)

The flexed LFP baby becomes an ROA.

Orientation of the baby to the mother's pelvis

The long axis of the sinciput is aligned with the left oblique diameter, while the brow occupies the left posterior corner of the brim. The shoulders are aligned with the right oblique diameter.

Long-arc rotation of the LFP baby (movements not illustrated)

***1.** Spontaneous conversion to a fully extended face (LMP) or a flexed vertex (ROA) presentation may take place at any point before or during labor. Conversion may be necessary before further descent is possible.

Unequal forces: Conversion can occur due to obliquely directed uterine force or variations in soft-tissue resistance or both. This can occur after engagement and anterior rotation. However, conversion to vertex usually occurs at or above the brim, with descent proceeding as an ROA position.

Impaction of the vertex: After anterior rotation, when the head is deeply descended, the vertex can become lodged against the maternal sacrum. Force from contractions presses the face downward, converting it into an LMP position, which may undergo long-arc-rotation to MA.

Conversion to a more favorable brow position: The baby's head and body may rotate 45° into an LFT position before entering the brim, which allows the long axis of the head to enter a longer diameter of the brim. Descent proceeds as for an LFT position.

When partial extension persists, progressive labor usually requires a small baby, a large pelvis or both. Labor may progress if conditions are optimal. However, arrest of descent could occur at any time due to an inability of the partially extended head to pass through the birth canal, frequently as a result of the open fetal mouth lodging against the pelvis. Considerable moulding may be required before the head can descend further.

***2.** The baby descends with difficulty throughout labor because one of the longest diameters of the head is presenting.

***3.** The head engages as the biparietal diameter passes slowly through the brim, a process made more difficult by the trouble the vertex has moulding past the pubic bone.

***4.** The brow rotates internally a total of 135°, from LFP to FA, as it adapts to the loop-shaped opening of the levator ani sling. Rotation consists of a downwardly spiraling movement, which facilitates descent. It usually occurs after dilation is complete and the brow is firmly pressed against the pelvic floor. The brow rotates 45° from the LFP position to LFT, then 45° to LFA and finally 45° to FA.

5. The baby's body moves with the shoulders as they undergo their first internal rotation. Following the rotation of the brow from LFP to LFT, the shoulders rotate 45° from the right oblique diameter to align with the anteroposterior diameter. As the brow rotates from LFT to LFA, the shoulders rotate 45° to align with the left oblique diameter. As the brow rotates from LFA to FA, they rotate another 45° to align with the transverse diameter of the brim, 135° in all.

6. The shoulders engage when the bisacromial diameter enters the transverse diameter of the brim, as the brow passes through the ischial tuberosities. The attitude of the shoulders shifts during descent as the torso accommodates to the shape of the birth canal.

7. The spine extends as the head enters the pelvis more deeply.

8-1. The second internal rotation of the shoulders begins between the time the brow distends the perineum and is born. As the midchest and spine enter the curve of the birth canal near the level of the ischial spines, they rotate 45°, moving the shoulders from the transverse into the left oblique diameter. This adjustment allows the spine to flex laterally. The neck twists as this occurs, allowing the brow to remain FA.

***9.** The lower face is now under the pubic bone, and the brow and most of the very moulded head is in the soft birth canal. The head crowns slowly as the lower neck and upper spine flex into the sacrum, causing the chin to tip forward slightly. The perineum retracts over the brow and vault of the skull. When the vault is almost free, the head straightens slightly and the lower face is born. The head is no longer held back in an attitude of extension, and the vertex now leads the way.

***10.** Restitution occurs as the neck untwists, allowing the head to rotate 45° from OP (FA) back to the ROP (LFA) position, restoring the long axis of the vertex to a 90° angle with the long axis of the shoulders.

8-2. The chest completes its second internal rotation, moving the shoulders 45° from the left oblique into the anteroposterior diameter before or during the next contraction. This brings the anterior shoulder under the pubic arch.

***11.** The head follows the internal rotation of the shoulders by rotating externally 45° from ROP (LFA) to ROT (LFT).

12. The anterior shoulder braces against the pubic bone as the posterior shoulder is born first by a process of lateral spinal flexion, after which the anterior shoulder slips past the pubic bone and emerges.

13. The torso and legs are born by a process of lateral flexion and a spiraling motion.

Moulding is similar in all anterior brow positions; any caput will form over the upper left forehead and bregma.

LFP orientation, head partially flexed	Internal rotation to LFT: Descent to engagement	Internal rotation of head and shoulders: LFT to LFA	Internal rotation: LFA to FA; chest rotates to transverse and engages

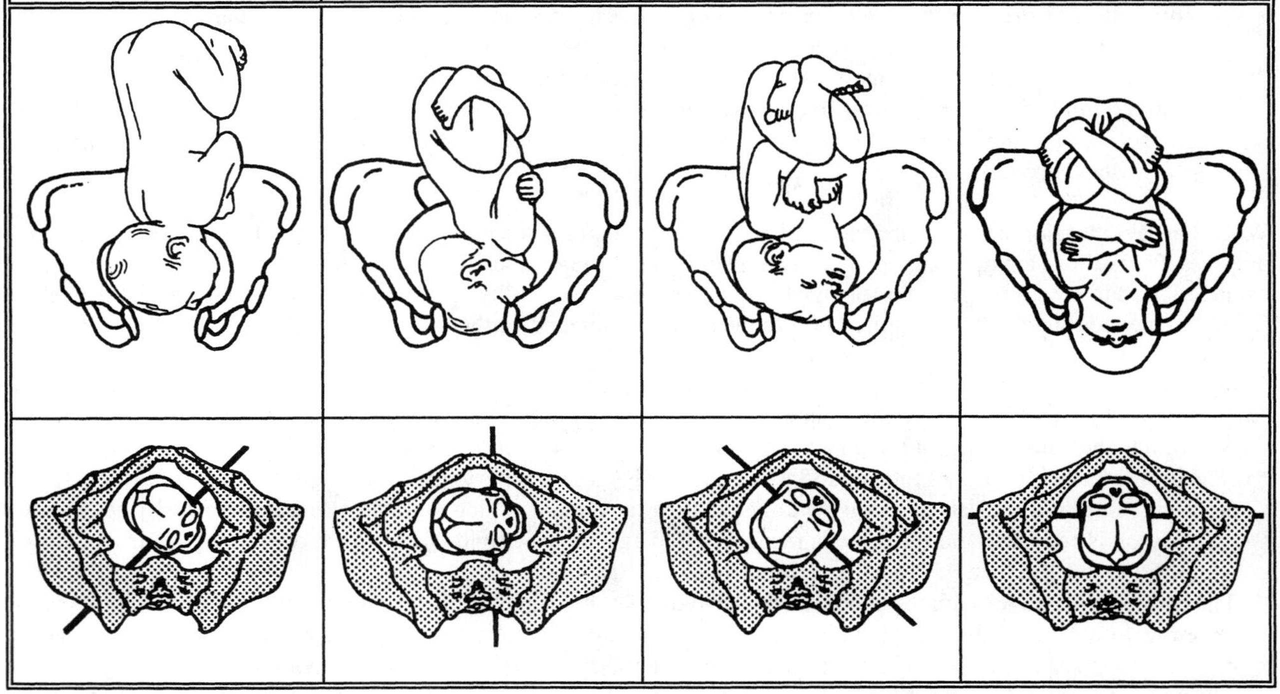

Midchest rotates as descent proceeds; bringing shoulders oblique. Upper spine extends as head is born.	The head is born FA (OP).	The head restitutes 45° from OP to ROP (FA to LFA) as the spine realigns.	Shoulders rotate to AP diameter as head rotates externally 45°: ROP to ROT (LFA to LFT)
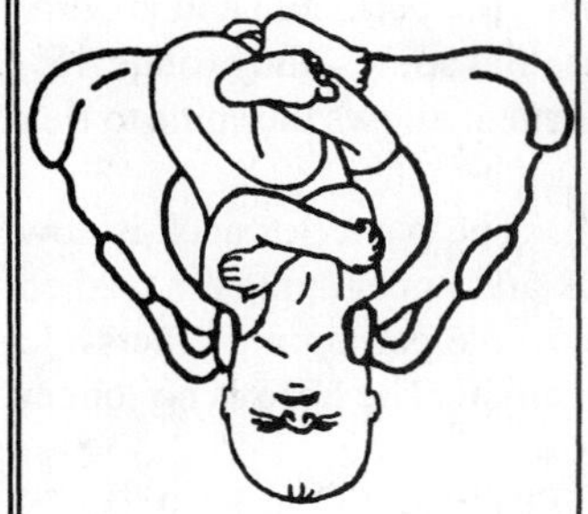	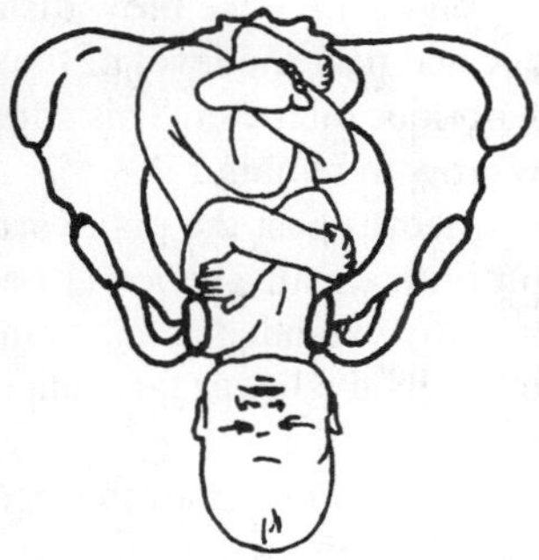	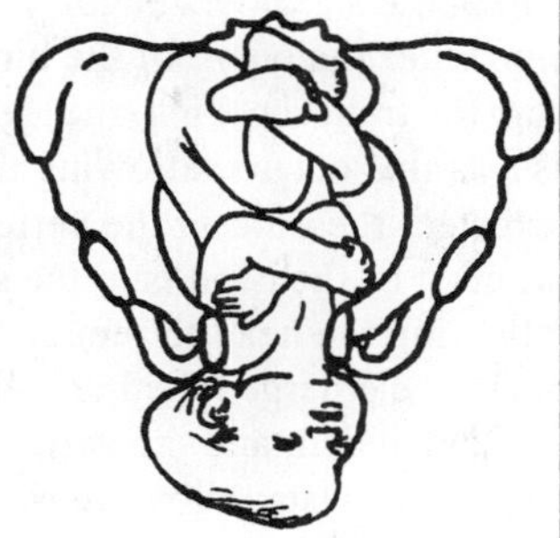	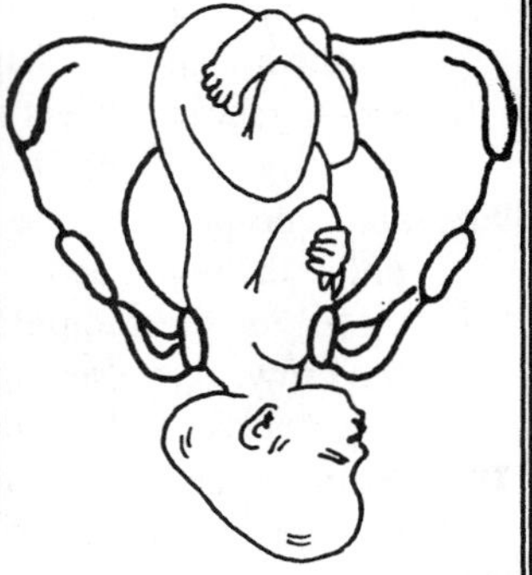
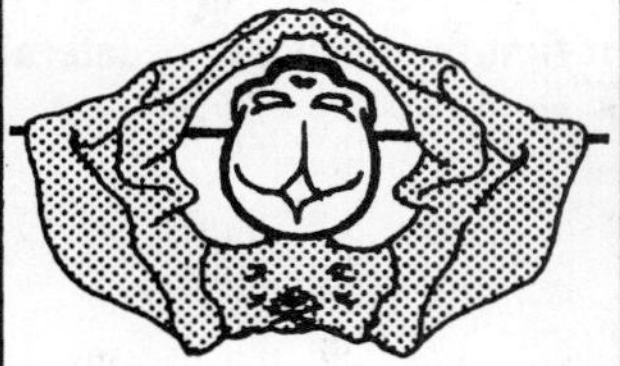	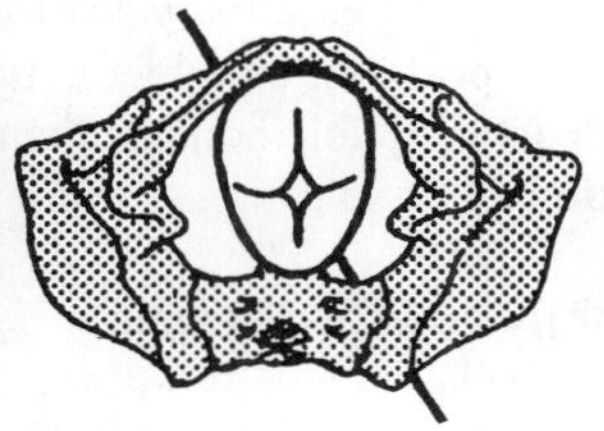	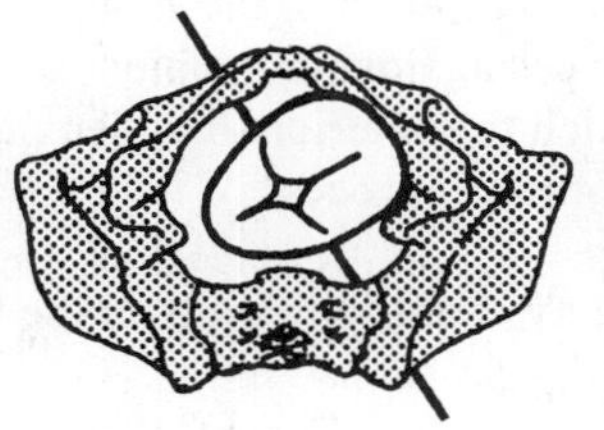	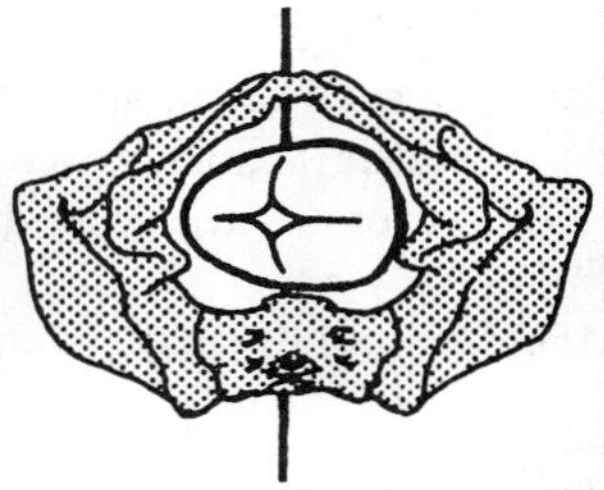

<u>Short-arc rotation of the LFP baby (movements not illustrated)</u>

***1.** Spontaneous conversion to a fully extended face (LMP) or a flexed vertex (ROA) presentation may take place at any point before or during labor. Conversion may be necessary before further descent is possible.

Unequal forces: Conversion can occur due to obliquely directed uterine force or variations in soft-tissue resistance or both. This can occur after engagement and anterior rotation. However, conversion to vertex usually occurs at or above the brim, with descent proceeding as an ROA position.

Impaction of the vertex: After anterior rotation, when the head is deeply descended, the vertex can become lodged against the maternal sacrum. Force from contractions presses the face downward, converting it into an LMP position, which may undergo long-arc-rotation to MA.

Conversion to a more favorable brow position: The baby's head and body may rotate 45° into an LFT position before entering the brim, which allows the long axis of the head to enter a longer diameter of the brim. Descent proceeds as for an LFT position.

When partial extension persists, progressive labor requires an small baby, a very large pelvis or both. Arrest of descent could occur at any time because of the difficulties of posterior descent, as a result of the open fetal mouth lodging against the pelvis or other reasons. Considerable moulding may be required before the head can descend further.

***2.** The baby descends with difficulty throughout labor because one of the longest diameters of the head is presenting.

***3.** The head engages as the biparietal diameter passes slowly through the brim, a process made more difficult by the trouble the vertex has moulding past the pubic bone.

***4.** The brow rotates internally 45°, from LFP position to FP, as it adapts to the loop-shaped opening of the levator ani sling. Rotation consists of a downwardly spiraling movement, which facilitates descent. It usually occurs after dilation is complete and the brow is firmly pressed against the pelvic floor.

5. The baby's body moves with the shoulders as they undergo their first internal rotation. Following the rotation of the brow from LFP to FP, the shoulders rotate 45° from the right oblique diameter to align with the transverse diameter of the brim.

6. The shoulders engage when the bisacromial diameter enters the transverse diameter of the brim, as the brow passes through the ischial tuberosities. The attitude of the shoulders shifts during descent as the torso accommodates to the shape of the birth canal.

7. The spine extends as the head enters the pelvis more deeply.

8-1. The second internal rotation of the shoulders begins between the time the brow distends the perineum and is born. As the midchest and spine enter the curve of the birth canal near the level of the ischial spines, they rotate 45°, moving the shoulders from the transverse into the right oblique diameter. This adjustment allows the spine to flex laterally. The neck twists as this occurs, allowing the brow to remain FP.

***9.** If labor does not become arrested, the bulk of the vertex squeezes past the pubic arch. The posterior neck is now under the pubic arch and most of the head is in the soft birth canal. The lower neck and upper spine are pushed up behind the occiput, allowing the head to remain partially extended as it advances; the perineum retracts and the brow, vertex and upper face emerge together followed by the lower face and occiput. The head is no longer held back in an attitude of extension, and the vertex now leads the way.

***10.** Restitution occurs as the neck untwists, allowing the head to rotate 45° from OA (FP) back to the ROA (LFP) position, restoring the long axis of the vertex to a 90° angle with the long axis of the shoulders.

8-2. The chest completes its second internal rotation, moving the shoulders 45° from the right oblique into the antero-posterior diameter before or during the next contraction. This brings the anterior shoulder under the pubic arch.

11. The head follows the internal rotation of the shoulders by rotating externally 45° from ROA (LFP) to ROT (LFT).

***12.** The anterior shoulder braces against the pubic bone as the posterior shoulder is born first by a process of lateral spinal flexion, after which the anterior shoulder slips past the pubic bone and emerges.

13. The torso and legs are born by a process of lateral flexion and a spiraling motion.

Moulding will be severe with any caput forming over the left forehead and bregma.

Summary of the Cardinal Spiraling Movements: Frontum Posterior (FP)

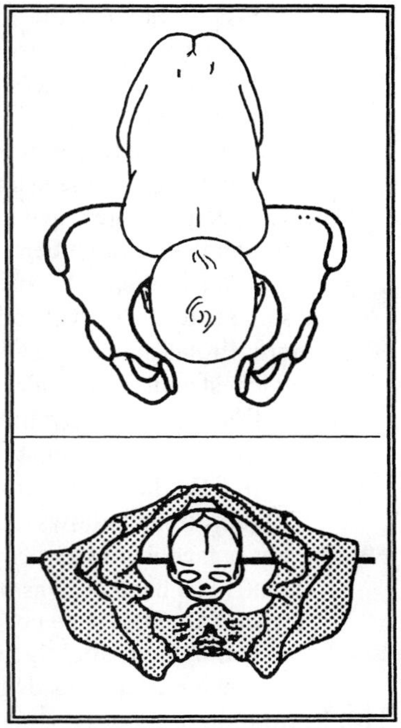

Theoretically, it is possible for a brow baby to present and descend with the sinciput directly posterior; however, this is unlikely to occur because the long presenting diameter accommodates best to an oblique or transverse pelvic diameter.

Orientation of the baby to the mother's pelvis

The long axis of the sinciput is aligned with the anteroposterior diameter, and the brow is directly posterior, in front of the spine. The shoulders are aligned with the transverse diameter.

Long-arc rotation from of the FP baby to FA (movements not illustrated)

Internal rotation of the shoulders may not occur before the shoulders enter the pelvic cavity when the baby is directly frontum posterior. When it does occur, it may occur in either a left or a right direction. Subsequent movements of the brow will follow according to the direction of shoulder rotation, as noted.

***1.** Spontaneous conversion to a fully extended face (MP) or a flexed vertex (OA) presentation may take place at any point before or during labor. Conversion may be necessary before further descent is possible.

Unequal forces: Conversion can occur due to obliquely directed uterine force or variations in soft-tissue resistance or both. This can occur after engagement and anterior rotation. However, conversion to vertex usually occurs at or above the brim, with descent proceeding as an OA position.

Impaction of the vertex: After anterior rotation, when the head is deeply descended, the vertex can become lodged against the maternal sacrum. Force from contractions presses the face downward into an MP position, which may undergo long-arc-rotation to MA.

Conversion to a more favorable brow position: The baby's head and body may rotate 45° into an RFP or LFP position before entering the brim, which allows the long axis of the head to enter a longer diameter of the brim. Descent proceeds as for an RFP or LFP position.

When partial extension persists, progressive labor requires an unusually small baby, a very large pelvis or both. Arrest of descent could occur at any time due to an inability of the partially extended head to pass through the birth canal, frequently as a result of the open fetal mouth lodging against the pelvis. Considerable moulding may be required before the head can descend further.

***2.** The baby attempts to descend with difficulty throughout labor because one of the longest diameters of the head is presenting.

***3.** The head engages as the biparietal diameter passes slowly through the brim, a process made more difficult by the trouble the vertex has moulding past the pubic bone and the trouble the brow has moulding past the sacral promontory.

***4.** Because the brow is directly FP, internal rotation can proceed in either a left or right direction, a total of 180° as it adapts to the loop-shaped opening of the levator ani sling. Rotation consists of a downwardly spiraling movement, which facilitates descent. It usually occurs after dilation is complete and the brow is firmly pressed against the pelvic floor. Beginning from an FP position, the brow rotates internally:

4-A. 45° to LFP, 45° to LFT, 45° to LFA and 45° to FA. (Follow "A" entries below.)

4-B. 45° to RFP, 45° to RFT, 45° to RFA and 45° to FA. (Follow "B" entries below.)

5. The baby's body moves with the shoulders as they undergo their first internal rotation.

5-A. Following the rotation of the brow from FP to LFP, the shoulders rotate 45° from the transverse diameter to align with the right oblique diameter. As the brow rotates from LFP to LFT, the shoulders rotate 45° to align with the anteroposterior diameter. As the brow rotates from LFT to LFA, the shoulders rotate 45° to align with the left oblique diameter, and as the brow rotates from LFA to FA, the shoulders rotate another 45° to align with the transverse diameter of the brim, 180° in all.

5-B. Following the rotation of the brow from FP to RFP, the shoulders rotate 45° from the transverse diameter to align with the left oblique diameter. As the brow rotates from RFP to RFT, the shoulders rotate 45° to align with the anteroposterior diameter. As the brow rotates from RFT to RFA, the shoulders rotate 45° to align with the right oblique diameter, and as the brow rotates from RFA to FA, the shoulders rotate another 45° to align with the transverse diameter of the brim, 180° in all.

6. The shoulders engage when the bisacromial diameter enters the transverse diameter of the brim, as the brow passes through the ischial tuberosities. The attitude of the shoulders shifts during descent as the torso accommodates to the shape of the birth canal.

7. The spine extends as the head enters the pelvis more deeply.

8-1. Internal rotation of the shoulders begins between the time the brow distends the perineum and is born. As the midchest and spine enter the curve of the birth canal near the level of the ischial spines, they rotate 45°, moving the shoulders from the transverse into:

8-1-A. the left oblique diameter.

8-1-B. the right oblique diameter.

This adjustment allows the spine to flex laterally. The neck turns as this occurs, allowing the brow to remain FA.

***9.** The lower face is now under the pubic bone, and the brow and most of the very moulded head is in the soft birth canal. The head crowns slowly as the lower neck and upper spine flex into the sacrum, causing the chin to tip forward slightly. The perineum retracts over the brow and vault of the skull. When the vault is almost free, the head straightens slightly and the lower face is born. The head is no longer held back in an attitude of extension, and the vertex now leads the way.

***10.** Restitution occurs as the neck untwists, allowing the head to rotate 45° from OP (FA) back to:

10-A. the ROP (LFA) position.

10-B. the LOP (RFA) position.

This movement restores the long axis of the vertex to a 90° angle with the long axis of the shoulders.

8-2. The chest completes its internal rotation, moving the shoulders 45° from:

8-2-A. the left oblique diameter

8-2-B. the right oblique diameter

into the anteroposterior diameter before or during the next contraction. This brings the anterior shoulder under the pubic arch.

***11.** The head follows the internal rotation of the shoulders by rotating externally 45°:

11-A. from ROP (LFA) to ROT (LFT).

11-B. from LOP (RFA) to LOT (RFT).

12. The anterior shoulder braces against the pubic bone as the posterior shoulder is born first by a process of lateral spinal flexion, after which the anterior shoulder slips past the pubic bone and emerges.

13. The torso and legs are born by a process of lateral flexion and a spiraling motion.

Moulding is similar in all brow positions. Any caput will form between the anterior upper forehead and bregma.

Summary of birth from a direct FP position (movements not illustrated)

***1.** Spontaneous conversion to a fully extended face (MP) or a flexed vertex (OA) presentation may take place at any point before or during labor. Conversion may be necessary before further descent is possible.

Unequal forces: Conversion can occur due to obliquely directed uterine force or variations in soft-tissue resistance or both. This can occur after engagement and anterior rotation. However, conversion to vertex usually occurs at or above the brim, with descent proceeding as for an OA position.

Impaction of the vertex: After anterior rotation, when the head is deeply descended, the vertex can become lodged against the maternal sacrum. Force from contractions presses the face downward, converting the face into an MP position, which may undergo long-arc-rotation to MA.

Conversion to a more favorable brow position: The baby's head and body may rotate 45° into an LFP or RFP position before entering the brim, which allows the long axis of the head to enter a longer diameter of the brim. Descent proceeds as for an LFP or RFP position.

When partial extension persists, progressive labor requires an unusually small baby, a very large pelvis or both. Arrest of descent could occur at any time due to an inability of the partially extended head to pass through the birth canal, frequently as a result of the open fetal mouth lodging against the pelvis. Considerable moulding may be required before the head can descend further.

***2.** The baby attempts to descend with difficulty throughout labor because one of the longest diameters of the head is presenting.
***3.** The head engages as the biparietal diameter passes through the brim, a process made more difficult by the trouble the vertex has moulding past the pubic bone and the trouble the brow has moulding past the sacral promontory.
***4.** Internal rotation of the brow does not occur.
5. The shoulders remain aligned with the transverse diameter of the brim.
6. The shoulders engage when the bisacromial diameter enters the transverse diameter of the brim, as the brow passes through the ischial tuberosities. The attitude of the shoulders shifts during descent as the torso accommodates to the shape of the birth canal.
7. The spine extends as the head enters the pelvis more deeply.
8-1. Internal rotation of the shoulders begins between the time the brow distends the perineum and is born. As the midchest and spine enter the curve of the birth canal near the level of the ischial spines, they rotate 45°, moving the shoulders from the transverse into:
8-1-A. the right oblique diameter. (Follow "A" entries below.)
8-1-B. the left oblique diameter. (Follow "B" entries below.)
This adjustment allows the spine to flex laterally. The neck turns as this occurs, allowing the brow to remain FP.
***9.** If labor does not become arrested, the bulk of the vertex squeezes past the pubic arch. The posterior neck is now under the pubic arch and the head is in the soft birth canal. The lower neck and upper spine begin to extend more, allowing the head to remain partially extended as it advances. The perineum retracts and the head is born. The head is no longer held back in an attitude of extension, and the vertex now leads the way.
***10.** Restitution occurs as the neck untwists, allowing the head to rotate 45° from OA (FP) back to:
10-A. the ROA (LFP) position.
10-B. the LOA (RFP) position.
This movement restores the long axis of the vertex to a 90° angle with the long axis of the shoulders.
8-2. The chest completes its second internal rotation, moving the shoulders 45° from:
8-2-A. the right oblique diameter
8-2-B. the left oblique diameter
into the anteroposterior diameter before or during the next contraction. This brings the anterior shoulder under the pubic arch.
11. The head follows the internal rotation of the shoulders by rotating externally 45°:
11-A. from ROA (LFP) to ROT (LFT).
11-B. from LOA (RFP) to LOT (RFT).
***12.** The anterior shoulder braces against the pubic bone as the posterior shoulder is born first by a process of lateral spinal flexion, after which the anterior shoulder slips past the pubic bone and emerges.
13. The torso and legs are born by a process of lateral flexion and a spiraling motion.

Moulding is similar in all brow positions. Any caput will form between the anterior upper forehead and bregma.

THE BIRTH PROCESS WHEN THE BABY IS BREECH

BREECH PRESENTATION: GENERAL PRINCIPLES

Incidence

Breech presentation is a variation on longitudinal lie wherein the buttocks (podalic pole) rather than the head (cephalic pole) present. The incidence of breech presentation varies among studies. Hickok and colleagues (1992) found a rate of 20.6% early in pregnancy (up to 25 or 26 weeks gestation). The rate declined steadily from 28 weeks on, dropping to 1.7% at 40 weeks gestation. Most studies agree that the overall percentage of women who enter labor with a breech baby at term (37 to 42 weeks) ranges from 3 to 4%.

Associated factors

Maternal factors contributing to breech presentation include anything that reduces the available space in the upper or lower uterus, such as the presence of tumors, cornual implantation of the placenta, uterine anomalies and pelvic contraction. Fetal factors include oligohydramnios (lessening the likelihood that the baby will rotate), polyhydramnios (which increases the mobility of the baby as well as the possibility of premature labor), fetal anomalies, placenta previa, multiple gestation, short or entangled cord (preventing rotation to a cephalic presentation) and a frank breech attitude. Many babies naturally assume a breech position prior to term; if labor begins prematurely, they will often remain breech.

Fetal parts relevant to breech birth

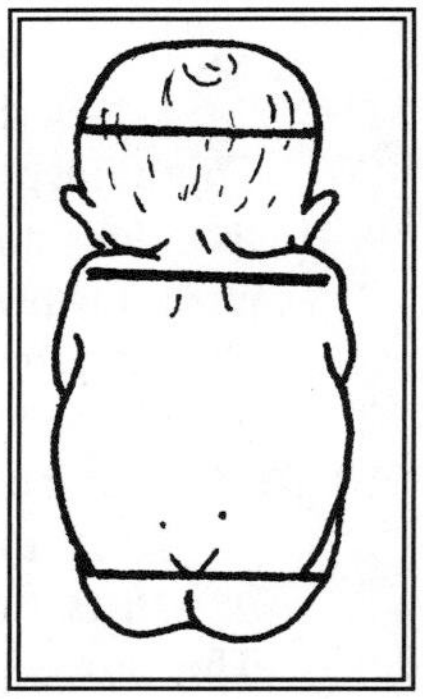

In cephalic presentations, the movements of two regions, the head, and the chest and shoulders, must be considered. In breech birth, however, there are three regions of the baby to consider: the legs, pelvis and lower torso; the shoulders, arms and upper torso; and the head. The fetal pelvis becomes clinically important as the first large, transverse bony diameter of the baby to descend through the birth canal. (Review the material on the shoulders, spine, pelvis and extremities in the chapter entitled "Features of Fetal Anatomy Pertinent to the Birth Process.")

Fetal planes and diameters relevant to breech descent: The transverse diameters relevant to breech descent are illustrated in the box to your right (from the top down: biparietal; bisacromial; bitrochanteric). When the plane of the pelvic girdle is viewed from above, it is basically a lima-bean-shape, with the dent toward the pubic bone (including both the soft and bony tissues). The bitrochanteric diameter spans the long axis of the pelvis and averages at least 9 cm (3.5 in) in a well-grown term baby, about the same as the 9.5 cm biparietal diameter. The shape of this diameter depends upon the position of the legs. When the legs are flexed or splinted up along the torso, the thighs contribute bulk in the anterior region, causing the presenting diameter to be more round. Leg flexion makes this pelvic diameter compressible by a inch or more. When the legs are extended downward, the lima-bean-shape prevails. The long axis of the bisacromial diameter of the ummoulded shoulders averages 12 cm, which is readily compressible by at least 2.25 cm (1 in). The flexible rib cage is also quite compressible. As always, actual measurements will vary, depending upon the size of the baby.

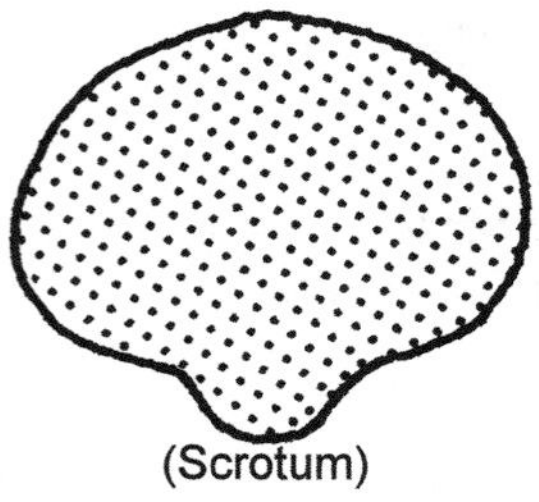

Bitrochanteric plane (thighs flexed)
Diameters: Transverse: 9 cm
AP: (sacropubic) 5.5-11 cm

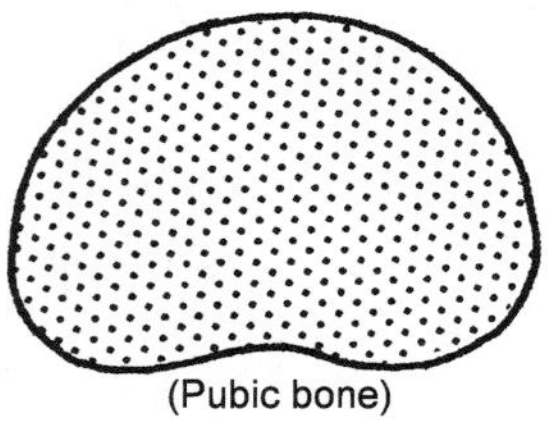

Bitrochanteric plane (thighs extended)
Diameters: Transverse 11 cm
AP: (sacropubic) 5.5-11 cm

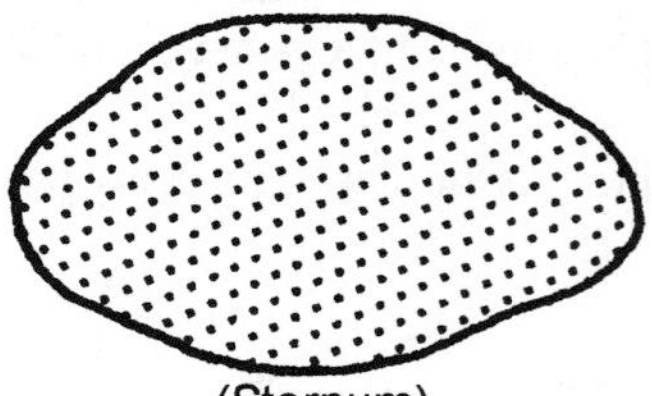

Unmoulded bisacromial (shoulder) plane
Diameters: Transverse 12 cm
AP: (dorsosternal) 9.5 cm

The other important diameters are those of the aftercoming head. The aftercoming head emerges as increasingly larger diameters pass through the introitus starting with the nape of the neck and ending with the vertex. In the well-flexed head, the suboccipitomental diameter is the first to present followed by the suboccipitofrontal. The last significant transverse diameter is the biparietal, which is intersected by the suboccipitobregmatic, just as in a well-flexed vertex presentation (Burns & Marshall, 1934). If the head is deflexed, the occipitomental diameter of 12 cm presents.

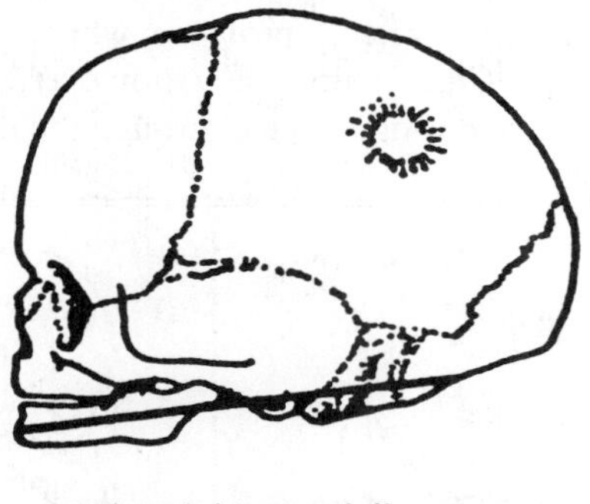

Suboccipitomental diameter

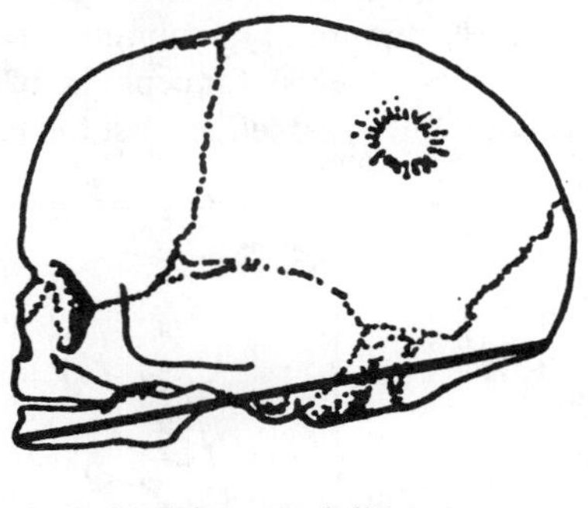

Occipitomental diameter

Keep in mind that the long axis of the pelvis is always at right angles with the genital cleft. When the baby descends with the sacrum anterior oblique, the long axis of the baby's pelvis lines up with one oblique diameter, and the genital cleft lines up in the opposite oblique diameter of the mother's pelvis. When the baby descends sacrum anterior, the long axis of the baby's pelvis lines up with the transverse diameter, and the genital cleft lines up in the anteroposterior diameter of the mother's pelvis.

Attitudes in breech presentation

When the baby presents breech, the denominator is always the sacrum, regardless of the position of any other part. The attitude of the fetus is distinguished according to the positions of the legs, arms and head. It is most frequently defined by the position of the legs, feet or knees, which can be situated in a variety of ways. Most commonly, the legs are splinted up against the baby's anterior torso. The legs may also be flexed at the hip, the knee or both, or they may be extended downward toward the cervix. Their position is highly significant as it impacts the suitability of the podalic pole as a dilating wedge.

The attitude of the head and arms is also significant. The head may be flexed with the chin against the chest, as it can be in vertex presentations, or it may be in any attitude of extension corresponding to the other cephalic presentations (median vertex, brow or face). The position of the arms, the legs and feet (as in a frank breech) or the presence of a loop of cord around the neck, can influence the attitude of the head. The arms are usually flexed across the anterior chest. However, one or both arms may be extended alongside the torso, raised near the head, extended over the head or raised and flexed at the elbow, with the forearm behind the fetal neck.

The attitude of the breech baby is stated as that of the legs followed by that of the head: for example, a "frank breech with an extended head" or a "single (or double) footling breech with the head flexed." While the attitude of the head can be identified with abdominal palpation or ultrasound, the attitude of the arms is usually identified only after the baby is born to the chest or scapulae.

There is almost no information available as to the relative frequency of these postural variations at the onset of labor. Castallo (1948), Gaskin (1992) and Mukhopadhyay and Arulkumaran (2002) are among the very few authors to offer any such statistics. Their numbers match closely and are quoted in the following descriptions.

Frank breech: Some 60 to 70% of all breech babies present frank, or buttocks first, with the legs extended straight up against the baby's torso so that the feet are near the neck. This type of breech is most common because having the legs splinted against the uterine wall in a jack-knife position limits the mobility of the torso, preventing rotation to a cephalic presentation during pregnancy. This, combined with the firm muscle tone of primigravidas, make first-time mothers the most likely candidates to present frank breech as term approaches. During labor, the attitude of the legs greatly influences whether descent can occur. Rigid splinting may delay descent, as the fetal spine is restricted in its ability to rotate or flex from side to side or forward and backward, although the limited ability of the knees to flex laterally does assist in descent. The position of the legs also tends to straighten the spine and may encourage the head to become extended, especially if the feet are tucked under the neck. However, if the buttocks of a good-sized, term baby can navigate and stretch the birth canal, it bodes well for easy passage of the head. This, coupled with the passage of increasingly larger skull diameters as the head descends, causes the flexed head to emerge easily and quickly in many frank breech births.

The smooth, essentially uniform contour of the fetal buttocks forms an effective dilating wedge, filling the pelvis and minimizing the risk of early rupture of membranes as well as the chance of cord prolapse, which occurs in about 0.5% of these labors (in comparison, the risk for cephalic babies is 0.4%). Cord compression, however, is somewhat more of a concern, as the legs are tightly pressed against the baby's abdomen during passage through the pelvis.

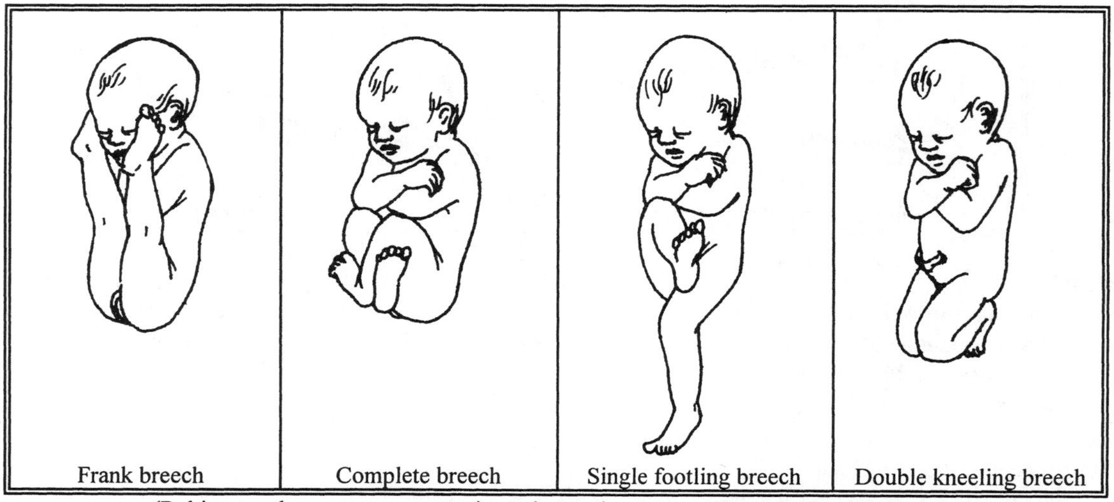

(Babies are shown sacrum posterior to better demonstrate the attitude of the legs.)

Incomplete breech (footling or kneeling): This refers to breech presentations in which one or both lower extremities extend downward into the yoni. Positioning is described as for any breech presentation (e.g., LSA, RSA, SA, SP) and the denominator is still the sacrum; however, these small, irregular parts lead the way.

Modern textbooks report footlings as rare; however Castallo (1948) states that 29% of all breeches are incomplete. Gaskin (1992) states that 10 to 20% of breeches present footling. An explanation for these varying figures lies in this attitude being the most common among preterm singleton breeches, occurring in 20 to 25% of preterm infants weighing over 2500 g (5 lb 8.5 oz) (Mukhopadhyay & Arulkumaran, 2002). As term approaches, the incidence goes down. A footling breech has more maneuvering ability because the legs are not splinted, allowing the baby to convert to a complete attitude or to turn to vertex more easily, which may be another reason why the incidence of footlings is widely variable among different studies.

Footling breeches carry an overall 15 to 18% risk of cord prolapse because small irregular parts lead the way through the pelvis, leaving room for the cord to wash down when the water breaks. Cord prolapse is most likely to occur when the baby is premature or small or in multiparous women, since their tissue tone is less firm. Even so, the risk of severe cord compression is less because the baby's torso is softer and leaves more room between the cord and the pelvic walls than is possible when the legs are extended against the body. The risk of prolapse is reduced after the membranes rupture but can still occur if the baby's or mother's movements shift the baby's lower body around and allow a low-lying cord to slip downward. Footling babies are also more likely to poke a hole through the intact membranes with a foot. There are two types of footling breeches. In a single footling breech, one foot is extended into the yoni. In a double footling breech, both feet are extended into the yoni.

At less than 5% of all term breeches, kneeling attitudes are the rarest of all and carry the same risks as footling breeches. Again, there are two types: single kneeling breech, where one knee extends into the cervix, and double kneeling breech, with both knees extended into the cervix (Gaskin, 1992).

A number of other attitudes are also possible, such as one leg extended up along the torso in a frank position and one leg extended down in a footling position, one foot and one knee presenting, one leg bent at the knee and flexed at the hip in a complete position with the other leg extended downward or in a frank attitude, etc. In reality, however, these contorted attitudes rarely occur. The particulars regarding clinical support for breech births with the legs in a variety of attitudes will be addressed in the chapter entitled "Assisting at the Birth of a Breech Baby."

Complete or flexed breech: This is the least common attitude, type, making up 10% of all preterm and term breeches. The baby's legs are completely flexed; that is, the legs are flexed at the hip, with the knees flexed as well. The knees may be up against the lower abdomen, or the lower legs are either flexed at the hip and knee with the feet under the buttocks or the legs are in a crossed "tailor sit" position with the feet against the underside of the thighs. The spine is usually well flexed. Here, the buttocks and legs form a reasonably uniform dilating wedge, although it is more irregular than the frank breech, making engagement less likely and cord prolapse more common, with an overall risk of prolapse ranging from 4 to 6%. The complete breech does a good job of stretching the birth canal, making room for the aftercoming head. The baby is illustrated in a complete breech attitude in the summarized descriptions of fetal descent in the various positions (LSA, RSA, LSP, etc.) that follow this chapter.

Frequency of breech positions

Documentation regarding the frequency of breech babies in various positions is hard to come by. Mayes (1959) states that LSA is most frequent (45%), followed by RSA (30%); no references could be found regarding the exact frequency of posterior breech positions, although several sources state that posterior positioning is relatively rare.

Risks of breech birth

Several unique aspects of breech birth render it potentially more dangerous for the baby and therefore call upon the midwife to be highly knowledgeable and skilled. In cephalic presentations, the largest and hardest part of the baby is born first, followed by successively softer and more malleable parts. If the head won't come out, at least the rest of the baby is still inside. In breech presentations, the opposite is true; the largest and hardest part of the baby is born last. If the head is too large to pass safely through the pelvis, this may not be known until after the rest of the body is born. If the baby is term, the size of the buttocks is such that it usually provides a good "test" of the pelvis (Cronk & Evans, 2002); that is, if a large breech passes easily, this bodes well for an easy birth of the head. The overall risk of cord prolapse is 3.7% (versus 0.3% in vertex births). The risk varies with the positioning of the legs, as previously discussed.

As with any birth, however, the size of the head may be appropriate in relation to the mother's pelvic structure, but if the head is deflexed, larger diameters will be presenting and birth of the head may be problematic. The head may get hung up (especially at the jawline and chin) if it tries to pass through a poorly prepared birth canal or a partially dilated cervix, either of which will encourage the head to deflex, thereby further increasing its presenting diameter. This complication most frequently arises when the baby is early. The head of a preterm baby is relatively larger in proportion to its body than that of a term baby. The small lower body parts may slip through a partially dilated cervix or birth canal with ease, leaving the passages insufficiently stretched to allow easy passage for the head. The risk of these problems developing is greatest if one or both of the lower limbs is extended downward.

In addition, in a cephalic presentation, once the shoulders are born, the rest of the body usually follows quickly. Even if it does not, the head is born and breathing is possible. In a breech, the baby may be born to the umbilicus for some minutes before the head has descended enough to create an airway for the baby. At the same time, the length of the cord extended from the umbilicus, past the upper torso and between the baby's body and head and the pelvic wall will inevitably undergo a certain amount of compression as the upper body is born.

Babies with malformations have a tendency to present breech more often than those who do not. This may not be recognized prior to birth, whether the mother has had any ultrasound exams or not. The baby is also at risk for a variety of injuries that are discussed in more detail in the chapter entitled "Assisting at the Birth of a Breech Baby."

Aside from the physiological risks, the biggest risk the practitioner brings to breech birth is unfamiliarity with observant attendance and an inability to limit the use of hands-on techniques to *only when necessary*. These deficiencies are due, in part, to the relative rarity of breeches coupled with the enormous amount of fear that the Western medical model brings to the process. These iatrogenic factors, as well as ways to minimize the inherent risks of breech birth, will also be discussed in more detail in the chapter entitled "Assisting at the Birth of a Breech Baby."

The Process of Birth in Sacrum Anterior Breech Presentations

Breech births are relatively infrequent, therefore theoretical mastery of the normal cardinal movements become crucial. Descent is potentially quite variable and complex in breeches. Therefore, it is important to have a thorough, working understanding of the basic principles of fetal anatomy and cephalic descent before studying this material. The movements of breech birth are more complex than those of cephalic presentations because the body presents three semi-independently mobile regions as it descends: the legs and breech (or lower torso), the chest and shoulders (or upper torso), and the head. These three regions are joined by two "hinges," the waist and the neck, and are connected by the long, flexible spine, making a variety of movements possible as the baby passes through the pelvis. Spinal mobility has always been recognized as an important component of breech descent. The descent and rotation of the pelvis and then the upper torso closely resemble that of the chest and shoulder girdle in a cephalic presentation and occur primarily for the same reason (as an accommodation to spinal flexion).

The shape of the first two regions is much more irregular than is that of the head. When the head leads the way, the motion of parts behind it do not usually affect its rotation or descent because the head is large, uniformly shaped and hard and can move relatively freely at the neck. In a breech, as small parts begin to be born, much of the baby is still inside. The weight and position of these irregular parts as they emerge shift as the baby's and mother's bodies change position and the freedom or impairment of motion afforded the baby by the mother's position (permitting him more or less ability to facilitate his own birth), all greatly impact the timing and direction of rotation. Even so, the basic movements of descent, internal rotation, and disengagement still apply to each of these anatomical regions successively.

During descent, the legs and pelvis, shoulders and arms, and head each represent an increasing degree of potential difficulty in passing through the pelvis. A sacrum anterior position lessons the likelihood of problems, as the small parts are directed toward the roomy posterior pelvis, while the smooth back passes through the shallow anterior pelvis. The shoulders are slightly wider than the hips, although moulding of the shoulder girdle tends to minimize this difference. The head is harder and less compressible than the pelvis or torso and has less time to mould than in a cephalic presentation because it passes through the pelvis relatively quickly. Whereas downward movement in vertex births tends to encourage head flexion, the downward movement of the aftercoming head and other parts may encourage extension. The mobility of the arms creates the possibility that they could become swept up beside or over the head. All this makes maintaining optimal fetal positioning during descent vitally important.

Notes on the Descriptions of Breech Descent

The movements described here represent a compilation of descriptions. Many of these details were gleaned from older textbooks by authors who had extensive clinical experience with breeches. English midwives Mary Cronk and Jane Evans (2002) are experienced hands-off breech practitioners. They collaborated and sent me notes on their observations of spontaneous breech descent and rotation, which have been incorporated into the descriptions that follow. The text assumes that the mother is in some sort of upright position such as standing, hands and knees or kneeling but not on her back, semi-sitting or lying on her side. Many of the differences among descriptions of breech descent are apparently due to intrinsic differences in the way birth occurs when the mother is in a supine versus a more or less upright position. The influence of gravity and fetal mobility appear to account for most of these discrepancies.

Most of what is known about how the breech descends and rotates comes from what can be observed during labor. I could find no X-ray studies of breech descent to inform us regarding the movements of parts still unborn. Therefore, the missing pieces, aside from what Mary and Jane have shared, have been filled in based on other research and my understanding of what is known about cephalic descent, spinal flexion, and the effect of splinted versus extended legs on torso mobility, as well as, in some cases, my own best guesses about how these factors will interact when the baby is in a particular position. Such extrapolations were necessary, for example, for the summaries describing sacrum transverse descent, which gets no attention in the existing obstetric literature. Nevertheless, if you study these descriptions and really understand them, you will have an excellent foundation from which to judge normal breech descent and rotation and the wide variations that can normally occur.

The process of breech birth can be more easily understood if the three relevant anatomical regions are focused upon in sequence. A "B" will be used to designate primary movements of the breech, including the lower torso (below the waist) and the sacrum (the denominator for the breech), an "S" designates primary movements of the upper torso and bisacromial diameter of the long axis of the shoulders (the denominator for the upper torso or chest) and an "O" designates primary movements of the occiput (the denominator for the flexed head). A sacrum anterior oblique orientation will be used as a template for discussion, since it is most common. The descent of the breech and torso for frank and complete/incomplete breech presentations are described separately because the attitude of the legs can significantly impact the way movements occur. Descent and birth of the head is essentially the same regardless of the attitude of the legs, so it is discussed last. Frank breeches are presented first, as they are most common. Have your doll and pelvic model in hand. Start by going through the table below, matching the movements with your doll. Once you feel comfortable with that, move on to the detailed explanations that follow. Do the same as you study each step throughout the chapter.

Descent and Birth of the Breech and Shoulders in Anterior Frank Breeches

THE CARDINAL MOVEMENTS OF BIRTH IN SACRUM ANTERIOR-OBLIQUE FRANK BREECH DESCENT

BREECH (LOWER TORSO) AND LEGS	SHOULDERS (UPPER TORSO)	HEAD
1-B. Spinal flexion (may be impaired because legs are splinted)	*1-S. Spinal flexion (may be impaired)*	**1-O. Flexion of the head (may be impaired)**
2-B. Descent	*2-S. Descent in concert with breech*	*2-O. Descent in concert with upper torso*
3-B. Engagement–sacrum anterior oblique or directly anterior		
4-B. Internal rotation to sacrum transverse • Dilating the soft birth canal	*3-S. First internal rotation with breech, to bring long axis AP*	*3-O. First internal rotation with torso, to bring occiput transverse*
5-B. Extension and lateroflexion of spine (as possible) • Dilating the perineum • Rumping (crowning) of the breech		
6-B. Birth of anterior and posterior buttock by lateral spinal flexion		
7-B. Restitution does not occur.		
8-B. First external rotation with upper torso, to bring sacrum anterior	**4-S. Second internal rotation to bring long axis of shoulders to transverse**	*4-O. Second internal rotation with torso to bring occiput anterior*
	5-S. Engagement as umbilicus is born *S. Flexion of shoulders*	
9-B. Second external rotation with upper torso, to bring sacrum transverse	**6-S. Third internal rotation to left or right to bring long shoulder axis AP**	*5-O. Third internal rotation with torso to bring occiput transverse*
B. Birth of legs (may occur at any point before/during birth of arms) *B. The baby may flex his legs, which aids head flexion.*	**7-S. Birth of anterior arm and shoulder by lateral spinal flexion**	*6-O. The head engages as the shoulders reach the outlet.*
10-B. Third external rotation with head, to bring sacrum anterior	*8-S. Slight movement to left or right as posterior arm is born–then shoulders rotate externally with the head to bring their long axis transverse*	**7-O. Fourth internal rotation begins before and completes after posterior arm is born to bring occiput anterior.**
		8-O. Birth of head by flexion

The cardinal movements as conceived by obstetrical writers can be applied to any type of longitudinal lie. However, envisioning them in breeches is more challenging because three regions of fetal anatomy are frequently moving in concert. The tables in this chapter provide a visual reference regarding movements that occur simultaneously. For all the tables, movements appearing in the same row occur together, with likely orientations. Each numbered movement in the tables matches those in the descriptions below. Cardinal movements of the descending part prior to its birth are shown in bold. Cardinal movements of parts that occur as a consequence of movements of the descending part appear in italics. Other pertinent changes appear in regular type. Read through the description, ignoring the italicized entries, to gain a more simplified understanding.

Descent and birth of the breech and lower torso in frank breech babies

1-S, 2-S, 1-O & 2-O. Flexion and descent of the upper torso and head: *Flexion of the head usually occurs prior to labor and influences the degree of flexion along the entire spine. (Flexion in the breech baby is discussed in detail on page 196.) Descent of the upper torso and head occurs in concert with that of the lower torso.*

1-B. Flexion of the lumbar spine: *Prior to labor, flexion of the lower spine occurs primarily as a secondary consequence of flexion of the head. If the cervical spine is not well flexed, the rest of the spine is not likely to be either. During labor, flexion or extension can be enhanced by the downward force from the fundus during uterine contractions. Spinal flexion is not really necessary to facilitate descent until the torso reaches the curved portion of the birth canal, when lateral flexion becomes important. Splinting of the legs against the torso will impair anterior and sometimes lateral flexion.*

2-B. Descent of the breech: The somewhat softer and more irregularly shaped breech is a slightly less efficient dilator than the head, even in first-time mothers. Even so, the bottom of a well-grown term baby approximates the size and shape of the term head. A less efficient dilating wedge plus the rigidity of the torso often causes the frank breech baby to remain high in the pelvis until the cervix is fully dilated and the membranes have ruptured, although it is just as normal for the breech to descend progressively as labor advances. In all breech babies, once the legs emerge, small parts hang dependent from the introitus, thus gravity and maternal positioning become critical influences over how birth proceeds as the baby descends further.

Anterior asynclitic descent: The pelvis often descends at an anteriorly-directed angle, with the anterior buttock leading the way (corresponding to the anterior asynclitism of Nägele in cephalic presentations [Greenhill, 1951]). This facilitates descent because the direction of slant points the baby's anterior tuberosity downward and toward the rear of the mother's pelvis, encouraging the anterior hip to descend easily past the upper border of the pubic bone without becoming hung up. If the pelvis is in an attitude of posterior asynclitism, the baby's anterior tuberosity is lifted up, toward the front of the mother's pelvis, making it easier for it to become caught against the upper border of the pubic bone.

3-B. Engagement of the frank breech: The baby usually begins labor with the sacrum in either an anterior oblique position, which may be only slight, or in a directly anterior orientation. Engagement occurs when the bitrochanteric diameter, the widest external transverse diameter of the fetal pelvis, descends through the brim. After engagement, the lowermost portion of the buttocks is still high in the pelvis, usually between –4 and –2 station.

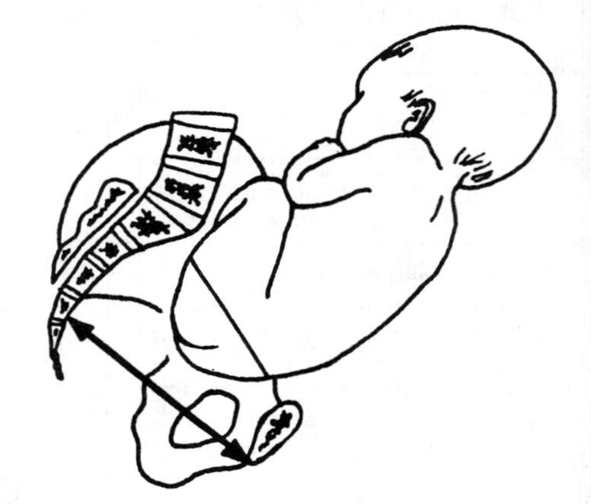

Anterior asynclitic engagement of the breech baby

4-B. Internal rotation of the lower torso and breech: As the breech reaches the curve of the birth canal, the lower torso usually rotates so that the long axis of the pelvis is in the anteroposterior diameter, to allow the spine to flex laterally. In most cases, internal rotation happens just before or during the pushing phase of labor and is encouraged as the baby's pelvis meets the resistance of the mother's pelvic floor muscles.

If the sacrum is already anterior oblique, it moves 45° to a sacrum transverse position. If the baby has engaged in only a slightly oblique orientation, the distance of travel to transverse will be between 45 and 90°. If the sacrum engaged directly anterior, it moves 45° to anterior oblique and then rotates an additional 45° to transverse, 90° in all.

Splinting of the legs may impair full rotation of the sacrum to transverse if the torso is quite rigid. It may also prevent or impair twisting at the waist. Because of this, frank descent is described as though the waist does not twist. If twisting does occur, descent is the same as for a baby with the legs in a complete or incomplete attitude.

3-S & 3-O. First internal rotation of the upper torso and head: *In frank breeches, splinting of the legs usually prevents twisting at the waist, thus the upper torso and the head undergo their first internal rotation in concert with the sacrum, moving the long axis of the shoulders into the anteroposterior diameter and the occiput to transverse.*

• **Dilating the soft birth canal:** Most full-term frank breeches do a good job of this, as the presenting part approximates the size of the head.

5-B. Extension and lateroflexion of the spine and torso: In frank breeches, the attitude and mobility of the legs greatly influences the ease with which lateral spinal flexion, and therefore descent, can occur. There is some lateral and some anteroposterior flexibility at the lumbar-sacral joint, which allows the pelvis to enter the curve of the birth canal. When the baby's pelvis rotates to the anteroposterior diameter and the legs are bent to either side of the torso, as illustrated on the left, sufficient descent results in the application of pressure to the lateral aspect of the anterior thigh, pushing the leg toward the midline, allowing the anterior hip to slip past the pubic bone. As the posterior hip approaches the deepest curve of the canal, the side of the posterior leg is similarly pressed toward the midline. However, if the baby rotates sacrum anterior, descent can be impaired if the knees bend at the level of the sacral promontory and the torso becomes bent. If the knees get past the promontory, rigidly splinted legs may bridge the sacral hollow, preventing spinal flexion into the curve of the canal because the knees can't hyperextend to allow it. This means the extended spine must work its way through the shallow anterior pelvis.

Even when the legs can move to facilitate spinal flexion, the torso is still stiffer than it would be if the legs were not splinted. Thus, the tendency is for the buttocks to be driven downward and more posteriorly against the coccyx and perineum as they meet the pelvic floor before they enter the deepest curve of the birth canal at the level of the tuberosities. This posteriorly directed descent is more pronounced when the mother is on her back with her legs up, which impairs sacral mobility, exaggerates the curve of the birth canal, and, if her knees are elevated, pivots the pelvic floor up, creating a barrier to descent. Thus, the birth of the frank breech baby is greatly facilitated when the birth canal is as straight as possible, which occurs when the mother is kneeling and leaning forward with her pelvis tilted forward or is standing upright. The term fetus is quite pliable, and when the legs have some mobility and the birth canal is made straighter by an optimal maternal position, descent may proceed with minimal difficulty.

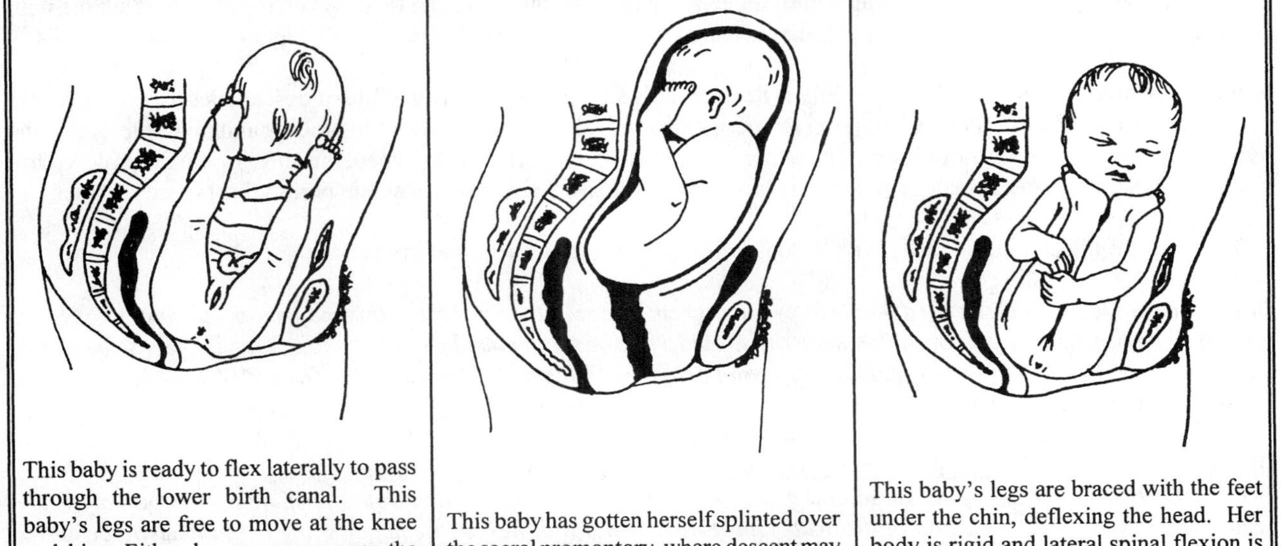

This baby is ready to flex laterally to pass through the lower birth canal. This baby's legs are free to move at the knee and hip. Either leg can cross over the torso during descent as pressure is applied from the pelvic side walls, allowing the spine to flex more easily.

This baby has gotten herself splinted over the sacral promontory, where descent may be arrested. Maternal position changes may help dislodge the baby and facilitate descent.

This baby's legs are braced with the feet under the chin, deflexing the head. Her body is rigid and lateral spinal flexion is going to be difficult, if not impossible. Wrapping of her arms around her knees locks her into this posture even more.

However, when the legs are rigidly splinted against the torso, which can occur if the feet are lodged in the anterior creases of the axilla, if they flank the head next to the ears, if they are wedged under the chin, or if the legs are crossed, mobility is minimized or prevented entirely. Cord entanglement could also limit leg mobility. When the legs are fixed, the only joints that may have limited lateral mobility are the knees and possibly the lumbar-sacral joint. Inflexibility of the legs reduces spinal flexion and maneuverability in all directions, impairing and sometimes arresting descent.

• **Dilating the perineum:** The breech moves down, stretching the perineal tissues by rocking back and forth with contractions just as the head does in a cephalic presentation. Rocking is always less pronounced, however, when the mother is upright, as gravity assists with descent.

• **Rumping or butting (crowning of the frank breech):** "Rumping" is sometimes defined as visualization of the breech at the introitus. However, it usually refers to the point when the presenting part no longer recedes between contractions during the pushing phase of labor. A "full rump" occurs when the widest diameter of the pelvis is encircled by the mouth of the introitus. In frank breeches, rumping is very much like crowning of the head because the bottom is large and round.

6-B. Birth of the frank breech: In most cases, the mother's pushing efforts, the walls of the birth canal and the forward-tilted angle of fetal pelvis result in the anterior buttock emerging first. Lateral flexion of the torso in an anterior direction causes the perineum to retract and the posterior buttock is born. Then the torso straightens and both hips advance.

Many textbooks state that the posterior buttock is normally born first, such as Castallo (1948), McNeile (1939) and Oxorn (1986), to name a few. Cronk, Evans (2002) and Myles (1968) as well as Mayes (1959) are among those who state that the anterior buttock comes first. I suspect that rampant obstetrical interventions of various kinds, including the use of anesthesia (which relaxes the soft tissues), as well as pushing in a supine position with the knees elevated as well as giant clitorotomies account for the perception that the posterior buttock is normally born first.

As the breech is born, the splinting of the legs results in the torso emerging at a forwardly directed angle of about 45° in relationship to the introitus. Imagine trying to insert your entire arm into a gently curved, somewhat flexible tube. The only places your arm can bend are at the wrist (just above the baby's sacrum) and at the elbow (the baby's lower neck). Your fist (the baby's pelvis) and forearm (the baby's torso) advance straight downward into the curve of the tube, then you must work your fist around the curve by flexing your wrist, stretching the tube and finally getting your elbow to the level of the curve. Once your elbow enters the curve, your forearm sticks out of the tube at an angle. In much the same way, the baby's torso has limited flexibility where the sacrum joins the spine, and again in the region of the cervical spine. The rigid body descends toward the posterior pelvic floor until it works its way around the curve, at that point the body sticks out of the introitus at an angle until the legs are free and the spine can flex. When the mother is supine with her knees elevated, the curve of the birth canal is exaggerated and the angle of the baby's torso is more pronounced.

Alternative birth of the breech: Especially if the mother is supine, the posterior angle of descent described above, the rigidity of the baby's torso and the barrier of the perineum may result in the anterior hip bracing and pivoting against the pubic bone, causing the posterior buttock to be born first as the perineum retracts. Then, the anterior hip drops down and out from under the pubic bone by a process of lateral spinal flexion and emerges as the periurethral tissues retract.

7-B. Restitution: Restitution of the breech does not occur when the waist is not twisted.

B. Birth of the legs: *The extended legs will eventually emerge spontaneously, but this may not occur until most of the torso is born because the feet are often near the shoulders. The torso must be out far enough for the feet to be free of the birth canal and drop down. Once the legs are born, the torso can rotate and flex. The birth of the legs does not constitute a cardinal movement.*

Descent and birth of the upper torso, arms and shoulders in the frank breech baby

1-S & 1-O. Flexion of the upper torso and head: *Prior to labor, flexion of the thoracic spine occurs primarily as a secondary consequence of flexion of the head. If the head is not well flexed, the upper spine is not likely to be either. However, pronounced spinal flexion is not really necessary to facilitate descent until the torso reaches the curved portion of the birth canal, when lateral spinal flexion becomes important. Flexion or extension will be enhanced by the downward force of uterine contractions.*

2-S, 2-O. The upper torso and shoulders descend throughout labor: *As the breech is born, the upper torso, shoulders and head continue to descend.*

4-S. Second internal rotation of the upper torso and shoulders: After the buttocks are born, the upper torso and shoulders are aligned with the anteroposterior diameter of the brim. As the upper torso moves into the pelvic cavity, it rotates internally, moving the shoulders 45° to an oblique diameter and then 45° to transverse, 90° in all, positioning the back under the pubic arch. Sometimes, the shoulders only rotate as far as the oblique diameter and descend from there.

8-B. First external rotation of the breech: *The just-born breech simultaneously undergoes its first external rotation, following the movement of the shoulders to sacrum anterior oblique and usually on to directly anterior.*

4-O. Second internal rotation of the head: *The head continues to follow the torso as it descends.*

5-S. Engagement of the shoulders: As the lower torso fully emerges to the umbilicus, the shoulders engage as the bisacromial diameter descends through the transverse or oblique diameter of the brim, whichever they have just rotated to occupy.

S. Flexion of the shoulders: *The shoulders accommodate to the shape of the birth canal as the baby moves down. The scapulae are pressed together, and the shoulders will tend to either curl forward, be pressed down along the torso or be hunched as the upper torso enters the curve of the birth canal. Moulding reduces the diameter of the shoulders by as much as 33%. Normally, the arms are folded over the chest; the elbows may be as high as the nipple line.*

6-S. Third internal rotation of the upper torso and shoulders: The upper torso arrives at the opening of the levator ani sling, near the level of the ischial spines, and is prompted to rotate internally by the need for the spine to flex laterally. Typically, the upper torso and shoulders rotate from the transverse diameter 45° to an anterior oblique orientation and then 45° to anteroposterior, 90° in all.

Sometimes, the upper torso only rotates 45°, stopping to descend through the oblique diameter. If splinted legs render the torso particularly rigid, the upper torso may not undergo any internal rotation in the pelvic cavity. Superrotation can occur as well, where the torso and occiput move from their original anterior-oblique orientation to the other (for example, if the baby began labor LSA and the shoulders rotated and engaged SA, she might then rotate to RSA and finally to RST).

9-B. Second external rotation of the breech: *The pelvis matches the movement of the upper torso, bringing the sacrum to an anterior oblique orientation and usually all the way to transverse.*

5-O. Third internal rotation of the head: *The occiput, following the movement of the upper torso, internally rotates to an anterior oblique orientation and then, in most cases, to transverse.*

7-S. Birth of the anterior arm and shoulder by lateral flexion of the upper spine: As the shoulders descend, typically the anterior shoulder presents under the pubic arch and, by a process of lateral spinal flexion, emerge first.

B. Birth of the legs: *If the feet have not been born yet, they usually drop out as the shoulders emerge.*

6-O. Engagement of the head: *The head engages when the shoulders reach the outlet (see page 197 for details).*

8-S . Birth of the posterior shoulder and arm and external rotation of the shoulders: *Once the anterior arm is born, the weight of the baby shifts. The shoulders may undergo a slight movement to the left or right as the posterior arm and shoulder work their way down. The perineum retracts as the shoulder is born. Once the posterior arm is out, the shoulders are free to rotate externally, following the head as it completes it fourth internal rotation to OA (7-O). Details regarding the descent and birth of the head (8-O), are found in the section beginning on page 196 entitled "Descent and birth of the head in all sacrum anterior breech babies."*

Alternative shoulder birth: Especially if the mother is supine, the anterior shoulder may become temporarily pressed against the pubic bone, causing the shoulder axis to be angled in such a way that the posterior arm and shoulder present and, by a process of lateroflexion, are born first as the perineum retracts. Then the weight of the baby shifts, allowing the anterior shoulder and arm to be released from beneath the symphysis.

10-B. Third external rotation of the breech: *Once the posterior arm is born, the torso moves in concert with the internal rotation of the head, externally rotating the sacrum from transverse, to anterior oblique, to sacrum anterior.*

Descent and Birth of the Breech and Shoulders in Complete or Incomplete Anterior Breeches

The cardinal movements of birth are even more complex in complete and incomplete breech babies because the spine is more free to move and the baby can twist at the waist or neck. Thus, both twisting and restitution are likely movements as the breech descends. The following chart summarizes the cardinal movements in these types of breeches.

THE CARDINAL MOVEMENTS OF BIRTH IN COMPLETE AND INCOMPLETE SACRUM ANTERIOR BREECH DESCENT		
BREECH (LOWER TORSO) AND LEGS	**SHOULDERS (UPPER TORSO)**	**HEAD**
1-B. Spinal flexion	*1-S. Spinal flexion*	*1-O. Flexion of the head*
2-B. Descent	*2-S. Descent in concert with breech*	*2-O. Descent in concert with torso.*
3-B. Engagement–sacrum anterior oblique or directly anterior (or waist twists to allow SA descent)	• *If waist does twist, upper torso remains oblique*	• *If waist does twist, occiput remains anterior oblique*
4-B. Internal rotation as waist twists as sacrum moves to transverse (or, internal restitution occurs as waist untwists to allow breech to move back to anterior oblique–then waist twists again as sacrum moves to transverse.) • Dilating the soft birth canal	*3-S. Internal rotation does not occur–the upper torso remains oblique*	*3-O. Internal rotation does not occur–occiput remains anterior oblique*
5-B. Extension and lateroflexion of spine • Dilating the perineum *B. Incomplete: birth of legs* • Complete: rumping of the breech		
6-B. Birth of anterior and posterior buttock by lateral spinal flexion *B. Complete: birth of legs*		
7-B. Restitution (waist untwists as sacrum returns to anterior oblique)		
8-B. First external rotation with upper torso to sacrum anterior	**4-S. First internal rotation–long axis of shoulders to transverse**	*4-O. First internal rotation with torso to bring occiput anterior*
B. The baby may flex his legs, which aids head flexion.	**5-S. Engagement as umbilicus is born** *S. Flexion of shoulders*	
9-B. Second external rotation with upper torso to bring sacrum transverse	**6-S. Second internal rotation to left or right to bring long shoulder axis AP**	*5-O. Second internal rotation with torso to bring occiput transverse (or neck twists to allow occiput to lag behind in anterior oblique position)*
	7-S. Birth of anterior arm and shoulder by lateroflexion of upper spine	*6-O. The head engages as the shoulders reach the outlet.*
10-B. Third external rotation with head to bring sacrum anterior	*8-S. Slight movement to left or right as posterior arm is born–then shoulders follow head, rotating externally to transverse*	**7-O. Third internal rotation begins before and completes after posterior arm is born to bring occiput anterior.**
		8-O. Birth of head by flexion

Descent and birth of the breech and lower torso in complete or incomplete anterior breech babies

1-S & 1-O. Flexion of the upper torso and head: *Flexion of the head usually occurs prior to labor and influences the degree of flexion along the entire spine. Spinal flexion is easier to accomplish and often more pronounced when the legs are not splinted up against the torso.*

2-S & 2-O. Descent of the upper torso and head. *Descent of the head occurs in concert with the torso.*

2-B. Descent of the breech: The softer and more irregularly shaped complete breech does not fill the birth canal as fully and is more compressible than the frank breech. These differences make it a somewhat inefficient dilator. In an incomplete breech, the feet or knees are extended toward the os; so there is really nothing sizable to serve as a dilating wedge except the intact membranes. These factors often cause the baby to remain high in the pelvis until the cervix is fully dilated and the membranes have ruptured, although progressive descent can also occur. Extended legs may project down through the partially dilated cervix, putting pressure on the posterior wall of the birth canal, creating a premature urge to push, prompting rupture of membranes and, possibly, cord prolapse, or all three.

In incomplete breech babies, if the membranes do rupture, the legs may emerge from the introitus prior to full dilation. Whenever small parts hang dependent from the introitus, gravity, and with it maternal positioning, become very important influences over how birth proceeds as the baby descends further.

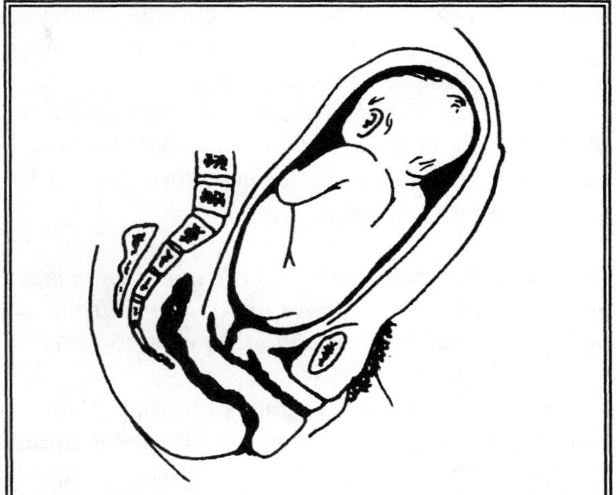
RSA complete breech descending (2-B) to engagement (3-B) (mother upright, kneeling)

3-B. Engagement of the breech: Regardless of the attitude of the legs or their level of descent, engagement is marked by the descent of the bitrochanteric diameter, the widest transverse diameter of the pelvis, through the brim. This usually occurs with the sacrum in an anterior oblique orientation, which may be only slight or directly anterior. Alternatively, before the breech enters the brim, the lower torso may undergo internal rotation as the fetus turns at the waist, moving the sacrum 45° to SA, which leaves the upper torso and head in an anterior oblique orientation. After engagement, the lowermost portion of the buttocks is still high in the pelvis, usually between –4 to –2 station.

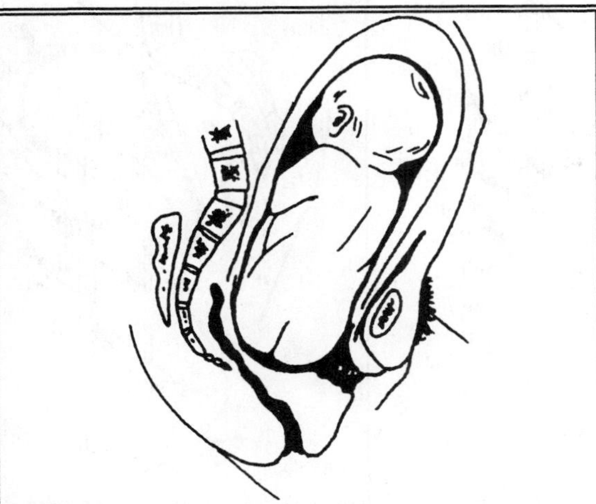
Descent (2-B) continues; internal rotation to RST by twisting at waist (4-B); spinal lateroflexion begins (5-B)

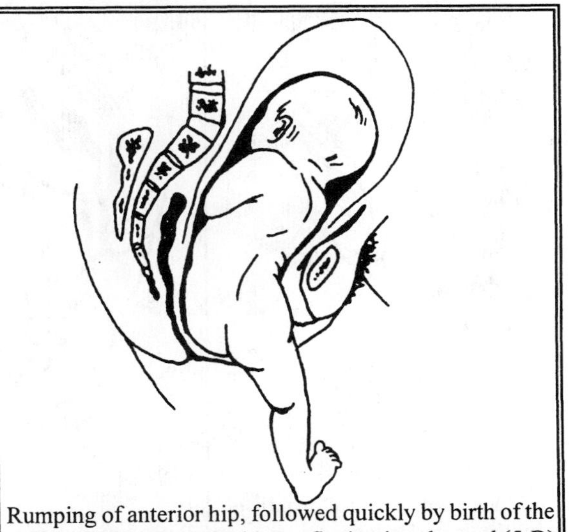
Rumping of anterior hip, followed quickly by birth of the anterior leg (6-B); spinal lateroflexion is enhanced (5-B)

• **Dilating the soft birth canal:** Intact membranes play an important role in ensuring adequate dilation of the passages.

Should the forebag rupture, the irregularly shaped small parts will have to do the dilating on their own.

4-B. Internal rotation of the lower torso and breech: Internal rotation takes place as the baby's torso and spine accommodate themselves to the sling-shaped levator ani muscle, as well as to the curve of the birth canal. In most cases, internal rotation happens just before or during the pushing phase of labor.

Further descent to the curve prompts the lower torso to rotate so that the long axis of the pelvis moves into the anteroposterior diameter. If the lower torso engaged through the anterior oblique diameter, it moves 45° to a sacrum transverse position by twisting at the waist, leaving the head and shoulders in an anterior oblique orientation. If the sacrum starts from only a slightly anterior oblique or a directly anterior orientation, the distance of travel to sacrum transverse would be between 45 and 90°.

If the sacrum rotated to direct anterior before entering the brim by twisting at the waist, it **internally restitutes** 45° by untwisting at the waist as it moves back to the anterior oblique quadrant it originally occupied (restoring the anatomical alignment with the upper torso and head). The sacrum then rotates internally 45° to transverse often by, once again, turning at the waist.

3-S & 3-O. Internal rotation of the upper torso and head: *These movements usually do not occur as the breech rotates because rotation of the lower torso is typically accomplished by twisting at the waist, leaving the upper torso and head in their original anterior oblique or directly anterior orientation.*

5-B. Lateroflexion of the spine and torso: Babies presenting as complete or incomplete breeches have the advantage of a more complete range of spinal movement, limited primarily by the confines of the birth canal as they descend. The spine straightens so that it can flex laterally, allowing easy passage through the deepest curve of the birth canal.

• **Dilating the perineum:** Dilation of the soft tissues is less efficient because smaller, more irregular parts are presenting.

• **Rumping or butting (crowning of the breech):** With the legs leading the way, rumping of the breech does not occur in the same way that it does when a large round part is emerging, but still takes place as the widest diameter of the pelvis passes through the introitus. Depending upon the exact positioning of the legs, the presentation of the complete breech at the vulva may approximate rumping in a frank breech, because the bottom will tend to present before the legs are born.

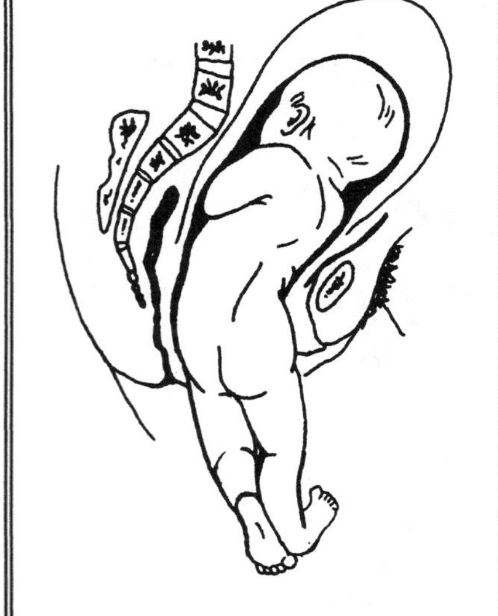

Posterior hip is born (6-B) followed quickly by the posterior leg

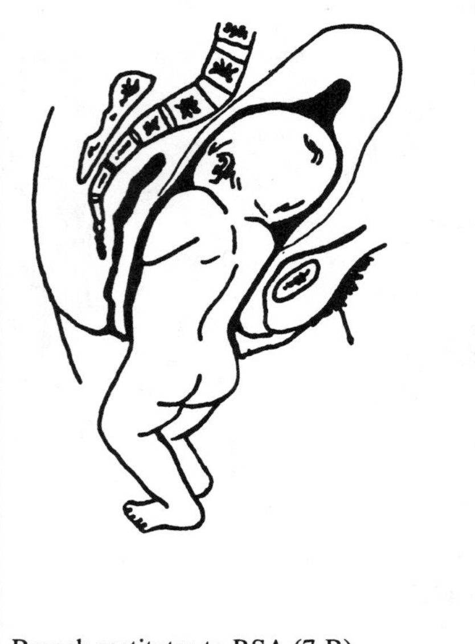

Breech restitutes to RSA (7-B)

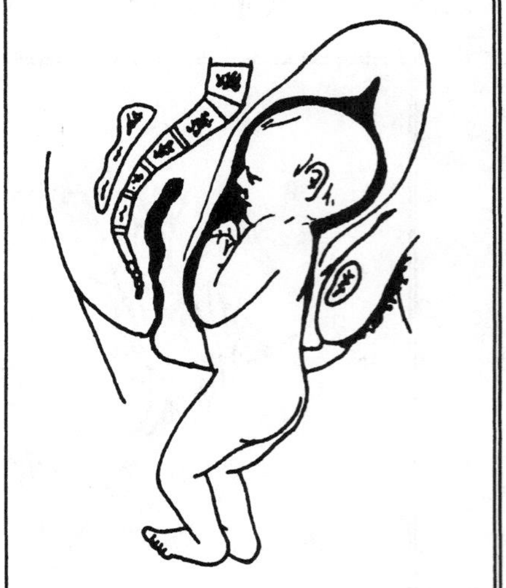

1st internal rotation of shoulders (4-S) and engagement in transverse diameter (5-S)

6-B. Birth of the breech: Especially when the mother is upright, the anterior buttock is usually born first, followed by the posterior buttock. The posterior buttock may also present first, at times, a variation that may be influenced by the position of the baby's legs or the mother's body.

B. Birth of the legs: *The birth of the legs varies, depending upon the attitude of the baby.*

Incomplete breech: *If the legs are extended down into the yoni, they will emerge before the breech is born.*

Complete breech: *If the legs are flexed, they will fall out, usually one after the other, along with or just after the birth of the buttocks.*

7-B. Restitution of the breech: The Latin root of "restitution" refers to the act of restoring. In modern textbooks, this term is reserved for discussing cephalic descent and refers to the return of the rotated head to its natural, anatomical position in relation to the shoulders after its emergence from the vulva. Older textbooks, however, used this term when referring to the return of any body part to its normal anatomical relationship with another. The term "restitution" can thus be applied to the movements of the upper and lower torso in relationship to each other as well as to the head.

Restitution of the lower torso occurs when internal rotation involves turning at the waist. Once the breech is born, the waist untwists, allowing the sacrum to restitute 45° from the transverse position from which it emerged back to its original anterior oblique orientation. This restores the parallel relationship of the long axis of the baby's pelvis with the long axis of the shoulders.

Descent and birth of the upper torso, arms and shoulders in the complete and incomplete breech baby

1-S, 2-S, & 1-O. Flexion of the upper spine and head and descent of the torso and head*: The upper spine flexes as a result of head flexion. The head descends in concert with the torso throughout labor.*

4-S. First internal rotation of the upper torso and shoulders: As the upper torso accommodates to the shape of the brim, the shoulders may remain oblique; however, they usually rotate 45° to a transverse orientation.

8-B. First external rotation of the breech: *The just-born breech simultaneously undergoes its first external rotation, following the upper torso to an anterior oblique and then, in most cases, to a sacrum anterior position.*

4-O. First internal rotation of the head: *After the breech has fully emerged, the head usually moves in concert with the shoulders as they rotate and descend. As the shoulder axis moves to the transverse diameter of the brim prior to engagement, the occiput usually follows, rotating 45° to anterior oblique and usually another 45° to become directly anterior.*

5-S. Engagement of the shoulders: After the lower torso has fully emerged to the umbilicus, the shoulders engage as the bisacromial diameter descends through the transverse diameter of the brim. If the upper torso and shoulders did not undergo first internal rotation, they will enter the brim through the oblique diameter they currently occupy.

S. Flexion of the shoulders: *The shoulders flex and move as necessary to facilitate passage through the birth canal.*

6-S. Second internal rotation of the upper torso and shoulders: The upper torso and spine arrive at the opening of the levator ani sling, near the level of the ischial spines, and are prompted to rotate internally by the need for the spine to flex laterally. The upper torso and shoulder axis rotate from the transverse diameter 45° to an oblique diameter and then 45° to anteroposterior, 90° in all.

If the shoulders entered the brim oblique, they rotate only 45° to anteroposterior. Superrotation is also common at this point when the entire baby is aligned in a directly anterior position, because it easy for him to rotate either way (for example, if the baby started labor LSA and the shoulders rotated and engaged transverse (SA), he might then rotate to RSA and finally to RST).

9-B. Second external rotation of the lower torso: *As the upper torso rotates, the breech follows, moving the sacrum to transverse.*

5-O. Second internal rotation of the head: *As the shoulders rotate, the occiput follows their movement, traveling with them to become transverse. Alternatively, the neck may twist, allowing the occiput to rotate only part way, lagging* *behind the upper torso by 45° in an anterior oblique orientation.*

<u>7-S. Birth of the anterior arm and shoulder by lateroflexion</u>: Most commonly, the anterior shoulder and arm are born first, by a process of lateroflexion of the spine.

6-O. Engagement of the head: *The head engages as the shoulders reach the outlet.*

8-S. Birth of posterior arm and shoulder and external rotation of shoulders: *Once the anterior arm is born, the weight of the baby shifts. The shoulders may make a slight movement in either a left or right direction as the posterior arm and shoulder are released from the perineum and born. The shoulders are then freed to rotate externally as they follow the third internal rotation of the head to OA (7-O).*

Alternative shoulder birth: Especially when the mother is supine, the anterior shoulder may become temporarily pressed against the pubic bone, causing the shoulder axis to be angled in such a way that the posterior arm and shoulder present and, by a process of lateroflexion, are born over the perineum first. Once they are born, the weight of the baby shifts, allowing the anterior shoulder and arm to be released from beneath the symphysis.

10-B. Third external rotation of the breech: *As the head undergoes its third internal rotation to occiput anterior, the lower torso moves with it as soon as the posterior arm is born, bringing the sacrum directly anterior.*

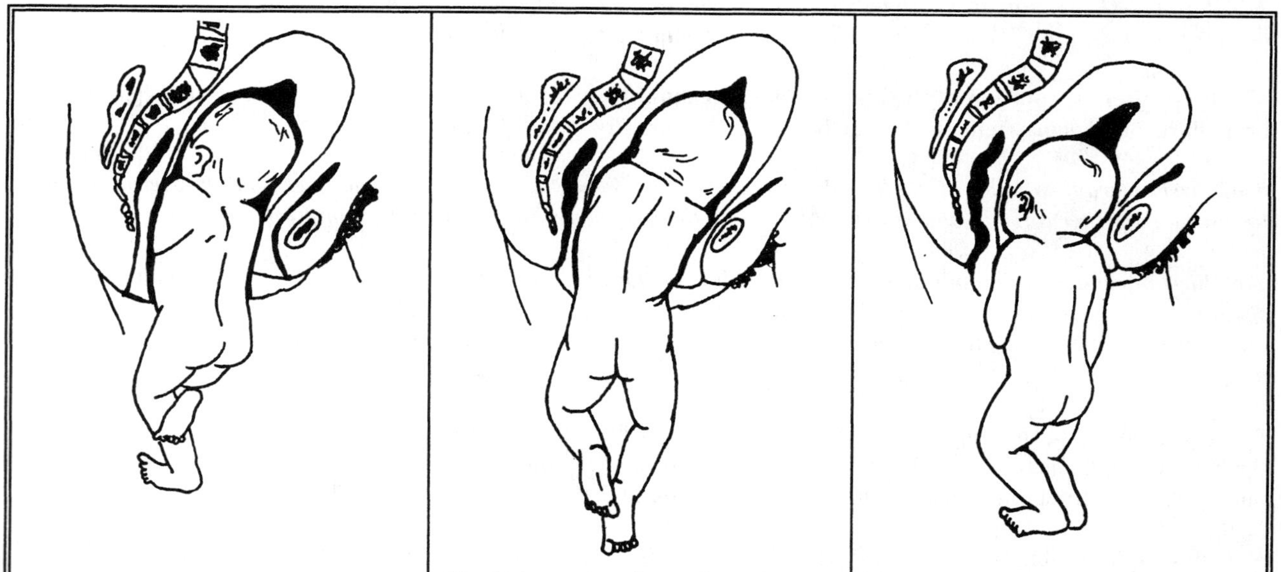

Upper torso rotates internally to RSA (6-S), lower torso and head follow (8-B, 5-O)

Shoulders continue internal rotation to AP (6-S); lower torso and head follow (8-B, 5-O)

Anterior arm has been born (7-S); posterior shoulder emerging (8-S), head ROA rotating to OA (7-0)

<u>Descent and Birth of the Head in All Sacrum Anterior Breech Babies</u>

1-O. Spinal flexion in the breech baby: The baby's head may be in any attitude from full flexion to full extension prior to or during descent. Spinal flexion in the breech must begin prior to labor and is prompted by flexion of the head. If the head is not flexed, the rest of the spine is not likely to be either. As with all anterior babies, the lordosis of the maternal spine encourages the fetal back to curve into the cradle created by the maternal abdominal wall, which also enhances flexion, although spinal flexion will be hampered in the breech baby with fully splinted legs.

As descent proceeds, however, the spine must straighten as the baby moves down to allow for lateral flexion through the curve of the birth canal. As is true for vertex descent, spinal extension can occur while the head remains flexed, although in breeches the direction of descent does not itself encourage head flexion (as it does in vertex descent where counterpressure from the birth canal helps the head stay flexed while the spine extends above it). However, research done by Borell and Fernström (1967) revealed that both toning and labor contractions help to flex (or extend) the head more as the fundus presses down on it, again demonstrating the importance of axial pressure in fetal flexion. Fortunately, it is most common for the head to be well flexed as it enters the pelvis.

Maintaining head flexion is of vital importance to the safe descent of the breech baby. As the head approaches the pelvic floor, flexion is encouraged by pressure from the soft tissues as the head leaves the cervix and enters the yoni and by uterine contractions as the fundus gathers itself around the aftercoming head. Flexion is also encouraged as the occiput is pressed toward the chest as it passes the pubic arch. After the legs have emerged, the baby will often lift his legs up to his belly. This tightens the abdominal muscles and curls the spine forward, which also helps the baby to keep his head flexed (Cronk & Evans, 2002). A deflexed head often requires correction via manual assistance from the midwife.

2-O. Descent of the head: *The head descends in concert with the lower body throughout labor. As the tip of the scapulae reach the outer border of the pubic arch, the head is entering the pelvis.*

3-O, 4-O and 5-O. Internal rotations of the head: *The head rotates internally, following the torso or lagging behind if the waist or neck twists, as previously described.*

6-O. Engagement of the head: *The head engages when the biparietal diameter passes through the brim, which occurs as the shoulders reach the outlet. The biparietal diameter typically engages in an anteroposterior orientation (occiput transverse) or aligned with one of the oblique diameters of the brim. Once the shoulders have fully emerged, their position should reflect that of the head, maintaining the natural 90° angle between the long axes of the two.*

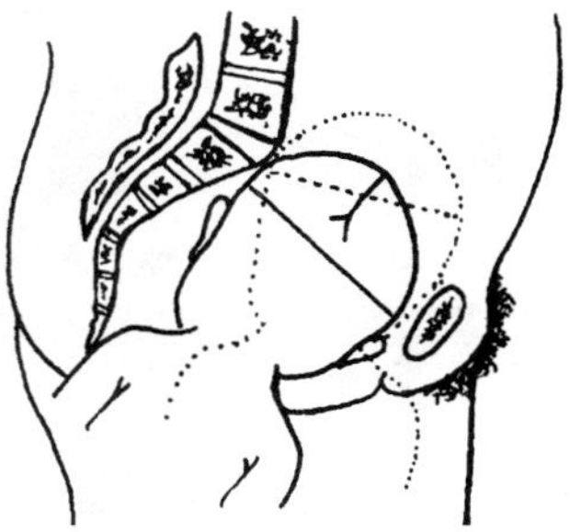

Descent of the head via a process of posterior asynclitism.

(after Williams, 1903)

Asynclitic descent of the head to engagement: *The breech baby may, at times, take advantage of asynclitic cephalic engagement by wiggling her head through the pelvis at an angle. This chance will be best afforded the baby whose mother is upright during pushing. Early editions of WILLIAMS OBSTETRICS (1917) are the only texts that mention asynclitic engagement of the aftercoming head. At that time, all types of asynclitic engagement were believed to be exclusively associated with descent through a contracted brim. In fact, it may be just as normal a movement for the breech baby who is born to an upright, mobile mother and is therefore also able to move and participate in her birth as it is for the occiput transverse baby in a vertex presentation.*

7-0. Final internal rotation of the head: Beginning prior to the birth of the posterior arm, the head begins its final internal rotation when it reaches the pelvic cavity. If the occiput entered the brim transverse, it begins to rotate 45° to an anterior oblique orientation. While this occurs, the posterior arm is born. After the posterior arm emerges, the occiput continues to rotate to OA, 90° in all, bringing it under the pubic bone and the face into the hollow of the sacrum. If the occiput engaged in an anterior oblique orientation, it rotates only 45° to become directly anterior. Either way, once the posterior arm is born, the torso is free to follow this movement.

8-O. The birth of the flexed head: The flexed head is born most easily when the upright mother leans forward. This causes the well-descended occiput to pivot against the pubic bone, allowing the flexed chin to emerge first. The perineum retracts as the mouth, nose and forehead follow posteriorly and the occiput and vertex emerge anteriorly. The pelvis, shoulders and arms work to dilate the soft passages for the head, which is born in reverse relative to a cephalic presentation (when the largest and hardest part of the baby dilates the soft passages first and the widest transverse diameter of the skull emerges first). As the head descends, the narrow planes of the neck lead the way, followed by increasingly larger planes through the biparietal. This process of increasingly wider diameters dilating the already stretched soft tissues often results in the well-flexed and unobstructed aftercoming head being born quickly and easily.

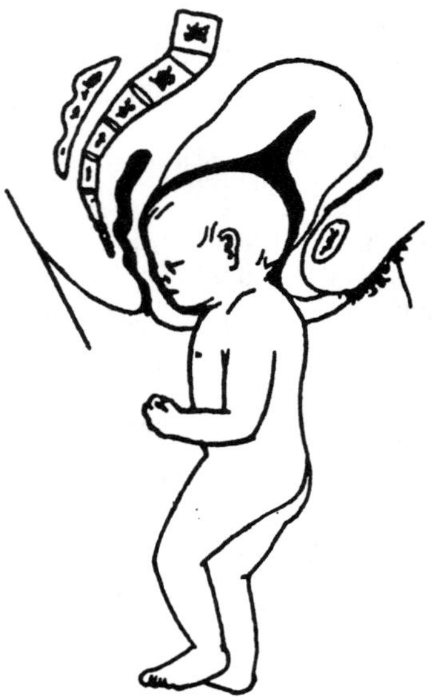

Flexed head is now OA, occiput is moving past pubic bone, perineum is stretching.

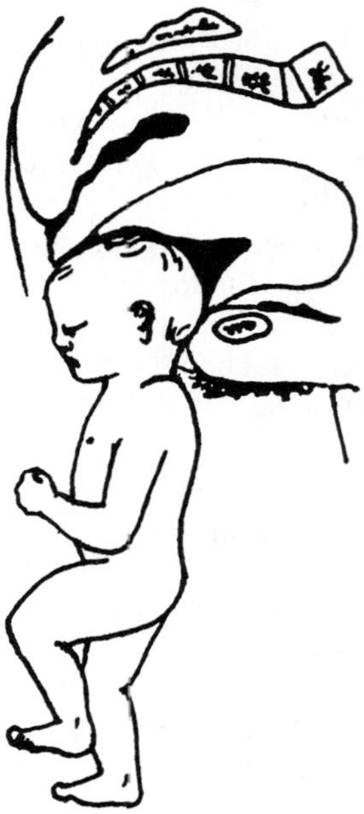

The mother leans forward when the nape of the neck is visible. The occiput pivots around the pubic arch, the face is born and the crown of the vertex is almost born.

Moulding of the Pelvis and Head in Breech Births

The baby's pelvis is not completely ossified at term rendering it compactible during descent. Most such moulding will resolve once the pelvis is freed from the birth canal, although minor joint misalignments should be expected and the baby should see a chiropractor or osteopath after birth for evaluation and adjustments, if required. Breech babies do not form caputs on their heads, but the anterior buttock may develop a caput-like swelling and the genitals may be swollen, especially if the baby descended frank breech. If an extended leg was the leading part, it may be swollen or bruised.

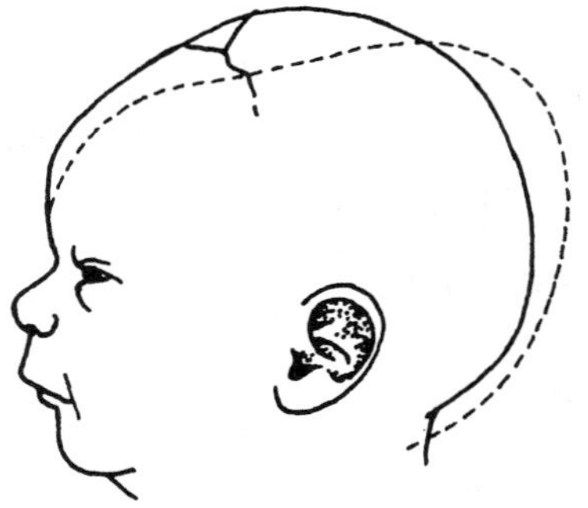

Flattening of the vertex

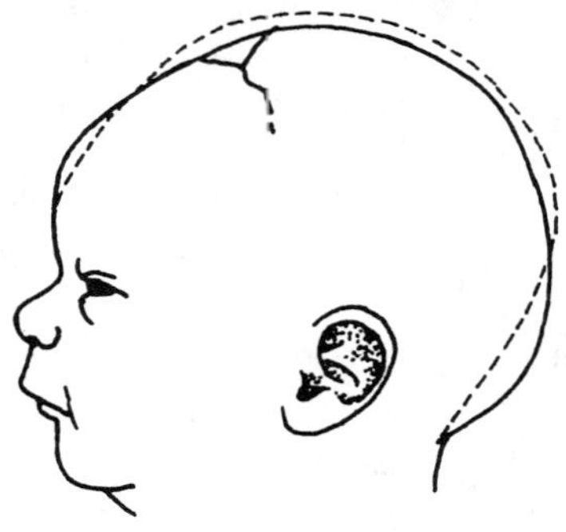

Rounding of the vertex

Cephalic moulding may begin prenatally or with the force of labor contractions, especially in primigravidas with good muscle tone. In such instances, the pressure from the fundus flattens the vertex. However, in most cases, compression from above does not result in obvious flattening, and cephalic moulding is otherwise minimal due to the rapidity with which the head passes through the pelvis. The baby's head is often slightly rounded as a result. This type of moulding usually elongates the submentovertical diameter, so that the crown of the head is slightly elevated, but such moulding may not be obvious.

Master Table of Sacrum Anterior Breech Descent

Master Table of Cardinal Spiraling Movements in Sacrum Anterior Breech Descent		
Sacrum (Lower Torso) and Legs	**Shoulders (Upper Torso)**	**Head**
1-B. Spinal flexion prior to labor *Frank: may be impaired*	*1-S. Spinal flexion prior to labor* *Frank: may be impaired*	**1-O. Flexion of the head prior to labor** **Frank: may be impaired**
2-B. Descent	*2-S. Descent in concert with breech*	*2-O. Descent in concert with torso*
3-B. Engagement sacrum anterior oblique or directly anterior **Complete-incomplete: waist may twist to orient sacrum**	• *Complete/incomplete: Internal rotation does not occur*	• *Complete-incomplete: Internal rotation does not occur*
• Dilating the soft birth canal		
4-B. Frank: Internal rotation to sacrum transverse **Complete/incomplete: internal restitution if waist is twisted and/or waist twists as sacrum rotates to transverse.**	*3-S. Frank: Internal rotation with breech* *Complete/incomplete: Internal rotation does not occur if waist twists*	*3-O. Frank: Internal rotation with torso* *Complete/incomplete: Internal rotation does not occur if waist twists*
5-B. Lateral flexion of spine (as possible) • Dilating the perineum *B. Incomplete: birth of legs* • Frank/complete: Rumping of the breech		
6-B. Birth of the anterior and posterior buttock by lateral spinal flexion *B. Complete: birth of legs*		
7-B. External restitution (if waist is twisted)		
8-B. First external rotation with upper torso to sacrum anterior	**4-S. Internal rotation–to bring long axis of shoulders transverse**	*4-O. Internal rotation with torso to bring occiput anterior*
	5-S. Engagement (as umbilicus is born) *S. Flexion of shoulders*	
9-B. Second external rotation with upper torso to sacrum transverse	**6-S. Internal rotation to left or right to bring long axis of shoulders AP**	*5-O. Internal rotation with upper torso to bring occiput transverse* *Complete/incomplete: neck may twist to allow occiput to lag behind in an anterior-oblique orientation*
B. Frank: birth of legs (may occur as shoulders are born) *B. Once the legs are born, the baby may flex them, which aids head flexion.*	**7-S. Birth of the anterior arm and shoulder by lateroflexion of upper spine**	*6-O. Engagement (as shoulders reach outlet)*
10-B. Third external rotation with head–to sacrum anterior	*8-S. Slight movement to left or right as posterior arm is born–then shoulders follow head, rotating externally to transverse*	**7-O. Internal rotation begins before and completes after posterior arm is born to bring occiput anterior**
		8-O. Birth of head by flexion

A Note to Students

To facilitate your grasp of the summaries that follow, make a copy of the tables of the cardinal spiraling movements in anterior frank breeches and anterior complete/incomplete breeches to use as guides as you study. Numbers in the tables correspond to the numbers in the summaries. In all the breech summaries, movements that occur as a consequence of the descending parts are in italics. Once you are familiar with the movements for each attitude, you can use the master table given on the previous page for reference. You may find it helpful to create a blank table for yourself and fill in the blanks with each movement from the summaries for each type of descent. In writing the summaries it has been a challenge throughout to find the balance between enough details and too many; therefore every possible movement is not included.

The cardinal movements are lettered and numbered (i.e., B-1) as shown in the tables. Particulars relevant to the attitude of the legs are noted as appropriate. These summaries also include a variety of options for movement at different points to impress upon you the variability of breech descent, which are listed from most to least likely, based on my understanding of fetal descent in general (most of these nuances have not ever been discussed in a text, therefore, what is known about fetal descent was applied hypothetically). Options are suggested for frank versus complete/incomplete descent, and are given according to probability, not absolutes. Because of their complexity, the summaries for breech descent use a somewhat different system of designation than do those for cephalic descent. Because letters are already used to indicate the denominators in the cardinal movements, when options are listed, cardinal movement are shown by a number in parentheses to indicate different options, for example 3-S(1). When relevant, these are further defined by a hyphen and an L (for leftward movement) or a R (for rightward movement). If no distinction is made regarding the attitude of the legs, that step is valid for all types of attitudes. If an L or R is lacking on a numbered step, it is either irrelevant or written in such as way that it can be . Even in a series which includes numbered steps, if no number is shown, that step is universally applicable as well. Focus on one series of options through each read-through to obtain a more simplified understanding. For example, follow the entire explanation for frank descent, choosing only one set of options (when applicable, for example, only leftward rotation). Assuming that the student is already familiar with how to follow optional movements from the other summaries and because these descriptions are so complex, notations such as "follow the '1' entries below" have been eliminated to simplify the text as much as possible.

The serial illustrations of breech birth in the summary chapters have been depicted with the baby in a complete attitude because it does not impair spinal flexion, thus descent is more complex. Frank breech descent is illustrated in the chapter entitled "Assisting at the Birth of a Breech Baby" with drawings rendered from actual photographs of breech births.

Once you have a working understanding of breech descent, see the chapter entitled "Variations in Breech Descent and Rotation" for more details. You may be wondering why I have included so many details regarding options for descent. It may seem unnecessarily confusing. You will see relatively few breech births in your career. Becoming *fluent* in the many possibilities for breech descent will help you not to freak out and intervene when birth is, in fact, proceeding normally.

Summary of the Cardinal Spiraling Movements: Left Sacrum Anterior (LSA)

Orientation of the baby to the mother's pelvis

The sacrum occupies the left anterior corner of the mother's pelvis (LSA), and the occiput is situated in the left anterior corner of the fundus (LOA). The long axes of the pelvis and shoulders are aligned with the left oblique diameter of the brim. The genital crease and sagittal suture are aligned with the right oblique diameter of the brim.

Descent and birth of the LSA breech

1-B, 1-S & 1-O. *Flexion of the lower torso begins prior to labor and is prompted by flexion of the head.*

1-B. Frank: *Splinting of the legs may impair flexion until the feet are born.*

2-B. The breech descends through the birth canal as labor progresses.

2-S & 2-O. *The entire baby moves down as the breech descends.*

3-B. The breech engages as the bitrochanteric diameter passes through the left oblique diameter of the brim, with the anterior hip frequently leading the way. After engagement, the breech often remains high in the pelvis until the membranes rupture or dilation is nearly complete.

4-B & 5-B. The breech rotates internally a total 45° from LSA to LST, as the lower torso descends through the deepest curve of the birth canal, requiring the spine to flex laterally. Rotation consists of a downwardly spiraling movement, which facilitates descent.

3-S & 3-O. Frank: *Because the legs are splinted, the entire torso and head undergo their first internal rotation as the breech moves to LST.*

3-S & 3-O. Complete/incomplete: *Internal rotation may occur as the baby turns at the waist, allowing the upper torso and shoulders to remain aligned with the left oblique pelvic diameter and the head to remain LOA.*

- **Frank/complete:** As pushing proceeds, the breech rumps.

6-B. Frank: The breech is born as the spine flexes laterally. The anterior buttock emerges, followed by the posterior buttock.

6-B. Complete/incomplete: The buttocks emerge during or after the birth of the legs.

B. *The legs are born according to their attitude.*

Frank: *Spontaneous emergence of the legs may not occur until the shoulders are being born.*

Incomplete: *The extended legs emerge before the breech.*

Complete: *The flexed legs usually disengage as the buttocks are born or immediately thereafter.*

7-B. Frank: No restitution occurs if the waist is not twisted.

7-B. Complete/incomplete: Restitution occurs if the waist is twisted to allow the breech to rotate 45° from LST back to the LSA position, restoring the long axis of the pelvis to a parallel relationship with the long axis of the shoulders.

Descent and birth of the upper torso, shoulders and arms

1-S & 1-O. *Flexion of the upper torso begins prior to labor and is prompted by flexion of the head.*

2-S & 2-O. *The upper torso and head continue to descend throughout labor.*

4-S. Frank: The entire torso undergoes its second internal rotation as the shoulders move 45° from the anteroposterior to the left oblique and then 45° to the transverse diameter, 90° in all.

8-B. Frank: *The breech rotates externally from LST to LSA to SA.*

4-O. Frank: *The head follows the torso by rotating internally from LOT to LOA to OA.*

4-S. Complete/incomplete: If the buttocks have restituted, the upper torso and shoulders undergo their first internal rotation by moving 45° from the left oblique to the transverse diameter before they enter the brim.

8-B. Complete/incomplete: *The breech follows the upper torso by rotating externally from LSA to SA.*

4-O. Complete/incomplete: *The head follows the upper torso by rotating internally from LOA to OA.*

5-S. The shoulders engage when the bisacromial diameter passes through the transverse diameter of the brim as the umbilicus is born. The attitude of the shoulders changes as necessary during descent.

6-S. The final internal rotation of the upper torso and shoulders occurs as they move a total of 90°. Beginning in the transverse diameter, the shoulders first rotate 45° to the left oblique diameter and then 45° to the anteroposterior diameter. This movement allows the thoracic spine to flex laterally as it passes through the deepest curve of the birth canal.

9-B. *The breech follows the upper torso by rotating externally from SA to LSA to LST.*

5-O. The head usually follows the torso by rotating internally from OA to LOA to LOT.

Note: Final internal rotation of the upper torso and shoulders could just as easily move to the right. (Follow summary for RSA, beginning with 6-S.)

7-S. The spine flexes laterally as the anterior shoulder and arm emerge from under the pubic arch.

6-O. The head engages LOT when the biparietal diameter passes through the anteroposterior diameter of the brim, as the shoulders reach the outlet.

8-S & 7-O. The shoulders may now make a slight movement to the left or right as the posterior shoulder and arm emerge. Simultaneously, the head begins its final internal rotation from LOT or LOA to OA. Once both shoulders are born, the torso is freed to rotate externally as it follows the head.

10-B. The breech makes its final external rotation, moving from LST or LSA to SA with the upper torso and head.

<u>**Descent and birth of the head**</u>

1-O. The head begins labor in an LOA orientation. It is usually flexed prior to the onset of labor. Flexion is often enhanced as the fundus gathers around the head during descent of the torso, as the baby lifts his legs after they have emerged, and finally as the occiput passes under the pubic bone.

2-O. The head descends continuously throughout labor as the lower body moves down.

8-O. The head is born as the nape of the neck and chin emerge, followed by the face, occiput and vertex.

Most pelvic moulding resolves upon release from the introitus. Cephalic moulding is usually minimal. Any caput that forms will develop over the left buttock.

LSA orientation, head and spine partly flexed	Internal rotation of the anterior hip, as sacrum rotates LSA to LST	Descent and birth of anterior hip and leg	Birth of posterior leg and restitution of breech, LST to LSA
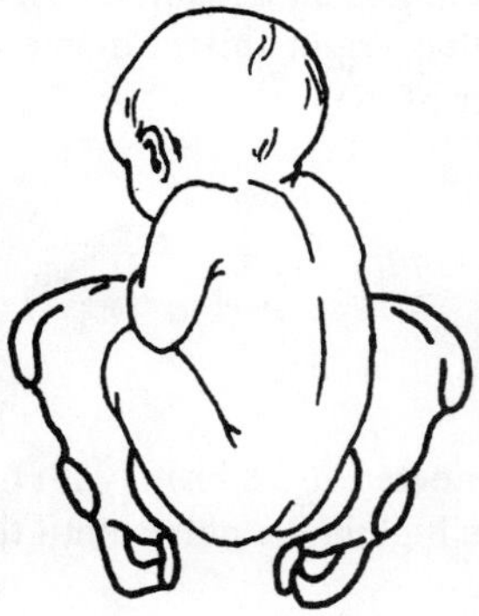	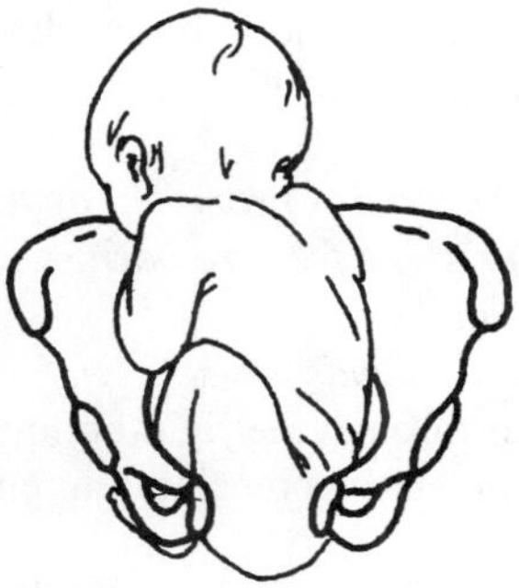	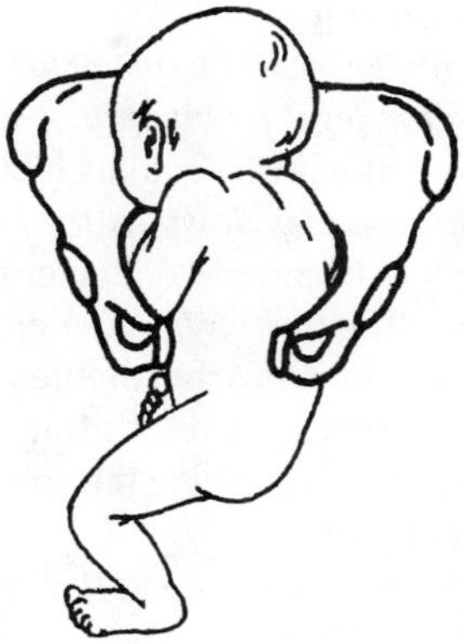	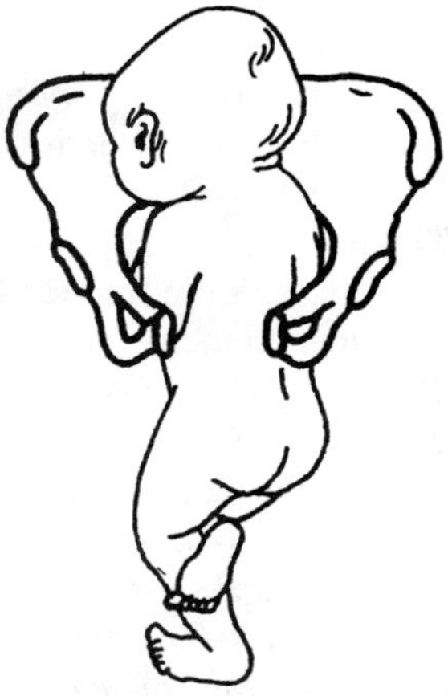
Internal rotation of shoulders to transverse for engagement: breech rotates LSA to LST	Shoulders rotate to AP, head engages, anterior arm is born	Posterior arm is born, head begins internal rotation to OA	Head finishes rotation to OA and is born by flexion.
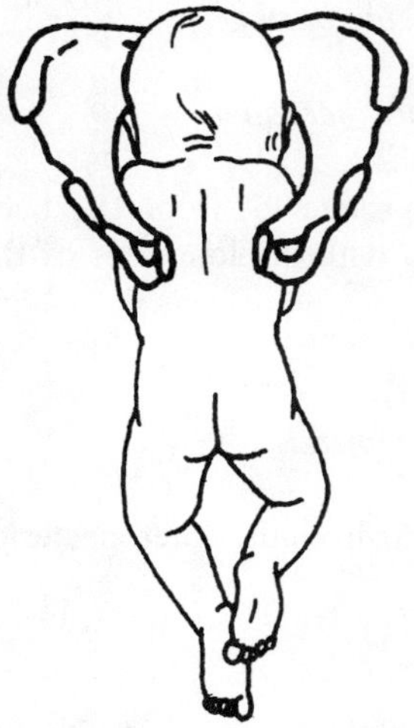	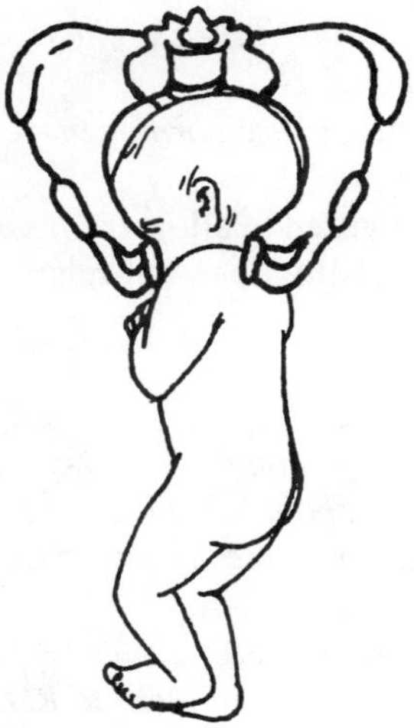	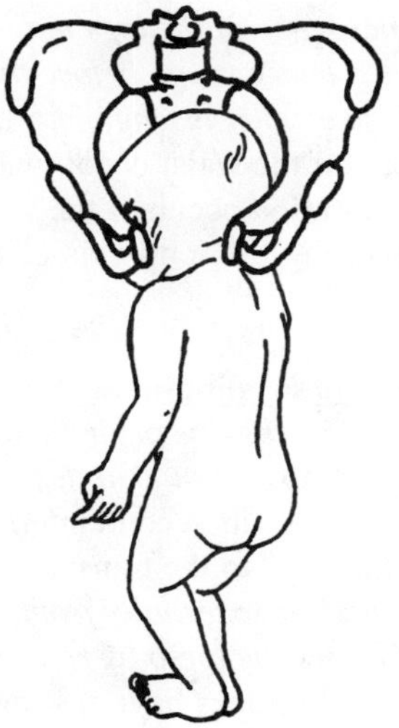	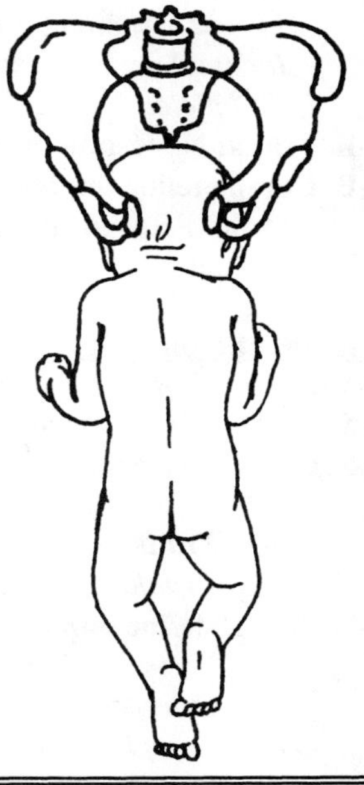

Summary of the Cardinal Spiraling Movements: Right Sacrum Anterior (RSA)

Orientation of the baby to the mother's pelvis

The sacrum occupies the right anterior corner of the mother's pelvis (RSA) and the occiput is situated in the right anterior corner of the fundus (ROA). The long axes of the pelvis and shoulders are aligned with the right oblique diameter of the brim. The genital crease and sagittal suture are aligned with the left oblique diameter of the brim.

Descent and birth of the RSA breech

1-B, 1-S & 1-O. *Flexion of the lower torso begins prior to labor and is prompted by flexion of the head.*

1-B. Frank: *Splinting of the legs may impair flexion until the feet are born.*

2-B. The breech descends through the birth canal as labor progresses.

2-S & 2-O. *The entire baby moves down as the breech descends.*

3-B. The breech engages as the bitrochanteric diameter passes through the right oblique diameter of the brim, with the anterior hip frequently leading the way. After engagement, the breech often remains high in the pelvis until the membranes rupture or dilation is nearly complete.

4-B & 5-B. The breech rotates internally a total of 45°, from RSA to RST, as the lower torso descends through the deepest curve of the birth canal, requiring the spine to flex laterally. Rotation consists of a downwardly spiraling movement, which facilitates descent.

3-S & 3-O. Frank: *Because the legs are splinted, the entire torso and head undergo their first internal rotation as the breech moves to RST.*

3-S & 3-O. Complete/incomplete: *Internal rotation may occur as the baby turns at the waist, allowing the upper torso and shoulders to remain aligned with the right oblique pelvic diameter and the head to remain ROA.*

- **Frank/complete:** As pushing proceeds, the breech rumps.

6-B. Frank: The breech is born as the spine flexes laterally. The anterior buttock emerges, followed by the posterior buttock.

6-B. Complete/incomplete: The buttocks emerge during or after the birth of the legs.

B. *The legs are born according to their attitude.*

Frank: *Spontaneous emergence of the legs may not occur until the shoulders are being born.*

Incomplete: *The extended legs emerge before the breech.*

Complete: *The flexed legs usually disengage as the buttocks are born or immediately thereafter.*

7-B. Frank: No restitution occurs if the waist is not twisted.

7-B. Complete/incomplete: Restitution occurs if the waist is twisted to allow the breech to rotate 45° from RST back to the RSA position, restoring the long axis of the pelvis to a parallel relationship with the long axis of the shoulders.

Descent and birth of the upper torso, shoulders and arms

1-S & 1-O. *Flexion of the upper torso begins prior to labor and is prompted by flexion of the head.*

2-S & 2-O. *The upper torso and head continue to descend throughout labor.*

4-S. Frank: The entire torso undergoes its second internal rotation as the shoulders move 45° from the anteroposterior to the right oblique and then 45° to the transverse diameter, 90° in all.

8-B. Frank: *The breech rotates externally from RST to RSA to SA.*

4-O. Frank: *The head follows the torso by rotating internally from ROT to ROA to OA.*

4-S. Complete/incomplete: If the buttocks have restituted, the upper torso and shoulders undergo their first internal rotation by moving 45° from the right oblique to the transverse diameter before they enter the brim.

8-B. Complete/incomplete: *The breech follows the upper torso by rotating externally from RSA to SA.*

4-O. Complete/incomplete: *The head follows the upper torso by rotating internally from ROA to OA.*

5-S. The shoulders engage when the bisacromial diameter passes through the transverse diameter of the brim as the umbilicus is born. The attitude of the shoulders changes as necessary during descent.

6-S. The final internal rotation of the upper torso and shoulders occurs as they move a total of 90°. Beginning in the transverse diameter, the shoulders first rotate 45° to the right oblique diameter and then 45° to the anteroposterior diameter. This movement allows the thoracic spine to flex laterally as it passes through the deepest curve of the birth canal.

9-B. *The breech follows the upper torso by rotating externally from SA to RSA to RST.*

5-O. The head usually follows the torso by rotating internally from OA to ROA to ROT.

Note: Final internal rotation of the upper torso and shoulders could just as easily move to the left. (Follow summary for LSA, beginning with 6-S.)

7-S. The spine flexes laterally as the anterior shoulder and arm emerge from under the pubic arch.

6-O. The head engages ROT when the biparietal diameter passes through the anteroposterior diameter of the brim, as the shoulders reach the outlet.

8-S & 7-O. The shoulders may now make a slight movement to the left or right as the posterior shoulder and arm emerge. Simultaneously, the head begins its final internal rotation, from ROT or ROA to OA. Once both shoulders are born, the torso is freed to rotate externally as it follows the head.

10-B. The breech makes its final external rotation, moving from RST to RSA to SA with the upper torso and head.

Descent and birth of the head

1-O. The head begins labor in an ROA orientation. It is usually flexed prior to the onset of labor. Flexion is often enhanced as the fundus gathers around the head during descent of the torso, as the baby lifts his legs after they have emerged and finally as the occiput passes under the pubic bone.

2-O. The head descends continuously throughout labor as the lower body moves down.

8-O. The head is born as the nape of the neck and chin emerge, followed by the face, occiput and vertex.

Most pelvic moulding resolves upon release from the introitus. Cephalic moulding is usually minimal. Any caput that forms will develop over the right buttock.

RSA Orientation, head and spine partly flexed	Internal rotation of the anterior hip, as sacrum rotates RSA to RST	Descent and birth of anterior hip and leg	Birth of posterior leg and restitution of breech, RST to RSA
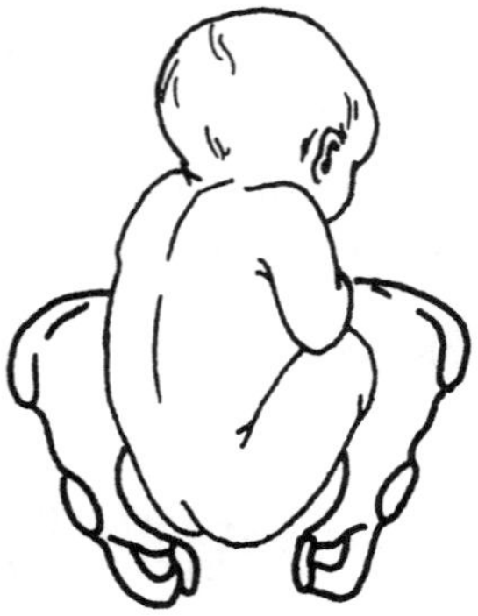	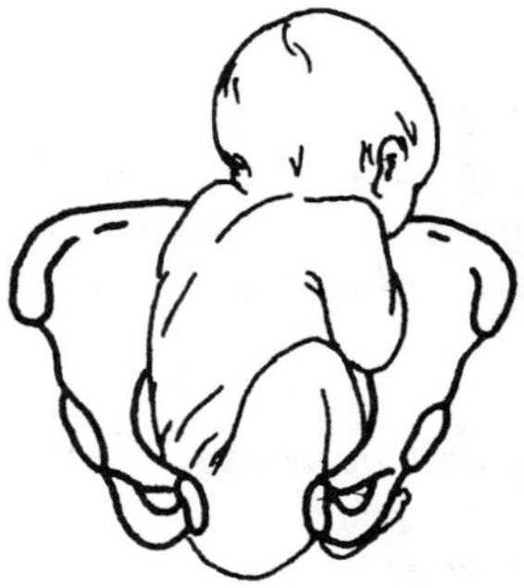	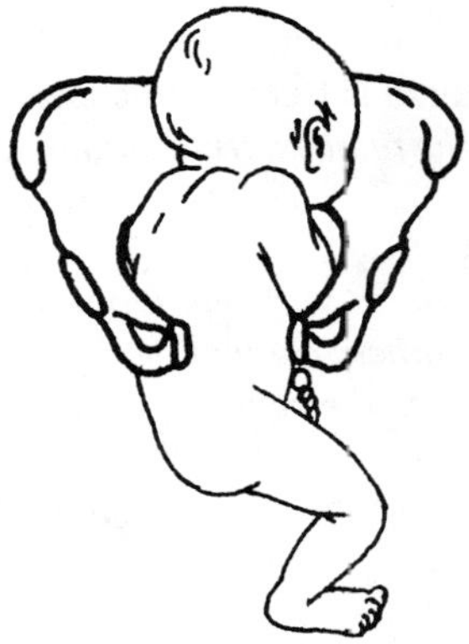	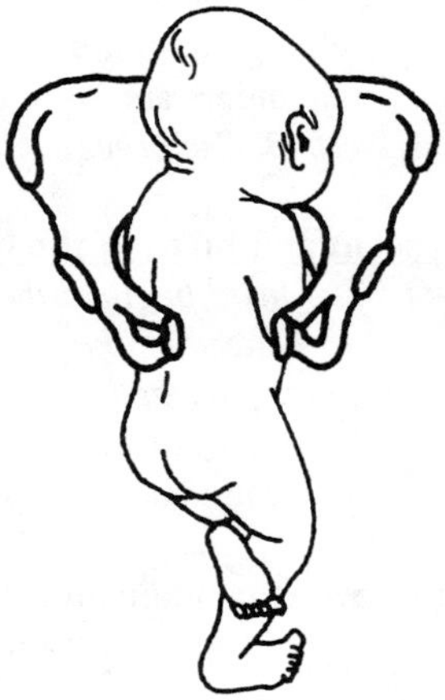
Internal rotation of shoulders to transverse for engagement; breech rotates RSA to RST	Shoulders rotate to AP, head engages, anterior arm is born	Posterior arm is born, head begins internal rotation to OA	Head finishes rotation to OA and is born by flexion
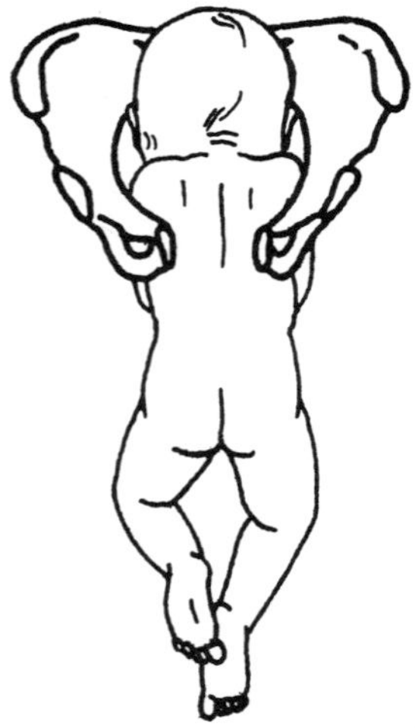	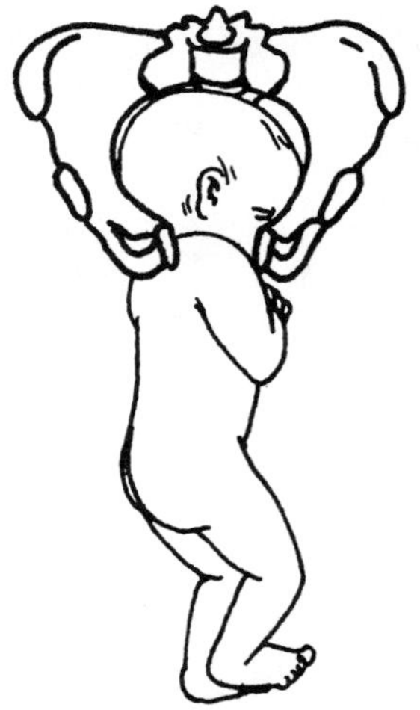	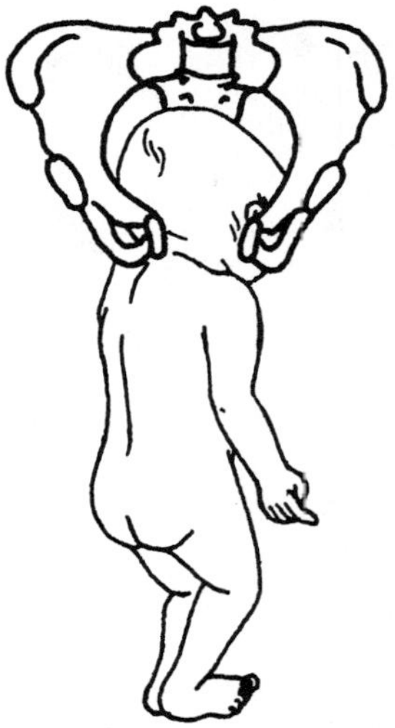	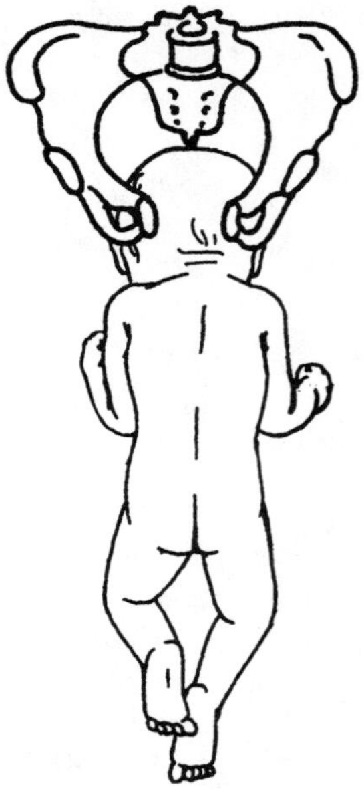

SUMMARY OF THE CARDINAL SPIRALING MOVEMENTS: SACRUM ANTERIOR (SA)

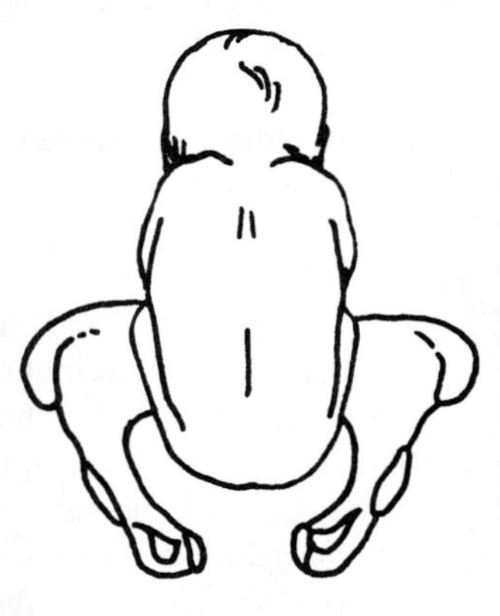
SA baby in a complete attitude before descent begins.

Birth with the baby SA is similar to other anterior breech births. Direct sacrum anterior birth is quite common, unlike directly anterior cephalic presentations. Therefore, this summary is placed in order with the other most common anterior positions. Because of the complexity of this description, no attempt was made to provide illustrations. Before studying this chapter, you should have a thorough, working knowledge of the cardinal movements in LSA and RSA descent. It is possible for the breech, shoulders and head to engage and descend transverse, without undergoing any significant internal or external rotations. This is most likely to occur if the baby is on the small side and the pelvis is large.

Orientation of the baby to the mother's pelvis

The sacrum is directly anterior (SA) (under the symphysis), and the occiput is situated in the anterior midline of the mother's torso (OA). The long axes of the pelvis and shoulder are aligned with the transverse diameter of the brim. The genital crease and sagittal suture are aligned with the anteroposterior diameter of the brim.

Descent and birth of the breech (movements not illustrated)

1-B, 1-S & 1-O. *Flexion of the lower torso begins prior to labor and is prompted by flexion of the head.*

1-B. Frank: *Splinting of the legs may impair flexion until the feet are born.*

2-B. The breech descends through the birth canal as labor progresses.

2-S & 2-O. *The entire baby moves down as the breech descends.*

3-B. The breech engages as the bitrochanteric diameter passes through the transverse diameter of the brim. After engagement, the breech often remains high in the pelvis until the membranes rupture or dilation is nearly complete.

4-B & 5-B. Internal rotation may occur as the lower torso descends into the deepest curve of the birth canal, requiring the spine to flex laterally. Rotation consists of a downwardly spiraling movement, which facilitates descent. Rotation may occur to the left or right or not at all, as follows:

To the left (1-L): The breech rotates internally 45° from SA to LSA.

3-S & 3-O(1-L). Frank: *Because the legs are splinted, the entire torso and head may undergo their first internal rotation as the breech moves to LSA.*

3-S & 3-O(1-L). Complete/incomplete: *Internal rotation may occur as the baby turns at the waist, allowing the upper torso and shoulders to remain aligned with the transverse pelvic diameter and the head to remain OA.*

Conversion to LSA may occur:

Frank: The entire baby rotates 90°, from SA to LSA to LST.

Complete/incomplete: Beginning from SA, the breech, upper torso and head undergo their first internal rotation of 45° to LSA. The baby may turn at the waist as the breech rotates another 45° to LST, which allows the shoulders to remain aligned with the left oblique pelvic diameter and the head to remain LOA. (Follow LSA summary, page 201, beginning with 6-B.)

To the right (2-R): The breech rotates internally 45° from SA to RSA.

3-S & 3-O(2-R). Frank: *Because the legs are splinted, the entire torso and head may undergo their first internal rotation as the breech moves to RSA.*

3-S & 3-O(2-R). Complete/incomplete: *Internal rotation may occur as the baby turns at the waist, allowing the upper torso and shoulders to remain aligned with the transverse diameter and the head to remain OA.*

Conversion to RSA may occur:

Frank: The entire baby rotates 90°, from SA to RSA to RST.

Complete/incomplete: Beginning from SA, the breech, upper torso and head undergo their first internal rotation of 45° to RSA. The baby may turn at the waist as the breech rotates another 45° to RST, which allows the shoulders to remain aligned with the right oblique pelvic diameter and head to remain ROA. (Follow RSA summary, page 204, beginning with 6-B.)

The baby may remain SA (3). Internal rotation does not occur. The baby remains in the SA position, taking advantage of the anteroposterior flexibility of the spine, which bends backward as the lower torso passes through the deepest curve of the birth canal.

3-S(3) & 3-O(3). The upper torso and head do not rotate internally, remaining in anatomical alignment with the breech.

- **Frank/complete:** As pushing proceeds, the breech rumps.

6-B. The breech is born by a process of spinal flexion. The direction of spinal flexion varies according to the orientation of the back.

6-B(1) or 6-B(2). Frank: The birth of the breech occurs as the spine flexes laterally. The anterior buttock emerges, followed by the posterior buttock.

6-B(2). Complete/incomplete: The buttocks emerge during or after the birth of the legs.

6-B(3). The breech is born as the buttocks emerge more or less simultaneously.

B. *The legs are born according to their attitude.*

Frank: *Spontaneous emergence of the legs may not occur until the shoulders are being born.*

Incomplete: *The extended legs emerge before the breech.*

Complete: *The flexed legs usually disengage as the buttocks are born or immediately thereafter.*

7-B. Restitution occurs only if the waist is twisted to restore the long axis of the pelvis to a parallel relationship with the long axis of the shoulders.

7-B(1) or 7-B(2). Frank: No restitution occurs.

7-B(1-L). Complete/incomplete: Restitution occurs if the waist is twisted to allow the breech to rotate 45° from LSA back to the SA position.

7-B(2-R). Complete/incomplete: Restitution occurs if the waist is twisted to allow the breech to rotate 45° from RSA back to the SA position.

7-B(3). No restitution occurs.

<u>Descent and birth of the upper torso, shoulders and arms when the sacrum descends SA</u>

1-S & 1-O. *Flexion of the upper torso begins prior to labor and is prompted by flexion of the head.*

2-S & 2-O. *The upper torso and head continue to descend throughout labor.*

4-S. Internal rotation may occur before the shoulders engage.

4-S(1-L). Frank: The upper torso undergoes a second internal rotation as the shoulders move 45° from the left oblique to the transverse diameter.

8-B(1-L) & 4-O(1-L). Frank: *The breech follows, externally rotating from LSA to SA and the head follows, internally rotating from LOA to OA.*

4-S(2-R). Frank: The entire torso undergoes a second internal rotation as the shoulders move 45° from the right oblique to the transverse diameter.

8-B(2-R) & 4-O(2-R). Frank: *The breech follows, externally rotating from RSA to SA and the head follows, internally rotating from ROA to OA.*

4-S(1) or 4-S(2). Complete/incomplete: No internal rotation occurs as the shoulders are already aligned with the transverse diameter of the brim.

8-B(1) & 4-O(1) or 8-B(2) 4-O(2). Complete/incomplete: *No rotation occurs. The breech remains SA and head remains OA.*

4-S(3). No internal rotation occurs as the shoulders are already aligned with the transverse diameter of the brim.

8-B(3) & 4-O(3). *No rotation occurs. The breech remains SA and the head remains OA.*

5-S. The shoulders engage when the bisacromial diameter passes through the transverse diameter of the brim as the umbilicus is born. The attitude of the shoulders changes as necessary during descent.

6-S. Internal rotation of the upper torso and shoulders may occur as the upper torso descends into the deepest curve of the birth canal, to allow the spine to flex laterally. The baby could convert to another position during internal rotation, as follows:

To LSA: (Follow LSA summary, page 201, beginning with 6-S.)

To RSA: (Follow RSA summary, page 204, beginning with 6-S)

When the baby does not convert to another position, internal rotation of the upper torso and shoulders may take place in one of the following ways:

6-S(1-L). The upper torso and shoulders rotate 45°, moving the shoulders from the transverse to the left oblique diameter.

9-B(1-L). *The breech follows the upper torso by rotating externally 45° from SA to LSA.*

5-O(1-L). *The head usually follows the upper torso by rotating internally from OA to LOA.*

6-S(2-R). The upper torso and shoulders rotate 45°, moving the shoulders from the transverse to the right oblique diameter.

9-B(2-R). *The breech follows the upper torso by rotating externally 45° from SA to RSA.*

5-O(2). *The head usually follows the upper torso by rotating internally from OA to ROA.*

6-S(3). No internal rotation occurs as the upper torso and shoulders descend through the transverse diameter of the outlet, taking advantage of the anteroposterior flexibility of the spine.

9-B(3). & 5-O(3). *The breech remains SA and the head remains OA.*

7-S(1) & 7-S(2). The spine flexes laterally as the anterior shoulder and arm emerge from under the pubic arch.

6-O(1-L). *The head engages LOA when the biparietal diameter passes through the left oblique diameter of the brim as the shoulders reach the outlet.*

6-O(2-R). *The head engages ROA when the biparietal diameter passes through the right oblique diameter of the brim as the shoulders reach the outlet.*

7-S(3). The arms emerge more or less simultaneously as the spine flexes and the shoulder axis adjusts as necessary.

6-O(3). *The head engages directly OA.*

8-S(1), 8-S(2) or 8-S(3). The shoulders may make a slight movement to the left or right as the posterior shoulder and arm emerge. Once the posterior arm is born, the torso is freed to follow any movement that the head may make.

7-O(1-L). As the posterior arm emerges, the upper torso follows the head as it undergoes its final internal rotation from LOA to OA.

10-B(1-L). *The breech follows the movements of the upper torso, rotating externally to SA.*

7-O(2-R). As the posterior arm emerges, the upper torso follows the head as it undergoes its final internal rotation from ROA to OA.

10-B(2-R). *The breech follows the movements of the upper torso, rotating externally to SA.*

7-O(3). No internal rotation occurs. The head is already OA.

10-B(3). *No external rotation occurs. The torso is already SA.*

Descent and birth of the head

1-O. *The head begins labor in an OA orientation. It is usually flexed prior to the onset of labor. Flexion is often enhanced as the fundus gathers around the head during descent of the torso, as the baby lifts his legs after they have emerged, and finally as the occiput passes under the pubic bone.*

2-O. *Descent occurs continuously throughout labor as the lower body moves down.*

8-O. The flexed head is born OA as the nape of the neck and chin emerge, followed by the face, occiput and vertex.

Most pelvic moulding resolves upon release from the introitus. Cephalic moulding is usually minimal. Any caput is likely to be over the central portion of the buttocks.

SUMMARY OF THE CARDINAL SPIRALING MOVEMENTS: LEFT SACRUM TRANSVERSE (LST)

The baby rarely presents with the sacrum transverse, almost always choosing the more favorable oblique angle to accommodate the long axis of the pelvis. In fact, transverse positioning is considered so rare, that textbooks old and new do not describe its movements. The explanations in this chapter and the next are derived from a general understanding of the process of breech descent.

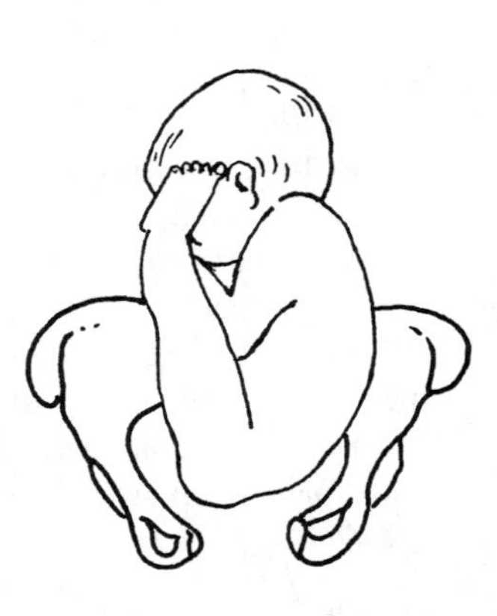

LST baby in frank attitude before descent begins.

Orientation of the baby to the mother's pelvis

The sacrum occupies the left side of the mother's pelvis (LST) and the occiput is situated to the left of the mother's torso (LOT). The long axes of the pelvis and shoulders are aligned with the anteroposterior diameter of the brim. The genital crease and the sagittal suture are aligned with the transverse diameter of the brim.

Descent and birth of the breech (movements not illustrated)

1-B, 1-S & 1-O. *Flexion of the lower torso begins prior to labor and is prompted by flexion of the head.*

1-B. Frank: *Splinting of the legs may impair flexion until the feet are born.*

2-B. The breech descends through the birth canal as labor progresses.

2-S & 2-O. *The entire baby moves down as the breech descends.*

3-B. The breech engages as the bitrochanteric diameter passes through the brim, with the anterior hip frequently leading the way.

3-B. Frank: The breech descends through the anteroposterior diameter (LST).

3-S & 3-O. Frank: *The upper torso and head do not rotate internally, remaining aligned with the breech.*

3-B. Complete/incomplete: The breech rotates internally 45°, from LST to LSA, as it enters the brim. Internal rotation is accomplished as the baby turns at the waist.

3-S & 3-O. Complete/incomplete: *Twisting of the waist allows the baby's upper torso to remain aligned with the anteroposterior diameter of the brim and the head to remain LOT.*

After engagement, the breech often remains high in the pelvis until the membranes rupture or dilation is nearly complete.

Conversion to LSA may also occur: The entire baby rotates 45° to LSA. (Follow LSA summary, page 201, beginning with 4-B.)

4-B & 5-B. Frank: If the baby engaged LST, no internal rotation occurs because the spine is already poised to flex laterally through the deepest curve of the birth canal.

4-B & 5-B. Complete/incomplete: Internal rotation is replaced by internal restitution if the waist untwists, moving the breech 45° from LSA back to LST, restoring the long axis of the pelvis to a parallel relationship with the long axis of the shoulders. This movement allows the lower torso to flex laterally as it descends through the deepest curve of the birth canal.

- **Frank/complete:** As pushing proceeds, the breech rumps.

6-B. Frank: The breech is born as the spine flexes laterally. The anterior buttock emerges, followed by the posterior buttock.

6-B. Complete/incomplete: The buttocks emerge during or after the birth of the legs.

B. *The legs are born according to their attitude.*

Frank: *Spontaneous emergence of the legs may not occur until the shoulders are being born.*

Incomplete: *The extended legs emerge before the breech.*

Complete: *The flexed legs usually disengage as each buttock is born or immediately thereafter.*

Descent and birth of the upper torso, shoulders and arms

1-S & 1-O. *Flexion of the upper torso begins prior to labor and is prompted by flexion of the head.*

2-S & 2-O. *The upper torso and head continue to descend throughout labor.*

4-S. After the buttocks are born, one of the following may occur:

4-S(1). No internal rotation occurs and the shoulders remain aligned with the anteroposterior diameter of the brim.

8-B(1) & 4-O(1). *The breech remains LST and the head remains LOT.*

4-S(2). The first internal rotation of the upper torso and shoulders begins as they move 45° from the antero-posterior to the left oblique diameter before they enter the brim.

8-B(2). *The breech follows the upper torso by rotating externally from LST to LSA.*

4-O(2). *The head follows the upper torso by rotating internally from LOT to LOA.*

5-S. The shoulders engage when the bisacromial diameter passes through

5-S(1). the anteroposterior diameter of the brim,

5-S(2). the left oblique diameter of the brim,

as the umbilicus is born. The attitude of the shoulders changes as necessary during descent.

6-S(1). The upper torso and shoulders continue to descend through the anteroposterior diameter. No internal rotation occurs because the spine is already poised to flex laterally through the deepest curve of the birth canal.

9-B(1) & 5-O(1). *The breech remains LST and the head remains LOT.*

6-S(2). The second internal rotation of the upper torso and shoulders occurs as they rotate 45° from the left oblique to the anteroposterior diameter. This movement allows the thoracic spine to flex laterally as it descends through the deepest curve of the birth canal.

9-B(2). *The breech rotates externally from LSA to LST.*

5-O(2). *The head rotates internally from LOA to LOT.*

7-S. The spine flexes laterally as the anterior shoulder and arm emerge from under the pubic arch.

6-O. *The head engages LOT when the biparietal diameter passes through the anteroposterior diameter of the brim as the shoulders reach the outlet.*

8-S & 7-O. The shoulders may now make a slight movement to the left or right as the posterior shoulder and arm emerge. Simultaneously, the head begins its final internal rotation, moving from LOT to LOA to OA. Once both shoulders are born, the torso is freed to rotate externally as it follows the head.

10-B. *The breech makes its final external rotation, moving from LST to LSA to SA with the upper torso and head.*

<u>**Descent and birth of the head**</u>

1-O. *The head begins labor in an LOT orientation. It is usually flexed prior to the onset of labor. Flexion is often enhanced as the fundus gathers around the head during descent of the torso, as the baby lifts his legs after they have emerged and finally as the occiput passes under the pubic bone.*

2-O. *Descent occurs continuously throughout labor as the lower body moves down.*

8-O. The flexed head is born from the OA position as the nape of the neck and chin emerge, followed by the face, occiput and vertex.

Moulding is essentially similar for all breech positions. Any caput will form on the left buttock.

SUMMARY OF THE CARDINAL SPIRALING MOVEMENTS: RIGHT SACRUM TRANSVERSE (RST)

RST descent is the mirror image of LST descent.

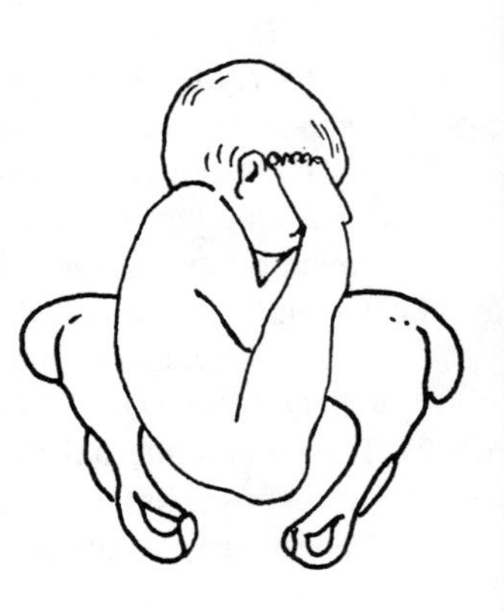

RST baby in frank attitude before descent begins.

Orientation of the baby to the mother's pelvis

The sacrum occupies the right side of the mother's pelvis RST) and the occiput is situated to the right of the mother's torso (ROT). The long axes of the pelvis and shoulders are aligned with the anteroposterior diameter of the brim. The genital crease and the sagittal suture are aligned with the transverse diameter of the brim.

Descent and birth of the breech (movements not illustrated)

1-B, 1-S & 1-O. *Flexion of the lower torso begins prior to labor and is prompted by flexion of the head.*

1-B. Frank: *Splinting of the legs may impair flexion until the feet are born.*

2-B. The breech descends through the birth canal as labor progresses.

2-S & 2-O. *The entire baby moves down as the breech descends.*

3-B. The bitrochanteric diameter engages through the brim, with the anterior hip frequently leading the way.

3-B. Frank: The breech descends through the anteroposterior diameter (RST).

3-S & 3-O. Frank: *Internal rotation does not occur. The upper torso remains aligned with the anteroposterior diameter of the brim and the head remains ROT.*

3-B. Complete/incomplete: The breech may rotate internally 45°, from RST to RSA as it enters the brim. Internal rotation is accomplished as the baby turns at the waist.

3-S & 3-O. Complete/incomplete: *Twisting of the waist allows the baby's upper torso to remain aligned with the anteroposterior diameter of the brim and the head to remain ROT.*

After engagement, the breech often remains high in the pelvis until the membranes rupture or dilation is nearly complete.

Conversion to RSA may also occur: The entire baby rotates 45° to RSA. (Follow RSA summary, page 204, beginning with 4-B.)

4-B & 5-B. Frank: If the baby engaged RST, no internal rotation occurs because the spin is already poised to flex laterally through the deepest curve of the birth canal.

4-B & 5-B. Complete/incomplete: Internal rotation is replaced by internal restitution if the waist is twisted, moving the breech 45° from RSA back to RST, restoring the long axis of the pelvis to a parallel relationship with the long axis of the shoulders. This movement allows the lower torso to flex laterally as it descends through the deepest curve of the birth canal.

- **Frank/complete:** As pushing proceeds, the breech rumps.

6-B. Frank: The breech is born as the spine flexes laterally. The anterior buttock emerges, followed by the posterior buttock.

6-B. Complete/incomplete: The buttocks emerge during or after the birth of the legs.

B. *The legs are born according to their attitude.*

Frank: *Spontaneous emergence of the legs may not occur until the shoulders are being born.*

Incomplete: *The extended legs emerge before the breech.*

Complete: *The flexed legs usually disengage as each buttock is born or immediately thereafter.*

Descent and birth of the upper torso, shoulders and arms

1-S & 1-O. *Flexion of the upper torso begins prior to labor and is prompted by flexion of the head.*

2-S & 2-O. *The upper torso and head continue to descend throughout labor.*

4-S. After the buttocks are born, one of the following may occur:

4-S(1). No internal rotation occurs and the shoulders remain aligned with the anteroposterior diameter of the brim.

8-B(1) & 4-O(1). *The breech remains RST and the head remains ROT.*

4-S(2). The first internal rotation of the upper torso and shoulders occurs as they move 45° from the anteroposterior to the right oblique diameter before they enter the brim.

8-B(2). *The breech follows the upper torso by rotating externally from RST to RSA.*

4-O(2). *The head follows the upper torso by rotating internally from ROT to RA.*

5-S. The shoulders engage when the bisacromial diameter passes through

5-S(1). the anteroposterior diameter of the brim, as the umbilicus is born.

5-S(2). the right oblique diameter of the brim, as the umbilicus is born.

The attitude of the shoulders changes as necessary during descent.

6-S(1). The upper torso and shoulders continue to descend through the anteroposterior diameter. No internal rotation occurs because the spine is already poised to flex laterally through the deepest curve of the birth canal.

9-B(1) & 5-O(1). *The breech remains RST and the head remains ROT.*

6-S(2). The second internal rotation of the upper torso and shoulders occurs as they rotate 45° from the right oblique to the anteroposterior diameter of the brim. This movement allows the thoracic spine to flex laterally as it descends through the deepest curve of the birth canal.

9-B(2). *The breech rotates externally from RSA to RST.*

5-O(2). *The head rotates internally from ROA to ROT.*

7-S. The spine flexes laterally as the anterior shoulder and arm emerge from under the pubic arch.

6-O. *The head engages ROT when the biparietal diameter passes through the anteroposterior diameter of the brim as the shoulders reach the outlet.*

8-S & 7-O. The shoulders may now make a slight movement to the left or right as the posterior shoulder and arm emerge. Simultaneously, the head begins its final internal rotation, moving from ROT to ROA to OA. Once both shoulders are born, the torso is freed to rotate externally as it follows the head.

10-B. *The breech makes its final external rotation, moving from RST to RSA to SA with the upper torso and head.*

Descent and birth of the head

1-O. *The head begins labor in an ROT orientation. It is usually flexed prior to the onset of labor. Flexion is often enhanced as the fundus gathers around the head during descent of the torso, as the baby lifts his legs after they have emerged, and finally as the occiput passes under the pubic bone.*

2-O. *Descent occurs continuously throughout labor as the lower body moves down.*

8-O. The flexed head is born from the OA position as the nape of the neck and chin emerge, followed by the face, occiput and vertex.

Moulding is essentially similar for all breech positions. Any caput will form on the right buttock.

THE PROCESS OF BIRTH IN SACRUM POSTERIOR BREECH PRESENTATIONS

Posterior breech positions are rare. When they do occur, labor often does not progress, the breech remains high in the pelvis and transport is the best and safest option. When labor does progress, rotation to the anterior is the desirable outcome. Although posterior breech positions of any type seldom occur, RSP breeches are more common than LSP. As with posterior positions in other presentations, the sacrum can either undergo long-arc rotation to become directly anterior or, more rarely, short-arc rotation to become directly posterior.

The cardinal movements of birth in long-arc rotation of the sacrum posterior oblique breech

The following tables combine probable movements for frank, complete and incomplete attitudes. (Explanatory notes on the soft tissues have been omitted.)

BREECH (LOWER TORSO) & LEGS	**UPPER TORSO (CHEST) & SHOULDERS**	**HEAD**
Descent begins with the sacrum posterior. The first 3 movements are the same, regardless of when anterior rotation occurs.		
1-B. Spinal flexion (may be impaired) *Frank: further limits flexion*	*1-S. Spinal flexion (may be impaired)* *Frank: further limits flexion*	*1-O. Flexion of head (may be impaired)* *Frank: further limits flexion*
2-B. Descent	*2-S. Descent in concert with breech*	*2-O. Descent in concert with chest*
3-B. Engagement–sacrum posterior oblique		
The baby may undergo long-arc rotation in either a left or a right direction as the breech descends.		
4-B. Long-arc internal rotation begins, bringing the sacrum transverse	*3-S. Long-arc internal rotation begins following breech to bring long axis AP*	*3-O. Long-arc internal rotation begins following upper torso to occiput transverse*
5-B. Lateral flexion of spine (as possible) *B. Incomplete breech: birth of legs* • Frank/complete: Rumping of breech		
6-B. Birth of the anterior and posterior buttock by lateral spinal flexion *B. Complete breech: birth of legs*		
7-B. Restitution does not occur		
Descent continues as for a LSA, LST, RSA or RST position, picking up at movement 4-S.		
If the breech descends posteriorly (as below), long-arc rotation may occur with the upper torso.		
4-B. Frank: No internal rotation, sacrum descends posterior oblique **Complete/incomplete: Internal rotation to transverse may occur as waist twists**	*3-S. Internal rotation does not occur.*	*3-O. Internal rotation does not occur*
5-B. Lateral flexion of the spine *B. Incomplete breech: birth of legs*		
6-B. Birth of the anterior and posterior buttock by lateral spinal flexion *B. Complete breech: birth of legs*		
7-B. Restitution (if waist is twisted)		
8-B. Long-arc external rotation with upper torso from posterior oblique to transverse to anterior oblique to SA	**4-S. Long arc internal rotation–to bring long axis from oblique to AP to oblique to transverse (with back up)**	*4-O. Long arc internal rotation to bring occiput from posterior oblique to transverse to anterior oblique to OA*
Descent proceeds as for a LSA, LST, RSA, or RST position, picking up at movement 5-S. (Table continued on next page.)		

Breech (lower torso) & Legs	Upper torso (chest) & Shoulders	Head
If anterior rotation does not occur with the upper torso, the entire torso descends sacrum posterior and long-arc rotation is postponed until the head is ready to undergo internal rotation.		
1-B. Spinal flexion (may be impaired) *Frank: further limits flexion*	*1-S. Spinal flexion (may be impaired)* *Frank: further limits flexion*	*1-O. Flexion of head (may be impaired)* *Frank: further limits flexion*
2-B. Descent	*2-S. Descent in concert with breech*	*2-O. Descent in concert with chest*
3-B. Engagement– posterior oblique		
4-B. Frank: No internal rotation, sacrum descends posterior oblique **Complete/incomplete: Internal rotation to sacrum transverse may occur as waist twists**	*3-S. Internal rotation does not occur.*	*3-O. Internal rotation does not occur.*
5-B. Lateral flexion of the spine *B. Incomplete breech: birth of legs* • Frank/complete: Rumping of breech		
6-B. Birth of the anterior and posterior buttock by lateral spinal flexion *B. Complete breech: birth of legs*		
7-B. Restitution (if the waist is twisted)		
8-B. External rotation, when it occurs, matches the movement of the upper torso.	**4-S. Internal rotation may not occur, with the shoulders descending oblique, or the shoulders may move to transverse, with the belly up.**	*4-O. Frank: Internal rotation, when it occurs, matches the movement of the upper torso.* *Complete/incomplete: The neck may twist, allowing the occiput to remain posterior oblique*
	5-S. Engagement (as umbilicus is born) *S. Flexion of shoulders*	
9-B. External rotation, when it occurs, moves the sacrum to posterior oblique.	**6-S. Internal rotation may not occur if the shoulders are already oblique. If the shoulder are transverse, they may internally rotate from transverse to oblique, with the belly up.**	*6-O. Frank: Internal rotation, when it occurs, moves occiput to posterior oblique.* *Complete/incomplete: Internal restitution occurs if the neck untwists, allowing the occiput to remain posterior oblique.*
B. Frank breech: Birth of legs may occur at any point before/during birth of shoulders	**7-S. Birth of anterior shoulder and arm by lateroflexion of upper spine**	*6-O. Engagement as shoulders reach outlet*
10-B. Long-arc external rotation with head to bring sacrum from posterior oblique, to transverse, to anterior oblique to SA	*8-S. Slight movement to left or right as posterior arm is born–then shoulders follow internal rotation of the head, rotating externally from oblique, to AP, to oblique to transverse.*	**7-O. Long-arc internal rotation begins before and completes after posterior arm is born to bring occiput from posterior oblique to transverse, to anterior oblique to OA**
		8-O. Birth of head by flexion

<u>Observations on the movements of long-arc rotation of the posterior breech</u>: As variable as rotation can be in breeches, and as rare as posterior breeches are, it is impossible to predict exactly how and when the baby will rotate to the anterior. As with any breech birth, much depends upon the attitude of the baby and the position of the mother. There are three opportunities for anterior rotation to occur: as the lower torso descends, as the upper torso and shoulders descend or, failing that, when the head reaches the pelvic floor. Once anterior rotation begins, it is likely to continue as each part is born, with the head rotating anteriorly as well. An upright, forward-leaning maternal position greatly facilitates anterior rotation; conversely, supine positions increase the likelihood that the baby will remain posterior.

The cardinal movements of birth in sacrum posterior breeches that undergo short-arc rotation

When the baby remains persistently posterior, birth is likely to proceed as described in the following chart (keep in mind the extreme variability of breech descent). While additional rotational movements are possible, for example, the entire torso and head could move with the breech toward an anterior orientation and then return to a posterior orientation, or the baby could twist at the waist or the neck to bring the lower body more anterior while leaving the head posterior as descent proceeds, these movements seem less likely because anterior rotation of any part will probably take the rest of the body along with it, therefore the description assumes that parts remain pretty much posterior throughout descent.

BREECH (LOWER TORSO) & LEGS	UPPER TORSO (CHEST) & SHOULDERS	HEAD
1-B. Spinal flexion (may be impaired) *Frank: further impairs flexion*	*1.S. Spinal flexion (may be impaired)* *Frank: further impairs flexion*	*1-O. Flexion of head (may be impaired)* *Frank: further impairs flexion*
2-B. Descent	*2-S. Descent in concert with breech*	*2-O. Descent in concert with upper torso*
3-B. Engagement–sacrum posterior oblique or directly posterior		
4-B. Frank: Internal rotation may not occur. **Complete/incomplete: Internal rotation to transverse may occur as waist twists**	*3-S. Internal rotation does not occur*	*3-O. Internal rotation does not occur.*
5-B. Lateral flexion of spine (as possible) *B. Incomplete: birth of legs* • Frank/complete: Rumping of breech		
6-B. Birth of anterior and posterior buttock by lateral spinal flexion *B. Complete: birth of legs*		
7-B. Restitution (if waist is twisted)		
8-B. External rotation, when it occurs, matches the movement of the upper torso, bringing the sacrum posterior.	**4-S. Internal rotation may not occur, with the shoulders descending oblique. When it occurs, the shoulders move to transverse, with the belly up.**	*4-O. Internal rotation, when it occurs, matches the movement of the upper torso, moving the occiput to directly posterior.*
	5-S. Engagement (as umbilicus is born) *S. Flexion of shoulders*	
9-B. External rotation, when it occurs, matches the movement of the upper torso, bringing the sacrum posterior oblique.	**6-S. Internal rotation, when it occurs, moves the long axis of the shoulders to an oblique diameter, with the belly up.**	*5-O. Internal rotation, when it occurs, matches the movement of the upper torso.* *Complete/incomplete: The neck may turn, allowing the head to remain OP.*
B. Frank: birth of legs may occur at any time before/during birth of the arms	**7-S. Birth of the anterior shoulder and arm, by lateroflexion of upper spine**	*6-O. Engagement (as shoulders reach outlet)*
10-B. External rotation, when it occurs, follows the head to bring sacrum SP	*8-S. Slight movement to left or right as posterior arm is born–then, if the head rotates internally, the shoulders follow, rotating externally from oblique to transverse.*	**7-O. Internal rotation, when it occurs, begins before and completes after posterior arm is born to occiput OP (rotation will not occur if the head is already OP).**
		8-O. Birth of the head by flexion or extension.

Comments on short-arc rotation of the posterior breech: When the breech baby rotates so that the belly is under the pubic arch, progress is challenged throughout descent by the possibility of arrest.

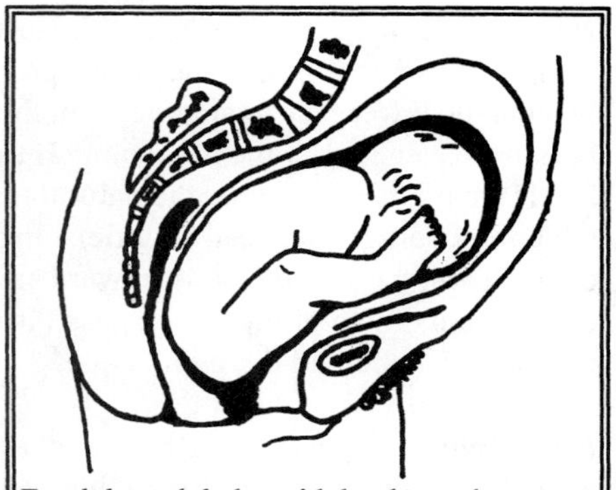
Frank breech baby with her knees bent over the pubic bone.

Descent and birth of the legs and lower torso: As in posterior cephalic presentations, the spine is poorly situated to flex very well prior to labor. As with any posterior position, neck and spinal deflexion may be encouraged because the fetal spine is next to the lordotic maternal spine. This is one reason the posterior breech often fails to descend. If the baby is frank breech, the splinted legs only compound this difficulty. The posterior region of the mother's torso above the brim) offers far less space for lateral mobility, and her spine interferes with forward flexion.

However, once descent begins, the baby who remains sacrum posterior is actually poised to flex more easily than one who rotates SA. As the anterior pelvis passes the pubic arch, the spine can curl forward if the legs don't interfere. If the baby is frank breech, direct SP descent of the torso to the point where the inner knees are level with the pubic arch may result in bending of the knees which, in turn, allows the spine to curl forward and thus could make passage easier, especially if the baby is small. For this reason, the preterm sacrum posterior baby may slip down rather quickly once the passages are sufficiently dilated to admit the small body, without sufficient cervical dilation to allow passage of the relatively larger head. However, the baby could just as easily become hung up with the knees flexed at the pubic arch and descent could be arrested, particularly if the baby is of good size at term.

Birth of the flexed or extended legs can present difficulties as well. If descent does occur, a flexed anterior leg can get hung up on the upper border of the pubic arch, preventing further descent. If the legs get past the pubic arch, they can usually be born without any particular problems, although it is still possible for a foot to get hung up at the brim, especially if the baby is in a frank position.

Descent and birth of the upper torso, arms and shoulders: Likewise, if anterior rotation does not occur with descent of the breech, as the upper torso moves down, the arms can become hung up on the pubic arch at the elbow or axilla, preventing engagement of the shoulders. Should that occur, one or both arms may be trapped and swept up near the head as the baby descends further, resulting in one or both extended arms developing in the shallow anterior pelvis, where there is less room to maneuver them into a better position and get them out. If the arms remain well down on the chest, their birth should not present any particular difficulty. Once the arms are out, the shoulders are usually born easily.

Birth of the occiput posterior aftercoming head: If the occiput does not rotate to become anterior prior to its birth, descent of the chin through the shallow anterior pelvis past the upper border of the pubic arch is a setup for dramatic extension of the head and subsequent difficulty with getting the head out, should the chin catch on the bone. In the worst case, the head may become so hung up in this position that instrumental intervention is the only thing that may save the baby, although this too places the baby at risk for additional injury. While passage of the occiput by the sacral promontory may encourage flexion, this will not take place if the chin gets stuck at the brim above the pubic arch, before engagement can occur. Even as the occiput is descending past the promontory, if the head is already deflexed, the chin may become hung up on the pubic bone as the occiput attempts to enter the hollow of the sacrum.

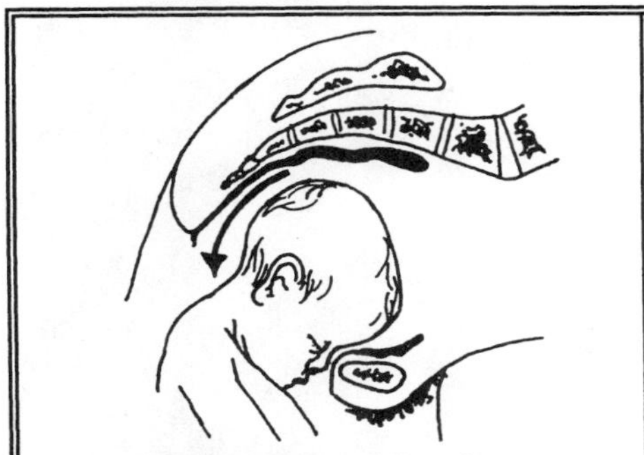
Posterior head flexed

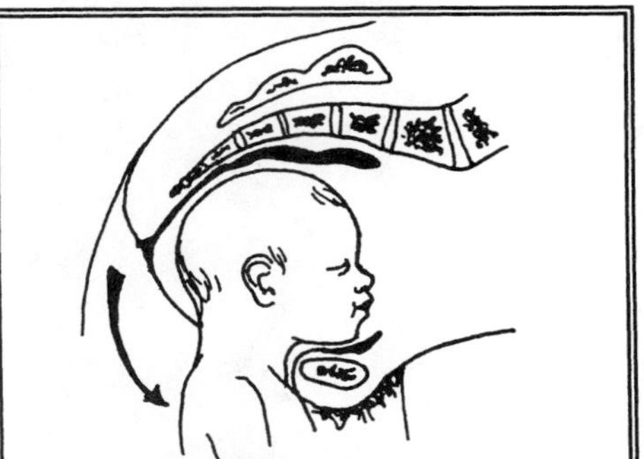
Posterior head extended

(Mother in a hands and knees position to facilitate rotation.)

If the head is flexed: If the head is in an attitude of flexion and the mother is upright, the best outcome is for the occiput to tip forward as it passes the sacral promontory and for the chin to descend past the upper border of the pubic arch, leaving the lower face to emerge from the periurethral area as the nape of the neck, occiput and crown of the vertex are born in sequence over the perineum. If the mother is upright, having her go to hands and knees may help birth the head.

If the mother is supine, the natural tendency is for the weight of the baby's body to fall backward toward the floor, which encourages the head to deflex. In order to maintain flexion, the midwife must first support the baby's body as the chin is born, then lift the body upward so that the bridge of the nose pivots under the pubic bone as the nape of the neck, occiput and crown of the vertex pass through the perineum as it retracts. Once the occipital eminence is born, the face emerges from behind the pubic bone.

If the head is extended: Birth is rendered still more difficult if the head descends in an extended attitude or becomes extended as it tries to engage. In this case, the chin becomes lodged against the pubic bone and the anterior neck serves as the pivot point as the occiput and vertex are born over the perineum. Delay may occur if the occiput catches on the lower sacrum during this process. Birth is facilitated by supporting the baby's body in a forward position if the mother is upright or lifting the body if she is supine.

SUMMARY OF THE CARDINAL SPIRALING MOVEMENTS: RIGHT SACRUM POSTERIOR (RSP)

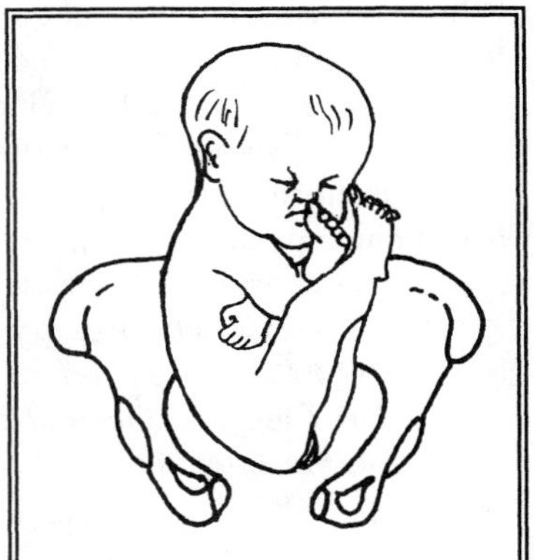

RSP baby in frank attitude before descent begins.

Orientation of the baby to the mother's pelvis

The sacrum occupies the right posterior corner of the mother's pelvis (RSP) and the occiput is situated to the right posterior corner of the mother's torso (ROP). The long axes of the pelvis and shoulder are aligned with the left oblique diameter. The genital crease and the sagittal suture are aligned with the right oblique diameter.

Summary of Long-arc Rotation of the RSP Baby (movements not illustrated)
Birth of the breech when long-arc anterior rotation occurs as it descends:

1-B, 1-S & 1-O. *Flexion of the lower torso begins prior to labor and is prompted by flexion of the head. Flexion is often impaired when the baby's back is adjacent to that of the mother.*

1-B. Frank: *Splinting of the legs may further impair flexion until the feet are born.*

2-B. The breech descends through the birth canal when labor progresses.

2-S & 2-O. *The entire baby moves down as the breech descends.*

3-B. The breech engages as the bitrochanteric diameter passes through the left oblique diameter of the brim. After engagement, the breech often remains high in the pelvis until the membranes rupture or dilation is nearly complete.

4-B & 5-B. Anterior rotation begins with the breech rotating internally a total of 45°, from RSP to RST as the lower torso enters the deepest curve of the birth canal, requiring the spine to flex laterally. Rotation consists of a downwardly spiraling movement, which facilitates descent.

3-S & 3-O. *The upper torso and head follow the breech, rotating internally from ROP to ROT.*

- **Frank/complete:** As pushing proceeds, the breech rumps.

6-B. Frank: The breech is born as the spine flexes laterally. The anterior buttock emerges, followed by the posterior buttock.

6-B. Complete/incomplete: The buttocks emerge during or after the birth of the legs.

B. *The legs are born according to their attitude.*

Frank: *Spontaneous emergence of the legs may not occur until the shoulders are being born.*

Incomplete: *The extended legs emerge before the breech.*

Complete: *The flexed legs usually disengage as each buttock is born or immediately thereafter.*

7-B. No restitution occurs.

From this point the birth of the baby proceeds as for a RSA (follow RSA summary, page 204, beginning with *1-S & 1-0.*)

When anterior rotation does not occur during descent of the breech, birth of the breech proceeds as for a persistent RSP. (Follow summary of short-arc rotation of the breech in the RSP baby on page 220, from 1-B to 7-B, then switch to the summary below describing anterior rotation of the upper torso.)

Descent, anterior rotation and birth of the upper torso when the breech has descended RSP and long-arc rotation has not yet occurred:

1-S & 1-O. *Flexion of the upper torso begins prior to labor and is prompted by flexion of the head.*

2-S & 2-O. *The upper torso and head continue to descend when labor progresses.*

4-S. Frank: Internal rotation may not occur with the shoulders descending through the left oblique diameter of the brim.

8-B & 4-O. Frank: *The breech remains aligned with the left oblique diameter and the head remains ROP.*

4-S. Complete/incomplete: Internal rotation may occur as the upper torso moves 45° to the transverse diameter of the brim.

8-B. Complete/incomplete: *The breech follows the upper torso by rotating externally from RSP to SP.*

4-O. Complete/incomplete: *The neck twists, allowing the head to remain ROP.*

Long-arc rotation may also occur: Starting from the left oblique diameter, the entire baby rotates 45° to the antero-posterior diameter, 45° to the right oblique diameter and 45° to transverse, RSP to RST to RSA to SA. (Birth proceeds as for a RSA, beginning with 5-S.)

If long-arc rotation does not occur: After step 4-S birth proceeds as follows:

5-S. The shoulders engage when the bisacromial diameter passes through

5-S. Frank: the left oblique diameter of the brim,

5-S. Complete/incomplete: the transverse diameter of the brim,

as the umbilicus is born. The attitude of the shoulders changes as necessary during descent.

6-S. Long-arc internal rotation begins as the upper torso and shoulders move 45° from the left oblique to the anteroposterior diameter. This movement allows the thoracic spine to flex laterally as it approaches the outlet.

*9-B **Frank:** The breech follows the upper torso by rotating externally from RSP to RST.*

*5-O **Frank:** The head follows the torso by rotating internally from ROP to ROT.*

*9-B. **Complete/incomplete:** The breech follows the upper torso and head by rotating externally from RSP to RST.*

*5-O **Complete/incomplete:** The neck untwists as the head follows the upper torso, rotating internally from ROP to ROT.*

At this point, birth of the shoulders proceeds as for a RSA. (Follow RSA summary, page 205, beginning with 7-S).

When anterior rotation does not occur during descent of the shoulders and upper torso, birth of the breech and upper torso proceeds as for a persistent RSP. (Follow summary of short-arc rotation of the breech and upper torso of the RSP baby on the this page from 1-B through to 6-O. Then switch to the summary below describing anterior rotation of the head.)

Descent, anterior rotation and birth of the head when anterior rotation did not occur during descent and rotation of the breech or upper torso and shoulders:

8-S & 7-O. The shoulders may now make a slight movement to the left or right as the posterior shoulder and arm emerge. Simultaneously the head begins long-arc internal rotation, moving from ROP to ROT to ROA to OA. Once both shoulders are born, the torso in freed to rotate externally, as it follows the head.

10-B & 8-S. The breech makes its final external rotation, moving from RSP to RST to RSA to SA.

8-O. Birth of the head by flexion allows the chin to emerge, followed by the occiput and vertex. Birth of the head by extension results in the neck pivoting under the pubic arch as the occiput passes through the perineum. Either way, the birth of the head usually requires some sort of manual assistance.

Short-arc Rotation of the RSP Baby

Rarely, anterior rotation does not occur and birth of the baby proceeds as for a persistent RSP.

Descent and birth of the posterior breech:

1-B, 1-S & 1-O. *Flexion of the lower torso may begin prior to labor and is prompted by flexion of the head. Flexion is often impaired when the baby's back is near that of the mother.*

1-B. Frank: *Splinting of the legs may further impair flexion until the feet are born.*

2-B. The breech descends through the birth canal if labor progresses.

2-S & 2-O. *The entire baby moves down if the breech descends.*

3-B. The breech engages as the bitrochanteric diameter passes through the left oblique diameter of the brim. After engagement, the breech often remains high in the pelvis until the membranes rupture or dilation is nearly complete.

4-B & 5-B. Frank: Internal rotation probably will not occur, with the breech remaining RSP. The spine takes advantage of lateral flexion to the extent possible as it moves through the deepest curve of the birth canal.

3-S & 3-O. Frank: *The upper torso remains aligned with the left oblique diameter and the head remains ROP.*

4-B & 5-B Complete/incomplete: Internal rotation may occur as the baby turns at the waist as the breech rotates 45° from RSP to RST to allow the spine to flex laterally as it descends through the deepest curve of the birth canal.

3-S& 3-O. Complete/incomplete: *Twisting at the waist allows the upper torso to remain aligned with the left oblique diameter and the head to remain ROP.*

- **Frank/complete:** As pushing proceeds, the breech rumps.

6-B. Frank: The breech is born as the spine flexes laterally. The anterior buttock emerges, followed by the posterior buttock.

6-B. Complete/incomplete: The buttocks emerge during or after the birth of the legs.

B. *The legs are born according to their attitude.*

Frank: *Spontaneous emergence of the legs may not occur until the shoulders are being born.*

Incomplete: *The extended legs emerge before the breech.*

Complete: *The flexed legs usually disengage as each buttock is born or immediately thereafter.*

7-B. Frank: No restitution occurs if the waist is not twisted.

7-B. Complete/incomplete: Restitution occurs if the waist is twisted to allow the breech to rotate 45° from RST back to RSP, restoring the long axis of the pelvis to a parallel relationship with the long axis of the shoulders.

Descent and birth of the upper torso, shoulders and arms:

1-S & 1-O. *Flexion of the upper torso begins prior to labor and is prompted by flexion of the head.*

2-S & 2-O. *The upper torso and head continue to descend if labor progresses.*

4-S. Frank: Internal rotation may not occur. The shoulders remain aligned with the left oblique diameter of the brim.

8-B & 4-O. Frank: *The breech remains RSP and the head remains ROP.*

4-S. Complete/incomplete: Internal rotation of the upper torso and shoulders may occur as they move 45° from the left oblique to the transverse pelvic diameter before they enter the brim.

8-B. *The breech follows the upper torso, rotating externally to SP.*

4-O. *As the torso rotates, the neck may twist, allowing the head to remain ROP.*

Conversion to SP may occur: The entire baby may rotate from RSP to SP before the upper torso enters the brim. Birth proceeds as for a direct SP birth. (Follow summary for a persistent SP, page 227, beginning with 5-S.)

5-S. The shoulders engage when the bisacromial diameter passes through the

5-S. Frank: transverse diameter of the brim,

5-S. Complete/incomplete: left oblique diameter of the brim,

as the umbilicus is born. The attitude of the shoulders changes as necessary during descent.

6-S. Frank: Internal rotation does not occur; the upper torso descends through the left oblique diameter of the brim.

9-B & 5-O. Frank: *The breech remains RSP and head remains ROP.*

6-S. Complete/incomplete: Internal restitution may occur as the neck untwists, allowing the torso to rotate 45° from SP to RSP, restoring the long axis of the shoulders to a 90° with the long axis of the head. This movement of the torso allows the spine to flex laterally as the shoulders are born.

9-B & 5-O. Complete/incomplete: *The breech rotates externally from SP to RSP while the head remains ROP.*

7-S. The spine flexes laterally as the anterior shoulder and arm emerge from under the pubic arch.

6-O. *The head engages ROP when the biparietal diameter passes through the left oblique diameter of the brim, as the shoulders reach the outlet.*

8-S & 7-O. The shoulders now make a slight movement to the left or right as the posterior shoulder and arm emerge. Simultaneously, the head begins short-arc rotation, moving from ROP to OP. Once both shoulders are born, the torso is freed to rotate externally as it follows the head.

10-B. *The breech makes its final external rotation, moving from RSP to SP, with the upper torso and head.*

Descent and birth when the head undergoes short-arc rotation to the posterior:

1-O. *The head begins labor in an ROP orientation. It is usually somewhat flexed prior to the onset of labor. Flexion is often enhanced as the fundus gathers around the head during descent of the torso, as the baby lifts his legs after they have emerged and finally as the occiput passes by the sacral promontory.*

2-O. *Descent occurs continuously throughout labor as the lower body moves down.*

7-O. The head rotates internally from ROP to OP as the shoulders and arms are born.

8-O. Birth of the head by flexion allows the chin to emerge, followed by the occiput and vertex. Birth of the head by extension results in the neck pivoting under the pubic arch as the occiput passes through the perineum. Either way, the birth of the head usually requires some sort of manual assistance.

Summary of the Cardinal Spiraling Movements: Left Sacrum Posterior (LSP)

Orientation of the baby to the mother's pelvis

The sacrum occupies the left posterior corner of the mother's pelvis (LSP) and the occiput is situated to the left posterior corner of the mother's torso (LOP). The long axes of the pelvis and shoulder are aligned with the right oblique diameter. The genital crease and the sagittal suture are aligned with the left oblique diameter.

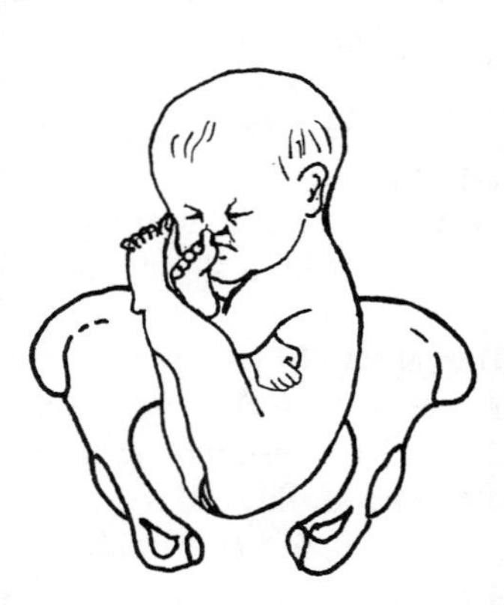

LSP baby in frank attitude before descent begins.

Summary of Long-arc Rotation of the LSP Baby (movements not illustrated)
Birth of the breech when long-arc anterior rotation occurs as it descends:

1-B, 1-S & 1-O. *Flexion of the lower torso begins prior to labor and is prompted by flexion of the head. Flexion is often impaired when the baby's back is adjacent to that of the mother.*

1-B. Frank: *Splinting of the legs may further impair flexion until the feet are born.*

2-B. The breech descends through the birth canal when labor progresses.

2-S & 2-O. *The entire baby moves down as the breech descends.*

3-B. The breech engages as the bitrochanteric diameter passes through the right oblique diameter of the brim. After engagement, the breech often remains high in the pelvis until the membranes rupture or dilation is nearly complete.

4-B & 5-B. Anterior rotation begins with the breech rotating internally a total of 45°, from LSP to LST as the lower torso enters the deepest curve of the birth canal, requiring the spine to flex laterally. Rotation consists of a downwardly spiraling movement, which facilitates descent.

3-S & 3-O. *The upper torso and head follow the breech, rotating internally from LOP to LOT.*

- **Frank/complete:** As pushing proceeds, the breech rumps.

6-B. Frank: The breech is born as the spine flexes laterally. The anterior buttock emerges, followed by the posterior buttock.

6-B. Complete/incomplete: The buttocks emerge during or after the birth of the legs.

B. *The legs are born according to their attitude.*

Frank: *Spontaneous emergence of the legs may not occur until the shoulders are being born.*

Incomplete: *The extended legs emerge before the breech.*

Complete: *The flexed legs usually disengage as each buttock is born or immediately thereafter.*

7-B. No restitution occurs.

From this point the birth of the baby proceeds as for an LSA position (follow LSA summary, page 201, beginning with *1-S & 1-O.*)

When anterior rotation does not occur during descent of the breech, birth of the breech proceeds as for a persistent LSP. (Follow summary of short-arc rotation of the breech in the LSP baby on the next page, from 1-B to 7-B, then switch to the summary below describing anterior rotation of the upper torso.)

Descent, anterior rotation and birth of the upper torso when the breech has descended LSP and long-arc rotation has not yet occurred:

1-S & 1-O. *Flexion of the upper torso begins prior to labor and is prompted by flexion of the head.*

2-S & 2-O. *The upper torso and head continue to descend when labor progresses.*

4-S. Frank: Internal rotation may not occur with the shoulders descending through the right oblique diameter of the brim.

8-B & 4-O. Frank: *The breech remains aligned with the right oblique diameter and the head remains LOP.*

4-S. Complete/incomplete: Internal rotation may occur as the upper torso moves 45° to the transverse diameter of the brim.

8-B. Complete/incomplete: *The breech follows the upper torso by rotating externally from LSP to SP.*

4-O. Complete/incomplete: *The neck twists, allowing the head to remain ROP.*

Long-arc rotation may also occur: Starting from the right oblique diameter, the entire baby rotates 45° to the anteroposterior diameter, 45° to the left oblique diameter and 45° to transverse; LSP to LST to LSA to SA. (Birth proceeds as for a LSA, beginning with 5-S.)

If long-arc rotation does not occur: After step 4-S, birth proceeds as follows:

5-S. The shoulders engage when the bisacromial diameter passes through:

5-S. Frank: the right oblique diameter of the brim,

5-S. Complete/incomplete: the transverse diameter of the brim,

as the umbilicus is born. The attitude of the shoulders changes as necessary during descent.

6-S. Long-arc internal rotation begins as the upper torso and shoulders move 45° from the right oblique to the anteroposterior diameter. This movement allows the thoracic spine to flex laterally as it approaches the outlet.

9-B. Frank: *The breech follows the upper torso by rotating externally from LSP to LST.*

5-O Frank: *The head follows the torso by rotating internally from LOP to LOT.*

9-B. Complete/incomplete: *The breech follows the upper torso by rotating externally from LSP to LST.*

5-O. Complete/incomplete: *The neck untwists as the head follows the upper torso by rotating internally from LOP to LOT.*

At this point, birth of the shoulders proceeds as for an LSA position. (Follow LSA summary, page 202, beginning with 7-S).

When anterior rotation does not occur during descent of the shoulders and upper torso, birth of the breech and upper torso proceeds as for a persistent LSP. (Follow summary of short-arc rotation of the breech and upper torso of the LSP baby on this page, from 1-B through to 6-O. Then switch to the summary below describing anterior rotation of the head.)

Descent, anterior rotation and birth of the head when anterior rotation did not occur during descent and rotation of the lower torso or upper torso and shoulders:

8-S & 7-O. The shoulders may now make a slight movement to the right or left as the posterior shoulder and arm emerge. Simultaneously the head begins long-arc internal rotation, moving from LOP to LOT to LOA to OA. Once both shoulders are born, the torso in freed to rotate externally, as it follows the head.

10-B & 8-S. *The breech makes its final external rotation, moving from LSP to LST to LSA to SA.*

8-O. Birth of the head by flexion allows the chin to emerge, followed by the occiput and vertex. Birth of the head by extension results in the neck pivoting under the pubic arch as the occiput passes through the perineum. Either way, the birth of the head usually requires some sort of manual assistance.

Short-arc Rotation of the LSP Baby

Rarely, anterior rotation does not occur and birth of the baby proceeds as for a persistent LSP.

Descent and birth of the breech:

1-B, 1-S & 1-O. *Flexion of the lower torso may begin prior to labor and is prompted by flexion of the head. Flexion is often impaired when the baby's back is near that of the mother.*

1-B. Frank: *Splinting of the legs may further impair flexion until the feet are born.*

2-B. The breech descends through the birth canal if labor progresses.

2-B & 2-O. *The entire baby moves down if the breech descends.*

3-B. The breech engages as the bitrochanteric diameter passes through the right oblique diameter of the brim. After engagement, the breech often remains high in the pelvis until the membranes rupture or dilation is nearly complete.

4-B. & 5-B. Frank: Internal rotation probably will not occur, with the breech remaining LSP. The spine takes advantage of lateral flexion to the extent possible as it moves through the deepest curve of the birth canal.

3-S & 3-O. Frank: *The upper torso remains aligned with the right oblique diameter and the head remains LOP.*

4-B. & 5-B. Complete/incomplete: Internal rotation may occur as the baby turns at the waist as the breech rotates 45° from LSP to LST to allow the spine to flex laterally as it descends through the deepest curve of the birth canal.

3-S& 3-O. Complete/incomplete: *Twisting at the waist allows the upper torso to remain aligned with the right oblique diameter and the head to remain LOP.*

• **Frank/complete:** As pushing proceeds, the breech rumps.

6-B. Frank: The breech is born as the spine flexes laterally. The anterior buttock emerges, followed by the posterior buttock.

6-B. Complete/incomplete: The buttocks emerge during or after the birth of the legs.

B. *The legs are born according to their attitude.*

Frank: *Spontaneous emergence of the legs may not occur until the shoulders are being born.*

Incomplete: *The extended legs emerge before the breech.*

Complete: *The flexed legs usually disengage as each buttock is born or immediately thereafter.*

7-B. Frank: No restitution occurs if the waist is not twisted.

7-B. Complete/incomplete: Restitution occurs if the waist is twisted to allow the breech to rotate 45° from LST back to LSP, restoring the long axis of the pelvis to a parallel relationship with the long axis of the shoulders.

Descent and birth of the shoulders and arms:

1-S & 1-O. *Flexion of the upper torso begins prior to labor and is prompted by flexion of the head.*

2-S & 2-O. *The upper torso and head continue to descend if labor progresses.*

4-S. Frank: Internal rotation may not occur. The shoulders remain aligned with the right oblique diameter of the brim.

8-B & 4-O. Frank: *The breech remains LSP and the head remains LOP.*

4-S. Complete/incomplete: Internal rotation of the upper torso and shoulders may occur as they move 45° from the right oblique to the transverse diameter before they enter the brim.

8-B. Complete/incomplete: *The breech follows the upper torso, rotating externally to SP.*

4-O. Complete/incomplete: *As the torso rotates, the neck may twist, allowing the head to remain LOP.*

Conversion to SP: The entire baby may rotate from LSP to SP before the upper torso enters the brim. Birth proceeds as for a direct SP birth. (Follow summary for a persistent SP, page 227, beginning with 5-S.)

5-S. The shoulders engage when the bisacromial diameter passes through the:

5-S. Frank: transverse diameter of the brim,

5-S. Complete/incomplete: right oblique diameter of the brim,

as the umbilicus is born. The attitude of the shoulders changes as necessary during descent.

6-S. Frank: Internal rotation does not occur; the upper torso descends through the right oblique diameter of the brim.

9-B & 5-O. Frank: *The breech remains LSP and head remains LOP.*

6-S. Complete/incomplete: Internal restitution occurs as the neck untwists, allowing the torso to rotate 45° from SP to LSP, restoring the long axis of the shoulders to a 90° with the long axis of the head. This movement allows the spine to flex laterally as the shoulders are born.

9-B & 5-O. Complete/incomplete: *The breech rotates externally from SP to LSP while the head remains LOP.*

7-S. The spine flexes laterally as the anterior shoulder and arm emerge from under the pubic arch.

6-O. *The head engages LOP when the biparietal diameter passes through the right oblique diameter of the brim, as the shoulders reach the outlet.*

8-S & 7-O. The shoulders now make a slight movement to the left or right as the posterior shoulder and arm emerge. Simultaneously, the head begins short-arc rotation, moving from LOP to OP. Once both shoulders are born, the torso is freed to rotate externally as it follows the head.

10-B. *The breech makes its final external rotation, moving from LSP to SP, with the upper torso and head.*

Descent and birth when the head undergoes short-arc rotation to the posterior:

1-O. *The head begins labor in an LOP orientation. It is usually somewhat flexed prior to the onset of labor. Flexion is often enhanced as the fundus gathers around the head during descent of the torso, as the baby lifts his legs after they have emerged and finally as the occiput passes by the sacral promontory.*

2-O. *Descent occurs continuously throughout labor as the lower body moves down.*

7-O. The head rotates internally from LOP to OP as the shoulders and arms are born.

8-O. Birth of the head by flexion allows the chin to emerge, followed by the occiput and vertex. Birth of the head by extension results in the neck pivoting under the pubic arch as the occiput passes through the perineum. Either way, the birth of the head usually requires some sort of manual assistance.

Summary of the Cardinal Spiraling Movements: Sacrum Posterior (SP)

A baby may very rarely assume a directly posterior position. Descent of the SP baby, with all the possible options for rotation, constitutes a graduate course in fetal descent. Be thoroughly familiar with all preceding descriptions before tackling this.

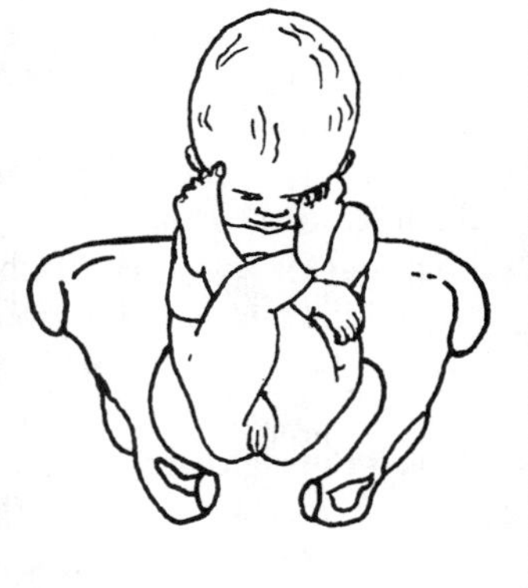

SP baby in a frank breech attitude before descent begins.

Orientation of the baby to the mother's pelvis

The sacrum is directly posterior, in front of the mother's sacrum (SP) and the occiput is situated in the posterior midline of the mother's torso (OP). The long axes of the pelvis and shoulders are aligned with the transverse diameter of the brim. The genital crease and the sagittal suture are aligned with the anteroposterior diameter of the brim.

Summary of long-arc rotation of the SP baby (movements not illustrated)
Descent and anterior rotation of the breech:

1-B, 1-S & 1-O. *Flexion of the lower torso begins prior to labor and is prompted by flexion of the head. Flexion is often impaired because the baby's back is up against that of the mother.*

1-B. Frank breech: *Splinting of the legs may further impair flexion until the feet are born.*

2-B. The breech descends through the birth canal when labor progresses.

2-S & 2-O. *The entire baby moves down as the breech descends.*

3-B. The breech engages as the bitrochanteric diameter passes through the transverse diameter of the brim. After engagement, the breech often remains high in the pelvis until the membranes rupture or dilation is nearly complete.

4-B & 5-B. Internal rotation of the lower torso begins the process of anterior rotation as the breech descends through the deepest curve of the birth canal, requiring the torso to flex laterally. Rotation consists of a downwardly spiraling movement, which facilitates descent. Regardless of the attitude of the legs, the entire baby may internally rotate:

To the left: from SP to LSP to LST. (Follow LSA summary, page 201, beginning with 6-B.)

To the right: from SP to RSP to RST. (Follow RSA summary, page 204, beginning with 6-B.)

When anterior rotation does not occur during descent of the breech, birth of the breech proceeds as for a persistent SP. (Follow the summary a persistent SP that begins on page 227, from 1-B to 7-B, then switch to the summary below describing anterior rotation of the upper torso.)

Descent, anterior rotation and birth of the upper torso when the breech has descended SP and long-arc rotation has not yet occurred:

1-S & 1-O. *Flexion of the upper torso begins prior to labor and is prompted by flexion of the head.*

2-S & 2-O. *The upper torso and head descend when labor progresses.*

4-S. Internal rotation does not occur because the shoulders are already transverse, poised to descend through the most favorable diameter of the brim.

4-B & 3-O. The breech remains SP and the head remains OP.

5-S. The shoulders engage when the bisacromial diameter passes through the transverse diameter of the brim as the umbilicus is born. The attitude of the shoulders changes as necessary during descent.

6-S. Anterior rotation of the upper torso and shoulders begins as they rotate internally a total of 90° to allow the thoracic spine to flex laterally as it descends to the deepest curve of the birth canal. Beginning from the transverse diameter, movement of the shoulders prompts long-arc rotation of the entire body. Regardless of the attitude of the legs, the baby rotates:

To the left: from SP to LSP to LST. (Follow LSA summary, page 202, beginning with 7-S.)

To the right: from SP to RSP to RST. (Follow RSA summary, page 205, beginning with 7-S.)

When anterior rotation does not occur during descent of the shoulders and upper torso, birth of the breech and upper torso proceeds as for a persistent SP. (Follow the summary for a persistent SP baby on this page for the breech and upper torso [1-B to 6-O]. Then switch to the summary immediately below describing anterior rotation of the head.)

Descent, anterior rotation and birth of the head when anterior rotation did not occur during descent and rotation of the breech or the shoulders:

8-S. Frank (1): The shoulders emerge more or less simultaneously.

8-S. Frank (2) & Complete/incomplete: The shoulders may now make a slight movement to the left or right as the posterior shoulder and arm emerge. Once both shoulders are born, the torso is freed to rotate externally, as it follows the head.

7-O Frank (1): Just after the shoulders are born, the head undergoes long-arc internal rotation to the left or right:

To the left: Starting from OP, it rotates to LOP, to LOT, to LOA, and finally to OA.

10-B(1-L) Frank: *The torso externally rotates 180° as it follows the head from SP to LSP, to LST, LSA and finally SA.*

To the right: Starting from OP, it rotates to ROP, to ROT, to ROA, and finally to OA.

10-B(1-R) Frank: *The torso externally rotates 180° as it follows the head from SP, to RSP, to RST, LSA and finally SA.*

7-O Frank (2) & Complete/incomplete: As the posterior arm is emerging, the head begins long-arc internal rotation to the left or right:

To the left: Starting from LOP, it rotates to LOT, to LOA, and finally to OA.

10-B(2-L). *The torso externally rotates 135° as it follows the head from LSP to LST, LSA and finally SA.*

To the right: Starting from ROP, the head rotates to ROT, to ROA, and finally to OA.

10-B(2-R). *The torso externally rotates 135° as it follows the head from RSP, to RST, RSA and finally SA.*

8-O. If the head is flexed, it is born from the OA position as the nape of the neck and chin emerge, followed by the face, occiput and vertex.

In rare cases, the SP baby may remain persistently posterior

Descent and birth of the persistently SP breech:

1-B, 1-S & 1-O. *Flexion of the lower torso begins prior to labor and is prompted by flexion of the head. Flexion is often impaired because the baby's back is against that of the mother.*

1-B. Frank: *Splinting of the legs may further impair flexion until the feet are born.*

2-B. The breech descends through the birth canal if labor progresses.

2-S & 2-O. *The entire baby moves down if the breech descends.*

3-B. The breech engages when the bitrochanteric diameter passes through the transverse diameter of the brim. After engagement, the breech often remains high in the pelvis until the membranes rupture or dilation is nearly complete.

4-B & 5-B. At this point, internal rotation may or may not occur.

4-B & 5-B. Frank: Internal rotation may not occur, with the breech descending SP. The spine takes advantage of anteroposterior flexion to the extent possible as it passes through the deepest curve of the birth canal.

3-S & 3-O. Frank: *The upper torso remains transverse and head remains OP.*

4-B. & 5-B. Complete/incomplete breech (1): Internal rotation may occur as the breech enters the curve of the birth canal, requiring the spine to flex laterally. The lower torso may rotate from transverse in a left or right direction:

To the left (1-L): to the right oblique diameter as the baby twists at the waist.

To the right (1-R): to the left oblique diameter as the baby twists at the waist.

3-S (1)& 3-O(1). *Twisting at the waist allows the shoulder axis to remain aligned with the transverse diameter of the brim and the head to remain OP.*

4-B & 5-B. Complete/incomplete breech (2): Internal rotation may occur as the breech enters the curve of the birth canal, requiring the spine to flex laterally. The entire torso may rotate as the baby twists at the neck, moving 45° in a left or right direction:

To the left (2-L): from SP to LSP.

3-S(2-L) & 4-O(2-L):. *The upper torso moves from transverse to the right oblique diameter. Twisting of the neck allows the head to remain OP.*

To the right (2-R): from SP to RSP.

3-S(2-R) & 4-O(2-R)*. The upper torso moves from transverse to the left oblique diameter. Twisting of the neck allows the head to remain OP.*

- **Frank/complete breech:** As pushing proceeds, the breech rumps.

6-B. Frank breech: The buttocks are born more or less simultaneously.

6-B. Complete/incomplete breech: The buttocks emerge during or after the birth of the legs.

B. *The legs are born according to their attitude.*

Frank: *Spontaneous emergence of the legs may not occur until the shoulders are being born.*

Incomplete: *The extended legs emerge before the breech.*

Complete: *The flexed legs usually disengage as each buttock is born or immediately thereafter.*

7-B. Restitution occurs only if the spine is twisted.

7-B. Frank: No restitution occurs.

7-B. Complete/incomplete (1): Restitution occurs as the baby untwists at the waist to allow the breech to rotate back 45° into the transverse diameter.

7-B. Complete/incomplete (2): Restitution occurs as the baby untwists at the neck to allow the torso to rotate back 45° into the transverse diameter.

Restitution restores the long axes of the breech and shoulders to a parallel relationship with each other and to a right angle with the long axis of the head.

Descent and birth of the upper torso, shoulders and arms in the persistently posterior SP baby:

1-S & 1-O. *Flexion of the upper torso begins prior to labor and is prompted by flexion of the head.*

2-S & 2-O. *The upper torso and head continue to descend if labor progresses.*

4-S. No internal rotation occurs. The upper torso and shoulders are already transverse, poised to descend through the most favorable diameter of the brim.

8-B & 4-O. *The breech remains SP and the head remains OP.*

5-S. The shoulders engage when the bisacromial diameter passes through transverse diameter of the brim as the umbilicus is born. The attitude of the shoulders changes as necessary during descent.

6-S. Internal rotation may or may not occur. Regardless of the attitude of the legs, one of the following may occur:

6-S(1). Internal rotation may not occur, with the upper torso descending transverse.

9-B(1) & 5-O(1). *The breech remains SP and the head remains OP.*

6-S(2): Internal rotation may occur as the entire torso rotates 45° to the left or right:

To the left (2-L): from the transverse to the right oblique diameter.

9-B(2-R) & 5-O(2-L). *The breech and head follow, moving the breech to LSP and the head to LOP.*

To the right (2-R): from the transverse to the left oblique diameter.

9-B(2-R) & 5-O(2-R). *The breech and head follow, moving the breech to RSP and the head to ROP.*

6-S(3): Internal rotation may occur as the baby twists at the neck, allowing the shoulders to rotate 45° to the left or right:

To the left (3-L): from transverse to the right oblique diameter.

9-B(3-L) & 5-O(3-L). *The breech follows the upper torso, moving the breech to LSP. Twisting of the neck allows the head to remain OP.*

To the right (3-R): from transverse to the left oblique diameter.

9-B(3-R) & 5-O(3-R). *The breech follows the upper torso, moving the breech to RSP. Twisting of the neck allows the head to remain OP.*

Internal rotation allows the thoracic spine to take better advantage of lateral flexion as it passes through the deepest curve of the birth canal.

7-S(1). The shoulders and arms are born more or less simultaneously.

6-O(1). *The head engages as the biparietal diameter passes through the transverse diameter of the brim as the shoulders reach the outlet.*

7-S(2). The spine flexes laterally as the anterior shoulder and arm emerge from under the pubic arch.

6-O(2). *The head engages when the biparietal diameter passes through:*

6-O(2-L). *the right oblique diameter of the brim as the shoulders reach the outlet.*

6-O(2-R). *the left oblique diameter of the brim as the shoulders reach the outlet.*

7-S(**3**). The spine flexes laterally as the anterior shoulder and arm emerge from under the pubic arch.

__6-O(3-L) or 6-O(3-R).__ The head engages when the biparietal diameter passes through the transverse diameter of the brim.

8-S & 7-O(1). No further rotation occurs because the shoulders are already transverse and the head is OP.

8-S & 7-O(2). The shoulders may now make a slight movement to the left or right as the posterior shoulder and arm emerge. Simultaneously, the head rotates internally:

7-O(2-L). from LOP to OP.

7-O(2-R). from ROP to OP.

Once both shoulders are born, the torso is freed to follow the movement of the head.

__10-B.__ The breech follows the upper torso:

__10-B(2-L).__ externally rotating from LSP to SP.

__10-B(2-R).__ externally rotating from RSP to SP.

8-S & 7-O(3). Once both shoulders are born, restitution occurs if the baby's neck is twisted, allowing the upper torso and shoulders to move back 45° from:

8-S(3-L). the right oblique diameter back to the transverse diameter of the brim.

__10-B(3-L).__ The breech follows the upper torso, restituting back from LSP to SP.

8-S(3-R). the left oblique diameter back to the transverse diameter of the brim.

__10-B(3-R).__ The breech follows the upper torso, restituting back from RSP to SP.

This movement restores the long axis of the shoulders to a 90° angle with the long axis of the head, which is OP.

Birth of the persistently SP head:

__1-O.__ The head begins labor in an OP orientation. It is usually somewhat flexed prior to the onset of labor. Flexion may be enhanced as the fundus gathers around the head during descent of the torso, as the baby lifts his legs after they have emerged and finally as the occiput passes by the sacral promontory.

__2-O.__ Descent occurs continuously throughout labor if the lower body moves down.

8-O. Birth of the head by flexion allows the chin to emerge, followed by the occiput and vertex. Birth of the head by extension results in the neck pivoting under the pubic arch as the occiput passes through the perineum. Either way, the birth of the head usually requires some sort of manual assistance.

VARIATIONS IN BREECH DESCENT AND ROTATION

Extension of the posterior leg and breech descent

Extension of the posterior leg affects the way the breech rotates during labor. In all labors, the lowermost portion of the presenting part tends to slip under the pubic arch. Thus, in cases where the anterior leg is extended, the side of the baby's body glides past the pubic arch without difficulty. Short-arc rotation of the anterior hip takes place through an arc of 45° (from an anterior oblique position to direct anterior), as it normally would.

However, when the posterior leg is extended into the yoni and the anterior leg is flexed at the hip and knee, the posterior leg almost always undergoes long rotation through an arc of 135° to arrive directly under the symphysis pubis before further descent proceeds. For the moment, consider the extended posterior leg to be the denominator, rather than the sacrum. If the extended leg is in a posterior oblique quadrant of the pelvis, it will have to rotate 45° forward to the nearest transverse position, then 45° to the nearest anterior oblique position then 45° to the directly anterior position (135° in all). This moves the extended leg under the symphysis and places the sacrum in a transverse position in the mother's pelvis.

Occasionally the extended posterior leg rotates in the opposite direction, moving 45° from one of the posterior oblique quadrants to a directly posterior position over the sacrum, then 45° to the opposite posterior oblique quadrant then forward 45° to the nearest transverse position, then 45° to the nearest anterior oblique position, and finally 45° to a directly anterior position (225° in all). This super-long-arc rotation places the sacrum in a transverse orientation as well.

The above explanation takes into account that the flexed anterior leg tends to splint the anterior side of the fetal torso somewhat, which hinders lateral flexion. The flexed leg is also more likely to get hung up on the upper border of the pubic rami, preventing descent of the posterior leg to the level of the inclined pelvic floor. Lateral flexion is not hindered on the side of the extended leg, a phenomenon that encourages the posterior hip to rotate all the way around to the symphysis pubis, where the uninterrupted length of the baby's body navigates past the pubic bone more easily. The posterior hip is also encouraged to rotate to the front by virtue of the forward-slanted construction of the anterior pelvis and the arrangement of the sacrosciatic ligaments and the levator ani sling. When propelled from above by contractions, any movable part that contacts these inclined planes tends to rotate in an anterior direction. In the exceedingly rare event that the posterior hip does not rotate to the anterior, the flexed anterior leg can project over the edge of the pubic bone and prevent descent.

Variations in internal rotation of the breech, upper torso, arms and shoulders

As discussed throughout this section, internal rotation of the sacrum or shoulders can vary a great deal in breeches. Just about any combination is possible with the entire body and head rotating together, the whole torso moving by turning the neck or the upper and lower torsos moving semi-independently by turning at the waist. The shoulders may superrotate to the opposite oblique diameter or may not rotate at all.

Problems with the birth of the arms: Aside from the problems with the birth of the arms described in the chapter entitled "The Process of Birth in Sacrum Posterior Breech Presentations," there are a few other ways the arms can pose a problem. When one or both fetal arms are extended, the same problems arise as in the case of a compound vertex presentation. One or both arms beside the aftercoming head increase the overall diameter as the head descends. This can delay descent of the head through the brim or pelvic cavity and result in the head getting stuck. In most cases, the midwife must manually dislodge the arms to complete the birth. Spontaneous extension of the arms is rare; extension is encouraged by inappropriate manipulation of the torso or legs before the shoulders are born.

When an arm is extended, bent at the elbow and positioned behind the fetal neck (a nuchal arm), it can cause even more difficulty with descent of the head. This is because the forearm may form a horizontal brace across the anterior pelvic brim. Manipulation by the midwife is required to free the arm.

Extension of the head: Whether the baby is sacrum posterior or anterior, if the head descends deflexed or becomes deflexed before it is born, the larger occipitomental diameter presents, making the birth of the head difficult. This is a dangerous situation for the baby, as cranial or cervical spinal injuries can occur during attempts to rectify this problem.

The Process of Labor When the Pelvis Is Contracted or the Baby Is in a Nonlongitudinal Lie

The Process of Labor for Women with Contracted Pelvises

A woman may give birth through her yoni regardless of the shape of her pelvis, provided it is large enough or the baby is small enough. When assessing the prospects of normal birth for a particular woman, a distinction must be made between pelvises that are simply distorted, but with little or no reduction in capacity, and those that are truly contracted or so distorted that actual contraction exists. Prenatal signs such as pendulous abdomen or the uterus riding high in the torso can be associated with a contracted pelvis because the presenting part cannot enter the brim. However, these conditions are usually related to other factors in well-nourished North American and European women.

True pelvic contraction that will impede yoni birth is hard to predict, since various factors determine whether labor progresses. Such factors include the overall health and psychological disposition of the mother, the strength of her contractions, her actual pelvic dimensions, the flexibility of her pelvic joints and soft tissue and her positions and activities during labor. As far as the baby is concerned, the size and mouldability of the fetal skull, the degree of flexion, and the position that the baby chooses during descent can influence the course of labor. Given optimal circumstances, women often give birth when their pelvic dimensions are seemingly far from ideal.

When a baby presents breech and a woman's pelvis is contracted, a natural birth is likely to result in arrest of the head once the body is born. This disaster is best avoided by opting for a surgical birth if contraction is suspected by internal exam or medical history. Characteristics indicative of significant pelvic contraction should be noted during the initial pelvimetry exam.

As surgery, anaesthesia and infection control advanced, the obstetrical tendency to do the best to get the baby out though the normal route gave way to a belief that surgical delivery was the safer option in some cases (which is certainly the case). Then, in the mid-1980s, the pendulum swung widely in that direction, and babies started to be cut out if they weren't falling out, leading to epidemic numbers of women and babies undergoing unnecessary surgery for presumed cephalopelvic disproportion when time, patience and a better understanding of normal birth would have remedied the situation. One outcome of this easy reliance on surgery has been that the detailed descriptions of labor through a contracted pelvis that once appeared in textbooks have now vanished. The 16th edition of WILLIAMS OBSTETRICS (Pritchard & MacDonald, 1980) was one of the last modern texts to discuss labor with various types of pelvic contraction, and even so, the descriptions of the processes of labor were reduced to mere generalities.

This chapter reviews what might happen when labor is allowed to progress naturally in women with various types and degrees of pelvic contraction. How labor will actually progress will vary according to the individual situation. Knowing how labor might progress in a woman with a truly contracted pelvis will help in recognizing an actual problem, in determining what types of assistance may encourage labor to progress and in deciding when transport is in order. The following explanations cover extreme examples of a variety of pelvic types. These descriptions are largely based upon those found in BIOLOGICAL PRINCIPLES AND MODERN PRACTICE OF OBSTETRICS (Greenhill & Friedman, 1974), which was the last edition of De Lee's obstetrics textbook, but they have been augmented with details found in other historical works. In most such cases, transport for a surgical birth would be warranted, unless the fetal condition is excellent, and steady, albeit slow, progress is being made. These examples are included to help in gaining an understanding of the problem and its timely recognition during labor. You should have a thorough grasp of pelvic anatomy and the normal process of birth before studying this chapter.

Labor in a woman with a contracted flat (platypelloid) pelvis

The anteroposterior diameter of the inlet is reduced and often causes delayed or arrested descent through the brim. The sacral promontory juts forward, which may prohibit the head from entering the pelvis through an anteroposterior or oblique diameter. The anatomic transverse pelvic diameter is measured from side to side through the center of the cavity. Since the jutting promontory forces the head forward, the available transverse diameter at the brim lies in front of this diameter. This reduces the actual space for the head to descend. This may result in abnormalities of attitude or presentation or both. As a result, the head may override the pubic bone or slide off to one side even before labor begins. Labor with a pronouncedly flat pelvis usually results in high transverse arrest, and even with a moderate degree of contraction, surgical delivery is often required.

Synclitic descent through a flat pelvis: Most often, the occiput will be transverse since the brim has a long transverse diameter and a short anteroposterior diameter. The head attempts to enter the pelvis in a flexed position, but the biparietal diameter is too large to pass through the true conjugate, which is the narrowest diameter in a platypelloid pelvis. The jutting sacral promontory diminishes the available space in the posterior pelvis, forcing the head to try and navigate the narrowed anteroposterior space left between the promontory and the pubic bone. As a result the head slides off to one side, so that the bitemporal diameter now lies over the true conjugate, and the parietal diameter lies in the larger space opposite the sacroiliac joint. As contractions apply pressure to the head, the parietal eminences impinge on the pelvic brim. Pressure from above causes the parietal eminences to catch at the brim. This causes the head to pivot, tipping the occiput backward and causing the forehead to be pressed downward, resulting in a deflexed position (Michaelis' obliquity). This tips the bitemporal diameter downward into the true conjugate. The bitemporal diameter (8 cm) is not only smaller, but quite compressible because of the coronal sutures on either side. The forehead now tries to engage, which may result in a persistent, nonprogressive brow presentation. The cord may prolapse in the space created when the head does not fill the pelvic inlet.

The head usually gets stuck in this position, as it cannot descend further, and a large caput forms. If labor does progress, the head gradually descends past the promontory as the bitemporal diameter passes through the brim. After the head enters the brim, the posterior vertex and occiput start to pivot downward. The head flexes and the occiput rotates internally toward the pubic bone when it meets the pelvic floor. The rest of labor progresses normally because the head is now past the plane of greatest contraction. However, inlet shoulder dystocia is more likely because the shoulders cannot enter the pelvic inlet at an oblique or anteroposterior diameter and are more likely to get stuck above the pubic bone. The pubic arch is also low in a platypelloid pelvis, further impeding proper descent of the shoulders.

Anterior asynclitic descent through a flat pelvis: Litzmann (1861) stated that anterior parietal presentations are three times more common than the posterior variety. In this situation, the head is in a position of exaggerated anterior asynclitism. Pronounced, persistent anterior asynclitism is more common in a flat, contracted pelvis. In the most extreme cases, the baby's posterior ear is in contact with his shoulder, and the anterior parietal bone occupies the diagonal conjugate with the sagittal suture *above* the level of the promontory. Acute anterior asynclitism occurs because the posterior parietal bone is held back by the jutting sacral promontory, causing the head to tilt sideways and the anterior parietal bone to attempt to descend. This negates the advantage afforded the head in entering the brim asynclitically because the acute angle of the head bypasses the narrow subsuperparietal diameter resulting in the broadside of the head presenting at the brim.

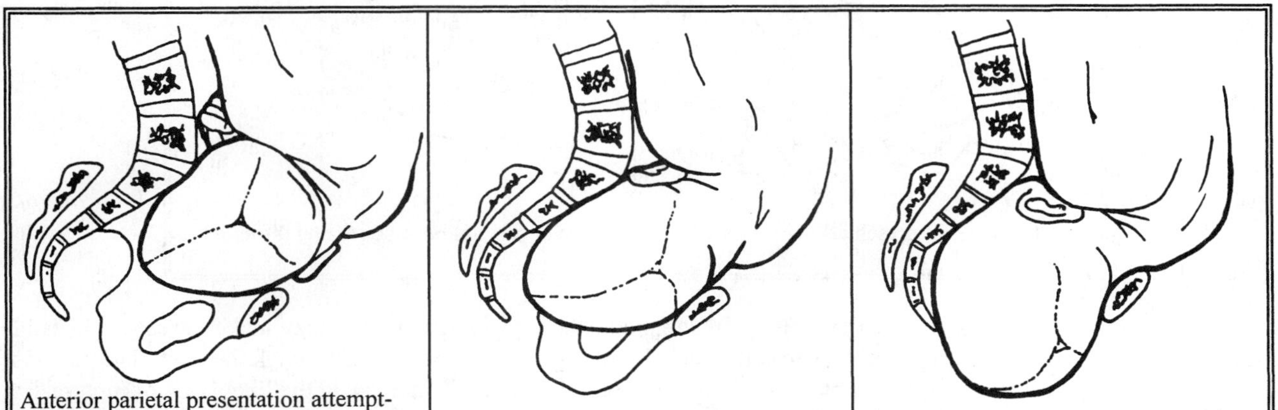

Anterior parietal presentation attempting descent through a wide, very shallow brim | Posterior parietal bone passes the promontory during engagement. | Head reaches the more spacious mid-pelvis and rotates OA.

You might suspect acute anterior asynclitism by noting straightening of the baby's spine during an abdominal examination in early labor. Lateroflexion at the neck, occurring because the baby's head is so deeply inclined toward her posterior shoulder, may also be noted.

On internal examination, the sagittal suture is aligned with the transverse diameter of the brim but is tilted backward, close to the sacrum, which may make it very difficult to reach. The anterior ear may be felt behind the pubic bone when the anterior asynclitism is very exaggerated. The fontanelles are often at the same level; however, if the brow is presenting, the anterior fontanelle will be lower. Excessive moulding renders the suture lines easy to find at first, but a caput overlies the suture lines as descent proceeds.

As labor progresses, the posterior parietal bone squeezes down past the sacral promontory, and the anterior parietal bone descends by a process of sliding and pivoting on the inside surface of the pubic bone. The length of time and amount of moulding required to allow further descent depends on the size and hardness of the skull and the size of the pelvic inlet, as well as the strength of contractions. The process may be completed within a few hours or active labor, may last for over a day. As soon as the largest diameter of the head passes through the inlet, or just as it is about to, the head flexes, the occiput moves down, and the anterior fontanelle moves out of reach. Anterior rotation often occurs immediately, and the birth proceeds with the normal movements of flexion, descent, spinal extension, restitution and external rotation.

Asynclitic posterior descent through a flat pelvis: The head is inclined toward the anterior shoulder in about 10% of exaggerated asynclitic presentations, with the posterior parietal bone occupying the rear of the pelvis. This occurs when the sacral promontory is positioned very low in relationship to the brim, thus allowing the posterior parietal bone to descend further than it can in the processes described above. The groove formed just above the pubis by the depression formed where the head is tilted toward the shoulder may be detectable during abdominal exam. The round anterior parietal bone may also be palpable externally, above the pubic bone. The contour of the uterus may be flatter, as the body of the baby is tipped toward the maternal spine. On internal exam, the sagittal suture is just behind the pubic bone, usually running transverse or slightly oblique. The fontanelles are at the same level, or the posterior fontanelle is out of reach due to head deflexion. If lateroflexion is pronounced, the posterior ear may be palpable near or above the sacral promontory on internal exam.

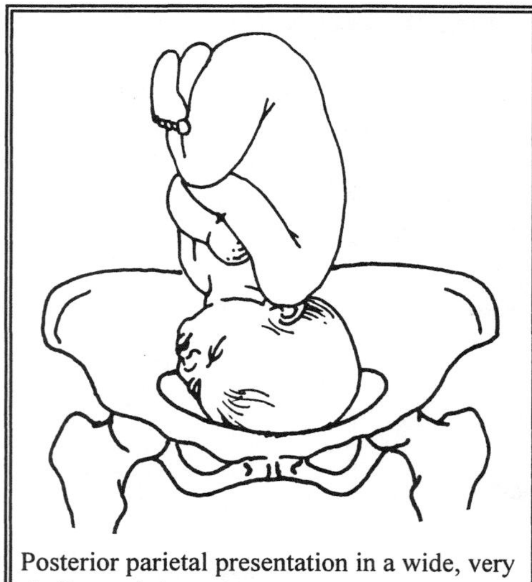

Posterior parietal presentation in a wide, very shallow pelvis.

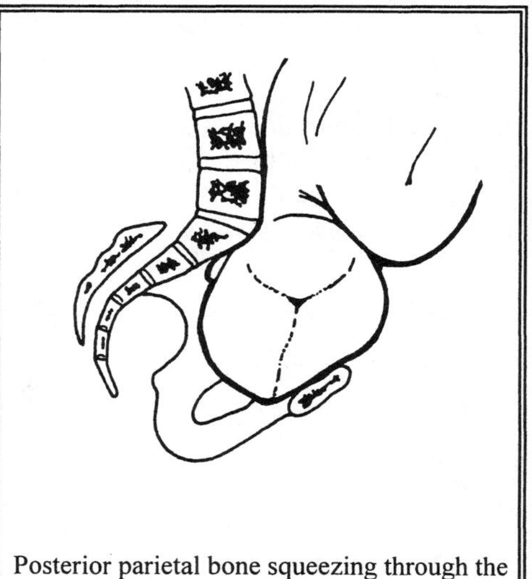

Posterior parietal bone squeezing through the brim.

Exaggerated posterior asynclitism in a flat pelvis renders labor more difficult and may make descent impossible because the baby is bent at nearly a right angle at the neck, impeding passage of the head through the inlet. The posterior wall of the uterus is prone to becoming excessively thin if labor is prolonged, increasing the likelihood of rupture.

If labor does progress, the posterior parietal bone pivots against the inside surface of the sacral promontory, and the anterior parietal bone slides down past the pubic bone into the pelvis as the head engages. As the head descends, the sagittal suture moves to a more central position and the head rotates to an oblique diameter. Sometimes lateroflexion continues until the head is born, and complete internal rotation does not occur. In this case, the head is born in an oblique diameter, with the nape of the neck passing under one of the rami of the pelvis.

Breech presentation in a platypelloid pelvis: The aftercoming head usually enters the transverse diameter of the brim, although a small head may enter the oblique diameter. The diameter at the base of the occiput is smaller than the succeeding diameters and, if the inlet is sufficiently contracted to prevent the descent of the engaged diameter, extension of the head will occur as the chin and jaw impinge on the brim.

However, when the transverse head can descend through the brim to the level of the biparietal diameter, the parietal eminences become hung up and act as a pivot point at the brim. Further descent encourages the bitemporal diameter to tip forward, and the head may flex to a degree. The posterior parietal bone becomes lodged against the sacral promontory. The anterior parietal bone acts as a pivot while the posterior parietal bone squeezes down past the promontory. A baby so stuck requires manipulation to pass through the pelvis, at great risk of fetal injury or death.

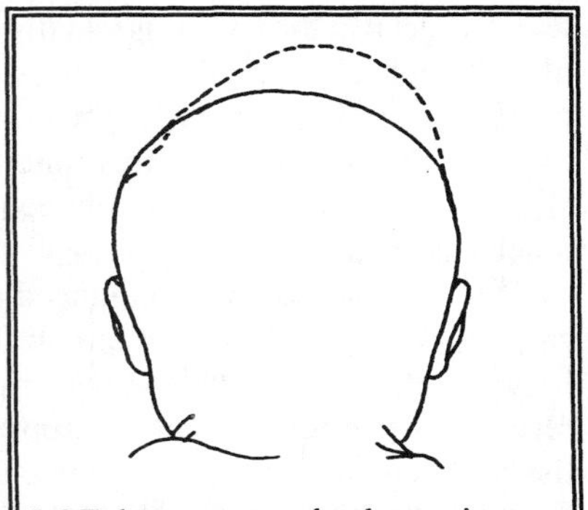
LOT descent: note the depression above the left parietal eminence.

Moulding after birth through a flat pelvis: Mild moulding may occur in the form of mismatching along the sagittal suture. The posterior parietal bone tends to be flattened with a compensating arching of the anterior parietal bone. However, descent through a flat pelvis involves localized pressure that often results in bruises or actual dents in the parietal bone that received the most direct pressure. When pelvic contraction is moderate, a gutter-like (or spoon-shaped) depression develops on the portion of the posterior parietal bone that passed over the promontory. When labor arrests, a pressure necrosis may develop in the overlying scalp. These lesions are usually found between the anterior fontanelle and the parietal eminence, often close to the sagittal suture. Typically a red streak runs from the depression. With more severe contraction, a succession of dents or a gutter-like groove may extend along the parietal bone. If the head was well flexed, the line extends anteriorly and downward in a curve paralleling the coronal suture, down past the temple, or it may terminate at the outer corner of the eye. If the head were extremely flexed, the line runs to the cheek. More rarely, similar marks appear on the portion of the head that has been in contact with the symphysis pubis.

In spite of these types of moulding, these babies tend to develop only a small caput. This is true for two reasons. First, prior to engagement, the head is above the long transverse diameter of the brim, where it is not impacted. This allows for plenty of scalp circulation, which minimizes caput formation. Once engagement occurs, the head is past the narrowest pelvic plane and descent often proceeds rapidly. The result is that a large caput does not have time to form. If descent becomes arrested after engagement, a large caput may develop, as always whenever descent is halted and the head becomes impacted in the pelvis.

In the case of the aftercoming head in a breech baby, a characteristic gutter-like indentation forms where the posterior parietal bone passed the promontory. It runs from the lowermost anterior corner of the parietal bone up and back toward the parietal eminence. When pelvic contraction is more severe, a funnel-shaped dent is produced where the parietal bone was lodged against the promontory.

The movements of birth in a generally contracted gynecoid pelvis (occiput presentation)

In this situation, the head fits the inlet well; abnormal attitudes, presentations and positions are not as frequently found as in the case of a flat pelvis. The risk of early rupture of membranes and cord prolapse is not increased because the presenting part fits the brim so much better than in a flat pelvis.

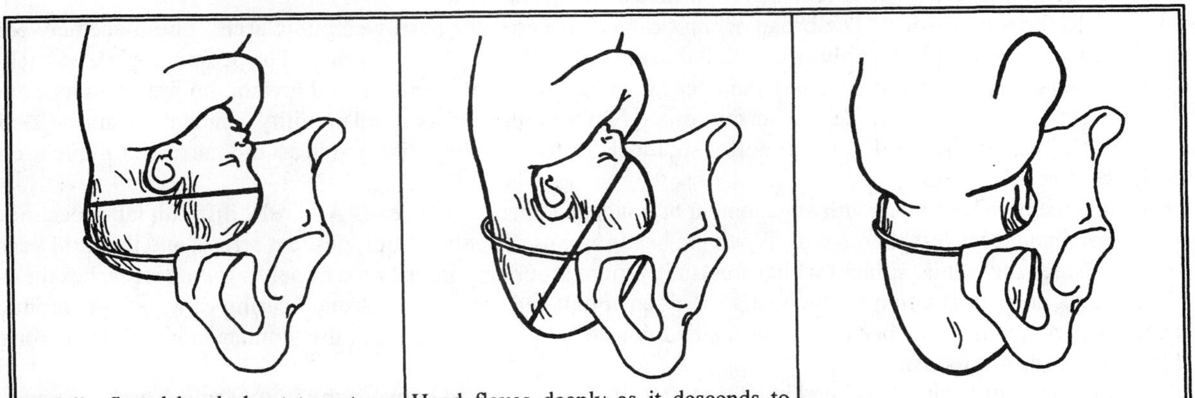

Partially flexed head about to enter a generally contracted pelvis.	Head flexes deeply as it descends to engagement.	Rotation complete.

Labor is characterized by extreme flexion of the fetal head (Roederer's obliquity), causing this type of labor to be called an "occiput presentation" in some historical texts. This extreme degree of flexion results from an exaggeration of the same process that produces flexion in normal labor, and affords the best opportunity for progress when the pelvis is contracted in all diameters. The actual degree of flexion corresponds to the degree of pelvic contraction. The head is well flexed in early labor and flexion increases with descent, bringing the posterior fontanelle within easy reach. Extreme flexion causes the sagittal suture to be almost perpendicular to the angle of descent, running in an oblique direction across the pelvis. Abdominal examination reveals the high forehead, which is easily felt over one pubic ramus. The occiput, which is deep in the pelvis, is usually not palpable externally even when a hand is pressed deeply into the lower abdomen near the pubic bone.

The head typically enters the brim via an oblique diameter. Thus, anterior asynclitism rarely occurs in these labors, as the sacral promontory is not pronounced. Slight posterior asynclitism may occur, with the posterior parietal bone being slightly low. However, a pronounced degree of posterior asynclitism is unfavorable. Descent through the brim is usually much easier than in a flat pelvis.

Moulding becomes pronounced as labor advances. The posterior fontanelle lies almost in the center of the pelvic cavity. Pressure around the circumference of the head impairs circulation to the scalp and leads to the formation of a large caput, which covers the posterior fontanelle. This extremely tight fit combined with strong contractions may also result in the cervix becoming trapped between the skull and the pelvic wall. This impairs circulation to the maternal tissues lying below the presenting part, may interfere with dilation and possibly lead to cervical amputation. Generally contracted pelvises, unlike those that are flat, are narrowed all the way to the outlet; therefore progress is slow throughout labor. Contractions are often not very effective and may stop altogether before the head reaches the perineum. High transverse arrest may occur.

With a normal pelvis, internal rotation may be delayed until the head is well placed against the pelvic floor. In a small pelvis, internal rotation tends to occur early because further descent depends upon optimal accommodation of the head to the bony space of the narrowed pelvic cavity. Therefore, internal rotation takes place as the vertex reaches the level of the ischial spines and usually must be complete before further progress can occur.

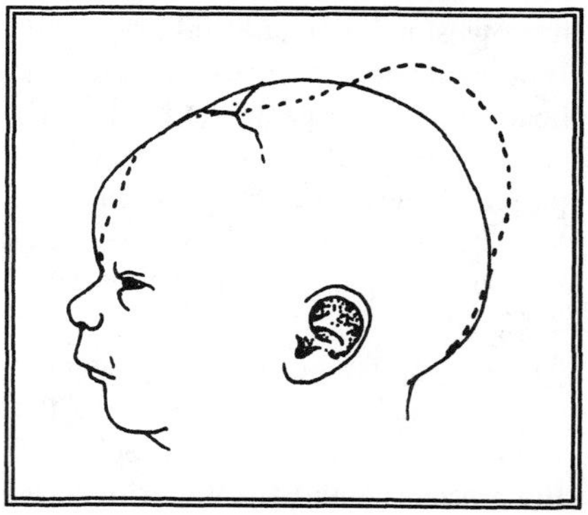

Moulding: Pressure marks are unusual because the resistances met are broad rather than sharp. When found, these marks are due to extreme head flexion and typically appear on the frontal bone that was nearest the sacral promontory. The occipitofrontal diameter is excessively elongated, the occiput is peaked, and the neck is almost in a line with the back of the head. The forehead and face are flattened, and the chin is buried in the chest. Extreme overlapping of suture lines and upward displacement of the parietal bones commonly occurs.

Movements of labor in an extremely android (funnel-shaped) pelvis

The resistance to descent begins at the pelvic outlet when the pelvis is funnel-shaped, and descent becomes arrested at this point. Extreme flexion occurs, and labor resembles that of a generally contracted gynecoid pelvis.

The funnel-shaped pelvis is often most contracted transversely, at the outlet between the tuberosities. The broad occiput cannot fit under the narrowed pubic arch. The space between the tuberosities and the coccyx is the only space available through which the head can pass. The occiput is pressed backward into the perineum and against the sacrum and coccyx. As a result, the perineum and levator ani are often torn and the coccyx fractured during labor. If the sacrum curves too far forward and maximum mobility cannot compensate, delivery will be impossible. If the head is born, outlet shoulder dystocia is very likely due to the narrowed pubic arch and generally contracted outlet.

The outcome of labor varies with engagement or nonengagement of the head. As a rule, difficult labor occurs when the bi-ischial diameter is less than 8 cm. When the head reaches the pelvic floor, descent arrests and the head becomes impacted between the ischial spines (which are usually quite prominent in this type of pelvis) when it reaches the pelvic floor. Even so, anterior rotation of the occiput is often completed. However, strong bearing-down efforts produce no advance. The perineum does not stretch or distend nor does bulging occur, and the woman soon recognizes that her pushing efforts are ineffective.

Internal examination finds the head in exaggerated flexion, squeezed between the ischial spines and covered with a large caput. The occiput is usually anterior, but sometimes the sagittal suture lies in the transverse diameter, indicating that the baby is in deep transverse arrest. The more reduced the space from the central point between the tuberosities to the tip of the coccyx (the posterior sagittal diameter of the pelvic outlet), the less likely it is that further descent will occur. (See the chapter entitled "Basic Principles of How the Mother's Soft and Bony Pelvic Structures Influence Fetal Descent" in this volume and the chapter entitled "Pelvimetry" in Volume I for more details.)

Labor in a transversely contracted pelvis

Mild degrees of contraction in the transverse diameter of the brim will not pose serious problems if the inlet is sufficiently large overall. A circular pelvis has the largest area for any given diameter, and a small round inlet may have more available room than a large one that has sides that are compressed or into which the sacral promontory projects.

In android and anthropoid pelvises, the head fits better when entering in a median vertex attitude with the occiput posterior; the baby naturally seeks to place his occiput in the larger posterior portion of the inlet.

If the sacrum projects forward, the whole head is also pushed forward; it then rotates to the transverse or even to the posterior once it is engaged. The head descends until it arrests between the prominent ischial spines. There are three possible progressions from this point:

- Flexion and anterior rotation of the occiput
- Natural or assisted flexion and posterior rotation of the occiput, or
- Surgical birth for arrest of labor.

Note that flexion is always required to complete this type of birth. Once flexion occurs, two possibilities present themselves:

- Flexion is enhanced, the occiput rotates posteriorly, the posterior portion of the vertex advances over the perineum, and the forehead emerges from between the pubic rami; or
- After posterior rotation, the head is less flexed, causing the central vertex to crown and the somewhat deflexed head to pass under the pubic bone.

Labor in an obliquely contracted pelvis

Oblique contraction refers to a pelvis that is unequally proportioned so that actual contraction exists in one or more planes. How labor progresses with this type of pelvis depends upon the amount of contraction in the true conjugate and, of course, the prominence of the sacrum. When the sacral promontory projects at an angle toward one ileopubic tubercle, that half of the pelvis is usually rendered impassable for the normally sized term fetus. Such a pelvis is equivalent to one that has an extreme degree of general contraction. The occiput usually descends on the opposite side in the larger portion of the pelvis, but may occasionally enter pointing toward the contracted half. Birth proceeds normally in some cases.

A breech labor through an obliquely contracted pelvis is very difficult. If unavoidable (a surprise breech in a location remote from medical assistance), it is most desirable for the occiput to come through the side that is least contracted. However, surgical birth is, by far, the safest option and should be planned for when the pelvis is known to be contracted in any way.

Dangers to mother and baby

Nonprogressive labor through a contracted pelvis is fraught with dangers for both mother and baby. Here is a rundown of major maternal problems from Stander's 9th edition of WILLIAMS OBSTETRICS (1945):

Abnormalities of dilation: A poorly fitting presenting part coupled with early rupture of membranes can lead to delay in dilation because the presenting part is not well applied to the os. This reduces or eliminates the counterpressure that the cervix needs to dilate most readily.

Abnormal uterine contractions: Abnormally weak or ineffective contractions can occur with obstruction or prolonged labor, both of which tire the uterine muscle.

Early rupture of membranes: When early rupture of membranes occurs, it increases the chance that infection will set in, that the cervix will not dilate in a timely fashion and that the cord will prolapse.

Intrapartum infection: Prolonged labor, rupture of membranes, multiple internal exams, tissue necrosis and exhaustion set the mother and baby up for infection.

Uterine rupture: Unrecognized obstructed labor for any reason presents the same danger of ruptured uterus as with a transverse lie. The character of uterine action is basically the same. See the chapter entitled "Transverse Lie" for a full description of this gruesome complication.

Production of fistulae and necrotic lesions in the maternal birth canal: Extreme pressure from the presenting part against the maternal soft tissues combined with lack of progress impairs circulation to the compressed tissues, eventually leading to tissue death and the formation of holes through the wall of the birth canal into the urinary or bowel tract. A tight fit between the presenting part and the pelvic wall can produce uniform pressure against the remaining portion of cervix, resulting in arrest of dilation. This can eventually result in annular detachment of the cervix as the compressed ring of cervical tissue that lies between the os and the neck of the cervix necroses and falls off.

Rupture of pelvic joints: The pelvic joints may separate on rare occasions. When this occurs, it is usually in cases of a contracted outlet, the symphysis and sometimes one or both sacroiliac joints giving way as the mother's body makes a maximum effort to accommodate passage of the baby.

Postpartum hemorrhage: Heavy bleeding is much more likely to occur after a prolonged and exhausting labor.

Here is a summary of major problems for the baby:

Cord prolapse: This life-threatening complication is more likely to occur when the presenting part fits poorly, which can contribute to rupture of membranes during early labor.

Enlarging caput: An increasing caput is dangerous, especially when it goes unnoticed and is mistaken for descent. Impaired scalp circulation may also occur leading to the formation of lesions, necrotic areas or sloughing of scalp tissue, leaving the baby more vulnerable to infection.

Severe moulding: Moulding can be so severe as to produce intracranial hemorrhage from tearing of the membranes of the dura and associated vessels, and skull indentations or actual fractures, either of which can lead to brain damage or death.

Newborn complications: Distress, infection, brain damage and death are all possibilities for these babies when a labor which should have been transported is allowed to proceed at home.

It is obvious from these lists of dire consequences that labor in women suspected of having contracted pelvises should be carefully monitored. Indications of lack of progress that do not respond to midwifery interventions should be cause to transport well before both mother and baby are placed in jeopardy.

OBLIQUE LIE

Oblique lie represents a stage in the transition from longitudinal to transverse lie and is far more common than transverse lie. It occurs when the long axis of the fetus is in a diagonal relationship to the long axis of the mother. The presenting part (either the breech or the head) is in the lower pole of the uterus but not centered over the pelvic cavity. This lie has also been referred to as an "oblique presentation" as well as a "deviated breech" or "deviated cephalic presentation," depending upon which fetal pole is lowermost in the uterus. It is important to distinguish between the entire uterus being tipped to one side (obliquity of the uterus, which is very common with the fundus tipped to the right), but with the fetus lying longitudinally within it, and a true oblique lie. A true oblique lie finds the baby lying at an angle in relationship to the long axis of the uterus.

Oblique lie may preexist labor, or it may develop during early labor if the head or the breech deviates from the inlet and lies in one of the iliac fossae. In the latter case, something may be preventing direct engagement, such as a small pelvic inlet or an anomaly of uterine structure, such as a septum. Other causes include a pelvic tumor, a fetal defect, placenta previa, a cord presentation or a fetal limb as well as an impacted rectum or an extremely distended bladder (especially in multiparas). Lax uterine tone also favors oblique as well as transverse lie. An oblique lie is typically somewhat unstable, moving to a longitudinal or transverse lie. However, it may be quite stable if a tumor or uterine anomaly is holding the baby in position.

If the baby in an oblique lie is left to his own devices, conversion to either a longitudinal lie or a transverse lie is likely to result. If the baby cannot or will not realign himself with the pelvic inlet and descend, a surgical delivery becomes necessary.

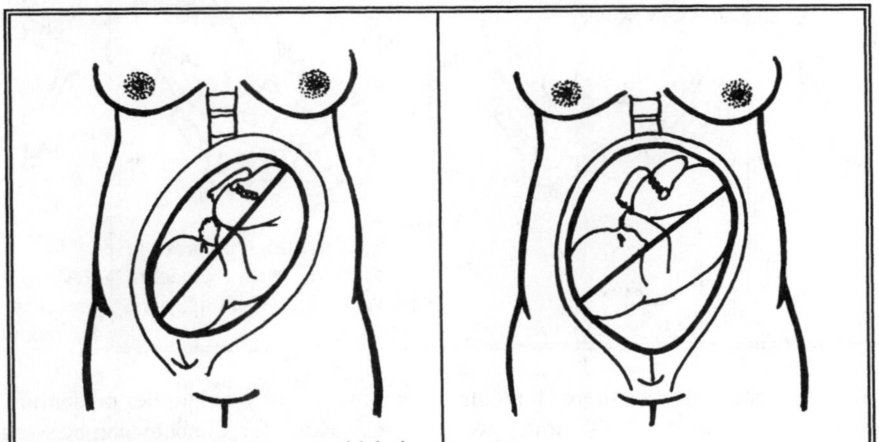

Marked obliquity of the uterus, which tips the baby to the side.

True oblique lie

TRANSVERSE LIE

The long axis of the mother and fetus are at roughly right angles to one another when the baby is lying transverse. The incidence of transverse lie is approximately one in every 500 births. Most transverse lies are established before labor begins and are therefore primary. On rare occasions, the onset of contractions results in rotation of a longitudinal lie into a transverse lie.

Reasons for its occurrence include pendulous abdomen, multiparity with associated lax abdominal and uterine muscles, abnormalities of the position of the uterus, abnormalities of uterine shape (such as arcuatus, septate, didelph [doubled] or bicornous) or the presence of fibroids or other tumors. In addition, multiple pregnancy, pelvic or fetal abnormality, prematurity, fetal demise, directly fundal or very low implantation of the placenta or placenta previa (any of which reduce the vertical space in the uterus) or abnormal mobility of the fetus are all associated with transverse lie.

A stable transverse lie is unlikely to go undetected prior to labor in women who receive prenatal care. Midwives working in very rural areas or in developing countries may encounter cases of undetected transverse lie in which labor has begun and may have the unhappy occasion to deal with a labor that has attempted to progress. It is also possible for a baby to take a notion to change from a longitudinal to a transverse lie prior to or during labor. Knowing the details of what is happening to the baby and the dangers to both mother and baby will assist you in knowing how to help these women.

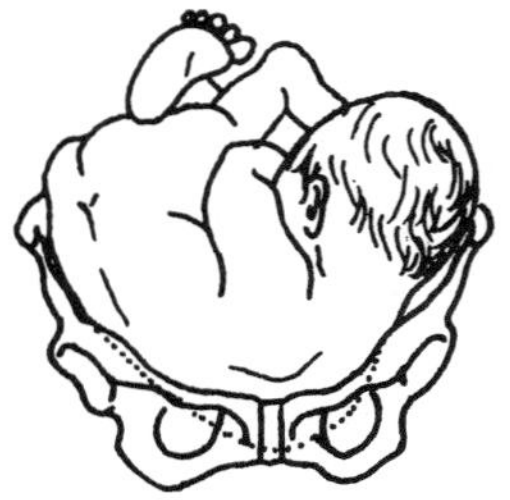

LAA

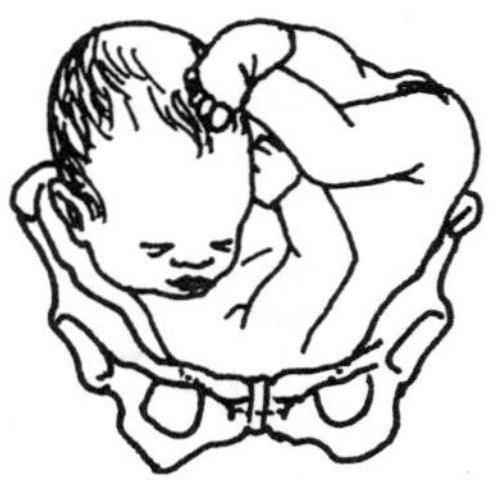

RAP: head in iliac fossa

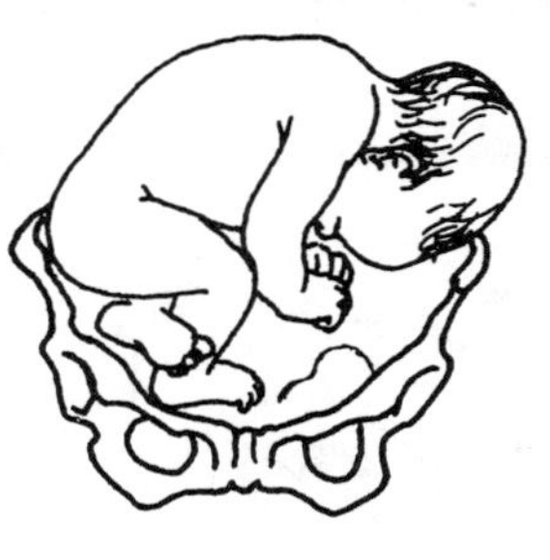

LAS, extremities presenting; associated with placenta previa; high risk of cord prolapse

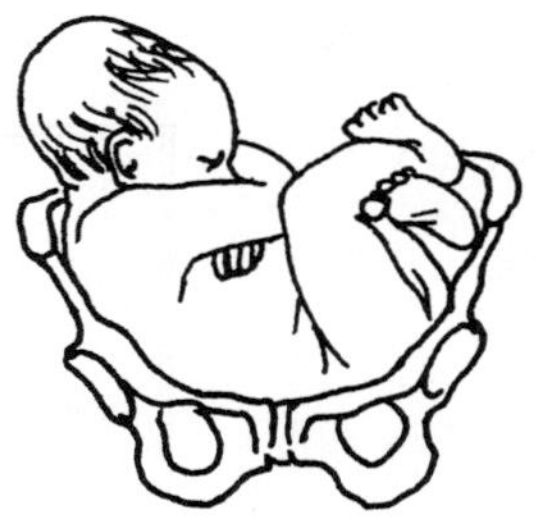

RAI, presenting the back, breech in iliac fossa; lessens the risk of cord prolapse

The breech is usually higher up in the uterus than the head, with the baby's shoulder presenting at the inlet, leading to this lie being commonly referred to as a "shoulder presentation." However, the baby can be so situated that her belly (complete with cord prolapse), back, flank (side of the body between the pelvis and ribs), or chest present. Alternatively, the back may be uppermost with one or more limbs extending downward toward the pelvic inlet. The fetal torso can become twisted so that the shoulder is in the pelvis, the abdomen is directed toward the fundus, and the legs extended upward. The neck may be twisted or the head can become deflexed. If the baby is lying on his side, he may extend an arm into the birth canal. The baby may lie directly across the maternal abdomen but is more likely to lie at an extremely oblique angle with either the head or the breech cradled in one of the iliac fossae. That the baby is more sideways than longitudinal is what distinguishes a transverse from an oblique lie. Understanding the wide variety of possible positions will assist you, should you examine a woman with a baby in a very unusual posture.

In any event, the denominator is the tip of the scapula, or more specifically, the acromion (A). The location of the fetal head determines whether the baby is left or right relative to the mother, and the location of the back determines if the baby is anterior or posterior. Thus RAA means that the lie is transverse, the head is on the mother's right side and the baby's back is anterior. The back is anterior and the head to the mother's left twice as often as not (Hirst, 1918). Sutton (2001) points out that the transverse baby prefers to rest her back in the hammock of the mother's abdomen, just as do babies in a longitudinal lie. There are no formal designations for babies presenting their back directly up or down. Therefore, I have assigned "S" for "superior" to designate a baby presenting his back directly up. I have assigned an "I" for "inferior" to designate a baby presenting his back directly down. Upon examination of a baby in a transverse lie, no distinct presenting part is felt in the birth canal, unless a limb or the cord has prolapsed.

Movements of birth in transverse lie

The successful culmination of labor in a transverse lie with a viable fetus is impossible. If the baby has died or is extremely small or premature (usually less than 800 grams [1 lb 12.5 oz]), it may be pliable enough to allow birth to occur through a large pelvis but not without risk of uterine rupture, infection or hemorrhage for the mother, as well as damage to the infant if she is still alive. Descent may occur by several processes.

Spontaneous rectification and version: In both of these rare cases, the transverse lie converts into a longitudinal lie at the onset of or during labor. Uterine contractions press the fetal pole nearest the pelvis further downward while the uppermost pole is simultaneously moved higher toward the fundus. Spontaneous rectification refers to movement of the head into the pelvis and may occur near term or during early labor. Since the breech is usually higher in the uterus than the head, the head most commonly moves toward the inlet.

Spontaneous version is far less common and refers to movement of the breech into the mother's pelvis. It tends to occur in multiparous women with weak contractions prior to rupture of the membranes and in situations in which the child is freely mobile, such as in the presence of polyhydramnios or prematurity. Version also occurs after the membranes rupture in women with strong contractions. In both cases, version is facilitated when the presenting part cannot easily enter the pelvis. For example, the cervix may be closed, preventing engagement. Instead, the lowermost fetal pole meets resistance from the cervix and begins to work its way up toward the fundus. This causes the pole of the baby nearest the fundus to be forced downward toward the brim, resulting in a vertex or breech presentation. Version requires a strong, resistant, living fetus and fundal contractions.

However, even in cases of fetal demise, awaiting spontaneous rectification or version is an unpredictable and dangerous gamble and should never be relied upon to remedy the situation.

Spontaneous evolution (birth from the transverse position): This occurs in rare cases in which the situation is neglected and labor proceeds with the baby lying transverse, at great risk to both mother and baby. It has been called nature's least likely and most dangerous effort. Spontaneous evolution was originally thought to occur via three possible mechanisms, any of which are highly prone to arrest of descent and impaction. In order to progress at all, exceptionally favorable conditions must prevail, including strong uterine contractions, a large pelvis, a soft, mouldable baby who is either quite small, premature, or dead and macerated. A full-term, living baby cannot be born by any of these mechanisms.

Roederer's method: The baby's body doubles up and is expelled in one mass (*conduplicato corpore)*. The baby is folded in on himself in a V-shape, and the scapula and back advance downward as the baby's head presses deeply into his chest and abdomen. The arm is usually not prolapsed.

Douglas' method: The second mechanism occurs most often when the back is anterior and an arm is prolapsed. The baby rotates and is born with the anterior surface of her body leading the way. The baby's body is forced into a pointed shape. It doubles in on itself laterally, with breech and head approaching each other. The head is arrested above the inlet, and the occiput rotates to the nearest anterior quadrant of the pelvis, greatly stretching the neck, which is pressed against the brim. The torso twists to allow the sacrum to rotate to the opposite posterior quadrant of the pelvis. The prolapsed arm and shoulder descend into the pelvic cavity.

The arm and shoulder emerge, leaving space for the rounded side of the thorax to become forced into the pelvis. The chest is born first, followed by the abdomen, breech and legs, which slide down, squeezing past the shoulder. After the legs drop out, the other arm and finally the head are born.

Denman's method: The last, and most rare, mechanism is a sort of spontaneous version that occurs in the pelvic cavity. The occiput rotates posteriorly and, as the breech descends, the shoulder ascends with the head. The breech finally comes down and out. This was said to be most common when the back is posterior.

Many historical authors believed that there is only one mechanism of spontaneous evolution in the transverse baby and that the these three distinct processes developed only because of early confusion about what was taking place. The illustrations on the next page present what are considered the "usual" movements during spontaneous evolution. With the many possible fetal positions, the exact process whereby the baby could get squashed down through the pelvis will vary accordingly.

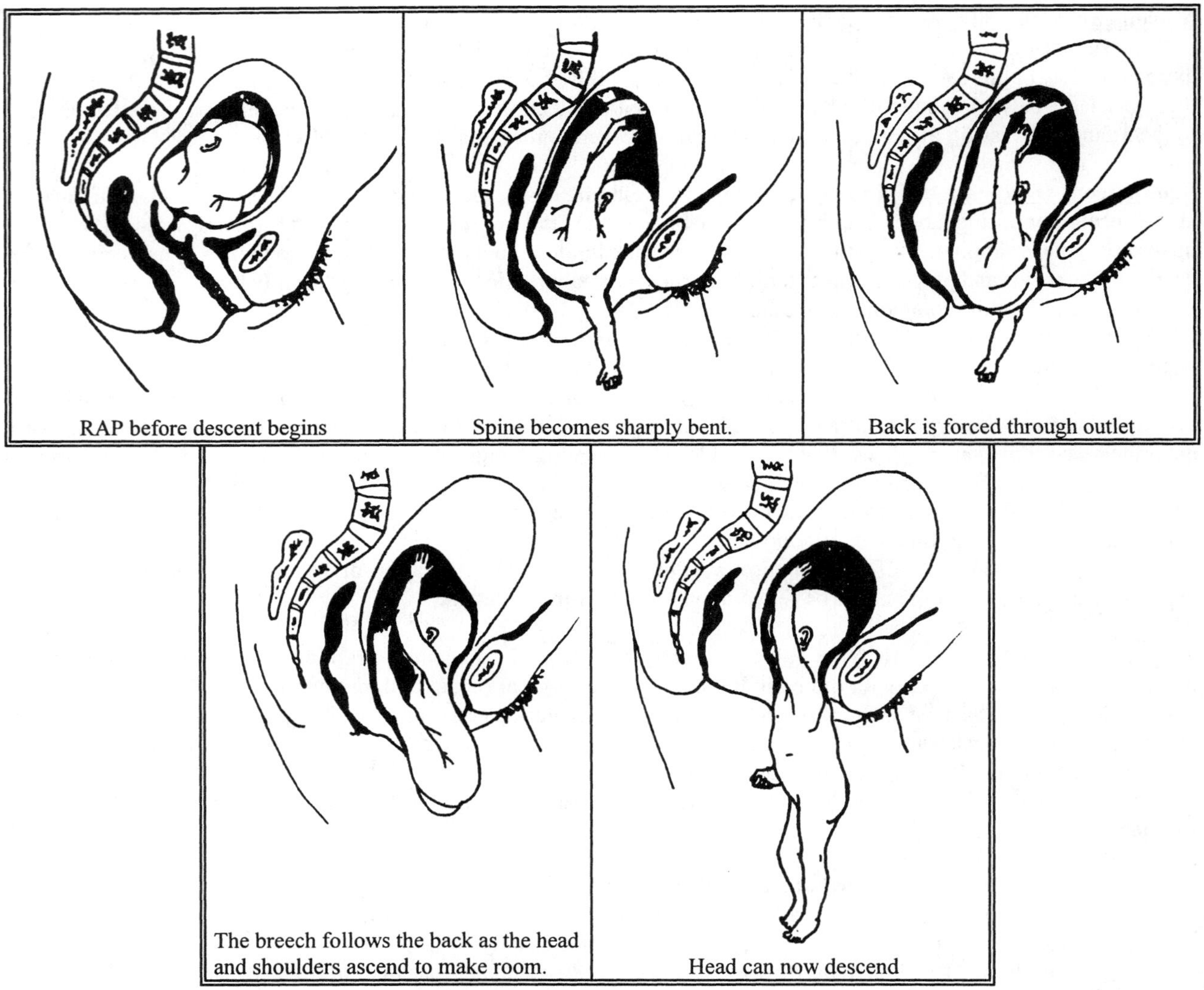

RAP before descent begins

Spine becomes sharply bent.

Back is forced through outlet

The breech follows the back as the head and shoulders ascend to make room.

Head can now descend

Spontaneous, neglected labor in transverse lie: Labor with a viable fetus in a transverse lie is a recipe for disaster. The baby cannot be born naturally, and if labor is allowed to proceed without appropriate intervention, the baby is likely to die and the uterus to rupture as it tries to get the baby out to no avail. The risks to both mother and baby are greatly increased should such a labor proceed undiagnosed or neglected.

In cases left to nature, the onset of labor is sporadic with slow, weak contractions because there is no hard presenting part pressing against the cervix. The membranes often give way as the force of contractions increases due to irregular pressure being exerted upon the forewaters and the lack of a presenting part to equalize the pressure. All the fluid tends to drain out at once, since no presenting part fills the pelvis. As a result, a fetal limb or the umbilical cord is often flushed out as well. The abrupt reduction in uterine volume causes the uterine walls to become temporarily slack, just as is the case when full dilation is reached in a vertex birth.

At this point, there is often a rest in uterine activity. This cessation of contractions may last from a few to many hours during which the uterine wall lies loosely against the baby. Whether a period of uterine quietude occurs or not, as time passes, either by virtue of spontaneous progression of uterine activity or due to manual attempts to turn the baby, contractions are likely to resume and become increasingly violent, tightly gripping the baby and rendering version unsafe and likely impossible. The presenting shoulder is forced into the pelvis, and the fetal body folds in on itself, with the breech pressed against the head, causing the uterine contour to become more globular. Prolapsed limbs become edematous and eventually black and gangrenous. The baby dies as a result of compression of the vital organs of the chest and head or as a result of interruption of the placental circulation by the almost constant uterine contractions of advanced obstructed labor or by abruption of the placenta due to extreme retraction of the upper uterine segment.

Contractions become increasingly irregular, tumultuous and continuous with great tenderness in the lower abdomen. A groove forms between the excessively thickened upper uterine segment and the extremely thinned lower uterine segment. This groove marks the location of a pathologic retraction ring and is often visible through the abdomen. The mother's pulse and temperature rise. Uterine rupture is imminent, and the mother often goes into shock and may die. If rupture does not occur, the contractions become weak and irregular, and the uterus is likely to become infected, leading to the death of the baby, if he has managed to survive this long. The baby and the small amount of amniotic fluid remaining begin to decompose, gas forms and the uterus becomes paralyzed and distended. (My discussion is based on Oxorn, 1986; Greenhill, 1951; Hirst, 1918; King, 1886.)

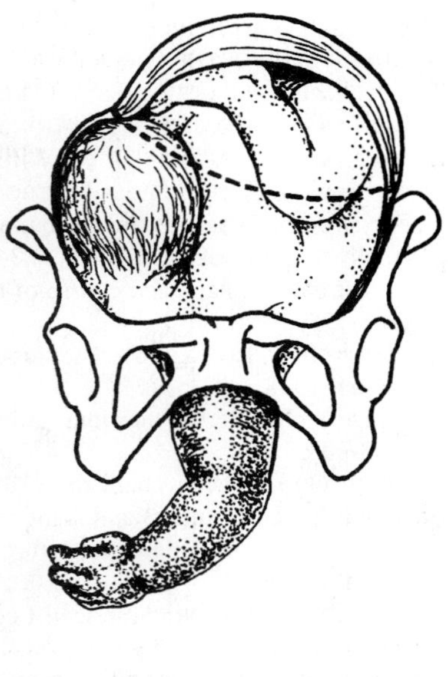

Neglected transverse lie (RAA) with an edematous prolapsed arm, thinned lower uterine segment (below dotted line) and excessively thickened upper uterine segment. A pathologic retraction ring (dotted line) separates the upper and lower segments. Most of the baby is now contained in the lower segment. (Mother is lying supine.)

Fetal compaction, moulding and caput formation: In the exceedingly rare event that a baby is born via spontaneous evolution, the vital organs of the chest and abdomen are likely to be severely damaged by the head being pressed into the viscera during descent. Such extreme compaction may kill a living baby during labor or may cause the baby to die shortly after birth. In addition, cord compression may occur during descent, and oxygen deprivation may result in brain damage, if not death.

If an arm has prolapsed, it will be grossly swollen and bruised. Sloughing of skin and even gangrene may be present. A caput-like swelling develops over the presenting shoulder, which is also bruised. Generalized bruising also occurs in areas where pressure was exerted on the mother's and baby's bodies during labor.

REFERENCES AND FURTHER READING ON ALL TYPES OF FETAL PRESENTATIONS

REFERENCES USED IN MULTIPLE CHAPTERS

Bard S. A COMPENDIUM OF THE THEORY AND PRACTICE OF MIDWIFERY, 1st ed. Collins & Perkins, New York NY, 1807. Cited in Jarcho J. THE PELVIS IN OBSTETRICS. Paul B Hoeber, New York NY, 1933.

Beard, R. THE OCCIPITO-POSTERIOR POSITION: ITS MECHANISM AND TREATMENT, 2nd ed. FW Peece & Sons, Adelaide Australia, 1937.

Beck A. OBSTETRICAL PRACTICE, 2nd ed. Williams & Wilkins Co, Baltimore MD, 1939.

Bennett VR, Brown LK, eds. MYLES TEXTBOOK FOR MIDWIVES,13th ed. Churchill Livingstone, Edinburgh UK, 1999.

Borell U, Fernström I. "The movements in the mechanism of disengagement with special reference to the attitude of the foetal head," ACTA OBSTET GYNECOL SCAND, 36(3);347-355, 1957a.

Borell U, Fernström I. "Shape and course of the birth canal, a radiographic study in the human," ACTA OBSTET GYNECOL SCAND, 36(2);166-178, 1957b.

Borell U, Fernström I. "Radiographic studies of the rotation of the foetal shoulders during labour," ACTA OBSTET GYNECOL SCAND, 37(1);54-61, 1958.

Borell U, Fernström I. "Internal anterior rotation of the foetal head: a contribution to its explanation," ACTA OBSTET GYNECOL SCAND, 38(1);103-108, 1959.

Borell U, Fernström I. "The mechanism of labour," RADIOL CLIN N AM, 5(1);73-85, Apr, 1967. (Summarizes all previous research on this topic by these authors and is the best single article for students.)

Calkins L. NORMAL LABOR, American Lecture Series, No. 246, American Lectures in Gynecology and Obstetrics. Charles C Thomas, Springfield IL, 1955.

Calkins L. ABNORMAL LABOR, American Lecture Series, No. 325, American Lectures in Obstetrics and Gynecology. Charles C Thomas, Springfield IL, 1958.

Castallo M. THE MECHANICS OF OBSTETRICS. FA Davis Co, Philadelphia PA, 1948.

Creasy R, ed. MANAGEMENT OF LABOR AND DELIVERY. Blackwell Science, Boston MA, 1997.

De Lee J. THE PRINCIPLES AND PRACTICE OF OBSTETRICS, 3rd ed. WB Saunders Co, Philadelphia PA, 1918.

De Lee J. THE PRINCIPLES AND PRACTICE OF OBSTETRICS, 7th ed. WB Saunders Co, Philadelphia PA, 1938.

Eastman N. WILLIAMS OBSTETRICS, 10th ed. Appleton-Century-Crofts, New York NY, 1950.

Eden T, Holland E. A MANUAL OF MIDWIFERY, 7th ed. J & A Churchill, London UK, 1931.

Edgar J. THE PRACTICE OF OBSTETRICS: DESIGNED FOR THE USE OF STUDENTS AND PRACTITIONERS OF MEDICINE, 5th rev. ed. P Balkiston's Son & Co, Philadelphia PA, 1916.

Gabbe S, et al., eds. OBSTETRICS: NORMAL AND PROBLEM PREGNANCIES, 3rd ed. Churchill Livingstone, New York NY, 1996.

Gaskin IM. "Assisting a Vaginal Breech Delivery," Farm Video Productions, Summertown TN, 1992.

Greenhill JP. THE PRINCIPLES AND PRACTICE OF OBSTETRICS, 10th ed. WB Saunders Co, Philadelphia PA, 1951.

Greenhill J, Friedman E. BIOLOGICAL PRINCIPLES AND MODERN PRACTICE OF OBSTETRICS, new ed. (14th ed. De Lee's PRINCIPLES AND PRACTICE OF OBSTETRICS), WB Saunders Co, Philadelphia PA, 1974.

Hirst B. A TEXT-BOOK OF OBSTETRICS, 8th ed. WB Saunders Co, Philadelphia PA, 1918.

Javert C, Steele KB. "The transverse position and the mechanism of labor. A historical collective review," INTERNAT ABSTR SURG, 75;507, 1942.

Kerr J Munro, et al. A COMBINED TEXTBOOK OF OBSTETRICS AND GYNOECOLOGY. E & S Livingstone, Edinburgh UK, 1923.

King A. A MANUAL OF OBSTETRICS, 3rd ed. Lea Brothers & Co, Philadelphia PA, 1886.

King J. BACK LABOR NO MORE!! WHAT EVERY WOMAN SHOULD KNOW BEFORE LABOR. Plenary Systems, Inc, Dallas TX, 1993.

Lemay G. "Birth like a flowing river" workshop, MIDWIFERY TODAY conf., Springfield OR, Mar 22-26, 2001.

Litzmann C. Die Geburt bei engem Becken, Leipzig, Breil kopf und Härtel, 1884; Die Formen des Beckens, insbesondere des engen weiblichen des Beckens, insbesondere des engen weiblichen Beckens, nach eigenen Beobachtungen unde Untersuchungen, Berlin, G. Reimer, 1861. Cited in Greenhill JP. THE PRINCIPLES AND PRACTICE OF OBSTETRICS, 10th ed. WB Saunders Co, Philadelphia PA, 1951.

Mayes B. A TEXTBOOK OF OBSTETRICS, rev ed. Australasian Publishing Co, Sydney Australia, 1959.

McCormick C. A TEXTBOOK ON PATHOLOGY OF LABOR, THE PUERPERIUM AND THE NEWBORN. CV Mosby, St. Louis MO, 1944.

McNeile L. OBSTETRICAL MANIKIN PRACTICE. Williams & Wilkins Co, Baltimore MD, 1939.

Miller A, Callander R. OBSTETRICS ILLUSTRATED, 4th ed. Churchill Livingstone, Edinburgh UK, 1989.

Morison CR. "Mechanism of labor: 1. normal labor," NURS MIRROR MIDWIVES J. 133(16);34-38, Oct 15, 1971.

Myles M. A TEXTBOOK FOR MIDWIVES, 6th ed. E & S Livingstone, London UK, 1968.

Oxorn H. OXORN-FOOTE HUMAN LABOR AND BIRTH, 5th ed. Appleton-Century-Crofts, Norwalk CT, 1986.

Peterson R, Miller N. A MANUAL FOR A DEMONSTRATION COURSE IN OBSTETRICS, 3rd ed. Edwards Brothers Inc, Ann Arbor MI, 1940.

Pritchard J, MacDonald P. WILLIAMS OBSTETRICS, 16th ed. Appleton-Century-Crofts, New York NY, 1980.

Rydberg E. THE MECHANISM OF LABOUR. Charles C Thomas, Springfield IL, 1954a.

Rydberg E. "The two hundred years' teaching of the mechanism of labor; a medico-historical sketch," AM J OBSTET GYNECOL, 68(1);236-244, July, 1954b.

Scott J, et al., eds. DANFORTH'S OBSTETRICS AND GYNECOLOGY, 6th ed. JB Lippincott Co, Philadelphia PA, 1990.
Sellers P. MIDWIFERY: A TEXTBOOK AND REFERENCE BOOK FOR MIDWIVES IN SOUTHERN AFRICA, VOL. I: NORMAL CHILDBIRTH. Juta & Co, Ltd, Kenwyn So Africa, 1993.
Smellie W. A TREATISE ON THE THEORY AND PRACTICE OF MIDWIFERY. D Wilson, London UK, 1752. Reprinted in Classics in Obstetrics and Gynecology Library, Gryphon Editions, New York NY, 1990.
Stander H. TEXTBOOK OF OBSTETRICS, 3rd ed. (9th ed. WILLIAMS OBSTETRICS). D Appleton-Century Co, New York NY, 1945.
Steer C. MOLOY'S EVALUATION OF THE PELVIS IN OBSTETRICS, 3rd ed. Plenum Medical Books Co, New York NY, 1975.
Stern D. COMYNS BERKELEY'S PICTORIAL MIDWIFERY: AN ATLAS OF MIDWIFERY FOR PUPIL MIDWIVES, 5th ed. Baillière, Tindall & Cox, London UK, 1956.
Sutton J. LET BIRTH BE BORN AGAIN! REDISCOVERING AND RECLAIMING OUR MIDWIFERY HERITAGE. Birth Concepts, Bedfont UK, 2001.
Sutton J, Scott P. UNDERSTANDING AND TEACHING OPTIMAL FOETAL POSITIONING, Bay Print Ltd, Tauranga NZ, 1996.
Sweet B, ed. MAYES' MIDWIFERY, 12th ed. Baillière Tindall, London UK, 1997.
Varney H. VARNEY'S MIDWIFERY, 3rd ed. Jones and Bartlett, Sudbury MA, 1997.
Vaux N. EDGAR'S PRACTICE OF OBSTETRICS, 6th ed. P Blakiston's Son & Co, Philadelphia PA, 1926.

THE CARDINAL SPIRALING MOVEMENTS: LEFT OCCIPUT TRANSVERSE

Baudelocque J. PRINCIPES SUR L'ART DES ACCOUCHEMENTS, Méquignon, Paris France, 1775.

REFERENCES SPECIFIC TO FACE AND BROW PRESENTATION

Arthure H. "Brow presentation; spontaneous rectification to a vertex in the pelvis," J OBSTET GYNAECOL BRIT EMP 64(6);909-910, Dec, 1957.
Benedetti T, et al. "Face presentation at term," OBSTET GYNECOL, 55(2);199-202, Feb, 1980.
Borell U, Fernström I. "The mechanism of labour in face and brow presentation, a radiological study," ACTA OBSTET GYNECOL SCAND, 39;626-644, 1960.
Cruikshank D, Cruikshank J. "Face and brow presentation: a review," CLIN OBSTET GYNECOL, 24(2);333-351, June, 1981.
Cruikshank D, White C. "Obstetric malpresentations: twenty years' experience." AM J OBSTET GYNECOL, 116(8);1097-1104, Aug 15, 1973.
Cucco V. "Face presentation," AM J OBSTET GYNECOL, 94(8);1085-1091, Apr 15, 1966.
Donald I. PRACTICAL OBSTETRIC PROBLEMS, 5th ed. Lloyd-Luke, London UK, 1979.
Ingolfsson A. "Brow presentations," ACTA OBSTET GYNECOL SCAND, 48(4);486-496, 1969.
Jennings P. "Brow presentation with vaginal delivery," AUST NZ J OBSTET GYNAECOL, 8(4);219-224, Nov, 1968.
Lachapelle ML. PRATIQUE DES ACCOUCHEMENTS, JB Baillière, Paris France,1821.
Schwartz Z, et al. "Face presentation," AUST NZ J OBSTET GYNAECOL, 26(2);172-176, Aug,1986.
Tucker BD, et al. "A study of face presentation in the normal mature fetus," SURG GYNECOL OBSTET, 90;199-203, 1957.
Williams JW. OBSTETRICS: A TEXTBOOK FOR THE USE OF STUDENTS AND PRACTITIONERS. D Appleton & Co, New York NY, 1903.

REFERENCES SPECIFIC TO BREECH PRESENTATION

Banks M. BREECH BIRTH WOMAN-WISE. Birthspirit Books, Hamilton NZ, 1998.
Burns J, Marshall C. "Breech, its etiology, diagnosis, prognosis and treatment with special reference to the treatment of the after-coming head," (sect Reports of Societies), BMJ, (1);820-821, May 5, 1934.
Cronk M, Evans J. Written and verbal editing comments on cardinal movements of breech labor, personal communications, Apr, 2002.
Ramin S., et al. OPERATIVE OBSTETRICS, 2nd ed. McGraw-Hill Medical Pub, New York NY, 2002.
Hickok DE, et al. "The frequency of breech presentation by gestational age at birth: a large population-based study," AM J OBSTET GYNECOL, 166(3);851-852, Mar, 1992.
Mukhopadhyay S, Arulkumaran S. "Breech delivery," BEST PRACT RES CLIN OBSTET GYNAECOL, 16(1);31-42, Feb, 2002.

NOTES:

ADDITIONAL MATERNAL CONSIDERATIONS

HOW AND WHY LABOR BEGINS

From a midwifery perspective, labor begins when mother, baby and external circumstances are poised to allow the process of opening and letting go to unfold. The birth process involves complex physiological, as well as psycho-emotional, sexual and spiritual, aspects. The biochemistry background necessary to understand the physical aspects of this process is complicated and beyond the scope of daily midwifery knowledge. This chapter is intended to give you an overview of this extremely intricate subject.

Science has not yet discovered the exact physiological means by which human labor begins. The uterus must remain relatively quiet and unresponsive during pregnancy, and the cervix must remain closed so that the conceptus can be retained. At the time of labor, the uterus is transformed into a coordinated, forcefully contracting organ, the lower end of which softens and opens to allow for birth. The biochemistry of these two uterine states differs among species. Current research into human labor focuses upon two general lines of investigation. The first postulates the retreat from a state of pregnancy maintenance wherein one or more agents are withdrawn, allowing labor to begin. The second, the uterotonin induction hypothesis, postulates that one or more agents which initiate labor are produced. Most theories involve both of these ideas.

Theories

Two independent observations have dominated the scientific study of the onset of labor for the past 40 years. One recognizes the important role of estrogen in maintaining pregnancy and focuses on the placenta as the primary source of this hormone. (Estrogen was previously thought to be produced almost entirely by the corpus luteum.) The second realization is that the fetus may play a role in initiating labor.

There are several specific hypotheses regarding why labor starts when it does, although all the data needed to determine their relative importance are not yet in. Of the theories discussed below, the first two hold the most promise. It is highly likely that uterine quiescence during pregnancy is maintained by a complex interaction of independent but cooperative mechanisms and that withdrawal of these agents at term allows the uterus to become more active.

The possible role of the fetus: Some animal research suggests that the onset of labor is regulated, at least in part, by the fetus, although how this works is not fully understood. It has been shown that sheep fetuses provide the initial signal that leads to the start of labor in ewes. However, a similar mechanism has not yet been proven in humans.

The rise in estrogen levels throughout pregnancy appears to influence myometrial changes that enhance the ability of the muscle to produce strong contractions. It also promotes progesterone activity. The placenta cannot synthesize estrogen without C_{19} steroids, which the fetus produces in copious amounts. As the onset of human labor draws near, the fetal membranes step up production of estrogen, an event probably triggered by the release of chemicals from the maturing fetal brain. Maturation of other fetal organs also leads to the urinary excretion of substances that stimulate prostaglandin synthesis in maternal and fetal tissues. Evidence suggests that when the baby has an anomaly that affects the normal functioning of the fetal adrenal glands (which produce C_{19} steroids), pregnancy is often, although not invariably, prolonged. The way that fetal influences upon labor combine with maternal triggers, however, is still unclear.

The progesterone withdrawal hypothesis: Until term, the uterine muscle is relatively quiet throughout pregnancy due, in part, to the influence of high levels of progesterone. However, progesterone administration does not prevent, delay or stop labor in either preterm or term pregnancies, nor does a fall in progesterone cause uterine contractions. Therefore, most researchers have decided that progesterone withdrawal is not a basic prerequisite for labor to begin. An unexplored possibility may be that the interruption of only certain types of progesterone activity by one or more specific agents through a progesterone-receptor-independent, gene-specific process may somehow be involved in the onset of labor. If such a process exists, it may manifest on a molecular, biochemical or cellular level.

The prostaglandin hypothesis: Prostaglandins were first identified in human amniotic fluid in 1967. Since that time, their relevance to the process of labor has become increasingly apparent. The activity of certain forms of these phospholipids increases in intrauterine tissues and in maternal plasma during labor. In many hospitals in the United States, the use of prostaglandins has replaced IV oxytocin infusion to initiate labor. PGE_2 gel or misoprostol (PGE_1) can be applied directly to the cervix to ripen it, followed by amniotomy once the uterus is responding with contractions. In some cases, the use of prostaglandin synthesis inhibitors such as indomethacin have been used to curtail preterm labor.

However, many researchers now consider the release of prostaglandins the result, rather than the cause, of labor, since prostaglandin concentrations in amniotic fluid increase as the cervix dilates. It is well understood that PGE_2 production is activated by inflammatory responses such as that which occurs when the forewaters are exposed to the nonsterile yoni environment during cervical dilation, resulting in a high concentration of prostaglandins in the forewaters. Prostaglandins may contribute to the effectiveness of uterine contractions once labor begins. Further research may clarify the exact role of prostaglandins as well as the ways in which hormones and other substances cooperate in the initiation of labor.

Corticotropin releasing hormone (CRH): CRH, an amino acid peptide secreted by the hypothalamus, stimulates the secretion of ACTH (adrenocorticotropic hormone) and beta-endorphin. CRH, which may also be secreted by the placenta, rises from undetectable levels prior to pregnancy to very high levels at term. The pituitary does not recognize this elevation, due to the presence of a binding protein (CRH-BP), the levels of which also increase throughout pregnancy. The CRH-BP binds with the CRH, rendering it inactive. At term, the production of CRH-BP falls off, causing the level of biologically active CRH to rise.

There are several observations that suggest that CRH may play a role in starting labor. CRH levels rise sharply in both preterm and term labor, as well as in cases of multiple gestation, but are low in postterm pregnancies. CRH stimulates amnion cells to produce prostaglandin and potentiates the contractile response of myometrial tissue to oxytocin, while oxytocin stimulates placental cells to produce CRH. Cytokines (proteins that mediate inflammatory responses) stimulate the secretion of CRH and may assist in starting labor in the presence of infection. The key to understanding how CRH may contribute to the onset of labor involves further research into why and how CRH-BP levels are triggered to fall at term.

Nitric oxide: Nitric oxide is an epithelial-derived relaxing factor (EDRF) and a potent vasodilator that relaxes vascular smooth muscle. Nitric oxide from the uterine epithelium may cause the uterine myometrium to relax during pregnancy; thus a reduction in nitric oxide levels may lead to the onset of labor. The nitric oxide donors nitroglycerin and amyl nitrate are known to relax the uterus, and nitroprusside inhibits CRH production. However, current research on animals does not fully support the principle role of nitric oxide as a uterine relaxant in pregnancy or its withdrawal in the initiation of labor.

Theories regarding how and why labor starts are constantly being proposed. Those mentioned here will, no doubt, undergo considerable modification in the years to come. While much is known regarding uterine physiology of late pregnancy, the exact biochemistry is still unclear in this area as well. The factors discussed in the next chapter come into play in the complex changes that precipitate the beginning of labor.

Anatomy and Physiology of Uterine Changes during Late Pregnancy and Labor

NOTE: This chapter expands upon material presented in Volume I, focusing on changes that lead up to and support the process of labor. (Uterine anatomy outside of pregnancy is covered in Volume I.)

The nonpregnant uterus of a woman who has never been pregnant is shaped like an inverted, flattened, hollow pear. Its shape, weight and dimensions vary somewhat among individuals and are particularly influenced by the number of babies a woman has had. A multiparous uterus is shaped somewhat less distinctly because it has been stretched. The uterus, at term, is the strongest muscle in humans. This specialized organ must be able to protect and support the baby during pregnancy and then produce powerful contractions and open up to allow the birth of the baby.

The uterus has several different regions that have distinct roles in the process of pregnancy and labor. The dome or **fundus** sits above the level where the uterine or egg tubes attach to the uterus. The body or **corpus**, which is the largest region, extends from the lower border of the fundus to the uterine isthmus. The **isthmus** begins where the body of the uterus narrows and is a transitional region between the corpus and the **cervix**.

The uterine wall

The wall of the uterus is composed of three primary layers: the outer peritoneal surface or serous epithelial layer (perimetrium), the middle, thicker layers of unstriped muscle (myometrium), and the membranous inner lining (endometrium). The anterior and posterior walls of the uterus are thicker than the lateral walls.

Perimetrium: The peritoneum lines the abdominal cavity. The perimetrium is the portion of the pelvic peritoneum that drapes over the uterus. The perimetrium is continuous with the folds of peritoneum on either side of the uterus, forming the broad ligaments. It is continuous anteriorly, covering the bladder at the level of the cervical isthmus, and is most firmly attached to the fundus. The cervix is covered by peritoneum only on its posterior aspect, just above the yoni. From here the perimetrium extends over the posterior yoni wall, becoming the peritoneum as it bends back onto the rectum, forming the rectouterine pouch. This pouch may be filled with loops of small intestine.

Parametrium: The parametrium originates from the subserous coat of the uterus and consists of loosely woven connective tissue that separates the suprayoni portion of the cervix from the bladder in front. It covers the sides of the cervix and extends laterally on either side between the layers of the broad ligaments. The uterine arteries reach the margins of the cervix in the parametrium, and the ureters run downward and forward in it at a distance of about 2 cm from the cervix on either side.

Myometrium: Sources vary as to the basic anatomy of the uterine muscle. This explanation reflects a composite of opinions. The myometrium makes up most of the uterine wall. It consists of three muscle layers composed of interlaced longitudinal, circular and oblique fibers, which are not well organized in the nonpregnant uterus. During pregnancy, they become more differentiated and organized so that effective contractions can take place in labor. Individual myometrial cells are arranged in interconnected bundles of 10 to 50 partially overlapping smooth muscle cells laid down in a mesh of collagen tissue known as **ground substance**. This matrix of connective tissue transmits the contractile force from individual myometrial cells along the muscle bundle.

The muscle cells of the inner layer are the least numerous and least compact. These muscles consist of mostly longitudinal and some oblique fibers arranged in circular spirals running both clockwise and counterclockwise, perpendicular to

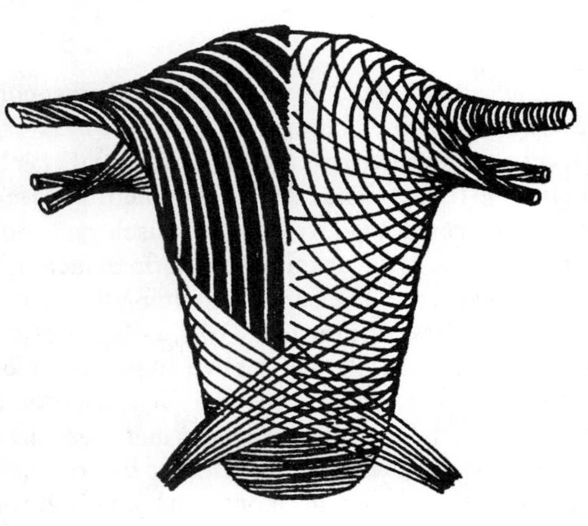

Inner and outer layers of uterine muscle

the long axis of the uterus. These fibers form sphincter-like closures at the openings of the egg tubes, the isthmus, and the cervix, where they are most abundant. This arrangement keeps the cervix closed during pregnancy and allows dilation during labor.

The middle layer is made up of fibers that run obliquely and are most abundant in the body and fundus. This layer facilitates the birth of the baby, as well as forming a network around the blood vessels that supply the placenta. After birth, these fibers contract around these vessels, preventing hemorrhage.

The outer layer comprises two-thirds of the myometrial thickness in the upper segment but only one-third of the thickness of the lower segment, with 10% in the cervix itself. This layer is most responsive to the hormones of labor that stimulate contractions.

Relatively few new muscle cells appear during pregnancy. Instead, existing muscle cells in the body and fundus stretch and enlarge as pregnancy advances. There is no significant change in the cervix. New fibrous tissue–along with new elastic tissue–does develop, especially in the external muscle layer, adding considerable strength to the uterine wall. The size and number of blood and lymphatic vessels also increase. The uterus has relatively few nerves in comparison to other smooth muscle cells, but these also enlarge as pregnancy advances. Their role is poorly understood.

Endometrium: The endometrium lines the uterus. It is a velvety pink mucous membrane containing surface epithelium, uterine glands, supporting connective tissue and numerous blood vessels. The endometrium is directly attached to the myometrium and is perforated by openings that lead to the uterine glands. These tubular glands form pockets, resembling the fingers of a glove, which extend down into the myometrium. The inner endometrial surface has patches of single-layered, columnar, ciliated cells surrounded by secretory tissue. The endometrium varies in thickness from 0.5 to 5 millimeters; depending primarily upon where a woman is in her menstrual cycle.

After conception, the endometrium receives the blastocyst and allows it to implant, transforming the nonpregnant endometrium into the **decidua**, the endometrium of pregnancy. The decidua is immunologically specialized so that the conceptus is neither rejected nor destroyed. It functions as endocrine tissue, producing a number of hormones and proteins that facilitate reception (called "apposition") and implantation of the blastocyst. It provides agents that support placental growth while the endometrium and underlying spiral arteries accept and then limit trophoblastic invasion.

The decidua has three functionally different regions. The decidua spongiosa is the innermost lining, attached directly to the myometrium. The decidua basialis or serotina is the area of endometrium between the implanted embryo and the myometrium; it underlies and attaches to the maternal side of the placenta. The decidua parietalis or vera is the altered endometrium that underlies the fetal membranes.

Changes in the uterine wall during pregnancy: In early pregnancy, the walls of the uterus become thicker than they were before conception. By term, however, the walls have thinned to a depth of ⅝ in (1.5 cm) or less. The fundus is the portion that undergoes the greatest degree of enlargement and thinning as pregnancy progresses.

The cervix

The cellular structure of the cervix differs considerably from that of the rest of the uterus. Only 5 to 25% of the cervix is made up of muscle fibers, all of which extend downward from the body of the uterus. The thickest portion of the cervical myometrium contains additional elastic and fibrous tissue (chiefly collagen and relatively resistant fibrous connective tissue). The cervical endometrium is much thinner than that of the body of the uterus. It contains connective tissue, or **stroma**, that overlays the muscle and collagen of the cervix and that is lined with tall, ciliated, columnar cells. Portions of the cervical epithelium form branching racemose glands, which secrete mucus and penetrate deeply into the underlying tissue. The nerves supplying the cervix are part of the autonomic nervous system.

During most of pregnancy, the collagen of the cervix is well organized in a longitudinal fashion in the ground substance (the gel-like connective tissue in which cells and fibers are embedded). Progesterone inhibits cervical softening. Near-term enzyme activity causes the collagen to break down. Hyaluronic acid levels rise and dermatan sulfate levels fall, chemical changes that cause the cervical tissue to retain water. Smooth muscle may also be involved in this process. According to current theory, the cervix becomes softer and more stretchable, or ripens, as a result. Catecholamines (stress hormones), which trigger the release of prostaglandins from nerve endings, may also play a part in cervical changes. Even though topically applied synthetic prostaglandins will ripen the cervix, the role of prostaglandins in the natural ripening process appears to be minimal (contrary to what has been thought). Relatively little is understood about the sequence or regulation of the ripening process.

The uterine tissues and hormonal interactions

The contraction-stimulating effect of various hormones and numerous other agents on uterine tissue is complex and not fully understood. For example, the role of oxytocin and prostaglandins, although studied for many decades, still has not been fully elucidated. Previously unrecognized hormones and other chemicals that influence these intricate processes are being identified all the time. The following represents a very simplified overview of this involved process, focusing on the aspects that are believed to be best understood as of this writing.

The uterus is relatively quiet during pregnancy, and the cervix remains closed so that pregnancy can progress without disruption. As pregnancy advances, several agents act upon the myometrium. **Uterotropins** are hormones and other agents that act on the myometrium and the cervix. They enable the synthesis of other agents, called **functional elements**, which prepare the uterine tissues for labor. **Uterotonins** are a class of agents including smooth muscle contractants that act directly on responsive myometrial cells, causing them to contract. They include oxytocin, prostaglandins, and endothelin-1, which may be produced in the myometrium or may be transported there from elsewhere in the body.

At the onset of **parturition** (the bringing forth of young), complex biochemical changes enhance the tendency of the uterine muscles to contract and stimulate the cervix to soften or ripen. It seems likely that a fail-safe process involving overlapping and possibly redundant biochemical interactions produce the timely onset, continuation and safe conclusion of labor. A central player in this process is intracellular free calcium found in the uterine muscle tissues, the amount of which is limited during most of pregnancy. As labor nears, the amount of available calcium ions within myometrial cells rises, stimulating the interaction of actin and myosin, two proteins that cause the cell to contract. During contractions, calcium levels fall causing the actin and myosin proteins to separate which results in cellular relaxation.

Oxytocin is a hormone that has been thought for decades to play a pivotal role in initiating labor; however, there is currently no evidence that it does. Intrauterine oxytocin synthesis is confined to the endometrium and has not been noted in uterine muscle. However, each myometrial cell does have oxytocin receptor sites. As pregnancy advances, estrogen acts in concert with uterine distention to increase the number of these sites. Oxytocin receptor sites are concentrated most heavily in the fundus, with four times fewer sites in the lower uterine segment and almost none in the cervix. When labor begins, estrogen triggers the number of oxytocin receptors in the uterine muscle tissues to rise by two to three times. Oxytocin levels are relatively constant before and during most of labor, rising only during pushing, postpartum and breast feeding. However, the increased number of oxytocin receptors facilitates uterine labor activity by directly increasing the availability of cellular calcium. This causes the uterine muscle to respond more vigorously, even during preterm labor.

Circulating oxytocin levels are fairly constant during pregnancy. The mother's pituitary gland secretes oxytocin in a pulsed pattern that varies rhythmically throughout the day, increasing at night and also influenced by factors such as maternal dietary intake, stress and nipple stimulation. All these factors complicate the accurate measurement of oxytocin in the body. With so powerful a hormone, a small rise has a significant effect. The pulse frequency of oxytocin is known to increase during labor; although it may not influence uterine activity directly until pushing, it primes both mother and baby to bond at the time of birth (see the chapter entitled "Ecstatic Birth: The Maternal Response to the Pain and Stress of Labor" for details). The fetus also secretes oxytocin, which helps prepare the baby for bonding; however, there is no evidence that oxytocin can pass through the placenta unchanged and enter the maternal circulation.

Oxytocin frees arachidonic acid from cell membranes, which enables the synthesis of prostaglandins. Prostaglandins are another class of hormones that appear to play a vital role once labor is underway. Of the several types, PGE_2 and $PGF_{2\alpha}$ are apparently the most important. All uterine tissue can synthesize prostaglandins, which are present in small amounts throughout pregnancy, although production is inhibited prior to the onset of labor.

The membranes and amniotic fluid produce a significant quantity of prostaglandins, but the total amount in amniotic fluid is tiny, about 1 μg. During labor, the amniotic cavity becomes functionally divided into upper and lower (forebag) compartments. During early labor (2.5 cm of dilation or less), prostaglandin concentration in the amniotic fluid of the upper compartment does not change. After 3 cm of dilation, although the prostaglandin concentration of the upper compartment remains low, the level in the forebag becomes much higher than prior to labor and continues to rise as labor progresses. By the time the cervix is 3 to 5 cm dilated, the level in the forebag is much higher than that in the upper compartment, although from 5.5 cm on, no further increase occurs. It is at this point that the presenting part tends to engage (if it has not already done so), resulting in more complete separation of the two compartments. (Prior to engagement, the fluids in the amnion can mix.)

Fragments of decidua parietalis attached to the surface of the forebag appear to be the main source of prostaglandins that enter the amniotic fluid. Decidual tissues are torn from the lower uterine segment during cervical ripening and remain attached to the forebag, which overlies the cervix. Exposure of these fragments to the unsterile yoni environment results in an inflammatory response. The inflammatory mediators produced, including cytokines and prostaglandin F_{2a}, are now thought to facilitate cervical dilation. The decidua is the primary source of $PGF_{2\alpha}$, which affects calcium availability in the cells and lowers the threshold at which the muscle cells contract. This helps to stimulate stronger contractions in labor (MacDonald & Casey, 1993).

Again, this represents a brief summary of the current scientific understanding of this process. If this copy of this book is more than 5 years old, I suggest you refer to a more current edition of this text or of WILLIAMS OBSTETRICS or a recent review article for the latest understanding of this rapidly evolving field of knowledge.

Uterine muscle activity in labor

The myometrium contains transcellular membrane channels, called **gap junctions**, which serve as conduits for the exchange of small molecules and electrical currents. These are relatively few throughout most of gestation, however the number and size of these gap junctions increases as pregnancy reaches term and again when labor begins (either prior to or at term). They start to disappear soon after birth. Adequate numbers and distribution of gap junctions are believed to enhance the production of coordinated uterine contractions by establishing electrical synchrony within the myometrium during contractions. This results in the sporadic toning contractions (or contractures) of pregnancy developing into the more frequent, mild contractions of early labor.

A pacemaker is a region of tissue that establishes a pace of activity. The existence of specialized, regionally located cardiac pacemaker cells is well established. Contractions originate in what are apparently pacemaker regions of the uterus–usually located in the cornua, near the egg tubes. However, unlike the pacemaker cells in the heart, myometrial cells in these regions have no discernible specialized features, and it is now believed that all uterine muscle cells have pacemaker capacities. Thus, the physiological basis for the theory of a pacemaker region in the uterus is unclear.

An integrated uterine contraction originating in the mother's left uterine cornual region.

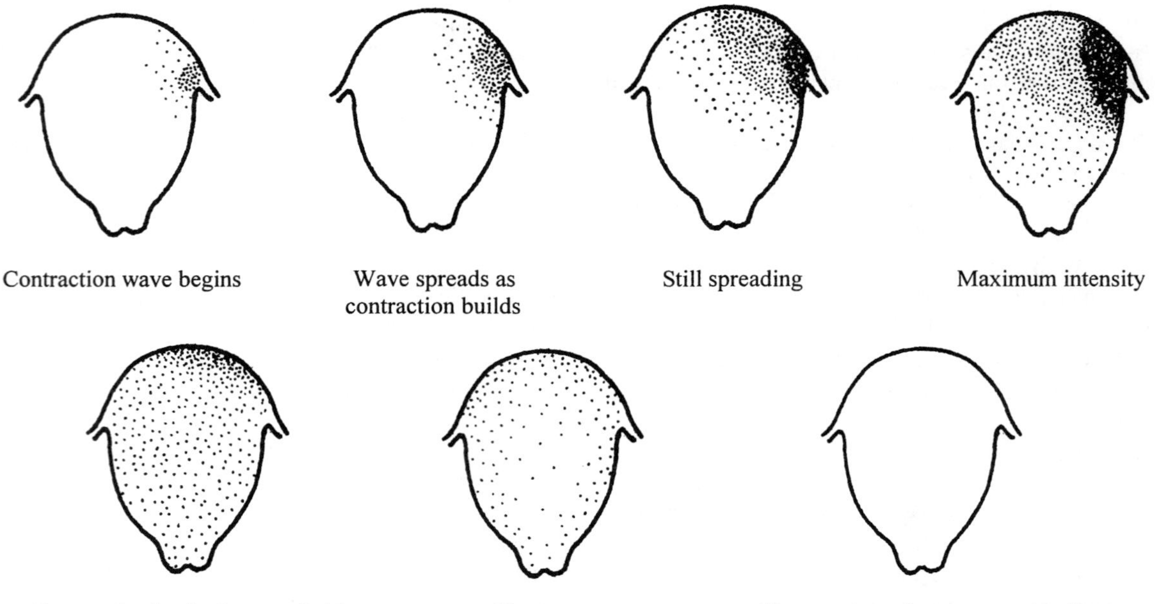

Contraction wave begins — Wave spreads as contraction builds — Still spreading — Maximum intensity

Contraction beginning to subside — Almost over — Uterus relaxes between contractions

(Relative strength of contraction indicated by depth of shading)

Nevertheless, an impulse usually arises from either the left or right cornual region, moving in a wave through the muscle sheet of the uterus. The wave sweeps upward slightly, toward the fundal area, then moves across and down the body of the uterus. This results in a coordinated uterine contraction approximately 15 seconds after the impulse is released. The contraction diminishes as the wave moves away from the pacemaker. Although the impulse reaches some areas of the uterus earlier than others, when uterine activity is coordinated, the contraction reaches its peak throughout all regions of the myometrium at the same time. The regions reached later by the wave peak more rapidly, so at the height of the contraction, the entire uterine muscle is acting in concert.

Should new pacemakers start springing up at different locations in the uterine muscle, the resulting contractions are not effective. The physiologic reason why new pacemaker regions develop is unclear. However, a mother's distressed emotional state is often reflected in nonproductive labor.

The outer myometrial coat of the upper uterine segment contains the most muscle fibers and oxytocin receptors; therefore, during any contraction, the upper portion of the uterus is active longer than the lower, which only contains one-third as many responsive muscle fibers. Although the entire uterine muscle responds to the stimulus to contract at the same time, normal contractions are most pronounced in the fundus, gradually diminish down the walls of the uterus, and are least intense near the isthmus. This is because the inner muscle layer, which makes up the entire cervix and two-thirds of the isthmus, has less contractile potential and is relatively unresponsive to oxytocin. (Sensations of pain are felt in the passive lower segment because the cervix is being pulled up from above as the upper segment works to thin and open the os.) Relaxation tends to take place throughout the uterine muscle simultaneously as the contraction subsides.

The way in which different areas of the uterus respond to contractions results in the formation of two distinct regions during labor. The actively contracting upper segment gets thicker as labor advances, while the lower segment is more passive as it thins and opens. While the tension throughout the uterus remains relatively constant, between contractions the myometrium of the upper segment does not relax completely, rather it becomes relatively fixed at a shorter length. This is called retraction. As the fundus contracts down on its contents, it takes up slack in the uterine walls, keeping the uterus in contact with the baby. Each contraction begins where the last left off, so that the upper segment becomes progressively thicker and the upper uterine cavity slightly smaller. Retraction requires the contents of the uterus to progressively decrease. For this to occur, especially in early labor when the cervix is still almost closed, the muscles of the lower segment must stretch, allowing more of the baby to occupy the lower segment. Thus, in normal labor, the upper segment retracts only to the extent that the lower segment distends and the cervix dilates.

Between contractions, the relaxation of the muscle walls of the lower segment undergo the opposite of retraction. They become stretched and do not return to their former length, rather, they remain relatively fixed at a longer length. This stretching is accompanied by thinning, usually to only a few millimeters in the thinnest part. As these two segments develop during labor, a boundary is formed, marked by a horizontal ridge on the inner surface of the uterus called the **physiologic retraction ring** (Cunningham et al., 2001).

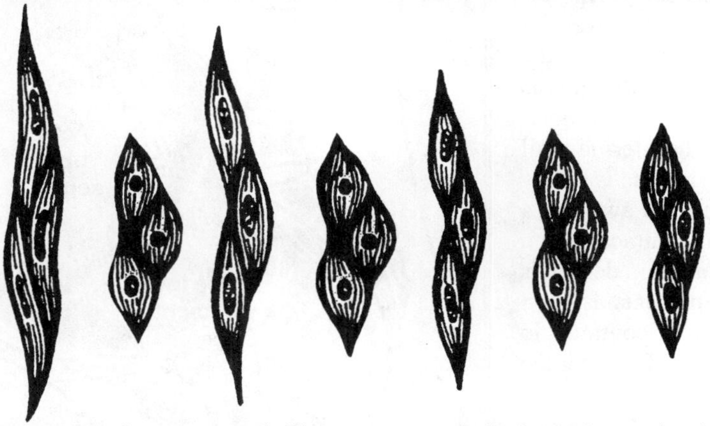

In the upper segment, each uterine muscle fiber gets progressively shorter (retracts) as labor advances. The first and longest cluster represents muscle cells relaxed, prior to labor. The rest, from left to right, alternate with contracted clusters (the short ones) followed by progressively shorter relaxed clusters as the muscle remains retracted between contractions. The opposite occurs in the muscle fibers of the lower segment (follow the sequence right to left).

These specialized activities of the uterine muscle assist in fetal descent into and through the cervical opening and the pelvic passageway as the upper segment shortens and thickens while the lower segment thins. When the cervix is fully dilated and the cervical barrier is gone, the uterine action in the thicker (and consequently stronger) upper segment changes from pulling up to actively pushing down, causing the baby to move through the birth canal.

The abdominal muscles assist labor by supporting the uterus in an upright, forward-tilting position but play no active role in birthing the baby until the mother begins pushing. The round ligaments contain muscles that contract at the same time as the upper segment of the uterus and anchor it, preventing it from ascending into the abdomen, thus helping to move the fetal presenting part downward.

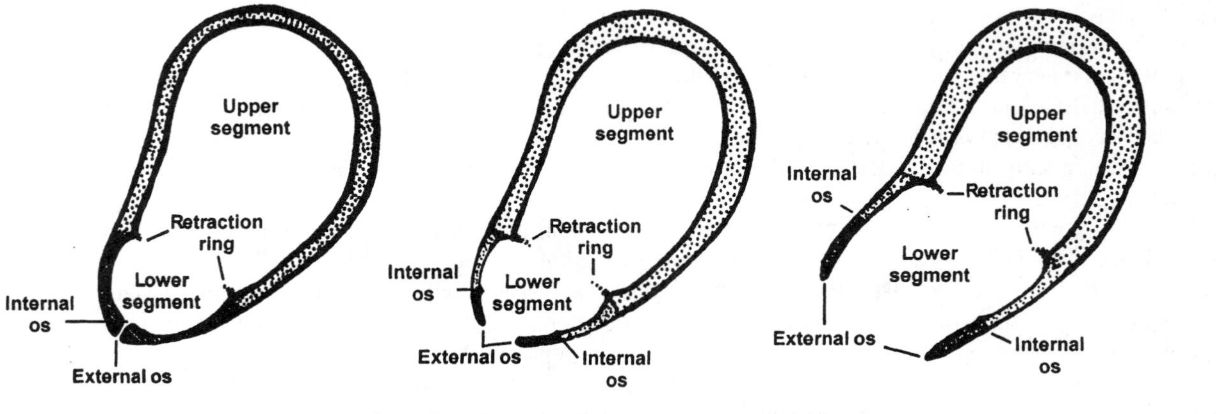

The development of the lower uterine segment occurs as labor progresses.

The birth of the placenta: The uterine cavity becomes progressively smaller as the baby moves down and emerges. This causes the uterine wall to shrink and thicken from a layer of less than 1 mm to 3 to 4 mm. After birth, ultimately, the wall collapses in on itself in innumerable folds. The size of the placental implantation site is thus reduced and the placenta becomes compressed, a process that assists in pushing placental blood into the newborn circulation, thus reducing the size of the placental mass. The placenta begins to shear off the uterine wall. Shortly thereafter, the uterus begins contracting again, accelerating placental detachment. As this occurs, the open maternal blood vessels in the placental site become ligated by the surrounding muscle fibers as the uterus continues to contract. The placental membranes remain attached to the uterine wall until the separation of the placenta is nearly complete. They are then peeled away by a combination of myometrial contraction and the weight of the placenta as it descends through the cervix. The placenta is born intact, allowing the uterus to continue to contract and complete its task of closing the open blood sinuses in the placental bed.

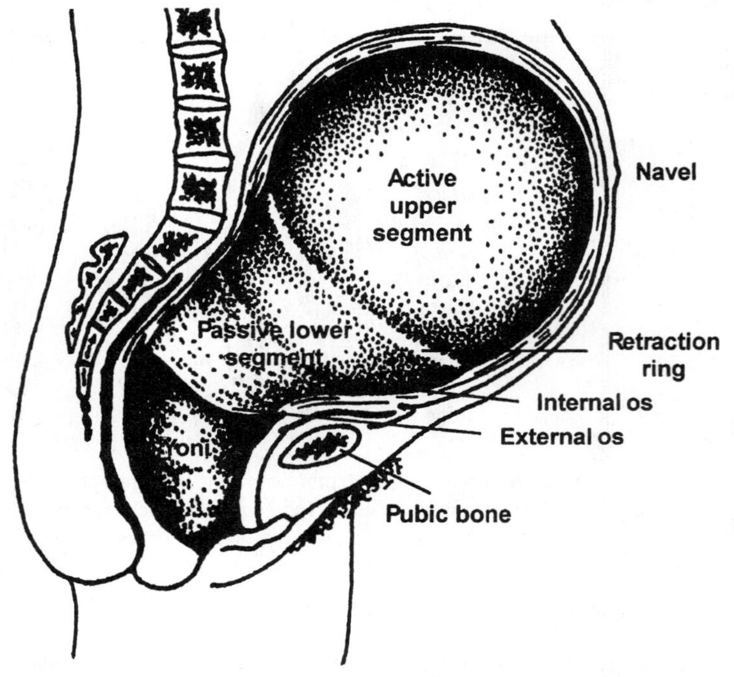

Cross section of uterus at full dilation (yoni shown partially dilated)

Nursing begins

The baby may begin to lick and nurse at the breast at any time after birth. This sends a physiological signal to the mother's body that the baby is out. Hormonal responses to stimulation by the newborn cause the uterine muscle to clamp down, preventing excessive bleeding from the placental site. The baby has moved from being nourished within the mother to being nourished at her breast. The cycle of new life is complete.

Nerves of the Female Reproductive System and Pelvis and the Pain of Labor

Note: Review the chapter entitled "The Nervous System" in HOLISTIC MIDWIFERY, Vol. I before reading this chapter.

Autonomic nerves of the sympathetic and the parasympathetic systems supply the pelvic organs. The sympathetic nerves inhibit muscles around the orifices and lumina of organs, thus causing sphincters to contract and blood vessels to constrict, holding the contents in. The parasympathetic nerves have the opposite effect; they cause the organs to expel their contents by relaxing sphincters and dilating blood vessels. Afferent, usually sensory, nerves conduct impulses from the peripheral nerve endings to the central nervous system, while efferent, usually motor, nerves conduct impulses away from the central nervous system to the periphery.

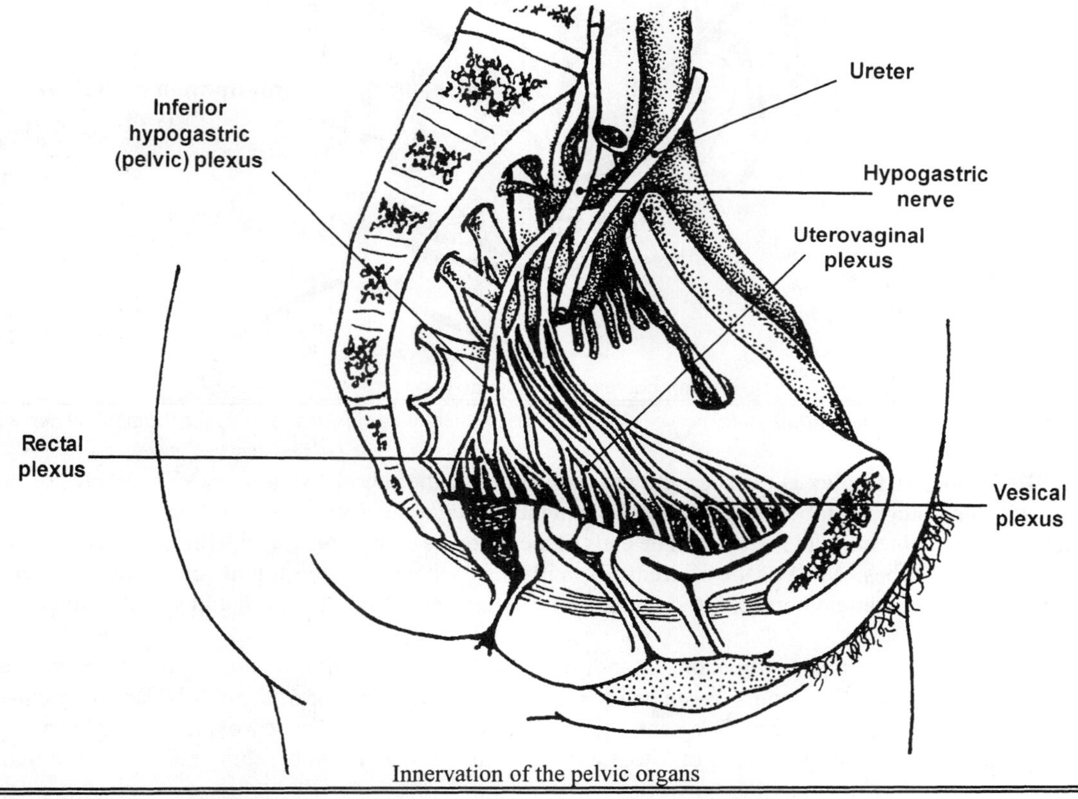

Innervation of the pelvic organs

Anatomy of the nerves of the pelvic organs

The sympathetic nerve supply of the pelvis is primarily a continuation of the large abdominal sympathetic plexuses, those chiefly involved being the celiac (solar) plexus, the aortic plexus and the renal plexus. From the underside of the celiac plexus, at the level of the superior mesenteric artery, two to three interconnected aortic (intermesenteric) nerves pass downward over the anterolateral surface of the aorta, receiving fibers from the inferior mesenteric and lumbar sympathetic ganglia. These nerves continue downward to below the point where the aorta divides, where they form a large network known as the **superior hypogastric plexus**. This plexus lies in front of the last lumbar vertebra and the promontory of the sacrum. This network, also referred to as the "presacral nerve," receives nerve fibers from the parasympathetic system and is joined by branches from the lumbar sympathetic chains. The lumbar splanchnic nerves consist of two to four short branches of the lumbar sympathetic trunk at the level of the first, second and third lumbar vertebrae; these nerves may play a part in the release of the sacrum that occurs as the upper fetal spine begins to extend during pushing (Sutton, 2001).

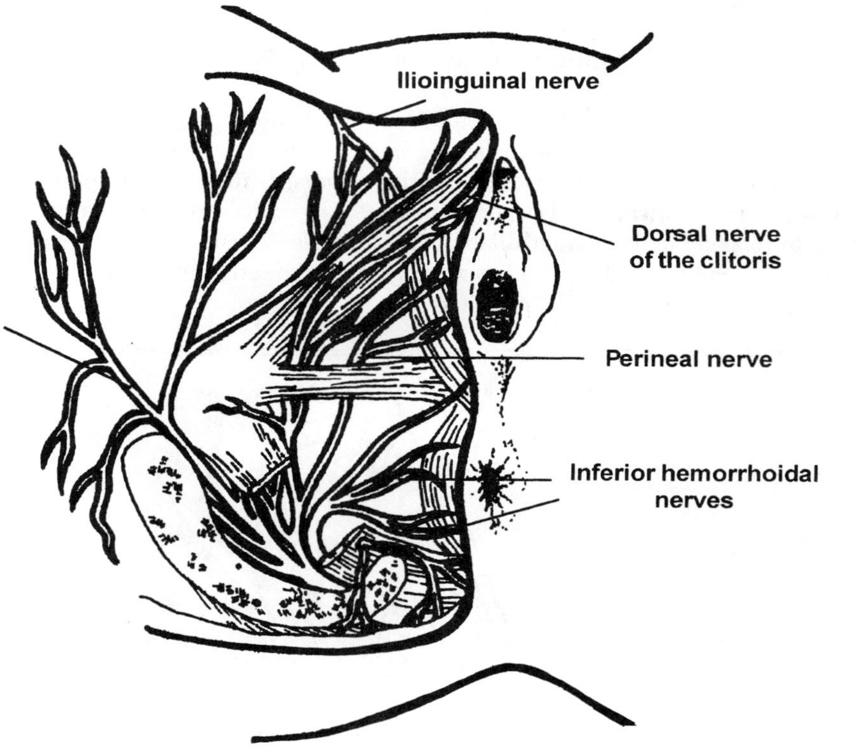

Major nerves supplying the perineum

(The course and distribution of the genitofemoral nerve is similar to that of the ilioinguinal nerve; only the ilioinguinal nerve is shown.)

The **middle hypogastric plexus** overlies and passes just below the sacral promontory. The nerves of this plexus supply the ovary, the outer egg tubes and the broad ligaments. They branch off into bundles, called fascicles, which supply the common and external iliac arteries. The ends of these nerves communicate with the uterine fibers innervating the inner end of the egg tubes. Most of the afferent fibers in these nerves enter the spinal cord through the dorsal roots of the tenth and eleventh thoracic nerves, although several may enter through the ninth and twelfth thoracic nerves as well.

The superior plexus forms two or three long strands of nerves that divide prior to entering the **inferior hypogastric** (or **pelvic) plexus**. These branches end in more pelvic plexuses lying in the floor of the cul-de-sacs on each side of the rectum, in the region of the uterosacral ligaments. Each pelvic plexus is composed of interlacing nerve fibers and numerous tiny ganglia, spread over an area of 2 to 3 cm (0.75 to 1.15 in). From here, the nerves extend to the pelvic organs, where they subdivide into smaller networks.

Secondary plexuses arising from the inferior hypogastric plexus follow the course of the hypogastric vessels. They include the **vesical plexus**, which arises from the anterior part of the inferior hypogastric plexus and supplies the bladder; the **rectal plexus**, which is formed by fibers from the upper part of the inferior hypogastric plexus and supplies the rectum; and the **uteroyoni (uterovaginal) plexus**, which supplies the egg tubes, uterus, yoni and erectile tissue of the vestibular bulb (also referred to as the "plexus of Lee-Frankenhäuser"). These nerves enter the cervix, uterus and yoni directly, often running alongside branches of the uterine and yoni blood vessels, supplying filaments to the uterine body and fundus as well as to the uterine artery and its branches. The ends of these nerves supply the inner end and isthmus of the egg tubes, where they communicate with nerves from the middle hypogastric plexus. The uterine nerves spread throughout the myometrium. Their fibers are distributed predominantly around the uterine end of the egg tubes, in the cervix and near the arterial branches of the uterus.

The nociceptive (pain-transmitting) nerve supply of the uterus, including the lower segment and the cervix, courses through the hypogastric plexuses, then through the lumbar sympathetic chain, finally connecting to the nerves of the spinal cord at T10, T11, T12 and L1 (Bonica, 1994). (This contradicts other textbooks, which state that the lower segment and cervical nerves transmit impulses through the spinal segments of S2, S3, and S4. Bonica's research demonstrated that the innervation described here is correct.) Many of these nerves are on the surface of the uterine muscle, broad ligaments and egg tubes. The portion of the uteroyoni plexus nearest the cervix is often referred to as the "paracervical plexus"; here specialized cervical nerve endings, called stretch receptors, signal changes in tone, volume and tension. These nerves are the source of most of the painful sensations of labor as the cervix is stretched and pulled open. Thus, spinal anesthesia administered above T10 minimizes or eliminates the woman's perception of labor pain. Pain is also absent in women whose spinal cord has been severed at T10 or above.

Innervation of the periurethral area and perineum: The muscles and skin of the perineum are primarily supplied by the **pudendal nerve,** which branches from the second, third and fourth sacral spinal nerves. The pudendal nerve is a mixed nerve, meaning it contains both afferent and efferent fibers. The sacral roots join together to form this peripheral nerve, which then exits the pelvis via the greater sciatic foramen (opening). The nerve then loops around the ischial spine to reenter the pelvis through the lesser sciatic foramen, traveling along the internal surface of the obturator internus muscle and passing through a split in the fascia known as Alcock's canal. As the pudendal nerve exits Alcock's canal, it divides into three branches:

- The **inferior hemorrhoidal nerve**, which supplies the anal canal, the external anal sphincter, skeletal muscle and perineal skin in the area of the anus
- The **perineal branch**, which supplies the urethral sphincter, the muscles and nerves of the perineum and the labia majora
- The **dorsal nerve of the clitoris**, which passes through the urogenital diaphragm to the glans of the clitoris

Major nerves supplying the perineal skin include the anterior labial branches of the **ilioinguinal nerve** (connected to the spinal nerves at L1), which supplies the mons veneris and the upper portion of the labia majora; the **genitofemoral nerve (genitocrural** or **nervus genitofemoralis)**, which is connected to the spinal nerves at L1 and L2, running through the inguinal canal and also suppling the labia; and the perineal branches of the **posterior femoral cutaneous nerve** (connected to the spinal nerves at S1, S2 and S3), which runs forward and medially in front of the ischial tuberosity to the lateral margin of the perineum and labia majora. The triggering of these sexual nerves during labor stimulates production of oxytocin and prompts the fetus ejection reflex. (This process is further explained in the chapter entitled "Ecstatic Birth: The Maternal Response to the Pain and Stress of Labor.")

The perforating cutaneous branches of the second and third sacral nerves pass through the sacrotuberous ligament and wrap around the lower border of the gluteus maximus muscle to supply the buttocks and perineum. The anococcygeal nerves (S4, S5, and the coccygeal nerve) unite along the coccyx and then pierce the sacrotuberous ligaments to supply the anococcygeal area.

The urethral sponge is a cavernosal neurovascular bundle that runs parallel with the urethra along the pelvic aspect of the anterior yoni wall (O'Connell et al., 1998). It is supplied by the pelvic plexus of the inferior hypogastric nerve, clitoral nerves and the pelvic splanchnic nerve. Sutton (2001) states that pressure from the presenting part on this area during descent triggers both voluntary and involuntary nerve pathways which, in turn, trigger the backward motion of the sacrum, the "opening of the back," that occurs prior to birth and as part of the fetus ejection reflex.

Adjacent nerves

Many of the nerves that supply the lower body pass through the pelvis to reach their destinations. Large nerve pathways, or trunks, emerge anteriorly from the four sacral foramina on either side, then divide and unite to form the sacral plexus. The sacral plexus is joined from above by the lumbosacral nerve trunk (originating at L4 and L5), which reaches the plexus by passing in front of the sacroiliac joint and leaves the sacral plexus through the greater sciatic notch. Note that the lumbosacral trunk can be damaged during difficult labors due to their placement in front of the sacroiliac joint; damage may lead to sciatic pain or paralysis of the perineal and anterior tibial muscles.

Why is labor painful?

The actual cause of labor pain is unknown. Possible sources include: oxygen deprivation in the contracted myometrium; compression of nerve ganglia in the cervix and lower uterus by the interlocking of muscle fibers during contractions; cervical stretching during dilation; stretching of the peritoneum that overlies the fundus; traction and stretching on the egg tubes, ovaries and supporting ligaments, pressure on the urethra, bladder and rectum and distension of the pelvic floor and perineum. Of these, compression of the nerve ganglia of the cervix and lower uterine segment is most likely to be the primary source of painful sensations. Additional regionalized pains occur when the fetus and pelvis are not working together perfectly, sending signals to the mother that she needs to move or change something so the baby can find her way down more easily.

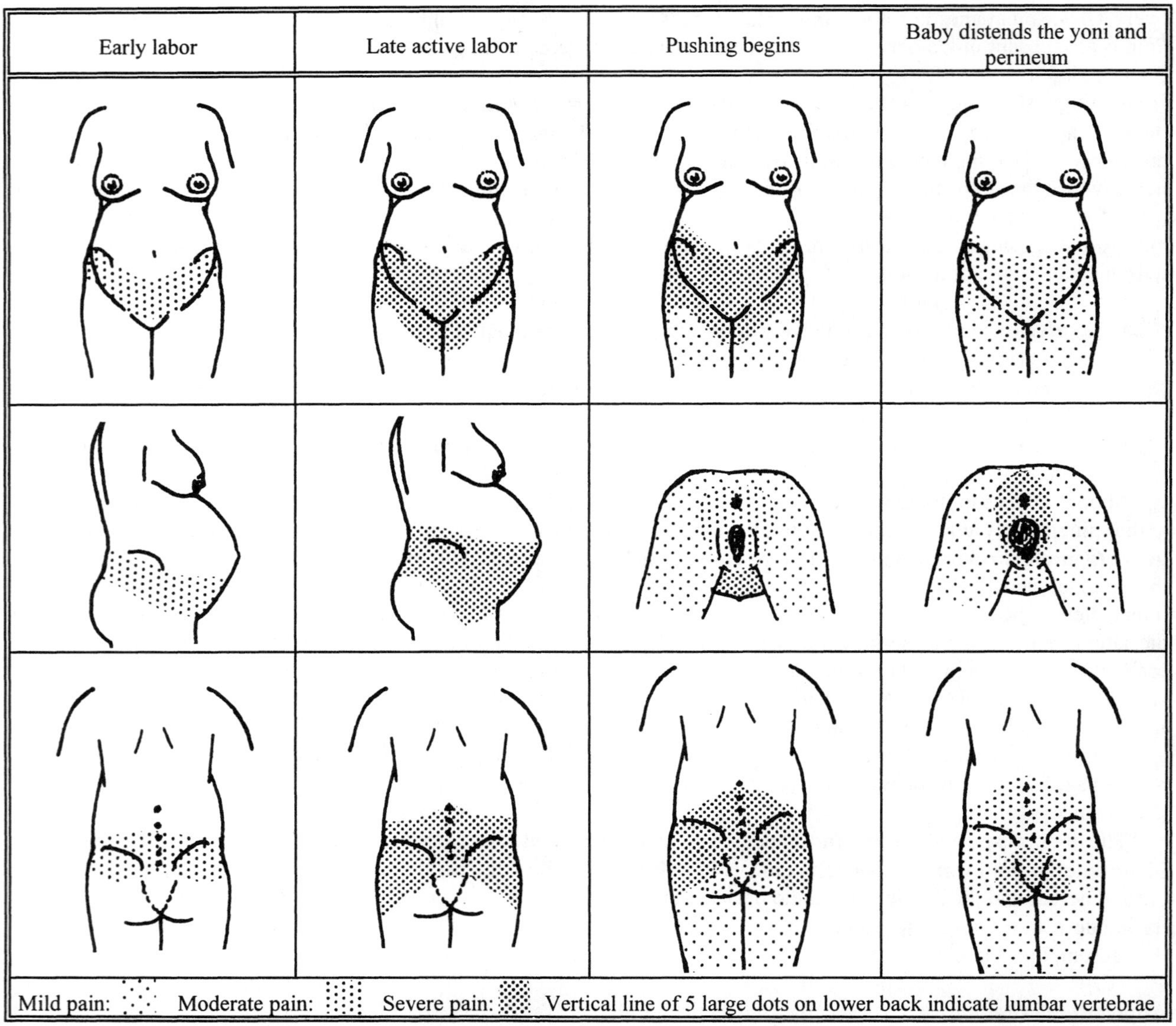

<u>The neuropathways triggered during labor</u>: Pain during labor follows a fairly predictable progression, although the nature and degree of pain reported by individual women varies widely. The periodic, rhythmic pain that occurs with uterine contractions is transmitted from the body and fundus of the uterus via the large uteroyoni plexus. The pain impulse passes along the hypogastric nerves and the lower aortic postganglionic sympathetic fibers to the paravertebral sympathetic chain at the level of the second and third lumbar vertebrae. It continues upward via the gray rami of T10, T11, T12 and L1, entering the communicating system of the four dorsal root ganglia at each of these vertebrae. From there it moves up the spinal cord to the thalamic pain center and its cortical radiations in the brain.

Cervical dilation is responsible for the majority of painful sensations during the first phase of labor, which intensify as uterine contractions become stronger and the cervix opens wider. Low suprapubic pain and low backache associated with cervical dilation are products of stimulation of these pathways as well. Pain progresses from aching to cramping to a sharp and intense sensation during contractions, that usually subsides as the contraction fades. However, unusual pressure from the presenting part can cause significant pain that persists between contractions.

Near full dilation, the messages carried by the local stretch receptors in the cervix override those carried by the hypogastric nerves. This leads to the complex sensations the woman experiences as full dilation approaches. Intense cervical stretching appears to trigger the long, strong contractions of late labor. Once the cervix is fully dilated, the amount of stimulation arising in the cervix decreases. However, in some women, uterine contractions and distension of the lower segment continue to cause pain in the same regions as during the first stage of labor.

Many women experience aching, burning or cramping in the thighs or legs during late labor and pushing. It is probably a result of the stimulation of pain-sensitive structures in the pelvic cavity by indirect traction on the uterine ligaments, the ligaments and fascia of the pelvic muscles, stretching of the bladder, urethra and rectum, and pressure on nerve roots from the lumbosacral plexus. This usually involves the nerve pathways of the sacral segments at L2 and L3.

As the perineum stretches during descent and pushing, pressure on the bladder, rectum and perineal tissues sends pain signals from local ganglia to the central nervous system via the pudendal and sacral nerves.

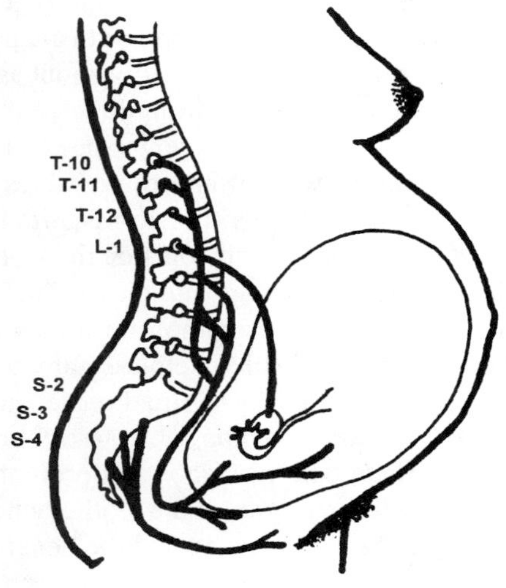

Spinal connections to the uterus

How painful stimuli are handled by the body

The relationship between a stimulus and the perception of pain is highly variable. Harmless or minimal stimuli may, at times, produce pain; the perceived location of pain may differ from the actual location of damage or stimulation (referred pain). Pain may also persist in the absence of stimulus or after healing (phantom pain), and the nature and location of pain can change over time. Some types of pain lessen with treatment; for others, there is no adequate relief. Any explanation of pain must take all these variables into account.

The perception of pain: Myelinated fibers in the peripheral nervous system are classified as "Aβ" (A beta) and "Aδ" (A delta) fibers, whereas unmyelinated fibers are referred to as "C" fibers. In general, the larger the diameter of the nerve fiber, the faster it transmits impulses. However, myelinated fibers transmit signals faster than C fibers, even if their diameters are identical, because myelination permits more rapid transfer of nerve impulses. A fibers give rise to acute, sharp pains, while C fibers are associated with longer-lasting aching or dull types of pain. The peripheral nerve pathways that supply the uterus, cervix and perineum contain both Aδ and C fibers, which accompany sympathetic nerves supplying the uterus in a specific sequence. Thus, as labor advances and neural pathways are stimulated sequentially, the location of the painful sensations move and spread in a predictable pattern.

All pain is transmitted via dermatomes consisting of areas of skin supplied by cutaneous branches from a single spinal nerve. Pain in early labor is felt in the T11 and T12 dermatome regions of the lower belly, back and sides. As labor advances, painful sensations intensify and spread from the T11 and T12 regions, eventually involving the T10 and L1 dermatome regions of the lower and midbelly, upper thighs, sides and back. During pushing, as the baby descends, pain from the cervix eases off and the sensation is transferred to the yoni canal and perineum via S2, S3 and S4 (Moore, 1997).

The gate control theory: A theory regarding the perception of pain was first proposed in 1965. It posits a physiological "gating mechanism" within the substantia gelatinosa, which is located in the gray matter of the spinal cord's dorsal horn. It suggests that sensory signals can only pass through the cells in this substantia gelatinosa when the "gate" is open. When closed, sensory information is blocked, forming the basis of a kind of physiological pain relief.

The gating effect is produced by simultaneous processes balancing excitatory and inhibitory sensory information. The gate opens when nerves are stimulated, prompting the release of neurotransmitters, which excite the neurons, transmitting pain signals within the ascending nerve pathways. When the gate mechanism is activated, descending signals from the brain that modulate pain are transmitted along the Aβ fibers, stimulating inhibitory interneurons in the dorsal horn. Since Aβ fibers are larger than Aδ and C fibers, they transmit signals faster and therefore these signals become dominant. Aβ fibers also release their own inhibitory neurotransmitters. Aβ fibers are activated when touch receptors are stimulated via massage, warm water or other means. The gate closes when nerve cells involved in pain modulation produce inhibitory neurotransmitters and endogenous opioids, causing the pain signals to be inhibited.

The limbic system: The limbic system consists of numerous groups of nerve cell bodies located deep within areas of the brain, including the hypothalamus. Although not fully understood, it is known that stimulation of limbic regions gives rise to emotions such as fear, anger, pleasure and satisfaction and possibly the emotional response to pain. The hypothalamus is believed to be involved with the memory of sensory experiences and learned emotional responses.

Understanding the pain of labor in context

With rare exceptions, labor and birth are painful. Cultural beliefs cause women to relate differently to the sensations of labor. Western culture is probably about as afraid of pain as it is of death, both of which are issues that the pregnant and birthing woman must confront directly as she prepares to give birth and become a mother.

The pain of labor has many advantages. It is important for us to understand these benefits so we can understand how to support laboring women and their babies as well as to educate women and families to realistically prepare for childbirth. The pain of labor transforms birth into a large and challenging event that the laboring woman moves through to arrive at caring for her baby outside the womb. The pain of labor thus helps elevate the physical process of birth into an initiation, a rite of passage into mothering. Having accomplished the enormous task of giving birth, the woman feels empowered. It is not uncommon for a new mother to report feeling that she is now able to do just about anything, including caring for this tiny, helpless baby that has just emerged from her body.

This is not only true in a spiritual sense; but in the biochemical realm as well. Active physical stress and pain trigger the body to release endorphins, which are not released when these triggers are absent. Endorphins enhance the mother's ability to continue with her labor and promote feelings of achievement and satisfaction, helping to ensure a positive receptive attitude on the part of the mother when she first greets her newborn. When drugs are used to ease pain in labor, the woman and her baby are denied the benefits of endorphin release.

The natural pain of labor can thus be seen as healthy pain. The sensations of labor let the mother know that birth is close, allowing her time to retreat to a safe location. In addition, Jean Sutton (2001) points out that the specific localized aches and pains of labor help guide the mother to assume positions and engage in activities that assist in fetal repositioning, rotation and descent, which, in turn, relieve excessive pain. Unusually severe pain signals a problem, another reason strong sensations are necessary. When drugs indiscriminately remove all sensation, the mother doesn't have her own body's cues to follow and is left dependent on the opinion of experts as to what her body is doing.

One of our jobs as midwives is to recognize that laboring women, regardless of risk status, require the same type of environment for baby-having as they do for baby-making: quiet, private, with little or no disturbance from outside forces. Even when hospitalization is needed, the environment should retain as many of these elements as possible. In such a setting, the pain of labor will usually be bearable because the mother will be able to focus inwardly. She will be guided by her sensations, resulting in a labor and birth that are much more likely to proceed without problems. The hormonally mediated "high" of labor will offset its discomfort, and the mother will be perfectly primed to welcome her newborn. Techniques to ease labor pain with minimal interference in this delicate process will be discussed throughout the text.

Long-term physical and emotional consequences of the use of pain-mitigating drugs during labor

To date, there have been no well controlled investigations to examine the short or long term effects of potent narcotic and other nervous-system dampening drugs on the rapidly developing fetal brain either during administration to the mother or for an indeterminate period afterward. Nor is the possible interaction between numerous drugs given many mothers taken into account. (Haire, 2004a, 2004b)

The emotional impact of drug use in labor has been studied in more depth. Jacobson and colleagues (1987, 1990), found that children of mothers who received opiates during labor have an increased risk of opiate addiction as teenagers. In essence, these babies learned right away that, in the face of stress, drugs are a viable option. The use of anesthesia as well as labor induction have also been linked to autism, which Michel Odent (1999) characterizes as the impaired capacity to love the self, others or both.

While such studies have been poorly received by a medical community unwilling to hear that its standard operating procedures are suspect, we, as midwives, should heed these warnings and support women in avoiding drug use during pregnancy and labor whenever possible. When drugs are necessary, using the smallest possible dose and supporting as much continuous mother-infant interaction as possible at the time of birth will help to minimize these negative effects.

ECSTATIC BIRTH: THE MATERNAL RESPONSE TO THE PAIN AND STRESS OF LABOR

This chapter explains some of the purely physical aspects of birthing energy. As you read this, keep in mind that the totality of birth is much more than the sum of its parts. Buckley (2002) points out that four major types of hormone groups come into play during pregnancy, birth and thereafter. These are:

- •Oxytocin, the hormone of love and attachment, is secreted by the posterior pituitary gland during all human sexual activity, including orgasm, labor, birth and breastfeeding.
- •Beta-endorphins, the hormones of pleasure and transcendence, are released in response to a variety of different types of stress, particularly painful stress. These opioid peptides are found in the brain and many other parts of the body. In the nervous system, endorphins bind to the same receptors that bind exogenous opiates.
- •Epinephrine and norepinephrine, also known as adrenaline and noradrenaline, are catecholamine hormones secreted by the adrenal medulla during fear and excitement.
- •Prolactin, known as the "mothering hormone," is secreted by the anterior pituitary gland. It is the primary hormone governing milk synthesis and secretion. Levels increase during pregnancy and labor and peak at birth. Prolactin is also the hormone of submission and surrender and contributes to feelings of anxiety. This helps the mother put the baby's needs before her own during early mothering when she nurses her baby.

These hormones are secreted in all live-bearing mammals by the middle, or limbic, brain, a more primitive part of the brain than the rational neocortex, which is dominant in modern humans.

Studies conflict regarding when, if and how stress-hormone (catecholamine) release stimulates or inhibits uterine activity. Understanding of the interaction between catecholamines and oxytocin is also vague, as is the relationship between stress hormones and other birth-related hormones. The explanations given here are, therefore, rudimentary and incomplete at best and are based on compiled research from several sources. Much is unknown about the female response to stress in general and the maternal response to stress during labor in particular. While the basic core of stress responses does not seem to vary greatly between human males and females, Taylor and colleagues (2000) postulate that women have adapted by developing an oxytocin-influenced "tend and befriend" response to stress, while an androgen-mediated "fight or flight" response has been found in studies focusing predominantly on men. Socially and biologically, this makes sense, as primitive women (whose life span was much shorter than modern humans) were often pregnant or tending dependent offspring and may not have been able to fight or flee in the same way as might an unencumbered male. This research suggests that the stress of labor may ready the mother to protect and bond with her newborn in ways previously unrecognized. Much work needs to be done to more fully understand the unique ways in which men and women respond to stress and the ways various hormones work for mother and baby during labor.

The effect of stress hormones on labor and their interaction with labor hormones appear to be a matter of timing and degree. Maternal catecholamine levels normally remain at prelabor levels throughout early labor as long as the mother is not unduly anxious or afraid. As labor progresses, catecholamine levels rise, but they do not necessarily impair the progress of labor. This is interesting in light of the large amounts of oxytocin that are released as part of the stress response in women. Elevated levels of adrenaline are evidenced by an increased respiratory rate, faster pulse, elevated blood pressure and slightly decreased peristalsis. As Gay Hendricks, a body-centered psychotherapist, points out, "fear is excitement without the breath." When the woman lets go to her hormonally mediated emotions and breathes into them, she lets the energy of birth flow through her, and labor tends to move along.

However, if fear, anxiety and stress become extreme during early to midlabor, the resulting prolonged and excessive rise in catecholamines has an overall inhibitory effect on uterine activity, resulting in weaker and more widely spaced contractions. This occurs because adrenal hormones prepare humans to engage in self-protective activities, diverting blood flow from nonessential organs (including the uterus) to the heart and skeletal muscles, preparing the body to protect itself. (This also reduces blood flow to the baby and may eventually lead to fetal distress.) Inhibition of uterine activity gives the mother an evolutionary advantage–if labor slows, she is more free to respond to danger by seeking support from others in her social network or moving to another location. Niles Newton refers to this as the "fetus-withholding phenomenon" (Newton et al., 1966).

Late in labor, a woman's fear for her environmental safety may also trigger a release of maternal catecholamines, which act in a very different fashion, leading to efficient uterine contractions and a rapid pushing phase. This response is well known to birth attendants who have assisted women in the midst of crises such as war or earthquakes. Birth attendants have also been known to say or do things to incite fear in the mother as a way of avoiding other interventions.

Rapid delivery when birth is imminent also offers an evolutionary advantage–the mother is readied by her hormones to become alert, give birth quickly, communicate with her social network to strategize protective activities, and perhaps grab her baby and move to a safer location.

Beta-endorphins are the body's natural response to hard work and serve as a defense against pain. These morphine-like chemicals are produced by the pituitary gland. A rise results in pain reduction and a heightened sense of well-being, pleasure, euphoria and dependency while reducing anxiety and irritability. The brain has specific receptors for these opioid peptides (morphine and heroin act on the same receptor sites). Noradrenaline and ACTH (adrenocorticotropic hormone) suppress endorphin production during early to midlabor. When the mother is relatively free of anxiety, endorphin levels rise in response to the increased sensations of pain as labor progresses. Labor support in the form of massage, acupressure, warm-water immersion and other means stimulates endorphin production, thus promoting the "altered state of consciousness" or "birth ecstasy" that women who have effective labors often experience. Endorphins cross the placenta and enter amniotic fluid. Thus, on a biochemical level, it appears likely that maternal well-being translates to fetal well-being and less pain for the baby during labor. Endorphins also promote the secretion of prolactin, a hormone that enhances maternal-infant bonding and also contributes to feelings of well-being. It is also associated with the "high" many women report during late labor and immediately after birth.

Michel Odent, a French physician who has pioneered research in the physiology of uninterrupted labor, theorizes that, if labor has been normal and the mother relatively free of fear, a physiologic catecholamine surge near the end of labor produces strong pushing contractions. Odent applies Niles Newton's term "fetus ejection reflex" (Newton et al., 1966) to this physiological phenomenon. The timing of this response varies among individual women and has no strict correlation with the descent of the presenting part, suggesting that it is not simply a matter of pressure on the pelvic floor. Odent observes that women who labor free of anxiety in private surroundings (low lights, minimal interference from attendants) usually have intense, rapid labors (3 to 5 hours in primigravidas at term).

During a rapid dilation phase of labor, there is often minimal muscular activity in the mother, a response consistent with low levels of catecholamines. As the undisturbed woman approaches full dilation, she will exhibit symptoms of a surge in catecholamines, including goose bumps, dilated pupils, thirst, and verbal expressions of euphoria, anger or fear, sometimes with references to being afraid of death. Such physiologically triggered emotional responses pass quickly as long as the birth attendants do not try to engage the woman with an intellectual response. The mother will suddenly become active, often assuming an upright posture while flexing her knees and grasping with her hands. These activities are often correlated with the onset of strong and efficient pushing contractions during which the baby descends and is born very rapidly. The mother will remain alert for 10 to 15 minutes after birth, tending to maintain a vertical position while making contact with her newborn. Maternal catecholamines return to normal levels within 3 to 21 minutes following birth, particularly if the ambient temperature is warm. Newborns have correspondingly high catecholamine levels and are alert and quick to find the breast and suck.

A catecholamine surge that hinders progress in early labor and facilitates progress at the end of labor appears paradoxical. Two theories have emerged to explain this phenomenon. The first centers on the lipolytic effect of adrenaline, which triggers the release of free fatty acids, particularly arachidonic acid (AA), the most abundant of the three precursors of prostaglandins in tissue lipids. The resulting metabolites, synthesized in the amnion and decidua vera, stimulate contractions. This effect is rapid and transitory, as the half-life of prostaglandins is approximately 30 seconds. The main effect of sudden lipolysis on uterine contractility should be excitatory. This effect is augmented during labor by an increased plasma level of cortisol, which blocks the biosynthesis of the inhibitory myometrial prostaglandins (prostacyclin). Thus, if the body is otherwise prepared to give birth, a catecholamine surge facilitates the pushing phase of labor. This effect passes quickly, however, and, if birth is not imminent, will not result in an acceleration of labor as explained previously.

Another theory involves receptors in the smooth muscles. The activation of *beta* receptors is usually inhibitory, while the activation of *alpha* receptors is usually excitatory. It is possible that, above a certain threshold, *alpha* receptors predominate. The ratio of adrenaline and noradrenaline released may also be a factor in the activation of *alpha* receptors. The ratio between *alpha* and *beta* receptors tends to increase near the end of pregnancy. This may be one reason why an authentic fetus ejection reflex is rare in preterm labors but commonly seen in the birth of small-for-dates babies born at term. Finally, the complexity of interaction between catecholamines and uterine activity may also be related to the varied responses of different regions of the myometrium, particularly the cervix.

When the mother-baby pair are left undisturbed during the hour following birth, maternal oxytocin levels peak as the mother meets her newborn. This high level of oxytocin is accompanied by a high level of prolactin, a perfect hormonal milieu for the mother to fall in love with her baby. This hormonal interplay results in prompt placental release and the uterus clamping down to minimize bleeding (Odent, 2002).

Your job

Strive to create an environment for every birthing woman that optimizes her chances of having a fully instinctive hormonally balanced response to labor. Holding that intention for a woman, seeing it in your mind's eye for her and knowing what is possible for all women can go a long way to creating the space where such births can occur more easily. This mental space is especially important for us as midwives to hold, since the wider culture we live in fears birth and has twisted the concept of normal birth so profoundly. However, each woman brings to her labor a variety of beliefs, cultural and religious mandates, personal experiences, relationships, fears, concerns and survival strategies that may be at odds with creating this ideal for herself. You must hold the space and then tune in to what she needs to achieve her own best birth experience. You must then support her needs, with no judgement, regardless of what they may be.

Additional Fetal and Neonatal Considerations

The Baby's Journey through Labor to Birth

NOTE: The content of this chapter compliments the chapter entitled "Placenta-to-Newborn Transfusion, Physiologic Closure of the Umbilical Vessels and Severance of the Cord." Reading both will give you the most complete understanding of this complex topic.

During the process of labor the baby is being prepared for the transition from life within the womb to life as a physically independent being. Uterine contractions massage and stimulate the baby, letting him know big changes are afoot and readying him for the complexity of stimulation he will encounter at birth. After birth when the cord is left intact, a series of circulatory changes take place as placental respiration continues while pulmonary respiration begins.

Fetal Stress Responses

The changes that the fetus experiences just prior to and during labor are initiated once the baby receives both psychic and hormonal messages that labor is about to begin.

Much of what we know about fetal stress in labor is based upon research performed on fetuses whose labors were disturbed and invaded in various ways in order to monitor the fetus and obtain fetal blood samples; this confounding factor no doubt alters fetal hormone levels outside the normal range. These infants were also very likely to have been subjected to cord clamping soon after birth, another factor that raises the stress level. For all these reasons, the findings of Lagercrantz and Slotkin [1986], upon which this section is based, are likely to be skewed accordingly. It is crucial to keep this in mind while studying this section.

Fetal endorphin and stress hormone levels during gestation

The fetus produces copious amounts of endorphins and stress hormones. As the end of pregnancy nears, the newborn's endorphin levels are three times higher than their baseline. This helps prepare the baby for dealing with any stresses the cramped quarters of the uterus may impose as labor draws near (Csontos et al., 1979). In contrast, stress hormone levels in the circulating blood volume are low because the rate of intrauterine catecholamine production and clearance are two to four times higher in the fetus than in the adult. Clearance occurs by means of reuptake, enzymatic breakdown, conjugation and secretion. Reuptake is the primary means of clearance, with the placenta accounting for over 50% of the reuptake that occurs. This protects the fetus from the adverse effects of chronically high levels of stress hormones and keeps the hormones in balance. Thus, fetal life is characterized by low circulating catecholamine concentrations accompanied by a high degree of sympathetic tone in the nervous system, meaning that the fetal nervous system is always poised for a stress response. The high rate of catecholamine production and clearance also prepare the fetus at the time of labor for successful transition to life outside the womb.

Fetal response to the stress of labor

The fetus is uniquely prepared to deal with the normal stresses of labor. In fact, these healthy stresses not only prepare the baby for the immediate transition to an air environment, but for life in general. Successfully navigating the journey to birth physically and psychologically lays the groundwork for the baby to meet challenges throughout life.

The physical aspect of this preparation is largely due to the stress hormones the fetus secretes before, during and after labor. As labor nears, the catecholamine levels in the resting fetus rise dramatically. Life-threatening stress from hypoxia, hypoglycemia, thermal variations and hemorrhage, either prior to term or during labor, also causes them to rise. Fetal catecholamines contribute to the synthesis of prostaglandins, helping both mother and infant prepare for labor to begin. The rise of stress hormones that occurs prior to and during labor is mediated, in large part, by pressure on the fetal head, as well as by the intermittent oxygen deprivation that is a normal accompaniment to uterine contractions. Even in very early labor (2 to 3 cm of dilation), the concentration of catecholamines in the fetal scalp is about five times higher than that found in an adult at rest.

The sympathetic nervous system of the fetus is immature. As a result, the fetal adrenal gland releases catecholamine hormones as a direct response to stress throughout most of gestation (whereas in an adult the release of catecholamines is dependent upon the activation of nerve impulses). Nerve-mediated release in adults results in the release of more adrenaline than noradrenaline. In contrast, the medulla of the fetal adrenal gland is larger than that of an adult and produces more noradrenaline than adrenaline throughout most of gestation. The fetal paraganglia, specialized tissues that appear as red-brown nodules scattered on the outside of the aorta, also serve as extra sources of this hormone. The paraganglia disappear during childhood.

While adrenaline (epinephrine) increases the heart rate and shunts blood to muscles in adults so they can actively respond to danger, noradrenaline (norepinephrine) is much more suited to the survival needs of the fetus. Fetal noradrenaline elevations protect the baby from asphyxia by redirecting blood flow to the heart, brain, adrenal glands and placenta during the fluctuations in oxygen saturation that normally occur during uterine contractions. These changes prompt a vagal response that leads to a rise in blood pressure; they may also result in a fall in heart rate, thereby reducing the demand on the heart and thus conserving oxygen. This assures that the fetus has access to as much oxygen during labor as she does prior to labor, even though less oxygenated blood is available during contractions. Thus the fetus, who cannot respond in a fight-or-flight fashion, is exquisitely equipped to deal with oxygen deprivation in utero. This response is similar to the diving reflex present in marine animals. (See the chapter entitled "Hydrotherapy and Waterbirth" for more information on the mammalian diving reflex in human babies.)

In the fetus, release of noradrenaline does not counteract the parasympathetic slowing of the heart during hypoxia, as adrenaline could. The immature heart is also less responsive to the effects of adrenaline than it will be in later life; therefore a higher level of adrenaline is necessary to produce heart rate increases, so a catecholamine surge is less likely to cause an irregular heart rate. If hypoxia is prolonged, however, a baby's adrenaline level may rise to levels that produce variable increases or decreases in the fetal heart rate during labor.

Additional fetal catecholamine surges occur during pushing and again at the time of birth, a product of increasing compression of the head during descent as well as in response to the slight hypoxia that normally accompanies birth. Adrenaline, which becomes more active in the hours immediately preceding birth, facilitates the transition the fetus must make once he is out of the womb. Adrenaline suppresses the production of lung fluid and stimulates the lungs to absorb fluid in the alveoli as well as to release adequate surfactant to help keep them inflated during exhalation once breathing begins. Catecholamines dilate the bronchioles; they also improve the ability of the lung to stretch and to efficiently exchange carbon dioxide and oxygen in the capillaries of the alveoli.

A catecholamine surge also speeds up the baby's metabolism, accelerating the breakdown of stored energy that can nourish cells once the infant no longer receives a steady supply of nutrients from the placenta. This includes the breakdown of normal fat into fatty acids and the breakdown of glycogen into glucose in the liver. Fetal catecholamines thus provide some protection against fetal hypoglycemia even if the mother is hypoglycemic. These benefits are sustained throughout the first hours after birth, when catecholamine levels in the newborn often remain relatively high, particularly when she is born into a stressful institutional environment. Catecholamines also alter blood flow, directing blood to vital organs and restricting flow to the peripheral circulation. This is especially important for babies who have experienced oxygen deprivation in utero or those who have difficulty breathing at birth. Asphyxiated infants (pH below 7.25) have been found to have catecholamine levels between 500 and 1000 nanomoles per liter of plasma, a level that would cause a stroke in an adult. Correlation of APGAR scores of distressed infants with their catecholamine and pH levels demonstrates that those babies who have higher catecholamine levels generally compensate much better than those who do not when faced with oxygen deprivation and asphyxia. However, excessively high catecholamine levels may lead to fetal heart rate abnormalities, susceptibility to respiratory distress, reduced tolerance for cold and decreased plasma volume due to peripheral vasoconstriction, metabolic acidosis, jaundice, and necrotizing enterocolitis in a baby exposed to a prolonged period of hypoxia or asphyxia. How high a level is too high is still not fully understood. Generally speaking, though, high levels of stress hormones are more protective than not, even when the baby is significantly compromised. Cord blood has also been found to contain a high level of oxytocin, which is known to be secreted along with stress hormones in adults (Gluckman, 1996). Oxytocin surges and catecholamine levels drop rapidly when the baby is with his mother and the room is warm. A high oxytocin level at the time of birth increases the baby's receptivity to bonding with his mother.

Normally elevated levels of stress hormones are likely to result in a baby who is alert and responsive at birth. Tests show that newborn catecholamine levels are often double or triple what they were in early labor. Levels typically start to decline about 30 minutes after birth, returning to prelabor resting levels by approximately two hours postpartum. A more rapid drop is greatly facilitated when the baby has uninterrupted contact with her mother and a warm environment, both of which support the rapid reduction of catecholamine levels and a corresponding rise in oxytocin. Newborns also receive additional endorphins as soon a nursing begins, as both colostrum and breast milk contain significant amounts (Gray et al., 2002; Zanardo et al., 2001a; 2001b).

Preterm babies are less prepared to deal with labor for a number of reasons. It is likely that they exhaust their capacity to deal with stress more quickly and succumb sooner to the adverse effects of high catecholamine levels than do term infants. This may in part be due to the fact that their catecholamine production is not fully established. Likewise, surgically born babies, especially those whose mothers have elective surgery prior to the onset of labor, are at a significant disadvantage because they have not experienced the stress or head compression that stimulates a catecholamine surge. Therefore the advantages described above are less available to these infants. The frequent incidence of respiratory problems in these babies may be contributed to by a low catecholamine response prior to birth.

Fetal and Adult Circulation and Respiration

The most dramatic physiological transformation that the newborn undertakes is the transition from dependence on the placenta to dependance on his lungs for oxygen. This change is reflected in the major difference between the fetal and adult circulatory routes. In the fetus, most blood is routed away from the lungs to be oxygenated in the placenta while in adults blood is transported to and from the lungs for oxygenation and for the discharge of waste gases.

Adult circulation

In adult human circulation, the cardiovascular system is divided into "right" (venous) and "left" (arterial) sides (although both arteries and veins are located throughout the body). The inferior vena cava, located on the right side of the body, carries deoxygenated blood coming from the systemic circulation (all other arterial and venous channels in various organs and regions of the body) into the right atrium of the heart. From there, it flows into the right ventricle, through the pulmonic valve, into the main pulmonary trunk and then on into the lungs. Gas exchange occurs in the alveoli; this oxygenated blood then flows through the pulmonary veins into the left atrium of the heart. It then enters the left ventricle; from there it exits the heart via the aorta for distribution to the rest of the body via the arteries. The only connections between the venous and arterial circulatory avenues occur in the capillary beds and in the lungs. Thus, there is a clear demarcation between the venous and arterial systems. The ventricular pumps operate in series; their output is equal. (Adult circulation, especially with regard to blood flow through the heart, is covered in more detail in Volume I of this text. Review that material before studying the section on fetal circulation.)

Pulmonary circulatory route: In the adult systemic circulation, the arteries carry oxygenated blood and the veins carry deoxygenated blood. Only in the pulmonary circuit is this relationship reversed, with the pulmonary arteries (consisting of a large arterial trunk and lateral branches leading to each lung) delivering deoxygenated blood to the lungs and the pulmonary veins (consisting of lateral branches connecting each lung to the heart) carrying oxygen-saturated blood back to the heart for distribution to the body.

Unique features of the fetal circulation

"Mature" fetal circulatory patterns are established by the 8th gestational week, although changes in the percentage of blood that enters and leaves the cardiac chambers and in the amount of blood that flows to various regions of the body changes as the fetus grows. The timing of these changes and the degree of blood flow variation that occurs are being researched extensively as ultrasonic diagnostic techniques become ever more refined.

Parallel ventricular action: The fetus is said to have two arterial systems and no true venous system in the adult sense because both of the ventricular pumps of the fetal heart work together, in parallel, to perfuse the systemic circulation with partially oxygenated blood. The left ventricle sends partially oxygenated blood into the ascending aorta while the right ventricle sends partially oxygenated blood into the pulmonary trunk and the ductus arteriosus (Allan et al., 2000).

Oxygen requirements of the fetus: Fetal circulation differs from that of the adult in that it is designed to deliver mixed blood (i.e., containing varying amounts of oxygenated and deoxygenated blood) throughout the body. The arterial oxygen tension in the fetus of 20 to 25 mm Hg is quite low by adult standards (104 mm Hg in the child and adult), but keep in mind that both oxygen reserve and availability during stress are more dependent upon the amount of oxygen delivered by the perfusing blood and the requirements of the tissues than on oxygen tension alone. Plus, fetal tissues are perfused at a higher rate than in the adult. This increased rate of delivery compensates for the low oxygen saturation in the fetus. In addition, the unique oxygen-retaining characteristics of fetal hemoglobin allows the fetus to take up large quantities of oxygen via the placenta, resulting in an arterial oxygen content that is only mildly diminished.

Equally important, the fetal demand for oxygen is less than that of the newborn. Intrauterine life requires little work as thermoregulation is unnecessary and the work of respiration, which requires about 30% of an adult's oxygen consumption to maintain, is essentially passive when it takes place in the placenta. If the fetus were truly in an hypoxic environment, oxygen extraction by the tissues would be greatly increased. However, in spite of the lower oxygen delivery in the fetus compared to the newborn (on average 22 ml O_2/kg/min versus 60 ml O_2/kg/min), oxygen consumption is also much less (7 ml O_2/kg/min compared to after birth, when the newborn consumes twice that of an adult in relation to weight), resulting in a remarkably constant rate of oxygen extraction that averages about 30% (Teitel, 1998).

PCO_2 (carbon dioxide) production in the fetus is slightly higher than in the adult, with an umbilical venous level ranging from 35 to 45 mmHg. Elimination of fetal carbon dioxide is enhanced by physiologic increase in the maternal ventilatory rate during pregnancy. Because of the lower carbon dioxide level in the mother's blood, a gradient is created favoring the transfer of fetal carbon dioxide across the placenta to the mother. A lower oxygen level in the fetus helps keep pulmonary vascular resistance high, while a lower carbon dioxide level and fetal prostaglandin production keep the ductus arteriosis open (Bloom, 2002).

Fetal hemoglobin: An important aspect of the fetal ability to do well in a low-oxygen milieu has to do with the unique characteristics of fetal hemoglobin. The term fetus has a hemoglobin count 50% higher than that of an adult. In addition, fetal hemoglobin has a higher affinity for oxygen than adult hemoglobin. Adult hemoglobin binds oxygen less efficiently because it binds well to organic phosphate, 2,3-diphosphoglycerate (2,3-DPG), reducing its affinity (holding power) for oxygen. Fetal hemoglobin cannot bind 2,3-DPG as well as adult hemoglobin. This means that it can carry as much as 20 to 30% more oxygen than adult hemoglobin at certain oxygen pressures. The oxygen-carrying capacity of the fetus rises throughout the course of gestation. Early on, the mother's oxygen-carrying capacity exceeds that of her baby; near term, the reverse is the case. However, fetal hemoglobin releases oxygen less readily than that of adults. This benefits the fetus because oxygen must travel all the way from the placenta via the cord to reach the body. Although oxygen release to the tissues is reduced, the fetal peripheral tissues require less oxygen in utero, and the brain, heart and other vital organs are the first to receive the most oxygen-rich blood. Fetal hemoglobin is high in the term newborn and decreases gradually over the first year of life. The baby's ability to bind oxygen usually matches that of the adult by 6 months of age as fetal hemoglobin production declines and is replaced by adult hemoglobin (Blackburn & Loper, 1992).

Anatomic variations unique to fetal circulation: Fetal circulation is best understood if studied with reference to the schematic drawings that appear on the page following this description. Healthy fetal circulation differs from that of the stabilized neonate and the adult in seven important respects:

1. The fetus has three unique circulatory structures that allow her to rely on the placenta rather than the lungs for gas exchange while in utero. These are:

The ductus venosus: The ductus venosus connects the umbilical venous circulation to the inferior vena cava and also serves as a liver bypass. It extends along the posterior surface of the liver, its inlet is a little more than halfway up the width of the liver and its outlet is level with the diaphragm. Blood flowing though the umbilical vein divides into two streams: one which supplies the liver and another which enters the ductus venosus. Both streams reunite in the inferior vena cava and then flow into the right atrium of the heart.

The exact anatomy and function of the ductus has been the least understood of the fetal circulatory structures. Research on 13 to 17 week fetuses shows that the ductus venosus has unique structural features, which previous studies suggest are also present at term. An anatomical "shelf" or rim is located at the inlet, but no evidence of a sphincter is found. The rim is made up, in large part, of elastin fibers that also extend along the vessel walls. There are several nerve bundles and fibers in the tissue surrounding the inlet; the number of these diminishes as the ductus approaches the diaphragm. This rim suggests that the ductus, unlike other veins, acts as a high-pressure system, generating a persistently high velocity blood flow that minimizes the mixing of blood from the placenta with less-oxygenated blood and that propels incoming blood toward the foramen ovale. The shelf may also reduce backflow into the portal vein during atrial contraction. The lumen narrows just above this rim, and the surrounding tissues are thicker. The lumen then widens from this narrow point as it approaches the outlet (about four-fifths of its length), making the ductus a tall, thin hourglass shape with a short lower end.

Above the inlet, the inner walls of the ductus are longitudinally corrugated. Its shape, as well as the structure of the vessel wall, may assist in dilation. The newest research postulates that innervated smooth muscle along the length of the vessel may vary the vessel diameter along its entire length, rather than just at the inlet, in response to physiological stimuli (Mavrides, et al., 2002). Shunting of blood through the ductus diminishes as gestation advances: 30% of the blood enters the ductus at 20 weeks; by 32 weeks, only 18% does so. This suggests that the maturing liver receives a higher prioritization in early gestation than was previously realized (Kiserud, 2000). The decrease in blood flow through the ductus as term approaches may also provide protection against cardiac overload during labor, when blood will be entering the umbilical vein under increased pressure during uterine contractions.

The foramen ovale: The foramen ovale, an opening or hole in the wall (septum) between the right and left atria of the heart, allows blood to flow in a right-to-left direction. The crescent-shaped upper and lower borders of the foramen ovale are both called the **septum secundum**. The lower free edge of the uppermost septum secundum is called the crista dividens; it helps to divide the blood into streams as it enters the right atrium.

The valve flap of the foramen ovale (the **septum primum**) is attached to the side of the left atrium. From here, it projects upward from the lower septum secundum. This thin flap of tissue acts like a one-way swinging door into the left atrium. Blood pressure in the right atrium is higher than in the left during fetal development due to the high pulmonary vascular resistance. This pressure causes the flap to open, permitting most of the well-oxygenated blood from the inferior vena cava to flow from the right atrium into the left through the foramen ovale.

The ductus arteriosus: The ductus arteriosus is a short fetal vessel with a diameter that almost matches that of the pulmonary artery. It serves as a conduit for blood exiting the right ventricle of the heart via the pulmonary artery, directing the majority of the blood to the aorta instead of the lungs. This duct remains open during fetal life due to the low oxygen content in the blood passing through it as well as to locally produced prostaglandins that cause the muscle cells of the vessel to remain relaxed.

The ductus arteriosus has classically been described as a vascular shunt. This concept is based on the tendency to view postnatal circulation as the norm. However, the designation of the ductus arteriosus as a shunt is incorrect when fetal circulation is viewed as a unique parallel arterial system. It is, instead, a necessary part of the normal vascular outlet of the right ventricle, allowing the appropriate amount of blood to enter the lungs and the remainder to move into the aorta. The ductus arteriosus is thus a vital structure unique to the fetus, which, together with the pulmonary trunk and descending aorta, forms the main pulmonary arch during most of gestation (Allan et al., 2000).

2. **The aortic isthmus:** An isthmus is a narrowing or constriction. This is a slightly funnel-shaped segment of the fetal aorta that begins to taper at the level of the left subclavian artery and reaches its narrowest point at the upper border of the outlet of the ductus arteriosus. It is normally no less than one-third of the diameter of the ascending aorta. It receives blood coming from the right ventricle via the ductus arteriosus and from the left ventricle via the aortic arch. Thus it serves as a connector between the two parallel arterial systems of the fetus. This portion of the aorta works as a true fetal shunt, permitting blood mixing to occur between the right and left ventricles. Each ventricle contributes a portion of blood to the flow through the aortic arch; thus forward and backward movement occurs as the heart contracts and relaxes. Therefore, hemodynamics in the isthmus reflect normal ventricular activity, maintaining a balance between the outgoing flow to the upper body and that of the outgoing flow to the lower body (Allan et al., 2000).

3. A number of veins in the adult, particularly those in the arms and legs, have valves placed just before (distal to) the point where branches merge. The fetus has many additional valves, especially in the upper body, where they assist in maintaining blood pressure when the rate and pressure of blood flowing into the umbilical vein fluctuates, which might occur with variations in maternal blood pressure and during uterine contractions. Most of these valves consist of two folds in the lining of the vein that meet in the middle in a peak. (To get an idea of the shape of most venous valves, put your hands in a prayer position. Now separate the heels of your hands, while you press your fingers together firmly. The backs of the heels of your hands form two cups that curve up on either side and attach to the wall of the vessel. Your fingers form pointed flaps. Blood flows between the heels of your hands, then out through the flaps formed by your fingers. Blood attempting to backwash from above is prevented from doing so.) The following valves are of particular interest:

Valve of the inferior vena cava (valvula venæ cavæ inferioris [Eustachii]; Eustachian valve; semilunar

valve of the inferior vena cava): This is a large valve formed by a fold of the membrane that lines the atrium and contains a few muscular fibers. It is situated just outside of and below the outlet of the inferior vena cava. The valve is "semilunar," shaped like a crescent moon (similar in shape to the web of skin between your stretched thumb and forefinger). Its outer convex border is attached to the anterior border of the vena caval orifice; its inner concave margin, which partially extends over the outlet of the vena cava, is unattached. The left tip of the crescent is continuous with the anterolateral edge of the foramen ovale while the right merges into the wall of the atrium. This valve directs the blood from the inferior vena cava through the foramen ovale, into the left atrium (Lewis, 1918; Goss, 1973; Williams, 1995).

Valves in the tributaries of the hepatic portal vein: The tributaries of the portal vein include the splenic, superior mesenteric, left gastric, right gastric, para-umbilical and cystic veins. The valves of these veins help to regulate blood pressure, maintain adequate circulation in the liver and lessen blood loss from the upper body during a traumatic fetal-to-neonatal transition (Morley, 2002c; Williams, 1995).

4. The placenta, the fetal organ of oxygenation, is outside the main body of the baby. At term, some 30% of the fetal blood moves through the cord and placenta at all times, resulting in fetal circulation being described as an "open system." The term is employed in comparison with adult circulation, which is defined as a closed system; this does not imply that blood ever leaves the fetus' circulating vessels.

5. Three umbilical vessels–two arteries and one vein–connect placental and systemic circulations.

6. The umbilical vein, the upper portion of the inferior vena cava and the pulmonary trunk and its arterial branches carry the most highly oxygenated blood to the heart and lungs (whereas in the adult, these pathways carry deoxygenated blood to the lungs for gas exchange). In the fetus, the pulmonary venous branches carry deoxygenated blood from the lungs back to the heart (in adults, the pulmonary veins carry fully oxygenated blood to the heart).

   The systemic arterial circulation in the fetus carries mixed, partly deoxygenated blood from the upper body to the lower body, and the umbilical artery carries deoxygenated blood back to the placenta for gas exchange (in the adult, the systemic arterial pathways carry the most highly oxygenated blood to the tissues). The fetal pulmonary arterial branches carry partially oxygenated blood to the lungs for nourishment (in the adult, they carry deoxygenated blood to the lungs for gas exchange).

7. There is minimal blood flow through the lungs (about 8% of cardiac output near term versus 45% in adult circulation).

The circulatory pathway in the fetus: Relatively well-oxygenated blood (PO_2 55 mm Hg) leaves the placenta through the umbilical vein; this vessel traverses the cord and enters the fetal abdomen at the umbilicus. It runs between the right and left lobes of the liver, where it meets the inlets of the ductus venosus and the portal sinus (which joins the portal vein). Here the incoming blood divides into two unequal streams. By 32 weeks, about 18% goes directly into the ductus venosus, while the larger stream flows into the liver through branches of the umbilical vein. The liver's stream enters the left and then the right branch of the portal vein, flowing through the liver sinusoids into the hepatic veins.

The two streams meet at the outlet of the ductus venosus at a point just below the diaphragm, where they enter the inferior vena cava and continue to flow more or less side by side, preventing the incoming umbilical venous blood from completely mixing with the blood returning from the lower body. The inferior vena cava now contains:

- Highly oxygenated blood coming straight from the umbilical vein via the ductus venosus
- Somewhat less well saturated blood that has already supplied the liver
- Deoxygenated blood returning directly from the abdominal organs and the lower half of the body

Maintaining two parallel streams results in only partial mixing of the ductus venosus stream with that coming in from the lower body, rendering it only slightly less well oxygenated than the blood coming directly from the umbilical vein.

As these streams exit the inferior vena cava, they are propelled against the valve of the inferior vena cava. The position of the outlet of the inferior vena cava and that of the valve itself cause the blood to be directed at an angle into the right atrium. Both streams shoot across the right atrial cavity and hit the lower border of the interatrial septum (the crista dividens), where they again enter different circulatory pathways.

About two-thirds of this blood becomes the left stream, which is propelled directly through the open flap of the foramen ovale into the left atrial cavity. The flap is held open by the right-to-left flow of blood. In the left atrium, the blood mixes with blood returning from the lungs via the pulmonary venous outlets in the upper wall of the left atrium.

The flap over the foramen ovale is pushed closed as both atria contract, forcing blood out of the left atrium into the left ventricle. This well-oxygenated blood then leaves the left ventricle via the ascending aorta, enters the aortic isthmus, mixes with a small amount of blood exiting the ductus arteriosus and flows into both the coronary arteries supplying the heart and the aortic arch vessels supplying the head, neck and upper limbs. This blood has a 60% oxygen saturation.

To summarize: The "left" stream, called the via sinistra ("the left way") follows this path:
inferior vena cava ➜ inferior vena cava valve ➜ right atrium + 2% from superior vena cava ➜ foramen ovale ➜left atrium + pulmonary veins ➜ left ventricle ➜ ascending aorta + aortic isthmus + small amount from ductus arteriosus ➜ coronary arteries + aortic arch vessels ➜upper body
(+ indicates combining of blood from different sources; ➜ indicates where the blood goes)

About one-third of the stream of blood exiting the inferior vena cava is deflected by the crista dividens so that it is retained in the right atrium; this becomes the right stream. The right stream mixes with most of the desaturated blood returning from the head and upper body via the superior vena cava, as well as with blood returning from the vessels supplying the heart muscle via the coronary sinus. The resulting mixture is moderately saturated with oxygen (about 38%). This blood is pumped into the right ventricle as the atria contract.

The right ventricle then contracts, pumping the right stream into the pulmonary trunk. There a small portion of it enters the pulmonary arterial branches and supplies the lung tissue with oxygen and nutrients. This now-deoxygenated blood then returns to the left atrium via the pulmonary veins. The majority of the right stream continues through the pulmonary trunk into the ductus arteriosus, into the aortic isthmus and then into the descending aorta, where it mixes with some blood from the aortic arch and proceeds downward to the lower body.

To summarize: The "right" stream, called the via dextra("the right way") follows this path:
remaining blood in right atrium + superior vena cava + coronary sinus ➜ right ventricle ➜ 8% pulmonary trunk + 92% pulmonary arterial branches ➜ ductus arteriosus ➜ aortic isthmus ➜ descending aorta ➜ lower body

Blood flow to the lower limbs and placenta: Most of the right stream travels through the descending aorta into the lower torso where it enters the right and left iliac arteries. Forty to fifty percent of this blood passes into the two hypogastric arteries that branch off the iliac arteries. The hypogastric arteries curve around the bladder to become the umbilical arteries, through which partially oxygenated blood travels to the placenta for reoxygenation.

The other 50 to 60% of the partially oxygenated blood continues downward through the descending aorta to supply the organs of the abdomen, pelvis and lower limbs. It then drains into the inferior vena cava as it journeys back to the heart. (Allan et al., 2000; Moore & Persaud, 1993; O'Rahilly & Müller, 2001; Walsh et al., 1974)

***Pulmonary circulation in the fetus*:** The blood vessels that supply the fetal lungs have a high degree of vascular resistance throughout gestation. This means that the blood vessels in the lungs are tightly constricted and compressed, allowing them to resist the entry of large amounts of blood, an amount said to be no more than 8 to 10% at most by term. This, in turn, maintains systemic blood flow in the proper direction and at pressures necessary to keep the ductus arteriosus and foramen ovale open. Most of the blood flowing from the right ventricle into the main pulmonary artery meets resistance as it tries to enter the pulmonary vessels, causing it to enter the ductus arteriosus instead. Fetal pulmonary circulation is further minimized by diversion of a major portion of inferior vena caval blood into the left atrium by way of the one-way valve of the foramen ovale.

One study challenges the long-held notion that a maximum of only 8% of cardiac output enters the fetal lungs, a figure derived exclusively from studies done on fetal lambs. Doppler research suggests that blood flow to the human lungs increases as pulmonary vasculature matures. According to Rasanen and colleagues (1996), at 20 weeks, the lungs receive about 13% of total cardiac output. By 30 weeks, they receive 25% of cardiac output as a result of mid-trimester vasodilation in the fetus. Could this be connected with the drop that occurs in maternal blood pressure? By 38 weeks, pulmonary vasoconstriction reasserts itself and pulmonary perfusion falls slightly to about 21%. Because this research has not been duplicated or confirmed, I adhere to the traditional 8% limit in this text. This study is interesting, however, in light of current theories regarding fetal-to-neonatal transition, which will be discussed later in this chapter.

Umbilical/placental circulation: Placental circulation begins when deoxygenated blood leaves the baby's body through the two umbilical arteries, traverses the cord and passes into the placenta. The umbilical arteries enter the body of the placenta at the base of the cord, then branch again as they enter the cotyledons. These branches further divide into smaller and smaller branches until they become capillary loops within each chorionic villus. Villous blood releases carbon dioxide and other wastes into the mother's bloodstream across a thin membrane, picks up oxygen, and then returns via the capillary loops to placental venules. From here, it flows into larger veins that merge together as they leave each cotyledon. These vessels merge to become one large vein that runs from the placenta through the umbilical cord to the body of the fetus.

Coiling of the umbilical cord assists in pumping venous blood from the placenta. Although the action of the fetal heart (which propels the blood through the arteries), painless uterine contractions and probably even the maternal heartbeat assist in pumping blood into the umbilical vein, blood flow through a coiled cord augments fetal cardiac preload by optimizing venous return from the placenta. Umbilical arterial and venous pulsations alternate with one another. The umbilical arteries expand longitudinally rather than circumferentially during fetal systole (the height of cardiac contraction), creating a relative negative pressure in the vein. During diastole (when the heart is at its most relaxed), the umbilical arteries contract, causing venous pressure to rise. Coiling provides multiple pressure variations that work together in a cumulative fashion, resulting in a milking action that moves blood from the placenta to the baby via the vein. The presence of two arteries tends to multiply this effect by a factor of two. Pressure throughout the length of the umbilical vein is enhanced by the resistance created at the ductus venosus and at the portal vein as blood enters the fetal body (Reynolds, 1952, 1978a, 1978b; Strong, 1997; Walsh et al., 1974).

Fetal lung development

During fetal development, the vasculature of the lungs is constricted and the alveolar capillaries are minimally perfused. Perfusion increases as the pulmonary structures mature, although the degree to which this occurs has not been definitively established. The increasing perfusion that occurs as gestation advances nourishes the tissues and allows the lungs to grow.

The cells in the fetal respiratory tract secrete fluid into the alveoli at a consistent rate. Near term, this amounts to 300 to 400 ml daily. The pressure exerted by this fluid holds the alveoli and other respiratory pathways open so that proper development can proceed. It also provides counterpressure, which serves to keep the pulmonary vessels and the alveoli inactive. The fetus swallows about half of the lung fluid expelled during breathing movements and passively expels a portion of it into the amniotic fluid (O'Rahilly & Müller, 2001). The larynx, aided by inhibition of the cephalad inspiratory abductor muscles, acts as a valve to keep a significant amount of fluid in the lungs. Only a small amount of amniotic fluid enters the fetal lungs during breathing movements because fetal breathing movements are primarily isometric; that is, they produce muscular activity that does not cause the lungs to fill and empty, even though some chest movement occurs (Johnson, 1996).

Mature fetal lungs contain a substantial amount of fluid (about 30 ml per kilogram of body weight or a little more than 1 oz per 2 lb 3.5 oz). While amniotic fluid has a pH of 7.20, lung secretions have a pH of 6.3, close to that of stomach acids. Lung fluid also has a high chloride content, less viscosity and a lower protein concentration than amniotic fluid. The production of lung fluid diminishes dramatically in the 48 hours prior to the onset of labor at term. Cells within the fetal lung switch from secreting to absorbing fluid, a shift prompted by fetal release of catecholamines and arginine vasopressin (AVP). Some of this fluid, sometimes as much as 35 ml, is pushed up and out of the baby's nose and mouth during a landbirth (for details regarding what happens during waterbirth, see the chapter entitled "Hydrotherapy and Waterbirth"). While some fluid is no doubt swallowed, usually over 100 ml (about 3.5 oz) remains in the lungs and must be reabsorbed into the bloodstream and the lymphatic system within a few minutes of birth.

The lungs also contain surfactant, a complex combination of phospholipids that lowers the surface tension forces of the alveolar walls. The principal constituent of surfactant is lecithin, which makes up 50 to 75% of surfactant phospholipids; its level rises as the baby nears term. A sufficient amount of mature surfactant assists in sustaining alveolar expansion during breathing.

If the preterm baby's membranes rupture, the lungs are stimulated to step up their maturation process during the next 35 hours or so (although surfactant maturation alone does not occur sufficiently to allow for air breathing if the baby is too early). Hypovolemia at birth (due to early cord clamping) leads to a deficiency of blood in the alveolar capillary framework. This, coupled with insufficient surfactant, results in widespread alveolar collapse (atelectasis) with each exhalation, requiring the baby to expend enormous energy to essentially reinflate his lungs with each breath. This effort uses oxygen quickly and rapidly tires the baby. (See page 277 for more details about surface tension and surfactant.)

Color-by-number key for this drawing:

1. Bright red (high oxygen content)
2. Blue (low oxygen content) (including 4 arrows in left atrium)
3. Purple-red (medium oxygen content)

3+. Deep purple-red (medium-low oxygen content)

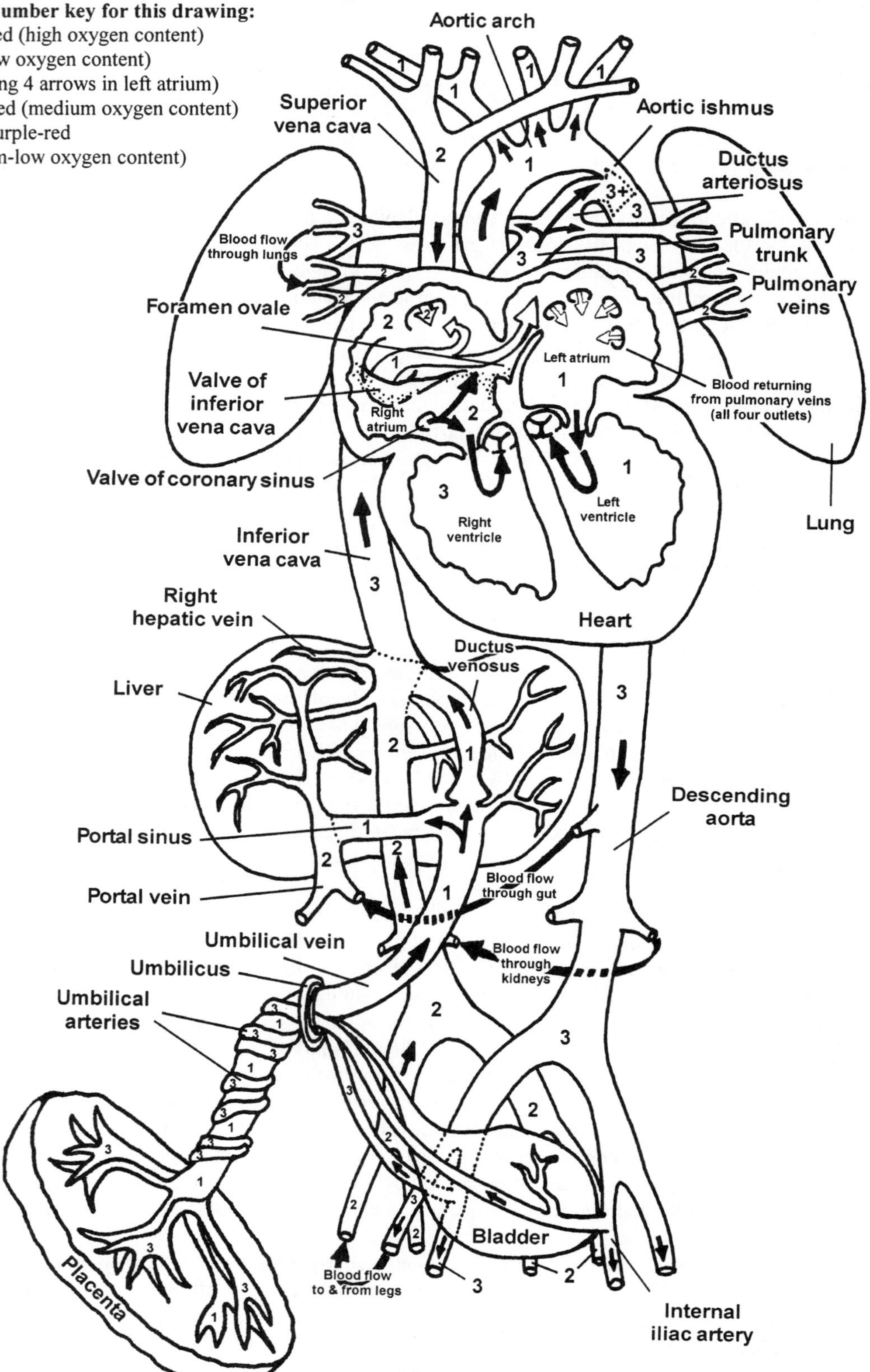

Pathways of fetal circulation

Color-by-number key for this drawing:
1. Bright red (high oxygen content)
2. Blue (poor oxygen content)
3. Burgundy red (medium oxygen content) (including 4 arrows in left atrium)

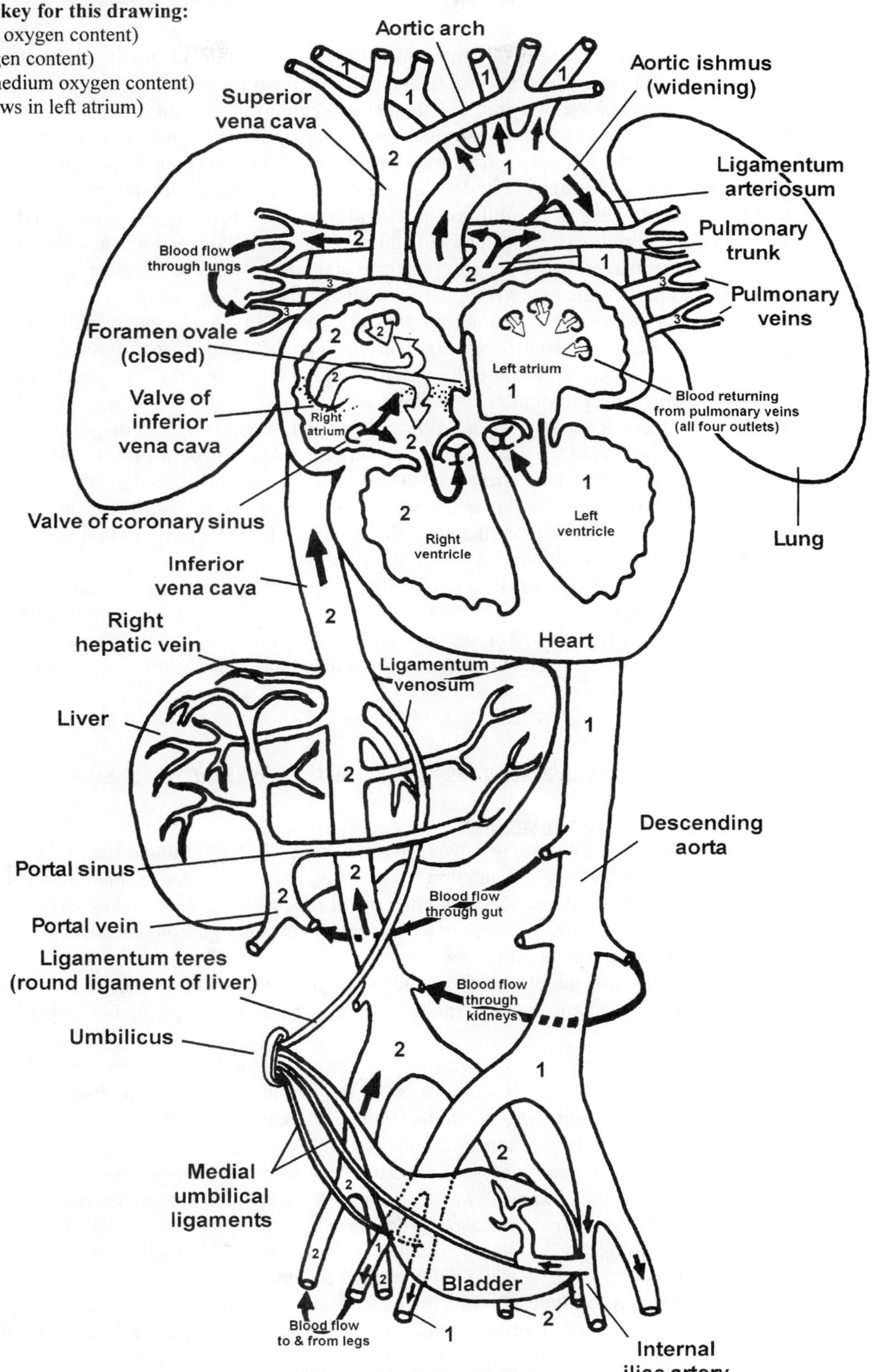

Pathways of neonatal and adult circulation

Fetal breathing movements: Fetal breathing movements are stimulated by a rise in the level of oxygen that reaches the fetus. The fetal hemoglobin level rises as term approaches, which gradually raises the oxygen-carrying capacity of the blood. Fetal breathing movements are normally intermittent and incoordinate, occurring about 40% of the time during both active periods and quiet sleep in the near-term fetus. These sternal movements occur due to fluid dynamics as well as inhibition and lack of coordination of upper airway inspiratory muscles. Although called "fetal breathing," these movements are not really practice for breathing air, because the fetal pulmonary pathways are thought to be completely obstructed at the larynx and at the hypopharynx during inspiration; however, breathing movements are believed to be important to airway development and may help develop the muscles involved in breathing.

Fetal breathing movements seem to be inhibited in several ways. The low oxygen tension in the resting fetus is one inhibiting factor. Hormonal inhibitors include prostaglandin E_2, adenosine and endorphins. Fetal breathing movements stop 48 hours before labor begins, probably due to a rise in prostaglandin E_2, although sleep cycles, heart rate variability and behavior patterns continue. Acute hypoxia in utero inhibits fetal breathing as carbon dioxide levels rise. If hypoxia is severe and prolonged; it will eventually prompt gasping. However, in experiments with lambs, sustained sublethal hypoxia lasting 8 to 12 hours led to recurrent breathing, heart rate variability and rest/activity cycles. Only the basal heart rate remained elevated, reflecting continued poor oxygenation. This shows that the fetus can override normal breathing inhibition mechanisms in ways not fully understood (Johnson, 1996).

The fetus apparently prepares for air breathing by involuntarily exercising her diaphragm via hiccuping, which produces a spontaneous contraction of the diaphragm. The untraumatized newborn exclusively practices diaphragmatic breathing, where the belly expands and the chest wall falls slightly. After birth, as the baby matures, she can select to breathe by either elevating the sternum or expanding the diaphragm, as can the adult (Morgan, 1995). Diaphragmatic breathing maximizes oxygenation, since more than two-thirds of the pulmonary circulation occurs in the lower third of the lungs. (In chest-breathing adults, less than a teacup full of blood passes primarily through the upper lungs. During diaphragmatic breathing over a quart passes through the lungs, especially the lower two-thirds.) Thus, sternal or chest breathing, which favors the upper third of the lungs, dramatically reduces pulmonary perfusion. Chest breathing is associated with high levels of stress, anxiety or unexpressed emotions, which may or may not be conscious (Hendricks & Hendricks, 1991). The Hendrickses call diaphragmatic breathing "happy baby breathing." A newborn who practices chest breathing is unduly stressed or traumatized.

The Transformation from Dependence upon the Placenta to the Lungs for Oxygenation

Fetus-to-newborn cardiorespiratory adaptation

The transition to pulmonary respiration involves the absorption of lung fluid and the redirecting of blood flow to allow the lungs to receive all the blood for oxygenation. During intrauterine life, gas exchange occurs between two liquid media, the mother's and baby's bloodstreams, across a thin membrane within the cotyledons of the placenta. After birth, this exchange occurs across the alveolar membrane in the lungs between a gaseous medium (room air) and the liquid blood flowing in the capillary beds surrounding the alveoli.

The fetal cardiovascular system adapts to life outside the womb with changes that occur during the infant's first minutes of life. Several things must happen either simultaneously or in close succession before the lungs can assume and maintain their functions. Ideally:

1. The intact pulsating umbilical cord delivers an adequate transfusion from the placenta to the newborn circulation. An adequate infusion of red cells raises the amount of oxygen the baby receives, which also stimulates and then helps maintain respirations (Mercer & Skovgaard, 2002).
2. A greater influx of blood into the pulmonary circulatory pathways begins the process of absorbing lung fluid and expanding the constricted pulmonary vessels. It is theorized that this may begin prior to the first breath.
3. Spontaneous respirations begin. Exposure of the wet newborn to the air and a sudden reduction in temperature may contribute to stimulating the baby to gasp and begin breathing. In some babies, this cold crying reflex results not only in breathing but in crying, which also triggers a gasp followed by breathing (Morley, 2002a). Crying, however, is not necessary for normal breathing to commence.
4. As the placental transfusion continues flowing in under pressure, left arterial pressure rises. This increases the blood pressure against the septum primum, thus closing the foramen ovale. This transforms the heart into a two-sided pump and shifts the circulation from a dual arterial to a venous and arterial circuit. The lungs begin to oxygenate the blood as breathing is established and the baby turns rosy pink (Morley, 2002a).

5. Some air remains in the alveoli at the end of expiration so that the lungs do not collapse (i.e., functional residual capacity is established). Adequate pulmonary blood flow assists in this process by erecting the capillary framework around each sac, helping sustain it in an expanded state as the baby exhales.
6. Pulmonary blood flow increases to full newborn levels as pulmonary vascular resistance is further reduced.
7. Cardiac output is redirected completely from the placenta to the lungs.

These events occur as efficiently and as atraumatically as possible when the flow of blood from the placenta is maintained, ensuring that the total volume of blood required to increase perfusion of the lungs and to maintain perfusion of other vital organs is available. Effective simultaneous pulmonary and placental respiration have been demonstrated to occur under experimental conditions; at birth, an intact cord allows the newborn to temporarily maintain two routes for oxygenation until the placenta has fully separated from the uterine wall (usually for at least 3 minutes after birth). During this adjustment, perfusion of the vitals organs, particularly the brain, is maintained. This is protective against brain damage, even in the presence of hypoxia as hypovolemia is more dangerous to the brain than is all but the most severe hypoxia (Morley, 2003).

A baby whose cord is cut before the placenta is born is thus experiencing a pathological transition. Aside from the physical insult, these babies take their very first breaths in an overwhelming state of fear and panic, thus imprinting them with negative messages about having support cut off, helping to form the basis for life philosophies based upon survival and scarcity rather than abundance and wholeness.

Why does the baby begin to breathe? To read the current medical literature one can easily get the impression that immediate cutting of the cord is a primary trigger for breathing (this is true only in that it makes breathing imperative for survival). As you delve deeper into the current literature, it becomes apparent that the exact reasons why breathing movements are intermittent in the fetus and continuous in the newborn are currently unknown. For many decades, the initiation of air breathing was thought to be triggered by the mild asphyxia (oxygen deprivation) present in most infants during the moments surrounding birth (which is, of course, transformed into total asphyxia by immediate cord clamping). In utero, the term fetus normally receives cord blood with an oxygen saturation that averages 70% (compared with an adult whose oxygen saturation is normally 94 to 98%). However, during late pushing, the oxygen content (saturation) of venous cord blood among individual babies varies widely before the baby begins to breathe. In a large number of newly born infants, oxygen saturation levels are less than 10% at the time of birth. Although there is usually an absence of metabolic acidosis (that is, the buffer base is normal), mild respiratory acidosis is present due to high Pco_2, a fall in serum pH, often to 7.28, and a low arterial Po_2. This brief period of reduced oxygen availability is part of the normal birth process. Some compression of the umbilical vein as the lower torso passes through the pelvis probably contributes to this fall in oxygen (Dunn, 1966). (Mercer [2002] points out that rushing the birth of the shoulders by not waiting for the next contraction after the birth of the head may deny the fetus her final bolus of placental blood which is transferred via high-pressure uterine contractions. This, in turn, may result in the baby having an artificially low blood oxygen level at birth.) One hypothesis postulates that mild hypoxia at birth stimulates the carotid and aortic chemo-receptors to initiate impulses that are then transmitted to the respiratory control center in the medulla. However, research shows that when the nerves to the carotid and aortic chemoreceptors are severed, breathing proceeds as usual. It may be that respiratory acidosis plays a part in this process in a way not yet understood (Tietel, 1998). See the subchapter entitled "Understanding Fetal and Neonatal Asphyxia" for more details.

On a contrary note, Mercer and Skovgaard (2002) believe that the increased red cell volume from the placental transfusion raises the level of oxygen in the newborn system, which stimulates the pulmonary vasculature to begin relaxation and the respiratory center to begin breathing. (The placental transfusion also helps to correct acidosis.) Another current theory postulates that breathing is triggered in part by the release of as yet unidentified chemicals or hormones.

Although the pressure exerted on the fetal thorax is significant during its passage through the birth canal, the resulting expansion that occurs upon birth probably does not contribute significantly to the initiation of breathing. However, it does assist in pressing some of the pulmonary fluid up and out of the upper airway, which seems to enhance both the volume of the first inspiration as well as the development of functional residual capacity (Vyas et al., 1986).

It has also been postulated that the abrupt drop in temperature the baby experiences when going from his mother's body into room air provides stimulus for the newborn to breathe. Exposure to air by itself may prompt biophysical triggers that initiate gasping followed by regular respirations, especially because the baby is born wet, which heightens the effect of a drop in temperature. In animal studies, it appears that environmental temperature chiefly determines the arousal threshold of the fetus and the effectiveness of breathing once it is established. Generally speaking, ambient temperature plays a major part in both inhibition and stimulation of breathing. Overheating causes panting. Even minimal cooling by as little as 1.8 to 3.6°F (1 to 2°C) stimulates breathing and nonshivering thermogenesis, and synchronizes the alae nasae and genioglossal muscles of the nose and tongue with diaphragmatic inspiratory activity.

The degree of temperature change newborns experience at birth varies widely. The baby leaves an intrauterine fluid environment of 100°F (38°C). If the baby is born into a near-body temperature pool of water, the mammalian diving reflex is operative and the baby will not try to breath. In a very hot climate, the temperature change may be minimal; however, exposure to air alone is a very dramatic shift. At a homebirth with the room temperature set at 80 to 85°F (21 26.6 to 29.5°C), there may still be a drop of 15 to 20°F (7.5 to 10°C). Having never experienced a temperature drop before, the effect must be dramatic. In an air-conditioned hospital delivery room, there may be as much as a 30 to 35°F (22 to 25°C) drop in temperature. Temperature variations may influence how abruptly the infant makes the transition to breathing on her own and may also contribute to the sought-for chemical or hormonal changes that let the baby know it is time to begin breathing. Morley (2002a) theorizes that the cold crying reflex is stimulated when the wet baby is exposed to air, which causes the baby to gasp and then begin crying and breathing. However, even with a drop of 20°F (16°C), many babies simply start breathing and never cry unless separated from their mothers. It seems that exposure to air is a good candidate for a respiratory trigger, but the possibility needs much more research.

When does the baby start to breathe? Fetal respiratory movements help the lungs grow and mature, and may prepare the surrounding musculature for more vigorous respiratory efforts at the time of birth. In the US, it is considered normal for mature, healthy babies to start breathing regularly within 30 seconds of birth into air. In a UK study (where the cord tends to be left intact longer than in the US), 75% of surviving babies were breathing regularly by 60 seconds, while 20% of normal babies took between 60 and 180 seconds to start breathing regularly (Chamberlain et al., 1975). Babies whose cords are left intact have the luxury of starting to breath when they are ready, and therefore may take a bit longer than babies whose cords are clamped early.

Pulmonary vascular resistance (PVR) before and after birth: During gestation, pulmonary vascular resistance is maintained by a complex balance of vasoconstrictive and vasodilator modulators, which include a variety of hormones and other biochemical agents, as well as by the thick muscular coat on the pulmonary vessels. Pressure both from the fluid within the alveoli and from active muscular constriction work together to mechanically compress the vessel walls and keep their radii small–a key component of pulmonary vascular resistance. Another key factor is the relatively low oxygen saturation of the fetal blood in general and that delivered to the lungs in particular. This results in a low oxygen tension in the fetus. The specific ways in which this contributes to PVR remain uncertain; however, a temporary increase in maternal oxygenation has been noted to cause a 10-fold increase in pulmonary blood flow in experiments on sheep fetuses who are three-quarters of the way to term. Vascular resistance returns to normal fetal levels when the mother once again breathes room air.

A central component of normal newborn transition is the relaxation of the pulmonary vasculature to allow all the blood to pass through the lungs for oxygenation. The initiation of rhythmic breathing causes vasodilation, even if the oxygen saturation of the blood does not rise. This is due, in part, to the mechanical expansion of the lungs, which increases the vessel radius. The carbon dioxide tension, or level, falls as the slight asphyxia of late labor reverses when breathing is initiated, a process that also helps reverse vasoconstriction. This effect is enhanced when the placental transfusion is available to help balance blood gases (see below).

Enlargement of the lungs may also directly enhance the synthesis of vasodilator agents. Even in the absence of ventilation, increased oxygen tension at birth also causes a reduction in PVR, which is partly due to the loss of the hypoxic component of PVR.

The placental transfusion hypothesis of alveolar expansion: Judith Mercer and Rebecca Skovgaard (2002) have proposed a new paradigm for neonatal transition, which is described in detail here. Newborn breathing is greatly facilitated when the cord remains intact to carry blood from the placenta into the pulmonary circulation. During pushing, uterine contractions pump blood toward the baby at an average pressure of 80 to 100 mm Hg, which easily exceeds the pressure required to expand the fetal pulmonary vessels. The placental attachment site is not constricted while the baby's body is still contained within the uterus, and the high uterine pressure has an indirect influence over the pressure at which blood is delivered through the cord to the baby. As each contraction subsides, pressure is temporarily relieved and blood can flow freely back into the placenta.

During pushing, the uterus gets smaller as the baby emerges, and the pressure from each contraction is increasingly brought to bear directly on the placenta. Rhythmic uterine contractions gather around the placenta, squeezing it and then partially releasing it, causing placental blood to be pushed into the fetal circulation in a step-wise fashion via the fetal circulatory pathways. Peter Dunn (1986) believes that the soft, elastic umbilical vein becomes pressed against the side-wall of the birth canal as the lower torso descends into the birth canal, temporarily reducing the flow of blood into the baby; the umbilical arteries continue to pump blood back toward the placenta. (This same phenomenon may also occur as the thorax is squeezed when the chest moves through the pelvis.) This causes the placenta to become engorged.

As soon as the pressure on the cord (or chest) is relieved, the uterine contraction that pushes the body out sends a bolus of oxygenated blood through the now patent umbilical vein into the baby's circulation. As a result, the infant's corporeal blood volume increases dramatically. The portal vein and ductus venosus become flooded with blood that cannot backwash unimpeded to the placenta (especially during uterine contractions). Instead, blood distends the portal veins of the liver, fills the heart, and flows through the pulmonary artery into the constricted pulmonary capillaries. Thus increased blood volume coming in under such high pressure may begin the process of overcoming pulmonary vascular resistance, causing the capillaries to begin expansion.

Mercer (2002) hypothesizes that, whereas 8 to 10% of the blood volume may enter the fetal lungs at term, the transitional newborn lungs receive a slightly larger infusion of blood before breathing even starts. (She also believes this may happen, to a small extent, prior to birth in many babies). Each infusion of blood into the partially dilated capillaries makes the next easier, thus allowing the percentage of blood flow to increase gradually and atraumatically while producing symmetrical erection of the capillaries in the alveoli walls. An increase in blood flow results in the immediate clearing of lung fluid via osmotic transfer from the alveoli. As this fluid, which held the alveoli open from the inside during fetal life, is absorbed, the increasingly engorged and erect capillaries form a framework, maintaining the expansion of the alveoli from the outside. Properly distended capillaries bulge into the lumen of the alveoli, fostering adequate gas exchange. The emptying of fluid from the well-supported alveoli effectively produces negative pressure within the alveolar sacs, which probably helps initiate breathing. Negative pressure is increased as the diaphragm descends during the first breath. In addition, the influx of red blood cells raises the oxygen level in the newborn, stimulating the respiratory center to initiate breathing, the same process that triggers fetal breathing movements prior to birth (Jäykkä, 1957, 1958).

With the partially engorged pulmonary capillaries holding the alveoli open in readiness to receive air in a calm, well-oxygenated baby, the net result is the familiar easing into breathing so typical of homeborn babies whose cords remain intact for many minutes or hours longer than ever occurs in the typical hospital setting (Mercer, 2002). These untraumatized babies often do not cry and, if they do, it is often only briefly. The first few breaths and cardiac rerouting result in more blood moving from the placenta into the circulatory pathways surrounding the alveoli. The capillary framework around each sac helps to hold them open during expiration.

The research to prove this "blood volume" model of lung expansion has yet to be completed. Some details, particularly regarding how an increased flow of blood might be allowed to go into the pulmonary vessels prior to the first breath, need to be more fully addressed. This theory is included here because it is the most exciting theory of physiologic neonatal transition to be found in the medical literature that matches what is seen clinically in babies with intact cords. All other theories are predicated on rapid or immediate cord clamping or "late" cord clamping (often within 3 minutes of birth), which may terminate the natural process, thus skewing the results.

It just makes sense that a purely physiologic transition would not require doing anything such as clamping and cutting the cord. Who had clamps or string eons ago, when this process was being perfected? An unclamped, open cord bleeds out; all the babies would have died! Even if the blood rushing in at high pressure is not sufficient to overcome pulmonary vascular resistance prior to the first breath, that the blood is waiting and available under high pressure when breathing does commence probably makes taking the first and each subsequent breath much easier. If the cord is cut or not pulsating at the time of the first breath, the baby must work much harder to draw blood into the pulmonary circulation by drawing blood from other vascular compartments to expand the alveoli. This causes the capillaries to expand irregularly at first (Jäykkä, 1957) and makes initiating and maintaining alveolar expansion much more difficult, especially if the baby is preterm.

The first respiratory activity of the newborn creates lower air pressure within the lungs than in the external atmosphere, or negative intrathoracic pressure. The pressure differential required to initially expand the lungs can be substantial but appears to be influenced significantly by adequate perfusion of the pulmonary circulation. When uterine contractions are allowed to do the work of filling the pulmonary capillary beds, the effort required of the newborn is much less. The first breathing efforts generate an intraesophageal pressure change averaging the equivalent of –20 to –40 cm

H_2O in studies done on infants whose cords remained intact (Karlberg, et al., 1962). The relationship between volume and intraesophageal pressure changes through a whole breath is often used for analysis of the mechanics of breathing since the intraesophageal pressure change represents the sum of forces acting on the lung in producing the respiratory volume change. A wide range of tidal volume (12 to 67 ml) during the first visible inspiration is larger than in resting infants with established respiration [15 to 20 ml]. Karlberg and associates also found a total pressure change ranging from 40 to 100 cm H_2O, which decreased during succeeding breaths. In most infants, significant lung inflation took place only after pulmonary resistance was overcome by creating a negative opening pressure of –20 to –40 cm H_2O; after that, inflation accelerated rapidly. These babies first breaths had short inspiratory phases and long, irregular high-pressure expiratory phases.

An opening pressure as high as – 100 cm H_2O has been noted when the baby is born preterm (and therefore has an even lower blood volume than a term infant), when breathing is initiated under the duress of early cord clamping, or when the cord is limp and the baby is born asphyxiated and makes no spontaneous efforts to breathe. When the cord transfusion is terminated, the baby must create all the force necessary to inflate the lungs.

Air enters the airways and lungs as soon as intrathoracic pressure falls and the diaphragm contracts (Karlberg et al., 1962). Air entering the upper respiratory tract must reach the alveoli by overcoming forces that obstruct its free flow. Three such forces are the constriction of the alveoli, frictional forces within the tiny neonatal airways and the viscosity of lung fluid in the respiratory tract. In all lungs, surface tension forces are minimized by the presence of an expanded capillary bed and, to a lesser extent, by the presence of adequate surfactant in the alveoli. However, fetal lung fluid also presents a major opposing force to the initial entry of air into the lungs; by term, the newborn whose cord is clamped rapidly must inhale into the equivalent of a bag of water. In the baby whose cord is intact, a significant quantity of this fluid is cleared more rapidly because of the additional blood flow. The volume of lung fluid (30 to 35 ml/kg) is roughly equivalent to the volume of functional residual capacity (explained in the next section) that begins to be established either before or after breathing begins. Birth via the yoni creates pressure on the baby's thorax and serves to expel a portion of these fluids, between 20 to 35 ml, from the respiratory tract. Thirty ml, however, constitutes only one-third of the total lung volume of a 6 lb 6 oz (2892 g) baby.

A large positive intrathoracic pressure (averaging 70 cm H_2O) is produced during the first expiration when the baby closes his glottis and pushes his first breath out of his airway. This high expiratory pressure distributes the air from the first breath throughout the lungs. (It is very likely that the babies with intact umbilical cords do not expire at such a high pressure because lung expansion is greatly assisted by the capillary expansion that occurs with placental transfusion.) The majority of the remaining fluid is actively removed by adrenaline-induced passive reabsorption across the alveolar epithelium by osmosis as increased blood flow brings more proteins to attract the fluid. An adequate placental-to-pulmonary transfusion provides plenty of blood to begin this process, possibly prior to the first breath. Fluid is also mobilized into the interstitial spaces and the lymphatic system. Respiratory activity massages the surrounding lymphatic vessels, helping the lymph to carry fluid away. Alveolar expansion, which stretches the sac walls and thus increases permeability, also facilitates this process.

It is common for the lungs to be "stiff" in the days following birth. At term, the lungs are in a semimature saccular phase of alveolar development, with relatively small air spaces surrounded by thick intrasaccular septa containing multiple capillaries. After the first seven days, typical mature alveoli begin to develop, characterized by thinner intra-alveolar walls in which a single capillary is in contact with the air space on each side of the septum. Mercer and Skovgaard believe these thick vascular walls play an important role in structurally supporting the newly opened alveoli in the first days of life. As the capillaries spread out over the course of the first hours or days, they eventually form a one-layer framework around the sacs, and the stiffness resolves. Muscles in the arteries also stretch, thin and straighten out as the lungs expand, a gradual process that is usually complete by 6 to 8 weeks of age. This stiffness may or may not produce symptoms; when it does, it is probably the cause of some cases of transient tachypnea of the newborn.

Establishing functional residual capacity (FRC): During normal respiration, some air must remain in the alveoli at the end of each expiration in order to maintain them in a partially inflated state. The volume of air retained is the lungs' "functional residual capacity" (FRC). The ability to retain the air is referred to as "alveolar stability."

In normal term lungs, the first expansion may require an opening pressure as high as 60 to 80 cm H_2O. At the end of each expiration the pressure is again zero; that is, intrathoracic pressure and pressure in the surrounding air are equal. The newborn compensates for stiffness in her lung tissue by partially closing her glottis during the expiratory phase of her first few breaths, an action that maintains a relatively a high positive pressure (20 to 30 cm H_2O) as long as possible.

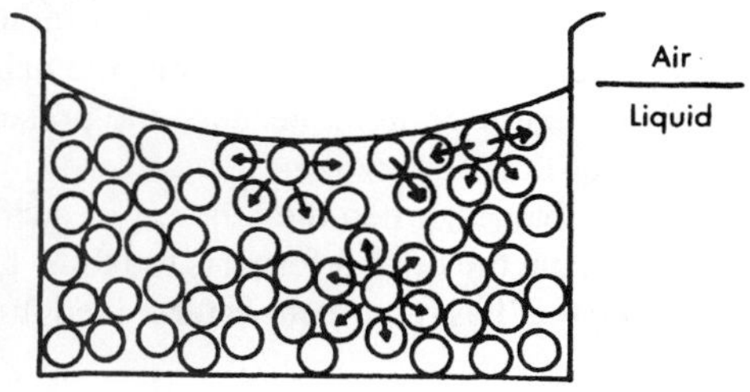

Surface tension in a glass of water

Less opening pressure is required during subsequent inhalation cycles, since the lungs are already partially expanded at rest and the alveoli remain more inflated after each breath. An FRC averaging 15 ml is usually established within the first breath or two when the baby achieves an adequate inspiratory volume (averaging 38 ml) and a prolonged inspiratory pressure (Vyas, et al., 1986). When FRC is fully established, the lungs may retain 25% of their fully expanded volume. In combination with surfactant, FRC makes the retention of air possible by minimizing surface tension.

FRC may be established more smoothly and quickly and maintained with less effort when the placental transfusion infuses the pulmonary circulation during and after the first breaths, holding the alveolar capillaries erect. In addition, FRC is smaller when the cord is left intact. Low pulmonary resistance is present during the first breath in some infants, and a residual volume is not detected during the first hour of life, supporting its development prior to the first breath (Karlberg et al., 1962).

If the lungs are not mature, inadequate surfactant levels contribute to more effortful breathing, as the alveoli have a tendency to deflate with each expiration. This is thought be due to the lesser pulmonary capillary filling that occurs in early clamped infants (Oh et al., 1967). If the alveoli cannot retain enough air to remain expanded after the first breath, every breath must be as forceful as the first. The combination of hypoxia (oxygen deprivation) and excessive effort quickly tires the preterm infant with immature lungs and compromises oxygen exchange (Korones, 1986).

Understanding surface tension: Surface tension is defined as the cohesive quality of the surface of a liquid. It is the property of liquids that makes their surfaces slightly elastic and enables the formation of separate drops by the interaction of molecules at or near the surface that tend to cohere and contract the surface into the smallest possible area. A glass of water can be used as an example. Below the surface, the water molecules are completely surrounded by other water molecules, resulting in equal pressure from all sides. The surface layer of water molecules is in contact with the air. The pressure exerted by the air molecules is less than that exerted by the surface water molecules. Therefore, the air above the water exerts little upward pull; the balance of force thus favors downward and horizontal directions. In fact, the molecules on the surface of the water are so cohesive that the water can stand up slightly above the rim of the container without spilling because the air does not overcome their cohesion.

The phenomenon of surface tension applies to the surface area of the alveolar wall, which is primarily liquid. When air enters the lungs, this liquid forms an envelope around the inhaled air. In the absence of sufficient surfactant, the liquid in the alveolar walls coheres when the air is expelled on exhalation, causing the alveoli to revert to a state similar to a big drop of water after each breath. This tendency is greatly enhanced when the pulmonary vasculature suffers from inadequate blood flow, allowing for more complete collapse of the alveoli with each exhalation. Air is retained more easily and alveolar collapse is less likely when the capillary framework of each alveoli is symmetrically expanded because the alveoli cannot revert to the "drop of water" state as readily (Korones, 1986).

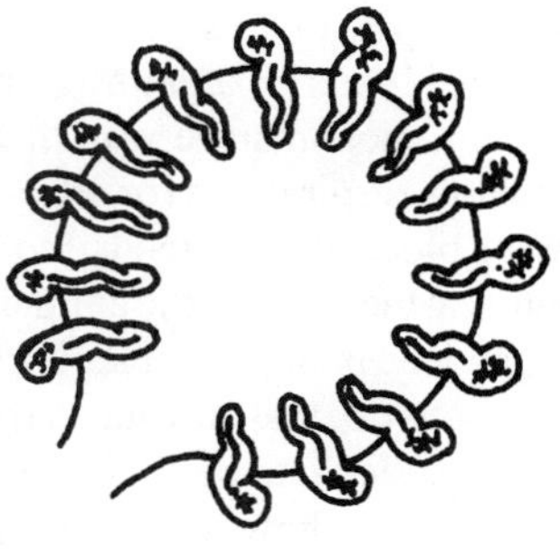
Inflation separates the surfactant molecules.

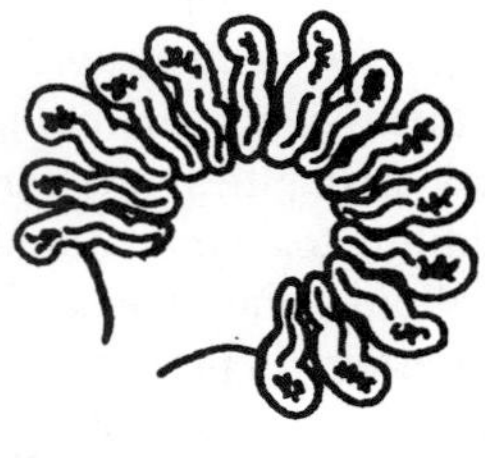
Deflation closes the gaps between molecules.

How surfactant facilitates breathing: Any substance that reduces the surface tension of liquids so that the liquid spreads out, rather than collecting in droplets, is a surfactant. It breaks the surface tension of water, causing the molecules to disperse, become more slippery and more permeable. Soap is the most familiar surfactant; it functions similarly to surfactant in the lungs.

In normal mature lungs, surfactant contributes to lessening the surface tension of the fluid alveolar walls. When a baby whose surfactant ratio is mature begins to breath, air inflates the alveoli and the lung fluid is absorbed, leaving the surfactant behind. The surfactant gets blown up like a soap bubble, forming an elastic lining on the inner walls of the alveoli that separates the inner walls from the air. During inspiration, the layer of surfactant molecules becomes thin enough to create tiny spaces between the molecules, allowing air to contact the surface of the alveolar wall directly. As alveoli shrink during expiration, the surfactant becomes thicker causing surface tension forces to diminish rather than increase. This thickening also helps prevent the alveoli from collapsing when the baby exhales. Thus the baby can breathe normally, and oxygen exchange can take place, even if blood volume is not optimal, because the presence of the surfactant can largely make up for poor capillary erection (Korones, 1986).

In preterm babies, when the amount of surfactant is inadequate, the surfactant that is present attempts to line the alveolar walls, but the layer it forms is too thin. Lacking sufficient elasticity, it collapses when the baby expires, just like a soap bubble that has too much water mixed in. If the baby has a low blood volume as well, he is in serious trouble.

Hemodynamics in the hours following birth and the relative importance of surfactant, blood volume and lung maturity: The unofficial age of viability is currently considered to be about 20 postovulatory weeks of gestation, although such tiny babies rarely survive because of the immaturity of their systems, particularly their lungs. By 24 weeks gestation, however, enough primitive, thin-walled, well-vascularized alveoli have developed that some of these babies stand a much better chance of surviving, especially if adequately sophisticated care is available to them. Air breathing is possible even though the lungs are not fully mature as long as the lung tissue is well perfused with blood and there is some surfactant present.

Mainstream neonatology views the presence of mature surfactant as the pivotal factor governing the baby's ability to maintain her lungs in a partially inflated state during expiration. However, there are experienced practitioners who feel strongly that the importance of surfactant to pulmonary function is secondary to the much more crucial issue of adequate pulmonary perfusion. Peter Dunn, a renowned and widely published English pediatrician of 40 years, and George Morley, a US obstetrician of 40 years and also a published author, are both strong proponents of physiologic newborn transition. In their own practices, both have noted remarkably mature respiration in preterm infants who have been allowed to receive their placental transfusion (Dunn, 1986, 1993; Morley, 2002c).

Morley points out that respiratory distress syndrome (RDS) can be induced at any age in conjunction with prolonged hypovolemic shock. Microscopic examination reveals that the hyaline membranes produced by a lack of sufficient placental transfusion in neonates is identical to those produced in an adult who has bled severely. Morley (2002b) explains that, while proteins do not normally leak through the capillary walls, in hyaline membrane disease the capillary walls are dying due to lack of oxygen and nutrients secondary to an inadequate blood volume. The breakdown of the vascular walls allows protein to leak through into the alveoli (which are also dying); this shows up as hyaline membranes under the microscope. Thus hyaline membrane disease is a condition of pulmonary shock or lack of adequate tissue perfusion in the lungs, a problem that can occur at any age, whenever blood flow is inadequate.

Morley goes on to say that a preterm infant born at 34 weeks gestation has a low level of surfactant in his lungs, yet the baby readily cries and turns a ruddy pink color when he receives an optimal placental transfusion at birth; the lungs behave in a most mature way that conflicts with the current idea of lung maturity. Under these ideal conditions, as spontaneous respirations (or artificial ventilations) are established, the pulmonary arterioles relax, resulting in a massive inflow of blood that distends the left atrium, presses closed the foramen ovale and expands the capillary framework surrounding the alveoli–the child turns pink. When the placental transfusion is allowed to fully and symmetrically distend and expand the pulmonary capillaries, the alveoli are assisted in remaining partially inflated during expiration by the erect vascular network that surrounds them like a frame, thus compensating for a surfactant ratio that is still immature. In the presence of adequate perfusion, any surfactant present helps prevent alveolar collapse and lessens the force needed to inflate the lungs; however, marginal levels of surfactant are much less useful if the blood volume is inadequate.

When blood volume is insufficient, alveolar vascular expansion occurs in a piecemeal and asymmetrical fashion as the baby struggles to initiate and maintain inflation almost entirely on her own. The air-filled alveoli tend to compress the inadequately erected capillaries that lie between them. This impedes gas exchange as well as capillary distension and prevents them from functioning as a framework. Thus, while early cord clamping predisposes all babies to increased respiratory difficulties, it is particularly detrimental to preterm babies (Jäykkä, 1958; Morley, 2002b, 2002c).

In addition to an immature level of surfactant, extremely preterm babies have a low serum albumin and thus a lower plasma colloid osmotic pressure than do more mature babies. Initially this may result in pulmonary edema because the osmotic pressure in preterm blood is too low to dry out the lungs, particularly when the lungs are minimally perfused. Recall that osmotic absorption is the result of proteins drawing water from fluids of lesser solute concentration into fluid that has a greater solute concentration. In this case, the solutes consist of the minerals and proteins in the bloodstream (see the subchapter entitled "Intravenous Equipment and IV Therapy" for a more complete explanation of the basics of osmosis). Removal of water causes the protein and mineral content of the plasma to rise proportionately. The higher the protein concentration in the plasma, the greater the osmotic action.

When the preterm infant receives a full placental transfusion, the high-pressure pumping action of the left ventricle (which is stronger than the right) forces the additional blood through the systemic arterial circulation. While the veins and arteries only function as blood transport vessels, the tiniest vessels, the capillaries, are semipermeable and allow the movement of fluids back and forth across their walls. When the additional blood reaches the arterial side of the capillaries, the force at which the fluid enters the vessels is such that water is literally pushed from the bloodstream through the capillary walls into the extracellular spaces as well as into the kidney's filtration system. This reduces the amount of water in the circulating blood volume, resulting in the rapid concentration of blood proteins, thereby increasing the otherwise low osmotic pressure in the preterm baby's blood. As this protein-rich blood passes into the venous (and pulmonary) side of the capillary beds, the increased osmotic action draws fluid across the alveolar walls into the circulation. Pulmonary edema is quickly resolved and the lungs "dry out" physiologically.

There are many reasons why preterm babies are more dependent than term babies upon an adequate placental transfusion to accomplish this hemoconcentration while maintaining an adequate blood volume. They have a lower serum albumin; furthermore, more of their blood volume is circulating through the placenta at any given time (about 50% versus 30% at term). Term babies also shift fluids in the fashion described above but to a lesser extent. This explains, in part, the rapid hemoconcentration and blood volume shifting that is a recognized result of allowing a placental transfusion to occur. (Postnatal hemodynamics are further discussed in the chapter entitled "Placenta-to-Newborn Transfusion, Physiologic Closure of the Umbilical Vessels and Severance of the Cord.")

In summary, surfactant works to help prevent alveolar collapse once breathing is initiated. It may, by lowering surface tension, lessen the force needed to inflate the lungs initially and to maintain functional residual capacity once breathing commences. However, surfactant is of little value if the child's blood volume is insufficient to maintain pulmonary capillary expansion and to facilitate hemoconcentration, as here described, to remove fluid from the lungs. Surfactant does not cure RDS, and its absence does not cause RDS. The normal functioning of the lungs (lung "maturity") depends much more on adequate blood volume and plasma colloid osmotic pressure than on surfactant alone.

Fetal and newborn systemic vascular resistance: The placenta and cord are vital parts of the fetal circulatory system. Placental vessels are generally relaxed and offer little resistance to blood flow. The fetal lungs require a small percentage of the blood flow to nourish them while they grow; therefore, the blood vessels of the lungs are constricted, resulting in high pulmonary vascular resistance. This helps maintain the pressures required to keep the ductus arteriosus and foramen ovale open, directing most of the blood away from the lungs. Blood leaves the baby's body via the umbilical cord, a process that prevents a build-up of pressure within the fetal body. These factors, in particular the high pulmonary vascular resistance, contribute to the low systemic vascular resistance of the fetus.

At birth, the pressure exerted by uterine contractions forces blood into the baby's body. This, coupled with air breathing, expands the lungs, resulting in an 80% drop in pulmonary blood pressure (vascular resistance) by stimulating arteriolar relaxation within minutes after birth. The dramatic decrease in pulmonary vascular resistance causes an equally dramatic 5-fold increase in pulmonary blood flow. Cord circulation slows and the cardiovascular shunts start to close down. These changes result in a rise in systemic vascular resistance. Thus the systemic vascular resistance is high in the newborn compared to that of the fetus, although it is still low when compared to an adult (Sagady, 1995). Immediate cord clamping requires the cardiovascular switch-over to happen almost instantaneously and raises the aortic blood pressure suddenly. An intact cord allows the baby to maintain placental circulation while initiating breathing efforts and provides a gentle transition. Remember that the intact cord also allows the baby to reverse transfuse blood back toward the placenta via the umbilical vein; although the question of whether central venous pressure can rise too high or too fast is debated among practitioners, leaving the cord intact makes either impossible, as it allows the baby to equilibrate his blood volume as necessary (Dunn, 1986, 1993). Dunn believes this process is especially protective to the delicate preterm brain.

Corresponding cardiovascular adaptations

Cardiovascular adaptation occurs simultaneously with the cardiopulmonary changes that happen as the infant is born and takes her first breaths. Six major changes in fetal circulation must take place if mature cardiovascular function is to take over. These changes are not a sudden occurrence. While major changes begin with the first breaths at birth, others occur gradually over hours or days. These changes are initially functional; that is, they occur as blood is rerouted from the placenta to the lungs for oxygenation. Later, anatomical closure permanently seals off these fetal structures.

Closure of the foramen ovale: An increased volume of blood flows from the lungs into the left atrium of the heart as pulmonary blood flow and oxygenation are established. This causes a rise in left atrial pressure with a corresponding drop in right atrial pressure. The pressure relationship between the atria is thus reversed from its fetal configuration. This results in increased pressure in the left atrium against the one-way flap of the foramen ovale pushing it only partially closed, thereby balancing atrial intake and helping to provide a smooth transition from placental to pulmonary respiration. The whole volume of inferior vena caval blood now joins the superior vena caval blood in the right atrium and augments pulmonary blood flow. To this is added the blood from the ductus arteriosus. The flap becomes firmly pressed against the septum secundum as left atrial return rises, thereby functionally closing the foramen. Eventually a seal forms around the margins of the flap, eliminating this right-to-left flow. There may be some residual flow through the foramen ovale during the transitional period when the seal is forming, although an adequate blood pressure works to keep the flap closed.

The septum secundum becomes permanently adhered to the atrial septum at several weeks or months of age. The sealed foramen ovale is referred to as the "fossa ovale." Should right atrial pressure again rise above left atrial pressure prior to fusion, as might occur if the baby were to become asphyxiated, the foramen will reopen. Sometimes the foramen ovale never fuses, but as long as blood flow is normal, functional closure is maintained.

Closure of the ductus arteriosus: The substantial muscles in this vessel begin to constrict as breathing becomes established and oxygen tension rises. Closure appears to be mediated by bradykinin, a substance released from the lungs as they inflate. The ductus arteriosus remains slightly open during the first few hours of life and ductal blood flow continues, although at a greatly reduced rate. The direction of flow will usually be from the aorta (left side) to the pulmonary artery (right side), because the pressures on the left (systemic) side of the circulation become much greater than the pressures on the right (pulmonary) side after birth. The ductus arteriosus constricts more firmly, over the next few hours, primarily in response to elevated oxygen tension. Functional closure is achieved by 15 hours in term infants, although this vessel can stay open much longer in the presence of persistent hypoxia or prematurity. Anatomic closure (fibrosis) is usually complete by two to three months of age. The ductus arteriosus becomes a ligament (the ligamentum arteriosum) following complete constriction.

Closure of the ductus venosus: The ductus venosus constricts along its entire length at birth so that all the blood enters the liver though the hepatic vessels. Functional closure occurs during the first three to seven days of life; anatomical closure is complete by two to three months, when the ductus venosus becomes the ligamentum venosum. The exact mechanism of anatomical closure is not fully understood.

Expansion of the aortic isthmus: After blood flow through the ductus arteriosus ceases, the aortic isthmus carries only fully oxygenated blood coming from the left side of the heart. The isthmus begins to enlarge following birth; by three to four months of age, it has reached the same diameter as the adjacent portions of the aortic arch (Lewis, 1918).

Closure of the umbilical vessels: The umbilical vein passes from the umbilicus to the porta hepatis, where it attaches to the left branch of the portal vein. Blood flow persists through the umbilical vein for a variable length of time after the baby starts to breathe. The umbilical vein remains open during very early infancy and may be used to give transfusions to the newborn. As the baby matures, the intra-abdominal portion of the umbilical vein gradually becomes the ligamentum teres, the round ligament of the liver.

The umbilical arteries consist of two hypogastric branches of the iliac arteries. They constrict shortly after birth, preventing blood loss. Their intra-abdominal portions fill with connective tissue; by the second or third month of life, they become the medial umbilical ligaments. The deeper ends of these vessels persist in the adult as the superior vesical arteries (sometimes still called the umbilical arteries).

Atrophy of some venous valves: The valve of the inferior vena cava occasionally persists in the adult and may assist in preventing the reflux of blood into the inferior vena cava during atrial contraction. More commonly, it is small and may present a cribriform (perforated) or filamentous appearance. Sometimes, it atrophies completely.

Valves present in other veins during gestation tend to reduce in number, especially those in the upper body. For example, the valves in the tributaries of the hepatic portal vein persist for a short while following birth, after which they disappear entirely. Some vessels only lose some of their valves; for instance, the greater saphenous vein, which runs from the groin to the foot, has an average of 14 valves in a child while that of an adult has 11 valves. Remnants of atrophied valves take the form of low crescent-shaped elevations on the inner wall of the veins (Burch, 1972).

Summary of fetus-to-newborn changes

The following table provides a simplified summary of cardiopulmonary changes, incoporating in the second step Mercer and Skovgaard's placental transfusion hypothesis.

ALVEOLI, CAPILLARY & LYMPHATIC VESSELS		DUCTUS ARTERIOSUS		FORAMEN OVALE	
1. In utero: Pulmonary vascular resistance is high; only 8% of blood flow reaches lungs. Alveoli are filled with surfactant–rich fluid. Constricted blood vessels minimize pulmonary circulation.		Wide open. Solid arrow shows blood flow through ductus to aortic arch. Dashed arrows show minimal flow to lungs.	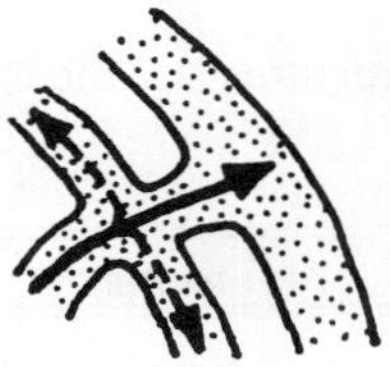	Blood flows from right to left atrium (solid arrow) through the foramen ovale. Septal flap is forced to baby's left by the higher pressure in the right atrium.	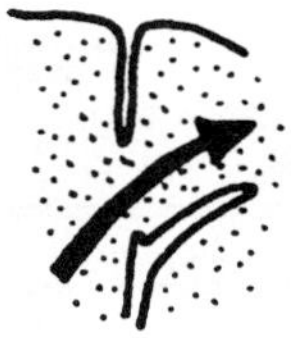
2. Placental transfusion begins process of expanding pulmonary capillaries. As the alveolar capillary framework begins to expand, plasma proteins start to pull fluid out.		Fetal circulation becomes distended with blood entering under pressure from uterine contractions.		Other cardiac changes may begin gradually as pulmonary vascular resistance falls.	
3. First inspiration or so: As first breath peaks, pressure builds in lungs. Fluid absorption continues as air enters alveoli. Surfactant coats new air-fluid interface. Blood vessels expand further as pulmonary vascular resistance keeps falling.	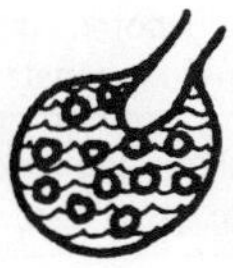	Ductus begins to constrict as increased blood flow is redirected into branches of the pulmonary arteries.	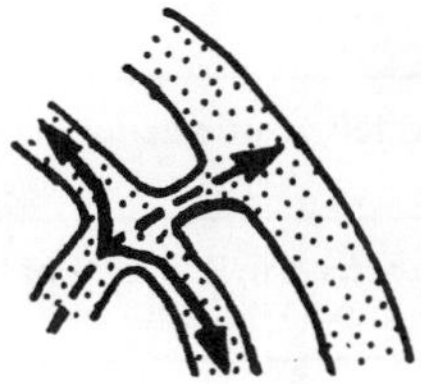	Flap over foramen moves right as right-sided cardiac pressure drops and left-sided pressure rises due to more blood flow being directed to the lungs.	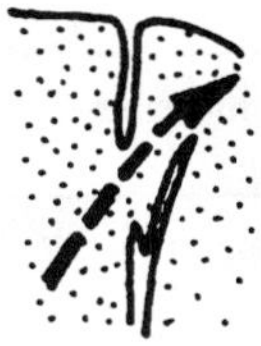
4. First expiration: Pressure drops as FRC begins to be established. Aided by capillary erection, alveoli retain air. Lymphatic flow increases by virtue of massaging action of respiration; more lung fluid is evacuated.	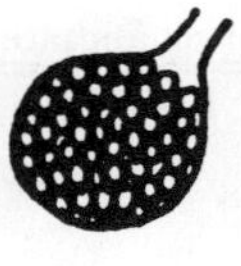	Little change.	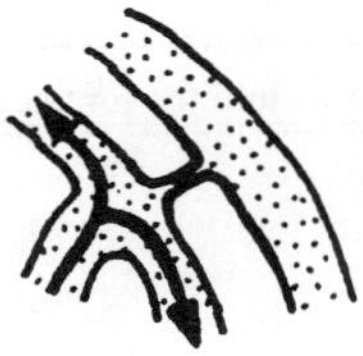	Little change.	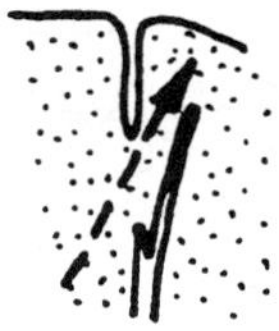
5. Subsequent breaths, full inhalation: Less and less pressure required as capillaries remain erect. Alveoli enlarge as more fluid clears. Surfactant molecules line the alveoli. Capillaries well distended, lymphatics slightly less dilated.	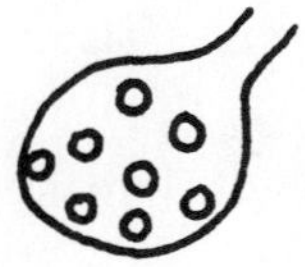	Ductal constriction is complete, eliminating blood flow from the pulmonary artery to the aorta.	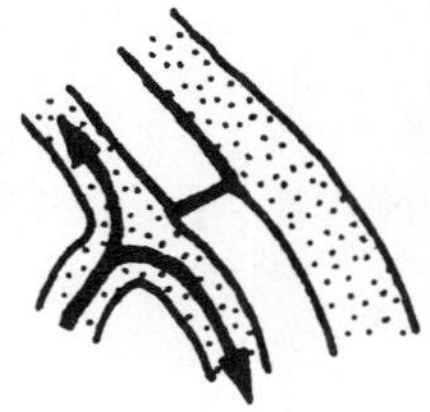	The flap of the foramen migrates further right and becomes plastered against the septum secundum.	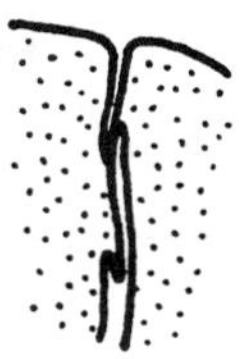

Alveoli, Capillary & Lymphatic Vessels		Ductus Arteriosus		Foramen Ovale	
6. Subsequent breaths: FRC maintained. Alveoli maintain FRC. Capillary flow is stable; flow of lung fluid to lymph vessels is further diminished.	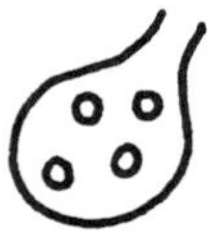	No change.	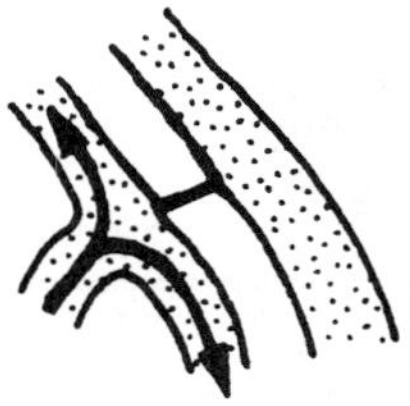	No change.	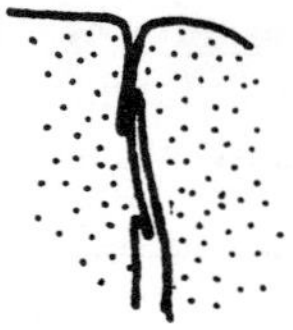

The following table summarizes fetal structures and the changes they undergo during the months following birth after newborn transition is complete:

Structure	Before Birth	After Birth
Umbilical vein	Brings oxygenated blood to the baby's body	Atrophies to become round ligament of liver
Umbilical arteries	Bring deoxygenated blood to placenta	Atrophy to become medial umbilical ligaments on anterior abdominal wall
Ductus venosus	Carries umbilical vein blood into inferior vena cava	Atrophies to become ligamentum venosum
Ductus arteriosis	Carries arterial and some venous blood from the pulmonary artery to the aorta	Atrophies to become ligamentum arteriosum
Foramen ovale	Connects right and left atria	Usually atrophies. May remain unfused but is functionally closed
Aortic isthmus	Connects right and left ventricular output	Widens to become continuous with aortic arch, carries only oxygenated blood from left ventricle
Lungs	Contain no air; only receive 8 to 10% of blood flow at term.	Filled with air and receive 45% of cardiac output for oxygen exchange
Pulmonary arteries	Bring little blood to lungs	Bring all the blood to the lungs
Aorta	Receives blood from both ventricles	Receives blood only from left ventricle
Inferior vena cava	Brings venous blood from body and oxygenated blood from placenta	Brings deoxygenated blood from systemic circulation to right atria
Valve of inf. vena cava	Helps direct blood flow into the foramen ovale	Of minor significance or atrophies entirely

PRODUCTION AND ELIMINATION OF MECONIUM DURING GESTATION

Meconium starts to appear in the fetal bowel between the 10th and 12th weeks of gestation. The fetus swallows amniotic fluid, along with any particulate matter that is floating in it. This fluid moves rapidly through the baby's body into the intestines, where most of the water is reabsorbed, leaving behind nondigestible residue such as lanugo and discarded cells. This debris mixes with mucus, bile and pancreatic secretions. The result is a thick and sticky, green-black substance made up of water, mucopolysaccharides, cholesterol and sterol precursors, protein, lipids, bile acids and salts (which impart its green color), enzymes, blood group substances, squamous cells, vernix and traces of certain chemical residues from our polluted environment.

Peristaltic movement in the gut is regulated by a variety of hormones; passage of bowel contents in adults is known to be under both hormonal and neural control. The blood level of motilin, a hormone that triggers peristalsis and defecation, rises significantly as the fetus matures. While motilin levels are highest in postdates babies, comparatively higher levels of motilin are found in babies who have amniotic fluid that is visibly stained with meconium near the time of birth. Progressive maturation of the gastrointestinal neuroplexus and parasympathetic nervous system are also thought to influence the passage of meconium. Because of these observations, it has been thought that the biological triggers for defecation are not really active in most babies until they approach term, but new research shows that fetal motilin levels are only part of the picture.

It has also been known for years that some apparently healthy fetuses pass meconium in utero before term. In the first study of its kind, Doppler investigations confirmed that the fetus experiences physiological defecation which begins between the 12th and 41st weeks of gestation (Ramón y Cajal & Martinez, 2003). The study used sophisticated ultrasound imaging techniques to observe babies between 15 and 41 weeks. Most were found to defecate at least once during a single 10 to 15+ minute observation period. The number of defecations was most frequent between weeks 28 and 33. After the 24th week, the anus remained closed between expulsions with the sphincter contracted. The anal activity decreased just prior to birth, and fetal defecation was of smaller volume at this time.

Thus, the passage of meconium in utero appears to be completely physiological. In light of this, Ciftci and associates (1999) postulate that visible meconium staining in the amniotic fluid at the time of labor is due to the suppression of fetal swallowing that occurs as a consequence of fetal distress, thus impairing clearance of the amniotic fluid (Ciftci et al., 1999). In addition to this, I theorize that an adrenalin surge prompted by maternal or fetal stress or during fetal hypoxia may cause the baby to expel more meconium than he normally would.

Body Temperature Regulation in the Fetus and Newborn

One of the most important physiological considerations in caring for the newborn is helping her maintain a normal body temperature. Leaving the cord intact so that the baby can receive an optimal transfusion of body-temperature placental blood maintains body warmth during fetal to neonatal transition. The maintenance of a steady supply of adequately oxygenated blood via normovolemia is the first and, in many ways, the most important way of ensuring the best possible thermoregulatory control in the baby throughout the transition period. (Oh & Lind, 1967; Morley, 2002, 2003)

This chapter will explore the physiology of temperature regulation in the newborn. Keep in mind that most research in this area has been done without consideration of the impact of immediate or early cord clamping versus physiologic closure of the cord vessels on the baby's ability to tolerate temperature fluctuations. Hypovolemic humans of any age are far less tolerant of temperature fluctuations and therefore more prone to develop hypothermia than those with an optimal blood volume. (Supporting the baby in maintaining a normal body temperature at the time of birth is covered in the chapter entitled "The Healthy Full-Term Newborn in the First Hours of Life.")

Basic Body Temperature Dynamics and Differences in the Fetus, Newborn and Adult

Heat production

Heat is produced by thermogenesis, the same metabolic process that provides energy.

Dissipation of heat

Blood flow from the body's core to the subcutaneous tissues serves as a heat dispersal mechanism, transferring the heat produced by metabolic activity from the body's core to its surface. Heat dissipation continues from the body surface to the environment. The difference in temperature between the warmer body core and the cooler body surface is known as the "**internal temperature gradient**" (ITG).

All babies have a thinner layer of subcutaneous fat than do adults. Less insulation means that heat is more easily transferred from the core of the body to the skin. Preterm infants, with even less body fat and less distance for the heat to travel from the core to the body surface, are at most risk for heat loss. In the smallest preterm infants, core temperature and surface temperature tend to approximate each other.

Posture also influences heat loss. Term babies typically hold their limbs against their body in a flexed position, which reduces the amount of body surface exposed to the environment. Preemies are again at a thermal disadvantage, tending to hold their limbs flaccidly away from their body because their muscles are not strong enough to maintain flexion.

The difference in temperature between body surface and the environment is known as the **external thermal gradient** (ETG). Various factors combine to determine the extent of this gradient: air temperature and movement (breezes and drafts), the temperature of surrounding surfaces, and the relative humidity of the ambient air. There are four ways heat loss can occur:

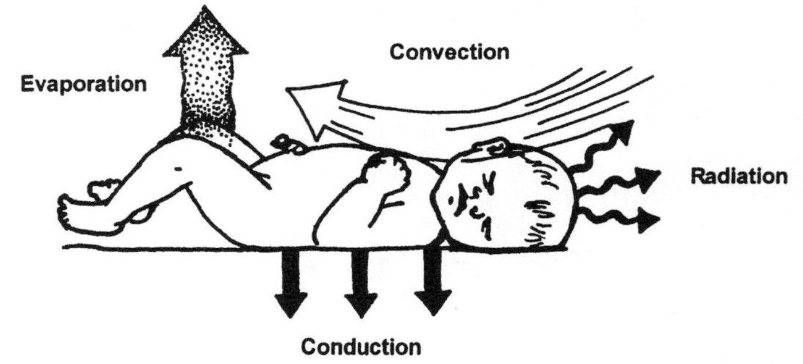

Four ways the newborn can lose heat to the environment.

Evaporation: Evaporative heat loss occurs during conversion of a liquid to a vapor; body heat and low humidity both encourage evaporation. Other types of evaporative heat loss include visible sweat and moisture lost from both the respiratory tract and exhaled gases. Evaporation of amniotic fluid from the baby's body is the primary cause of evaporative heat loss in newborns.

Conduction: Heat is also lost by conduction when the skin comes in direct contact with a cooler solid surface.

Radiation: Radiant heat loss occurs when heat is transferred from the baby to cooler surfaces that are near but not in direct contact with the baby's body (such as being near a cold wall).

Convection: This causes heat loss when the naked baby is exposed to cooler surrounding air. Air movement increases the rate of heat loss. If there is a draft, babies may get cold even at a room temperature of 86°F (30°C), especially those suffering from hypovolemia due to early cord clamping.

All these means of heat loss can also contribute to heat gain when the environment is too warm. For example, if the baby is near but not touching a hot object such as a radiator or lamp, radiation can contribute to heat gain (Korones, 1986; WHO, 1997)

Thermal equilibrium

Normal body temperature is maintained when there is a balance between the generation and dissipation of heat. Thermal equilibrium is present when the rate of heat generation equals the rate of heat loss. Passive temperature control is thus a by-product of metabolic heat production (via normal bodily activities such as protein breakdown and heart and lung activity) and heat transfer to the environment. If more heat is produced than is lost, heat storage ensues and body temperature rises. If more heat is lost than is generated, body temperature drops. Thus the normal, warm-blooded organism must continually lose and store heat to a variable extent, depending upon the rate of heat production within the body and the thermal influences of the environment.

Adult temperature regulation is also a product of dilation or constriction of surface blood vessels, involuntary muscular activity (such as shivering), voluntary muscular activity (such as movement), water loss (such as sweating), and behavior (such as seeking a more comfortable environment). Newborns have an additional means of temperature control called "**nonshivering thermogenesis**."

Humans are homeothermal, meaning we can maintain our body temperature at a very constant level due to a variety of regulating processes. The hypothalamus, especially its preoptic region, is the main integrating center for thermoregulation. Together, the heat-loss center in the anterior region and the heat-promoting central region of the hypothalamus comprise the thermoregulating centers of the body. The hypothalamus receives afferent input from both central and peripheral thermoreceptors. Peripheral receptors are located throughout the body's shell (skin layer), while the central thermoreceptors (receptors sensitive to the temperature of blood) are located in the vital organs (body core) and in the anterior hypothalamus itself. Much like a thermostat, the hypothalamus responds to this input by reflexively initiating appropriate heat-promoting or heat-dissipating activities via the autonomic nervous system. Although the central thermoreceptors are more critically located than the peripheral ones, varying signals from the cold and heat receptors in the skin alert the hypothalamus to the need to prevent temperature changes in the core based upon the average skin temperature, the rate and direction of temperature change and the size of the stimulated area.

The thermal environment is a composite of air (or water) temperature, ambient humidity, movement of air and the temperature of objects close to but not in direct contact with the body. A neutral thermal environment refers to the relatively narrow range of ambient environmental temperature at which the metabolic rate, and therefore oxygen consumption, is at a minimum. In this neutral range, temperature regulation is achieved and normal body temperature maintained only by control of sensible (dry, nonevaporative) heat loss, without regulatory changes in metabolic heat production or evaporative heat loss. If the temperature rises (requiring the body to dissipate heat) or falls (requiring the body to generate heat) outside of this range, oxygen consumption increases. The normal term newborn at rest consumes oxygen at a rate of 5 ml/kg/min. His metabolic rate, and therefore thermogenesis, does not increase if oxygen consumption does not increase as well.

Normal core body temperature ranges from 96.8 to 99.6°F (36 to 37.5°C) with well documented diurnal and menstrual variations of up to 1.8°F (1°C). In adults, a larger surface area provides more exposure to the environment, thus promoting heat loss. In babies, body surface is disproportionately large for body weight, and insulation in the form of fat is proportionately less relative to an adult. At birth, the term infant has only 5% of his adult body weight and only 15% of his adult body surface. The newborn thus has three times more body surface per kilogram of body weight than an adult. This discrepancy is even greater in preterm and low-birthweight babies. Because of the relatively small amount of tissue insulation in infants, the difference between core and mean skin temperature is considerably smaller than in an adult.

In adults, the thermoneutral range of the ambient air environment is 78.8 to 82.4°F (26 to 28°C). During water submersion it rises to 95 to 98.6°F (35 to 36°C) because the heat transfer coefficient is increased 200 times in water. Adults with a thick fat layer can have a thermoneutral zone during submersion as low as 87.8°F (31°C).

Unfortunately, there is very little data comparing babies who have received an optimal cord transfusion with those who have not. The thermoneutral range for infants whose cords are immediately clamped, the range in air is 89.6 to 95°F

(32 to 35°C) for the full-term naked newborn and may be as high as 95°F (35°C) for preterm infants. The exact range that can be tolerated will vary based on the size, weight and blood volume of each baby. Term and premature babies who have received their full placental transfusion via an intact cord are optimally prepared to cope with temperature variations within the physiologic limitations of their gestational age. Conversely, hypovolemic babies are less well equipped to cope with even minor variations, depending upon how hypovolemic they may be.

The increased body surface area to mass quotient in infants also results in the thermoreceptors in the skin and core being closer together than in an adult. This allows the baby to detect and adjust to changes in environmental temperature more rapidly, enabling babies to maintain their core temperature as accurately as an adult can. Even so, the narrower and higher thermoneutral range of the newborn is an ongoing challenge to the maintenance of normal body temperature. While a baby can become too warm, newborns are more vulnerable to hypothermia. Babies tend to lose heat more rapidly at a room temperature that is normal for adults, with this tendency more pronounced the more hypovolemic the baby is at birth. Such heat loss combined with a low blood volume may be life threatening, especially in small babies who are ill (Korones, 1986; WHO, 1997).

Body temperature in the fetus

Maternal temperature is the primary determinant of fetal temperature; both are tightly linked, a relationship that prevents the fetus from independently regulating her body temperature before birth. Fetal temperature normally ranges from 99.7 to 100.0°F (37.6 to 37.8°C). At term, the core temperature of the fetus, measured rectally, is 0.9°F (0.5°C) higher than maternal core temperature. The maternal-fetal temperature difference widens as gestation progresses and during uterine contractions (Korones, 1986). Fetal metabolic processes independently generate sufficient heat to maintain the body temperature at a higher level than that of the mother. Heat produced within the fetus accumulates until it reaches a level that causes it to be transferred into the mother's system. While some heat is lost through skin contact with the amniotic fluid and the uterine wall, most thermal regulation occurs when fetal blood circulates through the umbilical cord and intervillous space in the placenta, transferring heat to the mother's system for dissipation. Blood is an effective vehicle for heat transfer from the body core to its surface; its rapid flow through the placental villi delivers a significant quantity of heat, the total surface area of the villi being greater than the fetus' body surface. The placenta is normally capable of dissipating virtually all the heat produced by the fetus. Impaired placental perfusion will cause the fetus to lose heat more slowly.

If the mother's temperature is elevated due to increased activity or heat exposure, the difference between the maternal and fetal temperatures is reduced by a few tenths of a degree Celsius, thus offering the fetus a small margin of protection from overheating. Charles (1998) states that a modest rise in maternal temperature of up to 1.8° F (1°C) may benefit the baby by increasing oxygen transfer across the placenta. However, when the mother the mother's temperature rises higher than this, the flow of heat from the fetus to the mother is reversed, and the maternal-fetal temperature difference nearly doubles (Power, 1998) (however, we don't know how hot it too hot or how long overheating must go on to trigger this response). The fetus's metabolic activity increases because his core temperature rises, thus increasing oxygen consumption, leading to hypoxia. When maternal temperature falls, there is a lag time of unknown length before the baby's temperature returns to normal. The poor condition of babies born to severely febrile mothers is likely due to an increased demand for oxygen and overheating in the fetus beyond that which he can tolerate. If the baby is hypovolemic, he is poorly equipped to equilibrate his body temperature, especially if he is also septic.

Body temperature in the newborn

As a general rule, babies cool down and heat up much faster than do adults and are able to tolerate a more limited range of environmental temperatures. Although overheating can be dangerous, the tendency to lose heat rapidly is of primary concern in providing an environment that allows the baby to maintain a normal body temperature. Loss of heat per unit of body weight is four times greater in term newborns and five times greater in 3 lb 5 oz (1500 gram) premature infants whose cords are clamped too soon than in a normovolemic adult.

The smaller and earlier the baby, the less tolerance she has for temperature extremes. The thin skin of a preterm baby loses moisture rapidly; the distance from body core to surface is shorter; and there is little insulating fat. Thermal stability improves as the fetus gains weight and becomes more mature. This is in part because the term newborn has 70% of his blood volume in his body at birth, thus he is better able to withstand the blood loss represented by immediate cord clamping than the preterm infant who retains only 50% of her blood in her body. While a baby's capacity to regulate body temperature will always be limited compared to an adult's, babies whose cords are allowed to close physiologically are optimally prepared to deal with temperature fluctuations. Any baby having trouble establishing respirations or one whose cord is pulsing sluggishly or not at all at birth will be even more vulnerable to compromise. The use of anesthetic drugs during labor also reduces the baby's capacity to regulate his body temperature (Brück, 1998; Korones, 1986; WHO, 1997).

Responses to excessive heat: The newborn exposed to excessive heat cools herself off by dilating peripheral blood vessels in the skin. Dilation causes more blood to flow to the body surface carrying heat away from the body core. The baby appears flushed, especially in the limbs, may assume an extended posture and becomes irritable. The scalp, hands and feet are focal points of such heat loss with skin temperature exceeding core temperature and the feet no more than 2 to 3°C cooler than the abdomen.

Heat is also dissipated by evaporation of visible sweat and insensible water, which includes moisture lost through the skin and exhaled gases. Visible sweat, which appears on the forehead and temples, is first noted in preterm babies at 30 to 32 weeks gestation. Soon thereafter, visible sweating begins on their chest, and by 34 to 36 weeks sweating also occurs on the lower extremities. While neonates have dense sweat glands in some areas, sweating is a less responsive and less efficient means of heat loss than is vasodilation. This is even more true for preterm babies and those with central nervous system dysfunction (Power, 1998).

The same factors that account for rapid heat loss in newborns also tend to increase the rate of heat gain in excessively warm environments. Warmth receptors in the skin contribute to the stimulation of heat dissipation activities only when mean skin temperature is considerably increased over normal. Premature infants therefore develop hyperthermia very rapidly; this can lead to brain damage or death if the baby has no opportunity to cool himself off (Brück, 1998; Korones, 1986; WHO, 1997).

Physiology of hyperthermia: Once core temperature rises, hyperthermia exists. Even slight hyperthermia increases metabolic demands, with oxygen consumption rising dramatically, especially in preterm infants. Heart, respiratory and metabolic rates rise; insensible water loss leads to dehydration; and peripheral vasodilation eventually causes the blood pressure to drop, introducing the risk of metabolic acidosis and tissue hypoxia. Hyperthermia exacerbates brain injury following asphyxia.

Responses to a drop in temperature at birth: The normal term newborn experiences a drop in core temperature immediately after birth; temperature may fall to below 96.8°F (36°C) within the first three hours of life if care is not optimal. Even so, by eight hours the temperature usually has returned to the adult range, where it remains. The inevitable exposure of the wet newborn to the chill produced by an air environment after birth may be a primary trigger for breathing (Morley, 2002a).

Response to cold stress: When the healthy baby is exposed to cold, metabolism increases in an attempt to generate warmth. In this process, glucose consumption rises; glycogen stores are utilized and eventually depleted. Breakdown of brown fat commences. The respiratory rate rises as oxygen consumption increases. Eventually the amount of oxygen required exceeds the amount available and hypoxia ensues, leading to anaerobic metabolism and a fall in pH. Metabolic acidosis results in pulmonary vasoconstriction, hypoxia deepens and respiratory distress develops as the infant runs out of resources to cope with chilling.

Responses to excessive cold: The normal infant becomes restless and hyperactive when first exposed to cold, but this activity is not a significant source of heat. Heat conservation is one important means of maintaining core temperature. Body fat serves as an insulating barrier to core heat loss when an infant is exposed to cold. Restriction of blood flow to the skin surface increases the effectiveness of this insulating layer. This response is most pronounced in the hands and feet. This capacity to restrict blood flow is present at birth, but it is not as effective in the first 24 hours of life as it is afterward and is even less so when the baby is hypovolemic. She can achieve maximum thermogenesis to maintain her normal core temperature at an ambient temperature of 73.4°F (23°C) but can only sustain this effort for periods of 30 to 60 minutes. Age and blood volume affect the response to a low environmental temperature. Infants are more resistant to cold-induced cardiac arrhythmias and can survive much more severe chilling than an adult but not without a corresponding stress on the baby's thermoregulating capacity (Lean & James, 1986).

Physiology of hypothermia: Hypothermic responses begin when the body's core temperature starts to fall. Metabolism is tightly associated with body temperature in mammals. There is a 6 to 8% drop in metabolic activity for every 1.8° F (1° C) reduction in body temperature. Heart rate drops linearly with temperature as well. Mild hypothermia has been shown to increase or decrease cardiac output, depending upon the study. Low temperature increases vascular resistance in the lungs; thus the development of pulmonary hypertension is a feared consequence of prolonged hypothermia. Hypothermia also causes oxygen to become more tightly bound to hemoglobin, leading to tissue hypoxia even in the presence of sufficient oxygen saturation. Tissue hypoxia causes a reduction of oxygen supply to the tissues involved in heat production (skeletal tissues, muscles and brown fat) and significantly alters thermoregulation. A cold baby will thus have less oxygen available for tissue use. This understanding is the source of the strong admonitions to keep babies warm during revival efforts. A reduction in the partial pressure of carbon dioxide by 4.5% per degree Celsius of temperature makes it even more difficult for the hemoglobin to release oxygen to tissues; low PCO_2 is therefore particularly undesirable. Conversion of glycogen to glucose proceeds under hypoxic conditions, and the alternate chemical pathway (anaerobic glycolysis) that must be utilized dissipates glycogen at about 20 times the normal rate. Anaerobic glycolysis generates extra lactic acid, and metabolic acidosis develops. Hypoglycemia develops more quickly in babies with intrauterine malnutrition because glycogen stores are already low.

Technically, hypothermia exists when the newborn's core temperature drops below 96.8°F (36°C). Hypothermia inhibits ADH (antidiuretic hormone) production, increasing diuresis as well as interfering with reabsorption of sodium. Hypothermia also affects various enzymes; some of their effects are beneficial and others deleterious. For example, the enzymatic reaction of blood coagulation is dependent on temperature. Coagulation is prolonged at temperatures below 91.4°F (33°C). Hypothermia increases blood viscosity, with a 2 to 4% increase per 1.8°F (1°C) of cooling. This may impair perfusion, and possibly oxygenation, if the hematocrit is high. There is conflicting evidence regarding whether mild hypothermia increases susceptibility to infection or not. It reduces the number of circulating white blood cells, especially neutrophils; this effect reverses on rewarming. An increased risk of clinical pancreatitis that reverses with rewarming has also been seen in hypothermic adults. The least adverse changes seem to occur with mild hypothermia.

***Nonshivering thermogenesis**:* The baby's primary means of maintaining body temperature occurs via a metabolic process called **nonshivering thermogenesis**, which involves burning a unique type of fat. The onset of nonshivering thermogenesis is stimulated by the response of thermal nerve endings in the skin, not by a fall in core temperature. Nonshivering thermogenesis is more biologically economical than shivering, which increases convective heat loss and interferes with movement. Although the ability to shiver is well developed at birth, it is normally suppressed by nonshivering thermogenesis; the newborn shivering threshold appears to be displaced to a lower body temperature in comparison with the adult. In addition, babies may not be able to shiver long enough or intensely enough to produce substantial amounts of heat.

Nonshivering thermogenesis requires that the newborn have adequate levels of ATP, glucose, red blood cells and oxygen so that he can metabolize brown fat, which rapidly produces additional heat. This process is stimulated when the infant's skin temperature drops to between 95 and 96.8°F (35 to 36°C) (or when the temperature difference between the environment and the baby's skin exceeds 21.6° F [12° C]) (Gunn et al., 1991). This prompts the release of noradrenaline from sympathetic nerve endings that stimulate liposis (the breakdown of body fat). Catecholamines from the adrenal medulla and thyroxine (T_4) enhance this process. The term infant can increase the thermogenic rate two and one-half times over her resting rate, reaching a level almost equal to that of an adult. Heat production corresponds to the degree of cold to which the infant is exposed.

***The characteristics of brown fat*:** About 90% of a newborn's heat is generated by burning brown fat, a tissue unique to newborns. In the 1960s it was discovered that metabolic activity in brown fat is considerably greater than that in white fat. Primitive brown fat first appears at 26 to 30 weeks gestation. At term, brown fat is widely distributed, accounting for 2 to 7% of total newborn body weight. The areas of brown fat continue to enlarge as late as the third to fifth week after birth; most major deposits disappear some weeks later, unless cold stress depletes them sooner.

Sources vary as to the amount and distribution of brown fat. Most agree that the largest deposits are located along the posterior sides of the neck below the ears and in the axillary regions; together, these areas represent about 50% of the total brown fat mass. Large deposits also extend along the iliac crests and are gathered in the posterior abdominal cavity around the kidneys and adrenal glands, extending down toward the posterior abdominal cavity and pelvis. There are also relatively distinct masses in the body's core running along the thoracic and abdominal aorta, between the trachea and esophagus, and adjacent to the pancreas. Thin fingers of brown fat follow the intercostal arteries, beginning at the sternum and extending between each rib. A thin, jagged, kite-shaped sheet of brown fat lies within the shallow connective tissue of the posterior neck and upper thoracic spine, extending transversely between the scapulae. This region of distribution is unusual in not being located deep within the body or in association with major blood vessels. It is a relatively small mass that disappears a few weeks after birth.

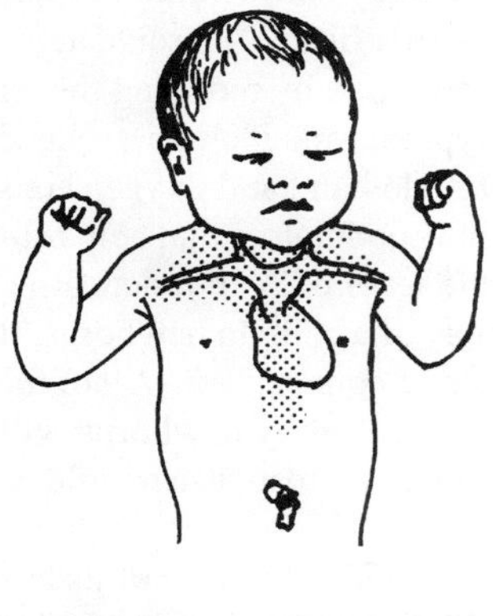

Brown fat distribution: anterior

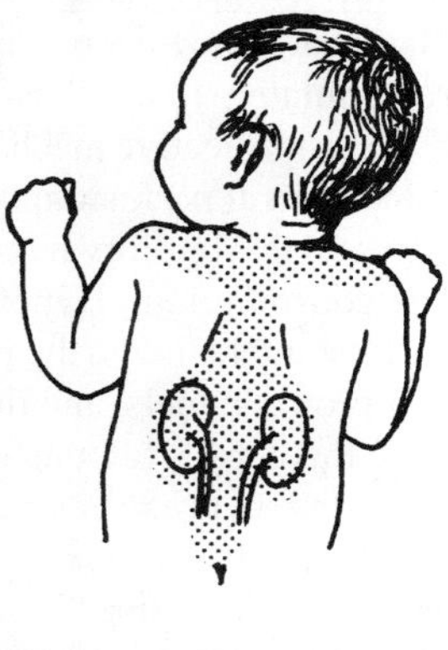

Brown fat distribution: posterior

More small deposits of brown fat are also located in the anterior mediastinum below and to either side of the xiphoid process, along the anterior abdomen from below the ribs to above the umbilicus, and in a small urachal patch that lies between the umbilicus and the bladder. Interior epigastric patches are found to either side of the lower abdomen, and small patches lie to either side of the symphysis pubis. Small deposits are also found posteriorly behind the shoulders, over the deltoid muscles and along the trapezial muscles on either side.

The cells of brown fat differ considerably from those of white adipose tissue. They contain a central nucleus, with numerous mitochondria and small lipid inclusions dispersed throughout the cytoplasm. (White fat cells have a peripheral nucleus and a single fat globule.) The buff to brownish-red color of brown fat is imparted by a copious blood supply, dense cellular content and a profusion of sympathetic nerve endings that terminate at the cell membrane. When cold stress stimulates these nerves, they release norepinephrine. This stimulates brown fat metabolism and activates lipase, which breaks down intracellular fat to form triglycerides. Triglycerides are broken down to form glycerol and nonesterified fatty acids. These substances become combusted within the mitochondria of brown fat cells as a result of the presence of the uncoupling protein thermogenin (UCP),[1] and heat is produced. This heat is transferred via the blood circulating through the brown fat to the skin surface (Bennett & Brown, 1999; Lean & James, 1986; Merklin, 1974; Power, 1998).

Factors that alter the infant's cold stress response: The newborn's ability to respond to cold stress is altered in the presence of hypovolemia, symptomatic hypoglycemia, hypoxia, intracranial hemorrhage, severe cerebral malformation, and other conditions producing severely disrupted central nervous system responses. Weight and the percentage of body fat are also factors. Babies who are sleeping deeply are also less capable of responding to cold stress. Even healthy term infants who experience prolonged exposure to cold eventually deplete their brown fat stores and are left with no reserves.

Differing opinions regarding cold stress: Research has shown that the threshold ambient temperature at which normal body temperature is maintained for certain animal species can be influenced by long- or short-term exposure to environmental temperatures outside the thermoneutral range, although how this may apply to human newborns is not fully understood. According to Russian homebirth practitioners, brief exposure of the newly born infant to extreme cold stimulates the immune system. It is thus the standard practice of many Russian midwives to immerse the baby in cold water briefly before handing her to the mother for skin-to-skin contact and warming after birth. This is done whether the

---

[1]Scientific effort has led to the identification of UCP as the key enzyme regulating nonshivering heat production. Because this research has been done by several groups, the UCP has been variously referred to in the literature as the "nucleotide-binding protein" (NbP), the "32-kDa protein of brown fat," the "guanosine 5' diphosphate (GDP)–binding protein" and the "proton conductance pathway of brown adipose tissue mitochondria."

baby is vigorous or depressed. Morley (2002a) also recommends the brief application of a cold, wet cloth to the baby's skin as a means of stimulating a gasp to initiate respirations. Chinese practitioners, in contrast, abhor the use of cold therapies for the mother or the baby because they feel it weakens the system in the long run.

The protective effects of mild hypothermia following asphyxia: The body temperature of asphyxiated infants tends to be 3.6°F (2°C) cooler than that of healthy babies for the first 20 hours after birth. Neuronal activity decreases in these babies as inhibitory neuromodulators rise. These changes induce hypothermia by reducing the temperature sensitivity of hypothalamic neurons. Neuroprotective mechanisms triggered by hypothermia include a reduced cerebral metabolic rate associated with a fall in cerebral perfusion, cytotoxic edema, energy demand and oxygen consumption. Metabolic depression results in an increase of inhibitory neurotransmitters and neuromodulators that help bring about this decrease in brain activity and energy consumption. Hypothermia also lowers the level of ATP (adenosine 5′-triphosphate), the immediate precursor of adenine nucleotides, the primary energy currency of a cell. In newborns, the neurons are small, the membranes contain fewer ion channels, and there are far fewer synaptic connections. All of these factors reduce the energy demand and increase the baby's tolerance for anoxia. Thus, while healthy newborns will try to increase their metabolism to counteract cooling, hypoxic newborns do not mount a metabolic response to cold because cold enhances their ability to survive neurologically intact.

It has long been known that the human brain generates a great deal of heat because of its large size. In adults, the brain is warmer than the rest of the core body temperature by 0.9 F (0.5 C). The body has elaborate ways of dissipating cerebral heat. As much as 85% of body heat is removed through the scalp. Although it had long been thought that brain damage always occurs concurrent with oxygen deprivation, since 1994 research has indicated that brain cooling can reduce or eliminate brain damage from asphyxia. It now seems there is a lag time, anywhere from a few hours to 100 hours, before such an insult leads to permanent brain damage in term infants and that babies born early may still be experiencing progressive brain damage at six weeks of age.

Perinatal hypoxic-ischemic brain injury is now understood to occur in two phases. The first phase takes place during the peripartum period when the fetal brain is exposed to asphyxiation because of inadequate blood flow that reduces oxygen delivery to the brain. The second phase occurs in the hours following birth and is due to secondary energy failure.

Hypothermia is now used therapeutically to try to preserve asphyxiated babies intact. Infants born at 36 weeks or more with evidence of an acute moderate to severe perinatal hypoxic-ischemic event are considered candidates for treatment. Cooling must be initiated within 6 hours of birth and preferably as soon as possible. Induced hypothermia aims to minimize the damage or prevent infants from experiencing the second phase of brain injury. Protocols vary. Various types of equipment are used to carefully control and maintain the temperature of the whole body and selective head cooling. The body is cooled to approximately 92.3 to 94.1 F (33.5 to 34.5 C) for 72 hours and then gradually warmed. Hypothermia is not entirely protective, however. The development of brain damage is also believed to be influenced by various inflammatory processes that hypothermia tends to aggravate. For prolonged therapeutic hypothermia to be used safely, the baby must be carefully monitored and equipment calibration must be precise. Babies are monitored for complications of asphyxia (such as seizures) with amplitude-integrated electroencephalogram (aEEG), serial neurological examinations, and laboratory and imaging studies before, during and after the procedure to ensure that the body is able to maintain normal functioning in the cooled state. Hypothermia is no magic cure and some impairment of compromised infants may persist. This therapy has not been in use long enough for long-term outcomes to be fully known.

From an evolutionary standpoint, it has been postulated that perhaps the baby's head was always meant to remain cool, but the body kept warm, to prevent systemic hypothermia. During most of human evolution, the baby, drenched in amniotic fluid, would have been born in the open air to a naked mother who gave birth in an upright position, speeding the transfusion of body-temperature placental blood. Once the mother picked up her infant, his body would be held against her own and kept warm while his head would have likely been exposed to the air for many millennia before (and likely after) clothing was developed. With his full placental transfusion on board and thus optimally perfused, the baby would have been well prepared to deal with the temperature disparity between his body, his head and the ambient air, thus reaping the apparent benefits of keeping a cool head.

Note that none of this research has been done with babies who have been allowed to receive their full placental transfusion. See the subchapter entitled "Understanding Fetal and Neonatal Asphyxia," for a look at how hypovolemia and poor perfusion contributes to brain damage.

REFERENCES AND FURTHER READING ON ADDITIONAL ANATOMICAL AND PHYSIOLOGICAL CONSIDERATIONS RELEVANT TO LABOR AND BIRTH

HOW AND WHY LABOR BEGINS

Cunningham, F et al., ed. "Chapter 11: Parturition," WILLIAMS OBSTETRICS, 21st ed. McGraw-Hill, New York NY, 2001.

ANATOMY AND PHYSIOLOGY OF UTERINE CHANGES DURING LATE PREGNANCY AND LABOR

Creasy R, ed. MANAGEMENT OF LABOR AND DELIVERY. Blackwell Science, Boston MA, 1997.

Cunningham FG, et al. WILLIAMS OBSTETRICS, 21st ed. McGraw-Hill, New York NY, 2001.

MacDonald PC, Casey ML. "The accumulation of prostaglandins (PG) in amniotic fluid is an aftereffect of labor and not indicative of a role for PGE_2 and PGE_{2a} in the initiation of human parturition," J CLIN ENDOCRINOL METAB, 76(5);1331-1339, May, 1993.

Oxorn H. OXORN-FOOTE HUMAN LABOR AND BIRTH, 5th ed. Appleton-Century-Crofts, Norwalk CT, 1986.

Smith R, ed. THE ENDOCRINOLOGY OF PARTURITION: BASIC SCIENCE AND CLINICAL APPLICATION, Vol. 27 of FRONTIERS HORMONE RES, Karger, Basel Switzerland, 2001.

Stables D. PHYSIOLOGY IN CHILDBEARING: WITH ANATOMY AND RELATED BIOSCIENCES. BaillièreTindall, New York NY, 1999.

NERVES OF THE FEMALE REPRODUCTIVE SYSTEM AND PELVIS AND THE PAIN OF LABOR

Anderson M, ed. THE ANATOMY AND PHYSIOLOGY OF OBSTETRICS, 6th ed. Faber & Faber, London UK, 1979.

Bennet VR, Brown LK, eds. MYLES TEXTBOOK FOR MIDWIVES. Churchill Livingstone, Edinburgh UK, 1999.

Bonica J. "Labour Pain," in Wall P, Melzack R, eds. TEXTBOOK OF PAIN, 3rd ed. Churchill-Livingstone, Edinburgh UK, 1994.

Brubaker L. Saclarides T, eds. THE FEMALE PELVIC FLOOR: DISORDERS OF FUNCTION AND SUPPORT. FA Davis Co, Philadelphia PA, 1996.

Goss C. ANATOMY OF THE HUMAN BODY BY HENRY GRAY, 29th American ed. Lea & Febiger, Philadelphia PA, 1973.

Haire D, "Improving the outcome of pregnancy through science," http://www.AIMSUSA.org, accessed Jan 7, 2004a.

Haire D, "Obstetric drugs: their effects on mother and infant," www.AIMSUSA.org, 2001, accessed Jan 7, 2004b.

Hattori R, et al. "Autistic and developmental disorders after general anaesthetic delivery" letter to the editor, LANCET, 337;1357-1358, June 1 ,1997.

Jacobson B, et al. "Perinatal origin of adult self-destructive behavior," ACTA PSYCHIATR SCAND, 76(4);364-371, Oct, 1987.

Jacobson B, et al. "Opiate addiction in adult offspring through possible imprinting after obstetric treatment," BMJ 301(6760);1067-1070, Nov 10, 1990.

Lieberman A. EASING LABOR PAIN, rev ed. Harvard Common Press, Boston MA, 1992.

Moore S, ed. UNDERSTANDING PAIN AND ITS RELIEF IN LABOUR. Churchill Livingstone, New York NY, 1997.

Netter F. CIBA COLLECTION OF MEDICAL ILLUSTRATIONS, VOL. 1, NERVOUS SYSTEM. CIBA Pharm. Products, Summit NJ, 1953.

Netter F. CIBA COLLECTION OF MEDICAL ILLUSTRATIONS, VOL. 2, REPRODUCTIVE SYSTEM. CIBA Pharm. Products, Summit NJ, 1954.

O'Connell H, et al. "Anatomical relationship between urethra and clitoris," J UROLOGY, 159(6);1892-1897, June, 1998.

Odent M. THE SCIENTIFICATION OF LOVE. Free Association Books, London UK, 1999.

Sagady M. "Renewing our faith in second stage," MIDWIFERY TODAY, (33);28-31, Spring, 1995.

Stables D. PHYSIOLOGY IN CHILDBEARING: WITH ANATOMY AND RELATED BIOSCIENCES. Baillière Tindall, New York NY, 1999.

Sutton J. "Optimal Fetal Positioning" handout from workshop, Seattle WA, May 8, 2000.

Sutton J. LET BIRTH BE BORN AGAIN! REDISCOVERING AND RECLAIMING OUR MIDWIFERY HERITAGE. Birth Concepts UK, Bedfont UK, 2001.

ECSTATIC BIRTH: THE MATERNAL RESPONSE TO THE PAIN AND STRESS OF LABOR

Buckley S. "Ecstatic birth: the hormonal blueprint of labor," MOTHERING, (111);51-59, Mar-Apr, 2002.

Buckley S. "Drugs in labor: an overview," MIDWIFERY TODAY, (71);13-20, Autumn 2004.

Lieberman A. EASING LABOR PAIN, rev. ed. Harvard Common Press, Boston MA, 1992.

Newton N, et al. "Experimental inhibition of labor through environmental disturbance," OBSTET GYNECOL, 27(3);371-377, Mar, 1966.

Odent M. THE NATURE OF BIRTH AND BREASTFEEDING. Bergin & Garvey, Westport CT, 1992.

Odent M. THE SCIENTIFICATION OF LOVE. Free Association Books, London UK, 1999.

Odent M. "The first hour following birth: don't wake the mother!" MIDWIFERY TODAY, (61);9-12, Spring, 2002.

Odent M. "Fear of death during labour." MIDWIFERY TODAY, (67);20-22, Fall, 2003.

Robertson A. "The pain of labor," MIDWIFERY TODAY, (37);19-21, 40-42, Spring, 1996.

Simkin P. "Stress, pain and catecholamines in labor: part 1. A review," BIRTH, 13(4);227-233, Dec, 1986.

Stables D. PHYSIOLOGY IN CHILDBEARING: WITH ANATOMY AND RELATED BIOSCIENCES. Baillière Tindall, New York NY, 1999.

Taylor S, et al. "Biobehavioral responses to stress in females: tend-and-befriend, not fight-or-flight," PSYCHOL REV, 107(3);411-429, July, 2000.

THE BABY'S JOURNEY THROUGH LABOR TO BIRTH

Allan L, et al., eds. Chapter 3: "Fetal cardiovascular physiology," in TEXTBOOK OF FETAL CARDIOLOGY. Greenwich Medical Media, London UK, 2000.

Blackburn S, Loper D. MATERNAL, FETAL, AND NEONATAL PHYSIOLOGY: A CLINICAL PERSPECTIVE. WB Saunders, Philadelphia PA, 1992.

Bloom R. Chapter 25: "Delivery room resuscitation of the newborn," in Fanaroff A, Martin R. NEONATAL-PERINATAL MEDICINE: DISEASES OF THE FETUS AND INFANT, 7th ed., VOL. 1. Mosby, St. Louis MO, 2002.

Bonnin P, et al. "Quantitative assessment of circulatory changes in the fetal aortic isthmus during progressive increase of resistance to umbilical blood flow," CIRC, 88(1);216-222, July, 1993.

Brück K. Chapter 68: "Neonatal thermal regulation," in Polin R, Fox W, eds. FETAL AND NEONATAL PHYSIOLOGY, 2nd ed., VOL. 1. WB Saunders Co, Philadelphia PA, 1998.

Burch G. A PRIMER OF VENOUS PRESSURE. Charles C Thomas, Springfield IL, 1972.

Chamberlain R, et al. Chapter 4: "The first breath," pp. 89-117, in BRITISH BIRTHS 1970, VOL. 1: THE FIRST WEEK OF LIFE. Heinemann Medical, London UK, 1975.

Cowan F et al. "Origin and timing of brain lesions in term infants with neonatal encephalopathy," LANCET, 361;736-742, Mar 1, 2003.

Csontos F, et al. "Elevated plasma beta-endorphin levels in pregnant women and their neonates," LIFE SCI, 25(10);835-844, Sept 3, 1979.

Deivoria-Papadopoulos M, McGovan J. "Oxygen Transport and Delivery," in Polin R, Fox W, eds. FETAL AND NEONATAL PHYSIOLOGY, 2nd ed., VOL. 1. WB Saunders, Philadelphia PA, 1998.

Dunn P. "The placental venous pressure during and after the third stage of labour following early cord ligation," J OBSTET GYNECOL BR COMMONW, 73(5);747-756, Oct, 1966.

Dunn P. "Alterations in the distribution of blood between the fetus (and infant) and placenta during and after birth." Presentation Canadian Pediatric Society, Centennial Commonwealth Meeting, Toronto Canada, Sept 3-9, 1967.

Dunn P. Chapter 21: "Reservations about the methods of assessing at birth the predictive value of intrapartum fetal monitoring including premature interruption of the feto-placental circulation," pp. 130-137, in Rolfe P, ed. FETAL PHYSIOLOGICAL MEASUREMENTS, report of the 2nd International Conference On Fetal and Neonatal Physiological Measurements, Apr 2-4, 1984, Oxford, UK. Butterworths, London UK, 1986.

Dunn P. "Cardio-respiratory adaptation of the preterm infant at birth," PAEDIATRICA INDONESIANA, 28(5-6):133-140, May-June, 1988.

Dunn P. "Controversies in neonatal resuscitation," EMIRATES MED J, 1(S);5-8, 1993.

Fouron, JC, et al. "Flow velocity profile of the fetal aortic isthmus through normal gestation," AM J CARDIO, 74(5);483-486, Sept 1, 1994.

Ghanayem NS, Gordon JB. "Modulation of pulmonary vasomotor tone in the fetus and neonate," RESP RES, 2(3);139-144, 2001.

Gluckman P. "Vasopressin and oxytocin," pp. 515-519 in Gluckman P, Heymann M, eds. PEDIATRICS AND PERINATOLOGY, 2nd ed. Arnold, London UK, 1996.

Goss C, ed. GRAY'S ANATOMY OF THE HUMAN BODY BY HENRY GRAY, 29th American ed. Lea & Febiger, Philadelphia PA, 1973.

Gray L, et al. "Breastfeeding is analgesic in healthy newborns," PEDIATR, 109(4);590-593, Apr, 2002.

Hendricks G, Hendricks K. RADIANCE! BREATHWORK, MOVEMENT & BODY-CENTERED PSYCHOTHERAPY. Wingbow Press, Berkeley CA, 1991.

Jäykkä S. "Capillary erection and lung expansion," ACTA PAEDIATR, 45(S112);1-91, Jan, 1957.

Jäykkä S. "Capillary erection and the structural appearance of fetal and neonatal lungs," ACTA PAEDIATR, 47(5);484-500, Sept, 1958.

Johnson P. "Birth under water–to breathe or not to breathe," BR J OBSTET GYNAECOL, 103(3);202-208, Mar, 1996.

Karlberg P, et al. "Respiratory studies in newborn infants, II Pulmonary ventilation and mechanics of breathing in the first minutes of life, including the onset of respiration," ACTA PEDIATR, 51;121-136, March, 1962.

Kiserud T. "Fetal venous circulation--an update on hemodynamics," J PERINAT MED, 28(2);90-96, 2000.

Kiserud, T, et al."Ultrasonographic velocimetry of the fetal ductus venosus," LANCET, 338(8780);1412-1414, Dec 7, 1991.

Korones S. HIGH-RISK NEWBORN INFANTS: THE BASIS FOR INTENSIVE NURSING CARE, 4th ed. CV Mosby Co, St. Louis MO, 1986.

Lagercrantz H, Slotkin T. "The 'stress' of being born," SCI AM, 254(4);100-107, Apr, 1986.

Lewis W, ed. GRAY'S ANATOMY OF THE HUMAN BODY, 20th American ed. Lea & Febiger, Philadelphia PA, 1918.

Li CH, et al. "Synthesis and analgesic activity of human beta-endorphin," J MED CHEM, 20(3);325-328, Mar, 1977.

Linderkamp O. "Placental transfusion: determinants and effects," CLIN PERINATOL, 9(3);559-592, Oct, 1982.

Mavrides E, et al. "The human ductus venosus between 13 and 17 weeks of gestation: histological and morphometric studies," ULTRASOUND OBSTET GYNECOL, 19(1);39-46, Jan, 2002.

Mercer J, CNM. Multiple e-mail communications, 2002.

Mercer J, Skovgaard R. "Neonatal transitional physiology: a new paradigm," J PERINAT NEONAT NURS, 15(4);56-75, Mar, 2002.

Mielke G, Benda N. "Cardiac output and central distribution of blood flow in the human fetus," CIRC, 103(12);1662-1668, Mar 27, 2001.

Moore K, Persaud T. THE DEVELOPING HUMAN: CLINICALLY ORIENTED EMBRYOLOGY, 5th ed. WB Saunders Co, Philadelphia PA, 1993.

Morgan E. THE DESCENT OF THE CHILD: HUMAN EVOLUTION FROM A NEW PERSPECTIVE. Oxford U Press, New York NY, 1995.

Morley G. "Why do babies cry? the anatomical and physiological changes during the moments after birth," www.cordclamping.com, accessed June 24, 2002a.

Morley G. Ob-Gyn. Unpublished letter to the editor re Pramanik A, et. al. "Respiratory Distress Syndrome: an article presented by emedicine for CME credits," submitted to www.emedicine.com, Nov 7, 2002b.

Morley G. Ob-Gyn. Personal communications and review of portions of the chapter, Dec. 2002c.

Morley G. "Neonatal encephalopathy, hypoxic ischemic encephalopathy and subsequent cerebral palsy: etiology, pathology and prevention." http://www.cordclamping.com. Accessed Nov 23, 2003.

Oh W, et al. "The effects of placental transfusion on respiratory mechanics of normal term newborn infants," PEDIATR, 40(1);6-12, July, 1967.

O'Rahilly R, Müller F. HUMAN EMBRYOLOGY AND TERATOLOGY, 3rd ed. Wiley-Liss, New York NY, 2001.

Padbury J. "The Adrenal Medulla," pp. 530-532, in Gluckman P, Heymann M, eds. PEDIATRICS AND PERINATOLOGY, 2nd ed. Arnold, London UK, 1996.

Power, G. Chapter 67: "Perinatal thermal physiology," in Polin R, Fox W, eds. FETAL AND NEONATAL PHYSIOLOGY, 2nd ed., VOL. 1. WB Saunders Co, Philadelphia PA, 1998.

Rasanen J, et al. "Role of the pulmonary circulation in the distribution of human fetal cardiac output during the second half of pregnancy," CIRCULATION, 94(5):1068-1073. Sept 1, 1996.

Reynolds S. "The umbilical cord," SCI AM, 187(1);70-74, July, 1952.

Reynolds S. "Mechanisms of placentofetal blood flow," OBSTET GYNECOL, 51(2);245-249, Feb, 1978a.

Reynolds S. Chapter 4: "The physical forces of blood flow in the umbilical vein," in Longo L, Reneau D, eds. FETAL AND NEWBORN CARDIOVASCULAR PHYSIOLOGY, VOL. 2: FETAL AND NEWBORN CIRCULATION, Proceedings of Am Phyiolog Soc, Aug. 11-14, 1976, Bryn Mawr, PA. Garland STPM Press, New York NY, 1978b.

Sagady M. "The physiology of fetal transformation at birth," MIDWIFERY TODAY, (34);28-30, Summer, 1995.

Strang LB. "Fetal lung liquid: secretion and reabsorption," PHYSIOL REV, 71(4);991-1016, Oct, 1991.

Strong T. "The umbilical pump: a contributor to twin-twin transfusion," OBSTET GYNECOL, 89(5 Pt 2);812-813, May, 1997.

Teitel D. Chapter 81: "Physiologic development of the cardiovascular system in the fetus," in Polin R, Fox W. FETAL AND NEONATAL PHYSIOLOGY, 2nd ed., VOL 1. WB Saunders Co, Philadelphia PA, 1998.

Thoresen M. "Cooling the newborn after asphxia–physiological and experimental background and its clinical use." SEMIN NEONATOL, 5(1);61-73, Feb, 2000.

Vyas H, et al. "Determinants of the first inspiratory volume and functional residual capacity," PEDIATR PULMONAL, 2(4);189-193, Jul-Aug, 1986.

Walsh S, et al. THE HUMAN FETAL AND NEONATAL CIRCULATION: FUNCTION AND STRUCTURE, American Lecture Series, Pub No. 870. Charles C Thomas, Springfield IL, 1974.

Walters DW, Olver RD. "The role of catecholamines in lung liquid absorption at birth," PEDATR RES, 12(3);239-242, Mar, 1978.

Wardrop C, Holland B. "The roles and vital importance of placental blood to the newborn infant," J PERINAT MED, 23(1-2);139-143, 1995.

Williams P, ed. GRAY'S ANATOMY: THE ANATOMICAL BASIS OF MEDICINE AND SURGERY, 38th ed. Churchill Livingstone, New York NY, 1995.

Zanardo V, et al. "Labor pain effects on colostral milk beta-endorphin concentrations of lactating mothers," BIOL NEONATE, 79(2);87-90, Feb, 2001a.

Zanardo V, et al. "Beta-endorphin concentrations in human milk," J PEDIATR GASTROENTEROL NUTR, 33(2);160-164, Aug, 2001b.

THE PRODUCTION AND ELIMINATION OF MECONIUM DURING GESTATION

Baker PN, et al. "An assessment of the use of meconium alone as an indication for fetal blood sampling," OBSTET GYNECOL, 80(5);792-796, Nov, 1992.

Ciftci AO, et al. "In-utero defecation: fact or fiction?" EUR J PEDIATR SURG, 9(6);376-380, Dec, 1999.

Ciftci AO, Tanyel F. "In utero defecation: a new concept," Turk J Pediatr. 1998 Jan-Mar; 40(1); 45-53, Jan-Mar, 1998.

Ciftci AO, et al. "Fetal distress does not affect in utero defecation but does impair the clearance of amniotic fluid," J PEDIATR SURG, 34(2);246-250, Feb, 1999.

Galan H. "Meconum-stained amniotic fluid: meaning and management," OMG MANAGEMENT: CME ARTICLE, http://www.obgmanagement.com/799/cme/799.html. July, 1999, accessed Aug 3, 2001.

Ramón y Cajal C, Martinez R. "Defecation in utero: a physiologic fetal function," AM J OBSTET GYNECOL, 188(1);153-156, Jan, 2003.

BODY TEMPERATURE REGULATION IN THE FETUS AND NEWBORN

Anderson T. "Time to throw the waterbirth thermometers away?" MIDIRS MIDWIFERY DIGEST, 14(3);370-374, Sept 2004.

BBC News Health. "'Miracle' cap may beat brain damage," TOMORROW'S WORLD, Mar 2, 1999, http://news.bbc.co.uk/hi/health/289115.stm.

Bennett VB, Brown LK, eds. MYLES TEXTBOOK FOR MIDWIVES, 13th ed. Churchill Livingstone, Edinburgh UK, 1999.

Brück K. Chapter 68: "Neonatal thermal regulation," in Polin R, Fox W, eds. FETAL AND NEONATAL PHYSIOLOGY, 2nd ed., VOL. 1.WB Saunders Co, Philadelphia PA, 1998.

Boston Children's Hospital, "New induced hypothermia protocol," PEDIATRIC VIEWS, Feb 2008; www.childrenshospital.org/views/feb08/new_induced_hypothermia.html> accessed Sept 9, 2013.

Charles C. "Fetal hyperthermia risk from warm water immersion," BJM, 6(3);152-156, 1998.

Coad J, Dunstall M. ANATOMY AND PHYSIOLOGY FOR MIDWIVES, Mosby, Philadelphia 2001.

Geissbuehler V, et al., "Waterbirth: water temperature and bathing time--mother knows best!," J PERINAT MED, 30(5);371-378, 2002.

Gunn T, et al. "Factors influencing the initiation of nonshivering thermogenesis." AMER J OBSTET GYNECOL, 164(1, Pt 1);210-217, 1991.

Kattwinkel, J, ed. NEONATAL RESUSCITATION TEXTBOOK, 6th ed. Am Acad Pediatrics & Am Heart Assoc, 2011.

Korones S. HIGHRISK NEWBORN INFANTS: THE BASIS FOR INTENSIVE NURSING CARE, 4th ed. CV Mosby Co, St. Louis MO, 1986.

Lean M, James W. "Brown adipose tissue in man," in Trayhurn P, Nicholls D, eds. BROWN ADIPOSE TISSUE. Edward Arnold, Baltimore MD, 1986.

Merklin R. "Growth and distribution of human fetal brown fat," ANAT REC, 178(3);637-645, Mar, 1974.

Morley G. "Why do babies cry? the anatomical and physiological changes during the moments after birth," www.cordclamping.com, accessed June 24, 2002a.

Newman K. "Neonatal Hypothermia: a method to provide neuroprotection after hypoxic ischemic encephalopathy," NAINR, 11(3):113-124, 2011 http://www.medscape.com/viewarticle/749601_3, accessed Sept 9 2013.

Oh W, Lind J. "Body temperature of the newborn infant in relation to placental transfusion," ACTA PAEDIATR SCAND, 172S:137-145, 1967.

Power, G. Chapter 67: "Perinatal thermal physiology," in Polin R, Fox W, eds. FETAL AND NEONATAL PHYSIOLOGY, 2nd ed., VOL. 1. WB Saunders Co, Philadelphia PA, 1998.

Richmond S, et al. RESUSCITATION AT BIRTH: THE NEWBORN LIFE SUPPORT PROVIDER COURSE MANUAL. Resuscitation Council (UK), Rochester, Kent UK, 2011.

Sanders M. MOSBY'S PARAMEDIC TEXTBOOK. Mosby Lifeline Inc, St. Louis MO, 1994.

Shankaran S, et al. "Brain injury following trial of hypothermia for neonatal hypoxic–ischaemic encephalopathy," ARCH DIS CHILD FETAL NEONATAL ED, 97(6): F398–F404, Nov 2012.

Swan N. "Cooling Cap for Newborns," RADIO NATIONAL HEALTH REPORT, Jan 26, 1998, www.abc.net.au/rn/talks/8.30/helthrp/sotires/ s10303.htm. Accessed Feb, 2003.

Thoresen M. "Cooling the newborn after asphyxia–physiological and experimental background and its clinical use," SEMIN NEONATOL, 5(1);61-73, Feb, 2000.

WHO. THERMAL PROTECTION OF THE NEWBORN: A PRACTICAL GUIDE, Safe Motherhood series. Geneva Switzerland, 1997.

BEING AT BIRTHS

Supplies and Equipment for Labor and Birth

Basic and Emergency Equipment and Supplies Used during Labor and Birth

The midwifery equipment an individual midwife carries will be influenced by a variety of factors, including where and how "technically" she practices. Midwives practicing in rural areas far from a hospital or in the developing world may carry some items that city-dwelling midwives may not feel are necessary. This chapter discusses all the relevant equipment, with the assumption that the items will be tailored to each midwife's practice situation. Additionally, it assumes that the midwife will carry the prenatal equipment discussed in Volume I and the suturing equipment described in HEALING PASSAGE. (Tips on the use of basic instruments such as scissors, hemostats and needle holders may also be found in HEALING PASSAGE.) This chapter focuses upon equipment features. Most details regarding how and when to use equipment will be discussed in appropriate locations throughout the text.

It is important to buy good-quality equipment. With proper care, good tools should last a lifetime and are always a wise investment. Poor-quality tools often fall short of the task when needed most and inevitably wear out more quickly. The only exception to this buy-the-best guideline involves seldom-used instruments that need not be precision tools, such as ring forceps. With good care and infrequent use, such lesser-quality tools can last a long time.

Basic Birth Instruments, Equipment, Supplies and Additional Items for Birth

The following section describes both basic and rarely needed equipment that most midwives will want to carry in their birth bag.

Three curved Rochester-Pean (or other style) hemostats

A hemostat is a scissor-like device with thick, serrated jaws, used to occlude a bleeding vessel; it is designed to stop bleeding while minimizing tissue damage. Rochester-Pean hemostats feature longer serrated jaws than some others. Their extra length makes them ideal for clamping the umbilical cord in a hurry. A curved instrument may be easier to use on the rare occasion when the cord needs to be clamped before the birth of the shoulders. Three hemostats are a good idea, so that an extra is always on hand in case of multiple birth!

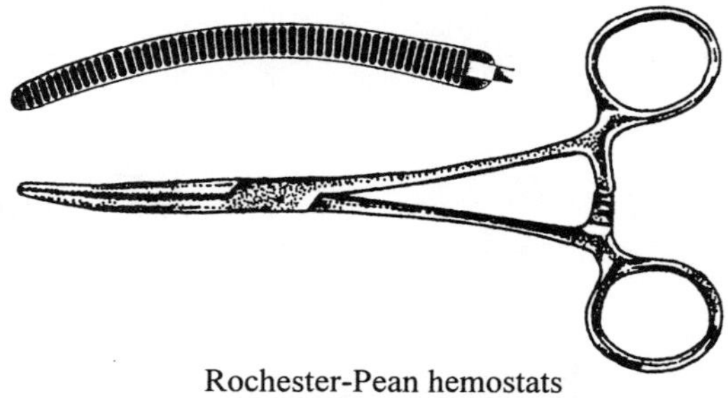

Rochester-Pean hemostats

Umbilical scissors

American-pattern umbilical scissors (by Miltex) have two inwardly curving blades that gather the cord into their jaws for cutting. Regular straight scissors tend to push the plump cord away as the jaws are closed, making the cutting of thick cords particularly challenging.

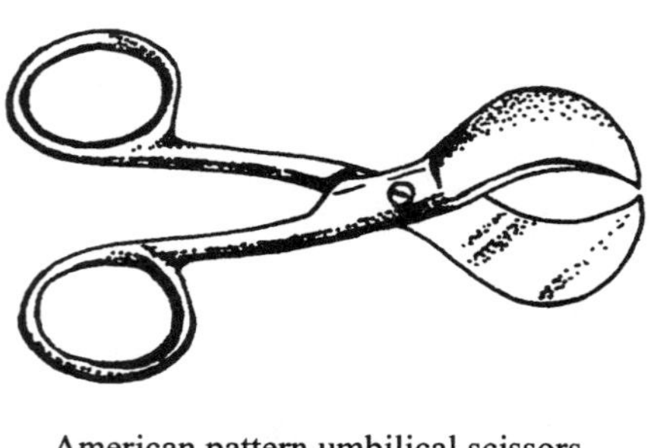

American pattern umbilical scissors

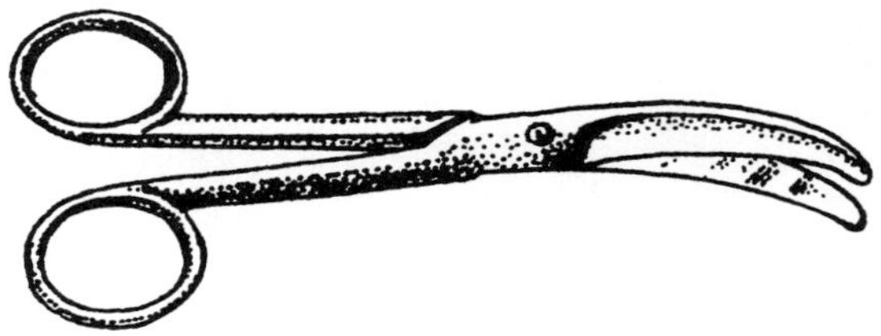

Busch umbilical scissors

Busch umbilical scissors (by Miltex) have straight, blunt-ended blades curved along their length, which means the tips will curve away from adjacent tissues, making them ideal for cutting a tight nuchal cord before the baby is completely born. Note that the blades of cord scissors should be somewhat dull. The dull edge produces a more serrated cut, which promotes vessel constriction and clotting.

Midwives on a tight budget can carry the less-expensive bandage scissors, which have large, blunt, triangular extensions at the tips.

Blunt-blunt surgical scissors

These scissors have two blunt-tipped sharp blades and may also be useful for cutting a tight cord around the baby's neck. They can also be used to cut clitorotomies or to incise the cervical rim in the very rare event that is necessary. Cutting the perineum requires a very sharp blade, while cutting the cord is best done with a dull blade. Therefore, it is best to have two separate instruments for these purposes. Surgical scissors are less expensive than umbilical scissors.

Scissor sharpener: Miltex makes a surgical scissor sharpener that works for nearly all types of scissors.

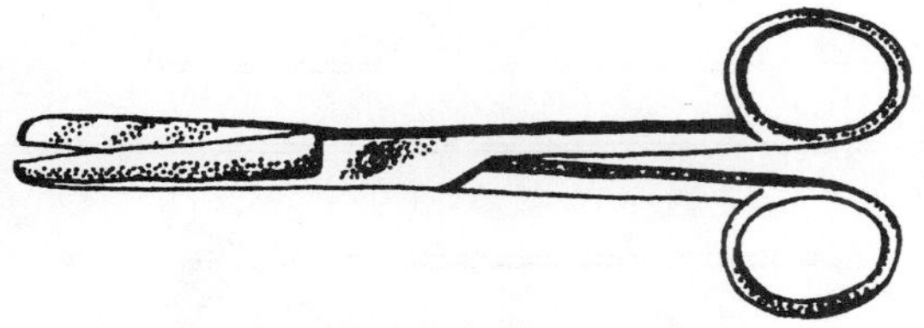

Blunt-blunt surgical scissors

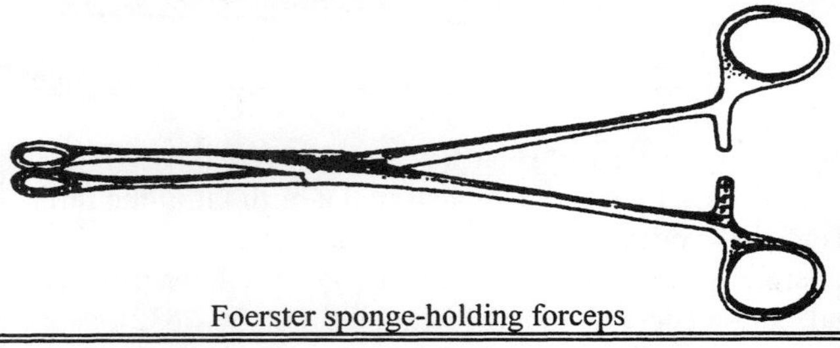

Foerster sponge-holding forceps

Foerster sponge-holding forceps or Kelly placenta forceps

Foerster forceps have a serrated open oval on the ends, and can be used for a variety of purposes, such as removing fragments of placental membranes, clamping off a tear in the cervix, and holding apart the yoni walls and grasping the edge of the cervix during examination of the upper vault of the yoni. Some midwives prefer to have two styles, a longer one (9.5 in or 24 cm) in the rare event that they need to manipulate the cervix, and a shorter one (7 in or 17.5 cm) which more easily assists with membrane removal.

Kelly placenta forceps are similar in design but are 12.5 in (31 cm) long with a slightly curved shaft.

Placenta previa tools

If you work where medical care is completely inaccessible, you might want to consider having a large package of sterile gauze bandage material, cord, tongue depressors and a pair of Teale Vulsellum forceps on hand. What these tools could be used for and the life-threatening risks involved in dealing with placenta previa without access to surgical birth are explained in the chapter entitled "Bleeding due to Placental Disruption."

Suturing instruments

Those midwives repairing all types of tears, including fourth degree, will need two pair of top-quality needle holders (one small, the other larger), a pair of stitch scissors, 4 to 5 small hemostats and two Allis clamps. A small needle holder and stitch scissors will suffice for minor repairs. Suture equipment also includes surgical thread with needles attached. (Suture material and the instruments used to cut and repair the perineum are discussed in full detail in HEALING PASSAGE.)

Amniotomy devices

A variety of instruments can be used to assist in rupturing the membranes. Rochester-Ochsner forceps have interlocking teeth on the end and will work in some cases, although a sharp-ended instrument is more efficient. A sterilized stainless-steel crochet hook can be used to puncture the bag. Disposable amniotomy hooks are quite long and feature a sharp, hooked, pointed tip; some have a curved shaft to adapt to the shape of the birth canal. Miltex makes the Beacham amniotome, a straight, stainless-steel amniohook that is 10.25 in (27 cm) long. Disposable amniohooks are long, curved and pretty scary looking, but have a sharp end and do the job. A pudendal needle and sheath can be used to create tiny punctures in the bag when trying to avoid

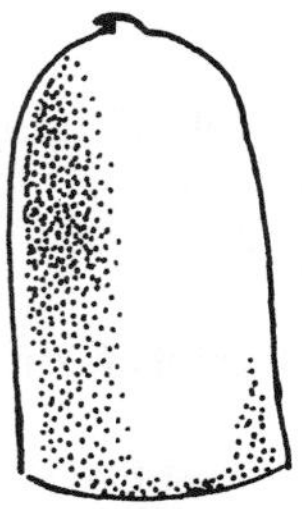

Memcot or Amni-cot

a big gush of fluid. (See the chapter entitled "Cord Problems and Emergencies during Labor.") Specialized nonlatex, disposable fingercots are available with a small plastic hook on the end, allowing finely tuned control of the process. The Memcot and the Amni-cot are two such devices: the Amni-cot is said not to slip during use. All of these tools can tear the baby rather than puncture a hole. Miltex also makes the Iowa membrane puncturing forceps with 6 × 6 teeth, which would tear a big hole in the membranes.

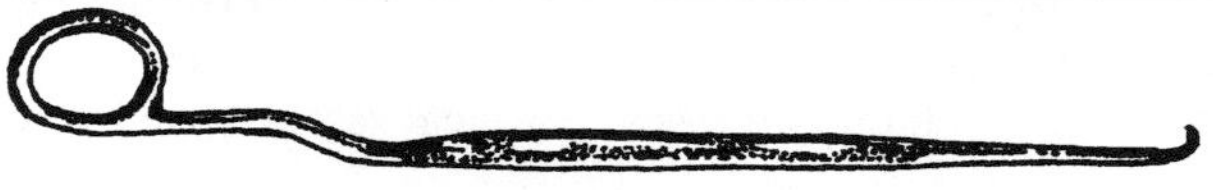
Beacham amniotome

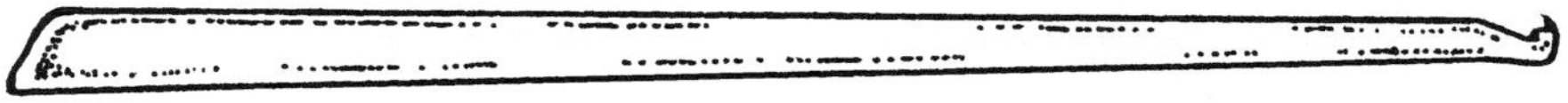
Disposable plastic amnihook

Pudendal needle and sheath

These items are included in the birth kit in the rare event that you need to rupture the membranes with tiny punctures to ease the waters out slowly. The Iowa trumpet pudendal needle guide (Miltex part no. 30-2632) is a stainless-steel sheath that is 5.5 in (14 cm) long. A long syringe needle and a length of IV tubing can be used as a substitute for these items. (See the chapter entitled "Cord Problems and Emergencies during Labor" for details.)

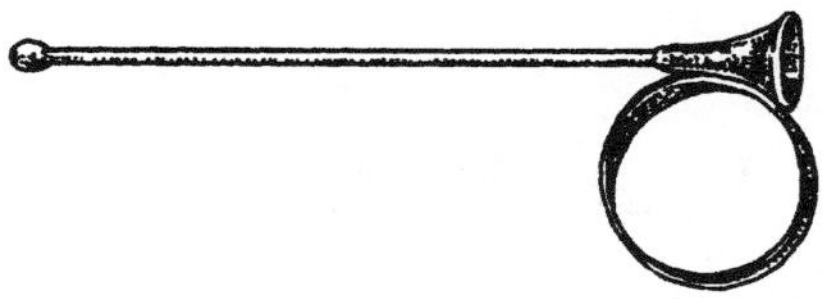
Iowa trumpet pudendal needle guide

Storage and care of instruments

Instruments should be thoroughly cleaned prior to sterilization. A scrub brush and a solution designed to clean instruments should be used, with particular attention given to any serrated edges and joints. Once clean, instruments should be packaged in one of the wide variety of materials designed to store sterilized equipment. The technique used for sterilization will influence the type of packaging used. Autoclavable, self-sealing, paper-backed plastic pouches are available, as are paper wraps and special tape that changes color once sterilized. Homemade wrapping made from white fabric can be used as an inner wrapper, followed by paper wrap suitable for use in autoclaves, pressure cookers and the oven. (However, note that fabric will become discolored from repeated dry sterilization techniques, such as baking.) Wrapped instrument packs can be sterilized in large, portable, steam pressure cookers designed to accommodate instruments, but a regular pressure cooker can also be used. Thirty minutes at 15 pounds of pressure is needed to kill all spores. Autoclaves are quite expensive but are a good investment and will help preserve your instruments.

Sometimes instruments must be cleaned immediately because of the need to go from one birth straight to another. Extra instrument wrappers, a scrub brush, and a cleaning solution should be included in your birth kit. Occasional use of a stain remover for stainless steel and a spray lubricant will maintain instruments in optimal working order. A cold sterilization solution such as Amerce, benzalkonium chloride, or 2% glutaraldehyde sterilant may be useful if you have a busy practice. Those midwives with very busy practices should consider purchasing two full sets of instruments. (Complete details regarding cleaning and sterilizing equipment can be found in HEALING PASSAGE.)

Oxygen monitoring and delivery and bag-and-mask resuscitation equipment

Carry a bag-and-mask resuscitator for the mother and the baby. The equipment used for oxygen delivery and resuscitation is discussed in detail in the subchapter entitled "Oxygen Delivery Devices and Resuscitation Equipment."

Pulse oximeter: Oximeters measure oxygen saturation; get one for use with both adults and neonates (not just infants).

Basic disposable items

With the exception of disposable varieties of amniotomy instruments, which are discussed above, the following constitute the basic list of disposable items you will want to have on hand.

Examination gloves: Most midwives carry both sterile and nonsterile gloves, and have both latex and nonlatex gloves available as well. Find a brand of glove that fits you well and provides a level of barrier protection with which you feel comfortable while still allowing for tactile sensitivity. Ordering singles (or pairs) of a variety of gloves in several sizes will allow you to experiment to find which fits you best. Be sure to have properly sized gloves on hand for each member of the birth team. Latex is broken down when it comes into contact with oil-based lubricants; vinyl gloves should be used whenever oil is the lubricant of choice. Have some nonlatex gloves on hand in case the mother is allergic to latex. Be sure to ask for samples to see if the gloves have sufficient tactile sensitivity, as many nonlatex gloves, in particular, are quite thick.

Nonsterile gloves are suitable for internal exams during labor with intact membranes. They are also used while examining the placenta, changing underpads, drawing blood, placing an IV and cleaning blood-contaminated equipment. Sterile gloves should be used once the membranes are broken during suturing and whenever manipulations require inserting your fingers or hands beyond the cervical os. Gloves with a wrist-level cuff will be fine for most uses; sterile elbow-length gloves (such as the Perry Xtenda brand sold through Cascade HealthCare Products) should be on hand in the event that you need to insert your hand into the uterus. (Since these gloves are not FDA approved for human use, some providers don the long gloves first and then place the surgical gloves over them to form a double layer, although this will decrease your tactile sensitivity.)

Some gloves come with the inside powdered with talc to facilitate putting them on. While powder significantly eases donning and removing gloves, talc is irritating to the respiratory tract (particularly in babies) and may be irritating to other tissues as well. The powder may also carry latex dust into the air, increasing the likelihood of allergic reactions. Unpowdered gloves eliminate all of these concerns. To don unpowdered gloves, however, your hands must be very dry. If your hands sweat a lot, carry a very small capped shaker of cornstarch to rub on your hands prior to donning gloves. An assistant can shake a small amount into your hands for you if you have just scrubbed. As long as the cornstarch is clean and does not touch the outside of the glove, you are still sterile once the gloves are on. (Donning sterile gloves is covered in HEALING PASSAGE and Volume I of this text. Issues regarding "clean" versus sterile technique are covered in HEALING PASSAGE.)

Sterile gauze squares: Four inch gauze squares come in handy for a variety of purposes and can be included as part of the birth kit the parents put together. It is a good idea, however, to carry some extra squares in your birth kit as backup.

Plastic-backed underpads: One popular brand is Chux pads in the United States. Any similar pad comes in very handy for absorbing birth fluids and keeping surfaces clean. For those who want a more ecologically friendly alternative, machine-washable underpads are available. Homemade pads can easily be created by sewing several layers of old sheets together with machine-washable plastic backing. (Check large fabric stores for ideas.) Regardless of type, you'll need around a dozen underpads for the birth. Some midwives like to get a dozen smaller pads (say 30 × 30 or 23 × 24 in) and some larger ones (23 × 36 in is a popular size) for different uses.

Antimicrobial solution: A hospital-grade antimicrobial solution for use on the skin, such as Betadine (iodine based, or Hibiclens) can be used to wash hands and for general cleanup. Beware of products which contain iodine; although they can be used, some mothers or babies may be sensitive to them.

Urinary catheters: Straight, flexible, all-purpose disposable urethral catheters with one flared end and a rounded tip with two eyes on either side on the other end can be used in the event that the mother cannot empty her bladder either during labor or postpartum. They are not used for this purpose on the baby, but they could be used for deep suctioning the baby if nothing else is available. Regular urinary catheters come in size 10 or 14 F ("F" refers to the French or Charrière scale, which is used to grade the size of sounds, tubes and catheters. It is based on a diameter of 1/3 mm equaling 1 F (e.g., 3 F = 1 mm). The smaller the number, the smaller the diameter. The size is written with an "F" but spoken by saying "a number one French.") Red rubber catheters are made of flexible latex, while red plastic catheters are slightly less flexible and are made of polyvinylchloride (PVC). Silicone catheters are also available. Since PVC is carcinogenic; silicone or latex products should be used whenever possible.

Indwelling or retention, double-lumen catheters, or Foley's, are designed for continuous bladder drainage. These have an inflatable balloon just below the drainage eyes which, when filled, causes the catheter tip to be retained in the bladder. A size 16 French Foley can be used to back-fill the bladder to elevate the presenting part in the event of a cord prolapse. (For details, see the chapter entitled "Cord Problems and Emergencies during Labor.") In addition to the Foley, you will need a needleless luer-lock syringe, a 60 cc catheter-tip (slip-tip) syringe, a disposable sterile bowl, sterile normal saline IV solution in a bottle (not a bag), and a catheter plug.

A very large 24 F Foley catheter can be used to induce labor. See the chapter entitled "Natural Augmentation and Induction of Labor" for details.

Syringes and needles: A variety of syringe and needle sizes will be needed to administer antihemorrhagic medication, local anesthetic or $RhoD_O$ immunoglobulin to the mother and to administer injectable Vitamin K to the baby. You should also carry a few large (20 cc) syringes for such tasks as aspirating orogastric tubing. The types of syringes needed for administering drugs and instruction on how to give an injection are covered in the subchapter entitled "Hypodermic Injections."

Sharps container: Various containers in a wide range of sizes are available for disposal of single-use sharp or potentially sharp objects after use. It is ideal to have at least one that will allow the disposal of a syringe with needle attached. Choose one that will fit in your birth bag. Do not attempt to cram sharps into a nearly full container or to empty and reuse it, as this defeats the purpose of avoiding puncture wounds. Have at least one back-up sharps container that can be put into service when the current one is almost filled.

IV equipment and supplies: The decision of whether to carry IV equipment or not will depend upon practice size and setting, as well as your personal beliefs regarding medical technology at births. You may have no desire to carry IV equipment since placing an IV can be risky and an IV is rarely needed at home. However, there are times when an IV can be used for stabilizing a shocky woman before transport or simply rehydrating a woman so she can continue to labor at home. Intravenous administration of antibiotics in the presence of Group B strep colonization is also possible. (Because IV equipment and its use is complex, it is covered separately in the subchapter entitled "Intravenous Equipment and IV Therapy.")

Blood-drawing equipment: Many midwives routinely collect a red (or gold) topped tube of cord blood at each birth. Some jurisdictions require syphilis testing for every baby. Blood is also collected from all Rh-negative mothers and their babies. Check with your local laboratory to confirm the color top needed for the tubes. (The equipment needed is discussed in detail in the chapter entitled "How to Draw Blood" in DIAGNOSTIC TESTS.)

Equipment to use for collecting maternal blood loss and receiving the placenta

Placenta pans: Although any pan or bowl from the parents' kitchen can be used to catch the placenta, it is quite nice to have a pair of stainless steel bowls that are shaped for the job. A wide-mouthed bowl with a shallow depth is perfect for slipping under the mother's bottom; it is deep enough to catch fluids and wide enough to allow you to visually monitor the amount of blood loss. Medical supply houses call these bowls "wash basins"; they are 12.25 in. in diameter and 3.5 in. deep (31 × 6.25 cm). Having two bowls makes it easier to keep track of initial blood loss, as the full pan can be replaced immediately with the second so that all the blood can be measured. These bowls also fit perfectly beneath the lid of a standard US toilet, in the event that the mother wants to sit on the toilet to deliver the placenta.

A fracture bedpan also allows good visualization of blood loss and placental birth; however, it may be harder to clean thoroughly due to the shielded end. It can be washed in a dishwasher after thorough hand cleaning.

Large, wide-mouth measuring cup: Get a large-mouthed measuring cup with metric and imperial measurements that can easily accommodate both liquid blood and clots, with sufficient capacity such that a quantity of blood can be measured without the need to empty it out. A plastic 6-cup (1.5 liter) or more measure with a lid can also be used for storage of equipment.

Placenta exam equipment: Many midwives examine the placenta on a plastic-backed underpad. However, a white acrylic cutting board measuring 15 × 12 inches (38 by 29 cm) or somewhat larger is an ideal surface for performing a placental exam. It will allow you to spread the placenta out on a neutral surface and will be an excellent background if photographs are desired. Try to find a board that is resistant to staining and scratching and that is as smooth as possible for ease in cleaning. Make sure it is dishwasher safe.

For those who are interested in gathering detailed placental data, it is nice to have a couple of carefully selected rulers to illustrate dimensions of placental features for photographs. These rulers should ideally be made of white plastic or metal (so that they are easy to clean) with black lettering and have both inch and centimeter scales. They should be at least 10 to 12 in (25.5 to 30.5 cm) long. Two rulers will allow you to place them at a right angle to each other to demonstrate length and width. For features longer than these rulers, you can also carry a 60 in (152 cm) plastic tape measure.

Professional-grade cutting boards, rulers, scales and scale holders designed specifically for this purpose can be obtained from Biomedical Instruments for Educational Photography, but they are quite expensive.

Sharp knife: A long, very sharp knife will assist when the need arises to cut the placenta during examination. Have some sort of protective shield for the blade for safe storage (a piece cardboard folded and taped to form a sheath will do) and remember to sharpen the knife periodically. An unserrated ham slicer or long filet knife may work well.

Dish-washing gloves: Rubber gloves are ideal for examining the placenta but should be used only for this purpose and for equipment clean-up after the birth. They can be cleaned by washing your hands in an antimicrobial solution with the gloves on, then carefully dry and store them. A hair dryer can be used to dry these gloves, which is particularly efficient if the inside of the glove becomes wet.

Additional items to have on hand

Magnifying glass: A fine-quality magnifying glass can come in very handy to examine very small, suspicious findings on the baby or the placenta.

Trays: Have some sort of surface on which to arrange your instruments and other tools to make your setup portable. Cookie sheets or similar items from the mother's home can be used. However, two breakfast-in-bed trays from any large variety store gives you two trays of the perfect size. Look for ones with two handles, collapsible legs, an easy to clean surface, a rim to keep things from falling off the tray (or to hold a folded towel for the baby) (Edmonds, 2004).

Space blanket: A regular-sized space blanket is a wonderful thing to have in case of maternal or newborn transport. Having two allows you to cover both mother and baby in the rare event of a double postpartum transport. You should have at least one sheet-style blanket as well as a bunting sized to fit a newborn. You need both because the bunting may not be suitable for babies with certain types of defects.

Hot-drink thermos: Pat Edmonds (2004), an experienced CPM practicing in Portland, OR, carries a thermos to keep hot water handy for use when herbs need to be administered quickly during labor or after the birth. For example, this would be very convenient if the mother were bleeding and you wanted to give her a powdered or tinctured herbal preparation mixed in hot water.

Pharmaceuticals: Drugs can be divided into two categories, those for the mother's use and those for the baby. For maternal use, many midwives carry a variety of antihemorrhagics, such as oxytocin, Methergine ampules and tablets; some carry misoprostol and a few have access to Hemobate. (Antihemorrhagic drugs are discussed in the subchapter entitled "Allopathic Pharmacologic Agents for Treating Uterine Atony.") Other drugs for maternal use include topical and injectable anesthetic without epinephrine, antibiotics for group B-strep prophylaxis and epinephrine for anaphylactic reactions. (Epinephrine is discussed at the end of the chapter entitled "Hypersensitivity Reactions and Anaphylactic Shock."). For the baby, you will want to have newborn eye prophylaxis, newborn concentration of injectable Vitamin K and an oral form of Vitamin K. Other drugs such as anticonvulsants and antihypertensives may be desirable and may be carried by midwives practicing in a very rural settings or in the developing world. The permitted use of pharmaceuticals varies widely among jurisdictions; those most used by independent midwives in the United States are the focus in this text.

Herbs, flower remedies and homeopathics: There are a large number of herbs and other remedies that midwives choose to use at births. This big subject is covered in a separate chapter in the subchapter entitled "Naturopathic Remedies."

Crock pot: A crock pot is ideal for keeping water or an herbal solution hot for use with compresses during pushing. Some midwives have the parents supply a crock pot; however, bringing your own means you do not have to wonder if theirs will work.

Thermometers: An indoor temperature gauge and an aquarium thermometer to test the water in a birthing tub or for a newborn bath will both come in handy.

Resealable plastic bags: A box of 1 quart and a box of 1 gallon resealable plastic freezer bags of your preference will come in handy for all sorts of things and are mentioned throughout this text. Freezer bags are more durable than others.

Miscellaneous maternal care items: You may want to carry a hot water/enema bottle and plug, enema hose and clamp, yoni and rectal tips, a small ice pack and a Fleet's enema. Other possible items include castor oil, flexible straws, cotton swabs, sterile cotton balls and cotton wool, and eye droppers.

Heating pads: An electric heating pad can be used to prewarm towels or receiving blankets for the baby. It can be used postpartum to relieve the mother's afterpains. Another can be used to wrap around an IV bag or oxygen tubing to warm the air during administration. Carry a few spring-closure clothes pins to secure the heating pad around the tubing.

Large hand mirror: A big hand mirror with a sturdy handle allows the mother and partner to watch the progress of crowning. If the mother is in an upright position, it can also allow you to check the mother's pushing progress without requiring her to move. It can also be used postpartum to show the mother a tear, etc.

Massage oil: A natural, general purpose massage oil or a special blend of oil for use on the perineum is a good thing to carry, although parents can also be encouraged to have a small, unopened bottle of olive oil on hand.

Cameras: Many parents supply their own cameras to take birth pictures; however, a midwife may want to carry a simple SLR camera, a bounce flash (to avoid lights in the eyes of mother or baby) and a Polaroid or digital camera. The Polaroid, with its advantage of on-the-spot developing, can be used in the event that a photo is needed right away. A regular 35-mm or digital camera can be used to record placental or newborn features as well as a perineal repair job or any unusual findings. Such photos become part of the medical record.

Quite aside from the medical advantage of having cameras, taking pictures at a birth can be a good way for a new apprentice to begin birth observation. Photography, however, can be very intrusive to the mother, invading her privacy and possibly prolonging labor; whoever is taking pictures should do so as quietly and unobtrusively as possible. Photography should cease if it seems to be affecting labor for the worse.

Spare parts and replacement power for equipment: Be sure to have additional batteries, light bulbs and other replaceable parts for the flashlight, Doppler, ophthalmoscope and any other battery-powered devices.

Personal items: Carrying a small supply of personal items will significantly increase your comfort level during marathon births or in the event you must leave one birth to go directly to another. This is also important so that you don't look (or smell) like something the cat dragged in if you must accompany a mother to the hospital during a transport. Items you may want include a toothbrush and toothpaste, dental floss, hair brush, shower cap, deodorant, shampoo, soap, nail file and clipper, contact lens solutions, back-up pair of glasses, reading glasses, clean underwear, a change of clothes, menstrual supplies, medications, vitamins and herbs.

Short fingernails: While not in your birth bag, your hands are a central part of your equipment. Midwives rely on their hands for many types of intrusive procedures and examinations. To prevent injury to the mother or baby and to facilitate the accuracy of your efforts, your nails should be clean and probably not longer than the tips of your fingers.

Protective clothing: A bib apron with pockets will protect your clothing as well as hold pens, extra gloves, etc. If you do not wear glasses, eye protection in the form of ordinary frames with plain glass lenses are an unobtrusive means of protecting your eyes from splatters. Commercial eye shields are also available. Each person attending the birth should bring some sort of eye protection.

Portable light source: The Snake Light by Black and Decker offers a bright, clear light; it can be twisted into virtually any position and directed where needed. It can even be hung around your neck and adjusted for suturing. Alternatively, some midwives use a "miner's lamp" on their forehead. A regular flashlight held by an assistant can also be used. Flashlights allow the midwife to visualize fetal head color or amniotic fluid, even in low-light situations. Midwives who practice in rural areas or anywhere that electric light may not always be available need multiple flashlights. This is important when open flame lamps are used for lighting (such as propane or kerosene lanterns), as they will have to be extinguished if oxygen is needed during the birth.

Folding stretcher: This may be essential for midwives working in remote locations.

Supplies and Equipment for Use in Baby Care

Baby exam equipment

Baby care includes routine physical exams as well as the support of both healthy and compromised newborns. To meet your needs in doing both, you should carry all the items described below.

Flexible tape measure: This is used to measure the baby's head, chest, abdomen and length during the baby exam. It should be made of plastic for easy cleaning and have both inch and centimeter scales. Stretchy, disposable circular tape measures are also available for measuring the head, chest and abdominal circumferences.

Neonatal stethoscope: A stethoscope specifically designed for newborns is an important tool. The newborn anatomy is so small that only a very small stethoscope is really effective at isolating sounds, particularly in the chest, where an adult scope will cover several ribs and produce static. It should have a reversible bell/diaphragm head.

Ruler: An easy way to measure the baby's length can be cheaply devised by taking a standard yard stick or easily cleaned ruler with both inch and centimeter measures (available in some hardware stores), and cutting it off to 25 in (83.5 cm). Caliper-style devices are also available but are expensive and bulky to carry.

Baby scale: A variety of baby scales are available. Table-top balance-beam or electric models can be used in an office, but these are cumbersome and prone to damage when carted around to births. A hanging scale is much more practical for this purpose. The Chatillon scale is a very accurate fish-scale type model, weighing up to 12 lb (5.45 kg) with 2 oz gradations. The Ultrasport digital fish scale weighs up to 25 lb in 1 oz gradations (10 kg × 0.01 kg); it has a tape measure on the side. The Salter baby weigher is similar to the Chatillon and has 100 gram gradations; it is widely used in England.

A sling in which to place the baby for weighing can be purchased or made. Remember to calibrate the scale to zero with the sling in place to accurately assess the baby's weight.

Infant rectal thermometer: Glass mercury thermometers have a column of silver liquid and are now no longer available. Glass alcohol thermometers have a blue or red column of liquid. Glass galinstan (gallium-indium-tin) thermometers have also been approved by the FDA. All types of glass thermometers can be used interchangeably and are read in the same manner. Any glass thermometers can be used to obtain either oral, axillary or rectal temperatures. However, rectal thermometers are made with a thick glass tip that minimizes the chances that the thermometer will break.

Digital electronic thermometers are considered accurate. Tympanic thermometers, on the other hand, are not only expensive but are less accurate. They require precise placement in the ear canal for an accurate reading and are not reliable in infants because their ear canal is so small.

Bright, cool light source: A small, bright flashlight that emits a cool light, with a small tip that seals flush against the skin, can be used for transillumination of newborn body parts. Use a light that is relatively small (the size of a pen light or somewhat larger) with the brightest, clearest, coolest beam you can find. A Wood's lamp can be useful in examining some skin lesions, but is not essential. (Transillumination is a diagnostic technique discussed in the subchapter entitled "Newborn Examination Techniques" and throughout the text as appropriate; see the Index.)

Goniometer and small clear protractor: A goniometer (go-knee-OHM-meter) is a tool used to assess angles during range-of-motion tests. It has a circular base with a mark for each degree and a movable arm. A newborn size is not available. A small clear protractor makes a reasonable substitute. The school supplies section of an office supply store should have one that has a movable arm to assist in finding angles, but one without an arm can also be used.

Additional baby items

Firm, portable surface: A long cookie sheet, serving tray, breakfast-in-bed tray (as already discussed) a cutting board or similar item can be used to provide a firm surface for infant resuscitation and transport. The best thing to purchase is a tray or pan which has a 1 in (3 cm) lip around the edge. This will allow the placement of a towel in the depression for padding and will prevent the towel from slipping. (Use of the tray is explained in the chapter entitled "Setting Up Equipment and Preparing the House for Birth.") All newborn care and transport protocols in this text assume you have some sort of portable transport surface such as this.

Suction devices for the baby: Suction devices include an ear syringe, a nasal syringe, and mucus-trap suction devices in a variety of styles, as well as feeding tubes, which can be used with large syringes to aspirate mucus and air during artificial ventilation. (These tools are discussed in detail in the subchapter entitled "Clearing the Baby's Airway.")

Umbilical cord clamps: Many devices are available for occluding the cord vessels after birth. The pros and cons of cord clamping are discussed elsewhere in this text; however, even those midwives who do not intend to clamp most cords will always want to have something on hand with which to do so. The simplest items are new, clean string or shoe laces tied in a tight square knot. These can be sterilized by boiling and placing them in a new pill bottle sealed with tape or in a new resealable plastic bag.

Metal cord clamps are reusable and can be sterilized in a birth equipment pack (birthwithlove.com). Metal clamps are easier to remove than the plastic cord clamps used in most hospitals. Disposable plastic clamps can be removed with a plastic clamp remover after 24 to 48 hours. Both types are more uncomfortable for the baby than a cord band.

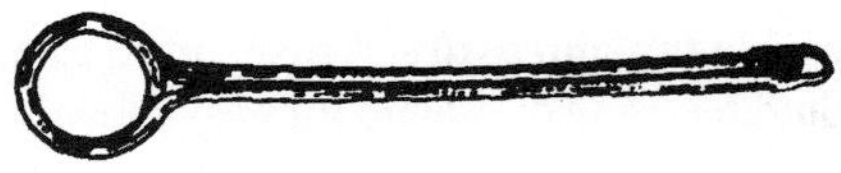

Hasseltine metal clamp (closed)

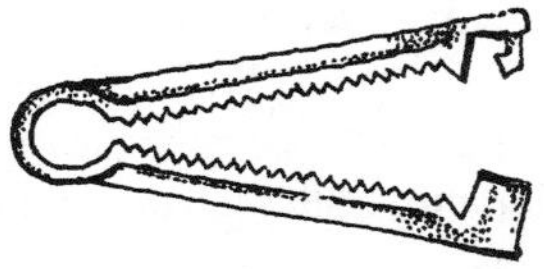

Plastic clamp (open)

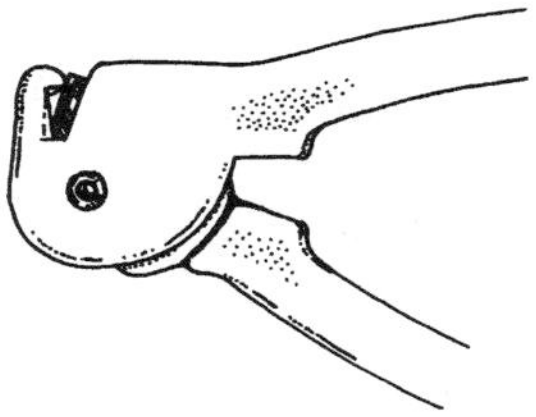

Close-up of cutter on a plastic cord clamp remover

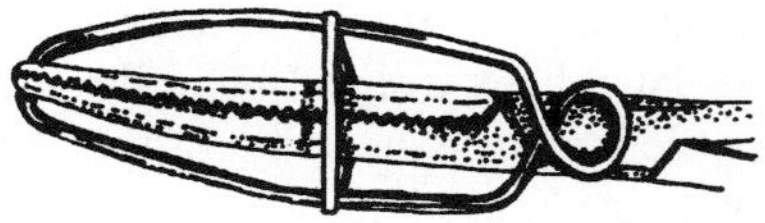

Close up of the unique features of the Averbach cord bander with a cord band in place

Tiny orthodontic rubber bands (the kind used for braces) can also be used. These are applied with an instrument called an Averbach cord bander, which is only available through Cascade HealthCare Products. It is a regular hemostat modified to include a lever device that is used to transfer a band from the instrument to the baby's cord stump. These bands are unobtrusive and work well in most cases. AVA cord bands are loaded onto snap-in-two plastic rings, no instrument required. Always have back-up cord clamps available as well. (See the chapter entitled "Placenta-to-Newborn Transfusion, Physiologic Closure of the Umbilical Vessels and Severance of the Cord" for information about using the cord bander.)

Burn box/tin foil/candles: Burning the cord is the most hygienic way to sever it. You can use two candles alone or shielded from the baby with tin foil or heavy cardboard but having a burn box makes it safer and provides an easy place to stretch the cord across and then hold the candles on either side, perpendicular to it. Burn boxes are available from www.cordburning.com.

Stamp pad: While footprints of the baby and fingerprints of the mother are unnecessary for identification purposes at home, parents may want baby footprints as a keepsake. Foot and palm prints should always be taken in the event of a fetal demise. Easy-to-use Kleen Print disposable stamp pads specially designed for newborn use are available from Cascade HealthCare Products.

Birth certificates: Pretty, printed certificates of homebirth with places for palm and foot prints can be obtained from Cascade or other suppliers. This might be something you want to provide for your clients or have them get themselves.

Materials to make hand or foot casts: A mold of the baby's hand or foot can be a valuable keepsake for any parent, but especially if the baby is born with a lethal defect or you attend a labor for a fetal demise. You will need dental alginate and dental plaster (die stone peach) both of which can be obtained from a dental supply house. You will also need paper cups (or another container large enough to accommodate the hand or foot plus a portion of the limb), tongue depressors, an electric mixer or a small whisk for mixing the casting materials and a small, sharp paring or pocket knife.

Seldom-needed emergency supplies and equipment for the baby

Elastic-support bandage: A long elastic band, 1 to 2 in (2.5 to 5 cm) wide (such as those used for athletic injuries) is useful for stabilizing a baby's injured limbs after a difficult birth.

Saline solution or salt tablets: Sterile, unpreserved saline solution prepared for IV or contact lens use is ideal to use in the event that a baby is born with defects requiring continuous moisture during transport. Plain salt tablets can also be used to make saline solution. Homemade saline solution should taste no more salty than tears.

Laryngoscope: This device, when used correctly, opens the glottis, allows visualization of the vocal cords and can be used when placing an endotracheal tube during infant resuscitation. It is a matter of controversy whether midwives should use a laryngoscope. Midwives working in rural areas and those with hospital experience that includes laryngoscopy may feel inadequately equipped without one. However, proper, safe technique requires frequent practice and use; a laryngoscope can cause serious damage. Midwives will rarely be faced with situations where visualizing the vocal cords is necessary; they may not be able to maintain the level of proficiency required to perform laryngoscopy safely. Alternative techniques will be found in the subchapter entitled "Digital Endotracheal Intubation of the Newborn."

Doppler fetoscope: Standard fetoscopes are discussed in Volume I of this textbook. Each midwife must decide for herself whether to carry a Doppler fetoscope or not. Ultrasound is still an unproven technology; exposing the baby to any amount of ultrasound unnecessarily seems imprudent.

Reasons midwives give for using a Doppler include listening to the fetal heart without requiring the mother to change positions, convenience during a water birth, the ability to listen to the heartbeat through a contraction easily, the ability to hear clearly in a woman-of-size or a woman with a posterior baby or an anterior placenta, and rapidity of assessing the heart rate. However, mere convenience seems a poor reason to expose the baby to an unnecessary risk, especially as ultrasound's potential negative effects are enhanced by water. Many who have honed their skills with a regular fetoscope are able to hear the heartbeat with the mother in a variety of positions. You can almost always hear heart tones with a fetoscope, even through crowning, if you have a practiced ear and are not hearing impaired.

On the other hand, if there is a real question as to the baby's well-being and all other means of assessing the baby still leave the question of well-being unanswered, it makes sense to have a Doppler on hand since it is a given that ultrasound will be used freely in the hospital upon transport for further fetal evaluation. (For a full discussion of this issue, see the chapter entitled "Ultrasonography and Doppler Diagnostic Techniques" in DIAGNOSTIC TESTS).

If you choose to purchase a Doppler, look for one that is easy to carry, easy to use and lightweight and that delivers the least possible amount of ultrasound to the baby and mother. Some models may have both speaker and headphone options. Some have digital displays and printed readouts. A waterproof cord and probe may be another desirable feature. Once you have settled on a Doppler, put it in its case at the bottom of your birth bag. Rely on your fetoscope and consider your Doppler as a backup of last resort. Also keep in mind that a Doppler could stop working for any number of reasons. If you are skilled with a fetoscope, you will not be at a significant disadvantage should this occur.

Miscellaneous, rarely needed and emergency baby equipment: The following equipment should also be on hand:

- •Infant blood pressure cuffs in 2.5 cm and 7 cm sizes (a detachable blood pressure gauge can be used with compatible cuffs)
- •21 and 23 gauge butterfly IV needles with at least 12 inch extension tubes; a 3-way stopcock that is compatible with the butterfly needles; 20, 40, or 60 cc syringe; and a 1.5 in, short-bevel spinal needle. Put these things in a box or resealable plastic bag and label it "pneumothorax venting supplies."
- •Infant airways in preterm and neonatal sizes (see the subchapter entitled "Selecting and Using an Infant Oropharyngeal Airway"). Also include several baby bottle nipples of different sizes and shapes with a large hole cut out of the tip. Put all of these in a resealable plastic bag marked "infant airways."
- •Infant feeding tubes in sizes 8 F, 10 F and 12 F; put these together in a labeled, resealable plastic bag.
- •Infant resuscitation equipment (bag-and-mask resuscitator, infant and preterm masks, additional masks to give blow-by oxygen and a neonatal nasal cannula if you practice in a moderately high altitude area.
- •The smallest long-handled, plastic-coated infant feeding spoon you can find (see the subchapter entitled "Clearing the Baby's Airway" for use of this item.)
- •A few small tongue depressors or new, wooden ice cream bar sticks.
- •Precurved (no stylet, no shoulder), endotracheal tubes in sizes 2.5, 3 and 3.5 ml and/or a laryngeal mask airway
- •Two dozen or so Telfa™ nonadherent dressings (any brand of nonwicking, absorbent, nonadherent, lint-free dressing will do)
- •Small unopened roll of clear, uncoated plastic food wrap
- •Three 36 in (91.4 cm) straps with velcro closures, or straps obtained from an outdoor supply house with click and cinch closures, and four 6 in (15 cm) soft cloth straps and 10 large safety pins. Put these things in a resealable plastic bag and label it "baby stabilization straps."

Most of these items will rarely, if ever, be needed, but you will be glad you thought ahead. Most of them are not expensive and will not require replacement. (Use of these items will be explained in the subchapters entitled "Complicated Respiratory Distress," "Externalized Organs and Neural Tube Defects," and "Birth Injuries [Other Than Cranial Injuries].")

Transporting Equipment: The Birth Bag

The birth bag can be anything that will work for you: a suitcase, a backpack, an old doctor's bag or a tackle box. Fabric bags designed especially for midwives are available on the retail market, or you can sew a bag yourself. What you select will depend upon how you want to organize and access your equipment and, to a certain extent, the environments in which you practice. For example, a suitcase allows you to store different types of items in labeled plastic freezer boxes (such as those made by TupperWare or Rubbermaid). Each box can have a label with a header such as "Baby Care Equipment" and an inventory of items that the box contains. This system makes it easy for someone unfamiliar with midwifery equipment to go to your bag and pull out a designated box. It also allows you to easily inventory items in each box as you reorganize your birth kit after the birth, when you are tired. A bag with pockets allows you to assign each pocket to a specific type of tool, so you and your assistants know where it is. Some bags can be opened and hung from a door knob or dresser drawer, revealing pockets with equipment ready to use. This setup is ideal for someone who often attends births in small spaces where it is hard to take equipment out and set it up in the birth room. Give some thought as to what system will work best for you. Check housewares, hardware and sporting goods sections at the store for containers. Ask to see the birth bags of other midwives to get ideas.

A Note to Students

Your head is, no doubt, reeling by now as you contemplate this vast list of supplies and equipment. While I have tried to break down these items according to those that are most useful and those seldom required, it may help immensely to talk to other midwives, your mentor or instructors at school and other students about what you need to start out. Generally speaking, buy the most used equipment first. Make do with items that can be borrowed from the parents rather than investing in common household items, such as a crock pot, right away. Look over the list and decide on which rarely needed and specialty items you might want to get first; for example, you might decide to purchase most of the inexpensive little items (such as rulers to measure the placenta and a coated baby spoon) just because they are cheap, even though you may rarely need them. Wait on cameras and the more expensive, exotic tools until you get more of a feel for clinical practice and can decide if they make sense for you to buy, given your practice setting and your clinical style.

POSITIONING-ASSIST EQUIPMENT AND MATERNAL COMFORT ITEMS

When birth takes place in a private environment, and the mother's feelings of security are fostered, she often gives birth quickly and easily, and birthing-assist equipment is nothing more than extraneous paraphernalia. Nevertheless, recognizing that anything can happen, many midwives carry a variety of tools. Survey the available tools and then figure out which, if any, seem right for your practice. When such an item is needed, it can be very useful in helping a woman sustain a position or activity that allows the birth to proceed. Where to get each of these items is included in the chapter at the end of the text entitled "Product, Equipment and Educational Resources."

Birthing stools

For millennia, midwives have used a variety of specialized furniture fashioned specifically to assist women in maintaining positions that are intended to make birth easier. They typically feature a place for the mother to rest her bottom with room to spread her legs wide apart while maintaining an upright position. Some provide back support. There are a number of popular birthing stools and chairs on the market; however, many designs require the mother to sit, placing pressure on the sacrum, thereby canceling the benefit afforded by supporting the mother in an upright position.

The deBy birthing stool is a notable exception to this trend. The creation of Conny deBy, a Dutch midwife, it provides a wide, U-shaped seat. When padded, the seat resembles a toilet seat with an open front and allows the mother to rest the back of her thighs on the sides, leaving her bottom suspended inside the "U." It is constructed of two U-shaped pieces of stainless steel pipe with three 16 in upright, open-frame supports also made of pipe; it weighs about 14 pounds. When evaluating birthing stools, sit on it yourself, if possible, to determine if and how much pressure is placed on the sacrum. A well-designed birthing stool allows the pelvic outlet to open, the sacrum to move freely and the midwife to see what is going on. Sutton and Scott (1996) recommend a drop of 18 in (45 cm) from the seat to the floor to keep the tuberosities above the knees and allow forward movement of the pelvis; the distance to the floor that is ideal for an individual woman will depend on her height, especially the length of her legs.

Ergonomic computer chair (kneeling chair)

These unusual-looking chairs have an angled kneeling pad and an angled seat. They allow you to sit with minimal back strain even though the chair does not have a back support. They also place the knees lower than the tuberosities and are therefore perfect to use when a woman is tired of standing and wishes to rest and keep her spinopubic angle open at the same time. One Scandinavian design has a rocker bottom, perfect for helping realign the baby.

Meditation cushion

Any new-age bookstore and many health food stores have these small, round cushions that are about 6 in deep and about 18 in (15 × 45 cm) in diameter. They are designed to lift the bottom off a floor or chair. They can be used to maintain a forward pelvic tilt when the woman is seated and are more portable than a kneeling chair.

The push-and-pull

Diane Holmes, an Indiana midwife, has designed a cane with a hook on both ends. This allows the woman to hold onto one end and a support person to hold on to the other to assist the woman in sustaining a full squat. It can also be used to support the mother's top leg in a side-lying birth. The Second Stage Enhancer tool, a variation on this design, features two large loop-handles connected by a chain.

Rebozo

A rebozo, or Mexican shawl, consists of a long piece of strong, soft cloth, the ends of which have long, silky fringes. A traditional garment of Mexican women, it is used as a baby carrier and in a variety of ways during pregnancy and labor. Rebozos come in various lengths, typically 27 × 82 in (68.5 × 202 cm) for an average size and 30 × 104 in (76 × 262 cm) for a large size. Although traditionally handwoven, they can be made out of any strong, soft, washable fabric.

Chin-up bar

These tension rods made for athletic use are designed to fit in a door frame. The bar makes an ideal thing for a woman to grab hold of when going into a full, semi- or standing squat. Additionally, a large rope or a doubled-up sheet can be tied around the bar to give the woman something to pull against during pushing. Remember that a doorway will be blocked when the bar is in use; therefore, think carefully about traffic flow when choosing which doorway to block.

The doorway of a large closet, having the mother face outward as she uses the bar, may be a good option in many home settings. A padded area or low stool can be placed behind her so she can rest.

Trampoline

Bouncing on a small, round trampoline can be used to help realign a baby who is coming down crooked. These trampolines are available at variety, sporting goods or exercise equipment stores.

Bean-bag chair

While the style went out long ago, bean bags make great support tools for use in labor. They can be moved fairly easily and can conform to the shape of the mother's body, allowing her to rest in various positions. Unfortunately, they are hard for the midwives to cart around. Although certainly not essential, if the idea appeals the mother, she might borrow one if she doesn't have one on hand.

Two wooden combs

Lovely wooden combs can be obtained in just about any city that has a large Asian market. Small plastic combs about two-thirds the width of the palm can also be used. The combs can be held by the laboring woman to stimulate acupressure points in her hands that help strengthen contractions. (See the chapter entitled "Using Comfort and Positioning Aids in Labor" for more information.)

Inflatable items

Birth (gymnastics or physical therapy) ball: These large, sturdy, inflatable balls hold up to 300 lb and are great birth accessories. The appropriate ball is determined by the height of the woman. When seated on the ball, her hips and knees should be at a 90° angle with the floor and her knees should be directly over her ankles. Large balls can be slightly underinflated to adjust to the woman's height. Penny Simkin recommends a 65 cm (29 in) ball as being the best size for most women. The ball should be inflated to the point that it still gives with pressure and rolls easily. Do not overinflate, as the ball may burst while in use. If in doubt, check inflation by marking the advertized height of the ball on the wall and placing the ball next to the mark to see if it is at or below that level. If a woman wishes to buy her own ball, she can determine her size with the table.

WOMAN'S HEIGHT	BEST BALL SIZE
Under 5 ft 2 in	53 cm
5 ft 2 in to 5 ft 7 in	65 cm
Over 5 ft 7 in	75 cm

(Perez, 2000)

An egg-shaped ball and a peanut-shaped one are also available to assist with squatting. Both are lower to the ground and have a limited range of movement (back and forth and up and down), offering the seated mother more stability. However, they do lower the tuberosities below the knees, so they must be used only when deep squatting is desirable.

These balls can be cleaned with soap and water or with the same types of cleansers used to clean hospital mattresses. Avoid using bleach, which hastens the breakdown of the plastic. They should be protected from sharp objects, heat, and other potential sources of damage. The Gymnastick or Pezzi brands are very sturdy. These may be obtained through a local hospital's physical therapy department or from a well-stocked children's store. They can also be ordered from Cutting Edge Press.

Beach ball: A regular kid's beach ball or a small therapy ball can be used to prop up the mother's upper leg when she is in a side-lying position. Note that a beach ball is not strong enough to support an adult's full weight.

Bath pillow: An inflatable pillow with suction cups on the back is easy to carry and provides considerable comfort to women reclining in the tub.

Inflation device: Save your breath by carrying a birth ball inflator, which can be obtained from ICEA.

Tummy lift

This labor aid was inspired by the book BACK LABOR NO MORE!! It provides a way for a support person or the mother herself to change the angle of her uterus during a contraction with a minimum of strain. It consists of a strip of padded cloth, 20 in long and 3 in wide, with two sturdy, looped, fabric handles on either end. The pad is reinforced by bands that run its length to form each loop at either end. The padded side of the lift is placed against the belly and moved up as the contraction builds, just as the mother would do with her hands. (See the chapter entitled "Entering Pains and Back Pain in Labor" for more details regarding changing the angle of the uterus.)

Birth Sling

Penny Simkin designed this padded cloth sling to allow a woman to be completely suspended during pushing. The sling, eye bolt, other accessories, an instructional video and a manual are included in the kit. Additional eye bolts are sold separately so the homebirth midwife can give, rent or sell bolts to her families, have them install them and bring her sling to use at their births.

Thermal packs

Cold pack: Penny Simkin, physical therapist, recommends the Dura Kold (DK 201) pack. This is a large, pliable cold pack with stretchy velcro straps and is available at athletic supply stores and Cutting Edge Press. Having two of these allows you to use one while the second one is chilling in the freezer.

Hot rice pack: A commercial hot rice pack, the Bed Buddy, can be found in many department and drug stores in the United States. You may also order Hot Soxs which are dyed attractive colors, from Cutting Edge Press or make your own by filling an adult-size athletic tube sock with 1.5 or 2 pounds of uncooked white rice. You can mix in some lavender flowers for relaxing aromatherapy. To prevent leaking, sew the top closed with several rows of stitching on a sewing machine. Other shapes can be made using washcloths sewn into pillows on three sides, filled with rice, and stitched shut. Have several, as these come in handy for simultaneous use on different regions of the body. The packs can be heated in the microwave or a regular oven.

Belly binder

You may want to have some long pieces of cloth on hand in case you want to bind a belly during labor. Suitable materials consist of long pieces of soft, light-weight fabric, such as a bed sheet or muslin. A rebozo can also be used. Make a belly binder by cutting a strip about 12 in (30 cm) wide and about 3 to 4 yards long. Sew one side of a wide piece of velcro to one end and hem all sides. Carry safety pins and the other side of the velcro fastener with you to the birth. You cannot attach the other velcro strip permanently because the size of the woman will alter how a strip of fabric will wrap around her, so you cannot know in advance where the loose end will need to be attached along the strip. Also select two large hand towels and two small bath towels to carry as well. The binder alone can be used for women with pendulous abdomens in labor. The rolled towels are placed along the sides of the uterus and held in place by the binder to function as splints to maintain a baby in a longitudinal lie.

As an alternative to this rather cumbersome process, Coflex makes a 5 yard elastic support bandage for veterinary use called Vet Wrap, which comes in a 2 in or 4 in width. It is available at most feed or farm supply stores in the United States and costs about $3.00. It has a reusable self-adhesive feature that would allow easy use as a belly wrap. Motherhood, Inc, also has available abdominal supporters that have velcro on one end and are adjustable to size.

TENS unit

TENS stands for transcutaneous electrical nerve stimulation. These devices are discussed in the subchapter entitled "The TENS Unit."

Bass musical instruments

Carol Gautschi of Port Angeles, Washington (2002), learned from a bass musician that bass sounds can stimulate a bowel movement. She has found that loud, deep vibrational tones help laboring women to release inwardly. Sometimes women hum a primitive tone that helps promote their altered state of consciousness. She has also found that playing a low toned didgeridoo can help promote release in the same way during labor and especially during pushing. The didgeridoo is perhaps the oldest known musical instrument of any kind and is a wind instrument of the aboriginal Australian peoples. A wealth of information can be found about digeridoos on the internet.

OSHA Regulations and the Disposal of Biological Waste

If you live in the United States and have employees, you are responsible for meeting Occupational Safety and Health Administration (OSHA) regulations to protect your employees from being exposed to health hazards on the job. Get a current list of those items that you must provide as an employer to meet OSHA standards (such as gloves of the proper size and a selection of materials for those who are allergic to latex; masks; eye protection; aprons; facilities and supplies for hand washing; first-aid items in case of needlestick or splatter of body fluid).

Small clinics and other midwives in your community as well as your local hazardous waste authority can provide information on how to dispose of waste items properly and on disposal services available in your area. Items that must be disposed of in specific ways include sharps (needles, Vacutainer tubes, etc.), disposable products saturated with body fluids to the point of dripping, and the placenta (if the parents do not wish to keep it themselves). Failure to comply with OSHA regulations garners penalties in the thousands of the dollars.

If you have no employees, you will have to decide how stringently you wish to abide by OSHA regulations; but you are not required to do so for your own protection. Nevertheless, you still need to dispose of potentially hazardous items in a manner consistent with minimizing exposure for anyone else who may need to handle them, including waste disposal personnel (aka garbage collectors).

References and Further Reading on Supplies and Equipment for Labor and Birth

Basic and Emergency Equipment and Supplies Used during Labor and Birth

Donn S, Faix R, eds. Neonatal Emergencies. Futura Pub Co, Mt Kisco NY, 1991.

Edmonds P, CPM, personal conversation, Feb 2004.

Miltex Co. Miltex Surgical Instruments. Miltex Instrument Co Inc, Lake Success NY, 1986.

Positioning-Assist Equipment and Maternal Comfort Items

Gautschi C. E-mail communication, 2002.

Perez P. Birth Balls: Use of Physical Therapy Ball in Maternity Care. Cutting Edge Press, Johnson VT, 2000.

Simkin P. "The Birth Sling" An Old Idea Revisited," VHS instructional video, Penny Simkin Productions, Seattle WA, 2003.

INTEGRATING YOUR PRESENCE INTO THE MOTHER'S SPACE

THE BIRTH ASSISTANTS

Note: This chapter builds on the information presented in Volume I regarding practice styles and those with whom you work.

Each midwife must grapple with whether she will bring other people to a birth and, if so, in what role or capacity. It is ideal to have two experienced midwives at every birth–one to attend the mother and one to attend the baby–plus an additional pair of knowledgeable, if not skilled, hands to assist in the event of a major problem. Midwives vary, however, in their inclination to work with other midwives, and if you live rurally, you may be the only midwife for miles around. In such situations, the role of your apprentice or assistant is extremely important.

Working with other midwives

Even two experienced midwives who attend births together will need to designate responsibilities so that, in a crisis, they do not resemble a clip from an old Keystone Cops movie. These roles need not be rigid and can be changed, if need be, in the midst of the birth. However, having an idea of who does what helps a lot and lessens the chance that essential care will be overlooked, especially when the midwives are tired.

Birth presents a natural division of tasks. It makes the most sense for one midwife to care for the mother and one for the baby. An apprentice can assist in both sets of tasks, and as she gains more experience, she can assume one of these roles under the supervision of a senior midwife.

If the mother has a preference to be attended by one midwife rather than the other, respect her choice. If she does not, you will have to decide who is best suited for which job. A feeling of particular affinity for the woman, or the possession of exceptional skill, may be the deciding factor. For example, if labor has been long and slow and a hemorrhage is more likely, the midwife who feels most confident handling this complication should attend the mother. When those attending the birth work smoothly together or have worked together over a long period of time, these roles are often selected with little or no discussion prior to or at the time of birth.

Beware of falling into a rut and never changing roles. It is important to allow all members of the practice to assume each role some of the time, so that skills remain well rounded. However, it is best not to change roles at the time of birth. In early labor, either midwife or an apprentice can listen to the fetal heart rate, take the mother's vital signs, chart or explain things to the parents; however, during pushing, when the energy of birth is intense, it helps the mother to know whose voice to focus on if she needs specific instructions. Here is a good idea of how to start assigning duties:

Possible responsibilities of the midwife attending the mother:

- Charts the mother's activities as soon as it is practical to do so
- Charts midwifery care as soon as it is practical to do so
- Observes mother during labor and pushing and assists only as required
- Offers verbal guidance to the mother, if indicated
- Ruptures membranes, if necessary
- Supports the perineum, if necessary
- Assesses baby's skin color as presenting part emerges
- Suctions baby while on the perineum, if indicated
- Deals with nuchal cord, hand, shoulder dystocia, etc.
- Assists partner in receiving the baby
- Receives baby, if indicated, and hands it to mother or to the midwife attending the baby
- Observes and assists with placental delivery, if indicated
- Monitors blood loss
- Performs tasks for the baby's midwife if she is otherwise occupied in a crisis, for example, calling an ambulance while the baby's midwife is performing resuscitation
- Examines perineum and places sutures, if indicated
- Performs postpartum care for mother and baby
- Steps in and helps with emergencies that the baby's midwife is unable to resolve alone

•Performs postpartum care for mother and checks the baby at the same time
•Helps tidy the mother's home and clean, repack and otherwise prepare birth equipment for the next birth

Possible responsibilities of the midwife attending the baby:
•Charts mother's activities as soon as it is practical to do so
•Charts midwifery care as soon as it is practical to do so
•Auscultates the fetal heart rate
•Makes suggestions according to FHR findings, such as maternal position changes, oxygen use, etc.
•Takes mother's vitals during active pushing, when indicated
•Assists with upper support in the periurethral area, if indicated
•Observes mother and baby immediately after birth and offers assistance, if indicated
•Takes baby from receiving midwife and assists mother in holding her newborn, if indicated
•Suctions the baby while still on the perineum, if indicated and the mother's midwife is otherwise occupied
•Performs tasks for the mother's midwife if she is otherwise occupied in a crisis (for example, while the mother's midwife is providing bimanual compression, the baby's midwife can prepare and administer natural remedies or drugs to stop the bleeding)
•Performs postural drainage or suctions fully born baby, if indicated
•Ensures measures are taken to keep the baby warm (drying baby, changing wet blankets, covering the head, etc.)
•Performs neonatal resuscitation, if indicated
•Talks to the parents about the baby's condition
•Assists the baby in latching onto the breast, if indicated
•Performs APGAR scoring at 1 and 5 minutes and as indicated
•Performs postpartum care of baby and mother
•Performs the newborn exam
•Steps in and helps with emergencies that the mother's midwife is unable to resolve alone
•Performs postpartum care of baby and assesses maternal status at the same time
•Helps tidy the mother's home and clean, repack and otherwise prepare birth equipment for the next birth

Once the birth is over, it is respectful to keep interference to a minimum, therefore the postpartum assessments of both mother and baby can be performed by one midwife at a time.

These lists are suggestions only and are intended to spark your own discussion of how to best work together. In the rare event that both mother and baby experience a crisis simultaneously, both midwives must be prepared to direct support persons and apprentices to perform other necessary tasks such as locating and handing them equipment, calling an ambulance or preparing a vehicle for transport.

Other aspects of labor care to discuss are policies and protocols for each type of birth situation and emergency, when to arrive during labor, hands-on versus hands-off approaches and when to consult or transport in various situations. Try to find out ahead of time those areas where strong differences of opinion exist regarding how to handle certain situations; perhaps one of you feels more comfortable staying at home in certain circumstances in which the other would transport. If there are personality differences or disagreements about practice style or protocols between you, these are likely to surface most abrasively during the high energy time of birth, especially if decisions must be made quickly. If you and your partner have had similar training backgrounds, this should help. However, just as it is hard to know how a woman will respond to labor, it is difficult to predict how another midwife will react until the stress is on.

Beware of pushing away good advice out of defensiveness or fear that you are inadequately trained. If your partner clearly has more experience than you or has skills that you lack, by all means take advantage of the opportunity to learn all you can. You'll not only be a more clinically competent midwife for it but will hone one of a midwife's most important character traits: humility.

Likewise, beware of choosing to work with a midwife who is obviously far less skilled than you or whose stated experience level does not match her responses at a birth. Listen to your intuition. If your partner has exaggerated her level of experience or training, it may not become apparent until you are working together under pressure during a birth. Regardless of how much you may like her as a person, do not let a dangerous or unskilled practitioner ruin your reputation as a midwife or entangle you in a tragic outcome that could have been avoided.

Finding a partner who is roughly at your level of skill and experience, with whom you communicate well both verbally and nonverbally and whose approach to practice closely matches your own is truly a blessing. It will serve you well at wonderful births as well as during close calls.

Working with apprentices

Apprentices can take on any of the tasks as outlined above whenever they are ready. However, when working with apprentices, you want to make sure you do not have unrealistic expectations regarding how much assistance she is able to offer. The pace at which information is incorporated and skills are developed varies among individuals. These differences do not, of themselves, reveal whether a particular person will make a good midwife.

A careful review of basic procedures with an apprentice before she attends any births will help her to be of optimal use. She should be familiar with the contents of your birth bag, how to set up equipment, and how to clean and repack equipment after the birth. Prior to attending any births, have apprentices go through your prenatal and birth bags at least once while you explain each item you carry and why. When relevant, show her how each piece of equipment works and is used. As well, make sure you know her background; an apprentice who has some formal training under her belt may know many basics, at least in theory. Nevertheless, make no assumptions; what may be obvious to you after years of experience may not be at all obvious to her. Walk through setting up at a birth while the woman is in early labor. A laminated checklist or chart describing or illustrating setup procedures may be helpful. Don't expect an apprentice to know or remember everything you told her about handling, setting up or using your equipment right away.

The first few times you give an apprentice a task, look over what she has done with her present to be sure all is in order or to remind her if she has forgotten anything. It is best to add tasks and skills one by one rather than expecting her to master several things at once. Ask your apprentice how she best learns and take this into consideration as you impart information. Remember, these things are quite routine to you, but she is integrating the experience of being at the birth on many levels. Don't expect too much, too fast. Once she has been to a few births, pass on some routine tasks such as charting, with your supervision.

Some apprentices are eager to get their hands in, while ignoring the other less glamorous aspects of being a midwife, such as cleaning up and staying centered in a crisis. Receiving the baby when the birth is going smoothly is really the least of what there is to learn. Be sure you are not being pressured by an apprentice to have lots of hands-on experience at the birth itself if you feel her overall comprehension of or interest in what is entailed is lacking.

Passing on tasks to an apprentice as she seems ready to expand her skills and responsibilities can be hard for some seasoned midwives. Seeing your student prepare to leave you and, at times, surpass you in certain areas can be difficult, but her skill is testimony to your good teaching. Likewise, it can be difficult at times to incorporate the input of an apprentice, but often a lot can be learned. Be respectful of your apprentice's point of view and welcome her fresh insights concerning your routines. Many apprentices go through a phase that could best be described as their "teenage" stage. During this time, they are evaluating your practice in light of how they plan to practice on their own. This is an ideal time to review the rationale for various aspects of your standard operating procedure. However, don't allow a cocky apprentice to jeopardize your relationship with your clients and don't put up with a know-it-all. Invite her to check out other apprenticeship options if you have trouble working together smoothly; it may be that you are simply incompatible.

Likewise, if you are apprenticing with a midwife whom you sincerely believe is practicing in a reckless or dangerous manner or who withholds vital information from you, remove yourself from the situation as soon as possible. Before doing so, talk with her in general terms regarding the procedures or techniques you believe to be a problem. Make sure you are not simply misinterpreting what you are seeing because of your lack of experience.

Here is an example: an apprentice with a solid theoretical background is left to labor sit a woman in moderately active labor in whom signs of infection become apparent (rapid fetal heart rate, fever in the mother). She immediately reports these findings to the senior midwife, who dismisses her concerns. Much later, the senior midwife reveals that she had given the mother quinine to stimulate labor and that the apparent signs of infection were really side-effects of the drug. She had not explained to the apprentice that the woman had received a drug, did not alert her as to what side-effects to expect and basically left her in the dark as to what was really going on, yet left her responsible to labor sit a medicated mother. This is a prime example of the type of dangerous situation I am advising you to remove yourself from as soon as possible.

Working with doulas

Midwives vary in their opinions regarding the role of doulas. Many feel that a midwife provides all the support a woman needs. However, others feel a doula offers a valuable service, especially when the midwife has a very busy practice. More about doulas will be discussed in the following chapter.

Issues that may arise with any attendants

Restimulated birth trauma: During labor, apprentices and primary attendants alike can have strong feelings that may relate to prenatal, labor or early infancy issues or their own labor experiences as mothers. Acknowledging this to your birth team is an important avenue to gaining insights, healing some of this past history and building a solid working relationship.

Keeping healthy boundaries: Birthing women want to know who will attend them at birth, and they prefer continuity of care. However, realistically, midwives are people too, with special events that are important to them, including vacations. To accommodate that you are only human, make arrangements, as much in advance as possible, for another midwife to cover for you in the event that a woman is due near the time of one of your special occasions. Have the mother meet this midwife in advance. Have a prearranged time that you will transfer care to the back-up midwife, even if that turns out to be in the midst of labor. Should this occur, call the other midwife so that she can arrive at the labor at least an hour or two before you must walk out the door. This will allow an overlapping time when you are both present together, allowing for chart review, giving the mother the security of continuity and you the security of knowing the woman is fully covered before you leave. Then, leave at the preappointed time, which should be planned so that you have time to ready yourself for the event or the trip without a frantic rush.

There will always be a few women who, because of a history of abuse or abandonment, will need the assurance of knowing exactly who will attend them at their labor; for these women, being able to depend on a specific individual with whom they feel bonded is a vital part of their healing and may make the difference in how they can open to birthing energy. However, in most cases, women can give birth with any competent midwife. It doesn't have to be you. It is, after all, the woman who is having the baby. Let go of any lingering notions that you are indispensable and enjoy your life. You deserve it.

Birth etiquette: As birth attendants, you and your apprentices know the most about what helps labor progress. Therefore you will not only be respecting those needs yourselves but serving as models for anyone else present. The birth room (the room where the mother is laboring) should be respected as sacred, private space. You are in the home of someone who is making love with the universe, truly a rare and privileged invitation. Casual conversation in the birth room, even if whispered, should be avoided. If prodromal labor is taking a while, those not directly involved in the mother's care should move to where conversation can be carried on out of the mother's ear shot or even leave the birth and be summoned by pager or phone (although I am personally strongly in favor of apprentices sitting out labors so that they learn to read the often subtle changes that reflect progress). One midwife or apprentice should stay in the room or near the door of the birthing room to monitor by listening, tuning into the energy and responding to any expressed or perceived needs of the mother. If a student wants to be there as well fine, but both attendants should make themselves as invisible as possible. Traffic in and out of the birth room should be minimal. Instruct others to knock gently or listen intently before entering the room softly and quietly if they must come and go.

Part of birthing etiquette includes respecting a woman's religious, ethnic and personal norms. On the way to the birth, remind each other of this woman's background and cultural context and be aware of household rules (such as removing your shoes on entering or the use of certain dishes for certain types of foods). These considerations should have been researched during prenatal care and reviewed at the prenatal home visit.

Discuss every birth: Be sure to discuss each birth shortly after it occurs. While it is fresh in your mind, review what happened, how each one of you responded appropriately, and what you could have done differently or more effectively. Even going over straightforward births will provide valuable information for you and your apprentice, as one of you may have a valuable insight that will inform the other. Many midwives have their apprentices fill out a birth log that includes a birth report and a list of what she has learned at each birth.

Take your apprentices with you to peer review, where they will learn many valuable things. It is helpful to hear other midwives comment on birth stories and to see integrity in action as midwives in a group setting discuss what could have been done differently at a birth. Hearing others discuss how to handle various emotional situations and unexpected problems that arise during labor will broaden your perspective as well.

When discussing births, everyone needs to be vigilant about respecting the confidentiality of information shared. Rumors, like wildfire, quickly blow out of proportion. Indeed, any formal peer review process should include a confidentiality policy. If everyone had a policy of not discussing a birth unless she was there or unless she is talking with someone who was, a lot of strife among midwives would be eased.

ARRIVING AT THE HOME OF THE LABORING WOMAN

Ours is a society in which women commonly give birth in institutions, where they are received and processed into a foreign and dominant system: the hospital. By contrast, the homebirth midwife enters the domain of the woman. This fact represents a fundamental difference in the midwife's approach to care during labor. The midwife is a visitor in the birthing woman's home and is, in essence, received as part of her extended family. The woman retains control over when the midwife is notified of her labor and when she invites the midwife into her own familiar surroundings, where her cultural context remains dominant. The midwife adapts herself to the woman's norms and must be sensitive to how her arrival and her presence affect the course of labor.

Once the pregnant woman or her support person calls to alert you that labor has begun, the decision of when you will arrive will be mutually worked out. Stay in periodic phone contact until either you or the mother feel it is time for you to join her. The timing of your arrival will vary, depending upon the mother's desire for your presence, her experience of labor, whether it is her first baby, what complications, if any, you feel might come up during early labor for this particular woman or baby, and the quantity and quality of support the woman has from her significant others. It will also be colored by your other obligations, such as appointments (which can, of course, be changed), other women who may be in labor and how long it will take to get to her home (taking into account such variables as the weather, traffic and time of day). Additionally, your style of practice prenatally, as well as your opinion regarding how much support women require in very early labor or prodromal labor, may influence when you arrive.

Once you and the mother decide it is time for you to leave for the birth, you will want to take all your birthing equipment with you. Labor may move at an unexpectedly rapid pace, necessitating all of your equipment, or you may need to go immediately from one birth to the next. You also may need to leave a labor in progress to attend another birth that is more imminent.

Sending an apprentice to labor sit

If you have other obligations, such as wrapping up prenatal appointments, that must be attended to prior to going to the birth, then sending an experienced apprentice ahead of you may be appropriate. First, recall this mother's particular emotional milieu (it may not be appropriate for every woman). If you think it is okay, then clear it with the mother. The apprentice to be sent should be sufficiently skilled to monitor labor, to oversee the basics of supporting maternal well-being, to check maternal and fetal vital signs, and to make recommendations to the mother. You must feel confident that your apprentice is able to recognize the early warning signs of a problem and will report any unusual findings to you immediately. Less-experienced apprentices should not be expected to take on responsibilities that they simply are not prepared to handle. To send such a person may not only result in early signs going unnoticed, but it may also undermine the confidence of the parents in your practice style. The parents hired you, an experienced primary attendant, for their birth, and that level of care is what they should receive.

Doulas

Doulas can be a wonderful asset to labor, particularly for women birthing in the hospital. If the parents have hired a doula, you should know when the doula is expected to arrive. If she is to get there before you, explain to her at what point you want to be called to the birth. It should, however, be primarily the responsibility of the parents, not the doula, to make sure you are called when the mother feels she wants you there. Doulas offer emotional and physical support, advice about comfort measures and position changes, and information concerning options during decision making (most relevant in the hospital since you will be discussing options in a home setting). Their training does not allow them to palpate the baby, assess the fetal heart rate, perform internal exams, check maternal vital signs or provide any other aspects of clinical care or advice. However, an experienced doula is often adept at reading the external signs of progress during labor.

A doula who attends one of your clients should understand your philosophy of birth as well as the woman's preferences. Ideally, the doula and your assistant or yourself should arrive at about the same time during labor. If the doula is present in prodromal or early labor while the woman awaits stronger labor, the doula, as well as the parents, can be instructed to call when contractions are spaced at a pace you designate (usually when contractions last 45 seconds, come at least every 5 minutes or when the mother first reports feeling any pressure in her pelvis).

Getting there from here

Generally, you will have already done at least one home visit during the prenatal period and will therefore know where you are going. If you have not yet had an opportunity to do a home visit, take a moment to sit down with a map and review your route before you leave. If there is any doubt, call the house and talk to someone to get accurate directions. This is a more efficient and safer plan than getting on the road and having to stop to ask directions along the way, or driving in a panic when a birth is imminent while trying to read a map or talk on a cell phone.

Aligning yourself with the task of midwifing

Before you get in the car, scan the mother's chart quickly to remind yourself of any special characteristics of her medical history or prenatal care. On the way to the birth, turn off the radio and center yourself by breathing deeply. Tune into the mother and her baby. Do whatever feels right to you to prepare yourself mentally, emotionally and spiritually for the birth. To some this may mean meditating, to others prayer, to others opening themselves to whatever information they may receive from spiritual sources about how to best help this woman and baby make this enormous transition. Prepare yourself to enter the sacred space of what Jean Sutton calls the "everyday miracle."

Easing yourself into the birthing energy

When you get to the woman's home, enter with as little fanfare as possible. The energies of birth are disrupted whenever new people, even the midwives, arrive at a labor in progress. It usually takes the mother a little while to settle back down into her labor. Bringing your equipment into the house and leaving it near the doorway allows you to enter quietly and unencumbered, able to observe both the mother and the setting (unless, of course, you think labor is far advanced and you need to set up quickly).

It is best not to rush in and immediately begin checking the mother's vitals and the fetal heart rate, unless you have been summoned to come now because of a suspected problem. These things can wait until you have had a chance to be there for 15 to 30 minutes or so, tuning into the situation, the mother and the feel of her labor. And remember, if the mother was checking into a hospital and there was no emergency, admissions procedures, shift changes and the like would often delay the first examination at least this long, if not longer.

Apprentice's arrival at the birth

If your apprentice has not gone ahead of you to monitor early labor, is very important for her to arrive at the birth when you do. Not only does this minimize the number of times the laboring woman must integrate the arrival of new people in her space, which is usually in the best interests of good progress in labor, but it gives you another pair of hands to set up as well as offering the apprentice valuable exposure to early labor. She is thus gaining an understanding of the totality of labor and has the opportunity to perform clinical tasks under your supervision. I believe midwives do their apprentices a great disservice when they only call them at the end of labor. However, there are always exceptions. If you feel that one more person will seriously disrupt a particular mother, wait to call the apprentice until labor is much more active; just don't make it your routine practice.

Setting Up Equipment and Preparing the House for Birth

Once the energy has settled after your arrival and you have performed your initial assessment of the mother and baby, you will want to set up the house for the birth. Some things are likely to be set up already. The contents of the birthing kit that you had the parents order and any additional supplies provided by the parents should be arranged as discussed at the home visit. Baby things will probably be laid out somewhere or at least gathered in one place. (Remember that some religious groups believe it is a bad omen to even purchase baby things prior to the birth. This is true, for example, of Orthodox Jews.) If supplies have not been taken out, locate and arrange these items yourself. If furniture has not yet been rearranged or other preparations have not been attended to, have the mother move to another part of the house temporarily so that the birthing room can be prepared. You will already have an idea of how you want things to be arranged from your home visit and may have given instructions over the phone to remind the parents what needs to be done.

If the mother is not birthing in water, the birthing surface should be firm and simultaneously accessible on either side by at least two of the midwifery care providers and one additional support person. Even when a waterbirth is planned, a suitable "dry birth" area should be prepared in the event that the mother exits the water.

Make sure there is appropriate food in the house as well as other necessities. If not and labor is early, send someone out now, if possible, so that folks won't be going in and out during heavy labor. When there are too many people hanging around for this point in labor, it is good to give them something to do away from the house.

Synchronize time pieces and hide the clocks

Rely on your cell phone for accurate times when recording activities and procedures in the labor record and to get the most exact time of birth, an important criterion if the parents want an astrological horoscope for their baby. All other time pieces should be synchronized and then put away, covered or turned to face the wall so that the mother can more easily enter the timeless altered state of consciousness conducive to birth.

Setting up your equipment

You will want to set up your equipment so that the things you use most frequently are at hand, the things you use for emergencies are taken out and set up discreetly but within easy reach and the things you use only rarely are accessible but still packed away. You do not want to transform the birthing room into a surgical suite. Make sure the logistics of traffic flow in the birthing room and the placement of your equipment are going to work and are portable, remembering that plans can change and the mother may not wind up birthing in that room. You will need a place to set up the equipment where it will not be disturbed, walked over by the dog or carried off by children. You will also need a place to put your birth bag, a location for the oxygen tank where it won't get knocked over (it can be placed on its side if you have a gauge that allows it), and access to the equipment you seldom use (such as an adult resuscitator).

How you set up your equipment is a very personal affair. Some midwives have birth bags with compartments that can be accessed when the bag is opened and hung from a dresser drawer. Others have tackle-box-type containers that can be opened and accessed on the floor. I set things up on two trays: on one I place a clean field (usually a new, Chux pad), over which I place the sterile field that the instruments are wrapped in or a wrapper from a package of sterile gloves. On this are placed scissors for cutting the perineum, cord scissors, a cord-clamping device, hemostats, and ring forceps. These are covered with another sterile field. Depending upon the size of the tray, sterile gauze, olive oil and toilet paper or facial tissue can be placed beside these, on another tray, or in a container.

Beside this tray can be placed another tray or container that holds your antihemorrhagic agents, such as Chinese and North American herbs, homeopathic remedies, drugs and syringes. Designate an assistant who will be responsible for drawing up a syringe if it becomes necessary. If no one who can do so is present, keep in mind that you may have to do this if the mother bleeds heavily after the birth and arrange these items accordingly.

In addition, you will want to set up a crock pot or similar warming device for soaking hot compresses to apply to the perineum during pushing. Fill it with filtered water, place it out of traffic, put on the lid and turn it on low. If you plan to use fresh ginger in the compress water, cut it up and put it in the water to gently steep during labor. Ginger promotes circulation to the area. If you use herbs for bleeding, boil some water and fill your thermos so you can dilute tinctures or powdered herbs in hot water, should the need arise.

Supplies such as Chux or towels that will be placed under the mother's bottom should be easily at hand and kept folded so as to keep them as clean as possible.

Setting up for the baby: Another area is set up for the baby. In most cases, any assistance that the baby needs after birth can be provided at the bedside or on the mother's chest. However, if the baby has a serious problem that requires full-scale resuscitation or transport, you will want a surface that is flat, firm, warm and portable on which to place the baby. This can be easily accomplished by preparing a baby tray. Use a breakfast-in-bed tray with foldable legs or, if one is not available, a cookie sheet or similar item that is large enough to support the full length of a term baby (at least 20 inches [50.8 cm]) and that is wide enough to eliminate worry about rolling the baby off the edge but not so wide as to prevent efficient resuscitation efforts if the baby must be moved while positioned on the tray.

1. First, place a heating pad on top of the tray.
2. Wrap the pad and the tray in a towel, taping the ends underneath the tray so they don't come undone.
3. Place receiving blankets on the towel-covered tray so they can be warming next to the heating pad. Place an infant stethoscope on top of the towels. Beside these place a bulb syringe and a deep suction device. Do not place instruments or suction devices directly on a heat source. A stocking hat can be kept handy, but need not be heated.
4. Plug in the heating pad and turn it on low or medium.

Near this tray, place another deep, flat, open container (such as a baking pan lined with a Chux pad or wrapped in a clean towel and taped) and place two infant airways (40 mm and 60 mm), a bag-and-mask resuscitator, a neonatal-and-infant-sized face mask, a space blanket and infant space bunting, a simple infant face mask for use with the oxygen tank, and a small bath towel to use as a bolster to stabilize the baby's head in a sniffing position if resuscitation is needed. If you have all these things in an easily accessible grab bag or box, so much the better. Just place it where it needs to be. If you ever plan to use an endotracheal tube, place it with these other supplies. If you do not have precurved tubes, form a curve in the indwelling wire through the packaging and place the tube in a resealable plastic bag and then in the freezer. Be sure to show the other birth assistants where you have put them. The cold will help them retain their shape during use (see the subchapter entitled "Digital Endotracheal Intubation of the Newborn" for details). If you do not wish to have them this stiff, place them with your other suction devices. Find the baby thermometer in the birth kit and place it with the other baby care equipment. Find and organize your rarely needed baby equipment, such as lint-free, nonadherent dressings and a bottle of sterile saline.

Laying out the most frequently used equipment on a tray and in a container makes it highly portable in the event that the mother moves from room to room in late labor or during pushing.

Cleanliness of linens and sanitary napkins: All linens should be freshly laundered. All supplies such as plastic backed absorbent underpads and sanitary napkins should be kept out of reach of pets and children but close at hand. They should remain wrapped or folded until ready to use. It is entirely unnecessary to sterilize sheets, blankets, towels, sanitary napkins, diapers and baby clothes; only things introduced inside the mother's uterus or bladder or baby's mouth need be sterile. If the membranes are intact and the mother is group B-strep negative, new, clean gloves can be used for internal exams. If the exam will require entry into the uterus (for example, during sweeping of the membranes), gloves should be sterile.

Setting up your oxygen: Prepare your oxygen tank for use as described in the subchapter entitled "Oxygen Delivery Devices and Resuscitation Equipment." Oxygen tubing should be attached to the port on the oxygen tank. A heating pad to heat the oxygen can be wrapped around the tubing and secured with clothespins (do not turn the heating pad on until oxygen is needed). The free end of the tube can then be attached to the oxygen port of a bag and mask or used to provide blow-by oxygen. A mask should be attached to the mask port on the bag. Both an airway and a tube for orogastric placement should be ready for use. You may want to do this in another room to avoid blatantly displaying medical equipment. Once it is set up, return to the birthing room, either placing the tank on a stand or laying it flat in a place where the gauge can be easily read by yourself or an assistant. One possible location is under a bed, with the gauge end out. It can also be wedged into a corner. The main thing is to put it somewhere where you can get to it easily but it won't fall, get knocked over or be kicked.

Setting up IV equipment: Hang or arrange your bag of IV supples in a discrete but accessible location in the birth room. Be sure to check the temperature where you plan to place everything, as the fluids will need to be at body temperature if they are to be used. Placing one bag of solution on a towel-padded heating pad set on low will gently warm it through the birth. Tape a thermometer to the top of the bag and cover it with an additional towel to hold in the warmth.

Setting up culturing supplies if an infection is suspected: If you know or suspect that the mother has an infection, or if membranes have been ruptured for some hours prior to birth and no prenatal group B-strep screening has been done, you may want to obtain cultures at the time of birth. If so, take out a sterile De Lee and three culturette tubes. These should be labeled now with the name of the mother, her birth date and Social Security number, as well as the source of the specimen. The two culturettes will be used to obtain specimens from the newborn ear canal and the fetal side of the placenta. One or two additional culturettes can be used to obtain a specimen from the maternal side of the placenta and the umbilical base if desired. To avoid mix-ups, use a highlighter or differently colored pens to indicate which tube is intended for which culture. The De Lee is used to obtain a sample of the baby's stomach secretions. Leave room on the labels to add the baby's name, time and date of birth, and the time the specimen was collected.

Make the bed: The bed is likely to have been made prior to your arrival. Many midwives advise parents to make the bed with a clean fitted sheet and top sheet tucked in all around. These are covered with a plastic fitted sheet or a plastic table cloth or large shower curtain. Then the bed is made a second time with old fitted and flat sheets to use during labor and the immediate postpartum period.

Preparing the birth tub: If this is to be a labor where water immersion is used, the birth tub should have been set up before you arrived. A sheet explaining how to do so is presented in a 2nd or later edition of Volume I.

Brew the herbal compress and herbal bath mixtures: Ask someone to oversee the brewing of the herbal mixtures for the birth. This is often a good job for friends or relatives. Water should be boiled in a large nonaluminum pan and taken off the heat. The herbs can be placed loose in the water or tied up in a piece of cheesecloth or one layer of a clean, old diaper or thin dish towel (to make a big tea bag) and placed in the water to steep for 6 to 8 hours or the duration of labor. See the chapter entitled "The Herbal Bath," for complete details.

Assign someone to monitor the environmental temperature

When you first arrive, the house can be kept at a temperature comfortable for the laboring woman. However, as birth draws near, the house should be warmed sufficiently to accommodate the more limited thermal tolerance of the baby. An apprentice can be assigned to adjust the temperature accordingly. Instruct her to ask where the thermostats are in the house and how they are adjusted or where the wood pile is in a home that has no electronically controlled heating system. She should also be responsible for seeing that drafts from open windows and doors are minimized at the time of birth. A space heater can kept handy in case it is needed then as well.

There is no thermal environment that is perfect for all sizes, gestational ages and conditions of newborn babies. What is appropriate for a term baby is too cold for a preterm baby. As a general rule, if term newborns are left wet and naked and have their cord clamped soon after birth, they cannot cope with prolonged exposure to a room temperature less than 87.8°F (31°C). In contrast, if the baby receives his full placental transfusion, he can tolerate a room temperature as low as 70°F (21.2°C) (Morley, 2002). However, to promote an optimal oxytocin level in both mother and baby, 80°F (26.6°C) or more is best. Eighty degrees is, of course, too warm for most adults. If the temperature cannot be measured, the guiding rule is that when adults (besides the mother) are slightly warm in short sleeves, the room is appropriately warm for the physiologically transfused baby.

Double-check emergency numbers and maps

Ask someone to check beside each phone to be sure that the numbers of all emergency personnel are in place. If not, assign one of the support people to prepare this list and double-check it before it is posted. Be sure the map to the hospital is with the birth supplies, and post it in some convenient place for review prior to transport. Also place a copy in the driver's seat of the proposed transport vehicle.

Partners, Friends and Family Members at the Birth

Read the chapter in Volume I entitled "Who Should Be at the Birth?" before studying this chapter.

Communications central

Unplug the phones in most of the house and have one phone that can be allowed to ring without disturbing the mother. Turn down the ringer on this phone, if necessary. A midwife, an apprentice or the woman's partner should answer this phone unless labor is very early or the mother is expecting a specific call. Otherwise, it is best to screen calls so that she can focus on her labor. It is best for the parents not to call every friend and relative they can think of to announce the onset of labor. While in some circles this may work out just fine, in many cases this produces a whole bunch of anxious people who will then call throughout labor to find out how things are going. If the parents have already called a lot of people by the time you arrive, enlist one of those present to report to the others regarding labor progress to cut down on calls to the house. Be sure whatever you tell this person is simple and straightforward, as news tends to get distorted as it is passed along.

Other people at the birth

Nonrelated guests and support people: Ideally, the parents will call you first when they suspect the mother is in labor. In most cases, it is best to postpone the arrival of additional people until you can get to the home, set up and assess the labor for yourself. At that point, a decision can be made about when to call whom and the best person or people to have in the house at that point. Women do not need an audience. Therefore, it is best to keep guest traffic to a minimum, regardless of how well prepared or well intentioned the guests may be. Factors such as the size of the mother's home, the availability of sleeping space and the logistics of the support people being able to entertain themselves without intruding upon the mother's privacy are important considerations when evaluating who and how many people should come and at what point. As people come and go at a birth, carefully observe the mother for changes in her demeanor as well as her labor pattern. While some disruption of labor is inevitable when new people come into her space, it often becomes obvious very quickly if someone should leave because labor has slowed down, the woman's pain threshold is lower or she is obviously distracted or self-conscious.

Related support people: It is much trickier to manage the comings and goings of relatives. If family members live nearby, you may already have asked about their house serving as an at-a-distance "waiting room" where friends and relatives can hang out while waiting for the baby. Keep them posted with updates every two to three hours. Try to call them before they call you, but be clear that you are involved in assisting the mother and cannot be calling every half-hour.

Partners: The woman's partner plays an important role in understanding the normal process of birth including the hormones involved, the woman's need for internalization and privacy and in holding an overarching belief that she can do it. It is likely that most primitive women gave birth without a partner present, therefore the role of the partner is new in our evolutionary experience. As much as possible, help the couple to understand that labor is primarily a mother-baby event and that the intrusive presence of anyone else can be disruptive, particularly during pushing and immediately afterward before the placenta is born (Odent, 1999, 2002). Many partners will feel excluded by these concepts, and some women may not grasp their importance. As well, each woman is an individual and some will be able to let go better with their partner fully involved. You must work with each couple to find a balance of partner involvement that is right for them and that affords the mother as much of what she needs as possible.

While much work has been done in the mainstream to make partners feel involved, often partner involvement is encouraged to the point that it distracts the woman from these basic needs. That said, the partner can help provide support in a variety of ways mostly by being a loving, intimate, unobstrusive presence for the woman. As for the specifics, you can model what to do for the partner and then step back and let him do it, only reinvolving yourself as needed to help them if he become confused or overwhelmed or it becomes obvious to you that something else is needed. This text assumes you will do this as appropriate. If you feel that he will be receptive, explain that being physically close to a laboring woman draws one into the vortex of energy coming through her, especially during late labor and pushing. Talk to him about channeling the energy in his own body (from the top of the head, through the center and out his feet to the floor).

Children at birth: Any children present should have a care provider whose sole responsibility is to look after them, taking them out of the house if the need arises. Children who have been well prepared for the sights and sounds of labor usually do well. If their own birth has been traumatic, however, being at a birth is likely to bring up fears and concerns for them; the child care provider should be aware of this possibility from prenatal conversations with you. Ideally, the house is large enough so that the children can remain at the end opposite of the one in which the mother is laboring. The mother's preferences should be the final word regarding the presence of children in the birth room at any time. If you arrive at the house and find that, for whatever reason, the designated care provider is not present and is not coming, do your best to recruit another person to fill this role. Meeting the children's needs is important for their future attitudes about birth and for the mother's peace of mind. Whether transport is required or not, someone will need to be responsible for the emotional and physical needs of the child; this person cannot be you.

Dealing with interpersonal dynamics

With any luck, most of the potential problems regarding support people will have been discussed, processed and worked out well before the onset of labor. However, this does not always happen for a variety of reasons. As well, unexpected guests do sometimes arrive on the scene. Furthermore, what was discussed during the prenatal period and supposedly worked out may present itself again during labor.

Nervous friends or relatives who have been invited and who understood about labor at home in theory may manifest some real fears as labor begins to unfold, especially if it does not move along rapidly. You can try to address their concerns, but keep in mind that most of these concerns probably stem from unresolved issues around their own birth experiences or those of their children. These types of issues will not be resolved by your kind and gentle explanations that everything is fine with the mother you are working with now. Be as positive as possible, but let them know that easy and safe homebirth *requires* maternal privacy and quiet and that you will let them know when things change or the baby is born. If their anxiety is still apparent, you (or the woman's partner) may have to politely ask them to leave. It is usually easier for you to be the bouncer, since you have some "medical" authority as the midwife. It is also less complicated for the parents from an interpersonal point of view.

Creating an Environment in Which a Woman Can Open Up and Let Go

The midwife's job is to guard the sanctity of the birth experience for the mother and baby. In doing so, you foster an environment that favors the natural process, one where birthing energy can flow, allowing labor to unfold gracefully, optimizing maternal and fetal well-being, minimizing complications and trauma and avoiding needless intervention. In her latest book, Ina May Gaskin (2003) explains her sphincter law concept. Noting that women in Western cultures tend to be most at ease relaxing other sphincters (anal, urinary) in private (unobserved), safe surroundings, she points out that the environment of birth should foster the same level of privacy and safety for relaxing the uterine sphincter (the cervix). Remembering, as well, the sexual nature of the birth experience, the environment needed is identical to that needed for a totally free sexual encounter. Use low lighting, keep the curtains or blinds closed, maintain personal modesty by replacing covers and clothing until the mother herself chooses to shed them. Minimize company from well-meaning support people and avoid obtrusive monitoring. The safer the mother feels, the less intrusive her environment, and the more sensitive her caregivers are to her emotional and psychological needs, the more likely it is that she will give birth without problems.

A peaceful, private environment decreases neocortex activity (the "smart" or intellectual part of our brain) and allows the midbrain and brain stem to dominate. These areas of the brain are the seat of the emotions and more primitive mammalian brain activities. The proper environment sets in motion the hormones of labor, which enhance progress, and endorphins, which help women deal with pain and enter the altered state of consciousness common to labors that progress easily and without complications. Immediately before, during and after birth, privacy allows oxytocin levels to soar, producing strong contractions that protect the mother from bleeding and allow her to fall in love with her baby.

When these environmental needs are met and the woman can allow herself to let go into her primitive, instinctive brain, where her knowledge of how to give birth resides, she usually does not require active support. She simply opens to the energy and has the baby. However, due to intensive cultural programming regarding the dangers of labor and the response to labor of individual women, some will require more active support than others in order to let go sufficiently to allow labor to advance.

Environments featuring bright lights, intrusive procedures, milling in and out by numbers of people, intellectual stimulation in the form of chitchat or a battery of questions, and strange sights, sounds and smells all work to keep the neocortex active and stimulate the release of stress hormones (catecholamines such as adrenalin, norepinephrine and cortisol). All these factors can contribute to a considerably prolonged and painful labor. Obviously, birth-inhibiting intrusions are most likely to occur in the hospital, but a house full of excited friends who have been invited to the birth can produce the same type of distraction. When an instinct is interrupted, it takes at least 4 seconds for the person to recover (Enning, 2003); if this is happening constantly during labor, it puts both mother and baby at a great disadvantage.

Not insignificantly, tension and stress influence how the woman perceives and responds to her experience. She may become more externalized, seeking to engage with her support people as she follows her female response to stress. She often begins to negatively interpret feedback from her care providers. High levels of stress hormones mobilize females to engage in specific protective strategies, including strengthening alliances and protecting self and offspring, the "tend and befriend" response; thus women can be easily led into interventions that they do not really want when stressed during labor. (For more details, see the chapter entitled "Ecstatic Birth: The Maternal Response to the Pain and Stress of Labor.") Stress causes blood to be shunted to the most vital organs, reducing blood flow to the uterus (and, therefore, the placenta), resulting in a diminished supply of oxygen to the baby, and, eventually, hypoxia reflected in abnormal fetal heart rate patterns. Uterine contractions slow down but may be perceived as more painful because catecholamine production interferes with the release of endorphins, which minimize pain.

Taking her cues

Be sure to ask the mother what she wants and what feels most supportive to her throughout labor. Just because she had a notion of what she wanted during her prenatal period does not necessarily mean that her ideas will match what she needs or wants as labor unfolds. Tune into where she is and respond accordingly. The more you learn to do this, the less you will feel compelled to examine and analyze her. For example, do not attempt to increase the strength of labor based on some arbitrary timeframe if she needs rest and the contractions have quieted down.

Let her know when things are going well

Labor is a tremendous unknown for every mother, but especially for a woman having her first baby. Your presence is reassuring to her, and sometimes all that is needed is your being there and a kind look, a nod of assurance, or a comforting, affirming nonverbal vocalization or even a hand signal (such as the okay sign or a thumbs-up), when things are going well. Not using words minimizes stimulation of her neocortex, thus facilitating the mother to let go to her primitive brain.

For women who require more definitive, verbal feedback, it is important to let her know what is going on from your experienced perspective. Each time you do anything to her (such as check her abdomen or the fetal heart rate), let her know when your findings are reassuring. "The baby sounds great." "What you are feeling now is normal." Do not elaborate on the clinical details or make specific predictions regarding how long labor is going to take. Offer general, affirmative feedback. This helps the woman stay grounded in a huge experience that can be quite overwhelming without skilled guidance and reassurance that what is happening should be happening. Your positive support will help to reduce her anxiety and to enhance production of the hormones that keep labor moving. If a woman is past early labor, avoid a long-winded dissertation on the academics of labor; this will only serve to engage her neocortex too much and hinder, rather than help, the process.

Let her know when things need to change

If you are concerned regarding the fetal heart rate or the mother's condition, you must let her know right away. This does not mean you must sound an alarm, unless the situation is suddenly dire, but you should tell her what your findings are and immediately offer suggestions of things that can be done, especially what she can do, to get things back on track. You need not belabor the technical intricacies of your concern, a simple "The fetal heart rate is a little slow; let's get you off this side and listen again" will be adequate to communicate such a problem. Only if things progress or persist would a more intellectual discussion regarding options and transport be warranted. Of course, as always, your choice regarding how to communicate must take into account the individual woman and her family. It will be obvious to you who requires more details than others for transient, correctable concerns.

Use hypnotic suggestion

Laboring women are exquisitely sensitive and therefore ripe to receive hypnotic suggestions. Use this to advantage with frightened or insecure women by explaining in simple terms what should be happening as labor progresses. For example, when you do something for the woman (such as massage her back), give her the suggestion that this helps her relax. Use phrases like "This contraction is melting your cervix away." Such suggestions should not be detailed, lengthy or technical but rich in visual and sensual imagery. They should be brief and to the point. Use a low, quiet, soothing voice. Speak in a well-modulated, even fashion; the more consistent your speech pattern, the more it will bypass her neocortex and speak directly to her subconscious.

Hypnotic suggestion can be particularly valuable during pushing as the baby is coming down, especially for women who have not fully entered into an altered state of consciousness. "The baby is rocking back and forth under your pubic arch, massaging your perineum open. The baby will crown, and the head will be born. The head will turn and we will wait for the next contraction to rotate the shoulders. The baby will come out and breathe right away." Once the baby is out, continue by suggesting a normal placental delivery. "You will continue to have contractions, and the placenta will detach and be born, then your uterus will clamp down, closing off the blood vessels that supplied the placenta." Remember that the subconscious mind does not hear negatives; it only takes active suggestions. The phrase "you will not bleed" is interpreted as "you will bleed" or simply "bleed." Therefore, make sure you use only positive phrases ("stop bleeding" counts as such a statement) which communicate what you want to happen, not what you don't want to happen!

Have faith in the process yourself

It is easy to get discouraged or doubtful when labor takes a peculiar or unfamiliar turn, especially when you lack lots of experience to back up an intuitive sense that everything is ultimately fine. Should this occur (and it will!), tune into your bodily sensations and take a reading of the birthing energy. Perhaps the mother is blocking it, which can be addressed. If you detect no such blockage, focus on the clinical evidence that things are fine while watching and waiting for signs that things either need to change or are once again flowing smoothly. Trusting birth is one of the most important things you can do as a midwife to ensure that each birth goes well.

Conversely, it is equally important not to be so starry-eyed that you miss obvious warning signs that something is truly not right. Pay attention to your gut reaction and pursue suspicious clinical indications of problems until you are satisfied that what is going on is not dangerous or, if it is, until it is resolved or safe transport has occurred.

References and Further Reading on Integrating Your Presence into the Mother's Space

Arriving at the Home of the Laboring Woman
Sutton J, Scott P. Understanding and Teaching Optimal Foetal Positioning, Bay Print Ltd, Tauranga NZ, 1996.

Setting Up Equipment and Preparing the House for Birth
Morley G, MD. Personal e-mail communication, 2002.

Partners, Friends and Family Members at the Birth
Odent M. The Scientification of Love, Free Association, London UK, 1999.
Odent M. "The first hour following birth: don't wake the mother!" Midwifery Today, (61);9-12, Spring, 2002.

Creating an Environment in Which a Woman can Open Up and Let Go
Enning C. "Birth on Demand," all day workshop on waterbirth, Midwifery Today conf., Springfield OR, March 2003.
Gaskin IM. Ina May's Guide to Childbirth. Bantam Books, New York NY, 2003.
Odent M. The Scientification of Love. Free Association Books, London UK, 1999.
Simkin P, Ancheta R. The Labor Progress Handbook. Blackwell Science, Oxford UK, 2000.

Monitoring Maternal and Fetal Well-Being during Labor

Record-Keeping during Labor

Keeping written records during the labor, birth and postpartum period is every bit as important as keeping good prenatal records. Recording activities and procedures when they occur allows you to assess what is helping and what is not, how long a problem is persisting or whether it is recurring, and to keep track of time (which can become distorted in long labors). You will be able to note patterns (such as contractions slowing down each time a certain person comes into the room) and discern subtle cues more easily when careful record keeping is the rule. Detailed records also provide valuable information for the mother in future birthing situations and if a question about your competence or style of care arises in the future. (This chapter assumes you know the basics covered in Volume I; review the chapter entitled "Charting and Record Keeping" before studying this one.)

Your birth record forms should be clear, designed for your practice and easy for others to read and understand. Pages should include spaces to record initial labor findings and ongoing labor notes. You should also have forms for postpartum care and newborn assessment. Fill-in-the-blank forms are not only handy, but become essential when you are tired and may overlook important components of care. You will also want to complete your statistics forms as soon as possible after the birth, when the details are fresh in your mind.

Record keeping during labor differs in some respects from charting during prenatals. You will probably not do full SOAP charting for each entry, since labor takes place during a condensed period of time. Commonly performed procedures can be charted as such, without detailing each step regarding how they are performed. For example, you can record "catheterized bladder: 500 cc clear, pale urine, trace ketones, all else negative."

However, when a problem arises, such as labor becoming prolonged, more careful notes are necessary to ensure that discussions of options and choices made by the parents are duly recorded. Labor can move along rapidly; if things are not recorded when they occur, the chances that they will be recorded correctly are slim. Make sure times and dates are accurate and avoid multiple entries of the same data by different attendants, which can lead to misinterpretations regarding the care provided if your records must be reviewed. Deviations from your protocols should be recorded and explained. This is particularly true if, for example, you recommend a course of action and the parents choose against it.

Use care when charting maternal responses, since emotions can run high during labor, and do not vent your own frustrations in the chart, unless it is clearly in the context of the situation. You might record, for example, "Mother refuses transport, wants to push another half-hour to see if she can get the baby out here. Explained serious concerns regarding fatigue and contraction pattern in relationship to history of postpartum hemorrhage." Quotation marks should used only when a direct quote is being recorded. Have the mother sign, date and time the labor note if you have a serious discussion regarding your desire to transport or an unforseen event or complication which has arisen during labor. Also record important phone calls or consultations with other practitioners during labor, keeping in mind the confidentiality of the client when communicating with other providers.

Record keeping is an excellent task to assign to a new apprentice who has observed a few births and reviewed enough charts to get a feel for the job. Her very first task might be to fill in the statistics form after the birth. Be available to answer questions she may have about anything that is unclear. She can take notes as she becomes more familiar with labor and your way of attending births. Double-check from time to time to make sure she knows what to write and to add your own notes, if necessary, to fully document any problems that have occurred. Keep in mind that an apprentice who has not witnessed a particular problem before will be absorbed in the experience and may not get down all the details. Be sure that each of you initial your individual entries in the chart.

Charting normal labor

In the best of circumstances, when all is well and the baby is born without any problems, the following things should be recorded, along with the time, date and initials of the recorder and the name of the attending (or examining) midwife. Always check to see what was written last before you start to make a note to avoid making duplicate entries; if you are uncertain regarding an entry, ask before you make your note. Duplicate entries later appear as though something happened twice, which can be problematic if your records are ever reviewed. Include the following:

- Telephone conversations with the mother or other parties prior to your arrival
- Your arrival

•Initial labor exam results
•Maternal vital signs, as indicated
•Fetal status, including movement and heart rate, as indicated
•Contraction pattern
•Status of the membranes
•Gastrointestinal distress (nausea, vomiting)
•Time of rupture of membranes, exact color of fluid, presence of particulate matter, amount and odor
•Excretory function
•Mother's emotional state and response to labor
•Food and drink intake
•Internal exam results, if performed
•Follow-up on questionable fetal or maternal status and results

Charting the fetal heart rate

The most specific aspect of fetal care during labor involves listening to the fetal heart rate. Initially, the fetal heart rate should be recorded with notes regarding the following:

•Concurrent uterine activity, such as the strength, duration and time between contractions
•At what point in relation to contractions did listening begin
•For how long listening was continuous and during how many contractions
•The position of the mother and palpated position of the baby
•The rate, rhythm and any changes noted in the FHR

Once the normal fetal heart rate pattern has been confirmed, periodically recheck as above. In the interim, a quick listen with a "sounds good" or a notation of the actual heart rate is frequently used to indicate that the heart rate is remaining within normal limits for that baby; this is especially handy during pushing, when prolonged listening is often not practical.

Charting other parameters

As labor progresses, you will want to record assessments of maternal parameters such as blood pressure or cervical status on internal exam, as well as the use of remedies of any kind, the mother's food and fluid intake, and bowel and bladder output (for example, "voided about ½ cup light yellow urine"). In addition to noting the fetal heart rate, you should record any other assessments of the baby, such as fetal movement or changing maternal position to correct the fetal heart rate.

Maternal position changes should be recorded, noting whether the mother spontaneously assumed another position or whether you suggested she do so. If the mother communicates things about her labor, note this in the chart and add your comments. (For example, "Mother says contractions are stronger. Contractions now 4 minutes apart, lasting 45 seconds, fundus firm at peak.") A note should be made in the chart at each change in the strength or character of the labor. It is good to make a note at least every half-hour even if there are no apparent changes.

Note when the mother's first bearing-down sensations begin and when and for how long she pushes effectively. This is very important because effective pushing is the only thing that births most babies. Be sure to properly record the resting phase of labor and the mother's activities at that time so there can be no confusion regarding whether or how much she was pushing during that period. If establishment of the urge to push is intermittent or delayed, be sure to record periods of nonpushing contractions accurately.

At the time of birth and immediately after make the following entries in the record:

•Length of time the head crowns
•Position of the mother at time of the birth of the head and if she changes position, the position of mother as the body is born
•Time of the birth of the head
•Position of the head at birth (OA, LOA, etc.)
•Appearance of the head at birth–any retraction? normal restitution?
•Progressive notes on appearance until birth of the body, such as color, grimace response and any other changes in the baby's appearance

•APGAR scores at 1 and 5 minutes (note why points were subtracted)

After the birth, note details regarding the placental delivery and the condition of the mother:
•Time of onset of contractions after the birth
•Blood loss between the birth of the baby and the placenta
•Characteristics of blood loss, such as dark red gush, trickle, intermittent, pulsing, clots, amount, etc.
•Position of the uterus before, during and after the placenta is born
•Time of placental delivery
•Mother's vital signs and level of consciousness

Vocabulary

It is important to chart things you can actually see or detect during a physical exam. Avoid using words that could be interpreted as diagnoses or medical opinions. Also avoid using terminology that is ill defined or suggests that you know what the problem may be, such as describing the baby as "asphyxiated," "depressed" or "hypoxic." Instead, report what you see: trunk pale, face purple-pink, slight movement in extremities. Record the APGAR score and note what you gave points for, but draw no conclusions on paper about what this might indicate. Write honest, straightforward notes in such a way that you would feel fine about having them reviewed by attorneys or government authorities unsupportive of midwifery or homebirth.

Charting emergencies

One of the most important aspects of charting during labor is to properly and completely record any problems that arise, especially unforeseen emergencies that cannot be thoroughly discussed with the parents prior to the need to take action. Prime examples of such crises are shoulder dystocia, postpartum hemorrhage and a baby in poor condition at birth. In addition to the notes described above, the following things should be reflected in the records of a woman whose baby has had a shoulder dystocia. This list can be modified to accommodate other types of problems and outright emergencies:

•Fetopelvic interactions such as retraction of the head, restitution or failure to restitute
•Decision to wait for the next contraction before intervening, if such a decision was made
•Position of shoulders
•The nature, timing and sequence of any interventions used to facilitate birth, such as:
  -Maternal position changes
  -Requests made of mother to assume a particular position or to push
  -Internal and external manipulations
•Appearance and care of baby at birth:
  -APGAR scores (1, 5 and 10 minute or more if indicated)
  -General appearance
  -Remedies given to baby
  -Resuscitative efforts (stimulation, oxygen, CPR)
  -Description of arm and hand movement, bruising, etc.
•Summary of any postpartum discussions with parents

For postpartum hemorrhage, you would record:
•Any remedies or drugs given to hasten the birth of the placenta
•Manual interventions used to hasten the birth of the placenta, control bleeding or both
•Amount of blood loss before, during and after placental delivery
•Estimated amount of amniotic fluid mixed with blood loss, if it proves impossible to differentiate blood from other fluids

Similar detail is relevant for any problem that occurs during labor, birth or the postpartum period. Additional things to include would be:
•Remedies or drugs given and maternal response
•Maternal vital signs
•Fetal heart rate during and between contractions during labor or vital signs of baby after birth

•Decision to transport
•Name, phone number and location of the person(s) with whom you spoke regarding transport
  -Time, date and length of the conversation
  -Topics discussed and parents' responses

Chart forms

The following initial labor exam form is taken from my personal chart archives. The second form, the "Labor Record," was inspired by the work of Yvonda Hedrick (1999), creator of a set of midwifery record forms that can be purchased for a one-time fee and copied for your practice. This labor record form offers many of the advantages of the partograph type of charting, without reducing labor to a standard curve. (See the chapter entitled "Product and Equipment Sources and Educational Resources" for information on how to obtain these forms.) You may want to enlarge this form to fill an 11 × 17 in piece of paper so that the boxes are larger. This can be folded in half, making it the same size as two regular 8.5 × 11 in pieces of paper. If it must be photocopied, be sure to copy both sides of the page and tape them together for the next practitioner.

The third form is intended for use in documenting additional details that you have no room to write on the chart. You can assign a reference number to each labor record entry that is linked to further details on the "Detailed Labor Notes" sheet. This reference number is entered in the left-hand column, along with the date and time of the note. Initial the detailed notes as well.

INITIAL LABOR EXAMINATION RECORD for____

History of labor prior to examination:

Date	Time	Comments

Preexamination observations: Time_______am/pm. Date _______ Place________________________________

Contractions every ____ min, lasting ____ seconds. Intensity______________________________________

Emotional state__________________________ Show__________________ Membranes ruptured? ______________

(Date_______ Time ______ Color of fluid _____________ Nitrazine test ____________)

Comments:____

Abdominal examination: Time______ am/pm. Date __________ Place _____________________________________

Fundal height _____ cm. Fetal position _____ Fetal motion ____

FHR (+) ___________/5 sec Variability _______ Placental sounds (o)___________________________________

Comments:____

Internal examination: Time______ am/pm Date ____________ Place ____

Show _______ Dilation ____ cm. Effacement ____% Cervical placement/consistency ______________________

Station ___ Membranes: Amnion _______ Chorion ______ Fetal position ________________________________

Comments:____

Maternal vital signs: Blood pressure_____ Pulse ____/min. Temperature _____°

Reflexes ______ Respirations_____/min. Hemoglobin _____ g last checked on _________________

Blood type & factor_______ Last bowel movement on ________ in the (am/pm evening)

Last full meal eaten was (breakfast/lunch/dinner/snack at ________ am/pm. on ___________.

Urine analysis: Color_____ Clarity ____ Protein ___ Glucose ____ Ketones ____ Pain ______

Difficulty voiding? ____

Labor record of ____________________ **Date**________________ **Page** ____ **of** ______

TIME/ DATE	MOTHER'S STATUS:		Contraction pattern			Internal exam				Vital signs				BABY's STATUS		OTHER FINDINGS/ SUGGESTIONS (remedies/meds/IV/etc. assign ref. # for detailed notes)	Initials
	Activity	Intake/ Output	Freq	Dura	Strength	S	D	E	Other findings:	BP	T	P	R	Activity	FHR		

Detailed Labor Notes of ______________________________ **Page ___ of ___**

Time/Date Ref. #	Notes/comments/elaborations/initials of midwife

ASSESSING AND SUPPORTING THE MOTHER'S WELL-BEING DURING LABOR

Assuming that you do not arrive in the midst of an emergency or when the mother is about to begin or is already pushing, you will be able to spend time getting settled and unobtrusively observing how the mother is coping with her labor. Tune into her response; is she resisting the energy or opening to it? Estimate how much progress has taken place; note the type of support she is receiving from whomever else is present and if it seems to be helping. Once the mother is accustomed to your presence, you can start to gently ask questions about how she is doing and what she is feeling. Try to avoid a barrage of complicated, technical questions, especially if she seems to be in active labor. Keep your questions short and simple, asking only what is really necessary.

Initial labor assessment

You will want to make an initial assessment of the mother and baby and follow up with periodic assessments, as indicated, throughout the labor and birth. Unless labor is obviously advanced, your first assessment should be done prior to setting up your equipment, to make sure setting up is warranted. Review the mother's medical and prenatal history, referring to her records as necessary and noting any significant history or prenatal findings that may impact either the mother or baby during labor or at the time of birth. Ask about the mother's level of energy, her emotional state and her perception of the baby's well-being.

Assist the mother in getting comfortable: Ask the mother to urinate; then have her arrange herself so that she can remain in the same position for the next 5 to 10 minutes as comfortably as possible. You should be able to access her belly for palpation as well as for listening to the fetal heart.

General physical condition, diet and elimination: Assess the mother's energy level. How long has she been "dealing with" contractions? (Which is to say, how long has she been focusing on contractions, breathing with them, etc.?) How much sleep has she had? What is her overall emotional state? Determine what she has been eating and drinking, if anything. If she has had any nausea or vomiting, or difficulty with urinating or in moving her bowels (either exceptionally liquid stools or constipation), take care of these problems sooner rather than later (see the chapter entitled "Nausea and Vomiting"). Removing all extraneous discomforts will give her more emotional space to deal with her labor. Remind her to urinate every 1 to 2 hours, as well as to eat and drink. Even a woman who has not experienced any nausea may sometimes avoid eating and drinking for fear that this will produce nausea (even if you have told her prenatally that this is not the case). Therefore, you may need to remind her that eating and drinking during labor are okay.

Assess the strength of contractions: Observe the mother's abdomen for evidence of labor-quality contractions (that is, does the uterus lean forward, become narrow on the sides and flat on the top with every contraction?). Palpate the fundus to assess the strength of contractions. To do so, press your fingerpads over the fundus between contractions and keep them there throughout a contraction. (See the chapter entitled "Abdominal Examination Techniques for Use during Labor" for full details on monitoring contractions with touch.)

Palpate for fetal lie, presentation, variety, attitude and position: Assess how the baby is situated and the volume of fluid while the uterus is quiet. If you have any doubts about your findings, perform an internal exam.

Listen to the fetal heart: Listen through at least two contractions beginning during the resting period between contractions and continuing through to the resting period after the second contraction. If you hear anything of concern, listen through several more contractions to ascertain whether there is a worrisome fetal heart rate pattern. (See the chapter entitled "Assessing and Supporting the Baby's Well-Being during Labor" for more detailed information.)

Assess any yoni discharge or bleeding: If the mother has passed any blood, ask to see any underwear, pads or tissue she caught it on so that you can see for yourself the amount, color and any mucus it contains. There is usually some intermittent bleeding that occurs as the cervix begins to dilate, particularly in first-time mothers. This is the most likely reason for blood to appear at the onset of or just prior to the time that labor began. This bloody show is a sign that cervical changes are taking place. Show that begins again in late labor as full dilation approaches is a good sign of progress. It occurs because small capillaries break as the cervix thins and opens. The amount of normal bleeding can vary widely and may, at times, be so copious that you must rule out serious causes before you can relax.

The bloody show produced by normal cervical changes is usually scant but at times can be thick, mucilaginous, gelatinous, stretchy (similar in texture to fertile cervical mucus but more copious), stringy or ropy, and medium to darkish red. Occasionally, it will appear dark brown and may at times have very small clots mixed in. A clump of mucus streaked with medium to dark red blood may be passed early on in labor but is often retained in the os until dilation has progressed and may come out all at once. It is often mixed with clear mucus from the cervix and appears intermittently. It is quite common for the amount of bloody show to increase when labor starts to progress rapidly or when cervical rigidity or scar tissue is broken up. Bright red streaks in otherwise mucusy show may indicate that cervical scar tissue is being stretched; more blood may indicate that the cervix is actually tearing.

Be on the alert for signs and symptoms that blood loss may be from the placenta or a torn fetal vessel. (For more information on bloody show and to differentially diagnose dangerous from benign bleeding, see the part entitled "Abnormal Bleeding during Labor.")

Passage of fluid: Ask about rupture of membranes and examine any linens used to catch fluids for color, vernix, quantity and odor. Try to differentiate light urine from amniotic fluid by smelling it and looking at it closely under good light. Sometimes it is very hard to differentiate the two, especially if the urine is very dilute. Urine left to stand will take on that characteristic "old urine" ammonia smell, which will not be present with amniotic fluid. (If you are not familiar with this smell, pick a day you will be home for a while, drink plenty of water, catch some of your urine on a paper towel, put it in a jar, and smell it at half-hour intervals.) It is also possible for some women to produce copious, clear yoni secretions near term that can come out in a gush and therefore mimic the passage of amniotic fluid. You can catch some drips on a piece of Nitrazine paper or swab or apply a sample to a Healthcrest Fertility Awareness Lens. (For more details, see the chapter entitled "The Placental Membranes and Amniotic Fluid during Labor" in this text and the chapter entitled "Rupture of Membranes before the Onset of Labor" in Volume I. Also see the chapters concerning identifying amniotic fluid in DIAGNOSTIC TESTS.)

Assessing maternal vital signs: Maternal vital signs are generally altered by labor. The extent to which this occurs is somewhat dependent upon the strength and length of labor as well as her emotional state. Additionally, a woman's carbohydrate metabolism rises progressively during early labor, as a result of both anxiety and increased muscular activity. This leads to an increase in temperature, pulse, respirations, cardiac output and fluid loss. However, the mother who is calm and centered will be less likely to display a major variation from her prelabor state than one who is more fearful or for whom labor becomes more physically challenging.

Here, the term "vital sign" is applied broadly to all of the following assessments. For an accurate assessment, consider the baseline established during late pregnancy when evaluating your findings during labor. When indicated, vital signs are assessed during labor in the same manner as during prenatal care. (Refer to the chapter entitled "The Physical Examination of the Woman" in Volume I for details about how to conduct each of these assessments.) The following is a review of each vital sign and its normal variations during labor. If and how often to check them is discussed at the end of this list.

Body temperature: A woman's temperature is slightly higher during normal labor due to the increase in metabolism, with the highest readings occurring during and immediately after the actual birth. Temperature normally rises as labor progresses but should not exceed 100.0°F (37.8°C). The rise is usually 1 to 2°F (0.5 to 1°C) above the woman's late pregnancy norm. (Keep in mind the normal diurnal fluctuation of approximately 1.8°F [1°C] in temperature throughout the day. The lowest value occurs in the morning and the peak in the late afternoon or early evening.) Temperature should never be assessed independently of other possible influencing factors. For example, an elevated temperature can be due to sitting in a bath that is too hot as well as dehydration or infection. Cooling or hydrating the mother should cause her temperature to return to normal after 30 minutes or so. Infection will also cause an elevation in temperature. A significant fever from infection may fluctuate somewhat but it will not normalize, regardless of what the mother does. No drugs such as aspirin should be given to reduce a fever during labor, as this will confuse the symptom picture. Aspirin also interferes with clotting.

The baby dissipates heat into the mother's system via the placenta during pregnancy and labor. The mother's body thus becomes accustomed to a reduced need to generate its own heat. After the birth, the sudden removal of the baby as a heat source causes an abrupt shift in maternal core temperature. In addition, the catecholamine surge during late labor contributes to the shivering that commonly occurs in women after they give birth, especially when the birthing room is not sufficiently warm.

Cardiac and blood pressure changes: The dilation phase of labor is associated with a progressive rise in cardiac output during each contraction. This occurs because the circulating blood volume varies rapidly during labor. It is temporarily increased by 300 to 500 ml as the blood that normally perfuses the uterus is displaced into the circulation as the uterus contracts and falls again when this blood returns to the uterine vasculature as the contraction tapers off. This results in a cumulative rise in cardiac output over the course of labor by 12 to 31% over the near-term baseline during dilation and up to 50% during pushing, leading to improved venous return and transient tachycardia. Supine positioning lowers cardiac output, increases heart rate and decreases stroke volume. Lateral positioning increases cardiac output and stroke volume while lowering the pulse. Cardiac changes are less dramatic when the mother is calm and relaxed. Epidural anesthesia appears to prevent the progressive increase in cardiac output (Blackburn & Loper, 1992).

Blood pressure elevations that occur during early labor see a rise of 5 mm Hg systolic before a contraction begins and a return to baseline after it ends. As contractions get stronger, blood pressure changes follow the same pattern and typically range from 10 to 20 mm Hg systolic (an average of 15 points) and 5 to 10 mm Hg diastolic. However, systolic pressure may rise as much as 35 mm Hg during contractions in some healthy women. The diastolic pressure can rise 25 mm Hg during first phase and as much as 55 mm Hg during active pushing. Pain, anxiety and fear also can cause a rise in catecholamine levels, with a corresponding rise in blood pressure due to an increase in sympathetic tone in the cardiovascular system.

There is normally no increase in blood pressure between contractions over a woman's late pregnancy baseline. Because of this, only assess blood pressure between contractions. However, if the mother is unduly stressed, fearful, apprehensive or angry, the blood pressure may rise between contractions as well. Expect women who demonstrate labile blood pressure when not in labor to have more pronounced fluctuations during labor.

Pulse: The elevation in pulse rate that most women experience during pregnancy will persist throughout labor and often increases slightly because of the increase in metabolism. The pulse rises slowly but progressively as labor advances but usually does not exceed 100 bpm. Once again, let prenatal values be your guide as to normal parameters for an individual woman during labor. The woman's pulse usually rises as a contraction builds and then drops back down to her pregnancy baseline as the contraction tapers off. There may be a drop in her pulse rate at the peak of a contraction if she is supine. The pulse will rise higher when labor is prolonged or when dehydration, hemorrhage, extreme pain, infection with fever or environmental overheating are present. The pulse may also rise in response to the administration of certain medications, especially those that inhibit contractions.

Respirations: During pregnancy the respiratory rate typically ranges between the normal nonpregnant average of 12 rpm or to as high as 15 rpm. The volume of each inspired breath is increased about 40% to meet the extra oxygen demands of pregnancy by the 7th week. The respiratory rate may increase slightly over the near-term range during labor. However, hyperventilation, characterized by dizziness and tingling in the extremities, is abnormal and may lead to alkalosis. It is difficult, if not impossible, to accurately count respirations during active labor, as women usually alter their breathing pattern in response to contractions. Therefore, counting maternal respirations is usually reserved for those situations in which the mother appears to be unusually stressed or in which a maternal complication is suspected. Respirations should return to normal after the birth. Painful or difficult breathing is a warning sign and may be associated with shock, amniotic fluid embolism, cardiac arrest, spontaneous pneumothorax or other physiologic crises. Thankfully, most of these events are rare in healthy childbearing women. Respiratory distress of unidentifiable cause that does not resolve quickly or that is recurrent, is cause for immediate transport.

Skin color and temperature: The woman's skin should be soft, warm, and dry with warm perspiration breaking out, especially on her upper lip and brow, as labor intensifies. Some women become hot and flushed as they work during hard labor and pushing. If her skin is bluish (cyanotic), pale, cold and clammy, look for causes of shock such as bleeding.

Dietary intake: For many years it was thought that gastric motility is so reduced during labor that digestion is virtually arrested. motility, the absorption of solid foods, and the secretion of gastric juices are only somewhat delayed, and gastric emptying time is only mildly prolonged over what it was near term. This tendency toward delay is enhanced by the use of analgesic agents. Gastric acidity rises somewhat. Fear and pain, as well as the ingestion of foods high in fiber and fat, also prolong digestion. The digestion of liquids is not affected by labor. A heavy meal may produce discomfort during labor, but it is important that women eat in order to keep their energy up. Soft, partially digested foods such as smoothies, cottage cheese, yogurt, kefir, and protein drinks, electrolyte-balancing fluids such as ReCharge and nourishing fluids such as miso soup, are good foods for labor. It is best to keep sweet foods to a minimum. Sugars tend to lower the pain threshold and cause more fluctuations in blood glucose levels (Stables, 1999).

However, women can and do eat all kinds of things during labor and should be encouraged to eat whatever nonsugary things they feel they can keep down, especially if nausea or vomiting have been a problem. If she only wants a sweet item, choose the most nutritious option and switch to less sweet foods when her stomach settles. As labor becomes more active and the woman more internalized, her desire for food will naturally diminish. This is not a concern as long as labor is progressing well.

Hydration: The mother should drink at least 4 ounces (half a cup) of fluid every hour during early labor, with a goal of 96 ounces (3 quarts or liters) in a 24 hr period. The woman's desire for fluids may decrease as labor becomes more active. This is a normal, hormonally mediated response and not a concern if labor is progressing well. However, women with long labors require periodic hydration. Dry mouth, acetone breath (which smells fruity or like an overripe apple) or urine that is concentrated, scant or dark are all indications that clinical dehydration is an impending problem. A rectal implant of fluids via a retention enema or an IV should be considered if the woman cannot keep down oral fluids. Nausea, vomiting and loose stools will accentuate dehydration, which will, in turn, trigger more nausea and vomiting. You must act to break this downward spiral. See the chapter entitled "Nausea and Vomiting" for details.

Urine production: This usually increases during labor due to a combination of factors, such as increased cardiac output, increased glomerular filtration rate and increased renal plasma flow. Women may test positive for ketones and often spill a trace to +1 of protein in their urine as a result of the muscular activity of labor or contamination from bloody show. If labor is prolonged, it is a good idea to test the urine every couple of hours or so. To obtain a sample for urinalysis, either place a placenta pan under the toilet seat, have the mother catch a random specimen in a paper cup or, at least, stick a urine dip stick in a stream of urine. The stream method is least desirable since it can easily become contaminated with yoni secretions, and the flowing urine tends to muddy the reagents on the stick, but it will do in a pinch. Minimally, use sticks that test for glucose, protein, ketones and specific gravity. See my text DIAGNOSTIC TESTS for a complete discussion of the meaning of these and other positive findings during labor. (Also see the chapters entitled "Protecting the Bladder during Labor" and "Understanding and Preventing Maternal Exhaustion" in this text for more details.)

Signs and symptoms of infection: Be alert for signs of infection during labor, especially in women whose membranes rupture early or who have a long labor. An elevated temperature, or persistent fetal tachycardia or both are often early signs of infection. As infection becomes more established, uterine tenderness, foul-smelling amniotic fluid and flu-like symptoms such as aches and pains may develop. Dysfunctional labor may be an associated factor. Take a woman's oral temperature if you suspect infection. If membranes have been ruptured for more than 10 hours, recheck her temperature every hour or two, being sure to wait at least 15 minutes after she emerges from a hot shower or bath before doing so.

The initial values obtained during the first examination in labor should be compared to any recorded during prenatals, taking into account the strength of labor and how hard she is working. If the membranes are ruptured, internal exams should be avoided whenever possible, which will help prevent infection.

Hematologic changes: Hemoglobin rises about 1.2 g/100 ml (12 g/l) during labor. It returns to normal prelabor levels by the first day after birth if blood loss has been within normal limits. Blood coagulation time decreases during labor, with a further increase in plasma fibrinogen above the normally elevated levels of late pregnancy. These changes reduce the risk of postpartum bleeding in healthy women. It can be normal for the white blood count to rise as much as 30 $\times 10^3/\mu l$ ($30 \times 10^9/l$) during the dilation phase of labor; however, you should rule out infection when the WBC rises over $15 \times 10^3/\mu l$ ($15 \times 10^9/l$). Blood glucose levels fall during labor, dropping quite a bit if labor is prolonged. More information on laboratory results can be found in my text DIAGNOSTIC TESTS.

How often should maternal vital signs be reassessed?

In the hospital, medical protocols dictate the regular assessment of blood pressure, pulse, temperature, respiratory rate and urinary output during labor as necessary components of care regardless of how smoothly or quickly labor may be progressing and regardless of how healthy the mother has been during pregnancy. This rote reassessment of maternal vital signs at frequent intervals is a product of fragmented prenatal care, protocols that are institutionally rather than individually based, and that labor is, in the end, still treated like a presurgical crisis in contemporary obstetrics. Routine assessments are intended to make up for no one practitioner on the hospital staff knowing the woman well enough to forgo them. This point must be emphasized when discussing the midwifery versus the medical standard of care with legislators and other regulatory bodies.

While at times it is advisable to regularly assess maternal vitals at home as well, how often this should be done and whether it is always necessary for a healthy woman who has demonstrated no problems during pregnancy is debatable. In fact, for a healthy woman who is involved in the intense work and altered consciousness of labor, taking a blood pressure is about as relevant or as helpful as doing so while she is making love. Multiple assessments tend to distract and medicalize a perfectly normal experience. Let the prenatal history, your initial labor assessment and ongoing evaluation of the mother's overall status be your guide. How often to reassess vitals at home depends upon what you know about a woman's medical and prenatal history, your current sense of the mother's and baby's well-being, and changes that occur during labor, such as rupture of membranes, changes in fetal movement or heart rate patterns, the onset of the urge to push, etc. Unfortunately, most state regulations do not allow for totally intuitive monitoring during labor.

However, if you are a relatively inexperienced midwife, having some sort of guideline regarding how often to reassess vitals, when it must be done, can be helpful. Start by checking vitals every 3 to 4 hours during early labor and every hour or so during active labor, depending upon the individual situation. This will help teach you the parameters of normal. As you become more experienced and your intuition and understanding of normal birth parameters becomes more refined, you will be able to forgo a rigid schedule and tune into each unique situation, assessing the mother as indicated, to the extent that the regulations in your local jurisdiction allow. Sometimes this means not assessing any vitals at all because you know the woman's prenatal history well, and her labor is moving along so smoothly and rapidly. At other times, it may mean checking as often as every 10 minutes if you or the mother have a concern. At still others, you may perform only one or two assessments throughout the entire labor. Listening to the woman and her labor, rather than rigid rules, will help you to know when a problem truly exists and lead you to respond appropriately. If you are in a situation in which you find you cannot tune in, where nothing is coming through, you can always fall back on scheduled checks.

ASSESSING AND SUPPORTING THE BABY'S WELL-BEING DURING LABOR

Labor represents work for both the mother and the baby. The baby cannot be seen and cannot communicate directly about how she feels, making ongoing clinical assessment of primary importance. When clinical signs cause you to question the status of the baby, palpation, scalp stimulation, or other means of prompting accelerations of the fetal heart rate can help clarify the picture. Whenever the mother is uncertain about the baby's status, you must rely on your own instinct and the clinical evidence at the time.

WAYS OF ASSESSING FETAL WELL-BEING OTHER THAN FETAL HEART RATE

There are six ways to monitor the condition of the baby: being aware of the connection between maternal and fetal well-being; acknowledging the mother's and midwife's intuitive sense of fetal well-being; paying attention to the mother's and midwife's awareness of fetal movement; assessing the amount and clarity of amniotic fluid upon rupture of membranes (discussed in the chapter entitled "The Placental Membranes and Amniotic Fluid during Labor"); once the presenting part is visible, monitoring the baby's skin color and monitoring the fetal heart rate, which, due to its complexity, will be discussed last.

Maternal Well-being Usually Equals Fetal Well-being

Always remember that the baby's well-being is directly related to that of the mother; what supports the mother almost always supports the baby. Providing the mother with a psychologically and emotionally calm and safe environment, keeping her well nourished and hydrated, encouraging position changes, and allowing her to rest when she can will all go a long way to supporting a healthy fetal response to labor.

The Mother's Intuitive Sense of the Baby's Well-being

Encourage each woman to tune into her baby's movements and her overall sense of how the baby is doing during prenatal care. By the end of pregnancy, a woman so instructed will know a lot about what is normal for her baby. In many cases, this type of attention fosters a highly refined intuitive link between mother and fetus. It can be very useful to ask a mother who has developed a strong intuitive link with her baby how the baby is doing during labor. This way of assessing fetal well-being is especially helpful if there are clinical signs that might indicate a problem, but nothing is definitive. In most cases, truly intuitive responses come quickly, with little thought and no analysis, and are usually accurate. If the mother is certain that the baby is fine, this is a good indication that all is well. If the mother is not certain or clearly states that the baby is in trouble, it is important to heed this concern, regardless of what the clinical signs indicate, especially if your intuitive sense of things also indicates a problem.

While the mother's intuition is a valuable guide to fetal well-being, be careful not to make a mother feel completely responsible for monitoring her baby. She may be in denial or just plain out of touch with what is going on, she may feel everything is fine when it isn't, or fears may cause her to think there is a problem when nothing is wrong. You must go by the overall feel of the situation when evaluating intuitive perceptions. Beware, also, of heeding the warnings of relatives or friends who may mean well but who may simply be frightened by the idea of homebirth. Hopefully, you will have addressed any fears they may have during the prenatal period; however, the intensity of labor can bring hidden fears to the surface.

Fetal Movement

One of the most tangible and easily monitored indications of fetal well-being is the fetal movement that occurs between contractions. The same quantity and quality of movement as that felt prenatally continues right up through labor in a healthy fetus with good reserves. The mother can often detect this movement. Ask her if she can feel the baby moving. If she cannot feel as much movement due to its having become subtler (because the intrauterine space is more restricted), you may be able to observe or feel movements that the mother cannot detect. Watch or palpate her belly for movement periodically during labor; this is an excellent way of keeping an eye on the status of the fetus. In some cases, movement will slow down as the baby descends deeply into the pelvis during late labor.

Note that fetal movement that occurs during the contractions of active labor may indicate that the baby is hypoxic. A series of sudden, rapid, jerky movements followed by little or no movement is an ominous sign suggesting that the baby has undergone a period of acute, severe hypoxia (such as might occur due to cord compression or placental abruption). Such movements often reflect last-gasp efforts prior to entering secondary apnea; the baby is likely to be in serious trouble or on the verge of death.

Skin color

Once the presenting part is visible, the color of the fetal scalp (or buttocks) offers a good gauge of fetal well-being and oxygenation. When the fetus is well oxygenated, the presenting part (usually the scalp) is pink to pink-lavender. Move the hair aside, wipe off any vernix or meconium, and observe the scalp in good light. A flashlight works fine for this purpose.

If the skin is frankly lavender or a slightly darker, bruised color, it may or may not reflect fetal problems. Edema, a caput in a vertex presentation, or bruising of the buttocks in a breech baby or of the face in a face presentation may confuse findings but if firm pressure is applied to blanch the cheek or buttock, some pink color should be seen as it returns to its usual shade. (Take care not to apply pressure to the eyes or genitals.) Return to normal color should take no more than three seconds. If fetal heart tones are also good, the baby is probably fine.

A purple hue can also indicate the onset of hypoxia. As moderate hypoxia develops, the baby's skin color becomes a fairly bluish purple. The heart rate may show variable decelerations at this point. As hypoxia worsens, the fetal heart rate becomes more variable and slow to return to a normal baseline after a drop. The scalp color progresses to a deep, inky blue. As lack of oxygen becomes severe, the heart rate slows and the scalp color becomes pale gray, lacking any pink color. The gray baby is in serious trouble, as a gray color indicates that circulation is not reaching the skin.

Skin that is very dark, or more white than pink, is an ominous sign. An increasingly dark color in a vertex presentation usually means that there is congestion in the baby's head from impaired blood return to the lower body. During pushing, this is likely to be due to a very tight cord or fetal parts pressing against the fetal neck. Once the head is out, a dark color may be due to a tight cord or shoulder dystocia. However, note that bruising alone can also cause the scalp to appear dark. A dark bruise may not blanch at all with pressure. A white scalp may indicate hypovolemia from cord compression, fetal bleeding, severe anemia, or absent fetal heart beat, any of which spell serious trouble.

If heart tones are somewhat slow, giving the mother oxygen can help them return to a normal baseline after contractions. Have the mother stop pushing to breathe oxygen through a contraction or two or after every pushing contraction, or change maternal position. Since fetal hemoglobin retains oxygen longer than that of adults, worrisome heart tones may appear before the scalp color changes. Good scalp color lets you know that the fetus has not been in prolonged distress. However, while a good scalp color is a reassuring sign, you must still act if heart tones begin to show compromise.

Whenever the skin color is questionable, be sure fetal heart tones are truly reassuring and that you are not listening to a flat baseline (i.e., lacking variability) or even to the mother's pulse. To differentiate the maternal from the fetal pulse, feel for the mother's radial (wrist) pulse as you simultaneously listen to the fetal heart.

When scalp color is alarming, transport if birth is not immediate. Lay the mother on her side or in whatever position maintains the best fetal heart rate and administer oxygen to her by nonrebreather mask at a rate of 8 to 10 liters per minute. Have her visualize her baby as pink and breathing normally when he is born.

The Fetal Heart Rate in Labor

Normal Exchange of Gases between Mother and Baby

The most important placental function is the exchange of circulating gases between the mother and fetus. Expanding gases exert pressure (expressed in torr or mm Hg). When two or more gases mix, the pressure exerted by each is referred to as "partial pressure." When moving across a membrane, the difference between the partial pressures of gases determines the directions in which they move. Gases move from a region of higher pressure to one of lower pressure until the pressure is equalized within the space the gases fill.

Diffusion of gases across the thin placental membrane is similar to that which occurs across cellular membranes in other organs; the main difference is that the exchange takes place between two independent circulatory systems. Fetal respiration occurs when oxygen diffuses from the mother's blood into the intervillous space of the uterine wall and then through the villous capillaries of the placenta into the fetal bloodstream. Carbon dioxide transfers in the opposite direction from fetus to mother. The flow of gases depends on their partial pressures in maternal and fetal blood and on unrestricted blood flow within the placenta, both of which help maintain normal pressures of the gases.

Oxygen transfer from maternal to fetal hemoglobin is regulated by the oxygen tension in the umbilical vessels, which is usually much lower than that of maternal vessels. Thus, oxygen moves from the maternal blood to fill the lower pressure space in the umbilical vein, and from here is distributed to the rest of the fetus. During labor, fetal oxygenation is likely to be disrupted. However, the fetus is adapted to compensate for low oxygen tension in the following ways (Tucker, 2000):

- The fetus' cardiac output, which is three to four times higher than that of a resting adult per kilogram of body weight, is based on the heart rate. Unlike adults, fetuses cannot increase cardiac stroke volume (the amount of blood the heart moves per beat), so raising their heart rate is the only means they have of compensating for a sudden lack of oxygen.
- Fetal blood has a greater oxygen carrying capacity due to a high hemoglobin count (compared to normal adult levels).
- Fetal hemoglobin binds oxygen more easily than adult hemoglobin. This means that the fetus has a higher capacity for oxygen saturation at the same PO_2 level as an adult. (For example, when the fetal hemoglobin is 15 mg/dl [0.15 μmol/l], the fetal oxygen carrying capacity is 22 ml/100 ml of blood, compared to an adult whose hemoglobin is 15 ml/dl [0.12 μmol/l] and whose oxygen-carrying capacity is 19 ml/100 ml of blood).
- The fetus has anatomical circulatory adaptations that direct blood to the placenta for oxygenation.

Similarly, the flow of carbon dioxide (CO_2) from fetus to mother occurs because the partial pressure of CO_2 in the intervillous space is lower than that in the umbilical vessels.

Maintenance of these pressure gradients and normal gas exchange are complex processes depending on many physiological and biochemical factors, including normal maternal blood gas levels and normal blood flow to and from the placenta. Fetal oxygenation also depends upon umbilical blood flow and the high affinity of intact fetal erythrocytes (red blood cells) for oxygen. In labor, intrauterine pressure increases during contractions and placental blood flow is slightly reduced–by about 2 mm Hg. At the same time, the intervillous spaces below the placenta retain blood to make more blood available for gas exchange. Accumulation of blood occurs because the uterine veins that drain the intervillous spaces constrict to a greater degree than the spiral arteries that supply them. Veins have thinner walls and are more easily compressed than arteries. This process apparently minimizes the impairment of gas exchange during contractions. Normal blood flow resumes between contractions.

Animal studies suggest that the normal placenta has a safety factor of about 50% of the uterine blood flow. That is, the uterine blood flow must drop to half its normal volume before oxygen uptake falls off and severe fetal acidosis develops. However, fetal compromise can occur during placental abruption of less than half the placental surface because of additional complicating factors that often accompany abruption, such as hypertonic contractions.

Cord compression, a marginally expanded maternal blood volume and problems with the connection between the placenta and the wall of the uterus (such as abruption), may all result in decreased oxygen flow to the fetus and lead to fetal distress in labor.

How the Fetal Heart Responds to Stress and Distress

The fetal heart rate arises from the sinoatrial node, a region of specialized cardiac muscle fibers supplied by the vagus nerve. These fibers normally act as the pacemaker of the cardiac conduction system, their intrinsic rate of activity being regulated by the sympathetic and parasympathetic nervous systems. Sympathetic stimulation increases the heart rate, and parasympathetic stimulation causes it to drop.

Since the fetus' sympathetic nervous system develops earlier than the parasympathetic system, the fetal heart rate is higher in early pregnancy, often ranging up to 180 bpm at 15 weeks and up to 150 bpm at 30 weeks. Continuous interplay between the sympathetic and parasympathetic systems accounts for the baseline variability of the fetal heart rate and demonstrates a healthy nervous system. Fetal circulation is dependent upon cardiac output and is directly related to the heart rate; thus, a fall in cardiac output results in a falling fetal heart rate. This is reflected in a decrease in baseline variability and a reduction in the amount of blood the heart pumps, thus lessening the amount of oxygen reaching the vital organs.

The fetal heart rate is modulated by other means as well. The region of the autonomic nervous system that regulates cardiac function is controlled by the cardioregulatory center in the midbrain. Chemoreceptors in the aorta and the midbrain are sensitive to oxygen and carbon dioxide tension. A drop in oxygen tension or blood pressure results in stimulation of sympathetic activity via the cardioregulatory center. This, in turn, prompts the release of adrenaline, which raises the heart rate, resulting in baseline tachycardia. Such tachycardia is not necessarily related to acidosis; however, prolonged hypoxia will cause the liver to release glycogen (stored glucose) as an alternative source of energy. In the presence of hypoxia, the glycogen is anaerobically metabolized, giving rise to the production of lactic acid and acidosis, which inhibits cardiac activity.

Labor produces for the baby a progressive state of mild hypoxia that the healthy fetus and placenta are well prepared to tolerate. A gradual decrease in fetal oxygenation occurs throughout normal labor. A transient fall in fetal oxygenation occurs with each contraction, reaching its lowest point about 90 seconds after a contraction peaks and normally taking another 90 seconds to recover. How long a baby can compensate for this relative hypoxia is dependent upon his glycogen reserves. The well-grown and well-nourished fetus will have adequate reserves to tolerate the intermittent reduction in cord blood flow that commonly occurs in normal labor. However, if oxygen levels continue to drop once the contraction is over, or if the fetus is unusually stressed or impaired, or if she enters labor with suboptimal reserves, cardiac output will fall due to a lack of oxygen, and glycogen reserves will become depleted. Fetal blood pressure will rise to compensate for this decreased output. Baroreceptors (stretch receptors found in the large aortic arteries) are sensitive to arterial blood pressure. These receptors trigger the vagus nerve, stimulation of which results in a fall in the fetal heart rate.

If the hypoxia is severe enough, vasoconstriction occurs, which redirects blood from the gut, liver and kidneys to the heart and brain, a protective mechanism to maintain oxygenation of these most vital organs. The early stages of this process are reversible. Less than 2% of babies with normal heart rates are acidotic at birth; only about 50% of those with severely abnormal heart rates have significant acidosis. Leaving the cord intact provides continued oxygenation and helps quickly reverse any acidosis that may have developed. Conversely, interruption of the placental transfusion by premature cord clamping at birth significantly impairs blood volume and prolongs any preexisting asphyxia. Asphyxia at the moment of birth (reflected in blood pH values) is therefore a poor indicator of nervous system damage. However, iatrogenically induced hypovolemia may aggravate hypoxia, resulting in significant damage once the baby is born.

Listening to the Fetal Heart during Labor

The basics of fetal heart rate assessment are covered in Volume I of this text. (Review the chapters entitled "Fetal Heart Rate Assessment and Locating the Placenta" and "Fetal Heart Rate Abnormalities" in Volume I before studying the material that follows.)

The careful assessment and thorough documentation of the fetal heart rate that you recorded during prenatal care will serve you well as you evaluate fetal well-being during labor. Since each fetus is an individual, your knowledge of the individual baby's heart rate is very helpful when contractions are added to the baby's environment. The following chart summarizes what you will be looking for. (Each of these parameters is covered in detail in this chapter with the exception of assessing uterine activity, which is covered in the chapter entitled "Additional Noninvasive Techniques for Assessing Progress.")

Preparing to listen

Have the mother empty her bladder. She may be unable to assume an ideal position for auscultation with a fetoscope; you therefore must become adept at listening with the mother in a variety of positions. This problem is eliminated when a Doppler fetoscope is used, but I urge you to reserve the use of a Doppler for those rare occasions when the heartbeat cannot be heard any other way. You will continue to hone your listening skills, avoid needlessly exposing babies to a technology not conclusively proven safe, and obtain more subtle information than if you rely on the electronic translation of the heart sounds through a machine.

ASSESSING THE FETAL HEART RATE DURING LABOR
Listen to the fetal heart periodically throughout labor. The following is the medical model guideline: **Early labor: every 30-60 minutes** **Active labor: every 15-30 minutes** **Pushing: every 5-15 minutes or after every contraction** Also listen after the mother makes major position changes, before and after any intervention, when uterine or maternal activity changes, upon rupture of membranes, and when otherwise clinically or intuitively indicated. Listen more frequently when a suspicious FHR is detected until the pattern resolves. **How long to listen:** From near the end of one contraction straight through until well after the end of the next contraction. Listen through two or three contractions, or as long as necessary to accurately assess the pattern. **What is the baseline rate (FHR between contractions)?** Normal: 110 to 160 bpm Tachycardia: >160 bpm Bradycardia: <110 bpm **What is the baseline variability?** •Absent •Minimal: undetectable to $\leq$ 5 bpm •Moderate or average: 6 to 25 bpm •Marked or saltatory: >25 bpm •Undulating (sinusoidal pattern) (Listen for several minutes if you suspect an undulating baseline or if you hear peculiarities such as skipped beats, abrupt rises or abrupt falls.) **Are there any significant variations in the FHR during or between contractions?** Accelerations: note associated findings (fetal movement or stimulation, uterine contractions, maternal hyperthermia or dehydration) Decelerations: Transient, early, late, variable: Reassuring decels: <30 to 45 sec, abrupt return to normal baseline with moderate variability, with or without shouldering Nonreassuring decels: >60 sec, slow return to rising baseline with absent variability, with or without overshooting Prolonged decelerations: >15 bpm below baseline, >2 min to <10 min Are they isolated or repetitive? Are they associated with late or variable decelerations? **What are the characteristics of uterine contractions?** •Frequency (time from onset of one contraction until the onset of the next) •Duration (time from the beginning to the end of an individual contraction) •Strength by abdominal palpation (mild, moderate, strong) •Resting period (time from the end of one contraction to the beginning of the next) **How is the baby generally responding to labor?** (movement patterns, fetal heart reactivity, color of presenting part)

Finding the point of maximum intensity

Once the mother is positioned as comfortably as possible, listen between contractions to find the region of her belly where you can hear the fetal heart most clearly. When the baby is occiput anterior, the point of maximum intensity is usually over the baby's upper back in the region of the anterior scapula. If the baby is posterior, it may be more to the side of the mother's belly or closer to the midline on the opposite side. When assessing where to listen, take into account that the best spot will move downward and rotate forward or backward in relationship to the mother's anterior midline as labor progresses and descent proceeds. These changes follow the rotation and descent of the fetus. Therefore, it is possible that you will have to reassess the point of maximum intensity, possibly each time you listen, if labor is moving along rapidly. You might find it helpful to track the location of the heartbeat by drawing a belly on the chart and marking the spot each time you listen. See Volume I for more details.

Try to find a listening spot that is not directly over one of the uterine arteries, which are located on either side of the lower to mid uterus. Be aware of the sound of your own cerebral blood flow in your ears as you try to listen, as it will obscure your ability to hear the baby. This loud pulsing sound will increase if your head is in a dependent position, which increases the cerebral blood flow. Listening to the baby is also more challenging when the placenta is implanted anteriorly. In this case, the additional sound of the swooshing of the placenta means you must really concentrate to hear the fetal heart during a contraction, when the placental sounds will be even louder. When the fetal back underlies the placenta, the point of maximum intensity may not be accessible to auscultation. Experiment with listening for an area where the fetal heart sounds are most clear between contractions. This will usually be over to the side, just past the edge of the placenta. Also try to find a location that allows you to hear the heart, not the cord. The softer, more diffuse sound of the cord will become obscured more easily during a contraction.

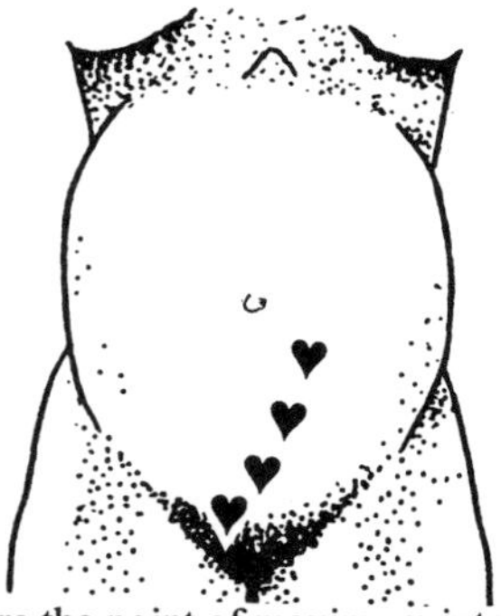

Where the point of maximum intensity moves during descent of a cephalic baby with the back in the left anterior quadrant

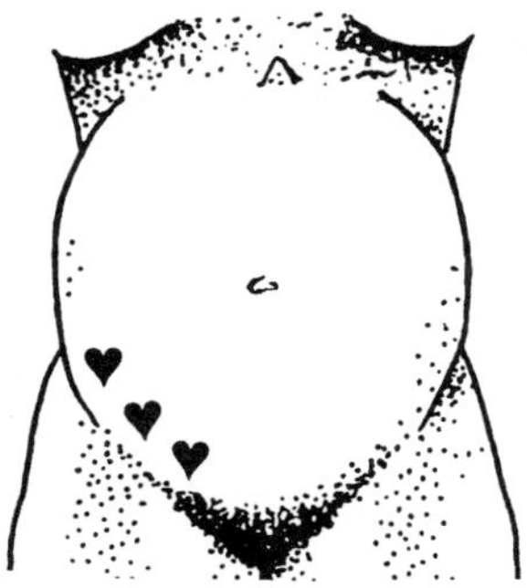

Where the point of maximum intensity moves during descent of a cephalic baby when the back is in the right posterior quadrant.

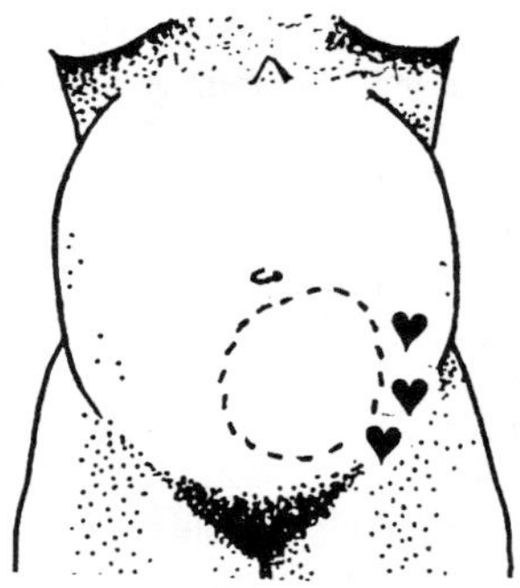

Listening past the edge of an anterior placenta (dashed line indicates borders of placenta); baby is LOT

How to listen in labor

Have a stop watch or a watch with a second hand readily available to keep track of each 5 sec count. Begin to listen between contractions, ideally as soon after a contraction subsides as possible. Press firmly into the abdomen if you are using a fetoscope with a bell-shaped head (such as an Allen). Remember to keep your hands or fingers off the headpiece of the fetoscope, as touching it will interfere with the transmission of sound and may result in a muscular "hum" from your hand that overlies and obscures the sounds coming from the uterus. Continue to listen through the next contraction, then for at least 30 sec to 1 min after it subsides completely. Contractions cause the uterus to become quite firm, and you will have to focus your attention to hear the heart continuously. Closing your eyes may help you focus as you locate the sound, although this obviously interferes with counting the rate.

During toning contractions and early labor, uterine activity tends to dampen the quality of fetal heart sounds, but the contraction itself produces no interfering sounds. As active labor kicks in, a soft, increasing, continuous roaring or rushing sound is heard as the contraction builds and peaks. This is similar to the sound you hear when you hold a spiral seashell to your ear, but it does not pulsate. The fetal heart sound will be behind the sound of the contraction, and will sound increasingly distant as the contraction intensifies. As a result, you may have to press the fetoscope quite firmly into the mother's belly to continue to track the heart sound. When using a fetoscope, you're hearing the roar of the contraction as it builds and peaks; this provides the perfect opportunity to assess the heart rate as it varies in relationship to the building, peaking and diminishing of the contraction, thus mimicking a primary function of an electronic fetal heart monitor.

If the heart is difficult to hear during the peak of the contraction, note that the heart rate patterns that are most likely to spell trouble are almost always detectable just after the peak or as the contraction subsides and thereafter. Listen as far into the contraction as possible, and remain in position so you can begin listening again as soon as possible after the peak and for 30 to 60 seconds after the contraction ends. When you note distinct discrepancies from one listening session to the next, listen more often, for a longer period, and through several contractions to better determine what is going on. When listening, be aware of whether the baby is moving in relation to contractions or not: movement during strong contractions often indicates hypoxia.

It is especially important not to confuse the maternal with the fetal pulse. If you are inexperienced or in doubt, palpate the mother's wrist for her radial pulse while you search for and listen to the fetal heart sounds. This is especially important if you suspect either severe distress or fetal death.

When an awkward position is required in order to locate the fetal heart rate, you may find that holding up a watch or a light to see the dial is difficult or impossible. If this happens, a good alternative is to hold the wrist of an assistant and tap out the heart rate with your finger while she does the counting. This is a very useful technique, especially when you want to communicate the rate and rhythm of the heart rate, but neither of you can record the information because both of you are occupied with the birth.

If the mother cannot tolerate your listening: Some women may complain about the amount of pressure required to listen to the fetal heart with a fetoscope during a contraction or about the positions they must maintain for you to be able to hear clearly. Try to find another place on her belly where you can hear the heartbeat so that she can arrange herself more comfortably; such an adjustment in the mother's position will usually resolve this conflict. If there are no signs of a problem with the baby, discontinue listening for a couple of contractions to give her a break.

In reality, women who are used to having you listen with a fetoscope throughout pregnancy very rarely complain about this during labor. When they have been informed that ultrasound's risks are uncertain, they are usually quite willing to do whatever it takes to prevent unnecessary fetal exposure.

How often to listen? This is truly one of the most difficult questions debated by homebirth midwives in North America. The use of constant electronic fetal heart monitoring during labor in North American obstetrics has fostered an atmosphere of hysteria and hypervigilance concerning the fetal heart rate, an attitude warranted only in very high-risk populations.

Although constant monitoring has become the unofficial standard, it has been shown to increase the use of interventions while failing to reduce fetal and newborn mortality or morbidity in low-risk pregnancies. Intermittent auscultation during labor, while popularly viewed as less than adequate, has been acknowledged as entirely adequate in the medical literature and even by ACOG. Underlying the hospital preference for electronics is the lack of the one-on-one nursing staff necessary to use intermittent auscultation with a fetoscope as well as the desire for printed documentation of the fetal status in the form of a monitor strip in case of later litigation.

This puts the home- or birthcenter-based midwife practicing in North America in a dilemma. If you are inexperienced or have mothers with whom you have not had an opportunity to build a strong relationship (and therefore feel less connected with the baby), you can always fall back on listening as often as is recommended in standard medical literature (Tucker, 2000):

Phase of Labor	Normal Labor	Difficult Labor or Risk Factors Noted
Early/latent	Every 30 to 60 min	Every 30 min
Active	Every 30 min	Every 15 min
Pushing	Every 15 min	Every 5 min or after every contraction

Whenever you undertake an intervention, such as artificial rupture of membranes or stimulating contractions, listen before as well as after the procedure. If your findings cause you concern, delay the use of any interventions until you are satisfied that the baby is doing well. If you have any reason to suspect fetal compromise, listen every 15 minutes or more often during active labor and during every contraction while pushing (as soon as you can hear). It is ideal if only one person is responsible for listening to the heart rate, as this reduces variation in the interpretation of what is heard. As a practical matter, however, this may be difficult; in such cases, thorough charting helps minimize discrepancies in findings.

The problem with scheduled listening is that the schedule can take precedence over your gut sense of what is needed and therefore can distract you from individualizing your care. Listening frequently when you are just learning is problematic because it can interfere with the development of these intuitive skills. To counter this, always try to tune into the baby before you listen, then see if your clinical findings confirm your intuitive impressions. As you gain more experience and develop your intuitive sense during labor, you can probably listen less often, depending upon the mother's activity, the strength of her labor and her stress level. Periodically ask the mother about her sense of fetal well-being and if the baby is moving normally. Normal fetal movement is a good indication that all is well. Use common sense. If a woman is napping, with mild, short, widely spaced contractions, and everything has been fine up until that point, you need not listen every 30 minutes. Instead, listen when she gets up for any reason or when more intense contractions resume. If contractions are coming back to back, if there is bleeding, if labor is prolonged, if there is meconium in the fluid, or if you have any reason to think that the baby is at increased risk (including an intuitive sense that things just aren't quite right), listen as frequently as necessary to determine if the heart rate is remaining within a normal range.

The Basics of Detecting Early Fetal Distress and Differentiating it from Transient Stress

Normal variability of the fetal heart rate is a hallmark of fetal well-being, indicating that the overall level of oxygenation is adequate and demonstrating the baby's ability to adapt to the normal oxygen fluctuations of labor. A healthy fetus can undergo periods of stress, reflected in changes in variability, baseline rate, or the appearance of periodic and nonperiodic patterns that are transient or that can be corrected by interventions such as maternal position changes, hydration and oxygenation. Fetal distress, on the other hand, occurs when hypoxemia progresses to hypoxia (decreased oxygen in the tissues) and acidosis.

Consider the fetal heart rate both independently and in combination with the length, strength and timing of contractions when the uterus is active. When evaluating the fetal heart rate, you assess four parameters: baseline rate, reactivity, variability and the association between any changes and uterine activity. Count the fetal heart rate in 5 sec consecutive intervals to gauge beat-to-beat variability. In general, fetal distress is very likely if the heart rate drops to less than 100 bpm during the first phase of labor, even if it recovers to a normal range before the next contraction. This is true for babies whose heart rates range within the average normal limits of 110 to160 bpm; there are, however, a small minority of perfectly normal babies whose heart rate is slower than 110 or whose upper range extends a little beyond 160. This is where careful prenatal records of the fetal heart rate, counted in 5 sec intervals and recorded as such, are invaluable in determining what is truly normal for a particular baby. Counting the fetal heart rate in 5 sec intervals should be continued and recorded as such during labor.

Electronic fetal heart monitoring has given us a specific way of thinking about and visualizing the fetal heart rate. The monitor simultaneously tracks the fetal heart rate and uterine contractions and charts each of them using parallel printouts on graph paper. The lower graph traces uterine activity, while the upper graph shows fetal heart activity. Viewed this way, one can readily see how the fetal heart rate responds to contractions, and one can detect fluctuations that create characteristic patterns on the graph paper. Electronic monitoring has also expanded the recognized types and degrees of fetal heart rate variations that may occur. These are reviewed below. All currently recognized patterns are included for completeness and to serve as a knowledge base should you need to transport the mother to the hospital, where she is likely to be put on a fetal heart monitor if she is still in labor, even though not all of them can be detected with a fetoscope or Doppler alone.

The examples of FHR patterns in this text use a stylized monitor strip. They are designed to give the reader a visual aid to understanding the concepts being discussed. They are not exact replicas of monitor strips and therefore only symbolically represent the timing of contractions and the strength of uterine activity. Spacing should be interpreted as proportional only: the closer the spacing, the closer the occurrence of the phenomena discussed; the higher the wave representing the uterine contraction, the stronger the contraction. Note that the fetal heart rate scale shown to the right of the examples changes depending upon what type of pattern is illustrated.

Fetal heart rate findings can be evaluated according to the following criteria:

Reassuring findings: Ideally, the fetal heart rate during labor should remain in the same range it was in during late pregnancy. In simplest terms, fetal well-being is demonstrated by a baseline heart rate that remains within the average range of 110 to 160 bpm, without tachycardia or bradycardia, with moderate variability around the baseline and the detection of short-term variability when using an electronic fetal heart monitor. The heart rate should be reactive, showing accelerations with fetal movement or stimulation, with no nonreassuring variable or late decelerations detected.

During active pushing, the heart rate may drop abruptly with head compression but should return to its normal baseline range within 5 to 20 seconds when the mother is not pushing.

Concerning findings: There is reason for concern if you detect a progressive increase, decrease or shift in the baseline fetal heart rate, tachycardia of 160 bpm or more, or decreasing baseline variability without an identified cause. A heart rate that repeatedly drifts down to 120 bpm or less immediately after contractions or that has a baseline that is gradually creeping upward into the 155 bpm range may also be of concern when these ranges are outside the normal parameters for a particular baby. (A discussion of the possible significance of these findings is included below.)

When you hear a heart rate pattern that leaves you wondering about the well-being of the baby, it is important to continue to listen to discover more about what might be going on. What you are hearing may be an isolated event of no clinical significance, or it may portend the development of periodic changes that reflect fetal compromise.

Nonreassuring findings: Distress is suspected if the heart rate is less than 110 bpm or more than 160 bpm, if a decrease of 20 bpm from baseline is heard following a contraction, or if the cardiac rhythm is irregular. Be alert for loss of variability; periodic or episodic changes, such as severe late or variable decelerations; a series of prolonged decelerations; severe bradycardia; or a true sinusoidal pattern. Any such changes can be associated with acidosis, which may be metabolic, respiratory, or both and which, when uncorrected, may lead to fetal damage or death.

Explore the overall situation whenever you hear a pattern that prompts concern. Do you feel intuitive forebodings or notice other clinical signs or symptoms that suggest something is amiss with fetal well-being? Listen through several contractions in a row, asking the mother to change her position as indicated. Once you have a good idea of what you are hearing, proceed with remedies discussed later in this chapter, and continue to listen until you are satisfied that the situation has corrected itself or until transport is accomplished.

Fetal Heart Rate Variability in Labor

Variability is defined as irregular fluctuations in the fetal heart rate and is a characteristic of a normal baseline. As is true during pregnancy, normal variability is the most important single indication of fetal well-being during labor. **Short-term variability (STV),** also called "beat-to-beat variability," refers to the variation in the interval between one heartbeat and the next. This is normally between 5 and 15 bpm, and usually ranges from 3 to 8 bpm. Short-term variability is evidence of an intact autonomic nervous system responding appropriately to nerve impulses. STV can be often be detected while listening with a fetoscope as a variation in the time between individual heartbeats, but there is no way to accurately record it without a continuous monitor.

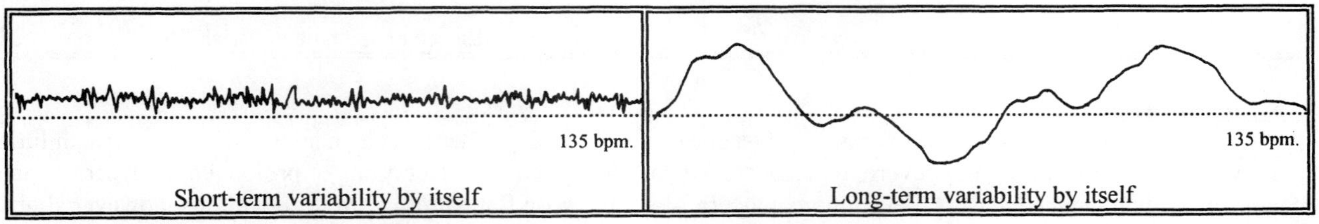

Long-term variability (LTV) is the rhythmical fluctuation of the heart rate during a 1 minute period. It is defined as the rise and fall of the rate, as well as the frequency with which the fetal heart rate crosses the imaginary baseline. LTV typically ranges from 3 to 25 bpm (or 3 to 5 bpm in a repeating cycle of 3 to 5 times per minute). It reflects adequate fetal oxygenation. Short- and long-term variability are usually considered together because they usually increase or decrease together. Instances when they change independently are described below. LTV can also be detected and will be reflected in a variation from one 5 sec count to the next. Variability may be classified according to the parameters discussed next.

Decreased variability

Diminishing variability is noted with:

- •Fetal sleep cycles (on average persisting 20 to 30 minutes and occasionally up to 80 minutes)
- •The immature nervous system of the extremely preterm fetus (less than 24 weeks gestation)
- •Hypoxia and acidosis
- •Uteroplacental insufficiency
- •Drugs such as narcotics, tranquilizers and anesthetics, which depress central nervous system responses
- •Congenital anomalies that affect the central nervous system, such as anencephaly
- •Certain heart defects

Fetal compromise should be suspected when fetal tachycardia accompanies a loss of baseline variability.

Loss of long-term variability: There is a loss of long-term variability when beat-to-beat changes around the baseline continue, but the long-term, rhythmical variations of the baseline between 3 and 25 bpm over a minute are lost. Most of the time, what appears to be a loss of long-term variability is really a normal reduction in reactivity due to fetal sleep.

Loss of short-term variability (wandering baseline): This rare pattern occurs when the range of variation is within the normal 110 to 160 bpm, but beat-to-beat variability is lost. It is associated with fetal anemia and occurs late in the development of fetal distress. When it persists, it is a very ominous sign, often noted prior to fetal death. Loss of short-term variability may be present when a normal baseline has been hard to establish. This type of fetal heart rate abnormality is the most difficult to detect without a fetal heart monitor in place. A wandering baseline with blunt, slow and irregular waves with a flat baseline may be associated with anencephaly.

DEGREE OF VARIABILITY	RANGE IN BEATS PER MINUTE (BPM)
Absent	Undetectable (no change)
Minimal	Possibly undetectable to $\leq$ 5 bpm
Moderate (average)	5 to 25 bpm
Marked	over 25 bpm

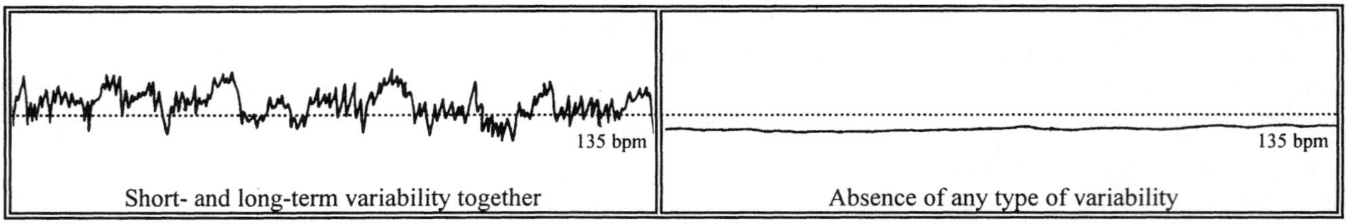

Short- and long-term variability together

Absence of any type of variability

Absence of variability

When both short- and long-term variability disappear, the heart rate pattern has a characteristic flatness with little or no variation. This is a sign of severe hypoxia. A flat baseline without decelerations or prolonged bradycardia may be associated with anencephaly. Of even more concern is an otherwise flat pattern with decelerations, however slight. A flat baseline with late decelerations and bradycardia is seen with severe neurological disorders.

Increased variability

Fetal stimulation and mild hypoxia may both increase variability. Maternal ingestion of stimulant or sympathomimetic drugs such as ritodrine and terbutaline can also cause variability to rise. At times, babies respond to mild hypoxia by temporarily raising their heart rate with a corresponding increase in short-term variability.

Saltatory pattern: This is a type of marked variability defined as rapid variations in the FHR, with excessive baseline variability of 25 bpm or more, producing a pattern of abrupt accelerations and decelerations that occur over the course of every 3 to 6 bpm. In a previously uncompromised fetus who had moderate (average) variability, a rise in stress hormones in response to a brief, acute hypoxic episode may result in the development of a saltatory pattern, indicating that the baby is compensating for early hypoxia. Shortly thereafter, the heart rate should calm down. This pattern may be noted during a period of bradycardia secondary to abnormally intense uterine activity, especially if the mother is pushing hard. It may be followed by more severe hypoxia if measures to decrease uterine activity are not successful (Van Geijn & Copray, 1994).

Reactivity

Reactivity is the type of variability that directly results from fetal movement or stimulation. The healthy fetus is constantly responding to his environment, and this response is reflected in a reactive fetal heart rate pattern. What may appear at first to be a problematic pattern may, in fact, be a perfectly normal response to activity or stimulation from an examination. Continue to listen to get an idea of what is really going on.

Decreased reactivity: When the fetus is asleep or the mother has received sedation or analgesia, the fetal heart rate temporarily loses reactivity. This may be confused with loss of long-term variability. When either fetal sleep or maternal drug intake is the reason for a decrease, the heart rate will return to normal reactivity after 30 to 80 minutes. Reactivity can be induced by several methods midwives use to stimulate the sleeping baby, such as palpation. Reactivity can be reduced in a fetus that otherwise shows normal variability in drugged mothers. The effects of maternal drug intake usually wear off as the drug is excreted, with a return of normal fetal heart reactivity.

Fetal Heart Rate Patterns You May Hear during Labor

There are three types of heart rate patterns you may hear during labor, all of which are described in detail below. These are the baseline rate, episodic, and periodic changes.

Episodic (nonperiodic or sporadic) changes: A fluctuation in the FHR that may occur at any time, unrelated to contractions. This means it may occur either during or between contractions but presents no predictable pattern of repetition. Episodic changes include accelerations and variable decelerations.

Periodic change: A repetitive fluctuation of the FHR that is consistently associated with uterine contractions and lasts less than 10 minutes; for example, early and late decelerations.

The baseline fetal heart rate during labor

The **baseline heart rate** is the normal heart rate for a healthy fetus who is at rest but not asleep, in the absence of uterine activity or stimulation such as loud noise, external palpation or internal exams. The baseline heart rate is determined by averaging the FHR when measured over the course of at least two full minutes (and preferably over a 10 minute period) rounded up or down in increments of 5 beats per minute. When averaging, exclude periodic or episodic changes, periods of marked variability and portions of the baseline that differ by more than 25 bpm.

Changes in the baseline rate: Any change in the heart rate that persists for more than 10 minutes constitutes a change in the baseline. A number of changes can occur; the baseline can rise or fall, which may or may not indicate a problem. Such a change may be transient or permanent.

Tachycardia: "Tachycardia" in a term fetus is defined as a sustained acceleration of the normal baseline to a rate of 160 bpm or more for 10 minutes or longer. Moderate tachycardia falls in the 160 to 170 bpm range; severe tachycardia is greater than 170 bpm. However, changes of 20 bpm or more from baseline represent relative tachycardia and may also reflect a problem. The high fetal heart rate increases the rate of oxygen distribution in the body. Moderate, uncomplicated tachycardia with good variability is not a problem, especially if the fetus is preterm (32 weeks or less).

However, when the baby is early (when organ systems are immature) or dysmature (of low birth weight) or whenever placental perfusion is impaired, tachycardia needs to be watched carefully to assure that other, more problematic patterns do not develop. Tachycardia may reflect hypoxia when reduced fetal motion, decreased variability, or prolonged variable or late decelerations, however slight, are also present. Transient tachycardia with diminished variability may also occur as the fetus recovers from an acute episode of distress that may initially have been associated with bradycardia. In this case, the heart rate should recover to its normal baseline with moderate variability. Baseline tachycardia may develop due to:

Fetal activity: Baseline variability is normal or increased in an active healthy baby. Accelerations prompted by fetal activity, most properly referred to as increased reactivity, may be mistaken as baseline tachycardia. Continue to listen until the baby calms down to see if the baseline returns to normal. Reactivity is an excellent indication of fetal well-being. Fetal hiccuping produces a short-term baseline increase.

Maternal anxiety and pain: Release of maternal catecholamines stimulates the sympathetic nervous system of both mother and baby. The result is an increase in both maternal and fetal heart rate.

Rise in maternal temperature: Dehydration or a hot bath can both result in a rise in maternal temperature, with a corresponding rise in fetal heart rate. Fever can also be related to intrauterine infection, a cold, the flu, a kidney infection, epidural anesthesia or prolonged labor in which the mother shows signs of distress, usually accompanied by an increase in both the maternal and fetal heart rate. Whenever persistent fetal tachycardia occurs, maternal infection should always be considered and ruled out as a possible cause. Changes in metabolism within the fetal myocardium can result in tachycardia up to two hours before the infected mother spikes a temperature.

Fetal infection and fever: Persistent fetal tachycardia may reflect an intrauterine infection that is not obviously affecting the mother.

Preterm gestation: A baby who is 32 weeks gestation or younger may develop baseline tachycardia due to immaturity of the vagus nerve. At 20 weeks, for example, a normal baseline range can be 150 to 170 bpm. The sympathetic nervous system is dominant in these babies, which can result in a persistently high normal heart rate.

Fetal hypoxia: Acute hypoxia or other stresses associated with impaired blood flow to the placenta can result in an increase in sympathetic stimulation, a rise in adrenal hormones (the catecholamines epinephrine and norepinephrine), or both. This results in a rise in heart rate, often in the high normal range early on, with a reduction in variability as the hypoxia persists.

Maternal hyperthyroidism: It is postulated that fetal tachycardia is prompted when long-acting thyroid stimulating hormones cross the placenta.

Fetal anemia: The fetal heart rate increases in the presence of anemia to raise cardiac output and improve tissue perfusion.

Drugs given to the mother: Parasympathetic blockers (such as atropine) or *beta*-sympathomimetic agents (such as ritodrine) disrupt parasympathetic and sympathetic control of heart activity in the fetus, leading to tachycardia. Recreational drugs often prompt the release of stress hormones, which can cause an increase in both maternal and fetal heart rates.

Fetal heart anomalies: The fetus with certain birth defects attempts to compensate by increasing both the cardiac rate and output, resulting in tachyarrhythmia; such anomalies may stress the heart to the point of failure.

Extreme tachycardia: The fetus cannot tolerate a heart rate that rises dramatically above baseline for long. Persistent, extreme elevation of the heart rate may lead to cardiac failure and is an emergency requiring transport unless birth is imminent. Extreme tachycardia can be divided into these types:

Sinus tachycardia: Defined by a FHR >160 bpm, this condition may result from maternal drug intake at term or infection. It is not necessarily a sign of fetal hypoxia unless seen with repetitive late decelerations, a lack of variability or both.

Supraventricular tachycardia (SVT): Defined by a FHR >200 bpm, SVT is the most frequently seen fetal tachyarrhythmia. Short periods are not significant. Longer periods are associated with cardiac output failure, nonimmune fetal hydrops, ascites, hydramnios and fetal death.

Atrial flutter/fibrillation: Defined by a FHR of 300 to 450 bpm; associated with a high mortality rate.

Bradycardia: Baseline bradycardia is defined as a sustained deceleration of the normal baseline rate below 110 bpm for 10 minutes or longer. Mild bradycardia (100 to 110 bpm) with good variability and no late decelerations is usually not a problem, especially in term babies. Some healthy postterm babies have marked vagal tone and may show a baseline bradycardia of 90 to 110 bpm, as do some babies who present persistently occiput posterior or occiput transverse.

Baseline bradycardia that accompanies any of the risk factors below can be particularly problematic if the heart rate drops below 100 bpm for more than 10 minutes. A rate below 80 bpm does not provide sufficient cardiac output and will result in asphyxia unless it corrects itself or is attended to promptly. Risk factors associated with a reduction in the baseline include:

Prolonged hypoxia: Persistent hypoxia causes the normal baseline to drop into a bradycardic range. Prolonged and severe bradycardia can also lead to chronic hypoxia. Profound fetal hypoxia depresses myocardial activity and lowers the heart rate.

Inadequate uterine blood flow: Problems with uterine or placental blood flow may be caused by maternal hypotension due to compression of the inferior vena cava, as well as a poorly expanded maternal blood volume, an unhealthy placenta, placenta previa or an abruption, any of which can lead to a compensatory drop in the fetal heart rate to conserve oxygen.

Maternal drug intake: Anesthetics may produce bradycardia because of a reflex response or as a result of maternal supine hypotension. *Beta*-adrenergic blocking agents (propranolol) block adrenaline receptor sites in the myocardium, permitting unopposed vagal stimulation, resulting in a fall in heart rate. Oxytocin reduces blood flow to the uterus during contractions.

Maternal hypothermia: This condition reduces fetal and maternal cardiac activity, lowers oxygen requirements and decreases heart rate.

Prolonged maternal hypoglycemia: This leads to fetal hypoglycemia and hypoxemia with a depression of cardiac activity.

Cord compression: Especially when prolonged, cord compression, or compression of a vasa previa, triggers sensitization of fetal baroceptors, resulting in vagal stimulation and a fall in the heart rate.

Fetal cardiac arrhythmias: When complete heart block is the cause, the heart rate may drop to between 50 to 90 bpm with no variability.

Amniotic fluid embolism (AFE): Bradycardia may occur by itself or be preceded by the abrupt onset of severe variable decelerations leading within minutes to bradycardia, a fetal heart rate response seen in all women who experience AFE prior to birth (Clark et al., 1995). Look for signs and symptoms of embolism in the mother (see the chapter entitled "Amniotic Fluid Embolism [Anaphylactoid Syndrome of Pregnancy]" for more details).

Relative bradycardia is any drop of 20 bpm or more from the baby's normal baseline. Its significance depends upon what the baseline is; if the baseline is well within the normal range and relative bradycardia does not push it into an abnormal range, it is an indication to watch the heart rate closely to see if it persists or has a pattern.

In general, bradycardia is a late sign of hypoxia, reflecting progressive acidosis when seen with periodic changes and decreasing baseline variability. When baseline variability is absent, especially for a prolonged period, expect current or impending fetal asphyxia which may result in neurological damage or death. Whenever a decrease in the baseline rate is noted, it is important to monitor for variability as well as periodic changes; also note how long these changes last from the onset of labor and whether they are transient or not.

Sinusoidal (si-nu-SOYD-all) pattern: This unusual pattern is most easily identified visually on a monitor strip; detecting it with a fetoscope will require careful, prolonged and experienced auscultation. It is defined as an extremely regular and smooth, undulating, repetitive pattern that ranges 30 bpm above or below the average baseline. It lasts at least 10 minutes, with 2 to 6 undulations of long-term variability per minute and shows little or no short-term (beat-to-beat) variability. The pattern is not correlated with the contraction pattern or fetal movement, nor does fetal movement result in heart rate accelerations. The extreme smoothness and regularity of the pattern distinguishes it from the changes produced by normal variability, which are ragged and irregular.

It is believed that this pattern, when pathological, results from cord compression or fluid build-up in the fetal peritoneal cavity (ascites), which impairs umbilical venous return. It has also been associated with hydrocephalus. The causes of a sinusoidal pattern fall into two categories:

Fetal anemia: A sinusoidal pattern is associated with fetal anemia resulting from Rh incompatibility, twin-to-twin transfusion or chronic fetal bleeding. In mothers known to be Rh-sensitized, the baby is usually anemic with a hematocrit below 30%. The presence of hydrops suggests a fetal hematocrit of 15% or less. Many severely Rh-affected babies do not display a true sinusoidal pattern but a rather rounded, blunted pattern without any accelerations.

Hypoxia: This may be indicated by an amplitude (range) of 20 beats or more and a frequency of 1 to 2 undulations per minute. This is suggestive of severe asphyxia and fetal anemia from fetomaternal bleeding (which can be confirmed by a positive Kleihauer-Betke test). It is an indication for immediate birth. Babies with a sinusoidal heart rate pattern due to hypoxia have a very poor prognosis, with a 75% mortality rate.

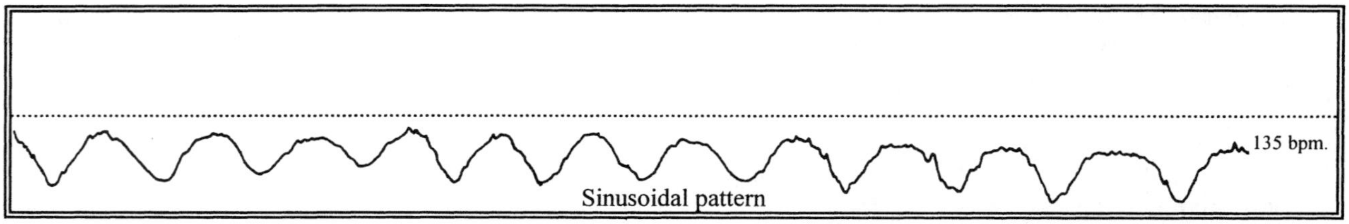

Pseudosinusoidal pattern: This is a benign variant of the above pattern; it is usually temporary and is not associated with poor fetal outcome. The wave pattern is intermittent, less uniform than a true sinusoidal pattern, and short-term variability is present. The pattern is preceded and followed by normal fetal heart rate findings. Benign findings do not usually persist for more than 20 to 30 minutes before the heart rate returns to normal variability. A pattern that meets these criteria, with no intervening periodic decelerations, is unlikely to indicate fetal compromise. The fetal heart often displays a pseudosinusoidal pattern after the mother is given narcotic or analgesic drugs, an effect that can be reversed with a dose of Narcan. Some practitioners feel that this pattern is also associated with fetal mouthing movements such as sucking.

Unless the pattern is clearly benign, consider all apparent sinusoidal patterns ominous until proven otherwise. If the pattern persists or the findings are unclear and the birth is not imminent, it is best to transport.

Episodic fetal heart rate patterns

Episodic (nonperiodic) accelerations: An "episodic acceleration" is defined as an increase in the fetal heart rate of 15 bpm or more that peaks in less than thirty seconds, and lasts for at least 15 seconds but less than two minutes from onset to return to baseline, and is unrelated to contractions. Episodic accelerations are determined in relationship to the most recently noted baseline rate. Most are not linked to uterine activity and are associated with average variability. Healthy episodic accelerations usually occur in response to:

- Fetal movement (reactivity)
- Fetal stimulation of any kind (reactivity associated with internal exams, abdominal palpation, scalp stimulation or environmental stimuli such as noise or voices)
- Breech or occiput posterior presentation

Accelerations in early babies: Prior to 32 weeks gestation, accelerations are defined as peaks of more than 10 bpm over baseline that last longer than 10 seconds.

Prolonged accelerations: A prolonged acceleration lasts longer than two minutes but fewer than 10. Any acceleration that lasts longer than 10 minutes represents a change in the baseline (see "Tachycardia").

Episodic (nonperiodic) decelerations: A deceleration is a temporary reduction in the fetal heart rate that lasts 15 seconds or more and produces a decrease of 15 bpm below the most recently established baseline. This term is also used when referring to any transient drop in the heart rate. Even slight decelerations, which drop less than 15 bpm, may be highly significant if repetitive or if there is an accompanying loss of baseline variability.

Transient decelerations: A single deceleration in the fetal heart rate is usually not indicative of compromise and is often related to factors such as supine hypotension in the mother. Stimulation of the baby via abdominal exam or during digital contact with the presenting part will sometimes produce a slight, very brief, deceleration, which occurs prior to a reactive acceleration. If the fetal heart rate returns to a normal baseline quickly once the stimulation is removed or when the mother changes position, there is no cause for concern.

Variable (Type III) decelerations: A fall in the heart rate that fluctuates and displays no consistent pattern or timing in relationship to uterine activity is called a **variable deceleration**. Variable decelerations represent the most commonly observed change in the fetal heart rate during labor. There is a decrease of 15 bpm or more below the baseline, often causing the heart rate to fall below 100 bpm, that lasts at least 15 seconds but less than two minutes from onset to resolution. Variable decelerations are characteristically abrupt; fewer than 30 seconds elapse from the onset of the deceleration to the lowest point. The heart rate then quickly returns to the baseline, with the deceleration typically lasting a total of 30 to 45 seconds. These decelerations are not necessarily repetitive, but when they are, the timing of onset, depth and duration varies from contraction to contraction. The pattern of deceleration also varies from occurrence to occurrence and may be described as either V-, U- or W-shaped.

There are two associated findings that may occur with variable decelerations:

Shouldering: This describes a pair of transient accelerations, the first of which occurs just before a variable deceleration and the second of which occurs at the end, before the FHR returns to baseline. Each instance of acceleration rises above the baseline and looks like a shrugged shoulder on a monitor printout at the beginning and again at the end of the deceleration. Each of these accelerations lasts fewer than 20 seconds. Shouldering is thought to reflect normal compensation for a transient lack of oxygen.

Overshooting: This phenomenon is an unpaired (singular) transitory acceleration that occurs at the end of a variable deceleration, prior to the return to baseline. Overshoots are associated with hypoxia. They usually follow moderate to severe variable decelerations, are accompanied by a lack of variability and persist for more than 20 seconds before returning to a baseline rate (which results in a rounded shape to the pattern of the acceleration).

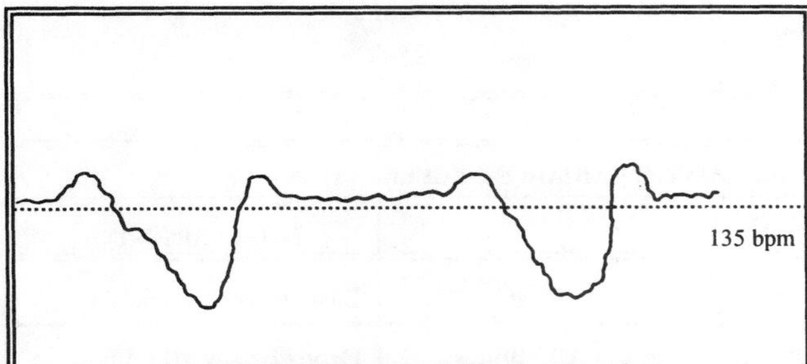

Shouldering with a variable deceleration

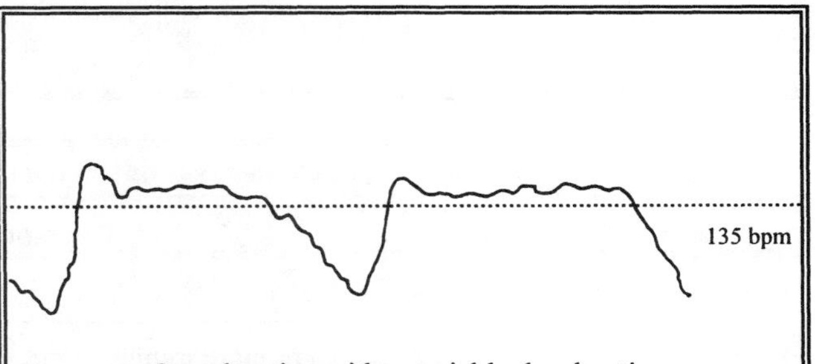

Overshooting with a variable deceleration

To distinguish shouldering from overshooting, you must listen carefully for an acceleration before the heart rate drops (the drop may take place during a contraction) and again at the end, before it returns to a normal range.

Many textbooks on fetal heart monitoring do not explain shouldering and overshooting very well. The definitions given here are based on those of the National Institute of Child Health and Human Development (NICHD, 1997).

Causes: Variable decelerations primarily result from any type of cord compression. Transient cord compression occurs during contractions in about 40% of all labors, and most fetuses can compensate for such brief periods of circulatory interruption between contractions. Persistent compression may occur due to more consistent pressure, tension on a short cord, a true knot, prolapse, entanglement or maternal position. Fetal movement in the presence of little to no amniotic fluid also frequently produces transient cord compression and variable decelerations. This type of variable deceleration is considered reassuring.

Mild variable decelerations: A mild variable deceleration occurs as a sudden drop to any level for less than 30 seconds with rapid return to baseline with average variability. While this pattern often reflects mild, intermittent or transient compression of the umbilical artery that does not compromise the baby, it requires careful monitoring to make sure it does not become severe. These decelerations are sometimes seen late in labor and with pushing because of stretching or compression of the cord as the baby moves down. Healthy babies can tolerate such decelerations if the total time from the onset of the pattern to the time of birth is short, if the baseline rate does not rise and if variability is maintained. This type of variable deceleration is considered a sign of well-being.

Moderate to severe variable decelerations: Variable decelerations that repeatedly decrease to a slow rate, last a long time, and show a progressively slower recovery to baseline are concerning, indicating worsening hypoxia. This is especially true if accompanied by other heart rate abnormalities, such as a decrease in baseline variability.

Moderate to severe variable decelerations are often the result of more severe cord compression from entanglement, knots, or prolapse. Severe, uncorrectable variable decelerations with absent variability and a rise in the baseline rate are seen with fetal hypoxia, acidosis and neurological depression at birth. Bradycardia by itself or preceded by the abrupt onset of severe variable decelerations leading within minutes to bradycardia is seen in the fetuses of all women who experience amniotic fluid embolism prior to birth (Clark et al., 1995). Look for signs and symptoms in the mother (see the chapter entitled "Amniotic Fluid Embolism [Anaphylactoid Syndrome of Pregnancy]," for more details). Below is a summary of how to judge the degree of severity with variable decelerations.

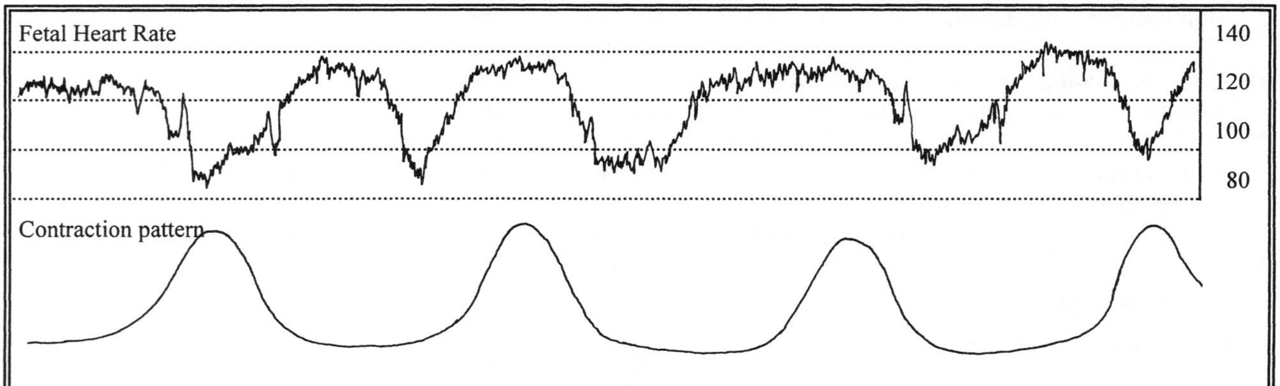

Variable decelerations

Distinguishing Compensatory from Problematic Variable Decelerations		
Parameter	**Reassuring**	**Nonreassuring**
Duration	Lasts less than 30 to 45 seconds	Lasts over one minute
Degree of drop	Falls 15 bpm or more from baseline, often falling below 100 bpm	Drops below 70 bpm
Variability	Normal	Absent
Associated findings	Shouldering	Overshooting
Return to baseline	Abrupt	Prolonged
Baseline rate	Normal	Rising

The Severity of Variable Decelerations (based on the duration of the nadir)	
Degree	**Findings**
Mild	Any decrease sustained for less than 30 sec Decrease to 70-80 bpm that lasts for less than 60 sec Decrease that remains over 80 bpm for any length of time
Moderate	Decrease below 70 bpm for 30 to 60 sec Decrease below 70 to 80 bpm for over 60 sec
Severe	Decrease below 70 bpm for over 60 sec

Prolonged decelerations: Prolonged deceleration of the fetal heart rate is defined as an episodic drop of more than 15 bpm which lasts at least two minutes but no longer than 10. A prolonged deceleration of more than 10 minutes duration reflects a change in the baseline rate.

Prolonged decelerations frequently involve a drop below 110 bpm and are often associated with a loss of variability, rebound tachycardia (where the heart rate rises before returning to baseline–similar to overshooting) or recurrent late decelerations, a pattern associated with maternal hypoxia, hypotension or tetanic contractions. (A fetus with baseline tachycardia may show a drop to a normal range.) Prolonged decelerations are usually isolated events that are commonly preceded by variable decelerations. Occasionally late decelerations follow prolonged decelerations. Prolonged decelerations may occur as a result of:

- Any other decrease in oxygenation
- Sudden cord compression or prolapse (most frequent cause)
- Vagal stimulation from internal exam or artificial rupture of membranes resulting in direct pressure on the fetal head
- Unphysiologic maternal pushing efforts that have the mother hold her breath and push for as long as she can
- Rapid descent of the head
- Maternal hypotension due to an epidural or being supine
- Paracervical anesthesia
- Uterine hypertonia or tetanic contractions
- Severe uteroplacental insufficiency
- Maternal hypoxia due to seizures or acute respiratory distress

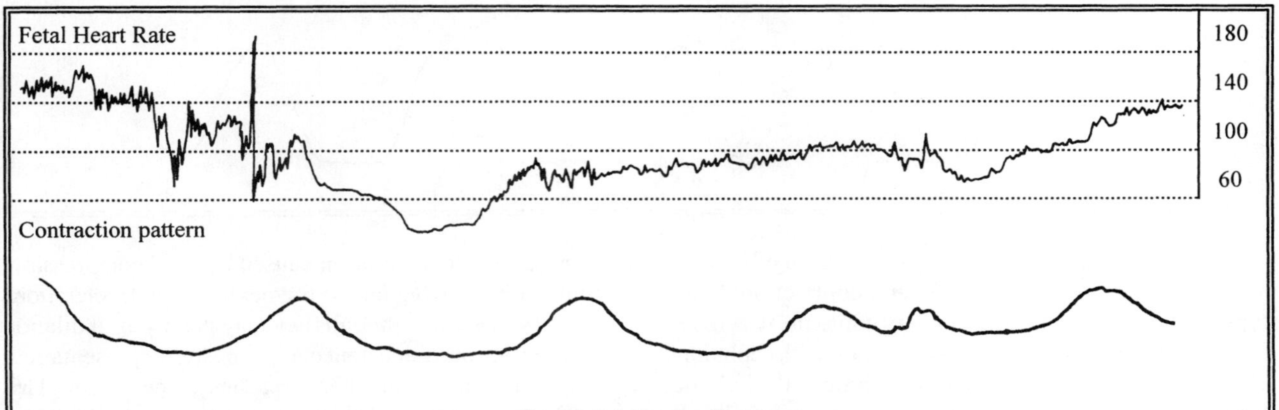

Prolonged decelerations

If a prolonged deceleration is an isolated event, assume the placenta has been able to compensate for the stress. A prolonged deceleration that occurs after a series of severe variable decelerations is much more serious. Prolonged decelerations that appear after a series of late decelerations may lead to severe bradycardia (30 to 60 bpm) just before fetal death.

Periodic fetal heart rate patterns

Periodic accelerations: Acceleration patterns that occur with uterine contractions typically resemble the shape of the contraction. Such accelerations begin either before or after the height of the contraction. The rise usually takes less than 30 seconds to reach its peak, and returns to baseline as the contraction is subsiding or just afterward. These accelerations last longer than 15 seconds but less than two minutes. Accelerations that are associated with uterine contractions may be the earliest sign that the umbilical cord is partially compressed or may reflect other early types of fetal distress, especially when seen with decreasing or absent baseline variability. Periodic accelerations are seen most often with variable decelerations and with breech presentation. The healthy fetus raises her heart rate in response to hypotension and decreased cardiac output. Be watchful that this pattern does not persist into tachycardia. When the cause of accelerations is unclear or when they are consistently associated with contractions, listen more frequently to assess whether fetal distress is present.

Lambda pattern: The lambda pattern is a temporary periodic change commonly seen in early labor that occurs in relationship to uterine contractions. It consists of an acceleration followed immediately by a deceleration that may occur over a span as long as two minutes with a return to a normal baseline. This pattern is considered benign, regardless of the timing of the deceleration. Why it occurs is not understood. Careful monitoring must be done to make sure it is not repetitive and to distinguish it from truly problematic patterns, especially late decelerations.

Periodic decelerations: There are two types of periodic decelerations that can occur during labor: early and late.
Early (Type I) decelerations: Early decelerations are characterized by as a mirror-image drop in the heart rate that matches the wave of the contraction. An early deceleration begins as the contraction builds, takes 30 seconds or longer to reach its lowest point as the contraction peaks and promptly returns to a normal baseline as the contraction tapers off. The degree of deceleration correlates with the strength of the uterine contraction. Normally the fetal heart rate rarely drops below 100 bpm (20 to 30 bpm below baseline). The total period of deceleration is usually less than 90 seconds. The baseline rate and variability remain within normal limits.

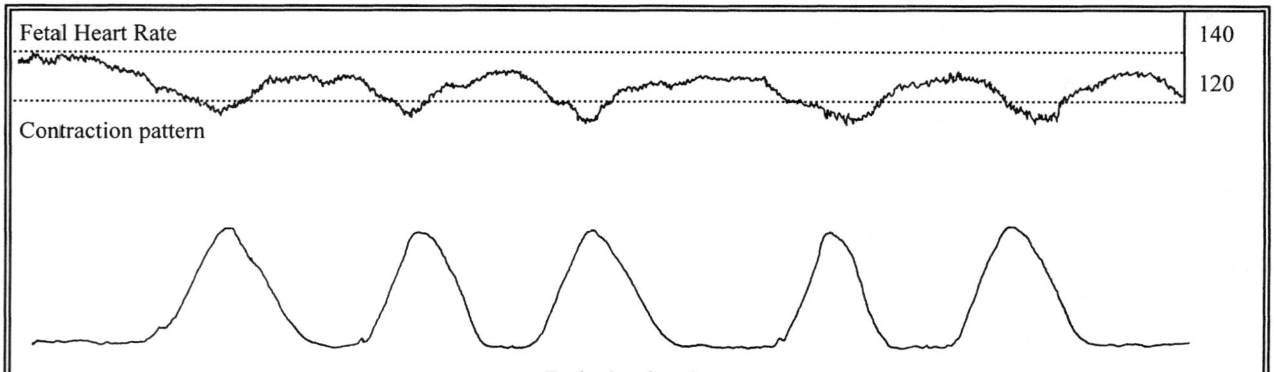

Early decelerations

In cephalic presentations, the appearance of early decelerations is a normal variation caused by head compression. Type I decelerations occur with each contraction, with only slight variation from one to the next. Early decelerations typically occur in first-time mothers while the cervix is dilating from 4 to 7 cm, although they may persist until dilation is complete. They also occur in association with cephalopelvic disproportion and persistent occiput posterior presentation. They often reappear during active pushing as the head descends through the pelvis or when it reaches the perineum. This is thought to be the result of direct vagal stimulation of the temporal baroreceptors due to increased pressure on the sides of the head as it passes through the birth canal.

Early decelerations *are* concerning if they occur:

•When a woman is not in labor, in association with toning contractions
•In very early labor, before the head has descended into the pelvis
•Along with other potentially problematic changes in the fetal heart rate, such as loss of baseline variability

Repetitive, *severe* early decelerations need careful observation, as they may lead to fetal acidosis. What constitutes a "severe" early deceleration is not well defined. (See also the discussion of prolonged decelerations in this chapter.)

Late (Type II) decelerations: Late decelerations are also associated with uterine contractions, presenting with a gradual decrease in the FHR and a gradual return to baseline. However, these decelerations reach their lowest point after the contraction peaks, taking more than 30 seconds after the drop begins to reach their nadir. After the contraction ends, the FHR then takes more than 20 seconds to return to baseline. Type II decelerations may or may not occur with each contraction. The fetal heart rate may remain within a normal range, and the drop can be as small as 3 to 5 bpm below the baseline rate. Late decelerations rarely dip below 100 bpm; the degree of deceleration usually matches the strength of the contraction.

Causes: Late decelerations occur due to a decrease in blood flow (and therefore oxygen) to the uterus. This leads to fetal hypoxia and depression of the fetal cardiac muscle, which activates the vagal response. This, in turn, leads to anaerobic metabolism and the production of lactic acidosis. The result is a fall in the heart rate. Late decelerations occur after the contraction peaks because oxygen levels are not adequate during the contraction. The contraction must ease off for normal uterine blood flow to resume, and it then takes time for the newly oxygenated blood to travel from the placenta to the fetal heart. During this interval, the fetal heart rate responds to the poorly oxygenated blood supply by decelerating. Once the deceleration has ended, the baseline rate and variability return to normal.

If the baby is compromised for any reason, the reduction in oxygen supply during contractions may result in impaired cardiac function as well as stimulation of the vagal nerve. The rate of oxygen transfer between contractions may not be sufficient to maintain adequate oxygenation, leading to a decrease or disappearance of variability and, eventually, baseline tachycardia. Variability may increase or decrease during the nadir of the deceleration. The longer it takes for the heart rate to begin to drop after the onset of the contraction, the more concerning the pattern. How much (or how little) the fetal heart rate falls from its normal rate has little to do with fetal status. It is the regularity and duration of the decelerations that indicate the severity of compromise.

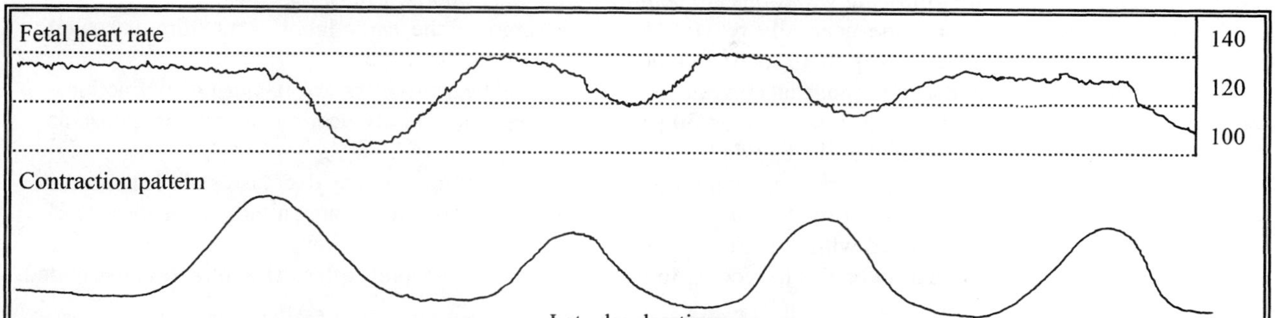

Late decelerations

Late decelerations are associated with:

- •Maternal hypotension or hypertension
- •Hypertonic uterine action due to oxytocin stimulation, prostaglandins, etc.
- •Inhibition of placental or fetal blood flow from cord compression (this usually produces variable decelerations)
- •Fetal anemia resulting from Rh sensitization, nonimmune hydrops or fetal-maternal hemorrhage
- •Maternal conditions such as anemia, cardiac disease, sickle-cell crisis, shock, collagen vascular disease, kidney disease and sclerotic arterial and venous changes (more common in older mothers)
- •Amnionitis, which reduces placental function and leads to oxygen deprivation
- •Intrauterine growth retardation resulting from chronic maternal hypertension, lupus, hyperthyroidism or intrauterine infection
- •Abnormal placentation, including placenta previa, vasa previa, infarction, or placental problems are associated with poorly controlled maternal diabetes
- •Abruption
- •Postmaturity
- •Regional anesthetics (spinal, epidural)

Late decelerations are extremely serious if seen with any of the following:

- •Every contraction
- •Only short intervals between decelerations
- •Decreased variability (no matter how slight the deceleration)
- •A slow recovery to normal baseline, giving a U-shape to the pattern of deceleration.

Fetal cardiac arrhythmias

Episodic cardiac arrhythmia occurs in many fetuses. Aside from tachycardia and bradycardia, you may note:

Skipped beats: Isolated extrasystoles, most of which are supraventricular in origin, are the most common fetal arrhythmia and are of little clinical significance. This sounds like a skipped beat but is usually a pause in the cardiac rhythm or an undetectable heartbeat.

Abrupt accelerations or decelerations above or below the baseline: These are associated with premature atrial or ventricular contractions. Such arrhythmias usually have no clinical significance.

Abrupt decelerations followed quickly by an abrupt return to the previous baseline: These have been seen during the nadir of severe variable decelerations and may reflect transient fetal cardiac asystole.

When listening intermittently, an arrhythmia will only be detected if you are listening exactly when such isolated events occur.

Fetal Heart Rate Variations during Active Pushing

It is important to understand the kinds of fetal heart rate variations that may occur in a healthy fetus when the mother is pushing. During dilation, the reference for interpreting fetal heart rate patterns is contractions. During pushing, maternal bearing-down efforts are superimposed upon the combined effects of uterine contractions and fetal descent through the pelvic and perineal birth canal. Thus, the usual classification of fetal heart rate changes may not accurately reflect what is going on. The following variations are commonly noted (Roberts, 1989):

Baseline changes: The baseline generally remains within 20 bpm of the early labor rate, although vagal stimulation often causes a drop of 10 to 20 bpm below the previous baseline.

Spikes: These are abrupt accelerations that correspond with maternal bearing-down efforts during contractions. They drop rapidly and usually last less than 30 seconds. These most likely occur as a vagal response as additional pressure is applied to the baby's head.

Accelerations: Sporadic accelerations that are not associated with contractions may decrease. While sporadic accelerations are always reassuring, they do not necessarily reflect fetal well-being, although an absence of any acceleration is associated with hypoxic babies.

As a general rule, expect healthy babies to recover to baseline within 15 seconds after the contraction has ended.

Next are changes that may reflect fetal compromise and require close listening and a confirmation of fetal status, which can be ascertained using scalp stimulation:

Decreased variability: If the range of variability drops to less than 5 to 10 bpm, especially if accompanied by a lack of accelerations, variable decelerations or bradycardia, the baby may be in trouble.

Decelerations: Prolonged late decelerations lasting more than 1 to 3 min that develop during pushing, or variable decelerations with a long recovery that were first noted during the dilation phase are both concerning.

Terminal bradycardia: This type of bradycardia occurs with the pushing efforts just before birth. If the fetal heart rate has been good prior to this point, it seldom reflects a compromised baby. It is thought to be due to a combination of head compression, vagal stimulation and possibly cord compression.

Moderate bradycardia: Defined as a rate of less than 100 bpm that persists for more than 10 minutes.

Finally, severe bradycardia of less than 60 to 80 bpm that persists for more than 10 minutes with minimal variability is an ominous sign requiring immediate birth or transport, whichever can be accomplished first.

What to Do in the Event of Concerning or Nonreassuring Heart Rate Patterns

Whenever the fetal heart rate is abnormal, the aim is to assist the return to a normal baseline before fetal metabolic acidosis develops. Measures must be taken to eliminate fetal hypoxia and maximize placental circulation. The midwife must attempt to rule out cord compression as well as maternal factors that may influence the baby's heart rate. Dealing with the heart rate pattern as outlined below will correct many transient or isolated abnormalities. When the suspicious pattern is persistent or multiple abnormalities are evident, more careful evaluation and follow-up with more frequent checks of the fetal heart rate are warranted.

It is always best to transport when questionable fetal heart rate patterns persist. During transport, aim to support the fetus in maintaining as normal a heart rate as possible.

Elevated baseline heart rate or a pattern involving suspicious accelerations

The following recommendations are not necessarily given in order of importance; all should be taken into account.

- Stop doing or giving anything intended to cause stronger contractions.
- Rule out prematurity (gestation prior to 32 weeks). It is unlikely that a singleton pregnancy at such an early gestation would be mistaken for a pregnancy at term; however, an unrecognized twin pregnancy could be present. Review the chart with special attention to the certainty of dates, quickening, fetal growth pattern, length of previous pregnancies, fundal height near the time of previous births and the size of previous babies at birth. Review these parameters with the mother. Listen again and palpate carefully both to determine if multiple gestation may be the issue and to rule out prematurity. For details, see the chapters entitled "Assisting at Multiple Births" and "When the Baby Is Early".

•Remember that the heart rate rises with normal fetal activity. Continue to listen frequently to determine if the baseline has risen or if the baby may simply be active or trying to find the right position for coming out, with the heart rate returning to baseline when the fetus takes a break.

•If the mother is afraid, calm her down. When the mother is afraid, the baby is afraid as well. On a physical level, her stress hormones are transmitted to the baby via the cord. Offer her Rescue Remedy. Have her take slow, deep abdominal breaths, help her to relax completely and have her talk to the baby. Recheck the heart rate to see if this resolves the problem. The baby may also be afraid independent of the mother.

•Change the mother's position to relieve any cord compression and recheck the heart. Cord compression can cause the heart rate to rise.

•If the mother is in a hot bath, have her get out, and recheck the heart rate several times over the next 15 to 30 minutes. If environmental heat is the cause, the heart rate should drop to a normal level over this interval.

•Hydrate the mother and check her blood glucose level, if indicated. Have her eat light foods and drink 8 to 16 oz of water or an electrolyte-balancing fluid, or give her an IV or retention enema. If she is dehydrated or hypoglycemic, the FHR should normalize 30 to 45 min after the fluid balance or glucose level normalizes.

•Dipstick the urine. (See my DIAGNOSTIC TESTS for what to do if findings are positive on urine or blood tests.)

•Take her temperature. An elevated temperature after cooling and hydrating may indicate an infection.

•Are the membranes ruptured? If so and the above measures do not cause the heart rate to drop to a normal baseline or normalize an elevated maternal temperature, the possibility of infection is increased. If the heart rate is still high and birth is not imminent, transport.

•If indicated, ask about recreational drug use. Find out what, if anything, she has taken, how much and when.

In the hospital, the staff will probably perform a fetal scalp blood test to determine pH and base deficit, although the value of this test is lessened if the mother has a fever.

Heart rate is slow, shows reduced variability or is otherwise bradycardic

•Stop doing or giving anything intended to cause stronger contractions.

• The depression might be transient due to sudden pressure on the baby's head from an internal exam or sudden rupture of membranes. Listen carefully and follow the steps below to try to rule out other causative factors.

•If the membranes have ruptured, perform an internal exam to feel for the cord. Feel high up around the presenting part to rule out occult cord prolapse to the best of your ability. Be mindful that a high exam may dislodge the presenting part and result in prolapse if you are not careful; go slow. If you have a high index of suspicion regarding the possibility of prolapse, prop the mother's hips up before you perform the exam.

•Stimulate the fetus by using abdominal palpation, your voice or the mother's voice, or by rubbing the fetal scalp for at least 30 seconds during an internal exam. Listen for accelerations during this process and for the next 5 minutes or through the next contraction (whichever comes first). Healthy babies respond to stimulation quickly, often within 10 seconds. If the heart rate rises at least 15 beats per minute for 15 seconds, this is an indirect indication of a good blood pH (i.e., no fetal acidosis). The baby should do fine in labor for at least another hour and a half. (See the chapter entitled "The Fetal Reactivity Test" in my text DIAGNOSTIC TESTS for more details on this procedure.) Continue to listen frequently and perform the test again in an hour and a half if the baby has not yet been born and the FHR is once again questionable.

•After ruling out cord prolapse, change the mother's position and continue to listen. Place the mother on her left side to optimize blood flow to the placenta, unless you have determined that the left side-lying position is actually contributing to the poor heart patterns. In that case, experiment with maternal positions while continuing to listen to find the one best suited to the baby. If fetal parts are putting pressure on the cord, a maternal position change will usually correct the problem. Record which positions caused the problem. If the mother wants to assume those positions later in labor, be sure to listen long enough to satisfy yourself that the fetal heart rate is remaining normal. A position that is problematic at one point during labor may pose no problem later because the fetus rotates and descends and can move away from the cord or placenta.

•If indicated, there is a technique you can use to try and confirm a nuchal cord described in the chapter entitled "Abdominal Examination Techniques for Use during Labor."

•Test urine and blood glucose. Hydrate the mother and correct dehydration, as above. If the problem is inadequate placental profusion, hydration via a IV, by mouth or with a retention enema should help.

•Give oxygen via a nonrebreather mask. If this improves the fetal heart rate, let the mother breathe the oxygen

for a few minutes, then remove the oxygen and continue to listen.
- Check the mother's blood pressure to see if hypotension is a factor.
- If indicated, question the mother about recreational drug use. Find out what, if anything, she has taken, how much and when.
- Fetal distress is an early sign of significant maternal compromise from blood loss or other reasons. Amniotic fluid embolism will also result in fetal distress as the mother becomes shocky.
- Fetal distress is an early indication of impending uterine rupture.

Maternal hyperoxygenation for fetal distress

Giving the mother pure oxygen is a technique commonly used to correct nonreassuring fetal heart patterns in labor. Although there are no good studies to date that demonstrate a clear advantage, maternal hyperoxygenation is widely used and does appear to affect the fetal heart rate for the better in many cases, although the reasons why are poorly understood.

The best theory recognizes that when a high concentration of a particular gas is inhaled, the gas goes into solution in the blood more quickly than usual. While each molecule of hemoglobin can carry a maximum of four oxygen molecules, plasma has the capacity to carry a much higher than normal concentration of oxygen. Arterial blood levels rise when one breathes pure oxygen. Thus, more oxygen is available for uptake by the mother's and baby's hemoglobin (Egan, 1973). A fetus' hemoglobin is normally higher than an adult's, which raises his capacity to carry oxygen above that of an adult with the same PO_2 level. Adding additional oxygen to the mother's bloodstream maximally saturates her red cells and loads her plasma, making more oxygen available to the fetus. This is especially helpful if the mother's oxyhemoglobin falls below normal levels. Maternal hemoglobin is normally about 95% saturated but can drop as low as 70% during labor (Reed et al., 1989).

Oxygen therapy causes similar increases in the oxygen content of both maternal and fetal blood. In some cases, when the baby has become hypoxic secondary to maternal hypoxia, for example, hyperoxygenation may result in the oxygen level in fetal blood rising even higher than that in the mother's (Meschia, 1977). Giving oxygen to the mother can improve her PO_2 within 16 seconds, followed by a variable but favorable response in the fetal heart rate. Maximum transfer potential from mother to baby is realized after the mother breathes 100% oxygen for about nine minutes (McNamara et al., 1993), although I have observed an almost immediate apparently positive response in the fetus to giving oxygen to a mother. However, another study found that administering oxygen to the mother produced only small increases in fetal arterial PO_2. For example, as maternal PO_2 increased from 91 mm Hg to 583 mm Hg, fetal arterial PO_2 rose only from 11 mm Hg to 16 mm Hg. In spite of this, because of the enhanced ability of the fetus to take up oxygen, even small changes in the fetal arterial levels produce a significant increase in fetal oxygen saturation, presumably benefitting the marginally hypoxic fetus (Clark, 1990; Wulf et al., 1972).

One study did show that cord blood pH drops significantly if the mother is given oxygen when there is no indication of fetal distress. Therefore, once the fetal heart rate normalizes, take the mother off the oxygen and monitor the fetal heart rate closely (Enkin et al., 2000). If the heart rate does not remain within normal limits with the mother breathing room air, keep her on oxygen until the baby is born.

Prolonged inspiration of pure oxygen for more than a few hours can be harmful to the lungs. Oxygen therapy of only short duration increases the production of free-radical molecules. Breathing 50% oxygen (8 to 10 lpm) at atmospheric pressure is considered safe. At this level, there is also no concern that maternal hyperoxygenation will increase fetal oxygen saturation to unsafe levels, as long as oxygen use is discontinued when fetal distress resolves. As soon as it is practical to do so, give the mother 1000 units of Vitamin E and 1000 mg of Vitamin C with bioflavonoids to help counteract the effects of free-radical production prompted by breathing oxygen-enriched air.

How the timing of concerning heart rate patterns influences options for treatment

During early or active labor: Fetal heart rate changes that are within normal limits can be taken as a sign of fetal well-being. However, if the pattern is at all suspicious, continue to listen through the next several contractions, with the mother in various positions. It is best for her to be standing, on her hands and knees, or side-lying. If you hear problematic heart sounds while she is lying on one side, have her roll onto the other side and listen again. If the heart rate changes are due to cord compression, changing the maternal position can clear up the problem right away.

Be warned that if the pattern is truly concerning, poor fetal heart tones in early labor usually indicate a baby that will not withstand the stress of active labor very well; it may be best to transport now. It is imperative that you make it very clear to the staff why you transported when you arrive at the hospital. If you feel the situation is ominous, tell them so.

You can offer the woman oxygen by nonrebreather mask to see if the fetal heart tones respond favorably. However, if the mother must breath oxygen to keep the heart rate in a normal range and birth is not imminent, you will very likely run out of oxygen well before labor is over. Keep the mother on oxygen while you take her to the hospital, if that is what is required to keep the baby stable. There, they will have a sufficient supply of oxygen, if need be, while the fetal status is evaluated on a fetal heart monitor.

Concerning fetal heart rate findings during pushing: The heart rate very often drops during pushing, even if it has been normal throughout labor. These drops are hard to monitor precisely, because listening with a fetoscope during active pushing is, in most cases, almost impossible due to the uterus contracting and the abdominal muscles tensing with maternal pushing efforts. Decelerations are most often caused by head compression as the baby moves through the pelvis. Dips in the form of rapid drops in the heart rate during spontaneous bearing-down efforts usually last about 30 seconds, quickly recovering to a normal baseline.

The important thing to evaluate is whether and how rapidly the heart rate returns to a normal baseline as the contraction eases off and maternal bearing-down efforts cease. At this point, the fetal heart should return within 15 seconds to a normal baseline. This is easy to monitor if you are counting the heart rate in 5 sec intervals. If fetal heart tones concern you during pushing, proceed as follows:

- Give the mother oxygen. This can help immensely, and you are not likely to run out of oxygen before the birth if pushing is proceeding well.
- Keep in mind that a mechanical problem may be the culprit. An increasingly tight cord around the neck will cut off circulation as the baby descends, which is likely if there is no recovery, if decelerations are increasingly severe or if the baby's head recedes inside dramatically between pushes (to be distinguished from the normal rocking motion of the presenting part during and between pushes). A few women also seem to have a point during descent where all their babies experience an alarming drop in heart rate. This is probably a tight point in the mother's pelvis triggering the temporal baroreceptors and causing a vasovagal response. Once past that point, the heart rate dramatically returns to normal. A careful review of previous records and the parents' recollection of previous births may bring such a pattern to light. The partner may be more aware than the mother that the care providers were concerned.
- Have the mother stop pushing for a contraction or two and breathe deeply, with or without supplemental oxygen, while you listen. This relieves acute pressure on the baby's head and often the heart rate returns to normal.
- Be sure the mother is using exhale pushing–short pushes with breaths between–rather than holding her breath.
- Change the mother's position. This can help dramatically.
- It is possible that a woman's loud vocalizations during pushing may frighten the baby. Have the mother talk to the baby about what is going on or do so yourself.
- Get the baby out. If the heart rate does not recover and it appears that birth can occur quickly, get the baby out as soon as possible. Consider cutting a clitorotomy, especially in a first-time mother with a tight hymen or perineum. If birth is not imminent, have the mother breathe through contractions, put her on oxygen, and transport. It may help to position her so that pressure on the head is reduced (knee-chest or hands and knees).

Imminent or Suspected Fetal Demise during Labor

Labor is not the time to decide to stay home with a baby who may have just died. If you are monitoring a woman in labor and believe her baby is in serious trouble or that death has occurred, you must transport. This is true even if the mother states that she wants to stay home and accepts that the baby has died. She will be in a certain degree of emotional shock and will likely be incapable of making a truly rational decision. Additional evaluation at the hospital is the best insurance that the parents will not later regret not having done everything that could have been done, as well as covering your bases as a practitioner. You may not be able to detect that the baby is still alive, although she might be found to be so when sophisticated technologies are used to assess the situation. Saving such a baby may require an immediate emergency surgical birth. If the death of a baby is confirmed and medically documented, the parents still have the option, if they so desire, of going back home to labor, if necessary by signing out AMA (against medical advice).

If you detect severe fetal distress, believe the baby is in danger of death, but she is coming so quickly that birth at home is unavoidable, complete the birth, provide resuscitation to the best of your ability and transport if indicated.

FINDING	CHARACTERISTICS	RELATED TO CONTRACTIONS?	TIMING	DURATION	ASSOCIATED WITH
Baseline findings in labor					
Normal	110 to 160 bpm (as during late pregnancy)	No	Fetus at rest between contractions	Throughout labor	Healthy fetal status
Tachycardia FHR > 160 bpm for 10+ min (or ≥ 20 bpm above baseline)	Moderate: >160 to 170 bpm	No	Onset varies with fetal condition	Change in baseline rate	Early response to hypoxia
	Severe: >170 bpm				Dehydration; infection; if seen w/reduced fetal motion and variability or w/prolonged variable or late decelerations, the baby is compromised.
	Extreme: >200 bpm				Fetal heart abnormalities
Bradycardia FHR < 110 bpm for > 10 min (or 20 bpm below baseline)	Mild:100-110 bpm	No	Baseline change; onset varies with fetal condition	Change in baseline rate	Good variability & no late decels at term, fetus is healthy.
	Below 100 bpm for ≥10 min				Significant fetal hypoxia
Sinusoidal pattern	Changes 30 bpm over or under baseline with 2 to 6 undulations per min of LTV only	No	Uniform undulating baseline (wave pattern)	≥10 min	Fetal anemia or hypoxia
Pseudosinusoidal pattern	Less uniform, with STV preceded and followed by normal baseline	No	Undulating baseline	20 to 30 min	Maternal drugs, fetal mouth movements (thumb sucking)
Normal & abnormal variability					
Types of variability	Short-term variability (STV)	No	Beat-to-beat variation of FHR	Changes with every heart-beat	Considered together, STV and LTV are hallmarks of fetal well-being.
	Long-term variability (LTV): rhythmical fluctuation, 3-25 bpm		3-5 bpm, cycle repeats 3-5 times per min	Successive 1 min intervals	
Absent	Undetectable	No	Baseline variation	Onset w/hypoxia	Severe hypoxia
Minimal	Undetectable to ≤ 5 bpm				
Moderate (average)	5 to 25 bpm	No	Baseline variation	Throughout labor	Fetal well-being and adequate oxygenation
Marked variability	over 25 bpm	No	Baseline change	Onset w/hypoxia	Hypoxia

FINDING	CHARACTERISTICS	RELATED TO CONTRACTIONS?	TIMING	DURATION	ASSOCIATED WITH
Episodic (nonperiodic) FHR patterns: FHR changes completely unrelated to or that do not consistently occur in relation to contractions					
Reactive accelerations	**TERM:** Rise of ≥15 bpm for >2 min but <10 min **<32 WKS:** >10 bpm over baseline, lasting >10 sec	No; occurs w/fetal movement or stimulation	Episodic	≥ 15 sec	Healthy, physiologic response to movement, stimulation; breech or posterior presentation
Decelerations	FHR falls ≥15 bpm lasting 15 sec or more	No	Episodic	≥ 15 sec	Fetal stress
Variable decelerations (Type III):U-shaped, V-shaped or W-shaped decelerations	**Reassuring:** Falls of 15 bpm rate, often >100 bpm w/normal variability & baseline, with shouldering	Not consistently	Considered episodic >30 sec to nadir	Any drop for <30 sec, 70-80 bpm for <60 sec or >80 bpm for any duration	Mild compression of cord with good fetal compensation
	Shouldering: Paired accelerations; one at beginning and one at end of the deceleration	No	Before & after decelerations	<20 sec for each acceleration	Good fetal compensation for temporary lack of oxygen
	Nonreassuring: Fall to <70 bpm, no variability, overshoots	Not consistently	Prolonged return to a rising baseline	>1 min	Severe cord compression, hypoxia and acidosis
	Overshoot: Acceleration after contraction at end of deceleration	No	Prolonged	>20 sec for single acceleration	Hypoxia
Prolonged decelerations	FHR fall of ≥15 bpm that lasts at least 2 and no more than 10 min	No; isolated event	With head compression	1 to 2 min	With recovery to normal baseline & variability, fetus is compensating well.
	FHR drops 15 or more bpm	No	Episodic	>2 min and <10 min	Serious w/loss of variability or after a series of late or variable decelerations
Cardiac arrhythmias	Skipped beats	No	Random	Sporadic	Supraventricular origin; benign
	Rises or falls of the rate around the baseline	No	Baseline variation	Abrupt changes	Premature atrial or ventricular contractions, benign
	Sharp deceleration with return to previous baseline rate	No	Often seen at nadir of severe variable decelerations	Abrupt fall and rise	Fetal cardiac asystole, probably benign. Cord prolapse, rapid cephalic descent.

FINDING	CHARACTERISTICS	RELATED TO CONTRACTIONS?	TIMING	DURATION	ASSOCIATED WITH
Periodic changes: FHR changes that are consistently associated with contractions					
Lambda pattern	Acceleration followed by a deceleration with a return to normal baseline	Occurs during contractions	Early labor	Short, not repetitive	Unknown why this occurs; a benign finding.
Repetitive Accelerations	Rises $\geq$15 bpm with <30 seconds from onset to peak of acceleration	Returns to baseline just before or after the end of the contraction	Periodic	At least 15 sec but < 2 min	May be earliest sign of cord compression
Early decelerations (Type I)	Falls $\geq$15 bpm below baseline; rate rarely falls to <100 bpm.	Mirrors contractions w/nadir at peak or within 15 sec of peak	Gradual decrease and recovery	Usually < 90 sec	Head compression w/descent and w/crowning (dangerous prior to descent)
Late decelerations (Type II)	Decelerations with nadir occurring after peak of contractions	Reaches lowest FHR > 15 sec after contractions peak	Gradual decrease and recovery	Usually < 90 sec	Placental insufficiency or previa; vasa previa; abruption; maternal diabetes, hypo- or hypertension; hypertonic contraction; sickle-cell crisis

References and Further Reading on Monitoring the Mother's and Baby's Well-Being during Labor

Record-keeping during Labor

Hedrick Y. "The pregnancy pack, midwifery chart forms for midwives in all practice settings." Angel Dance Midwifery Service, Floral City FL, 1999.

Assessing and Supporting the Mother's Well-Being during Labor

Blackburn S, Loper D. MATERNAL, FETAL AND NEONATAL PHYSIOLOGY. WB Saunders Co, Philadelphia PA, 1992.

Marieb E. HUMAN ANATOMY AND PHYSIOLOGY, 4th ed. Benjamin/Cummings, Menlo Park CA, 1998.

Stables D. PHYSIOLOGY OF CHILDBEARING: WITH ANATOMY AND RELATED BIOSCIENCES." Baillière Tindall, Edinburgh, UK, 1999.

Assessing and Supporting the Baby's Well-Being during Labor

Clark S. "Shock in the pregnant patient," SEMIN PERINATOL, 14(1);52-58, Feb, 1990.

Clark S, et al. "Amniotic fluid embolism: analysis of the national registry," AM J OBSTET GYNECOL, 172(4 Pt 1);1158-1169, Apr, 1995.

Clyman R, Heymann M. "Fetal cardiovascular physiology," in Creasy R, Resnick R, eds. MATERNAL-FETAL MEDICINE, 4th ed. WB Saunders, Philadelphia PA, 1999.

Egan D. FUNDAMENTALS OF RESPIRATORY THERAPY, 2nd ed. CV Mosby Co, St. Louis MO, 1973.

Enkin M, et al. A GUIDE TO EFFECTIVE CARE IN PREGNANCY AND CHILDBIRTH, 3rd ed. Oxford U, Oxford UK, 2000.

Gauge S, Henderson C. CTG MADE EASY. Churchill Livingstone, New York NY, 1992.

Goodlin R, Lowe E. "A functional umbilical cord occlusion heart rate pattern. The significance of overshoot," OBSTET GYNECOL, 43(1);22-30, Jan, 1974.

McKay S, Roberts J. "Second stage labor: what is normal?" JOGNN, 14(2);101-106, Mar-Apr, 1985.

McNamara H, et al. "The effect on fetal arteriolar oxygen saturation resulting from giving oxygen to the mother measured by pulse oximetry," BR J OBSTET GYNAECOL, 100(5);446-449, May, 1993.

Meschia G. "Transfer of oxygen across the placenta." in Gluck L, ed. INTRAUTERINE ASPHYXIA AND THE DEVELOPING FETAL BRAIN. Year Book Medical, Chicago IL, 1977.

National Institute of Child Health and Human Development Research Planning Workshop: "Electronic fetal heart rate monitoring: research guidelines for interpretation," AM J OBSTET GYNECOL, 177(6);1385-1390, Dec,1997.

Parer J. HANDBOOK OF FETAL HEART RATE MONITORING, 2nd ed. WB Saunders Co, Philadelphia PA, 1997.

Reed P, et al. "Maternal oxygenation during normal labour," BR J ANAESTH, 62(3);316-318, Mar, 1989.

Roberts J. "Managing fetal bradycardia during second stage of labor," MCN, 14(6);394-398, Nov-Dec, 1989.

Tucker S. POCKET GUIDE TO FETAL MONITORING AND ASSESSMENT, 4th ed. Mosby, St. Louis MO, 2000.

Van Geijn H, Copray F, eds. A CRITICAL APPRAISAL OF FETAL SURVEILLANCE. Excerpta Medica, Amsterdam, the Netherlands, 1994.

Varney H. VARNEY'S MIDWIFERY, 3rd ed. Jones & Bartlett, Sudbury MA, 1997.

Williams J, Blanchard J. ELECTRONIC MONITORING OF THE FETAL HEART. Books for Midwives Press, Hale UK,1996.

Wulf K, et al. "Clinical aspects of placental gas exchange," in Longo, L, Bartels H, eds. RESPIRATORY GAS EXCHANGE AND BLOOD FLOW IN THE PLACENTA. National Institute of Child Health and Human Development, Bethesda MD, 1972.

Understanding and Monitoring the Flow of Labor

Assessing the Progress and Strength of Labor: An Overview

Stages or phases?

The labor process is divided into stages by the medical model, a concept that has fostered rigid ideas about what does and does not happen at various points as labor moves along. In fact, the rhythm of labor is very much like the rhythm of women's sexuality in general. In this text, the various turning points during labor are designated as phases and focus on what is happening: preparatory labor, dilation, resting, pushing, birth, postbirth rest, placental birth. This honors the gradual and rhythmic, fluid and female melding of one process into another with no precise beginning or end points at any time.

Is the woman really in labor?

(The identification of labor is covered in detail in Volume I in the chapter entitled "The Onset of Normal Labor at Term.") Once you are at the mother's home, you will want to reconfirm your impressions that labor has begun. Definitions of labor in the medical literature vary widely. Friedman (1967), the guy we can thank for the North American medical definition of normal labor, says the onset of labor is simply when the woman first feels regular uterine contractions. Well, that covers most well-nourished women near term who are having bouts of regular toning contractions (felt as a tightening in the fundus and frequently lasting over a minute). The team led by O'Driscoll (1993), an Irish obstetrician who has popularized active management of labor, feels that labor has not begun until painful contractions are coming at least every 10 minutes and are accompanied by bloody show, rupture of membranes or 100% cervical effacement. In this book, labor is considered established if contractions are progressing in intensity, duration and frequency and are accompanied by cervical changes. Especially in first-time mothers, these changes are accompanied by contractions that alter the shape (not just the firmness) of the uterus and are felt low down in the suprapubic area. Labor contractions cause the uterus to lean forward, the sidewalls to narrow and the fundus to flatten. These changes are usually best detected in an unclothed, upright woman, although the uterus will rear up if the mother is lying down (Simkin & Ancheta, 2000; Sutton, 2001). Multiparas can have contractions that change the cervix internally but that may not cause these types of uterine contour changes early on.

Learning to observe women in labor

There are many ways a midwife can evaluate the progress and strength of labor. First of all, she can watch the mother's reactions, listen to her as she describes how her contractions feel, and see how she reacts as she experiences contractions. Underpinning these clinical observations, the midwife consciously opens herself to feeling the energy of birth as it moves through the mother. As you observe her on all these levels, you should remain as unobtrusive as possible. Sitting in the room doing needlework or reading keeps you occupied yet able to hear and see everything.

There are many ways to assess progress. Progress in "normal" labor is defined by the medical model according to rigid objective criteria regarding the number of centimeters the woman dilates and the amount of cervical effacement that occurs within a given timeframe. This type of definition, at best, detracts from individualizing a woman's care and, at worst, often leads to numerous, and cumulatively dangerous, interventions to try to make labor conform to artificially constructed parameters of "normal." When we use only two physical parameters to assess progress, not only do we limit our view of what is normal but we tune out the many other indications that labor is moving along. We tend to lose sight of the individual woman when we reduce her labor to plotted lines on a graph.

A mother easing out of fear and into dealing with her labor in a centered fashion is definitely progressing. Descent and rotation of the presenting part, movements of the os from a very posterior to a more normal position, and changes in cervical consistency are all signs of progress according to the midwifery model care. These things cannot happen unless birthing energy is flowing.

The many subtle signs of progress will only become obvious to you if you labor-sit from early labor through birth for significant numbers of women. There is no substitute for continuity of attendance to hone your assessment of labor until it is second nature. Hospitals often must rely on internal exams because institutional care is set up to provide discontinuous attendance; the presence of those in attendance at any particular labor is often so fragmented that tuning into the flow of labor is hampered or impossible. Also, the many disruptions that occur in a hospital setting frequently alter the mother's behavior and her delicate hormonal balance and thus confuse the signs of progress.

When a woman labors, her body language, her vocalizations, the way her uterus looks during and between contractions, the changes in her lower abdomen and pelvis, and the contours of her abdomen as the baby rotates all offer information about progress. The woman's sense of emotional and psychological well-being is equally important when assessing how labor is advancing and what support she may require.

It is extremely important to remember that every mother-baby pair is unique. While the progress of normal labor has many similar characteristics, every labor has different nuances and a woman's needs can vary widely based on a huge array of factors. The discussions of labor throughout this text are only a guide. It is possible for labor to begin at any of the points listed below, for labor to skip from one point to another, and for women to move back and forth among behavioral responses with no clear pattern. As a general rule, women having their first baby have a tendency to overestimate the advancement of their labor while women having their second baby are more realistic about the progress of labor. As parity rises, labor patterns become more variable and women may either be right on or may sometimes underestimate the progress of their labor. Never allow what any book says is "supposed to happen" override your respect for the individuality of each woman's experience of her labor. Respond to the woman and her needs above all else.

What to watch for: As a midwife, you learn how to assess labor on many levels. Internal exams can give you valuable information and are an essential component of good care whenever there is a question about what is going on. However, you should develop an ability to simply be with laboring women and, by watching and listening to what is going on, tell how labor is progressing. Keep in mind that grand midwives, with thousands of births behind them, often sit in the corner of the room without performing even one internal exam. They rely instead upon their highly refined intuitive sense of the birth process and the flow of birthing energy coupled with years of experience in quietly observing women's behavior during labor to know exactly what is happening.

There are numerous specific techniques for assessing progress, many of which have never been documented. I have managed to glean some of these from my sister midwives, and they are described in the chapter entitled "Additional Noninvasive Techniques for Assessing Progress." General, observational impressions are covered in this chapter. When you are just starting out, it can be helpful to assess the progress of labor to the best of your ability and then confirm your impressions with infrequent internal exams.

The length of truly undisturbed, physiologic labor

Once labor becomes established in a healthy, well-nourished, psychologically open woman who is upright, mobile and leaning forward and in an environment that respects her need for privacy with a baby who is already in an LOA position, labor takes around 4 to 8 hours in a first-time baby and 2 to 4 hours for subsequent babies (Sutton, 2001). The overview that follows encompasses parameters considered normal within a wide range of variations.

The dilation phase of labor: During most of the labor process the cervix is thinning (effacing), opening (dilating) and being pulled to a more central position in the yoni canal so the baby can descend and be born.

Preparatory uterine activity: It is possible for both mother and midwife to be convinced that a woman is in early labor when she is not. A woman can have regular contractions that do not go away with a change of activity or exhibit other characteristics of the prelabor contractions, but neither do they increase in frequency, duration or intensity. Nevertheless, the mother is acutely aware of them. These contractions may go on in long bouts for many hours or even days before cervical dilation begins. Often, preparatory uterine activity can be distinguished because the energy feels "flat," which is to say, not very strong and not building.

In such a case, stay in close touch with the mother, reminding her that these contractions are preparing her cervix for the work ahead by softening and effacing it and, in some cases, moving it forward. Sometimes these changes must occur before the cervix can even begin to dilate. They are not a waste of effort, there is nothing "false" about them, and each preparatory contraction moves her closer to having her baby.

Tell her that, while these changes are a necessary component of progressive labor, she should think of this as a preliminary to progressive uterine activity. It is unwise to call it "early labor" as this will only discourage the mother, who may begin to think her labor will never end. You must state very clearly that labor has not yet begun and that it is imperative for her to eat, rest, sleep and go about her daily activities without wearing herself to a frazzle. At night, she should sleep and rest as much as possible on her left side (see detailed descriptions of positioning in the chapter entitled "Positions and Activities for Labor"), and she should remember that early labor could begin at any time. She should have someone stay with her who is calm and understands the normalcy of this, the last part of pregnancy. This person can support her in taking care of herself until labor kicks in.

When preparatory uterine activity or early labor results in long, painful contractions, the baby may be trying to rotate into a more optimal position so he can enter the brim (Sutton calls these "entering pains"). See the chapter entitled "Entering Pains and Back Pain in Labor" for more details.

Early (latent phase or prodromal) labor: Early labor begins with the onset of regular, increasingly intense contractions that are coordinated with lower abdominal sensations and that do not go away with a change in maternal activity. The mother may be excited and sometimes uncertain whether "this is it." Early labor lasts until the first-time mother reaches 3 to 4 cm of dilation. For multiparas, the duration of early labor has a wider variation because their cervices open more easily with mild, early labor contractions. For them, early labor may continue until they reach 5 or 6 cm of dilation. Typically, these contractions begin by lasting anywhere from 15 to 40 seconds and are spaced 15 to 30 minutes apart and change the shape of the uterus with every contraction. Normal early labor contractions are short, sharp and well spaced (Simkin, 2001; Sutton, 2001).

The object of early labor is to prepare the cervix for more rapid progress as contractions become more intense. Progressive early labor contractions efface the cervix and begin the process of dilation. When the cervix is very posterior, these contractions help bring it around to a more normal position. Because of these cervical changes, mucusy bloody show occurs at this phase. When the cervix is soft and ideally positioned and the baby is occiput anterior and low in the pelvis, much of the work of early labor has taken place during periods of toning contractions. Early labor will therefore be shorter. When things vary from these ideal circumstances, early labor can take much longer. It will also be prolonged if the mother is afraid, as a high catecholamine level will slow early labor (Simkin, 2001).

Generally, the less the woman has to concentrate directly on her contractions to get through them, the earlier she is in labor. However, take note that women who have had babies before will behave as though they are in early labor for a longer period of time than those having their first baby, even though they may be far more advanced in terms of dilation.

One way to assess the strength of labor is to try to distract the woman. Have a support person engage her to keep her mind off her contractions at this point. Cards, other games, television, reading, movies, light outdoor recreation such as a walk or picnic, or similar activities are good distractions that are not too tiring. If these tend to ease the labor down or ease down her responses to it, she is probably overreacting to her sensations.

Women may also want to clean house (the nesting instinct). Smiling, walking and talking are often easy at this point. A woman may feel restless and is often hungry. She should eat whatever she likes, but encourage foods easily digested and high in protein or complex carbohydrates for the work ahead. Loose bowels and a slightly runny nose are also often a part of the juicy loosening-up that is going on at this time. Forward-leaning positions are often chosen instinctively from this point on.

Once contractions last at least one minute from start to finish (peaking usually after about 30 seconds) and come every five minutes or more frequently and the mother can no longer be distracted from them, the first-time mother is probably entering active labor. Thus, it is more the character of the contractions, how the woman must respond to them and the overall feel of the energy than the actual amount of dilation that signals the gradual transition from early to active labor. However, if the cervix is quite firm at the onset of contractions, the baby is high in the pelvis, there are scars on the cervix, reproductive hormone balance has been off in the past, or hormone-based contraception has been used for a while before conception–sometimes even for unidentifiable reasons–contractions can continue to build without much change in the cervix. In these cases, additional assistance is often called for. Remedies for a long, slow early labor can be found in the chapters entitled "Natural Induction and Augmentation of Labor" and "Endless Early Labor."

Banks of New Zealand (2000) has noted that yawning in laboring women can be a sign that they are gearing up for another "level" of labor activity.

Active labor: This phase typically covers the period of dilation between 4 or 5 cm and about 7 or 8 cm. Some women have a characteristic flush over their cheekbones around 4 cm dilation. It doesn't last very long but signals that active labor is beginning (Flint, 1986). Susan Claypool (2001), a midwife in California, notes that when women are about 5 to 6 cm dilated, their body odor takes on a smell similar to amniotic fluid. This is only reliable if the bag is intact because, obviously, you will be able to smell amniotic fluid throughout labor if the membranes have ruptured early.

The mother now accepts that she is in labor and, if not overly afraid, appears confident and committed to the work ahead. Talking and other nonlabor-related activities will gradually give way to deeper breathing and focused attention, which may be directed internally or externally toward a support person. Contractions typically last at least 1 minute and are spaced 4 to 5 minutes apart. A heightened awareness in the midwife often indicates that the birthing energy is starting to take off. The woman may be able to continue talking through contractions at this point, but it takes more effort. The cervix responds to the contractions by dilating more readily, since most of the effacement has already taken place during early labor. Active labor may last anywhere from 20 minutes to six hours, but sometimes takes considerably longer, especially during first labors. Conversely, when women who have given birth before have steady contractions every 3 to 4 minutes, the baby will usually be born in about an hour. Some women have flushed cheekbones at 6 cm, while others will throw up at 6 centimeters and then become very serious about their labor, often progressing rapidly to pushing, sometimes within two hours.

The mother may still be hungry, depending upon the length of her labor up to this point. Always allow her to eat if she wants to. Drinking is also important. She feels many changes occurring in her body and may settle into one position or activity that helps her cope with labor. She often feels increasing pressure and fullness in her pelvis at this point, and may experience backache, cramping across the lower back, or sensations similar to menstrual cramps low down in front. She also may feel stretching in her pelvis, and her symphysis pubis may be sore. All these sensations are related to the baby moving lower into her pelvis. Also watch for early decelerations in the fetal heart rate, another sign that the head is well applied to the cervix or pressing against the pelvic floor.

Hard labor: When hard labor begins varies among women, but usually occurs as they are dilating through their 7th to 8th or 9th centimeter. Women often become less modest as active labor gets even stronger. They also become serious about the work they are doing. A woman may still walk, but her movements become slower and more deliberate. She may want to lie down. Caroline Flint, an English midwife, points out that as labor becomes more intense, many women tense their feet with every contraction, curling the toes and contorting the feet in various ways (Flint, 1986). The mother may doze between contractions and concentrate deeply during contractions. The mother may describe her uterus as being more "involved" during contractions. The pain may feel deeper or higher. The baby may start moving and squirming as she searches for the best position to facilitate further descent. This movement is particularly true of the presenting part.

As maternal prostaglandin and endorphin levels rise, the mother's lips may swell slightly, her nipples may darken, and her breasts may fill so that she looks full and sensual. Some women even glow. Her voice becomes deeper and softer. She may seek to hide her face or in other ways create more privacy as she focuses her attention internally. If the mother is lying in bed, she may need to shift from side to side more often. Women may either move around a lot or stay in one position at this point in labor (Busch, 2000).

The woman often assumes a variety of positions as labor advances. She may appear to be working harder. Some women will prefer to keep busy between contractions in early hard labor. However, note that the inability to stay still at all (a sense of agitation to her movements) may indicate that the mother is trying to "move away" from the sensations of labor, a process that can be distinguished from effective position changes by observing her overall body language and demeanor as well as her response to the contractions themselves. Rising on tip toes, tightening her buttocks, closing her legs are all signs of moving away from her contractions. Moving into the sensations usually means leaning forward, opening the legs, rhythmic pelvic movements, deep vocalizations, and bending the knees as the contraction builds and peaks. As you become experienced, you will begin to identify corresponding clues in your own body that birthing energy is building or is blocked.

As the mother nears 8 cm, she may begin to feel hot or cold, trembly and cranky. Contractions are often back-to-back at this point, usually following a regular pattern and lasting 60 seconds or longer. The mother may report that one contraction is not over before the next begins. She may complain of pain even without contractions; it is important to distinguish pain related to fetal descent from complications such as abruption or uterine rupture. The mother's desire to urinate may increase as the descending presenting part puts pressure on her bladder. She is working intensely now and may find labor to be almost overwhelming. Losing track of time at this point is common for the woman as well as her midwives. She must concentrate on relaxing, because tension increases her pain. She feels intense pelvic pressure. Full relaxation and rest between contractions feels great.

Transition: This covers the period of active labor from about 8 to 9 cm to complete dilation. If labor has been uncomplicated, expect this phase to last between 5 and 20 contractions (Simkin, 2001). The woman's contractions may become irregular, may have two peaks, may come back-to-back, and may even stop completely for a time. Transition represents a turning point in labor. As the cervix moves more and more out of the way, the baby can more easily descend to the pelvic floor, where internal rotation will eventually take place if it has not already occurred.

The woman enters into an altered state of consciousness as labor becomes more intense–inhibitions fall away, and the most modest woman may shed clothing, use harsh language, yell or become irritated with comfort measures that she had enjoyed earlier in labor. You may notice huge beads of sweat on her upper lip and lots of moisture on the back of her neck. The mother may complain of feeling hot or she may have hot and cold flashes. Some women become increasingly internally focused. Rapid physical changes may produce panic, disbelief and fear. She may express doubt that she can go through with the labor. She may become insecure and afraid, expressing the desire for it "just to be over" and may feel like giving up. Women need simple, preferably non- or minimally verbal encouragement at this point that what is happening is normal and that they are, in fact, doing a good job. Nods, smiles, affirming vocalizations that do not involve speech and brief phrases such as "You're doing so well," "This is just what should be happening," "Bring your breath to your cervix and open it wider" will usually suffice. Do not, however, belabor a mother's fears by trying to rationalize with her too much. Some of this response is purely hormonal and will pass with your gentle presence and support.

A variety of physical signs and symptoms may continue to come and go as labor advances, including perspiration, flushed cheeks, nausea, vomiting, and shakes or tremors, especially in the legs and jaw. These responses are due to the energy of birth moving through a woman rapidly and are often exaggerated if the mother is attempting to block the energy. Abdominal breathing will help smooth them out, as will breathing while channeling (consciously directing) the energy of the breath out through the feet and into the earth.

As the baby descends, the woman will start to feel increasing pressure in her pelvis, if she hasn't felt it already. The membranes often rupture right about now. The mother is likely to feel some lower back discomfort as the head moves past the sacral promontory on its way down, even if the baby is in an ideal position. This discomfort is often pronounced if the baby is occiput posterior or breech. This pain will move lower down her back and sacrum as the baby moves through the pelvis. Eventually she begins to feel pressure in her pelvic floor. This may occur either before or after complete dilation. Many women have another bloody show around eight centimeters, particularly first-time mothers. This may last until dilation is complete. Also watch for slight labial swelling as pushing draws near. Be aware that it is possible for an anterior cervical lip to be stretched way down, even as far as the introitus; being able to see the head on the perineum is not always a guarantee that full dilation has occurred.

Complete dilation to full emergence of the baby: The mother's uterus begins to transition from actively pulling up to bearing down as the cervix nears full dilation, usually beginning around 9 centimeters or just afterward. This process often takes time. If the baby is low enough in the pelvis, the cervix tends to recede behind the presenting part once it has pulled up past the largest presenting diameter.

Resting phase: It is normal, especially in first-time mothers, for there to be a space between complete dilation and the onset of effective pushing. Frequently, contractions are less frequent and less intense once full dilation is reached. The mother has an opportunity to rest and gather strength for the rest of labor. Now the uterus must take up slack, as it gathers itself around the baby (for details, see the chapter entitled "The Resting Phase of Labor"). This pause in maternal effort may be so short as to be undetectable or it may last for several hours. Simkin (2001) notes that, after the tumult of transition, the woman suddenly becomes more clear headed, less withdrawn and more optimistic. A long rest at full dilation is not a problem, and women who are relaxed and unafraid may doze off. Once the baby reaches the pelvic floor at about +2 station or lower and rotates (if rotation has not already occurred), a spontaneous urge to push will usually begin. Gloria Lemay (2000) of Canada comments that full dilation and unobstructed descent may be signaled by either passage of stool as a contraction builds or a spontaneous bearing-down urge that starts at the beginning of a contraction rather than only at the peak. Maggie Banks (2000) notes that women sometimes hiccup as they draw close to pushing.

Active pushing: This occurs when uterine contractions begin spontaneous bearing down and the baby descends further, flexion is enhanced, the presenting part becomes pressed firmly against the pelvic floor, and internal rotation occurs (if it has not already done so). The urge to push may begin gradually only as the contraction peaks, it may appear sporadically at first, or the woman may have a sudden, distinct and overwhelming involuntary urge to push. The uterus rises up dramatically and the fundus is quite hard during pushing contractions. The woman may come to her feet, reach up for something to grasp and express fears for her safety or that of her baby. Soothe her nonverbally whenever possible; remember that her fear is largely due to the surge of hormones she is experiencing at this time. Do not get into an intellectual discussion regarding these fears; they should subside. If she is insistent, however, talk to her about any gut concerns she may have, just in case her fears are founded in an intuitive understanding that something really isn't right; when a specific concern is brought to light, be sure to offer transport as one option among the others you present. This will usually ease her mind and get her back on track with having the baby. Pushing can take a varying amount of time.

When a full-fledged fetal ejection reflex occurs, the baby may descend from high in the pelvis all of a sudden and then be born quickly, in the space of one or two contractions. However, pushing can take longer than this, especially if the woman, for whatever reason, has not fully entered into a peak hormonal release. The overall length of time is not as important as maternal and fetal well-being and as the actual amount of effective pushing taking place.

The presence of an anterior cervical lip or compound presentation may present with classic signs and symptoms. See the chapters entitled "Cervical and Other Soft-Tissue Problems during Labor" and "Assisting a Woman Whose Baby Is in a Compound Presentation" for recommendations on how to deal with these problems.

There are some women who can give birth without adding any voluntary effort to the spontaneous work of the uterus. These women simply relax their pelvic floor as the uterus pushes the baby out. They will appear to be breathing deeply; you will see the uterus rise up and bear down, but the woman will be quite relaxed. Most women, however, will need to put at least some effort of their own into getting the baby out.

Crowning to birth: The birth is a process that spans the time from when the baby's presenting part no longer recedes between contractions until the emergence of the rest of his body. During this process, the mother continues to have contractions and push according to her urge to do so. Once crowning begins, the lower neck and upper spine start to extend beneath the pubic bone. The mother may report a burning sensation as the presenting part stretches the perineum. Women often announce that the baby is coming; this happens more often with multiparas. Whenever you are told that the baby is coming, recheck, even if you have checked recently and found her nowhere near ready. She is probably right! Women often move around as the baby is coming out, thrusting their hips forward to maximally open the spinopubic angle and may change positions between the birth of the head and the shoulders.

Postbirth resting phase: After the baby is born the mother may need a short time to regroup and redirect her attention to her newborn. A second, usually much shorter resting phase occurs as the uterus adapts itself to its smaller size in preparation for the release of the placenta. A warm, undisturbed environment during the minutes following birth will increase the mother's ability to bond with her infant, thus promoting optimal hormone levels to assist in releasing the placenta and staying uterine bleeding.

The birth of the placenta: After a relatively brief resting phase, contractions resume, and soon thereafter the placenta is delivered. The woman may feel these contractions, but they are very different from labor contractions. A slight amount of pressure in the yoni will often precede the birth of the placenta. At this point, the uterus clamps down and bleeding from the open placental site stops.

The baby begins to nurse: Ideally the baby will be nursing by this time as well. A nursing baby is good insurance that the uterus will stay contracted and will not bleed.

ABDOMINAL EXAMINATION TECHNIQUES FOR USE DURING LABOR

This chapter builds on the information covered in the chapters entitled "The Fine Art of Palpation," "Assessing the Volume of Amniotic Fluid," "Measuring the Fundal Height and Girth of the Uterus" and "Overall Assessment of Fetal Size and Growth" from Volume I of this text. Review those chapters before studying this one.

The skills that you develop during prenatal care will serve you well when watching the mother's abdomen during and between contractions in labor. Visible evidence of contractions is an excellent indication that progressive labor is underway. The uterus will tense, rise up, become slightly narrower along its sides, and lean forward as the contraction peaks, and then settle back down and soften as the contraction subsides. Labor is established when these changes occur with every contraction, becoming more pronounced as labor advances. Their visibility will depend upon the thickness of the woman's abdominal wall, her height (which influences how "out front" she carries her pregnancy) and the depth of her pelvic inlet. A deep anteroposterior diameter of the brim will often cancel out, to an extent, the visible forward lean of the uterus during a contraction. If the woman has a thin pad of fat over her abdomen, the contour of the baby's body may be more apparent during contractions. This will be even more obvious once the membranes rupture and some fluid drains away.

Early labor

At this point the uterus is more round and slightly more pendulous than at any other point during labor. The head is usually higher up and situated more anteriorly than it will be later. If not engaged, the head tends to float near the pubic bone and is mobile at the inlet, especially in multiparous women. The baby's back is found over to one side if the body is transverse; it may be transverse or anterior oblique if the baby is LOA or ROA.

Established labor

Contractions become stronger and more regular. If the head was not engaged before labor began, the posterior parietal eminence now slips below the promontory of the sacrum as the head engages. The uterus tends to lengthen as the head descends and the baby's spine stretches out. The baby's back tends to either rotate toward the mother's anterior midline or turn further toward the mother's spine, depending upon whether the occiput is anterior or posterior.

Palpating fetal position during labor: Prenatal palpation skills can be used to determine the lie, presentation, attitude and variety of the baby during labor. Palpation should only be attempted between uterine contractions. Palpating during contractions is fruitless because the uterus is too firm for you to assess what you are feeling accurately. It is also painful for the mother, because you will invariably attempt to overcome the tension of the contraction with additional pressure. Finally, keeping a woman supine during contractions is uncomfortable, to say the least.

Palpation can provide useful information, especially if there is a question as to the lie or presentation of the baby. This is especially true if you are considering performing an internal exam during labor, whenever there appears to be a problem with progress, when the mother senses a large movement on the baby's part, or when you observe that the contour of the uterus has changed markedly, suggesting a change in fetal position. Remember that even though the baby may have been vertex at your last prenatal appointment, she can and sometimes does change lie or position between that time and labor. Although this doesn't happen often, it is a possibility that cannot be overlooked, especially in multiparous mothers. The baby's position can become altered, even if the baby is known to be dead.

Characteristics of uterine activity: Observing the pattern, intensity, frequency and duration of uterine contractions and how these affect the cervix is among the most important means of assessing labor on the physical level. There are several defined parameters you can assess:

Frequency: The frequency of contractions is assessed by measuring the time from the start of one contraction to the beginning of the next.

Duration: The duration is timed from the onset of a contraction until it ends.

Interval (resting time): The time between contractions is measured from the end of one contraction to the beginning of the next.

Amplitude (strength): Generally measured in the amount of pressure that builds inside the uterus during the peak of a contraction.

Each contraction has a **building phase (increment), peak phase (acme)**, and **easing-down phase (decrement)**.

The building phase lasts longer than the others combined. How all these factors work together is also important. Labor usually starts with mild, irregular or infrequent contractions lasting 15 to 20 seconds and coming every 20 to 30 minutes. As labor progresses, contractions become more frequent, longer, and stronger until they last 60 to 90 seconds and are spaced about 2 to 3 minutes apart. Note that women can begin labor anywhere along the continuum between very infrequent contractions and closely spaced, intense ones. Some women never develop particularly intense, frequent contractions, yet they give birth just fine. This is especially true with women who have had babies before.

Contractions that occur more often than every two minutes and last more than 90 seconds can be extremely stressful for the baby, since the uterine muscle is not able to relax sufficiently to restore full blood flow to the placenta before the next contraction starts. These intense contractions are likely to occur only during a labor that has been artificially stimulated with oxytocin or synthetic prostaglandins.

In addition to monitoring the frequency, duration and interval, the careful observer can gather clues as to the effectiveness of contractions. Each contraction follows what is known as a "normal gradient pattern." During effective labor, the uterus contracts in a synchronous pattern, with contraction activity that is strongest and lasts the longest in the fundus. The contraction tapers off in intensity in the midportion of the uterus, becoming minimal to nonexistent in the lower uterine segment near the cervix. This contractile pattern allows the muscles at the top of the uterus to pull up on the relatively passive lower uterine segment, resulting in cervical effacement and dilation.

It is not normally the contracting fundus that hurts but the cervix, which is being pulled open. Typically, women describe a low-down, pulling sensation in their anterior abdomen, just above and behind their pubic bone. Occasionally this pulling sensation radiates from the lower back, with no sensation in front. When this occurs, at times it can be related to a reversed gradient pattern, which renders contractions ineffective. (See the chapter entitled "Difficulties with Contractions" for details.)

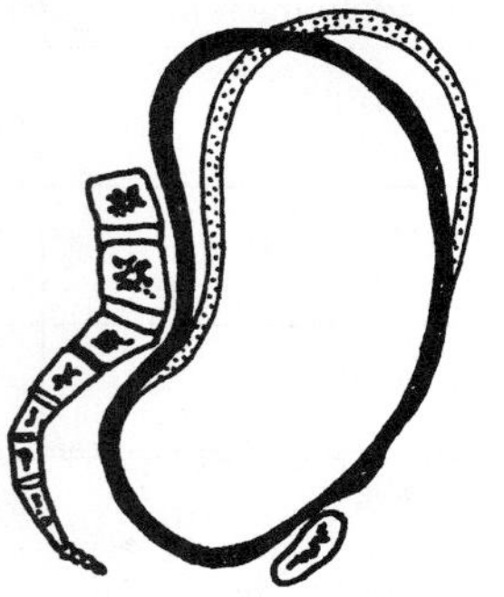

Lateral view of uterus during a contraction(dotted outline)

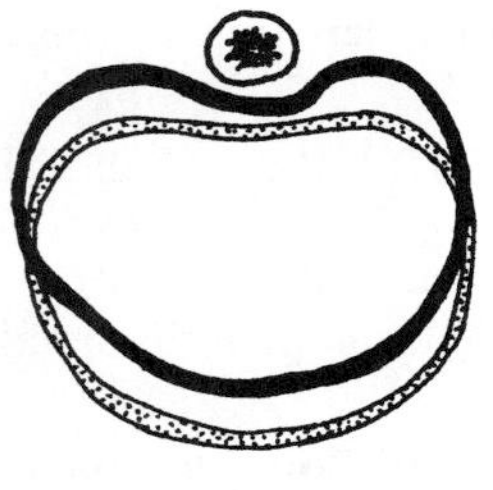

Looking down on the uterus from above

Changes in uterine shape: Once labor begins, each contraction causes the uterus to elongate, drawing the longitudinal fibers of the uterus taut. The lower segment and cervix are stretched thin as they are pulled upward over the lower pole of the baby. The corresponding decrease in the horizontal diameter of the uterus straightens the fetal spine some 5 to 10 cm, pressing the upper pole into the fundus and the lower pole downward. This produces **fetal axis pressure** on the lower segment and the os which also facilitates dilation (Cunningham et al., 2001)

These illustrations show the uterus at rest (solid line) compared to the uterus during contractions (dotted line). When uterine muscle tone is good and the baby is anterior, the uterus leans away from the spine to help direct the presenting part into the upper pelvic cavity. If muscle tone is poor, the uterus sags too far forward during and between contractions, and the thrust of contractions is directed toward the woman's spine.

The amplitude of contractions: A normal contractile wave starts in one of the cornual regions of the uterus. The impulse moves or propagates from one muscle cell to the next in a downward direction, spreading at a rate of 1 to 3 cm per second. Within 30 seconds the entire myometrium is active and the pressure within the amniotic fluid peaks and is then sustained for a varying number of seconds. Pressure then declines to the resting level of 6 to 8 mm Hg. During early labor, peak pressures of 20 to 40 mm Hg are created. In late first phase, pressures rise to 40 to 60 mmHg. During pushing, the uterus produces pressures of 60 to 80 mm Hg. When voluntary maternal pushing is added to that of the uterus, pressures rise to 100 mm Hg or so. However, it is important to note that there is no set pattern of uterine activity that constitutes normal labor. Research by Turnbull (1957) and, later, Schulman and Romney (1970) found no correlation between the amplitude of uterine contractions and the rate of cervical dilation. Thus, the degree to which the cervix yields or resists the contractions has a great deal to do with the progress of labor.

<u>Palpating the fundus to assess contractions</u>: When in doubt about the strength of contractions, the fundus can be palpated to determine their relative intensity. Press the pads of two fingers firmly into the abdomen near the fundus at a point not directly over the body of the baby. Begin when the uterus is quiet and palpate throughout the following contraction. The maximum degree to which the uterus becomes firm varies among individual women and with the strength of labor. As a rule, the firmer the uterus becomes at the peak of a contraction, the stronger the contraction. Continue to palpate during and between five or six contractions in a row to compare the maximum and minimum firmness of the uterus. The weakest contraction in such a series offers the most accurate information regarding their strength (Calkins, 1958).

Strength of Contraction	Sensation on Fundal Palpation
Between contractions	Fundus soft and easily indentable with fingerpad pressure
Mild	Abdomen easy to indent to feel the fundus underneath (like pressing your fingerpads into the cartilaginous tip of your nose)
Moderate	Abdomen firmer, some fundal indentation still occurs (like pressing your fingerpads into the front of your chin)
Strong	Abdomen and fundus are rigid and almost impossible to indent (like pressing your fingerpads against your forehead).

(Adapted from Tucker, 2000)

The midwife can usually detect the onset of a contraction before the mother does by the increasing firmness of the fundus. The midwife will also be likely to palpate the contraction as it tapers off, even after the mother has reported that the sensation of the contraction has subsided.

Although it is widely stated that the contracting uterus is rock-hard during active labor, this is generally true only for contractions stimulated by drugs. In fact, natural contractions usually produce an extremely firm uterus but does not feel quite as rock-hard on firm finger pressure unless the uterus is actively pushing.

Monitoring rotation and descent externally: In an LOT presentation, the baby's back is first positioned to the mother's left side. As labor progresses, the baby's back can be followed as it moves from the mother's left, around and down in a slight downward spiral toward the mother's midline, just above the pubic bone. However, you may find it easier to monitor the location of the anterior shoulder than the entire back because it presents a smaller, more specific landmark.

Using the anterior shoulder as a gauge of internal rotation and descent of the head: The rotation of the anterior shoulder during labor often matches the descent and internal rotation of the head. The height of the shoulder above the symphysis is a direct indication of cephalic descent. If the shoulder axis rotates to transverse as the head completes internal rotation, the anterior shoulder will move past the midline and to the side. If the shoulder axis remains oblique, the anterior shoulder will remain just off the midline as it descends. Thus, the relation of the anterior shoulder to the midline of the mother's abdomen is a direct indication of internal shoulder rotation and an indirect indication of internal rotation of the head.

The position of the shoulder should be noted in the labor record on a simple drawing of the mother's belly in the chart such as this: (·). An inverted capital "T" can be used to indicate the location of the shoulder and a "+" can be used for the location of the fetal heart sounds. A marker can also be used to draw on the mother's belly, especially if a problem with descent is suspected. When using an inverted "T" to indicate the shoulder, the transverse line is marked along the top of the shoulder and the vertical line extends upward through the center of the shoulder. Another horizontal line can be used in the mother's midline to designate the upper border of the pubic bone. This creates an easy and minimally invasive way of monitoring

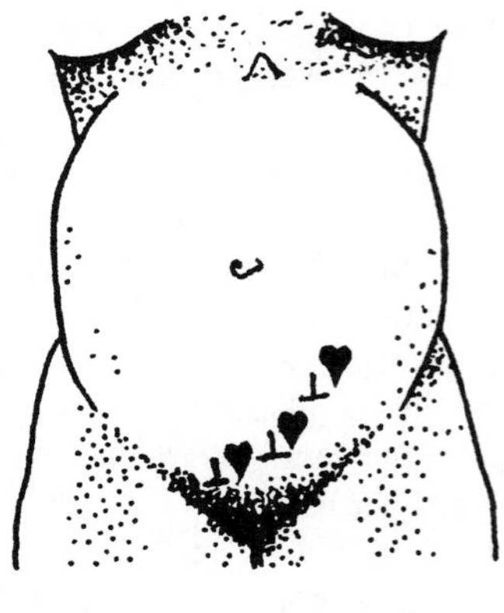

Location of shoulder (inverted "T") and FHR (♥) as baby descends LOT or LOA

descent. While marking the mother's belly may sound silly, paying close attention to these external signs when there is a question regarding fetal position or descent will minimize the number of much more intrusive internal exams. It will also help you hone your ability to watch a mother's abdomen and note changes in the contour that indicate changes in the fetal position.

In most cases, when the shoulder reaches the top of the symphysis, the head will be beginning to distend the perineum, unless the baby is smaller than average or the pelvis is unusually deep. This method of monitoring descent is useful with a cephalic baby in an anterior or transverse position. It is also helps when there is a significant degree of moulding or caput formation because the shoulder will not descend unless the head is descending as well. It is less useful when the baby is posterior (because it will be harder to find the shoulder unless the baby is rotating anteriorly) or when the placenta is implanted on the anterior uterine wall.

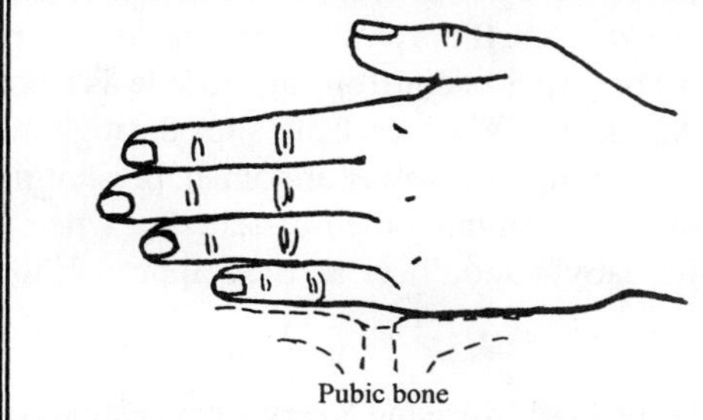

How to hold your hand to gauge station externally

External assessment of the station of the head: The next chart illustrates how the head can also be palpated externally to determine descent. This is particularly helpful if the baby has developed a caput, making absolute identification of the skull difficult on internal exam. This method as well as tracking the position of the shoulder is also very helpful when the membranes are ruptured making internal exams unadvisable. The two techniques can be used simultaneously to arrive at a more exact assessment.

Descent of the head is gauged in "fifths" in relationship to its passage through the brim. The width of all five fingers of one hand, held together straight out, parallel to and with the border of the lowermost finger level with the upper border of the symphysis is used as a guide to determine how many fifths of the head are above the brim. The width of each finger represents one-fifth. For example, when the head is mobile above the brim (floating), it occupies all the space above the upper border of the pubic bone, accommodating the full width of five fingers. As the head descends, the portion remaining above the brim is represented by fewer fingers. Generally speaking, the head is engaged (that is, the biparietal diameter has passed through the brim) when the portion remaining above the brim is represented by two fingers or less.

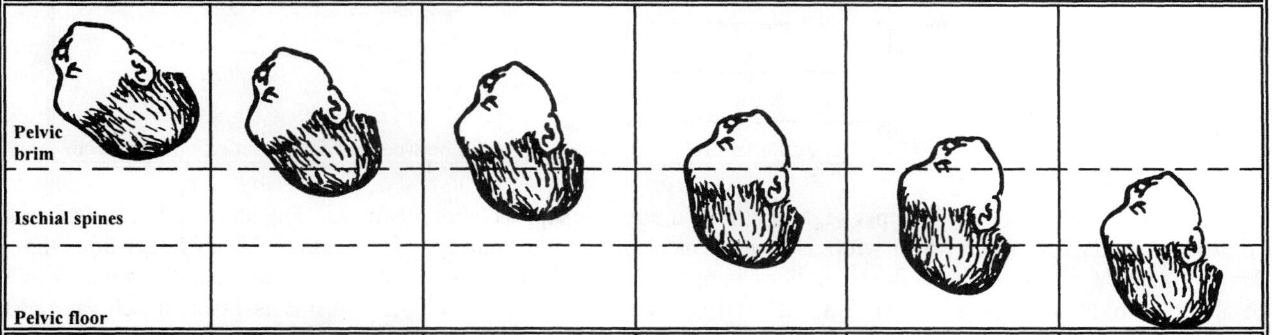

5/5	4/5	3/5	2/5	1/5	0/5
Sinciput and occiput both above brim	Sinciput prominent; occiput easily felt but descending	Sinciput rising as head flexes more, occiput still just palpable	Sinciput not so prominent; little or no occiput felt	Sinciput barely felt or not felt; occiput not felt	Head on pelvic floor; not palpable above brim

S=sinciput; O=occiput

Monitoring descent and rotation by the location of the fetal heart sounds: The location where the fetal heart sounds are the loudest will change position during labor as the baby rotates and descends into the pelvis. Search for this point on the mother's abdomen each time you listen to the fetal heart. When you are learning, you can make little "+" marks on the mother's belly or on a drawing in her chart. This point will descend and move across the belly as the baby moves down and rotates, arriving at a more or less midline position well down on the belly as transition nears. This is, of course, more difficult to follow if the placenta is on the anterior wall of the uterus or the baby's back is posterior. Note that this phenomenon is only detectable with the use of a regular fetoscope. A Doppler amplifies the sound too much, making locating the point of maximum intensity less clearly defined.

Checking descent at the pubic bone: Diane Barnes, (2000), a CNM in Missouri, shares that she looks for a change in the contour of the abdomen just above the pubic bone to check descent. Prior to about +1 station, there is a slight bulge in this area, which smooths out as the baby descends further. She refers to this as the "ski slope effect" and checks for it while she is listening to the fetal heart. Be sure, however, that the slight bulge is not due to an overfull bladder!

Development of a crease above the pubic bone: Descent can be assessed fairly well by watching for the line or crease that forms on the mother's lower abdomen parallel to the symphysis as dilation advances. If the mother is quite thin, there might not be any crease at all at the beginning of labor. The crease develops and becomes wider from side to side as labor progresses. Near transition, it is usually three-quarters of the width of the lower belly. When the head slips through the cervix and settles into the birth canal, the crease usually spans nearly the entire width of the lower abdomen, presenting a visible sign that the onset of pushing is imminent. This crease cannot always be seen in women-of-size, but when it can be observed, it is quite reliable. It may be produced by the bulk of the baby's shoulders as they approach the symphysis (Gentlebirth midwifery archives, 2001).

Indirect assessment of dilation by monitoring fundal height: Kathy Deol (2001) of Iowa and Kerry Lizon (2000) of Michigan have shared a technique learned from Russian midwives to assess dilation. The width of the fingers, held together, straight out and perpendicular to the longitudinal axis of the mother's body, is used as a guide. With the mother lying flat, measure the space between the height of the fundus and the xiphoid process during the peak of a contraction using your fingers. As the space between the xiphoid and the fundus shortens (becomes narrower), dilation advances.

FINGER-BREADTHS BETWEEN FUNDUS & XIPHOID	APPROXIMATE DILATION
5	none
4	2 cm
3	4 cm
2	6 cm
1	8 cm
0	Full dilation

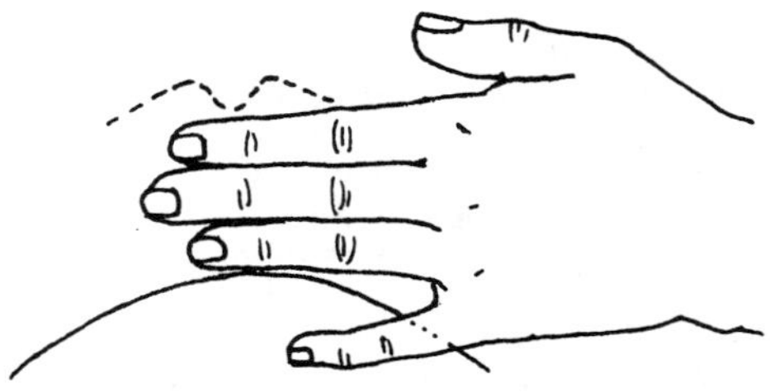

Three fingers fit between the fundus and xiphoid at 4 cm.

This occurs, in part, because the upper segment of the uterus thickens as labor advances. The uterus also rises more as contractions intensify. Each finger width is counted as 2 cm. The formula is as follows: number of finger-breadths × 2 = Y; 10 cm − Y = number of cm dilation. For example, if you can fit four fingers in the space, then the mother would be about 2 cm dilated (4 × 2 = 8, 10 − 8 = 2 cm dilation.) Of course, the accuracy of this assessment will vary a bit depending upon the size of your hands, the length and depth of the mother's torso and the depth of her pelvis. The chart above will help you perform this assessment without having to calculate.

Checking for the ascension of the retraction ring: Another method used by Russian midwives to detect progress in dilation is monitoring the development of the lower segment by palpating the retraction ring as it rises above the pubic bone. The lower segment is 3 to 4 inches in length (7.5 to 10 cm) by the end of pregnancy. This places the retraction ring at approximately the same level as the pubic bone. As labor advances, the lower uterine segment becomes thinner and longer as the upper segment thickens, producing a ridge where the two segments meet. Although this ridge is not visible unless labor is obstructed, the line of demarcation between the upper and lower uterine segments can often be palpated as it rises above the pubic bone as labor advances.

To locate the ring, make sure your hand is warm and the mother's bladder is empty. Have the mother lie down on a firm surface. Use the palmar surface of your fingers to gently palpate the lower abdomen during a contraction. Starting at the pubic bone, move your hand over the lower segment, making a gentle pressing or rocking motion to distinguish the line of demarcation between the upper segment, which is quite firm, and the lower segment, which is much less so; it can feel elastic and almost fluctuant (Hellman & Pritchard, 1971).

Once you have identified the retraction ring, you may be able to find it at the onset of contractions or even, in some cases, between them, although it will be easiest to distinguish the ring when the upper segment is contracted because the soft lower segment will contrast with the firm upper segment. As labor progresses, the ring rises to about one-third of the way between the pubic bone and the mother's navel by the time the cervix is fully dilated. Its actual location at this point will vary depending upon the length of the mother's torso. For example, a woman who is short-waisted will likely have a retraction ring that is halfway between her pubic bone and her navel; a long-waisted mother's retraction ring will be closer to her pubic bone. Once the cervix is fully dilated and the upper segment can move the baby down through an unobstructed passageway, the retraction ring stops rising.

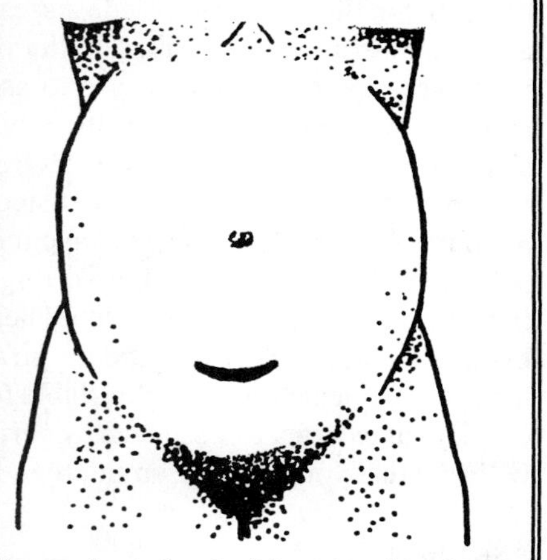

Approximate level of the retraction ring at full dilation during normal labor.

A pathologic retraction ring may be visible as high up as the umbilicus, with the upper uterine segment appearing bulky and thickened in contrast to the very thin and tender lower segment. The line of demarcation between the two segments is very pronounced, and a distinct ridge may be visible and can be felt on palpation. See the chapter entitled "Recognizing and Dealing with Obstructed Labor" for more details.

Checking for a nuchal cord: See the chapter entitled "Cord Problems and Emergencies during Labor" for a method of checking abdominally for a cord around the neck.

ADDITIONAL NONINVASIVE TECHNIQUES FOR ASSESSING PROGRESS

Some of the less quantifiable methods of assessing labor progress via observation and physiological findings are discussed in the chapter entitled "Assessing the Progress and Strength of Labor: An Overview." Techniques involving abdominal exam are described in the preceding chapter. This chapter focuses on additional techniques that various midwives, doulas and nurses use to assess progress in labor without performing an internal exam. While all these methods give approximate results only, they carry the advantage of being noninvasive. These techniques have been shared by midwives and practitioners from around the world, and credit has been duly given, and permission to print them has been obtained. Watch for the listed changes as labor progresses. If the expected signs are not occurring or if they are but something seems amiss, take this as an indication that an internal exam may be warranted.

The following methods of detecting progress all rely on external signs that will vary among women depending upon the length of their torso, their overall height, the size of their baby and the depth of their pelvis. Be sure that the mother's bladder is empty before you attempt an assessment requiring palpation near the pubic bone. Not only does a full bladder make assessment more uncomfortable for the mother, but it may confuse your findings. Remember that you can always check your external assessments by performing an internal exam. As you become an astute birth observer, however, you will find that you will rely on internal exams less and less to verify your clinical and intuitive impressions.

Ask the mother

Jill Cohen (2001) reports that she asks mothers how far along they are and finds that women invariably respond that they do not know. She then asks them to tune in during a contraction and show her how far along they are by spreading their fingers. Internal exams to verify the mothers' impressions have confirmed the accuracy of the mothers' assessments.

Monitoring the pituitary reflex point

In her book POLLY'S BIRTH BOOK: OBSTETRICS FOR THE HOME, Polly Block, a Utah midwife, describes a technique that she relies upon to monitor and enhance progress during labor. A point that she calls both the pituitary and the uterine reflex is located at the center of the top of the pad of the heel. This spot can be massaged with the thumb in a circular pattern. Use olive oil to reduce friction. As the uterus contracts, a mild, sphincter-like sensation can be detected in this spot. The spot "opens" when the contraction puts pressure on the cervix to effect dilation, producing a rather deep, fluid sensation in this area. The reflex point "closes" and becomes firm again as the contraction subsides. Monitoring this spot allows the midwife to detect a contraction 3 to 5 seconds before the mother becomes aware of it. After 5 cm dilation, the uterine reflex no longer firms up between contractions, but remains soft and open.

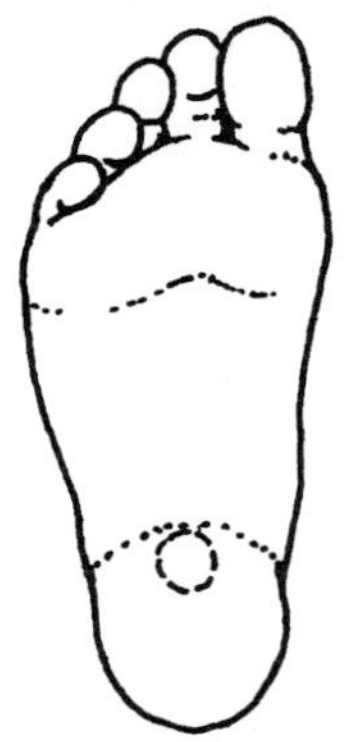

Locating the pituitary reflex point

You will notice that the cervical-uterine reflex spot on one foot feels different than the spot on the other. Upon closer inspection, you will note that one side of the uterine reflex on one foot is thicker. The circular opening is round and full on one foot and irregular on the other. The foot on which the irregular area appears is the side of the mother's body on which the placenta is located. The approximate site of placental attachment is indicated by the location of the irregularity on the circle. A small round knot in the center of the reflex on the opposite foot represents the baby (Block, 1984).

Monitor the mother's anterior fontanelle

If you place your palm over the top of your own head, you will note a distinctly warm region where your anterior fontanelle once was. In eastern religions, this is known as the Crown "chakra," or energy center. The mother's anterior fontanelle gets increasingly warm as labor advances and will heat up dramatically as she reaches full dilation. Begin by checking it early in labor and periodically as labor advances.

Assessing dilation by monitoring temperature changes in the lower leg

Allison Radcliff (2000) shares a technique she learned from a traditional Mexican midwife in Austin, Texas. It involves noticing temperature changes on the surface of the mother's leg between the ankle and the knee. Most (but not all) women experience a temperature change in their calf when they labor.

When the woman is not yet dilated, the toes and feet may be cold, but the rest of the leg is warm. As labor progresses, the line of demarcation between the cold region and the warm region moves up the leg from the ankle toward the knee. This means that when the coolness extends halfway between the ankle and the knee and the leg is warm above that point, a woman is about 5 centimeters dilated. When the entire calf is cold, but the knee is warm, the urge to push should follow shortly. Your findings will be thrown off by extra warmth from external sources such as blankets or a hot bath. It takes about 15 to 20 minutes after a woman comes out of the bath or blankets are removed before this sign once again becomes reliable.

Watch for changes in the sacrum and coccyx

You may notice the sacrum bulge (or appear to broaden) over the region of the promontory as the biparietal diameter moves past that point. You can then follow progress by watching the bulge move lower on the mother's backside. The coccyx will be pressed outward as the baby descends. As pushing begins in earnest, the sacroiliac joints widen and the sacrum moves back 1 to 2 cm, creating more room at the outlet. If you cannot see the sacrum contours change, you can usually use the palm of your hand to locate the bulge of the head and follow it down. You may be able to feel the baby's face moving beneath your hand when your palm is placed over the sacrum. As you get more practiced you will be able to detect this movement visually in most women. Maggie Banks (2000) of New Zealand also comments that a phenomenal amount of heat builds up over the mother's sacral spine in late labor just prior to and at the onset of pushing.

Watch for changes in the gluteal (or natal) cleft

Midwives Maggie Banks (2000) of New Zealand and Karen Valcourt (1996) of Hickory, North Carolina, both note changes in the color of the skin in the cleavage of the buttocks as labor advances. They are not alone in this observation; it was first officially reported in the LANCET (Byrne & Edmonds,1990) and later by Leslie Hobbs (1998). According to these sources, a solid red line starts to appear in the gluteal cleft when the cervix begins to dilate, beginning at the upper border of the anal opening. The distance between the upper anal margin and the nape of the buttocks (top of the butt crack, the point just below the sacrococcygeal joint where the coccyx begins to curve inward in most people) is visually divided into tenths. A 2 mm wide line climbs up the center of the cleavage as labor advances, reflecting both dilation and descent in the station of the presenting part. The research states that the line terminates at the nape of the buttocks; however, both Banks and Valcourt have observed that the line often continues upward until it reaches the flat portion of the sacrum.

The research reported in the LANCET included 102 women, 89% of whom developed the line and 10.4% of whom showed no line; it was initially absent in 6.25% of those who later developed it. The researchers found a correlation between the length of the red line and dilation but an even more significant correlation with station. The study speculated that the line develops as a result of vasocongestion in the basivertebral and intervertebral veins around the sacrum due to the increasing intrapelvic pressure as the fetal presenting part descends. The correlation between the length of the line and dilation may be due to the relationship between the degree of dilation and the station of the fetus.

As labor becomes more active, the line not only becomes longer, but its color deepens. Karen notes that, in Caucasian women, the color ranges from deep red to bluish purple. She has observed that in women-of-color, it deepens to a dark brown with a red tinge. The deepest color comes in the accelerated phase of labor when the woman is entering transition.

Maggie notes that, in some women, the deepening color will extend upward beyond the solid line above the top of the gluteal cleft either before they have an urge to push or until they begin pushing effectively. This extension presents as tiny filaments of color, similar in appearance to spider veins but along tiny wrinkle lines, causing the lines to look almost like long hairs. In one case, Maggie noticed an unusually expanded region of color at the top of the line, which turned out to be due to an old scar from a pilonidal sinus. In that case, it did not correlate with the woman being nearly ready to push.

Other changes in the sacrococcygeal region: Jill Cohen (2001) as well as many other midwives, has noted other characteristic changes in the cleft of the buttocks during late labor, prior to pushing. The cheeks of the buttocks begin to flatten out and separate from the middle outward due to the underlying pressure exerted by the baby's head. The lower end of the cleft also widens from the perineum toward the back as the presenting part descends and presses out on the tissues below the coccyx. A widening inverted V-shaped area, the color of the mother's perineum, becomes increasingly apparent just above and around the anus as this occurs. The anus also opens and flattens as the baby reaches the pelvic floor but before the presenting part is visible. These changes are, of course, most apparent when the woman is bending over.

Goose bumps on the buttocks

A well-seasoned labor and delivery nurse shares that a reliable indicator of the baby's descent through the cervix and into the birth canal is the appearance of goose bumps on the mother's bottom. Women will announce an urge to push or spontaneous grunting or pushing begins only minutes after these appear. She has found this correlation to be 100% accurate. Note that goose bumps are associated with catecholamine release.

Watch how the mother moves and positions herself late in labor

Caroline Flint (1986), an English midwife, notes that women begin to spontaneously rotate their pelvis as active labor becomes stronger. This brings the baby into position for birth. Jill Cohen (2001) notes that a woman begins to spontaneously rock her bottom, open her legs more, and lean forward as transition nears its end, just prior to pushing.

Watch for the fetus ejection reflex

A burst of muscle activity, the need to grasp onto something (often overhead), dry mouth, upper-chest breathing, dilated pupils, flexing of the knees, accompanied by a rush of anger or euphoria and a fleeting expression of fear all typically herald the onset of strong contractions that soon lead to pushing, especially in women who have had optimal privacy during labor.

Bloody show

Bloody show at the beginning of labor usually signals that significant cervical changes have begun. Many women have a second bloody show as the presenting part passes through the fully dilated cervical os. This show should be quite mucilaginous and stretchy; a trickle of brighter blood near the end of dilation, accompanied by lots of suprapubic pain, can also mean a cervical lip is being pulled down with the presenting part (see the chapter entitled "Cervical and Other Soft-Tissue Problems during Labor" for details).

PERFORMING INTERNAL EXAMS DURING LABOR

The chapter entitled "Assessing Cervical Changes during Pregnancy" in Volume I of this text covers a great deal of basic information on this topic. Please review that chapter before studying this one. In this chapter, I will cover additional variables to consider when performing internal exams during labor. The presenting part assumes different positions in relationship to the pelvis as the cervix opens and the baby moves down. Thus an internal exam is more than checking dilation: it includes parameters such as fetal lie, position, synclitism, attitude and station as well as cervical position, effacement and consistency. Understanding the many subtle ways that these factors can change and interact allows you to more accurately assess how the mother is progressing in labor.

Some of the techniques and findings described in this chapter may be rarely, if ever, relevant to your practice. They are included here for completeness and for that once-in-a-career time when they are needed. Although some are exceedingly rare, such findings are described throughout the chapter at whatever point they are likely to be detected as you proceed through the exam. Just knowing the possibilities of what you may be feeling is sometimes a great help.

An internal exam can, at times, be an invaluable assessment. However, because it is an intrusive intervention, it should be used prudently and only after all other means of assessing the situation have been exhausted or when definitive information that can usually be gathered via an internal is needed quickly. As you become attuned to the energy of birth as it manifests during labor and pay attention to the myriad physical signs that labor is advancing, you will find that you rely on internal exams less and less to know how a woman's labor is progressing. Her behavior and the feel of the energy in the room will be enough, in many cases, to help you judge how far along she is and what help she needs at the moment. An internal exam is an interruption of the flow of energy outward, as you push your fingers inside to see what is going on. It can, at times, impede the progress of labor, as well as encourage the development of infection. Nevertheless, if you are unsure what is happening, if the external signs are simply absent, inconsistent or contradictory, if you need to confirm an unusual fetal position, if the woman has a prove-it-to-me attitude or if labor appears to have stalled, an internal exam can often offer much valuable information to help you determine how best to assist the mother and baby.

Preparing for the Exam

Positioning the mother for an exam

Have the mother urinate and arrange herself comfortably on a firm, padded surface, lying on her back with her knees flexed and feet apart, or soles together and knees flopped to either side. Place pillows under her knees to lessen the strain on her hip joints and help relax the perineum. If you have short fingers, have the mother assume a McRoberts position or have her tip her pubic bone upward to flatten her lower back against the bed. One of these positions will assist you in reaching everything more easily. Having the mother lie down for an exam allows her to relax her pelvic muscles completely and is usually the best way to perform a thorough exam. It also relaxes the abdomen, which makes it easer to palpate the baby externally if necessary while doing an internal. The drawback to this position is that it narrows the spinopubic angle. As you perform your exam, keep in mind that the mother's position may have changed the position of the baby. If the waters are intact and the head was not seated in the pelvis before she reclined, it may float up out of the pelvis slightly or even a great deal. Wait for a contraction to subside before proceeding.

Other positions of the mother during an exam: Most findings from internal exams, including those given here, are described as if performed on a woman lying on her back. However, there may be times when examining the mother who is in a standing, squatting or in a hands-and-knees position is most appropriate. Turn this book in order to rotate the illustrations to match the mother's position. Keep in mind that the mother's position may alter your ability to reach landmarks, sometimes rendering them easier to find but often making them harder to distinguish, as well as shifting the baby's position or degree of descent. If your have serious questions regarding what may be affecting a mother's progress, having her lie down is usually the best position to use, especially if your hands are small or fingers are short.

Palpate the abdomen

Observe the mother's abdomen when she is upright and walking for clues regarding fetal position (this is covered in Volume I of this text). Abdominal palpation should also be performed between contractions prior to an internal exam, unless you suspect a complication, such as cord prolapse, in which case you should confirm what is going on immediately. (See the chapter entitled "Abdominal Examination Techniques for Use during Labor" for more details.) Thorough palpation will guide you regarding what you might feel during an internal exam. It can serve as a preliminary guide to locating the sagittal suture and the fontanelles. For example, if the abdominal exam indicates that the baby's back is to the mother's anterior left side, you would first check for the sagittal suture running from two to eight o'clock, with the posterior fontanelle at two o'clock and the anterior fontanelle near eight o'clock. In a transverse lie, your abdominal exam should reveal no fetal pole in the fundus or at the brim, guiding you to be particularly careful not to rupture the membranes as you attempt to confirm the fetal position internally. If you suspect that the presenting part is not in the brim, prop the mother's bottom up with several folded sheets or blankets before proceeding in order to elevate her lower body slightly. This will help protect against cord prolapse if the membranes rupture during your exam.

Note that the position of the baby's body as palpated externally does not guarantee the position of the presenting part. For example, it is possible for the back to be anterior and for the head to be twisted at the neck, presenting occiput posterior. You could also find the baby to be transverse externally, yet you detect a small, well-engaged head in the pelvis. In this case, the mother may be carrying twins. Discrepancies such as these provide useful information regarding things you need to investigate further and clues as to how to proceed during labor.

Performing the Exam

Don a nonsterile glove if the membranes are intact, or a sterile glove if they are not or you are unsure of their status. Apply a small amount of sterile, water-based lubricant if necessary.

What to Check for during an Internal Exam

The following is a list of questions you will want to ask yourself as you perform an internal exam. Some of these assessments overlap; however, they are addressed separately for the sake of clarity.

- Are there any unusual symptoms such as bleeding?
- Are there any unusual findings on or near the external genitals?
- What is the condition of the walls and musculature of the yoni?
- Where is the cervix?
- How effaced is the cervix?
- How dilated is the cervix?
- Is the cervix evenly dilated or is the dilation lopsided?
- Is the cervical opening anterior, posterior, pulled to one side or centrally located?
- What is the consistency of the cervix? (Rigid, soft, edematous? Is the surface regular or irregular? Does it hang like an empty cuff or is it well applied to the presenting part?)
- Are the membranes intact?
- What is the presentation? If cephalic, has the baby developed a caput?
- Where is the presenting part? (Floating anteriorly, well fitted into the midpelvis or dipping posteriorly?)
- Is the head moulded?
- What is the presenting part and how is it situated in relationship to maternal pelvic landmarks? Can you identify suture lines and fontanelles?
- Does the presenting part feel normally formed?
- At what station is the presenting part?
- Is there any change in the cervix, the position or station of the presenting part, the consistency of the membranes (if intact) or any other feature during contractions?

As you can see, an internal exam can tell you much more than how dilated a woman is. We shall now review each of these items in detail. You will not always perform every type of exam listed here with each and every internal. You will pick and choose among them based on previous findings and current necessity.

Touch pictures

Throughout this chapter, an old convention known as a "touch picture" is used to show the landmarks you will be searching for during an internal exam. The presenting part is shown well applied to a widely dilated cervix to best demonstrate all the landmarks. When you perform an exam, what you can touch directly will be influenced by the depth of descent, the amount of forewaters and the size of the cervical os. You may need to reach past the edges of the os to identify these landmarks if the membranes allow.

Assessing your findings

As you review this material and gain experience, it is important not to dismiss findings or impressions because they do not match what you think you should be feeling or what you have always felt. Don't automatically assume it is due to a lack of skill. The first time you palpate something unusual, it will probably throw you for a loop. You might be feeling a face, genitals, a bottom, a foot, a knee, ribs, an arm, an umbilical cord, a placenta, an ear, a hand or even a defective fetal part. You may be palpating a variation in maternal anatomy, such as a cervical polyp. Keep your mind open to what you might be feeling rather than making hasty assumptions.

Relating to the baby during your exam

The baby is aware of whatever is going on in the environment. When you contact the baby directly, as you do when you examine the baby's presenting part, it can help to talk to the baby. If a position change needs to occur, explain to the baby, in simple language, what needs to take place. Often, when I have done an exam during long labors, I have found the baby turning his head this way and that, as if trying to find his way out or as if he is being disturbed by the exam. Be mindful of how you express your findings to the mother, because the baby is also listening.

If there is bleeding

Slight bleeding is usually show, a result of the normal birth process. However, the two most likely sources of dangerous bleeding, previa and abruption, must always be kept in mind. Other, reasons for abnormal bleeding are cervical tears, stretching cervical scars or, much more rarely, either a ruptured maternal varicosity high in the yoni or a ruptured vasa previa. All types of abnormal bleeding in labor are further discussed in the part entitled "Abnormal Bleeding during Labor."

Regardless of the source, if bleeding has been heavy you may encounter a clot when you attempt to perform an exam. It is rare for a complete previa to go undetected all the way into labor, but it can happen, presenting with bright red bleeding. In such cases, disruption of an overlying clot or the placenta itself may lead to massive hemorrhage. If you think that abruption or previa, may be the source of bleeding, see the chapter entitled "Bleeding due to Placental Disruption" for how to proceed. If you seriously suspect previa, your safest option is to forego an exam and transport immediately.

However, assuming that neither previa nor abruption or a ruptured vessel is the cause, bleeding from cervical trauma or even bloody show can, at times, be more than you would expect, but is intermittent. It usually has a characteristically mucusy feel and is not very bright red. Cervical bleeding is rarely dangerous and would only be of concern if it signaled that a cervical tear was extending into the lower uterine segment or the bladder. Much less commonly, yoni bleeding may indicate that a uterine rupture is occurring (see the chapter entitled "Uterine Rupture during Labor" for more details.)

Are there any unusual findings on or near the external genitals?

Look carefully to determine if any varicosities have become apparent or if lesions of any kind have developed since your last prenatal genital exam. If the woman has had genital mutilation in the past, reassess the scars now and again late in labor when you first suspect the baby is approaching the perineum to help you determine how to proceed. This woman may need to have the scars separated (cut open) to allow for birth (see my text HEALING PASSAGE for details).

If the membranes have ruptured, check to see if the fluid has the characteristic salty, subtle ocean smell of healthy fluid. Sometimes the smell will be stronger because normal yoni odors can be pronounced in women at term. Foul-smelling fluid is a sign of intrauterine infection, and transport is your safest alternative.

Insert your fingers

Gently insert your two examining fingers (index and middle) into the yoni, index finger uppermost. Occasionally, if landmarks are difficult to reach and there are problems in labor demanding more information, a thorough exam may require inserting your entire hand. Insertion may be difficult or impossible if the woman has been infibulated. In this case, take extra care, use plenty of lubricant, and proceed very slowly, beginning with one finger.

What is the condition of the walls and musculature of yoni?

The yoni should feel warm and moist with soft, stretchy walls. A hot, dry yoni is a sign of prolonged obstructed labor. This is caused by a tight-fitting presenting part that is impeding circulation in the pelvis. If the woman's temperature is elevated, the yoni may be hot but should not be dry. If the walls are normally warm and moist but firm and rigid, anticipate a long labor. The presence of scar tissue from a previous clitorotomy or bad tear may resist stretching, causing a delay during pushing. A full bowel, which feels lumpy and encroaches on the space in the canal, can be detected by palpation along the posterior wall of the yoni (Bennett & Brown, 1999). Indentable lumps in the yoni walls may be varicosities. The muscles of the yoni should be assessed as well. Using the information from the chapter entitled "Examining the Muscles of the Perineum and Explaining Perineal Stretching" in Vol I of this text, compare both sides for tension and talk to the mother about your findings. Soft-tissue tension is a primary cause of slow labor.

Herniations and the progress of labor: Large herniations into the yoni (cystoceles, rectoceles, etc.) appear as an outpouching of the wall overlying the hernia. If such a prolapse exists, be sure to check it periodically during labor, as it may become trapped in front of the presenting part. (For details on how to handle this, see the chapter entitled "Cervical and Other Soft-Tissue Problems during Labor.")

Recheck pelvimetry

If indicated, this is a good time to reassess any unusual findings from your initial pelvimetry exam. The hormones of late pregnancy will make the pelvic tissues softer than ever, meaning that any features you previously had questions about will be easier to palpate.

Checking the cervix

Where is the cervical os? Once a woman is in labor, the cervical os is usually pointed toward the sacrococcygeal joint, directly in line with the force of the uterine contractions. Therefore, to find the os, first follow the anterior yoni wall up to the central, most anterior region of the anterior fornix, where the curve of the distended cervix meets the canal. Begin to advance your fingers down and around the bulge of the cervix toward the sacrum until you run into an indentation, a soft (or firm) ring of tissue that admits your finger; this is the os. If dilation is more advanced, you may encounter a portion of the cervical lip rather than a ring. If so, follow it around until you are satisfied you have identified the complete circular orifice. Note that an extremely anterior cervix (high in the anterior fornix) may be associated with an sacculated uterus, a very rare event at term. See the chapter entitled "Recognizing and Dealing With Obstructed Labor."

It is easy to mistake a thin cervix with a barely dilated, very posterior os for complete dilation, especially if the examiner is inexperienced or hasty. It is also possible for a roll of yoni tissue to be created by pressure from the descending presenting part. This compressed roll of tissue may be mistaken for the cervical lip with the presenting part behind it. A ring of tissue can, on rare occasions, form a band all the way around the yoni wall and obscure findings. A prolapse of the urethra or rectum, which produces a bulge into the yoni canal, can become flattened and lodge next to the presenting part, also mimicking the cervical lip.

Feel all the way around the circumference of the cervix. Once you think you have found the rim of the cervix, advance your fingers straight back in the midline to make sure there is not a less dilated, internal os that you are missing. Be sure to evaluate all these factors before you declare that the mother has reached a particular dilation. If you still have not found the os with these techniques, starting at the upper anterior fornix, sweep your fingers from side to side as you advance them backward in a systematic search, as the os could be pulled off to one side.

The surface of the undilated or partially dilated cervix will most likely feel uniformly smooth and convexly curved. (To the get a sense of what the presenting part feels like when palpated through a partially effaced cervix, use your finger to feel the inside of your cheek while applying pressure against your face with your other hand.) If the cervix is quite thin (effaced), it may be mobile over the surface of the presenting part (or the bag of waters) between contractions.

If the membranes are intact, the opening of the os will contain a portion of the very smooth, probably somewhat firm, fluid-filled membranes, which is often slightly fluctuant between contractions. If the membranes are ruptured, the presenting part, if it is the baby's head, will most likely feel very firm and somewhat textured, from the presence of hair. If another part of the baby is presenting, the skin will feel exceptionally smooth, often smoother than the membranes and, of course, will not be fluctuant in the normal circumstance.

How effaced is the cervix? Most of the thinning of the cervical canal usually takes place prior to significant dilation in a primigravida and along with dilation in a multigravida. Effacement requires a lot of uterine effort when the cervix has never been opened before; thus first-time mothers often have longer periods of early labor. This is also true of women who have had babies via surgical births before their labor began.

Assessing effacement is a very subjective process. The length of the uneffaced cervix varies but averages about 2 in (2.5 cm). To get a feel for cervical effacement, press your lips together and stick them out as far as you can. Now, insert a fingertip all the way to your teeth. This is the equivalent of about 50% effacement. Now, with your finger still in place, slowly draw your lips back to a normal closed position, keeping them pressed against your finger. This movement mimics cervical thinning (which does not happen so fast!). Now pull your closed lips into a wide tense smile. The edges of your lips feel very much like 100% effacement in most women, although few will reach the "paper- thin" quality that is often mentioned. In reality, the cervix rarely gets that thin. Multiparous mothers usually don't efface completely, even at full dilation.

How dilated is the cervix? Once you have located the os, determine how dilated it is. Insert your two fingers into the os (if possible) and spread your fingertips across the center of the opening until you contact the edges. Take care not to stretch it, as this will increase your estimate of dilation. The distance between the outer border of your two fingertips is the measure of dilation. If there is a discrepancy between the dilation of the internal and external os, the "official" dilation is that of the internal os, but note the dilation of the external os as well.

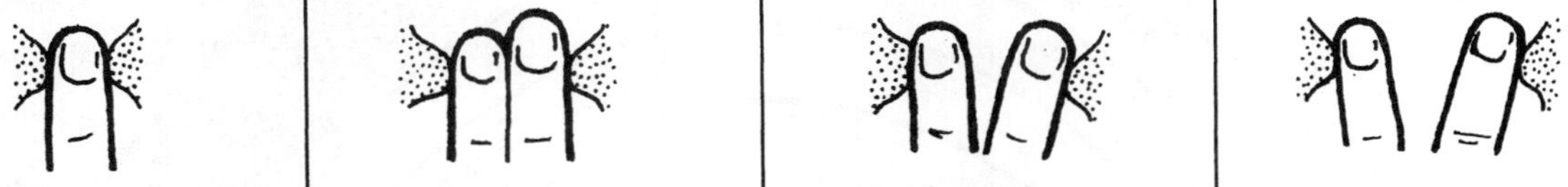

1 finger (2 cm) | 2 fingers (3-3.5 cm) | 3 fingers (5-5.5 cm) | 4 fingers (7-7.5 cm)

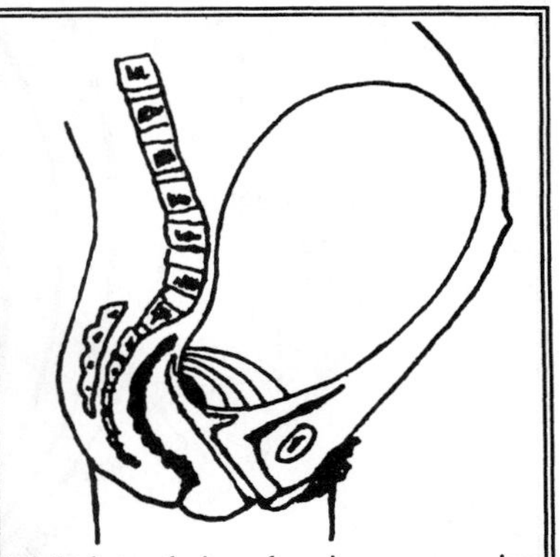

Right lateral view showing progressive dilation.

These drawings illustrate checking early dilation with finger breadths. Since the size and length of your fingers affect how early dilation is estimated, measure your own fingers with a centimeter tape and compare your findings with those above. In early labor, the os may barely admit a fingertip or two. As labor advances, you will need to stretch your fingers apart to reach its edges. Progressive cervical changes are an excellent indication that a woman is in active labor.

Most explanations of dilation assume that the cervix is centered between the walls of the yoni and show the cervix dilating in uniformly round progressions from the center outward. In fact, since the cervix is pointed posteriorly in most women, it more typically dilates from the back of the yoni forward in an elliptical shape (Sutton, 2000). In early labor, up to about 3 or 4 cm, the os is posterior but more or less circular, although it can be oblong side-to-side if the head is quite asynclitic. As dilation progresses the cervix becomes more oval or egg-shaped, with the wider part of the egg most posterior. The posterior rim tends to remain more stationary and undergoes less retraction and is taken up sooner, while the anterior cervix widens and stretches over the baby's head. As a result, it is quite common to palpate a broad rim of cervix anteriorly and laterally with little or no rim felt posteriorly (see the drawing on the following page).

Dilation is assessed from 0 (zero) to 10 cm which is considered full dilation (colloquially referred to as "fully" in the United Kingdom and as "complete" in the United States). It is best to assess dilation across the widest transverse opening of the cervix. Once dilation is well underway, assessing the amount of rim left to dilate is just as valid as noting the amount of opening the os has undergone (and much easier if your fingers are short); either way, the remaining rim of the cervix must move out of the way. Be sure to record exactly what you assessed in your notes, a particularly important part of charting if more than one midwife will be performing internal exams during labor.

Ten centimeters is the standard measurement for "full dilation" because the widest diameter of the flexed, term infant skull is 9.5 cm; however, the 0-to-10 scale represents only an average. Full dilation occurs when the presenting part has descended through the os or when no cervix can be felt around the circumference. In a premature birth, if the head is quite low and passes through, this may occur before 10 cm. If the mother's pelvis is quite large, the woman may still have a rim of cervix even though she is past the 10 cm point. Even so, unless the baby is in trouble, you typically do not need to instruct a woman that she is ready to push. When she is ready, she will push with no instruction. Many women experience a resting phase once they are fully dilated, thus full dilation by itself does not mean that pushing should begin.

In some cases, even though you can still feel a rim of cervix, the uterus can push the baby past it without any cervical trauma when a spontaneous urge to push triggers involuntary bearing down. As long as the pushing urge is involuntary and the uterus can push the baby through without dragging down an edge of cervix with the head, she is, for all practical purposes, fully dilated if the presentation is cephalic. In breeches, the entire cervical rim should be taken up before pushing begins to avoid entrapment of the aftercoming arms or head during descent.

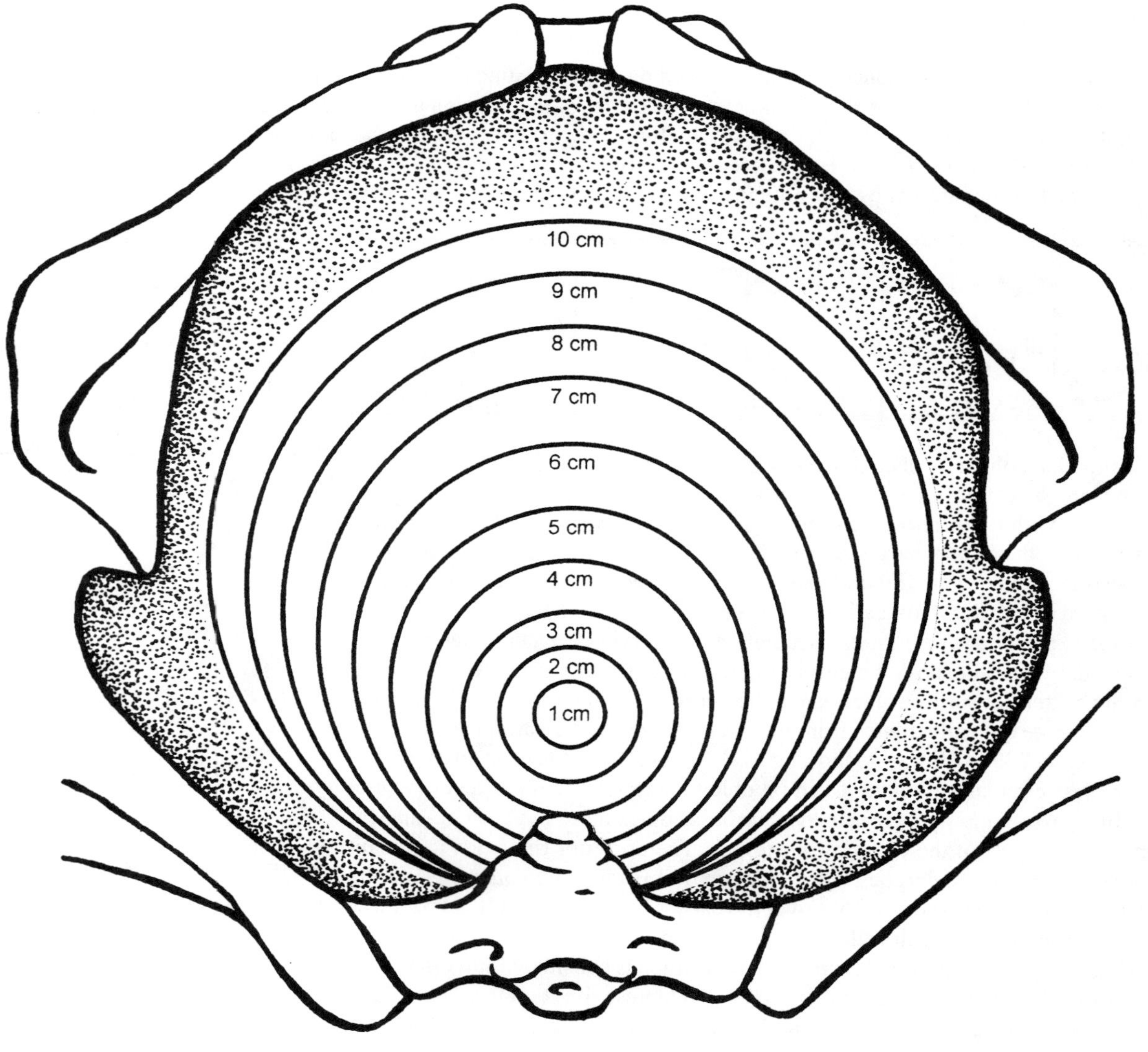

Dilation proceeds from the midposterior yoni forward. The first few centimeters of dilation are more nearly circular. Then, as the posterior cervix is almost entirely dilated, the os becomes more elliptical. A narrow edge of the posterior cervix will often persist until dilation is complete (life size).

Learning to assess dilation is greatly facilitated by making a dilation chart and by carrying a small centimeter ruler with you. When you are learning you can "check the dilation" of round objects such as jars or jar lids with your fingers and then double-check your assessment with the ruler. This way your fingers will learn how to tell dilation. Also, if you hold your examining fingers inside the edges of the cervix and then open the fingers of your other hand, they will automatically match the angle of your internal fingers. An assistant can then hold up a ruler to your external hand to double-check your assessment.

Is the cervix evenly dilated or is the dilation lopsided? Uneven dilation can offer clues as to how the presenting part is trying to come through the pelvis, especially when labor is not progressing well. Both the contour of the os and the amount of effacement can vary around the circumference of the cervix. Sometimes this is due to the way the uterus is contracting. More often, however, it has to do with the way the presenting part is positioned, pulling the cervix off center or placing uneven pressure on different areas of the cervix. A presenting part that is poorly applied to the cervix or factors such as asynclitism, nuchal cord, cervical polyps, a partial placenta previa, variations in pelvic anatomy, uneven muscle tone or tension in the pelvic floor, or a hand or foot stuck up under the chin or near the head (thus impeding direct head flexion) can all cause the cervical opening to be off center.

Is the cervical opening anterior, posterior, over to one side or centrally located? (Placement of the cervix is thoroughly explained in Volume I in the chapter entitled "Assessing Cervical Changes during Pregnancy.") The os may be quite posterior at the onset of labor, especially in women with long cervical canals who are more than 60% effaced. Pulling the cervix into a more central position can help the contractions work most efficiently. (See the chapter entitled "Cervical and Other Soft-tissue Problems during Labor.") The reasons why this may occur are the same as those given above. When the cervix is pulled over to one side, lopsided dilation frequently occurs as well.

What is the consistency of the cervix? Ideally, the cervical lip is applied to the presenting part and is soft and yielding to your examining finger between contractions. It becomes well applied to the bag of waters or the presenting part during contractions, when it opens slightly more than when relaxed.

However, both Dr. John Stevenson (2001), an Australian homebirth physician, and I have observed that it can be quite normal for the cervix to have a characteristic tight, leathery feel up to about 5 cm of dilation. This is especially true of first-time mothers who have not taken evening primrose oil during the last weeks of pregnancy. As labor progresses, dilation may remain slow until the cervix suddenly undergoes a remarkable change from being thin, tight and tough to being thicker, very soft, elastic and mucusy. It is important not to confuse this normal shift in the consistency of the cervix with cervical edema. It is difficult to reach the posterior rim of the cervix while the anterior rim is easily palpated. The surrounding soft tissues of the yoni become soft and stretchy as well. After this change, the cervix yields to contractions much more readily, and some women can push through such a cervix after they have reached 8 cm.

However, at times the cervix may feel rigid and unyielding, even to the point of feeling as though there were a tight ring inside its edge. An edematous cervix often does not yield to stretching and has an enlarged border that may feel anywhere from spongy to taut and rigid. A very swollen cervix will feel puffy or even like bread dough and may bleed slightly during an exam. The entire cervix or only a portion may feel rigid due to previous scarring.

A cervix that is not well applied to the presenting part during a contraction indicates either that the woman is not in labor or that some problem exists with the descent of the presenting part (either due to the position of the presenting part or one of the problems suggested in the section on uneven dilation above). There may be a problem with the quality of the uterine contractions. In multiparas, the cervix may not be as well applied to the presenting part as in a primigravida until labor is advanced. If this seems to be the case, leave your fingers in place and wait to see if the cervix becomes better applied with the force of a contraction. If the woman is really in labor, some type of change should be detectable in the cervix during a contraction in the form of either tensing or pulling back.

Examining the placental membranes

Are the membranes intact? You will probably ascertain whether the membranes are intact simultaneously with your other assessments. Healthy membranes typically feel strong and sturdy, like a thick, slippery plastic bag; they are somewhat fluctuant between contractions and normally very taut during a labor contraction. (They usually do not tighten up during toning contractions or, if they do, it is only slight.) In a typical vertex presentation, the membranes feel like a watch glass, slightly rounded and pressed against the inside the cervical opening. They have a distinctly smooth feel, although you may sometimes find soft ragged bits of membranes overlying a uniformly intact bag. The ragged pieces are most likely tags of ruptured chorion, with the amnion still intact. More rarely, you may be able to detect fluid trapped between the two bags or the somewhat slack chorion loosely overlying the more taut amnion.

Feel the entire surface of the membranes exposed within the open os to rule out any irregularities of texture or structure that may indicate either an edge of placenta or a blood vessel (see below).

Grape-like structures with the membranes intact are more likely to be small polyps or other growths attached to the mother's upper genital track. Such growths can be pressed out from inside the cervical canal during dilation and therefore not found during internal exams performed prior to labor. Confirm attachment to maternal tissue by following the outlines of the growth all around; if small growths are found, these can usually be pushed back up through the os and out of the way so the baby can bypass them without difficulty. Similar structures may also be present if there are hydatidiform formations on a portion of placenta overlying the os. A viable baby can develop in the presence of a partially molar placenta.

Another reason for an irregular membrane surface would be the septum of fused membranes in a multiple gestation, although the bags rarely present side-by-side like this. This feels like a subtle, flat ridge of tissue running across the membranes. You may also find two pouches, from the separate bags of waters of multiples. Thoroughly repalpate the abdomen and listen for two babies. (See the chapter entitled "Assisting at Multiple Births" for more details.)

If you are unsure if the membranes are intact, palpate for fetal scalp hair and try to catch a lock of hair between your fingers, or attempt to wrinkle the scalp with your fingers. Note, however, that a lax forewater can also wrinkle slightly at times. Pushing the presenting part up will cause water to leak out if the membranes are ruptured. Likewise, finding vernix on your glove after your exam is diagnostic. The presence of meconium is usually indicative of membrane rupture; however, on rare occasions, meconium can seep through into the mucus plug and confuse your findings.

The membranes may be in close contact with or directly applied to the presenting part, particularly if it is low in the pelvis. This gives the presenting part a uniformly slick feel. Such close application of the forewaters may make it difficult to tell if the membranes are intact. If the membranes do not bulge with a contraction, you can have the mother bear down or you can apply pressure to the fundus, which will often move water downward to create forewaters and cause the membranes to bulge if they are intact. Conversely, when the forewaters are deep, they, not the harder presenting part, act as the cervical dilator. Rupture of the membranes in these cases will often cause dilation to recede unless the presenting part drops down to fill the space previously taken up by the forewaters.

The bag may also assume an hourglass shape, with half of the hourglass slipping down through the os and presenting as a soft, fluctuant pouch of water. This may occur in any woman having an otherwise normal labor and is usually a by-product of the tissue quality of the membranes coupled with a presenting part that is not well-seated in the pelvis, allowing fluid to seep around the sides so that the forebag and the hindwaters communicate. Hourglass membranes do not, in any way, aid dilation. Be aware, however, that it is sometimes associated with uncommon cephalic positions, contracted pelvis and transverse lie.

(Various tests to identify amniotic fluid are described in my text DIAGNOSTIC TESTS. For more information regarding the membranes and fluid also see the chapter entitled "The Placental Membranes and Amniotic Fluid during Labor" in this volume and the one entitled "Rupture of Membranes before the Onset of Labor" in Volume I of this text).

Identifying a vasa previa: Very rarely, you may feel a peculiar, long, soft, rounded, pulsating feature that traverses the membranes overlying the os. This is a vasa previa, a fetal blood vessel that passes through the presenting portion of intact membranes on its way from the cord insertion point to the placenta or between two placental lobes. A very careful speculum exam with a flashlight can be used to confirm this finding if the os is anterior and sufficiently dilated. You will note a dark vessel passing through the membranes, although you must look carefully if a baby with a full head of dark hair is close behind the forebag. Meconium in the forewaters may also make a vasa previa difficult to see. Such a vessel may be compressed as the presenting part descends and can rupture along with the membranes. This can result in fatal fetal bleeding. If you strongly suspect a vasa previa, it may be most prudent to forego confirmation, which increases the risk of rupturing the membranes, place the mother in a position that relieves pressure on the bag and transport.

Identifying a cord presentation or prolapse: Take the opportunity to rule out cord presentation or prolapse whenever an internal exam is performed. Feel over the surface of the presenting part, the external cervical os, up through each yoni fornix, and over the swell of the thinned lower segment for evidence of occult prolapse.

In cord presentation, the umbilical cord is contained within an intact forebag. There will be no firm presenting part within the bag, and, depending upon the quantity of forewaters, you may or may not be able to detect a subtle, lumpy, pulsating mass through the membranes. Cord presentation may be confused with a vasa previa, if the vessel traversing the membranes is quite thick. Rarely, the belly of a baby with an omphalocele can be positioned directly over the internal os; loops of encapsulated intestines may be mistaken for a cord. In this case, abdominal palpation may have alerted you to a transverse lie; additionally, there will be no pulsations in the intestinal parts, although you may feel the pulsing umbilical cord as well. An "intact bag" may be felt, even though amniotic fluid has apparently escaped; this is really the membrane overlying the defect. It may also be an intact cord-filled amnion behind a ruptured chorion, so assess carefully.

Once the forewaters break, the cord can prolapse with a loop extending into the yoni canal. In such a case, the cord should be identifiable as such. However, the cord can also feel bunched up and indistinctly soft, which may cause confusion. Pulsations cinch the diagnosis, although a compressed cord may not pulse or may pulse only weakly. Pulsations may be present between contractions when prolapse first occurs and become weak, irregular or disappear entirely during contractions. In addition, on very rare occasions, what initially feels like a straightforward cord prolapse can also be a loop of fetal intestines with or without accompanying umbilical cord in a transverse or breech baby with a gastroschisis defect that has prolapsed through the cervix. Such a defect does not pulse like a cord and may feel soft and doughy, since it is full of meconium. A loop of maternal intestines that has prolapsed through the posterior fornix may be also be mistaken for a cord. Such a catastrophe may accompany uterine rupture. In either event, transport, as both situations require immediate medical attention.

The pulsing cord is warm, firm, and full of blood. A cord that is cool, flaccid, pulseless and empty of blood is an ominous sign. To detect a pulse, gently press the cord against the presenting part, wall of the maternal pelvis or between the two examining fingers. Care must be taken to distinguish the cord pulse from your own or the mother's; gentle palpation should take place between contractions. If you are still unsure as to what you are feeling, keep pressure off the prolapsed cord and transport immediately. (Read the section in this chapter entitled "Does the presenting part feel normally formed?" and see the chapter entitled "Cord Problems and Emergencies during Labor" for more details.)

A flattened, pedunculated submucous myoma (a benign muscular tumor of the uterus) attached near the cervical os can mimic a short loop of cord and can be very difficult to distinguish from a prolapse if the woman is of large size and the presenting part still high in the pelvis. If suspected, gently but thoroughly palpate the mass to determine if it is actually a loop of tissue (confirming cord) or if it is attached to the mother (Kerr et al., 1923). Even a good prenatal internal exam may not identify such a mass prior to labor, as its prolapse may require cervical dilation and pressure from above to force it downward where is can be palpated.

What is the fetal presentation?

Ideally you will perform abdominal palpation prior to an internal exam. If the part is low enough to reach, confirm the fetal presentation by ascertaining which fetal pole is in the pelvis. Although most fetuses maintain the same lie that they assumed in late pregnancy throughout labor, this is by no means always the case; babies can and do change their polarity before and during labor.

If the presenting part is too high to reach, you must rule out a nonvertex presentation. The most likely possibilities are floating vertex, followed by a face, breech or transverse lie and, lastly, brow presentation. It can help to palpate the mother's abdomen and try to press the presenting part down into the pelvis with your external hand (taking care not to rupture the membranes) while keeping a hand inside.

The fetal head feels hard and uniformly rounded. The buttocks will feel exquisitely smooth and slightly less regular, although this subtle difference may escape you if you are inexperienced and the membranes are intact. The skin of the face is equally smooth; the face itself is very soft and somewhat irregular and fills the space if labor is advanced. A rounded, elongated irregular shape may be an arm or a thigh. An arm, hand or foot may be felt in a longitudinal, compound presentation. Ribs may confuse you, primarily because you've probably never felt them before. The skin covering the ribs is thin, like that of the skull, and overlies long, narrow, closely spaced bones with a "washboard" texture.

VERTEX	BREECH	FACE
Hard, uniformly bony feel	Softer, except over sacrum, anus	Soft, irregular, indentations to either side of nose, over eyes, mouth
Uniformly thin tissue layer over a hard surface	Thicker layer of more irregular padding over surface	Thicker layer over cheeks, thin over forehead, chin, orbital ridges
Round and regular circumference	Oval, somewhat irregular circumference	Nearly round and regular circumference
Textured surface due to hair	Absolutely velvety smooth with no other texture	Velvety smooth.

The palpable difference between the hard, smooth dome of the skull and the soft, irregular face is great enough to diagnose a face presentation or at least suspect it or a breech presentation. However, the feel of the vertex and the forehead are similar, and moulding and swelling may confuse you. If in doubt, go back and do a thorough abdominal examination looking for deflexion, especially if there is failure to progress. Additionally, take the time to assess for any suture lines or fontanelles. The table on the last page summarizes the distinguishing cephalic and breech features.

If the baby is dead

If the baby has recently died, the landmarks of the presenting part can feel fairly normal; however, reflex responses will, of course, be absent. The longer the baby has been dead, the more signs become apparent. A fetus that has suffered intrauterine death some days prior to labor has skull bones that are soft and freely movable at the suture lines (in some cases, a sensation similar to the crackling of an egg shell can be elicited with a fingertip); you may feel them grate against or overlap each other. The scalp may feel soft and flabby. The head of the deceased baby is a less effective dilator. No caput will form because circulation has ceased. In breech presentations, the anus is relaxed and does not contract around the examining finger. The mouth and lips are flaccid. A prolapsed arm or leg will hang limply. An extended limb or the presenting part may be white but is often dark due to pooling of blood or bruising of the dependent part. Even if the baby is dead, repositioning or even a change in the lie does occasionally happen prior to or during labor; lack of muscle tone may facilitate such shifts.

Identifying a fetus papyraceus or acardiac fetus: If the presenting part feels highly unusual, a fetus papyraceus may be overlying the presenting part of a normal baby. By definition, such a fetus is shriveled and compressed (like a mummy), although it can be moist and may or may not be encased in membranes. The body texture ranges from that of a firm mass of fibrin-like material to one more rigid with a drier, leathery feel. The texture may not be distinguishable from that of a thin succenturiate lobe or mass of dense blood clot. On rare occasions a dead baby is retained for months and becomes excessively calcified; a fetus of this type is referred to as a "lithopedion," and presents as a fairly rigid mass that may also feel grainy. A wax-like material which may appear to you to be vernix, may also coat the skin of a dead baby retained for many months (Singer & Macpherson, 1998). For details, see the chapter entitled "Assisting at the Labor and Birth of a Mother Whose Baby is Known to Have Lethal Defects or to Have Died Prior to the Onset of Labor."

An acardiac fetus may feel like a mass of normal fetal tissue without definition or normal bony landmarks. However, some acardiac fetuses have partially developed bodies and skeletons, particularly in their lower half. Perform a thorough examination of the entire palpable mass to determine whether gross defects are present. This will be best accomplished if the woman is at least 5 centimeters dilated, with ruptured membranes (Schuler-Maloney, 2000).

Where is the presenting part?

The degree of descent of the presenting part can vary widely during labor. Generally speaking, first-time mothers enter labor with the head engaged or nearly so, and multigravidas enter labor with the head higher in the pelvis. However, when labor is not well established, it is not unusual to find the head high and only partially palpable, even in first-time mothers. The head may float high in the anterior portion of the pelvis, be well fitted into the pelvic cavity, or dip into the posterior pelvis. Often, if the head is still high in the pelvis, you will have a sense that the head is asynclitic, although this is not easy to confirm (asynclitism is probably normal at that point). The degree of descent and the tenseness and quantity of forewaters greatly influence your ability to determine which part is presenting and its position.

What is the presenting part and how is it situated in relationship to maternal pelvic landmarks?

Once you believe you have determined the presentation, feel the presenting part of the baby. The way it is positioned in relationship to the maternal pelvis is part of this assessment. When the mother reclines for the exam, the head often floats up, and it is found floating high near the pubic bone, especially in early labor. This may occur even if the head seems to be deeper in the pelvis when the mother is upright. Until uterine retraction is established and fixes the baby in the pelvis, shifts in maternal position will continue to have a dramatic effect on head position when she reclines. When the head is floating, there is usually a large forewater in front of the head filling the posterior pelvis, making detection of specific landmarks difficult or even impossible.

The fetal landmarks you feel with the baby in various positions is called the "touch picture." The ones included in this chapter show landmarks when the baby is well down in the pelvis, surrounded by a ring of soft tissue. However, earlier in labor the os will not reveal so much of the presenting part and you will have to feel up inside the undilated edges to find unexposed landmarks. For example, at 4 cm dilation, you may only be able to feel one fontanelle; a cheek, nose or eyebrow ridge; or a single buttock, depending upon the presentation.

In vertex presentations, the touch picture consists of the firm skull and suture lines, the location of which will indicate the position of the head. When another part of the baby presents, or the head is deflexed, other regions are within reach.

If the baby's head is further down and you hold your finger against it for a few minutes, you can often feel the baby moving his head, flexing, deflexing and lateroflexing, rotating a few degrees this way and that, to find the best way out. If you have an idea about what might help, you might tell the baby what you want him to do regarding head position. However, remember that the baby may be aware of something on his side of the pelvis that you cannot feel!

Take the time to find identifying landmarks, especially when the breech or shoulder presents, because these presentations are relatively rare. If the lie is longitudinal, you will feel either the buttocks or the head; however, it is possible to have a hand, foot or cord alongside either presenting part. Detecting a brow presentation can be difficult, since the feel of the forehead is more similar to the feel of the vertex.

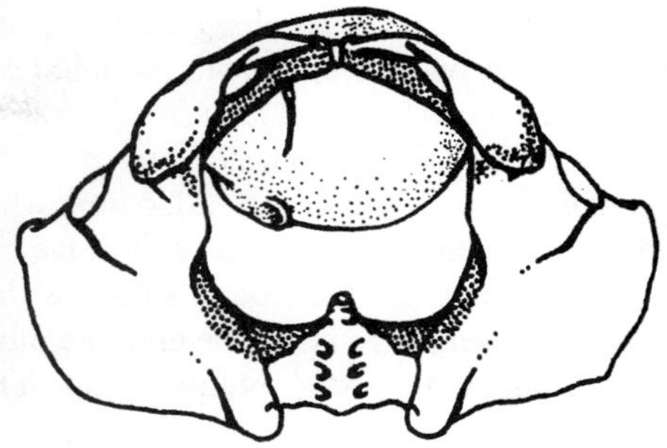

LOT head floating above the pubic bone when woman lies down for the exam.

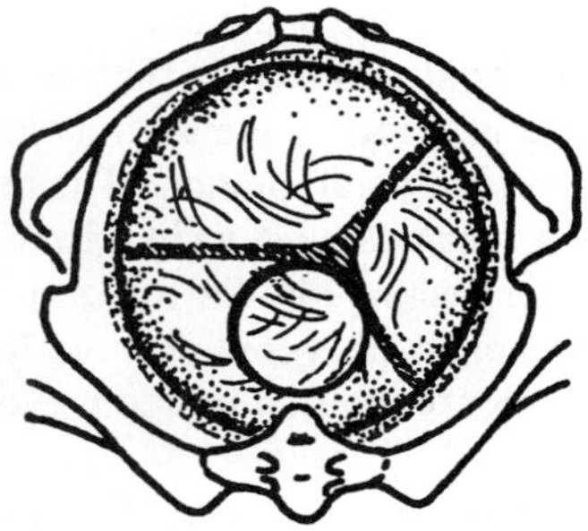

Touch picture of a well-flexed LOT baby showing what can be felt through the os during early dilation. In this case, fetal hair and the skull could be identified, but no sutures are exposed.

Identifying a caput: If you are having trouble determining what you feel even though the membranes are ruptured and the presenting part is reasonably low in the pelvis, the baby may have a caput. While a caput usually forms on the head, a similar swelling may develop on any other part of the baby that presents. A caput has a soft, swollen feel to it and makes palpation of the features beneath it difficult, if not impossible. Note that a scrotum can sometimes mimic a caput. If a caput has formed on the head, you must feel around its margins to try to locate where the suture lines extend out from under it. Firm pressure into the caput can help identify landmarks beneath it. This, however, will likely be uncomfortable for the baby; explain to her why you feel the need to do it. Massaging around the edges may also reduce swelling, making palpation easier. Formation of a caput in the presence of intact membranes is a sign of significantly impaired descent.

With a well-established cranial caput, you must gauge the position of the head, the way labor is progressing and what, if anything, can be done to correct a position that is not ideal before the caput becomes any larger and further impedes repositioning. It is very important to judge descent only by the advancement of the bony skull because an enlarging caput can mimic advancement when, in fact, descent is impeded. Also keep in mind that excessive moulding may force the top of the skull lower in the yoni while the biparietal diameter remains unengaged; real descent is not occurring in this case either. You can attempt to reduce the caput by applying arnica cream or oil directly to the baby's head or by giving the mother homeopathic arnica in a 30C or 200C potency.

When the head is down: If the head is at 0 station or below, you will first feel the hard, rounded surface of the skull upon touching the presenting part. Note that the head can feel remarkably distant, small and buoyant if it is at the brim or dipping and the membranes are still intact. It will often be floating in the anterior portion of the brim, up above and behind the pubic bone. Having the mother lie down will cause the head to rise up further and accentuate these findings. When the head is lower and the forewaters are not pronounced, the things described below will be easier to distinguish.

Identifying suture lines: Slowly sweep your fingers along the scalp until a suture line is located. The suture lines will feel like long thin slightly depressed areas or shallow clefts in the surface of the skull. When palpating suture lines, use the same rocking or gently sliding finger movement that you would use to test the edge of a knife for sharpness.

Identifying the sagittal suture: Findings from your abdominal exam offer guidance as to where the suture is likely to be. As soon as you identify the sagittal suture, you can be sure that the presenting part is the head with the occiput either anterior or posterior. It cannot be a face, breech, foot, arm, shoulder, or rib cage, and the baby cannot have anencephaly.

Next, slide your finger along the length of the sagittal suture. The sagittal suture forms a long, narrow indentation that terminates on both ends with fontanelles that have bone around and beyond their borders (more about identifying the fontanelles can be found later in this chapter). Identification of the sagittal suture confirms the diameter of the pelvis in which the head is situated. Note whether the edges of the suture lines feel quite pronounced, a signs that indicates an excessive degree of moulding. Also note whether the sagittal suture recedes sharply upward into the pelvis. If so, the head is very deeply flexed. These findings may be associated with a contracted pelvis.

You may confuse the frontal suture with the sagittal suture in a baby who is presenting her brow. Although the anterior fontanelle will be at one end, the other end will terminate at the brow line. Identification of the orbital ridges confirms that the vertex is not presenting. The anterior fontanelle may be nearly centered in the cervical opening.

Determine the synclitism of the head: If the baby is vertex, the touch pictures on pages 394 and 395 will give you an idea of what an asynclitic head feels like in labor. During your exam, note the location of the sagittal suture in relationship to the symphysis pubis; the nearer the two, the more posterior the asynclitism. The further back it is, the more anterior the asynclitism. In other words, the sagittal suture is difficult to reach in anterior asynclitism and tipped anteriorly (toward the pubic bone) in posterior asynclitism. The head usually enters the pelvis via a moderate degree of posterior asynclitism and then tips the other way to become moderately anteriorly asynclitic as it descends further. If the baby's head is synclitic, the sagittal suture will be found centered in the transverse diameter of the pelvis. All of this occurs prior to internal rotation. The head can be cocked at any point in labor, no matter how it is otherwise positioned.

A head deep in the pelvis in a pronounced anterior parietal attitude may indicate twins with the second baby behind the first one, pushing him far forward. Extreme degrees of asynclitism prior to engagement are also associated with a nuchal hand or a pelvis contracted in its anteroposterior diameter. It is also normal for the sagittal suture to be slightly asynclitic prior to internal rotation, even if the head is not occiput transverse.

Finding the posterior fontanelle: You should find a fontanelle at either end of the sagittal suture. The posterior fontanelle is easiest to reach when the head is well flexed. If the posterior fontanelle is almost centered, flexion is extreme. If the head is not well flexed, applying only enough fundal pressure between contractions to produce more flexion may bring the posterior fontanelle within reach. However, this does not always work, and if the head is in a really cocked position, it may jam it in more. If you have not located the sagittal suture, follow whatever suture you find until it terminates in a fontanelle or another distinct feature.

The posterior fontanelle is a small triangular opening formed by a Y-shaped angle where the sagittal suture meets the center of the lambdoidal suture. Since this small membranous area is not easy to feel, especially when the head is moulded, confirm your finding by feeling for the blunt tip of the occipital bone. The wide, blunt tip of the intraparietal occipital bone is felt at the very end of the sagittal suture, where it terminates at the lambdoidal suture. If the head is moulded, the occipital bone will be slightly recessed below the level of the two softer parietal bones, which also meet at the edge of this wedge. Certain identification of the occipital bone confirms a more or less flexed attitude.

Finding the anterior fontanelle: If the posterior fontanelle has been accurately identified, you really do not need to find the anterior fontanelle. Ideally, it is not easy to palpate the anterior fontanelle because the head is flexed.

The anterior fontanelle is at the end of the sagittal suture opposite the posterior fontanelle (if the posterior fontanelle is at the 10 o'clock position, the anterior fontanelle should be found at 4 o'clock, confirming that the head is ROA). If you feel you do need to identify it, glide your finger along the sagittal suture. Continue to feel around in this area to locate the anterior fontanelle, which is formed at the meeting points of the sagittal, coronal and frontal sutures, which converge at right angles to create a relatively large, open, diamond-shaped membranous space, with its longer point directed toward the face (this nuance can be difficult to detect during a typical internal exam, especially if any moulding is present). Unlike the area surrounding the posterior fontanelle, the bones bordering the anterior fontanelle have more "give" to them and may feel slightly springy to pressure. Loss of flexibility suggests that the baby is past due. Move across the anterior fontanelle to find the suture opposite the sagittal to locate the frontal suture, which intersects the two frontal bones, and follow it ½ to ⅞ in (1 to 2 cm) beyond the membranous border of the fontanelle. Identification of the frontal suture ensures that you have found the anterior fontanelle.

Locating a sagittal fontanelle or parietal foramina: Occasionally you may encounter a baby with a smaller, diamond-shaped sagittal fontanelle along the sagittal suture, usually nearer the posterior fontanelle. Not only is such an opening smaller than the true anterior fontanelle, the distance between it and the true posterior fontanelle is suspiciously short. If you think you have found a sagittal fontanelle, continue to search beyond it, along the sagittal suture, for the anterior fontanelle. Even more rarely, to one or both sides of the sagittal suture, you may find round openings which are large parietal foramina. These openings are usually 3 mm in diameter, and therefore cannot be palpated, but can range up to 3 cm in diameter, although this is rare. The finding of an opening unconnected to the suture line confirms that it is not a normal fontanelle. A sagittal fontanelle or large parietal foramina indicate that the skull is less ossified than usual.

Checking for flexion: The location of the fontanelles and suture lines gives you information regarding head flexion, synclitism, and the location of the occiput. If the fontanelles are at roughly the same level in the pelvis or if the anterior fontanelle is easily reached, the head is not well flexed. In a flexed vertex presentation, the posterior fontanelle is lower in the pelvis and more centered. The anterior fontanelle is higher and harder to reach, and the sagittal suture is nearly parallel to the axis of the fetal body. Refer to the touch pictures to guide you in identifying various positions. Note that intact membranes, moulding and swelling add to the difficulty of determining the degree of flexion.

Checking the density of the fetal skull: You can get an idea of the firmness of the skull by palpating it near the sagittal suture. The edges of the sutures of a normal, term infant will have a firm, slightly springy feel. A postmature skull feels dense where the two parietal bones meet. A premature baby's skull is softer and more elastic along the suture lines. Craniotabes (soft skull) can develop in an otherwise normal baby who has been subjected to unusually intense and prolonged pressure during late gestation. The parietooccipital region is most often affected and tends to be soft and is often indentable, with a feel like pressing your finger into a ping-pong ball or aluminum soda can. Crackling or fluctuant sensations may be detected in the hydrocephalic skull (most easily detected on rectal exam). The skull of a baby with achondroplasia (a disorder of the cartilage that produces dwarfism) may also be fluctuant on palpation. Babies with anencephaly have exposed brain tissue, which will be soft and often bleeds on palpation. You may feel irregular skull features where the dome of the skull should be and may detect a bony edge at the brow line.

Identifying hydrocephalus: If hydrocephalus is diagnosed prior to labor, the birth should take place in the hospital. However, hydrocephaly may have eluded detection during pregnancy. Severely affected babies may die shortly before labor, but many enter labor alive. The baby usually presents longitudinally, with breeches making up 35% of the total. In vertex presentations, the head typically remains above the brim and feels bulkier and softer than a normal head that is still floating (the same abdominal findings will prevail if the baby is breech, except that the head will be in the fundus). This softness can only be detected if you insert your fingers deeply into the yoni, although in some cases a portion of the moulded skull may distend through the partially open os, especially if the baby is dead and the head is not massively enlarged with fluid. The bones of the skull feel elastic and the sutures and fontanelles feel very widely spaced. Don't jump to conclusions, however, if the sutures, especially the anterior fontanelle, feel somewhat large; if the skull feels otherwise normal, hydrocephalus is unlikely. The head is usually fixed, as the walls of the uterus are overstretched and hold it in place. The head does not descend even though labor goes on for many hours (Kerr et al., 1923). Although a minor degree of hydrocephalus may allow descent, if it is suspected, transport.

Checking for moulding: Assess whether the parietal sutures are unevenly matched and, if so, to what extent. As the head moulds, the parietal bones become elongated and the intraparietal occipital bone usually slips beneath the parietal bones posteriorly. The following scale, modified from Sellers (1993), can be used to grade moulding:

0: Bones normally spaced at suture lines, sutures easily identified with no detectable moulding
+1: Bones just touch each other
+2: Bony edges elevated but can be separated easily with finger pressure
+3: Bony edges elevated and possibly staggered and cannot be separated with finger pressure

Excessive moulding usually indicates a tight fit or a poorly positioned head. It can confuse your findings when you attempt to determine the station; the head can be stuck, with the skull pressed down into the pelvis. This is even more confusing if the baby has a caput, which she may if descent is arrested. If you detect +3 moulding, you may have difficulty assessing station even if there is no caput because the parietal bones are likely to be displaced downward. Palpation of the lower abdomen above the pubic bone may give you more information about station. (Also see the chapter entitled "Abdominal Examination Techniques for Use during Labor")

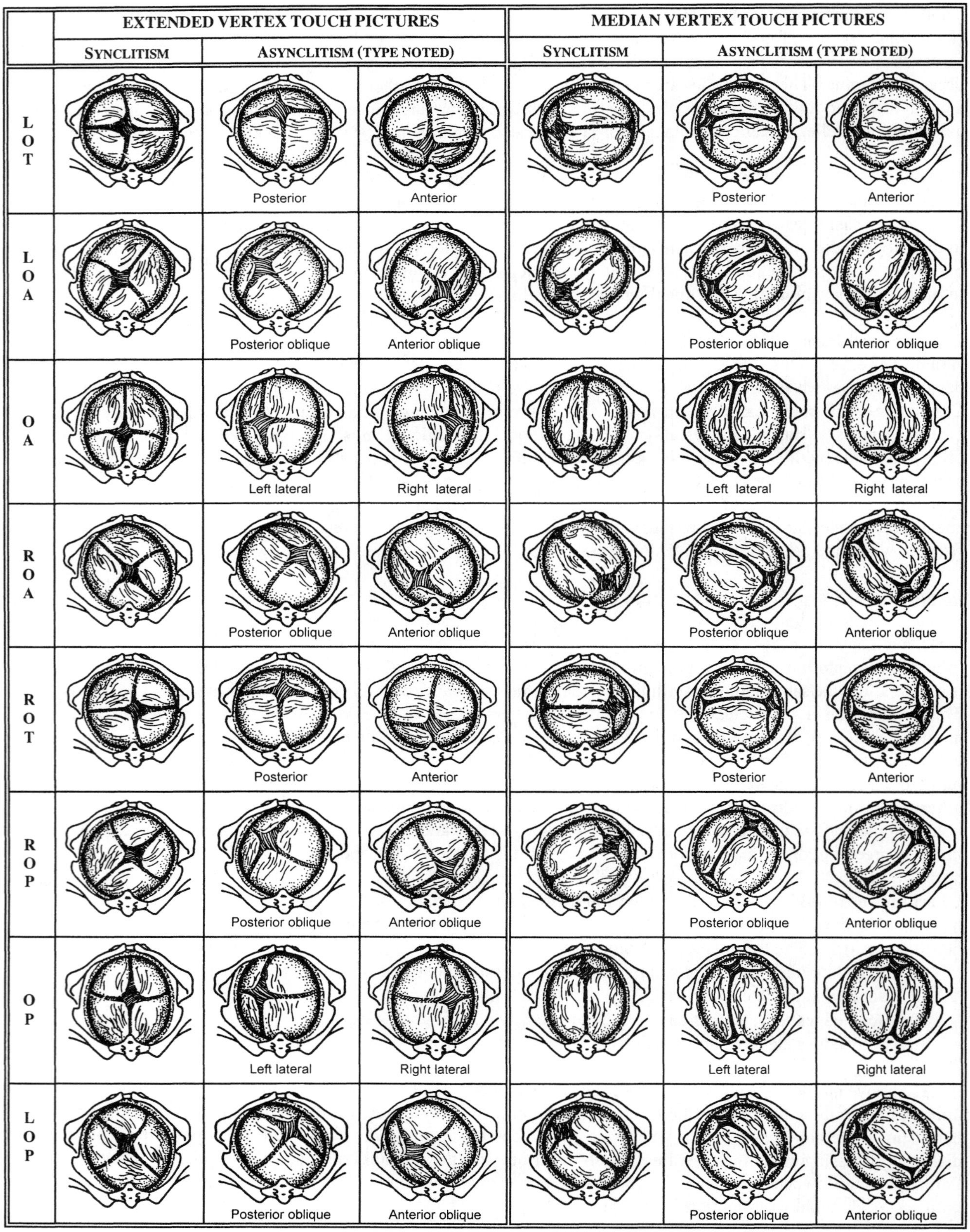
EXTENDED VERTEX TOUCH PICTURES
MEDIAN VERTEX TOUCH PICTURES
SYNCLITISM
ASYNCLITISM (TYPE NOTED)
SYNCLITISM
ASYNCLITISM (TYPE NOTED)
LOT
Posterior
Anterior
Posterior
Anterior
LOA
Posterior oblique
Anterior oblique
Posterior oblique
Anterior oblique
OA
Left lateral
Right lateral
Left lateral
Right lateral
ROA
Posterior oblique
Anterior oblique
Posterior oblique
Anterior oblique
ROT
Posterior
Anterior
Posterior
Anterior
ROP
Posterior oblique
Anterior oblique
Posterior oblique
Anterior oblique
OP
Left lateral
Right lateral
Left lateral
Right lateral
LOP
Posterior oblique
Anterior oblique
Posterior oblique
Anterior oblique

	MODERATELY FLEXED VERTEX TOUCH PICTURES			WELL FLEXED VERTEX TOUCH PICTURES		
	SYNCLITISM	ASYNCLITISM (TYPE NOTED)		SYNCLITISM	ASYNCLITISM (TYPE NOTED)	
LOT	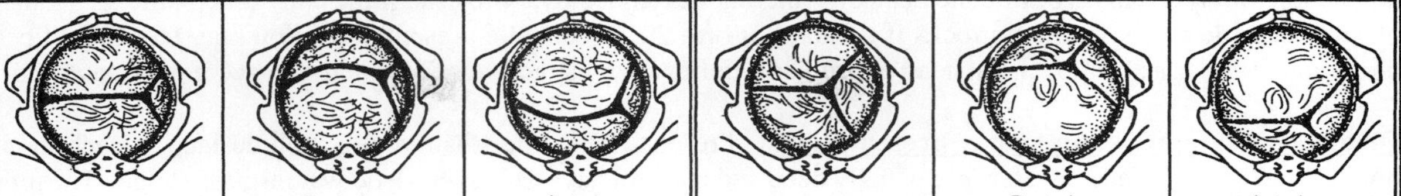	Posterior	Anterior		Posterior	Anterior
LOA	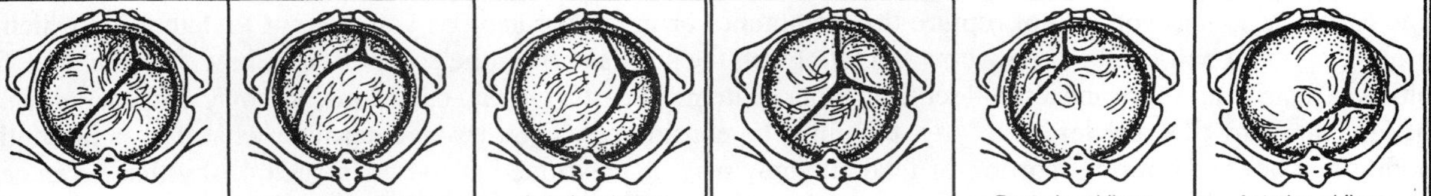	Posterior oblique	Anterior oblique		Posterior oblique	Anterior oblique
OA	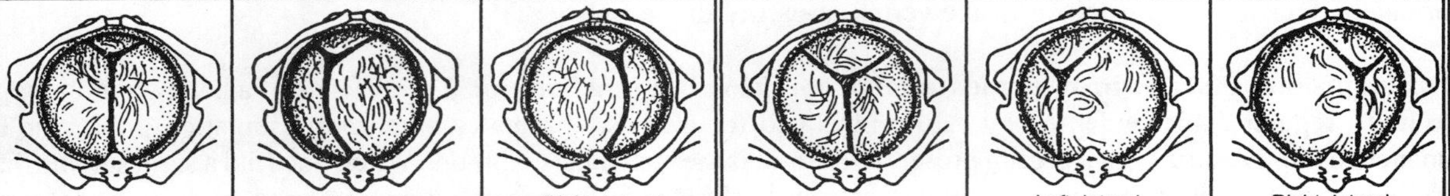	Left lateral	Right lateral		Left lateral	Right lateral
ROA	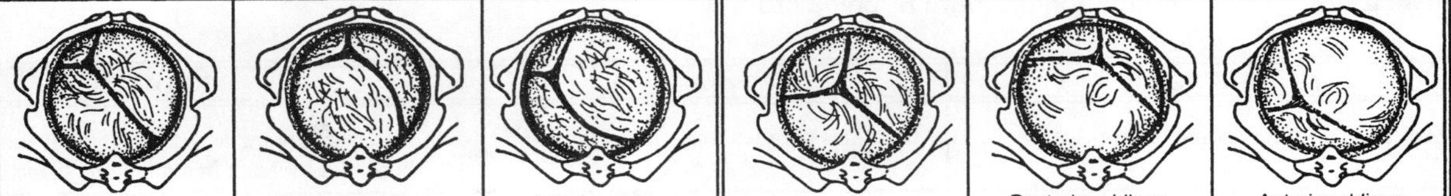	Posterior oblique	Anterior oblique		Posterior oblique	Anterior oblique
ROT	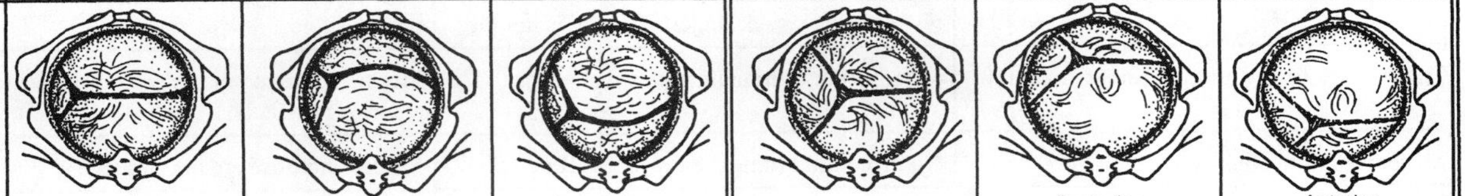	Posterior	Anterior		Posterior	Anterior
ROP	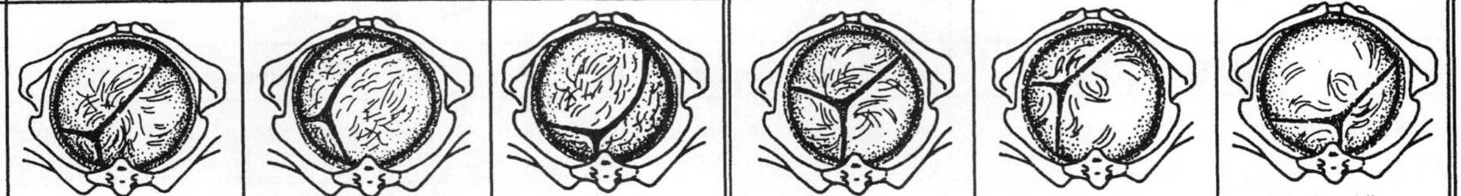	Posterior oblique	Anterior oblique		Posterior oblique	Anterior oblique
OP	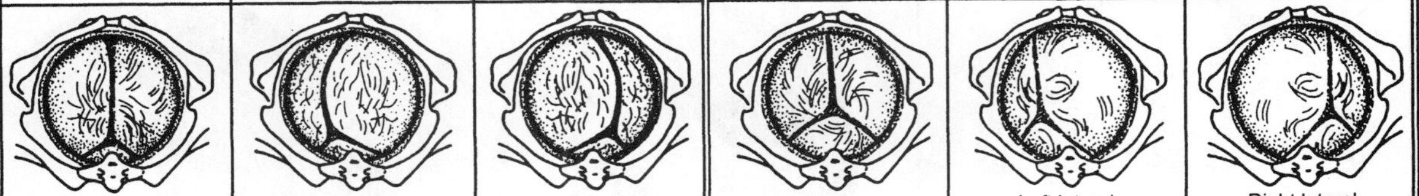	Left lateral	Right lateral		Left lateral	Right lateral
LOP	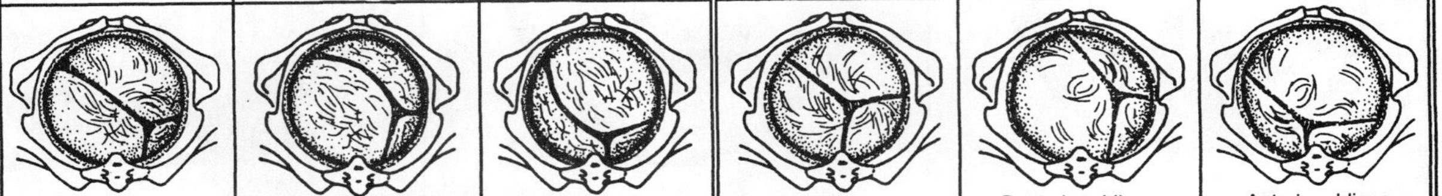	Posterior oblique	Anterior oblique		Posterior oblique	Anterior oblique

Nuchal and compound presentation: A minor form of compound presentation occurs with a nuchal hand or foot, most commonly a fist, is under the chin, preventing flexion. A true compound presentation typically occurs when a hand (or much more rarely a foot) is beside the head or sometimes extended over the head if the baby is cephalic, or a hand or foot extended beside or above the buttocks if the baby is breech. In cephalic presentations you may feel fingertips or toes beside the head or an arm over the head as well as a deflexed or asynclitic head due to the accompanying limb.

Distinguishing other-than-vertex presentations: Presentations other than vertex include face, breech, transverse, oblique and brow. The forewaters are usually deep and may not have a characteristic watch-glass shape. The presenting part is typically high until labor is advanced. Internal palpation is difficult at best. It is important that you proceed slowly and carefully so that you do not rupture the membranes or injure the baby as you attempt to determine which part is presenting. You will need to know how to distinguish the soft face from the soft buttocks, how to tell a knee from an elbow, a hand from a foot and a shoulder from other anatomical parts. On rare occasions, you may also encounter regions of fetal anatomy that are defective. All this must be considered as you try to determine what part is presenting. In addition, a perfectly normal portion of fetal anatomy may be positioned at the os in such a way that it can easily be mistaken for another; for example, the crease of the leg at the hip may be mistaken for the posterior axilla of the shoulder or one buttock may be mistaken for the vertex or part of the face.

Distinguishing a face or brow presentation from the vertex or a bottom: The absence of a hard, slightly rough (due to hair), regular dome, indented by suture lines and fontanelles, eliminates a vertex presentation unless the baby is anencephalic. Next rule out a breech presentation, as it is the next most common. When you find a satin smooth, hairless, irregular surface with prominences and depressions perforated by an opening, you will know at once the baby is either in a face or breech presentation or, more rarely, a brow.

BREECH	FACE	BROW
Anus has no surrounding bony ridges.	Mouth has parallel bony ridges (gums).	Anterior fontanelle is unperforated and bordered by bone in a diamond shape.
Anus is closed and firm or grips finger.	Lips are soft and lax and may suck, mouth is wide and may suck finger. Tongue is unique.	Eyes form two soft depressions below the orbital ridge.
Tuberosities form a straight line with anus.	Mouth forms a triangle with cheekbones.	Frontal suture connects orbital ridge and anterior fontanelle.
Meconium from anus on glove.	No meconium (unless baby has a GI defect).	Mouth and nose are out of reach.
Tuberosities separated by soft perpendicular genital cleft.	Cheekbones separated by flat nasal bridge.	Forehead separated by slightly depressed frontal suture.
Nothing feels like the orbital ridge.	Orbital ridge forms a straight line.	Orbital ridge forms a straight line.
Spines of sacrum (row of bumps above anus).	No bumps. Frontal suture forms a perpendicular depression above orbital ridges.	No bumps. Frontal suture forms a perpendicular depression above orbital ridge.

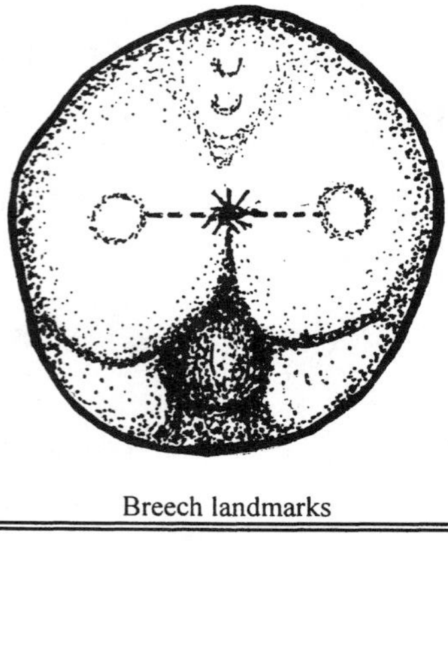
Breech landmarks

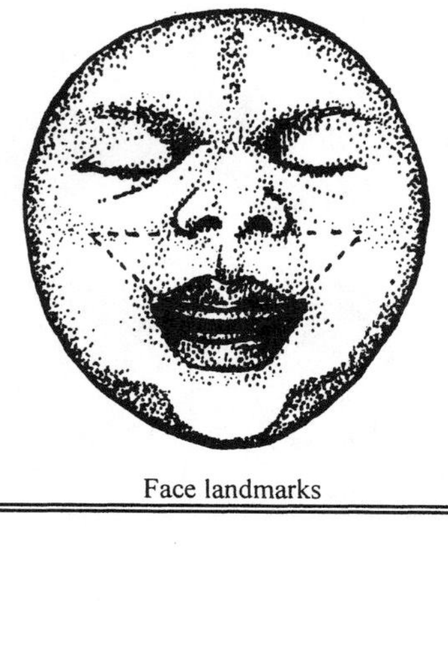
Face landmarks

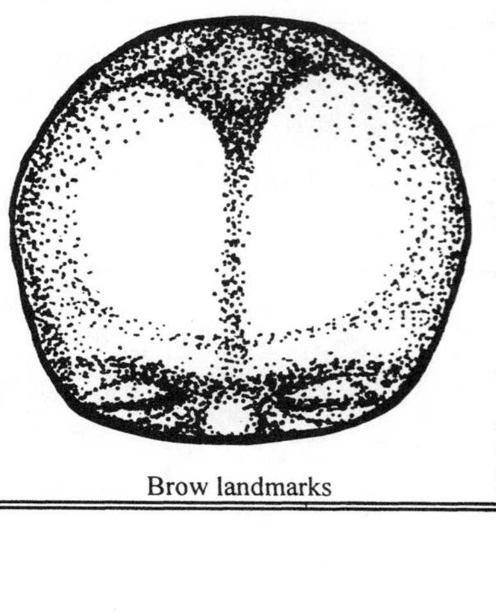
Brow landmarks

A frank breech presentation may confuse you, as the bottom of a term baby can feel nearly as firm as the head and the scrotum can sometimes mimic a caput. Compared with the vertex, the shape of the breech is more oval and the surface softer and more irregular, with a bony area over the sacrum. (The bottom of a preterm baby feels skinny and bony because his fat layer is not well developed.) The pad of tissue overlying the bottom and the face is thicker than that on the scalp. The skin of the buttocks or face also feels incredibly soft and smooth, unlike the vertex, which often has hair and therefore a textured feel even through intact membranes.

If you think the baby is frank breech, feel for bony landmarks, such as the tuberosities and sacrum, as well as the anus. The tuberosities are separated by a groove of soft tissue, the genital crease. The tuberosities and the anus will be in a straight line at right angles to the genital crease. There are no hard edges around the anus that resemble the gums. The sacrum is a row of nodules that are centered above the anus and between the buttocks. These nodules are continuous with the vertebrae above. The baby's genitals will, most likely, be swollen from the pressure during descent. Labia may feel like lips at first touch. The scrotum may be quite enlarged and full of fluid. Take care not to injure these delicate tissues.

Avoid inserting your fingertip into the anus, but, if you do so accidently, it will grip your finger, and your glove may have a bit of meconium on it after you complete your exam. (This stimulation may prompt the baby to pass meconium.)

Touch pictures for frank breech presentations are shown below.

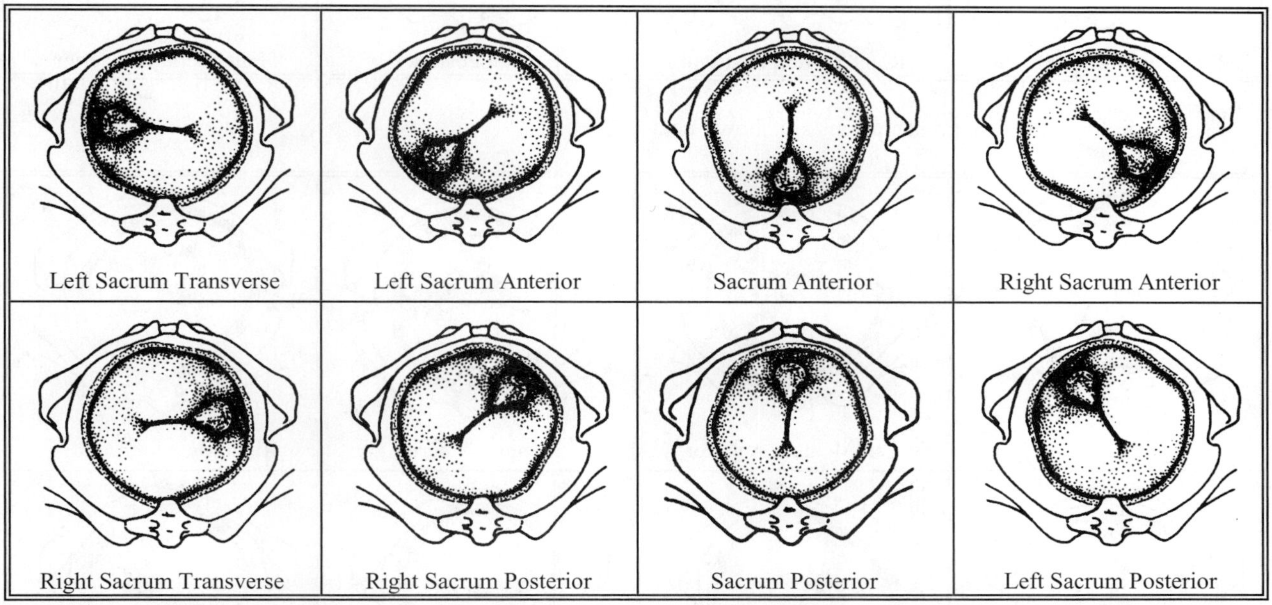

What you feel in the case of a complete, kneeling or footling breech is more complex. Jane Evans (personal communication, 2012) has noted that when one or both knees are applied to the perineum, the perineum has a noticeably irregular contour (also note that pressure often causes the knee to the pressed to the side). In a complete breech, feet and thighs may be palpable alongside the buttocks; otherwise, the touch picture is similar to a frank breech. When extremities are extended, you need to be able to distinguish between a hand, foot, knee and elbow. The sacrum is still the denominator as far as breech presentation goes, but you have to take extra care not to rupture the membranes when small, irregular parts present first. If you cannot reach the sacrum because the membranes are intact, your careful assessment of the position of the legs will assist in determining the position of the sacrum. Be careful not to rupture the membranes.

The next series of touch pictures show the baby in a complete breech presentation.

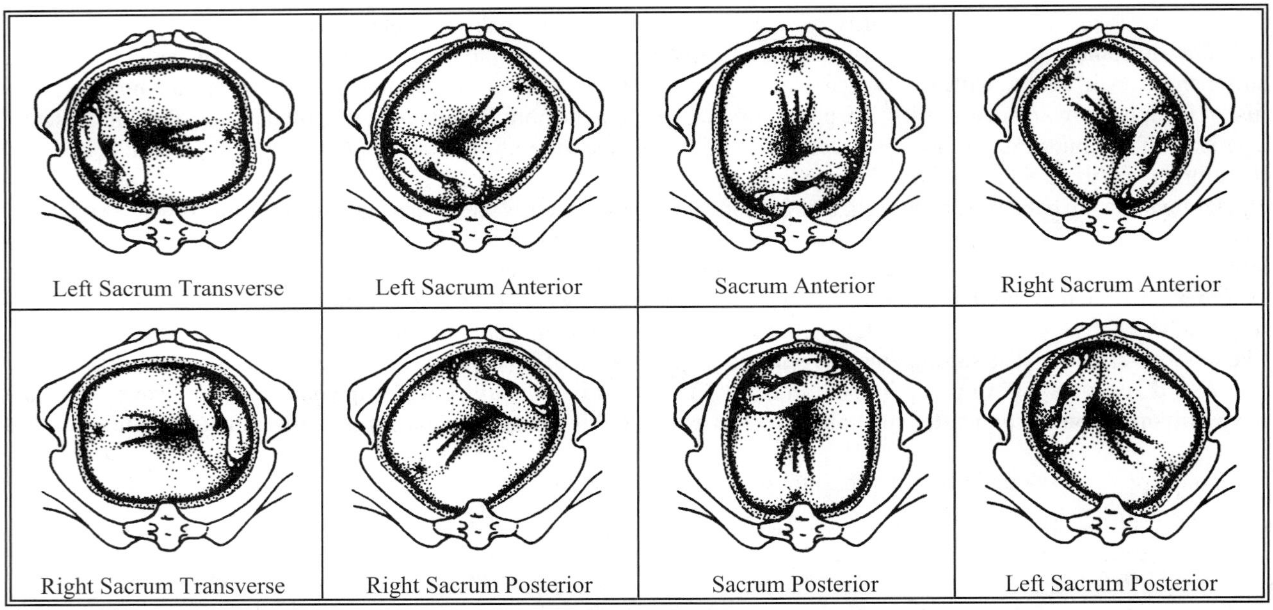

Touch pictures for face presentations are shown next:

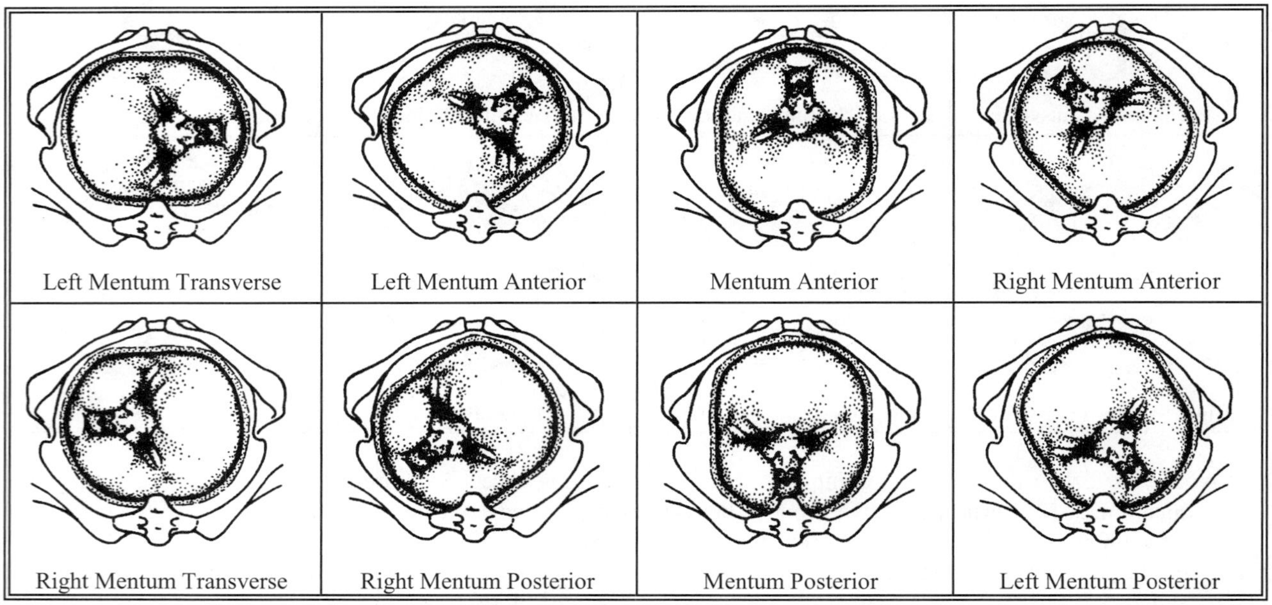

Distinguishing a face presentation may be less difficult when the face is still high in the pelvis and the membranes have ruptured rather than later when descent and increasing pressure have produced facial edema. However, regardless of the amount of swelling, two areas will always be palpable: the bridge of the nose and the gums. The bridge of the nose is quite firm and forms a flat area between the eyes and cheekbones just below the orbital ridge. The nose itself feels rubbery. The lips have a decidedly lax feel as compared to the anus, but their laxity may be obscured by edema. The gums feel hard. It is common for babies presenting their faces to open their mouths between contractions and close them firmly during contractions, probably a response to the contraction's downward pressure. The baby may even suck your finger. The cheekbones are connected by a bony ridge across the face. The cheekbones and mouth form a triangle.

Whatever the position, your ability to tell what is presenting will be much hampered if the cervix is not widely open. In such cases, the os will typically encircle a portion of the presenting part that fits into the opening most easily.

This is frequently a parietal bone if the baby is vertex, a buttock if the baby is breech, a cheek if the baby is in a face presentation, the forehead if the baby is in a brow presentation, or the tip of a shoulder if the baby is transverse.

Identifying fetal small parts: On rare occasions you may need to distinguish various fetal small parts, which will be vary unfamiliar. The following will help you prepare for such an event.

Distinguishing a knee or heel from an elbow: The newborn knee can be confused with the heel, the elbow or the tip of the shoulder. The knee is rather blunt with two blunt, bony protrusions (tuberosities) and a depression where the patella (kneecap) protrudes in an adult because the patella is quite undeveloped in the newborn. The elbow has a single, sharper point at the bend of the forearm (the olecranon process) and a depression on each side of this tip. The heel and shoulder each have only one blunt-pointed end. When doing a baby exam after birth, note these differences.

KNEE	HEEL	ELBOW	TIP OF SHOULDER
Two blunt tips on each side	One blunt tip	One sharp tip	One semi-blunt tip
Central depression	No depression	Lateral depressions on each side	No depression

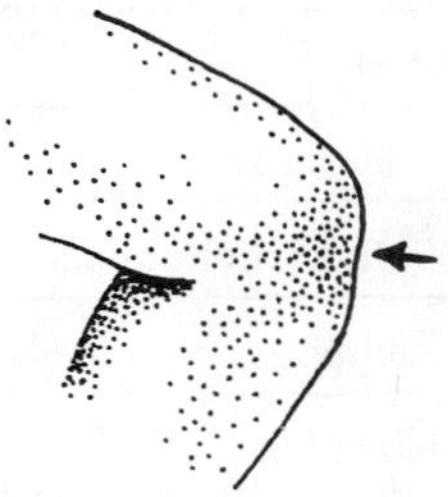

The region of the knee-cap feels hollow.

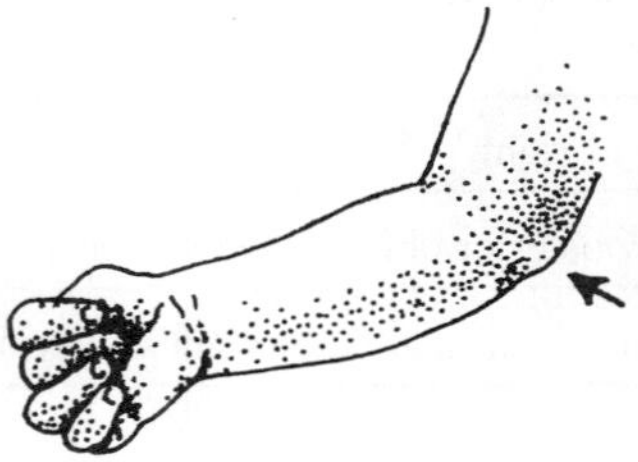

The tip of the elbow is sharply pointed.

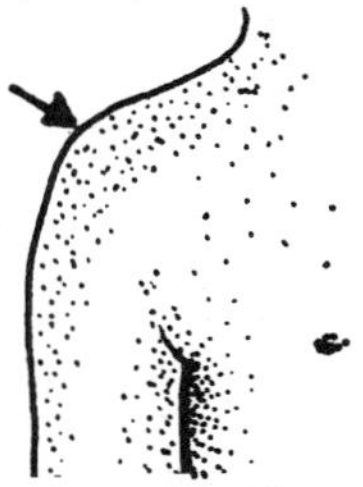

The point of the shoulder presents a semi-blunt tip.

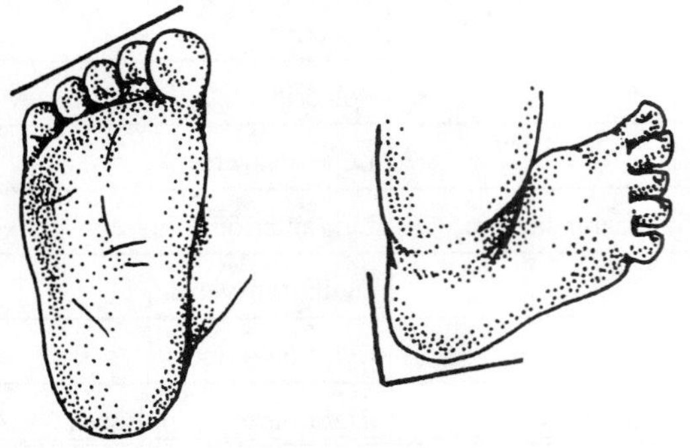

FEATURES OF THE FOOT

The heel makes a right angle to the leg
The foot cannot be straightened at the ankle; the heel remains
The sole is oblong, and longer than it is wide
The inner border of the foot is thicker than the outer border
The toes are roughly the same length, forming a straight line
The toes may flex and grip, but cannot really grasp
The big toe cannot flex over the sole

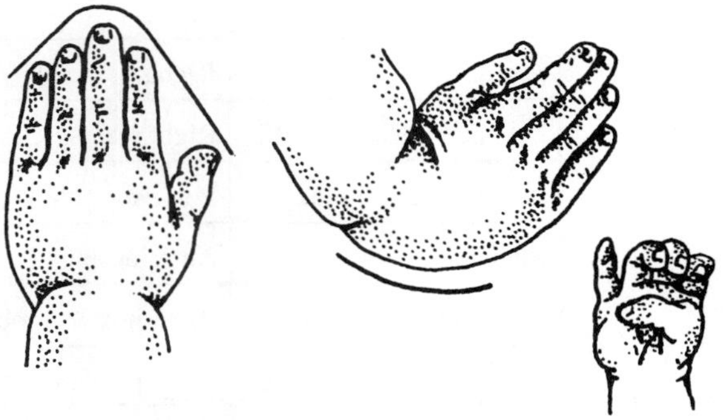

FEATURES OF THE HAND

The hand can be moved in line with the forearm
The heel of the hand disappears when the wrist is straightened
The palm is square and short
The palm is of uniform thickness
The fingers are longer and unequal in length, forming a curve
The fingers may flex and grasp yours
The thumb can flex over the palm

Distinguishing a foot from a hand: A hand may prolapse into the yoni if the baby is in a transverse lie or in a compound presentation with the arm extended over the head. Much more rarely, a hand could extend beside the torso and the fingers may be palpable in a frank breech baby. A foot is most likely to extend downward if the baby is presenting footling breech. This can also occur, although much more rarely, if the foot is positioned beside or over the head or if the legs are extended with the baby in a transverse lie. Also, in rare cases, a breech twin may straddle her transverse sibling, presenting one or both hands or feet at the cervix. Use a doll with distinct hand and foot features or ask a baby or small child to let you practice feeling her hands and feet as you review this material.

The sole of the foot is oblong and longer than it is wide. The inner border is thicker than the outer. Identification of the heel is the most important landmark when distinguishing a hand from a foot. In its normal, anatomical position, the foot is at a right angle to the lower leg. If you move your fingers along the plantar surface (sole) from the posterior ankle along the sole to the toes, the heel is still apparent; pointing the toes in a ballerina attitude does nothing to reduce the heel. The hand, in contrast, can move into a direct line with the forearm. When you run your fingers from the wrist to the palm, the heel at the base of the hand (below the little finger) disappears, differentiating it from the foot. These differences are illustrated in the table on the following page.

Telling a right from a left foot: The foot can also be distinguished by the position of the big toe, the heel and the sole.

Presenting Foot	Baby's heel to mother's	Baby's big toe to mother's	Location of Sacrum (if breech)
Right	Symphysis	Right	Anterior
	Sacrum	Left	Posterior
	Left side	Anterior right	Left transverse
	Left anterior oblique	Right posterior oblique, toe nearer hip	Left anterior oblique
	Left posterior oblique	Left posterior quadrant, toe nearer symphysis	Left posterior oblique
	Right side	Left rear	Right transverse
	Right anterior oblique	Left posterior oblique, toe nearer hip	Right anterior oblique
	Right posterior oblique	Left posterior oblique, toe nearer symphysis	Right posterior oblique
Left	Symphysis	Left	Anterior
	Sacrum	Right	Posterior
	Left side	Right rear	Left transverse
	Left anterior oblique	Posterior oblique quadrant, toe nearer sacrum	Left anterior oblique
	Right side	Anterior left	Right transverse
	Right anterior oblique	Right posterior oblique, big toe nearer hip	Left transverse
	Right posterior oblique	Right posterior oblique, big toe nearer symphysis	Right posterior oblique

Telling the right hand from the left hand: A right or left hand can be distinguished by the position of the palm and thumb. Note that the thumb points to the head *unless* the arm is twisted.

If the back of the baby's hand is facing you, another way to identify which hand is presenting is to "shake hands" with the baby. If you must use your right hand, it is the baby's right, if you must use your left, it is the baby's left. Also see the chart below. Study these variations using a doll with distinct hands and feet and a pelvic model.

Presenting hand	**Baby's thumb to mother's**	**Relationship of baby's palm to maternal landmarks**	**Most likely fetal position**
Right	Right	Anterior	Transverse–head to mother's right
	Left	Posterior	Transverse–head to mother's left
	Anterior	Facing left thigh	Compound presentation most likely, rarely transverse lie with head directly anterior
	Posterior	Facing right thigh	Compound presentation most likely, rarely transverse lie with head directly posterior
Left	Left	Anterior	Transverse–head to mother's left
	Right	Posterior	Transverse–head to mother's right
	Anterior	Facing right thigh	Compound presentation most likely, rarely transverse lie with head directly anterior
	Posterior	Facing left thigh	Compound presentation most likely, rarely transverse lie with head directly posterior

If two limbs are presenting: It is possible for a breech baby to extend both legs. In other cases, you might discover an arm and a leg, two arms, or a hand and a foot, extended into the yoni. If you should find two limbs, you must ask yourself if they might belong to two different babies. Refer to the sections immediately above to help you figure out if you have two right or left limbs, which will usually confirm two babies unless a single baby has a strange anomaly. If you still aren't sure, try to determine if more than one baby is involved by following each limb as high as possible to see if the related anatomy is consistent with one baby or two. Finding limbs from two different babies means they are either both contained within one ruptured membrane or they have separate bags, both of which are broken. (See the chapter entitled "Assisting at Multiple Births" for more details.)

Identifying a shoulder presentation: Any part of the fetal anatomy along the trunk can present when the baby is lying transverse: arm, thigh, hip, back, rib cage, belly or, most commonly, the area near the shoulder. The front or back of the shoulder may be palpable. Thus the touch picture for a transverse lie can vary more than for any other presentation. The tip of the shoulder is more rounded than either the knee, elbow or heel. It has only one prominence from which three bony ridges extend: the spine of the scapula (acromion), the humerus and the clavicle. However, very little of the baby's anatomy is usually within reach unless the presenting part is impacted in the pelvis or an arm has prolapsed. If an arm emerges, the thumb should direct you to the side where the head is located, unless the arm is twisted. An irregular mass without a uniform shape, no orifices and no suture lines tells you that you have a very unusual presentation (rule out a knee) or a baby with a very unusual structural abnormality. This could also be a hip presentation in a transverse lie or a breech baby lying somewhat oblique.

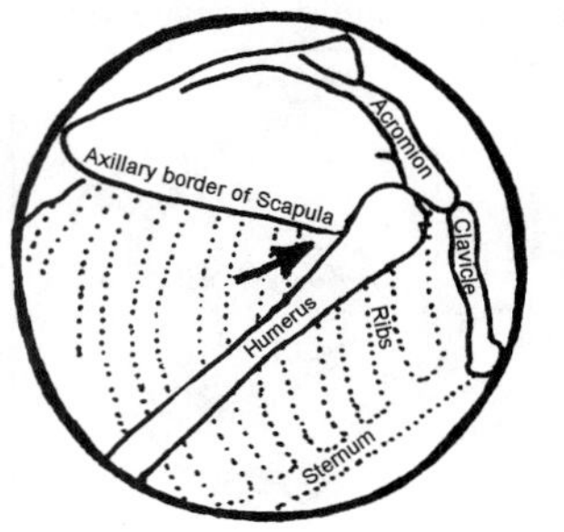

Arrow points to the axillary fold and toward the baby's head

Distinguishing the spine from the ribs and shoulder: The long, narrow ribs and intercostal spaces present a distinct "washboard" feel, closely spaced ridges interspersed with indented spaces, and with a thin overlying skin layer. The rib cage feels unlike any other part of the fetus you normally palpate. The spine presents a narrow, horizontally ridged area. If the posterior surface of the shoulder presents, the tip of the acromion process may be palpable, as well as the radiating bony ridges of the humerus, scapula, spine and clavicle. The "arrow" formed where the arm joins the body at the angle of the armpit points in the direction of the fetal head. The location of the head is what orients the lie of the baby to the mother's left or right side (the left or right designation never refers to the baby's left or right side). The back may also be positioned directly up toward the fundus (I call this superior–S) or directly toward the cervix (inferior–I).

The following touch pictures are for a baby in an transverse lie who is presenting her shoulder.

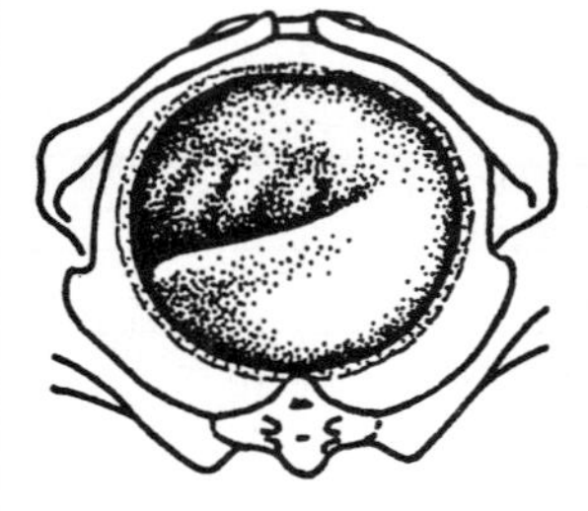
Left Acromion Anterior

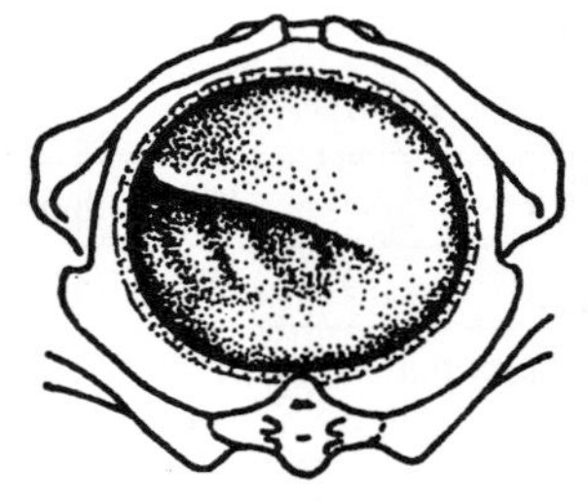
Left Acromion Posterior

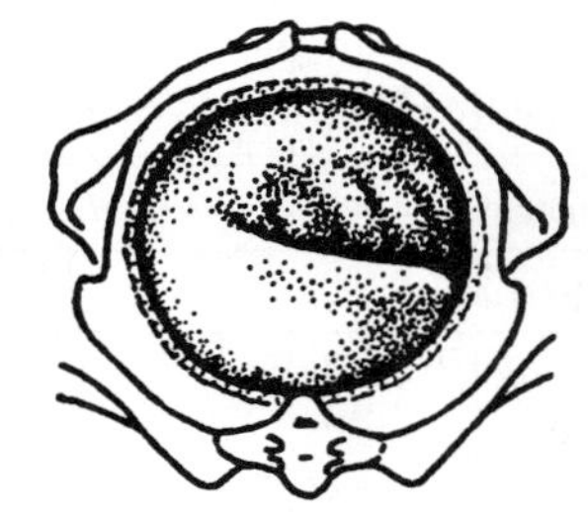
Right Acromion Anterior

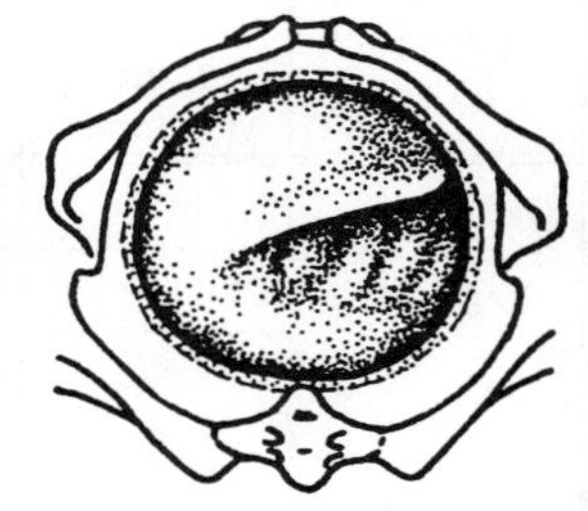
Right Acromion Posterior

Detecting a brow presentation: Brow is the rarest of all presentations. The forehead is the lowest presenting feature and occupies the center of the pelvis. You can feel the anterior fontanelle on one side and the root of the nose and the orbital ridge on the opposite side of the head. The nose, mouth and chin are out of reach. The frontal suture usually runs in the transverse diameter or a little obliquely. The length of the frontal suture is palpable toward the face and indicates the degree of deflexion; that is, the more of the frontal suture you can feel, the more deflexed the head. In a true brow attitude, you cannot feel the nose because the orbital ridge is in the same plane as the posterior border of the anterior fontanelle (Greenhill, 1951).

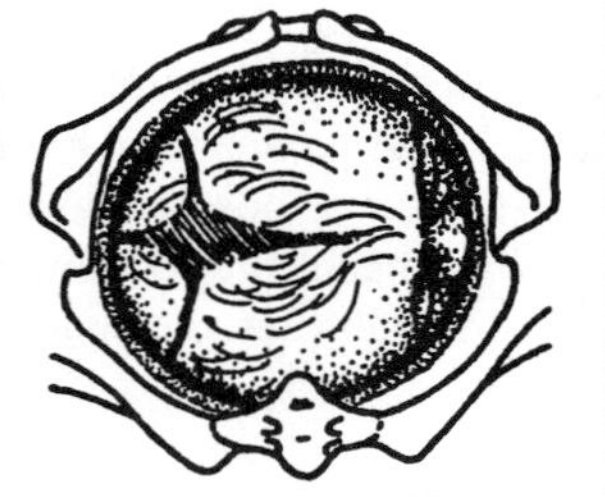
Left Frontum Transverse

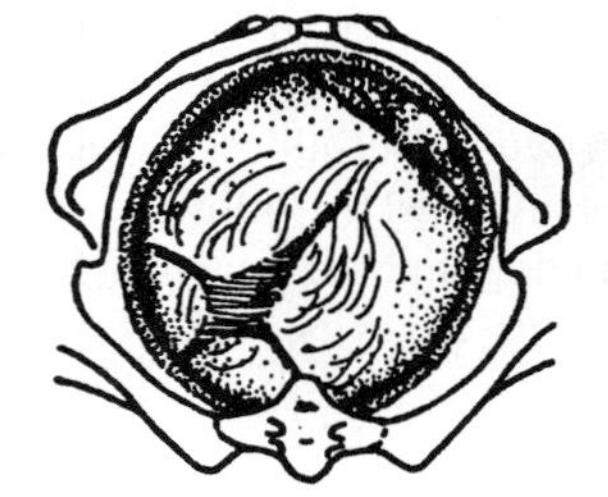
Left Frontum Anterior

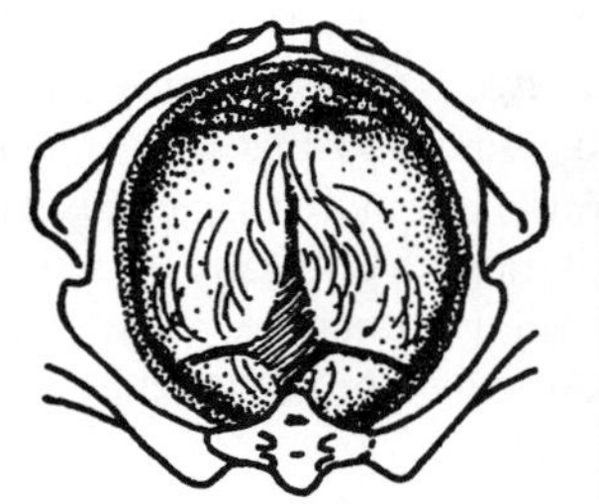
Frontum Anterior

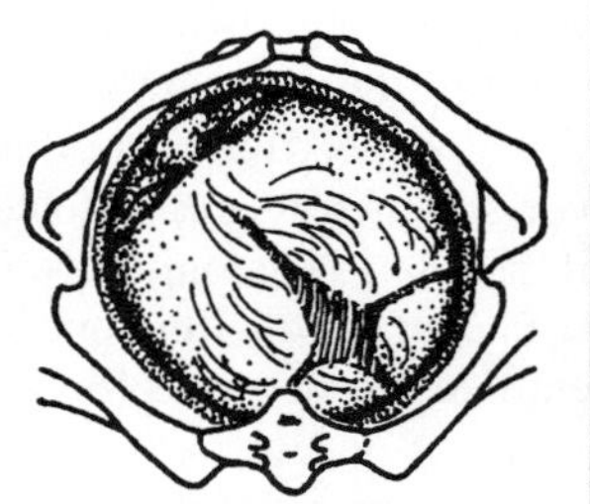
Right Frontum Anterior

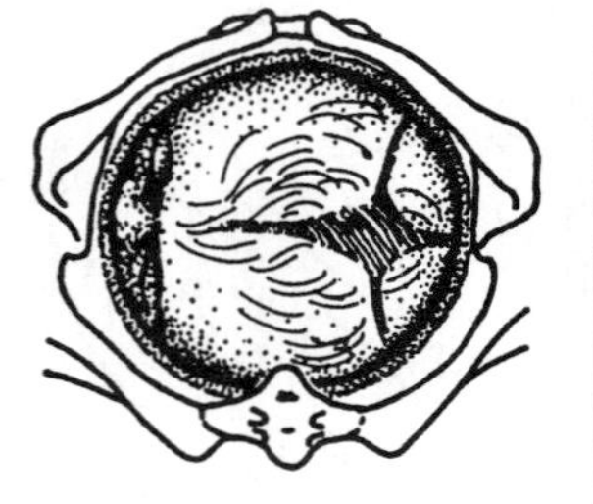
Right Frontum Transverse

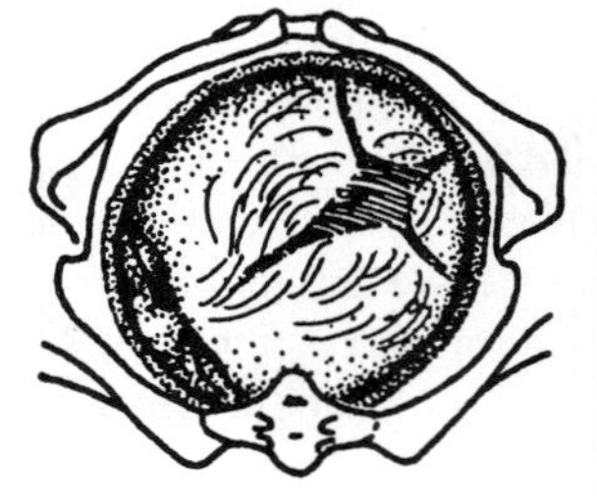
Right Frontum Posterior

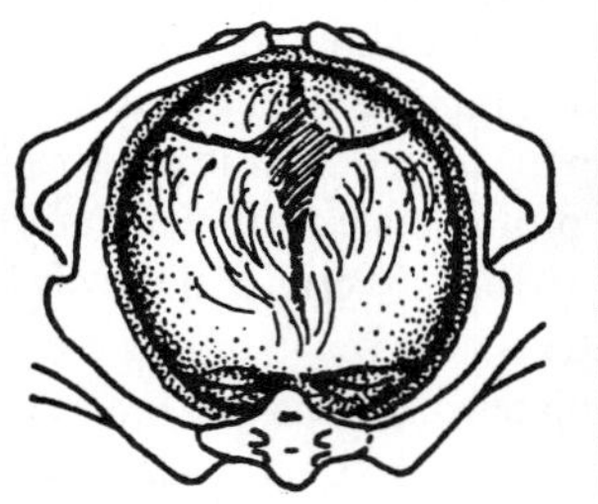
Frontum Posterior

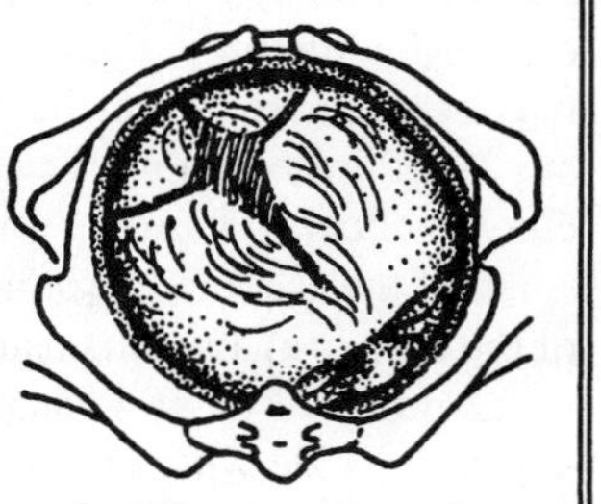
Left Frontum Posterior

Identifying an ear: There may be rare occasions when identification of an ear is useful; for example, if the baby has a large caput, labor is stuck and other attempts at identifying the fetal position have been unsuccessful. To do this, you must insert your whole hand into the yoni, unless the position of the head is quite asynclitic. The cervix must be nearly fully dilated, the membranes ruptured, and the pelvic musculature must be very relaxed. Identification of an ear using this method requires unseating the head in the pelvis to allow you to place your hand beside the head. This technique carries a risk of cord prolapse; to minimize this risk have the woman lie on a flat surface with her hips gently elevated and have an assistant monitor the fetal heart rate during the procedure.

The pinna points to the back of the head. By placing your index and middle fingers on either side of the ear, you can readily determine its orientation. You may become confused as to the direction if the ear is folded forward; the use of two

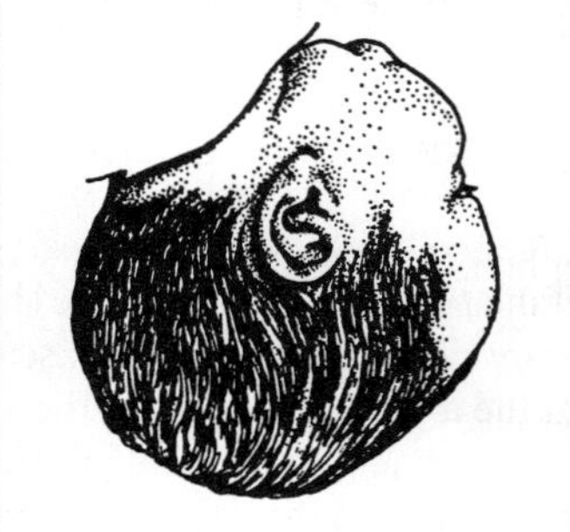
The head will be oriented like this when you palpate an ear.

fingers on either side should eliminate doubt as to which ear you are feeling. The anterior border of the ear is irregular while the posterior border is continuous. It is rarely necessary to go higher than the ear to confirm position, but if still in doubt, palpate the nape of the neck and the lower border of the jaw to further confirm direction. Once you are finished, flatten your hand against the head and gently withdraw it slowly enough to make sure that contractions move the head back into the pelvis enough to prevent cord prolapse. Listen to the fetal heart rate to confirm the cord is not compressed before the mother changes her position (Mayes, 1954).

Does the presenting part feel normally formed?

Finding a fetal defect on exam is a rare occurrence. It is important not to make ill-thought-out comments should you palpate the presenting part and note something unusual. However, you do need to be thinking about what part you are feeling and if abnormalities might be involved. Seek confirmation with additional abdominal palpation or ask your midwifery partner to perform another internal so you can get her opinion. Something that, at first, leads you to think the baby has a defect, may, in fact, be a normal region of fetal or maternal anatomy that you are not used to feeling. For example, you may have discovered that the baby is in an unusual position. Something you may think is attached to the fetus may be a previously unidentified part of the mother's anatomy, such as a swollen cervical lip or a polyp.

On the other hand, don't dismiss what you feel. If you are certain that the baby is vertex but you feel an unusually soft region, you could be feeling the placenta or an anencephalic baby (either of which, by the way, may produce some bleeding on exam). If you thought the waters broke and you still find what feels like a bag, you may be feeling an intact encephalocele. Be careful! If you can't locate normal sutures or fontanelles, the baby may have a defective skull.

What is the station of the presenting part?

Determining station requires that you first locate the mother's ischial spines. Using the techniques given to find the spines in Volume I, locate one, then the other. If the spines are not parallel with each other, gauge station by the lower of the two. Place your middle finger on a spine and reach out with your index finger toward the center of the birth canal to locate the lowermost portion of the presenting part. (If the baby is breech with a leg or knee extended into the yoni, the lowermost border of the presenting part–in this case, the pelvis– is used when assessing station.) Assess how far down into the pelvis it is in relationship to the ischial spine and translate that into the number of centimeters it is above or below the level of the spines. Be sure your finger contacts the scalp against the skull if the baby is in a cephalic presentation. The station of a caput is not relevant unless the head is stuck and the caput is getting bigger; if so, note the station of the skull as well as that of the caput, to be sure that what appears to be advancement is not actually increased swelling in the caput or extreme moulding. The same principle applies for breech or face babies; gently palpate to be sure your finger is against one of the baby's tuberosities, sacrum, cheekbones or chin, not her swollen genitals or cheeks. Remember that station can move up or down as labor progresses and the baby finds his best way out.

Is there any change in the cervix, the position or station of the presenting part, the consistency of the membranes (if intact) or change in any other feature during contractions?

The cervix should be pulled up and become more tense with the force of each active labor contraction. Ideally, the os draws up and opens slightly while the membranes tighten up and the presenting part is pressed downward. The cervix may tighten up with contractions if it is scarred or the mother is tense. The baby in a cocked position may not move down with contractions. Often a strong bag of waters buoys the baby up just out of reach, and the bag is really the only thing acting as a cervical dilator.

A change in the consistency of the membranes from loose to taut during a contraction is one excellent indication that a woman is in labor, progressive cervical changes being the other excellent indication.

Recording Your Findings

Record all the information you obtain during your exam, as it will prove very useful later if you must do additional exams to assess progress. For example, note the date and time along with: "Baby feels LOA per abdominal exam, internal: 3 cm dilated, cervix soft, central, slightly posterior, 40% effaced; station -1, bag intact, bulges w/contr, baby appears to be vertex, sutures not within reach, large forewaters."

How Often Should Internal Exams Be Performed?

You may need to perform one or more internal exams in a variety of situations; for example, if you are not very experienced at reading the external signs of progress, if you have another woman in labor, if there are concerns about a variable fetal position or if you suspect obstructed labor. As a rule, an internal exam no more than every four hours will help you assess progress without being overly intrusive. Four hours is not too long for lack of progress with dilation or descent to go on without detection in most cases. It gives you time to do what might be needed to get a hung-up labor back on track without exhausting the mother. However, once you have detected a problem with progress, more frequent exams may be warranted until things are flowing smoothly again.

The number of internal exams you feel the need to do will diminish as you become more experienced. However, you should never hesitate to perform multiple exams when any of your findings are unusual or uncertain. The point is not to avoid exams, but to avoid unnecessary exams. Foregoing exams in the case of an odd presentation could land the mother in the hospital unnecessarily because you didn't do what was needed to thoroughly assess what was going on and assist in resolving the problem. Furthermore, to allow a woman to labor with a dangerous situation that goes unrecognized because you do not have the skills (because you never learned to do a good exam) or because you have a misplaced attitude regarding interfering with labor is negligence. If you have a question, explain your concerns to the mother, what they might indicate and the need for more frequent or more thorough exams. Virtually every mother who is adequately informed in this way will go along with exams you deem necessary to keep labor on track and out of trouble.

If you are working with a partner and are uncertain about your findings, it is always a good idea to have your partner check as well. This gives two opinions on the spot and often provides valuable additional information. At the very least, it may confirm your own findings and offer more certainty regarding how to proceed. If neither of you can figure out what is going on, you can wait through a few contractions, have the mother move around to see if the fetal position will shift (depending upon what you think the problem may be) and try again. Continue to monitor with frequent exams until you are satisfied that all is well. If you truly cannot figure out what is going on and there are any problems whatsoever with the progress of labor, transport.

Maternal Reaction to Your Exam

Sometimes, the news obtained on internal exam is positive and the woman can go back to the work of labor much encouraged. However, a woman can become very discouraged upon learning that the baby's head is in an odd asynclitic posture or dilation is not nearly what she hoped it would be. It is important to allow her to express her discouragement openly and to cry if necessary. This, alone, can change the energy. Remember to emphasize that having more information about what is going on with her labor ultimately lets you know what techniques can help correct the problem.

Finally, finding a truly unusual or abnormal situation can help finalize the decision to transport before labor takes a dangerous turn for mother, baby or both.

THE PLACENTAL MEMBRANES AND AMNIOTIC FLUID DURING LABOR

NOTE: This chapter builds on the chapter entitled "Rupture of Membranes before the Onset of Labor" in Volume I of this text. Review it before studying this one.

Labor When the Membranes Are Intact

Intact membranes and the baby

It is to the mother's and baby's great advantage for the membranes to remain intact for as long as possible. The intact membranes provide protection from organisms that may ascend into the uterus from the cervix or yoni. The forewaters cushion the presenting part as it descends, protecting the head from stress and preventing or minimizing caput formation. While downward pressure from the fundus on the long axis of the fetus assists with dilation (Borell & Fernström, 1967), a sufficient quantity of amniotic fluid contained within intact membranes and surrounding the fetus helps to evenly distribute the pressure from the uterine contractions on the baby, cord and placenta to a certain extent. The forewaters also protect against cord prolapse when the head is not engaged. Finally, amniotic fluid provides support and cushioning around the cord during contractions, thus minimizing compression.

When the baby is breech, the forewaters provide a more uniform dilating wedge, particularly if the baby is in a complete or footling presentation. The forewaters buoy the presenting part up, facilitating rotation as well as any needed correction in the angle of descent.

If the volume of fluid is less than optimal or the membranes rupture before or during labor, the force applied to fetal parts above the presenting part during a contraction may still be equalized to a varying degree, depending upon the size of the pockets of fluid that remain, but the presenting part itself comes in direct contact with the internal os and must bear the brunt of the pressure with no cushioning.

Intact membranes and the course of labor

During contractions, the thick muscle walls of the upper uterine segment contract before those of the lower uterine segment. This pushes amniotic fluid into the lower part of the uterus, thus reducing the diameter of the upper segment. The fetal spine straightens and the downward movement of the amniotic fluid causes the lower segment to balloon, reinforcing the transmission of fluid pressure to the presenting part and the os (Narik, 281 in Carey, 1963).

Formation of the forewaters: The chorion becomes detached from the lower uterine segment as the cervix thins and stretches during labor. The increased intrauterine pressure from contractions usually causes the loosened portion of the lower end of the bag to bulge downward into the mouth of the dilating os to a depth of ¼ to ½ inch (6 to 12 mm) or more. The well-flexed fetal head fits snugly into the cervix, thus separating the fluid in front of the presenting part (the forewaters) from that above or behind the presenting part (the hindwaters).

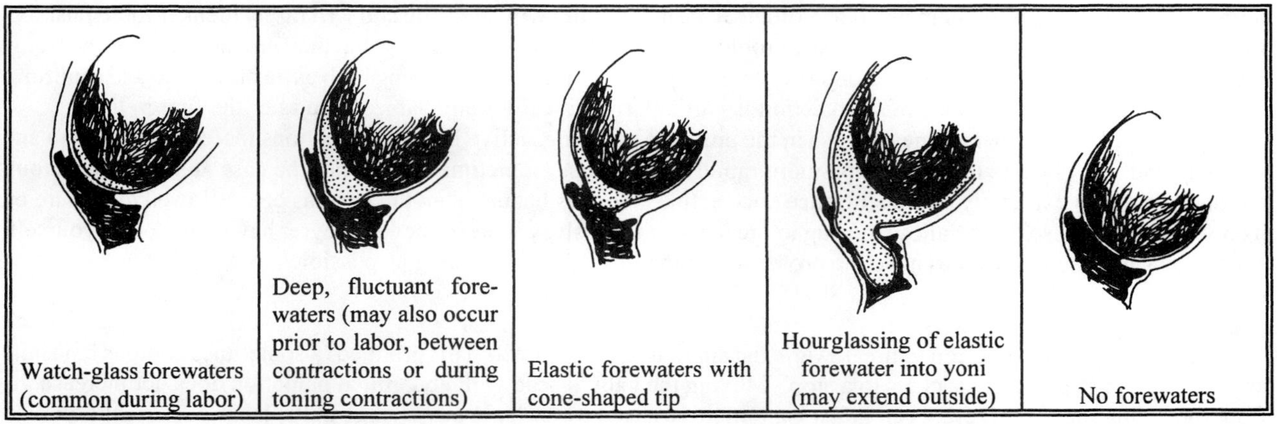

Watch-glass forewaters (common during labor)

Deep, fluctuant forewaters (may also occur prior to labor, between contractions or during toning contractions)

Elastic forewaters with cone-shaped tip

Hourglassing of elastic forewater into yoni (may extend outside)

No forewaters

The protruding portion of the membranes in front of a presenting head often takes the shape of a watch glass because the membranes are strong and contain only a relatively small amount of fluid and because the head blocks the descent of additional water from above. In other cases, the membranes form a soft, round-tipped cone that extends through the cervix. The bag may also be so elastic that a pouch of fluid, the size of which can vary greatly, may hang down into or outside the yoni; this is called an "hourglass forewater." It often forms when the presenting part is not fully sealing off the forewaters from the hindwaters, and the force of contractions pushes water into the forebag and stretches it. Finally, the membranes of the forebag may be so tightly applied to the presenting part that they contain no forewaters at all. In this case, the head is bearing the brunt of the pressure of descent almost as if the membranes are ruptured.

Identifying an intact bag

The bag of waters feels very much like a plastic bag with a thin application of lubricant over its surface. The distinctly smooth, slippery, uniform feel of the membranes will usually inform you that the bag is intact, even if no forewaters have formed. However, be aware that if the baby is not vertex, you can be fooled into thinking the bag is intact by the smooth feel of the fetal skin. Also, the surface of an intact bag should have no topical features. This is not as true of the baby's anatomy if you are touching it directly, although a small area of the bare fetal skin can feel quite smooth and featureless as well, and a very tight bag may feel slightly irregular as it conforms to the contour of the part it is covering. If you are unsure if the membranes are intact, place the mother in a Trendelenburg position or have her turn on her side, and try to buoy the baby up during an internal exam. If the bag is intact and there is any fluid in the lower uterine segment, a small amount may trickle down into the forewaters, confirming an intact bag. If any water trickles out of the yoni, this confirms that the membranes have ruptured.

Meconium staining of adjacent tissues, mucus and fluids prior to membrane rupture

Meconium staining that is long-standing or extreme can absorb through the intact membranes and stain the mucus plug or yoni mucus. This indicates that the baby has passed quite a bit of meconium prior to labor, possibly in the presence of little or no amniotic fluid and impaired swallowing, in a time interval sufficient to allow it to soak through both membranes. This rare event often indicates severe compromise in the infant, although it is not necessarily related to concurrent fetal distress per se (which is to say that the fetal heart rate may be normal at the time this is discovered). Anecdotally, midwives have reported such staining in a small number of cases. One baby had a spinal defect; another had renal agenesis. In two other cases, concurrent fetal distress was severe; one of these babies lived and the other did not. Seepage of meconium through the membranes should be interpreted as a "red flag" warning that the baby is in trouble; if you detect such staining and birth is not imminent, immediate transport is recommended.

Spontaneous Rupture of Membranes

Timing of spontaneous rupture

Membranes that are left alone will spontaneously rupture either early on, just before or as labor starts, or much more commonly, about the time active pushing begins. If the woman has taken 500 mg of Vitamin C with bioflavonoids daily during her pregnancy, as recommended in Volume I, the membranes will be strong and will rarely break prior to pushing. In fact, you may sometimes have the opposite problem; membranes that are so strong that they prevent descent! A strong, intact bag is especially important for mothers carrying breeches or multiples, offering both extra protection and a uniform dilator. In the case of multiples, this protection is particularly critical for any babies born after the first in line.

Typically, once the membranes release in the presence of strong, active labor, contractions increase in duration and intensity and labor begins to move along more rapidly. Of course, sometimes this is not the case and labor stalls out, although this is an extremely rare occurrence once active labor has begun when the bag has been allowed to rupture on its own. In either case, if you allow the bag to break spontaneously, you never have to regret having broken it yourself. This allows mother and baby to have the protection of the intact bag for as long as possible.

When only the chorion breaks

It is possible for the chorion to break while the amnion remains intact. This produces a sometimes copious but finite amount of fluid that usually trickles to a stop. Moving the baby's head with abdominal palpation does not increase the flow and an internal exam reveals an intact bag. In this case, you won't see any change in the labor because the amnion isn't ruptured. You also don't have to worry about an increased risk of infection.

Frank rupture

A frank rupture occurs when both the chorion and amnion break. This releases a variable amount of fluid depending upon the amount of fluid in the forewaters, whether the baby's presenting part has descended sufficiently to prevent hindwaters from escaping, and the amount of fluid in general. Anything from a slight trickle to a substantial flow can be normal. If the waters break suddenly with force behind them, as might occur at the peak of a contraction or during active pushing, a forceful out-splashing will typically occur.

At this point, the clock starts ticking because you must be on the alert for the possibility of infection. If labor is advanced, you probably have little to be concerned about. However, though rare, the baby can become infected with group B-strep, even if the baby is born within an hour or two, if the mother has a high colony count in her yoni. Once the membranes are ruptured, watch for fetal heart rate variability, which, if severe, probably reflects cord compression. If the membranes are ruptured for some hours before birth listen to the fetal heart rate more often. If an infection is known or suspected, cultures can be taken from the baby and placenta at the time of birth (details about doing so can be found in my text DIAGNOSTIC TESTS).

Crying in utero (vagitus uteri)

After rupture of membranes, babies have been heard crying in utero on very rare occasions (Thiery and associates reported three such incidents [1973]). This occurs when air enters the amniotic sac and the baby breathes enough to start crying. This is most likely to occur during some sort of invasive procedure such as an internal exam or manipulation or the introduction of a device, as might occur in a hospital birth.

Characteristics of Amniotic Fluid

Healthy fluid should smell like fresh, clear, warm sea water: heavy, salty, and clean. The smell of healthy yoni secretions is also mixed in. If the mother's hygiene is less than ideal, the odor will be stronger. A penetratingly foul smell is suggestive of an infectious process and transport is in order. The consistency should be like thick water, fluid but more substantial than plain water, less so than blood. It is also more slippery between your fingers than water. The color is normally clear, but the fluid may be flecked with vernix. If stained, the color is highly significant.

COLOR	MOST LIKELY CAUSE	OTHER CAUSES
Brown	Old meconium staining	Could be due to old blood. The fluid is sometimes murky and greenish brown if the baby has died some time before labor.
Green	Recent meconium staining	Hemolyzed blood
Port (red) wine	Concealed abruption produces dark red fluid into which the blood is well mixed. Most likely, when abruption occurs high in the uterus, adjacent membranes rupture and blood empties into the amniotic sac	Ruptured umbilical vessel (rare) or other fetal bleeding (unlikely)
Yellow to gold	Light meconium staining	Fetal bilirubin–suspect blood incompatibility or a liver disorder

Meconium-stained fluid

(Physiological considerations regarding meconium are covered in the chapter entitled "Production and Elimination of Meconium during Gestation." That chapter will provide background on the following discussion.) Seven to 22% of all babies born between 36 and 42 weeks have visible meconium in the amniotic fluid prior to birth. This may be the result of impaired swallowing, fetal hypoxia prior to or during labor, stress unrelated to hypoxia (such as a traumatic prenatal or intrapartum experience that frightens the mother, her baby or both), or fetal maturation, since nearly 50% of all babies born past 42 weeks gestation have visible meconium in their birth waters. Whether the presence of meconium-stained fluid in labor reflects acute fetal distress or not, the presence of meconium, by itself, can be problematic. If the fetus becomes stressed to the point of gasping, meconium can be aspirated into the tracheobronchial tree and lungs. This is now thought to happen while the fetus is still in utero, due to the development of prolonged asphyxia and not after the birth, when she takes her first breaths. Therefore, suctioning on the perineum or after birth does not prevent meconium aspiration syndrome. In addition, meconium has a potentially toxic effect on the myocyte cells in the umbilical cord and, postnatally, on the lung tissue. Further concerns about meconium will also be discussed at the end of this chapter.

Detecting meconium: Meconium is usually first detected upon rupture of membranes. The water is visibly stained, appearing on a continuum from barely stained green or gold transparent fluid to a thick, opaque sludge. White tissue or towels can be used to catch the first fluid passed so it can be examined right away under good light. If you are not present when membranes rupture, ask the woman to both save her underwear and catch some fluid on a white cloth or tissue for you to examine when you arrive.

However, meconium may not always be easy to detect, depending upon what you are examining and the quantity of fluid you have. For example, a small amount of fluid or a mucus plug streaked with dark blood may not clearly show a greenish tinge. To get a clearer picture, place the sample from your glove or fabric directly into a small glass of tepid water and gently stir it around. If meconium is present, the water will become stained green.

Assessing the degree of staining: Any meconium in the fluid should be noted for color, viscosity and quantity. Light meconium presents as a greenish yellow, greenish or occasionally brownish discoloration of otherwise watery, translucent fluid with no particulate matter. It can be so light as to be barely detectable. When the fluid is smeared across newsprint, the print can be read easily. Lightly stained fluid is less likely to produce airway blockage should it be inhaled, and the healthy fetus is better prepared to cope should this occur.

Moderate staining presents as darker fluid that is watery and may or may not also contain particles. When smeared across newsprint, the print is difficult to read. Thick meconium is often described as "pea soup" consistency; that is, particulate, thick, sometimes viscous and opaque, usually pea green to medium dark green or brown. When smeared across newsprint, the print is impossible to read. While it is often assumed that particulate matter means chunks or flakes floating in otherwise relatively thin fluid, homogenized fluid that is thoroughly saturated with meconium to the point of a creamy sludge also describes particulate material. While it may be reasonable to speculate that thick meconium is more hazardous than thin, there are currently no clinical studies that warrant basing care guidelines on meconium consistency (Kattwinkel et al., 2011).

Pure, undiluted meconium (frank meconium) can be passed when a breech baby is descending. This occurs due to pressure on the fetal abdomen and does not, by itself, indicate distress. It is also common for the baby to pass meconium just as it is being born (terminal meconium). In this case, the meconium is usually behind the head in a cephalic birth.

The thickness of the fluid is affected not only by the quantity of meconium passed but also by the amount of fluid there is to dilute it. A reduced volume of amniotic fluid can be related to insufficient maternal hydration. It may also be associated with chronic fetal hypoxia, which, in turn, lowers fetal urinary output and results in low amniotic fluid volume. Little or no amniotic fluid upon rupture of membranes is associated with the finding of thick meconium in the hindwaters 50% of the time, as well as with a sharp increase in perinatal mortality.

Also note that the forewaters may be clear while the hindwaters are stained with meconium. In this case, the head acts as a cork, sealing off the hindwaters when the forewaters rupture. The staining becomes apparent only as labor progresses and the presenting part changes position to allow escape of the hindwaters; this may not occur until the head is born. Meconium that is only in the hindwaters has probably been passed during labor, unless the baby has been well engaged prior to the onset of labor (otherwise it would have had a chance to become mixed into the forewaters). If you suspect there is meconium in the hindwaters or have questionable findings, you can prop the mother's bottom up and gently push the baby's head up slightly to see if distinctly stained fluid escapes.

Clinical significance of meconium-stained fluid: The significance and clinical ramifications of meconium-stained fluid have long been debated. The presence of meconium in amniotic fluid has been associated with vasoconstrictive effects on the umbilical cord that may result in vasospasm and impaired fetal-placental blood flow (Altshuler & Hyde, 1989). This is apparently due to the toxic effect of meconium on myocytes in the vessels on the placental surface and in the cord after prolonged exposure (exceeding 18 hours). Necrotic changes may be noted in one or more of these vessels on microscopic exam. Meconium staining exceeding 16 hours duration has also, on rare occasions, been associated with ulceration and vascular necrosis in the cord. Meconium also has necrotic and erosive effects on the amnion. Such damage may be due to the bile acids in the stool, although this has not been firmly established (Altshuler et al., 1992). Meconium can also inhibit the bacteriostatic properties of normal amniotic fluid. Meconium concentrations over 1%

enhance the ability of amniotic fluid to sustain bacterial growth, which may also be linked to an inhibition of neutrophil activity (Clark & Duff, 1995) or alterations of zinc concentration (Hoskins et al., 1987). (One percent would appear as light staining if the total volume of amniotic fluid is average.)

Meconium staining noted during labor has been associated with abnormal fetal heart rate patterns in several studies. However, the relationship between the presence of meconium during labor, low APGAR scores and fetal acidosis remains controversial. Many studies that noted an association did not take into account variables that affect the fetal heart rate and APGAR score, such as vigorous suctioning at the time of birth (which can trigger a vasovagal response and produce an artificially depressed baby). Likewise, the best studies of neonatal acidosis did not find meconium staining to be predictive of neonatal acidosis (Steer et al., 1989).

It has long been assumed that meconium staining, by itself, is a sign of current fetal distress, regardless of all other factors. If this is so, then all babies with meconium-stained fluid would have adverse perinatal outcomes, whether they had other evidence of current compromise or not. However, studies and clinical experience show that outcomes of babies with meconium-stained fluid who had normal heart rate patterns in labor are the same as those who passed no meconium and had normal fetal heart rate patterns. Likewise, when a group of babies who passed meconium and had abnormal fetal heart rate patterns was compared to babies who did not pass meconium but had abnormal heart rate patterns, the outcomes were similar. The incidence of meconium passage was similar in asphyxiated and unasphyxiated infants as well (Galan, 1999). Furthermore, it is now known that the fetus experiences periodic defecation throughout most of pregnancy. Thus, meconium staining alone may or may not reflect fetal compromise at some point and does not, by itself, indicate that the baby is currently having a problem (Miller et al., 1975; Bochner et al., 1987; Baker et al., 1992).

For many years, the color and consistency of meconium in the fluid was thought to reflect the degree of fetal compromise. Passage of meconium during early labor may carry a greater correlation with associated fetal distress than meconium first noted during pushing when clear fluid was noted previously (Meis et al., 1978). Even so, studies have been inconsistent in showing a reliable pattern of association between signs of fetal compromise and the degree to which the fluid is stained and current protocols do not recommend altering care based on the consistency of the meconium.

There is also the issue of when and how meconium aspiration occurs. Meconium-staining occurs in approximately 12% of live births. About a third of these infants have meconium below the vocal cords. However, meconium aspiration syndrome (MAS) develops in only 2 of every 1000 live-born infants. Ninety-five percent of infants with aspirated meconium are able to clear their lungs spontaneously. Those that can't are now believed to have lung damage due to pulmonary vascular changes that have occurred due to an episode of prolonged intrauterine asphyxia. These blood vessel changes have also been found in babies born through clear fluid. In the most severe cases there is right-to-left shunting and persistent fetal circulation with subsequent death (Katz, et al., 1992). Meconium staining may therefore only be a marker in some babies for asphyxia-related lung damage, which may be the real cause of MAS. Thus suctioning at birth (which can depress respiratory efforts) to prevent meconium aspiration is no longer recommended in the UK (Richmond, 2011). (Suctioning of the mouth and nose to clear out meconium using a bulb syringe or catheter as necessary after birth is still acceptable according to US/NRP guidelines [2011].)

Given that you cannot be sure if or when fetal distress may have occurred, the midwife is advised to view meconium-stained amniotic fluid as an indication to check the fetal heart rate more frequently, with the understanding that thick meconium probably means that the volume of amniotic fluid is significantly reduced. Unresolvable fetal distress with or without meconium stained fluid (rather than the presence of meconium per se except as otherwise noted in this chapter) when birth is not imminent is cause for transport. After birth, the midwife should be prepared to suction babies who have meconium staining, if indicated (Vain et al., 2004; Velaphi et al., 2006).

References added in 2013:

Kattwinkel, J, ed. Neonatal Resuscitation Textbook, 6th ed. Am Acad Pediatrics & Am Heart Assoc, 2011.

Katz V, et al. "Meconium aspiration syndrome: reflections on a murky subject," Am J Obstet Gynecol 166(1, Pt 1):171-183, Jan 1992.

Richmond S, ed. Newborn Life Support, 3rd ed. Resuscitation Council, UK, 2011.

Vain N, et al. "Oropharyngeal and nasopharyngeal suctioning of meconium-stained neonates before delivery of their shoulders: multicentre, randomized controlled trial," Lancet, 364(9434):597-602, Aug 14-20, 2004.

Velaphi S., et al. "Intrapartum and postdelivery management of infants born to mothers with meconium-stained amniotic fluid: evidence-based recommendations," Clin Perinatol, 33(1):29-42, Mar 2006.

References and Further Reading on Understanding and Monitoring the Flow of Labor

References used in multiple chapters

Banks M. Personal e-mail communication, Mar 6, 2000.

Flint C. Sensitive Midwifery. Heinemann Professional, Oxford UK, 1986.

Hellman L, Pritchard J. Williams Obstetrics, 14th ed. Appleton-Century-Crofts, New York NY, 1971.

Myerscough P. Munro Kerr's Operative Obstetrics, 9th ed. Williams & Wilkins Co, Baltimore MD, 1977.

Oxorn H. Oxorn-Foote Human Labor and Birth, 5th ed. Appleton-Century-Crofts, Norwalk CT, 1986.

Sellers P. Midwifery, A Textbook and Reference Book for Midwives in Southern Africa, Vol. 1: Normal Childbirth. Juta & Co, Ltd., Kenwyn South Africa, 1993.

Tucker S. Pocket Guide to Fetal Monitoring and Assessment, 4th ed. Mosby, St. Louis MO, 2000.

Assessing the Progress and Strength of Labor: An Overview

Busch J. Personal communications, 2000.

Claypool S, midwife. Personal communications, Oakland CA, 2001.

Flint C. Sensitive Midwifery. Heinemann Professional, Oxford UK, 1986.

Friedman E. Labor: Clinical Evaluation and Management. Appleton-Century-Crofts, New York NY, 1967.

Hathaway M, Hathaway J. "The Bradley method: overview of labor and birth," class handout, Amer Assoc Husband Coached Childbirth, 1989.

Lemay G. "Pushing for first-time moms," Midwifery Today, (55);9-11, Autumn, 2000.

O'Driscoll K, et al. Active Management of Labor: The Dublin Experience, 3rd ed. Mosby Year Book, London UK, 1993.

Simkin P. The Birth Partner: Everything You Need to Know to Help a Woman through Childbirth, 2nd ed. Harvard Common Press Inc, Boston MA, 2001.

Simkin P, Ancheta R. The Labor Progress Handbook. Blackwell Science, Oxford UK, 2000.

Sutton J. Let Birth Be Born Again! Rediscovering and Reclaiming Our Midwifery Heritage. Birth Concepts UK, Bedfont UK, 2001.

Abdominal Examination and Palpation Techniques for Use during Labor

Barnes D. Personal communication, 2000.

Calkins L. Abnormal Labor, American Lecture Series, No. 325, American Lectures in Obstetrics and Gynecology. Charles C Thomas, Springfield IL, 1958.

Cunningham, F et al., ed. "Chapter 11: Parturition," Williams Obstetrics, 21st ed. McGraw-Hill, New York NY, 2001.

Deol K. Personal e-mail communication, recd. Mar 1, 2000.

Gentlebirth midwifery archives, http://www.gentlebirth.com, accessed 2001.

Lizon K. E-mail communication, recd. Mar 2, 2000.

Marshall M, Buffington S. Life-Saving Skills Manual for Midwives: Module 9: Vacuum Extraction; Module 10: Other Emergencies, 3rd ed. American College of Nurse-Midwives, Washington DC, 1998.

Porritt N. The Abdomen in Labour: Being a General Practitioner's Clinical Study of the Parturient Abdomen. Humphrey Milford, London UK, 1926.

Roberts J. "Managing fetal bradycardia during second state of labor," MCN, 14(6);394-398, Nov/Dec 1989.

Schulman H, Romney SL. "Variability of uterine contractions in normal human parturition," Obstet Gynecol, 36(2);215-21, Aug 1970.

Turnbull A. "Uterine contractions in normal and abnormal labour," J Obstet Gynaecol Br Emp, 64(3);321-33, June 1957.

Additional Noninvasive Techniques for Assessing Progress

Block P. Polly's Birth Book: Obstetrics for the Home. Hearthspun Pub, American Fork UT, 1984.

Byrne D, Edmonds D. "Clinical method for evaluating progress in first stage of labour," Lancet, 335(8681);122, Jan 13, 1990.

Cohen J. Personal communication, 2001.

Davis-Floyd R, Davis E. "Intuition as authoritative knowledge in midwifery and homebirth," in Davis-Floyd R, Arvidson P, eds. Intuition: The Inside Story, Routledge, London England, 1997.

Hobbs L. "Assessing cervical dilatation without VE," Practicing Midwife, 1(11);34, Nov 1998.

Kirkham M. "Bodily knowledge: the wisdom of nausea," Midwifery Today, (52;15,Winter, 1999.

Radcliff A. Personal e-mail communication, recd. Mar 2, 2000.

Valcourt K. Personal fax communication, recd. Sept 15, 1996.

Performing Internal Yoni Exams during Labor

Bennett VR, Brown LK, eds. Myles Textbook for Midwives, 13th ed. Churchill Livingstone, Edinburgh UK, 1999.

Hamlin RHJ. Stepping Stones to Labour Ward Diagnosis. Rigby Ltd, Adelaide Australia, 1959.

Greenhill J. Principles and Practice of Obstetrics, 10th ed. WB Saunders Co, Philadelphia PA, 1951.

Kerr J Munro, et al. A Combined Textbook of Obstetrics and Gynæcology. E & S Livingstone, Edinburgh UK, 1923.

Mayes B. A Textbook of Obstetrics. Australasian Pub Co, Sydney Australia, 1954.

Playfair WS, Harris R. A Treatise on the Science and Practice of Midwifery, 3rd American ed. Henry C Lea, Philadelphia PA, 1880.

Schuler-Maloney D, Lee S. The Placenta: To Know Me Is to Love Me. DSM Pathworks, Inc, St. Mary's IO, 1998.

Schuler-Maloney D. E-mail communication, recd. Nov 24, 2000.

Singer D, Macpherson T. "Fetal death and the macerated stillborn infant," in Wigglesworth J, Singer D. eds. Textbook of Fetal and Neonatal Pathology, 2nd ed. Blackwell Sciences, Malden MA, 1998.

Stevenson J. Personal communication, Nov, 2001.

Sutton J. "Optimal fetal positioning" workshop handout, Seattle WA, May 8, 2000.

The Placental Membranes and Amniotic Fluid during Labor

Altshuler G, Hyde S. "Meconium-induced vasoconstriction: A potential cause of cerebral and other fetal hypoperfusion and of poor pregnancy outcome," J Child Neurol, 4(2);137-142, Apr, 1989.

Altshuler, G, et al. "Meconium-induced umbilical cord vascular necrosis and ulcerations: A potential link between the placenta and poor pregnancy outcome," Obstet Gynecol,79(5 Pt 2);760-766, May. 1992.

Baker PN, et al. "An assessment of the use of meconium alone as an indication for fetal blood sampling," Obstet Gynecol, 80(5);792-796, Nov, 1992.

Bochner, C, et al. "The role of antepartum testing in the management of postterm pregnancies with heavy meconium in early labor," Obstet Gynecol, 1987 Jun;69(6);903-907, Jun, 1987.

Borell U, Fernström I. "The mechanism of labour," Radiol Clin N Amer, 5(1);173-85, Apr, 1967.

Carey H. Modern Trends in Human Reproductive Physiology–1. Butterworths, London England, 1963.

Clark P, Duff P. "Inhibition of neutrophil oxidative burst and phagocytosis by meconium," Am J Obstet Gynecol, 173(4);1301-1305, Oct, 1995.

Galan H. "Meconium-stained amniotic fluid: meaning and management," OMG Management: CME article, http://www.obgmanagement.com/799/cme/799.html, July 1999, accessed Aug 3, 2001.

Hoskins IA, et al. "Effects of alterations of zinc-to-phosphorus ratios and meconium content on group B Streptococcus growth in human amniotic fluid in vitro," Am J Obstet Gynecol, 157(3);770-773, Sept, 1987.

Meis PJ, et al. "Meconium passage: a new classification for risk assessment during labor," Am J Obstet Gynecol, 131(5):509-13, July 1, 1978.

Meis PJ, et al. "Late meconium passage in labor–a sign of fetal distress?" Obstet Gynecol, 59(3);332-335, Mar, 1982.

Miller FC, et al. "Significance of meconium during labor," Am J Obstet Gynecol, 122(5);573-580, July 1, 1975.

Schneider K, neonatal respiratory therapist, Providence Hospital, Portland OR. Personal communications, July, 1999.

Steer PJ, et al. "Interrelationships among abnormal cardiotocograms in labor, meconium staining of the amniotic fluid, arterial cord blood pH, and APGAR scores," Obstet Gynecol, 74(5);715-721, Nov, 1989.

Thiery M, et al. "Vagitus uterinus," J Obstet Gynecol Br Commonw, 80(2);183-185, Feb 1973.

SUPPORTING THE WOMAN DURING LABOR AND BIRTH

INDIVIDUALIZING CARE DURING LABOR

Continuity of care

A fundamental difference between the care provided by a homebirth midwife and that provided by a practitioner in an institutional setting is the ongoing relationship the midwife develops with the mother and family over the course of the pregnancy. When prenatal care takes place with only one to two providers, when the course of care is communicated between providers sharing care and when the woman knows her midwives well, a relationship of trust, caring and partnership grows. This partnership with the woman is the foundation of good midwifery care and is a big part of what makes our care fundamentally different.

Continuity of care allows the midwife to develop an in-depth knowledge of the parameters of well-being unique to each pregnant woman and baby. She has the opportunity to observe and converse with the mother at length during unrushed prenatal visits and home visits. Repeated, careful assessment of the mother's physical status during pregnancy gives the midwife a wealth of information to use during labor. Likewise, the midwife cultivates her special relationship with the unborn baby through talking to the baby, palpating, listening to the fetal heart with a fetoscope (rather than a Doppler), monitoring fetal growth and amniotic fluid volume, and getting familiar with fetal movements.

Attitude

The midwifery attitude toward care is fundamentally different as well. The partnership developed over the course of pregnancy continues to evolve during labor as mother and midwife work together with the energy of birth. Midwives view themselves as experienced facilitators of a process while continuously recognizing that the birth is happening within the woman's body. The woman holds the locus of control and information about what is taking place. The midwife advises and recommends based on feedback (both verbal and nonverbal) from the woman but does not tell the mother what to do in most circumstances. The only time when this shifts is during a true emergency, when the midwife's clinical skills become of paramount importance in navigating the situation.

Individualization of care during labor

All the time and energy spent during the pregnancy in getting to know the woman and her unborn baby pays off during labor. The intuitively alert midwife is exquisitely attuned to the woman in her care. Routinized, rote care, which is a standard in institutions, becomes absurdly invasive at home. The midwife watches, listens and speaks to the mother, already well known to her, regarding her well-being as the need arises. A history of good nutrition during pregnancy and a well-grown baby allay concerns regarding the sudden appearance of toxemia. The midwife's assessment skills are thus at the service of the birthing woman, not imposed upon the woman when it is obvious that everything is fine.

Individualization of care for the unborn baby is slightly trickier, as the baby cannot be seen and talked to. However, the woman's and the midwife's sense of the baby's well-being, the baby's responsiveness to stimulation, and the history of fetal heart findings gathered during pregnancy greatly assist in providing individualized care for the baby during labor.

When the midwife finds herself attending women whom she knows less well, periodic assessments become more important because the depth of the partnership relationship and knowledge of normal parameters is lacking. The midwife must use her own judgment regarding when and if a particular intervention is warranted.

Individualizing care also extends to the nature and amount of support that is appropriate for each woman. While some women will blossom during a labor in which they are allowed complete privacy, others will interpret this as abandonment and will need more hands-on support to achieve the depth of focus required to let go.

Every action is an intervention

The homebirth midwife recognizes that any and all her actions regarding the woman or her unborn baby are, in the end, interventions. Therefore, each action must be carefully weighed as to its potential benefit and the possible problems that may ensue if it is carried out. The anticipated benefit must always outweigh the potential risk when an intervention is to be used. Remember that there are no guarantees. Proceeding with any intervention may produce undesirable results. Likewise, failing to intervene when it is called for can have dire consequences.

TUNING INTO BIRTHING ENERGY

At the risk of quantifying and therefore reducing a centrally important midwifery concept to the sum of its parts, let me introduce ways to tune into birthing energy. The central requirement for a smooth, progressive labor is free-flowing birthing energy. The mother's body forms a conduit for birthing energy, opening her to the spiritual world so that she can channel her baby through to this physical plane of existence. While many people not familiar with birth may not be able to relate to this concept, almost everyone knows the difference between having sex with a free flow of sexual energy versus without it. This creative energy carries you away, expands the experience and creates a state of euphoria. The hormones that promote psychic openness during sex function the same way during labor. Unless and until this energy is building and carrying the woman along, labor will not really progress. In essence, the same type of energy that gets the baby started also gets the baby out. It's that simple.

Perhaps the most important and yet ineffable thing midwives do is be fully present at the birth as they monitor the energy. This is most possible when the environment is undisturbed and the midwife can, without distraction, tune into the mother, who herself feels free to unselfconsciously experience her labor. The following description attempts to give the reader a starting point for understanding birthing energy and how it can be accessed and utilized in the labor situation. There is no right way to do this. As you gain experience, your own unique relationship and response to birthing energy will make itself known and eventually will become second nature to you.

Much of what is wrong with hospital birth has to do with the total absence of the concept of birthing energy and how its flow is enhanced; instead birth is treated as a purely physical event. Personnel shift changes, lack of privacy, beeping monitors, bright lights and the like are just not conductive to the easy flow of this energy or to reading it, although birthing energy is powerful and manifests even under the most adverse conditions (were this not true, the surgical birth rate in the hospital would be 100%).

Reading birthing energy

In many cases, the presence of birthing energy can be felt at the onset of progressive labor and usually becomes increasingly noticeable as active labor moves along. Midwives monitor the energy in a variety of ways, learning to feel it rise in their own body as it builds and moves through the mother. Experienced midwives report that certain emotional, mental or physical signs and sensations of their own are reliable indications of the mother's progress in labor, particularly when it comes to the onset of pushing. For example, some midwives always have a loose stool just before pushing begins. Maggie Banks describes her experience of birthing energy like this:

> As far as the assessment of labor goes–I also work very much on the birthing energy. . . . For me there is a feeling of "thickness" which pervades the room when women are in well established labor and going with the flow. It feels like you are lying on your back in the middle of the ocean without any wharf or rocks to steady yourself against, and knowing that the swells and hollows will support you. I am surrounded by this and know that any of my moves will be synchronous with her movements. The ebb and flow comes with the woman's breathing. This part of labor is mesmerizing by its rhythm. There is an overwhelming feeling that "this is fine.". . . As labor builds, I [also] very much feel a dry heat in my cheeks. (Banks, 2000)

I have always felt a mild energy current coursing through my body at the point where labor really takes off. Note at what point such signs appear. Many times people attending a birth, including the midwives, begin to get antsy around 8 centimeters. This is an unconscious response to the energy of transition, reflected in everyone's emotional state. Some midwives experience specific physiological signs or symptoms at certain points during labor. Hilary Schlinger of Ithaca, NY, notes that she is often nauseous at births where complications such a hemorrhage or fetal distress later develop. Other indications may be more subtle. A nurse midwife says that her hands reach out and know what to do at a birth and finds that everything is fine if she steps out of the way. The energy of birth will instruct you when things are going smoothly and when it is time to jump in and lend a skilled hand. This is another way that birthing energy manifests in your own body.

As you gain experience, dreams, premonitions and intuitive perceptions will also come to you either before, during or even after the birth in the form of insights or symbolic messages. The more open you are to your chosen spiritual path, the more attuned you will be to receiving these messages and the better you will be at applying their content to clinical situations.

There will be many suggestions throughout this text regarding what to look for and how to help, including specific suggestions on assisting the mother to open to the energy of birth. The glue that pulls these disparate facts and suggestions together is the continuous, sensitive presence of the attuned midwife who can discern what might work for an individual woman. However, in reality the only way to get adept at this skill is by being present at many labors and births. Your awareness of what you are looking for and how the energy of birth makes its presence known will further your progress immensely.

Birthing energy and others present

Birthing energy will affect everyone present at the birth. Men may interpret these feelings as sexual, which they are in the sense that they are all part of the same flow of creative, life-sustaining energy. Women tend to recognize this feeling as familiar, as the same energy which is operative during menstruation and other female bodily functions, although to a lesser extent than it is during labor. Both men and women often relate unconsciously to birthing energy with increased anxiety and fear. Perhaps this is because feeling the energy of birth triggers unresolved issues from their own gestations and births. It is important to acknowledge that the energy of labor is affecting the others present; you can say something like "As the mother's labor becomes stronger, we will all start to feel more excited. Sometimes people sympathize with the mother and begin to feel afraid and anxious that the mother is in pain. We must all remember that the intense sensations of labor are what will complete the birth." Choose the words you use to discuss this concept carefully; some people can be offended by the word "energy" but will grasp the concept when explained in other ways. The important thing is for all present to acknowledge and respect the things that facilitate the unimpeded flow of labor.

DON'T JUST DO SOMETHING

Assuming that women are well prepared for labor with a good understanding of how their body, especially their pelvis, and their baby both work to facilitate birth, very often, when women need help in labor, they ask for it. Therefore, before you make a move to interfere with the mother's labor in any way, review and reflect upon why you want to do so and what you propose to do. This will keep you focused on *this* mother's labor and minimize the tendency to allow routines to slip into your practice style at births. Although "cookbook" midwifery can get you through in many cases, it is not in the best interest of the women you serve and also, ultimately, makes your job less rewarding. An in-depth knowledge of the way purely physiological labor proceeds and a trust in the process will result in a better understanding of when to interrupt the mother. There is no one right way to evaluate the need to intervene, as with the previous chapter; the following discussion is intended to offer the student a starting point. As you become more experienced, your own unique intuitive abilities will develop and you will find your own best way to evaluate women in labor.

Issues to consider

You will generally have time to make this assessment unless an obvious emergency which requires your immediate attention presents itself. Here are some suggestions that Holly Scholles (2003) has offered as a way of assessing what to do next.

What are you observing? Observe the support persons and the environment. Become conscious of the temperature and light level and sounds in the room. Be aware of what has taken place up until this point or what may have recently changed about the mother's environment. Look carefully at the woman. What is she doing (or not doing)? How is she holding her body, her legs and thighs, her arms, her lips, mouth and throat, her buttocks? Is she making any sounds? How is she moving? Is she remaining still? What is her position? What, if anything, is she saying? What are others saying to her? At this point, try to be as factual as possible; do not interpret your observations.

What is the context of these observations? How long have these things been going on? Is there a pattern to her behavior? Does it seem to relate to anything else going on in the room or the house? Review your chart notes.

What do you sense that the mother is feeling? What is your interpretation of her behavior or the behavior of others in the room? Realize that this is your interpretation and not necessarily what is going on for them

What are you feeling? Are you projecting your own feelings onto the mother? For example, is she making loud, sensual sounds that make *you* uncomfortable? Do you feel the need to do something because the energy of birth is getting stronger? Do you interpret her intense responses as unbearable pain? Is this the point in labor where your last client needed a particular type of help? Are you tired? Are you worried about a personal crisis? Are you feeling torn about how long you have been at this labor and other responsibilities that you have looming? Are you hypoglycemic? Does this woman remind you of a previous client who had a serious complication? Have you recently attended a birth that had *any* type of serious complication? Are you afraid? Does this mother have a history of a specific type of problem or labor pattern? Did a previous baby of hers have a problem at birth?

How is the birthing energy flowing? Now that you have considered all of the above and have that out of the way (or at least are more conscious of your own agenda), tune into the energy. Breathe into and through your whole body, your breasts, uterus, cervix and yoni and identify where in your body the energy is the strongest. Does the energy flow through you or does it stop anywhere? Flowing birth energy may manifest in a number of ways, including a sensation of well-being, sexual feelings, streaming feelings, breathing easy, a mental attitude that things are going well, optimism, premenstrual-like feelings, expansion and fullness in the pelvic area, or a pervading sense of change in the nonphysical environment such as Maggie Banks describes in the preceding chapter.

Do you feel that the energy is blocked? Blocked birthing energy is often reflected in feelings of agitation, fear, anxiety, frustration, despair, hopelessness, possibly even aches and pains and the overwhelming desire to manage and control the situation. If so, try to differentiate where it is blocked in your body. Look at the mother; does it appear that she is holding energy in this area? If not, discharge your own accumulation of birthing energy. Do this by breathing the energy from the top of your head and consciously breathing into any areas that you feel are blocked. Since you are not the one in labor, this should be easy for you to do. If you cannot do this, it may be that you are intuitively picking up on blocks that the mother herself is holding. Once you have discharged the energy from your body, reassess the situation.

Conversely, complications or dangerous situations can be read in the birthing energy as well. You may have a sense of foreboding, feel cut off from spiritual help or have a sense that there is a dark, cloud-like energy pervading the room. A gut-level, core fear should not be ignored and may signal serious problems; this may come up as you assess clinical signs, such as the fetal heart rate. (You can use your gut reaction as a barometer to help you decide if what you are hearing indicates a serious problem or a benign variation.) Of course, you would also continue to listen to the baby until the clinical picture resolved, but your intuition will help guide you regarding how to proceed.

What is your overall assessment of the mother's and baby's well-being? How is the mother? Is she coping well? Is she doing the basic things she needs to do to remain in good shape as labor progresses (eating, drinking, resting, moving, eliminating)? How is the baby? When did you last check the fetal heart rate? Is the baby moving?

If there is a question about fetal well-being, send the psychic message to the baby that you need a clear indication of his status. He can give you clues by becoming active, changing his heart rate, rotating or responding normally to a scalp stimulation test. If you know the babies you work with well, they will often let you know what is going on with them, for example, by moving or changing their heart rate on request (really!). If you get no messages from the baby, you must go by clinical evidence alone.

How does the mother feel about her labor? After careful reflection on the situation, you can approach the mother and find out what is going on from her perspective. While talking tends to activate her neocortex, you are less likely to impose conversation on her unnecessarily if you have taken the steps outlined here before you speak with her. Just as in love-making, sometimes talking in the context of the circumstances is quite appropriate. How does she feel labor is going? What does she think might help? Once you have the mother's feedback, you can reevaluate your impressions before you suggest anything.

What do you propose? By tuning into the mother as described, you are much more likely to come up with one or more options that will really help in the situation. Recall how this woman prepared for labor prenatally. Did she do stretching? Do you believe she has a good understanding of how her pelvis works with fetal descent? If she does not, and she is having a hard time coping, she is probably afraid because she does not know how to work with the energy. Once you have come to a conclusion about your perceptions, you can outline what, if anything, needs to change or what you propose that the mother do.

Increasing the intuitive skills you bring to the birth

The more skills you have to call on, the better. Training in any of the following will help you tune into and work with the energy in your own body and that of the mother.

- Hands-on healing techniques such as massage, Reiki, Therapeutic Touch and Shiatsu as well as many others
- Centering, meditative practices such as Buddhist meditation or prayer
- Moving meditative energy work such as Chi-gong
- Hypnosis techniques for use during pregnancy and labor

Positions and Activities for Labor

Creating an environment in which the woman feels free to choose her activity and position at any point during labor is a hallmark of the midwifery model of care. This chapter provides an overview of the different positions and techniques commonly used during labor. Many of them will be mentioned again in other chapters because so many are applicable in more than one situation. Variations and further details on many of these positions in specific applications, as well as additional activities and positions useful for stuck labors, are reviewed in the chapters entitled "Maternal Position during Pushing and at the Time of Birth," "Techniques Used to Help the Baby Descend during Labor," "Assisting a Woman Whose Baby is in a Posterior Position," and "Assisting a Woman Whose Baby Is in a Compound Presentation."

This chapter focuses on many techniques that enhance normal progress and also discusses why some positions don't. The information has been gathered from a variety of sources. Penny Simkin's work is referenced for many of the following descriptions. Penny is a well-known doula and childbirth instructor from Seattle, Washington. Initially trained as a physical therapist, she has worked as a labor support person for many years and is a founder of Doulas of North America (DONA). Penny has shared her wealth of experience in several fine books, in particular her 38 minute video COMFORT MEASURES FOR CHILDBIRTH and THE LABOR PROGRESS HANDBOOK, co-authored with Ruth Ancheta, both important references used in preparing this chapter. Jean Sutton, a New Zealand midwife, has produced LET BIRTH BE BORN AGAIN (2001), which outlines many points also reiterated here. Valerie El Halta, a US midwife, has shared many good tips in her workshops and articles. Guadalupe Trueba's video and accompanying booklet entitled COMFORT MEASURES FOR CHILDBIRTH: THE REBOZO WAY (2001) bring to North America the specifics about using this shawl, a trick of the trade of the traditional midwives of Mexico. Other contributions are credited as they appear.

The Concept of Available Space

Jean Sutton (2001) points out that, while the pelvic canal and the baby remain more or less the same size, changing the position of either can make maximal use of the available space. This can be dramatically demonstrated by filling a wide-mouthed jar half-full of water. Drop in a ball that will float; its diameter should be about three-quarters of the diameter of the jar. Look at the space in the jar when it is positioned upright (comparable to having a woman semi-sitting in bed with her knees up, which levels the brim). Then tilt the jar and see how the water level widens to fill the space and changes the relationship of the sidewalls (comparable to a woman standing, brim tipped forward, which lifts the level of the promontory high above the upper border of the pubic bone).

General Principles for Guiding Activities and Position Changes during Labor

1. Generally speaking, upright forward-tilted positions prompt the most rapid progress in labor and give the baby the best opportunity to position herself optimally.
2. The pelvis and sacrum must be relaxed and mobile for any position to work well.
3. Don't make suggestions unless the woman seems to need it.
4. Don't hesitate to make suggestions when a change seems called for.
5. There are no hard and fast rules that work for every labor, all the time; go with what works.

Ideally, women assume the positions that intuitively feel right to them. Very often these are the very positions that enhance labor progress. Keeping in mind that a private and secure setting is the primary element that supports successful birth, recommendations regarding activities and positions should be offered gently *only* when the woman seems to be foundering in her own sense of what is needed or seems to be stuck or afraid to let labor become stronger. What you suggest will also depend upon the birthing energy and what might help in this specific case. Generally speaking, suggestions regarding positions or activities are only needed to the point that a woman allows the birthing energy to fully flow through her. After that, you can unobtrusively step back and watch labor unfold. Allow your instinct and hers to be your guides. While some women give birth rapidly by laboring quietly, privately and mostly in one position, fearful women will remain in one position for extended periods of time if they are concerned about the strength of labor and wish to maintain the energy at a manageable level. Because of this, some midwives encourage women to change positions as often as every 20 minutes throughout active labor. I do not recommend this routinely, but it may be very helpful for an individual woman who is afraid or has many control issues. If you are tuned into the mother, the chances that your suggestions will be appropriate are much increased.

Commonly Used Positions and Activities for Labor

The rest of this chapter provides an overview of some basic positions that are commonly referred to in this and other textbooks. Some have been named, as usual, after the male doctors who first wrote about or popularized them. Regardless of the mother's position, make sure her buttocks, lower back and pelvic area are relaxed. This can be seen in loose, soft buttocks and slightly flexed thighs and knees. The mother can also be reminded to keep her internal tissues loose and open: if she has done yoni stretching, as described in Volume I, or worked with the Pink Kit, described in a recent edition of Volume I of this text, she will know exactly what you mean and be able to focus in internal relaxation as well.

Upright positions

In this text, any position that does not involve lying down is broadly referred to as an upright position

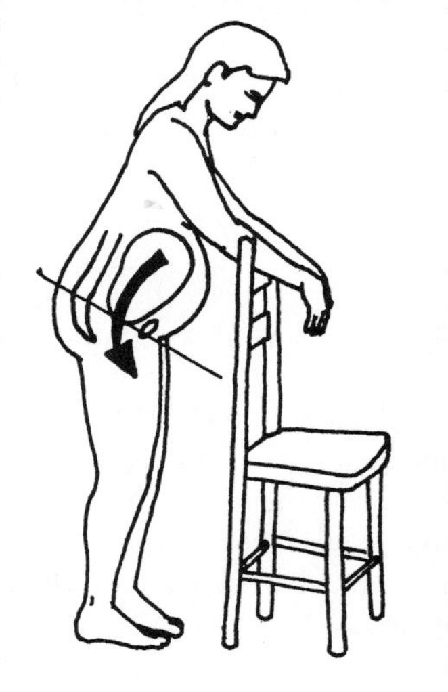

Leaning forward

(redrawn with permission from illustrations by Stella Cruz, © Ruth Ancheta 2000)

Leaning forward: Encourage any position in which the mother leans forward with her back straight, her pubic bone tipped forward and her tuberosities higher than her knees (i.e., not squatting). These postures open the angle between the spine, and the pubic bone, straighten the birth canal and help with rotation and descent (Sutton & Scott, 1996).

Tilting the pelvis forward: Tilting the pelvis forward from a standing or sitting position (in which the woman is sitting forward on her tuberosities) moves the woman's hip joints in front of her ankles and maximally opens the spinopubic angle, widening the inlet to its fullest extent. Birthing energy instructs the woman to open her pelvis for the baby in this way, pivoting the pubic bone down and the sacrum, coccyx and levator ani muscles up and out of the way. (In 1892, Gustav Walcher recommended a position to open the inlet in which the woman leaned back flat on a table with her bottom off the edge, her feet dangling toward the floor and her legs spread; an attempt to mimic nature for women who had received drugs.)

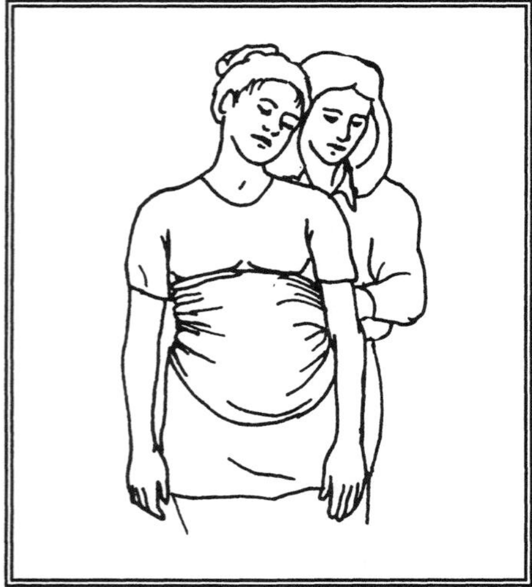

(Adapted with permission from photographs appearing in Comfort Measures for Childbirth: The Rebozo Way, © 2001, Guadalupe Trueba.)

Walking: Walking is one of the best overall activities for labor, especially if the woman stops to lean forward during contractions. An upright position allows gravity to assist in bringing the baby down, while the motion of the pelvis helps the baby find an optimal position for the descending presenting part.

Dancing: Slow, sensuous dancing with lots of big, undulating hip movements–the mother's version of belly dancing–can help the pelvis loosen up and move the baby down. Slow dancing with her partner is also nice. The woman should stand supported, with her arms around the neck and shoulders of her partner. Her partner can reach around to apply pressure or hot compresses to her lower back. Dancing may be particularly helpful for women with android pelvises (Simkin, 1995).

A rebozo can be used to gently rock the woman's belly as she sways. Wrap the center of the rebozo over the uterus and tighten it gently until the woman feels its support. Her dance partner can then wrap the ends around her back and make sure they stay put as she moves (Trueba, 2001).

Sway back (sagging forward): The woman who is upright and leaning forward who lets her belly sag forward and drops her lower back, creating a sway in her lumbar spine, is optimally opening her inlet and moving the sacrum up and out of the way to let the baby through. Her back and abdominal muscles and her buttocks are relaxed in this posture, and her lowermost lumbar vertebra does not lock against the sacrum as it might when she arches her back rigidly (see the section below entitled “Upright positions to avoid”).

Tilted tailor-sitting: Sitting with the legs crossed and the pelvis tipped forward is a good position in which the woman can rest off her feet for awhile. This position can easily be achieved by sitting on a meditation cushion or seat or any firm, round pillow about 6 in deep and 18 in across. As a variation, the woman can sit with the soles of her feet together, which will help to open the outlet a bit. This position takes advantage of gravity while keeping the mother still and is helpful when you want pressure down in a situation in which the risk of membrane rupture is increased (El Halta, 1998). Note that traditional tailor sitting in which the woman’s bottom is on the floor lowers the tuberosities slightly below the knees and therefore narrows the brim. It should not be used before the baby is well engaged and even then not for a long period of time (Sutton, 2001).

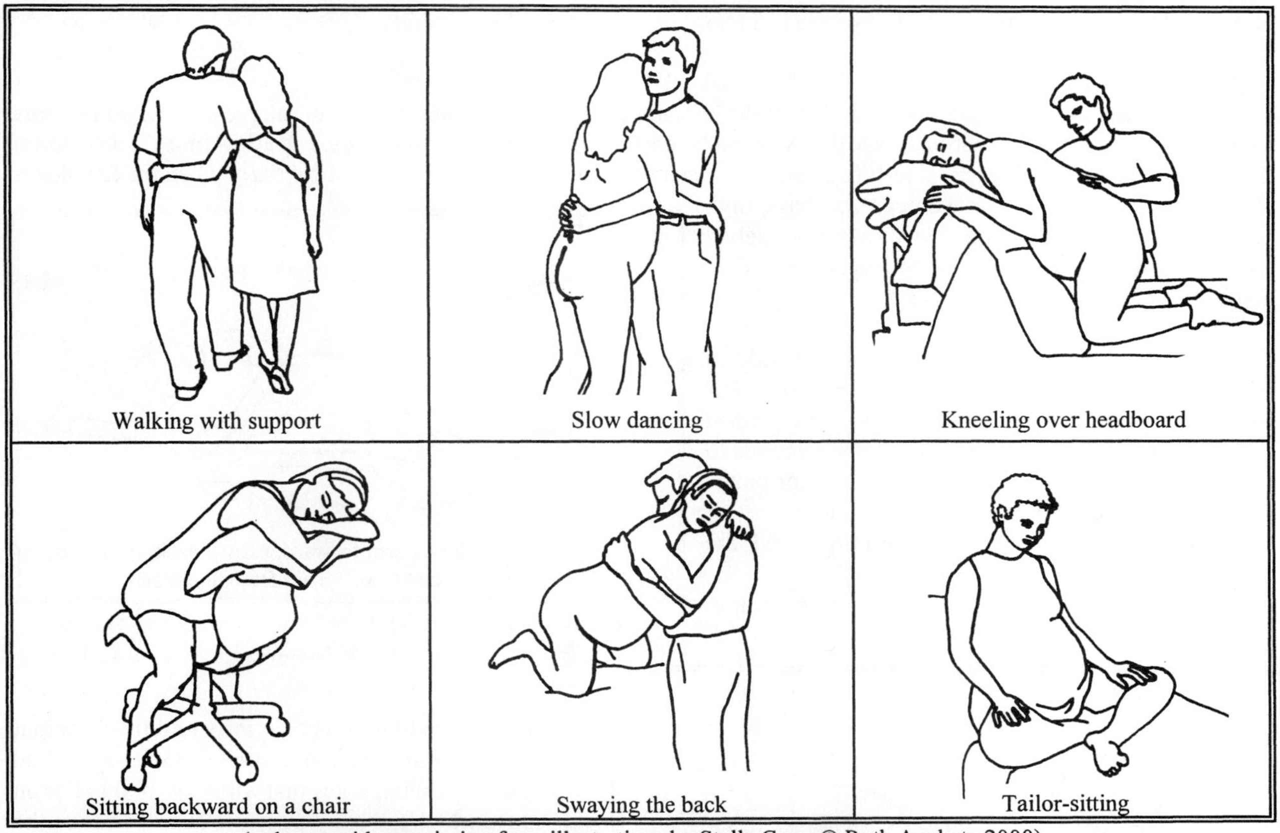

(redrawn with permission from illustrations by Stella Cruz, © Ruth Ancheta 2000)

Sitting backward on a chair or toilet: For this you will need a chair with no arms. The woman straddles the chair seat and leans over the back of the chair, moving her bottom back toward the edge of the seat to maximize the forward position of her belly. She can place a pillow under her belly for comfort and a meditation cushion or a folded towel under her bottom to allow her to tip her pelvis forward more easily. This position simulates what occurs in any forward-leaning position. Leaning forward can be used if she is standing; however, this is an excellent position to allow the mother to take a break if she is tired.

Upright positions to avoid:

Slouch sitting: This is the term I use for sitting in any furniture that requires the mother to sit with her tuberosities lower than her knees. This posture, commonly required by "comfortable" modern furniture, closes the spinopubic angle, exaggerates the curve of the birth canal and hinders engagement and rotation. It should be avoided throughout pregnancy and labor (Sutton & Scott, 1996).

Deep (full) squat: Deep squatting should be avoided during early and active labor. Its limited use, after complete dilation and during pushing, is discussed in the chapters entitled "Maternal Position during Pushing and at the Time of Birth" and "Assisting a Woman Whose Baby Is in a Posterior Position."

Arching the back: Note that a woman in an upright position who rigidly arches her back and tenses her buttocks is usually trying to move away from sensations low down in front. Arching the entire back may be a response to extreme pain in the pubic area; "moving away" from her pubic bone is a classic response during "entering pains" when the baby tries to rotate past the pubic bone or late in labor when there is an anterior lip being stretched and pulled downward. Women also arch backward in response to intense back pain (see the chapter entitled "Entering Pains and Back Pain in Labor" for details). Arching the back in this manner may lock the lowermost lumbar vertebra against the upper sacrum, impairing mobility at the level of the outlet. It also tightens the abdominal muscles over the uterus, limiting the abdominal space and requiring the baby who is attempting to rotate to do so uphill.

Side-lying positions

Lying on the side is a good position for rest during labor. Being gravity neutral, it can relieve downward pressure from premature pushing sensations, ease the stress on hemorrhoids and vulval varicosities, and allow time for an anterior lip to be pulled up. In addition, side-lying relieves pressure on the inferior vena cava (particularly when the left side is chosen), and so is good for women who have high blood pressure. This position also allows more pelvic mobility than other horizontal positions since there is no counter-pressure on the sacrum.

Simple side-lying: The woman lies on the side to which the vertex baby's occiput is directed. (For example, if the baby is LOT, LOA or LOP, the woman lies on her left.) This encourages the baby's occiput to remain transverse or move toward her anterior pelvis (Simkin & Ancheta, 2000). This is particularly true if the woman is having strong contractions and the presenting part is not yet engaged.

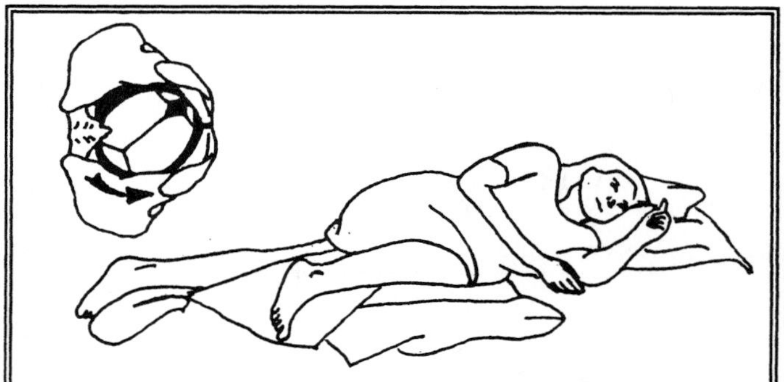

Simple side-lying, lower arm forward, baby's back to the bed, belly propped with a folded towel to aid fetal alignment.

(redrawn with permission from illustrations by Stella Cruz, © Ruth Ancheta 2000)

Lying on the side opposite the baby's occiput encourages him to rotate posteriorly or remain occiput posterior. Faith Hendrickson (1981), a retired Minnesota midwife, notes that when the mother lies on the side to which the baby's belly is directed before the head is engaged, the tends head to deflex during strong labor as gravity pulls the baby's belly toward the bed, causing the spine and neck to deflex. The only exception to this cautionary note regarding side-lying is the semiprone position, which, when used appropriately, will encourage flexion.

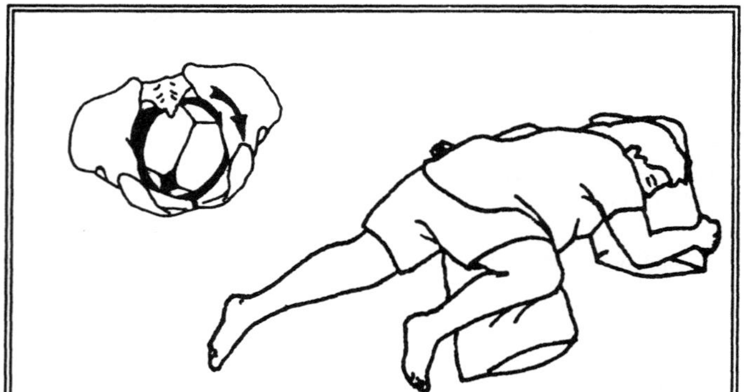

Semiprone, lower arm back, baby's back to ceiling.

(redrawn with permission from illustrations by Stella Cruz, © Ruth Ancheta 2000)

Semiprone (exaggerated Sims; semirecumbent; Bradley relaxation position): The woman lies on her side with her lower hip propped with pillows. Her lower arm and lower leg are stretched behind her torso. She bends her upper hip joint and knee to a 90° angle or more (which tends to pinch the brim on that side, a lesser angle leaves the brim more open). The upper knee may be propped up with a pillow. Her upper hip and torso are tilted toward the bed. Asymmetrical positioning of the legs brings the pelvic bones slightly out of their parallel alignment. This plus the forward position of the upper leg encourage the weight of the occiput to rotate in an anterior direction when the woman lies on the side opposite the fetal occiput (the side to which the baby is facing). If the baby is LOP, she lies on her right; if ROT or ROP, she lies on her left (Simkin & Ancheta, 2000).

Elevated semiprone (elevated Sims): Have the mother assume the semiprone position as described above (baby's back away from bed), but do not prop her bent leg. Elevate her buttocks by placing one or more pillows beneath her lower hip. This position floats the head up and out of the pelvis more effectively.

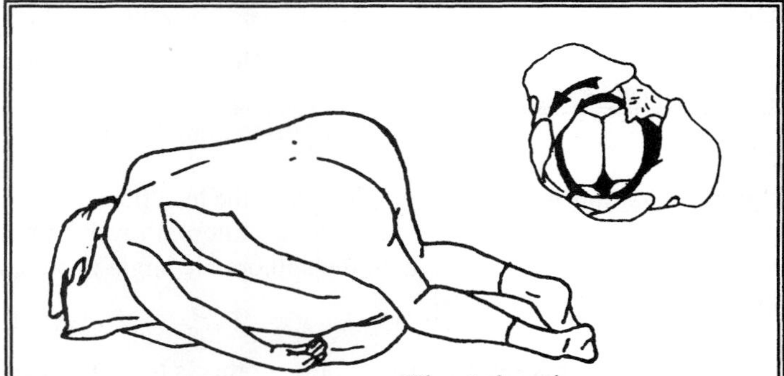

Elevated semiprone

Supine (dorsal) positions

This term denotes lying flat on the back, although the torso may be elevated slightly (less than 45°). The woman's legs may be flat on the bed or her knees may be bent with her feet flat on the bed. This position is gravity neutral. However, the weight of the uterus falls against the inferior vena cava, eventually resulting in supine hypotension (reflected in a fall in blood pressure). The placement of a wedge, such as a long, folded towel, under the woman's right torso and hip will assist in displacing the weight of the uterus to the side and thus offset the tendency of any supine position to lower blood pressure, especially if the woman remains in this position for a length of time.

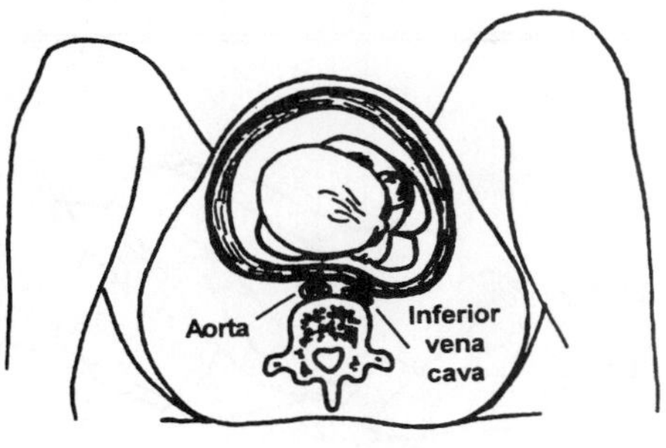

Direct pressure on large vessels

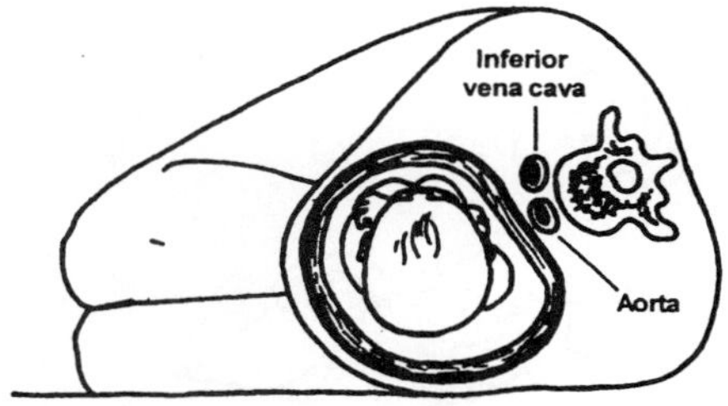

Pressure is relieved when the woman rolls to her side.

Supine positions also tend to reduce pelvic diameters. Women often want to bend their knees in this position for stability. With the knees higher than the tuberosities, the spinopubic angle is narrowed. Instead of her sacral promontory being 6.5 cm higher than the top of her pubic bone, it is only 1 to 2 cm higher (Sutton, 2001). This causes the brim to present a flat plane in relationship to the angle of fetal descent and tends to result in a median vertex attitude, even if the baby is LOA.

The mother's weight falls directly on her sacrum and coccyx, which prevents most, if not all, sacral movement. The inner surfaces of the ischia flare outward and forward, altering the soft-tissue dynamics and lessening the counterpressure that helps the baby's head stay flexed. Less than ideal flexion results in inadequate cervical pressure, with the parietal bones more likely to catch on the sides of the os, which can lead to an anterior cervical lip. Contractions may be more frequent and painful but are usually less effective than when the mother is upright in part because the contracting uterus must work against gravity to rear up and lean forward, causing the muscle to work harder and leading to both maternal and myometrial exhaustion (Sutton, 2001).

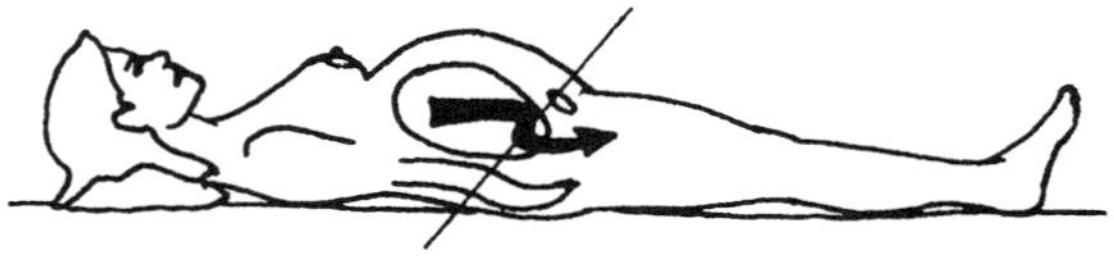

Lying flat creates a jog in the birth canal at the level of the sacral promontory

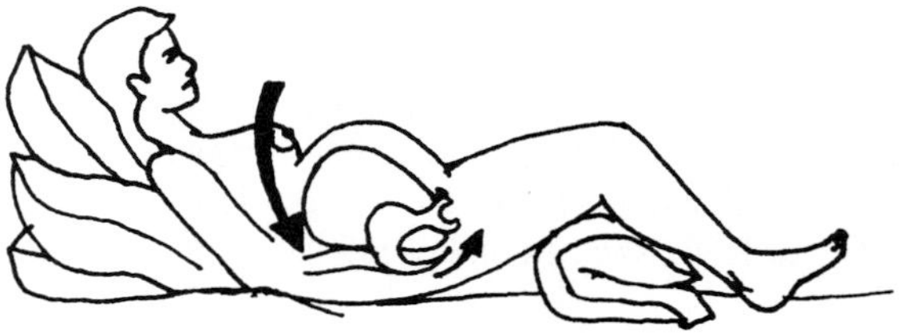

Elevating the knees levels and narrows the brim as well as the space immediately above it and exaggerates the curve of the birth canal

(redrawn with permission from illustrations by Stella Cruz, © Ruth Ancheta 2000)

Supine, legs flopped open: Lying flat with the legs flexed and the knees flopped to either side, perhaps supported with pillows, offers ideal access for a thorough internal exam. Otherwise, it is a position to be avoided. Note that this modified position will still tighten the spinopubic angle to a certain extent, often causing the head to lift up above the brim if it is not well engaged.

Semi-sitting: In this seated position, the mother's torso is elevated at least 45° but less than 90° in relationship to her lower body. Her legs are often flexed at the hip, with the knees bent. It allows more assistance from gravity and puts less pressure on the aorta and inferior vena cava than does a supine position, thereby improving oxygenation to the baby. Simkin and Ancheta (2000) feel that semi-sitting is an acceptable position for women to use during preparatory uterine activity and in very early labor, before the fetus has begun to descend. They find it often allows the woman to rest better than a more lateral position. They also like semi-sitting for women in early or early active labor who have a pendulous abdomen; it lifts the belly into a more vertical position and therefore brings the presenting part more directly over the pelvic inlet. A belly binder or lifting the abdomen, however, can also counteract the effects of a pendulous abdomen and allows the mother to assume forward-leaning positions that keep the brim open.

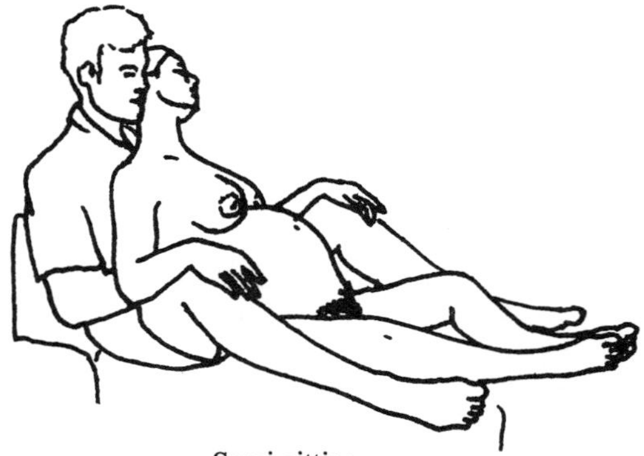

Semi-sitting

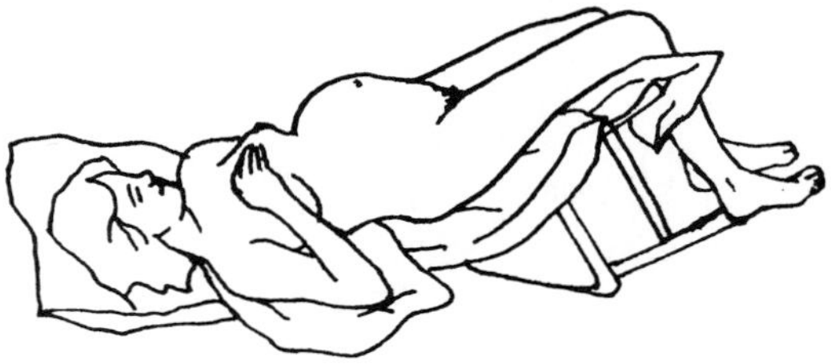

Trendelenburg

(Box on left redrawn with permission from illustrations by Stella Cruz, © Ruth Ancheta 2000)

Sutton (2001) and I believe that semi-sitting may be the worst possible position for any phase of labor (short of hanging by the heels), as it places undue pressure on the sacrum and reduces the spinopubic angle from 120° to less than 90° because the knees are elevated higher than the tuberosities, exaggerating all the disadvantages already detailed. Narrowing of the inlet favors occiput posterior engagement, if it occurs at all.

Slant-board (Trendelenburg): The woman lies on her side or flat on her back on a bed, inverted chair or table that is elevated at the foot end to raise her pelvis higher than her head. This position elevates the presenting part out of the pelvis for repositioning or for relieving pressure on a prolapsed cord. It should not be used for postpartum shock, as it encourages blood to pool in the uterus. (Proper positioning for shock is discussed in the chapter entitled "Hypovolemic

Shock due to Hemorrhage.")

Belly-down positions

This category includes all positions that allow the abdomen to hang suspended below the torso. These positions are generally contraindicated for women who have a pendulous abdomen because the downward pull of gravity will result in the baby "descending" uphill. However, some midwives report that placing several pillows under the mother's belly will lift a pendulous abdomen up, eliminating this problem. A pregnancy girdle or a belly binder could also be used.

Kneeling or hands and knees: These are ideal forward-leaning positions. A woman can balance her weight between her hips when she kneels or assumes a position on her hands and knees on a firm surface. This increases the transverse diameters of the pelvic cavity and maintains the space between the spine and the pubic bone at an optimal 120° angle when the pelvic brim is tipped down and away from the spine (pelvic rock position with the back slightly swayed). Side-to-side and figure-eight hip motions can be done in these positions and will take the ischial spines out of their parallel relationship, creating more room for the baby's head (Sutton & Scott, 1996).

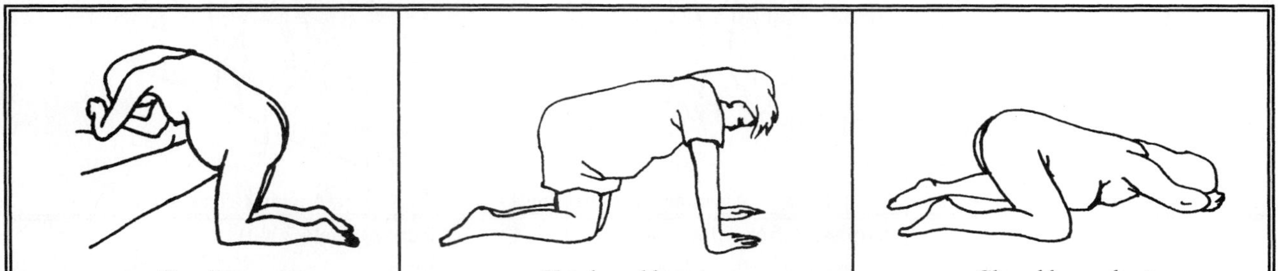

Kneeling | Hands and knees | Closed knee-chest

(redrawn with permission from illustrations by Stella Cruz, © Ruth Ancheta 2000)

Closed knee chest: In this position, the woman is in a knee-chest position with her knees together and her hips flexed and sharply abducted up under her abdomen. Her bottom is lower than in the open position described above, and the space between her spine and pubic bone is thus reduced, which tightens the inlet, making this a position best avoided prior to the point at which the baby is well engaged and internal rotation has already occurred. It can relieve back pain (but this may be because it pushes the unengaged head away from the brim, so it really does not help at that point). It can also take pressure off of hemorrhoids or an anterior lip, reverse the effect of gravity, and spread the pelvic bones from the midpelvis, at the level of the spines, down to the outlet (Simkin & Ancheta, 2000).

Open, exaggerated knee-chest: The woman is on her knees, with her bottom elevated high in the air. Her thighs and knees are flexed and her legs are spread and positioned somewhat more than 90° in relationship to the floor. Her fundus touches the floor or nearly so. Her shoulders are pressed as flat on the floor as possible, with her arms either down to her sides or bent at the elbow to either side of her head. A soft pillow placed between her belly and her chest makes this not-very-comfortable position somewhat more so. She tips her pelvic brim forward by swaying her back. This position floats the presenting part out of the pelvis and opens the brim, giving the baby the opportunity to reenter the pelvis in a more favorable position. It is tiring to maintain (although less so in early labor) and should only be used for specific therapeutic purposes, such as rotating the baby (El Halta, 1998; Simkin & Ancheta, 2000). See the chapter entitled "Assisting a Woman Whose Baby Is in a Posterior Position."

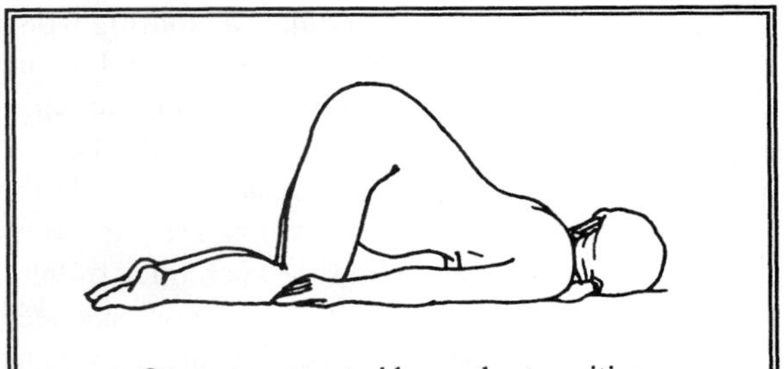

Open, exaggerated knee-chest position

Asymmetrical positions

Penny Simkin, as well as many midwives, has popularized a variety of asymmetrical positions for their effectiveness in overcoming problems with positioning and descent. These positions consist of postures that require the woman to raise, stretch or move one leg differently from the other. These postures open the pelvis on the side of the movement and create room in the pelvis on the stretched side for the head to turn or otherwise reposition itself. The direction of the occiput usually determines which leg to move. For example, if the baby is arrested in an ROT position, the mother should move her right leg. Moving that side often feels better than moving the other. Specifics regarding the variety of positions in this category are given in the chapter entitled "Techniques Used to Help the Baby Descend during Labor and Pushing."

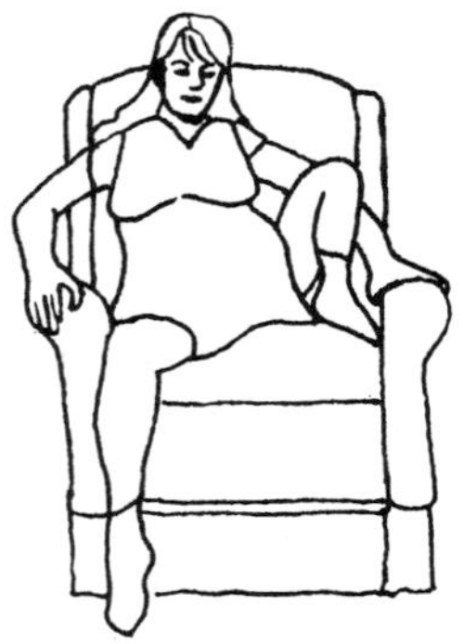
Asymmetrical sitting

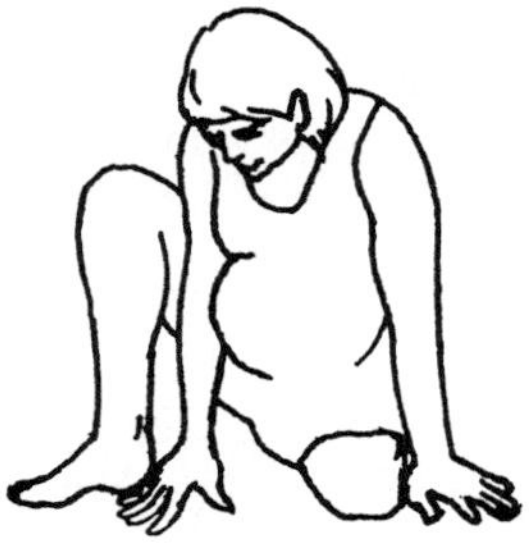
Asymmetrical kneeling

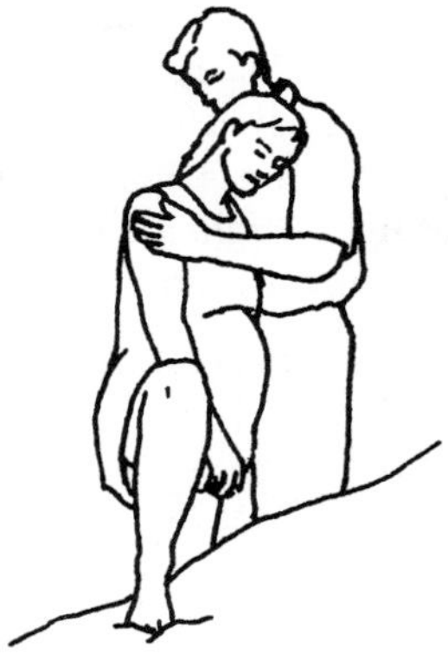
Asymmetrical standing

(redrawn with permission from illustrations by Stella Cruz, © Ruth Ancheta 2000)

Alternating, rhythmical movements: In any position, movements such as belly dancing, forming figure-eights with the hips or swaying side-to-side while standing, sitting on a birth ball or in a hands-and-knees position also change the relationship of the pelvic bones, move the ischial spines out of alignment in an alternating pattern and encourage the baby to find the most favorable position for her head (Simkin, 1995).

Using a rebozo: Many positions can be modified by using a rebozo to form a sling around part of the woman's body to gently rock her from side to side. Rhythmic movement can produce deep relaxation that will facilitate rotation of the baby when a change in fetal position is called for. Rebozo techniques will be mentioned throughout the text as appropriate.

Midwife's labor monitoring position

One of the best ways to monitor a laboring woman who needs to rest is to have her lie on her side. Her partner can lie down, facing her. The midwife lies behind the mother and spoons her, then lifts her upper arm over the woman and places her hand on the woman's belly. It is sometimes possible to feel fetal movement (reassuring you that the baby is doing well without having to jump up and listen to the heart rate). You can also monitor the intensity, duration and frequency of contractions as well as help guide the mother through them, if necessary. This position can be used whenever labor slows, when the woman requires physical contact for reassurance, when the need is for a quiet space and the midwife wishes to continue to keep track of labor or whenever constant physical monitoring might be useful and a side-lying position appropriate. This cannot and need not be done with all women, of course, but is a great option to keep in mind when the woman is receptive and the circumstances are right.

USING COMFORT AND POSITIONING AIDS IN LABOR

Comfort and pain relief in labor

It is important for midwives and doulas who attend birthing women–and for laboring women themselves–to keep in mind the overarching purpose of the sensations of labor and the incredible instinct at the disposal of laboring women. Part of the midwife's job is to assure that each woman has a quiet space and minimal distraction with limited intellectual input so that she can access her primitive brain, where the knowledge of how to give birth resides. This environmental milieu allows the optimal flow of hormones and other chemicals that will take a woman to the altered state that allows her to move through labor quickly and easily.

The wise midwife paves the way for this ideal response to labor by preparing the woman prenatally so that the woman has a solid understanding of how the baby comes down and how her pelvis and soft tissues work together to facilitate descent, including exercises to help her connect with her body and specifically her pelvis, including consciously learning to relax them. This goes far beyond mere schooling in comfort measures. They are essential ways the midwife can help the woman align her mental grasp of the birth process with what she experiences during labor. They tune her in, rather than pull her away, from her experience of her own body. Such preparation bridges the cultural gap created when birth is generally hidden, as it is in western industrialized countries. For many women, it is a tall order to expect them to trust their ability to be instinctively in-tune with a process of which they have no direct knowledge or experience, having never seen a birth. A well-prepared woman is more likely to be able to read her body's signals and go with the flow than one who is not, in large part because she is not nearly so afraid. There is a lot of ineffective childbirth education out there, but the proper kind of preparation puts women in control of their own experience and thus, paradoxically, creates more possibility for letting go. See Vol. I for more information.

Once a foundation is laid, the midwife creates the space for the well-prepared woman to find her own path to birth during labor, using the cues her body gives her to adjust her movements and posture so that the baby can find his own way through her pelvis. On the other hand, a woman who has merely been prepared to "deal with" the contractions may find herself in a constant search for "the most comfortable" whatever, which will usually slow labor down. This is because the focus needs to be on opening to birthing energy rather than on "dealing with the labor." Too much attention on "comfort" for its own sake and a focus on simply avoiding the pain mentally externalizes a woman and otherwise distracts her, interfering with the building momentum required to give birth.

Most of the attitudes and teachings regarding comfort in labor have grown out of the focus on labor as primarily a painful physical event. Western culture presents the laboring woman with only two prospects for the experience of labor: pain (the grit-your-teeth-and-get-through-it concept of natural childbirth) or the illusion of a pain-free, risk-free, consequence-free birth using drugs, instruments and, frequently, surgery. The other option, a hormonally mediated spiritually transformative experience (the requirements for which are, incidentally, not met in most hospital settings), goes completely undiscussed. Thus, the evolution of comfort measures has flourished with the work of childbirth educators and doulas who support women giving birth in a hospital. In this setting, comfort measures can play an important role. They provide something pleasant for the woman to focus on and help create an atmosphere of reassurance, familiarity and trust in an otherwise strange and artificial environment. Thus, comfort measures, to a point, increase the likelihood of a more normal labor in these settings. (Even so, they do not take the place of teaching a woman about how to consciously work with her body.) At home, much of this type of external reassurance is not necessary because the woman is in her own environment, surrounded by the things and people she already knows and trusts.

Assuming the woman is well-prepared, our job is to always return a woman to her experience and help her move through it. It is only within this context that we judiciously offer comfort measures and then only to the extent that they enhance the mother's efforts to follow her body through labor. Therefore, observe what is working in each labor and gently use or withdraw comfort measures as the mother's labor dictates. Used correctly, comfort measures do not distract a woman from her labor and can help her make a deeper connection with the energy flowing through her.

Specific (localized) pains mean something

While the general discomforts of dilation and the baby moving through the pelvis are part of the normal process, specific, localized aches or pains are usually signals that something needs to change, usually something having to do with the baby's position. It is important not to ignore these cues from the baby by arbitrarily attempting to relieve the pain. Talk to the mother, asking open-ended questions about exactly what she is feeling and where, including the type of pain and when it hurts. Does it ever go away and, if so, when? If the mother is having trouble figuring out how to respond to a pain, maybe you can help her interpret the pain and then come up with a plan that will really help move labor along.

Working with birthing energy

Repetitive, soft, relaxed, rhythmic and sensual movements tend to enhance the flow of birthing energy, especially in cases in which the woman is feeling overwhelmed or unable to channel the energy completely. Guidance from the tuned-in midwife can be a big help as well. Place your warmed hands over an area of her body where you sense the energy flow is blocked. As you do so, you will tune into your own body for confirmation that this is the area that needs attention. Ask the mother to consciously direct her breath to that area, seeing and feeling it expand and open as she exhales. At the same time, you can be affirming what should be happening with that low, soothing, hypnotic tone of voice that you have been cultivating, with phrases such as "This contraction opens you wider," "Breathe into and through my hands" and whatever else seems appropriate to the situation. These kinds of direct support methods will often obviate the need for using equipment. The more the mother can turn to her own inner resources to handle her labor, the more likely it is that her hormones will surge to optimal levels.

Positioning aids

A variety of items can used at births to increase the mother's ability to deal with labor. These aids are introduced in the chapter entitled "Positioning-Assist Equipment and Maternal Comfort Items," where basics about each item are discussed. This section focuses on the use of these items.

Birth (physical therapy) ball: Inflate the ball so that it is firm but not rigid. Someone should steady the ball as the woman sits on it. She should place her feet flat on the floor in front of her, about two feet apart, before she plants her bottom squarely in the center of the top of the ball. If she feels unstable on the ball, her partner should stand behind her while she gets used to being on it. On the ball, she can bounce gently or rock her hips side to side. Someone should be nearby in case she loses her balance. You can place a chair in front of her with its back to her to give her something to hold on to. In forward-leaning positions with the woman on her knees (which are on the floor), the ball can be placed in front of her to support her upper body.

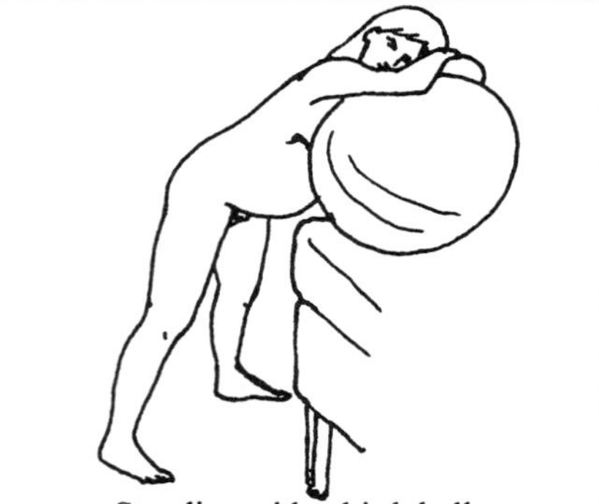
Standing with a birth ball

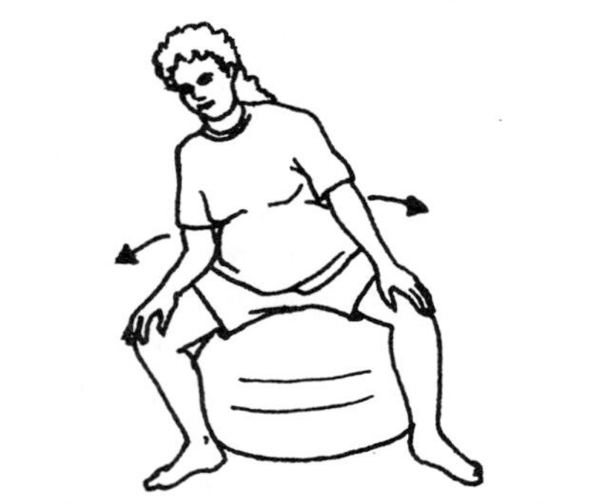
Sitting and swaying on a birth ball

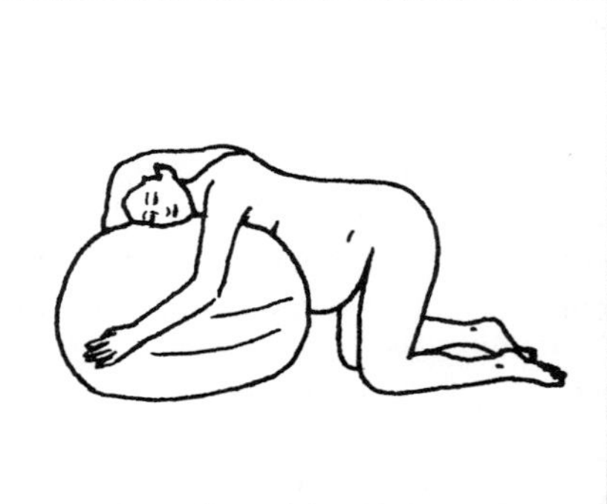
Kneeling with a birth ball

A rebozo can be wrapped around the woman's back and spread out to give broad support. An assistant stands in front of the woman, holding both ends. This provides a counterbalancing force for the woman to help her maintain her balance with less effort and allows her to sway slightly without worrying about falling off the ball. The support person must remain attentive so that she doesn't become unbalanced (Trueba, 2001). The rebozo can also be wrapped around the mother's belly, with someone standing behind her to rock her.

Meditation cushion: These little pillows are designed for maintaining a seated position on the tuberosities and are perfect for helping women achieve seated positions with the pelvis tilted forward.

Bean-bag chair: Although large, bulky and unwieldy to haul around, bean bags can be wonderful positioning aids if the parents have one in their home or can borrow one for the birth. They can be used in the same way that a birth ball can be used and are great for cradling the belly as the mother leans forward over it on her knees. However, do not encourage women to slouch down into one in a seated position, as this will raise the knees above the tuberosities and pinch off the pelvic brim.

Computer (kneeling) chair: This is a much more cumbersome device to carry with you but is very useful. It allows the woman to sit on her tuberosities; if her knees get tired, she can switch to a cushion for a while or try another position.

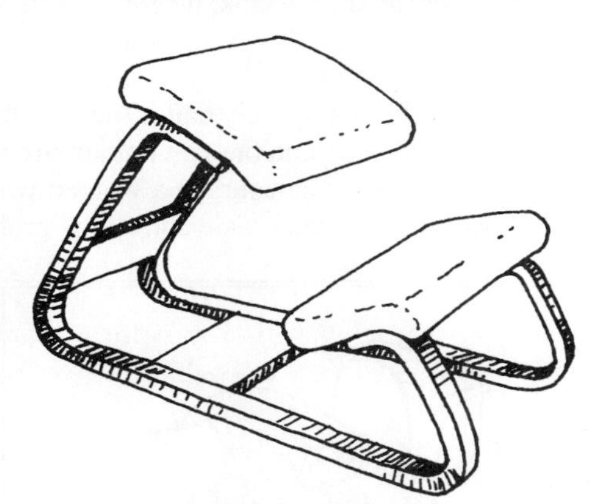
Computer chair

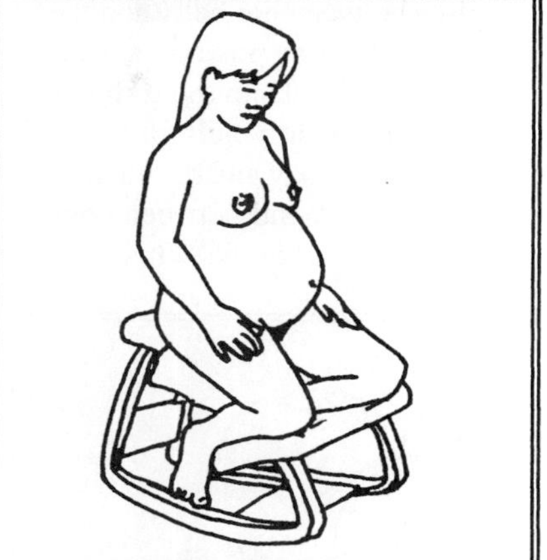
Woman seated on chair

Birth Sling: This padded, cloth sling designed by Penny Simkin can be used at any point throughout labor to get all the pressure off the pelvis by allowing the woman to be totally suspended from her upper body. As such, it is one of the most innovative and useful items to come on the market in many a day. It is wide enough to support the woman under her bent elbows, rather than under the arms, thus eliminating worries about damage to the radial nerve. It has a two-foot height adjustment range. It must be attached to a large eye-bolt that is installed into a ceiling beam. If parents are interested in this option, you could rent or sell them an eye-bolt to install, while you bring the sling.

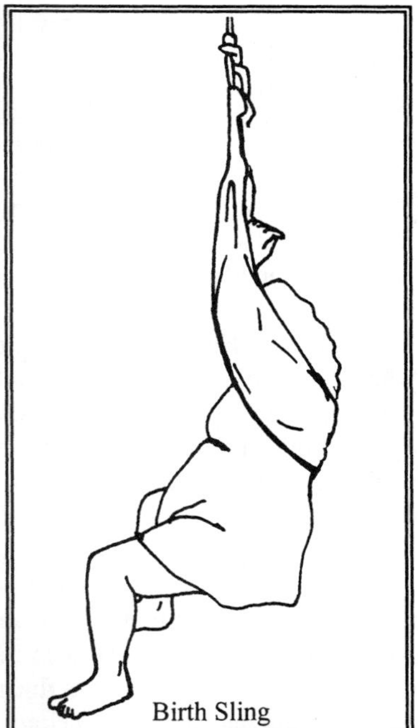
Birth Sling

(redrawn with permission from illustrations by Stella Cruz, © Ruth Ancheta 2000)

Chin-up bar: This is a metal bar sold at sporting goods stores. It has rubber ends and its length can be adjusted. Wedge the bar in a door frame to provide the woman something with which she can support herself while she squats during pushing. It can be positioned for either a standing or full squat.

Preventing radial nerve injury: When any long, thin object, such as a bar or the back of a chair, a strip of cloth or even the arm of a support person, is placed in front of or to the side of a woman for her to prop on, be sure she rests her forearms across the top of the object (both elbows out to the side) or holds onto it with her hands. Resting with upper arm or underarms over the object can result in serious radial nerve injury and is to be avoided (Roubal et al., 1996). The woman should not maintain any position that requires her arms to bear her weight for long periods of time nor should she keep her arms resting across anything narrow (be it the back of a chair, someone's arm or a metal bar). It is a good idea to have the woman stand and shake her arms out and otherwise change positions frequently when using her arms for support.

Push-and-pull: This device was invented by Diane Holmes, a midwife in Indiana. It comes in two styles: a double-handled "cane," consisting of a rod with a crook on each end, and two elongated loops of rigid plastic connected by a chain. Either style can be used to assist a woman in a standing or a full squat. The cane is best suited to support her upper leg during a side-lying birth. When used for squatting, a support person holds one end, and the mother holds the other, then both go down into a squat together, allowing the support person to provide a counterbalancing weight and thus help the mother maintain her position.

Sitting on the toilet: For many women, on the toilet is one of the few places where they feel free to let things out of their body. Therefore, the toilet is a perfect place to put women who have trouble relaxing and opening up. The woman can either sit face-forward and lean into someone's shoulders or can face the tank of the toilet (this often works best for smaller women) with a pillow between her belly and the tank and one on the top of the tank, where she can rest her head. This provides a restful, forward-leaning position and approximates the benefits of belly lifting, which is described in the chapter entitled "Techniques Used to Help the Baby Descend during Labor."

Note that sitting on the toilet is only helpful to a point. Prolonged toilet-sitting may cause the perineum to swell because the weight of the woman's body and the unequal pressure created by the hole in the seat impair circulation. After about a half-hour, have the mother stand between contractions. Do not, however, encourage a woman whose vulva is swelling to remain on the toilet indefinitely. This will increase the swelling and can create additional problems.

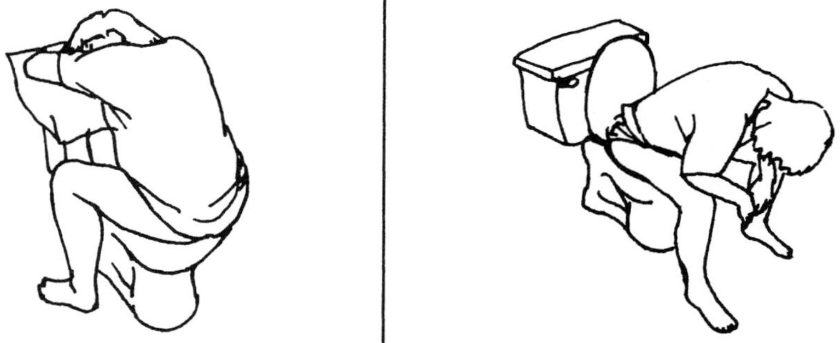

On toilet, facing the tank | On toilet, leaning forward

(redrawn with permission from illustrations by Stella Cruz, © Ruth Ancheta 2000)

The use of hot and cold packs in labor

Both heat and cold can be used in a variety of ways to relieve discomfort during labor. Some women prefer one over the other, and some types of pain are better treated with one than the other.

Precautions: Hormonal changes during labor increase a woman's pain threshold significantly; take this into account when using cold or hot packs or baths for pain relief. As a rule, never place anything directly on the woman's skin that you cannot hold in your bare hands. Packs used on a woman's back or abdomen may be reheated or rechilled and used again. However, packs that have come into contact with the woman's body fluids can contaminate the oven, microwave or freezer. If the item has been soiled with the woman's body fluids, throw it away, or put it in the laundry and use a clean item. If this is not possible, place the pack in an appropriate container or plastic bag prior to reheating or recooling.

Cold packs: Cold produces a numbing effect that slows the transmission of nerve impulses, effectively reducing pain and easing muscle spasms (Lehmann, 1982). Penny Simkin highly recommends cold packs applied to the lower back for back pain. Cold packs can also be helpful if the mother reports that she is overheated, if she is sweating, if she has external swollen hemorrhoids during pushing, if there is musculoskeletal and joint pain, or if there is a need to reduce perineal pain and swelling. (Note that sweating or feeling overheated in a bath means the bathwater is too hot; reduce the temperature. See the chapter entitled "Hydrotherapy and Waterbirth" for details.) A cold perineal compress may also help reduce pain and swelling if the woman has been sitting on the toilet for too long in labor. Cold can also be applied to the perineum after birth if swelling is severe (Simkin & Ancheta, 2000).

Cold packs can be fashioned out of wet, frozen towels or washcloths, exam gloves filled with water and frozen or filled with ice chips (use a rubber band or a knot to close the end), cold drink cans, ice packs or resealable plastic bags of frozen water. A commercial gel pack can also be used. The Dura Kold (DK 201) pack is large enough to strap across a woman's lower back and includes two velcro straps, allowing the woman to walk without an attendant to hold the cold pack in place. Rice socks can also be frozen for one and a half to two hours for use as cold packs. They will remain cold for about one hour or more. If you have a cold pack without straps, a rebozo can be used to hold the pack in place (Trueba, 2001).

According to Chinese medical theory, birth is a heat-losing experience for the mother, and practitioners generally advise against the use of cold therapies. Thus, if cold is to be used, make sure that the mother is warm everywhere else (including her nose, hands and feet) before using a cold pack. If she is otherwise cold, the pack will not help to relieve the pain. The cold pack can be used as long as it is effective. The mother will be able to determine how much relief she can expect within 20 to 30 minutes of application.

Never apply a cold pack directly to the skin, as the sudden cold is too shocking. In addition, the reduced sensitivity to pain that occurs during labor may lead to tissue damage if the cold pack is placed directly on the skin or left in place too long. Place one or two layers of cloth between the skin and the pack, allowing the tissue under the pack to cool gradually. If the pack is still too cold, add more layers and remove them as the item warms. Additionally, a cold, wet washcloth can be used to sponge down a sweaty woman's face, arms and hands (Simkin & Ancheta, 2000). Some women also like a cold washcloth draped on the nape of their neck.

Hot packs: Heat can also be very soothing in labor. Heat increases local skin temperature, stimulates the peripheral circulation and aids in removing metabolic wastes from the tissues. Muscle spasms often release when heat is applied, and the woman's pain threshold may be raised more than when a cold pack is used. Heat may also reduce catecholamine levels and help to mitigate the side-effects of elevated levels, such as goose bumps and shivering. This, in turn, may make a woman more receptive to touch that she would otherwise be too sensitive to tolerate. Heat applied to the fundus may also increase uterine activity (Khamis et al., 1983; Simkin & Ancheta, 2000).

Options for applying heat include: a moist, hot towel, an electric heating pad, a pressure-activated silica gel pack, a heated rice pack, or a hot water bottle. Wet items and dry rice packs can be heated in a microwave oven very effectively. Place the item in a microwave and set it on high for 3 to 5 minutes. Wet items can also be placed in a ceramic dish in a conventional oven set to 180°F (82°C) for 10 minutes. A crock pot set on low can be used in any room with electricity to keep wet packs warm. Dry hot towels or blankets can be used to drape over the woman's body. Heat towels and blankets in a paper bag in a warm conventional oven for 20 minutes. Wet or dry, any of these can be placed across the lower abdomen, in the groin area, on the thighs, lower back, shoulders or perineum. The heat source should not feel uncomfortable in the hand of the support person who prepares it. Women in labor may not react, even if a heat source is causing a burn. Wrap very hot items in two or more layers of unheated towels and remove the layers as the item cools.

Heat should be suggested when a woman is feeling cold, when she has pain in a specific location, when she is anxious or when there is muscle tension. Hot compresses feel good on the perineum to some women during pushing. Some midwives find hot packs effective in reducing perineal swelling after birth, a therapy supported by Chinese medical theory. Heat should not be used if you suspect that a woman has a fever or is already overheated (Simkin & Ancheta, 2000).

Hydrotherapy

The use of water is a time-honored means of relaxing and supporting the laboring woman, which in turn, often makes her labor more efficient. For a full discussion of the use of flowing water and water immersion during labor, see the chapter entitled "Hydrotherapy and Waterbirth."

Counterpressure techniques

Counterpressure is used against a body part that is being pressed upon from within and is most often effective in the pelvic area, frequently over the sacrum. However, pressing inward on a part that is trying to move outward to make space for the baby is really counterproductive. Counterpressure should therefore not be used continuously or for a long period of time. It is best used as a stop gap measure to help a woman cope while you help her decide how she wants to move her labor forward, with the use, for example, of sterile water injections, position changes or manual rotation of the baby.

Hand pressure: The heel of the hand or the fist of a sturdy support person can be used to apply pressure to the focal point of pain in the lower back. The mother can stand, lean forward and brace herself against a wall or piece of furniture; lean over a birth ball or assume a hands-and-knees position. To begin, the support person presses into a spot on either side of the spine, well below the waist. The mother can guide the person from there. The pressure should remain constant throughout the contraction and be as strong as necessary. The support person can stabilize the woman by holding onto one of her hips so the she won't fall over. Alternatively, the laboring woman can position herself to minimize becoming imbalanced. She should not have to tense up to prevent herself from falling. While very effective, counterpressure quickly exhausts the person doing the pressing. Therefore, it is important to take turns with others at the birth and alternate with other techniques. When back pain is extreme, a less-than-ideal fetal position is usually the culprit. Sterile water papules can be offered as a pain-relief option, and activities and position changes can be employed to try and rotate the baby. (Also see the subchapter entitled "Sterile Water Injections for the Relief of Excessive Localized Pain" and the chapter entitled "Techniques Used to Help the Baby Descend during Labor.")

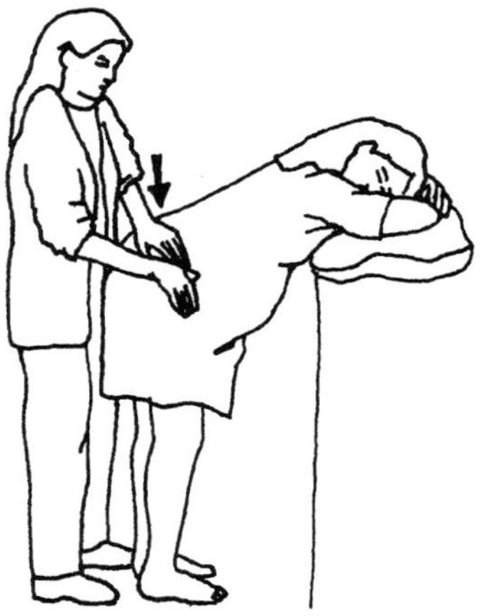
Hand pressure and massage on one hip

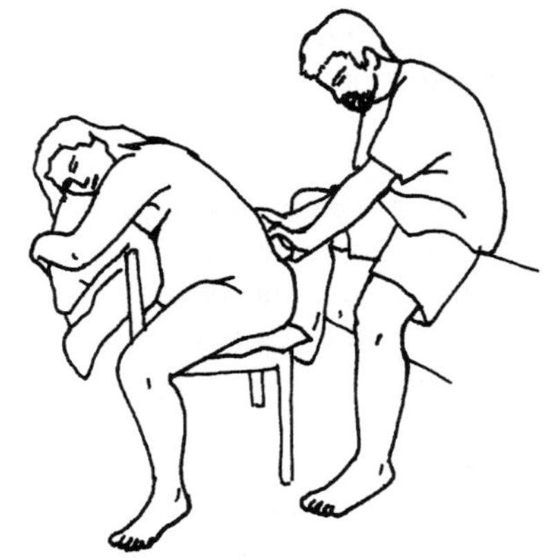
Counterpressure using a tennis ball

Rolling pin or ball: A rolling pin or a ball (like a tennis or baseball) can be used to apply counterpressure to the lower back. Another option is a full, chilled drink can, which provides both pressure and cold. A support person should press the can or roll the rolling pin into the area of the woman's back that hurts most.

The knee press: Kristi Ridd taught Penny Simkin (1995) this valuable technique. As pressure is applied through the femur into the flexed hip joints, the dimensions of the pelvic cavity are altered, and the sacroiliac joints are released and low back pain is often relieved. Do not use this technique in women who have joint disease, inflammation, pain or damage to their knees. Unlike counterpressure, this can be used to give the mother a break from other activities and will not be counterproductive to the progress of labor.

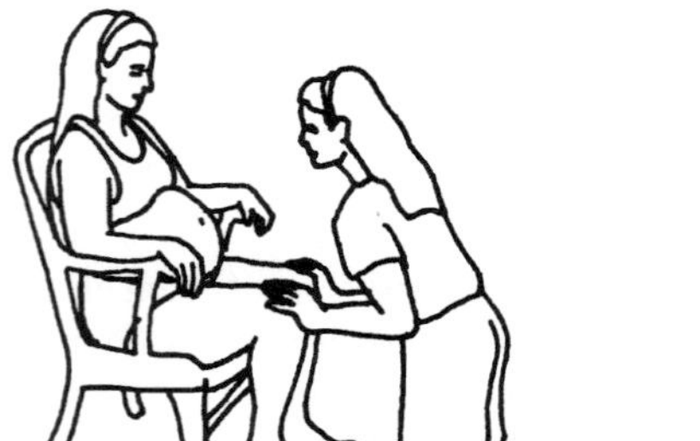
Knee-press, woman seated

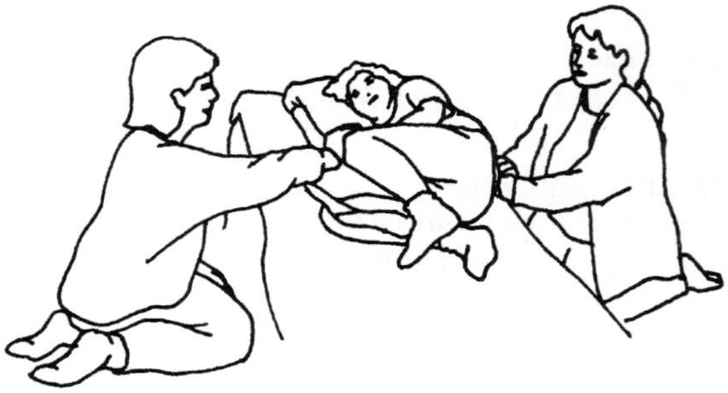
Knee-press, woman side-lying

(All drawings on this page redrawn with permission from illustrations by Stella Cruz, © Ruth Ancheta 2000)

If the woman is sitting: The mother sits upright in a straight-backed chair; sitting on a meditation cushion will keep the spinopubic angle open. She places her feet flat on the floor and her knees a few inches apart. If her feet do not reach the floor, support them with something so that they are planted flat. A support person kneels in front of her, placing the heel of his hands on the area just below the mother's knee caps on either side. During contractions, the support person rises up off his haunches, locks his elbows in close to his trunk and applies pressure to the knees by leaning forward so that her upper body (not just her arms) supplies the pressure as the force is conducted through her hands to the front of the knees, up the femur and to the hip joints. The pressure should remain constant during the contraction. The knee press can also be done with the woman lying on the same side to which the baby's back is positioned.

If the woman is side-lying: The woman lies on her side with her upper knee and hip joint bent to 90° angles and supported by a couple of pillows. Two support people are needed, one positioned at the mother's back and the other in front of her to press the knee. During contractions, the back person presses on the woman's sacrum while the knee person cups his hand over the woman's upper knee and presses toward the woman's hip joint.

Rebozo technique: To use this technique with a rebozo, have the woman sit on the shawl so that it spans her body from under her upper thigh to above her lower back, forming a hammock for her pelvis. The support person kneels, facing the woman, and uses his upper torso to apply pressure to the woman's knees by leaning forward against the woman's upper legs. This frees his hands so that he can hold the ends of the rebozo and pull them toward himself. This can be tiring, so vary the mother's position and switch off support people frequently (Trueba, 2001).

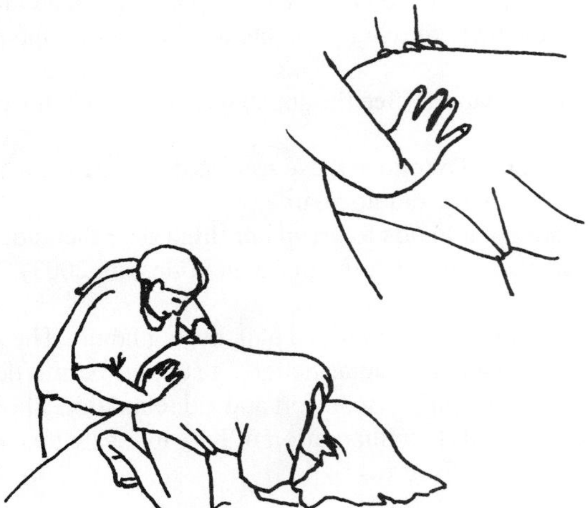

Double hip squeeze

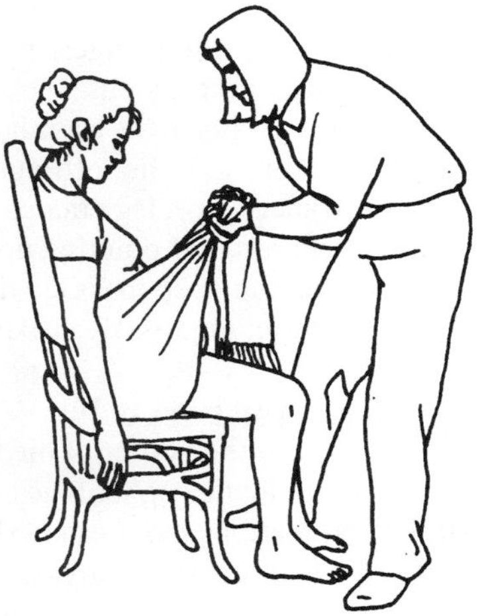

Double hip squeeze using a rebozo (to do the knee press, hold the rebozo like this, kneel in front of the woman and pull on the rebozo while pressing your torso against her knees)

(Left box redrawn with permission from illustrations by Stella Cruz, © Ruth Ancheta 2000; right box drawn with permission from photographs appearing in COMFORT MEASURES FOR CHILDBIRTH: THE REBOZO WAY, © 2001, Guadalupe Trueba.)

Double hip squeeze: This is a variation on back pressure that is very effective for some women. It is not certain why the hip squeeze works. It may slightly reduce tension on the sacroiliac joints. If extreme pressure is needed, it may indicate that the baby is deeply engaged and may, in fact, hinder rotation. Therefore, while useful at relieving pain, it should be used with caution and never at the expense of preventing rotation (Simkin & Ancheta, 2000).

Have the woman bend forward at the waist; she can lean over a bed, bean bag, or physical therapy ball or the seat of a chair or couch. The support person stands behind the woman and places his hands well below the iliac crests on the fleshiest part of her buttocks. During a contraction, he presses both of these areas constantly, as if pressing the hips together using the entire palms of the hands (not just the heels). Light pressure may be sufficient. This is a difficult technique to keep up it should be performed only to the point of effectiveness (Simkin, 1995).

The hip squeeze can also be performed with a rebozo. The center of the rebozo is first draped over a chair seat. The woman then sits on it, spreading out the rebozo to form a hammock for her pelvis (as described in the knee-press entry above). The support person holds both ends of the shawl in her hands and either gathers them together over the center of the woman's midline or holds each side of the rebozo parallel with the sides of the mother's body and pulls forward, thereby applying counterpressure to the hips. The support person should take instruction from the woman regarding the amount of pressure that feels good (Trueba, 2001).

Hip lift: If the baby is well engaged, this may help facilitate descent. Have the woman lie on her side. A support person kneels behind the woman, placing the heel of the hand closest to the mother's head firmly on her upper hip bone so that direct downward pressure can be applied. The woman assists the support person in finding her uppermost tuberosity (sit bone). The support person places the fingers of the other hand under the edge of the upper tuberosity. She then slowly applies pressure to the hip bone while lifting the mother's tuberosity. This moves the upper hip, opening the midpelvis and outlet (Wintergreen, 2004).

Massage

Massage of many different types has been used for ages to calm and relax the laboring mother.

- Classic effleurage is a Lamaze distraction technique using very light, repetitive touch, which can be soothing and pleasant. It is performed with the mother using the fingertips of both hands to lightly massage up the center of her belly over the top and down the sides in two large ovular patterns. However, a support person can use one hand to massage in the same kind of pattern, up the middle of the belly, over and around the fundus and down the sides of the belly in circular motions. Take care to avoid the navel, which will be sensitive in many women.
- To help stimulate contractions, use an open hand; press your palm over the belly and grasp and massage the uterus with your palm and fingerpads in a smooth, firm manner, moving your hand all over the upper segment, focusing on the fundus.
- Massage the pressure points in the rhomboid of Venus to stimulate labor. (See the subchapter entitled "Sterile Water Injections for the Relief of Excessive Localized Pain.")
- It is common for women to get leg cramps during labor and pushing. To relieve these spasms, have the woman flex her foot, with her toes pointing up, and then deeply massage the cramped area.
- If the mother is tense and deep massage does not help, use both open hands to grasp her thigh on either side. During a contraction, vigorously shake the tissue. This can also help relax the perineum (Gaskin, 2003).

Massaging the pituitary (uterine) reflex: Massaging this reflex point can help relieve pain during labor. The point is located at the top center of the border of the heel pad. Using olive oil and a circular pattern, a support person deeply and firmly massages this point throughout the contraction to lessen the woman's discomfort and aid relaxation, allowing her to handle strong contractions more easily (Block, 1984). See details and an illustration of how to locate this reflex in the chapter entitled "Additional Noninvasive Techniques for Assessing Progress."

Acupressure to enhance endorphin release

Stimulation of Jianjing (GB-21) and Ciliau (BL-32) are very effective when used as suggested by Debra Betts in the "Information for Midwives" section of her excellent manual ACUPRESSURE: PROMOTING A NATURAL LABOR AND PARTNER INVOLVEMENT:

> The most effective way to provide [pain relief during labor] with acupressure is to teach GB-21 and BL-32 to the woman and her support people prior to labour; around 36 weeks I find the ideal time. Although the points may feel tender when practicing the location, it is important to stress that during labour they are not to be used with gritted teeth! They should feel useful to the woman as she uses them, setting up a pain-relieving effect, a sense of well-being or a feeling of control that wears off when their support people stop using them. On using them correctly there is a distinct feeling around the site of pressure. This may be felt as a numbness, warmth, tingling, aching, or buzzing sensation. If they feel uncomfortable or painful try repositioning or select another point.
>
> These points appear to be most effective when used at the beginning of labour, rather than waiting till there is strong pain during labour. From feedback, it appears that using them early encourages the production of endorphins, as women report not only a reduction in the level of the pain of their contractions but also a sense of well-being, that they feel calm and relaxed, this disappears when the support people discontinue using the

acupressure. . . . Women report the effect equal to, or preferable to using a Tens machine, and then have the obvious advantage of being useful in water. (Betts, 2002)

Holding combs

The points located in the crease where the fingers join the hand can be stimulated by holding the teeth of a small, palm-width comb against them with the fingers. Combs are held tightly in both hands during contractions. This is said to help release endorphins (possibly because the technique itself produces a certain amount of pain). Some women have found holding combs in this manner very helpful in dealing with contractions, while others have not. For women who are having a hard time relaxing, having a place to direct their tension (such as their grip) can help them focus it away from the cervix and pelvis.

In addition to the techniques described above, ask the mother what would feel best to her. She may be have found a technique that worked for her in a previous labor or when she is under stress or in pain, or she may want to try a suggestion from a relative or friend. This provides an opportunity for you to learn a new technique as well.

Sexuality as an analgesic and labor enhancer

Birth is a very sexual experience. The hormones of birth, the sounds, the altered state of consciousness, even the anatomy of birth are all related to sex. This link, however, has been deemphasized over the decades. With the advent of the Victorian era followed by the institutionalization of birth and the switch to primarily male care providers, the obvious link between a woman's sexuality and the birthing process was discreetly swept under the rug, allowing a clinical approach to prevail. Manifestations of female sexuality were generally viewed as evidence of the disordered condition of being female and were treated accordingly.

The connection between the mouth and the birth canal: As Ina May Gaskin has pointed out numerous times in her writings, the mouth, cervix and yoni are connected. On an anatomical level, the upper and lower jaws mirror the pelvic girdle, with the hard palate reflecting the shape of the sacrum. The lips represent the mouth of the yoni, the oral cavity, the yoni canal and the throat and larynx, the cervix. When these structures are consciously kept loose and open, the "mouth" of the womb tends to follow suit. Watch women's mouths as they labor and think of gentle, encouraging ways to remind them to stay open and loose. Singing, sounding, kissing and blowing through loose lips so that they flutter on exhale are all good ways to accomplish this as well as enhance the production of labor hormones (Gaskin, 2003).

Sexual stimulation and pain relief: Mammals, including primates, are well known to lick their genitals during labor, especially as pushing approaches. In addition, there are many primitive images of laboring mother goddesses manipulating their genitals (for example, the Sheela-na-gig, a Celtic mother goddess, is depicted with her hands spreading her yoni wide during birth). While masturbation is a taboo subject in many cultures, clitoral or other vulval stimulation can be very pleasurable during labor and can provide some analgesic effects for the woman. Of course, orgasm is a terrific uterine stimulant as well. In fact, some women have reported powerful orgasms that have occurred as the baby expands the birth canal during late pushing. Many women instinctively express other behaviors associated with sexuality such as moaning or other vocalizations, moving their pelvis and other activities that help them deal with the intensity of labor as they open to the energy of birth.

As midwives, we can encourage couples or the woman herself to provide whatever genital stimulation feels good. Since there is still so much stigma around the word "masturbation," the use of phrases like "Feel free to massage your vulva or touch yourself" might be better received. Some midwives (Gaskin, 1978) have provided clitoral stimulation for the woman during pushing; however, in light of the heightened awareness of sexual abuse issues, it would probably be best for you to encourage the mother to stimulate herself. If the partner provides stimulation, it is important that he or she be willing to do so purely for the comfort of the laboring woman, with no other goals in mind. The labor environment must be as private as possible in order for a woman to feel free to touch herself. However, your comfort with the idea and your encouragement to consider this as an option will create an atmosphere of permission in which the mother can experiment. The really great thing about using sexual stimulation in this manner is that it will directly stimulate the production of the hormones that enhance the progress of labor (Field, 1985). If the woman seems willing, leave the room, while waiting quietly outside or, if the space allows, withdraw to a very obscure location within the room, remembering to make your presence known before engaging with her again.

PROTECTING THE BLADDER DURING LABOR

A full bladder during labor may become injured as the baby descends. It can also influence the position and descent of the fetal head by holding it up or causing it to maintain an unfavorable attitude, especially in multiparous women. Therefore, it is important for the mother to urinate every hour or two throughout labor. Give the woman some privacy and offer the following tried and true tricks if she is having difficulty voiding:

•Place a few drops of spirits of peppermint in the toilet to stimulate urination (the fumes help relax the urethra). *Never* apply spirits of peppermint to the woman's body.
•Have either a support person or the mother lightly stroke her sides and thighs. This may relax her enough to let go.
•Have the mother blow bubbles through a straw into a glass of water; for some women, this works immediately.
•Ask the mother to blow on her thumb, which should also work quickly.
•Place the mother's hand in a sink with warm running water flowing over it; often just the sound of trickling water will get things going.

However, none of this will work if the presenting part is obstructing the flow. Sometimes a horizontal position–for example, in a hot bath–helps reduce the pressure on the urethra if the baby is low. Swelling around the urethra may leave the mother unable to distinguish full bladder sensations from contractions. Aim to reduce the swelling, either by changing her position to relieve downward pressure, applying a cold pack or giving homeopathic arnica.

The full bladder appears as a fluctuant mass above the pubic bone. There may be a slight dip that falls between the pubic bone and the navel just above the fundus of the full bladder, giving the abdominal contour the look of a posterior presentation. This is most easily observed with the mother lying flat.

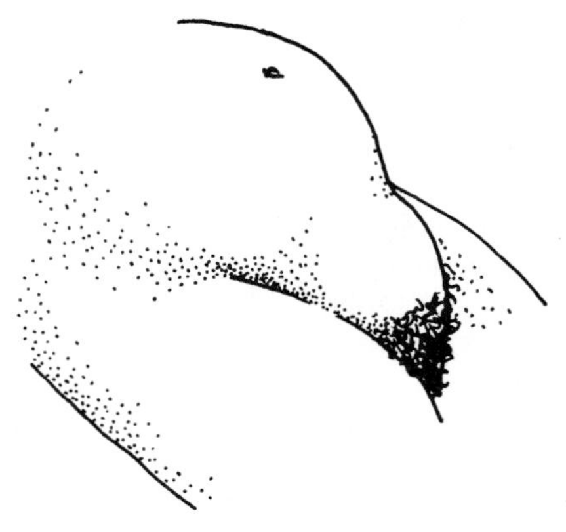
Contour of belly when the bladder is full

Although a full bladder can inhibit descent as well as uterine activity, it usually doesn't (Read et al., 1980). It may, on rare occasions, become a problem if it is extremely distended and the baby is not yet engaged. In this case, the mother may feel pain during fetal descent or rotation or during pushing, causing her to tense up and thus impede progress. The full bladder can be damaged from pressure as the baby descends or when a small fold of the lower bladder wall becomes caught between a low head and the pubic bone. Either of these problems can lead to a vesicoyoni (vesicovaginal [VES-eh-koe-VAJ-eh-nahl]) fistula (a hole between the bladder and the yoni) from pressure necrosis, even if the upper wall of the yoni is not visibly damaged after birth. Damage is more likely if forceful, sustained pushing takes place before the head reaches the pelvic floor. Fortunately, the actual incidence of this is extremely rare.

If the mother cannot void and the bladder is obviously full, catheterization before the baby gets any lower is the best solution. (See instructions given in the subchapter entitled "Urinary Catheterization.")

LATENT (PRODROMAL) AND EARLY LABOR

NOTE: The chapter entitled "The Onset of Normal Labor at Term" in Volume I of this text discusses how to tell if a woman is in labor. Also read the chapter entitled "Assessing the Progress and Strength of Labor: An Overview" in this text before studying the ones that follow in this section.

These phases are defined by the strength of contractions, the degree of cervical dilation and the rapidity with which labor is progressing. Prodromal labor occurs when contractions are continuing and primarily finishes ripening the cervix and produces effacement. Early labor then produces the first few centimeters of dilation, however, very often these occur together. Given this definition, the beginning and duration of latent labor varies widely; with most women (particularly multiparas) undergoing some of these changes over the four weeks preceding the onset of active labor. When the onset of latent phase is more easily identified, it consists of relatively mild contractions, which are typically only 15 to 20 sec long and may be spaced anywhere from 5 to 30 min apart.

The first-time mother's cervix has never opened before, thus providing more work for latent labor contractions. She is likely to experience a longer early labor, which may last anywhere from a few to 24 hours and occasionally longer. The cervix is more firm and must frequently be almost completely effaced before dilation can begin. Therefore, early labor often produces only 2 to 3 cm of dilation in many first-time mothers. However, when the baby is already engaged in an LOA position when labor begins, smooth, steady progress can be expected with short, sharp and well-spaced early contractions. If the mother stands and leans forward, all the energy of each contraction hastens progress by going straight to the cervix.

In contrast, the cervix of a woman who has given birth before responds more readily to preparatory uterine activity as well as to these early contractions, softening and effacing more quickly and usually dilating to 4 or 5 cm (and sometimes more) before stronger contractions begin and before the cervix is fully effaced.

In the hospital, women in latent labor often wind up with many interventions, including surgical birth, because they and their practitioners are convinced that the contractions are strong but no progress in the form of dilation is being made. This is especially true with first-time mothers, who have no idea how strong the contractions can be. Women who have had augmented labors or drugs for previous births may also have a distorted idea about what normal labor is like. It is your job to help each woman have a realistic perspective regarding what to expect from her entire labor.

Support the mother to pace herself

Once you have determined that a woman is experiencing uterine activity that is likely to lead to active labor, encourage her to pace herself. As much as you may have emphasized pacing during prenatal care, you will have to reiterate it now, especially with first-time mothers. In the excitement of early labor, a woman often anticipates how her labor will go. This often leads her to overreact to early labor and fear what lies ahead. She needs to eat, drink and rest as much as possible to prepare for the harder work she will face. Early labor usually lasts from two-thirds to three-quarters of the entire time it takes for a woman to reach full dilation (Simkin, 2001). Twelve to twenty-four hours is not unusual for a first-time mother. Tell women to be prepared for at least a 36 hr process from the beginning of labor through to birth.

However, there is no way to know in advance how long labor may last, particularly with first babies. If it lasts only a few hours, women usually give birth with no problems no matter how severely they may react to labor or how much energy they may expend coping with it. However, if early labor lasts 24 hours, active labor lasts 12 and pushing takes another 2, the mother will pay dearly for not pacing herself early on. A first-time mother does not know how much labor will demand of her and therefore needs guidance regarding this critical factor.

Nourishment and fluids in early labor: The work of labor requires 200 to 300 calories and 4 oz of fluid per hour. Normal labor produces minimal changes in plasma electrolyte levels, glucose concentration and osmolality, with fetal levels paralleling maternal levels closely but at slightly lower levels. Well-nourished women enter labor in a state of relative overhydration because they have a well-expanded blood volume. However, they lack the ability to excrete excess fluid loads. The mother and fetus are thus protected from dehydration during labor to a certain extent, which is why the mother doesn't require more than 4 oz of oral fluids an hour. In a normal labor, IVs are thus unnecessary and likely to produce fluid imbalance, leading to edema after the birth.

If early labor starts in the morning, advise the woman to eat and drink throughout the day. If labor starts at night, the woman should eat dinner as she normally would and have a light, protein-rich snack before going to bed early. Many midwives encourage a meal rich in complex carbohydrates as early labor begins to help move labor along. If labor lasts longer than expected, ongoing intake of fluids and food is an important part of maintaining energy levels. Women usually do not enter active labor if they are hungry. Being well nourished in early labor also helps reduce the catecholamine surge that occurs if the woman is excited or anxious at the beginning of labor.

Emotional responses to latent and early labor

Women can feel a wide range of emotions during this time, from excitement to fear or even panic. Contractions are probably the strongest many a first-time mother has ever felt, yet she is being told this is only early labor. This can lead a first-time mother to projecting that she is more advanced in her labor than she really is. Using breathing techniques and applying her focused attention to her contractions early on will exhaust her and make for a big let-down once she realizes that she is not progressing as rapidly as she hopes. In these cases, a look at her gluteal crease or an internal exam can be a reality check for both of you and can provide concrete evidence of how she is doing. This will prevent her from fantasizing and you from missing important cues, should she be progressing more rapidly than you expect based solely upon the amount of time she has been having contractions.

The presence of the midwife during latent and early labor

When should the midwife stay for the labor? If you arrive during early labor and choose to stay, make sure you have some activities to occupy your time while early labor progresses. It is important that the woman not feel she is a "watched pot" or that she has to "produce" active labor for you or anyone else. She may become discouraged because she equates your presence with the idea that labor should be moving along faster than it is.

Often the best choice is to assess the woman and baby, observe her labor pattern for a while, and leave. A nearby movie theater, park, library or mall provide good places to wait unless she lives close to you, in which case you can just go home. Remaining at her house and attending her as though her labor is far more advanced than it is, will wear both of you out. Leaving her alone can ease any performance anxiety she may have and provide the privacy she requires to allow strong labor to take over.

However, if the woman is coping poorly, is very afraid, is throwing up or has no other support people to stay with her, you or an assistant should stay until she can either settle into a realistic response to her physical sensations or until active progress is underway and she gives birth. If her condition is stable but she cannot rest and simply needs companionship, you can also opt to take her someplace nearby where she can engage in distracting activities, such as window-shopping, walking in the park, eating a light meal or watching a film.

Rest and sleep

If a woman begins labor early in the morning or midday, with active labor nowhere in sight, she should attempt to rest or nap in the afternoon and go to bed early. Chances are she will awake during the night or early the next morning in active labor.

The woman who begins early labor in the evening or the middle of the night should attempt to rest or sleep. It is quite possible for her to doze off between contractions that last less than a minute, followed by 10 to 15 minutes of relaxation. If she can talk through contractions, she can probably sleep as well. Hot baths, warm milk (containing the natural sedative tryptophan) and certain herbs, such as skullcap or catnip tincture, can be used as sedatives. Start out with 5 drop doses of one or both of these herbal tinctures every 15 minutes until relaxation creeps in. A back rub or massage can also help to ease her into sleep. While giving the mother a glass of wine to aid relaxation can be very effective, giving the mother alcohol also exposes the fetus to its effects as labor is about to begin. The psychological imprint on the fetus that results from an alcohol-induced altered state of consciousness should be kept in mind, especially in families in which alcohol abuse is a problem.

Breathing and relaxation techniques for early labor: A woman should breathe normally and, of course, relax as much as possible until she must focus on her contractions. Relaxation of the pelvic structures is of paramount importance to well-placed fetal descent at all points during labor; tight muscles can buoy the baby up as well as promote persistent asynclitism or deflexion. Premature use of the sort of breathing techniques that are sometimes needed in active labor will only tire the woman who is still in early labor.

Positions for early labor

The use of specific techniques to encourage contractions is generally ill advised at this point, unless early labor is much prolonged. (See the chapter entitled "Endless Early Labor" for suggestions.) The exception to this general rule is to keep the spinopubic angle open. Forward-leaning positions, with the knees placed below the tuberosities, will facilitate this. Likewise the mother should avoid sitting in furniture that allows her bottom to sink down below her knees, as this will pinch off the brim and impair normal descent and rotation.

Involving support people during latent and early labor

Whether the mother's chosen support people will be truly supportive at this point is always a matter for individual assessment. You should have discussed with the mother whom she wants at the birth as part of your prenatal care. However, support people may have been unavailable to attend a prenatal visit or may show up unexpectedly. Most of the time, they have never sat through an entire labor or witnessed a birth, let alone a homebirth. Some may have attended a hospital birth and thus have a very distorted idea about how labor should evolve. In either case, they are often excited and somewhat apprehensive about the whole affair.

With ideal relationship dynamics, one or at the most two support people (in addition to the primary partner) may be very helpful *if* they can remain low-key, not hover over the mother and encourage the mother to do what she needs to do. When you explain to them that the same atmosphere that promotes a satisfying sexual experience (or using the toilet, depending on whom you are talking to) promotes a progressive labor, they are more likely to truly understand what is needed. It is particularly important for these people to understand and trust that her labor is normal at this point. What she doesn't need is a bunch of people either settling in for a party marathon or encouraging her to relate to early labor as if it were transition. It is your job to assess how her support people are reacting, either to offer them guidance or invite them to leave if they are not proving helpful or if there are simply too many people around.

Active Dilation

The contractions of active labor become stronger and longer and gradually require increasing amounts of attention. The cervix is now soft and has been pulled forward somewhat by early labor contractions. The cervix has effaced in most primigravidas; multiparas may never fully efface, and the effacement they have usually occurs concurrently with dilation. The cervix is typically dilated to at least 3 cm and more often to 4 or 5 cm as early labor flows into active labor.

The woman becomes more psychically open and emotionally vulnerable as labor advances. She may already feel tired after being unable to sleep through the night during early labor. Her desire for outside distractions wanes; sounds and activities from others may become annoying She enters a hypnotically suggestible state that makes things that she is told or that are said in her presence potent suggestions to her subconscious. The midwife can make good use of this openness in the words and phrases she uses to encourage the woman to cope with and open to the energy of her labor. There are several other things you can do to help her make good progress.

Monitor the environment

Keep observers, and distracting sounds and lights to a minimum. Limit the number of people in the room. Side conversations and chitchat are inappropriate, as is audible entertainment from another part of the house. Set an example by having only one midwife stay with her at any given time. This midwife should be quietly occupied with needlework or a book, while she remains the strong, silent, unobservant but ever present presence that nearly every laboring woman needs. This will enhance the mother's production of endorphins and speed labor along.

Monitor the energy

If labor is really progressing, you can expect that evidence of this will become more palpable to you as a result. Physical sensations, a change in the vibes in the room, a certain emotional resonance with the mother's altered state any of these may occur for individual midwives as the energy of birth begins to really get going.

Support her to stay in the present

A woman can become quite discouraged after having gone through early labor, perhaps for many hours or even days, or she can become determined to get it over with as she enters active labor and senses how strong the contractions are becoming. Anticipating either how long labor will last or assessing how long it has been does not help labor to progress; it just engages her neocortex, which is counterproductive. What does help is for the mother to focus and be completely present with each contraction and then to completely rest in between. From here on out, labor becomes a real "be here now" experience. If a woman is fearful of her contractions, the best thing she can do to is to move *through* the fear, rather than resist it. She can do this by acknowledging her feelings verbally and locating the physical sensations connected with the emotion in her body. Encourage her to breathe into that area and open to her feelings as she goes through the contraction. Placing your hands where you feel the energy of her breath can be used to best advantage can be very helpful.

Resisting the fear will only make it harder to cope and will inevitably result in resistance to the labor process as well. Unusually strong fear reactions may arise for the woman who has experienced abuse; who has been frightened about labor as a result of the experiences of friends, family members, or previous births of her own; or who has body memories about her own birth process. At times, the sensations of labor will trigger the release of feelings that are overwhelming and that cannot be completely released at once. In these cases, techniques, such as classic Lamaze, which encourage the woman to use a visual focal point on a wall or engage in complicated breathing patterns designed to distract her from her internal process, can prove useful to individual women. However, I have found techniques that help the mother tune into and harmonize with her body and help her maintain her emotional equilibrium to be much more helpful for most women.

Techniques for helping women who have experienced extreme abuse in their lives are detailed in the chapter entitled "Understanding Physical, Emotional and Sexual Abuse Issues," in Volume I of this text. It is expected that you would have discussed strategies for dealing with emotions that might arise during labor with women who have a known history of abuse during their prenatal care. That chapter also offers suggestions for supporting women who have body memories come up that they are unaware are connected to a history of abuse.

Food and fluid needs

The catecholamine surge of early labor drops once active labor is rolling along. Women become increasingly internalized and often do not wish to eat or drink very much. As labor gets stronger, the skeletal muscles and the neocortex tend to reduce their activities, with the uterine muscle, the hypothalamus and pituitary gland being the most active parts of the body. The pituitary produces oxytocin, endorphins, prolactin and antidiuretic hormone, which helps prevent water loss. When the mother is unafraid and labor advances quickly, she will desire to eat little or nothing and will probably only want water to drink. Forcing fluids is not necessary, as long as progress is steady (Odent, 1994).

Support her to relax

Once active labor begins and the mother starts to focus on her contractions, relaxation becomes something that she must consciously strive to achieve. The natural tendency is to clench up with the uncomfortable, if not downright painful, sensations from the cervix as it opens.

Place her in warm water: I consider a bathtub to be an almost essential requirement, especially for first-time mothers. A body of water can do worlds of good to help a woman relax and internalize her focus so that labor can progress. (The use of water is discussed in detail in the chapter entitled "Hydrotherapy and Waterbirth.")

Encourage her to change positions and activities regularly

It can be tempting not to intervene when it looks as if what a woman is doing is working, and this is valid to a certain extent. Keep in mind, however, that what works at one point in labor may keep the energy from building as contractions grow stronger. Tune into the energy. If it seems to be blocked, having the mother change positions is an excellent way to keep the birth energy moving, to move the mother's pelvis around, and to encourage the baby to move down.

Apply a hot pack to the lower abdomen

The application of heat is soothing and can help relax the cervix as well as the rest of the body. Hand towels or cloth diapers soaked in hot water can be used for this purpose, as can an electric heating pad wrapped in a towel. A hot water bottle also works, although some women will not want to feel the weight of anything on their bodies. Applications of heat are also helpful when placed on the lower back for back pain. (For details, see the chapter entitled "Using Comfort and Positioning Aids in Labor.")

Aches and pains during labor

Almost every woman's back hurts at some point in late labor. This is due to the pelvic joints stretching and opening as the baby comes through. A woman can have pain in front at the symphysis pubis and in back in her sacroiliac joints, especially when the biparietal diameter passes through the midpelvis. Sometimes the pain is referred to the center of the sacrum, or it may feel like a band of pain all the way around her hips. This discomfort is normal and women need to be reminded that it represents good progress. Back labor from a posterior presentation is experienced in the same regions but typically is much more severe. It is discussed in the chapter entitled "Assisting a Woman Whose Baby Is in a Posterior Position." Other types of pain, particularly localized pains, can be caused by specific difficulties. Suprapubic pain may be caused by a compound presentation (see the chapter entitled "Assisting a Woman Whose Baby Is in a Compound Presentation"). Side pain may be due to persistent asynclitism (see the chapter entitled "Techniques Used to Help the Baby Descend during Labor").

Transition

This period of labor starts at about 8 cm of dilation through to full dilation. It is a time of intense work and concentration for the mother. The energy of birth builds rapidly now, and everyone involved will feel it on some level. This is often when the woman proclaims that she can't do it, that she wants to go to the hospital, or that she wants drugs. The simple fear that she can't cope any longer is the one you are most likely to hear at a homebirth. The midwife needs to reassure the mother in transition that her birth energy is strong and about to shift gears and can, therefore, feel very overwhelming, but all that is normal.

Coping techniques that have worked up to this point may cease to offer comfort, and touch that soothed before may become intolerable. Even modest, quiet women may strip off their clothes and make quite a bit of noise. Other women may drift into an altered state of consciousness, even dozing between contractions. If a woman has not used sexual stimulation or vocalizations up to this point and is having trouble integrating the energy, this would be a good time to remind her of these options.

Go with the flow of the mother's preferences at this point and give her lots of encouragement regarding her ability to deal with the labor. Do not, however, make specific estimates regarding the duration of the rest of the labor, when she will be able to push or how soon the baby is likely to be born, as anything can happen as labor moves along. Predictions such as these only make for disappointment later if they do not pan out.

You may notice that you or others present at the birth get antsy during this time. You may feel agitated or suddenly start wondering if something is wrong or why labor is taking forever. This is the way midwives sometimes manifest the energy of transition, especially when they have allowed themselves to become distracted from consciously tuning in. Take a deep breath or two and relax yourself. Channel the energy through from the top of your head down through your feet, especially if you are working closely with the mother. This will help ground the energy in your own body.

BREATHING AND RELAXING DURING LABOR

A woman's ability to relax and to breathe in a way that enhances relaxation makes a huge difference in how well she is able to conserve her energy and cope with labor. While many sources recommend learning various breathing techniques during pregnancy, some women find it hard to implement what they have learned once labor arrives. Just about anything can be taught to a woman on the spot in labor with no problem. In my practice, it has seemed that spur-of-the-moment instruction is just as effective as prenatal practice. The exception to this is specific techniques that involve relaxing specific muscle groups in the pelvis and the cervix. These types of breathing exercises can begin prenatally to prepare the woman to release her pelvis during labor.

Since the process of labor is a very sexual experience, privacy alone helps the mother relax. So, too, does sitting in a warm bath or shower, or lying in a tub while a support person pours warm water over her belly during contractions. Listening to soft music of the woman's preference can also be helpful, as well as changing positions periodically. Music that has a gentle ebb-and-flow rhythm is ideal for laboring women as are deep bass tones. Music with a regimented pace (such as compositions based on the sound of the fetal heart heard through a Doppler) can result in the woman's labor becoming regulated as well (Banks, 2002).

In addition, any form of relaxation that the woman uses on a regular basis can also be used during labor. Many women are also aware of what helps them get through challenging experiences from other physical pursuits. For example, Schlinger (2003) describes a rock climber who did not want any conversation until she arrived at the summit of her climb. In labor, she needed the same quiet space to concentrate. Women who have been abused may need a constant stream of vocal encouragement to help them stay present during a sexual or a birth experience.

When considering relaxation techniques, remember that the pelvis is the most important part that needs to be relaxed. A woman can be limp as a dishrag, but if she is rigidly tightening her pelvic area, it won't help. Likewise, a woman can carry tension is other parts of her body, but if she can manage to keep her buttocks, birth canal and cervix soft and yielding, labor should move along just fine.

Breathing

Penny Simkin has noticed that, during labor, women often accumulate tension without being aware of it. Any spot where a woman usually holds her tension is likely to be a trouble spot during labor as well. Rather than trying to relax her entire body at once, have a support person help the woman identify and relax especially tense areas of the body. Penny calls this technique the "Roving Body Check." The mother breathes in slowly, while the support person places one or both hands firmly on the part to be released, assessing whether there is tension in that area. The mother then exhales, focusing on relaxing that area as the partner gradually releases the pressure. During the next breath, the support person moves her hands to another area and repeats the process. The mother should state whether this is helpful; some women may find it more useful to relax their bodies region by region rather than all at once, but without verbal or tactile assistance (Simkin, 1995). This type of interactive relaxation may be most useful when the midwife or the mother feels that the birthing energy is blocked; having the woman breathe into your hands can smooth this out and expand that area to channel more of the energy of birth.

Many breathing techniques have been recommended to women for use in labor, the best of which is simply deep abdominal breathing at a rate of 5 to 12 breaths per minute. Focusing on filling the belly rather than the lungs with air requires moving the diaphragm downward. This lifts abdominal muscles away from the uterus. Breathing this way greatly enhances oxygen exchange because it causes the lungs to fill with more air than does chest breathing. It calms the mother and promotes relaxation as well as a sense of well-being. It is the kind of breathing that relaxed babies use.

Tension causes humans to breathe shallowly, high in the chest. A woman who breathes this way during labor may feel restless and more fearful. Even so, as labor becomes very intense, some women find it helpful to shift to lighter, higher breaths during contractions, breathing as quickly as 30 to 60 breaths per minute. The inhalation should be silent and the exhalation audible. She should try breathing in through her nose and out through her mouth. If this is not enough, touching the tongue lightly to the roof of the mouth, just behind the front teeth, during mouth breathing will stimulate the flow of saliva and help prevent a dry mouth. The face, shoulders and back tend to tense up as the mother breathes in this manner; help her pay particular attention to relaxing these areas.

Another breathing technique involves a series of pants and blows, a combination of slow and light breathing. Three or four light breaths are followed by a slower breath. The more complicated the pattern, the more the breathing distracts a woman from what is going on in her body, which takes her away from being with her labor. Most of the time, women birthing at home do not require such complex breathing patterns to get through labor. However, any technique that works to assist a particular woman to get through her labor is preferable to transport for drugs.

Hyperventilation: Respirations that are faster than necessary lead to elevated oxygen levels in the blood. This presents with lightheadedness, dizziness and tingling in the hands and feet. When this occurs, have the woman try to move less air in and out of her lungs either by slowing her breathing or by breathing more shallowly. She can also revert to deep abdominal breathing. She should make sure her face and upper body are relaxed and that her inhalations are silent. If hyperventilation persists, have the mother slow her breathing and breathe into a paper bag placed over the nose and mouth for a few contractions. A drop of pure frankincense oil can be applied to the bag, when can help correct hyperventilation. Breathing into a bag temporarily increases the amount of carbon dioxide in the air. This helps rebalance the blood gases and correct the problem (Simkin, 1995).

Rebozo relaxation techniques

A rebozo can be used in a variety of ways to enhance relaxation in labor, as Guadalupe Trueba explains in her excellent video and accompanying booklet COMFORT MEASURES FOR CHILDBIRTH: THE REBOZO WAY (2001).

Rebozo effleurage: Have the woman assume a comfortable side-lying position. The fringe of the rebozo is then lightly drawn over her entire body as she breathes and relaxes. To enhance this effect, a tiny bit of lavender essential oil or another relaxing oil that is pleasant to the woman can be sprayed on the cloth or rubbed on the hands and then the hands lightly rubbed over the rebozo.

Tailor sitting and rocking: The woman assumes a tailor position (sitting up, legs crossed, her bottom can be propped on a meditation cushion or a couple of folded towels). The rebozo is passed across her upper chest (above the breasts) and under each arm to form an upper body sling. A support person stands behind the woman, holds the ends of the rebozo, and slowly moves it back and forth, rocking the woman's upper body passively as she relaxes and breathes into the sensation. The woman's weight should not be supported in this position as this may lead to nerve damage.

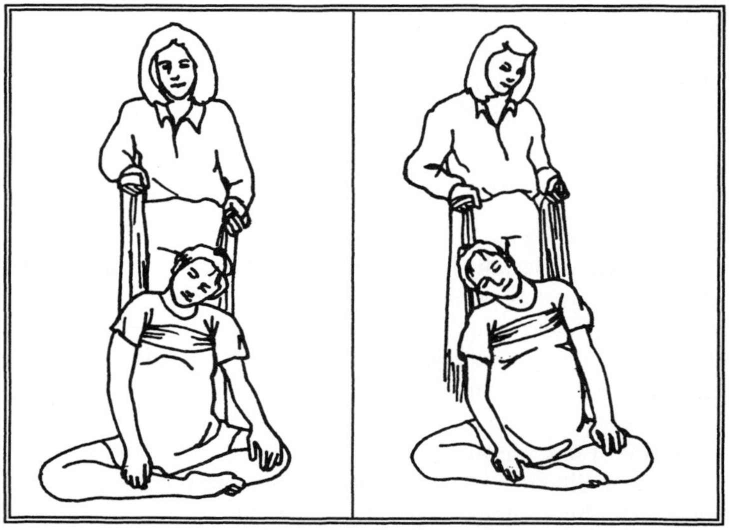

(Adapted with permission from photographs appearing in COMFORT MEASURES FOR CHILDBIRTH: THE REBOZO WAY© 2001, Guadalupe Trueba)

Head wrap: The woman assumes whatever position she is most attracted to at the moment. The center of the rebozo is widened and placed over her eyes, forehead and ears; the ends are then drawn behind the head and crossed. Gentle pressure is created as a support person pulls on the ends in opposite directions. This muffles outside sights and sounds and can be very centering. This may not appeal to all women, so be sure to discuss it beforehand.

The use of acupressure for relaxation

Stimulating KI-1 promotes general relaxation and is very effective at relaxing the perineum during pushing. It is also helpful if the woman feels frantic or afraid. Apply deep pressure at an angle toward the big toe. KI-1 is easily accessed when the woman is in a position that exposes the soles of her feet (for example, if she is in a hands-and-knees position).

To relax the pelvis and bring the baby down, the following is quoted directly from Debra Betts' excellent manual ACUPRESSURE: PROMOTING A NATURAL LABOUR AND PARTNER INVOLVEMENT, on the use GB-30 and BL-32:

> When you place your hands on the woman's hips [during labor] you can push your thumbs into this point [GB-30], helping the woman to move in rotating movements during contractions. This point can also be used during transition, especially when combined with massage strokes, beginning at BL-32 and radiating out to this point [GB-30]. (Betts, 2002) (To locate these points, see the subchapter entitled "Traditional Chinese Medicine.")

The Resting Phase of Labor

One of the most important contributions midwifery care has made to the understanding of labor has been the recognition that after full dilation is reached there is often a period of uterine quietude that occurs prior to the onset of active pushing. During this time, which many midwives call the "rest-and-be-thankful-period," the woman's body prepares for pushing. Do not get the impression that she suddenly snaps out of her "labor trance," although she may become somewhat more alert. Instead, it reflects a shift in the energy. Often, especially if the baby is still high in the pelvis, the uterus will continue to contract but spontaneous pushing urges will not yet occur. With all the "rah-rah-push-push-push as soon as you are complete" coaching that is an integral part of institutionally based North American birth culture, it is important to understand why this phase is so important and a normal part of labor for so many women.

Special nerve receptors called "proprioceptors" (PRO-pry-oh-SEP-tors) are stimulated by the pressure and stretching that the presenting part exerts on the cervix during cervical dilation. Nerve stimulation causes the release of hormones that produces strong contractions (the Ferguson reflex), which stretch the uterus tightly around the baby. Once complete dilation is reached, the presenting part descends past the os, which is then no longer stimulated in the same way and which causes the uterus to become temporarily slack because the presenting part is no longer contained within it. As contractions continue, this flaccidity is gradually taken up by muscle retraction until the uterus hugs the baby firmly again. At the same time, the bladder and anterior soft tissues are drawn up along with the lower segment. Thus, the "resting" phase is actually a period of uterine tightening; as such it can be likened to the pause between the birth of the head and the birth of the shoulders that occurs in most labors. Trying to rush through or ignore it can actually create problems where none previously existed (Fairman, 1990).

During this period, contractions slowly move the baby deeper into the birth canal. The counterpressure provided by the resilient muscles of the pelvic floor assist in head flexion and rotation, and the resting phase allows for the shoulder axis to finish rotating to the transverse diameter of the brim as well, if this has not already occurred. This process of latent rotation and descent after full dilation is now referred to in medical circles as "laboring down." As time passes, the contractions change in character, and an urge to push gradually becomes established. (If the baby is tending toward a posterior position at this point in labor, see the chapter entitled "Assisting a Woman Whose Baby Is in a Posterior Position.")

The resting phase may last anywhere from a few minutes to several hours. During this time, women can eat, drink, rest and sleep, if possible, between contractions. Many European midwives report that the left-lateral position is best if the woman wishes to lie down during this time. A spontaneous urge to push will usually be the natural conclusion of this phase of labor. Pushing prior to the establishment of a spontaneous urge may jam the incompletely rotated head into the pelvis, producing a transverse arrest or asynclitic presentation, or may strain muscles and ligaments by forcing the as-yet unprepared uterus to bear down.

Women can go for 12 hours or more and not develop an urge to push. This in and of itself does not present a problem as long as mother and baby are fine. However, it is problematic if the membranes are ruptured (particularly when internal exams have been performed); if the mother is unable (or unwilling) to rest, eat, and drink; or if she is otherwise coping poorly or is psychologically blocked. (Long resting phases are often related to psychological issues.) A hot hip bath often relaxes the pelvic floor sufficiently so that the uterus can move the baby down, helping to establish a spontaneous urge to push.

Be prepared as pushing draws near

The resting phase gives you an opportunity to make sure all is in order for the birth. Check to see that your equipment is where you want it, towels are warming on the heating pad and any other special preparations are in place before active pushing begins.

Active Pushing

Ensure a warm environment for pushing

Adjust the room temperature in the birthing room so that it will be at least 80°F (27°C) at the time of the birth. If it is a hot summer day, assign someone to turn off any fans or air conditioners (or at least turn them down), and close doors and windows to eliminate drafts, and have a space heater ready to turn on, if appropriate, just before the baby is born. Having the room an appropriate temperature is important for both mother and baby. The baby dissipates heat into the mother's system via the placenta during pregnancy and labor. The mother's body thus becomes accustomed to a reduced need to generate its own heat. After the birth, the sudden removal of the baby as a heat source causes a small but abrupt shift in maternal core temperature. In addition, the catecholamine surge during late labor contributes to the shivering that commonly occurs in women after they give birth. Cold causes the mother to produce even more stress hormones. Warmth, on the other hand, causes the levels of maternal and newborn stress hormones to fall rapidly, followed by a surge of oxytocin to help the mother deliver her placenta, lactate and fall in love with her baby. The newborn, who is experiencing an abrupt change from an aquatic environment held at a constant temperature to an atmosphere subject to air movement, will be least traumatized by being born into a warm environment. He will also experience a faster drop in stress hormones and an equally rapid rise in oxytocin.

When does pushing begin?

Pushing begins when the uterus, the mother or both start to bear down. The trigger for spontaneous pushing is not necessarily full dilation. A hormonal surge, in the case of the fetus ejection reflex, or sufficient pressure on the floor of the yoni can also produce an urge to push, which is more a product of the station of the presenting part than the state of the cervix. Thus, the urge to push may develop prior to complete dilation or several hours afterward.

Women who have had hospital births in the past may ask you if they can push. Your response to this should be "Do you feel like pushing?" If a woman asks, she is often not quite there yet; however, some women who have been admonished to wait for an internal exam in the past may ask even if the urge is strong. A woman who is fully in tune with her hormones will naturally move into spontaneous pushing, no questions asked.

The physiological response to pelvic pressure may be "turned off" in women whose stretch receptors in the pelvic region have been ignored outside of pregnancy, for example, in those who regularly put off urination. This phenomenon may be in play with a woman who has a very low baby and no urge to push. Likewise, highly sensitive stretch receptors may be a factor when women have a strong urge to push well before full dilation and significant fetal descent (Sagady, 1995).

Reading the signs of pushing urges: Gloria Lemay (2000) offers some insightful tips regarding watching women as the urge to push builds. Avoiding internal exams whenever possible, she prefers to take cues from the woman's behavior. The woman still has some dilating to do when pushing urges occur only at the peak (rather than the beginning) of a contraction. Pushing urges that vary in intensity or that are not present for every contraction are another clue that the cervix is not fully out of the way. In addition, bloody show continues as long as the cervix is still opening and usually ceases once it is gone, resuming only if a laceration occurs as the presenting part distends the birth canal and perineum.

What pushing feels like

The first urges to push are often described as a downwardly directed sensation in the abdomen. A sensation of fullness in the rectum, similar to having a full bowel, is added to this abdominal feeling as descent continues. Pressure is transmitted through the posterior yoni wall to the floor of the rectum. It is important to remember that the focus of descent and bearing down is in the yoni. At this point, if any guidance is necessary, the woman is best advised to let the sensation build as the baby stretches the pelvic floor. She can do this by allowing the uterine contractions to do their work while not adding any pushing efforts of her own until her urge to push becomes irresistible. As the baby descends, some mothers report a sensation of "splitting in two." The sensations of pushing often feel extremely intense but are perfectly normal and mean the pelvic bones as well as the muscular floor are stretching as the head moves past the tuberosities. Finally, the sensations transform into a pins-and-needles or burning feeling as the mouth of the yoni opens wide to let the widest part of the presenting part emerge. Hilary Schlinger (2002) points out that these terms are quite inadequate to describe what many women go through during crowning. She describes a sensation like stretching your lips until they are tucked behind your ears or like a bowling ball trying to come through. This sensation has also been called the "ring of fire"; and often prompts the woman to reach down and provide her own perineal or labial support.

Within the next contraction or two, the head is born. The following contraction usually brings the shoulders and the rest of the baby's body (Lemay, 2000).

Schlinger (2002) observes two basic pushing patterns: fast and often quite painful, with the baby moving down and being born quickly, or slower and more pleasurable, with characteristic rocking of the presenting part back and forth with contractions. This takes longer but may be less painful than a superfast pushing phase. However, I have known women who had a very fast and relatively painless pushing phase as well.

The fetus ejection reflex

In the best of all circumstances, the woman will experience a surge of catecholamines and oxytocin, which triggers a fetus ejection reflex, prompting her to stand, reach for something above her waist to grasp, and sag her body forward. (Reaching up tends to lengthen the torso.) Her uterus begins to have strong, effective contractions which release the baby from her body. This is not pushing in the traditional sense but an involuntary expulsion of the baby from her body. She opens her knees and after only a few contractions the baby emerges. The baby may descend, rapidly and all at once, from high in the yoni to crowning. As this occurs, the mother may tip her brim forward as her sacrum moves backward 1 to 2 cm, widening the pelvis in all dimensions. Odent (2000) points out that "second stage" is something that happens when physiologic labor is interrupted to the point that this reflexive birth of the baby does not occur.

Physiologic pushing

When labor is disrupted to the point that the fetus ejection reflex is impaired or when it happens more slowly for whatever reason, the woman can still have a physiologic pushing phase. The pressure that results as the presenting part moves down stimulates the proprioceptors in the wall of the yoni, the rectum, the floor of the yoni and finally the perineum. In turn, the uterus begins bearing-down efforts as it rises, high and firm, with contractions. Research on uterine pressure during pushing provides a graph depicting a bell-shaped contraction with pressures of 70 to 80 mm Hg at the peak. Within this period are 3 to 5 surges of energy that intermittently raise the intrauterine pressure to 140 to 160 mm Hg; these surges may reflect the work of the abdominal muscles being added to the strength of the contractions (Sagady, 1995).

Once the uterus starts bearing down, a truly involuntary pushing urge begins. This is the best kind of pushing because the uterus is working just as it should to bring the baby through the lower pelvis. Coupled with the mother's voluntary efforts, this free-flowing birthing energy is what is needed to bring babies down and out, even when the presenting part is not in an ideal position. Women often announce the onset of uterine pushing with a comment like "It's pushing!"; a catch in the throat or a throaty groan as a contraction builds also signal the completely involuntary nature of the uterine action. Involuntary bearing down may start prior to full dilation. When this occurs, have the woman go with the energy but not add any voluntary effort.

Women who are allowed to push spontaneously, with no direction from their care providers, push in a way that is effective in moving the baby down, that does not exhaust them, and that maximizes the oxygen that the baby receives. Physiologic pushing also places less stress on the perineal muscles and ligaments and results in less tearing.

Bearing down often begins with the gradual building of the urge to push, which takes place over several contractions. If instruction seems necessary, tell the mother to bear down only when and for as long as she feels the need to do so. If there is still a cervical lip when this urge begins, have the mother breathe through the urge without adding anything to it. This will allow her body to take up the last bit of cervix without resisting this natural, involuntary sensation. (See the chapter entitled "Cervical and Other Soft-tissue Problems during Labor" for ways to deal with a cervical lip.)

Spontaneous efforts consist of both open- and closed-glottis pushing. **Open-glottis pushing** is defined as bearing down while making sound or releasing breath, whereas **closed-glottis pushing** involves holding the breath. Women instinctively use a combination of both styles of pushing, favoring open-glottis pushing or holding their breath for only 6 seconds or less. As the contraction builds, the woman will bear down when she feels the need to do so and may take several breaths (usually three or so) between bearing-down efforts. Open-glottis pushing has the advantage of maximizing placental profusion and minimizing variations in maternal blood gases.

During pushing, the woman can be encouraged to assume different positions if she appears to need orientation regarding how to deal with the energy. If not, just provide her with your supportive presence and encouragement to find her own way through this part of labor.

The process of descent during pushing

Once pushing by the uterus, the woman or both becomes established, the head starts to descend further, first dilating the levator ani muscles of the pelvic floor and then the more shallow muscles of the urogenital diaphragm to pass beneath the pubic bone. If internal rotation of the head and shoulders has not yet occurred, it will take place around this time.

The anterior yoni wall is vulnerable to damage once active pushing begins. During this part of labor, the initial build-up of the contraction results in a tautening of the anterior yoni wall. This tightening smooths out the anterior canal and pulls the bladder out of the way prior to actively pushing down on the baby. The mother who is following her body will not begin experiencing pushing surges until after this tautening has occurred. However, if the mother is instructed to push from the onset of a contraction, pressure from the presenting part applied to the slack anterior yoni wall can result in the formation of a wrinkle of yoni tissue in front of the presenting part. This not only has the potential for impeding progress, but also for damaging the fascia of the bladder, leading to later complications such as incontinence and bladder prolapse (Sagady, 1995).

The head rocks down into the floor of the yoni as the woman pushes. The head tends to move back inside between contractions, sometimes by as much as a whole station or more, especially in a first-time mother with good muscle tone. This rocking pattern is minimized when the mother is upright but will still occur to a certain extent, although it may not occur at all during a fetus ejection reflex because the baby descends so rapidly. Rocking of the head is most pronounced when the woman is in a horizontal position, as the force of the contraction must overcome not only tissue resistance but also gravity to advance the presenting part.

The rocking of the head massages and softens the muscles, enabling them to open and embrace the head as it descends. The head rocks into the muscles, which thin and open, eventually dilating to allow the head to pass through. During crowning (the point when the head no longer rocks backward), slow, steady stretching of the introitus by the head between contractions accomplishes the same kind of thinning for the outer tissues.

This mechanism is poorly understood in North American obstetrics and is often misinterpreted as backsliding between contractions. Lack of understanding leads to forceful coaching of the mother, urging her to keep the baby's head low the entire time she is pushing, which, in turn, results in strained pushing efforts, little time between pushes and often a fluctuating fetal heart rate pattern due to inadequate oxygenation.

Distinguishing effective pushing: Effective pushing is judged by how far down the head rocks during a contraction, not how far back inside it rocks between them. It is quite normal to see the head rock down to the same station for several contractions and then suddenly make significant and permanent advancement forward. If you believe progress is impaired because certain muscles are exceptionally tight, use your fingers to help the mother identify where to relax. If the mother seems to have rocked the baby to a certain point but is not getting beyond it, encourage her to push past that point with her contractions; i.e., to rock the head a little further down each time she pushes. Changing her position can also be helpful, as can having her put her hand on the baby's head and push the baby into her own hands.

In almost every case, truly effective pushing will result in fetal descent. However, on rare occasions, this will not be the case. It then becomes imperative to be able to distinguish lack of descent due to faulty technique from a labor that is truly obstructed. To determine if effective pushing is taking place, insert two fingers into the yoni to feel how the pelvic floor is responding to maternal efforts. Look at the mother to make sure she is not stopping the push higher up in her body. Bulging in the vulval area, tension in unruptured membranes or both can be clues that the energy is being directed to the right place. A sense of bulging around the presenting part during active pushing may also be obvious, even if no descent takes place. Bulging of the vulva that persists between contractions and that is not related to perineal distention from the presenting part may in fact be swelling, a sign of obstruction. Once you get a feel for what the tissues feel like during effective pushing with descent, you will be able to tell if a woman is pushing effectively even if no descent is occurring. Effective pushing without descent is an indication of obstruction of some type. Experiment with different positions. Monitor the duration of effective pushing carefully. If nothing is working to bring the baby down, you may need to transport.

How long should women push?

The medical model places much emphasis on the speedy conclusion of labor, due, not in small part, to the institution's need to clear the room for the next laboring woman and professional pressure to clear the slate of patients for the next shift of staff. For many years, the medical model has defined the outside limit of "normal second stage" as two hours for first-time mothers and one hour for multiparas (although ACOG added an additional hour if the woman has an epidural). Averages are said to be 50 minutes for primigravidas and 20 minutes for multigravidas. In practice, "second stage" is usually assessed from complete dilation until birth, not accounting for the resting phase or periods when pushing is not happening or is not effective. In addition, hospital-based pushing protocols often involve forceful, sustained, directed pushing throughout contractions (which compromises mother and baby if continued for too long).

Menticoglou and colleagues (1995) found that pushing lasted more than 2 hours in a quarter of 6041 nulliparas at term and that a second phase that exceeded 6 hours was not related to fetal outcome (they attributed this to careful fetal monitoring and scalp pH assessments). They concluded that there is no compelling reason to intervene just because a certain amount of time has passed. They also found that the rate of instrumental or surgical intervention increased after the 3 hr mark and that only 10 to 15% of women gave birth spontaneously when pushing exceeded 6 hours.

While a fetus ejection reflex can be over in a few minutes, normal variations include active pushing that can start and stop or develop slowly; in rare cases, a woman will need to be taught how to push effectively. When this is true, the time spent pushing will not be continuous. How the mother and baby are faring, whether or not a caput or excessive moulding are developing, and the amount of descent are good criteria to use when evaluating how long is too long. In general, as long as the mother and baby are doing well and progress is being made during the contractions when effective pushing does take place, labor can take as long as it needs to take, rest periods included. However, you must be vigilant to make sure that everything is really okay when the pushing phase is prolonged.

Keeping records during pushing

The period of time the mother spends actively and effectively pushing is the most important factor in determining the length of the pushing phase of labor. Careful chart notes should reflect when the woman is really pushing and when she is resting or simply having nonexpulsive contractions and not pushing. You should also differentiate between effective pushing and noneffective pushing and make careful notes on the nuances of progress in terms of fetal descent. The regulations in some jurisdictions dictate an arbitrary amount of time pushing should take, counted from when complete dilation is determined. In these cases, postponing or eliminating internal exams can help to push the time frame back for these women. (If you haven't done an internal, you certainly can't chart complete dilation, now can you?) This strategy is already popular among hospital based nurse midwives who are navigating strict guidelines for practice.

Common difficulties that can arise during pushing

Helping the urge to push develop: If the mother has rested sufficiently and the presenting part is not well applied to the pelvic floor, place the mother in a tub of warm water with her hips and lower belly fully submerged. This often helps soften the perineum and allows the contractions to bring the baby down. Be sure to tell the mother to consciously relax her perineum and birth canal as she relaxes in the water. Playing a didgeridoo may also work wonders for developing more downward movement. Whenever there is a problem with pushing, simple remedies such as these should be tried before resorting to other, more aggressive interventions.

Unfocused or diffused pushing: A woman whose hormonal milieu is less than ideal may not understand how to center the effort of pushing in her yoni. She may be vocalizing with each urge and breathing well; however, it is obvious that her efforts are not bringing the baby down, as no progress is evident after 30 minutes or so (Simkin & Ancheta, 2000). The woman may be "getting ahead" of her labor and needs to be told to stop adding anything to the push.

Placing her in a bathtub of hot water, hips submerged, can help the uterus bring the baby down far enough to create more downward pressure in the yoni and stimulate a better urge to push within an hour or so. She may be too mentally involved in "trying to do it right" and need a dark, private space (like the bathroom) where she can better access her primitive brain.

Mixed messages regarding pushing: Sometimes the baby is very low, but the woman does not interpret the pressure as an urge to push. At one birth of a first-time mother, I could see the head but she walked and rested for quite a while with no pushing urge in sight. She finally said, "If only I wasn't so constipated, maybe I would feel like pushing." Once I explained to her that it was the baby she was feeling, she slowly figured out how to work with the sensation and push the baby out. Having a woman touch the baby's head can help her integrate what she is feeling.

Unphysiologic pushing: Forceful, sustained closed-glottis pushing is still the rule in many hospital settings. Caregivers may demand that the woman "hold-her-breath-and-push-push-push" while someone counts to ten (or more). She is then told to exhale, take another breath and push again, with a total of three or more efforts throughout each contraction. The woman is instructed to push in this fashion from the onset of each contraction until the baby is born. She may be told to push like this whether her uterus is pushing or not; the criterion for pushing in many institutional settings being complete dilation rather than the readiness of the body to begin active descent. The woman is often instructed to push as though she were having a bowel movement, which can leave her confused about where to direct the energy.

Holding the breath while straining to push utilizes the Valsalva maneuver, which was originally devised to expel pus from the middle ear. This type of pushing is detrimental for both mother and baby. Its emphasis on maximal maternal effort was introduced by natural childbirth educators in the 1950s as a way to "work" with the unphysiologic lithotomy position required during births in hospitals, in hopes that the baby would be born quickly enough to avoid a forceps delivery (Simkin & Ancheta, 2000).

The rationale for this approach is to get the baby out faster, thus theoretically minimizing maternal and newborn stress. In fact, pushing may or may not take longer if the woman pushes physiologically, following her body's cues. However, when physiologic pushing does take longer, no adverse effects have been noted in babies. Ironically, the hospital environment is not conducive to purely physiologic labor, which produces the fastest pushing phase of all, with an uninhibited fetus ejection reflex.

There are more disadvantages to unphysiologic pushing. Holding the breath creates a closed high-pressure system in the chest, decreasing both venous return and arterial blood pressure as well as lowering cardiac output. This decreases the amount of blood flowing to the heart when oxygen intake is already dramatically reduced. Arterial pressure is the force that delivers blood to the uterus; the longer sustained pushing goes on, the more arterial pressure continues to fall, and the longer the baby's oxygen supply is compromised. Blood flow to the uterus stops at intrauterine pressures above 50 to 60 mm Hg. While the healthy infant is well prepared for the temporary lack of oxygen that occurs during physiologic pushing, the sustained lack of oxygen resulting from sustained unphysiologic pushing is unduly stressful. The baby also suffers because unphysiologic pushing prolongs head compression; as a result, the fetal heart rate may drop dramatically. These effects can be tolerated by most term fetuses, but the preterm or small-for-dates baby may fare worse, as will the baby experiencing some cord compression. In short, unphysiologic pushing is not related to better neonatal outcomes and may contribute to poor ones.

Unphysiologic pushing also directly compromises the mother because blood flow returning to her heart is impeded; the woman's head, face, arms and legs become congested with blood. When an IV is in place, blood can often be seen backing up into the catheter. Maternal carbon dioxide levels rise until the mother lets her breath go and gasps, which causes her blood pressure to shoot up. Eventually, blood vessels burst in her face, neck and the sclera of her eyes. Rapid distention and stretching of the pelvic soft tissues leads to perineal edema and trauma, resulting in damage that increases the chance that the woman will develop urinary incontinence in later life. Maternal exhaustion is common with this type of pushing as well.

Some hospital practitioners recommend sustained open-glottis pushing following the same basic pattern described above except that 3 or 4 second breath-holding periods are followed by bearing down as the woman lets her breath out slowly. This approach, while far from ideal, involves less sustained intrathoracic pressure, reducing some of the detrimental effects of sustained closed-glottis pushing.

Forceful, sustained pushing, especially if begun before a spontaneous urge to push is established, may severely strain the pelvic supportive tissue and cause undue stress to upper yoni tissues, resulting in tears even before the head is visible at the introitus. The risk is even higher if active pushing is started before the presenting part reaches the pelvic floor. It can also cause trauma to the pelvic muscles (particularly if no progress is being made).

Sometimes women have an urge to push prior to complete dilation. (For details see the chapter entitled "Cervical and Other Soft-Tissue Problems during Labor.") Frequently, hospital staff misinterpret lack of descent during premature (and thus ineffective) pushing to be the result of cephalopelvic disproportion and perform an unnecessary surgical delivery (Cosner & deJong, 1993; McKay & Roberts, 1985; Sagady, 1995; Simkin & Ancheta, 2000).

Physical impediments to pushing: An excessively long and exhausting labor may complicate pushing by leaving both the mother and uterine muscle tired. The position of the baby's head may not be ideal. A full bowel or bladder may also inhibit descent or cause pain during pushing. Of course, lack of progress may be due to an obstruction (such as a cyst or tumor), as well as true cephalopelvic disproportion (CPD). However, CPD is extremely rare in mature women with no history of rickets or pelvic bone injury. (When assessing progress via internal exams, always be sure the skull is advancing and you are not merely monitoring a caput or extreme moulding that is becoming more severe.)

Weak, widely spaced or absent contractions: Spontaneous bearing down is not going to occur if the uterus is not contracting. Most of the time contractions do not stop completely during the resting phase. When they do, a delay of many minutes or hours may go by while the woman rests and eats. In most cases, contractions spontaneously resume. Sometimes, however, they do not. Often when they do not, there are underlying psychological issues impeding the flow of birthing energy. Sometimes it seems that the baby is resisting birth. If so, once these issues are acknowledged (including talking to the baby), the mother can make a decision to transport for oxytocic augmentation or attempt augmentation with nipple stimulation, herbs, homeopathic remedies, and effleurage at home (see the chapter entitled "Natural Induction and Augmentation of Labor"). Once contractions have resumed, they will build into spontaneous pushing (with any luck).

Occasionally, contractions will be good and strong in one position, only to peter out when the woman changes position. If this occurs, keep experimenting with positions until the woman finds a good position for pushing with good contractions. If contractions do not pick up, you can attempt to assist fetal descent and help the mother learn how to push as described above. *Do not attempt to complete the birth without the reestablishment of good, regular contractions.* No contractions during pushing can forebode lack of contractions for getting the placenta out, which is a set-up for postpartum hemorrhage.

Directed pushing

If the suggestions offered above do not produce any changes for the better and the woman still cannot focus her energy or if her pushing efforts seem to dissipate into nonproductive effort, you can gently guide her. Have her insert her fingers into her yoni to identify the baby's presenting part. Help her to assume a more upright position, as gravity will assist her in directing her pushing energy. It often helps to ask the woman to push as though she were trying to expel a tampon from her yoni. Having her cough forcefully between contractions while noticing how her perineum opens can also help her direct the pushing energy when a contraction occurs. Never tell a woman to push as though she were having a bowel movement because the energy needs to be centered in the yoni, not the rectum. Rectally centered pushing may move the baby down as a by-product but will also aggravate hemorrhoids and be unduly stressful for the pelvic floor.

Teaching the mother to push effectively: If a long resting phase has come and gone, absolutely nothing else is working to bring on an urge to push, the baby is at least +1 station, the mother cannot rest and regroup and psychological issues have been discussed, you can try to teach the mother to push. (This also helps if the mother is disoriented, is moving away from the pressure in her pelvis or has a history of abuse.) First, have her get on a birthing stool that allows full sacral mobility or into the Birth Sling. Don gloves and place two fingers of each of your hands inside the yoni at 4 and 8 o'clock. As the contraction builds, use the length of the first two fingers of both hands to apply deep bilateral pressure into the urogenital diaphragm (the muscular ring about a third of the way inside the introitus). This stimulates the proprioceptors in the yoni, triggers the release of oxytocin, and simulates the pressure of the presenting part, which prompts an urge to push. As the mother pushes, gradually draw your fingers outward while maintaining pressure. Then, if necessary, reinsert your fingers and repeat this massage.

Have her push *through her yoni* into the pressure while consciously relaxing her birth canal. She can hold her breath to get a feel for where she is focusing the energy of the push, but since it is the direction of the push that moves the baby, (rather than hard pushing with breath holding), long periods of pushing with sustained breath holding should not be instructed beyond what is necessary for the mother to get a sense of what she needs to do. Physiologic breath holding for no more than 6 seconds is usually sufficient for her to learn where to push. Place a mirror between her legs or invite her to insert her own fingers to see and feel if her pushing efforts are effective. If no progress is made after a few contractions, do not continue. She will only exhaust herself and exert undue strain on her uterine and cervical ligaments.

Simultaneously monitor how the mother is relaxing and if her introitus is bulging as she pushes (or if the head is rocking). If the head is not visible, keep a finger inside to tell her when you feel the head advance with her efforts. Very often it helps tremendously when you tell her she is pushing correctly and ask her to note what was different during that push. Watch her mouth and shoulders as well as her introitus. If she is holding all of her pushing effort above the diaphragm, she is pushing ineffectually. (This "high" pushing is frequently seen when women are afraid of the pressure, have been sexually abused or are afraid of tearing.) Ask her to redirect the energy downward.

If she has not been successful in learning to push in an upright position, have her lie flat on the floor with her legs held up, widely apart. Although this constitutes pushing uphill (down, around, and up under the pubic bone and up the perineum), it can help to increase the pressure on the perineum by tightening it, and therefore can assist in stimulating an urge to push. After pushing is established and the baby is lower, she can try another position.

Teaching the mother to push works best if the uterus is contracting well but simply not bearing down. Some women, by sheer force of will and an intuitive understanding, can overcome the lack of a pushing urge and move the baby down.

MATERNAL POSITION DURING PUSHING AND AT THE TIME OF BIRTH

The position that the mother chooses during pushing depends upon her instincts and her hormonal milieu at the end of dilation as well as her strength and stamina. She should choose the position that best enhances the quality of her contractions and her ability to push; if she is experiencing a fetus ejection reflex, she will do so instinctively. The midwife needs to ensure that whatever position the mother assumes preserves fetal well-being as reflected by a normal fetal heart rate and the skin color of the presenting part.

An ideal position allows the mother's sacrum and coccyx the freedom to rotate backward, the rest of the pelvis room to open to optimal dimensions to allow for birth, and contractions to remain strong and close together. It is amazing how often what appears to be an otherwise ideal position slows contractions down. Whatever position works for a particular woman is the correct position for her. It is quite natural for women to change positions several times in the course of pushing. Some women even change positions after the head is out.

Understanding How the Pelvis Works during Pushing

As you read the following discussion of positions used for pushing and for birth, I suggest that you assume these positions yourself and check your own pelvic bones to gauge whether they are free to move and how much movement occurs when you shift your legs. Keep in mind that any movement you detect will differ from that experienced by a laboring woman because the hormones of late pregnancy and labor soften her ligaments and cartilage. It is also helpful to have a pelvic model on hand so you can see clearly which bones receive the most pressure and are afforded the most mobility in different positions (Robertson, 1998).

If some of the pelvic diameters are snug or the head is not ideally positioned, changing positions every two or three pushes will often help work the baby down past the tight spot. Some women will do this instinctively, while others may need guidance. Women also tend to reach up and grasp something above their waist during late pushing when experiencing a fetus ejection reflex. This lengthens the torso and makes it easy to sag the belly forward as the sacrum moves backward. Some general tips to avoid problems:

Be sure the surface below the woman is firm: A firm surface provides stability for upright positions and very little give for more horizontal positions. A soft, squashy bed into which the woman's bottom sinks is never helpful for any part of labor. If you believe that a soft surface makes her more comfortable and affords more sacral mobility, think again. What little sacral mobility it may afford is more than negated by having the mother's bottom sinking into an indentation that exaggerates the curve of the birth canal, making moving to another position extremely difficult and affording less access to the baby should you need to provide hands-on assistance.

Be sure her bladder is empty before pushing begins: If pushing takes some time, have her urinate again, before the head becomes too low.

Be sure the mother is accessible from the front and at least one side: Do not let the mother corner herself into a tight space to give birth, especially if pushing is taking a while. Birth in a tight space will impair your ability to assist her should that be required.

Positions for Pushing

Horizontal positions

I begin with horizontal positions of all kinds not because they are the best but because they are still frequently used by many practitioners both in and out of hospital.

Semi-sitting (approximately 45° angle or so) positions: Semi-sitting positions with the sacrum, rather than the tuberosities, supporting the mother's weight are employed to get pressure off the inferior vena cava. However, other than hanging head down by the ankles, semi-sitting is the worst possible position for pushing. The angle of the seated position and the position of the legs may or may not permit the tuberosities to move to a limited extent. For example, a reclining position of 30° to 45° allows the most tuberosity movement because they are not resting on the bed. However, movement of the sacrum and coccyx is impossible since all the mother's weight is transferred to these bones. If the mother's coccyx is fused and immobile due to a previous injury, this limits the space at the outlet even more.

Semi-sitting also narrows the brim, reducing its angle in relation to the spine from a tilt of 120° to a level plane of about 90°. This leveling effect occurs throughout the pelvic cavity, reducing the space available for the baby to maneuver. All seated postures with the feet flat and legs raised also exaggerate the curve of the birth canal, which is made worse when a woman forms her back into a "C" shape and holds her legs or knees up against her torso, as is so often advised in hospital births because this reverses the lordosis of late pregnancy (Sutton & Scott, 1996). The mouth of the outlet is now directed upward, greatly exaggerating the curve of the birth canal and requiring the mother to work against gravity to bring the head under the pubic arch. Whereas normally the baby's spine straightens out during late labor as the baby prepares to pass directly down and out through the open, gently curved birth canal of the upright mother, now the baby must contort his spine to navigate through this convoluted passageway.

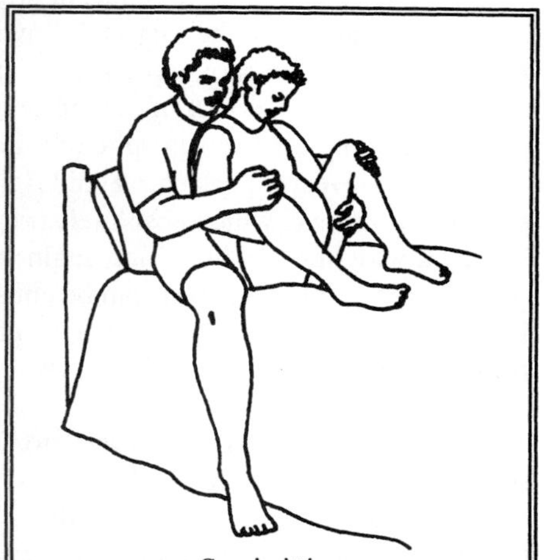

Semi-sitting

(Redrawn with permission from illustrations by Stella Cruz, © Ruth Ancheta, 2000)

Leveling the pelvic brim can also hinder shoulder rotation. If the chest and shoulders have not yet undergone their first internal rotation, this can jam the shoulder axis against the sacral promontory as the brim catches the anterior shoulder, thus hindering rotation to the transverse. This invites the anterior shoulder to get stuck behind the pubic arch. Reduced space at the outlet may hinder the second internal rotation of the shoulders and make it harder for the midwife to see if shoulder rotation is occurring normally. Finally, the contracting uterus must work against gravity to "rear up" from a reclining position, wasting some of the energy of the contraction and making the mother's work that much harder.

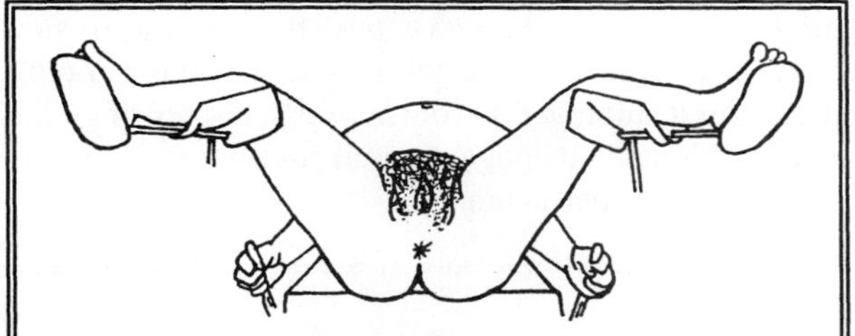

Lithotomy position on hospital delivery table

<u>Supine positions</u>: Supine positions of any kind are not recommended. Both the lithotomy position (where the woman is flat on her back, with her legs spread, bottom hanging halfway off the table and feet high up in stirrups) and the dorsal position (where she is flat on her back with her feet flat on the birthing surface, no stirrups). Supine positions allow more movement of the tuberosities and coccyx than semi-sitting. However, neither position allows for much sacral movement. Many hospitals have the woman move her bottom to the end of the delivery table, then elevate and widen her legs by placing her feet in stirrups (the wider the legs are spaced, the tenser the perineum will be) making access easier for the birth attendant. This adjustment also widens the pelvic outlet, although the large pelvic bones are, for all practical purposes, immobilized in all types of dorsal positions. Also, the curve of the birth canal is somewhat exaggerated (although less so than in a semi-sit). In addition, the heavy uterus is pressing on the inferior vena cava, resulting in hypotension in the mother and decreased blood flow to the uterus. For other problems with supine positions in general, see the section on semi-sitting, above.

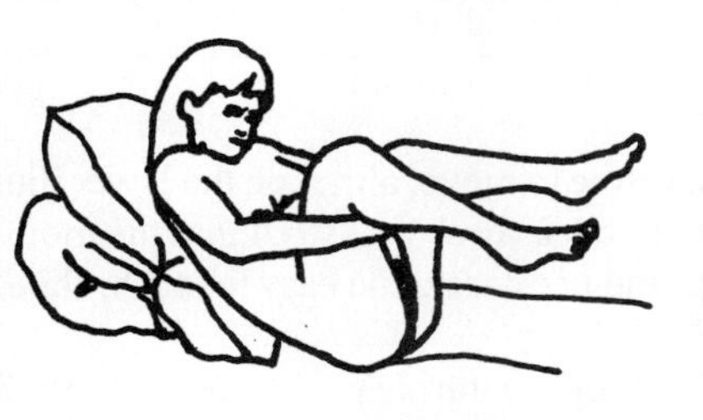

Semi-seated, lithotomy style

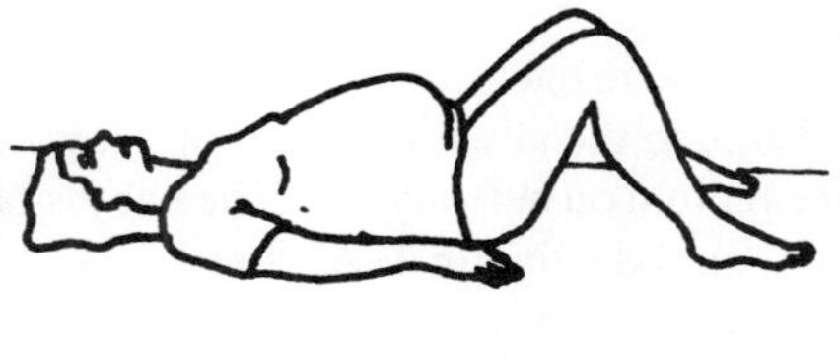

Dorsal position

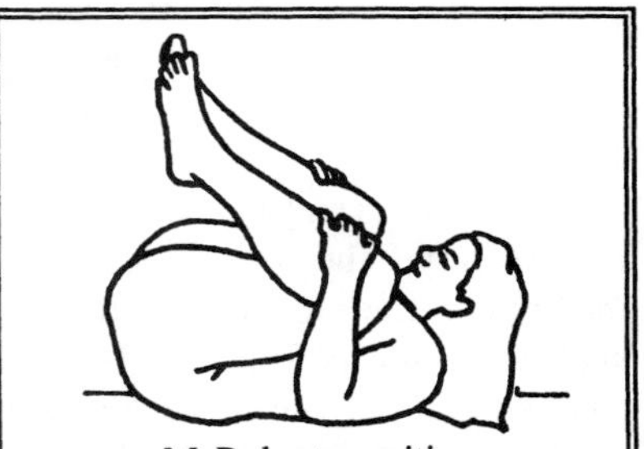

McRoberts position

(Redrawn with permission from illustrations by Stella Cruz, © Ruth Ancheta, 2000)

As Sutton and Scott (1996) and Robertson (1998) point out, women in seated or reclining positions instinctively raise their bottoms off the bed, lift a leg, or attempt to roll to one side during pushing. This is an unconscious response aimed at getting pressure off the sacrum, allowing more pelvic mobility and increasing the angle between the pubic bone and the spine to give the baby more room to descend as the head comes under the pubic bone. That many women manage to give birth in some sort of supine or semi-sitting position is only testimony to the incredible tendency of the birth process to complete itself in spite of unphysiologic interventions.

It is, however, important to avoid rigidity in midwifery, never say never and instead focus on whatever works. I have seen a few births in which absolutely no position worked to bring the baby down other than having the mother lie flat on her back with her legs held high against her belly (McRoberts position). When this is what it takes to bring the baby down, often another position can be chosen once the presenting part is well under the pubic bone and the pushing urge is established. In one case in which the mother had previously broken her coccyx, the baby was not born until the mother pushed in this position while lying flat on a hard surface.

McRoberts position: This is a variation on the supine position, where the mother lies on a firm surface, flat on her back, with her legs hyperflexed and her knees brought up as high as possible to either side of her abdomen. This position tilts the pubic bone upward, narrowing the inlet but widening the pelvic outlet; it is used in the medical model as a measure to prevent shoulder dystocia and to pivot the pubic bone up when shoulder dystocia has developed. It is intended to release the anterior shoulder and widen the pelvic outlet.

Sutton (2001) states that bringing the knees to the belly for pushing is the worst thing you can do because it narrows the brim and thus is likely to interfere with shoulder rotation and descent. It also stretches and tightens the large gluteal muscles of the buttocks, which will impair movement of the coccyx as well as increase tension in the pelvic floor. The pros and cons of the McRoberts position are discussed in greater detail in the chapter entitled "Shoulder Dystocia."

Side-lying positions:

Top-leg supported: A left, side-lying position works well for many women, especially if labor has been long or if the mother, for any reason, feels unable to sustain her weight in an upright position long enough to push the baby out. A side-lying position provides some of the benefits of an upright position because it allows some pelvic mobility. It is a gravity-neutral position, taking the weight off the inferior vena cava and making it suitable for women with a history of genital wall prolapses or varicosities of any kind, weak perineal muscles, sphincter damage, genital mutilation or uterine inversion because it slows the birth down and puts less direct pressure on the perineum.

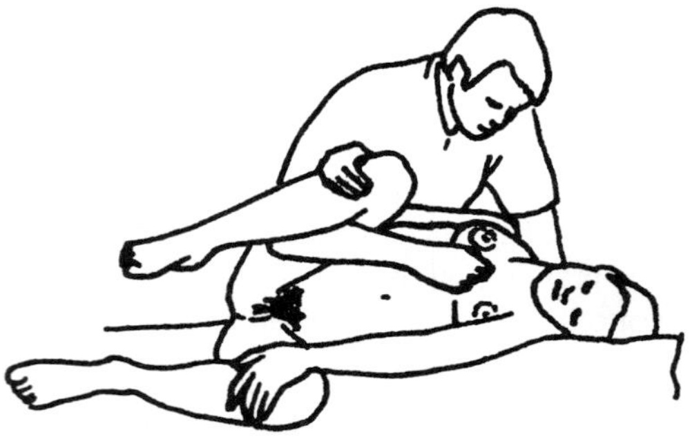

Side-lying with top leg supported

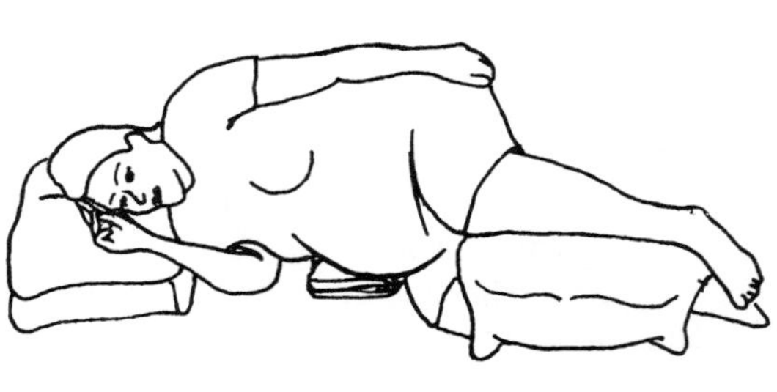

Side-lying legs together with knee and belly support

(Redrawn with permission from illustrations by Stella Cruz, © Ruth Ancheta, 2000)

The sacrum and coccyx are also free to rotate backward, and the upper ilium is free to move, although the lower ilium is stationary. The perineum is quite visible to the attending midwife. It is easy to clear away any stool that the mother may pass as the baby presses against the rectum on her way out. The baby's face and neck are quite easy to reach, should suctioning or cord disentanglement be required (Simkin & Ancheta, 2000).

While side-lying either the laboring woman or a support person can hold up her top leg during pushes and as the baby emerges. Alternatively, the leg can be supported by placing an underinflated beach ball between the woman's knees. Some midwives also use pillows to support the upper leg. The cane-style Push-and-Pull device can be used to elevate the mother's upper leg as well: have a support person hold one end, the mother hold the other and rest the upper leg on the straight bar between the hooks. Instead of supporting the top leg, it often works better for the mother to raise the top leg, bend it at the knee and plant the foot on the bed. This creates more room in the uppermost portion of the pelvic cavity. If the baby is engaged or lower and the occiput is still transverse or anterior oblique, the mother can roll to the side opposite the back (if the baby is ROA, she rolls her left side), and bend her upper leg forward to slant her pelvis. This can help complete the process of rotation to OA.

Legs together: It is also possible for the mother to give birth with her legs completely together if they are sufficiently flexed at the hips and knees, with the top leg flexed slightly further forward than the bottom. This was a favored position in Victorian times because it maintains the woman's modesty. It also places minimal strain on the perineum. In fact, some midwives recommend keeping the legs as close together as possible, as this allows maximal anteroposterior stretching of the perineum, which they feel is much reduced when the top leg is supported (Gentlebirth midwifery archives, 2001). A thin pillow can be placed between the knees for comfort and a folded towel can be placed under the abdomen for support.

Side-lying McRoberts: In this position, the mother assumes a McRoberts position, as described above, and then rolls over on her side. This arrangement is recommended by some as a good position for preventing shoulder dystocia, although it tightens the brim (see the chapter entitled "Shoulder Dystocia" for a discussion of this position).

Upright postures

Upright postures include standing, squatting and kneeling. An upright posture lessens the amount of rocking the presenting part does during pushing, creating more continuous pressure on the perineum between contractions, which in turn facilitates stretching. Most upright postures involve an angle greater than 90° between the spine and the thighs, which keeps the spinopubic angle open. With no pressure on the sacrum and coccyx, these bones are free to release and move out of the way. Leaning forward pivots the sacrum, coccyx and levator ani sling of the perineal floor up and back, so that the baby is passing more in front of the muscular sling than through it. Any postures that combine these features are generally the most conducive to a rapid pushing phase and will typically be chosen instinctively by a woman experiencing a fetus ejection reflex. Women often reach for something above their waists as the baby moves down, so having something in front of her to grab onto, such as someone's shoulders, is helpful.

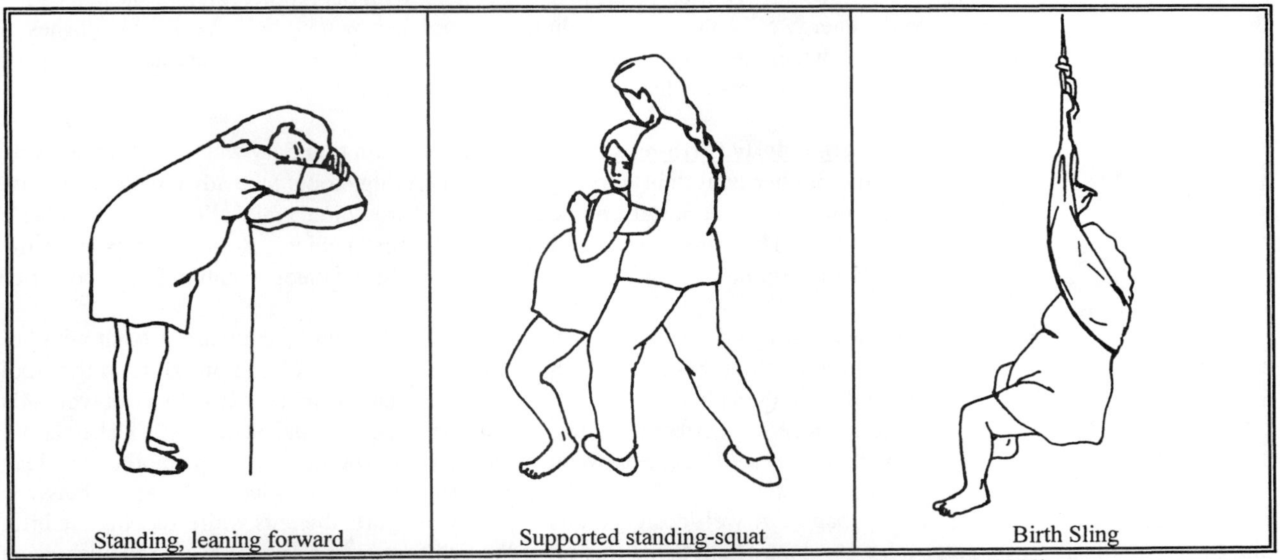

(Redrawn with permission from illustrations by Stella Cruz, © Ruth Ancheta, 2000)

Standing, leaning forward: An ideal position for birth, as described above. The woman can allow her back to sway forward, which brings the angle between the pelvis and the uterus into a straighter line for descent. Some women even choose to stand completely unsupported to give birth.

Supported standing-squat: This position, popularized by Michel Odent, is great for a woman who needs or wants support but wishes to give birth fully upright. A standing support person bends his elbows and passes his forearms under the arms of the mother, interlocking his fingers with hers. The support person uses his forearms to support the woman under her armpits. The back of the support person should be against a wall, with his knees bent slightly to avoid back strain. During a contraction, the woman bends her knees to drop her bottom down and pushes, supported by the strength of the person holding her up. The angle of her thighs should never be less than 90° in relationship to her spine. Between contractions, she can stand, giving the support person a break; however, she will probably want to remain in a standing squat once crowning begins. Obviously, the support person must be bigger and stronger than the mother and, even then, may tire quickly.

The Dangle: An alternative way to support the mother that works equally well for her and demands less of the support person involves an adaptation called "the dangle," which was devised by Penny Simkin. The support person sits on a high, firm surface, such as a kitchen counter top with her legs supported so that her thighs are at a 90° angle to the floor and her bottom is part-way off the surface to make plenty of room between her legs (you will have to search for furniture and books that can make the supports the proper height). The mother places her back between the support person's legs, with her forearms resting on her thighs. The support person grips the mother's torso with his thighs and supports her weight with his legs as the mother drops down and hangs free, using her feet to balance while pushing. Between contractions, the mother can stand.

Penny has also designed the Birth Sling (see the drawing on the last page) to allow the woman to be fully supported in the dangle position. The Sling allows her to move her torso and pelvis in a variety of ways and lift her feet entirely so that she is freely suspended. The mother can also place her back against a wall and use the Sling as support to stand and squat without other assistance, although the mother must then support herself with her legs, so she does not get the benefit of being suspended.

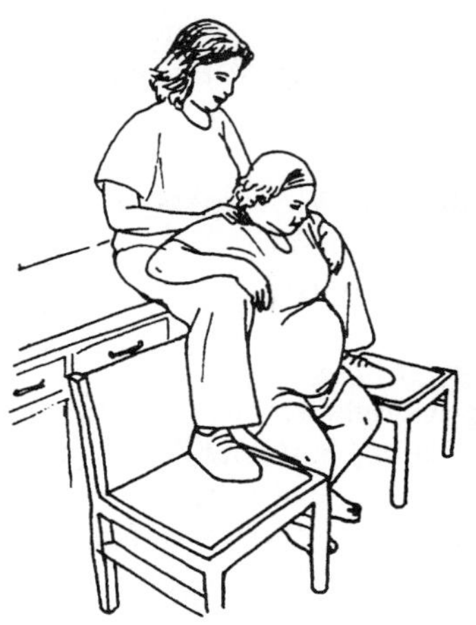
The Dangle

Amplifying the birthing energy: Anytime a support person is in direct contact with the mother's torso, she can add to the mother's efforts by opening to the energy of birth and channeling it through her own body as the woman pushes. I have seen this technique work very well when the mother was tired and stronger pushing efforts were needed or when the mother needs psychic assistance in grounding and channeling the energy of birth.

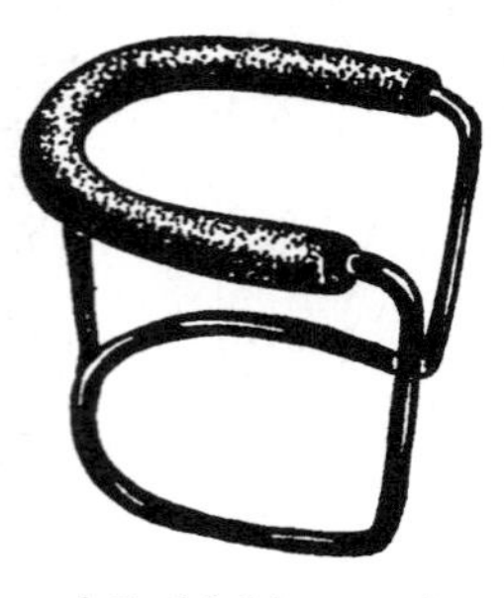
deBy birthing stool

Birth with a deBy birthing stool: Generally speaking, gravity works most effectively when the mother is upright during pushing. Birthing stools take advantage of gravity, helping the baby move past the pubic bone toward crowning, while allowing the mother's legs to rest. They are especially helpful with first babies. Stools can increase the efficiency of contractions and encourage the baby's spontaneous rotation from a posterior position.

A well-designed birthing support, such the deBy, allows the woman to sit with her feet flat on the floor, her back straight and her sacrum free of compression. If the stool is too tall, telephone books or other large supports can be placed under a short woman's feet to achieve the correct posture. According to Sutton and Scott (1996), she should maintain at least a 90° angle between her spine and the pubic bone. The mother may lean forward or back to push and then rest backward into someone's arms between contractions (see drawings on the next page). A well-designed birthing stool supports the legs while keeping the brim and the outlet open. Sitting on such a stool may help the uterus bring the baby down and create an urge to push, even if the baby is higher than 0 station.

Deep (full) squat: This position only works well after the baby is well positioned and well engaged. If used before this, it is likely to hinder engagement or encourage engagement in an undesirable position. Even after engagement, it reduces the spinopubic angle from 120° to between 45 and 65°, making descent and rotation of the shoulders and chest more difficult. Exaggeration of the pelvic curve requires the fetus to maximally flex his spine to maneuver around the pubic arch. Deep squatting done before the biparietal diameter passes the brim (and, in some women, prior to its reaching the ischial spines), or if the baby is above 0 station, will not facilitate progress (Fairman, 1990).

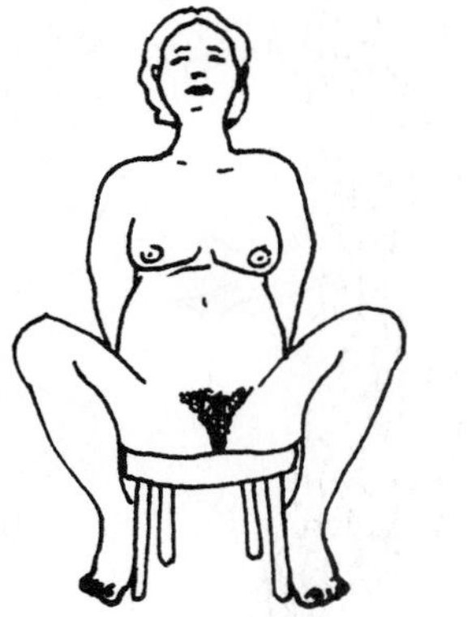

Poorly designed birthing stool (knees too high, seat putting pressure on sacrum)

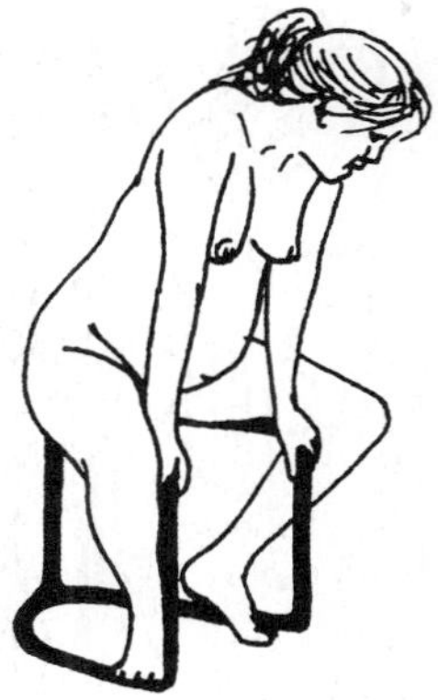

The deBy birthing stool (knees correct height, no pressure on sacrum if woman leans forward, moves up or if she sits on the stool with the opening to the rear.)

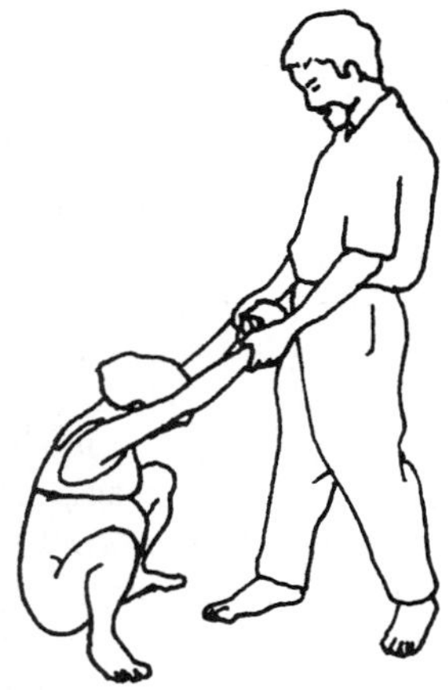

Deep (full) squat with support

(Left and right boxes redrawn with permission from illustrations by Stella Cruz, © Ruth Ancheta, 2000)
(Center box drawn from a photograph provided by deBy Birth Supports and Cilia Bannenberg, with permission, 2004)

If the baby is at a plus station and engaged in a desirable position, squatting can stimulate the urge to push by exaggerating the pressure on the perineum. It can also help a woman who is resisting the sensations of pushing by moving her down into the energy or a woman whose baby is receding dramatically between contractions (Schlinger, 2003).

Although many midwives find deep squatting after the baby is well into the pelvis quite useful, Sutton and Scott (1996) advise against deep squats, even after engagement, because of the narrowing of the brim. If the woman does not seem to benefit from a deep squat position, abandon it in favor of positions that place the knees lower than the tuberosities and thus maintain a wider spinopubic angle.

To do a deep squat properly, the woman should have her feet flat on the floor, with her knees directly in line with her toes and her bottom low to the ground. Two people should be on either side of the woman to help her maintain her balance and provide support. Alternatively, one support person can sit on a stool or on the edge of a low bed with her legs spread wide; the woman can then squat facing outward and use the knees for support. To avoid stiffness in the legs, the woman (and support person) should stand and walk frequently, interspersing walking with squatting. In cultures where squatting is not a commonly used position, prolonged squatting compresses blood vessels and nerves behind the knees, impairing circulation, and may lead to entrapment neuropathy. Standing or leaning back between contractions also avoids these more serious problems (Simkin & Ancheta, 2000).

One of the best tools for assisting a woman to maintain any kind of squat is the Push-and-Pull device. One end of this device is held by the mother and the other is held by a support person. Both then go down into a squat. The counterbalance of the support person helps the mother maintain her position. Be sure the support person is at least the same size as the mother. Another option for squatting of any type is to use a chin-up bar installed in a doorway, the level of which can be altered according to the mother's height and depth of squatting.

Suspended rear squat: This position can be used any time maximal opening of the midplane and pelvic outlet is required in a woman whose baby is deeply engaged. Have a support person sit in a sturdy chair with no arms (such as a kitchen or dining room chair) with their bottom near the edge of the chair and knees spread widely apart. Have the mother straddle the legs of the seated person, with her knees approximately next to the support person's hips and her toes pointing toward the back of the chair. The mother lowers her bottom so that it hangs suspended between the support person's thighs (which reduces the spinopubic angle). The support person can wrap his arms around the woman's back and interlace his fingers to support her firmly or hold the hands of an additional support person, as illustrated (Simkin

& Ancheta, 2000).

Suspended forward squat: A support person sits in a chair, as above. The mother then sits on her lap, with her back to the support person. During pushes, the support person holds the mother and spreads her legs, so that the mother's bottom is suspended between the support person's legs, with her thighs on top of and supported by the support person's thighs. The mother can rest her feet on stable surfaces on either side of her that are approximately half the height of the chair. The support person wraps her arms around the mother to hold her during pushing or reaches under her arms, to apply pressure to the mother's thighs during pushing, removing her arms between contractions so the mother does not have to rest her arms on those of the support person, thereby avoiding radial nerve compression. This position allows more pelvic mobility; the mother can tip her pelvis forward.

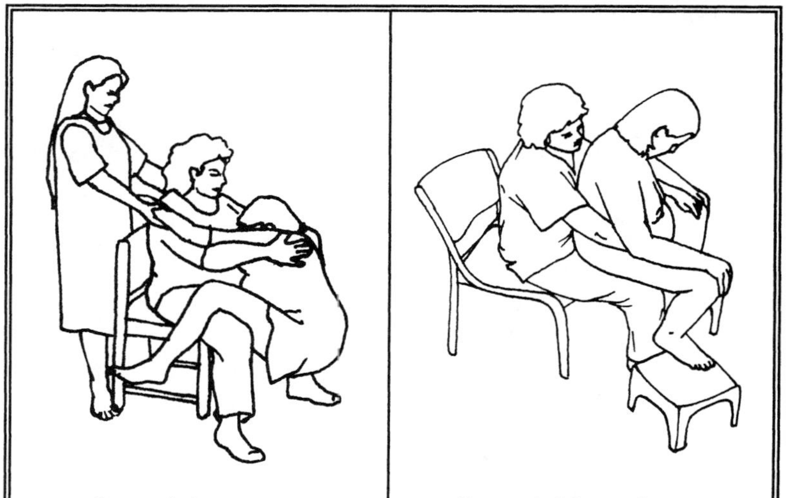

Suspended rear squat — Suspended forward squat

(Left box redrawn from illustrations by Stella Cruz, © Ruth Ancheta, 2000; right box drawn from a photograph by Ruth Ancheta, 2004; with permission.)

It also allows the spinopubic angle to stay more open because the mother's bottom does not drop down as far as in a suspended rear squat. It can be adapted to a squat when the mother lets her bottom drop further downward, using the support person's thighs to rest her arms.

Supported extended squat: Irena Sotelo (2001), a traditional Mexican midwife, uses a modification of the same basic position described above. The support person sits in a sturdy chair. The birthing woman sits on his lap, facing forward, then leans back and stretches her legs straight out on either side. Two other support people hold the mother's feet up at about a 45° angle. Irena finds that this position can help when nothing else has worked to bring the baby out.

One-sided upright kneeling: The mother gets on her knees with her spine straight, then brings one leg up so that her foot is flat on the floor in front of her. Alternatively, she can lean forward on a support person or a piece of furniture. This position rotates the pelvis, helping the baby's shoulders rotate, come beneath the pubic bone and emerge without getting stuck. (For more details, see the chapter entitled "Shoulder Dystocia.")

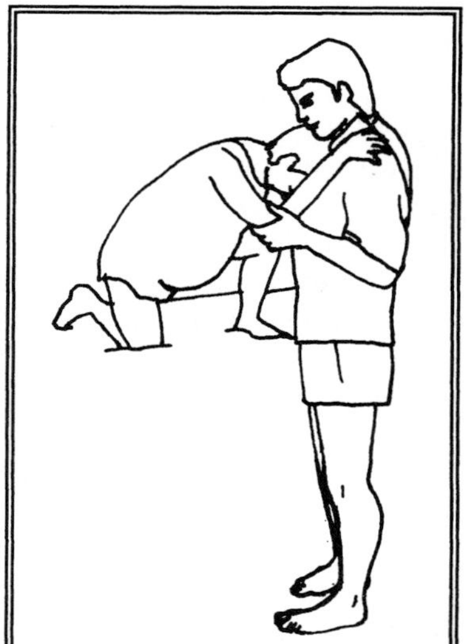

One-sided kneeling

(Redrawn with permission from illustrations by Stella Cruz, © Ruth Ancheta, 2000)

Full kneel, knees spread, leaning forward: The mother pushes while supporting herself on her knees and leaning forward with her spine straight and her thighs spread apart. She can brace her hands on her thighs. Or, she can quite comfortably elevate her bottom and support her upper body with her arms resting on the side of the bed, which is a good height for many women. Note that moving back to "sit" on the feet with hands planted on the bed makes tearing more likely. The mother may lift her torso, reach up and thrust the pelvis forward as the baby moves down and the sacrum releases (Sutton, 2001).

Hands-and-knees: The mother is on her hands and knees, or on her knees with her upper body supported by someone's lap, a birth-ball, a bean-bag chair or the back of someone who is also in a hands-and-knees position. This position opens the pelvis, gives the midwife excellent visualization of the perineum, and helps some women develop a stronger urge to push. The transverse diameter of the midpelvis is increased, the spinopubic angle remains open and the ischial spines can easily be moved out of alignment if the mother moves her hips. Swaying her back raises the sacrum and coccyx out of the path of descent. The woman may remain on her knees while raising the back as the baby emerges.

This is not a good position for women with a pendulous abdomen nor should it be used during the birth of a first baby in a multiple birth. In both cases, the abdomen is distended forward, which may make pushing harder. With a multiple birth, the extra room created in the uterus by the birth of the first baby can result in the second baby floating into an unfavorable position. If the mother with lax abdominal muscles really wants to try this position, some of these risks may be lessened by placing a couple of large pillows under the abdomen for support or by using a belly binder. See the chapter entitled "Shoulder Dystocia" for a more thorough discussion of the hands-and-knees position.

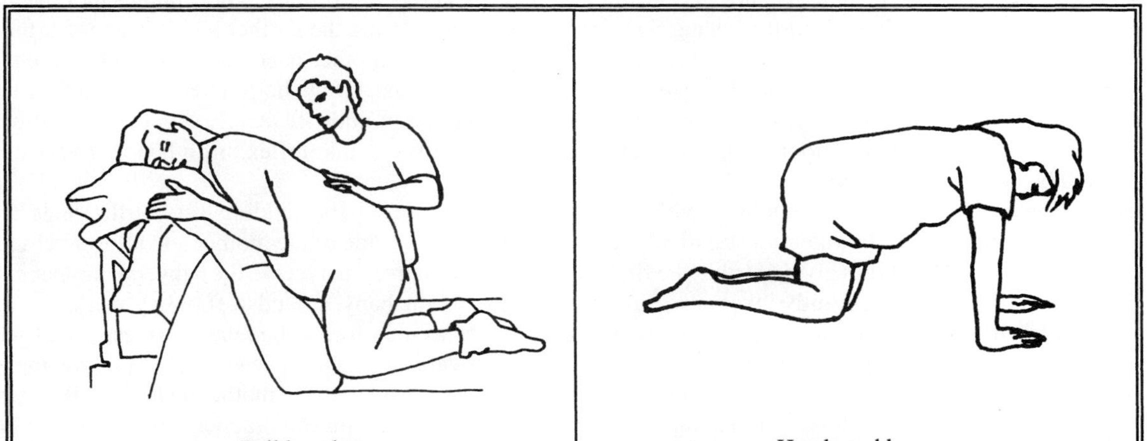

Full kneel | Hands and knees

(Redrawn with permission from illustrations by Stella Cruz, © Ruth Ancheta, 2000)

Assisting at the Birth of a Vertex Baby

How, or even if, a midwife needs to assist the emergence of the baby as the head distends the perineum will depend upon both the position of the mother and her willingness to actively assist the birth herself. Either of these factors may change several times during pushing, crowning and birth. Regardless of the mother's position, ensure that she is undistracted, which will make the need for assistance much less likely. Place a soft "landing pad" beneath her in case the baby should unexpectedly fall out.

There are many opinions on how to best receive the baby as he emerges, varying from a completely hands-off approach to specific hand maneuvers that are used for every birth and modified according to maternal position and fetal presentation. The idea that manual assistance is necessary has been fostered in hospitals, where babies have been born to women lying on a table with their bottoms hanging over a tile floor, rendering the mother helpless to assist the birth herself and a hands-off approach by the care provider dangerous. When the mother is not constrained to assume such an unnatural posture, it is best to assess each birth individually and decide what, if any, help is needed as each part of the baby is born. *Most of the time, no hands-on assistance is needed,* the mother or midwife merely supports the baby as she emerges so she doesn't drop to the floor. If the mother experiences a fetus ejection reflex, birth happens very quickly and there will be no time to do anything else!

Cornelia Enning (2003), a German midwife with a totally hands-off approach to attending waterbirths, feels her tear rate is low for this reason. While watching attentively, Cornelia stands to the side of the mother and allows her to do as much as she will to assist herself in giving birth. She finds if she positions herself to receive the baby, the mother expects her to do so and is likely to be less fully involved. Since water supports the baby, a hands-off policy works well.

This chapter will discuss procedures appropriate for all births, such as monitoring the fetal heart, as well as what to do in the event that hands-on assistance is needed during the straightforward emergence of a vertex baby. Drawings were rendered from photographs showing the birth of the head from the LOA position with the mother on her hands and knees. It is extremely helpful to have a life-size doll and pelvic model on hand so that you can practice how you might handle the baby as he comes out with the mother in different positions.

Assessing fetal well-being during pushing

Attend to the condition of the baby throughout pushing efforts by auscultating the fetal heart rate and evaluating the scalp color. How to do so and the normal variations to expect are covered in the chapter entitled "Assessing and Supporting the Baby's Well-Being during Labor."

The perineum

Observe the condition of the perineum before the head is born. (More details about perineal care during birth can be found in the chapter entitled "Caring for the Mother's Soft Tissues at the Time of Birth" in this section of the book.) If a fetus ejection reflex occurs, the baby will come out quickly. If not, the head rocks forward with a push and then recedes between contractions. This process massages the pelvic floor open, making more and more room for the head beneath the curve of the pubic bone. This rocking process is less pronounced when the mother is upright because the head tends to stay more forward between contractions than it does when she is horizontal. Once the pelvic floor is sufficiently softened, the biparietal diameter will stay beneath the pubic arch, and crowning will begin.

Passage of stool by the mother

Any stool in the rectum is pressed out as the head moves down against the perineum and is a good sign of progress. Be sure to tell the mother that she is doing well. Removing stool can cause a reflex contraction of the pelvic floor and may inhibit progress (never remove stool when the baby is breech). If you or she deem it necessary, warn her, be very gentle, directing wiping efforts away from the opening of the yoni. Use either toilet paper or facial tissue rather gauze, since they are less abrasive. Apply a little oil before you wipe, to ease discomfort, especially if she has hemorrhoids.

Intact membranes

If the membranes are still intact and you are of the opinion that it is better to break the bag prior to the birth of the head, then do so between contractions or just as a contraction is building, when the head starts to distend the perineum and the bag is bulging at the introitus. Be sure it is the head and not just a large forewater before you break it or you may interfere with progress. Press your gloved fingertip or an instrument into the bag to break the waters. See the chapter entitled "The Placental Membranes and Amniotic Fluid during Labor" for details on examining the fluid.

If you or the parents are of the opinion that the bag should be left alone to allow the baby to be born in the caul, then don't do anything, but be prepared for a "splashdown"; the bag is likely to rupture suddenly during active pushing. Also discuss the possibility of breaking the membranes before the head is out if the color of the forewaters leads you to suspect meconium-stained fluid.

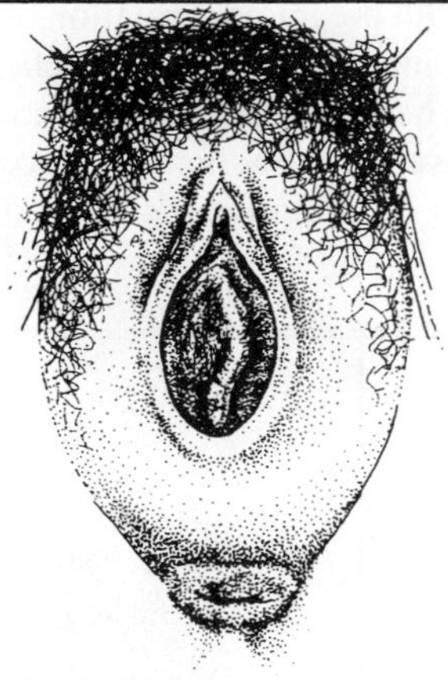

Characteristic scalp wrinkling: occiput anterior

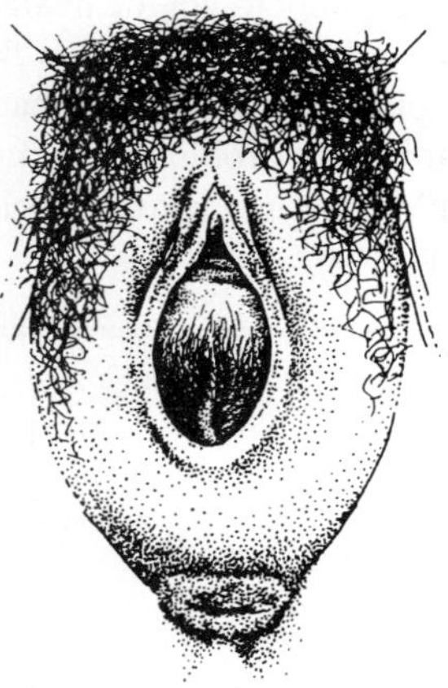

Characteristic scalp wrinkling: occiput posterior

(The forewaters are ruptured and the mother is standing; you are below her, looking directly up between her legs.)

Anterior or posterior presentation?

The scalp, when visible through hair, and the forehead have a characteristic pattern of wrinkling depending upon whether the occiput is anterior or posterior, which can be quite pronounced. Anterior wrinkling produces deep longitudinal folds over the vertex (reminiscent of a walnut shell and sometimes as deep as walnut meat), while posterior wrinkling produces a few shallow horizontal wrinkles across the bregma. This wrinkling will smooth out as crowning begins. Knowing the wrinkling pattern can help you decide which way to apply pressure if you think the techniques in the following sections would be useful.

Assisting flexion of an occiput anterior baby: The idea of maintaining flexion stems from the mistaken notion that the head extends during birth, as well as the still-prevalent practice of cutting the perineum, which removes some of the natural counterpressure supplied by the tissues. Typically allowing the birth of the head to occur spontaneously realizing that any number of things may influence the degree of flexion and trying to affect it may not always be wise, most home-based midwives do not attempt to influence head flexion. For example, if a hand is under the baby's chin (a common reason the head may be somewhat deflexed) and the midwife tries to force greater flexion, she may actually impede descent. Assisting flexion is also difficult or impossible to do unless the mother is in a supine position.

However, if assistance with flexion seems warranted for any reason, here is how to go about it: as the head of a baby in an occiput anterior position moves outward toward a full crown, provide some counterpressure directly to the region of the upper vertex downward (toward the mother's anus) to ensure that flexion is maintained until the occiput clears the pubic arch. The mother can do this herself; it is especially effective for lessening burning sensations in the periurethral and clitoral area. Alternatively, you can provide counterpressure by covering the head with your entire hand, including the length (not just the tips) of your fingers. If the baby is anterior, direct pressure toward the mother's sacrum, pressing the baby's chin to her chest. (You will want to be sure the baby is occiput anterior before doing so!) Using the length of your fingers provides more generalized and even pressure, which will minimize the chance of intracranial hemorrhage. Never push over a fontanelle. It may be easiest to use your nondominant hand for this purpose, leaving your dominant hand free to grab any equipment that may be needed. Sutton (2001) suggests simply placing two fingers on either side of the perineum to assist flexion.

Assisting flexion of an occiput posterior baby: It probably makes more sense to attempt to flex the head of a posterior baby if the appearance of the emerging head suggests that it is somewhat deflexed and the perineum is very tense and not retracting. To do so, use the same kind of hand maneuver described above to apply pressure to the vertex, however, direct it up toward the pubic bone and inward. Leave the head alone to extend on its own once the occiput has cleared the perineum. Again, this is usually unnecessary.

Pushing between contractions

The head will emerge on its own, usually during a contraction. It is my belief that active maternal pushing efforts should always be coordinated with contractions, allowing shoulder rotation to take place normally. Pushing between contractions in an attempt to get the head out without a tear may interfere with the internal rotation of the shoulders and create a problem with their birth. Allow the crowning head to stretch the perineum between contractions, and then allow the uterus to complete the birth of the head with the next contraction. If the head should emerge spontaneously between contractions, that is not a problem, just don't encourage active pushing between contractions (not every midwife agrees with this opinion). Having the mother blow or pant to ease the head out during contractions does not seem to interfere with normal shoulder rotation.

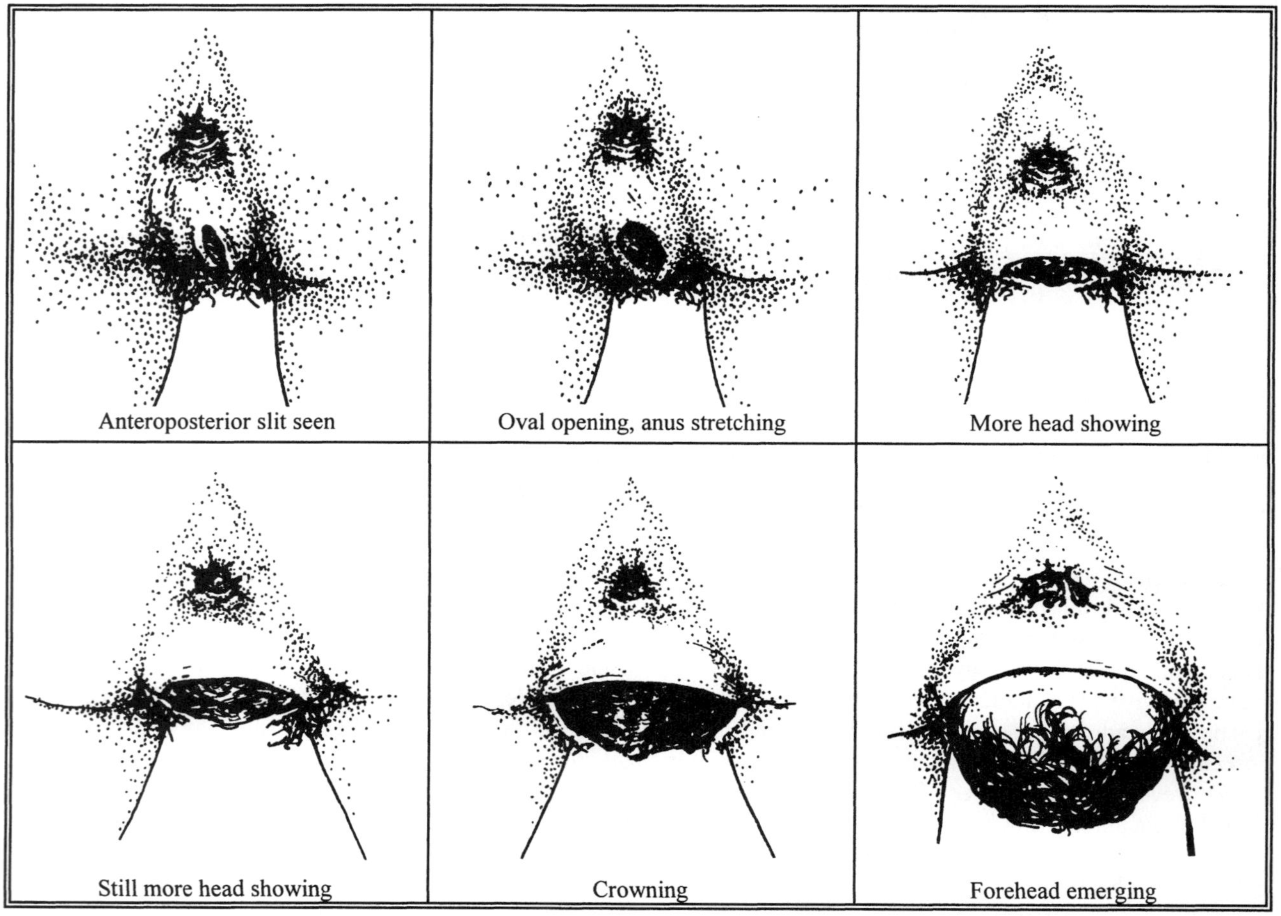

Anteroposterior slit seen | Oval opening, anus stretching | More head showing
Still more head showing | Crowning | Forehead emerging

Maternal bleeding before the head is out

A small amount of bright red to medium red bleeding that occurs as the perineum stretches is usually due to a perineal or labial tear; an external tear may be visible and usually occurs as the tissues undergo their maximum stretch. However, slightly darker bleeding with no evidence of tissue trauma is more likely to be from a cervical or cord tear or a placental abruption. Unless the fetal heart rate drops dramatically, there will be no way distinguish whether bleeding is affecting fetal well-being. The best course of action is to get the baby out as quickly as possible. Encourage the mother to push, perhaps alter her position to facilitate more rapid descent, and, as a last resort, do a clitorotomy.

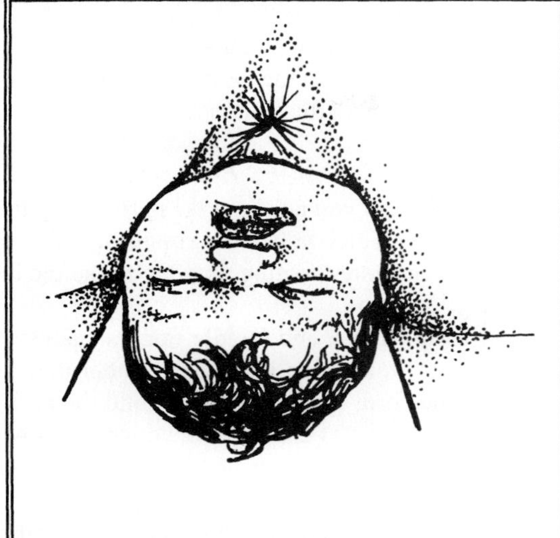

Head is born OA, perineum is intact

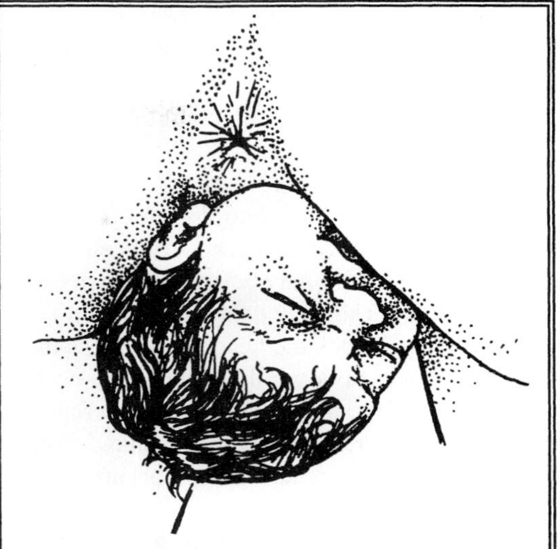

Restitution has occurred from OA to LOA.

Watch the sacrum

If you are behind the mother, watch her sacrum for the appearance of asymmetry of the bone or lumps which indicate that the baby may have a hand (or foot) beside the head.

Encourage the mother to assist the birth

Encourage the mother to reach down and feel the baby as she is emerging. If there is a hand up by the head, the mother, especially if she is upright and kneeling, is in an excellent position from which she can check to see if the baby has a hand up. She can then push the baby's hand back inside herself and can best gauge the effect her manipulations have on her tissues.

Restitution

Normally, restitution occurs very quickly, in many cases almost instantly, once the head is born.

Supporting the baby when the mother is upright

Many, if not most, of your births will be with the mother in some variation of an upright position; it is therefore useful to have a hand maneuver that can help support the baby after the head is out. Which hand you use will depend upon your relative dexterity with your left as opposed to your right, the position of the baby and the position of the mother. Hold one hand rigid with the fingers together and spread the crotch of your index finger and thumb into a wide "C." Place the crotch of your thumb and index finger around the baby's neck (taking care not to apply pressure against the neck) with the palm directed toward the mother. This allows you to gently support the shoulders as they emerge rather than letting the baby's body fall out. You don't need to do this until the body is actually coming.

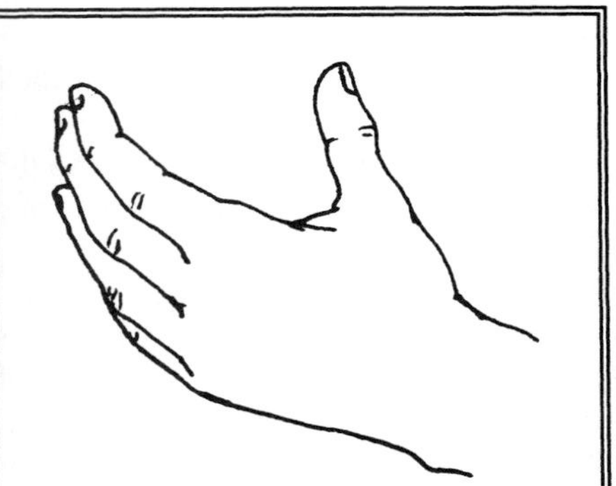

How to shape your hand

Wiping the face

Once the head is born you may, if it seems needed, gently wipe the baby's face and head with a soft towel or cloth. Drying the head and face minimizes heat loss and removes fluids that may interfere with breathing. However, drying the baby thoroughly is not critical in homebirths because the birthing room should be at least 80°F (27°C) during late pushing (unlike a hospital delivery room, which is often kept quite cold to minimize the proliferation of bacteria and to promote the comfort of the care providers). The baby will also be allowed his placental transfusion, which will greatly assist with thermoregulation.

Should you clear the baby's airway?

If there is meconium staining, once the head is born, the question of whether to suction on the perineum arises. It is no longer recommended in the US or the UK (see references below) to suction on the perineum, regardless of whether meconium has been passed or not. Meconium is also discussed further later in this chapter.

Checking for a nuchal cord

You can check for the umbilical cord if you feel it is necessary, although you need not do so routinely if things are proceeding smoothly. Variable fetal heart rate decelerations during labor will alert you to the possibility of a nuchal cord. Of course, sometimes the cord may be around the neck with no fetal heart rate warning, in which case the birth of the shoulders will probably be slightly delayed.

To check for the cord once the head is out, press the nail side of your index and middle fingers against the baby's neck and slide the fingertips down the nape of the neck; this will cause you to run into or slip under the cord as you advance your hand. Use the tips and pads of your fingers to feel for the cord, which may be around the neck in one or more loops, over a shoulder, or draped like a shawl over both shoulders. If you do find cord, your fingers will already be positioned so that you can bend them to curl around the cord to move it out of the way.

Dealing with a nuchal cord without cutting it: Leave the cord intact whenever possible. Even a cord that appears to have stopped pulsing will usually resume pulsing again after birth, once tension on it is relieved. There are several options for dealing with the cord. Let the baby's color and the fetal heart rate determine how to proceed. If the heart rate is dropping precipitously and the color is poor and you cannot somersault the baby out quickly, you may have to cut it.

- If the cord is loose enough, slip it down over the shoulders like a shawl, so that the baby is born through the loop. This maneuver may create a loose knot in the cord when there was no knot to begin with.
- Bring a loose loop of cord up, out and over the head.
- If the cord is too tight to slip over the head but not so tight as to delay the birth, somersault the baby out by supporting the baby around the neck from below (against the perineum). Do so by spreading your thumb and forefinger widely in the shape of a "C" and fitting the crotch of these fingers around the baby's neck. If necessary, keep the head close to the mother by pressing the baby's face into the mother's thigh. Allow the shoulders and body to be born as you continue to support the neck. Holding the neck lets the baby's body advance outward while minimizing tension on the cord. Once the shoulders are born, continue to flex the head by pushing the face toward the mother's thigh to allow more room as the body is born. Use your other hand to support the body as it emerges, especially if the mother is upright.

  This sounds impossible in theory, but in fact a newborn's body is extremely flexible and this works very well. This technique can be used with the mother in any position and usually allows the cord to remain intact and resume pulsations after the birth.

Once the baby is out, quickly unwrap the cord from around the baby so as not to produce undue strain and break it (see the section at the end of the chapter for details about less common cord problems at birth.).

When a nuchal cord must be cut: It is extremely rare for the cord to be absolutely too tight to permit any of the above options. You should always attempt to somersault the baby before deciding to cut the cord. If the cord is too tight to allow this, immediately clamp it in two places, making sure to clamp along the same visible length of cord. Be sure about this because otherwise you could remove a section of wrapped cord, leaving the baby's end or the placental end open and bleeding. Remedying the situation at that point and in a timely fashion may be difficult or impossible, plus it will be impossible to tell if the baby's end is the one bleeding.

Place the clamps about 2 to 3 in apart, as space allows. Cut the cord between the clamps. Unwind the cord (which may have several loops) before the head is born. Have someone help the mother to pant during this process and explain to the mother and the baby what is going on. Cutting the cord in this manner always presents the risk of accidently nicking the baby or mother; it also means that the baby's oxygen supply is being abruptly cut off, eliminating a gradual transition from intrauterine to extrauterine life and necessitating getting the baby out as soon as possible.

This baby will be hypovolemic from cord compression and will not receive any of the placental blood

---

Kattwinkel, J, ed. NEONATAL RESUSCITATION TEXTBOOK, 6th ed. Am Acad Pediatrics & Am. Heart Assoc, 2011.
Richmond S, ed. NEWBORN LIFE SUPPORT, 3rd ed. Resuscitation Council, UK, 2011.

intended to fill his pulmonary circulatory system. Therefore, he will be suffering what is, in effect, a hemorrhage. He may be slow to begin breathing and should be watched carefully, and, if indicated, assisted promptly.

If you find a nuchal hand or foot

When you check for a nuchal cord, you may discover a small body part near the baby's neck. Most commonly you will find a nuchal hand; you will want to control its emergence in order to prevent a tear. To do so, use your free hand to try to tuck it back under the chin and hold it in place. The room in the sacrum should allow this. Support the arm as it emerges to keep the elbow close to the chest during the rest of the birth.

If the hand is by the face or the birth occurs so rapidly that repositioning the hand is impossible, do your best to hold the arm close to the baby's body so that the elbow does not slice down into the perineum. Alternatively, as the baby's body begins to be born, grasp the hand and bring it out, attempting to keep the elbow close to the baby's body on the way. This procedure risks a tear from the elbow as well but is less apt to cause a tear than an uncontrolled delivery of the flexed nuchal arm. If the arm is more fully extended so that the elbow is at the level of the neck, do not try to bring the arm out; the depression formed by the neck allows the elbow to be pressed inward where it less likely to cause a tear.

Much more rarely, you may find a foot near the head; this could interfere with the lateral flexion of the body during the rest of the birth. Fortunately, it is a rare occurrence. The baby should come out, regardless, just as in a frank breech birth. Leaving the foot where it is, have the mother push while you grasp the baby around the upper arms and work the baby out slowly by gently wiggling him from side to side to bring his body through the pelvis. Once the chest is freed, the baby should be able to breathe. If the baby does not advance with this maneuver, you can also try pushing the foot back up toward the chest to flex the leg, but this may be difficult to do with the leg pinned in the birth canal.

Wait for external rotation of the head

Now you wait, sometimes a few minutes, for the next contraction. During this time, the head will be snug against the perineum and the face will be pink to pink-lavender; the baby may grimace or even start breathing. As the next contraction begins, the head will rotate externally if it has not already done so, signaling that the shoulders have undergone their second internal rotation and are now ready to be born and you will see the neck start to appear. It is very important to give the baby a chance to spontaneously rotate her shoulders unless signs of shoulder dystocia are apparent and you are choosing a prophylactic intervention to avoid this (see the chapter entitled "Shoulder Dystocia" for full details). If the mother is upright, shoulder rotation may occur quickly, before the next contraction. If the baby is coming, let her come.

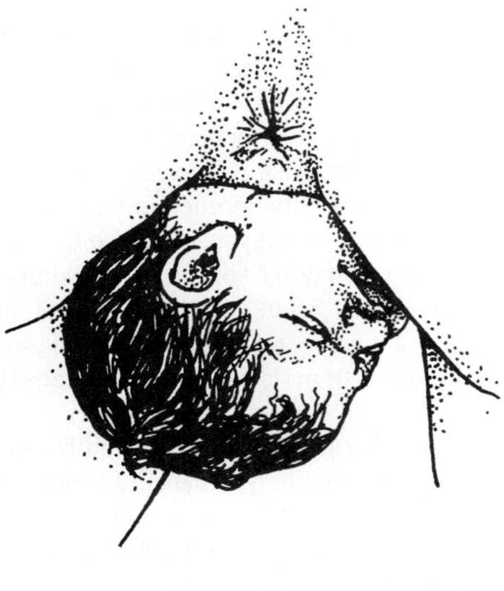

The head rotates externally, signaling that the shoulders have rotated internally to the antero-posterior diameter.

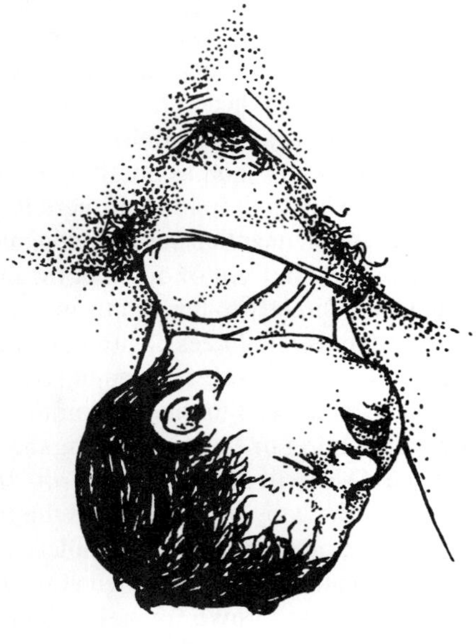

The posterior shoulder is born first.

The birth of the shoulders and arms

If the birth is not manipulated and the shoulders have rotated normally, the posterior shoulder is likely to come first, even though the anterior shoulder may be visible. First note, however, that the normal birth of the shoulders can vary; as long as they are coming, there is no problem. It is fine for your hands to be poised but off the baby until the next contraction starts, although the baby may come very quickly. Not providing support allows the weight of the head to assist internal rotation and the birth of the posterior shoulder, especially when the mother is upright. Once the posterior shoulder has cleared the perineum, in most cases, the anterior shoulder will be born with the mother's spontaneous pushing efforts. If the mother is reaching down to receive her baby, do not interfere.

The birth of the shoulders: *If the mother is upright* and does not reach to assist the birth herself, form a collar for the baby's neck by holding the fingers of one hand in the shape of a "C" and poise that palm at the back of the baby's neck. Be prepared to apply your palm to the upper back and support the shoulders with your fingers as they emerge, directing support against the back and shoulders, rather than the side of the neck. Alternatively, gently place your palm over the crown of the head, taking care not to apply pressure to the head as the baby advances.

If the mother is lying belly-up, you can help guide the shoulders out, if indicated. Shift your body so that you are on the same side of the mother as the baby's occiput. Poise both hands near the head so that your fingers point toward the baby's face and your little fingers are nearest the mother's genitals, to prevent you from accidently touching the anus. The shoulders should emerge spontaneously. If they do not, assess which shoulder wants to come first. To assist the birth of the posterior shoulder; guide the shoulder by applying gentle upward and outward pressure to the side of the head with your lower hand. To assist with the anterior shoulder, gently direct downward and outward pressure on the side of the head with your top hand until the anterior shoulder appears. Do either as the mother bears down during a contraction. *Do not pull on the head or apply excessive force.*

If the birth of the shoulders seems delayed, check again for a tight cord or a nuchal hand that might hinder their emergence. Some guidance, as above, may be necessary to effect birth when these problems exist. Shoulder dystocia is dealt with in the chapter entitled "Shoulder Dystocia."

Supporting the birth of the arms: If the woman is in a more or less reclining position, you can slide your hands down along the baby's upper arms as they emerge. Keep your hands there until the elbows and hands are free. This controls the birth of the arms and prevents the arms and elbows from jabbing into the perineum and causing a tear. Do not try this if the mother is upright, as you are likely to drop the baby.

Receiving the rest of the baby's body

If the mother is upright: The woman may or may not be able to reach down, depending on her balance and whether another person is supporting her under her arms. You may have one hand forming a collar around the baby's neck or on the head. Your other hand should be poised, ready to support the baby's body as it emerges by applying your palm to the torso, sliding down the back to the crotch and wrapping your fingers around the lower legs as soon as possible. Do not try to reposition your hands to grasp the baby under the arms as you are likely to drop him. If there is a soft landing pad below the mother and she is in a position that brings her bottom near that surface, you may not need to support the baby at all. Once the baby is born, place him on his side in front of or under the mother and let her reach down for the baby. Alternately, you can hand the baby directly to her, if this will not cause her to lose her balance and the cord is long enough.

If she is in a hands-and-knees position, you can receive the baby and pass it between her legs as she rises to her knees. She can then be assisted to turn over and lie down or to maintain her upright position, while holding the baby and awaiting the birth of the placenta.

If the mother is side-lying or belly-up: Bring the mother's hands to her perineum as the head is emerging and stand by to see if she will complete the birth. If not, once the arms emerge, you can slide your hands under the arms and lift the baby, facing toward the mother's belly, up to her. Simultaneously encourage her to reach down and grasp the baby to complete the birth. How possible this will be will depend upon the mother's position and emotional milieu at the time the baby emerges.

If the mother cannot reach down for her baby and she is more or less belly-up: If you need to receive the remainder of the baby's body and then hand the baby to the mother do the following: after the shoulders are born, one hand will form a collar with the crotch of your thumb and forefinger forming a semicircle around the baby's neck. Your thumb will be near the nape of the baby's neck and your fingers on the neck above the chest with your palm over the shoulder. Slide your free hand down the baby's back or chest. Insert your index finger between the legs after the buttocks are born. Continue moving your hand down the legs toward the ankles as the legs emerge. Touch your thumb and middle finger to your index finger, to produce a grasp that firmly holds both ankles. This way, you are very unlikely to drop the baby. Extend your arms to hand the baby to the mother. Do not try this if the mother is upright because the baby will emerge much more quickly, with gravity fully assisting the process.

Assisting the partner to receive the baby: Often the partner will wind up next to the mother, supporting her physically, emotionally or both during pushing. However, there are many couples who want the partner to receive the baby. When this is desired, midwives have various ways of participating, usually limiting their hands-on help to getting the head out without tears and dealing with any problems such as nuchal cord, shoulder dystocia or the need to resuscitate the baby after birth. The midwife should be right beside the partner, placing her hands over the partner's hands, if necessary, to guide them. The partner can hand the baby to the mother in the same way that the midwife would.

Cord care at birth

Look at the length of the cord and, if there is a true knot, loosen it to allow blood flow. Additional information regarding the issue of how the cord and placenta should be cared for at this point is thoroughly discussed in the chapter entitled "Placenta-to-Newborn Transfusion, Physiologic Closure of the Umbilical Vessels and Severance of the Cord."

Other special circumstances

If the head is born in the caul: This may occur if the bag remains intact or, much more rarely, when the bag has a hole in it but is otherwise so strong that it does not pull back over the baby's head as it descends. Take a breath and look carefully at the head. It can look quite peculiar and you may be confused at first as to the orientation of the baby's face. This is especially true because being born in the caul is a relatively uncommon event. The safest way to break the bag is to locate the baby's mouth. Use your fingertip to poke a hole into the bag over the mouth and use your hand to grasp under the edge of the bag (which will be very slippery) and pull the bag off the baby's face by pulling it up over the face and the vertex. I suggest using only your finger, rather than, say, a bulb syringe, because your blunt finger will produce the least trauma if you accidently try to break the bag over some part other than the mouth. It is possible for the membranes to be so stretchy that the entire baby emerges encased in the membranes. Gently puncture the bag over the mouth or the crease of the neck, lift the bag over the baby's head and remove it.

Soft tissue dystocia: Sometimes the descent of a big baby will be delayed as it squeezes through the healthy, well-padded soft tissue of the birth canal, like frozen orange juice slowly oozing from the can. (This can, at first, appear to be a bigger problem when it occurs before the shoulder emerge, namely bone-on-bone shoulder dystocia. True shoulder dystocia is addressed in the chapter entitled "Shoulder Dystocia.") At times the baby may even be born to the waist and then stop. Inserting a couple of fingers along the baby's back to break the suction will often result in advancement without any other manipulation. This is less likely to occur when the mother is upright (Scholles, 2001).

If the cord breaks during birth: See the chapter entitled "Cord Problems and Emergencies during Labor."

If intrauterine infection is suspected: If you know or suspect that the baby is at risk for infection, use a cotton-tipped culturette to swab the external ear canal as the head emerges. Rub for 30 seconds and place the swab in the culture tube immediately. Have an assistant break the liquid medium in the tip of the tube, complete the labeling of the tube with baby's name, birth time and date and refrigerate. Use a sterile De Lee to aspirate some stomach secretions for culture as well. (See my text DIAGNOSTIC TESTS for more details about when, how and why to culture at birth.)

If the baby was born through meconium-stained fluid: Aggressively clearing the airway of meconium- stained babies at birth has been practiced for decades in an attempt to reduce the incidence of meconium aspiration syndrome (MAS). However, because deep asphyxial fetal gasping in utero appears to account for almost all of the meconium aspiration that develops into a problem, it is likely that suctioning at birth may actually do more harm than good. Dr. John Stevenson (1988?) (an Australian physician who attended about 1200 homebirths from 1976 to 1984) feels that suctioning itself may either push meconium farther down into the baby's airway or precipitate aspiration and favors postural drainage as a gentler and safer approach when airway clearance is necessary. (See the subchapter entitled "Clearing the Baby's

Airway" for details on a variety of methods.)

In fact, it is known that severe MAS can even occur in the absence of meconium staining and in spite of suctioning. Even so, there is still no universal standard regarding the care of the meconium-stained infant. The UK resuscitation manual (Richmond, et al., 2011) states that most babies born through meconium-stained fluids have not inhaled any particulate matter and that there is no evidence that extensive airway clearance of the nose and mouth reduces the number of babies who get sick. In addition, pediatric experts agree that it is useless and perhaps dangerous to attempt to restrict respiratory efforts in any way (for example by compressing the chest while suctioning) in an attempt to clear the airway prior to the first breath. In contrast to the UK guidelines, US resuscitation guidelines (Kattwinkel et al., 2011) base suctioning on the condition of the baby is at birth. If the baby is vigorous (breathing well, muscle tone is good and the heart rate is above 100 bpm) only shallow suctioning of the mouth and nose with a bulb syringe or tube is advised after the baby is fully born if there is meconium staining or obvious airway obstruction. Deep suctioning the vigorous, struggling baby is now felt to pose more risk of injury than anything else. If the baby is not vigorous after birth, laryngoscopy with deep suctioning of the trachea for meconium prior to beginning resuscitation is still recommended in the US.

It is now generally accepted that meconium-stained fluid does not require extensive airway clearance prior to the birth of the shoulders. A randomized control trial of 1,245 infants which looked at the issue of whether to suction before birth of the shoulders concludes that MAS occurs at identical rates whether this is done or not (Boschert, 2003). They point out that the research used to support this practice, first done in 1976, found only a nonsignificant trend in its favor. Similar studies in 1988 and 1992 found no benefit at all. Neither the most recent US nor UK resuscitation guidelines (Kattwinkel, 2011; Richmond et al., 2011) recommend suctioning on the perineum.

Ideally, the most current protocols are being implemented in your local medical community. If not, midwives must pick their way through any prevailing conflicting opinions in her area because local practices do not always match what the research shows. (When practitioners have believed for many years that meconium must cleared at all costs this can make it very difficult to change practices.) After birth, when the airway is to be cleared, postural drainage can be used to clear any obstructing fluids. Meconium can also be removed from the oral cavity and nose gently by wiping it away with a finger covered with gauze or with the tube from a mucus-trap suction device such as a De Lee fitted with a 10 or 12 F catheter, which Gage and colleagues (1981) found to be more effective and less traumatic than the use of a bulb syringe. The most recent US and UK resuscitation guidelines (Kattwinkel, 2011; Richmond et al., 2011) state that there is no research that supports basing suctioning guidelines on the consistency of the meconium. As always, the umbilical cord should remain intact to ensure that the alveoli are maximally expanded and to create a less stressful transition for the baby.

Deep suctioning has also been used after the baby has stabilized for five minutes or so to clear from the stomach any meconium that the baby may have swallowed. This initial period of stabilization reduces the chance that deep suctioning will trigger a vasovagal response. (Deep suctioning is explained in the subchapter entitled "Clearing the Baby's Airway.") While clearing meconium from the stomach by passing a feeding tube or using a mucus-trap suction device does makes more room for colostrum, it is not necessary and is both invasive and frightening to the baby. Nursing will help the baby clear mucus from his nose and upper respiratory track and will help the stomach contents pass through his gastrointestinal tract more quickly.

Note that green staining in the oral secretions or vomitus of a baby who has been born through clear fluid is highly associated with gastrointestinal defects. See the subchapter entitled "Abdominal Distention and Vomiting at Birth: Detecting Gastrointestinal Anomalies" for more details.

If the head or the body won't come out: There are several reasons the head may come down but not come out, some of which are relatively benign and easy to remedy and some of which involve serious complications. Here is a rundown of what could be causing the delay and what you might do about it.

Mother's fear of tearing: Delay in the birth of the head could be due to maternal fear of tearing. In this common situation, you simply need to provide support and encouragement and possibly change the mother's position to one that is more upright, which will help to move the baby down more quickly.

Mother's fear of pressure: This is akin to fear of tearing but is more likely to be subconscious and could easily be related to a history of childhood sexual abuse, whether remembered or not. Gentle guidance to focus on the present moment will help the mother center on what the pressure is about right now. Having her touch the presenting part can also be very helpful, as it focuses her on her body and brings her into the moment in a very powerful way. You may need to guide her hand while you tell her what you are doing and what she is feeling; she may resist at first, so do not force her but gently encourage her to feel the head. Once women have a hand on the head, their attitude is usually transformed.

Cessation of contractions after the head is born: While this problem may be related to maternal fear, it presents a real physical risk of malrotation of the shoulders; in some cases, cessation of contractions at this point signals severe shoulder dystocia (Schlinger, 2003). See the chapter entitled "Shoulder Dystocia" for details. If the shoulders are already well positioned, the rest of the baby will usually emerge even without additional contractions, but that does not address the need for contractions to deliver the placenta and clamp down the uterus. Therefore, the first thing to do is stimulate more contractions, whether the rest of the baby is born spontaneously or not. The following things have all proven effective, and may be used individually or in combination until contractions resume:

- Reach up and using the open-handed grasping massage described in the chapter entitled "Natural Induction and Augmentation of Labor," which will often stimulate another contraction in short order.
- Tell the mother to focus on her baby and on having contractions; having her touch the baby's head will help.
- Have her partner or your assistant stimulate her nipples.
- Give her a dropperful of cotton root bark tincture.

If contractions do not resume, either change the mother's position to facilitate birth or reach in and get the baby (or both) and be prepared for bleeding. Continue to try to stimulate the uterus as above (see the chapter entitled "Birth of the Placenta, Cord and Membranes" for full details).

Compound presentation: Another reason for delay could be a hand beside the head or near the chin. A hand beside the head will increase the diameter of the presenting parts and cause the head to come out slowly. A careful digital exam around the perimeter of the head might reward you with finding fingers. If you do and the head is coming, albeit slowly, allow the birth to continue. If the head is truly arrested, you can try to reposition the hand by using your fingertips to push the hand back up. Tell the baby what needs to happen. You can also try repositioning the mother so that her bottom is elevated to give the baby room to withdraw her hand. Also see the chapter entitled "Assisting a Woman Whose Baby Is in a Compound Presentation." Once the small part is out of the way, be prepared for rapid progress!

Shoulders stuck at brim before the head is born: Sutton (2001) states that the posterior shoulder can get jammed beside the sacral promontory, causing the anterior shoulder to become lodged above the brim in front, preventing descent of the head. This is most likely to occur in posterior labors when the spine, and therefore the shoulder axis, is extended (rather than flexed). See the chapters entitled "Assisting a Woman Whose Baby Is in a Posterior Position" and "Recognizing and Dealing With Obstructed Labor" for details.

Less common cord problems: See the chapter entitled "Cord Problems and Emergencies during Labor."

Contraction of the pelvic outlet: If the pubic arch is too tight, descent can become arrested even though the station of the presenting part is quite low. Change the mother's position. If that doesn't work, the subchapter entitled "Opening the Pelvis (or the Midwife's Forceps)" discusses other techniques aimed at opening the outlet. If the baby won't come, you will need to transport. Keep in mind that performing a clitorotomy will not remedy the situation if the bony pelvis is holding things up.

Head is born but shoulders will not come: See the chapter entitled "Shoulder Dystocia" for a complete discussion of the most likely reason for this serious birth emergency.

Rare causes of arrested birth: The following list covers all the rare reasons that birth may be delayed or arrested. Unless otherwise noted, these topics are covered in the chapter entitled "Recognizing and Dealing with Obstructed Labor."

- Abnormal shortening of the umbilical cord

•Maternal tumors
•Fetal abnormalities such as hydrocephalus, enlarged abdomen or body-stalk anomaly
•Rupture of the uterus with part or all of the unborn portion of the baby's body extruded through the tear into the abdominal cavity (covered in the chapter entitled "Uterine Rupture during Labor")
•Constriction ring
•Problems related to multiple births such as fetus papyraceus or conjoined twins or locked twins (covered in the chapter entitled "Assisting at Multiple Births")
•Incompletely dilated cervix clamped down around a cephalic baby's neck, which mimics shoulder dystocia.

Bonding and Nursing after Birth

When women give birth relatively undisturbed and have received no drugs the issue of "facilitating" bonding does not often arise. Full access to the baby and an absence of interruption set the stage for the organic, hormonally-mediated process that brought labor to its conclusion to continue seamlessly as the mother meets her baby as a separate being. It may take a minute or two for a woman to shift from the process of having given birth to relating to her baby. Even so, it will be obvious that she is ripe to do so and that nothing need be done. She reaches for her baby, brings her to her chest and is thoroughly engaged in falling in love with her. Nursing can begin whenever the mother and baby seem ready and will further enhance the bonding taking place. To the extent possible, at least the first 20 minutes or so should remain as undisturbed as possible by anyone, including family members (who should have been prepared for this prenatally).

However, in cases where the mother gives birth and then seems to recede into a state of shock (possibly reflecting a history of abuse) or is much more concerned with the logistics of the immediate postpartum period than she is with her baby, you need to step in to try and bridge the gap. Number one, *never* separate the baby from the mother unless a life threatening situation demands hospital transport. Even if resuscitation is required, it can and actually must be done at the bedside if the cord is to stay intact. Most women will become engaged if given the space to do so. Secondly, when a mother cannot muster the emotional reserve to relate to her baby on a purely emotional level, she is still usually capable of nursing. Since nursing is something the mother does for the baby, rather than something she feels, she can be engaged in the process of positioning the baby correctly and getting the baby to latch on. These activities bring the baby close to her and stimulate the release of oxytocin which will, in turn, help her become more receptive to her baby and is, at the same time, calming to the baby. The physical act of nursing can help ground a woman and center her on her baby and should be encouraged soon after birth in such women, sooner than you might otherwise encourage nursing if the maternal response were optimal. Nursing will also facilitate the release of the placenta.

Note that the expression of maternal interest and involvement or distress with the newborn may vary for a number of reasons. In one extreme example, a mother of several sons who desperately wanted a girl threw herself on the bed and wept when she discovered that her newborn was also a boy. Such afterbirth disappointment may be related to the sex or condition of the baby, events that occurred during the labor or birth, or relationship issues, to name a few reasons. The only thing to do is to avoid judgement, make sure another family member welcomes and holds the baby (preferably skin-to-skin) while you help the mother to feel her feelings and come to terms with the present circumstance as best she can in the moment. She will no doubt, have to go through a process of grieving, accepting and moving on to bonding with the baby, over the days or even weeks following birth. The process of human bonding as well as difficult postpartum situations, including depression and psychosis, will be addressed further in Volume III of this text.

Nursing

Have the mother get comfortable. Check the baby's oral reflexes (see the description that begins on page 739) and then help the mother get him on the breast. Watch to make sure things are going well. The numerous details about how all this is accomplished will be thoroughly reviewed in Volume III of this text. Also see the most recent edition of THE BREASTFEEDING ANSWER BOOK by La Leche League International for more details.

HYDROTHERAPY AND WATERBIRTH

Laboring and giving birth in water has become increasingly popular in Western industrialized countries since about 1985; there are now many midwives who attend births where the baby emerges under water on a regular basis. Interestingly, while home landbirth is still viewed as dangerous by many hospital practitioners, waterbirth has been accepted in many hospitals both in North America and in Europe. This chapter will address issues that are unique to the use of water immersion during labor and birth and augments the basic information found elsewhere in this text that applies to all births.

Human Birth into Water and the Mammalian Diving Reflex

Is the baby likely to drown if born under water?

This is one of the two primary concerns of those who question the safety of waterbirth. Knowing that the fetus makes respiratory movements in utero, which is a liquid environment, one may logically wonder if the baby will try to breathe and aspirate fluid once born into warm water.

In the normal situation, when the baby is not distressed, the answer is no. A number of factors contribute to this: first, fetal breathing movements are not sufficient to cause the baby to inhale significant quantities of amniotic fluid during pregnancy; secondly, there is a normal inhibition of these respiratory movements that begins just before the onset of labor. Furthermore, birth into a slightly cooler water environment and differing composition of amniotic fluid and water both enhance an intact mammalian diving reflex, which protects the baby from inhaling water. (See the section below and the section entitled "Fetus-to-newborn cardiopulmonary adaptations" in the chapter entitled "The Baby's Journey through Labor to Birth" for more details regarding fetal and newborn respiratory activity and why this is so.)

The other primary concern that arises is whether there is an increased risk of maternal infection with waterbirth; the answer to this question is "no" as well.

The mammalian diving reflex

The diving reflex conserves oxygen during periods of water submersion via a variety of physiologic adaptations. This reflex, which is most well developed in water-dwelling mammals, is present to a lesser extent in a variety of other animals including amphibians, reptiles, birds and land mammals. It is well known that newborn mammals of all kinds are extremely resistant to drowning. In humans, the diving reflex provides limited protection against asphyxia and is more pronounced in infants than in adults. Stimulation of this reflex at birth and restimulation throughout infancy enhances this reflex and increases the likelihood that it will remain intact as the child matures.

The diving reflex in humans: The trigeminal nerve (the 5th cranial nerve), supplies the chief sensory nerves of the face and the motor nerve controlling the muscles of mastication. The diving reflex is triggered when the facial branches are activated by water touching the face, particularly the lips. When temperature receptors, also located in the face, mainly around the eyes and forehead (Laitman & Reidenberg, 1988), sense that the water temperature differs from that of the air, the diving reflex is further potentiated. These triggers produce either voluntary or reflex apnea (cessation of breathing). Activation can even be triggered to a lesser degree by touching a wet cloth to the face. If water should enter the pharynx or larynx, the glottis tends to spasm, which prevents water from entering the trachea. Water entering the pharynx also helps stimulate the vagus nerve, which prompts the cardiovascular adjustments to diving. (To trigger the apneic response of the diving reflex, submerge your face in water with a snorkel in place for at least one minute. If you don't have a snorkel, use a soda straw. Unless you are a diver and are acclimated to breathing underwater, it should prove somewhat difficult to take a breath through the snorkel.)

Inhibition of the respiratory mechanism also triggers a profound redistribution of blood flow. Peripheral vasoconstriction increases between 26 to 33%. This reduces oxygen consumption by shunting blood away from tissues that are relatively resistant to the effects of asphyxia, such as the limbs, and rerouting it to the organs most vulnerable to oxygen deprivation: the heart, brain, liver and kidneys. In addition, both humans and diving mammals have a specialized red pigment called **myoglobin**. Myoglobin is similar to hemoglobin, but stores oxygen within muscle cells, where it is immediately available to the tissues during a dive. The capacity to shunt blood to vital organs and extract oxygen from myoglobin is much more pronounced in diving mammals.

Simultaneous stimulation of the vagal nerve (which supplies the supraventricular region of the heart) is responsible for the development of bradycardia, which decreases the cardiac output. In combination with peripheral vasoconstriction, this results in the maintenance of arterial blood pressure at or near normal levels for a period of time. Unlike diving mammals, humans will progressively develop hypertension the longer they are completely submerged. Vasoconstriction eventually develops in most vascular beds as submersion continues.

The diving reflex is triggered by only a slight difference between the air and water temperature and is heightened considerably when the water temperature drops below a critical level or when the person is afraid. In adults, the overstimulation threshold is reached when water temperature drops below about 68°F (20°C). The temperature at which overstimulation occurs is higher for infants, whose cold tolerance is less than that of adults. When the diving reflex is hyperstimulated for too long, fatal bradycardia and cardiac arrhythmias can occur.

The diving reflex at birth: The cardiovascular adjustments of the diving reflex are elicited by the process of labor, which appears to protect the fetus against asphyxia during late labor and pushing. With the diving reflex partially triggered, the unstressed newborn is uniquely adapted to emerge under water. The inhibition of respiratory motions that is normal in the hours prior to labor is further potentiated as his head is born and his face contacts the water, especially when the water is slightly cooler than the intrauterine environment. After birth, the baby with an intact, pulsating cord is still respirating via the placenta. As a land mammal, he is in the unique position of being underwater and still fully oxygenated, therefore he is not truly apneic. Because of this, pronounced bradycardia does not occur, although some rerouting of the blood flow enhances oxygenation to the heart, brain, liver and kidneys, leaving the limbs less perfused. Stress hormones are also lower as well. These changes are reflected in the prolongation of the normal newborn lavender-pink peripheral color often noted in waterbirth babies.

Hydrotherapy in Labor

The benefits of water immersion

Laboring in water is a good choice for many women, whether they wish to give birth in water or not. The basic principles that make hydrotherapy beneficial for other therapeutic uses also apply to laboring and giving birth. These benefits include buoyancy, hydrostatic pressure, heat, and decreased blood pressure. In addition, the use of a variety of routine interventions such as medications and continuous monitoring are reduced when hydrotherapy is freely available in the hospital.

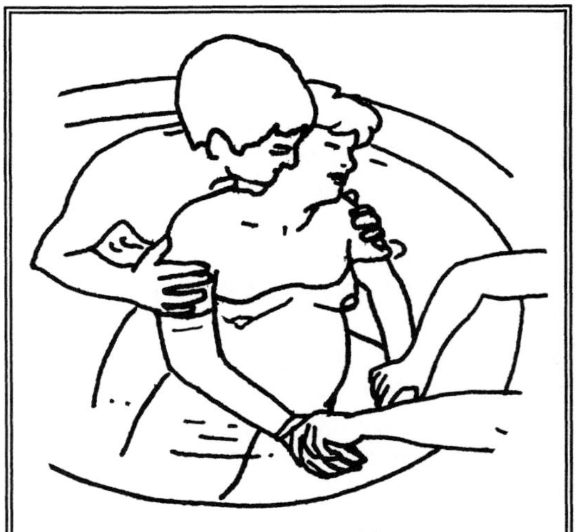

Laboring in a hot tub with support

(Redrawn with permission from illustrations by Stella Cruz, © Ruth Ancheta, 2000)

A body immersed in water loses weight equal to the weight of the water that is displaced. When the body is immersed to chest level, about 75% of the body weight is displaced. Water immersion relieves the woman of supporting her full weight, facilitates her movements and allows her to relax more deeply. It can create more space in the pelvis because the mother's ability to move is enhanced and muscles tend to work more efficiently under water. Buoyancy assists in the spontaneous rotation of the baby, and equalizing of pressure usually means that perineal tearing is reduced. Pressure on the cervix from the baby's head is decreased because gravity is not operative. (While this sounds like a disadvantage, and otherwise would be, it is usually balanced out by the other benefits.) Relaxation minimizes pain and decreases anxiety as adrenalin levels fall and oxytocin levels rise. After 20 to 30 minutes of water immersion, there is an increase in endorphins that results in a drop in mean arterial pressure and a consequent decrease in blood pressure. Those women who choose to use whirlpool jets during labor may also benefit from the gentle nipple stimulation afforded by the moving water, thus further enhancing oxytocin release.

When the body is immersed in water, the pressure is the same in all directions and equally distributed at any given depth beneath the surface of the liquid. This phenomenon is known as "hydrostatic pressure," which is proportional to the depth of the water. It is partly responsible for the noted reduction in pain that most women experience upon entering the water. Submersion also induces a redistribution of body fluid (see section below on the physiology of waterbirth). Enning (2003a) estimates that edema is reduced by 600 to 1000 ml.

Showers and baths

Flowing water also provides some degree of pain relief for many women. The woman can sit on a stool or plastic lawn chair in the shower. Warm running water from a shower head or a mobile shower spray can be directed over the belly, lower back or shoulders. When labor is long or a woman is tense, a hot shower can help her relax and feel refreshed. As a general rule, the temperature of running water should not exceed 98.6° (37°C). However, a few women will request the water to be hotter than this. If the water is not being allowed to pool beneath the mother (i.e., the drain is open), let the mother's comfort and the fetal heart rate be your guide. If the water is pooling beneath the mother do not allow the water temperature to rise over body temperature to prevent overheating, fetal tachycardia and the myriad adverse effects of hyperthermia. (See recommendations below for water temperatures at various points during labor.)

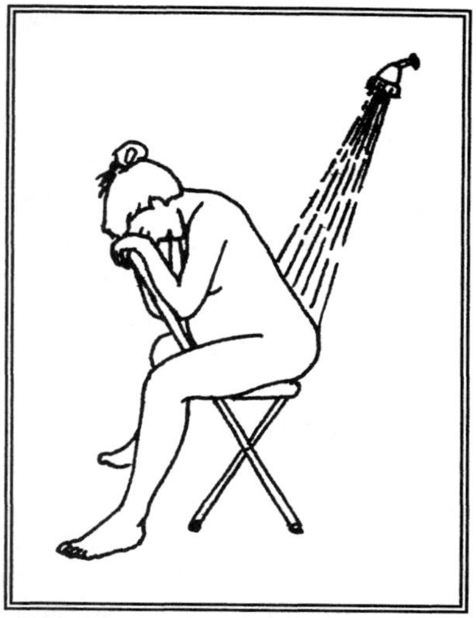

(Redrawn with permission from illustrations by Stella Cruz, © Ruth Ancheta, 2000)

A bath also helps in a variety of situations such as helping a woman get comfortable so she can rest between contractions. If a woman is fully dilated but the baby is high, placing her in warm water helps relax pelvic soft tissues, allowing the baby to descend so that a pushing urge is established. Many women find it relaxing to rest in a warm tub of water with someone pouring warm water over their belly during and between contractions. This has an almost hypnotic effect and helps with focusing and internalizing during labor. A woman should not be left alone in hot water, as she may become faint or lose her balance. Someone should remain unobtrusively present, out of sight in a corner of the bathroom, just in case she needs help. If her partner can join her in the water, so much the better; then they can be left alone together.

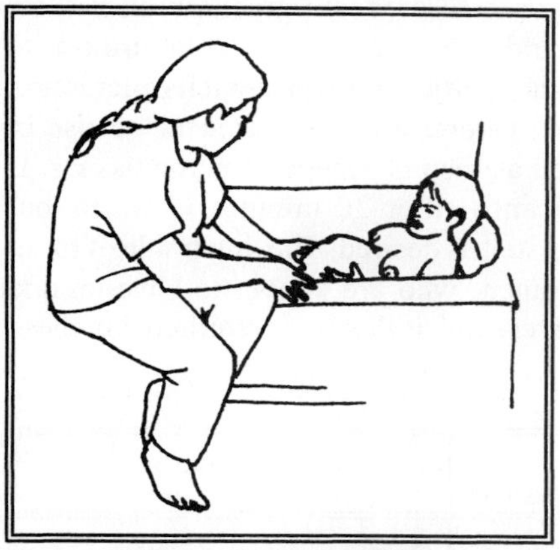

(Redrawn with permission from illustrations by Stella Cruz, © Ruth Ancheta, 2000)

Water Temperature and Its Impact on the Physiology of Labor

In the United States, water for birthing has traditionally been kept at a temperature of about 99 to 100°F (37.2 to 37.8°C), hotter than anywhere else in the world, according to Enning. Cornelia Enning is a German waterbirth midwife and author of the text WASSERGEBURTSHILFE, which includes her research on the physiology of waterbirth. She observes that water temperature has a profound effect on the mother's and baby's response to labor. She finds that optimal water temperature varies according to the phase of labor. She advocates mildly cool water as the ideal temperature range for active labor and cephalic births. Enning emphasizes the following benefits (2003a, 2003b):

- It slows neural transmission by lowering body core temperature slightly.
- Slowed neurotransmission lessens pain as well as contraction of the skeletal muscles.
- Oxygen uptake via the uterine vessels is enhanced.
- Glucose metabolism is more economical.
- Core blood volume is balanced with peripheral circulation and viscosity improved.
- Muscle tone is normalized as the level of stress hormones fall.
- Uterine muscle contraction is enhanced, making contractions more efficient in labor and after birth, minimizing bleeding and speeding placental delivery.

These biochemical changes occur because the mother's core body temperature drops slightly in cool water. When the water line is above the breasts, the core temperature is affected most rapidly. Enning uses a water temperature between 86 and 91°F (30 and 32.5°C) for active labor with head-first babies and finds that this results in a fall in maternal core temperature of no more than 3.6°F (2°C) at a water temperature of 86°F (30°C) (cooler water can cause late placental abruption, or the placenta to come on the heels of the baby). The chart on the next page compares the risks and benefits of hot versus cooler water. Water temperatures of 98.6°F (37°C) or less tend to produce mild to moderate changes.

However, at a water temperature of 102.2°F (39°C), maternal heart rate and cardiac output are significantly increased, stretching the heart walls and triggering the release of ANP (the significance of this is explained below). The fetal heart rate responds to overheating by rising as well, and maternal core temperature is maintained at about 101°F (38.3°C), which is a bit too hot.

Under all circumstances, water immersion produces a redistribution of blood volume that increases blood flow into the infrathoracic space. This occurs as the result of increased venous return to the thorax, which is due to the hydrostatic pressure gradient and is dependent on the depth of water immersion. Tissue fluid is also pushed into the circulating blood volume, reducing edema and increasing plasma volume. This stimulates the posterior pituitary gland to release oxytocin. This increase in blood volume stretches the heart walls as well, increasing both the heart rate and cardiac output and eventually causing specialized heart cells to release **atrial natriuretic peptide** (ANP).

ANP inhibits the pituitary gland's release of vasopressin, a water-retention hormone that is closely related to oxytocin and has a wide range of effects, including antidiuresis. It even has an oxytocic effect on nonpregnant women. In midpregnancy, vasopressin and oxytocin are about equipotent in stimulating uterine contractions. As pregnancy advances, the response to vasopressin remains relatively stable while the response to oxytocin gradually increases. Vasopressin can theoretically be used to induce labor, and water immersion could conceivably be used to turn off its effects. However, even though the effects of ANP on vasopressin are well established, little is known about its interaction with oxytocin, although water immersion is known to result in a balancing of vasopressin-oxytocin levels, a rise in endorphins, and the activation of oxytocin receptors in the myometrium as well as insulin receptors in the tissues. If drinking is not permitted, vasopressin release seems to be decreased significantly after 30 minutes in water, but vasopressin levels remain unchanged after an hour of submersion if fluids are ingested as desired. The down side of these research studies is that most were performed on adult males, not laboring women, who are known to have unique physiological responses in just about every way that has been studied; much more research is therefore required, but these studies can be used as a starting point for understanding water's effects.

System effected	**Hyperthermia (95-102°F/35-38.8°C)**	**Mild hypothermia (86-91/91-95°F) (30-32.7/32.7-35°C)**	**Hypothermia (77-86°F/25-30°C)**
Central nervous system	Induces flushing; sweating; increased metabolic rate	Reduces the metabolic rate	Causes shivering, stalled labor, premature exhaustion
Cardiovascular system	Increases blood pressure, pulse rate and dehydration; increases heat production in the mother	Reduces blood pressure and pulse rate; assists heat conduction (cools the mother); inhibits thrombocyte production	Lowers heart rate, decreases core body temperature, causes peripheral vasoconstriction
Respiratory system	Increases respiratory rate, resulting in hyperventilation and leading to oxygen deficiency	Decreases oxygen demand; normalizes respiratory rate, which balances respiratory gases	Produces apnea, reduces energy consumption and results in acidosis
Hormonal effects	Adversely affects contraction pattern; increases anxiety, thirst; lowers stress tolerance; prostaglandin$_2$ and free thyroxine both rise	Balances vasopressin-oxytocin levels; elevates endorphins; activates oxytocin receptors in the myometrium and insulin receptors in the tissues	Elevates glycogen consumption and vasopressin production with resulting diuresis, leading to a loss of body fluids.
Fetus	Causes tachycardia; raises adrenalin levels; increases glucose consumption and risk of intracranial bleeding in the baby, leading to distress and lethargy at birth	Regulates fetal heart rate; protects against hemorrhagic disease of the newborn by normalizing clotting response; stabilizes primitive reflex responses; activates fetal movements	Fetal movement and heart rate slows; baby is likely to be hypoglycemic at birth and slow to begin breathing due to a reduced prostaglandin$_2$ level.
Placenta	Increases rate of cellular death; raises progesterone levels; increases risk of retroplacental clotting; delays placental separation	Improves placental blood flow and efficiency of contractions; speeds separation of the placenta (usually separates within 4 min after birth)	Inhibits oxytocin synthesis, produces metabolic acidosis; encourages abruption

(Enning, 2003a; 2003b)

Interesting research by Geissbuehler and colleagues (2002) studied 47 healthy women, 30 of whom chose waterbirth and 17 landbirth. Water temperatures were recorded every 2 minutes and maternal axillary temperatures were taken every 30 minutes. Mothers freely chose their water temperatures, which ranged widely from as low as 73.4°F (23°C) to as high as 102.0°F (38.9°C), averaging 96.2°F (35.7°C) at the time of birth with an ambient air temperature of 73.4 to 77°F (23 to 25°C). The average time each woman spent in the water was 98 minutes, with a range of 28 to 364 minutes. Despite the wide variation in water temperature, maternal body temperature did not vary significantly, averaging 97.4°F (36.3°C) upon entering the water, 98.4°F (36.9°C) at birth and 98.4°F (36.9°C) one hour postpartum; all within normal core range. Neonatal temperatures remained similarly stable, ranging from 98.2 to 98.6°F (36.8 to 37°C) at all times. They concluded that women know what temperature will work for them and that they should be the ones to dictate the temperature of the water. Further, they warned that external guidelines may disrupt the physiologic control of core temperature regulation. These data support the notion that cooler water temperatures are fine at the time of birth and that hysteria about the precise regulation of water temperature at near body temperatures or slightly higher is misplaced. These researchers did not, however, look at the overall physiology in the same depth as has Enning or Odent. They did not consider the effect of water temperature on minimizing problems with such things as placental delivery with a midwife's eye. Therefore, while these data are interesting, I believe Enning's observations are worth noting. Therefore, her more specific recommendations are included here so you can form your own opinion about what is best.

Effects of anticipating water immersion on the laboring woman

Michel Odent (1997) has observed that the time during which a laboring woman is anticipating the bath is often associated with rapid progression in dilation. The sight and sounds of the water seem to prompt this response. He speculates that water may reduce neocortical inhibitions. The midwife can use this knowledge by making sure the laboring woman is near the pool or tub while it is ceremoniously prepared, helping the woman enter the pool ideally primed to move through her labor more rapidly.

General Considerations for Midwifery Care during Labor and Birth in Water

Risk factors and waterbirth

Any maternal condition involving high blood pressure will greatly benefit from water immersion as water at the right temperature lowers blood pressure. Water immersion also lessens the risk of uterine rupture for YBAC labors, reduces edema and bleeding, enhances fetal oxygenation and facilitates birth (especially when pelvic dimensions are marginal). Thus a baby remaining persistently occiput posterior or presenting by the face or brow may birth more easily under water. A postdates baby benefits from the enhanced placental circulation that occurs when the mother is immersed.

If the baby has a known defect: Stimulation of the nerve pathways mediating the diving reflex may produce serious or fatal cardiac arrhythmias in persons with certain preexisting organic disorders. Therefore, underwater birth is not advisable for babies known to have defects involving systems supplied by the vagus nerve, such as certain cardiac disorders or defects of the larynx, respiratory or abdominal organs. These adverse effects may be maximized when the water temperature is too hot as the baby emerges. Also, any baby known to have exposed internal structures such as open spinal cord defects should not be born in water, as these structures are highly susceptible to contamination and infection. While one could argue that waterbirth will protect such structures from trauma, the risk of contamination and water absorption though exposed structures makes waterbirth ill advised.

When the baby's condition is assumed to be healthy, bring her to the surface within 10 seconds of birth to minimize any ill effects if there are unrecognized organic disorders that may be adversely affected by further stimulation of the diving reflex.

Preparing and filling the tub

Whenever possible, the waterbirth tub should have been obtained and prepared prior to labor. Because of this, the instructions regarding how to do so are included in the second or later editions of HOLISTIC MIDWIFERY, Vol. I.

Ambient temperature

Enning (2003b) recommends a room temperature that is 1.8 to 5.4°F (1 to 3°C) warmer than the water in the tub, to simulate a steamy tropical environment. This can be easily accomplished by placing the tub in a small room. A very warm environment enhances oxytocin levels and eliminates any worries that the constantly wet baby will become chilled after the birth. At the time of birth, fans should be turned off and windows and doors kept closed to prevent drafts.

Prepare a birthing area beside the tub for the mother

A place should be prepared on the floor beside the tub with a padded surface, pillows and other comfort and support devices so that if the mother needs to leave the tub rapidly during labor or birth, there will be a comfortable place for her to go. A stack of dry towels should also be available to dry the mother and anyone who has been in the tub.

When to change the water

The water should be changed if feces or other debris expelled into the water cannot be removed with a medium-sized fish net or kitchen strainer. The prompt removal of solid waste is sufficient to maintain an adequate level of cleanliness. If the woman should release enough loose fecal matter to render the water muddy, she should get out and the tub should be emptied, cleaned and refilled. If this happens at the time of birth, bring the baby up immediately.

Adding salt to the water

The addition of salt is *not necessary* for a safe waterbirth. The vast majority of midwives in the United States use plain water. However, Enning (2003a) prefers to add sea salt to mimic a more physiologic fluid and recommends a salinity between 0.25 and 0.9%, depending upon the anticipated risk of cord prolapse or the emergence of small parts prior to birth (such as might occur during breech descent). The higher the risk of such problems, the closer the solution should be to the normal salinity of blood, which is 0.9%.

CAPACITY OF TUB*		AMOUNT OF SEA SALT TO ADD*	
LITER	GALLON	0.25%	0.9%
200	53	500 g	1.8 kg
300	79	750 g	2.7 kg
379	100	948 g	3.41 kg
400	106	1 kg	3.6 kg
416	110	1.04 kg	3.74 kg
436	115	1.09 kg	3.9 kg
454	120	1.14 kg	4.1 kg
500	132	1.25 kg	4.5 kg
600	158	1.5 kg	5.4 kg
700	185	1.75 kg	6.3 kg
800	211	2 kg	7.2 kg
900	238	2.25 kg	8.4 kg
1000	264	2.5 kg	9 kg

*Rounded off to nearest whole number (adapted from Enning, 2003a)

Here is her formula to figure out how much salt to use:

quantity of water in liters X desired salt concentration (either 0.25 or 0.9 or something in between) ÷ 100 = quantity of salt in kilograms. To arrive at the amount of salt in grams, multiply the kilogram value by 1000.
Example: 0.25% salt concentration in a tub containing 300 liters of water
Solution: (300 X 0.25 = 75) ÷ 100 = .75 kilograms. To convert to grams: .75 × 1000 = 750 grams of salt

Approximate conversions: 1000 grams = 1 kilogram = 2 lb 3.5 oz; 1 liter = 33.8 oz; 1 gallon = 128 oz
To convert gallons to approximate number of liters: Number of gallons × 128 = no. of oz;
Number of ounces ÷ 33.8 = equivalent no. of liters.

The average birthing tub holds between 100 and 120 gallons (378.70 to 454.43 liters) of water.

Saline helps to buoy the mother's weight, minimizes body fluid loss from sweating and more closely simulates amniotic fluid. Salt is also a natural antimicrobial. It should be noted, however, that women resting in salt water will become dehydrated eventually. Enning estimates this occurs after 5 hours of continual submersion.

Timing considerations regarding immersion

Enning (2003b) has noted a definite pattern to a woman's response to immersion during labor. She finds that women must be in mildly hypothermic water for 30 minutes before the maximum effect will be realized. Aside from the hormonal responses prompted by submersion, these effects include a rapid drop in heart rate and blood pressure after 20 minutes in water (there is a consistent fall of up to 20 mm Hg in only the diastolic reading) and a drop in core temperature when the water is sufficiently cool (but no less than 86°F [30°C]).

These effects are maintained for 2 hours, sometimes 3; after that there is no additional benefit as far as enhancing hormonal release because the pituitary stops responding. Once the mother leaves the water, it can take 30 minutes to an hour and a half for the effect of the water to subside; the longer the woman remains in the water, the less time it will take for her metabolism to return to "dry land" normals. She should therefore stay out of the water for 1.5 to 2 hours before returning to water to achieve the maximum effect.

Early labor: The use of water immersion during early labor is controversial. While showers are fine at any point, some studies and some individual practitioners have noted that labor can slow down in some women if they enter the water before active labor is established. Contractions often stop temporarily and may not resume until the woman exits the water. Because of this, a bath is sometimes used to try to stop preterm labor or to give a woman a break from one of those long, slow, early labor marathons. Other women enter the water in early labor and make significant progress during the first couple of hours, after which labor slows down. Barbara Harper (2001) suggests that the midwife evaluate the woman's contraction pattern and overall level of birthing energy. If the uterus is quite active, even though dilation is just beginning, immersion may move things along rapidly. Some women enter a bath in early labor and progress continuously to birth. However, if early labor is slow, use water to relax the woman so she can sleep, but don't expect rapid progress.

Enning (2003b) reports that preparatory uterine activity, which primarily promotes effacement, often spaces out when the mother is immersed in water. Thus, immersing a woman who may or may not be in labor can help these toning contractions ease off, clarify the fact that she is not yet in progressive labor and allow her to rest. However, even though toning contractions may ease off, thus prolonging early labor, she finds that effacement is often enhanced. When early labor contractions are painful, submersion them less so. During early contractions, she advises a water temperature between 95 to 98.6°F (35 to 37°C). She finds that warmer water has an enhanced effect until about 3 cm of dilation.

Active labor: Once active labor is well underway, reduce the water temperature to between 92 and 94°F (33.5 to 34.7°C). As pushing nears, lower the water temperature again to about 86°F (30°C) until the placenta is out. The water will be cooling naturally over the course of labor. Cooling the water results in active babies who participate in their own birth; water which is too hot results in lethargic, limp babies who are slower to come around and may require resuscitation more often. Following all of her protocols, Enning finds that primigravida labors average 5 hours and multigravida labors average 3 hours.

Based on our current, albeit incomplete, understanding, Odent (1997) draws the following conclusions regarding submersion in active labor:

- There is a short-term response to immersion at body temperature that involves immediate and dramatic pain relief. This is probably associated with a reduced level of catecholamines, which facilitates the release of hormones that enhance dilation. Women often fall asleep once they enter the water. Blood volume redistribution contributes to the release of oxytocin through a direct effect on the hypothalamic-pituitary axis.
- After time passes, the activity of the posterior pituitary is gradually suppressed by the release of ANP. This appears to occur sometime after one to two hours of submersion and is most pronounced if the water is too hot or if woman does not drink freely while immersed. As pituitary activity subsides, contractions may also become weaker and less efficient.

Full dilation: Odent (1997) has observed that women who enter the water in active labor may easily progress to complete dilation in a hour's time, after which contractions may become less productive, often prompting the woman to leave the water spontaneously (Eriksson et al., 1997; Katz et al., 1990). This slowing of labor after full dilation represents the resting phase also observed during many labors in women who are not immersed.

Postpartum: Rewarm the water to the mid-90s° F (mid-30s°C) if the mother stays in the water while nursing.

When to get out of the tub: As a general guideline, have the woman get out of the water at least every one to two hours to ambulate even if she is having no problems in the tub. The mother should also leave the tub if she experiences lightheadedness, dizziness, faintness, weakness, or needs to use the toilet.

As with any birth, individualized care and assessment are the hallmark of good midwifery practice. If the woman wants to get into the tub, evaluate the effect of immersion for a hour or so. A mother who is concentrating deeply and whose labor is active, should be left alone to go with the flow, as with any other laboring woman. Unless labor is quite early, dramatic progress can be anticipated during the first hour or so in the water. Over time, oxytocin release may be suppressed, especially if the water temperature exceeds 98.6°F (37°C), leading to a possible decrease in labor activity in women who have been immersed continuously for more than two hours. If labor shows signs of slowing, change the energy, unless the mother is tired and needs to rest. If you note no significant change in the direction you were looking for, have the mother get out of the tub for a period of 15 to 30 minutes, and see what happens. Someone should be available to take the mother's hand, assist her in stepping out of the water and accompany her until she feels grounded. If labor stops, the woman was not really in labor yet, the water temperature could be hindering the process, or some other factor is interfering. As labor progresses, getting back in the water is always an option.

Listening to the baby

Auscultation of the fetal heart should take place as for any labor. A fetoscope or nonwaterproof Doppler can be used if the woman elevates her belly out of the water during listening. A piece of plastic wrap can be placed over the bell of a fetoscope and rubber-banded in place to minimize water entering the headpiece and interfering with auscultation.

If you cannot hear clearly with the mother in the tub, have her get out and continue to listen until you are satisfied that the fetal heart rate is normal, or use a waterproof Doppler. A nonwaterproof Doppler's head can be submerged if it is first covered with a plastic bag or a condom secured with a rubber band or tape to avoid water damage to the transducer. However, if water does get into the transducer, the Doppler could easily become inoperable. *Keep in mind that water enhances the effects of ultrasound*, so listening to the baby while the mother is in water delivers the potentially harmful ultrasound waves to the mother and baby even more efficiently.

Use of whirlpool jets

Water jets can be turned on during labor if the mother so desires, and in early labor they may be helpful as the circulating water provides some nipple stimulation. However, keep in mind that the sound of the jets will be very loud for the baby, even though the baby is still in utero. As labor advances, many women find the movement of the water too much as they deal with contractions. Even if the mother prefers the jets during active labor, it is best to turn them off during pushing so that the perineum, any fluids passed and color of the baby's scalp can be more easily assessed as well as to reduce the amount of noise to which the newborn is directly exposed at birth.

Maternal activity and movement

Almost every laboring woman benefits from movement and position changes that keep the circulation moving and the pelvis open. This is true for waterbirthers as well. Women can move about in the water and perform many of the specific corrective techniques found elsewhere in this book, if indicated. At times, however, removing the woman from the water is the best option. This is true if the woman's labor seems to have stalled out, if she seems to be holding the energy of labor back, or if gravity may help in correcting a problem that has arisen with fetal position.

Maternal hydration

Oral fluids must be encouraged, with the aim of keeping ketone output within normal limits, with a specific gravity of 1.020 or less. Enning (2003b) recommends that women have clear water only from the onset of pushing until birth. Water loss via sweating is lessened when women labor in saline. Mothers laboring in water that is too hot tend to sweat more and show an increase in diuresis; they may also rise out of the water, hang over the side of the tub and request a cold cloth or water. When this occurs, get her out for awhile and cool the water down.

Internal exams

Internal exams, when needed, can be performed with the mother immersed as long as she can position herself so that the necessary information can be obtained from the exam. She can raise her bottom up toward the surface of the water by lifting her pelvis and using her hands underneath her bottom for support. However, it may be more comfortable for both mother and midwife to perform an exam with the mother out of the water and may be essential if a thorough exam is indicated. Schlinger (2002) cautions against performing internal exams in water if the membranes are ruptured, as she feels this may introduce unsterile water into the upper yoni.

Urination in the water

Uninfected urine is sterile. Therefore, it is fine for the woman to urinate in the pool if she does not desire to get out of the water. However, getting out to go to the toilet is a good way to incorporate a change in the mother's activity. Even though urine is sterile in normal circumstances, it would be best if support people refrain from peeing in the tub.

When support people enter the tub

Some midwives feel that anyone entering the tub during the labor should shower beforehand to keep the water as clean as possible. However, water does not normally enter the yoni when a woman is immersed, and if the person is basically clean and chemical-free (perfumes, oils, and chemical deodorants should be washed off), he can get in. You should decide if you want to request that support persons wear bathing suits when entering the tub.

Altered states of consciousness and waterbirth

Most women experience an altered state consciousness in labor; this is no different for women laboring in water. Normal, endorphin-related responses must be differentiated from problems due to being in the tub. If the mother seems to be faint from overheating, add cold water to the tub, place a cold wet cloth on her face and give her a cold drink to bring her around before you have her exit the tub. Watch for shivering and blue lips (the water should never be allowed to get this cold; however, if the tub is outside, the woman may become chilled from the surrounding air). If the water is not cold but the woman's lips are blue, rule out concealed bleeding or shock from some other cause. If the woman becomes chilled, she is likely to remark on this and exit the tub herself.

Rupture of membranes

Rupture of membranes alone is not a reason to restrict the use of a tub during labor. In normal situations, water does not enter the yoni when the woman is relaxing in water. It is invasive procedures and exams that are associated with an increased risk of infection, not water immersion (Aderhold & Perry, 1991; Siegel, 1960).

How long to leave the baby underwater

The baby should be gently lifted from the water shortly after birth, usually within 5 to 10 seconds, either by the parents or the midwife. Turn the baby face down in the water, spread one hand under the baby's rib cage, cup your other hand over the buttocks for stability and lift the baby from the water at a slightly head-up angle. Alternatively, grasp the baby from behind under her arms, allow the head to flex forward and tip the body forward slightly to drain any water from the mouth and keep the nostrils down. This way, water will not pool in the baby's mouth and nose as she is exposed to air. Pay attention to the length of the cord as you lift the baby from the water; it may not allow you to lift her very far.

If the baby is distressed or the cord either broke or was cut during the birth and the mother did not exit the tub, bring the baby to the surface immediately and clamp the baby's end of the cord as soon as possible. Theoretically, the shock of the cord being severed and the loss of the placental transfusion may panic the baby into breathing.

Normal newborn responses during waterbirth

Cool water results in babies who are more actively involved in their own birth, exhibiting better muscle tone and more movement as they emerge. These babies seem optimally conscious and aware at the time of emergence from the water and stabilize more quickly than those born into body temperature water or hotter, who tend to be limp and lethargic.

Several newborn reflexes are elicited during emergence in slightly cool water. The baby will reflexively push himself out with his feet as he emerges. In addition to the diving reflex, the asymmetric tonic neck reflex (ATNR) is triggered as the baby reaches out with one arm and bends the other. The baby will also flex into a fetal position. The symmetrical tonic neck reflex is then triggered as the baby cross crawls with his head extended, all of which result in the baby spiraling out. If all is well, the midwife should not touch the baby as he emerges, allowing this dance to proceed.

At the time of birth, the undisturbed mother reaches down to touch the head as the baby spirals out and the baby, with the assistance of the ATNR, turns to face his mother as she touches him, they make eye contact, mother lifts the baby under the arms and brings him to her chest. A healthy, unstressed newborn, when gathered to his mother enface against her chest will turn his face and anterior body to his right and the mother's left side (over her heart). Unhealthy babies tend go to the opposite side (Enning, 2003b; Polin & Spitzer, 2001). After birth, immerse the baby to the nipple line with the heart under water; the increased water pressure helps increase the blood volume in the heart chambers.

The APGAR/Enning Score for waterbirths

It is typical for the waterborn newborn to have a bluish-lavender appearance and to take up to 60 seconds to begin breathing once the face is exposed to air. Babies born into air have received different stimuli prior to full emergence having already been exposed to air between the birth of their head and their shoulders. The waterborn baby does not receive the same stimuli and may be slower to start than a baby who has been born into air.

Based on her observations of hundreds of waterbirths, Enning (2003a; 2003b) has devised a modified APGAR score for waterborn babies, to be assessed at 1, 5 and 10 minutes. There are 6 parameters with a maximum score of ten. She strongly feels that the progress toward an optimal score of ten is slower in waterborn babies because the levels of stress hormones are lower as the baby is born, although cord blood gases are generally less acidic when compared to landborn babies. Because of these variations, APGAR scores are taken at 1, 5 and 10 minutes, with the 10 min score more closely approximating the same degree of adaptation reflected in the 5 minute score in landborn babies. Most of the parameters of the APGAR/Enning score are assessed as for a landborn baby, with the following special considerations:

Grimace: Enning notes that eye opening and blinking are good indications of grimace response in the waterborn baby. Since the baby is less stressed than many landborn babies, grimacing per se does not happen as often. More typical grimacing would also be assessed and receives the same score as for a landborn baby.

Muscle tone: Muscle tone is assessed by the degree to which the baby actively assists in her birth. Opening of the distal extremities occurs when the baby is actively "swimming," with the hands open (not clenched) and, in a breech, the toes splayed (not clenched or cramped).

Lung fluid expulsion reflex (LFER): The lung fluid expulsion reflex was named by Enning to describe what she sees during waterbirths. As the baby is born, he actively discharges fluid from the mouth, which can be seen jetting out into the water. At the same time, the baby's chest and diaphragm contract in a reflexive movement to help expel the fluid. Vigorous babies do this right away. They are not trying to breath and do not appear to be in distress as this occurs. The LFER and respiratory effort never occur simultaneously in a normal term newborn. The LFER can be used to assess the baby before bringing her to the surface. After that, this assessment is replaced by the more traditional observation of respiratory effort. According to Enning (2003c), while relaxation of the chest muscles between expulsive efforts would ordinarily allow water to enter the lungs, there are three reasons why this does not normally occur: the remaining fluid in the lungs, a mature level of surfactant and the diving-induced closure of the larynx between expulsions of fluid (which occurs when the receptors around the lips trigger the glossopharyngeal nerve). This means that a term or near-term newborn can have the LFER triggered and not inhale water.

PARAMETER	0	1	2	1 MIN	5 MIN	10 MIN
Appearance (color)	Pale/blue	Extremities blue	Pink all over			
Pulse (heart rate)	Absent	<100	>100			
Grimace (eye movement)	Closed or staring	One eye open	Eyes focusing and blinking			
Activity (muscle tone)	Floppy	Grasp reflex (hands or feet)	Swimming movements			
Lung fluid expulsion reflex (head under water)	Absent	Chest movement	Open mouth			
Respiratory effort (head above water)	Absent	Irregular	Regular			

Care of the baby after birth

It is ideal if the baby's face can be supported above the water's surface while most of the baby's body stays submerged. However, as long as the room is warm and the baby's body is at least halfway submerged in the tub, his core temperature should be maintained. Placing blankets and hats on the baby who is still in the water will result in getting the coverings wet, thus encouraging heat loss. Dry, warmed blankets and a newborn stocking cap should be available to wrap the baby once the mother is ready to leave the water.

Delivery of the placenta

Some practitioners prefer to remove the mother from the water for the birth of the placenta out of concern that birth of the placenta in the water will make assessing blood loss difficult or impossible and that an embolism may result from exposure of the placental site to the water. However, it is perfectly safe to deliver the placenta with the mother in the water. Since water does not travel up the yoni, the risk of embolism is not increased. Enning (2003b) finds that uterus clamps down rapidly after a waterbirth, especially when the water is around 86°F (30°C), although colder water can lead to premature separation. Conversely, if the water is too warm, the placenta can be retained for hours. However, waterbirth generally results in less bleeding, whether the water is too hot or too cold. A lower water temperature at the time of placental delivery also results in a shorter duration of lochial flow postpartum. She does recommend removing the mother from the water if a manual removal is required.

Those practitioners who regularly attend waterbirths learn to assess blood loss in the tub and to minimize blood flow into the water. To do so, hold the placenta pan beneath the mother or place it on the bottom of the tub. As the placenta is born, use the cord to gently guide the placenta out (but do not lift it up), allowing it to plop directly down into the bowl. As the placenta falls into the bowl, the membranes will come together behind it, sealing in the separation bleeding. This, of course, will not be so neat if the placenta slips out sideways. Gently bring the bowl to the surface and carefully hold the membranes in place as you drain off the water by tilting the opposite side of the pan, this way you do not dump the separation gush into the water (O'Conner, 2000). Leave the cord intact and elevate the placenta to the side of the tub, with the cord trailing down toward the baby. Otherwise, the heat from the water may encourage the cord vessels to remain fully patent, allowing blood to pool in the placenta.

Assessing bleeding after birth

Gently swish your hand near the mother's yoni to clear the water and visualize blood loss. You will be able to see it trickling out. Blood loss can be assessed by watching how dark the water becomes. If the tub itself is dark, placing a white towel beneath the mother prior to birth will make blood loss easier to assess. If you suspect that the mother is hemorrhaging, remove her from the water immediately, allowing you to have better access to her for providing care and for accurately measuring and monitoring blood loss. With a mildly cool waterbirth, there is 50 to 100 ml of blood loss, on average (Enning, 2003b).

Getting the mother out of the water

The mother who is not bleeding can remain in the tub as long as she desires. When she is ready to leave the water, the baby should be held by someone else while the mother is assisted out. Upon leaving the tub, about 30 minutes to 2 hours after the birth, the mother may bleed approximately 50 ml of "cleansing blood" (Enning, 2003b). Remember, exiting the water will restore the mother's relationship to gravity and may be disorienting for many women as they also are coming out of an altered state of consciousness. Someone should stay with her and assist her in drying off and moving to her bed.

Postpartum care

Care for the waterbirth infant and mother from this point on does not differ from that for any other.

Expert opinions regarding breech and twin waterbirth

Breech birth: Dr. Herman Ponette has pioneered breech birth underwater at his center in Belgium. His experience is mostly with multigravid women who have completed at least 37 weeks of gestation, who have begun labor spontaneously and who receive no augmentation. He screens women prenatally and selects those he anticipates will react calmly and cooperatively during labor and birth. He feels there is a great advantage to breech birth underwater due to the baby's body floating and being supported, usually eliminating the need for manipulation during the birth the head. The baby is also more able to move and facilitate her own birth. He feels it is less advisable to allow footling babies to be born in water, although he does not state why. He also uses a transparent birthing tub to afford himself full visibility during pushing. Finally, he recommends plenty of experience with "dry" breech births before proceeding to attend breeches underwater. The slightest problem or delay during labor is reason enough to get the mother out of the water. He also feels that a first baby that is breech is a contraindication for waterbirth. This is probably because the assistance of gravity is felt to be necessary to overcome the soft-tissue resistance of a previously undilated birth canal, although he does not say (Ponette, 1996).

Enning (2003b) also has quite a bit of experience with breech waterbirths. During prenatal care, she attempts external version, often with the mother herself doing the turning while in the water. If a version is painful, the version is subsequently unsuccessful, or the mother is fearful, Enning does not proceed with waterbirth.

During labor, breech babies benefit because fetal oxygenation is enhanced. Should the cord prolapse in the water, the blood flow is not as likely to become impaired, especially if this happens as the baby is emerging. Should this happen, Enning listens to the baby through the abdomen and simultaneously palpates for cord pulsations to see if the cord pulse has slowed. There should be no passage of meconium during labor: if there is, she assumes the baby to be in distress. As birth nears, Enning warms the water to 92 to 97°F (33.3 to 36.1°C) to reduce stimulation to the baby as he emerges. Unclenched toes and open hands indicate that the baby is relaxed, a reassuring sign. As the shoulders and arms are born, the body of the baby will tend to float upward, thus spontaneously pivoting the head around the pubic bone (a natural Bracht's maneuver). As the baby comes out, the mother can reach down to assist the birth, and the baby will actively move to do so as well.

As soon as the baby is out, add cool water to reduce the tub temperature back down to 86°F (30°C) until the placenta has been born.

Multiple birth: Likewise, Dr. Ponette is in the vanguard of practitioners who have worked with twin births underwater. The same basic criteria described for breech birth would also apply here (multigravidas who have reached at least 37 weeks of gestation, emotionally centered women being the optimal candidates; easy labor proceeding to an easy, spontaneous birth). He states that the time between the birth of the two babies should be no more than 10 minutes. (His feelings regarding the time limit between twins may be from a medical-model view that the second twin should be born quickly. See the chapter entitled "Assisting at Multiple Births" for more details.) Fetal maturity limits may relate to concerns about intracranial pressure changes from decompression upon leaving the birth canal coupled with the additional pressure changes the baby will be subjected to once she is brought out of the water (Ponette, 1996).

Enning (2003b), who also has considerable experience with multiples and waterbirth, feels that normal twins are most commonly vertex; other presentations suggest that there may be a problem with the nonvertex twin. Twins have generally better heart rate patterns when the mother labors in water. As with breeches, she warms the water to 92 to 97°F (33.3 to 36.1°C) until the last baby has been born. At this point, she adds cold water to reduce the water temperature back down to 86°F (30°C) until the placenta has been delivered.

When complications arise with the mother in water

Many practitioners ask women to leave the water if there is a problem during the birth itself such as the onset of fetal distress (as evidenced by poor fetal heart rate findings or poor scalp color), a tight nuchal cord or shoulder dystocia. However, many complications can be handled in the water. The midwife must decide if the problem is likely to cause sufficient fetal distress to stimulate gasping, which would place the baby at increased risk of drowning. Have the mother remove herself from the water if a complication that is not readily resolved arises.

Snags during labor: If a woman in early labor cannot remain immersed at 95°F (35°C), lower the water temperature to make it more tolerable by adding cold water to the tub or by having the mother stand up out of the water, which will produce a cold shock. If the mother has problems such as bleeding, engorgement or thrombosis in varicose veins, she is too hot (another indication of this is the mother wanting a cold cloth on her head). Get her out of the water or add cold water to reduce the water temperature no lower than 86°F (30°C).

If the mother wants to hold onto the solid edge of the pool, this may be a signal that she is afraid or is having other emotional or physiological issues come up (Enning, 2003a, 2003b).

If the baby's head is not engaged, have the mother exit the water to get her back into gravity, do walking laps around the house, and go up and down stairs or get on and off the bed alternating with walking to bring it down. Any other techniques found throughout this text to bring babies down may also be helpful.

Fetal distress: Sustained fetal heart rate decelerations without recovery would be reason enough to get the mother out if she is nearing birth. However, the types of remedies you would typically employ in a landbirth, such as position changes, giving the mother oxygen and having her breathe through a pushing contraction or two, can be used with the mother in the water as well and should certainly be tried in an effort to remedy the problem. Fetal distress must be quite severe for spontaneous gasping to overcome the apnea reflex that will be stimulated when the face contacts the water.

Cord complications: Cord problems can be handled in the same manner as with the woman out of the water and, in fact, may be easier to remedy with the baby fully submerged. However, if the cord is broken, contact between the open ends and the warm water will encourage more bleeding. Because of this, if the problem can be identified before the baby is born, the mother should, whenever possible, exit the water prior to birth.

Meconium staining: Generally speaking, even thick meconium staining can be handled without removing the mother from the water. Any meconium in the baby's mouth will be expelled into the water and immediately diluted as the head is born. To help clear the nostrils of meconium, the midwife can use two fingers on either side of the bridge of the nose to massage downward from the level of the corner of the eyes to the nostrils. If necessary, a finger can be placed in the mouth to scoop out thick meconium. All this can be done prior to the birth of the shoulders, with the baby still underwater. In term babies, postural drainage can be used to further clear the airway as they are brought out of the water. An assistant with a bulb syringe and a mucus-trap suction device should be standing by in case postural drainage does not sufficiently clear the airway (Harper, 2001).

Shoulder dystocia: While shoulder dystocia can sometimes be handled with the mother immersed, a change of position is often necessary to accomplish the birth. However, if this can be done without the mother lifting her bottom out of the water, then proceed with the head submerged. The cephalic circulatory congestion that often occurs with a severe shoulder dystocia is often less pronounced when the head is submerged because of the hydrostatic pressure on the head; this may lessen distress. Keep this in mind when using the baby's color to help assess the severity of shoulder dystocia.

Exposure of the baby's head to air during birth: What if, for example, when changing positions during pushing, the mother exposes the baby's head, which has already been born under water, to air? Is it safe to resubmerge the baby's head to complete the birth? If the head is crowning, resubmergence is not a problem. However, if the face is already exposed, it is probably best to err on the side of caution and avoid resubmerging the baby. Simply have the mother remain standing or lean over to complete the birth. Resubmergence is particularly undesirable if the baby is distressed or if there has been a shoulder dystocia, a tight cord or any other problem that can produce significant hypoxia, as a distressed baby's diving reflex may be impaired.

It is helpful to know that resubmergence of the fully born head has happened by accident on a number of occasions. For the nondistressed baby, brief exposure to air has not been proven to be significant; the mammalian diving reflex is restimulated when the baby is resubmerged to complete the birth.

If the baby is inadvertently resubmerged, have the mother lift herself out of the water as quickly as possible, which can usually be accomplished quite easily if she merely stands up. If this is impossible prior to birth, bring the baby up to the surface as soon as he is born.

Newborn resuscitation: If resuscitation is needed, support the baby's head with one hand and the body should float. Bag and mask or mouth-to-mask ventilations can be started in the tub. Leaving the baby in the tub will allow the pulsing cord to remain warm, maximizing oxygen delivery to the baby while she establishes spontaneous respirations. If the cord is not pulsing and the mother is stable, you can have her stand up to allow blood to gravity-feed into the baby. Have someone assist her to her feet and stay by her side while she is standing. Once the placenta is delivered, it can be held above the baby until breathing is well established. If cardiac massage is needed, three attendants may be required if the baby is to remain in water. One person holds a cookie sheet under the baby, another provides cardiac massage, while another ventilates.

CARING FOR THE MOTHER'S SOFT TISSUES DURING BIRTH

Midwives view birth as a sexual and physiological event that need not result in trauma to mother or baby. When a healthy woman's hormonal balance during labor is ideal, her tissues should be well prepared to open to the extent necessary to give birth without tearing. However, in Western cultures, a woman's perineum is far more protected than were those of her primitive foremothers, making hers more vulnerable to tearing because it is softer and less exposed to the elements. Western women do not squat and even use the toilet in an upright sitting position. These things make Western women somewhat more prone to tearing than they might otherwise be, even in the best of circumstances. Because of this, midwives the world over have discussed the ways in which genital trauma can be prevented or minimized for centuries.

There is nothing conclusive regarding what does or does not minimize tearing. Many experienced midwives feel that the more the woman is given the space to follow her own body's cues, the less likely she will be to tear. During a true fetus ejection reflex, the hormonal balance is optimal, aside from there being no time to try and prevent a tear.

Just about everything that is done to prevent tears involves focused attention and control on the mother's part, which distracts her from her inner experience. The only thing which does not is to encourage her to support her own tissues, which can be done instinctively if there isn't a lot of conversation about it.

Midwives have experimented with performing internal yoni massage during birth, with the intension of stretching the yoni tissue. However, yoni massage often seems to produce edema and make the tissue more friable; furthermore, many women find it extremely uncomfortable. Instead, you can use hot herbal compresses kept in a crock pot. (An herbal infusion of fresh ginger root or comfrey leaf works great.) Apply light, even pressure with compresses (one hand across the upper tissue and one on the perineum) to the entire periurethral and perineal area before and during crowning. An assistant can help by doing upper support, leaving the receiving midwife free to use one hand on the perineum and one to receive the baby. Apply oil to help the tissue stretch, but do not thin the perineum manually, since this may irritate and traumatize tissues.

Maternal positioning is also felt by many to be an important factor in preventing tears. An ideal position allows maximal sacral mobility with the least amount of tension on the perineum while encouraging strong, effective contractions; it also results in less elongation of the perineum as it does stretch, keeping the tissues from thinning too much. Positioning the mother's legs so that the knees and feet are about 14 to 16 inches (33.6 to 40.6 cm) apart prevents external stretching of the perineum and affords more give for the baby's head (Formato, 1985). Watch the perineum during pushing. If it seems unduly strained, you can try having the mother change position. Sutton (2001) states that keeping the back straight during pushing or rounding the back into a "C" shape increases the likelihood of perineal tears, as does birthing in a supine position, because they displace pressure posteriorly so that the head must dilate the perineum, rather than mostly passing above it, as occurs when the mother stands, sags her back and leans forward.

If pushing is resulting in a tightly stretched, taunt, and shiny perineum, have the mother refrain from pushing for one or two contractions. This can assist by giving the perineum more time to stretch. When offering verbal encouragement, emphasize a loose mouth and opening up, not pushing through (Kitzinger, 1990).

If a woman has painful hemorrhoids, she may involuntarily hold back and resist pushing because she fears increasing the pain. This tenses the perineum and makes tearing more likely. Applying counterpressure to the anus with a hot or cold compress (such as a gauze-covered ice cube) can help relieve the pain enough to get her past this resistance. Be especially careful not to contaminate the compress solution or the yoni area with compresses used for this purpose. One old text recommends that the midwife insert her lubricated thumb just inside the mother's anus to provide counterpressure to hemorrhoids. Do not attempt this without getting the mother's permission first, and be sure to change gloves when you remove your thumb.

Other midwives encourage the woman to push the head out between contractions, in the hope of minimizing tears by birthing the head slowly. However, this seems to increase the likelihood of sticky shoulders because the contraction is not working with the push to rotate the shoulder girdle correctly. Allowing the head to emerge spontaneously between contractions is not a problem.

Another option is to have the mother work with her breath and your guidance to ease the head and shoulders out. Blowing, or giving short pushes broken up by breathing, can help with this. The precision and timing of pushes and breathing must be more carefully tuned as crowning of the head increases. The more upright the mother is, the sooner pushing must be slowed down to avoid a rapid birth; this is determined by watching the tissue and talking to the mother. If she reports burning, these midwives have her blow and then push again.

Even though the head is born over an intact perineum, the shoulders, irregularly shaped as they are, can cause a tear as they are born. Some midwives continue perineal support as the shoulders birth, not so firmly, however, as to inhibit rotation. Jean Sutton recommends that no support be provided as the head and shoulders are born. She feels that as long as the mother assumes an upright position where she is leaning forward, with knees apart and lower than her hips, the baby will birth easily without undue perineal strain, and tearing will be minimal (Sutton & Scott, 1996).

If shoulder rotation seems delayed, check for a tight cord or (more likely) a hand near the face or shoulder inhibiting birth. A little elbow can cause a very big tear. If you can manage it, guide the baby out so the arm is kept as close to the body as possible. Bringing the hand and arm out as the shoulders begin to birth frequently jabs the elbow right down into the perineum, creating a deep pocket tear. This maneuver can cause the shoulders to malrotate as well. If you do decide to draw the hand out, wait to do so until the mother is pushing and keep the arm and elbow as close to the baby's body as possible (Feral, 1988; Tritten 1988).

To support the perineum with a woman in a suspended upright position, apply a warm, wet, wrung-out washcloth or piece of old diaper to the entire vulval area, holding it with one hand to contact the tissue but applying no pressure. Have the mother slow her pushing efforts when you can see about ⅓ of the top of the head (i.e., sooner than usual). This signals that the biparietal diameter is level with the lower pubic bone (or almost so). Have the mother blow through pushing to allow the uterus to complete the birth while you allow the head to emerge into the washcloth. Do not apply pressure with your fingers to any part of the perineum, as this may cause the tissue to spasm and encourage tearing. Be ready to support the baby around the neck and shoulders and expect the body to deliver in short order (deBy product brochure).

Learning to support the mother to birth without tearing, and adapting to a more hands-off approach to perineal support, may take some adjustment. Midwives experienced with the suspended upright position (either in a Birth Sling, on a birthing stool or with the mother leaning forward) report, after their initial adjustment period, a significant reduction in perineal tears and a somewhat more frequent occurrence of minor labial tearing (due to the pressure on the upper tissue from the mother leaning forward). To minimize tears in front, make sure the perineum is not stretched taut from side to side because of the way the mother is sitting.

As you can see, the recommendations for preventing tears are many and some of them conflict. Attempts to prevent tears impose a great deal of "midwifery" into the instinctive act of birth. You will have to talk to other midwives, as well as your clients, to come up with a way to deal with the issue of tearing for yourself.

There are times when other concerns override protecting the perineum. This may be the case when labor progress is slow due to weak contractions, when there is a problem with the fetal heart rate, or when a shoulder dystocia is anticipated. A change in the mother's position, having her breathe oxygen, or having her push with alternate contractions may remedy the situation without compromising the baby's well-being. However, if in doubt, a torn perineum is preferable to a very depressed baby.

Clitorotomy (episiotomy)

The need to cut the perineum is rare. It primarily depends upon the condition of the baby and, much less commonly, the condition of the perineal tissue itself. If the baby appears to be seriously compromised and you are convinced that birth would happen immediately if you cut the perineum, then do so. If the perineum is so very tight and unyielding that maternal attempts to push through it are tiring her excessively and beginning to be reflected in a worsening fetal response, have her change to a more upright, forward-leaning position to pivot the pelvic floor up and back; this may solve the problem. If not, cutting the perineum may be warranted. Usually, however, the need to cut the perineum has more to do with practitioner distress than anything else.

If the woman has undergone genital mutilation, her scar tissue will have to be watched closely during pushing, warm compresses and applying oil may help it to stretch (evening primrose oil with arnica tincture added would be helpful). She may also require an incision.

If you feel you must perform a clitorotomy (so called here because the perineum is filled with clitoral circulatory tissue), proceed as follows: if you have a pair of scissors with a fat, guarded blade, use two fingers to lift the edge of the perineum, open the scissor blades and guide the fat blade behind the perineum with your dominant hand. Feel to confirm that you have not overlapped either a fold of maternal or fetal tissue. Hold the scissor blades perpendicular to the skin surface and cut at a very slight angle to one side (essentially an off-center but midline cut to try and avoid a direct extension into the rectal sphincter). Cut only a small incision, say a quarter inch, and see if that is enough. Any cut is likely to extend. If you do not have scissors intended for this purpose, insert the length of two fingers behind the perineum and then insert one scissor blade between your fingers. Keep your fingers in place to guard the blade as you cut with the other hand. Once the cut is made, keep the blades of the scissors closed and remove them from the area.

Reopening the blades invites additional injury. (For full details on all topics relevant to the perineum and its repair, see my HEALING PASSAGE.)

Protecting the periurethral area

Take care not to focus so much attention on the perineum that your overzealous efforts push the head up and cause major labial or periclitoral damage while the perineum remains intact. Some midwives only recommend that the mother flex the head herself by pressing downward on the vertex to relieve tension on the upper tissues.

If there is a low or very steeply angled pubic arch, the head may be pressed further down into the perineal floor to compensate. This, in combination with a strong, resistant perineum, is a setup for labial tears. Positions that allow maximal sacral mobility are an important factor in reducing the chances of tearing.

If the head is large or is in a deflexed position, if there is a tight nuchal cord or a hand near the head or neck, if a cystocele or rectocele exists, or if the vulva is swollen or varicosed, have the mother lie on her side and guide her to birth the baby gently and slowly to help minimize structural damage. Try to ease the shoulders out one at a time.

When a tear seems likely

The appearance of a white line down the perineum frequently precedes a tear as the tissue becomes more strained. This line will be along the line of a previous scar, if one exists. The first thing to do is help the mother stop her pushing efforts by having her take deep breaths. Wait until the next contraction (or even for several contractions) to resume active pushing. This allows the perineum to adjust to the pressure and to stretch rather than tear. In the meantime, apply hot compresses and plenty of oil to assist this process. Changing maternal position may also help. If the perineum starts to tear, use the same tactics as well as supporting beneath the laceration to try and prevent more damage. Slow, gentle birth of the head and shoulders can minimize further trauma.

The same suggestions apply if periurethral or labial damage seems to be occurring. These tears are often heralded by bright red bleeding that, at first, may appear to come from behind the baby but is really from the labial area. (A slight trickle of blood may occur as the hymen is torn during the birth of a first baby.)

When there is a crisis (such as shoulder dystocia), protecting the perineum must be set aside for the more urgent need to get the baby out without delay.

Extreme perineal or periurethral swelling may occur in some progressive labors and, when they do, the tissue is very prone to tearing. Giving the mother homeopathic arnica (30C or 200C) by mouth or applying arnica gel directly to the swollen tissues along with a cold compress can help reduce the swelling. Having the mother lie on her side and proceeding as described for vulval varicosities may also minimize trauma.

Preventing trauma to vulval varicosities

Try to minimize pressure on vulval varicosities during pushing by having the mother birth in a more horizontal position. Be careful to ease the head out slowly. If the varicosities are only on one side, a lateral position with the mother lying so that the veins are uppermost can work well. Most women with problematic veins are also multiparas; their babies usually come out without the need for intense pushing, which is an advantage. As the head begins to crown, apply warm (but not superhot) compresses around the opening of the yoni, being sure to provide even support over the varicosed vessels. After the birth, be alert to the possibility of a developing hematoma from deeper tissue damage.

If support hose have been helpful during pregnancy, they can be worn during labor and continued throughout the first 6 weeks postpartum until the veins reduce to their prepregnant size.

Unhealthy tissue

Unhealthy tissue is, of course, attached to an unhealthy woman. A lifetime of poor nutrition and inadequate health care can leave a woman with very fragile tissue at the time of birth. Such tissue is often the consistency of wet newsprint or rotten meat. Sometimes an unhealthy woman has extensive tearing, despite an easy birth. The tissue cannot withstand much stress either from birth or your perineal inspection. Stitches tend to pull through the tissue, resulting in a more difficult repair.

Prenatal dietary improvement, vitamin supplements (C with bioflavonoids, E and zinc), and postpartum herbal therapy using comfrey poultices and sitz baths of rosemary infusion may help, as well as drinking comfrey infusion. But don't expect miracles in nine months after a lifetime of deficiencies.

References and Further Reading on Supporting the Woman During Labor and Birth

References used in multiple chapters

Betts D. Acupressure: Promoting a Natural Labour and Partner Involvement. http://home.clear.net.nz/pages/debra_betts/. Downloaded Feb 15, 2002.

Block P. Polly's Birth Book: Obstetrics for the Home. Hearthspun Pub, American Fork UT, 1984.

Davis-Floyd R, Davis E. "Intuition as authoritative knowledge in midwifery and homebirth," in Davis-Floyd R, Arvidson P, eds. Intuition: the Inside Story, Routledge, London England, 1997.

Fairman J. "Respecting the resting phase of labor," Clarion CPM Newsletter, 7(3);1-10, Ap, 1990.

Odent M. The Scientification of Love. Free Association Books, London UK, 1999.

Odent M. "Insights into pushing: second stage as a disruption of the fetus ejection reflex," Midwifery Today, (55);12, Autumn 2000.

Schlinger H. Editing notes, 2002, 2003.

Simkin P. Guide to Comfort Measures for Childbirth, accompanying manual for video tape Comfort Measures for Labor. Penny Simkin, Inc, Seattle WA, 1995.

Simkin P. The Birth Partner: Everything You Need to Know to Help a Woman through Childbirth, Harvard Common Press, Boston MA, 2001.

Simkin P, Ancheta R. The Labor Progress Handbook. Blackwell Science, Oxford UK, 2000.

Sutton J. Let Birth Be Born Again: Rediscovering and Reclaiming Our Midwifery Heritage! Birth Concepts UK, Middlesex UK, 2001.

Sutton J. Scott, P. Understanding and Teaching Optimal Foetal Positioning, 2nd ed. Birth Concepts, Tauranga NZ, 1996.

Trueba G. Comfort Measures for Childbirth: The Rebozo Way, The Rebozo Way, Calle 23, #40, Club de Golf, Mexicao, 14620 Mexico D F, Mexico, 2001.

Tuning into Birthing Energy

Banks M. Personal e-mail communication, Mar 6, 2000.

Davis-Floyd R, Davis E. "Intuition as authoritative knowledge in midwifery and homebirth," Med Anthropol Q, 10(2);237-269, June 1996.

Don't Just Do Something

Scholles H. Editing notes, 2003.

Positions and Activities for Labor

Balaskas J. Active Birth: The New Approach to Giving Birth Naturally, rev ed. Harvard Common Press, Harvard MA, 1992.

El Halta V. "Preventing prolonged labor," Midwifery Today, (46);22-27, Summer, 1998.

Hendrickson F. Midwifery in 10,000 Easy Steps, Part 1: A Critical and Constructive Look at Midwifery and Obstetrics by a Birth Attendant with over 20 Years Unlicenced Experience. Privately published, Hillman, MN, 1981.

Jarcho J. The Pelvis in Obstetrics. Paul B Hoeber, Inc, New York NY, 1933.

King J. Back Labor No More!! What Every Woman Should Know before Labor. Plenary Systems, Inc, Dallas TX, 1993.

Walcher G. "Die Veränderlichkeit der Conjugata," Verhandl d deutsch Gesellsch f Gynäk, (1891), 4;446, 1892.

Using Comfort and Positioning Aids in Labor

Edmunds J. "Serving our birthing sisters," Midwifery Today, (33);32-33, 43, 52, Spring, 1995.

Field M. "The jewel in the crown: clitoral massage as an analgesia for labor," Childbirth Alternatives Qtrly, VI(4);4-5, Summer, 1985.

Gaskin IM. Spiritual Midwifery, rev. ed. Book Pub Co, Summertown TN, 1978.

Gaskin IM. Ina May's Guide to Childbirth. Bantam Books, New York NY, 2003.

Khamis Y, et al. "Effect of heat on uterine contractions during normal labor," Internat J Gynaecol Obstet, 21(6);491-493, Dec, 1983.

Lehmann J, ed. Therapeutic Heat and Cold, 3rd ed. Williams & Wilkins, Baltimore MD, 1982.

Roubal P, et al. "Bilateral radial nerve palsies from use of the standard birthing bar," Obstet Gynecol, 87(5 Pt 2);820-821, 1996.

Wintergreen, presentation on "The Pink Kit," Portland, OR, 2004.

Protecting the Bladder during Labor

Donald I. Practical Obstetric Problems, 5th ed. Lloyd-Luke Ltd, London UK, 1979.

Read J, et al. "Urinary bladder distention: effect on labor and uterine activity," Obstet Gynecol, 56(5);565-570, Nov, 1980.

ACTIVE DILATION

Odent, "Pregnant women are not marathon runners," MIDWIFERY TODAY, (31);23-25, Autumn, 1994.

BREATHING AND RELAXING DURING LABOR

Banks M. "Breech Birth Women Wise," Pre-conf. workshop, MANA conf., Wakefield MA, Oct 24, 2002.

ACTIVE PUSHING

Aderhold K, Roberts J. "Phases of second stage labor. Four descriptive case studies," JNM, 36(5);267-275, Sept-Oct, 1991.

Cosner K, deJong E. "Physiologic second-stage labor," MCN, 18(1);38-43, Jan-Feb, 1993.

Lemay G. "Pushing for first-time moms," MIDWIFERY TODAY, (55);9-11, 13, Autumn, 2000.

McKay S, Roberts J. "Second stage labor: what is normal?" JOGNN, 14(2);101-106, Mar-Apr, 1985.

Menticoglou SM, et al. "Perinatal outcome in relation to second-stage duration," AM J OBSTET GYNECOL, 173(3 Pt 1);906-912, Sept, 1995.

Sagady M. "Renewing our faith in second stage," MIDWIFERY TODAY (33);28-31, 41-43, Spring, 1995.

MATERNAL POSITION DURING PUSHING AND AT THE TIME OF BIRTH

Bannenberg C, deBy birthing support representative, 2004.

Gentlebirth midwifery archives, http://www.gentlebirth.com. Accessed 2001.

Robertson A. "The Pelvis in Labor," MANA Conf., taped workshop, MANA98, #631, CAL Tapes, San Jose CA, 1998.

Sotelo I. 5-day midwifery intensive with Doña Irene Sotelo, traditional Mexican midwife," MIDWIFERY TODAY, Eugene OR, Aug 27-31, 2001.

ASSISTING AT THE BIRTH OF A VERTEX BABY

Boschert, S. "Suctioning doesn't alter meconium aspiration risk: intrapartum suctioning also did not change neonatal mortality rates (done before shoulder delivery)," OB/GYN NEWS, April 1, 2003.

Davis E. HEART AND HANDS: A MIDWIFE'S GUIDE TO PREGNANCY AND BIRTH, 2nd ed. Celestial Arts, Berkeley CA, 1987.

Dunn T, et al. "DeLee suction. Does it have clinical significance?" J REPROD MED, 46(10);905-908, Oct, 2001.

Enning C. "Birth on Demand," all day workshop on waterbirth, MIDWIFERY TODAY conf., Springfield OR, Mar, 2003.

Gage J, et al. "Suctioning of upper airway meconium in newborn infants," JAMA, 246(22);2590-2592, Dec 4, 1981.

Kattwinkel J, ed. TEXTBOOK OF NEONATAL RESUSCITATION, 4th ed. Am Heart Assoc & Am Acad Pediatr, Dallas TX, 2000.

O'Conner D, CNM. Personal communication, Sept, 2000.

Richmond S, et al. RESUSCITATION AT BIRTH: THE NEWBORN LIFE SUPPORT PROVIDER MANUAL. Resuscitation Council (UK), Rochester, Kent UK, 2001.

Schneider K. Neonatal respiratory therapist. Personal communication, 1999-2000.

Scholles H. "Some thoughts on shoulder dystocia," Unpublished notes, recd. Nov 8, 2001.

Stevenson J. Private correspondence, 1988?

Varney H. VARNEY'S MIDWIFERY, 3rd ed. Jones & Bartlett, Sudbury MA, 1997.

HYDROTHERAPY AND WATERBIRTH

Aderhold K, Perry L. "Jet hydrotherapy for labor and postpartum pain relief," MCN, 16(2);97-99, Mar-Apr, 1991.

Anderson T. "Time to throw the waterbirth thermometer away?" MIDIRS DIGEST, 14(3);370-374, Sept 2004.

Embrey MP, Moir JC. "A comparison of the oxytocic effects of synthetic vasopressin and oxytocin," J OBSTET GYNAECOL BRIT COMMONW, 74(5);648-652, Oct, 1967.

Enning C. WASSERGEBURTSHILFE. Hippokrates Verlag, Stuttgart Germany, 2003a.

Enning C. "Birth on Demand," all day workshop on waterbirth, MIDWIFERY TODAY conf., Springfield OR, Mar, 2003b.

Enning C. E-mail communications, Mar, 2003c.

Epstein M. "Renal effects of head-out water immersion in man: implications for an understanding of volume homeostasis," PHYSIOL REV, 58(3);529-581, July, 1978.

Eriksson M, et al. "Early or late bath during the first stage of labour: a randomized study of 200 women," MIDWIFERY, 13(3);146-148, Sept, 1997.

Fainer D, et al. "Resuscitation of dogs from fresh water drowning," J APPL PHYSIOL, 3(7);417-426, 1951.

Gooden B. "Drowning and the diving reflex in man," MED J AUSTRALIA, 2(11);583-587, Sept, 1972.

Geissbuehler V, et al., "Waterbirth: water temperature and bathing time--mother knows best!," J PERINAT MED, 30(5);371-378, 2002.

Harper B. Editing notes, 2001.

James L. "Acidosis of the newborn and its relation to birth asphyxia," ACTA PAEDIATR, 49(S122);17-28, Mar, 1960.

Katz VL, et al. "A comparison of bed rest and immersion for treating the edema of pregnancy," OBSTET GYNECOL, 75(2);147-151, Feb, 1990.

Laitman J, Reidenberg J. "Advances in understanding the relationship between the skull base and larynx with comments on the origin of speech," HUMAN EVOL, 3;101-111, 1988.
Lin Y. "Applied physiology of diving: review article," SPORTS MED, 5(1);41-56, Jan, 1988.
McGraw M. "Swimming behavior of the human infant," J PEDIATR, 15(4);485-490, Oct, 1939.
Metzker Coutinho EM, Vieira Lopes AC. "Response of the nonpregnant uterus to vasopressin as an index of ovarian function," AM J OBSTET GYNECOL, 102(4);479-489, Oct 15, 1968.
Morgan E. THE AQUATIC APE HYPOTHESIS, Souvenir Press, London UK, 1997.
Morgan M, English translation of portions of Enning C. WASSERURTSHILFE, Hippokrates Verlag, Stuttgart, Germany, 2003.
Norsk P, Epstein M. "Effects of water immersion on arginine vasopressin release in humans," J APPL PHYSIOL, 64(1);1-10, Jan, 1988.
O'Conner D, CNM. Personal conversation, MIDWIFERY TODAY retreat, Waldport OR, July, 2000.
Odent M. "Can water immersion stop labor?" JNM, 42(5);414-416, Sept-Oct, 1997.
Polin R, Spitzer A, eds. FETAL AND NEONATAL SECRETS, Hanley & Belfus, Inc, Philadelphia PA, 2001.
Ponette H. "Water-births, my experience of 1600 water-births, including breeches and twins, Henri Serruys Hospital, 1989-1995," Belgium, Jan, 1996.
Siegel P. "Does bath water enter the vagina?" OBSTET GYNECOL 15;660-661, May, 1960.

CARING FOR THE MOTHER'S SOFT TISSUES DURING BIRTH

Feral C. "Protecting the upper tissues," MIDWIFERY TODAY, 1(5);22-23, Winter, 1988.
Formato LS. "Routine prophylactic episiotomy, is it always necessary?" JNM, 30(3);144-148, May-June, 1985.
Kitzinger S. "Episiotomy," MOTHERING, (55);62-65, Apr-May-June, 1990.
Tritten J. "Preventing Tears," MIDWIFERY TODAY, 1(2);16, 44, Spring, 1987.

MISSING THE BIRTH

The best-laid plans of midwives and the women they care for can go awry. A woman may call you when she first thinks labor is beginning, but labor may pick up its pace more rapidly than either of you expect. Traffic may be bad, there may be a wreck on the only route to her home, or you may be at another birth halfway across the state when she calls. Dozens of unexpected events can delay your arrival. Regardless of how carefully you plan or how thoroughly you instruct women regarding when to notify you, you will miss births; it is part and parcel of doing births at home. And, remember that doctors must, at times, travel to the hospital, so they sometimes miss births too. It is also a product of women being truly undisturbed and following their bodies, which results in physiologically rapid labors. This is especially true of multiparas who are overdue and have been priming their uterus with herbs. No matter how imminent birth is, or whether the mother gives birth before your arrival, you should always get there as soon as you possibly can to reassure her that all is well.

Today, with cell phones in hand, most midwives will be able to provide telephone consultation while the birth is in process to whomever is there supporting the mother. If the mother is home alone and has a speaker phone, she can turn that on, if she desires, or she may wish to fully concentrate on her labor, knowing that you are on your way.

If pushing is starting, it is important for a woman to go with her body, whether you are present and ready or not. Under no circumstances should a woman be encouraged to do anything, such as crossing her legs, to forcibly hold back her baby, nor should anything, such as applying counterpressure to the presenting part, be done by an attendant to impede the birth, as such actions can lead to newborn brain damage. If the baby is being born while you are en route, all parties present should be told to just let the baby come, and you will arrive as soon as possible. Breathing through pushing contractions and assuming a position that lessens the effect of gravity (such as Trendelenburg or knee-chest) can help slow the birth without harm if, for example, transport is deemed necessary. Once the baby is born, remind those present not to do anything to the cord, to keep the baby warm and put her to the breast.

If a catastrophe should occur, such as sudden rupture of membranes with a cord prolapse, you should have the mother assume a knee-chest position and have a support person elevate the presenting part. Tell them you will meet them at the hospital. You can be the one to call for an ambulance or, if another person is present at the house, he can do so. Be sure they let you know to which hospital they transport.

Most of the time, when you are en route to a sudden birth, you will miss the baby but you will arrive shortly thereafter. Rarely will you miss a placenta. Contrary to dire predictions regarding precipitous labors in the medical literature, well-prepared and well-nourished women who have their babies rapidly usually do quite well. In the wake of it all, the woman often feels empowered and quite pleased with herself, as she truly knows she had her baby completely on her own. Often the partner is the one who is seriously distressed and may greet you at the door as white as a sheet while the mother is composed and holding her baby. Once you arrive, proceed with postpartum care as you normally would.

The Birth and Examination of the Cord and Placenta

Placenta-to-Newborn Transfusion, Physiologic Closure of the Umbilical Vessels and Severance of the Cord

The cord should be left intact after the birth at least until the placenta has been born and ideally until all pulsing has disappeared at the umbilicus. The cord can then be cut several inches from the baby and will not bleed. This chapter elaborates why this is so important, as well as why clamping the cord prematurely is so dangerous.

As you read, keep in mind that the research used to support much of what follows comes from studies that were trying to observe physiology by imposing most assuredly pathological conditions on the infant, such as clamping of the cord at various times rather than leaving everything alone and seeing what happened. I have attempted to make good use of the best research; however, discrepancies between the findings as originally published and the actual physiology of neonatal transition are highly likely.

This type of research is fraught with problems. Even today, there is no quick, reliable way to determine blood volume, and all existing methods are imprecise. In particular, estimating fetal blood volume is highly prone to errors because of rapid fetal development, the rapid processing of labeled blood indicators introduced into the fetal system, the inaccessibility of the fetus, and the fetal blood volume being distributed between the fetal body and his cord and placenta. The condition of the fetus or newborn at the time the samples are collected also affects the results. The blood volume values presented here are averages, as the results of various researchers differ somewhat as to the actual blood volume of the fetus and newborn based on the methods used to gather the information as well as the number and actual gestation of the babies involved. The following therefore represents a survey of the literature combined with the opinion of myself and other professionals who have observed physiologic infant transition in their own practices. I have endeavored to distinguish theory from fact or researched data as appropriate.

Umbilical Cord Care among Higher Primates and Indigenous Humans

Among some species of higher primates, the mother eats the placenta. If not, she makes no attempt to severe the cord (although it may break off). She carries both baby and placenta around over the first days of life; the cord atrophies and the cord and placenta separate naturally (Trevathan, 1987). Humans have referred to this practice of natural cord separation as **Lotus birth**. Atlee (1957) points out that, until humans began to fashion cutting tools from plants, stones or metal, there was no way to separate the cord other than cutting it with the teeth, rubbing it on a rock, or possibly cauterizing it with fire and nothing to ligate a bleeding, pulsating cord.

With the many taboos and beliefs about blood in all human cultures, it seems highly improbable that primitive humans would disrupt a part of the body that carried blood if they wanted the baby to survive. Therefore, for over 99% of our existence as a species, babies were born to mothers who usually delivered in an upright position, the baby stayed attached to the placenta until it was born and all blood had drained from it. Were this detrimental to the newborn, genetics would have fixed this long ago or we would have died out.

Today, in most indigenous cultures, the cord is usually left intact until the placenta has been delivered, in keeping with the belief that all the life from the placenta must be transferred to the baby or the baby may die. In some Asian and African cultures, the cord is stripped or milked, especially if the baby is not breathing, in order to bring the baby's soul back from the mother (WHO, 1999). These age-old practices are supported by what is currently known from a Western scientific viewpoint regarding the importance of the placental transfusion at birth.

Fetoplacental and Newborn Blood Volume

Prior to birth, the baby's "body" includes the cord and placenta. The cord is a specialized part of the baby's vascular system while the placenta is a vital fetal organ of great complexity that functions, in large part, as a transfer organ serving nutritional, excretory and respiratory functions. During gestation, the total blood volume is distributed between the fetal body, cord and placenta; however, the total blood volume is calculated using only the weight of the fetal body, not including that of the placenta and cord. Between 16 and 22 weeks, the total fetoplacental blood volume averages 162 ± 21 ml per kilogram fetal body weight (Morris et al., 1974). Total blood volume appears to adjust proportionately as gestational age advances and the baby gains weight. Sneeden (1955) found a similar value of 180 ml/kg of fetal weight at 18 weeks, which dropped to an average of 150 ml/kg by 26 weeks. By term, the blood volume averaged 120 ml/kg of fetal weight. The ratio between the fetoplacental blood volume and fetal weight remains constant throughout gestation, so the formula based on fetal weight is reliable until term. (Reminder: 1000 grams = 2.2 pounds = 2 pounds, 3.5 ounces; one ounce equals 28.4 ml; 1 ml = 1 cc.)

The distribution of the total blood volume between the fetus, cord and placenta also changes over gestation. At 30 weeks, about half of the total blood volume is in the cord and placenta at any given time and half is in the baby's body. By term, the placenta/cord-to-fetus volume ratio has changed, so that approximately 30% of the blood is in the cord and placenta and 70% is in the baby at any given time. All of this blood is the *baby's blood.* A term fetus weighing 8 lb 13 oz (almost 4 kg or 3997 grams) would have an average of 120 ml of blood volume per kilogram of body weight, giving her a total fetoplacental blood volume of about 480 ml (16.9 oz). A 33 week preterm baby weighing 3 lb 5 oz (1.5 kg) or 1500 grams would have an average 130 ml/kg of body weight, giving him a total fetoplacental blood volume of 195 ml (6.8 oz). The decrease in blood volume per unit of body weight as the fetus matures is probably due to the rapid increase in fatty tissue, which is relatively less vascular.

After birth, the blood volume of a term baby whose cord is left intact for at least a few minutes ranges anywhere from 110 to 115 ml/kg of body weight, with a hematocrit ranging from 50 to 65%. Using the average for this range, 112 ml/kg, the baby would have 3.9 oz of blood for every 2.2 lb (1 kg) of body weight. (Note: ranges of "normal" for newborn blood volumes are based upon studies that artificially terminated placental transfusion at various times.) However, among the general population of newborns in the United States (who are born in hospitals and whose cords are usually immediately clamped), blood volume ranges from 70 to 100 ml/kg, demonstrating the marked hypovolemia that can be produced by premature termination of the placental transfusion (Linderkamp, 1982).

The well-perfused baby shifts fluid from the intravascular to the extravascular spaces over the hours following birth, resulting in a temporary, relative hemoconcentration. These shifts make it hard to study the exact blood volume of the well-transfused baby. The resulting hemoconcentration has also confounded definitions of polycythemia (too many red blood cells). Poorly transfused babies do not shift fluids in this manner. Instead, they constrict less vital circulatory pathways and recruit blood from other regions of the body to try to maintain an adequate blood supply to the most vital organs, such as the brain, and maintain as stable a blood pressure as possible, as does any victim of hypovolemic shock (Morley, 2002d; Yao & Lind, 1982).

The Anatomy of the Umbilical Cord at Term

The umbilical cord at term is normally a trivascular conduit that carries corporeal blood to and from the placenta. The umbilical vessels are unique in several important respects. The vein carries oxygenated blood from the placenta to the baby. It has no valves, which means blood can flow freely back and forth as long as it is patent (Benirschke, 2002). The walls of the umbilical vessels consist of three layers, just like other large vessels. The vein has an intima (innermost) endothelial layer, the cells of which are longitudinally oriented. Next is the media (middle) layer, consisting of tiny longitudinal, obliquely oriented elastic fibers but having no true internal elastic membrane. It also has circularly and obliquely oriented muscle cells. These smooth muscle cells lie parallel to each other at right angles to the length of the vein and have a regular, circular arrangement held together by a ground substance that allows them to slide over each other, an important factor in producing effective postnatal contraction. The adventitia (outermost) layer is composed of sheet-like membranes of Wharton's jelly. As the intra-abdominal portion of the umbilical vein approaches the liver, the muscular and elastic tissues diminish as the structure transitions to one with more connective tissue and a thicker layer of Wharton's jelly.

The two umbilical arteries carry deoxygenated blood from the baby to the placenta. Their walls are similar to that of the vein, except the media layer consists of two separate layers–an outer strong layer of concentric muscle sheets similar to that of the vein, and an inner layer with longitudinal muscle cells; between these layers is a fine network of elastic fibers.

The venous lumen, when filled with blood, is larger along its entire length than that of the two arteries combined by almost 30%, making it the largest fetal vessel. This results in the blood volume in the vein equalling the blood volume of both arteries combined. The rate of blood flow in the vein is about one-half the velocity of flow through the arteries.

By term, the cord vessels transport about 125 to 150 ml/kg of fetal weight, or about 40% of fetal cardiac output each minute, with an average arterial pressure of 70 to 80 mm Hg and an average venous pressure of 10 to 20 mm Hg.

The umbilical cord has no skin or fat. While the portion of the vessels contained in the abdomen are innervated, the umbilical cord proper is generally agreed to have no nerve supply. (Although such a supply has been sought and some evidence for neural fibers has been found by various researchers [Benirschke & Kaufmann, 2000]). The vessels are surrounded by a layer of Wharton's jelly, a translucent semigelatinous connective tissue of varying thickness, which is covered by a tightly fused layer of amnion. Contrary to a commonly held notion, Wharton's jelly does not cushion the cord while it is fully functioning. Full distention of the vessels pulls the jelly tautly over the surface of the cord, where it serves as a strong, thin sheath, providing counterpressure to the vessels, thereby preventing ballooning of the cord and pooling of blood. This also means that cord blood must flow under pressure, or else the Wharton's jelly would expand and the vessels would collapse. As cord function starts to decline after birth, the gelatinous texture of Wharton's jelly becomes apparent as the vessels constrict and the jelly loosens up.

Some 95% of all cords have coiled vessels, most commonly due to spiraling of the arteries around the vein, although the reverse may also occur. Coiling occurs in a counterclockwise direction rather than a clockwise direction by a ratio of 7:1. The coils increase in length as their distance from the fetus increases. Coiling appears to reinforce the cord, making it strong and flexible, and assists in helping the cord to stretch in the same way that a coiled phone cord can stretch. However, although the vessels have some limited elasticity, the membranes that sheath the cord do not (Morley, 2002e). Coiling also assists in amplifying the pumping action of the blood as it moves through the cord, a process explained in more detail in the chapter entitled "The Baby's Journey through Labor to Birth" (Reynolds, 1952, 1978a, 1978b; Strong, 1997; Walsh et al. 1974).

Physiology of Placenta-to-Newborn Transfusion

The placenta is both a fetal and a newborn respiratory organ, although it is not widely acknowledged as such by mainstream obstetrics or neonatology. "Transfusion" means the process of passing from one to another; the fetus-to-newborn transition process is designed so that the fetus can transfer most of her placental blood volume into her body at the time of birth, maintaining continuous blood flow to the entire system and facilitating the transition to air breathing. The vessels supplying the fetal lungs are constricted in utero; thus, the lungs are minimally perfused prior to birth and receive only 8 to 10% of the total blood flow. The lungs of a term newborn baby of average size require approximately 45 ml (1.58 oz) of blood to expand the pulmonary capillary beds when breathing begins (this equates to 40 to 55% of the cardiac output).

Uterine activity and the placental transfusion

It has been theorized that the placenta-to-newborn transfusion may begin even before the baby is born. During pushing contractions, as the uterus becomes increasingly empty, more and more pressure is brought to bear directly on the placenta. The placenta is squeezed during contractions, forcing blood in the cord arteries toward the baby at high pressure. This high pressure may begin the process of dilating the alveoli capillaries prior to birth. Coupled with the inflow of blood, a fall in pulmonary resistance may be triggered by exposure of parts of the baby's body to air, causing hormonal and chemical changes that signal that birth is imminent (Mercer & Skovgaard, 2002). (Perhaps a certain percentage of the body must be exposed before this shift is triggered.) As Morley (2002a) points out, there is only one place for a large bolus of blood flowing under high pressure to go, into the nearest empty blood vessels, which are in the lungs. This pressure is temporarily relieved between contractions, allowing blood to return to the placenta for oxygenation as well as allowing the baby a gradual adjustment to the increase in lung perfusion.

Placental engorgement just prior to birth

Peter Dunn (1966) found that the placenta is extremely engorged with blood as the baby is emerging (he estimated that there is, on average, 66 ml of blood retained in the placenta when clamping is performed immediately). He felt that this degree of engorgement could not be the normal state of the placenta but was a temporary state brought about during the brief passage of the baby's body through the birth canal. He speculated that the umbilical cord becomes partially compressed when the lower torso is passing through the birth canal, temporarily impairing venous flow from the placenta to the baby; the arteries, which move blood under more pressure from the heart, still carry blood from the baby to the placenta. Dunn also postulated that the baby, who experiences the squeezing effect of passage through the birth canal, would be likely to sustain congestive hemorrhage if blood flow from the placenta were not somehow impaired during this brief interval (Dunn, 2002). Morley (2002e) does not agree on this point; although cord compression can cause placental engorgement, he observed that the large, hard fetal head has just dilated the birth canal, paving the way for the lower body to pass through with minimal compression. (Perhaps the engorgement that Dunn found is due, in part, to the thoracic squeeze the baby experiences when the chest passes through the canal, an event which impairs blood return to the baby and which is rendered more severe during an obstructed birth such as shoulder dystocia.)

Regardless of the mechanism of placental engorgement, I propose that the engorgement Dunn observed makes the placenta firm and resistant to bending, keeping the area of attachment on the uterine wall maximally spread out and minimizing the chance it will detach prematurely when the uterus becomes dramatically smaller as the baby's body exits the uterine cavity. Furthermore, when unimpaired blood flow resumes as the baby emerges, the engorged placenta has a large bolus of well-oxygenated blood with a normal pH ready to flow into the baby with the force of the contraction that delivers the baby's body. This is reflected in the majority of babies at birth having cords that are full of blood and pulsating strongly. The arteries are still carrying blood from the baby to the placenta for oxygenation and the vein is delivering oxygenated blood to the baby just as efficiently.

Pulmonary capillary expansion continues

As the baby emerges (possibly as the baby receives this bolus of blood and before breathing commences), a higher percentage of blood is forced through the fetal circulatory pathways into the lungs. There it continues the process begun during pregnancy of expanding the constricted capillary framework surrounding each alveolus and reducing the effort required of the baby to expand his alveoli. (These ideas regarding prebirth capillary expansion are primarily based on the research of Jäykkä [1957, 1958], who looked at the effect of the fluid pressures that are required to expand the pulmonary vasculature. He found irregular perfusion when adequate blood flow was lacking or when the baby was required to inflate the lungs with no simultaneous influx of blood [Mercer & Skovgaard, 2002].)

Reflexes that help trigger breathing

At birth, the baby is exposed for the first time to a dry environment that is colder than her mother's womb. Even in a hot climate, the air, evaporation, drafts, etc. (all of which would have been present millions of years ago) stimulate two reflexes: the cold crying reflex and the cold pressor reflex, both of which raise the blood pressure in the aorta and may be enough to cause the blood to become rerouted to the lungs (Morley, 2002d). Although a squalling baby is most certainly breathing, babies do not have to cry to begin breathing well on their own. However, the cold crying reflex may still come into play even when the transition is gentle enough to occur without active crying. Morley believes that these babies may take longer to dry out their lungs than those that cry vigorously. In studies of newborn transfusion variations immediately after birth, rapid transfusion seemed to result in a burst of crying (which Gunther noted was also common in babies receiving transfusions when the rate of flow was too fast). Most often, the rise in intrathoracic pressure during crying seemed to dam back inflow from the umbilical vein or even push blood into the cord vein at the umbilicus when the cord had previously been empty. Crying may therefore slow the transfusion in naturally born babies.

However, studies of transfusion dynamics on a few surgically born babies by Gunther (1957), suggested that lusty crying increased the amount transfused, while quiet babies received much less. This may have to do with incompletely understood processes operative for babies who are having an unphysiologic birth, as their placentas were removed from an atonic uterus and taken, with the baby, across the room for the transfusion to continue; large increases in weight, which exceeded those of naturally born infants, suggesting that these babies were lifted from the uterus in a state of relative hypovolemia compared to their naturally born counterparts.

The role of uterine contractions

The uterus continues to contract after birth. Dunn (1966) showed that the interval between birth and the peak of the first postbirth uterine contraction is, on average, 2 minutes and 15 seconds (135 sec). Contractions then continue at an average rate of one every 2 minutes, 38 seconds (158 sec). The placental venous pressure (the pressure in the umbilical vein) is 49 mm Hg between contractions; as the contraction peaks, it rises to as high as 102 mm Hg. High venous pressure during pushing and immediately after birth moves blood from the placenta into the baby. The spiral arteries of the uterus under the still-attached placenta supply oxygen as the blood is transfused in successive spurts with each uterine contraction. Thus an uninterrupted supply of oxygen-saturated cord blood continues to flow to the baby for as long as the placenta is attached to the uterine wall, normally at least three minutes after birth. The newborn is fully oxygenated at fetal levels (umbilical venous blood is about 70% saturated) and has time to gradually begin to breathe without any need to rush. The brain and other vital organs are continuously perfused with oxygenated blood while this occurs. The liver receives a large bolus of blood, which allows it to continue to synthesize glucose, keeping the brain and other vital organs adequately nourished. (Poor uterine contractility allows umbilical venous blood to flow in either direction. Thus, the baby should be held below the level of the placenta in these cases [Gunther, 1957].)

Gradual transition

When respiration begins, air fills the alveolar sacs. At the same time, blood is pushed by the heart into the capillary framework surrounding each alveolus (or, if Mercer is right, capillary expansion increases), as oxygenation is gradually transferred from the placenta to the lungs; that is, from the fetal organ of respiration to the newborn organ of respiration. (See the chapter entitled "The Baby's Journey through Labor to Birth" for a more detailed explanation of these cardiopulmonary changes.) The additional hemoglobin from the red blood cells the baby receives provide a reserve supply of oxygen while the baby's breathing becomes established. Blood pressure shifts also occur gradually as the placental transfusion diminishes and the cord vessels close down.

Blood volume and other organ systems: As the task of respiration shifts to the lungs, the placenta also transfers its alimentary and excretory activities to the gut and kidneys. These organs also benefit from continuously adequate perfusion and small amounts of additional circulating volume to help meet the new demands of digestion and filtration. The placental transfusion is also put to good use in maintaining optimal cellular nutrition as the baby becomes more active during the days following birth.

Optimal thermal regulation: An adequate blood supply makes the baby more resilient to variations in environmental temperature as the baby leaves the consistent temperature of the womb (Oh & Lind, 1967). Cooling of the skin during a normal birth does not result in hypothermia if the cord is pulsating because blood is circulating through the placenta (which is still inside a hot mother) and heating the newborn. While the cord does cool upon exposure to air, the cord blood remains close to body temperature when blood is flowing rapidly in the minutes following birth. After the cord vessels undergo physiologic closure, the newborn has enough blood volume to shift circulation back and forth from his core to the skin to regulate heat loss and retention more effectively than one who is hypovolemic. The term baby also has a layer of insulating fat (which preterm babies do not have) and, if the ambient temperature drops sufficiently, he is capable of metabolizing brown fat to produce heat and maintain a normal temperature (Morley, 2003).

The timing and quantity of placental transfusion

The expanded pulmonary circulation requires only about 45 ml of blood the placenta contains at least 125 to 150 ml of blood at the time of the baby's birth. It is not expected that every drop of placental blood would ever reach the infant; however, a cord left intact longer than just a few minutes affords the breathing newborn a more optimal transfusion. Full cord function carries blood to and from the placenta for a variable length of time after birth, with only intermittent slowing of blood return to the placenta during uterine contractions. The baby whose cord is pulsating strongly and who breathes almost immediately receives a substantial placental transfusion in the first 60 seconds of life, especially when she is held below the level of the placenta. Stembera and associates (1965) noted that about 248 ml of blood per minute coursed through the fully pulsating cord in the average 6 lb 10 oz (3 kg) baby during the first 4 minutes. This averages 75 ± 7 ml/min per kg of body weight. The flow was strongest during the first 100 to 120 seconds. The flow had dramatically decreased in most, but not all, of the 17 term babies studied after 1.5 to 2 minutes. Yao and colleagues (1969) found that a baby held at the level of the introitus receives a 50% transfusion within one minute and 100% within 3 minutes. (None of these researchers waited to see what happened if the cord was left intact after that.)

However, when the cord is not pulsating or when breathing is delayed, lung expansion theoretically takes place more gradually. Thin cords seem to go white sooner that thick ones, and transfer ceases soon after the cord turns white (Gunther, 1957). If pulsing is absent, the baby will have to rely almost entirely on breathing efforts to establish optimal lung perfusion because blood is not coming into the newborn circulation under pressure in the same manner. Stembera and associates (1968) found a cord flow of only 50 ml/min in babies born distressed and little or no flow if the cord was limp. Therefore, it is imperative that the cord remain intact until the baby has taken at least five breaths on his own. However, even in normal, unasphyxiated newborns, it seems that gas exchange in the lungs is established gradually, with the first five breaths or so providing minimal oxygenation to the normal newborn, who is still being oxygenated via his cord blood while his lungs continue to expand and clear of fluid.

Rhythmic regulation of the placental transfusion

In vigorous newborns, the placental transfusion proceeds in a rhythmic manner as breathing becomes established. This rhythmic pattern is first produced by the pressure of each uterine contraction propelling blood toward the baby at high pressure. Between contractions, intrauterine pressure on the placenta is relieved and the baby has an opportunity to backflow blood via the open, valveless umbilical vein. This transfusion process is further regulated by the sphincter-like action of the portion of the umbilical vein that is within the baby's abdomen (Morley, 2002d).

Blood flow toward the placenta via the umbilical arteries begins to diminish after several minutes due to arterial constriction, which is prompted by a rise in blood oxygen levels as the baby begins to breathe. The umbilical vein remains intermittently patent, continuing to bring oxygenated placental blood to the baby. This process tapers off as the placental blood volume drops, as fetal circulatory changes send blood to the lungs rather than to the placenta and as the placenta detaches. As blood flow slows, the coiling in the cord also begins to relax. While all this is occurring, passive back-and-forth flow of blood toward the placenta via the valveless umbilical vein can continue to take place.

Thus the transfer of blood is not simply a matter of turning the tap off with a cord clamp or allowing the transfusion to proceed by leaving the cord intact and holding the baby below the placenta. The natural process allows for an ebb and flow of blood between baby and placenta, allowing optimal perfusion if full equilibration is allowed to occur.

Systemic balance

The possibility of damage to the brain and other organs from temporary cardiovascular overload is eliminated when the baby is kept close to the level of the placenta during most of the time the cord remains intact (Dunn, 1966). This is true because the vein, which has no valves, allows any excess blood to backflow toward the placenta. The baby has an opportunity to continue to equilibrate her blood flow during the pauses between contractions, as well as after the placenta is born. If the newborn is kept well below the level of the placenta the entire time that the cord remains intact, the transfusion will occur rapidly and the healthy baby will reflexively close his umbilical valve within the abdomen after receiving enough cord blood (Morley, 2002d). Either way, a temporary overload cannot occur. However, the heart must work harder to push blood uphill, and a baby who has suffered asphyxia may be less capable of shutting off the flow at the umbilicus. For this reason, keeping the compromised baby below the placenta during stabilization and then level with the placenta while the cord remains intact allows the heart to return blood to the umbilical vein if necessary.

Physiologic closure of the cord vessels: A complex, incompletely understood series of hormonal, biochemical and mechanical processes govern the process of closing down the cord vessels. The vessels become increasingly sensitive to mechanical irritation during the last two weeks of pregnancy. Evaporative heat loss causes the cord to cool rapidly as soon as it is exposed to air. Tension on the cord that occurs during normal birth may help to trigger blood vessel contraction as well. A rise in oxygen saturation as breathing is established also contributes to vessel constriction.

The pulsations of the intact cord diminish, then gradually cease, and spiraling of the cord begins to relax as the bulk of the placental transfusion is accomplished. This occurs as numerous localized constrictions develop in the muscular layer of the umbilical arteries. The constrictions form at intervals in the circumference of the cord. They begin as a series of small, intermittently spaced indentations in the arterial wall nearest the surface of the cord and evolve into deep scallops along the length of the muscle. These scalloped constrictions gradually narrow and close the lumen. These constrictions appear to occur more gradually and are less pronounced when the cord is left intact. In addition, an inner longitudinal layer rich in ground substance, with loosely arranged cells and few contractile elements, serves as a plastic tissue that folds within the actively narrowing lumen of the artery to complete closure. Closure occurs when the tension of the constricting arterial walls exceeds the transmural pressure, which is reduced by diminishing blood flow after birth. (**Transmural pressure** is that which the blood exerts against the vessel walls as it flows.)

Umbilical artery closure may begin as soon as 45 to 60 seconds after birth, signaled by diminishing pulsation in the cord and indicating that the arteries have largely ceased to function. Arterial flow begins to diminish at the placental end first because the fetal heart is actively pumping blood out of the baby toward the placenta. Venous flow begins to diminish at the baby's end first, as the placental transfusion returning to the baby tapers off. (Keep in mind that these findings were derived from lengths of cord obtained at various times after birth. The cords were double-clamped and dissected, a highly invasive and unphysiologic process likely to trigger responses in the vessels similar to those that might occur when a cord ruptures during birth. Arterial and venous closure is quite likely to be more gradual in the intact cord.) If the cord is cut and the stump is examined at this point, the arteries will be constricted but blood will be clearly visible in the vein, which is still engorged with blood (Yao & Lind, 1982).

Like all veins, the umbilical vein, has a thinner muscular coat and is composed of more separate layers of longitudinal or circular fibers than the arteries, is more distensible than they are. At birth, the vein responds to all the same influences as do the arteries and in the same manner. However, because its diameter is more than double that of the arteries, even strong contractions of the muscle coat do not obliterate the lumen of the vessel. Thus, the vein remains patent much longer than the arteries, with most venous activity diminishing at 4 to 6 minutes after birth (again, timing is based on clamped and dissected cord sections), although some studies show minor fluctuations still occurring up to 20 minutes later in some babies. By the time most pulsating diminishes, the transfusion is nearly complete.

Leaving the cord intact beyond this point allows the baby to continue to equilibrate the amount of blood in his body via the valveless vein. Equilibration is regulated by reflexive response of the intra-abdominal portion of the umbilical vein, eliminating the possibility that central venous pressure will rise to a dangerously high level, which can occur when the placental transfusion is abruptly interrupted soon after birth (Born et al., 1954). This process will occur most effectively if the baby and the delivered placenta are kept at the same level; this is easily accomplished by wrapping the newly born placenta in a Chux pad or clean cloth and plastic bag and then placing it on the mother or beside the baby on the bed. Having the placenta close to the level of the baby is a neutral zone, that has little or no effect on the amount of blood that flows to or from the baby.

Lotus birth leaves the cord intact until it drops off on its own, usually at a few days postpartum. Its effects on the baby's blood volume are the same as for physiologic closure of the vessels.

Postnatal blood volume dynamics and the placental transfusion

The circulating blood volume of well-perfused babies changes dramatically over the hours following birth. The increase in total blood volume from the placental transfusion is soon decreased by hemoconcentration as fluid is transferred into the tissues; the hematocrit rises, as does the albumin concentration of the circulating blood volume, a process most pronounced in preterm babies, who have a lower blood albumin level at birth (for more details on this, see the chapter entitled "The Baby's Journey through Labor to Birth"). This temporary rise in hematocrit can be misinterpreted as polycythemia. Hemoconcentration increases plasma colloid osmotic pressure, which enhances the elimination of lung fluid and keeps the lungs dry (Morley, 2002d). The volume of blood received plus any hemoconcentration that occurs also increases blood viscosity. This helps keep the pulmonary vasculature erect and pulmonary vascular resistance low, resulting in increased pulmonary and systemic vascular dilation, which, according to a basic principle of physics, requires a higher viscosity (Mercer, 2001). The well-perfused baby urinates frequently after birth as she eliminates excess fluid volume, some of which has been transferred from the lungs as they dry out. By about 72 hours, the blood volume becomes more stable as transition is complete.

Medical Management of the Cord

Charles Darwin's grandfather Erasmus Darwin was a doctor, researcher and inventor. In 1801 in his book *Zoonomia*, he expressed his strong opinion as to why the cord should be left alone:

> Another thing, very injurious to the child, is the tying and cutting of the navel string too soon; which should always be left till the child has not only repeatedly breathed but till all pulsation in the cord ceases. As otherwise the child is much weaker than it ought to be, a portion of the blood being left in the placenta, which ought to have been in the child.

During the twentieth century, birth in the Western world was transferred more and more into medical hands. The use of various interventions mounted as institutionalized care was established. The practice of immediate or early clamping of the cord was first widely recommended in the 1930s as a way of reducing the amount of anesthesia that reached the infant. Even so, at that time and for the next 30 years or so, many doctors left the cord intact until pulsing had ceased in the midportion of cord, as is clearly evident by studying the textbooks of those decades. However, in the 1960s, rapid clamping was further promoted as a means of reducing the incidence and the then-thought ominous sequelae of, what turned out to be, physiologic jaundice. By the late 1970s, prevention of polycythemia was added to the list of presumed benefits derived from clamping the cord soon after birth.

The case for immediate cord clamping got an additional boost with the advent of specialized neonatal care. Newborn survival moved more to the fore as a sought-after outcome of birth starting in the early 1950s. In 1952, Virginia Apgar introduced neonatal scoring at 1 and 5 minutes of life. By the early 1960s, neonatal resuscitation protocols were revised and became more standardized. The health care provider for the mother-fetus pair began to routinely transfer newborn care to the pediatric staff, who took the baby across the room to be evaluated on a special warming table that housed newborn equipment. This resulted in almost immediate cord clamping, especially in the presence of preterm birth, neonatal distress or meconium staining of the amniotic fluid, when there was a perceived requirement for immediate intervention. (Ironically, this is when the baby needs his placental transfusion the most.) In addition, the rise in malpractice litigation during the 1980s and 1990s caused doctors to seek a means of documenting that infants were born healthy under their care. In 1995 the American Academy of Obstetricians and Gynecologists (ACOG) released an Educational Bulletin (No. 216) recommending immediate cord clamping in order to obtain cord blood for blood gas studies. This bulletin was quietly withdrawn in a small-print announcement in the February 2002 issue of OBSTETRICS AND GYNECOLOGY, the ACOG journal, an action that released ACOG from further liability. This followed an unpublished and unanswered letter sent to ACOG by Morley (Morley, 2002b).

Since the late 1990s, there has been increasing interest in harvesting cord blood to obtain stem cells for future use by the baby, her family or researchers. The net result of all these trends, policies and recommendations is that most doctors, some midwives and the general public have inferred that the cord blood is useless to the baby once she is born and that routine, immediate cord clamping does no harm. Actually, cutting the cord to provide resuscitative assistance or to collect cord blood immediately after birth very likely and ironically contributes to problems such as brain damage, which the practitioner is trying by these means to prove he had no part in (Morley, 2002b).

Immediate vs. early clamping

Immediate clamping is that performed as soon as possible after the birth, typically within the first several seconds, sometimes even before the buttocks have fully emerged. In the worst case, during surgical births, the doctor may reach in and clamp the cord even before lifting the baby from the uterus.

In this text, the term "early clamping" will refer to clamping that occurs at least several minutes after birth (usually 3 to 5), which often correlates with the cessation of cord pulsations halfway between the baby and the placenta. (Other sources label this "late" or "delayed" clamping. However, this action still prematurely terminates a physiologic process; therefore it has been renamed "early clamping" in this text. Waiting until the placental transfusion is complete will be referred to as physiologic clamping or closure.

When the placental transfusion is interrupted

When the cord is clamped too soon, the placenta is prematurely amputated, abruptly preventing or interrupting the transfusion process. As a result, the baby may suddenly be deprived of as much as one-third to one-half of her blood volume–a circulatory insult no adult could withstand–leaving the baby in a state of hypovolemic shock. A loss of 50 ml of blood in a baby weighing 7.5 lbs is the equivalent to 1000 ml of blood loss in an adult weighing 150 pounds (Atlee, 1957). Could this be why "sick neonates are one of the most heavily transfused groups of patients in modern medicine"? (Murray & Roberts, 2004)

Physiologic closure of the umbilical vessels occurs after the vessels are completely empty of blood throughout their length and cord pulsing has stopped at the umbilicus. The physiologic process dictates a stepwise transfusion of blood that is regulated in part by the timing of uterine contractions and in part by reflexive valve action in the umbilical vein within the baby's abdomen. Thus, clamping performed at the height of a uterine contraction could result in a temporarily overwhelming bolus of blood entering the baby that his system is not quite ready to integrate; clamping that occurs between uterine contractions can result in too much blood being retained in the placenta. Even after the placenta is born, equilibration continues by slight adjustments that occur via reflex action of the intra-abdominal portions of the vessels, eliminating the development of excessive central venous pressure and thus allowing the baby's system to gradually integrate the additional blood volume. While overtransfusion is ultimately impossible because all the blood is baby's blood to begin with, allowing physiologic equilibration to take place as it naturally occurs is the most gentle option as far as normal neonatal transition is concerned. Furthermore, even a temporary overload of the fetal circulation can cause vascular damage in the fragile germinal matrix of the preterm infant's brain; this is prevented when the cord is left intact and the baby is kept at a neutral level in relationship to the placenta (Dunn, 2002).

Immediate or early cord clamping thus produces what amounts to a significant loss of blood; the baby's compensatory response is to redirect blood to his pulmonary circulation and his most vital organs and away from other less essential areas. When the transfusion is interrupted before the baby has taken his first breath, it results in a decrease in the size of the heart during the first three or four cardiac cycles, after which the heart again increases in size, almost to the size of the fetal heart. This occurs as blood is recruited from the corporeal circulation to expand the alveoli, leaving the heart momentarily without enough blood and dramatically decreasing perfusion of the brain and other vital organs, a condition that improves as the baby struggles to reestablish circulatory equilibrium in the face of hypovolemia (Lind et al., 1959). The cord clamp thrusts the baby into a state of total asphyxia, as the flow of oxygenated blood from the placenta is cut off. This results in a dramatic rise in blood pressure partly due to the asphyxia and partly because the low peripheral circulatory resistance of the placenta is suddenly removed (Born et al., 1954). This extreme rise in blood pressure is particularly dangerous to the still-delicate vascular network within the preterm baby's brain.

While the normal term baby will almost always survive this hypovolemic insult, clamping the cord of a compromised infant prior to the onset of sustained respirations poses even more danger (DeMarsh et al., 1941). In the hypoxic fetus, compensatory vasodilation or constriction occurs, depending upon the duration of the hypoxia. Either adversely influences the amount of blood the baby receives even further. The baby is expected to revive without that critical pulmonary transfusion, meaning the baby is completely on her own to inflate her wet, poorly perfused alveoli, requiring higher ventilatory pressures and risking injury to the delicate lungs. After birth, these babies breathe more slowly and have a larger functional residual capacity than do those who receive their placental transfusion, reflecting the work involved to keep less optimally perfused alveoli inflated (Oh et al., 1967). Thus, the tendency of hospital personnel to clamp the cord immediately and rush the distressed baby away from the mother to another care provider in order to begin resuscitative efforts is both unphysiologic and self-defeating. Clamping the cord prior to the establishment of regular respirations in a preterm infant can pose a real threat to his survival.

The transfer of placental blood is also more critical for early babies, who have less blood in their systems than term babies and who may, even in the best of circumstances, experience difficulty in establishing or maintaining respirations if their lungs are not sufficiently mature. When the alveoli are not held erect by the blood from the placental transfusion, the effect is doubly damaging in the baby who must also cope with an immature level of surfactant. Not only are the lungs deprived of adequate circulating volume, but the lesser corporeal blood volume of babies born prior to 30 weeks leaves the brain and gut more vulnerable to necrosis, infection and permanent damage. Allowing the preterm baby to receive an optimal placental transfusion and the opportunity to equilibrate volume at the time of birth thus not only protects her from respiratory distress, but prevents hypovolemia, eliminating the need for transfusion in the first days of life as well as greatly increasing her ability to stabilize and maintain normal respirations (Dunn, 1966; Morley, 2002e).

Babies whose cords are clamped early tend to have stable blood pressures and show no significant changes in hematocrit or blood volume in the hours following birth. Some researchers have concluded that this indicates that their blood volume is adequate. In fact, at a minimum, these babies must recruit blood from other vascular compartments to ensure adequate blood flow to vital organs; they often appear pale after birth and have a more limited tolerance of temperature variations than well-perfused newborns. These hypovolemic babies are further compromised when multiple blood samples are taken for numerous neonatal tests, which, for some babies, may continue for days or even weeks after birth. This may eventually necessitate a transfusion, exposing the baby to the myriad risks that this intervention entails.

The very discussion and emphasis that the medical model places on clamping the cord, rather than simply cutting it, suggests the interruption of a process. It is well known that when the cord is cut too soon and the baby's end is not clamped, the baby hemorrhages; if the placental end is left open, it spurts blood. The necessity to use a clamp at all shows that the natural and spontaneous closure of the umbilical vessels within the baby's abdomen is incomplete.

Risks and benefits related to timing of clamping

While some research has been done to determine the effects of late clamping, much less has been done to look at the effects of early clamping. The following list summarizes and expands on many of the reasons why awaiting physiologic closure of the umbilical vessels is almost always a good practice:

- Allowing the placental transfusion to take place results in newborn retention of a 50% larger red cell volume dispersed through a slightly enlarged blood volume, with higher hematocrit values than in babies whose cords are clamped immediately. The iron in these cells is stored by the body, protecting the baby from anemia for months after birth as well as ensuring optimal oxygen transport to vital organs. Thus, deprivation of placental blood results in a large loss of iron to the baby (DeMarsh et al., 1941). All the fuss about breast milk lacking iron becomes irrelevant. This is particularly important for babies born at high altitudes, where the oxygen level in the air is reduced.
- Depriving the baby of his placental transfusion also deprives him of quantities of white blood cells, antibodies and platelets, as well as plasma proteins and other nutrient benefits that come with adequate perfusion.
- Early clamping can result in idiopathic respiratory distress syndrome (the earlier the cord is clamped, the more severe the distress) (Saigal et al.,1972). Morley (2002b) points out that inadequate pulmonary blood flow

leads to lung tissue necrosis, slow infarction and permanent loss of tissue if the baby survives at all.

- Leaving the cord intact is associated with a significant rise in pressure in the baby's vena cava and the right atrium of the heart that persists throughout the first few hours of life (Moss & Monset-Conchard, 1967). The longer the cord is left intact, the higher the systemic vascular resistance; likewise earlier clamping is correlated with a significant drop in systemic vascular resistance over the first hours of life. Thus, babies whose cords are clamped too soon may have poor circulation and bluish limbs, and have more trouble maintaining a normal temperature.
- Immediate clamping correlates with a higher incidence of cardiac murmurs in the first 14 days of life because blood volume is insufficient to produce full closure of the fetal circulatory pathways (Buckels & Usher, 1965).
- Hypovolemic circulation favors the brain and heart and affects blood flow to the gut. The resulting suboptimal blood flow to the gastrointestinal tract increases the risk of necrotizing enteritis in preterm babies; this severe condition involves ulceration and infection of the ilium and colon (Nelson, 1999).
- The baby receives an optimal transfusion of her own stem cells when the cord is left intact. These undifferentiated cells may contribute to lifelong well-being in ways not fully appreciated at this time. Conversely, denying the baby these valuable cells may make her more vulnerable to the development of cancers as well as other chronic diseases.

It is considered normal for some newborns to display a dramatic color difference between the upper and lower body immediately after birth. As circulation changes from fetal to neonatal status, oxygen saturation is significantly higher in the blood supplying the head, upper body and right arm than that supplying the lower body. Thus a diagonal line of demarcation is sometimes visible across the chest, with the upper body and face appearing pink, and the lower body and legs appearing pale or blue. This is thought to reflect a persistence of the fetal circulation, where unsaturated blood flows across a still-patent ductus arteriosus with a little mixing of oxygen-saturated blood from the left ventricle. This color differential disappears as the flow through the ductus venosus decreases, serving as a sign of the transition from fetal to neonatal circulatory pathways (Fletcher, 1998).

However, this has not been observed by Dr. Morley (2002e) or by me, nor have other experienced practitioners who await physiologic closure and with whom I have spoken observed this phenomenon. It may instead reflect the hypovolemic status of a baby who has been subjected to early cord clamping. It is also likely to be indicative of what amounts to an imbalance in perfusion, as the baby's body must distribute an inadequate amount of blood to compensate.

Recognizing Complete Physiologic Closure of the Umbilical Vessels

Since waiting for the complete placental transfusion to take place prior to cutting the cord is in the best interests of the baby, the question arises: how long should you wait? Typically, hospital-based midwives wait at least until the cord stops pulsing midway between the baby and the mother. Many homebirth midwives wait until the placenta is out before clamping the cord. Lotus birth advocates recommend waiting until the cord falls away on its own. They believe this purely physiologic approach honors the baby's bodily integrity and allows a transitional period of closure, as the fetal to newborn passage is allowed to take place naturally over the first days of life. True physiological closure occurs somewhere between these two extremes.

Several studies have looked at transfusion dynamics during and between uterine contractions by constantly monitoring the babies' weights immediately after birth (Allmeling & Haselhorst, 1930; Haselhorst, 1929; Gunther, 1957). They found a gain in the infant's weight with each postnatal uterine contraction, although the amount of gain diminished with each successive contraction. Pulsations in the cord were taken to indicate partial or complete patency of the arteries, which did not recur once it had ceased; after that point, blood was considered to flow only through the vein (Gunther, 1957). They also found that very strong umbilical vascular pulsations resulted in small transient decreases in weight. In nearly all of the infants studied, the weight had stabilized by 20 minutes after birth, often within 10 minutes or less. (It is interesting to speculate what they might have learned if they had waited even longer to cut the cord.)

Even today, little is understood about how much blood the newborn's body can accept. This may correlate with the size of both the newborn and his placenta. The amount of blood in the placenta is dependent on its size. Gunther (1957) found that cord pulsations continued in some cases without a corresponding gain in newborn weight, suggesting that a primary anatomical reservoir had already been filled in the liver, lungs and spleen. However, other cases showed that, after the cessation of pulsations, slight weight shifts continued at a rate of about 60 g of blood per minute, which were obviously venous.

In most cases, the cord is pulsing strongly when a baby is born. This pulse is due, in part, to the baby's heartbeat. The baby is still actively receiving oxygenated blood from the placenta via the umbilical vein. The force of each uterine contraction squeezes the placenta, producing a high-pressure infusion of cord blood; this temporarily subsides as each contraction eases off. This rhythmic process usually continues for the first 3 to 5 minutes after birth, and sometimes longer. Gradually, the cord becomes limp as the baby's breathing is established.

The arteries gradually empty of blood, becoming collapsed and then constricted, whitish strands in the cord. (Recall that the umbilical arteries carry blood from the baby to the placenta; as oxygen tension rises, the arteries are triggered to constrict.) The vein remains distended much longer. Although the vein appears reduced to a partially collapsed tube containing intermittent, sausage-like segments of blood interspersed with more collapsed areas, when the cord has completely ceased to pulse halfway between the baby and placenta, the cord at the base of the umbilicus is always still pulsing strongly. Some midwives, including myself, wait until the cord stops pulsing at the base of the umbilicus before cutting it. Cessation of pulsation is determined by using the pad of the thumb and forefinger to lightly palpate the skin-covered base of the cord where it enters the baby's belly. Typically, it takes one and a half to three hours (and occasionally longer) for pulsing at the umbilical base to completely disappear.

The rationale for waiting this long is that the baby will receive an optimal transfusion of blood and will have adequate opportunity to equilibrate her blood volume through the cord if necessary. The baby is handed to the mother, who is usually, by this time, lying down. Thus the baby is held at or slightly above the level of the placenta, which is a neutral zone that has no effect on the transfusion one way or the other. When pulsing has ceased at the umbilicus, all the cord vessels appear flat and white along their entire length in the intact cord. Examination of the cut end of all three umbilical vessels finds them collapsed and empty of blood, or almost so.

In my experience, awaiting full physiologic closure has two advantages. First, significant visible jaundice virtually disappears from this population of babies. Those who do experience jaundice clear it quickly. Theoretically, this may occur because any extra blood that initially enters the baby's system has an opportunity to backwash toward the placenta when the cord remains intact, giving the baby's blood volume a chance to fully equilibrate. Certainly, Allmeling, Haselhorst's, and Gunther's research supports this theory. Secondly, when the cord is drained dry, there is scarcely any blood left in the cord vessels. As a result, the cord dries up and falls off in less than a week, often within 2 to 3 days.

The placenta can be wrapped in a disposable underpad or a plastic bag and towel once it is born and placed next to the mother until the baby's umbilicus is completely quiet. You will notice that very little to no blood comes from the end when the cord is finally cut, and you will have to milk whatever blood is left in the vessels upward during examination of the cord stump to visually confirm the number of cord vessels.

If, for any reason, the cord must be cut before the placenta is born (or sooner than 20 to 30 minutes postpartum), Morley (2002c) advises checking for closure of the intra-abdominal umbilical vessels by trying to strip some of the blood remaining in the umbilical end of the cord back into the baby. If this proves difficult, the vessels are nearly closed. If this is impossible (you may even rupture a vessel in the cord), then the base of the cord vessels is closed, at least when subjected to positive pressure from the outside. Even at this point, however, most babies will still have some pulsing at the base of the umbilicus. Therefore, this test cannot detect whether the baby is still in the process of equilibrating his blood volume by reflexively releasing tiny amounts of his blood, but you can be sure that he has taken in all the blood he is going to get. At this point the cord can be cut if necessary.

Other Issues Regarding Placental Transfusion

Milking or stripping the cord

This term refers to actively forcing cord blood in one direction, usually into the baby. To strip the cord, position the baby below the level of the placenta. If the placenta is not yet born, use your thumb and index finger to compress the cord near the placenta end, as close to the mother as possible. Now slowly and deliberately slide your fingers down the cord to the baby's umbilical base. Repeat this process two or three times or more, especially if you find that the cord is still passively filling but the blood is sluggish in reaching the baby. Release the cord between each stripping to allow as much blood as possible to fill the vein before proceeding to strip it again.

Stripping the cord has been widely condemned in modern medical circles as a recipe for polycythemia resulting from overtransfusion. In previous decades, its routine practice mainly stemmed from a desire to hurry the placental transfusion so that the cord could be cut and the baby handed over to the pediatric staff. One of the few studies that examined the effects of cord stripping (Siddall & Richardson, 1953), found that the practice did not appear to be harmful, apparently transferred the maximum amount of blood to the baby and did not increase the rate of jaundice (some have expressed concern that stripping may damage red blood cells, but I could find no support of this myth in the literature [Colozzi, 1954; McCausland et al., 1949; Siddall et al., 1952]). However, normal babies will receive an optimal transfusion when the cord is left alone. Forcing blood into the well-perfused baby may produce temporary circulatory overload if the baby is not given the opportunity to equilibrate her blood volume via a continuously intact cord, although this caution is only based on theory.

However, stripping the cord should be considered if cord pulsations are sluggish or absent in a baby who is having a hard time getting started. Morley (1998) has found that stripping the cord is greatly beneficial to a nonbreathing baby born with a slow or absent heartbeat. Stripping sends a bolus of oxygenated blood from the placenta into the heart and is the ideal means of producing cardiac distention, which is a strong stimulus to cardiac systole. The human plasma protein fraction in the blood is an additional impetus to restart the heart. If the cord is still pulsating, simply lowering the baby below the placenta may accomplish the same thing. Cord stripping can be done in a few seconds while the newborn is being otherwise stimulated and positioned for additional resuscitative procedures.

Gravity

Gravity can help or hinder the process of placenta-to-newborn transfusion. Because the umbilical vein lacks valves, gravity can impact placental transfusion when the hydrostatic pressure created by the position of the baby in relation to the placenta is sufficient to alter the usual pressure gradient between the uteroplacental and the baby's vascular systems. There is no significant influence when the baby is held either 4 inches (10 cm) above or below the placenta. Raising the baby 20 to 24 inches (50 to 60 cm) above the placenta (which produces a hydrostatic pressure about equal to that of the resting uterine pressure) for 3 minutes prevents placental transfusion (Yao & Lind, 1982). However, hydrostatic drainage back into the attached placenta during elevation is reversed during uterine contractions, which can generate an umbilical venous pressure of about 102 mm Hg. Hypovolemia is especially likely when the baby is held high enough above the placenta to create a siphoning effect in the presence of a relaxed uterus, as typically occurs during surgical births. Lowering the baby by the length of the cord can speed the usual placental transfusion considerably, so that the entire transfusion may occur in as little as 30 seconds. Holding the baby below the level of the placenta is particularly beneficial when a baby is slow to start breathing.

However, overall, the combined effect of uterine contractions and newborn respiratory efforts are the most important determinants of how much blood the healthy, breathing baby will receive unless the baby is held statically at an extreme level in relationship to the placenta. In the normal course of birth, uterine contractions and changes in position that the baby naturally undergoes as the mother moves about will balance things out, especially if the cord is left intact. The exception is when the baby is born distressed; this is discussed under "Fetal hypoxia" below.

Placental implantation site

A placenta implanted high in the uterus will receive the most direct and efficient pressure from postpartum uterine contractions. One implanted in the lower uterine segment, where the uterine contractions are not as intense, results in less efficient delivery of the placental transfusion (Yao & Lind, 1982). Therefore, it is especially important to leave all cords intact at least until the placenta is born, to afford the baby the best possible advantage from receiving placental blood under as much uterine pressure as possible.

Cord limp and bloodless at the time of birth

A cord that is completely limp at birth can "jump start" as the baby comes around or as the uterus begins to contract, even when the baby was not distressed at birth. Any blood the baby can get from the cord will be important, so leave the cord intact whenever possible, at least until breathing is well established. Lowering the baby below the level of the placenta and stripping the cord (especially if the baby seems to be having trouble) help facilitate ongoing transfusion before the cord starts pulsing again.

Fetal hypoxia

Although the complex responses of the fetus and neonate to hypoxia as they relate to blood volume are not fully understood and extremely difficult to study in the human fetus, some basic things are known. Acute hypoxia first triggers peripheral vasoconstriction, which effectively reduces the size of the intravascular compartment. This helps perfuse vital organs, but the increased systemic vascular resistance can also result in blood being squeezed from the baby's system back into the placenta, thus lowering the baby's blood volume while he is still in utero. Furthermore, if intrauterine hypoxia is the result of cord compression, some or all of the normal blood flow between the baby and placenta may be impaired, especially during descent when tension on the cord increases. Thus blood becomes backlogged in the placenta, reducing the fetal blood volume even more. Any of these sequelae can cause the acutely hypoxic baby to be born in a state of hypovolemia. After birth, vasoconstriction will continue if breathing and heart rate do not normalize quickly. Clamping the cord prior to the establishment of normal respirations denies these babies the opportunity to retrieve this lost blood volume, as well as to receive a normal placental transfusion. It also prevents them from equilibrating their blood volume during recovery.

Initially, intrauterine hypoxia promotes extreme vasodilation in an effort to bring in as much oxygen as possible. Leaving the cord intact allows oxygenation to be restored, acidity to start to reverse, and affords the baby the opportunity to off-load extra blood via her umbilical vein. Chronic hypoxia can also cause the fetus to produce additional red blood cells in an attempt to compensate for a lack of oxygen. Thus, true polycythemia is precipitated by an adverse intrauterine environment. Allowing a potentially polycythemic baby to have her full placental transfusion will not increase the ratio of red blood cells in the whole blood; it will, however, greatly assist her in establishing respirations. Prolonged or chronic hypoxia leads to vasoconstriction and hypovolemia at birth, which can be quickly resolved when the cord remains intact.

Virtually every distressed baby born in the hospital today is subjected to immediate cord clamping, even though the evidence strongly supports the benefit of leaving the cord intact. However, whatever the birth setting, resuscitation can still be performed without separating the baby from his placenta. The unresponsive baby should be kept lower than the undelivered placenta until spontaneous breathing is well established. If the placenta delivers in the midst of resuscitation efforts, an assistant should hold it, fetal-side down, above the baby as high up as the length of the cord permits until the baby is breathing on his own and has fully recovered. This will prevent reverse transfusion, as blood will tend to passively drain toward the baby until the baby is stable, the compensatory vasodilation or constriction has resolved and the baby can take over reflexively balancing his own blood volume (Landau, 1953). (Also see the section below entitled "Chronic cord compression and dehydration.")

Surgical birth

Surgically born babies are typically lifted from an atonic uterus which interferes with and usually prevents placental transfusion and may even result in a loss of corporeal blood back into the placenta before clamping occurs as the baby is lifted out. How to prevent this is covered in the chapter entitled "Once You are in the Hospital."

When the Cord must be Clamped in an Emergency

Truly emergent reasons for clamping the cord quickly are rare. Even a cord that is around the neck can usually be left intact. Most of the time the baby can be born, even if she is quite entangled in her cord, which can then be unwound. On the rare occasion that a cord is so tight or short that it must be cut, be sure to place two clamps side by side on a single visible segment of cord and cut between them. Once the cord is clamped, time is of the essence as the baby's oxygen supply is now completely cut off.

If the cord breaks at the time of birth, it must be clamped on the baby's side or the baby will hemorrhage. If both ends are visible, you will not be able to tell which end is attached to the baby; clamp both until the baby is born, then remove the clamp on the placental end to allow drainage and facilitate placental detachment and descent. During your postpartum watch, keep in mind that this baby has lost a considerable amount of blood and monitor accordingly.

Cutting the Cord

Whenever possible, allow the mother to lead the question as to the appropriate time to cut the cord. Once she asks, ask the baby. Tell the baby that there are no nerves in the cord and cutting should not, at this point, produce physical pain (although it is easy to imagine that the baby can suffer physical discomfort if the pulsating cord is amputated). Cutting the cord may, however, produce great psychic distress if the baby is not ready or willing to let it go. Lotus birth advocate Shivam Rachana (2000), author of LOTUS BIRTH, recounts stories of asking babies at about the one and a half-hour point if it was okay to cut their cord. While some babies seemed fine, she says others squirmed, fretted, grabbed their cord or wrung their hands. These babies, she surmised, were not finished with their cords. (She does not mention checking the umbilical base for pulsations. Had pulsing ceased, some fretful babies may have responded differently.) She points out that the baby receives an influx of vital force from the placenta as it atrophies over the first days of life, underscoring that the placenta represents more than physical support for the baby. Recognizing that you are severing the baby from what has been his lifeline up until now and are amputating a part of his body are important aspects of respecting his physical and psychic integrity.

When the decision is made to cut the cord, you may or may not wish to clamp it. The stump will not bleed and clamping is superfluous if the cord is drained completely and cut long. However, if the mother wishes to take an herbal bath with her baby after cutting, clamp the baby's cord stump for the duration of the bath because the water will dissolve the clots in the end of the cord and cause it to seep a little. The clamp can then be removed after the bath or at the 24 hr postpartum home visit.

If the cord is to be clamped before cutting, place the clamp on the baby's side at least 2 or 3 cm from the base of the umbilicus (do not clamp normal skin, which may extend up the cord base for a variable distance, as this will hurt!). Plan to leave a 1 to 2 cm end beyond the clamp to avoid having the device slip off and to minimize the chances of introducing contaminants into the cord vessels. Place a gauze pad beneath the intended site of severance. You, the mother, or a significant other can cut the cord between the clamp and the placenta. To prevent bleeding, use scissors that have a somewhat dull blade, because the sawing motion required to cut the cord helps activate clotting factors and encourages platelet aggregation. Otherwise, simply cut the cord about 3 to 4 in (7 or 8 cm) long and forgo the clamp. If the cord actively bleeds or seeps without a clamp, either it was cut too soon or the baby may have a clotting disorder. If the baby is compromised and requires transport, insertion of an umbilical catheter at the hospital will be facilitated by leaving a minimum of 2 cm of translucent cord between the baby and the clamp.

If the umbilical base is swollen, it may simply be edematous. However, more rarely there may be associated fetal defects such as omphalocele, where loops of intestines are in the base of the cord, or a patent allantoic duct that is still connected to the bladder. Even more rarely, a length of intestine may traverse a portion of what appears to be a perfectly normal cord. If the baby's abdomen or the cord is swollen at or near the umbilical base, it is best to leave the cord intact and take the baby and placenta to the hospital for evaluation. If the cord must be cut, sever it at the placental insertion.

Cord clamping technology

Numerous devices can be used to clamp the cord. Boiled shoelaces are a fine choice. While thick string or wide dental floss will work, they much more easily slice through the cord, especially if the cord is fat and gelatinous, be careful! Cord tape, a heavy shoestring-like material, is also available in individually packaged sterile lengths. Metal clamps are reusable and are easy for parents to remove, both big advantages. The Averbach cord bander, an instrument that allows you to place a tiny rubber band on the cord, also works well. However, if the cord is thick and gelatinous, the little rubber bands will also tend to cut through the cord. Therefore it is best to use a plastic or metal clamp to ligate these cords. Plastic cord clamps are particularly effective because they have a wide serrated jaw. However, they require a special clamp cutter for removal. Tying the cord is accomplished as follows:

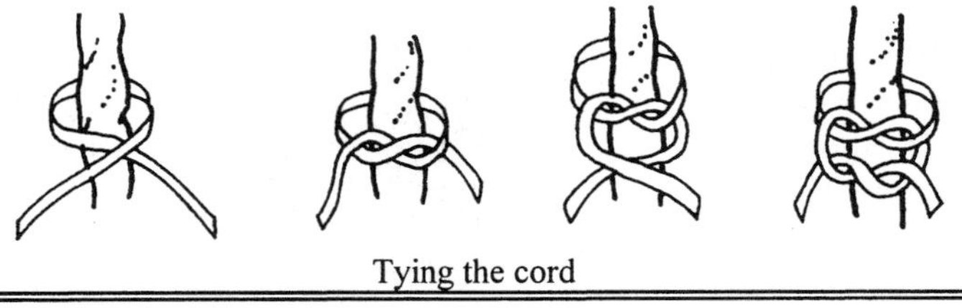

Tying the cord

Averbach cord bander: The cord bander is a handy tool used to place a tiny rubber band around the cord, making this the least obtrusive way to ensure that the cord stump does not seep. To load the band on the instrument, first wet the tip of the instrument and do either of the following:

1. Lock the rachet to close the tip of the instrument and have the lever down, with the circle tip toward the handle. Use your fingers to place the band over the tip and roll it half-way up the lever. It may help to brace the handle-end against your belly to help push the band down over the end.
2. Place the band over the tip of the a standard hemostat. Open the hemostat the stretch the band and place it over the tip of the closed cord bander. Angle the tips of the hemostat and pull it away; the band should remain in place.

With either of these methods, load the band far enough up the end of the instrument to allow for room for clamping the cord between the band and the tip end of the instrument. The instrument can be sterilized with the band in place. Bands are latex and should not be used if the baby is likely to be latex sensitive. Once loaded, apply the band as follows:

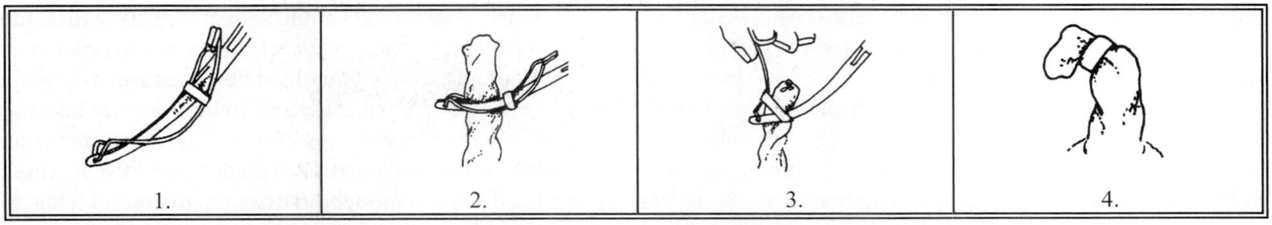

1. End of cord bander with cord band in place.
2. Use the finger-rings to open the tip of the instrument, making sure the spring is facing up (away from the baby). Place the jaws around the cord, at least 2 cm from the base and clamp, as you would any hemostat. Cut the cord 1 cm above the clamp. If the cord is white and limp, it can be cut before or after you use the clamp.
3. After the cord is cut, lift the lever up, over and down, so the band will slide off the tip and over the cord stump.
4. Once the band is in place, open the jaws of the instrument and remove it from the cord.

Burning the cord: Using a candle on either side of the stretched cord to burn it in two is the most hygienic way to severe it, especially in resource-poor areas. There will be sizzling and a loud pop; it takes 5 to 10 minutes and cauterizes the vessels. See www.cordburning.com for full details.

Real and Imagined Complications of Awaiting Physiologic Closure

Only one anecdotal case has been reported of a complication that was apparently a direct result of leaving the cord intact until the pulse disappeared at the umbilicus. An apparently normal baby became progressively paler and weaker. The baby was somehow losing blood through the intact cord. This pathophysiology was never explained, and the placenta was not held at an extreme level below the baby. However, this underscores that all newborns need observation. Use common sense. If you believe the baby's condition is deteriorating due to blood loss, hold the placenta up to transfuse as much blood as possible back into the baby, stripping the cord if necessary. When done, clamp the cord, reevaluate the situation, and prepare for transport, if indicated.

Polycythemia and hyperviscosity

The medical literature is filled with warnings about overtransfusion leading to polycythemia in newborns who have experienced cord clamping after 3 to 5 minutes or so. Although waiting for this period of time does raise the number of red blood cells, the count will not usually rise into an abnormal range. The well-transfused baby undergoes fluid shifts during the first hours of life; testing may reveal a high hematocrit at one point that later drops. Well-perfused babies urinate frequently and have a higher blood pressure than those who are not. A lack of understanding of these normal circulatory dynamics has led to a misinterpretation of findings in some studies (Mercer, 2001).

True polycythemia occurs when the fetus suffering from chronic intrauterine hypoxia compensates by producing an excess of red blood cells. It therefore preexists birth and has nothing to do with placental transfusion. Chronic hypoxia is associated with maternal diabetes, preeclampsia and hypertension. The normal baby will not have too many red blood cells after receiving her placental transfusion, especially if full equilibration is allowed to occur.

One aftermath of asphyxia in the presence of hypovolemia is capillary leak syndrome, which usually develops in the days following birth. It occurs when hypoxia causes the vascular endothelial walls to become more porous, allowing plasma components such as salt, water and albumin to leak from the circulating blood volume into surrounding tissues. This raises the colloid osmotic pressure outside the capillaries as more fluid is pulled from the circulation into the tissues. The result is an elevated hematocrit in the presence of a hemoconcentrated hypovolemia creating an apparent polycythemia that is, in fact, due to less fluid in the circulation (Jones et al., 1990; Mercer, 2001).

Polycythemia can be produced via simple dehydration that occurs when the cord is cut too fast. When the plasma volume is not in balance, there appear to be too many red blood cells; the same phenomenon is seen in dehydrated adults who display elevated hemoglobin levels. These babies jaundice more frequently and more severely because their liver function is compromised secondary to hypoperfusion (the liver processes the red blood cells).

Hyperviscosity refers to a change in the blood that increases its resistance to flow and often accompanies polycythemia; in plain English, babies with pathologic hyperviscosity have thick, dense blood and are even more severely dehydrated (Morley, 2003). How hyperviscosity occurs is generally poorly understood among neonatologists, with some studies linking it to poor neurologic outcomes, while others find no such correlation. Hyperviscosity is a byproduct of severe hypovolemia, which may occur in the presence of chronic cord compression when blood becomes sequestered in the placenta. Hypovolemia leads to peripheral vasoconstriction, which aggravates the effect of hyperviscosity because it narrows the vessels, leading to blood stagnation and reduced oxygen delivery to the tissues. While placental transfusion (as well as blood transfusion) does elevate blood viscosity, the additional blood volume is accompanied by a decrease in vascular resistance that results in increased pulmonary and generalized vasodilation, both essential to normal fetal-to-neonatal transition. (Mercer, 2001)

Jaundice

During the late 1970s, the era that spawned the hysteria about polycythemia, concern about the risks of jaundice in the otherwise normal term newborn was also on the rise. Since that time, the term "physiologic jaundice" has come into its own, with the recognition that bilirubin is an antioxidant (see the information on newborn jaundice in my text DIAGNOSTIC TESTS for full details). The best way to minimize jaundice and its risks is to let the cord stay intact for as long as possible so the baby can fully equilibrate his blood volume.

Preterm birth

It has been feared that allowing preterm babies to have their placental transfusions may overperfuse their systems, resulting in rupture of delicate blood vessels in the brain and in dangerously high bilirubin levels. Paradoxically, these babies need their placental transfusions *even more urgently* than do term babies because their lungs are less mature and because more of their blood is in the placenta at any given time. There is simply no research based on completely physiologic transition that substantiates these fears; early babies should be allowed to have their transfusion with the cord remaining intact so that they can equilibrate their blood volume.

Are There Exceptions to Allowing Physiologic Closure of the Cord Vessels?

Chronic cord compression and dehydration

Morley (2003) explains that, in situations involving prolonged partial compression of the umbilical cord in labor (such as oligohydramnios or rupture of membranes with the escape of almost all the fluid), the arterial flow, which pumps, continues more or less normally, while umbilical veinous return to the baby, which is passive, is impaired. This causes the placenta to become increasingly engorged with blood. As hydrostatic pressure in the villi beds rises, fluid is forced into the mother's system, resulting in gradual dehydration of the fetus. (When a venous tourniquet is placed on a limb, the limb becomes swollen; the placenta has no tissue space to accommodate displaced fluids.) When these babies are born, their cord vessels are constricted and may look like three strings of blood in a white cord. The placenta is packed with red cells but virtually empty of fluid; thus no placental transfusion can occur. These babies are usually born floppy and white, covered in thick meconium. They have hyperviscosity and may have polycythemia, both of which result from dehydration. They require immediate IV fluids, which, in essence, provides an artificial placental transfusion, making this the only circumstance which warrants immediate cord cutting to access the umbilical vein for transfusion. Skilled monitoring of the fetal heart rate during labor should identify babies who are headed for severe compromise and transport should take place before birth whenever possible. If transport is not possible prior to birth, all the midwife can do is resuscitate the baby below the level of the cord and hope for the best while someone arranges for immediate hospital transport for the baby. Do not attempt volume expansion at home. (See "polycythemia and hyperviscosity" above.)

Collecting cord blood

The question arises of how to allow a baby to receive an optimal transfusion when cord blood must be collected (for example, if the mother is RhoD negative). Waiting about 10 minutes would give the baby an opportunity to receive most of the placental blood, but at this point the cord flow is so significantly reduced that collecting enough blood is difficult. Therefore, it is best to collect blood shortly after birth. Although the following method creates a bit of a mess, it is one way to allow the baby to have as much blood as possible while still getting an adequate sample. Use a Vacutainer tube with an 18 gauge needle to collect the sample from a cord vessel. Have an assistant hold a length of cord between her two hands. Swab the proposed puncture site with antiseptic herbal tincture, allowing it to dry thoroughly, being sure all maternal blood is cleansed from the site. Draw the blood from the largest vessel, then apply a piece of sterile gauze to the puncture site. The puncture should seal up, allowing the cord to remain mostly intact. It is important to maintain sterility while collecting the blood so that pathogens are not introduced into the baby's bloodstream.

An alternative is to wait until the placenta is delivered and take blood from the base of the cord where it joins the placenta or from a placental vessel. However, this is much more difficult than taking blood from the middle of the cord while it is still pumping.

You can also try "clamping" the pulsating cord in two places by having a gloved assistant use the pads of the thumb and forefinger of each hand to occlude blood flow in a section of cord, draw blood from the engorged vessels between the "clamps" as described above and then release the cord without cutting it. Using fingers instead of clamps will lessen vessel trauma and reduce the likelihood of spasm so that the transfusion can resume most easily.

<u>Multiple births</u>

In multiple births in which both or all babies are roughly the same size and have a normal appearance, keep each baby in a neutral position (level with or slightly below the placenta) at birth; all cords can then remain intact. If the babies are obviously different sizes, with one appearing very puny and pale and the other very ruddy, this indicates chronic twin-to-twin transfusion has occurred during gestation. In such cases, it is generally recommended that the cord of each baby be clamped on both the placental and newborn side as soon as possible after each birth, although leaving the cord intact longer for the smaller, paler, hypovolemic baby may be the best way of allowing the babies to balance the blood volume between them (Yao & Lind, 1982). A massive amount of research is required in this area (Gilhooley, 2001). Gunther (1957) recommends leaving the first twin below the level of the placenta until the cord is white and the uterus has started to contract again. The rationale for immediate clamping with chronic twin-to-twin transfusion is discussed in the chapter entitled "Assisting at Multiple Births." Chronic TTT is a serious condition and requires transport.

<u>Blood incompatibilities</u>

It has been long recommended to clamp and cut the baby's side of the cord shortly after birth when the mother is known or suspected to be sensitized to a blood factor for which the baby is positive. The rationale for this approach is that the baby's liver is already overtaxed with processing damaged red blood cells, and the infusion of additional antibody-laden blood into the portal vein may overburden it unnecessarily, doing more harm than good. Therefore, the recommendation has leaned in favor of early or immediate clamping.

However, this fetus has been coping with antibodies throughout gestation. The total volume of antibodies transferred from the maternal system will not be appreciably increased in the time it takes to allow the baby to receive his placental transfusion. While placental blood does contain antibodies, it also carries all the other nutrients that the baby receives from a whole blood transfusion, thus bolstering the baby's ability to deal with sensitization and making a case for leaving the cord intact. Babies who develop anemia in utero (in this case, due to the destruction of red blood cells) tend to send more blood to the placenta in an attempt to gather more oxygen. Clamping the cord too soon will place the newborn at a disadvantage in initiating respirations by leaving this extra blood in the placenta. Rapid termination of the placental transfusion will add another stress to an already stressful transition. For all these reasons, Morley (2002e) recommends leaving the cord intact in these babies, even if jaundice or hydrops is apparent.

<u>Early Clamping and the Placental End of the Cord</u>

Regardless of when clamping occurs, the placental end should remain unclamped to allow the blood to drain from the cord, minimizing the chances of maternal-fetal blood mixing at the attachment site as well as hastening detachment. If the mother has torn, be sure to keep the bleeding end of the cord away from the open wound, as slight blood mixing may be possible otherwise. (See the chapter entitled "Blood Types and Incompatibilities" in DIAGNOSTIC TESTS for more information.)

BIRTH OF THE PLACENTA, CORD AND MEMBRANES

The birth is not complete until the placenta is born, the uterus has clamped down and the mother is engaged with her baby (with or without nursing). This is important to remember for the health of both mother and baby. The period of time between when the baby is born and the clamping down of the empty uterus holds the most risk for the mother because there is the potential for excessive bleeding.

The Physiology of Placental Detachment and Birth

The delivery of the placenta has seven basic phases:

1. **Optimal hormone release:** This facilitates strong pushing contractions and a normal third phase.
2. **Resting phase:** The uterus adjusts to its dramatic reduction in size by shrinking around the placenta. (This can happen quickly in the presence of an optimal hormonal balance.)
3. **Postbirth uterine contractions:** These facilitate the transfusion of placental blood to the baby, a process that empties the placenta of fetal blood, causing it to shrink and begin the process of detachment.
4. **Detaching contractions:** The mother becomes aware of stronger contractions.
5. **Complete detachment:** The placenta is released from the uterine wall.
6. **Descent:** The placenta descends through the uterine cavity, cervix and birth canal.
7. **Birth of the cord, placenta and membranes**

1. The hormonal milieu

During and after the birth, the mother's body releases a variety of hormones that supply the biological foundation for successful attachment to her newborn, for successful detachment and birth of the placenta and for clamping down of the uterus. This hormonal release occurs optimally when the mother has already entered an altered state of consciousness during labor and is left as undisturbed as possible afterward. Lights should remain low and the room should be quite warm, which will help her (and her baby's) catecholamine levels to fall rapidly and oxytocin levels rise. This, in turn, allows her oxytocin, prolactin and estrogen levels to rise and remain at optimal levels. As she makes contact with her baby, holds the baby skin-to-skin, attempts to nurse for the first time, gazes into her baby's eyes and listens to the baby's cooing, the mother is still completely engrossed in the altered state of consciousness that is the hallmark of an undisturbed labor. It is this optimal environment that prompts the mother to release sufficient oxytocin to produce a normal, physiologic third phase of labor (Odent, 2002).

Because the baby has been born, the energy shifts at this time and is much more confined to the mother-baby pair. For this reason, everyone else in the room tends to lose touch with the intense energy that was just flooding the room, and frequently the altered state and needs of the mother and baby are not fully respected. As the midwife, you must continue to hold the space for the mother so the birth can complete itself.

2-5. The detachment of the placenta

The following description assumes that the cord is either left intact or, if not, that the unclamped placental end is allowed to bleed out into a pan until the placenta is born.

The uterine cavity is gradually emptied of its contents as the baby descends during pushing. The muscles of the uterus continue to retract, as they have been doing throughout labor, causing most of the myometrial wall to thicken even more. The placental attachment site at term is about the size of a small dinner plate. The uterine wall beneath it remains thin compared to the adjacent myometrium; the placenta is still attached and fully functional.

Dunn has observed that the immediately clamped cord leaves the placenta hugely engorged with blood. To explain this phenomenon, he postulates that, as the baby's torso passes through the birth canal, the umbilical vein becomes compressed, impairing blood flow from the placenta, while the muscular, actively pumping umbilical arteries continue to transfer fetal blood to the placenta. This results in a momentary placental engorgement that maximizes oxygenation of the blood that is retained. As the baby is completely born, pressure on the umbilical cord is relieved and the last pushing contraction squeezes the placenta, sending a bolus of oxygenated blood into the baby as the entire uterine wall starts to shrink (Dunn, 1966).

Immediately following birth, the placenta and intact cord continue to function, providing oxygenated blood to the baby. As placental blood is transferred to the baby's lungs, the blood volume of the placenta falls and the placental mass shrinks, facilitating separation and eventually passage through the cervix. Placental shrinkage allows the uterus to clamp down more efficiently, shutting down the uterine sinuses beneath the placenta. Reduction in placental size is only achieved when the cord is left intact or remains unclamped on the placental side after the cord is severed. Blood draining from the placenta reduces placental blood volume, and therefore reduces uterine contents, by approximately 90 ml (3 oz) of blood. As the uterine wall continues to retract, each uterine contraction squeezes more blood out of the placenta in an ebb-and-flow rhythm, further reducing its size and increasing its flexibility while supplying the baby with her own blood via the intact cord. After birth, the mother's awareness of baby's sounds and movements (especially licking, suckling or sucking at the breast) trigger hormonal responses that let the mother's body know that the baby is out and that the placenta can be released.

Postbirth resting phase: The interval between the baby's birth and the first uterine contraction is typically about 2 minutes, 15 seconds. Thereafter, contractions continue at a rate of one every 98 seconds or so (Dunn, 1966). These are "resting phase" postpartal contractions of which the mother is usually unaware. The myometrial layer underlying the placenta begins to thicken from less than 1 cm to over 2 cm with each uterine contraction. The placenta becomes compressed and the blood in the intervillous spaces is forced back into the spongy layer of the uterine decidua. Constrictions of the oblique uterine muscle fibers put pressure on the maternal vessels, making them tense and congested, a state that prevents the blood in the decidua from seeping back into the mother's system. This decidual blood forms a network of fibrin over the placental implantation site, which aids hemostasis. The contractions also promote further placental separation by causing the distended uterine vessels to open and release a small amount of blood that seeps between the uterine wall and the maternal surface of the placenta. Microseparations are encouraged by shrinkage of the uterine wall beneath the placenta, as the placenta cannot reduce its surface area to the same degree. Thus, it begins to peel off the uterine wall. Additional contractions force the placenta into the still stretched and distended lower uterine segment and then toward the cervix.

6-7. Descent and birth of the placenta

Inverted separation–fetal side first (Schultz mechanism): Inverted separation tends to occur when the placenta is implanted on or near the fundus or on the upper sidewalls of the uterus. Placental separation usually begins in the center of the parenchyma (maternal side). Bleeding from the uterine wall and tiny tears in the surface of the parenchyma cause a retroplacental clot to form. This clot may aid separation because its weight exerts downward pressure, helping to detach the placenta from its implantation site. The combined weight of the clot and placenta also helps the membranes to peel away from the uterine wall and trail behind the placenta as it comes away and descends toward the cervix with the fetal surface advancing downward. In other words, the placenta and membranes turn inside out and the cord leads the way. Central cord insertion with placental inversion results in the largest possible diameter of the placental mass presenting at the cervix. The os must be about 6 cm dilated in order for a placenta drained of blood to pass through. (If the same placenta is engorged with blood, the os must be 8 cm dilated [Dunn, 1985].)

The process of placental separation by means of inversion was first formally described by Bernard S. Schultz, a German obstetrician (1827–1919). Since the shiny fetal surface leads the way, inverted separation is commonly referred to as "shiny Schultz." Inverted separation is associated with more complete detachment of the placenta and membranes than the sideways separation described next because the weight of the clot assists this process. There is also less blood loss because there are more ligating muscle fibers in the upper uterine segment, where the placenta was attached.

Sideways separation–maternal side first (Duncan mechanism): A placenta that is attached to the lower uterine sidewalls or nearer the os typically begins to detach unevenly along one of its edges. Blood escapes from under the detached edge so that separation is often not facilitated by a build-up of blood between the placenta and the uterine wall. The placenta descends by slipping out sideways, with the maternal surface visible during birth. Only about 5 cm of dilation is required when the edge of the drained placenta presents at the os (Dunn, 1985).

This type of placental separation, first formally described by Scottish obstetrician James M. Duncan (1826–1890), is called "dirty Duncan" because it is accompanied by visible blood loss and because the more textured and bloody maternal side presents as it emerges. Sideways separation takes longer and is more frequently associated with ragged, incompletely detached membranes and a greater volume of blood loss due to fewer oblique muscle fibers being present to close off maternal vessels in the implantation site on the uterine wall.

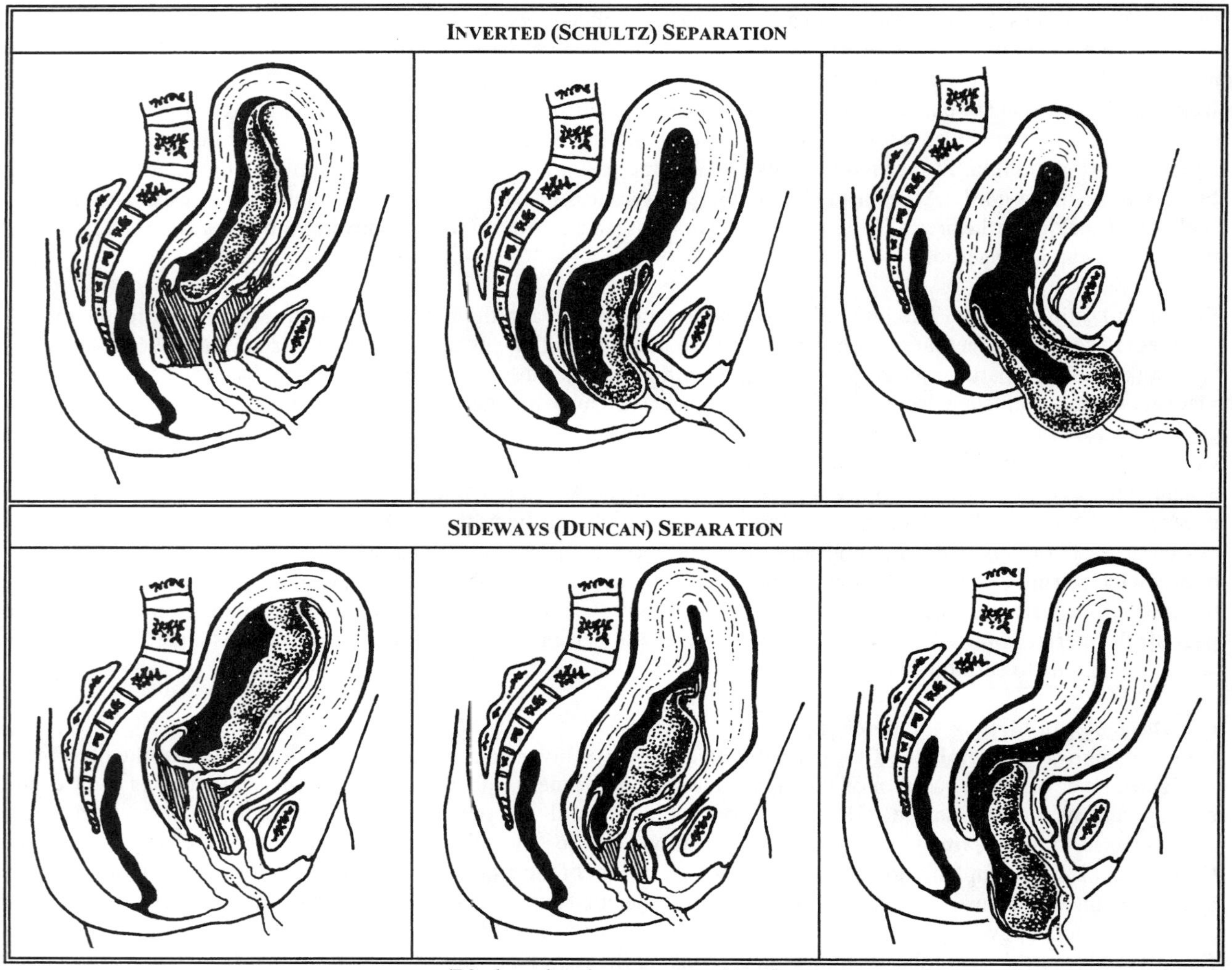

(Blackened regions represent blood)

The uterine vessels are closed off

The retraction of the upper uterine segment prevents massive maternal hemorrhage by constricting the blood vessels intertwined within the myometrium. Vigorous uterine contractions bring together the walls of the uterus in numerous folds and exert further pressure on the open placental site, activating the coagulation mechanism. Following separation, a fibrin web covers the now furrowed implantation site like a tapestry, minimizing additional blood loss and the formation of large clots. The placental site is reduced to a 2 in diameter region in the empty and fully contracted uterus.

Blood incompatibility issues

The chance of mixing of maternal and fetal blood is greatly reduced when the placenta empties itself of the baby's blood via the intact or open cord. This moves fetal blood away from the uterine wall to the benefit of mothers who are Rh-negative or who have other blood incompatibility issues. A higher rate of maternal sensitization occurs when the placenta remains engorged with fetal blood and its expulsion is either aggressively encouraged or allowed to delay. This happens because as each uterine contraction squeezes the full placenta, fetal blood has more opportunity to burst through on the maternal side where it will mix with the mother's blood (Doolittle & Moritz, 1966).

Normal Progress and Signs of Placental Separation

Note: Any actions on the part of the midwife during this time can interfere with the well-orchestrated interplay of mother and baby. Take care; observe them unobtrusively; do only what is necessary; otherwise, leave them alone.

Cues that the placenta has separated can be subtle, and not all signs are apparent in every birthing situation. Therefore, it is important to be familiar with all of them. It helps to be aware of what is occurring in each phase of birth and be in good rapport with the mother's process so you can tune into what is happening with her now.

Timing of contractions, uterine changes and fundal height

Typically the mother delivers the placenta during the first 3 to 30 minutes after the birth. The better the hormonal balance, the sooner the placenta is likely to deliver. After the baby is completely born, the mother usually has a short period that she perceives as uterine rest before contractions that she can feel resume. The uterus generally has resting-phase contractions for about twice as long as the length of time between the final pushing contractions before birth. For example, if the last several pushing contractions were about five minutes apart, expect the first noticeable "placental" contraction to occur about 10 minutes after birth. This resting phase, which correlates with the resting phase many women experience at complete dilation, allows the uterus to retract and gather itself together for its final job of expelling the placenta.

Once the resting phase is over, noticeable contractions recur with regularity. These strong contractions are palpable as the fundus firms up below the umbilicus. The fundus feels round or discoid, somewhat firm, and wide when the placenta is still in the upper segment. The placenta typically releases after three such detaching contractions, which will usually be spaced more closely than twice the time of pushing contractions once they begin.

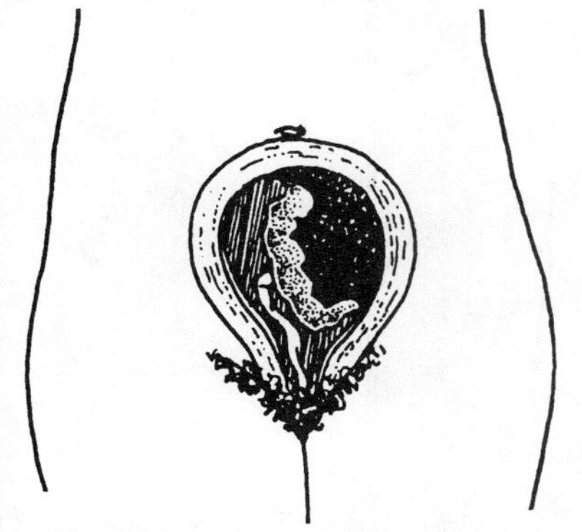
Placenta in upper segment

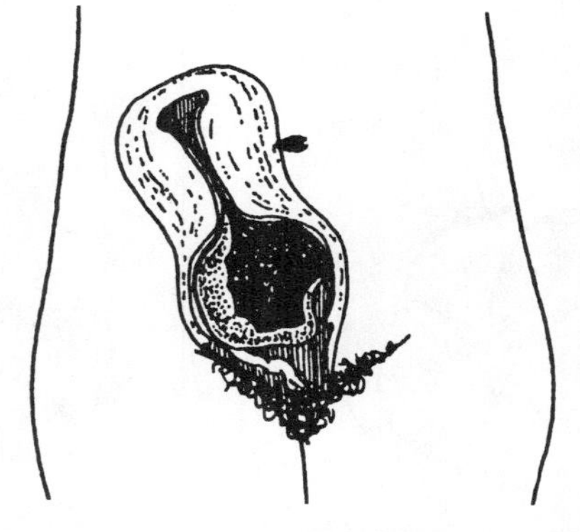
Placenta in lower segment

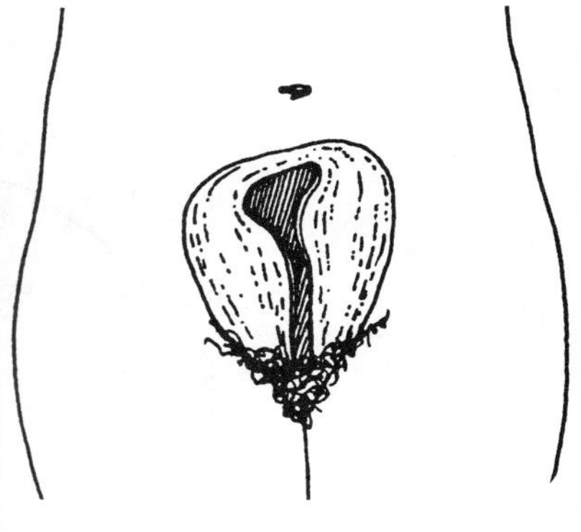
Uterus empty

Uterine Changes during Placental Detachment		
Timing of findings	**Uterine findings**	
	Consistency on palpation	**Fundal height**
After baby is born (placenta still attached)	Fundus feels wide, discoid & firm, like a small beach ball (not boggy)*	About 2.5 cm below the navel
Placenta separated & descended into lower uterine segment	Fundus feels round, smaller & hard, like a cricket ball or baseball; ballotable	At or just above the navel
Uterus just emptied, placenta in upper yoni	Fundus is about the size and density of a grapefruit, firm & semimobile (not boggy)	4 to 5 cm below the navel

*"Boggy" describes the relaxed postpartum uterus, which feels large, soft and squishy with indistinct borders. (Sellers, 1993).

The placenta separates and descends into the stretched out lower uterine segment; the fundus feels smaller, rounder and more mobile as the uterus continues to contract. Once empty, the upper uterine segment rises above the level of the placenta internally and can be felt above the level of the navel externally. The firm upper segment is now contracted above the softer lower uterine segment that is currently filled with the placenta. The fundus is therefore high and freely mobile at the junction of the isthmus, and may tilt to one side of the midline, usually to the mother's right. The contracted fundus will be located at, or just above, the navel. Once the placenta descends through the os into the upper vault of the yoni, the upper segment contracts down to meet it as the lower uterine segment is emptied; thus the fundus descends (Bennett & Brown, 1999; El Halta, 1989).

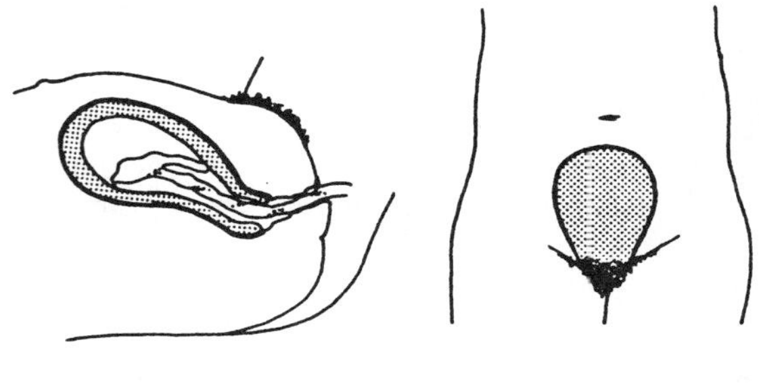

Contour of abdomen after birth, as placenta is detaching (mother supine)

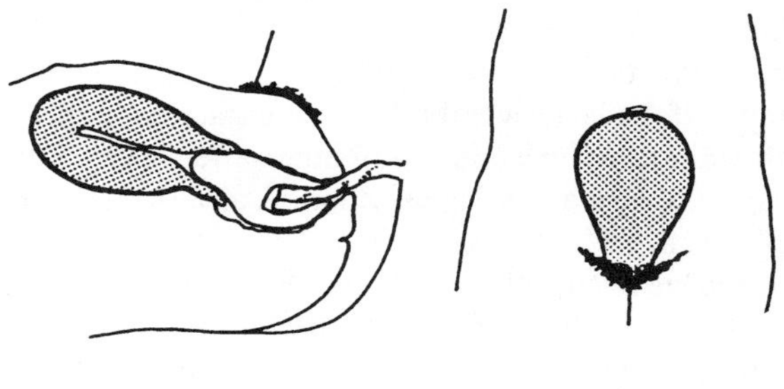

Contour of abdomen as placenta is descending out of the fundus (mother supine)

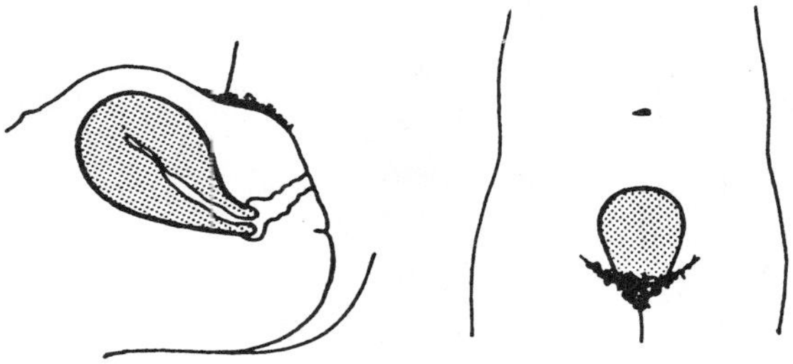

Contour of abdomen after the placenta is born (mother supine)

Additional signs of separation

Apart from these uterine changes, other clinical signs that placental detachment is occurring are listed below:

Diminished pulsing and blood pressure in cord vessels: Observe the cord for pulsations. If it is still obviously pulsing, complete separation has not yet occurred. Diminishing or absent pulsations indicate that the placenta is separated or almost so *unless* the baby is not breathing well, in which case cord pulsations or back flow are unreliable indicators of placental detachment. If you are unsure, you can pinch the cord between your fingers and milk it toward the introitus for a distance of 10 to 15 cm and then release. If separation is not complete, a distinct backflow of pressure will occur toward the baby. If separation is complete and the placenta is in the process of descending through the lower segment and os, reverse milking should result in a decline of pressure after each contraction. If separation is complete or nearly so, the backflow will be noticeably diminished or absent (Long, 1991).

Using the backflow test after the bulk of the placental blood has passed to the baby should not interfere with continued equilibration of the baby's blood volume, since that takes place in the portion of the umbilical vein nearest the baby. However, do not use this method of assessment if the cord is unusually short, if there is a knot in the cord or if it sports other uncommon features.

Newborn response: Enning (2003), notes that the behavior of the baby changes as the placenta detaches. She has observed that babies become irritable, often complaining that the cord transfusion has finished by crying three times as the placenta comes away from the uterine wall.

A sudden trickle or small gush of blood: The open uterine sinuses beneath the placenta bleed out as it detaches from the uterine wall because the uterus is not yet empty and cannot fully clamp down to squeeze the sinuses shut. This retroplacental bleeding leads to the formation of a soft clot. In some cases, a small amount of this blood leaks down and out. If the placenta is low lying, the amount of blood released at this point is usually larger because there are fewer ligating muscles in the lower uterine segment and because the placenta is not in a position to occlude the escape of blood. However, bleeding is an unreliable sign of full separation because blood loss may be trapped in the membranes of a separated placenta and thus not escape at all or bleeding may occur when the placenta has only partially separated.

Lengthening of the umbilical cord at the introitus: In most cases, the cord advances ahead of the placental disk as the placenta moves down from the uterine wall toward the cervix and beyond. This gives the appearance of the cord getting longer as the placenta descends. However, sometimes the pliable cord does not lengthen because it becomes bunched up in the upper yoni, even though the placenta has separated and begun to descend. This is especially true in low-lying placentas. At other times, what appears to be a lengthening cord is the unraveling of a long cord that had become bunched up in the yoni without accompanying placental descent.

Maternal vital signs during placental detachment

The mother's heart rate and blood pressure may rise slightly as the placenta is expelled but should return to normal ranges once the placenta is out. Forgo disturbing the mother with checking vitals during the birth of the placenta unless she is showing signs of blood loss or other distress or placental expulsion is unduly delayed. These signs could mean there is concealed bleeding taking place, which could be from the uterus or a hematoma.

Timing variations in the birth of the placenta

Most placentas are born within 30 minutes after the birth, although timing of detachment will vary. The placenta can begin to separate with the birth of the baby. When this occurs, you may see a gush of blood as the head is born. (A gush is also seen when periurethral tearing occurs.) Placental bleeding at this point is classified as an abruption and requires immediate delivery of the baby. The placenta may begin to separate within a couple of minutes of birth; this most commonly occurs when the mother is upright and experiencing a powerful fetus ejection reflex.

Normal detachment can also be delayed for an hour or more. The most common reason for delay in the birth of the placenta is that cues signaling its separation and readiness for delivery were missed by the midwife and the mother. Also be aware that the woman who does not want to let go of the pregnancy or who has been frightened with stories of hemorrhage related to third phase may, either consciously or unconsciously, hang on to her placenta. Talk to her about moving on to complete the birth and help her visualize placental detachment. The longer detachment takes, the more suspicious you should be of a physical problem preventing normal detachment from occurring. Most of these problems are rare; for details see the chapter entitled "Uncommon Problems That Can Interfere with the Birth of the Placenta."

Cord Clamping's Effects on Placental Detachment and Birth

Depending upon its timing, cord clamping causes a variable amount of fetal blood to be retained in the placenta, leaving it engorged, which renders it stiff and inflexible. Studies have shown that immediate cord clamping prolongs the average duration of placental delivery. The larger bulk of the placenta impedes the uterus' attempts to clamp down to detach and expel it and to close off the underlying uterine sinuses, which, in turn, increases maternal blood loss (Walsh, 1968). Partial separation is more likely in this case and often leads to more uterine bleeding for the same reasons. Additionally, the engorged placenta is larger in diameter and less pliable, so it may have more difficulty passing through the partially closed cervix.

The Spontaneous Birth of the Placenta

Most placentas will be born without any problem or excessive bleeding; however, you should always observe the mother as unobtrusively as possible and monitor to the extent necessary until the placenta is out and the uterus is empty and well contracted. The following recommendations are most applicable when a woman has not been able to enter the altered state of consciousness indicative of optimal hormonal levels during labor and is therefore at more risk for problems. Let your intuition be your guide as to how closely you follow the suggestions below. The trick is to be totally noninterventive when things are going well and still be ready to act immediately if not.

The mother's position immediately after birth

The mother will usually find herself in the position from which she delivered the baby right after birth. Most women desire to remain in a relatively upright position as the baby emerges and immediately thereafter. This naturally lessens compression of the inferior vena cava, thus (theoretically) minimizing blood loss. However, mothers who give birth upright usually experience a sudden, large gush of blood shortly after the birth. (Some midwives believe that women actually bleed more when they are upright. However, others feel that this is simply the expulsion of a normal separation gush that does not have an opportunity to pool in the uterus.) If the mother is upright and you know that she is very tired, encourage her to lie down at this point. Even if she doesn't bleed excessively, the rapid shifts in uterine content could make her feel unstable, which is not as likely to occur if she is supine.

Side-lying, hands-and-knees, squatting, kneeling or lying supine are other options for positions which the mother may assume once the baby is born. The worst position is lying back, bent at the waist (semi-sitting), which exaggerates the birth canal. The baby should not be placed on the mother's lower abdomen, as the weight of the baby plus the weight of the uterus tends to compress the inferior vena cava, inhibiting blood flow to the heart and encouraging the blood to flow out of the open uterine sinuses. After five to ten minutes, the adrenaline rush from the birth subsides and the mother often wishes to lie down. (Odent, 2002).

The position of the mother during placental delivery

The mother may use either a reclining, almost supine, or an upright position to deliver the placenta. A placenta pan, which fits beneath a standard US toilet seat can be used over the toilet bowl; it will rest on the porcelain rim. Lower the seat. Have the mother push her placenta out over the pan. The pan will catch both blood loss and the placenta. Alternately, have the mother sit on an open-bottom birthing stool and hold a pan beneath her.

The power of suggestion

Remind the mother that additional contractions will birth her placenta, clamp the uterus down and close off the site of placental attachment. Be aware that first-time mothers may not be aware of these contractions because they are so much less intense than labor contractions. Encourage the mother to relate to her newborn and, if the baby seems interested in nursing, put the baby to her breast. Even if the baby does not want to nurse right away, putting the baby near the breast will signal her body that it is safe to release the placenta.

Prepare for the birth of the placenta

The primary attendant or a skilled assistant should position herself between the mother's legs, if she is reclining, or at a convenient vantage point below and in front of the mother if she is upright. Use a clean dry gauze pad to wipe away any fecal matter expelled during pushing from the yoni in a downward (backward) direction. Change the pad beneath the mother to further clean the area. Then, wedge a shallow pan halfway under the mother's buttocks (or between her legs on the floor) to catch any blood. There should be sufficient light to see any blood that fills the pan. A Snake Light is useful because it provides ample light while allowing you to keep the room lights low. It can be formed into a collar around your neck, with the light directed into the pan.

Monitoring the fundus: If the mother is standing, watch below for blood loss. If the mother is reclining, rest your hand lightly on the mother's abdomen and find the fundus to monitor for uterine contractions. You want to make sure that the uterus is not ballooning with blood that is not being expelled because the placenta is blocking the way at the os. The uterine contour may feel somewhat indistinct immediately after the birth. However, it should not be so soft or so large that you cannot find its outline with your hand, nor should it be enlarging; any of these signs signals concealed hemorrhage. Your hand should not leave the fundus, or should leave it only briefly, until the placenta is born. Wait for contractions to resume on their own. Massage of the fundus prior to complete separation of the placenta is likely to produce weak, dysrhythmic contractions that only partially detach the placenta, raising the risk of postpartum hemorrhage.

If contractions are slow to start or if bleeding is concerning, the best course of action is to stimulate the uterus with nipple stimulation, herbs or oxytocin. Once noticeable contractions resume, the presence of your hand resting on the fundus may actually stimulate contractions.

You can learn to do a degree of fundal monitoring when the mother is upright. However, it is more difficult because the tension in the abdominal muscles will affect your ability to feel the uterus, and it is harder to make sure you are not pressing (risking uterine prolapse or inversion).

Rule out a second baby: A surprise twin is always a possibility. Thus, the person checking the fundus should always rule out another baby before encouraging the delivery of the placenta. In rare cases, the first placenta is delivered before the second baby. However, the placentas of twins are usually fused and, even if they are not, typically neither is born until all babies are out. How will you know if there is another baby? The fundus will be fuller than usual and you may feel fetal movement. The first baby may appear surprisingly small or early, given the mother's prenatal fundal height. If you have any doubt, use a fetoscope and listen for a fetal heart before proceeding any further. If you discover a second baby, see the chapter entitled "Assisting at Multiple Births" for a discussion of what to do at this point.

Wait for signs of separation

Ask the mother to inform you when another contraction comes on. Then wait patiently for contractions to resume. At this point, the only reason to intervene is if you believe excessive bleeding is occurring. You might suspect this if a significant flow of blood comes out, if the fundus enlarges rapidly, or if the mother exhibits signs of shock, however slight, without visible bleeding.

If you note a contraction with no comment from the mother, inform her that you believe she is having a contraction. She will usually confirm your impression. Once she knows what an afterbirth contraction feels like, she will be better able to tell when additional contractions occur. Keep your hand on the fundus.

How long to wait: The woman is in no danger as long as she is not bleeding. The trick is to be sure she is has no concealed bleeding behind the placenta. Recall her labor pattern. Sometimes delays or plateaus in progress during labor also occur during the labor for the placenta. If the birth of the placenta is much delayed, you can talk to the woman about how she is feeling and ask her about any thoughts she may have about this part of labor. Sometimes beliefs are revealed at this time that directly impact why there is a delay. For example, she may be waiting for you to finish the birth! Visualization can help; one mother whose placenta had been retained for three hours delivered it under guided visualization of ocean waves moving it down and out.

It is customary to wait at least one hour before intervening manually, unless the onset of blood loss or the mother's condition dictates acting sooner. Some blood loss may indicate that the placenta has separated and is about to be born. Most often, when the placenta does not come out, it is just sitting there, completely detached, and gentle cord traction, as described in this chapter, will bring it out and finish this phase of labor. Note that retained placenta with no bleeding whatsoever in the presence of good uterine contractions may be due to placenta accreta. In this case, transport is your best alternative.

Encourage maternal pushing

Once some or all the signs of placental separation and descent appear, encourage the mother to push *with a contraction* (as she did to bring the baby) to spontaneously birth the placenta. Pushing in the absence of a contraction increases the likelihood of uterine prolapse or inversion and should always be discouraged. Remind her that the placenta is small and soft compared to the baby and delivering it will not feel like having the baby.

Spontaneous placental delivery

The mother may have to push if she is lying down. If the mother is reclining, lift the placenta by the cord as it emerges and guide it out and slightly upward, following the curve of Carus. It will come through the cervix with a plop, squish through the birth canal and present as a bulge at the introitus, which will want to drop down; lifting the cord helps straighten the path of descent for the membranes which will follow. Make sure that the membranes are completely expelled by watching to see that they slip out easily, leaving no ragged fragments at the introitus. You can also allow the placenta to emerge into the pan without help. If the mother is upright, hold a placenta pan up to her introitus so the placenta does not have a distance to fall to the ground (instead of lifting the cord, as described above).

If uterine contractions are strong and the mother is upright, gravity alone is usually sufficient to birth the placenta. Hold a placenta pan up to her yoni as the placenta emerges or catch it in your gloved hands. The main thing is to avoid having the placenta fall a distance to the pan, which invites a messy splashdown as well as the tearing of any membranes that are not fully detached.

Culturing for infection

You may wish to culture one or both sides of the placenta if intrauterine infection is known or suspected. If only one culture is to be collected, swab the fetal surface with a cotton-tipped culturette as the placenta is coming out, but before it completely emerges. Try to touch only the placenta and not the mother. If the placenta delivers Duncan, carefully and quickly unfold it and swab the fetal side. When culturing both sides, always culture the side that presents first, then unfold it to culture the opposite side. Use two separate culturettes when swabbing both sides; first complete one, returning it to its culture tube, and then complete the other. Have an assistant break the liquid medium in the tip of the tube, complete the labeling of the tube with baby's name, placental birth time and date, and refrigerate the specimens. (For more details about when, what and how to culture for infection, see my text DIAGNOSTICS TESTS.)

Judging blood loss

Do your best to assure that excessive blood loss does not occur prior to, during and after placental delivery. Many texts set the upper limit of normal blood loss at 500 ml or 17.6 oz. (For those who think in terms of cups, 2 cups equals about 454 ml.) However, many well-nourished women can lose up to 1000 ml or about 4.4 cups and are fine. These women have an optimally expanded blood volume during pregnancy. In my experience, some women, particularly those with good, well-rounded macrobiotic diets, lose far less blood than the average.

These averages refer, however, to total blood loss in the first 24 hours postpartum. As you wait for the placenta to be born, you must assess how much blood was lost during labor (if any), how much is currently being lost and how much more the mother is likely to lose during and after the placental delivery. It is generally advisable to take some action to encourage placental delivery after one or two cups of blood loss with no signs of placental delivery in sight, even if the mother has no predisposing risk factors for increased bleeding. Base your judgement regarding when to intervene on the individual circumstances, taking the factors listed under "When to Actively Assist the Birth of the Placenta" (below) into account.

Differentiating uterine bleeding from other fluids: Some of the fluid in the pan may be amniotic fluid mixed with blood, causing the volume of blood lost to appear larger than it actually is. Of course, this will only be a factor when you have been very quick to get the pan in place immediately after the birth. Also, if the cord is cut and unclamped, some of the blood is from the placenta, not the mother. If you decide to cut the cord, you may want to catch the cord blood and dispose of it separately so that it does not confuse your findings regarding how much blood the mother has lost.

Transfer the blood from the pan to a measuring container. Allow the blood to stand for up to five minutes. The blood will start to clot and sink to the bottom, leaving other fluids on top. The blood loss can then be accurately measured. Once assessed, the blood can be disposed of down the toilet or saved for the mother to use as a valuable addition to her garden soil.

Measuring blood loss: The assistant should take a pan partially filled with blood and hand the midwife a clean one. The assistant then measures the collected blood in a wide-mouthed measuring cup and keeps the attending midwife apprised of how much total blood loss has occurred. The assistant should then rinse out the first pan in warm water and bring it back to the bedside, continuing to rotate pans and keep track of blood loss until the placenta is born and the uterus is firmly contracted. The amount of blood lost with the placenta should be recorded in the chart.

When to Actively Assist the Birth of the Placenta

Experience teaches the midwife when to assist the birth of the placenta. The list below is a useful guide:

Uterine atony (little or no contraction): Uterine atony frequently follows long labors because the uterine muscle is tired. Atony often leads to incomplete detachment as well as excessive bleeding before and after the placenta is delivered. The solution is to produce more effective contractions. Also see the chapter entitled "Immediate Postpartum Hemorrhage." Uterine atony accounts for 90% of all postpartum bleeding.

Significant bleeding: When bleeding is occurring and the placenta is not coming, act quickly, especially if you know that the placenta was low-lying.

Mother's nutritional status: Act more quickly if the mother did not eat as well as necessary during pregnancy because her blood volume will not be optimal.

Mother's hemoglobin at term: Even with an expanded blood volume, if the hemoglobin is below 10 grams (6.25 mmol/l or 100 g/l), the woman cannot tolerate much blood loss and may go into shock after losing less than 500 ml because her oxygen-carrying capacity is already so marginal.

Length of labor: A tired uterus will not contract as effectively.

Mother's stamina: Even with good contractions, a tired woman does not tolerate blood loss well.

Contraction pattern prior to birth: Lazy, spaced-out pushing contractions usually do not become close and strong once the baby is born. Thus, expect weak contractions and more bleeding. Act quickly if the birth of the placenta is delayed, with the administration of uterine stimulants as part of your plan.

Any signs or symptoms of shock: Regardless of how slight, take such signs seriously. Each woman's threshold for blood loss differs.

History of bleeding from past labors: If this woman has a history of heavy bleeding, act quickly.

Uterus contains tumors (fibroids, myomas, etc.) These make postpartum contractions less efficient at detaching the placenta and can interfere with clamping down afterwards. Both can lead to heavier bleeding.

Any history of bleeding during this labor: When bleeding has occurred prior to birth, the mother has already dipped into her pregnancy reserves and will be, to a varying extent, less tolerant of additional blood loss with the placenta. Due to the sporadic nature of most blood loss during labor and the possibility that it may be partially or completely concealed and that some of the blood may have mixed with amniotic fluid, it will be difficult or impossible to accurately judge how much she has already lost. Immediate birth of the placenta with little or no additional blood loss would be ideal.

Polyhydramnios, a very large baby or multiple gestation at term: Any of these may result in an overstretched uterus, leaving the myometrium with more work to do to return to a size that will effectively clamp off bleeding vessels.

Baby's enthusiasm for nursing: Nursing contributes to effective uterine activity and thus curtails bleeding. If the baby isn't interested, you may need to compensate with nipple stimulation. The woman's partner or a young sibling can suck at the breast, or manual stimulation can be used.

Gestational age of baby: The earlier the baby, the less blood volume the mother will have and the smaller and more firmly adherent the placenta will be. A small placenta coupled with a uterus that is not as full as it would be at term means less reduction in size and possibly incomplete detachment. (See the chapter entitled "When the Baby Is Early" for more details.)

Compromised newborn: When the baby has a problem, especially one necessitating transport, the emotional impact and distracting nature of this event make it difficult for the mother to focus her attention on her own well-being; expect more bleeding and third-phase problems.

What to do

Remind the mother that her uterus will continue to contract in order to birth the placenta. Have her lie supine. Wedge the edge of a placenta pan under her bottom, between her legs at an angle and place a hand on the fundus. If bleeding is concerning or the uterus is already boggy (indistinct shape, squishy and soft) and applying your open palm over the fundus and gently rocking it back and forth produces no change, proceed directly to the suggestions below, picking up along the list according to the seriousness of the situation. For example, if the uterus is indistinct and bleeding is heavy, go directly to acupressure, uterine tonic herbs or an IM injection of oxytocin. If one of these does not work in a timely fashion (defined by the mother's overall condition, the uterus becoming firmer and more easily outlined, the delivery of the placenta, cessation of blood loss and your clinical and intuitive sense of what is appropriate), move on to the next suggestion until the mother has effective contractions and the placenta is born.

Mother-baby contact: Let the mother hold the baby whenever possible. Even if you are interfering quite a bit at this point, contact with the baby will help the mother's body produce hormones that can help the placenta come.

Check the bladder: A full bladder can cause the uterus to produce ineffective contractions and interfere with normal retraction, thus increasing the likelihood of bleeding. It can also block the easy descent of the placenta through the cervix. Gently palpate above the pubic bone to determine if the bladder feels swollen. Also refer to your records to see when the mother last voided and how much urine she passed. If necessary, have the mother empty her bladder into the toilet, a pan or a towel. If she cannot do so, catheterize her. After birth, the pelvic area is numb to some extent; thus, women are commonly unaware of the need to urinate.

Stimulate the nipples: Either the mother or partner can use fingers to gently roll the nipple. Better, if the baby wants to, he can nurse. The partner or an older nursing sibling can also suck on a nipple. A breast pump is also effective. Nipple stimulation should prompt the release of oxytocin and uterine contractions.

Stroke the sides of the uterus: Do so firmly, on both sides with the palms of your hands in an upward direction. This technique, recommended by Gregory White, a homebirth doctor in Chicago, is said to trigger the round ligaments to activate the pacemaker regions in the cornua of the uterus and prompt uterine contractions (White, 1997).

Acupressure techniques: Zita West (2001) suggests three possible options for stimulating the uterus to release the placenta:

•Stimulate CV-4 with firm pressure if you can reach the point easily.

•GB-21 is the empirical point for treating placental problems. Stimulate it by itself or along with BL-60 to help move the energy downward.

•LI-4, LIV-3 and SP-6 can all be stimulated together using firm pressure to help expel the placenta.

A woman's energy level is quite vulnerable after the birth, and some women may not be able to tolerate the simulation of multiple points at all or for a prolonged period of time.

Give the mother cotton root bark tincture: Regardless of the mother's symptom picture, this is one of the best herbs for stimulating contractions and descending the placenta. A dropperful can be taken as often as every 15 minutes.

Allopathic drugs: If none of the above is adequate, give the mother an intramuscular injection of 5 to10 units of oxytocin (Pitocin or Syntocinon) using a 1.5 in needle. Oxytocin is the drug least likely to cause placental entrapment behind the cervix because it produces rhythmic contractions of the upper uterine segment. (See the subchapter entitled "Allopathic Pharmacologic Agents for Treating Uterine Atony" for details about this recommendation.) If there is no blood loss and the placenta fails to deliver after oxytocin administration, it may be because the placenta is accreted, especially if the woman has risk factors for accreta. See the chapter entitled "Uncommon Problems That Can Interfere with the Birth of the Placenta."

Manual stimulation of the uterus: Manually stimulating the uterus to actively encourage contractions should only be performed if bleeding is concerning with no placenta in sight, and the above measures are not working fast enough. Even then, it should only be done by *gently* moving the hand you have placed on the fundus in a back-and-forth or side-to-side motion. Increase this massage only to the point of effectiveness and provide cord traction (as explained under "Controlled cord traction" below). Vigorous massage of the uterus is not required. *Avoid fundal fiddling.* It is unnecessary because the uterus almost always contracts when a hand is cupped around the fundus and *gently* rocked. Uterine manipulation in the form of kneading, pressing, or squeezing causes weak, dysrhythmic contractions and is likely to result in partial detachment, crushing of the placenta and more bleeding without placental delivery. Once the placenta is born, vigorous manipulation is also likely to disrupt the clot that is trying to form in the placental site, thereby initiating more bleeding.

Incomplete detachment of the normal placenta: The placenta must be fully detached before efforts are made to extract it. Sufficient uterine activity is usually all that is necessary to accomplish this. Incomplete detachment can result from dysrhythmic contractions caused by the application of vigorous or poorly timed fundal massage or when the uterus is just not contracting sufficiently to fully detach the placenta. Thus, the first solution to try is to stimulate stronger contractions, which will probably detach the placenta and minimize the possibility of excessive bleeding. To stimulate effective contractions, see "What to do," above.

If the placenta does not birth after effective uterine contractions have resumed (or if effective contractions do not develop), follow the cord up to the cervix to check for detachment (below). The detached placenta could be inside the partially closed-down os. If neither uterine stimulation nor any of the tricks described in this chapter are successful in bringing the placenta down and out, consider other possible factors (see the chapter entitled "Uncommon Problems That Can Interfere with the Birth of the Placenta").

A build-up of blood behind the placenta: Excessive bleeding can occur behind the undelivered placenta if you are not watchful. This happens when the detached or partially detached placenta blocks the os and prevents the blood from coming out. Bleeding almost always means the placenta is at least partially detached (unless it is coming from a laceration), and very often it means that the placenta is detached. If you suspect concealed bleeding, do not hesitate to apply fundal pressure to expel the blood because the bleeding will only increase as long as the uterus is not empty. The expulsion of retained clots may facilitate placental detachment, both because clots collected behind the placenta will move underneath it and help separate it from the uterine wall and because emptying the uterus will stimulate more effective contractions.

A placenta pan should be under the mother's bottom. Cup your hand over the fundus, fingers behind and thumb in front so your hand overlies the fundus, do not, however, squeeze the fundus. Now press in, down and around the curve of the pubic arch slowly and steadily and watch the introitus for the appearance of a gush of blood. You can combine this pressure with keeping the cord taut with your other hand to see what happens with the placenta as you press. Ideally, this technique should be used during a contraction to avoid inverting the uterus. The entire uterus will move down slightly toward the pubic bone as you press. Remember you are trying to empty the uterus, not push it out of the mother! You must also be careful not to use excessive force, as this will place undue strain on the uterine and cervical ligaments, inviting later prolapse. Guarding the uterus (see below) will help to protect against this.

Checking for placental detachment: While going through the steps previously listed, signs of detachment are likely to develop. In some cases contractions occur, the placenta appears to have detached, the mother pushes, yet the placenta is not delivered. This often happens because the placenta is trapped in the lower uterine segment, inside the os, or because the placenta is only partially detached. Here are some ways to confirm that detachment has occurred.

Using suprapubic pressure: Suprapubic pressure is widely recommended to check for placental detachment. The mother should be supine. Stand to her side with your dominant side to her feet. First, take hold of the cord in your dominant hand and gently stretch the cord out (not upward) to take up any slack (you are not doing cord traction). You do not have to hold the cord in this manner, but it helps you tell what's going on. Now place the inner edge (thumb side) of your other hand above and parallel with the pubic bone (palm toward the woman's head) and apply pressure down toward her spine, then slightly upward, toward her head. If the placenta is still in the upper uterine segment, the cord is supposed to retract back into the yoni with this maneuver. You will feel the tension in the cord as this occurs; allow enough give to relax the cord as it retracts.

Unfortunately, this maneuver is fraught with pitfalls. One study found an 18% rate of false findings with this technique (Akiyama et al., 1981). If the placenta is still inside the os, retraction may occur even if the placenta is detached. If you don't take up all the slack, the cord may or may not retract (if it is bunched up in the birth canal, it may have enough slack not to) whether the placenta is still in the fundus or has descended into the lower uterine segment. This technique is most reliable only after the placenta has passed through the os. Furthermore, cord retraction can drag pathogens from the upper genital tract into the uterus, increasing the risk of intrauterine contamination.

Checking internally: Don a sterile glove on your dominant hand while you hold the cord taut with your other hand. Follow the cord up to the cervix with your dominant hand. Do you feel the mass of the placenta filling the os? If so, the placenta is probably completely detached and just sitting there (although in low implantations, a placenta at the os could still be partially attached). If following the cord leads you into the os and you do not feel any placental mass or if your hand is led to the fetal surface dangling from higher up in the uterine cavity, this probably indicates that the placenta is not fully detached. This technique is not definitive either, but is more reliable than suprapubic pressure.

Ways to assist the birth of the detached placenta: A fully detached placenta may be retained in the uterus due to lack of adequate contractions, a partially closed cervix that holds the placenta inside the uterus or, more rarely, a constriction ring. Retained placenta (whether detached or not) can produce variable consistency in the uterus, alternating between firm and soft. This is the uterus trying to clamp down with something still inside. To get it out, review the following options. (Entrapment by a constriction ring is discussed in the chapter entitled "Uncommon Problems That Can Interfere with the Birth of the Placenta.")

Fundal pressure: Fundal pressure can be used to push the fully separated placenta out of the lower uterine segment or the birth canal or to expel clots from the uterus after the placenta is born. *Fundal pressure should never be used in an attempt to detach the entire placenta or a portion of it from the uterine wall, nor should it be used if the mother is upright.*

To do so invites uterine inversion and strain on the uterine and cervical ligaments.

Controlled cord traction: A form of this technique was first formally introduced in 1940 as the "Brant-Andrews maneuver." Today, this technique has been refined and is now called "controlled cord traction." Cord traction can help remove the fully detached placenta from the uterine cavity, partially closed cervix or the yoni. *Cord traction should never be used in an attempt to detach the entire placenta or a portion of it from the uterine wall.* To do so invites partial detachment, cord breakage, uterine inversion, placental tearing, maternal-fetal blood mixing and postpartum hemorrhage.

The uterus usually expels the placenta on its own after adequate contractions have resumed. However, if the mother or the uterine muscle is very tired, this process may be helped along with controlled cord traction. Cord traction is also useful when the placenta is detached but is not descending past the cervix, which may have closed down just enough to make its passage difficult. Partial closure of the os may occur with or without the use of uterine stimulants. Cord traction is routinely used in institutions and some midwifery training programs to assist the birth of the placenta (although this isn't recommended). While careless cord traction poses significant risks, gentle, sensitive traction applied during a contraction when the signs of separation are favorable is relatively safe and can speed the emptying and therefore the clamping down of the uterus, thus minimizing blood loss.

Use cord traction *only* when the mother is in a position that allows you to have a hand well applied to the fundus. The woman should lie with her lower body flat on the bed so that the descent of the placenta is not impeded by an exaggerated curve in the birth canal or by becoming hung up on the pubic bone. *Never* apply cord traction if the mother is upright (standing, squatting, or even semi-sitting); it is impossible to adequately monitor the fundus when the mother is upright and pushing because her abdominal muscles will interfere with your efforts. Cord traction with the mother upright invites uterine inversion. The cord can be used to guide out the detached placenta when you are experienced.

Ideally, traction should only be applied when the uterus is contracting. However, once you are skilled with the technique, the detached placenta can be delivered with traction in the absence of a contraction if there is excessive bleeding and if the uterus is not very boggy (never use cord traction if the uterus is extremely boggy–too much risk of inversion). Using cord traction in the absence of a contraction does increase the risk of uterine inversion, so always guard the uterus when this is done.

Guarding the uterus: It is commonly recommended that one hand be used to guard the uterus whenever you are pulling from below or pressing on the fundus. Guarding the uterus is intended to provide enough support below the fundus to prevent undue strain on the uterine and cervical ligaments and to prevent pushing the fundus into the pelvis, which is likely to cause excessive bleeding and may precipitate uterine inversion. Guarding can easily be done while standing to the mother's side if she is lying down or more awkwardly when you are positioned between her legs. Avoid jamming your hand down toward the spine, as this will pinch off the lower segment and impede placental descent.

C guarding: This is the term I have coined for what I do. To guard while pulling on the cord, stand to the mother's side with your dominant side toward her feet. Form the index finger and thumb of your nondominant hand into a wide "C" shape. Now place the crotch of your thumb and forefinger above the pubic bone, palm toward the mother's head. Cup your palm and fingers around the upper segment so that the "C" shape forms a channel around the region of the retraction ring. Your palm can be pivoted in and up against the anterior uterus to straighten the cervical birth canal when you apply cord traction from below. (See modified Brant-Andrews maneuver.)

Modified Calkin technique: Stand to the woman's side with your dominant side toward her feet. Place the hand nearest her head flat over her abdomen with your fingertips directed toward and slightly beneath the upper border of the symphysis. Apply controlled cord traction with your other hand (Pastore, 1936).

Modified Brant-Andrews maneuver: Place your nondominant hand palm-down so that its heel is pressed against the upper uterine segment at the level of the pubic bone, where it can be used to gently displace the well-contracted fundus down toward the spine and slightly up toward the mother's navel. This straightens the cervical portion of the birth canal and the upper portion of the yoni, creating an easy passageway for the placenta to descend further. Be careful where you direct your pressure; if you cram the heel of your hand straight downward above the upper border of the pubic bone, you are likely to compress the lower uterine segment, thereby trapping the placenta and interfering with your traction efforts. Use your other hand to pull the cord taut and to apply cord traction.

If the cord does not retract when the uterus is elevated, this probably indicates that the placenta has separated (this sign is not fully reliable; see the discussion of suprapubic pressure earlier in this chapter).

Note that the primary intent of this maneuver is to straighten the birth canal while providing some fundal support.

Guarding the uterus during any type of cord traction can be counterproductive; in essence, the effort of each of your hands is working against the other. Also, these techniques may cause you to pull harder on the cord than is advisable to overcome the resistance created by the guarding hand. Therefore, you may find it much more helpful and informative to keep one hand on the fundus, as described below. However, if you do want to guard from below the fundus, follow the instructions above, as these techniques minimize compression of the lower uterine segment.

Keeping a hand on the fundus: This is my much preferred alternative to guarding the uterus from below the fundus. It is also easier to use this method if you are kneeling between the supine mother's legs. Keep one palm lightly cupped over the fundus when performing any manipulations from below. You will be able to feel if the uterus starts to recede en masse under your hand as you apply traction (which indicates that the placenta is probably not detached or that it is caught inside the os) or if a dimpling starts at the top of the fundus (which indicates that the fundus may try to invert).

How to do controlled cord traction: To start, place one hand on the fundus and monitor for the resumption of contractions (as described above under "Monitoring the fundus") and signs of separation.

How to grasp the cord: In the meantime, grasp the cord with your gloved dominant hand and wrap it around or between your fingers to achieve a firm grip (it will be quite slippery). If this does not allow you to achieve a good grip, apply a long-tipped hemostat (such as a Rochester-Pean) perpendicular to the cord so that the clamped end sticks out beyond the cord. Straddle the cord with your index and middle fingers, and hook your fingers over the hemostat to either side. It is important for your hand to be in direct contact with the cord, not just the instrument; there are subtle things you may otherwise miss.

Apply traction and monitor placental descent: Use the hand holding the cord to gently apply enough tension to extend the cord to its maximum length. If the cord is very long, reposition your grip or the hemostat further up the cord, closer to the yoni, so that you have better control of the placenta and greater sensitivity regarding what is happening inside the uterus. Move your nondominant hand down the front of the uterus to rest above the pubic bone. As you watch and feel for cord retraction at the introitus, make a gentle side-to-side "sawing" motion above the pubic bone with this hand. If the cord retreats back into the yoni, this suggests that the placenta is not yet through the os and may not be fully detached. In this case, wait for one more contraction, then reposition your hand on the fundus.

When you feel certain that separation is complete, wait for the next contraction and then ask the mother to push. Using your dominant hand, gently apply smooth, firm and steady cord traction while keeping your nondominant hand on the fundus (or reposition your abdominal hand to do the modified Brant-Andrews maneuver, described above). Tell the mother to let you know if she feels any pain. Pull no harder than you can pull on the end of your nose without your fingers slipping off (Hendrickson, 1981) no greater than 1 pound of tension (pulling force). The direction of pull should be at about a 45° angle downward in relation to the introitus until you see the placenta begin to fill the yoni. Then redirect your traction to a 45° angle upward in a smooth arch to follow the curve of Carus. If the placenta is through the os, traction should quickly produce a swelling at the introitus as the placenta distends the lower yoni. Once the body of the placenta is delivered, guide the emergence of the membranes by lifting the placenta up by the cord. As the edges of the membranes emerge, catch in the pan any trapped blood that escapes.

If cord traction fails to produce advancement but you are convinced that the placenta is detached, maintain steady, *gentle* traction, but do not increase it. Keep one hand on the fundus as you wait for the next contraction. At some point before or during the next contraction, a give may be felt as the placenta slides through the cervix. This is a smooth "ker-plunk," a gentle movement of squeezing through and release as the placenta passes through the partially closed os that is different from that which occurs if the placenta is being pulled off the uterine wall or if the membranes or the cord are tearing. It is smoother, more of a release or a bump. (The only way to know what this feels like is to practice, first with models and then eventually in a supervised birthing situation.) This give is followed by steady advance of the cord. If no progress is detected, stop and wait for the next contraction. You can also talk the mother through doing her own cord traction, as she is very unlikely to hurt herself.

If the placenta is coming but you see or feel that membranes are tearing on their way out, cease cord traction and immediately support the weight of the placenta in the pan under the mother's bottom. Dealing with trailing membranes is described below.

Getting the placenta past a partially closed cervix: Gently and slowly moving the cord side to side, up and down or in a wide circle while applying cord traction often helps work the placenta through the cervix. (Do not get so carried away with this that your overvigorous efforts cause you to miss any tearing sensations.)

In the rare event that none of this is productive, don a sterile glove and follow the cord up to the cervix. If the placenta is detached but the cervix has partially closed down, you may have to massage the cervix to help it let go. Have the mother visualize and focus on the cervix relaxing and the placenta slipping through. Apply hot towels to the mother's lower belly to help relax the cervix. Wait a few minutes, then try some fundal pressure to help expel a trapped placenta (Hendrickson, 1981).

Another rarely needed trick is to don a sterile glove and walk your fingers across the part of the placenta you can feel inside the os to get to an edge, loop your finger over the edge and work it down toward the os to allow the placenta to slide out sideways, which makes it less bulky. Be *very* careful if you do this because you don't want to disrupt a partially detached placenta. This technique raises the risk of infection and is only likely to be called for if an oxytocic drug has prompted too much closure of the os, preventing the placenta from easily passing through. Even so, moving the cord around should be sufficient to work the placenta through the os and is far less invasive.

Entrapment in a perineal pouch: If a long perineum has been very stretchy and distended during the birth, the fully detached placenta may descend into the yoni and become hung up in the pouch created by the distended tissues. In this case, the mother would probably be lying down, the placenta would be just inside the introitus, and cord lengthening would have occurred. Use the cord to lift the placenta and bring it out with gentle traction (Hendrickson, 1981).

<u>Precautions and danger signs</u>: Discontinue traction *immediately* in the event of any of the following:

Any pain reported by the mother: Most commonly, the placenta may still be partially attached; the uterus could also be trying to invert.

A give or jerk: Any sensations, however slight, of a sudden ragged give or a tiny jerk detected by the hand putting traction on the cord usually means the placenta is not fully detached and cotyledons or membranes are being torn. Once you are familiar with the sensation, it actually feels like tearing. Most rarely, it indicates that the cord is tearing, which is more likely to occur if the cord is thin or fragile. A similar sensation may be felt when the placenta is fully detached and the membranes are being torn off the uterine wall, whether from the weight of clots, from positioning during descent or from your traction efforts.

Distinct resistance: This often means the placenta is trapped above the os or a portion of it is still attached. To assess the situation, use the techniques already discussed.

The uterus retreats: The entire mass of the uterus starts retreating (moving downward) from under your hand. This occurs as the uterus is pulled upon from below while the placenta is still attached or is detached but retained inside the cervix. Should this occur, stop and assess whether the placenta is trapped in the os.

The uterus dimples: The top of the uterus starts to dimple under your hand, indicating that the fundus is trying to invert, probably with the placenta still firmly attached. Once this has started to occur, the possibility of inversion is high, even if you discontinue cord traction completely. It would be best to transport immediately with the mother in a Trendelenburg position.

The contraction has subsided: It is always most prudent to apply cord traction during a contraction to minimize the possibility of uterine inversion.

<u>Breaking of the cord</u>: Although the cord is fairly elastic, it can break during the birth of the baby or afterward during attempts to provide cord traction. Ghosh and colleagues (1984) found that the breaking strain of the cord averages 2.49 times the weight of the baby at birth. For example, if the baby weighs 8 lb 8 oz (3856 g), the tensile strength would be a little more than 21 pounds. The strongest part of the cord is usually near the placental insertion point. The average force of combined uterine and abdominal pressure brought to bear on the baby during pushing is about 40 lb (Oldfield, 1929). Therefore, if the cord is short or twisted, or if it is wrapped or positioned in a way that unduly strains it, breakage can occur during normal fetal descent, although this is relatively rare.

Cords that are prone to breakage are usually thin and fragile with little Wharton's jelly; breaking a thick cord requires quite a bit of tension. When breakage occurs, clamp any end you can reach immediately. If the rest of the cord is short, it may recede back inside the yoni, leaving you nothing to monitor or hold on to should the birth of the placenta require assistance. A good way to bring the placenta down is to get the mother upright, especially if the birth of the placenta seems delayed. Sit her on the toilet as described early in this chapter under "The position of the mother during placental delivery." If that doesn't work, try all the ways previously listed under "What to do" to get the placenta to come. You can also try to reach up into the yoni to find and clamp the end of the cord. If this is possible, you may be able to use cord traction, but it will be more difficult. If the placenta cannot be delivered and bleeding is concerning, timely transport is your best option.

If the placenta still has not been born: See the chapter entitled "Uncommon Problems That Can Interfere with the Birth of the Placenta," for additional information on less common problems with placental delivery and postpartum bleeding.

After the Placenta Is Out

Trailing membranes: Sometimes the placenta is born trailing a strand of membranes that appears to still be attached to the uterine wall. If a substantial portion of membranes are still attached to the edge of the placenta, grasp the entire placenta with both hands and slowly twist it around to peel the membranes off the uterine wall and cause them to slip out.

If trailing membranes tear completely away from the placenta during its delivery, securely grasp the widest portion of the membranes that you can reach at the introitus with sponge forceps and twist them out slowly, holding them in a straight line with the introitus. A ring forceps works well for this, as the ring can grasp and spread the membranes out for a secure grip. Do not clamp the very end of the membranes, as this is likely to result in ripping them during twisting. Reposition your clamp closer to the introitus as the membranes start to come out so that you maintain good control over this process. If you meet resistance, examine the edge of the placenta, as described next.

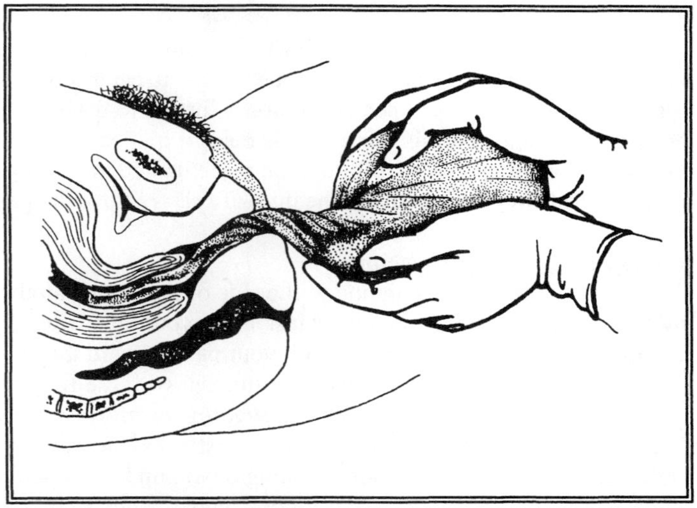

If the membranes are still attached to the edge of the placenta and are being very stubborn about coming (twisting the placenta does not seem to be working), use a pair of ring forceps to clamp the membranes about 1 in (2 cm) from the edge of the placenta. Then, leave the forceps in place. Use a pair of surgical scissors to trim the membranes between the clamp and the edge of the placenta as near the clamp as possible (take care not to cut the edge of the placenta or the mother). Carefully examine that portion of the cut membranes left on the placental edge to see if there are any cut blood vessels or other unusual features that would suggest the trailing membranes are attached to a retained succenturiate lobe. To distinguish blood vessels from streaks of blood, blot or wipe them gently with a gauze pad soaked in clear water. If there are no severed blood vessels, grasp the ring forceps and gently twist the membranes, which should peel them off the uterine wall and allow them to come out.

Blood vessels along the edge of the placenta running off into the membranes are evidence of a retained succenturiate lobe. Gail Hart (2003) points out that the end of the membranes could enclose blood, which may make passage through the cervix more difficult. Try gently rotating or seesawing the membranes back and forth or in circles to help the small lobe detach or to work the blood-filled sac through the cervix. However, be aware that a larger tissue mass is likely to be on the other end; therefore manipulate the membranes as though bringing out a very small placenta. Sudden sensations of giving may indicate that the membranes are tearing. Even if no blood vessels were found in the membranes, an extra placental lobe could still be a factor, as not all such lobes have vessels that lead to the main body of the placenta. Therefore, take care not to use undue force in trying to remove the membranes. When they come out, spread them, and check them carefully for holes or trailing blood vessels, which suggest a small lobe has been torn out and retained.

If you cannot retrieve all the membranes but are convinced no actual placental tissue has been retained, be aware that infection or delayed postpartum bleeding from retained membranes is very rare, unless perhaps you are in a tropical climate. Excessive postpartum uterine cramping is often absent, even when a large portion of membranes are retained.

Consider giving herbs or other agents that cause the uterus to contract and empty, such as angelica tincture or a series of Methergine tablets, especially if the postpartum lochia seems heavy. Explain to the mother what has happened and tell her to expect a fragment of membranes, which is likely to have a layer of congealed clot around it, to be expelled in the next few days.

If you are concerned about infection, insert a sterile speculum, visualize the cervix and use ring forceps to carefully remove any fragments of membranes you see hanging from the os. If there are fragments you can reach with your fingers, facial tissue can be used to collect them, as they will adhere to facial tissue. While you could do an intrauterine exploration to try and retrieve any remaining pieces, this is invasive and raises the risk of infection to the point that it is not worth it unless you suspect retained placental fragments. The mother will not be very pleased about this intervention.

Passage of a portion of tissue: If rigid maternal tissues (primarily the cervix) have impeded descent for some time prior to birth, a fragment of tissue may, on rare occasions, necrose and slough off and come out either before or after the birth. When such a thing occurs, it is usually a piece of cervix, which may be mistaken for placental tissue. Anything that appears to be something other than a blood clot should be saved and examined carefully once the mother is stable. Examination of the placenta should clarify whether the tissue is likely to be placental or maternal in origin. See the chapter entitled "Cervical and Other Soft-Tissues Problems during Labor" for additional information.

Immediate aftercare: The midwife who oversaw the birth of the placenta should remain nearby for the next 10 minutes or so and keep a shallow pan beneath the mother to catch any blood that follows the placenta. She should gently palpate the uterus by placing her open palm on the fundus to determine if it is contracting. She may apply fundal pressure to ensure that all the blood in the uterus is being expelled. Generally speaking, once empty, the uterus will clamp down; one or two small gushes will follow the placenta and then slow down to a sporadic, start-and-stop discharge of blood, much like a heavy period. Now the midwife can remove the pan and herself from her position as placenta catcher.

Fundal pressure to expel clots

Guard the uterus by standing to the side of the supine mother, with your nondominant side to her feet. Instruct the mother to relax her abdominal muscles. Form your thumb and forefinger into a "C," place the crotch of your thumb and forefinger above the pubic bone, with your palm toward the mother's feet.

Cup your dominant hand over the fundus, with the fingers directed toward the mother's spine. *Never dig your fingertips into the top of the fundus as that invites inversion.* Rest your palm over the fundus, leaving the thumb free. With a firm, quick, smooth, motion of the wrist, press the well-contracted uterus downward in an arch following the curve of Carus. The motion is one of scooping down, under the pubic arch and toward the outlet. This motion differs from direct downward pressure on the fundus, which tends to fold the upper segment over the lower segment and impede placental descent. Excessive pressure must be avoided, as it will unduly strain the uterine and cervical ligaments.

To Practice Controlled Cord Traction

Make a pillow by sewing around the edges of two 8 in (20 cm) circles of cloth, leaving a small opening. Fill with 1.3 pounds of fine bird seed and sew shut. Sew a macrame rope or upholstery cord in the center of one side of the pillow. You now have a cloth placenta with a central cord insertion.

To make a placenta with a lateral (Battledore) cord insertion (see the following chapter for details), cut cloth as above and construct, fill and sew the round part shut, as before. Sew through the surface in several places to quilt the placenta and hold the fill in place, then attach the cord to the edge.

Get together with other midwives or students. First practice how hard to pull by pinching your nose between your thumb and index finger and pulling until just before your fingers slip off. Also try pulling on each other's noses, as this will give you a much better feel of how hard you can pull. You can also tie a cord to a 1 lb weight (like a small bag of flour) and pull just enough to make the bag move. Then, with a partner, practice cord traction and bringing the cloth placentas through the os and out with one of you using your hands as the lower uterine segment and os. The central cord attachment mimics a Schultz delivery, while the Battledore attachment is more similar to a Duncan delivery. To practice bringing the placenta through the birth canal, trim a sock with a heel to an 8 in length, with the heel in the middle to mimic the curve of Carus and with the toe cut out.

Examining the Placenta

This chapter covers how to perform a thorough gross examination of the placenta, focusing on visual and manual inspection of the relevant anatomy, including normal variations and pathological findings. Placental examination is one of the most important assessments midwives perform because retained placental fragments place the mother at risk for excessive bleeding and infection.

The placenta often holds clues regarding the condition of the newborn. For example, a very pale placenta with ruptured vessels of a hard-to-start, hypotensive baby points to fetal anemia and blood loss. A baby who is difficult to resuscitate may have amnion nodosum plaques on his placenta, which are commonly associated with severe oligohydramnios and underdeveloped lungs. In addition, features of the placenta offer clues as to what may have impacted certain findings during pregnancy or labor. For example, you may discover a true knot in the cord or evidence of a twin gestation.

Preparing for the Exam

The placental exam should be performed prior to leaving the house and after the baby and mother are stable. However, if the mother is actively bleeding and the cause is unknown, examine the maternal side of the placenta as soon as possible to determine if any pieces, which might be the cause of the bleeding, are missing. Later, after the mother has stabilized, proceed with a more complete examination.

Parents are often very interested in the placenta; offer to examine it at the bedside. Explain to the parents that the primary reason for examining the placenta is to determine if it is complete and appears healthy. Use good, glare-free light; daylight is perfect. Wear exam or dishwashing gloves. Ideally, the placenta should be examined on a white surface such as an acrylic cutting board. A white background always helps in identifying unusual color variations. If one is not available, spread out a clean underpad or newspaper on a flat surface. Have a pan of water nearby to rinse your gloves during the exam and, if indicated, examine parts of the placenta underwater. Handle the placenta gently to avoid tearing membranes or tissue; such damage may confuse your findings.

The cord need not be cut in order to proceed. You can perform every part of the exam with the baby still attached. You may also wait until the cord has been cut to perform your full exam; the placenta will not significantly deteriorate in an hour or three. If the parents have chosen Lotus birth, perform a complete placental exam prior to the application of any herbal or salt preservatives.

Using placenta as an antihemorrhagic agent

When using a piece of placenta as an antihemorrhagic agent, first quickly examine the maternal side to ensure that it is intact before a piece is removed. Tearing a piece out of the parenchyma prior to inspection may make it impossible to determine whether a piece of placenta is still retained in the uterus. To avoid any doubt about the placenta's integrity during the full exam, take a photo of the maternal side for reference before you remove a chunk. A Polaroid or digital photo is best because it will develop immediately. Keep it in the mother's chart. If no camera is available, both you and your assistant should quickly examine the maternal side together to confirm that it is complete. Draw a picture of the placenta in the chart indicating the size and location of the piece that is removed. Note the time as well and who examined the placenta. Making these notes will eliminate any doubts that may arise later as to the completeness of the maternal side.

Recording your findings

See the end of this chapter for an example of a placental examination form.

General Anatomy of the Normal, Healthy Singleton Placenta at Term

Weight, size and shape

The placenta is made up of fetal tissue and normally weighs about one-sixth the weight of the newborn. This averages about 1 lb 2 oz (500 grams). It is usually a flat, circular or oval disc that is thicker near the center, tapers off to its thinnest at the edges, has an average diameter of 6 to 8 inches (15 to 20 cm) and an average thickness of ⅔ to 1¼ inches (1.5 to 3 cm). At high altitudes, the placenta is most often an ovoid shape.

Fetal side of the placenta

Although all placental tissue is of fetal origin, it has two distinct surfaces that are named according to the member of the mother-fetus pair with which the surface is in nearest contact. The fetal surface is covered with two layers of membranes. The exquisitely smooth **amnion** is the most superficial layer; in direct contact with the amniotic fluid and fetus; it is loosely adherent to the chorion. The **chorion** underlies the amnion and is very firmly fused to the parenchymal surface. This double layer of membranes extends in a continuous layer from the base of the umbilical cord over the entire fetal surface of the placenta, giving it a smooth, shiny appearance. The **chorionic plate** is that portion of the chorionic membrane overlying the region of the parenchyma's basal plate that is attached to the uterine wall. The villi underlying the chorionic plate contain poorly saturated hemoglobin, giving the fetal surface a blue-purple cast; the actual depth of color varies according to the extent to which the placenta has been drained of blood.

Under these membranes, the fetal surface is riddled with blood vessels that fan out from the base of the cord. The major arteries traverse the fetal surface toward the edge of the placenta. At this point, they take a 90° turn into the body of the placental tissue and are now called **truncal arteries**. From here, they branch to form capillaries. Each truncal artery supplies a cotyledon. Blood returns to the cord from the parenchyma through tiny venules that supply veins. The veins emerge on the fetal surface near the point where the corresponding artery entered the tissue. There is one artery for each vein in most cotyledons. As a rule, arteries almost always cross over veins, especially near the cord insertion point. These blood vessels will appear thin, pale and less engorged with blood when the cord has been left intact or been allowed to bleed out if it was cut.

Maternal side of the placenta

The other side of the placenta is designated the maternal side because it is directly attached to the uterine wall during pregnancy. The maternal side normally appears medium pale to deep blood red. The depth of color and flexibility of the tissue has to do with the amount of fetal blood it contains. Babies who have been allowed a full placental transfusion have paler, more flexible placentas.

The maternal side is covered by a thin, translucent, grayish film of decidua basalis that is soft and easily torn. The placental body or meat is called the **parenchyma** (pair-REN-ka-ma). The parenchyma lies between the chorionic plate and the decidua basalis. The entire thickness of the meaty maternal portion below the chorion-covered fetal surface is referred to as the **basal plate**, which comprises the villous layer. This tissue is organized into a series of discrete regions called cotyledons (or lobules) that are separated by grooves or septa composed of fibrous tissue. Each cotyledon contains a huge number of fetal blood vessels. The cotyledons fit together along these septa like the pieces of a puzzle. The body of the parenchyma is also divided horizontally into three parallel layers or zones of equal thickness when measured at the center of the basal plate. These are:

The fetal or subchorionic zone: This is located directly beneath the chorionic plate covering the fetal surface.

The intermediate zone: The tissue sandwiched between the fetal and maternal zones.

The maternal zone: A region made up of the most mature villi that are involved in gas transfer. This layer offers the most information regarding villus maturity and the general condition of the tissue when examined microscopically.

The **marginal** or **transition zone** is a vaguely defined cross-sectional region at the edge of the placenta's circumference where the basal plate, the chorionic plate and the extraplacental membranes separate. It is often visible on the fetal surface as a slightly elevated, opaque ring up to 1 cm wide called the **subchorial closing ring** (Schuler-Maloney & Lee, 1998). The basal plate at the marginal zone has characteristics of the other zones of the pachyemia and is itself distinguished by two boundaries:

The inner margin: This forms the inside edge of the transition zone, where the chorionic plate ends and the marginal zone begins. On the fetal surface, its circumference is defined by the line formed by connecting the points where the peripheral ends of the fetal vessels traversing the fetal surface become truncal arteries as they are redirected downward into the parenchyma.

The outer margin: This is the outermost border of the transitional zone where the attachment of the chorionic plate to the basal plate ends and the unattached "bag" portion of the membranous chorion begins.

The extraplacental membranes

The two layers of the placental membranes, the chorion and the amnion, extend beyond the border of the placental disc to form a continuous double-layered sac in which the fetus and amniotic fluid were enclosed during gestation. This sac is called the **extraplacental membranes**, which, when intact, should be large enough to cover the placenta approximately one and a half times. All regions of the membranes normally appear translucent and colorless with a pale gray white cast, transmitting the color of underlying structures. The chorion is less easily torn, slightly more opaque and thicker than the more fragile, transparent amnion; however, the tensile strength (i.e., the amount of stretching a material can withstand before breaking) of the amnion is greater. "Ghosts" are nonfunctional remnants of chorionic blood vessels; these traverse the chorion, appearing as widely spaced, fine lines that do not contain blood.

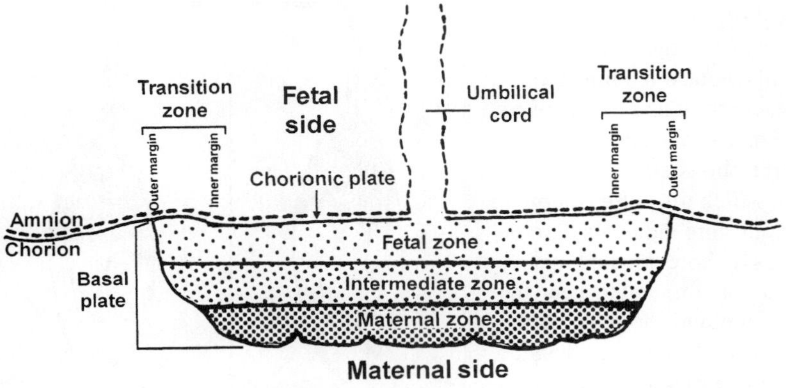

Landmarks of the parenchyma and fetal surface in cross-section

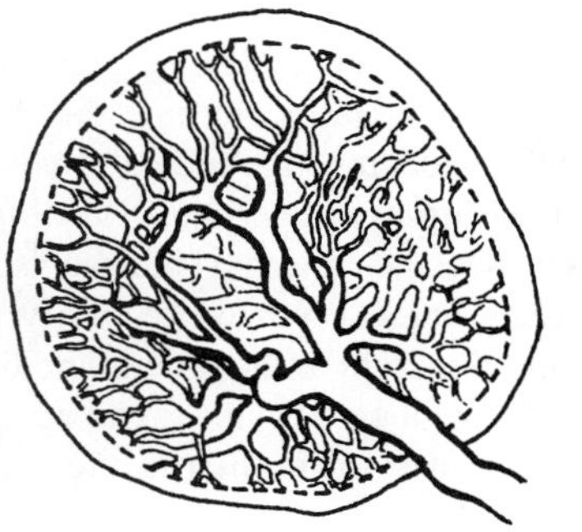
"Connecting" truncal arteries on the fetal surface to define the inner margin of the transition zone

Umbilical cord

The umbilical cord arises from the fetal surface of the placenta. It usually has a spiral or coiled appearance. Its insertion point varies and is typically located somewhere between the edge and the center of the fetal surface. Its length is thought to be related to the degree of fetal mobility and thus the stretching force to which it was subjected. Usually measuring between 21.5 to 24 inches (54 and 61 cm) long and averaging about 22 inches (55 cm), it is commonly slightly longer than the total length of the baby. At term, the cord contains three fetal blood vessels; two arteries and one vein. These vessels are surrounded by a clear, gelatinous protective substance called Wharton's jelly, the amount of which can vary considerably. A layer of amnion is fused with the Wharton's jelly and forms the outermost covering of the cord.

The Placental Exam

Smell

The healthy placenta has a fresh, rich, earthy, slightly pungent smell that is similar to the smell of fresh menstrual blood, only slightly stronger.

Vernix

Small or large lumps of vernix may be loosely adherent to the fetal surface or extraplacental membranes. Vernix presents as creamy white flakes resembling off-white cream cheese that are easily removed and may be stained with meconium or blood. Vernix and amniotic fluid can insinuate between the layers of membranes if the amnion ruptures during labor. Some lesions may appear at first glance to be vernix, but they are not easily removed nor do they have a cream-cheese-like texture. (See the section later in this chapter covering variations and anomalies of the placenta for more details.)

The membranes

Examine the membranes first because they may become torn during the rest of the exam. Handle the placenta gently to prevent disruption of the maternal side prior to its examination. You can hold the placenta by the cord and allow the membranes to hang down from the edges of the placenta. The vast majority of cords will be strong enough to allow this. Remember that if you are holding the placenta suspended by the cord you are looking at it inside out. However, if you suspect that the cord is too fragile, do not attempt to support the weight of the placenta by the cord alone. Instead, place your open hand flat against the maternal side and allow the membranes to drape down over your forearm. Alternatively, place the placenta maternal side up on the examining surface and hold the membranes up by the edges of the opening from which the baby emerged.

Size: The size of the extraplacental sac should be appropriate to the size of the baby and roughly one and a half times the size of the placenta. Polyhydramnios or oligohydramnios will both cause the bag to be larger or smaller, respectively, than usual.

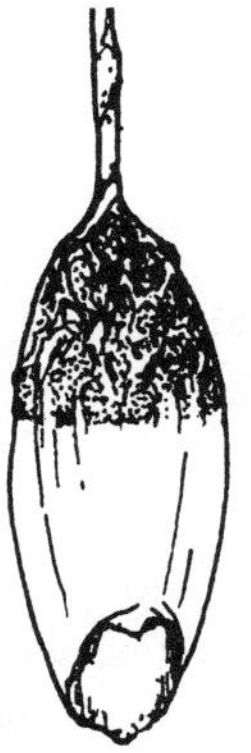

The hole is located near the "bottom" in this fundally implanted placenta

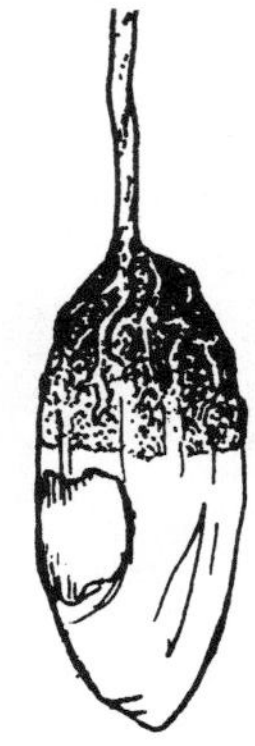

The hole is located near the placenta when the placenta is implanted near the cervix

Determining where the placenta was implanted: When there is a single, neat hole in the bag, the distance between the hole and the nearest placental edge indicates where the placenta was implanted in relationship to the cervix. Holding the placenta in any of the ways that protect the maternal side shows how the membranes were situated in utero and allows you to easily determine the distance from the placental margin to the hole in the bag from which the baby emerged.

A hole located close to the edge of the placenta indicates that the placenta was lower in the uterus, whereas a hole located nearly opposite the placenta indicates the placenta was implanted near the fundus. The typical distance between the hole and the edge of the placenta is about 2 to 3.5 inches (5 to 9 cm). When the distance measures over 4 inches (10 cm), it is likely that a fundal implantation occurred. A low-lying implantation site increases the risk of maternal bleeding postpartum because fewer ligating muscles are located in this region of the uterine wall. Placental location, determined by postpartum intrauterine examination, varies as follows: anterior uterine wall, 53%; posterior wall, 39%; side-walls, 8%; directly central fundal implantation, 2%; fundal implantation extending to upper segment, 42%; upper segment, 47%; implantation involving both the upper and lower segment, 9% (Benirschke & Kaufmann, 2000).

Determining if the membranes are complete: It is usually easy to see whether all the membranes are present if the opening in the bag is neat and without jagged edges. This will also be obvious when you hold the placenta suspended by the cord. If the opening is shredded or torn, bring the edges together to try to determine if the membranes are all there. A large ragged hole indicates that the membranes may have fragmented during detachment and delivery, making it more difficult to determine if they are all present. Friable (easily torn) membranes also suggest inadequate nutrition or inflammation. Gently spread any separate pieces out in an attempt to reconstruct the entire bag.

Examining the chorion and amnion: Note the consistency of the chorion (outer bag) and the amnion (inner bag). Normal membranes are slippery if wet, much less so if dry. Note as well the transparency and color as you examine them. The amnion is translucent, while the chorion is slightly less so. Either membrane may have small streaks of blood on them and very thin adherent clots. The fine ghost of a vascular network can be detected in the chorion. The bag may have a brownish, greenish or even a yellowish tinge if the baby passed meconium in utero. Look for areas of thickening or frank masses in both sacs.

The two bags are often fused or partly fused. Fully separating the extraplacental amnion from the chorion enables you to see if both the chorion and the amnion are complete. Although complete separation is usually not necessary, it should be done if a question arises about whether either bag is complete. Usually the bags separate easily right up to the edge of the placenta when one is peeled away from the other. From there, the amnion is easily separated from the surface of the placental chorion right up to the cord insertion point. However, separating the chorion from the fetal surface is basically impossible and need not be attempted.

Examine any holes in the membranes to see if any blood vessels lead into and away from them. Such vessels indicate that a succenturiate lobe may have been torn away and thus retained in utero. However, an accessory lobe can be torn away and leave no communicating vessels to give you a clue. Normally, isolated holes do not occur in the membranes; should you find a hole, not merely a tear, assume that a lobe is retained.

Sometimes, the remnant of the yolk sac is present near the placenta's edge, either in the extraplacental membranes or on the chorionic plate. It appears beneath the amnion as a 3 to 5 mm (rarely up to 15 mm) white to yellow ovoid disk that has a pasty consistency. You may also find a tiny remnant of a blood vessel running from the yolk sac to the cord insertion point.

The maternal surface

Next, examine the red, lobulated, meaty-looking maternal side of the placenta by placing the fetal side down on a flat surface.

Color: The color of the maternal surface varies and normally depends upon the amount of blood it contains. If the cord has been cut and the placental end clamped soon after birth, the placenta will be engorged with blood, resulting in a dark red color. If the cord has been left intact or the cut placental end has been allowed to drain out, the cotyledons will appear thinner, slightly deflated and paler in hue. Abnormal color variations are covered later in this chapter.

Assessing and removing blood clots: Before the maternal surface can be examined, it should be checked for fresh, red blood clots that may cling to the surface from its delivery. Remove these by gently lifting them up with gloved fingers or carefully rinsing them off with water over a closed container. That way, if tissue fragments are in a clot, they won't be lost. Do not remove clots with gauze or a towel, as rubbing may tear the maternal surface, confusing your findings. A tissue fragment that is discovered in association with an intact placenta is likely to be maternal in origin. See the chapter entitled "Cervical and Other Soft-Tissue Problems during Labor" for details regarding cervical detachment.

Dark, firmly adherent clots may have been formed in utero during gestation or during labor. Remove each clot by very gently insinuating your fingertips beneath one edge and carefully lifting it up. Be aware that a clot may be attached to a partially torn area of placenta beneath it. Once removed, look though the clot for tissue fragments. Remember that fibrin strands found in clots are not part of the placenta. Rinsing the clot gently with water will cause the fibrin strands to dissolve, revealing any actual tissue it may contain. Frequently clots form a smooth, thin covering over an area of placenta, and represent a localized region where a small abruption occurred at some point during pregnancy or labor. If the placenta was partially separated for a period of time before it was delivered, the clot that formed over the detached portion may be quite large and firm with distinct borders. Inspect the area beneath any clots to see if the underlying tissue is indented. An indentation indicates that the clot was there for a while. Clots that formed later, during the delivery of the placenta, do not, as a rule, leave such indentations and are brighter red in color.

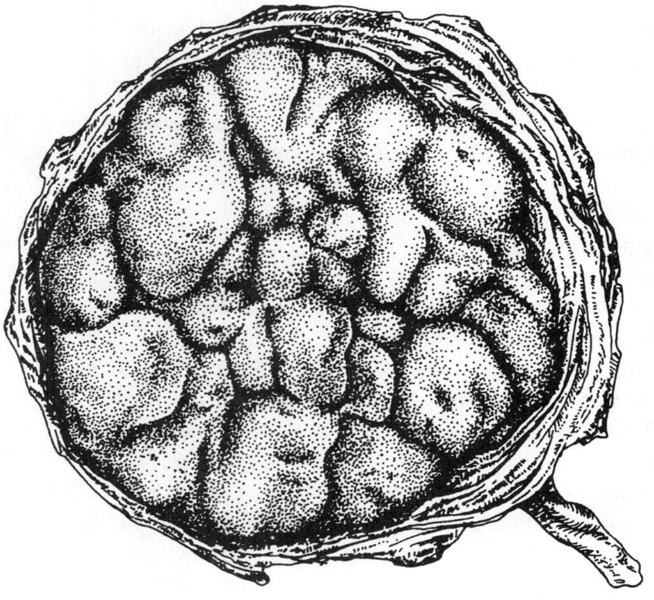

Maternal side of a completely intact placenta (membranes removed)

Initial assessment: Take an overall look at the maternal side of the placenta by cradling the placenta, mother's side up, in your open hands and spreading your fingers so that you support as much of the parenchyma as possible. Gently spread the tissues by opening your hands widely, which will part the septa between the lobes, and check the borders of the cotyledons for tears, shredding, and missing pieces. When entire cotyledons are torn away, they leave a thin, roughly textured, recessed defect in the maternal side of the placenta that should be readily apparent during the exam. Missing fragments leave frayed edges; the "puzzle" may appear incomplete at septal margins, or an otherwise intact lobe may have a ragged surface. Now gently cup your hands to bring the tissue together so that the cotyledons touch. All cotyledons should fit together nicely like pieces of a jigsaw puzzle, appearing smooth around their edges, complete across their surface and otherwise intact. Again, place the placenta, maternal side up, on a flat surface, avoiding stretching out or separating the cotyledons.

Examining the surface: Next, the entire maternal side should be systematically examined. Starting at a point along the edge, follow the periphery of the tissue with your fingerpads to check for smoothness, blotting the tissue with gauze or wiping gently, as necessary. Move toward the center until the entire surface is examined, using a pattern similar to that which you would use in examining a breast for lumps. The texture should be consistent, with relatively uniform, rounded cotyledon surfaces that are intact and unfragmented. Run your fingerpads over the surface; it should feel soft and somewhat firm. Firmness will vary, depending upon the overall health of the placenta; some allow your finger to easily puncture the surface. Others have a grainy texture in spots or over the entire surface, the result of mineral deposits.

Ragged areas on the surface of a cotyledon require closer inspection. Use the pad of your finger to gently move the torn edges together. Take care to put them back in the way they fit most easily. Do not force the tissue to fit, as this may obscure that a fragment is missing. If the torn and rough edges fit smoothly together without forceful closing of the gap, and if broken or jagged edges of the thin decidua fit into each other perfectly, nothing is missing in that area. The ragged portions of the placenta can also be submerged in still water. If villi are seen free and floating, this may indicate that a fragment of the placenta has been retained.

The fetal side

Turn the placenta over and place it on the exam surface, fetal side up. Do so carefully to avoid disturbing the maternal side.

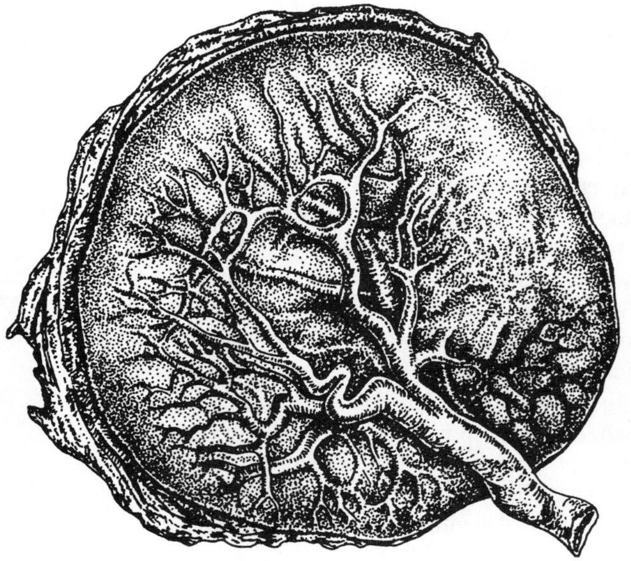

Fetal side of a completely intact placenta
(membranes removed)

Examining the marginal zone: The normal marginal zone (where the membranes attach to the edge of the chorionic plate) forms a ring around the edge of the fetal surface and is visible as an opaque border in 71% of all placentas; in 21%, it is an incomplete border, and in 8%, it cannot be identified at all. It normally measures 1 cm or less in width. A ruptured vessel (marginal sinus) along the edge reveals the source of otherwise unexplained bleeding during labor; this may occur with a low-lying placenta.

Placenta extrachorialis occurs when the circumference of chorionic plate is smaller than that of the basal plate. This is a developmental phenomenon present to some degree in as many as 25% of all placentas. The basal plate is often thicker than usual. The marginal zone does not form a 1 cm border at the placental edge. Instead, it develops a variable distance from the circumference of the chorionic plate. A rim of "naked" parenchyma projects beyond this boundary. The fetal surface appears normal within the marginal zone. The truncal arteries of the fetal surface dive into the deeper placental tissue before reaching this transitional boundary, as is normally the case. The exposed rim of parenchyma may appear weakened and worn away, giving the impression that an abruption occurred.

There are two forms of placenta extrachorialis, which can occur alone or in combination in different regions of the circumference of the same placenta. Extrachorialis may also develop along only a portion of the placental margin, with the rest appearing as usual.

Placenta marginata (circummarginate): This usually forms a flat to sightly elevated transition zone from villous to membranous chorion. The elevation is due to small amounts of fibrin trapped between the unadhered membranes and the basal plate. The membranes do not fold back on themselves.

Placenta circumvallata (circumvallate): The border of the villous placental membranes is folded or rolled, forming a rim on the basal plate a variable distance from the center of the chorionic plate. This raised rim gives the impression that the chorionic plate within its borders is depressed. The folded region may contain degenerated decidua and fibrin from old clots.

Except for the raised rim in the circumvallate variety, these two different variations present a similar appearance. The cause of these variations is unknown. A controversial theory links them to problems that occurred early in the pregnancy. Extrachorial placentation results in a smaller than normal amniotic cavity, increasing the risk of placental bleeding from exposed extrachorial villi. Circumvallate placentation is associated with multi-parity as well as an increased incidence of threatened abortion, antepartum hemorrhage, premature labor, abruption, prolonged oligohydramnios, postpartum hemorrhage and a more frequent need for manual removal of the placenta. There are no clinical repercussions to be expected once the placenta is out except that some babies may be slightly underweight for their gestation.

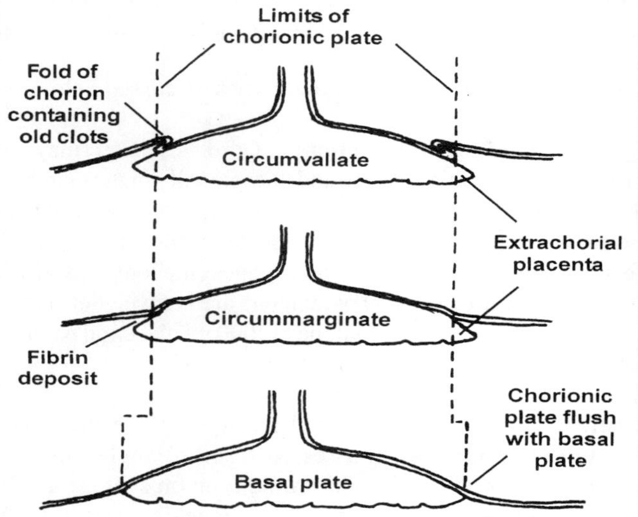

Extrachorial placental formation

Blood vessel distribution: The fetal surface is riddled with a network of blood vessels that form one of two charac-teristic patterns, although mixed patterns occasionally occur. In the **disperse pattern** (which occurs 63% of the time), a network of blood vessels spreads out in all directions from beneath the umbilical cord in a mostly uniform pattern. The disperse pattern is most often found with central insertion of the cord. In a **magistral** (MAJ-is-tral) **pattern** (which occurs 37% of the time), the vessels fan out over the fetal surface in more of a palm leaf pattern from the umbilical cord, which is inserted nearer the edge of the placenta. These vessels form many branches and are fairly uniform in diameter.

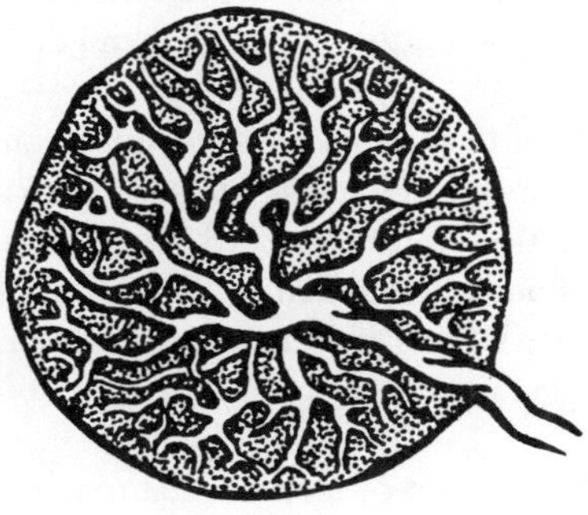

Disperse pattern with central insertion of the cord

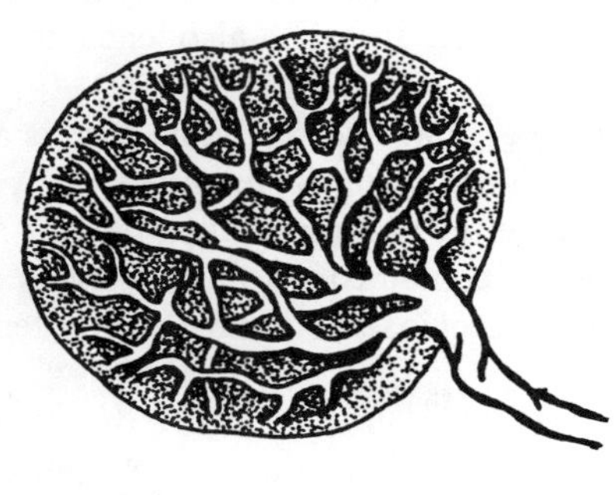

Magistral pattern with Battledore cord insertion

When inspecting the fetal surface, follow the major vessels as they leave the cord insertion point to where they dip down into the parenchyma. Look here for any lumps, lesions or other unusual characteristics. Typically, the membranes overlying the arteries appear whitish while the veins appear dark purple to black against the surrounding surface. The larger arteries cross over veins, especially near the cord insertion point. A reversal of this pattern–that is, the larger veins crossing over arteries–may be associated with abnormal fetal development and polyhydramnios. Check the vessels at the base of their placental insertion point and carefully investigate for tears, clots or other evidence of damage.

The cord

A normal cord appears translucent, pearly white and spiraled. The outer layer consists of inseparably fused amnion within which the vessels are surrounded by a protective coat of Wharton's jelly. The cord is quite firm to the touch and the Wharton's jelly tense and thin when the cord is fully pulsing. Only as the blood vessels relax does the jelly become apparent. At that point, the degree of springy firmness varies significantly, depending on the amount of Wharton's jelly that is present and the amount of blood that remains in the cord vessels. The thickness of the layer of jelly varies widely among normal cords and may vary along the length of the same cord. A nonpulsating cord feels limp, squishy and soft.

Examine the cord for the characteristics discussed below.

The point of cord insertion: Cord insertion may occur anywhere on the fetal surface and occasionally in the membranes. To identify the point of cord insertion, first locate the exact center of the placenta by measuring across the widest part of the fetal surface in two perpendicular planes (the longest and widest diameters). Cord insertion parameters are not well defined in the literature. Doris Schuler-Maloney (2000), a placental pathologist in Iowa, offers these guidelines:

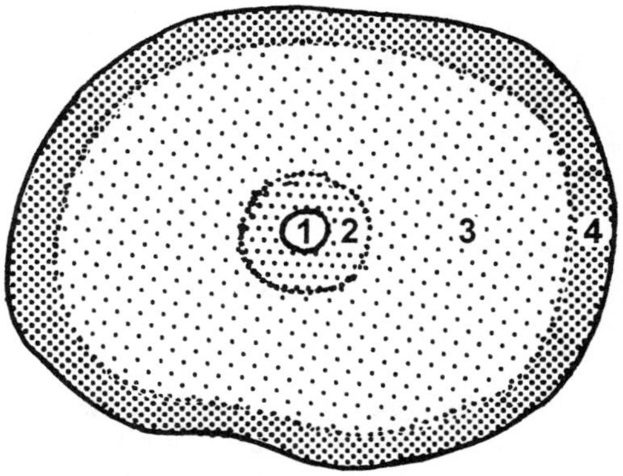

Cord insertion guidelines
1–Central; 2–Paracentral; 3–Eccentric; 4–Marginal

Central: The cord inserts in the center of the placenta and appears central when assessed from all angles and edges. The center of the placenta would span on average a 1 to 1.5 cm diameter, which is also the average diameter of the base of the cord.

Paracentral: The cord inserts outside the center but is within a 2 to 3 cm (1 to 1.25 in) radius of the center.

Eccentric: The cord inserts between paracentral and marginal locations. To distinguish between a paracentrally and eccentrically located insertion, measure from the center of the placenta to the edge closest to the cord insertion point. If the cord is closer to the center, but not exact, it is paracentral. If the insertion point is nearer the outer "half" from the center, it is eccentric.

Marginal (Battledore): The cord inserts at or within 1.5 cm (⅝ in) of the edge of the placenta. Some studies report an excess incidence of miscarriage, premature labor, neonatal asphyxia and congenital malformations related to this type of insertion. Battledore insertion also lends itself to sideways presentation of the placenta during its descent.

The type of cord insertion: Normally the cord is a discrete tube of tissue that passes from its insertion point at the umbilicus to its insertion point on the fetal surface. A sheath of normal skin of varying length may extend from the baby's abdomen at the base of the umbilicus; then there is an abrupt transition to normal cord. In the cord proper, the entire length of all vessels is contained within two layers of membranes and surrounded by Wharton's jelly. A variety of uncommon cord and vessel insertions have been noted. Since these variations are rare, they are described in the later part of this chapter.

An amniotic web (amniotic chorda): An amniotic web consists of a fold of amnion that extends from the placental surface along the umbilical cord for several centimeters. It arises from a base that is typically wide along the bottom edge, which is attached to the fetal surface of the placenta. One upright edge is attached to the cord while the parallel edge is free, altogether forming a thin, triangular web. The long bottom edge of the web may also attach to the fetal surface, forming a membranous anchor that holds the first few centimeters of cord horizontal to the placental surface. A web may be loose or relatively tight, binding the cord to the surface. Tight webs can limit cord mobility and blood flow.

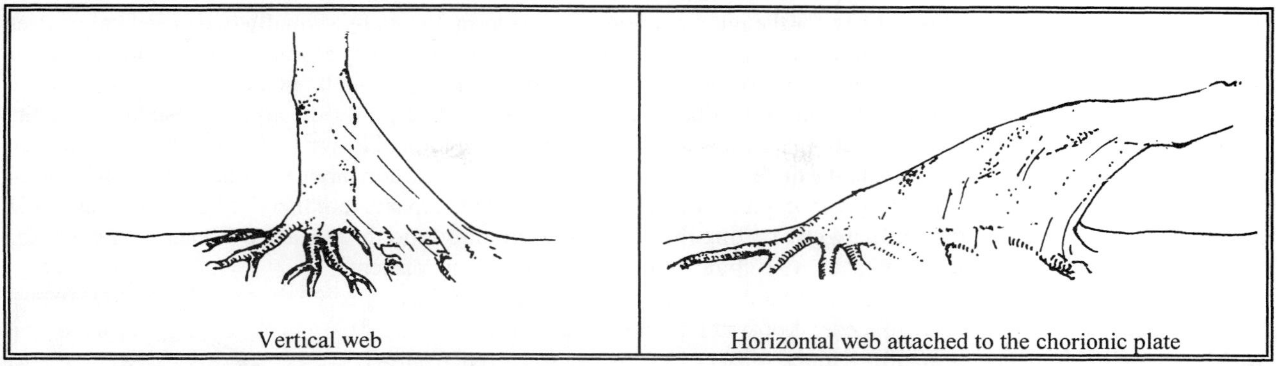

Vertical web | Horizontal web attached to the chorionic plate

Length: Measure the entire length of the translucent cord with a flexible measuring tape and record its length in both inches and centimeters. If the cord has been cut, remember to include any cord left at the baby's umbilicus in your measurement. If the cord has an unusual formation, measure the distance from the umbilicus to the point where the cord vessels become abnormal, then measure the length of each vessel to its end at the placenta. Be sure to illustrate the cord formation in your records. Next, measure the widest and narrowest diameters of the cord. To do so, gently lay the cord out straight and identify its widest and narrowest portions. Place your measuring device perpendicularly under each region and look straight down to get the most exact measurement.

Spiraling (helices or chirality): Most cords have a spiral pattern along their length. To assess the cord for spiraling, hold it up in front of you with the placenta below. If the baby is still attached, lay the baby "above" the placenta. Stretch the cord slightly to distinguish the upward direction of the twist, which is always toward the baby. The direction of the upward slant to your left or right determines if it is a left or right spiral. Left spiraling is seven times more frequent than right, probably because the right umbilical artery is usually larger than the left; the torque that results from the differing blood flows causes the cord to twist left. Less commonly, a single cord displays both right and left spiraling. The direction of spiral is not significant. Long cords tend to spiral more.

Spiraling is often absent in cords with only two vessels and in cases where fetal movement has been restricted (for example, when amniotic bands are present). Although it is unnecessary to count spirals, you should comment in your records if the number seems unusual in any way. Forty turns are the average, but much higher numbers have been described. In general, spiraling is associated with healthy fetal activity and therefore may be related to better fetal outcome. Strong and associates (1994) devised a coiling index by dividing the number of complete twists by the length of the cord, arriving at a average index of 0.21. Those fetuses whose coiling index was below 0.1 or above 0.3 had significantly increased rates of poor outcome, including chromosomal defects, fetal distress and meconium staining. Excessive coiling has also been linked to cocaine usage and a higher incidence of premature labor.

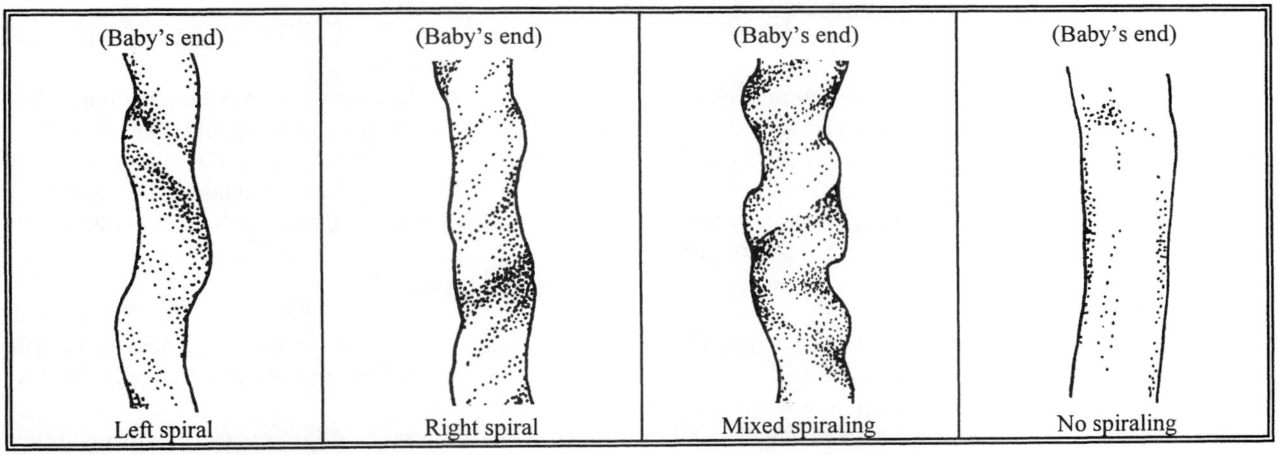

Left spiral | Right spiral | Mixed spiraling | No spiraling

The number of cord vessels: If the cord is to be cut, sever it in a region that is apparently normal, halfway between baby and the placenta. Check the cut end for the number of vessels. At term, there are normally two umbilical arteries and one umbilical vein. A second umbilical vein atrophies during the second month of gestation. The umbilical arteries of 96% of all babies have either a communication (hyrtlanastomosis) or are actually fused at some point. The anastomosis is usually located within 1.5 cm of the placental surface, although at times, the arteries fuse far above the placental insertion site. This communication is believed to provide an equalization of flow and pressure between the two arteries, ensuring balanced blood flow to the different placental lobes. Examine the cord above this level when evaluating the number of vessels to avoid misdiagnosing a missing vessel. Whenever it appears that there are only two vessels in a cord, make sure there are truly only two by cutting the cord and examining it in three places: (1) near the baby, (2) midway between the baby and placenta and (3) about 3 cm (1.25 in) above the placenta.

To examine the vessel stumps, hold the cord between your thumb and index fingers just below the cut end and squeeze. Look straight down into the end. The two arteries should appear as small, distinct orifices that, when squeezed from below, often telescope upward and look like two tiny tubes. The single vein is a less distinct tubular opening with loose sidewalls. The diameter of the arteries averages 3 mm, often widening slightly near the placenta. The opening of the vein averages 6 mm. Typically, a tiny bit of blood oozes out of the open ends of the vessels as you squeeze, which facilitates their identification. However, when the baby has been allowed to fully equilibrate her blood volume, the vessels are collapsed and empty of all but a trace of blood. If you cannot see the vessels, milk the cord to expel a small amount of blood. If you still have difficulty locating either the arteries or the vein, simply recut the cord a little closer to the placenta and recheck at the new cut.

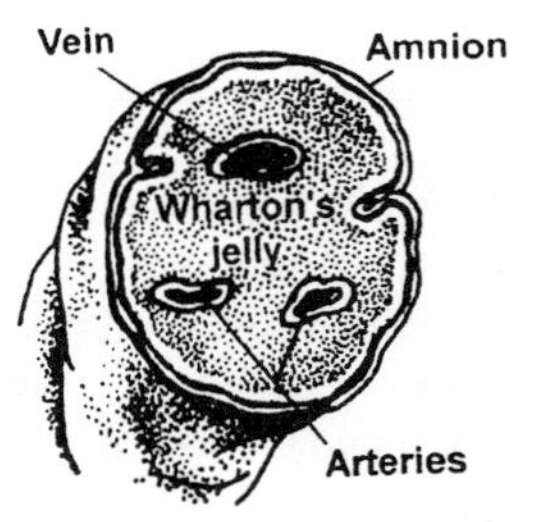

The stump of the umbilical cord

If the cord is intact at the time of the placental exam, transilluminate it. Darken the room and place a small, bright, narrow-beam flashlight under the cord at each of the three locations mentioned above. The vessels should be easily identified (Kravitz & Molina, 1966). This works best when the cord is fresh and the Wharton's jelly is still prominent.

<u>Preservation</u>: If there are changes in the mother's or baby's condition, it may become necessary to send the placenta to a lab for examination. It can be refrigerated at 7.2° F (4° C) for up to 7 days with minimal changes in its gross or microscopic features. Freezing and thawing produces artifacts that can confuse pathological studies (Schuler-Maloney & Lee, 1998). More about the pathological examination of the placenta can be found in a recent edition of my DIAGNOSTIC TESTS.

This concludes the basics of a complete gross exam. You may note a number of variations when performing your exam. The next part of the chapter covers a variety of visible lesions and other findings, and their possible significance.

General Variations and Abnormalities and What They May Mean

Unusual odor

Recent ingestion of garlic by the mother may produce a sulfide odor in the placenta. Foul-smelling amniotic fluid or placental tissue strongly suggests infection. A fetid-smelling placenta or amniotic fluid should alert you to the possibility of intrauterine infection with *E. coli* in the baby and possibly the mother. A sweeter smell is associated with *Listeria monocytogenes*. If you detect an odd smell, store the placenta at 39.2°F (4°C) for half an hour or so to enhance the growth and odor of these organisms; you may then recognize them more easily. If you suspect an infection, the mother and baby should be evaluated as soon as possible.

Abnormal size

Large and heavy placentas often correspond to a large baby. Babies infected with syphilis often have large, pale placentas with a greasy appearance. Erythroblastosis also causes large placentas; their villi become clogged with dead red blood cells, and more villi develop in order to continue nourishing the baby.

Smaller and lighter placentas may be seen with babies who have systemic diseases. A failure of adequate blood flow to the placenta, caused by inadequate blood volume expansion in the mother or localized variations in the uterine wall, may also result in small placentas. This usually occurs with growth restricted babies.

Unusual shapes and formations

The placenta may develop into a wide variety of shapes. Most shape variations are of no particular clinical importance unless they interfere with placental functions (for example, if it is too thin), result in abnormal adhesion, adversely influence fetal descent or the shape causes one or more pieces of placenta to be retained in utero. A placenta with multiple lobes may cause you to suspect that there was a multiple gestation. However, it may, in fact, be one placenta that formed as two or more regions in the membranes. This type of formation may be related to irregularities in blood flow to the decidua.

Accessory lobe: One or more accessory lobes of variable size may be found adjacent to the main placenta. They are often relatively small and thin. The overall incidence of these lobes is 3% to 6%. There are three different types of accessory lobes:

Placenta spuria: This accessory lobe forms an isolated island in the membranes and does not have a vascular connection with the main placental disc.

Digitate lobe: This type of lobe joins the main body of the placenta by a bridge of parenchymal tissue.

Succenturiate lobe: This lobe appears as an island of tissue in the membranes, with vessels running to it from the main placenta.

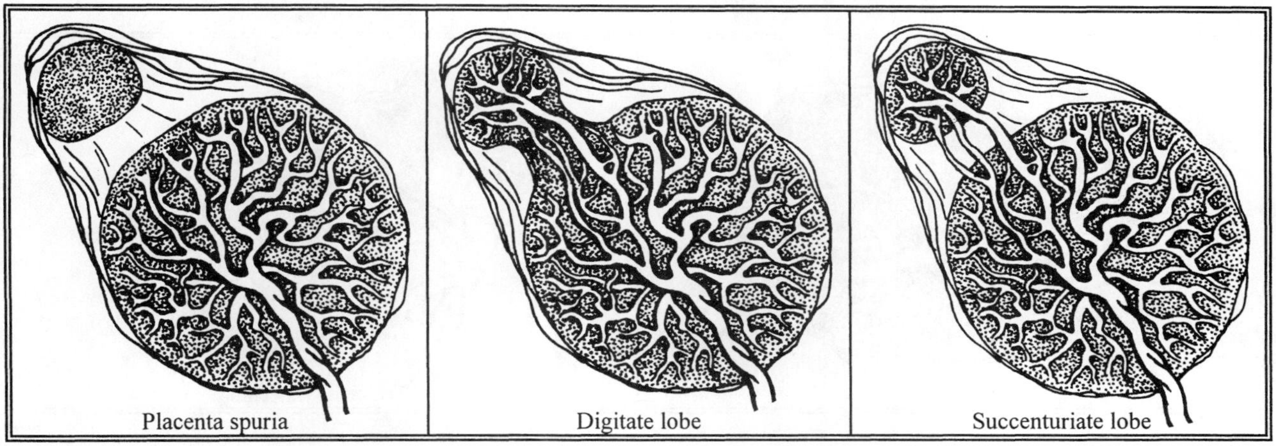

Because accessory lobes are typically small, they may not be of sufficient size or weight to detach normally from the uterine wall. Instead, they may tear out of the membranes, remaining adhered or retained within the uterus, where they can potentially lead to hemorrhage and infection. Therefore, if you suspect that a lobe has been retained, you should transport for a curettage.

Placenta membranacea (placenta diffusa): During normal early development, the entire surface of the chorion is covered with villi. Most of these villi disappear as gestation continues, leaving a clearly demarcated, thickened region of normal parenchyma. However, this rare defect occurs once in every 25,000 pregnancies when villi overlying the decidua capsularis fail to atrophy. The outer surface of the membranes is covered mostly or entirely by chorionic villi of varying thicknesses, usually averaging 1 to 2 cm. Rarely, there may be a localized thickening to form a placental disc.

Placenta membranacea has been associated with maternal immunization and infection during the first trimester (Naeye, 1990). It also has some correlation with maternal obesity, diabetes, fetal malformations, and motor disorders in parents or siblings. Other risk factors include disturbances of the endometrium such as atrophy, hypoplasia, endometriosis or poor decidual blood supply. Reports of the fetal consequences vary. Some babies experience growth retardation while others are normally sized. Preterm labor is more common. There is a high risk of bleeding as term nears and cervical ripening begins because placental villi usually overlie the os. The villi may abnormally attach to the myometrium (accreta) because they are so thin and diffuse. Even if they do not, fragments of tissues may remain adhered during separation, leading to postpartum hemorrhage.

Ring-shape: Also known as a “girdle,” “collar,” “zonary” or “annular” placenta, this rare anomaly is a variation of placenta membranacea, occurring about once in every 6000 births. The placenta may resemble a slice of a hollow cylinder, forming a complete ring. However, more commonly a portion of the ring atrophies, leaving a horseshoe-shaped placenta; in this case, fetal placental vessels will be found running across the gap in the atrophied portion. A ring-shaped placenta increases the risk of ante- and postpartum bleeding because a larger area of the uterine wall is involved and is often seen with low-birthweight babies.

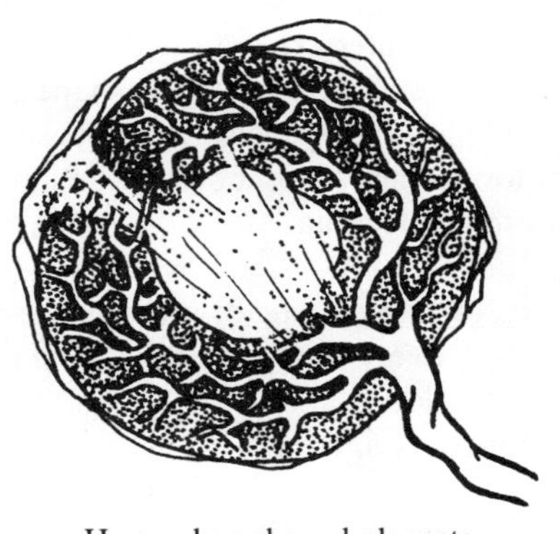

Horse-shoe shaped placenta

Bilobate placenta: Also known as "bipartite" or "duplex," this placenta is formed of two nearly equally sized lobes that may be marginally fused, connected by a bridge of chorion, or entirely separate. The umbilical cord is usually inserted between the two lobes. The cord may insert into the connecting bridge (often velamentously) or into the larger of the two lobes. Studies vary widely as to the frequency of its occurrence. Some report one in every 350 births (Fox, 1997). High gravidity, older mothers and a history of infertility seem to predispose to this type of placenta. It is associated with a higher frequency of both first-trimester bleeding and adherent placenta postpartum.

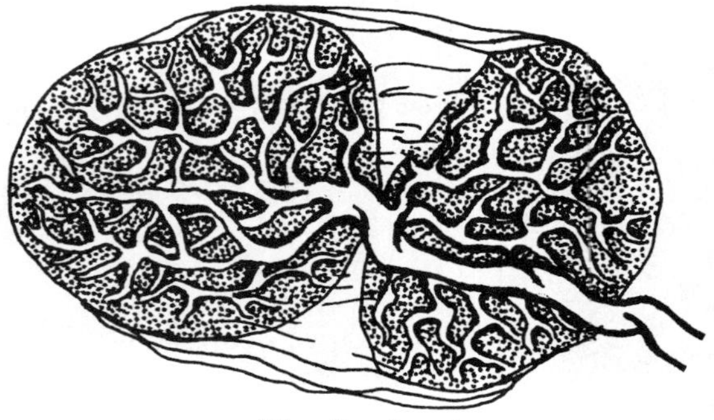

Bipartite placenta

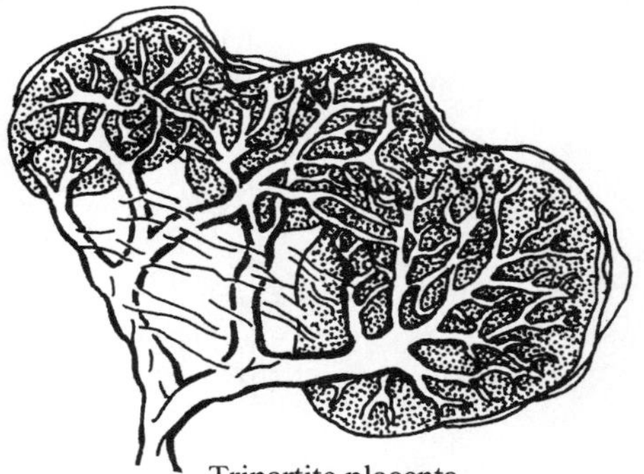

Tripartite placenta

Multilobate: Placentas formed from three or more nearly equally sized lobes are very rare, although there have been reports of placentas with four, five and even seven lobes. They may develop as the result of irregular atrophy of the villous shell. Multiple lobes are clinically significant only when one is torn from the membranes and retained within the uterus, when vessels that run through the membranes to supply the lobe or connect to the cord are torn (a rare occurrence that results in fetal hemorrhage), when a lobe overlies the internal os, creating a placenta previa, or when a blood vessel overlies the os, resulting in a vasa previa.

Fenestrate: In this very rare abnormality, a portion of the basal plate of a discoidal (round) placenta is very thin or missing entirely. The defect commonly presents as a lack of villous tissue with the chorionic plate present. The portion of the chorionic plate overlying the defect may be depressed on the fetal side and give the impression of a missing cotyledon on the maternal side. More rarely, no chorion overlies the area, leaving a hole. The appearance of such defects may be mistakenly interpreted to indicate that a portion of a cotyledon has been torn out. When there are smooth edges, no surface fragments, and a whitish chorionic plate under and around the area of the defect, nothing has been torn away.

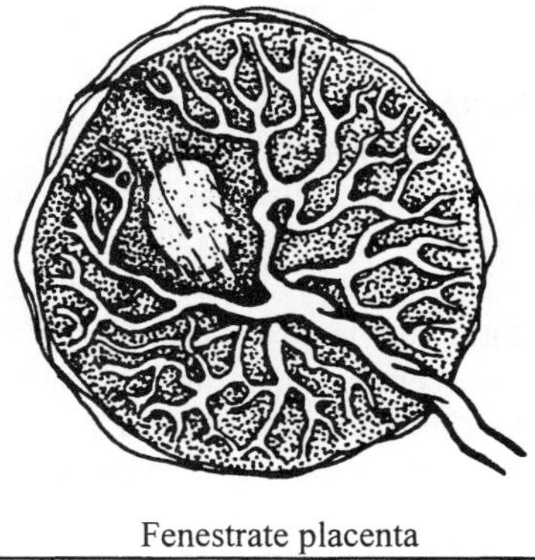

Fenestrate placenta

Capped: This very rare formation results in a cupped or bell-shaped placenta.

Variations and abnormalities of the membranes

The extraplacental membranes are continuous with those that overlie the fetal surface of the placenta; therefore, the abnormal findings below may appear on either the fetal surface, or the extraplacental membranes or on both.

Unusual color: The primary cause of discolored membranes is meconium staining, which can leave them green, yellow, golden or chocolate brown. The fresher the meconium, the more slimy and green it is likely to be. Listeriosis infection and hemolyzed blood can both stain the membranes green as well. Laboratory tests for iron stains can distinguish blood staining from meconium. There is a strong possibility that staining is a by-product of infection or bleeding when the baby is born prior to 34 weeks and has no major malformations.

Meconium staining may seep through the membranes and stain the fetal surface of a placenta that stands at room temperature for many hours via postpartum macrophage transfer. To minimize the development of this artifact, refrigerate the placenta if it is to be examined again at a later time or sent to a lab.

Reduced translucency: Opacity or a whitish appearance of the fetal surface occurs approximately 7.7% of the time. In one-third of these cases it is due to long umbilical cords, excessive fibrin beneath the chorionic plate, and other findings associated with vigorous fetal movements (suggesting that trauma may be the cause). Other cases are associated with preterm and postterm birth, major fetal malformations, fetal growth retardation, stillbirth and neonatal death. Meconium staining of more than 3 hours duration, severe oligohydramnios, and marked edema of the membranes may also reduce translucency. When all the risk factors are considered, an opaque fetal surface is also associated with a 40% higher than usual frequency of long-term motor disorders accompanied by mental retardation and nonfebrile seizure disorders.

Reduced translucency is also associated with infection. Early amnionitis does not lead to any visible changes; however, moderately severe infection leads to tissue infiltration by acute inflammatory cells, resulting in varying degrees of discoloration and opacity of the sac and membranes overlying the placental surface. The entire surface of the membranes or a localized region will appear dull and cloudy with a creamy pale yellow to off-white color. Progressive cloudiness and discoloration eventually leads to opacity and obliteration of the surface anatomy, obscuring visualization of underlying blood vessels on the fetal surface. While chorioamnionitis is associated with infection, it is not invariably so. Note that the suffix "-itis" connotes inflammation with white blood cell activity, which is not always prompted by infection.

Signs of infection: Most intrauterine infections do not produce visible changes in the membranes. However, they may smell foul. Infected membranes may appear gray tan and opaque due to tissue infiltration by acute inflammatory cells. If inflammation is long-standing, the fetal surface is yellow from accumulated leukocyte exudate, and clots may be present in the chorionic vessels (which normally appear as ghosts, containing no blood). Chorionic vessels may also appear to be in various stages of degeneration or calcification, usually without local inflammation. The amnion may be roughened or may have lost its normal luster; both membranes are often friable, edematous and slimy. In rare cases, chorioamnionitis is caused by *Candida albicans*. The membranes, especially those sheathing the umbilical cord, may be studded with pinpoint-sized yellowish white nodules or plaques.

Amnion nodosum: These small, slightly raised plaques or nodules appear on the fetal surface of the amnion, often near the cord insertion point. They may also develop in the extraplacental amnion or on the umbilical cord. They are often perfectly round or oval and slightly three-dimensional, measuring on average 1 to 5 mm across with a shiny surface and greyish yellow coloring. They easily detach from the amnion, leaving a ragged, saucer-like depression. The nodules often cluster to form irregular plaques. Soft, waxy and somewhat granular in texture, they consist of hair, squamous cells and sebum, which are the same materials normally found floating in the amniotic fluid and vernix. They are thought to form due to the close proximity of vernix to regions of amnion. These nodules become covered with new amnion as it regenerates without any tissue reaction or inflammation. A sufficient quantity of vernix must be present for the nodules to form; therefore, they are rarely seen prior to 28 weeks gestation. A single lesion is probably the yolk sac. It can be distinguished because it will not wipe off the membranes.

These nodules are clinically significant because they are most often associated with oligohydramnios. Thus they are often found with babies who have renal agenesis, congenital obstruction of the fetal urinary tract, extramembranous pregnancy or any other condition associated with profound oligohydramnios. However, they can also be found in the membranes of healthy babies.

Cysts: Round, firm, translucent, fluctuant, membrane-covered swellings are commonly found on the fetal side of the placenta. Most are a few millimeters in diameter. However, cysts with diameters up to 8 cm do occur. These are usually insignificant. Occasionally a cyst may contain a blighted ovum.

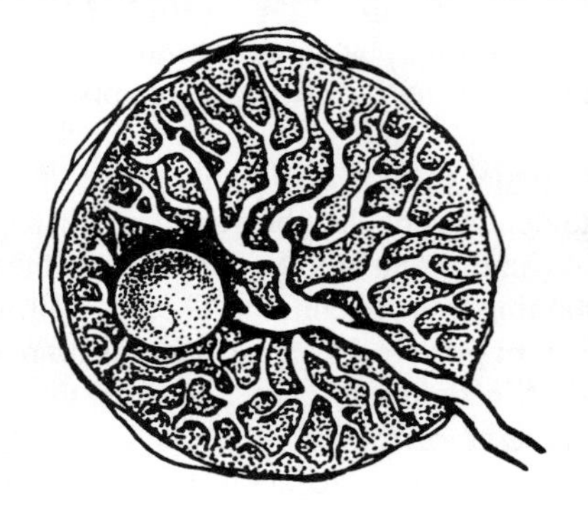
Cyst on fetal surface underlying amnion

Squamous metaplasia: This term is applied to gray or white concentric water-repellent plaques 0.5 to 3 mm in diameter that are generally flat or only slightly elevated. Usually localized near the base of the cord on the fetal surface, these plaques are tightly adherent and cannot be removed without disrupting the underlying amnion. They are seen in 25% to 60% of term placentas and represent focal keratinization of the normal squamous epithelium that makes up the amnion. They are a sign of pregnancy maturation but nothing more. The name is a misnomer, because there is no change in the cell type.

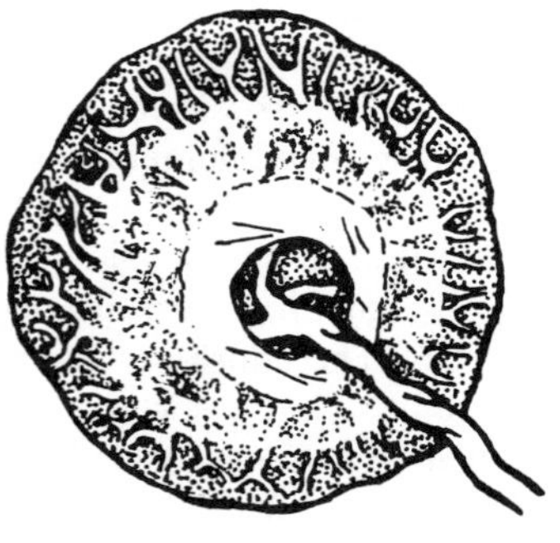
Extramembranous placenta

Discordant size between the baby and the sac: If the sac is very small in relation to the size of the baby, the baby may have developed in a chronically low volume of amniotic fluid. Conversely, an overly large sac may be related to polyhydramnios.

Extramembranous pregnancy is an extremely rare event in which the membranous sac is obviously too small to have contained the baby. The sac wall is rather firm and usually has a thick, rolled edge at the margins of rupture. Amnion nodosum may be present. Typically the membranes ruptured between the 11th and 23rd week of pregnancy, with birth occurring between the 27th and 35th weeks. There is a continuous leakage of fluid from the time of rupture. Many infants die from complications of severe compression, prematurity or infection. These pregnancies are associated with circumvallate placentas. However, it is unknown whether the circumvallate formation causes the membrane rupture to occur.

In an extra-amniotic pregnancy, the amnion ruptures, leaving the baby to develop in the chorion alone. The amnion presents as a small apron-like "cuff" or "collar" around the insertion of the cord or as amniotic strings (see below). Amnion nodosum may also be present in cases of scant amniotic fluid. Although the baby may go to term, this type of pregnancy is often associated with oligohydramnios and early miscarriage.

Subamniotic hematoma: These lesions, appearing as plum-colored swellings that lift the amnion away from the chorionic plate, are formed by collections of free blood trapped between the amnion and chorion on the fetal surface of the placenta. They are usually small and often have a roughly triangular shape. They appear to develop as the result of birth trauma to superficial venous vessels traversing the chorionic plate, usually a result of excessive traction on the cord. Therefore, they have no impact on fetal well-being. Older lesions may be associated with low birthweight.

Amniotic bands and strings: During fetal life, pieces of ruptured amnion may form into wide strips (bands) that may become rolled into strings. The incidence is 1 in 10,000 live births.

There are two main theories addressing the formation of amniotic bands. The first hypothesizes that, early in gestation, a primary abnormality of the limb buds occurs and the "amniotic" bands are, in fact, sloughed off, abnormal, redundant tissue.

The second, more popular theory involves rupture of the amnion in early pregnancy. A thick gel surrounds the amnion and fills the space between the extraplacental membranes prior to the fusion of the amnion and chorion sometime during the 12th to the 17th week of gestation. If the amnion ruptures before fusion takes place, the fetus is believed to escape into the chorionic sac. At this point, the amnion may fragment and shred or roll up into a rope-like structure extending from the base of the cord. In addition, the raw chorion absorbs fluid, resulting in oligohydramnios. As a result, the baby is subjected to undue pressure which can lead to various positional anomalies of the extremities. When the delicate fetal skin rubs against the rough chorion, abrasions occur. The strings may attach to these abrasions, producing fusion anomalies, or strings may encircle a fetal part, leading to stricture or amputation. Even if none of these accidents occur, the band can encircle and constrict the umbilical cord and lead to death. Although the baby does not always become entangled, finding a denuded placenta without fetal involvement is rare. The following table lists fetal defects that have been associated with amniotic band syndrome.

SYSTEM OR REGION AFFECTED	SPECIFIC ANOMALIES NOTED
Limb anomalies	Constriction rings, amputations, fenestrated syndactyly, club feet
Craniofacial anomalies (developmental disruption in these areas may be secondary to the stickiness of these regions in early embryos)	Facial & cranial clefting, encephalocele, anencephaly, cleft lip & palate, microphthalmia, nasal defects
Parietal (walls of body cavity) anomalies	Gastroschisis, thoracic wall defect
Umbilical cord	Strangulation

(Schuler-Maloney & Lee, 1998)

Teratoma: These very rare tumors are always located between the amnion and chorion and usually appear on the fetal surface, although they are sometimes found in the membranes adjacent to the edge of the placenta. They may be smooth, round or oval and measure between 2.5 to 7.5 cm (1 to 3 in) in diameter. Their arterial supply is usually from a branch of a fetal artery on the surface of the placenta. Teratomas frequently contain squamous epithelium, often with skin appendages, together with fat, muscle, mesenchyme, nerve, gastrointestinal tissues, cartilage and disorganized bone. There is no evidence that these legions are malignant, and they are of no clinical significance.

Variations and anomalies of the parenchyma

Unusual thickness: Remarkably thin placentas, with average thicknesses of less than 2 cm (¾ in), are associated with severe prematurity or retarded placental growth due to obstructed circulation. Thick placentas of a depth of 3 cm (1⅛ in) or greater are often very healthy. Babies with hydrops fetalis may also have an unusually thick placenta (Schuler-Maloney & Lee, 1998). Keep in mind that flexibility or lack thereof in an otherwise normal placenta has to do with the amount of fetal blood it contains and not thickness, although a flexible placenta may give the impression of thinness and an engorged placenta may be mistaken for being abnormally thick. (See also the previous part discussing placenta membranacea.)

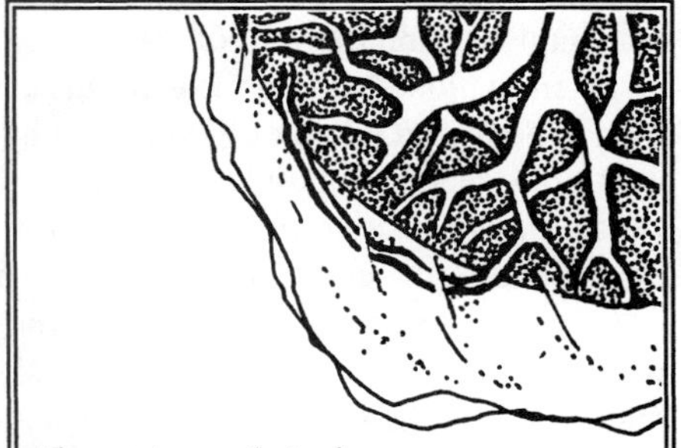

Aberrant vessel at edge (viewed from fetal side)

Aberrant vessels: Most aberrant vessels are tiny, run off the edge of the placenta, traverse the membranes for a short distance and then reenter the placenta. They are typically small and undamaged. While unusual, these vessels are complete and therefore do not indicate that anything is torn or missing. A larger, torn vessel may contain a clot and reveal a source of bleeding in labor.

Abnormal color: Uncommonly pale cotyledons are usually the result of fetal anemia, which may occur with erythroblastosis or fetal bleeding. A syphilitic placenta is typically pale and yellowish gray. A bulky, pale, edematous and heavy placenta is, on rare occasions, associated with fetal cancer. Metastases from maternal melanoma can cause the placenta to be firm with a brownish or grey tinge. Excessively dark areas of the placenta may indicate areas of trauma, where blood has clotted and become darkened. Dark areas may also be adherent clots on the surface or, more rarely, hemangiomas. A pale pink-white, stiff parenchyma may be seen after fetal demise.

Edema: The edematous parenchyma is thick, pale and mushy. It exudes fluid when pressed or squeezed. Edema is associated with maternal heart disease, diabetes, kidney disorders such as nephritis, and fetal disorders such as severe erythroblastosis and cancer. Severe placental edema is usually associated with intrauterine fetal demise.

Objects embedded in the parenchyma: Any object present within the uterus at the time of conception can become surrounded by and thus embedded in the placental tissue. Although much less likely, an object may also become embedded in the cord or membranes. I have heard reports of the obvious, such as an intrauterine contraceptive device, and the not so obvious, such as a tampon that had become lost through the cervix some time prior to conception. Babies have also been born holding an IUD.

Visible lesions on or in the parenchyma: The vast majority of visible parenchymal lesions are of no clinical significance. However, the following information is given to clarify language and dispel myths about the relative importance of various lesions detected during the exam. In addition, it is useful to have accurate information to give parents regarding any unusual features and to be able to reassure them if a finding is benign. Send the placenta in for a pathological workup if you are unsure.

Historically, the term "infarct" has been used indiscriminately to refer to a wide variety of parenchymal lesions that arise from very different causes. This has led to confusion and misclassification. Visible abnormalities of the placenta may be grouped in a variety of ways. Fox (1997) prefers classifying lesions by causative pathology:

- Disturbances of maternal blood flow to or through the placenta
- Disturbances of fetal blood flow to or through the placenta
- Thrombi (blood clots) and hematomas
- Nonvascular lesions

Fox offers the clearest definitions and explanations of various lesions; this text follows his nomenclature.

Lesions due to disturbances of maternal blood flow to or through the placenta

Perivillous fibrin deposition: Some degree of fibrin deposition occurs in the intervillous space in nearly all term placentas and appears as a fine speckling. When deposition is extensive, it is usually located along the periphery of the parenchyma, often filling in the marginal angle where the parenchyma tapers off to meet the membranes. When it occurs nearer the center of the parenchyma, it forms an irregular vertical strip between the maternal and fetal surfaces or a roughly circular or ovoid plaque near the chorionic plate or in the middle of the parenchyma. Although often irregular in outline, the lesion is hard and sharply demarcated from the surrounding normal tissue. The cut surface is usually white but may have a brown or slightly yellow tinge. Although often slightly granular, fibrin deposits may also be smooth and featureless.

Whether such lesions occur within the depths of the placental tissue or beneath the chorion, the way they form is essentially similar. Fibrin deposits result from the clotting of maternal blood within the closed spaces between the placental villi and the wall of the uterus. This clotting is produced by the turbulence, eddies, stasis and thrombosis that result from blood passing through this closed irregular space, as well as from the change in direction and velocity of the blood and the presence of the villi, which act as baffles. The villi are simply bystanders in this process; their inclusion within the plaque is purely accidental. The fibrin cuts off the oxygen to the syncytiotrophoblast of the trapped villi, causing this sensitive tissue to die. Enough oxygen is transferred to the villi themselves to keep them alive, where cytotrophoblastic cells are prompted to proliferate as a result of hypoxia.

In spite of this complex process, most fibrin plaques are of no clinical significance. Fibrin deposition is found in women who generally have good blood flow through the placenta; in fact, a well-expanded blood volume apparently predisposes to the formation of such plaques. Indeed, 20 to 30% of the placenta (possibly more) can be affected, usually without adverse consequences for the fetus. Perivillous plaques are found in 22% of term placentas from normal pregnancies. They are uncommon in premature births, though prolonged pregnancy does not show an increased incidence. They are found infrequently in the placentas of women with diabetes, toxemia or essential hypertension.

The functional reserve of the placental villi can be diminished in women whose blood volume is poorly expanded. When 70 to 80% of the placenta is involved, its normal reserve capacity is lost, resulting in fetal demise. Fetal growth retardation often occurs when the involvement is widespread but not severe.

Subchorionic fibrin plaque: This occurs in 20% of all placentas and seems virtually unaffected by maternal factors. It develops when a layer of maternal fibrin collects in the intervillous space beneath the chorionic plate on the fetal side of the placenta. Fibrin is derived from the clotting of maternal blood within the closed irregular spaces between the placental villi and the uterine wall. This process parallels the formation of perivillous fibrin deposition; the only difference is the absence of included villi in the subchorionic plaques. This may be due to the comparative lack of villi in this layer of the parenchyma, which also accounts for the relative ease with which the forming clots push the villi aside.

The fibrin forms a hard, white, shiny plaque of varying thickness. It is usually a roughly triangular or rectangular lesion with the base of one edge fused to the undersurface of the chorionic plate. The other edges protrude into the body of the parenchyma. It is not unusual to find fresh laminated clots in various stages of being transformed into fibrin where the plaque meets the intervillous space. These plaques are distinct from the surrounding normal tissue.

These lesions are of no clinical significance, and their presence does not interfere with fetal development or growth. In fact, a lack of subchorionic fibrin has been associated with a lack of fetal movement, short cord and an unduly high incidence of neurological handicaps and diminished intelligence (Naeye, 1990).

Massive basal plate fibrin deposition: This term coined by Fox (1997) refers to a phenomenon widely and imprecisely referred to as "maternal floor infarction." It is, in fact, not an infarct at all, because necrosis is not a feature of this lesion. (There is a vast difference between true infarctions and fibrin deposits; see the section on infarctions below.) Studies differ as to its occurrence, although it is rare. Part of the problem in data collection is the imprecise terminology.

The lesion consists of excess fibrin deposited on the basal plate of the intervillous space; as the fibrin deposits increase, basally situated villi become trapped in the enlarging fibrinous mass and undergo the same types of changes that occur in a plaque of perivillous fibrin. In many cases, there is also extensive perivillous fibrin deposition at sites more distant from the basal plate. Basal plate fibrin deposits cause the maternal surface to appear thick, stiff and grayish yellow. Some or all of the surface of the parenchyma may be smooth without distinct fissures between the cotyledons or may have a convoluted appearance that resembles the wrinkles of the brain, with prominent septa between cotyledons. In cross-section, the basal plate appears markedly thickened by firm white material that can reduce the height of the intervillous space considerably. The cord is typically quite long. Additional features related to these lesions include large fibrin deposits on the maternal surface and an increased number of septal and subchorial cysts.

Excessive fibrin deposits may reduce maternal blood flow into the parenchyma, leading to fetal malnutrition and subsequent fetal growth retardation. The lesions tend to recur in subsequent pregnancies and are associated with a 26-fold increase in fetal demise. They are associated with latent herpes simplex type II infection of the endometrium. Although many of these pregnancies end in stillbirth, live birth does occur. The resulting babies are at increased risk for neurological abnormalities due to impaired uteroplacental blood flow.

Although a placenta that has been retained in utero for a time after fetal death accumulates fibrin and becomes firm, basal plate fibrin deposition as described here does not occur with most stillbirths.

Infarcts: A wide variety of names have been assigned to this one type of lesion; however, an infarct is nothing other than a localized area of tissue that has suffered from an interrupted blood supply, become necrotic, and died. Researchers have hotly debated whether the villous blood flow disturbance is fetal or maternal in origin. The most likely culprit is some problem involving obstruction of flow to the uterine vessels underlying the placenta, since the mother's blood carries the oxygen and nutrients that supply the villi. When obstruction first develops, the villi crowd together in the affected area, where they become dilated and congested. Then they start to die, until the region consists of ghost villi with no evidence of maternal blood circulation through the intervillous space. Instead, this space is often filled with a thin layer of fibrin that has leaked from necrotic fetal vessels.

Infarcts are most commonly found around the placental edges rather than its center, but may occur in any part of the parenchymal tissue. They vary in size from small lesions of 4 to 5 mm to large ones that involve most of the villous tissue. They may be ovoid or spherical in shape on the surface. Most often, they are roughly triangular when viewed from the side with the base extending downward toward the basal plate and the point penetrating into the depths of the parenchyma. They may involve the full thickness of the placenta. In rare instances, an infarct is encased entirely within the parenchyma, not touching the basal plate. A fresh infarct is dark red and feels firmer than the surrounding tissue on palpation (which is often the only way to distinguish it at this early stage).

As an infarct ages, it becomes increasingly firm and its color changes successively from brown to yellow and, finally, to white. A 10- to 14-day-old infarct has a firm, brown, slightly waxy, smooth surface when sliced. A long-standing infarct appears white and hard with a smooth or slightly granular surface when sliced. The basal plate underlying the lesion may appear perfectly normal but is more often necrotic as well.

Minor degrees of placental infarction involving less than 5% of the villi are frequently seen in normal pregnancies and are of no clinical significance. However, extensive infarction is associated with an increased risk of fetal hypoxia, intrauterine growth retardation and death. This observation, coupled with the confusion generated by combining different types of lesions under the catch-all term "infarct," has led to the belief that the placenta has little, if any, ability to compensate for insults to the villi.

In fact, in most cases, a similar or greater loss of villi due to entrapment in maternal fibrin is benign (Fox, 1997). The placenta can compensate for the loss of 15 to 20% of its villous tissue as a result of ischemic necrosis (i.e., death of villi due to interrupted blood supply). Greater degrees of infarction indicate extensive thrombosis of maternal vessels below the placenta–a pathological development almost always the result of the blood volume contraction of toxemia and complicated hypertension during pregnancy. Therefore, extensive infarctions are the visibile hallmark of a grossly abnormal vascular tree and severely compromised maternal uteroplacental circulation. These factors are the real cause of the apparent adverse effect of infarctions on fetal growth and well-being, rather than simple destruction of villi. This finding does not deny that infarctions can make a bad situation somewhat worse, but the infarctions per se are not the primary cause of fetal compromise.

Parenchymal lesions related to disturbances of fetal blood flow to or through the placenta

Fetal artery thrombosis: An area of villous avascularity is produced when a clot blocks a fetal villous stem artery. Such clots (thrombi) develop in otherwise normal fetal arteries; there are no obvious factors that predispose to their development. The resulting avascular villi are nonfunctional, although the healthy, well-perfused placenta can easily compensate for this loss, especially since lack of function in a single fetal artery will deprive no more than about 5% of the villi that they supply.

Thrombi appear as sharply delineated regions of pallor; they are roughly triangular within the placental tissue, with the base abutting the basal plate. The normal texture of the cross-sectioned surface of the parenchyma is retained. An area of pallor of this type is fairly easily identified in placental samples that have been fixed in formalin (a laboratory tissue preservative), but is difficult to see in the unfixed placenta. Localized areas of pallor may also result from villous edema, focal villous immaturity or as an artifact of the fixation process. However, in these cases, the pallid area usually lacks the characteristic shape of the lesion resulting from a fetal artery thrombosis.

Approximately 4.5% of placentas from full-term, uncomplicated pregnancies have a fetal artery thrombosis. It occurs in about 10% of placentas of women who have diabetes mellitus. Placentas from stillborn babies show a 14% incidence, commonly with multiple thrombi that often include 40 to 50% or more of the villi. Severe toxemia (HELLP syndrome), protein C deficiency and both maternal as well as fetal coagulation disorders have been associated with this problem.

Thrombi and hematomas of the parenchyma

Massive subchorial thrombosis or hematoma (Breus' mole): This lesion is formed of a fresh-red blood clot measuring more than 1 cm in thickness that separates the chorionic plate from the underlying villous tissue over most of the area the clot occupies. It occurs in about 1 out of every 2000 births. The clot tends to elevate and distort the fetal surface of the placenta by forming bumpy, bulging protuberances but may also form a single, smooth mass. When the placenta is dissected, thick nodular masses can be stripped off the chorionic plate, revealing the underlying villous tissue. Sometimes the clot penetrates deeply through the parenchyma and may reach the basal plate to form a transplacental thrombosis. No villi are incorporated in such lesions.

How these clots form is poorly understood. It was once believed that they were exclusively related to spontaneous abortions. More recently they have been identified in placentas from more advanced pregnancies and those of babies born alive. Since these lesions consist of fresh clots, they may influence when labor begins. It has been suggested that small subchorial hematomas are more common than is generally reported but are often missed on exam. However, small clots are usually the precursors to a plaque of fibrin, not the lesion described here. The two conditions cannot be equated and are readily differentiated; they are almost certainly due to different causes.

Retroplacental blood clot: Acute abruption produces a retroplacental blood clot that may seep into the overlying parenchymal tissue. An abruption that occurs within minutes of birth, however, may leave no evidence on the placenta. An abruption that occurred some hours prior to birth produces an adherent blood clot that may leave evidence of compression in the underlying maternal surface in the form of a smooth indentation. An even older abruption can be identified by a drier, firmer clot that may leave a depression but usually includes infarction of the underlying villi. Associated findings include a long or short umbilical cord, chorioamnionitis, chorioangioma, and separation along the edge of a placenta previa.

Note that a retroplacental hematoma and a clot produced by an abruption are not the same, although both are the result of a degree of placental separation from the uterine wall. Abruption is a dramatic clinical complication that usually leads to birth and often leaves no pathological imprint on the placenta, whereas a retroplacental hematoma rarely gives rise to clinical symptoms and the pregnancy continues, even when the hematoma is quite large.

Retroplacental hematoma: These hematomas lie between the basal plate and the uterine wall. Usually a large hematoma is very obvious and can cover all or most of the maternal surface of the placenta. Smaller ones may be less easy to detect and may measure only 1 to 2 cm (⅜ to ¾ in) across. They are more easily recognized when the placenta is sliced in cross-section, revealing the hematoma bulging up toward the chorionic plate, compressing the overlying parenchyma, which is often infarcted.

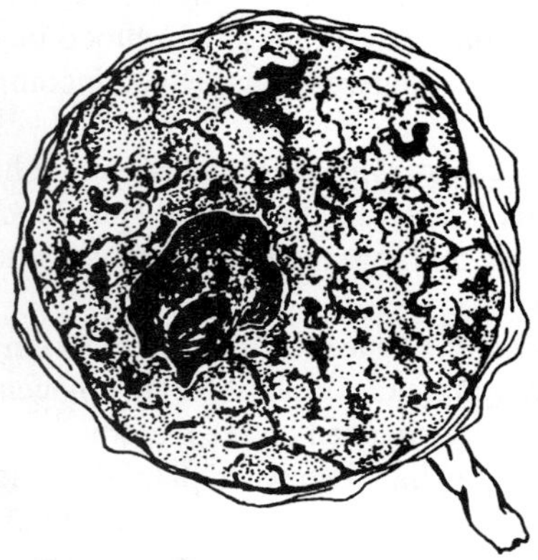

Site of clot formation on maternal side (clot removed)

Fresh hematomas are soft, red and easily separated from the maternal surface. Detachment of the clot may occur during the birth or the handling of the placenta prior to examination. Upon detachment, the clot leaves a crater-like depression in the maternal side. An older hematoma is hard, firmly adherent to the maternal surface and deep wine red to brown in color. It may appear to blend with an infarct that is underneath it, making it difficult to distinguish from the infarct itself. Retroplacental hematomas can be distinguished from simple adherent blood clots such as those produced during normal placental separation because adherent clots are easily stripped from the maternal surface and do not leave an indentation.

Retroplacental hematomas appear in about 4.5% of all placentas, with a 3-fold increase among women with toxemia. Even though retroplacental clots are the primary finding after an abruption, each can exist independently. Women with a clinical history of abruption have an accompanying retroplacental hematoma only about 30% of the time. Conversely, only about 35% of all women with retroplacental hematoma have a history consistent with abruption.

The reasons why hematomas develop are still not clear. It is understood that basal plate necrosis and villous infarction are a result, not a cause, of these lesions. Most researchers believe they develop when a maternal decidual arteriole becomes weakened from toxemia and ruptures; however, they also develop in perfectly normal pregnancies.

The impact of such lesions is largely dependent upon their size. Small lesions do not pose any risks. Large hematomas may result in extensive areas of placental infarction, as they separate a significant portion of the underlying villi from the uterine wall. The pregnancy may continue normally if it is otherwise healthy (since the reserve capacity of the placenta allows for 20-25% of the villi to be nonfunctioning), and the the fetus will suffer only if a huge hematoma develops. These hematomas pose much more risk to the fetus when the pregnancy is complicated by toxemia because the reserve capacity of the placenta is already reduced.

Marginal hematoma (subchorionic hemorrhage): This crescent-shaped blood clot runs along the edge of the maternal side of the placenta and adheres to the maternal side of the membranes. It may also spread out as a thin layer along the edge of the maternal surface of an adjacent cotyledon, where it does not leave an impression when removed. The depth of the clot is roughly triangular when the placenta is sliced in cross-section. One side of the clot typically adheres to the membranes while the other adheres to the edge of the placenta, with the apex adhering to the angle formed where the placenta and membranes meet.

It is not certain how these clots form. The most likely theory postulates that they result from a partial previa. As the uterine muscle works to take up the lower segment in labor and the cervix opens, the margin of the placenta is disrupted and bleeding occurs. While marginal hematomas that develop in the third trimester may result in prenatal bleeding, they are not usually associated with fetal or maternal distress.

Intervillous thrombosis: These villus-free nodular collections of coagulated blood in the intervillous space do not contain platelets, thus they lack the classical characteristics of a blood clot. Usually round or oval, they can occur in any part of the parenchyma. A small percentage are in contact with the basal plate. Occasionally there is only one, although more commonly there are a number of lesions of varying size and age in a single placenta. Their size ranges from 1 to 5 cm in diameter with most measuring 1 to 2 cm across. Fresh thrombi are soft and dark red. As they age, the color changes from brown to yellow to white, the clots become increasingly harder, and the red cells degenerate, progressively laying down fibrin in a linear, streaked pattern. Such streaks appear as fine light lines in or on the thrombi. Eventually a hard, white, sharply delineated, shiny deposit is formed.

Reports on the incidence of these lesions varies widely, from 3 to 50%. Their etiology appears to be related to fetal bleeding into the intervillous space via a rupture within the placenta. These lesions have no effect on placental function or fetal well-being; however, they do mark a site of fetal bleeding into the maternal circulation, which could lead to sensitization if the potential for blood incompatibilities exists. Interestingly, this lesion is accompanied by an increased incidence of maternal-fetal Rh_OD incompatibility.

Kline's hemorrhage: These lesions are hemorrhagic areas in the parenchyma consisting of nodular regions of semifluid or fluid blood within the tissue. The blood flows out when the placenta is sliced open, leaving a sharply delineated cavity. These lesions appear to be very fresh intervillous thrombi and are not really a separate entity.

Nonvascular lesions of the parenchyma

Calcification: Calcification of the placenta is a common occurrence. The deposits appear as small, hard, scattered flecks that are often located on the maternal side of the placenta and may be quite extensive. Sufficient calcifications produce a sandpaper-like texture on palpation and a gritty sensation as the placenta is sliced. The deposits are usually found in the basal plate and in the septa; calcification of the chorionic plate is uncommon. Healthy villous tissue is rarely visibly calcified, but considerable deposits may be present in old infarcts and fibrin plaques.

The incidence of reported placental calcification on gross examination ranges from 14 to 37%. X-ray studies show a range from 75 to 90% due to some deposits found on X-ray not being grossly detectable.

Two types of calcification can occur. Physiological or structural calcification develops as invisible granules during the first six months of pregnancy. Metastatic calcification, with easily visible plaque-like deposits, occurs during the later months of gestation. There is no evidence that the latter develops in dead or degenerate tissue.

Different types of calcium, including physiologic and metastatic as well as calcium en route from mother to baby and found in intracellular fluid, have been found by chemical analyses. Gross calcification is uncommon prior to 36 weeks but increases rapidly as term approaches. An increased incidence has been noted in primigravidas, in the placentas of babies born in the late summer and early autumn, and in those from higher socioeconomic groups. However, neither prolonged pregnancy, toxemia, essential hypertension, maternal diabetes, nor stillbirth are related to an increased amount of calcium deposits in the placenta from prolonged retention of an intrauterine demise. Calcification, in itself, does not represent any compromise to the infant. In my experience, calcification appears to be related to the intake of poorly assimilated calcium supplements or drinking highly mineralized (hard) water. I have also noted excessive granular deposits in the placentas of women who smoke.

Septal cyst: These cysts are round or oval and are sharply delineated from the surrounding tissue, usually measuring 5 to 10 mm across. The cyst wall is formed by a thin, smooth, glistening membrane; the contents are grey and gelatinous. Cysts are usually found below the chorionic plate, and their walls are often directly continuous with an underlying septum. Although they are commonly seen in edematous placentas, the areas where they appear are not edematous. The edema associates them with maternal diabetes or Rh_OD incompatibility. The way these cysts form is unknown. However, holistic medical theory attributes cystic formation to accumulations of toxins in the system. Because these cysts have no apparent affect on the mother or baby, they are considered clinically insignificant.

Placental tumors: A variety of growths and anomalies of development of the placental tissues may occur:

Hemangiomas (chorangioma, chorioangioma, fibroangiomyxoma, fibroma): Large vascular tumors, popularly known as "birthmarks," are the most common nontrophoblastic tumors of the placenta. The documented incidence varies widely, ranging between 1 in 100 to 1 in 9000 to 1 in 50,000. Small tumors, which may not be detectable on visual inspection, have been found in about 1% of all placentas and have no clinical significance. Large tumors (over 5 cm [2 in] in diameter) are associated with increased placental weight and may result from antepartum hemorrhage (either from retroplacental bleeding or directly from the tumor).

These tumors may appear as multiple or (more commonly) single lesions. Large hemangiomas usually appear as bulging protuberances on the fetal side of the placenta. Occasionally, the tumor is encased in membranes and attached by a vascular pedicle. Tumors that are small and contained within the body of the placenta may be invisible. Some, however, occur on the maternal surface, where they may appear to partially or completely replace a cotyledon.

Hemangiomas are composed of blood vessels, loose and immature cellular tissue, calcifications, infarcts, blood clots, occasionally necrosed tissue and, rarely, fat. They vary in size from a few millimeters to over 5 cm (2 in) in diameter and may weight to up to 1500 grams (3 lb 5 oz). Large, external hemangiomas typically have a purplish red, glistening, encapsulated surface. If the vascular component predominates, the inside will be fleshy, dark and congested. When the stromal component (framework of the lesion) predominates, the insides may be stringy. These lesions may be round, ovoid or kidney-shaped, and are frequently bumpy; sometimes they are deeply grooved by bands of fibrous tissue.

Intraplacental tumors are usually smaller, round and demarcated from the surrounding normal villous tissue by a visible capsule. The cut surface of the tumour may be brown, yellow, tan, plum, red or white, and is usually smoother and firmer than normal placental tissue. These small lesions may easily be mistaken for blood clots; however, they lack the characteristic layering that appears as stringy bands of fibrin when a clot is broken up.

Most of these lesions are clinically irrelevant. However, a variety of complications have been seen with tumors measuring more than 5 cm (2 in) in diameter. A high percentage of large lesions have been associated with polyhydramnios and, more rarely, oligohydramnios. Hemangiomas occasionally cause retroplacental bleeding or, due to rupture of the vascular pedicle of a pediculated tumor, fetal hemorrhage. Labor is usually normal. However, a large tumor may obstruct the birth canal. It may also separate and deliver prior to or after the birth of the baby but before the placenta. In other cases, it separates and remains in utero, raising the risk of postpartum bleeding.

Fetal death is slightly more frequent in babies whose placentas have hemangiomas because blood is circulated through the lesions. If the lesions are of sufficient number or size, the shunting of blood through this route results in unoxygenated, nutrient-poor blood being returned to the fetus, leading to growth retardation, distress, or cardiac failure and death. A number of minor fetal malformations, such as cutaneous nevi (a type of birthmark), single umbilical artery, deformed ear or strabismus, may be associated with the placental hemangiomas. Transitory complications may include enlargement of the heart (caused by the extra cardiac load required to pump blood through the additional vascular spaces), edema (which may indicate cardiac failure), low albumin levels, thrombocytopenia (low platelets) or anemia (which may be due to leakage of protein from the vessels of the lesion), blood cell damage (a result of cells passing through the tumor), consumption coagulopathy (triggered by the release of thromboplastic substance from the lesion) or massive, chronic fetomaternal bleeding.

Placental metastasis from maternal cancer: Metastases that migrate from a primary maternal tumor to the placenta are blood-borne. They occur only in women with widely disseminated malignancy. Malignant melanomas, common in young adults and spread by the vascular system, are the most common type of cancer involved. Carcinomas of the breast and bronchus are next, with intestinal and cervical cancers rarely involved. These placentas often show characteristic abnormalities such as tumor deposits, which appear as black or brown nodules of varying size within the parenchyma. Generally, the placenta itself is rather firm and has a brownish or greyish tinge. Placentas containing cancer cells from nonmelanotic lesions often appear normal; however, visible lesions are present in about 25% of these cases, with deposits ranging from the size of a pinhead to as large as 1 to 2 cm (⅜ to ¾ in) in diameter. Placentas suspected to contain such lesions should be refrigerated for microscopic examination. The baby should be examined by a pediatric oncologist if the placenta is found to contain metastases. In very rare cases, malignant melanoma spreads to the fetus.

Placental metastasis of fetal origin: A very rare occurrence, these placental tumors are most often associated with fetal neuroblastoma (cancer of the embryonic nerve cells) and, much more rarely, with hepatoblastoma (liver cancer), leukemia or melanoma. They are characterized by a bulky, pale, edematous, and heavy parenchyma (most weighing over 1000 g). All bear a close resemblance to the hydropic placenta found in severe erythroblastosis. This appearance may be due to mechanical obstruction of the venous return by a large tumor in the baby's abdomen. The cancerous areas of the placenta are only detectable on microscopic examination.

Hydatidiform mole: Many complete molar pregnancies will end in miscarriage well before term. Hydatidiform villi show visible molar changes, appearing as semitranslucent grape-like clusters. The entire placenta or only a portion may develop this way. In a complete mole, there is typically no evidence of normal placental tissue and no membranes are present. An incomplete mole may vary in size from a small, barely visible area to a few centimeters in diameter. It is possible for a pregnancy to continue in the presence of a partial hydatidiform mole.

In a partial mole, vesicles are scattered throughout normal placental tissue. Such placentas tend to retain a basic placental shape and are usually accompanied by normal villi and an identifiable amnion, chorion and cord. Sometimes a fetal remnant will be found or a viable baby may be born.

Placentas that appear to contain molar formations should be saved for microscopic examination. The mother will need to be monitored after the birth to detect persistent trophoblastic disease. For more information, see the chapter entitled "Hydatidiform or Vesicular Mole" in Volume I. An invasive hydatidiform mole occurs when the villi penetrate the uterine wall. This may lead to partial detachment of an otherwise abnormally embedded placenta. The embedded portion will require surgical removal.

Variations and Anomalies of the Cord

Whenever cord anomalies are found or suspected or when the baby has evidence of gastrointestinal or genitourinary tract or multiple anomalies, leave the cord intact or dissect it out of the placenta, leaving it as long as possible. By doing so, you minimize the chance of accidental damage to internal structures that may be displaced inside the cord.

Rare types of cord insertion: There are three variations on cord insertion that may be found.

Velamentous insertion: The cord vessels leave the placenta a variable distance from one another, course between the amnion and chorion and unite to form a normal length of umbilical cord at some distance from the edge of the placenta. The normal cord then inserts at the umbilicus. The branched portion of the vessels is surrounded only by the membranes; without the protective Wharton's jelly, they are left more vulnerable to damage. Velamentous insertion occurs about 1% of the time and is often associated with multiples.

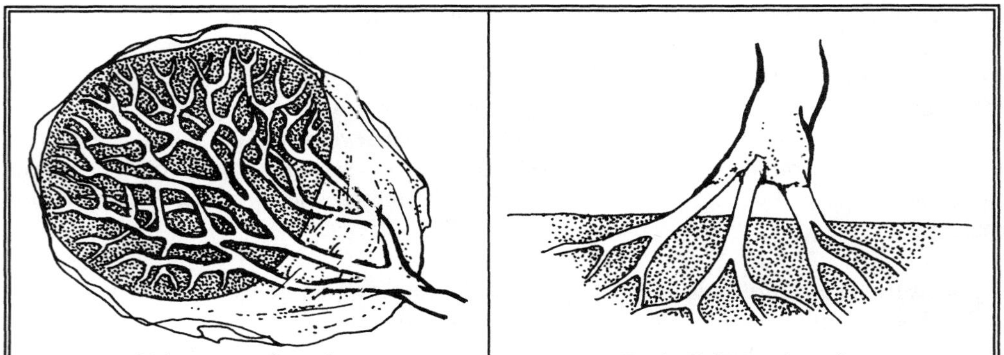

Velamentous insertion | Funiculi furcate insertion

Interposition (interposito velamentosa): This type of velamentous insertion forms exactly as described above but is distinguished by the Wharton's jelly that surrounds each branched portion of vessel. The vessels may traverse the chorionic membrane or the amnion before entering the normal portion of cord. Identifying the membrane into which the cord inserts may be difficult on gross examination.

Furcate insertion (funiculi furcata): Here, the cord is normal for most of its length. However, the vessels lose their protective covering of membranes and Wharton's jelly and then branch before they reach the insertion point on the placental surface. These fully exposed vessels are easily damaged.

Congenital absence of the cord: Complete absence of the cord–also known as "body stalk anomaly"–is rare. Characteristically, it occurs in conjunction with abdominal wall defects in which most of the abdominal organs are contained in a sac that is directly attached to the placenta. The labor would appear obstructed as the baby would not descend. Fetal problems will probably have been detected through careful prenatal exams, with ultrasound identification of this tragic problem during pregnancy. This anomaly is universally fatal.

Abnormal length of the cord: Cord length is related to the degree of fetal mobility. Thus, conditions that restrict mobility are often, although not always, associated with very short cords.

Cords that are 32 cm (12.75 in) or less are considered short. Their incidence is between 0.4 and 0.9%. While most babies with short cords are born healthy, a significant number experience fetal distress and neonatal asphyxia. This distress is generally believed to be the result of excessive traction during descent in labor, which produces tension on the cord vessels and thus a degree of vessel compression. However, this theory has not been proven. Babies with unduly short cords often show mental and motor impairment; this may reflect preexisting impairment, with the short cord the result, rather than the cause, of diminished fetal activity.

Very long cords have been associated with increased knotting, torsion and prolapse accidents. The definition of an abnormally long cord is not precise. Suggested maximum normal lengths are between 80 and 100 cm (31 to 40 in).

Variations in cord thickness and the quantity of Wharton's jelly:

Thick or edematous cord: The thickness of the cord normally depends on the amount of Wharton's jelly present. The quantity of jelly is linked to the amount of water it contains as well as to the amount of amniotic fluid. Edema of the cord exists when its diameter on cross-section is at least 1.3 cm (7/16 in). The edematous cord has a pale, loose, fat, jelly-like structure that is more translucent than normal Wharton's jelly. These characteristics are best evaluated by examining the cut end, but will be obvious in the intact cord as well. All or only a portion of the cord may be thickened or inflamed. Cord edema is present in up to 10% of all babies. Associated clinical findings include prematurity, abruption, Rh_OD isoimmunization, maternal diabetes, toxemia, maternal hypertension, elective surgical birth, abruption, cigarette smoking and macerated stillbirth. There is also a higher incidence with male babies. Infants with thick cords do not seem to suffer increased fetal distress or neonatal asphyxia. These babies are more prone to respiratory distress syndrome and transient respiratory distress due to the associated complications rather than to the edematous cord itself.

When the urachus does not close properly during fetal development, the baby will have a thick, glistening, hydropic and tense cord at birth. When the cord stump falls off, urine will drain from the umbilicus. This very serious problem needs to be distinguished from simple edema of the cord. If the cord stump drains clear fluid or, if clamped, continues to appear swollen during the days before the stump separates, have the baby evaluated.

Thin cord: A lack of Wharton's jelly is usually related to low amniotic fluid volume and makes the cord more prone to prolapse. Thin cords may be associated with fetal growth retardation, cord compression accidents, major fetal malformations, and postmature babies. However, by itself, a thin cord is not associated with any unfavorable outcome.

Absence of periarterial Wharton's jelly: In the medical literature, there have been described three examples in which Wharton's jelly was completely absent around the umbilical cord arteries but was found around the vein. In all three cases, this was associated with perinatal death.

Abnormal number of vessels in the cord: Occasionally, the cord may have only two vessels, an artery and a vein. This finding is associated in about 33% of these babies with a variety of related anomalies that do not seem to fall in any particular category. Many such babies have a low birthweight. Associated placental abnormalities often include circumvallate placentation, velamentous insertion of the cord and low placental weight. All babies with only two cord vessels should be assessed by a pediatrician as soon as possible. Remember that the two umbilical arteries may fuse into a single vessel at their lower end before they insert into the placenta. If the section of cord being examined is 3 cm (1⅛ in) or less from the placental surface, this normal variation may be mistakenly interpreted as a two-vessel defect. Examine the cord in the center and near the baby to confirm the absence of an artery.

The presence of more than three vessels in the cord has received far less attention from researchers, although this anomaly may be more common than too few vessels. Additional arteries or another vein may be present. True extra vessels are most commonly found in sections taken from the central portion of the cord. These may be due to a persistent right umbilical vein, which occurs infrequently in humans. They may also form as a result of the branching of normal vessels, which can be revealed by dissecting the cord longitudinally. In some cases, what looks like additional vessels may be due to vascular looping of an otherwise normal vessel in a false knot. Stillbirths and a history of maternal smoking have been related to an increased number of vessels.

While most studies find no correlation between additional vessels and fetal malformations, Karchmer and colleagues (1966) found four babies that had four vessels out of 40 infants with defects. However, most studies, including that of Karchmer's team, have suffered because the possibility that the extra vessel was an artifact from vascular branching or looping was not eliminated. Even though in most cases the presence of a fourth vessel is found to be insignificant, the possibility of a congenital defect should be followed up with a pediatric evaluation.

Vestigial remnants in the cord: Vestigial remnants are the remains of once functional structures that were required at some point during gestation. Several such remnants may mimic an extra cord vessel.

Vitelline duct: A very small, pinstripe of a vessel on the surface of the cord is a remnant of the vitelline (omphalomesenteric) duct. The vitelline duct connects the embryo to the yolk sac via the cord and gut and atrophies by the 7th to 16th week of gestation. Vitelline remnants may be straight, zig-zagged, or follow the length of the cord in the fashion of a barbershops's pole. They may begin at the baby's end of the cord, only to trail off and disappear after traversing the surface for a variable distance, or they can span the length of the cord. They have no muscular coat and are usually insignificant.

Very rarely, remnants of distended vitelline ducts have been associated with atresia of the small intestines, which may be the cause of abdominal distension. Small bowel may extend for a variable length within a cord that appears perfectly normal, although this is extremely rare. Vitelline cysts may rarely contain intestinal walls as well. These cysts are frequently surrounded by a network of small vessels. They usually develop near the baby's end of the cord and range from 0.4 to 6 cm (3/16 to 1.5 in) in diameter. They can also develop some distance from the baby and still contain intestinal tissue. They are four times more common in male babies. Other types of organ tissue, such as liver and pancreatic, is rarely found in cord lesions such as hemangiomas. (Benirschke & Kaufmann, 2000).

Allantoic duct: The allantoic duct is an early fetal connection to the bladder that usually atrophies by 15 weeks gestation, leaving a microscopic rudiment in the baby called the median umbilical ligament. Sometimes it can be seen between the two arteries as an epithelial cell collection without an opening in the fetal end of the cut cord. This channel may be patent in some babies, presenting with a dilated, tense and swollen umbilical cord which discharges urine when cut. This indicates that the allantoic duct has not closed as it should and the baby should be evaluated.

Cord inflammation (funisitis): Acute cord inflammation may not present any visible signs, although in some cases the cord may be swollen. Chronic inflammation produces necrosis and is indicated by the presence of chalky, yellow-white stripes that follow the spiral course of the cord vessels. If this stripe calcifies, it produces a barber-shop pole appearance. When the cord is cross-sectioned, these stripes look brownish- to creamy-yellow, appearing as rings or crescents around the circumference of the cord vessels. There may also be necrosis in the center of the cord. If calcification is severe, the cord may be so rigid that clamping is difficult. Funisitis is not diagnostic of fetal infection; however, the degree of cord inflammation is related to the degree of chorioamnionitis. Any baby with funisitis should be evaluated for infection.

Wedge-shaped greenish yellow, nodular (hard), granular plaques may be found just beneath the overlying amnion of a cord infected with *Candida albicans*. Most cases of cord candida are not associated with true fetal infection; however, when this occurs, it can be fatal. The infected baby may have a rash or present signs of sepsis. Syphilis is one of the most serious causes of necrotizing funisitis, and these cord findings may be the only obvious sign of infection at the time of birth (Fojaco et al., 1989).

Mechanical phenomena of the cord: A variety of different vascular formations of the cord as well as accidents can take place during intrauterine life.

False knots: Appearing to be knots, these bumpy areas in the cord are actually places where cord vessels have looped back on themselves, creating a lump. They may also be formed by dilated vessels or a lump of Wharton's jelly. Some cords have several false knots along their length. False knots are associated with minimal or absent spiraling of the cord. They have no clinical significance.

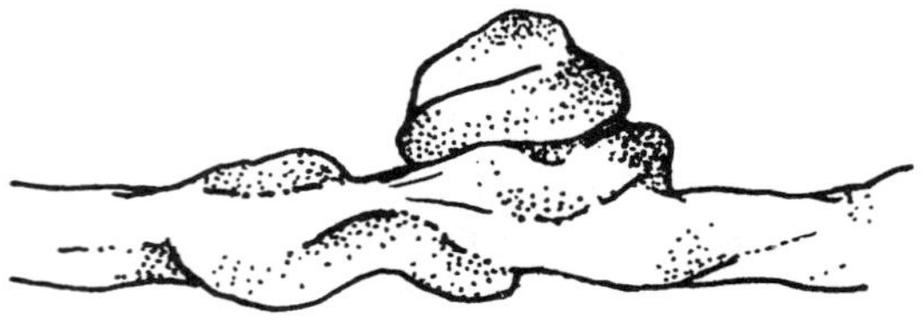

False knot due to looping of umbilical vessels

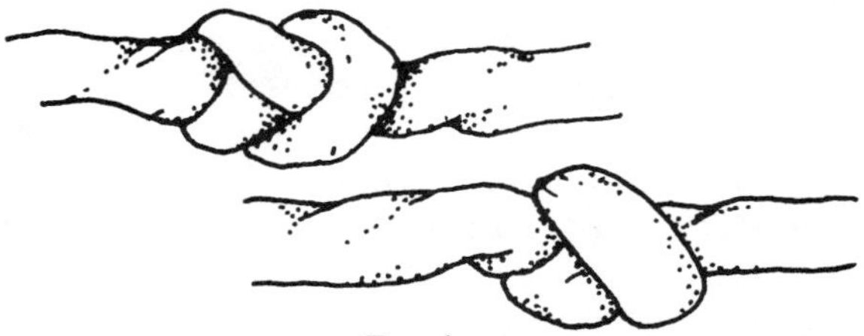

True knots

True knots: Typically, cords that have true knots are longer than average. Reasons for the formation of knots include movements of the young fetus, a ratio of amniotic fluid to fetal size that allows for large movements, and manipulation of the cord during the process of birth that results in knots being formed by removing a loop of cord from around the baby's neck or some other part of the body or by bringing the baby through a loop of cord without removing it. Other predisposing factors include a very vigorous fetus and monoamniotic multiple gestation.

A knot may not be life threatening. In most cases, the knot has been loose throughout gestation; if it hadn't been, the fetus would have shown compromise. However, if fetal descent during labor or fetal movement tightens an existing knot, fetal circulation can be impaired, producing fetal distress and possibly hypovolemia at birth. If circulation is cut off entirely, the baby will die. True knots are associated with a perinatal mortality rate ranging from 8% to 11%. Knots subjected to long-standing tightness can be distinguished by the following characteristics:

- Marked and permanent grooving of the cord at the site of the knot
- Loss of Wharton's jelly and constriction of the umbilical vessels at the site of the knot
- Persistent curling at the site of the knot when it is loosened or untied

Identify the ends of the cord leading to and from the knot prior to cutting the cord. Prepare one cord clamp labeled "placental side" and the another "baby side." Clamp the cord a couple of inches above and below the knot with these clamps (plastic or stainless steel clamps are fine), leaving the knot itself intact. Now, cut the cord above and below the knot, at least l cm (3/8 in) from each clamp, leaving enough of a cord stump on either side so the vessels can be examined. The knot itself should be left intact.

A knot that has compromised fetal circulation is tight with curling and compression grooving of the underlying Wharton's jelly; this will be obvious if you loosen the knot enough to examine its loops. Photograph the knot before exam and after it is loosened. Also examine each cord stump for vessel changes on either side of the knot and on the remaining ends still attached to the baby and the placenta. In long-standing cases, the vessels within the knot are constricted. The vessels on the baby's side are edematous with arterial distention while those on the placental end show venous distention. These changes indicate that blood flow through the knot was impaired. If no such changes are found, the knot was probably not the cause of any fetal distress. Take close-up photographs of the cut ends as they are being examined. Be sure the label on each clamp is visible for the photo. If the cord is to remain intact, transillumination may help to determine if the vessels on one side appear to be enlarged.

A cord with a true knot is often long enough to remain unaffected by changes in fetal position or descent during labor. A knot that has tightened during early labor will not have all the features of a long-standing knot but may also cause intrapartum distress or death, or result in neonatal asphyxia. A knot that has caused such problems will have some evidence of edema, congestion or thrombosis.

Torsion: Torsion or extreme twisting of the cord is very rare. It may occur throughout the entire length of the cord but is, more commonly, a localized feature. Torsion is more commonly associated with multiparity and male infants. Contributing factors may include cord stricture and excessive cord length. The twisted area lacks Wharton's jelly; however, loss of jelly may be a result of the torsion rather than a predisposing factor. Torsion can occur at either end of the cord but is most common near the fetus. Sufficient torsion can result in fetal death but may also develop after a baby has died for other reasons. Torsion that occurred prior to fetal death can be identified because the cord will remain twisted if that portion is cut away from the rest of the cord. Microscopic examination will show congestion, edema and possibly thrombosis at the site of torsion.

Stricture: Stricture of the cord is a very rare phenomenon that presents as a short, well-defined, usually singular narrowing of the cord diameter, most often near the fetal end. The umbilical vessels at the site of stricture may be markedly contracted, usually with a severe, localized deficiency of Wharton's jelly. Torsion often complicates stricture, although stricture precedes torsion and is never caused by it.

Vascular lesions of the umbilical cord:

Aneurysm: An aneurysm is caused by congenital weakness in a blood vessel wall leading to localized dilation of the vessel, usually an artery. Aneurysms of the cord are very rare. Rupture of the weak area will lead to fetal blood loss, hematoma formation or rupture of the cord. Rupture of an aneurysm presents with bleeding within the cord, leaving bloody streaks and possibly swelling, with accompanying red or dark purple discoloration. The baby can continue to lose blood from his circulation into the cord if it is left intact (in the same way that internal injuries allow blood to escape from the vascular system). If increasing swelling of the cord indicates that active bleeding is still occurring, raise the placenta above the baby as far as the length of the cord allows to drain as much blood as possible back toward the baby, then clamp the cord on the baby's side of the lesion to curtail additional blood loss.

Hematoma: A hematoma is a collection of blood beneath the surface of tissue caused by damage to blood vessels secondary to trauma. Iatrogenic cord hematomas may be caused by amniocentesis, umbilical blood sampling, or intrauterine blood transfusion. Weakness of musculature or elastic tissue, varicosed vein, and aneurysm account for some hematomas, although in most cases no obvious cause can be found.

Intrafunicular hematomas occur when the blood clot remains below the surface of the cord and leaks into the Wharton's jelly. This usually occurs at one site, although multiple hematomas have been seen. Hematomas most commonly occur toward or at the fetal end of the cord, and present as a rounded or sausage-shaped swelling that ranges from reddish purple to eggplant in color. Such hematomas vary considerably in size, ranging from 1 cm (3/8 in) in diameter to as thick as a child's arm. They typically span 4 to 40 cm (1.5 to 16 in) along the length of the cord, but can run the full length. Such hematomas are most commonly due to a rupture of an umbilical vein or, much less commonly, an artery. Even more rarely, bleeding is caused by a ruptured hemangioma of the cord.

Sufficient fetal bleeding will lead to death. However, it is not clear if the 40 to 50% rate of fetal demise is due to the hematoma or whether both the hematoma and fetal death result from some other causal factor. Extravascular bleeding of any type is life threatening. It is possible for the fetus to exsanguinate completely when a hematoma ruptures and bleeds into the amniotic sac, remembering that the total blood volume of a fetus amounts to about 16.9 oz in an 8 lb 13 oz baby at term. However, most such bleeding episodes represent minimal blood loss. While there are many theories as to how death may result, in most cases there is no clear relationship between the hematoma and the death.

Thrombosis: This rare finding refers to clots that develop in an undamaged umbilical vessel. It occurs in 1 of every 1290 births and is found during one out of every 938 perinatal autopsies (Heifetz, 1988). Most thrombi are associated with other cord accidents such as compression, torsion, stricture or hematoma. The remaining thrombi are largely associated with obstetrical complications and fetal abnormalities, although in a few cases the cause cannot be determined. Thrombi are usually located in the vein, but clots may form both in the vein and the arteries. While it may appear that fetal demise is the result of the thrombosis, in most cases the clot develops as a secondary complication of another problem. A thrombosis is unlikely to be the only cause of fetal demise in all but a small minority of cases. Some babies do survive vessel thrombosis. Thrombi of the cord are usually not visible unless they are quite large.

Rupture: Rupture of the umbilical vessels refers to tearing or other damage to an umbilical blood vessel that results in the formation of a cord hematoma (see above). Hematomas usually remain contained within the cord; however, sometimes the hematoma causes a rupture through the wall of the cord and bleeds into the amniotic fluid. Vessels within the umbilical cord may rupture at any time during pregnancy or the actual birth. Cord rupture rarely occurs during labor; when it does, it is probably related to a tight torsion of the cord, undue shortness, trauma or inflammation. Most complete ruptures occur immediately after the birth of the child in conjunction with precipitate births, especially those that occur in upright or squatting positions.

Ulceration: Ulceration of the umbilical cord is associated with congenital intestinal abnormalities. The ulcerated cord often hemorrhages severely. Leave this baby's cord unclamped or sever it at the placental base and transport for evaluation as soon as possible.

<u>Tumors of the cord</u>: Fetal death frequently results from the presence of large tumors that obstruct blood flow in the cord. Fortunately, significant tumors of the cord are rare. A few different types of tumors have been identified.

Cysts: There are several kinds of umbilical cord cysts. Vestigial remnants may give rise to cysts from remains of either the allantoic duct or the yolk stalk (omphalomesenteric duct). Cysts may contain smooth muscle and nerve ganglia as well as tiny blood vessels and are usually small and of no importance. However, they can reach the size of a hen's egg, and a cyst of sufficient size can compress umbilical vessels. Cysts derived from foreign material trapped in the amnion are uncommon and usually small.

Pseudocysts may be formed by degenerating Wharton's jelly. These are not true cysts but cavities that result from mucoid degeneration of the jelly.

Hemangioma (angioma): Hemangiomas of the cord are rare, although greater awareness and better examination efforts have resulted in the discovery of a larger number in recent years. They appear as rounded, ovoid swellings usually ranging from 3 to 17 cm (1.25 to 6.75 in) diameter, but in very rare cases may span the entire length of the cord. The clinical significance of this phenomenon is not well defined. In many cases, the fetus dies in utero. However, because it is highly possible that a lack of thorough examination has resulted in an underreporting of cord hemangiomas, there may be a higher incidence of harmless lesions of this type than is generally recognized.

Teratoma: Teratomas are always derived from germ cells originating from the yolk sac and contain tissues and features that are recognizable parts of the body such as hair follicles, epithelium of various kinds, glands of various kinds, fat, muscle, cartilage and bone. Teratomas of the cord are exceedingly rare and are typically benign.

Metastasis of fetal cancer to the cord: This is also a rare condition that usually does not produce a lesion that is detectable on visual inspection.

Examining the Placenta of a Singleton Baby That Has Died

After a baby dies, the placenta is still a functioning, viable organ that goes through a predictable series of progressive morphological changes. This is because the condition of the placenta is largely dependent upon maternal circulation and not upon that contributed by the fetus. Most of the changes that occur are only detectable in the laboratory and have to do with villous morphology. Death of the fetus results in cessation of the fetal circulation, leading to changes as the villi shut down and maternal blood flow to the placenta diminishes, although not enough to impair continued viability of the villi. Blood stagnates in the villi and edema develops. Infarcts may be obvious on gross examination, often involving more than 10% of the parenchyma. The membranes may thicken and become mineralized in as few as five days after death. Gross abnormalities of placental shape are seen in 12% of fetal deaths. It is much more common to find a velamentous or marginal cord insertion and seven times more common to find only one artery in the cord. Other findings associated with fetal morbidity and mortality are noted throughout this chapter. The examination of these placentas is of limited value. If from a fresh stillborn (less than 48 hours from demise) they are essentially like that of a live-born infant; after that, progressive changes can be detected that are the natural consequence of a cessation of circulation. Past 14 days, however, histological examination of the placenta is largely useless as a means of determining the timing of the death. The problem with normal postmortem placental changes is that they may be mistakenly thought to have been present and a contributing factor at the time of death.

Examining Placentas from a Multiple Gestation

Any of the above features may be present in the placentas from a multiple gestation. The primary additional features to consider pertain to the type of twinning that occurred and to whether vascular anastomoses run between the placentas.

Types of twin placentas

In general, twinning occurs as either monozygotic (derived from one ovum and one sperm) or dizygotic (derived from two ova and two sperm). However, there are many permutations of these two basic forms of twinning that have been discovered with the advent of assisted reproduction. These nuances are explained in a recent edition of Volume I of this text, in the chapter entitled "Multiple Gestation." Pertinent to this discussion is that, while it is usually the case that unlike-sex twins are dizygotic, it is possible for them to occur due to a variant form of monozygotic conception. Thus, sex and membrane configuration allow tentative assignment of zygosity only about 50% of the time. When more babies are involved, they may be of mixed monozygotic and dizygotic origins. The only definitive way to confirm the type of twinning is to perform genetic studies on all the babies.

Dizygotic placentas: Dizygotic twins occur when two eggs are fertilized by two sperm and are no more genetically similar than any two siblings. In most cases, two entirely separate placentas form, each with its own chorion and amnion (making them dichorionic and diamniotic), which may implant in separate locations on the uterine wall or so closely together that they fuse along one edge.

Monozygotic placentas: The structure of monozygotic placentas varies depending upon when a single fertilized ovum divides to create two babies. It is believed that two separate embryos, each with its own placenta, chorionic and amniotic sac identical to those seen in dizygotic twins, will develop if the single fertilized ovum divides during the first three days after fertilization, i.e. before the trophoblast differentiates. About 20 to 40% of monozygotic twins have a single dichorionic placenta. Most twins with a single chorion (monochorionic) placenta are monozygotic. However, it is important to recognize that the presence of two chorions does not exclude monozygosity and that a single chorion does not necessarily rule out dizygotic conception.

Examining the placental disks
Number of basal plates: The placentas may present as one large disk or two. If there are more than two babies, some placentas may be fused while others remain separate. Fusion or separation alone does not confirm the type of zygosity.

Separate disks: When there are two separate disks, each placenta will have two chorions and two amnions. However, the zygosity of unlike-sex twins cannot be determined by this finding alone. Examine each disk as for a singleton birth. What is certain about these babies is that there was no twin-to-twin transfusion because there was no vascular communication between the placentas.

Fused disks: Fusion of the disks calls for careful examination of the membrane layers to distinguish the number and types of membranes. Estimate and record the percentage of the whole disk occupied by each placenta. Finding a vascular equator, the central region of the line of fusion on the fetal surface that is devoid of blood vessels, reflects that dizygotic twins have separate circulations. Fusion may make it difficult to identify two chorions on visual inspection alone. You may want to save the placentas for microscopic analysis.

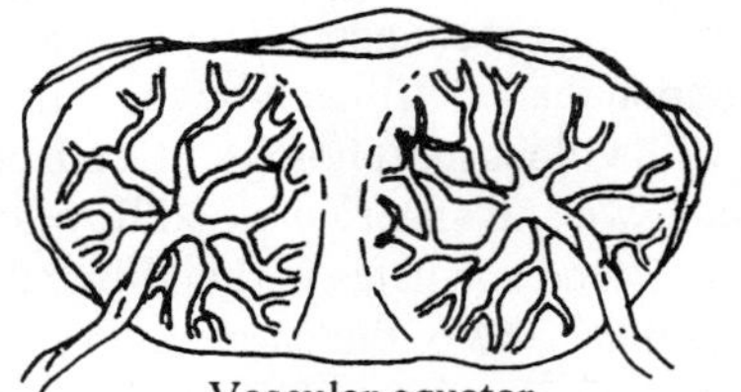

(after Schuler-Maloney & Lee, 1998)

Weight: The weight of each placenta offers information about fetal growth. When the disks are separate, the weight of each baby should be compared with that of their respective placenta. Fused disks usually weigh less than the total weight of separate disk placentas from similarly sized babies.

Shape: An unusually shaped disk may occur due to uterine structural abnormalities, the presence of a fibroid or the way the placenta implanted (e.g., previa).

Color and thickness: Note the color and thickness of each disk. Are they roughly the same color or is one disk much darker red than the other? Is there a significant difference in the thickness of one disk compared to the other? Disparity of coloration or thickness suggests twin-to-twin transfusion syndrome.

A portion of the parenchyma that is whitish with a firm texture may be an impression left by a fetus papyraceus retained in utero or you may discover a small, shriveled-up, leathery fetus adherent to the fetal surface.

Examining the membranes
There are four different types of placentation that can occur in multiple gestations. Since the membrane configuration is not definitive proof of zygosity, the terms for the number of membranes, such as "monochorionic," should not be used interchangeably with terms denoting zygosity.

Formation and fusion of membranes: The membranes may present in several different configurations.
Two chorions/two amnions (dichorionic-diamniotic): Two separate placental disks with two complete sets of membranes are usually associated with a dizygotic gestation. These placentas may be fused along one border or entirely separate. An intermediate form of twinning between dizygotic and monozygotic may occur, in which placentation is the same as for purely dizygotic twins. (For more information about this phenomenon see a recent edition of Volume I.)

One chorion/two amnions (monochorionic-diamniotic): A single placenta with two amniotic sacs and one chorion develops if splitting occurs at the blastocyst stage (between the third and eighth days after fertilization), when the trophoblast but not the amniotic cavity has differentiated. The babies are usually monozygotic (identical).

One chorion/one amnion (monochorionic-monoamniotic): It is thought by some that only one placenta and one amniotic sac will develop if the ovum splits after the amniotic cavity differentiates, which happens between the 8th and 13th days after fertilization. Others believe that two amnions form even then, but sometimes the septum breaks down and disappears, leaving the babies in one amniotic sac. However the phenomenon occurs, monoamniotic babies are at risk for cord and limb entanglement. The occurrence of either may make descent and birth difficult or impossible for one or both babies and may seriously jeopardize blood flow in one or both.

Splitting that occurs at or after the 13th day of development results in conjoined twins. These babies are contained in one large amnion surrounded by one large chorion. The most minimal type of conjoining is found when their two umbilical cords fuse into one before inserting into the placenta.

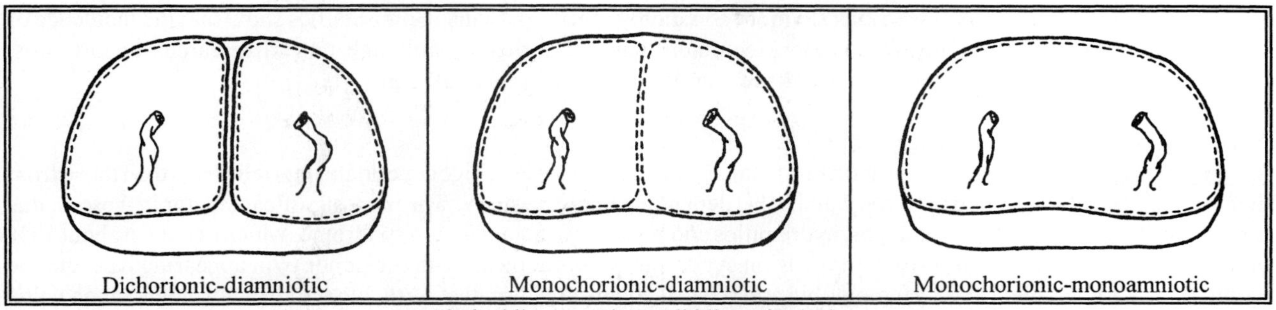

(dashed line =amnion; solid line=chorion)

Examining the membranous septum in fused placentas: The septum is the wall of membranes formed when the edges of the parenchymas are fused. When a septum is present, examining it is the best way to identify the number and types of bags present. Determining whether you have two chorions and two amnions, one chorion and two amnions, or one chorion and one amnion can be tricky, although sometimes it is quite obvious. To avoid confusion, remember that the extraplacental membranes arising from the periphery of the placental disc will always have both a chorion and an amnion. The difficulty arises when trying to distinguish the number of layers along the line of fusion.

To determine the number of amnions and chorions present, place the placentas with the maternal side down. Blot off or gently rinse any blood from the entire surface of both sides of the fused membranes. Hold the membranous septum vertically (like two ends of a sheet) and inspect it for remnants of blood vessels or chorionic tissue. Look for a place along the upper edge of the septum that appears as though it may be easily divided. Now gently peel the membranes apart. Next is a list of your likely findings:

- What appear to be three membranes, with two translucent sheets that can be peeled from either side of a centrally located, thicker sheet (Fig. A), is most likely two amnions on either side of a tightly fused pair of chorions. There will be a raised ridge of fibrin along the line where the dividing membrane inserts onto the chorionic plate. If two chorions are found, perform the remainder of the exam as for two separate placentas.
- A septum that is thick and relatively opaque, consisting of membranes that cannot easily be teased apart, is probably also from a dichorionic-diamniotic placenta.
- A thin, translucent septum that can be easily separated into two identifiable layers of amnion with no chorion in between (Fig. B). These amnions do not "insert" into the chorionic plate; therefore, the fused membranes can easily become detached from the fetal surface and move around, often resulting in a line of fusion that does not overlie the vascular equator of the placenta. Diamniotic-monochorionic membranes are usually derived from a monozygotic gestation.
- The complete absence of a septum indicates that there is only one amnion. In this case, one placenta and one set of membranes enclosed two babies. To be certain, carefully examine the fetal surface for fragments of membranes, which suggests that a double-layer septum was present but has been torn away.

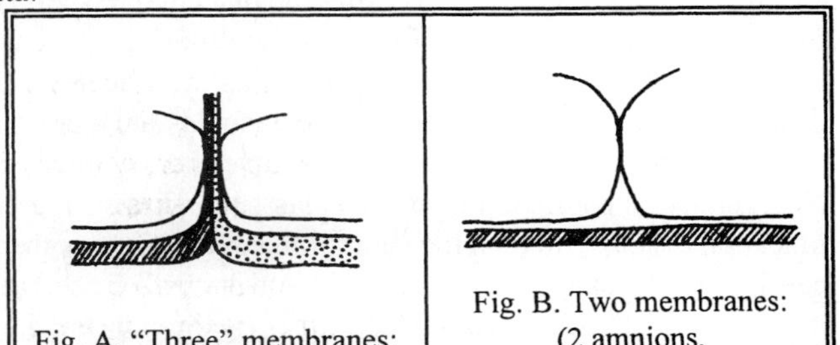
Fig. A. "Three" membranes: (2 amnions, 2 fused chorions)

Fig. B. Two membranes: (2 amnions, 1 underlying chorion)

(adapted from Schuler-Maloney & Lee, 1998)

If division of the membranes proves difficult, do not tear up the entire septum trying to separate them. To avoid damaging placental structures that may offer useful information, leave the membranes as intact as possible, perform the rest of the gross examination, and then take the placenta to a lab for definitive analysis.

The placement of the holes in the bags can provide clues as to how the babies were positioned during pregnancy.

If the babies were situated side by side, each forewater should have an escape hole. If the babies were situated one above the other, the second baby had to pass through the membranous division between the amniotic cavities on its way out. The hole in the bag for the second twin will be located in the septum that separated one amniotic cavity from the other.

Cord variations

Marginal and velamentous insertions are more commonly seen with twins. Some studies show that the incidence of a single umbilical artery in one twin is more common than in singletons, although not all research supports this. However, it is prudent to be certain that you have identified three vessels in all cords.

Notes on types of multiple placentation

Monochorionic-diamniotic: Twins with this form of placentation suffer a higher perinatal mortality rate than those from dichorionic placentas, ranging between 7 and 25%, depending upon the study. The most significant factor in these deaths is prematurity, often associated with polyhydramnios and twin-to-twin transfusion syndrome, which occurs in about 15% of all such twins. Acute twin-to-twin transfusion syndrome occurs at birth, with the donor twin appearing pale and the recipient twin ruddy (plethoric). Hemoglobin and red cell counts are normal at birth, but within a few hours blood value abnormalities become apparent in each baby. Chronic twin-to-twin transfusion syndrome represents a long-standing circulatory imbalance with a slow transfusion from one twin to the other. Classically described signs include an excess of fluid in the sac of the recipient twin and a lack of fluid in the sac of the donor; one twin is smaller, pale and anemic, while the other is ruddy and polycythemic, often with an enlarged heart. With deep artery to vein anastomosis, the donor placenta may display amnion nodosum, a pale parenchyma with small chorionic vessels and a thin cord. The recipient placenta shows a dark congested parenchyma with engorged chorionic vessels and an edematous cord. Hemoglobin and birthweight discrepancies are not as common as the other signs, thus polyhydramnios, edema and cardiac hypertrophy in the recipient twin and oligohydramnios in the donor twin are considered defining clinical signs of this syndrome.

An attempt should be made to determine whether vascular communication exists in any monochorionic-diamniotic placenta. This becomes especially important when the following situations are present: if, after gross and microscopic exam, the type of placentation is still in doubt, if there is evidence of twin-to-twin transfusion syndrome, if there is an abnormality in a surviving twin following death of one infant in utero, and if one twin dies for no obvious reason.

If the placentas are found to be monochorionic, look for anastomoses between the two disks. Generally, the further apart the cord insertions are, the smaller will be the anastomotic channels. Detecting vascular anastomoses, or communicating circulatory systems, may or may not be possible from a visual inspection alone. Large vessels that form links between cord insertion points are often visible on the fetal surface. These usually represent direct arterial connections between a chorionic artery of one baby and a chorionic artery of the other. Less often, superficial vessels communicate from vein to vein; a few placentas will show both types. There are more potential problems when anastomoses are present deep within the placental tissue. They can occur in shared lobules that are supplied by an artery of one twin that drains into a vein of the other via the capillaries. There are often multiple shared lobules; these are usually situated along the margin separating the placentas. These communicating vessels may or may not run in the same direction. Most monochorionic twin placentas have both deep and superficial anastomoses.

Anastomoses are identified in the lab either by injecting a radiopaque dye and tracing the communications with an X-ray study, or by injecting colored plastic into a vessel, preparing a corrosion specimen (which removes the surrounding placental tissue), and then looking for the plastic in the other side of a fused placenta. At home, milk, air or colored saline can be injected into a surface vessel and its path traced across the disk; the type of vessel may be identified because arteries almost always cross over veins. Again, don't make a complete mess of the vessels trying to inject solutions into them at home. The unfortunate reality is that none of these methods is very accurate. Since it is impossible to tell whether and to what extent communicating vessels may be present from a visual inspection alone, it is important to save all placentas from multiple gestations in the refrigerator in the event that laboratory inspection is warranted.

Monochorionic-monoamniotic: This type of placentation is related to a higher rate of mortality than any other because the babies are in a single bag. The cords may become entangled around the babies or they may twist and knot with each other. If one twin is entangled in the cord of the other, it may be impossible to tell whose cord is whose. Thus cutting the cord to facilitate the birth of the first may jeopardize the other twin. Surprisingly, twin-to-twin transfusion syndrome is not a significant cause of problems with this type of placentation, although vascular communications frequently occur.

Dichorionic-diamniotic: These should be considered the same as placentas of any siblings in most respects. Death among babies with this type of placentation is rarely placenta related. Very occasionally, such placentas may have vascular anastomoses, but twin-to-twin transfusion syndrome has not been shown to occur in these cases.

One unusual feature of some of these placentas is the phenomenon of irregular chorionic fusion. The chorions do not meet over the line of fusion between the two parenchymas. Instead, the path of membranous fusion may run diagonally from one placental surface over to the other across the line of placental fusion. This may occur even if the placentas are not fused, and a portion of one disk may be covered by the chorion of the other. This is theorized to occur as the fluid pressure of one sac expands, pushing the other away, resulting in the lifting of the edge of the chorion, similar to that which happens in circumvallate placentation. It has no clinical significance, and no vascular fusion occurs in the areas of chorionic overlap (Benirschke & Kaufmann, 2000).

Evidence of multiple gestation that did not reach term (i.e., death of one twin)

A phenomenon has been discovered via serial ultrasound exams in which a twin is noted at an early point in gestation and is found to have "vanished" in subsequent scans. Such a baby may disappear completely, leaving no detectable trace by the time of birth. Sometimes genetic evidence confirms that a second baby was present, as when both 46, XX and 46, XY cell lines are found in what appears to be a singleton placenta. Other evidence of the vanished twin may include a collapsed gestational sac, which appears as a plaque-like thickening within the membranes of the surviving twin's sac. Embryonic tissue may also be present and, with careful inspection, may be visible as small nodules or foci of thickening.

A consequence of vascular anastomoses is that the death of one twin may be associated with brain or organ lesions in the other (see the chapter entitled "Assisting at Multiple Births" for further details). These types of abnormalities are uncommon when the fetus dies very early gestation. If death occurs around 16 to 20 weeks, the development of a fetus papyraceus is the most likely outcome. The dead fetus becomes flattened and takes on a shriveled, mummified appearance. Fetus papyraceus is associated with anatomical defects such as intestinal atresia in the surviving twin. In these cases, the transfer of thromboplastic material or emboli through vascular anastomoses appears the most likely cause.

An acardiac fetus is believed to be the result of twin-to-twin transfusion syndrome; it only occurs in 1% of all monozygotic multiple gestations. These extremely abnormal fetuses vary considerably in their appearance and the degree to which their organs develop, ranging from a large, grossly anomalous fetus to a soft, amorphous mass. It is believed that a vascular malfunction in the placenta causes the abnormal twin to lack an individual placental circulation and yet have an arterial system that communicates with branches of the umbilical artery of the normal twin. The abnormal fetus has a reversed circulation, thus receiving unoxygenated blood that has already perfused the normal twin. This situation leads to altered cardiovascular development and secondary anomalies in other organs. Fetus acardius is therefore regarded as a form of conjoined twin in which the conjunction is via the chorionic circulation. The normal twin, who has to pump blood to the abnormal baby, may develop cardiomegaly and high-output cardiac failure as a result.

The discovery of evidence of another baby who did not survive will be a blow to the parents, who are likely to enter a state of grief for the loss of this baby; this is particularly true of the mother. The baby has also lost a sibling, and the emotional impact of this should be acknowledged by talking to the baby about the experience in the days following birth.

Placentation in higher-order multiples

Follow the same principles already outlined for twins when examining fused disks and their dividing membranes in the placentas of triplets, quadruplets and other multiple gestations. Examine each physically separate disk as you would any singleton placenta.

Photographing Unusual Placentas

You may wish to take pictures of unusual placentas or specific placental features for the medical record as well as for educational purposes. First, blot the placenta and membranes dry with a cloth towel or gauze which will not leave behind fragments of lint. If the features of interest do not include blood clots or other removable lesions, you might even wash the placenta with clear, slowly running water. Then, arrange it on a flat, white surface. If you want to record membrane opacity, hold up a portion of the membranes to allow light to shine through, then backlight the membranes using a flashlight or table lamp. Place two rulers at right angles along the placenta's edges, to aid in establishing the dimensions of your findings. When photographing a specific feature close up, place a ruler next to the feature and line the ruler up with the feature's longest diameter. Place another ruler at right angles to the end of the first to clarify your photo. Photograph both sides of the placenta.

REFERENCES AND FURTHER READING ON THE BIRTH AND EXAMINATION OF THE CORD AND PLACENTA

PLACENTA-TO-NEWBORN TRANSFUSION, PHYSIOLOGIC CLOSURE OF THE UMBILICAL VESSELS AND SEVERANCE OF THE CORD

Allmeling A, Haselhorst G. "Die Gewichtszunahme von neugeborenen infolge postnataler Transfusion," Z GEBURTSHILFE GENAEKOL, 98;103-104, 1930.

ACOG. UMBILICAL ARTERY BLOOD ACID-BASE ANALYSIS. ACOG Educational Bulletin No. 216, Washington DC, 1995.

ACOG. Withdrawal of Practice Bulletin No. 216, AM J OBSTET GYNECOL, 186(2);361, Feb, 2002.

Atlee HB. THE GIST OF OBSTETRICS. Charles C Thomas, Springfield IL, 1957.

Benirschke K, E-mail communication, 2002.

Benirschke K, Kaufmann P. PATHOLOGY OF THE HUMAN PLACENTA, 4th ed. Springer-Verlag, New York NY, 2000.

Born G, et al. "Changes in the heart and lungs at birth," SYMP QUANT BIOL, 19;102-108, 1954.

Buckels L, Usher R. "Cardiopulmonary effects of placental transfusion," J PEDIATR, 67;339-347, 1965.

Colozzi A. "Clamping of the umbilical cord: its effect on placental transfusion," NEJM, 250(15);629-632, Apr 15, 1954.

Darwin E. ZOONOMIA, 3rd ed. Vol. 3. I Johnson, London UK, 1801, p. 302.

DeMarsh G, et al. "The effect of depriving the infant of its placental blood," JAMA, 116;2568-2573, June 7, 1941.

Dunn P. "The placental venous pressure during and after the third stage of labour following early cord ligation," J OBSTET GYNAECOL BR COMMONW, 73(5);747-756, Oct, 1966.

Dunn P. "Alterations in the distribution of blood between the fetus (and infant) and placenta during and after birth," Presentation Canadian Pediatric Society, Centennial Commonwealth Meeting, Toronto, CANADA, Sept 3-9, 1967.

Dunn P. E-mail communication, recd. Oct 7, 2002.

Fletcher MA. PHYSICAL DIAGNOSIS IN NEONATOLOGY. Lippincott-Raven, New York NY, 1998.

Gilhooley J. Neonatologist. E-mail communication, 2001.

Gunther M. "The transfer of blood between baby and placenta in the minutes after birth," LANCET, 272(6982);1277-1280, June 22, 1957.

Haselhorst G. "Uber Art und Dauer der Blutstromung in den Nabelschmurgefassen post partum." Z GEBURTSHILFE GYNAEKOL, 96;487-499, 1929.

Jäykkä S. "Capillary erection and lung expansion," ACTA PÆDIATRICA, 46(S112);1-91, Jan, 1957.

Jäykkä S. "Capillary erection and the structural appearance of fetal and neonatal lungs," ACTA PÆDIATRICA, 47(5);484-500, Sept, 1958.

Jones J, et al. "Total circulating red cells versus haematocrit as the primary descriptor of oxygen transport by the blood," BR J HAEMATOL, 76(2);288-294, Oct, 1990.

Landau D. "Hyaline membrane formation in the newborn: hematogenic shock as a possible etiologic factor," MISSOURI MED, 50(3);183-185, Mar, 1953.

Lind J, et al. Film: ROENTGENCINEMATOGRAPHIC STUDIES ON THE AERATION OF THE LUNG AT BIRTH. Second Scandinavian Summer Meeting of Biochemistry, Medical Chemistry, Pharmacology and Physiology, Turku, Finland, Aug 27-29, 1959. Cited in Peltonen T. "Placental transfusion–advantage and disadvantage," EUR J PEDIATR, 137(2);141-146, Oct, 1981.

Linderkamp O. "Placental transfusion: determinants and effects," CLIN PERINATOL, 9(3);559-592, Oct, 1982.

McCausland A, et al. "Management of cord and placental blood and its effect upon the newborn, Part 1" CALIF MED, 71(3);190-196, Sept, 1949.

Mercer J. "Current best evidence: review of the literature on umbilical cord clamping," J MIDWIF WOMEN'S HEALTH, 46(6);402-414, Nov-Dec, 2001.

Mercer J, Skovgaard R. "Neonatal transitional physiology: a new paradigm," J PERINAT NEONAT NURS, 15(4);56-75, Mar, 2002.

Morley G. "Cord closure: can hasty clamping injure the newborn?" OBG MANAGEMENT, pp. 29-36, July, 1998.

Morley G. "How the cord clamp injures your baby's brain," www.cordclamping.com, Feb 26, 2002a.

Morley G. "Erasmus Darwin: the physiology and iatrogenic pathology of the third stage of labor," www.cordclamping.com, Feb 26, 2002b.

Morley G. "To clamp or not to clamp, this is the answer," www.cordclamping.com, March 8, 2002c.

Morley G. "Why do babies cry? The anatomical and physiological changes during the moments after birth," www.corclamping.com, April 11, 2002d.

Morley G. Multiple e-mail communications during 2002e.

Morley G. Multiple e-mail communications during Nov 2003.

Morris J, et al. "Measurement of fetoplacental blood volume in the human previable fetus," AM J OBSTET GYNECOL, 118(7);927-934, Apr 1, 1974.

Moss A, Monset-Conchard M. "Placental transfusion: early versus late clamping of the umbilical cord," PEDIATR, 40(1);109-126, July, 1967.

Murray N, Roberts I. "Neonatal transfusion practice," ARCH DIS CHILD FETAL NEONATAL ED, 89;F101-107, 2004.

Nelson C, CNM. "Intrauterine and intact cord resuscitation," workshop tapes, MAWS conf., Oct 22, 1999.

Oh W, et al. "The effects of placental transfusion on respiratory mechanics of normal term newborn infants," PEDIATR, 40(1);6-12, 1967.

Oh W, Lind J. "Body temperature of the newborn infant in relation to placental transfusion," ACTA PAEDIATR SCAND, 172-S;137-145, 1967.

Peltonen T. "Placental transfusion–advantage and disadvantage," EUR J PEDIATR, 137(2);141-146, Oct, 1981.

Rachana S. LOTUS BIRTH. Greemwood Press, Steels Creek Australia, 2000.

Reynolds S. "The umbilical cord," SCI AM, 187(1);70-74, July, 1952.

Reynolds S. "Mechanisms of placentofetal blood flow," OBSTET GYNECOL 51(2);245-249, Feb, 1978a.

Reynolds, S. Chapter 4: "The physical forces of blood flow in the umbilical vein," in Longo L, Reneau D, eds. FETAL AND NEWBORN CARDIOVASCULAR PHYSIOLOGY, VOL 2: FETAL AND NEWBORN CIRCULATION, proceedings of Am Phyiolog Soc, Aug 11-14, 1976. Garland STPM Press, New York NY, 1978b.

Saigal S, et al. "Placental transfusion and hyperbilirubinemia in the premature," PEDIATR, 49(3);406-419, Mar, 1972.

Saigal S, Usher R. "Symptomatic neonatal plethora," BIOL NEONATE, 32(1-2);62-72, 1977.

Siddall R, et al. "Effect on cesarean section babies of stripping or milking of the umbilical cords," AM J OBSTET GYNECOL, 63(5);1059-1064, May, 1952.

Siddall R, Richardson R. "Milking or stripping the umbilical cord," OBSTET GYNECOL, 1(2);230-233, Feb, 1953.

Smith C. THE PHYSIOLOGY OF THE NEWBORN INFANT, 2nd ed. Charles C Thomas, Springfield IL, 1951.

Sneeden V. Unpublished study cited in Osgood E. "Development and growth of hematopoietic tissues; with a clinically practical method of growth analysis," PEDIATR, 15(6);733-751, June, 1955.

Society of Obstetricians and Gynecologists of Canada. Policy statement No. 89. May, 2000.

Stembera Z, et al. "Umbilical blood flow in healthy newborn infants during the first minutes after birth,"AM J OBSTET GYNECOL, 91;568-574, Feb 15, 1965.

Stembera Z, et al. "Umbilical blood flow in newborn infants who suffered intrauterine hypoxia," AM J OBSTET GYNECOL, 101(4);546-553, June 15,1968.

Strong T. "The umbilical pump: a contributor to twin-twin transfusion," OBSTET GYNECOL 89(5 pt 2);812-813, May, 1997.

Trevathan W. HUMAN BIRTH: AN EVOLUTIONARY PERSPECTIVE. Aldine de Gruyter, New York NY, 1987.

Waldrop, et al. "Red cell physiology," pp. 868-876, in Gluckman et al., eds. PEDIATRICS AND PERINATOLOGY, 2nd ed. Arnold, London UK, 1996.

Walsh S, et al. THE HUMAN FETAL AND NEONATAL CIRCULATION: FUNCTION AND STRUCTURE. American Lecture Series, No. 870. Charles C Thomas, Springfield IL, 1974.

WHO, "Care of the umbilical cord: a review of the evidence," Maternal and Newborn Health/Safe Motherhood, 98.4, Geneva Switzerland, 1999.

Yao AC, et al. "Distribution of blood between infant and placenta after birth," LANCET, 2(7626):871-873, Oct 25, 1969.

Yao AC, Lind J. PLACENTAL TRANSFUSION: A CLINICAL AND PHYSIOLOGICAL STUDY. Charles C Thomas, Springfield IL, 1982.

BIRTH OF THE PLACENTA, CORD AND MEMBRANES

Akiyama H, et al. "An approach to detection of placental separation and expulsion with new clinical signs: a study based on hemodynamic method and ultrasonography," AM J OBSTET GYNECOL, 140(5);505-511, July 1, 1981.

Bennett V, Brown L, eds. MYLES TEXTBOOK FOR MIDWIVES, 13th ed., Churchill Livingstone, Edinburgh UK, 1999.

Doolittle J, Moritz C. "Prevention of erythroblastosis by an obstetric technic," OBSTET GYNECOL, 27(4);529-531, Apr, 1966.

Dunn P. "The placental venous pressure during and after the third stage of labour following early cord ligation," J OBSTET GYNECOL BR COMMONW, 73(5);747-756, Oct, 1966.

Dunn P. Chapter 7: "The third stage and fetal adaptation," in Clinch J, Matthews T, eds. PERINATAL MEDICINE: PROCEEDINGS OF THE IX EUROPEAN CONGRESS OF PERINATAL MEDICINE, DUBLIN, IRELAND, SEPT. 3-5, 1984, MTP Press Ltd, Lancaster UK, 1985.

El Halta V. ADVANCED MIDWIFERY SEMINAR: MOVING MIDWIFERY FORWARD: ESSAYS AND OUTLINES, privately published workshop manual, Garden of Life, Dearborn MI, 1989.

El Halta V. "Taking the fear out of third stage," SPECIAL DELIVERY, Fall, 1990 and MIDWIFERY TODAY, (48);18-22, Winter, 1998.

Enning C. "Birth on Demand," all day workshop on waterbirth, MIDWIFERY TODAY conf., Springfield OR, March 2003.

Ghosh KG, et al. "Tensile properties of human umbilical cord," INDIAN J MED RES, 79;538-541, Apr, 1984.

Hart G. Midwife, Portland OR. Personal conversation, Dec 2003.

Hendrickson F. MIDWIFERY IN 10,000 EASY STEPS, PART 1: A CRITICAL AND CONSTRUCTIVE LOOK AT MIDWIFERY AND OBSTETRICS BY A BIRTH ATTENDANT WITH OVER 20 YEARS UNLICENCED EXPERIENCE. Privately published, Hillman MN, Jan, 1981.

Long P. "Bleeding and the third stage of labor," NAACOGS CLIN ISSUES IN PERIN WOMEN'S HEALTH NURS, 2(3);385-395, 1991.

Odent M. "The first hour following birth: don't wake the mother!" MIDWIFERY TODAY, (61);9-12, Spring, 2002.

Oldfield C. HERMAN'S DIFFICULT LABOR: A GUIDE FOR STUDENTS AND PRACTITIONERS, 7th ed. William Wood & Co, New York NY, 1929.

Pastore J. "A study of the blood loss in the third stage of labor and the factors involved," AM J OBSTET GYNECOL, 31;78, 1936.

Sellers P. MIDWIFERY: A TEXTBOOK AND REFERENCE BOOK FOR MIDWIVES IN SOUTHERN AFRICA, VOL 1: NORMAL CHILDBIRTH. Juta & Co, Ltd, Kenwyn So Africa, 1993.
Varney H. VARNEY'S MIDWIFERY, 3rd ed. Jones & Bartlett, Sudbury MA, 1997.
Walsh, S. "Maternal effects of early and late clamping of the umbilical cord," LANCET 1(7550);996-997, May 11, 1968.
West Z. ACUPUNCTURE IN PREGNANCY AND CHILDBIRTH. Churchill Livingstone, Edinburgh UK, 2001.
White G. "Breech Roundtables" workshop, cassette tape, MIDWIFERY TODAY conf. New York NY, 1997.

EXAMINATION OF THE PLACENTA

Benirschke K, Kaufmann P. PATHOLOGY OF THE HUMAN PLACENTA, 4th ed. Springer Verlag, New York NY, 2000.
Fojaco RD, et al. "Congenital syphilis and necrotizing funisitis," JAMA, 261(12);1788-1790, Mar 24-31,1989.
Fox H. PATHOLOGY OF THE PLACENTA, 2nd ed. WB Saunders Co, Ltd, London UK, 1997.
Gall S, ed. MULTIPLE PREGNANCY AND DELIVERY. Mosby, St. Louis MO, 1996.
Heifetz S. "Thrombosis of the umbilical cord: analysis of 52 cases and literature review," PEDIATR PATHOL, 8(1);37-54, 1988.
Karchmer S, et al. "Anomalias del cordon umbilical y coexistencia de malformaciones congenitas," GINECOLOGIA Y OBSTETRICIA DE MEXICO, 21(124):831-837, 1966.
Kravitz H, Molina R. "A technique for improved visualization of the umbilical vessels," IMJ, 130(1);23-25, July, 1966.
Naeye RL. "The clinical significance of absent subchorionic fibrin in the placenta," AMERICAN J CLIN PATH, 94(2); 196-198, Aug, 1990.
Schuler-Maloney D. E-mail communications, 2000.
Schuler-Maloney D, Lee S. THE PLACENTA: TO KNOW ME IS TO LOVE ME. DSM Pathworks, Inc, St. Mary's IA, 1998.
Singer D, Macpherson T. "Fetal death and the macerated stillborn infant," in Wigglesworth J, Singer D, eds. TEXTBOOK OF FETAL AND PERINATAL PATHOLOGY, 2nd ed. Blackwell Sciences, Malden MA, 1998.
Strong TH, et al. "The umbilical coiling index," AM J OBSTET GYNECOL, 170(1 Pt 1);29-32, May, 1994.

EVALUATING NEWBORN WELL-BEING

THE HEALTHY FULL-TERM NEWBORN IN THE FIRST HOURS OF LIFE

Always keep in mind that the baby is a sensitive, sentient being who will be deeply impressed by her first experiences of life outside her mother.

The Baby's Arrival

The mother receives her baby

If the mother is assisting the birth herself or the baby is emerging close to a soft landing surface, do not touch the baby as he emerges. At the time of birth, the undisturbed mother reaches down to touch the head, the baby emerges, they make eye contact, the mother lifts the baby under the arms and brings him to her chest when she is ready. A healthy, unstressed newborn, when gathered to his mother enface against her chest will turn his face and anterior body to his right and his mother's left side, so that his right side is against his mother's left breast. An unhealthy baby will tend to turn to the opposite side (Enning, 2003). Babies prefer to turn their heads to their right by 39 weeks; 90% of newborns spend 80% of the time head turned toward the right. This behavior has been observed as early as 28 weeks and may reflect the normal asymmetry of cerebral function at birth (Polin & Spitzer, 2001).

Welcoming the baby

Concurrent with physical care and supervision, the newborn baby should be lovingly welcomed to the world. Observe the mother's response to her baby. It may be obvious that the mother is in a wonderfully altered state of consciousness and the atmosphere is one of quiet reverence, with the mother totally involved in receiving her newborn. In this case, you need only observe as unobtrusively as possible.

If this is not the case and the mother or both partners are not relating to the baby, phrases such as "We are so glad you are here," "You are loved and wanted," "We are so glad you are a (boy or girl)," should be expressed freely. If the parents are not doing this, you can provide a model for them by saying such things yourself and encouraging them to welcome their baby as well. Sometimes you will know in advance that these statements cannot come clearly from the parents, who may have wanted a baby of a different sex or may have had grave ambivalence regarding the pregnancy. In these cases, the midwife can make these into "I" statements, and the baby will have received an unequivocal welcome from at least one significant person at the birth.

Physical Care of the Newborn

If the mother is positioned so that she can reach for her baby and the room is sufficiently warm, you need do nothing once the baby is born. Even if the mother is on her hands and knees, she is likely to reposition herself and reach for the baby if she does not get the impression you are ready to do so for her. Whenever you do intervene, think of it as just that. These first minutes of mother-infant contact should be as pure and uninterrupted as is safely possible.

Keep the environment warm

It is ideal to have the room sufficiently warm so that drying the baby is not a big concern. Regardless of how warm the room may be, some normal evaporative heat loss will occur as the wet baby emerges into the air; this will be sufficient to help stimulate breathing. There is also no need to be overzealous in drying the term baby if the cord is intact and the room into which the baby is born is at least 80° to 90°F (26.2 to 32°C) and free of drafts. For a baby whose cord has been clamped early, a thermoneutral environment is generally considered to be between 87.8 and 93.2°F (31 to 34°C). The World Health Organization (1997) recommends a room temperature between 77 and 82.4°F (25 to 28°C). A warm environment enhances oxytocin release in both mother and baby, speeding the birth of the placenta and a fall in stress hormones and thus fostering bonding. If the baby seems cold, heat the room up. Humidity is recommended to be at 50%. If the environment is dry, increase the ambient moisture in the air by either putting large pot of water on the stove on a slow simmer or by starting a vaporizer that puts out warm mist (rather than cold, as would a humidifier).

Drying the baby

When the mother is fully engaged with her baby, do not interrupt this process to dry the baby off or instruct the mother to do so; rather, be sure the room is quite warm and have a warmed receiving blanket to open and hand to her when she is ready. If the room cannot be warmed adequately, if the mother is not in a position to bring the baby into her arms, or if she is not focused on the baby, a dry, warm receiving blanket should be placed over the baby's head and body. Then either lay the baby on her side between the mother's legs or knees or give the baby, loosely covered, to the mother. A baby placed in the mother's arms under a covering will be kept warm by the body heat from them both. Have another dry, warmed blanket ready to replace the first as it becomes wet. If the mother is still not fully engaged with her baby, gently dry the baby's head and continue to replace wet or damp blankets until the baby is more or less dry, depending upon the ambient temperature (the colder the room, the more you must be concerned about thoroughly drying the baby). There is no need to take the baby from the mother to dry him off, and the mother can certainly assist in this process. Do not attempt to remove vernix from the baby, as it provides a protective coating for the skin. Drying helps the baby maintain a normal body temperature and it provides gentle stimulation should the baby be slow to start breathing deeply.

Observe the baby for normal transitional signs and behavior

The transition period refers to the first 6 to 12 hours of life, during which the healthy baby goes through a series of dramatic physiologic changes reflected in her level of alertness, emotional responses, vital signs and gastrointestinal activity. With or without drying, all that most babies will need is to the quietly observed for normal responses and appearance. Have a neonatal stethoscope around your neck so that you can easily and unobtrusively check the heart rate, respirations and breath sounds if you have any doubt about the newborn's status. As long as the baby is breathing well, has a good color (that is, the rosy pink that indicates adequate circulation and oxygenation), displays good flexion in the extremities and you note no other problems that might require immediate hands-on attention, you can allow the parents to hold and bond with their baby undisturbed. The section below outlines what you can expect regarding the baby's normal transition.

Normal transition in homeborn babies: Neonatology has delineated a series of normal, adaptive changes and behaviors that occur immediately after birth and during the hours that follow. These changes comprise the transitional period when the baby is adapting to life outside the womb and are said to occur in all babies, regardless of gestational age or route of birth (yoni or surgical). However, it is obvious that homeborn babies were not included in the studied populations because transition occurs differently among babies born at home.

The big difference is that hospital-born babies have greater levels of stress. The normal transitional signs outlined below include a description of what you are likely to see at home contrasted with what is considered within the normal range for hospital-born babies. It must be remembered that hospital-based "normal parameters" are derived from populations of babies who have had routine early cord clamping, handling by several care providers, typically are separated from their mother at some point soon after birth and other interventions preceded by a labor during which the mother has often had drugs, instrumental delivery or surgery. Although most of the extreme physiologic responses described may be seen in any baby, they are usually not seen in homeborn babies who are not exposed to maternal drugs during labor, are given directly to and never separated from their mothers, whose cords remain intact and who are not handled by strangers. In short, the homeborn baby makes a smoother and more complete transition more quickly after birth than do those born in a medical setting.

I. The first period of reactivity: This period lasts at least one and usually two to three hours in normal babies born at home. (It is said to span the first 30 minutes among babies born in medical settings.) It may be marked by:

- A heart rate over 100 bpm at birth. In the hospital, a rapid increase in heart rate to 160 to 180 bpm for 10 to 15 minutes followed by a fall to 100 to 120 over the first 30 minutes is considered normal. This acceleration in the heart rate is more likely to occur when the baby is handled vigorously at the time of birth, when the cord is clamped too soon, and when the baby is otherwise generally stressed.
- Muscle tone, which varies at birth. It can be perfectly normal and is very common for babies to be born with limbs well flexed; however a brief period of transient floppiness may also be seen in otherwise normal infants who had slight hypoxia immediately prior to birth. Any floppiness quickly returns to flexion as breathing begins and the baby turns pink.
- Skin color transitions from lavender pink to rosy pink in the first minute or two of life. There may be a brief period of differential cyanosis in the seconds following birth during which the face, right arm and chest are

pink and the lower body is brightly blue. Brief periods of duskiness of the hands and feet, especially during crying just after birth, may be normal. Generalized duskiness may also occur but is less likely to be seen in babies whose cords are left intact (Fletcher, 1998).

- The tidal volume of the first breath ranges from 12 to 67 ml, with an average range of 31 to 67 ml. It is characterized by a distinct, short inspiration followed often without pause by a prolonged, irregular expiration associated with a high positive intrathoracic pressure. Although some babies have short, distinct expiratory phases with a definite pause at the end of expiration (Karlberg et al., 1962). Subsequent breaths follow the initial pattern during the first minute or so of life. Respirations continue and stabilize in an unhurried manner with increasing lung inflation on each inhalation. The undistressed newborn often gives the impression of one waking up abruptly from a deep sleep. There may be some crackling sounds from residual lung fluid on auscultation of the lung field. Respirations are likely to be more irregular for the first 15 minutes or so, with rates ranging from 60 to 80 rpm or briefly even higher. Respirations tend to smooth out sooner when placental transfusion is uninterrupted. Crackles (like Rice Crispies cereal in milk) and some grunting, flaring and retracting may be noted interspersed with periods of apnea, usually lasting less than 10 seconds each. Respiratory efforts may be increased when the baby is stressed, which could occur from fear or anger. Even homeborn babies may be born angry or frightened by the events of their birth.
- An infant who is usually quiet and alert, seldom crying at birth or crying only briefly. The baby often undergoes the first minutes of adaptation to breathing in a very restful state.
- A decrease in body temperature is expected in babies born into cold hospital environments. In babies who are born into a warm room, the temperature drop is less extreme.
- A baby who shows interest in nursing with rooting and sucking motions or sucking the hands or fingers. If offered the breast, the baby will often attempt to latch on.
- A baby who seeks eye contact and searches the faces of his parents and siblings as well as alerting to sounds, especially familiar voices.
- Bowel sounds being absent for the first 15 minutes. Birth fluids may drain from the mouth, but there is little saliva production.
- The passage of meconium and urine in this time period.

II. Deep postbirth sleep: After the initial period of alertness, the baby falls into a deep sleep that often lasts 4 to 6 hours and sometimes longer. This allows the baby to integrate the experience of birth.

- The baby is hard to rouse from this sleep and should not be disturbed to nurse. The normal newborn has enough stored glycogen to withstand a long period of sleep at this time, especially if she has had colostrum prior to falling asleep and a full placental transfusion has taken place.
- Heart rate and respirations should be within normal limits. Fast, shallow and synchronous breathing at a rate of 60 breaths/min may be observed.
- Color is excellent.
- Spontaneous jerks and twitches that are intermittent and fleeting are normal.
- Muscle tone is reduced and the baby is very relaxed but not flaccid.
- The abdomen will be rounded and smooth, with audible bowel sounds. Peristaltic waves may be visible.
- Minimal oral secretions are typical.

It is noteworthy that this period of deep sleep is not observed in hospital-born babies at this point. The normal second period of transition for those babies is a "decreased period of responsiveness," which lasts from 30 minutes to 2 hours. I suspect this is due to a hospital schedule that does not allow the babies to sleep well at this time as well as to the level of stress surrounding their birth, which interferes with their normal sleep pattern. It may also be due to how overwhelmed the baby feels from being subjected to the many routine procedures of hospital care. The interruption of this deep sleep period plus the additional stresses may be a primary reason why hospital-born babies frequently sleep very deeply for many hours in the two to three days that follow birth, a phenomenon not normally observed in homeborn babies.

III. The baby wakes up. After the postbirth sleep, the baby awakes and acts like a normal newborn with stable heart rate, normal gastrointestinal and kidney activity, and a desire to nurse.

- From here on, for the first weeks after birth, the baby should nurse, or be encouraged to nurse, every 2 hours or more frequently if he desires.

- •Activity results in brief periods of reactive tachycardia and rapid respiration. Changes in muscle tone and skin color and bowel sounds can all be normal as well.
- •Respirations normally remain irregular.
- •Oral mucus may increase, with some gagging and spitting up.
- •If the baby has not already done so, he should pass both urine and meconium.

Among hospital-born babies, the third period is described as a "second period of reactivity during which the baby's responsiveness returns and may become exaggerated." It is said to last 2 to 8 hours. As it diminishes, the baby becomes relatively stable and is ready to nurse (Thureen et al., 1999). That a baby may take this long to be "ready to nurse" is another indication that his birth was a traumatic experience.

Specific physical parameters

Heart rate

The vast majority of homeborn babies will have a heart rate over 100 bpm shortly after birth. The heart rate of an agitated baby may range as high as 160 to 180 bpm for the first 10 to 15 minutes, with a gradual drop over the first half-hour to a baseline rate between 100 and 120 bpm. It can be assumed that a crying baby or an alert, pink, breathing baby has a heart rate of 100 bpm or more. The time required for a healthy, term newborn's heart rate to return to her early labor baseline averages 17 minutes (± 7 minutes) when the mother has pushed physiologically, as opposed to an average of 50 minutes when the mother uses forced pushing (Gruener, 1982). The heart rate falls into the 100 to 120 bpm range and is relatively less reactive to any movement as the baby falls into her postbirth sleep. The heart rate may drop as low as 80 bpm during periods of diminished responsiveness. If there are no accompanying changes in color or respiration, this is very normal.

Color changes immediately after birth

Most babies are born a warm shade of lavender pink. This is reflective of the normally lower oxygen saturation of the fetus, which is further reduced to a small extent by the end of labor. All babies, regardless of race, become rosy pink in the first 30 to 60 seconds as breathing is established. The hands and feet may remain lavender pink for longer but should become rosy pink when warmed. Some duskiness may develop around the mouth in some normal babies, especially with exertion, but should not persist. If the baby is pale, blue, limp or not breathing, proceed with resuscitation.

Normal temperature variations at birth

Scalp temperature can fall from 96.8 to 93.2°F (36 to 34°C) as the baby's head emerges from the mother's body during birth, particularly when emerging in a cold delivery room, which is where all available studies were performed. Similarly rapid changes may occur as the rest of the body is born. In studies done of hospital-born babies who were not warmed after birth and whose cords were cut quickly, deep (core) body temperature of the term infant fell 0.2°F (0.1°C) per minute and skin temperature fell 0.5°F (0.3°C) per minute. The total drop in deep body temperature can be as great as 3.6 to 5.4°F (2 to 3°C). A dramatic decrease in skin temperature occurred within 10 minutes of exposure to cold room air. While some drop in temperature is physiologic, since postbirth body temperature is normally lower than that in utero, the unprotected, early-clamped newborn can lose enough heat to have a fall in temperature of 3.6 to 7.2°F (2 to 4°C), with even greater drops in the following hours if the baby is not warmed. A naked baby who has experienced early cord clamping and who is exposed to an environmental temperature of 73.4°F (23°C) at birth experiences the same degree of heat loss as does a naked adult at 32°F (0°C).

Mature babies who have been born into a sufficiently warm, draft-free room and have received an optimal placental transfusion are at less risk of becoming chilled even if naked, especially if they have been dried off and they remain in their mother's arms. While some term infants can handle an ambient temperature as low as 70°F (21.5°C), the room should be at least 80 to 90°F (26.5 to 32.5°C) to enhance oxytocin levels in both mother and infant. A stocking cap can be placed over the head to minimize heat loss. If you are still concerned, throw a blanket or, if it is a hot summer, a sheet over both mother and baby. There is a normal decrease in body temperature and an increase in motor activity and muscle tone after birth. If you suspect that the baby is becoming chilled, simply feel his extremities. If the baby feels cool or is not maintaining that rosy pink glow in his hands or feet, add more covers and a newborn stocking cap, if not done already.

If either the temperature of the room or the baby is still not optimal, take the baby's temperature. An axillary temperature is least invasive, but the tip of the thermometer must be carefully placed in the armpit and held under the closed arm for at least 5 minutes. Alternatively, a rectal temperature can be taken much more quickly. Gently insert the lubricated thermometer tip, angling it toward the umbilicus, and wait 2 minutes before reading. Expect that this will prompt the passage of meconium and be prepared. (See Volume I for detailed instructions on taking temperatures with a glass thermometer and the chapter entitled "Parting Instructions for the Parents" in this volume for more details.) A normal newborn kept in a near-neutral thermal environment and with a full placental transfusion on board should be able to restore her initial body temperature by 2 to 3 hours of age, and probably much sooner.

It is unusual for a newborn's temperature to become elevated unless the environment is overly warm. If the skin temperature is over 100.4°F (38°C) and remains high after the environment is cooled, a rectal temperature should be taken. Unless the temperature has been elevated for a while, the rectal temperature is less likely to be affected by environmental variations; if it is also high, infection or neurologic causes must be ruled out. Term infants sweat in response to thermal stress. Visible sweating at rest in a baby with a normal temperature is usually abnormal and may indicate distress, often from heart disease, although you may note mild sweating occasionally if the baby is quite large for gestational age.

Muscle tone

The baby should have good muscle tone at birth. To check for this, extend a limb and see if the baby draws it back. The baby is usually alert over the first few hours, exploring the faces of those around him, displaying spontaneous startles and Moro reflexes, tremors, increased muscle tone and purposeless movements of the arms and legs. These types of activities should be short, intermittent and not extreme. Spontaneous jerks and tremors are common but should be fleeting.

Respirations

Normal babies whose cords are still intact may take the first 30 to 90 seconds of life to fully transition from placental to pulmonary respiration, although most will begin breathing almost immediately. Nearly all healthy babies will be breathing regularly within three minutes of birth. Stay relaxed and observant as long as progress is being made in that direction and the baby is flexed and pink with a heart rate of 100 bpm or more. Irregular respirations during the first 15 minutes of life with rates ranging from 60 to 100 rpm are normal, with rates slowing to an average of 50 to 80 rpm. When listening through a stethoscope, the lungs may not sound completely clear for the first 30 to 60 minutes, but breath sounds should be audible and equal on both sides. As transition is completed, the baby's respiratory rate ranges from 35 to 70 rpm and continues to be irregular, particularly when the baby is awake. Regular breathing cycles lasting 10 to 18 seconds are interspersed with pauses lasting at least 3 seconds (a deep breath, several more shallow breaths, up to 3 seconds of apnea, a couple of rapid, deeper breaths, for example, is a very typical pattern).

Listen to the baby's chest with a newborn stethoscope if you have doubts about her respiratory status. Count the respirations for a full minute, to compensate for the irregular breathing all normal babies display. It can take a few breaths for the baby to fully expand her lungs and for most of the lung fluid to be pulled out. Breathing may be quite irregular immediately after birth, but is usually sufficient for adequate ventilation. However, gasping (occasional breaths with long pauses in between) is not adequate and may indicate that the airway is blocked or the baby is apneic (see the subchapter entitled "Evaluating and Assisting the Infant in Need of Resuscitation").

There should be no sustained evidence of true respiratory distress as described in the subchapter entitled "Evaluating the Apparently Normal Baby Who Develops Respiratory Distress." If the baby does not cry or breathe at all and does not respond to being handled or dried, or if you note other signs of respiratory distress, especially deep retractions, lower the baby below the level of the placenta (or raise the placenta above the baby if it has already been delivered), slowly and deliberately strip the cord several times, and begin resuscitation efforts immediately.

Babies born via surgery or after a very fast labor tend to grunt and experience other forms of true respiratory distress, including rapid breathing, during these first hours more than those born after several hours of labor. Fast labors do not give the baby's lungs much chance to dry out before birth. Surgical delivery is invariably accompanied by immediate cord clamping often before being lifted from the uterus, with additional blood loss because the uterus is usually atonic (thus no blood is forced into the baby prior to severing the cord). These babies usually have poorly perfused lungs and are struggling to expand their alveoli and maintain adequate oxygenation.

For very different reasons, healthy homeborn babies who have experienced physiologic cord closure may also continue to breathe shallowly and rapidly at a rate above 60 rpm up to 6 hours after birth. The higher respiratory rate (a form of transient tachypnea) is thought to be due to increased filling of the pulmonary vasculature, higher viscosity of the blood and a lower functional residual capacity. These variations stiffen the alveoli, causing babies to breathe shallowly and more rapidly than most of their quickly clamped counterparts. Unless experiencing true respiratory *distress*, a healthy baby with physiologic tachypnea appears comfortable and can slow his breathing to nurse without any compromise; his breathing is not labored and his color remains good (Fletcher, 1998). Fast, shallow, synchronous breathing is the rule until the baby falls into his deep postbirth sleep, when rates typically drop to about one-third of what they were when the baby was awake, when rates up to 60 breaths/min are normal. There may be increased barreling of the chest during this period of rest. Gasping (occasional breathes with long pauses in between) does not provide adequate ventilation and may indicate that the airway is blocked or the baby is apneic (see the subchapter entitled "Evaluating and Assisting the Infant in Need of Resuscitation"). Immediately clamped babies have been found to have significantly lower respiratory rates, ranging from 49 to 54 breaths/min by the 24th hour of life. By 2 to 5 days of age, the values were the same for both groups (Mercer, 2001; Oh et al., 1967; Yao et al., 1971). Some physiologically clamped babies also display mild grunting that begins in the first 30 minutes of life, peaks 30 to 60 minutes after birth and disappears gradually over the second to fourth hour of life (Oh et al., 1967). Normal newborns may present occasional mild retractions and slight flaring of the nostrils as well.

Abdominal changes

There are no audible sounds in the abdomen upon auscultation at birth. Bowel sounds begin to occur during the first 15 minutes of life as air enters the gastrointestinal tract for the first time. When the baby has been breathing for a few minutes, the upper abdomen will appear slightly more distended than the lower abdomen. It is very common to see multiple loops of bowel through the abdominal wall, especially in babies with little subcutaneous fat, such as early babies or those with lower abdominal muscle tone. (The same phenomenon may occur, but be less visibly apparent, in babies born closer to term who have a normal fat layer.) Peristaltic waves are seen carrying the air along the loops. These visible loops should recede after the first hour (Fletcher, 1998).

Bowel and bladder function

The baby is likely to pass meconium and urinate within the first hours of life. Passage of a large quantity of meconium is normal; however, the passage of several small silver-dollar-sized blobs may indicate a problem with stenosis in the rectum or anus. Whenever possible, passage of meconium should be observed to determine if it is coming from the anus or being extruded through a defect in the yoni, penis, urethra or perineum. Urination should occur in a forceful stream (more so in boys than girls) that is usually steady but can be normally intermittent. Urination should occur independent of crying or straining.

Newborn states of consciousness

The baby will have a period of alertness ranging from one to two hours after birth. This period can include spontaneous startle reactions, mouth movements, tremors, crying and side-to-side head movements. This is followed by deep sleep, providing a period of rest and integration of the enormous experience just undergone. This deep postbirth sleep may last for several hours; the baby should be allowed to rest undisturbed next to or on the mother.

Upon awakening, the baby will again be responsive, experiencing an increase in heart rate, brief periods of rapid respiration, and abrupt changes in muscle tone, color and bowel sounds. Oral mucus may become prominent. Gagging, vomiting (nonforceful spitting up) and sneezing are not unusual, but coughing should not occur. The baby becomes more responsive to internal and external stimuli and may have frequent changes in heart rate. This alert period may be relatively brief or last for several hours. The first meconium stool may be passed, if this has not yet happened.

Interest in and ability to nurse

Babies often show an interest in the breast shortly after birth. They may nuzzle and lick the breast if left completely undisturbed and remain skin-to-skin with their mother. All babies should be encouraged to nurse if they so desire. When a baby is believed to be at risk for hypoglycemia (early, small, IUGR and very large babies), nursing should begin within an hour of birth. Nursing sessions should be spaced no more than 4 hours apart when the mother and baby are sleeping; otherwise the baby should nurse a minimum of every two hours.

Blood glucose changes after birth

During gestation, the fetus receives a constant flow of glucose from her mother via the placenta. (If the mother's glucose is too high, the baby compensates by producing extra insulin to regulate her own blood sugar levels, meaning she will almost certainly be hypoglycemic at birth and will remain so until her insulin levels readjust.) After birth, all babies experience a postnatal fall in glucose levels. The fall will be greater in a preterm baby, those who undergo a stressful labor, those who do not receive a full placental transfusion and those who do not nurse soon after birth. Full-term babies who nurse within three hours of birth have an average glucose level of 70 mg/dl (3.9 mmol/l), a level well within normal limits. Nursing is the best way to ensure that a normal baby maintains a normal glucose level in the hours and days following birth.

APGAR scores

Use color, respiratory effort and heart rate to assess the need for resuscitation. The APGAR score reflects how the baby is responding to resuscitation efforts. After the initial scores, it can be repeated every 5 minutes up to 20 minutes.

Recognizing a Baby Who Is Having an Abnormal Transition

It is important be able to tell if the baby is in trouble during the postpartum stay. Sometimes this is obvious and dramatic; others times, it creeps up on you as the baby becomes less and less able to compensate for underlying problems. Any of the following indicate that the baby is having trouble making the fetus-to-newborn transition:

- Increasingly rapid breathing, grunting, retractions and rales
- Persistent central cyanosis or pallor
- Apnea, with or without bradycardia, lasting more than 10 seconds at term (20 seconds for preterm <35 weeks)
- Temperature instability
- Prolonged capillary refill time (>3 sec) and unstable blood pressure
- Unusual neurologic signs and symptoms
- Excessive quantities of saliva, drooling or choking episodes
- Persistently visible peristalsis
- Persistent hypoglycemia that does not resolve with treatment

Respiratory distress

Persistently rapid breathing, grunting, retractions and crackles: Any of these signs may be within normal limits during the initial neonatal transition. For example, if the baby becomes too cold, she may breathe rapidly and show some retractions; these signs should resolve if the baby is warmed. However, the persistence or worsening of any of these signs is cause for concern, as are signs of respiratory distress that resolve only to reappear later with no apparent cause. Any degree of respiratory distress that prevents the baby from breathing and nursing at the same time and that cannot be resolved is also cause for transport. (More details can be found in the subchapter entitled "Evaluating the Apparently Normal Baby Who Develops Respiratory Distress.")

Persistently visible central cyanosis or pallor: Although a red flag, visual assessment of central cyanosis is subjective and therefore not always reliable. Therefore an oximeter should be used to determine the O_2 saturation, which should be 89-100% in a baby more than 10 minutes old (mild fluctuations are normal) (O'Brien et al., 2000). If O_2 saturation is below 89% use blow-by oxygen to bring up it to 95-99%, remove oxygen and continue to test. If the baby is otherwise transitioning normally, monitor and observe. If not or oxygen saturation is not staying above 90%, consult. If you don't have an oximeter, go by the behavior and color of the baby. If in doubt, transport.

The persistence of pallor is also very concerning. Pallor often signals underlying anemia, peripheral vasoconstriction or both due to problems such as hypovolemia, asphyxia or cardiac shock. It will be hard to distinguish pallor caused by anemia from that caused by vasoconstriction; either way, transport is in order.

Apnea lasting more than 10 or 20 seconds: Normally, brief pauses in breathing last no longer than 3 seconds and certainly less than 10. Prolonged periods of apnea, with or without associated bradycardia, require prompt investigation. Twenty seconds is the outside limit of normal and is more typically seen in preterm babies than in those born at term. Possible causes include maternal drug intake, perinatal asphyxia, infection, shock and central nervous system disorders.

O'Brien, et al., "Oxygen saturation during the first 24 hours of life," ARCH DIS CHILD FETAL NEONATAL ED, 83(1):F35-F38, JUL 2000.

Cardiovascular events

Bradycardia: The baby's heart rate may drop as low as 80 bpm during deep sleep. However, whenever bradycardia is persistent, it requires careful evaluation; heart defects are a possibility.

Prolonged capillary refill time and unstable blood pressure: Pronounced vasoconstriction with poor capillary refill time (over 3 seconds) and generally poor perfusion are warning signs of serious underlying problems such as hypoxia, sepsis, cardiovascular instability or central nervous system injury.

Temperature instability

A persistently low body temperature less than 97.7°F or 36.5°C, or an inability to maintain a normal temperature in a reasonably warm room is usually due to early cord clamping. It may also be the result of maternal drug intake, perinatal hypoxia, metabolic disruption, central nervous system disorders or sepsis. A septic baby may not develop a fever. Warm the baby by placing her skin-to-skin between her mother's breasts and cover both with a blanket. Recheck the newborn's temperature in 20 minutes.

A persistently high body temperature, above 99.5°F or 37.5°C, is much less common; sepsis must also be considered and should be suspected first unless there are obvious reasons why the baby may be overheated. If that is the problem, cooling the baby by removing covering and cooling the room or bathing in water not more than 3.6°F (2°C) cooler than the baby's temperature should quickly result in a drop in temperature. If persistent hypo- or hyperthermia cannot be resolved, transport.

Unusual neurologic signs and symptoms

Marked depression or lethargy, decreased activity with marked and persistently poor muscle tone, irritability, and excessive, persistent or prolonged tremors all require further investigation.

Gastrointestinal events

Secretion of excessive quantities of saliva, drooling or choking episodes: Large quantities of oral secretions and drooling, especially if accompanied by choking or coughing spells, are all indicative of a compromised transition and require further evaluation. They may indicate a gastrointestinal obstruction.

Persistently visible peristalsis: If visibly distended loops persist in the same area, especially in an upper quadrant, this raises the suspicion of a bowel obstruction. When two distinct loop "bubbles" persist beyond the first hour, particularly when the rest of the abdomen is relatively less distended, an obstructed duodenum is the likely cause (Fletcher, 1998).

Persistent hypoglycemia

Babies who remain hypoglycemic despite nursing may have a rare pancreatic disorder. Babies born small for gestational age with persistently low blood sugar may have a degree of pancreatic dysfunction. Nesidioblastosis is a rare disorder characterized by large for gestational age growth (typically weighing 9 lb 11 oz or more [4.4 ± 0.3 kg]) in a baby whose mother is not diabetic. Nesidioblastosis is really a misnomer, as this term is used to describe the normal development of pancreatic tissue. More precisely, it is a poorly defined condition and may be best called **persistent neonatal hyperinsulinemic hypoglycemia (PNHH) of nesidiodysplasia** characterized by subtle cellular abnormalities in the neonatal pancreas (Ariel et al., 1988). These babies have physiques which resemble those of infants of mothers with poorly controlled diabetes. They also display jitteriness, myoclonic jerks, cyanotic episodes, apnea and seizures within hours of birth. A glucose level below which brain damage occurs has been a long-sought value, but has yet to be absolutely defined. At present, a level below 47 mg/dl (2.6 mmol/l) in both preterm and term babies has been found to acutely effect regions of the brain with high glucose demand and is now generally regarded as the lower limit of normal.

In any event, any baby who will not nurse before you leave the house should have a glucose test with a heel prick. Brain damage is believed to occur in some babies who remain asymptomatic in the presence of a low glucose level (remembering that this research only looked at early clamped babies). Note that capillary sampling is unreliable if the baby is poorly perfused. Be sure the baby is warm and pink to the extremities before testing. If hypoglycemia is detected, have the baby nurse or feed the baby molasses water (do not use honey, as it may carry botulism) and repeat the test after 45 minutes to an hour. In the meantime observe the baby for symptoms. If the baby's condition is worsening, transport without delay. More details regarding neonatal hypoglycemia can be found in my text DIAGNOSTIC TESTS.

Specific Underlying Problems That Are Associated with Abnormal Transition

Babies born via surgery

Abnormal transition is commonly seen after surgical delivery. The degree of this will depend upon the medications the mother was given prior to birth. Initially, these babies may be highly agitated, and the first period of reactivity for hospital babies (30 minutes) is prolonged, with the clinical symptoms described being more extreme. These babies often have a high volume of lung fluid because their cord is clamped immediately. The excess fluid results in tachypnea, nasal flaring, grunting, mild intercostal retractions and the may require supplemental oxygen during the first few hours of life (depending upon saturation levels). Allowing the baby to receive his full placental transfusion will help minimize the degree of respiratory distress (which can also occur due to fear and anxiety as well as for physical reasons).

Maternal drug intake producing neonatal depression

Drugs that cause neonatal depression include narcotics, barbiturates and magnesium sulfate. The condition of the drug-exposed baby at birth varies; some will require resuscitation. Evidence of general depression at birth requires monitoring the baby to determine whether there is a need for ventilatory assistance or IV fluids (if the baby cannot suck or swallow), whether the baby is hypoglycemic, and whether the effect of the drugs is wearing off. The baby who breathes on her own and makes it through the first period of reactivity may still display shallow breathing, temperature instability, poor sucking reflex, reduced spontaneous activity, delayed passage of meconium and urine, and poor increase in muscle tone during the hours that follow. This is relevant when caring for hospital-born babies whose mothers are transported and receive drugs prior to or during labor and who then leave the hospital shortly after birth.

Babies born to drug-addicted mothers: When the pregnant mother is addicted to nicotine, alcohol or drugs, so is the baby. After birth, these babies display moderate depression and evidence of drug withdrawal, which usually occurs after the first 30 minutes or so (withdrawal is probably further delayed in babies who receive their full placental transfusion). Withdrawal is marked by accentuation of the lability of heart rate and respiratory patterns normally observed at this point, and agitation with extreme irritability, jitteriness, tremors and inconsolable crying. The baby should be held as much as possible and verbally encouraged to express his fear and rage (Thureen et al., 1999).

Disorders involving the heart and lungs

Persistent pulmonary hypertension of the newborn (PPHN): Some newborns never switch over from fetal to newborn circulation at all. Others may have an initial period during which the blood is rerouted from fetal to newborn circulatory pathways, then have their transitioning pulmonary circulation revert to the in utero pattern. This may occur because the baby's pulmonary vascular resistance remains high due to not receiving a sufficient amount or any of her placental transfusion or due to a stressful insult such as hypoxia, hypotension, acidosis or hypercarbia (rise in arterial carbon dioxide tension). This results in reactivation of the fetal cardiovascular pathways, with blood flowing through the foramen ovale and ductus arteriosus leading to severe and progressive hypoxemia (poor delivery of oxygen to the tissues). PPHN may occur because of one of these conditions:

Inadequate blood volume: The baby is unable to maintain the alveolar vascular bed in an expanded state as a direct result of hypovolemia usually caused by premature termination of the placental transfusion.

Poor adaptation of the pulmonary vasculature to breathing: Vasoconstriction with normal cardiopulmonary anatomy may result from hypoxia, hypercarbia, acidosis or sepsis.

Excessive muscular development of the pulmonary arterioles during gestation: This is seen with chronic stress during pregnancy and premature closure of the ductus arteriosus but may also happen independently.

Underdevelopment of the blood vessels supplying the lungs: This is seen when the lungs are poorly developed and results in severe, unresponsive, fixed pulmonary artery hypertension.

Obstructed blood flow to the lungs: This may be caused by hyperviscosity, total anomalous pulmonary venous return, pulmonary vein stenosis, or left outflow tract obstructive lesions.

Clinical conditions associated with PPHN include meconium aspiration, sepsis, pneumonia, respiratory distress syndrome, congenital diaphragmatic hernia, heart disease, polycythemia and a number of other, as yet undetermined causes. Signs and symptoms include tachypnea, respiratory distress, acidosis, cardiovascular instability and rapidly progressing cyanosis and hypoxemia.

Respiratory distress may be present at birth or become increasingly obvious over the first 6 to 12 hours of life with cyanosis and tachypnea. Lability of the systemic arterial saturation with handling is a key clinical feature: at home, this would be detected by worsening cyanosis with handling if oxygen saturation falls to 85% or below. Lung sounds may also be reduced on auscultation.

Immature lungs: Preterm babies, especially those born before 34 weeks, are prone to breathing difficulties. Those that do experience uncomplicated respiratory distress have a persistently worsening level of distress that usually peaks at 2 to 3 days, with recovery beginning after 72 hours of life. Any early baby should be watched closely but can be expected to do much better in general when optimally transfused at birth.

Meconium Aspiration Syndrome (MAS): This refers to respiratory distress due to inhalation of meconium below the vocal cords. However, what is called "MAS" may occur in some babies who have no evidence of meconium aspiration. It may stem from mechanical obstruction of the large or small airways. Obstruction of the small airways can produce atelectasis (collapse) if the obstruction is complete or produce overdistension of localized regions of alveoli if some air gets through but cannot passively be exhaled past the partial obstruction (ball-valve effect). Chemical irritation can lead to inflammation of the lung tissue (pneumonitis) a few hours after birth. Overdistension of the lung tissue due to obstruction can lead to rupture of the lung in that region, resulting in an air leak (pneumothorax or pneumomediastinum). PPHN can result from MAS-associated hypoxia.

These babies are usually dysmature with a history of intrapartum distress. Presenting symptoms include tachypnea, retractions, cyanosis, nasal flaring and sometimes grunting. See the subchapter entitled "Meconium Aspiration."

Compromise due to perinatal asphyxia

Asphyxia is heralded during labor by fetal bradycardia, which indicates that the baby is trying to compensate for a reduced amount of oxygenation in the tissues. The mature hypoxic fetus reroutes blood to flow to the heart, brain and adrenal glands to ensure adequate oxygenation to these most vital organs. The impact of an asphyxial event upon neonatal transition after birth will vary depending upon its severity and whether the insult of immediate cord clamping is superimposed on the original compromising event. Commonly these babies have a poor or unsustained response to birth stimuli, and the transitional period is prolonged, delayed and compromised.

Multiorgan system injury may occur with severe asphyxia, particularly when complicated by hypovolemia. When the severity of the asphyxia exceeds the baby's adaptive and protective capabilities, the redistribution of blood to vital organs will fail, resulting in acute injury to the tissues. After birth, these organs will show varying degrees of impaired functioning. Such injury is enhanced when the placental transfusion is cut off prior to its completion. Sequelae include PPHN, reduced surfactant, MAS, low platelets, disseminated intravascular coagulation, necrotizing enterocolitis, liver dysfunction, seizures, edema of the brain, myocardial depression, tricuspid insufficiency, myocardial necrosis, hypotension and shock, oliguria, renal failure, acidosis, hypoglycemia, reduced blood levels of calcium and sodium, and the development of hypoxic-ischemic encephalopathy and eventually cerebral palsy in some children.

Hypoxic ischemic encephalopathy (HIE): This term designates the clinical and neurological findings believed to occur in full-term babies who suffer from intrapartum or postpartum asphyxia.

Stage I (Mild): May present with a brief period of lethargy immediately after birth or, more frequently, with signs of cerebral irritation. These babies spend most of their time lying quietly but only minor disturbances result in excessive jittery muscular activity. Hyperalertness, uninhibited reflexes, and overactivity of the sympathetic nervous system may also be noted. The eyes are often wide open and staring with decreased frequency of blinking and prolonged periods of wakefulness with an anxious or frowning expression. The baby may have a shrill, high-pitched dry that is noticeably different from the normal "hungry baby" cry. Rapid eye and tongue movements and short myoclonic twitching movements are sometimes seen. Head retraction and hyperextension present in some of these babies. Rhythmic alternating extension and flexion of the limbs, resembling bicycling or boxing motions which persist for long periods are occasionally noted to be distinguished from seizure activity, which is usually brief and presents with less complicated motion. These signs last less than 24 hours. When in doubt regarding seizure activity, an electroencephalogram should be obtained (Johnston et al., 2003)

Stage II (Moderate): Reduced responsiveness, lethargy, stupor, hypotonia, depressed respiration, abnormal muscle tone, suppressed primitive reflexes, difficulty with nursing and occasionally, seizures for the first few days of life with the infant becoming irritable when disturbed.

Stage III (Severe): A diminished level of consciousness or coma, profound flaccidity and immobility, suppressed brain stem function with depressed or periodic respirations from birth. Repeated seizures or either a clonic (repetitious jerking), myoclonic (single, sudden and large jerks) or tonic (stiffness) may occur. The baby suffers from increased intracranial pressure presenting with a tense or bulging anterior fontanelle. They baby has little or no responsiveness to stimulation. The baby cannot suck, displays poor thermal control with hypothermia, vomiting, abnormal cry and cyanotic attacks. Over the first 24 hours of life as intracranial edema occurs, cerebral irritability develops with increased extensor tone resulting in arching of the back, extension of the head, trunk and limbs and reflex responses now become brisk. The asymmetric tonic neck response can be elicited consistently and may present during spontaneous body movements. Exaggerated extension makes nursing difficult, and a rigid baby impairs the bonding process. These symptoms gradually subside with a slow return to a more normal pattern of behavior unless the cerebral injury results in permanent damage.

These stages are not applicable in preterm infants, who do not present in the same manner as do term infants. When neither the prenatal or the labor history nor the condition of the baby at birth suggest asphyxia, other causes of a decreased level of consciousness must be sought. This baby should be transported immediately (Thureen et al., 1999).

THE APGAR SCORE

In 1953, Dr. Virginia Apgar developed an objective clinical tool to assess and discuss the infant's vital signs during the first minutes after birth. Since then, the APGAR score has been used routinely as a shorthand way to provide a simple, systematic means of assessing the newborn, to communicate regarding the newborn's clinical status, and to monitor the status of the infant during the process of initial evaluation and providing assistance.

An overview of the APGAR score

An APGAR score is routinely performed at one and five minutes of age. The criteria for this scoring system rely heavily on cardiopulmonary function, reflexes and other central nervous system phenomena. Infants with a low APGAR score are assumed to be in jeopardy, requiring support to establish normal respirations and (at times) cardiac function.

The following table summarizes the parameters of the APGAR score. It uses the letters A-P-G-A-R as an acronym, put in order of the spelling of Apgar's name for easy recall. With experience, performing the APGAR score becomes automatic as you greet the newborn in the first minutes of life.

VITAL SIGN	SCORE (MAXIMUM OF 10 POSSIBLE POINTS)		
	0	1	2
Appearance (color)	Blue or pale	Pink with blue hands and feet	Pink all over
Pulse (heart rate)	Absent	Less than 100 bpm	Over 100 bpm
Grimace response (reflex irritability)	No response	Grimace reflexes weak or delayed (hard to rouse)	Prompt and vigorous (awake and alert or crying vigorously)
Activity (muscle tone)	Limp	Some flexion	Well flexed or active motion
Respiratory effort	Absent	Weak or gasping	Deep and regular or crying

The variables measured are essentially vital signs and neuromuscular responses that can be easily assessed and, when impaired, may reflect serious systemic disruption. The responses that the APGAR score evaluates fail in a predictable order, with color being the first to be compromised, followed by respiratory effort, a drop in heart rate, diminished spontaneous tone and reflex irritability, and finally the disappearance of the heartbeat. The discussion below ranks each parameter in order of relative importance.

Pulse (heart rate): Depression of the heart rate is the single most significant APGAR finding, reflecting the compromised status of the acid-base (pH) balance of the blood. Among all the APGAR parameters, the heart rate is usually the last sign to fall or disappear. A heart rate of 100 to 140 bpm is considered excellent and given a score of 2. A heart rate under 100 receives a score of 1; if no heart rate can be seen, felt or heard, the score is 0.

The heart rate can be determined by using a stethoscope, which should always be used to confirm a poor heart rate if there is any doubt. However, other methods can also be employed that avoid disturbing the mother and infant at this time. Observe the area below the xiphoid process or the lower rib cage for a visible heartbeat, or place your fingers lightly on the baby's midchest. The base of the cord may also be palpated by straddling it with two fingers lightly pressed against the abdomen. The midwife performing the APGAR score can tap out the heart rate for her partner if there is a question about the baby's status.

A normal pulse score is not always an accurate gauge of the neonatal status. For example, although tachycardia may reflect an abnormality or a drug reaction (if the baby has been born after transport, for example), it still receives a score of 2. Likewise, bradycardia may be caused by congenital heart block or certain drugs given to the mother and not reflect hypoxia per se, even though it can lower the score.

Respiratory effort: Respiratory effort is ranked next in importance, since without adequate oxygenation (either via the placenta or the lungs), hypoxia and cardiac compromise will rapidly follow. An infant who is apneic at 60 seconds of life gets a score of 0, while those who breath, or cry by one minute receive a 2 rating. All other types of respiratory effort, such as irregular, shallow breathing or a very weak cry, get a score of 1. A baby who has only gasped once at 30 to 45 seconds and who makes no further effort to breathe gets a score of 0, since he is apneic at the time of the first evaluation (one minute). Note that this is an evaluation of respiratory effort only; the respiratory rate is not counted. Note that respiration is certainly a reflex response, even though it is not considered as such for this assessment.

Grimace response (reflex irritability): This refers to response to some form of stimulation. The testing method used by the medical model involves routine bulb suctioning of every baby's mouth and nose. Very often babies grimace or move spontaneously during or immediately after birth, and an observed response can be assessed. The desired responses include facial grimacing or sneezing, which receive a score of 2. A slight grimace or weak cry is scored with a 1, and no response gets a 0. Apgar (1952) notes that, while elimination is not a reflex response to stimulation, urination or passage of meconium were originally considered to be good signs (although elimination does not add to the score). Both muscle tone and reflex irritability are acute measures of central nervous system integrity, which can be compromised by conditions other than asphyxia (such as traumas and maternal medications) and can artificially lower the score.

Activity (muscle tone): A completely limp infant receives a 0 score, while one who is born with good tone demonstrated by spontaneously flexed arms and legs that resist extension is given 2 points. Again, observation of mother-infant interaction may allow this assessment without interference with bonding. Maternal drug intake may either depress or increase muscle tone, depending upon the drug in question.

Appearance (skin color): Skin color, as a reflection of peripheral perfusion, is often the first sign to be compromised but is the least reliable indication of the overall status of the baby. This is because color can still be good in a baby who is rapidly losing ground. Assessment of the baby's color is also the most subjective of these measures, and color has the least correlation with umbilical pH, arterial carbon dioxide tension and base excess. Skin color is normally lavender pink at birth, a product of the normally lower oxygen saturation of the fetus. This is quickly transformed to rosy pink with the initiation of good respirations and the maintenance of a normal heart rate. A score of 1 is given when only the torso is pink; when the hands and feet are also pink, the score rises to 2. Few infants whose cords are clamped quickly can achieve a score of 2 by one minute.

A baby may be breathing well and still remain purplish or blue even when given 100% oxygen. The most common reasons for this are acidosis and pulmonary vasoconstriction. Other causes include cyanotic congential heart disease, methemoglobinemia (oxidation of hemoglobin, making it useless for oxygenation and causing the blood to have a brownish color, which can be mistaken for cyanosis), polycythemia and poorly developed lungs. The very pale baby may be hypovolemic or hypotensive. Some maternally administered drugs such as magnesium sulfate can cause peripheral vasodilation and a pink color in an otherwise hypotonic, lethargic baby.

When to do an APGAR score

The APGAR score is routinely performed at one and five minutes of age. When the five minute APGAR is less than 7, additional scores should be obtained every five minutes for up to 20 minutes or until two consecutive scores are 8 or above. Additional scores are used to record the effectiveness of life-support interventions and any corresponding changes in the baby's condition. The APGAR score may be noted at odd times (for example, at 3 minutes) as a way of recording improvement. The APGAR can be continuously assessed every five minutes until the baby is stable.

Assessing the APGAR parameters in untraumatized, healthy homeborn babies

Have a stethoscope on hand and listen to the lungs and heart, unless the baby is fully pink, well-flexed, active and alert with good respirations or crying. Note that homeborn babies are often quite relaxed at birth and many do not cry. This usually does not mean the baby is in trouble, especially if the cord is still intact. If the baby's limbs are not fully flexed at birth, check muscle tone by grasping a wrist or ankle, extending the limb and seeing if the baby offers resistance. You can also see if the baby will grip your finger. Grimace response is present if the baby responds to tactile stimulation (such as touching the lips or inserting a finger shallowly into the mouth). A baby who is pink, alert, inflating her lungs well on auscultation, and has a heart rate above 100 is in very good shape, with an APGAR of 9 or 10.

The meaning of the score

The score places babies with a value of 7 or above in the range of normal newborn variation, with scores less than 7 considered to reflect varying degrees of distress. The score is a discontinuous scale, with the "biological distance" between values of 1 and 4 being much larger than that between 7 and 10. As an APGAR score of 1 improves to 4, resuscitation has been successful at reversing the condition of a baby nearing death. In babies who have a one minute score of 7, an improving APGAR reflects shades of normal newborn response during the transition to breathing room air.

Although, generally speaking, the degree of asphyxia is worse when the APGAR score is lower, as mentioned earlier, this is not always the case. It is possible for an infant not to be asphyxiated and still have a low APGAR score, depending upon which signs are scoring low. It is also possible for babies to have a low score for reasons other than asphyxia. It is now well recognized that the APGAR score does not reliably predict the long-term outcome for the baby.

The limits of the APGAR assessment: The APGAR score is useful only to a point. For one thing, it is a subjective assessment and therefore is best performed by the most impartial birth assistant present, preferably not the midwife who received the baby. Criteria such as muscle tone, color and reflex irritability are partly dependent upon the gestational age of the baby; early babies, even those who have not experienced any oxygen deprivation, score lower in all these areas. Medications given to the mother and some conditions of the newborn may also skew the APGAR score.

Because the APGAR score assesses the depression of vital functions, abnormal conditions that cause an increase in respiration or heart rate may artificially improve the score. Some neuromuscular or cerebral malformations can increase muscle tone and respiratory effort. Thus, infants compromised with these types of disorders will not be accurately identified, and a high score may not accurately reflect the infant's status.

Likewise, certain cardiorespiratory conditions may depress the baby's heart rate, respirations and muscle tone. Infection may result in depression or irritation of the baby's muscle tone, color may be poor, and the baby's response to resuscitation depressed. Because of these kinds of underlying problems, it is inappropriate to assume that a low score automatically indicates that the baby has suffered from asphyxia or hypoxic insult.

Despite such limitations, the APGAR score is a universally applied evaluation of the baby in the minutes following birth and is useful as a way of communicating about the condition of the baby in your records and to other practitioners.

CLINICAL SIGNS AND TYPICAL APGAR SCORES OF BABIES WITH VARYING DEGREES OF DEPRESSION

PARAMETER	LEVEL OF RESPIRATORY DEPRESSION			
	None	Mild	Moderate	Severe
Color	1 to 2	0 to 1	0	0
Respirations	2	1 to 2	0	0
Tone	1 to 2	1 to 2	0 to 1	0
Reflex irritability	2	2	1 to 2	0 to 1
Heart rate	2	2	2	0 to 2
TOTALS	8 to 10	7 to 9	4 to 5	0 to 3

(Graves, 1988)

Responding to and understanding APGAR scores: The one minute score is most reflective of the baby's condition in utero. Most newly homeborn term infants are quite vigorous with APGAR scores of 8 to 10. These babies need no specific support other than to ensure a clear airway and that they are not chilled.

If the one minute APGAR falls between 5 and 7, the baby will have a varying degree of poor color, decreased respiratory effort, decreased muscle tone or all three, but good reflex irritability and a heart rate over 100 bpm. This baby usually responds well to stimulation but needs close observation.

A one minute APGAR of 3 to 5 represents moderate depression with poor color, decreased tone, and reduced reflex irritability. The baby's heart rate will probably be over 100 bpm. Cover the basics (clear airway, drying, warmth) and observe for steady improvement (assuming an intact cord). Offer a few ventilations with a bag and mask, if indicated. Observe responses carefully and proceed as indicated.

A baby with a 1 min APGAR of 3 or less is in serious trouble. He may be gray or blue gray, apneic with no response to stimulation and have a heart rate less than 100 bpm. This baby requires a full-scale resuscitation effort.

Are babies with low scores acidotic? It was long assumed that babies with low scores were acidotic at birth. This has been refuted with research that shows only a minority of babies with scores less than 7 at either 1 or 5 min to be acidotic. Likewise, of those who proved to be significantly acidotic, 73% had APGAR scores over 7 at 1 min and 86% had scores over 7 at five min. The score appears to be more reliable at ruling out acidosis than predicting it (Levinson et al., 2002).

However, the need for positive-pressure ventilation coupled with cardiac compressions are predictive of more unfavorable outcomes when the baby is also acidotic (pH < 7.00). Conversely, babies requiring the same degree of resuscitation who had normal cord blood pH tend to have a normal outcome (Volpe, 2001).

Can the APGAR score predict the likelihood of death? The APGAR score appears to be a useful prognostic tool in predicting short-term mortality for groups of infants, especially those of low birthweight, although it is less useful when trying to predict the outcome for an individual baby. The duration of delayed onset of breathing is an important prognostic sign, presumably because it reflects the severity of intrauterine insult. This is underscored by a study of 165 babies, 42% of whom had an increased rate of death or subsequent neurological deficits when breathing was delayed 1 to 9 minutes; 56% had similar outcomes when breathing was delayed 10 to 19 minutes and 88% of whom are thus compromised when breathing was delayed more than 20 minutes (Volpe, 2001).

Very low birthweight infants tend to have a higher mortality regardless of their score, although one study found significantly worse outcomes among babies whose scores were poor. In another study, APGAR scores of 0 or 1 at one min were associated with a mortality rate of 23% in the first 27 days of life, decreasing to 0.1% for infants with 1 min scores of 10. The 27-day mortality rate for infants with 5 min scores of 0 or 1 was 49%; this decreased with increasingly good scores. This study also showed that the APGAR score more accurately predicts death in the first 2 days of life rather than the period from 2 to 27 days and that the 5 min score is the most useful in this respect. This trend was most pronounced in babies with low birthweight and in babies weighing over 4000 grams, probably because some of these large babies were from diabetic mothers or because they suffered injury during a difficult birth. In additional studies, lower 5 min scores (0 to 3) were associated with a 10- to 15-fold increase in mortality during the first year of life than were high scores of 7 to 10. Among babies with a low score at 20 minutes after birth, 59% of term infants and 96% of low birthweight (less than 2500 g) died by the end of their first year. (Studies are summarized in Sniderman et al., 2002.)

Does a low APGAR score predict long-term neurologic problems? Hypoxic ischemic brain injury can cause a low APGAR score, and a low score implies the possibility of ongoing brain damage. Therefore, predicting the long-term outcome for babies with low scores has been attempted for many years. This approach is fraught with problems, however, because quantification of the score varies among practitioners, often dramatically. Second, each of the five criteria are given equal weight, even though the relevance of each to central nervous system integrity differs significantly. Finally, depressed scores may result from a variety of problems other than hypoxic-ischemic insult, including aspiration with laryngeal inhibition, suctioning (which triggers a vasovagal response with respiratory and cardiac depression) and preterm birth, all of which have a favorable prognosis if other complicating factors are absent (Volpe, 2001).

A low APGAR score at one minute does not predict an individual baby's future outcome, regardless of how low it may be. Even when the one minute score is 0 (apparent stillbirth), one study found a 40% rate of survival, with 60% of those babies surviving neurologically intact (Jain et al., 1991). The five minute assessment, and especially the change in the score from one to five minutes, is a useful index of the effectiveness of measures being taken to stabilize the infant. The studies summarized by Sniderman and colleagues (2002) that looked at short-term mortality were extended to look at long-term neurologic morbidity. At one year of age, neurologic assessments were correlated to one and five minute scores and birthweight. Of 14,155 infants, 1.9% had definite neurologic problems; 3.6% of these had one minute scores of 0 to 3. The incidence of problems dropped to 1.6% among infants with one minute scores of 7 to 10. When the five minute score was assessed, the disparity was greater, with abnormalities appearing in infants with low scores four times more frequently than among those in the high-score group. Birthweight was still highly significant, with a 6-fold rise in neurologic impairment in babies weighing 1001 to 2000 grams at birth when compared with those weighing over 2500 grams. However, note that even a five minute score of 0 to 3, which *may* be the result of a hypoxic insult, has limited usefulness as an indication of the severity of the problem, and correlates poorly with future neurologic well-being for individual babies.

The same studies also looked at the rate of cerebral palsy, mental retardation and other minor handicaps among these children up to 7 years of age. Although the incidence of cerebral palsy was higher among those with low APGAR scores, 73% of affected children had normal scores at birth. Even a score as low as 0 to 3 at five minutes correlated poorly with future neurologic outcome. However, a child with a 1 min APGAR of 0 to 3 but a ten minute APGAR of 4 or greater has a 1% change of developing cerebral palsy. Of those with a 15 minute score of 0 to 3, 53% die and 38% of the survivors will later develop cerebral palsy. Of babies with a 20 minute score of 0 to 3, 59% die and 57% of the survivors go on to develop cerebral palsy. Most children who develop cerebral palsy are not asphyxiated at birth (Polin & Spitzer, 2001).

A five minute score of 7 or above is considered normal. However, because the APGAR is a rather crude tool, subtle effects of perinatal asphyxia or maternal medication may be missed. Babies with normal scores may be found to have profound neurologic depression with the use of more sophisticated assessment techniques. Five-minute scores of 4, 5 and 6 are intermediate and are not high-risk markers of later neurological impairment. Therefore, a low APGAR score cannot be taken by itself as evidence of or as the result of substantial asphyxia and is not sufficient reason to assume, for example, that cerebral palsy developed as the result of prenatal asphyxia. The term "asphyxia" in a clinical context should be reserved to describe a combination of damaging factors including acidemia, hypoxia, and metabolic acidosis.

Correlation of the APGAR score with future neurologic health increases when the score remains between 0 and 3 at 10, 15 and 20 minutes after birth but still does not indicate the cause of any future disability. However, when the APGAR score is still zero at 10 minutes, the chances of survival are very slim (Volpe, 2001). A newborn who has had "asphyxia" near the time of birth severe enough to result in acute neurologic injury demonstrates all of the following:

- Profound metabolic or mixed acidemia (pH < 7.00) on an umbilical cord arterial blood sample. (This will be impossible to assess at home and interferes with placental transfusion, so it is not recommended.)
- Persistence of an APGAR score of 0 to 3 for longer than 5 minutes
- Neonatal neurologic signs and symptoms such as seizures, coma, and poor muscle tone *and* multisystem organ dysfunction reflective of neonatal neurologic damage (e.g., the cardiovascular, gastrointestinal, hematologic, or pulmonary systems must show evidence of compromise)
- Other possible causes of neurologic compromise include preexisting brain lesions and should be excluded before perinatal asphyxia is assigned as the cause.

The link between cerebral palsy and prenatal hypoxia is weak, and the causes of most cases remain unknown or unrecognized. In children without cerebral palsy, mental retardation and other neurologic disorders were not more commonly associated with low APGAR scores. While mental retardation and epilepsy sometimes accompany cerebral palsy, there is no evidence that they are caused by perinatal asphyxia unless cerebral palsy is also present, and even then the relationship of these conditions is still not certain (ACOG, 1986).

One aspect of routine contemporary care that was not addressed in this opinion is premature cord clamping, which, given all the previously discussed effects, may have a profound effect on the brain and neurological development over the first year of life. Even if the cord blood shows a normal pH, the clamping required to obtain the sample may, in fact, be the very thing that pushes a compromised infant over the line and eventually leads to brain damage (Morley, 2002). Thus, while obstetrical care during labor may not contribute directly to the development of cerebral palsy, routine early clamping of the cord very well may. Babies who have also experienced asphyxia or hypovolemia secondary to prolonged cord compression in utero would be even more vulnerable to these adverse effects.

Stages of recovery in depressed babies

The five minute score is most reflective of the infant's spontaneous adaptation to life outside the womb or to resuscitation efforts. The progress of recovery for the infant with an initially low APGAR score will generally begin with an increase in the heart rate (if it was low or absent). The heart should respond as soon as effective resuscitation efforts begin. If the heart rate was not particularly slow, the first sign of recovery will be an increase or return of reflexes such as the grimace response (the baby moves her mouth or screws up her face during ventilation), then a rise in respiratory effort, followed closely by increased heart rate and restoration of good color, which may take 3 to 5 minutes. At this point, grimace response will continue to improve, and finally muscle tone will return, but it will usually take longer to fully normalize than all the other parameters, often as long as 15 to 20 minutes. How long depends upon how long the baby was asphyxiated.

STATES OF NEWBORN CONSCIOUSNESS AND BEHAVIOR

The newborn has a predictable, directed repertoire of responses when interacting socially with a nurturing adult as well as when responding to both positive and negative tactile, visual and auditory stimuli. The intensity of these neurological responses as well as his interest in nursing and bonding is influenced by the baby's state of consciousness or behavior. **Consciousness** is the degree to which an individual is aware while **behavior** refers to responses. Although consciousness and behavior affect finding at all ages, they are looked at more formally together in newborns because of the immaturity of the nervous system at birth. In fact, most neuromechanisms in babies are dependent on the behavioral state, making it the most sensitive of all indicators of neurologic function. Thus, assessment of the newborn is only meaningful when the behavioral state is understood and noted in relationship to the response during assessment. The optimal behavioral state for any test is one in which a response of medium intensity is consistently elicited. Therefore, it is important to have an understanding of the clinical ranking of newborn states prior to interpreting newborn activity and response. These states may be self-evident to anyone who has had experience with newborns; however, the summaries below will help the student better understand how the baby might respond in different states, and will also illuminate the recommendations regarding behavioral states in the subchapter entitled "Developmental Reflexes and Other Neuromotor Evaluations" in this portion of the text.

NEWBORN STATES OF CONSCIOUSNESS AND BEHAVIOR	
SLEEP STATES	
Deep or quiet sleep	No spontaneous activity, except occasional startles, twitches or sucking motions at regular intervals. The eyes are firmly closed and still. Startles with some delay, only from intense external stimuli. Suppression of startles is rapid, and the baby quickly returns to deep sleep. Respirations are abdominal, deep, regular, smooth and relatively slow, averaging 36 breaths/min.
Light or active sleep	Eyes closed but may open briefly at intervals. Isolated rapid eye movements under closed lids, lasting several seconds, indicate dream activity. Some isolated body movement, with random startles, twitches, writhing and stretching, lasting several seconds. Movements are smoother and more monitored than in deep sleep. Sucking movements occur on and off; infant is responsive to internal and external stimuli, frequently with startles, often resulting in a change to a drowsy state. May occasionally smile, frown, grimace, move the mouth and make brief fussy or crying sounds. Breathing is irregular, costal, usually faster than in quiet sleep, averaging 46 breaths/min.
AWAKE STATES	
Drowsy; semi-dozing	Eyes open and close occasionally or flutter. Baby is heavy-lidded with dull, glazed appearance. Facial movement possible, but face often appears still. Activity varies, with interspersed mild startles; reactive to stimuli; movements are smooth but responses are delayed. State change after stimulation is frequently noted. Fussing may be present. Breathing is fairly regular, but faster and more shallow than during quiet sleep.
Quiet alert	Alert, bright, wide eyes with minimal body movements. Attentive to environment; focuses attention on any available stimuli. A few spontaneous startles, reactive to stimulation with increase in startles or activity level. Additional stimulus may draw the attention, but with some delay. Intermittent fussing does not result in change of state. Breathing is regular for a baby (all babies breathe somewhat irregularly).
Active alert; fussy	Same characteristics as for quiet alert, but mild, agitated vocalizations are continuous, or one burst of crying may occur. Much body activity with fussiness, eyes open with less brightening, face active, irregular breathing. Baby is increasingly sensitive to disturbing stimuli (hunger, fatigue, noise, excessive handling) and may fuss.
Crying	Same as for quiet alert, but generalized motor activity is more intense and there is intense crying that is difficult to break through with stimulation. Very responsive to all unpleasant stimuli. Increased motor activity, color changes in skin, eyes tightly shut or open, grimaces, breathing more irregular.

(Brazelton, 1973, 1999; Illingworth, 1970, 1987)

Each of these states is relatively distinct; however, the normal infant makes smooth, almost imperceptible transitions from one state to another. The ability to make these transitions smoothly on a regular basis is a hallmark of normal newborn behavior and neurologic well-being. These responses depend upon a number of physiologic variables including hunger, nutrition, hydration, timing within individual sleep-wake cycles and gestational age. Preterm babies are sleepier and less alert than those born at term, but all normal infants display the full range of behaviors listed in the table.

Typical newborn behavior

Behavioral responses also offer valuable clues about cerebral integrity. How the baby behaves and how competently he can maintain "organized" behavior are signs of neurological health. For example, if the baby is awake and resting quietly in your lap and is then gently transferred to your shoulder, does he make a smooth transition from one position to another or does the change prompt flailing of the limbs, crying or grimacing? These are important indicators of the status of neurologic function and can indicate if the baby is in pain or is ill. Examples of normal responses follow.

Irritability: The baby responds to aversive stimuli such as uncovering, undressing, being pulled to sit, being turned over, ventral suspension or elicitation of reflexes such as the Moro by audibly crying or fussing for at least 3 seconds. Normal babies react for several seconds but start to calm down almost as soon as the stimulus is removed. Relatively benign activities should prompt no intense response. Activities such as eliciting the Moro response are more irritating than undressing or the pull-to-sit maneuver. Observe for reactions as well as how strong a stimulus must be in order to elicit a response. Abnormal babies may have exaggerated responses to less irritating stimuli, a prolonged reaction or no reaction in spite of a strong stimulus. Preterm babies tend to have a less intense crying reaction to the same stimuli, especially when they have experienced a lot of discomfort in the course of care. They may respond with decreases in oxygen saturation, apnea or a mass reflex such as a startle rather than crying.

Cuddliness: A normal, alert infant should respond to being held in both vertical and horizontal positions. She may resist being held by pushing away, thrashing or stiffening or may nestle by turning her head toward the person holding her and molding her body to theirs. Do not confuse hypotonia with cuddliness.

Self-quieting activity: A crying baby should make observable efforts to calm himself. This ranges from making no attempt to quiet without the caregiver intervening to sustained self-quieting with no outside help needed. Such activities include rooting, mouthing an object such as a fist, modulating the intensity of his cry, shifting position or becoming visually attentive.

Visual and auditory response habituation (decrement): This is demonstrated when the baby is repeatedly presented with an aversive stimulus. The baby should be able to accustom herself to a specific stimuli, controlling startles by delaying and finally decreasing localized startle response. Full decrement is when the baby shuts out or ignores the stimuli altogether. Similar responses can be elicited with disturbing visual or auditory stimuli. After habitation is achieved, substitution of a new stimulus in a series results in the response returning. This is called dehabitation. Short-term memory, the ability to discriminate between two stimuli and the ability to respond are all necessary for this behavior. You need not formally evaluate for habituation or decrement but can watch for it as you relate to the baby postpartum. Habituation is discussed further in the subchapter entitled "Evaluating the Newborn with Suspected Neurological Compromise."

Visual and auditory orientation: The awake and alert baby should be able to fixate on and follow an interesting object with his eyes. This may occur only briefly or may extend to complex following. A similar response is observed with pleasant sounds. An absence of vertical head movement when following is not abnormal although side-to-side movement frequently occurs.

Defensive reaction: Normal term babies should actively participate in certain defensive reactions. For example, a cloth covering the face should be swiped away and directly removed. Other responses to such an obstruction include general quieting, twisting of the body, head turning or nondirected swipes. Babies may express a defensive reaction in other unpleasant situations, such as when they are held in an uncomfortable position, dislike their clothing, or feel smothered by bedclothes. (This chapter was based on Brazelton, 1999; Illingworth, 1987; Prechtl, 1977.)

Assessment of Gestational Age

A baby's physical characteristics, neuromuscular control, response and reflexes, sensory capabilities and general behavior all progress through predictable stages as the fetus grows. These stages, within certain limits, make it possible to assess the gestational age of the newborn. Conversely, knowing a baby's approximate gestational age is an important prerequisite to accurate physical assessment of the baby in every other respect. Thus, in this book, gestational age assessment is included before most other types of assessments are discussed. In many cases, you will not need to formally assess gestational age; however, these evaluations are important for midwives to know. You may need to assess the gestational age of an infant whose mother has not been seen prenatally throughout her pregnancy, or you may be surprised by two small babies rather than the large one you expected. This chapter is offered as a reference for when you are uncertain of the baby's age or for when you need to communicate intelligently with other professionals. If you have carefully attempted to assess gestational age during pregnancy, this evaluation is hopefully nothing more than a confirmation of what you already know.

There are five basic methods of estimating gestational age: having a known date of conception (the best); calculation of the due date based on the last menstrual period (approximate); evaluation of the progress of the pregnancy with palpation, fundal height measurement; quickening and timing of auscultating the fetal heart for the first time; and ultrasound examination and assessment of the fetus using physical and neurologic criteria (which is increasingly imprecise as pregnancy advances). Size is not one of the criteria used in assessing gestational age after early pregnancy because the health of an otherwise normal newborn can be greatly influenced by the mother's nutritional status. A well-nourished mother may give birth to an early baby who is substantially larger than data predict; likewise, her truly postdates baby may also appear plump and healthy. Tests for gestational age are therefore based on the baby's state of maturity, independent of weight and size at birth.

Gestational age is reckoned as the completed weeks of pregnancy after the onset of the last menstrual period. For example, a baby who has been in utero for 38 weeks and 3 days is in his 39th week of gestation. Babies born prior to 37 completed weeks of gestation (36 weeks and 6 days) are considered preterm. Those born between the beginning of the first day of the 38th week though the end of the last day of the 41st week are considered to be at term. Those born after 42 weeks (42 weeks plus 1 day or more) are considered postterm. Gestational age is counted from the first day of the last menstrual period, even though conception occurs two weeks later. Thus, the baby born at 40 weeks of pregnancy (right on time) is also considered to be at 40 weeks gestation for the purposes of this assessment (Fletcher, 1999).

The most widely recognized gestational age assessment tool is the Dubowitz scale, published in 1970. This system assessed 10 neurologic and 11 physical criteria. In 1979 a modified scale was introduced by Ballard. Both systems were criticized for overestimating the actual gestational age by about two weeks. The Ballard tool was modified twelve years later (Ballard, 1991) to better assess extremely preterm infants; it now overestimates gestational age by only 0.3 to 0.6 weeks (2 to 4 days) if the baby is 37 weeks or less, according to Ballard (1991), but recent studies found it to be off by 1.3 to 3.3 weeks in infants less than 28 weeks; thus there is no really accurate way to assess the extremely preterm infant (Sola & Chow, 1999). There are numerous other scales that are generally less well-known than these two. For the sake of simplicity, and because this book is for midwives and not neonatologists, the New Ballard score is presented here.

Note that, while I draw correlations between individual scores and gestational age in weeks, these are mentioned for study and not as part of the assessment. There was no reference that gave gestational estimations for every assessment, so these are best guesses. In addition, a single assessment is too limited to allow determination of a baby's age because of variations and overlap in the maturation of all the signs. The most accurate score is obtained when the entire assessment is performed. The scoring should be practiced once the basics of the exam are understood using the abbreviated forms found on the following pages and without reference to the gestational age parameters mentioned.

Circumstances of Assessment

Determining which babies to assess

Any baby who does not appear to fit into the physical and neurological limits of a normal term baby should be evaluated more closely. Any newborn whose weight is below the tenth percentile ("low birthweight," 2500 grams or less at birth) should be evaluated. These babies may have been born either early or at term but are truly small for gestational age. Likewise, a baby who is large for gestational age may be macrosomic or simply larger than average. A truly macrosomic baby could also be preterm. These size relationships are explained in detail in the chapter entitled "Assessment of the Baby's Size and Its Relationship to Gestational Age."

The following two charts are modified versions of the New Ballard score assessment forms. The physical findings are evaluated as part of every normal newborn examination; the neuromuscular criteria are added when there is further question regarding gestational age. The score is arrived at by taking the total from the physical criteria and the neuromuscular criteria and adding them together. The score is then used to approximate gestational age according to the scale provided at the end of this chapter.

PHYSICAL SIGN	PHYSICAL MATURITY SCORE							RECORD SCORE HERE
	-1	0	1	2	3	4	5	
Skin	Sticky, friable, transparent	Very thin, gelatinous, red, translucent	Thin, smooth, pink, visible veins	Smooth, medium thickness, superficial peeling or rash; few veins	Slight thickening, stiff, cracking, pale areas, very few veins	Dry, deep cracking, no veins visible	Leathery, cracked, wrinkled	
Lanugo	None	Sparse	Abundant	Thinning	Bald areas	Mostly absent		
Plantar surface of foot	Heel-toe: 40-50 mm: -1 <40 mm: -2	Heel-toe: > 50 mm No creases	Faint red marks	Anterior transverse crease only	Creases over anterior ⅔ of sole	Creases over entire sole		
Breast	Invisible	Barely perceptible features	Flat areola: no breast bud palpable	Stippled areola: 1-2 mm breast bud	Raised areola: 3-4 mm breast bud	Full areola: 5-10 mm breast bud		
Eye/Ear	Lids fused: loosely: –1 tightly: –2	Lids open; Pinna flat, stays folded	Soft, slightly curved pinna; slow recoil	Well-curved pinna; soft but ready recoil	Pinna formed & firm; instant recoil	Thick cartilage; ear stiff		
Genitals (male)	Scrotum flat, smooth, empty	Scrotum, empty; faint rugae	Testes in upper canal; rare rugae	Testes descending, few rugae	Testes descended, many rugae	Testes down; deep rugae		
Genitals (female)	Prominent clitoris; labia majora & minora flat	Prominent clitoris; small labia minora	Prominent clitoris; enlarging labia minora	Labia majora & minora equally prominent	Labia majora large; labia minora small	Labia majora cover labia minora & clitoris		
							TOTAL PHYSICAL MATURITY SCORE	

Neuromuscular Maturity Sign	Score							Record Score Here
	-1	0	1	2	3	4	5	
Posture	Limbs tend to stay wherever they are placed 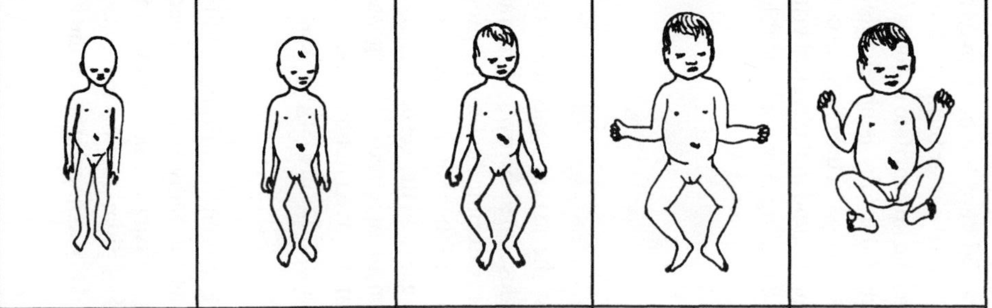							
Square window (wrist)	>90° 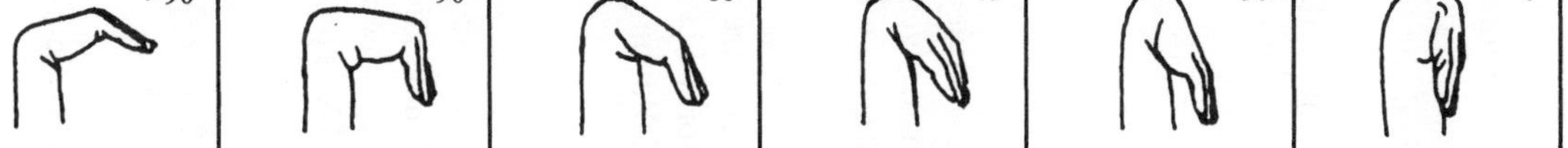	90°	60°	45°	30°	0°		
Scarf sign	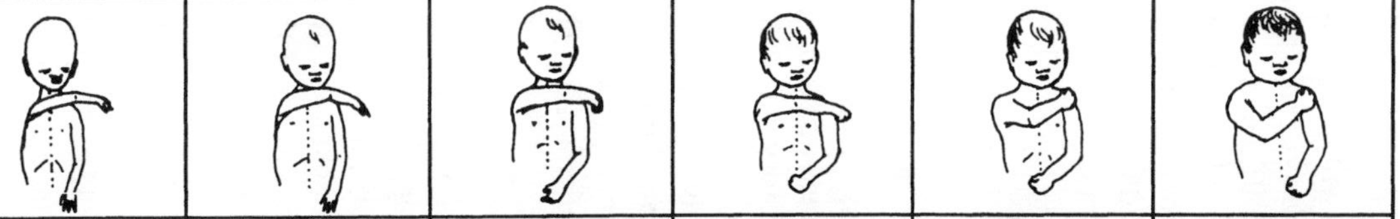							
Arm recoil	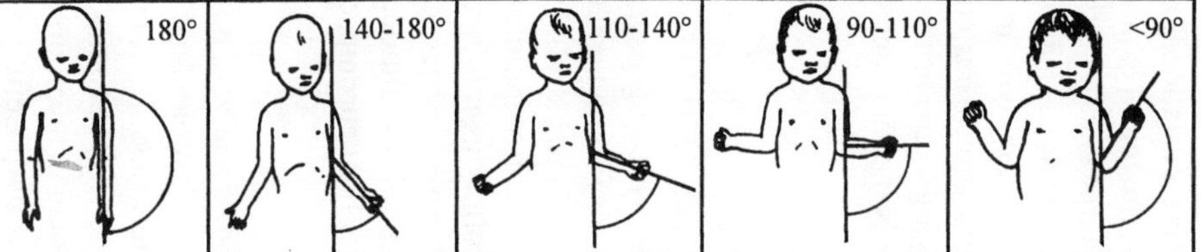	180°	140-180°	110-140°	90-110°	<90°		
Popliteal angle	180° 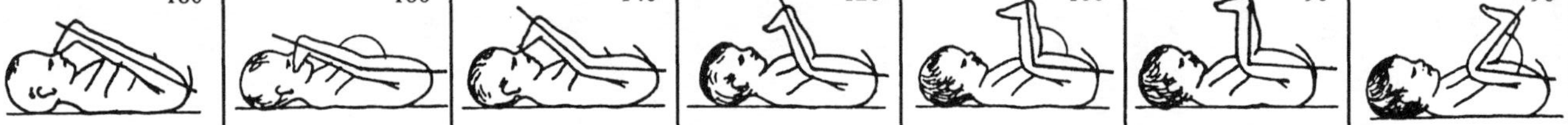	160°	140°	120°	100°	90°	<90°	
Heel to ear	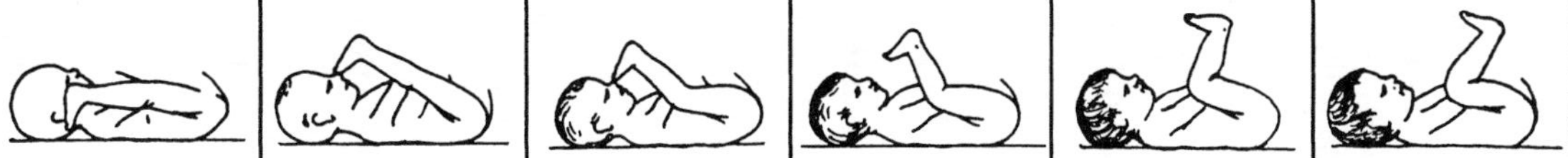							
							Total Neuromuscular Maturity Score	

Timing the gestational age assessment

The following criteria for the best time to perform this assessment have been suggested (Thureen et al., 1999):

20 to 26 week gestation: Perform the exam within 12 hours of birth.
More than 26 weeks gestation: The exam is valid if done during the first 96 hours of life.

However, there is debate regarding the ideal timing of the exam because the neuromuscular adjustment that the baby experiences following birth may alter the results. This adjustment is complicated by superimposed factors that may further alter the normal neuromuscular response of the baby. Such factors include fetal or neonatal asphyxia, maternal drug intake, and medications given directly to the baby. The most common reason for a midwife in homebirth practice to be performing this exam is to determine gestational age in order to assess what special care the baby may require and whether transport is in order. Thus, the initial exam will most likely be performed shortly after birth. Follow-up exams may be called for if the findings disagree significantly with other parameters, such as the known date of the last menstrual period, the date of conception, or other assessments. If the neurological condition of the baby is unreliable at birth for reasons such as those described above, Dubowitz and colleagues (1970) recommend assessing the physical criteria alone, multiplying that score by two, and assigning a gestational age based on the total. They found that physical criteria scored together were more reliable than trying to arrive at a total score when the neurologic findings are questionable; however, the total score using all parameters is the most accurate.

New Ballard Score

Physical maturity assessments

First, review the charts on the preceding pages, which offer an overview of the assessments used to determine gestational age. The technique for performing each examination or maneuver is described below. Accuracy requires experience as well as consideration of the baby's history and state of consciousness during the scoring process. Even very premature infants who are hooked up to monitors can be examined because none of these assessments require lifting the baby. Many midwives use the following minimally intrusive evaluations when gauging the gestational age of a baby. Since most of your babies will be born at or near term, these assessments are often sufficient to verify gestational age. The neuromuscular assessments that follow, although important to a formal evaluation, need not be done unless you are still uncertain about the baby's age or her neuromuscular health. The following descriptions are largely based on Ballard (1979, 1991).

Skin: Examine the skin over the abdominal wall both by picking up a fold of skin between your thumb and index finger and by visual inspection. The texture, color and opacity of the skin changes as the baby matures, because of the development of thicker subcutaneous tissue. Extremely preterm infants have sticky, transparent skin; they score –1. With age, veins become less visible as the skin becomes thicker and more opaque and as pigmentation increases. The soft subtle skin may begin to crack and peel in the hours following birth. This is most likely to happen when the baby is born with no vernix or when the vernix is purposefully removed with soap.

Scoring:
- –1: Dark red, sticky, easily damaged, transparent (20 to 28 weeks)
- 0: Red, very thin with a gelatinous texture (26 to 32 weeks)
- 1: Pink, thin and smooth, visible veins (32 to 36 weeks)
- 2: Smooth and of medium thickness; irritation, rash and superficial peeling may be present, few visible veins (36 to 39 weeks)
- 3: Pale areas, slight thickening and stiff texture with superficial cracking and peeling, especially of the hands and feet, very few indistinct veins are visible (40 to 42 weeks)
- 4: Thick and parchment-like texture with superficial or deep cracking, no veins visible
- 5: Leathery texture with cracks and wrinkles, no veins visible. (42+ weeks)

Lanugo: Examine the back between and over the scapulae for the presence and length of lanugo (baby body hair). It may help to shine a flashlight at an angle over the region being examined. Lanugo first appears at 19 to 20 weeks but is not usually obvious until a few weeks later. Development peaks at 28 to 30 weeks gestation, when it covers the entire back;

it then gradually falls out in patches of baldness, beginning on the lower back and moving up toward the shoulders as the baby matures. Lanugo may still be abundant over the upper back (especially between the scapulae) even at term, and it may be noted over the face, legs, arms and shoulders as well, especially in Hispanic babies or those of Southern European descent (dark-skinned Caucasians). The pigmentation and quantity of body hair correlate with the baby's race, sex and nutritional status.

Scoring:
- –1: No lanugo (–20 weeks)
- 0: Sparse distribution (appears at 20 to 21 weeks)
- 1: Abundant, long and thick over the entire back (21 to 30+ weeks)
- 2: Hair thinning, especially over lower back (30+ to 37+ weeks)
- 3: Small amount of lanugo remains with bald areas (38 to 41+ weeks)
- 4: Sparse lanugo remains, mostly over the upper back (41+ weeks)

Plantar creases of foot: The sole (plantar surface) of the foot is examined for length in very preterm babies. Foot length is measured from the tip of the big toe to the base of the heel. Foot length is primarily of academic interest for midwives, since you are unlikely to care for babies born early enough for this assessment to be relevant.

In babies born closer to term, the sole is examined for creases, which must be distinguished from wrinkles. Normal muscle activity and uterine compression result in plantar and palmar creases. Look for the presence and distribution of pronounced, indented creases that are deep and well defined. Wrinkles are more superficial and less distinct. Creases begin to appear between 28 and 30 weeks, starting from the top of the foot near the toes and progressing downward toward the heel with advancing age. Creases cover the anterior two-thirds of the sole at 36 weeks; by term, the entire sole is creased. The foot will wrinkle dramatically in the hours following birth, rendering this assessment more difficult. Therefore, an initial evaluation is best performed within the first two hours of life. If later, smooth the skin taut over the foot, which will reveal true creases as distinct lines (Ziai et al., 1984). Abnormal creases may be found with certain disorders; serious neuromotor defects of the lower extremities are associated with decreased creasing or only deep vertical creases, while oligohydramnios tends to increase creasing.

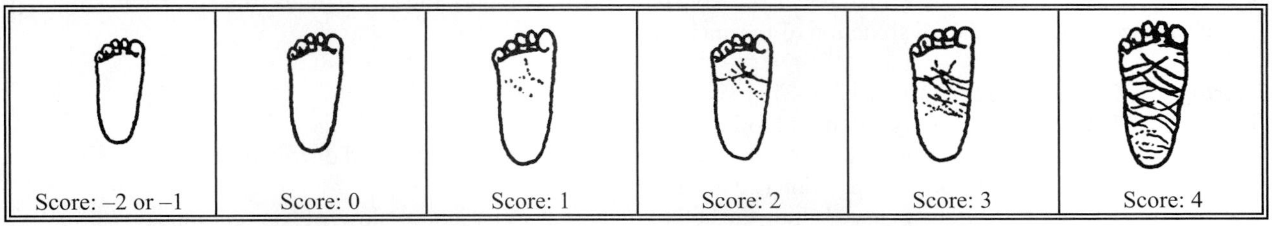

Scoring:
- –2: No creases. Heel to toe length of less than 40 mm (20 to 24+ weeks)
- –1: No creases. Heel to toe length 40 to 50 mm (20 to 28 weeks)
- 0: No creases. Heel to toe length greater than 50 mm (22 to 28+ weeks)
- 1: Faint red marks over anterior half of sole, no creases (28 to 30+ weeks)
- 2: Anterior transverse crease only (30+ to 35 weeks)
- 3: Indented creases over the anterior two-thirds of the sole (36 to 38 weeks)
- 4: Deeply indented creases covering the entire sole of the foot (38+ weeks)

Breasts: The areolae are assessed for color (pigmentation) and stippling (orange peel texture), which both become more pronounced as term approaches. The size of the breast bud is measured by gently grasping it at the edges with your finger and thumb and raising it very slightly up off the chest wall. When present, it feels like a lentil of varying size underlying the areola. All of the features of the breasts become more pronounced as gestational age advances. The nipple and areola can be identified prior to 34 weeks, but they are immature and unpigmented. The nipples becomes erectile between 34 and 36 weeks, and the underlying breast bud can be palpated. The breast bud begins to respond to maternal hormones around the 35th week. By 36 to 38 weeks the bud is more easily felt, and by term it has reached 5 to 10 mm in diameter. While the volume of breast tissue depends somewhat upon fetal nutrition and fat deposits, areolar development occurs with increasing gestational age, independent of these factors.

Scoring: –1: No perceptible breast tissue or areola (–26 weeks)
0: Flat, barely visible pigmenting of the areola (26 to 30+ weeks)
1: Flat, lightly pigmented areola with no underlying breast bud (30 to 33+ weeks)
2: Stippled areola with 1 to 2 mm breast bud (34 to 37+ weeks)
3: Raised, stippled areola with 3 to 4 mm breast bud (37+ to 39+ weeks)
4: Full areola with 5 to 10 mm breast bud (39+ weeks)

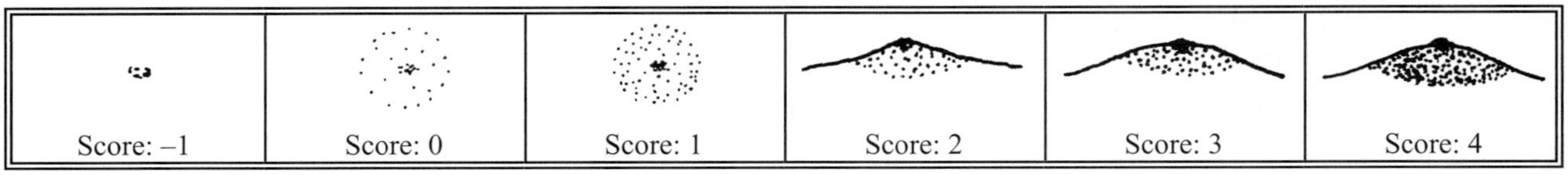

Eyelid fissure (opening): This evaluation is relevant only in very early babies. Hopefully, you will not be caught in an emergency with such an early baby at home. The eyelids are fused in early gestation. Opening starts at 22 weeks, and complete unfusing has usually occurred by 28 weeks. If the baby is very early, evaluate visually for unfused eyelids. Try to part the lids from above and below with *gentle* traction. Two points should be subtracted if the lids are tightly fused (no separation with gentle traction), with one point being subtracted for loosely fused eyelids (partial separation with gentle traction). If the baby is obviously far more mature by other parameters, eyelid fusion is not relevant in the evaluation of gestational age, as it represents an abnormality rather than an indication of maturity. Certain defects, notably anophthalmia (absence of the eye), may be associated with a fused lid at term. The scoring for eyelid fissure is combined with the score for ear cartilage (see below).

Ear cartilage: Ear cartilage becomes firmer with maturity as calcium is preferentially distributed in the last few weeks of pregnancy unless the ear is subjected to continuous pressure in utero or the auricular muscles lack normal anatomy or activity. Evaluate the formation and amount of cartilage in the ear auricle as well as the recoil when it is folded forward and released. The pinnae are flat in very early babies. Incurving of the border (helix) proceeds from the top down toward the lobes as the baby matures. Excessive intrauterine compression of the pinna (due to fetal positioning) may decrease firmness, as can dysfunction of the auricular muscles.

Scoring: (eyes & ears)
–2: Eyelids are tightly fused. (–27 weeks)
–1: Eyelids are loosely fused. (22 to 27 weeks)
0: Eyelids open (23 to 28 weeks); pinna feels soft and is easily folded and distorted without springing back into its original position (20 to 31+ weeks)
1: Pinna soft, slightly curved along the helix; easily folded but returns slowly to an anatomical position on its own (31 to 35+ weeks)
2: Ear cartilage formed and firm and can be felt to the edge of the pinna, which springs back readily after being folded. (36 to 39+ weeks)
3: Pinna is formed and firm with definite cartilage extending to the edge. It springs back instantly into an anatomical position after being folded. (39+ weeks)
4: Ear cartilage is thick and stiff. It springs back instantly when folded. (39+ weeks)

Genitalia: Normal maturation of the genitalia continues right up until term. Accurate assessment of gestational age is therefore essential when evaluating the relative normalcy of genital findings. It will also minimize the possibility of evaluating the genitalia as atypical when they are merely immature.

Female genitalia: With advancing age, the labia minora increase in size before the majora. Eventually, the labia majora fully cover the labia minora. At term, both pairs of lips completely cover the clitoris. Covering depends upon adequate fat disposition and appears abnormally immature with poor nutrition. It may also be increased in the presence of edema or bruising. Girls are assessed with the hips half abducted, based on the prominence of the clitoris as well as the development of the labia minor and majora. The clitoris reaches its term size before 30 weeks due to the influence of maternal hormones, so it appears large in otherwise normal preterm infants. The appearance of a pigmented vertical line, the linea nigra, above the pubis and extending toward the umbilicus suggests a gestational age of at least 36 weeks and is more likely to be seen in babies-of-color. The genitalia should be assessed with the hips partly flexed.

Scoring:

–1: Clitoris prominent and labia flat (–29 weeks)
0: Clitoris prominent with small, widely separated labia majora (29 to 35+ weeks)
1: Clitoris prominent with larger labia minora (32 to 36 weeks)
2: Labia majora are widely separated, labia minora protrude (in a lateral view, they project beyond the labia majora, labia minora and majora are equal in size (34 to 37 weeks)
3: Labia majora are larger than the labia minora, extending around the sides of the clitoris (36 to 39+ weeks)
4: Labia majora cover the clitoris and labia minora (39+ weeks)

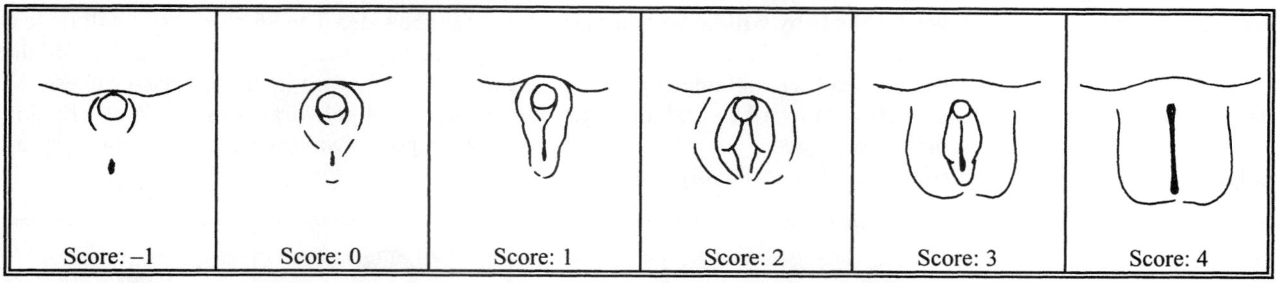

Male genitalia: Boys are assessed for the presence and the degree of descent of the testes into the scrotum. Precise timing of testicular descent occurs during the third trimester, making the testes' progress through the inguinal canal into the scrotum a marker of gestational age. Observe the suspension of the scrotum; it becomes more pendulous if the baby is postdates. Also note the amount of wrinkling (rugae) over the scrotum. Rugae are first visible at 28 weeks and become more pronounced as gestation advances, fully covering the scrotum at term. The testicles must be fully descended at some point for the scrotum to develop fully into its pendulous, ruggated term appearance even if the sac is empty at birth. The presence of edema, a hydrocele or testicular torsion may smooth out the rugae.

Scoring:
–1: Scrotum is flat against the body and smooth (–28 weeks)
0: Scrotum is empty with faint rugae (28 to 30 weeks)
1: Testes are in the upper inguinal canal; a very few scattered rugae appear on the scrotum (27 to 35+ weeks)
2: Testes are descending; a few rugae appear on the anterior scrotum (36 to 39+ weeks)
3: The testes are descended; shallow rugae cover the scrotum (40 to 41+ weeks)
4: The testes are pendulous with deep rugae covering the scrotum (41+ weeks)

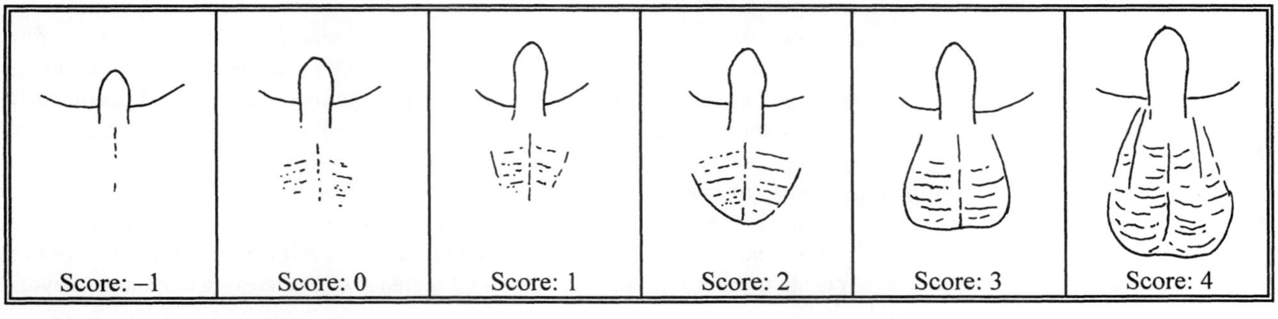

<u>Neuromuscular assessments</u>

Neuromuscular maturity is generally marked by increasing tone and flexion as the infant nears term; maturation of specific muscle groups and related joints results in predictable changes, although there is wide overlap as to when they occur in individual babies. All of the assessments below are based on the understanding that passive tone is more indicative of gestational age than is active tone. These tests are performed with the baby lying on his back (supine) fully supported by a soft, cradling examining surface, such as a feather pillow or a foam mattress, that is firm enough to allow the baby to lie relatively flat but not so firm as to require the baby's spine to be fully flattened against a hard surface.

Posture at rest: The infant is placed nude on her back; her posture is observed while she is quiet and relaxed. Scoring is based on the degree of flexion or extension of the arms, knees and hips. The degree of hip adduction or abduction is also noted. In general, a very preterm baby will lie with arms and legs either extended or in the position in which they are placed. Note that "full extension" of the arms usually involves slight bending at the elbow; because of this, if there is doubt about the score, base your assessment on the posture of the legs. The baby will assume an increasingly flexed posture as gestational age advances first in the legs and later in the arms. Thus, at 28 weeks, the baby lies with all the limbs extended and the legs spread. By 32 weeks, the baby lies with arms extended, but the legs flexed at the knee and spread at the hip. Up until 32 weeks, the baby will lie with her head turned to the side. The 36 week baby will lie less like a frog, primarily maintaining flexion in all limbs and holding the limbs at rest against gravity, that is, up toward the body, even when supine. At term, the head is maintained in line with the trunk, the arms are flexed against the chest, the hands are clenched, and the legs are flexed toward the abdomen. Compression from oligohydramnios accelerates flexion and artificially raises this score. Prolonged poor fetal motor activity or poor swallowing with accompanying polyhydramnios over a long period will also artificially lower the score.

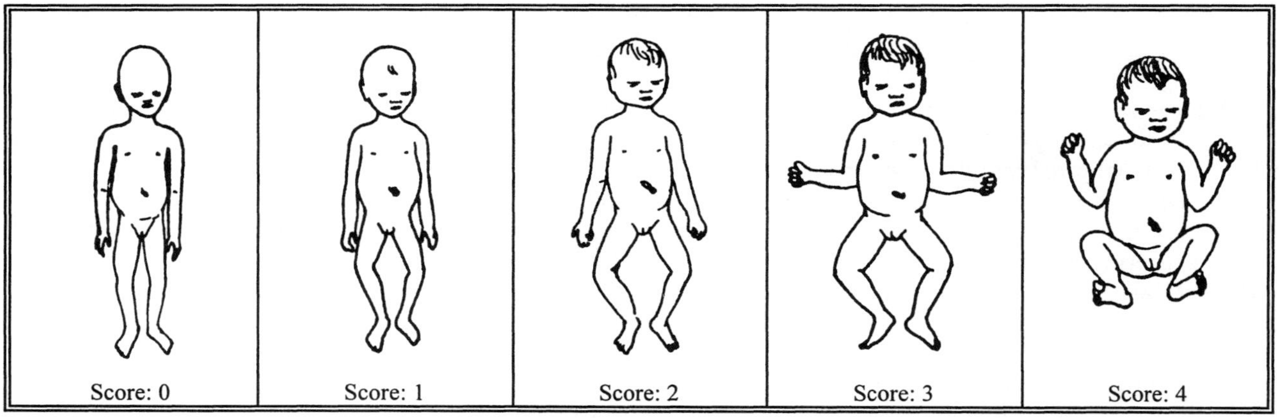

Scoring:

0: Arms and legs fully extended (–29 weeks)
1: Slight flexion of hips and knees, with arms still extended (29 to 31+ weeks)
2: Stronger flexion of legs, with arms extended (31 to 33+ weeks)
3: Legs flexed and abducted, arms slightly flexed (33 to 35+ weeks)
4: Arms and legs are fully flexed. (36+ weeks)

Square window (wrist): Place your thumb on the back of the baby's hand and your index finger on the outside of his wrist. Flex the infant's hand toward his forearm at the wrist, exerting enough pressure to achieve as much flexion as possible without rotating the wrist. The angle between the forearm and the heel of the palm is measured (technically, the angle measured is that between the hypothenar eminence, the fleshy mass on the heel of the palm, and the ventral, or inner, surface of the forearm). Preterm babies have limited flexion; they form a 90° angle with this test. The angle decreases with advancing gestational age; by term, the baby's wrist flexes completely, so that the heel of the palm can be pressed against the forearm. Normally, the response is symmetrical in both wrists, although the angle is somewhat dependent upon in utero positioning. Marked intrauterine pressure, such as might occur with severe oligohydramnios, will artificially increase wrist flexion. It is abnormal for there to be a marked increase or decrease in movement beyond that which is expected for gestational age.

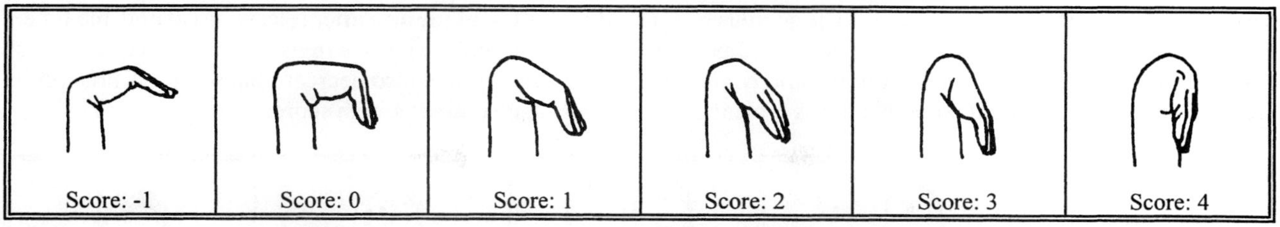

Scoring:

- -1: The heel of palm and forearm form an angle greater than 90° (–28 weeks).
- 0: The heel of palm and forearm form a 90° angle (28 to 31+ weeks).
- 1: The heel of palm and forearm form a 60° angle (31 to 35+ weeks).
- 2: The heel of palm and forearm form a 45° angle (35 to 38 weeks).
- 3: The heel of palm and forearm form a 30° angle (38 to 40 weeks).
- 4: The heel of palm and forearm touch and do not form an angle (41+ weeks).

Scarf sign: The performance of the scarf sign depends upon the maturity of the deltoids, terse major and rhomboid muscles, and indicates shoulder and upper axial tone. With the baby lying supine, position her head in the midline on her shoulders. Grasp one of the baby's hands and pull her arm across the chest and around her neck as far as possible, as though the baby was going to scratch her back over her opposite shoulder (i.e., the arm forms a "scarf" around the neck). You may assist this maneuver by lifting the elbow across the body. Make sure the baby's back remains flat on the mattress. Now assess the position of the elbow in relationship to the midline of the body. This finding uses the midline of the chest and the axillary line (a line drawn from the center of the underarm downward, parallel to the chest wall) as points of reference.

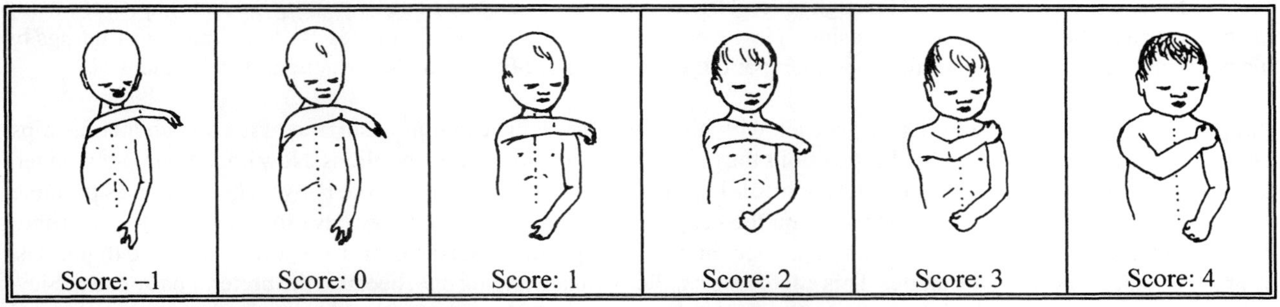

Scoring:

- -1: Elbow can be brought past the opposite axillary line. (–29 weeks)
- 0: Elbow can be brought just past the opposite axillary line. (30 to 35+ weeks)
- 1: Elbow stops at the edge of the border of the opposite axillary line. (36 to 38 weeks)
- 2: Elbow stops at midline of chest. (36 to 39+ weeks)
- 3: Elbow remains parallel with the axillary line on the same side. (39+ weeks)
- 4: Elbow cannot cross the axillary line on the same side. (39+ weeks)

The baby demonstrates increasing resistance to her elbow being pulled past the midline as gestational age advances. Another way to assess this sign is to see how far the baby's hand reaches in relationship to her opposite shoulder; in preterm babies, the hand reaches past the tip of the shoulder (acromion), while in the term baby the hand will reach to the acromion, so that the baby could hold her opposite shoulder, but no further. Obesity decreases the range and raises the score, as does chest wall edema, an abnormally shortened humerus, and hypertonicity of the shoulder girdle. Brachial plexus injury or generalized hypotonia will artificially increase the range of motion and thus lower the score.

Forearm recoil: The baby is placed in a supine position with the head centered on the shoulders. The baby's arms are flexed at the elbow and held against the upper arm. The flexed arm is then held alongside to the chest for five seconds. The arms are then gently but fully extended by bringing the hands down to the baby's sides to extend the elbows. Then release the hands. Do not attempt to simultaneously test for arm traction nor forcefully extend the arms, as other responses will interfere with the score. The score is based on the position of the arm after release. Also note the time it takes for the baby to replace her arm in the flexed posture. Early babies do not resist extension and display a sluggish response with little or no flexion. Any pathology affecting motor strength will also decrease the score. A brisk, fully flexed response that is equal on both sides is typical of a term baby and receives a high score.

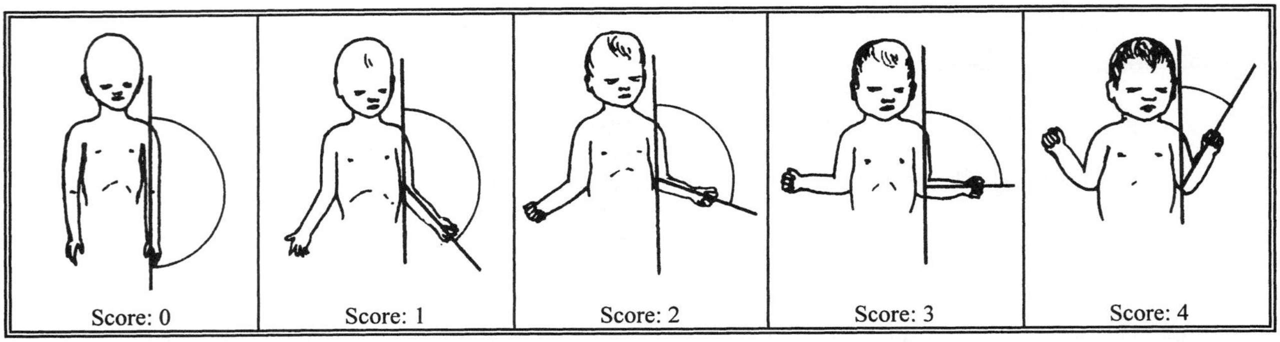

Scoring:

0: Arms remain fully extended. (–32 weeks)
1: Sluggish return to incomplete flexion with arms flexed between 140 and 180° (34+ weeks)
2: Slow return to incomplete flexion with arms flexed between 110 and 140° (36+ weeks)
3: More active return to nearly full flexion between 90 and 110° (38+ weeks)
4: Vigorous return to full flexion with arms flexed less than 90° (40+ weeks)

Abnormal responses include absent, delayed or weak recoil, forceful flexion with stimulation of a mass startle, and asymmetrical responses that persist through several trials. This test can also be done by pulling the hands up, thus raising the entire arm at the shoulder, and releasing. However, the method described eliminates confounding your findings by inadvertently adding traction to the assessment; and the responses to both methods are generally equivalent.

Popliteal angle: Lie the baby flat on his back with his pelvis flat on the examining surface. Flex and abduct the hips, placing the thighs on the abdomen; this positions the knees above the level of the umbilicus. Now hook your index fingers behind the ankles and gently extend (lift) the lower legs in an arch toward the side of the baby's cheek as far as possible, keeping the thigh over the lateral abdomen and the baby's hips on the bed. (You may have to assess one leg at a time.) The popliteal angle is that formed behind the knee, between the posterior surfaces of the lower leg and the thigh. Use your protractor to measure the angle. This angle gets smaller with advancing age, because the preterm baby can achieve greater extension than can the infant at term, as flexion becomes more dominant. Breech presentation, especially frank breech, tends to result in an angle that is greater than expected for age. Testing both limbs together allows you to assess whether the angles are symmetrical. The angle decreases as term approaches and then increases in the first 9 months of life. A posterior hip dislocation will prevent positioning the hip in abduction.

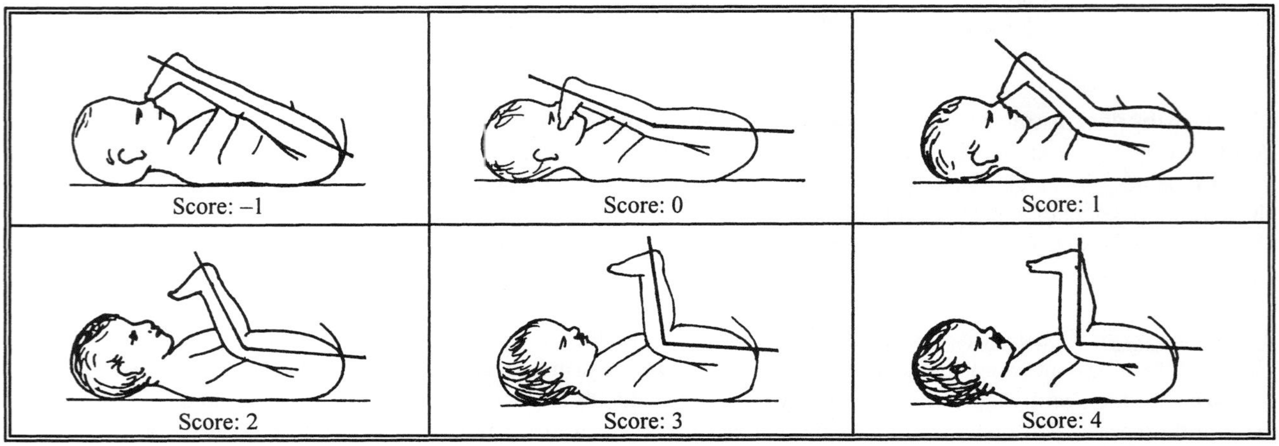

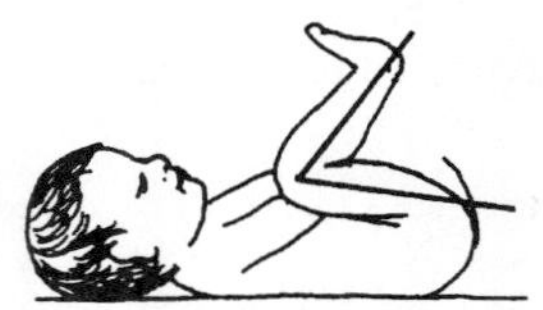

Score: 5

Scoring: --1: Extension is so extreme that the toes touch the baby's face (180° angle) (–28 weeks)

0: Easy but not quite full, extension of the lower leg creating a nearly straight line with the thigh (160°) (26 to 28 weeks)

1: More resistance to full extension, with the lower leg stopping at 140° (29 to 32 weeks)

2: Lower leg stops at 120° (32 to 34 weeks)

3: Lower leg stops just before the midline (100° angle) (33 to 38 weeks)

4: Lower leg stops with the foot straight up in the air (90° angle) (38 to 40 weeks)

5: Lower leg extends less than 90° (40+ weeks)

Heel-to-ear: Lie the baby flat on his back. Grasp a foot gently with your thumb and index fingers and press it as far as possible toward the baby's ear until the foot tends to slip from your fingers, while keeping the baby's pelvis against the table. The thighs and knees are not held in this maneuver and may bend down alongside the abdomen. Note the distance between the foot and the ear as well as the angle made by an arc formed behind the knee. Make your assessment quickly to avoid relaxation at the hip joint which will confuse your result. The baby is increasingly resistant to this maneuver as term approaches, making it difficult and then impossible to fully extend the knees; the angle again increases after birth as the baby matures.

Scoring: -1: Leg extends easily and fully with the heel level with the ear on the same side (–26 weeks).

0: Leg is fully extended with the foot stopping just in front of the face (30 to 34 weeks).

1: Lower leg slightly bent at the knee with the foot over the face (32 to 34 weeks).

2: Lower leg bent at the knee, forming a 120° angle, with the foot suspended over the upper chest (34 to 38 weeks).

3: Lower leg bent at the knee with foot straight up in the air (90° angle) (38 to 40 weeks)

4: Lower leg so flexed that the foot cannot even be brought to a full 90° angle (40+ weeks)

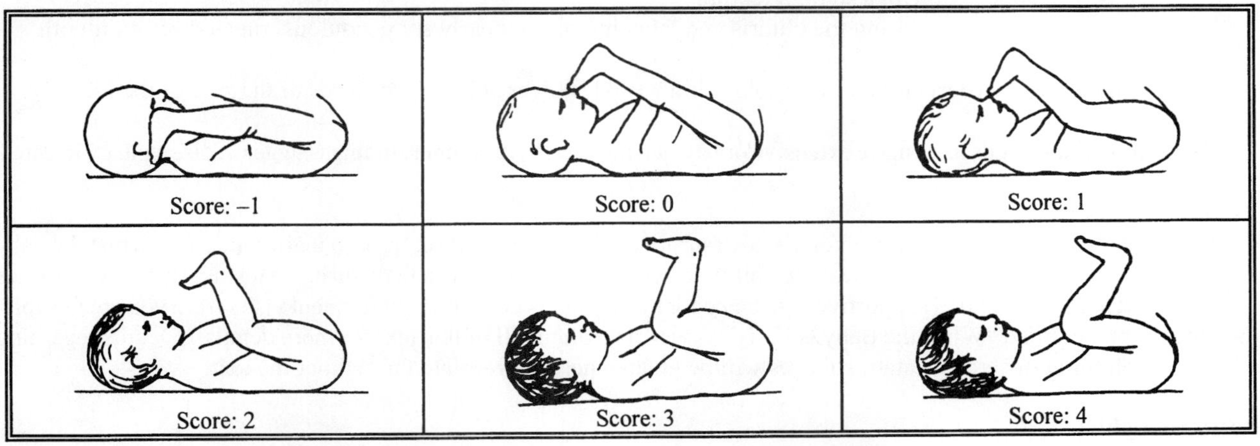

Term babies have increased flexor tone in the first few days of life; making it difficult or impossible to fully extend the knees. If this is the case, measure the angle created by an imaginary arc extended from the center of the upper leg

This maneuver assumes there is no hip dislocation, which will also interfere with rotation. Normally, the angles are equal for both legs and appropriate for age. Asymmetry is abnormal. An angle greater than expected for gestational age suggests hypotonia, and an angle smaller than expected for age suggests hypertonia.

The Total Ballard Score

The maturity rating uses the combined score from the neuromuscular and physical assessments for a formal assessment. For example, if the total maturity rating adds up to 15, the baby is assessed as being 30 weeks gestation. When the score falls between the numbers listed, an approximate interim gestational age must be assigned. For example, a score of 23 might receive an age rating of 33 weeks.

New Ballad Maturity Rating	Approximate Gestational age (By LMP)
-10	20
-5	22
0	24
5	26
10	28
15	30
20	32
25	34
30	36
35	38
40	40
45	42
50	44

Unexpected scores

Factors that may skew the score must be considered when there is a difference between the expected and the actual score. These include the timing of the exam, conditions that may influence joint mobility, and active and passive muscle tone. Have your midwife partner perform the assessment independently at the first day home visit, when the test is most accurate for babies near term. Variations in assessment may occur with even the most experienced clinicians. An unexpected score can be a clue to historical factors or abnormal conditions that may have otherwise gone unnoticed. Keep in mind that dating by this exam may not be any more accurate than the best dating derived from other methods used prior to the birth.

Confirming term gestation

You should be very familiar with the characteristics of both term and near-term babies, as those are the ones you are most likely to attend at home. Confirming term status via a brief evaluation is all that is necessary in the vast majority of babies. Term characteristics include:

- Stiff, springy ear cartilage
- Completely formed areola with a breast bud of 5 to 10 mm
- A resting posture of full flexion, limbs held against gravity
- Pink, mostly opaque skin with a smooth texture
- Genitalia: plump labia enclosing the clitoris and labia minora or nearly so; pendulous, rugated scrotum with descended testicles
- True plantar creases (deeper than just crinkly skin wrinkles) over at least two-thirds of the sole of the foot

The examination needs to be more extensive only when these criteria or other findings suggest a discrepancy in dates.

Preterm babies

Occasionally you may be caught at home with a surprise preterm baby. If so, the two main concerns are that the baby is able to breathe on her own and nurse. The ability to suck is a matter of muscle maturity. Most 35 to 36 week babies can be kept at home when good supportive assistance for the mother is available and frequent visits from you are feasible. (See the chapter entitled "When the Baby Is Early" as well as Volume III of this text for more details.) Details regarding what to watch for at different gestational ages will be given where appropriate throughout the text.

Postterm babies

These babies are healthy, alert and well grown, exhibiting all the characteristics of a normal, mature baby.

Dysmature babies

There is a difference between babies who are born past their due date (postterm) and those who are labeled

dysmature (formerly "postmature"). Dysmaturity occurs when a baby who has presumably been growing well during late pregnancy begins to lose weight and show other characteristic changes. This has been thought to be due to a falling off of placental efficiency when it occurs past term, brought about by the impending "death" of the placenta, which is believed to reflect the natural limits of the ability of the placenta to support a pregnancy. However, Fox (1997) absolutely refutes this theory of placental insufficiency as the cause, stating that villi growth continues right up until birth in the placenta, although it does slow down somewhat as term approaches.

In studying the placental villi of dysmature babies, he has found that circulation on the fetal side seems to slow down in a small percentage of postterm babies and may possibly be the cause of dysmaturity. However, no conclusive views about the causes of this phenomenon exist at this time, although in many cases, it most certainly has something to do with maternal nutrition at the end of pregnancy. While the condition of many babies presenting with signs of dysmaturity can be attributed to less-than-optimal maternal nutrition, not all can. Some anecdotal cases seem to be related to maternal hormonal imbalances that retard the timely onset of labor and sometimes milk production (Schlinger, 2003).

McLean and associates (1991) did a careful study of babies born past term and determined that weight increases as pregnancy progresses. Furthermore, the characteristics of "dysmaturity" can be seen in any baby who has suffered intrauterine growth restriction regardless of gestation; there is no evidence that this happens more frequently in postterm births.

The typical dysmature baby has some loss of previously laid-down subcutaneous fat, which results in soft, loose, baggy skin that has a dry, wrinkled, parchment-like texture with very little or no vernix or lanugo. He may also have increased hardness of the skull bones, long, thin arms and legs, and an apprehensive look. The nails are typically long and scalp hair is profuse. These babies often have mild to moderate oligohydramnios and are more prone to cord compression during labor for this reason. Not surprisingly, they are usually born quite hungry. Passage of meconium prior to birth is a frequent occurrence. These babies are at risk for lower APGAR scores, polycythemia and increased mortality, with 75 to 85% of these deaths occurring during labor.

ASSESSMENT OF THE BABY'S SIZE AND ITS RELATIONSHIP TO GESTATIONAL AGE

The pattern of normal growth is an important reference used to understand abnormalities in the newborn. "Normal" is defined by data gathered from large populations of babies and compiled into growth curves reflecting a broad range of variation. Once gestational age has been determined, the baby's size can be assessed in relationship to his age.

Intrauterine Growth and Development

Fetal and neonatal growth occur on a continuum. Growth during gestation is dependent upon both intrinsic (within the fetus) and extrinsic (outside the fetus) factors. If the baby is normal and healthy, the primary intrinsic influence on size at birth involves normal, hereditarily determined variations in stature. However, fetal growth potential may be negatively influenced by genetic abnormalities that are established at the time of conception or by fetal infection.

Extrinsic factors are outside the fetus and include the growth support systems provided by the mother's body and her environment such as her nutrition, adequate blood volume perfusing the placental bed, normal gas and waste exchange across the placental membranes, as well as a constant thermal environment. These maternal contributions may be altered as a result of maternal malnutrition, disease, toxemia, recurrent bleeding or other disorders as well as environmental exposures to chemicals or other toxins. Multiple pregnancy is also classified as an extrinsic factor. During pregnancy, the growth potential of the fetus is also limited to a certain extent by the capacity of the uterus itself (Korones, 1986).

Normal cell growth during gestation occurs in three integrated stages. Cell growth first begins when the fertilized ovum starts to divide. Nuclei are produced during cell division, or mitosis. Containing the DNA blueprint for the cell, nuclei are responsible for the early growth of any organ. They multiply rapidly during the first part of embryonic and fetal growth; up until about 25 weeks, cytoplasmic mass (the primary component influencing the size of the cells) remains relatively small and the cytoplasm-to-DNA ratio of each cell stays about the same. This period of rapid cell division is called **hyperplasia**.

After the first few weeks of pure cell division, cellular differentiation begins. The second stage of growth involves an increased production of cytoplasm as the cells that have been laid down to form each organ begin to enlarge and the rate of multiplication declines. Cell enlargement is called **hypertrophy**. Although hypertrophy and hyperplasia continue to occur simultaneously, the rate of hypertrophy increases, raising the cytoplasm-to-DNA ratio. The cells of various organs enlarge at different rates according to their individual genetic programing.

Overall, the most rapid period of fetal growth is in the 20 weeks between 12 and 36 weeks gestation (postconceptual age). The normal period of hyperplastic growth varies according to the organ involved. The third stage of growth occurs as hypertrophy accelerates and hyperplasia declines even more. Existing cells continue to enlarge while fewer new cells multiply. Cytoplasm-to-DNA ratio now increases even more. If there is an interruption in these normal processes, the stage at which such disruption occurs will influence how baby's development is affected.

The mother's nutrition is the primary extrinsic factor that supports normal fetal development in an otherwise normal pregnancy. Adequate protein intake supports normal hyperplasia and symmetrical growth both early on and throughout gestation. Continued optimal maternal nutrition during the last trimester supports the final stages of fetal growth, especially brain and nervous system development, that take place prior to birth. These nutritional factors influence the development of the fetus throughout gestation.

Criteria for Assessing Newborn Size and Growth

The term "anthropometric" refers to comparative measurements of the human body. The three criteria that have been established to evaluate fetal and newborn growth and well-being in relationship to gestational age are weight, occipitofrontal head circumference and crown-heel length. More details regarding taking these measurements are included in the subchapter entitled "Assessing the Infant's Body Weight, Measurements, Proportions and Temperature," but their relevance is explained below. As you read about each of these parameters (based on Korones, 1986), keep in mind that any patterns or rates of growth mentioned can vary among individual normal babies.

Weight

Weight is the most frequently performed measurement used to assess growth status because it is the most accurate, most easily obtained and is extremely sensitive to daily changes. Weight is a summary value because it shows changes in the content of protein, fat and water in the skeleton, brain and other organs. A well-defined pattern of fetal weight gain, especially during the third trimester, has been established using large populations of babies. In spite of normal individual variations, fetal growth is unrestricted during most of pregnancy. Between 32 and 36 weeks, the rate of weight gain peaks at 200 to 225 g/week and declines thereafter. Even though fetal growth slows a bit as term approaches, when her mother is well nourished, the baby will continue to gain weight and remain well padded with fat until birth occurs. The difference in average newborn weight can vary as much as 1500 grams, reflecting the influence of maternal nutrition on the growth of the fetus. The rate of fetal growth tends to individualize as the baby gets closer to term. Progressive changes are the cumulative effect of increases in water, fat and protein content.

Water: Water (and the minerals it contains) contributes the largest proportion of the weight of both the fetus and newborn. The body of a 1 g embryo is 93 to 95% water. The percentage of water weight falls as term approaches; by 26 weeks, it is 85% of body weight; at 30 weeks, it is 80%: at 38 weeks, it is 74%; and by 40 weeks, it has fallen to 71%. Distribution also changes as total body water falls. Extracellular fluid diminishes as the fetus matures, while intracellular fluid rises as the cells differentiate and increase in size. At term, extracellular water and minerals comprise 45% of body weight (about 2700 g); two months later, it is 30% of body weight. These changes influence the baby's ability to maintain body temperature as well as the fluid-electrolyte balance.

Fat: Body fat is minimal during the first 20 weeks of gestation, comprising only about 1% of total body weight. Laying down of fat deposits accelerates after that point; by the third trimester, subcutaneous fat is accumulating rapidly. The fetus produces fat from glucose and, to a lesser extent, from transplacentally derived essential fatty acids. Fat accumulates as body water diminishes and the organs enlarge. Brown fat deposits appear early during the second half of gestation. White fat is primarily laid down in subcutaneous tissues. Fat is used to store energy for later use, as might be required if the baby develops dysmaturity syndrome. The metabolism of white fat generates heat, but unlike brown fat, the newborn cannot use it to respond to cold stress. Most fetal fat develops in the last 8 weeks of gestation. During the first 20 weeks, fat accounts for only 1% of body weight. By 26 weeks, fat accounts for about 3% of total body weight; at 35 weeks, 8%; at term, 15% of weight, with 80% of it in the subcutaneous tissue (about 475 g in all) (Korones, 1986).

Protein: The only "ready-made" proteins transferred across the placenta in significant quantities are the immunoglobulins, predominately immunoglobulin G (gamma globulin). The fetus synthesizes all other proteins from amino acids, which do cross the placenta. Thus the fetus produces protein independently; the amino acid content of fetal protein molecules is similar to those of the adult. Since the mother cannot contribute complete proteins from her own tissues to the fetus, her diet must supply enough raw protein material in the form of amino acids to allow her to adequately expand her blood volume while simultaneously transferring sufficient quantities of amino acids across the placenta so the baby can make his own protein molecules. At term, the fetus has accumulated about 400 g of body protein.

Genetic influences on weight: About 20% of all variables influencing birthweight are due to genetic contributions of the mother; 20% are due to the fetus' genetic makeup and 60% depend on the fetal environment. Although genes from both parents contribute to their offspring's growth and final adult size, maternal genes appear to exert the main influence over the weight at birth in girls, while the presence of the Y chromosome seems to result in baby boys who grow faster in utero and weigh on the average 150 to 200 grams more than their female siblings. Birthweights tend to trend in family groups (that means, it is common for women in the same family to have babies of similar weights); however, dietary and cultural practices that also have a direct impact on the size of the baby may be partly responsible for such trends.

Problems with using weight as a parameter for growth: There are a few drawbacks to using weight as a growth assessment. One can be misled by weight as an estimate of lean body mass because it is affected by the total body water status of the baby. For instance, if the baby has excessive fluid accumulation from hydrops or congestive heart failure she will weigh more than she would without these conditions. It is difficult to assess what proportion of an infant's birth weight is excess water until they have undergone diuresis. Thus the assessment of the appropriateness of such a baby's lean body mass is virtually impossible at birth.

Occipitofrontal head circumference

Head circumference is measured at the level of the supraorbital ridges (just above the eyebrows) in front and at the level of the occipital eminence in the back. Head circumference reflects the growth of the brain and, in most babies, correlates well with brain weight. However, the relationship between the two is not entirely consistent.

Growth of the head is linear with maximal growth occurring between 30 and 32 weeks; the head circumference increases an average of 1.2 mm daily. Daily increments diminish gradually after 32 weeks, the head is growing only 0.2 mm daily by 40 weeks. Postnatally, head circumference begins to grow at a rate paralleling that of maximal gestational growth, with the cranium enlarging by about 1.1 mm daily. This apparent slowing of growth near term may be a genetically programed protection to ensure that the baby's head can pass through the maternal pelvis. Generally, head growth continues more or less normally relative to weight and length during mild to moderate intrauterine malnutrition, making it a less sensitive indicator of caloric restriction. Thus, a baby may have a normal occipitofrontal head circumference and still have suffered from intrauterine growth restriction, including suboptimal brain development.

The occipitofrontal head circumference can help determine the etiology of fetal growth anomalies. Isolated microcephaly or a head circumference that is disproportionately small compared to weight and length suggest severe brain pathology happened early in gestation. However, circumferences that exceed the normal range rarely indicate that the brain is bigger than average. In many cases, a large measurement will correlate with the baby's overall proportions, reflecting a baby who is larger than average but perfectly normal. When this is not the case, a large measurement usually indicates some abnormality of fluid balance within the brain, such as hydrocephalus.

Crown-heel length

Length is the most accurate indicator of linear growth and also reflects lean body mass. It increases by 1 cm per week beginning in the 25th week of gestation. Peak increases of 1.3 cm weekly occur between 31 and 34 weeks. After that, growth tends to slow; by 40 weeks, the incremental rate averages 0.5 cm weekly. After birth, the pattern of length growth is similar to that of weight and head circumference, returning to the rate that prevailed at 32 weeks gestation. Length is spared at the expense of weight if there has been mild malnutrition during gestation. This can be noted by comparing the length percentile to the weight percentile for a particular baby (Korones, 1986).

Standard One-Factor Growth Charts

Weight, length and head circumference are proportional for gestational age in a normal, healthy, well-nourished baby. This reflects normal cell growth and development and makes chance of problems unlikely. To establish proportionate growth, each of the three parameters: weight (in grams), length and occipitofrontal head circumference (each in centimeters) are compared to a standardized growth chart. An infant may be classified as either small, appropriate or large for gestational age for each of these measurements.

Problems with using growth charts

Since the early 1960s, a number of charts have been developed to try and quantify intrauterine growth up until the time of birth. The data from any such charts must be understood to be approximate, as there are many problems with gathering and standardizing such data. These curves represent percentiles of static perinatal measurements, and the growth of any particular fetus or groups of fetuses does not necessarily follow such curves. Measurements taken at birth represent a one-time, cross-sectional measurement of an individual baby (rather than a longitudinal measurement plotting the growth of each infant over time). Therefore, all the infants measured to arrive at a growth curve for 39 weeks are different from all those measured at 38 weeks. Connecting the averages of these two sets to create a "growth curve" is not entirely appropriate since growth was not measured in the same infants. While this can establish percentiles for the designated parameter at a given gestational age, dynamic continued growth for each baby, had he remained in utero, cannot be inferred from this data (Georgieff, 1995).

These growth charts are problematic for many other reasons as well. First of all, they rely on accurate pregnancy dating; however, the methods used for establishing dates are often iffy, at best. It has been suggested that the apparent slowing that occurs in the weight curve near term and thereafter results, not from a true biologic slowing, but from an artifact in the way data are collected. McLean and colleagues (1991) point out that the characteristic slowing of growth at 36 to 37 weeks, and the plateau in growth that is depicted in charts for babies born past 41 weeks, is because the curves are based on menstrual history and are distorted by errors in gestational-age assignment in postdates babies. Standards have likely been distorted by the inclusion of many growth-restricted fetuses and by cases in which monthly yoni bleeding in early pregnancy was mistaken for the last menstrual period. These growth charts show a wider spread of mean growth values in preterm than in term infants. Such values are clearly inaccurate, since it is known that individualization in fetal size becomes more prominent as term nears. (Naeye & Dixon, 1978).

Preterm birth is not the norm and although we rarely know all the reasons why a baby is born early, we do know that often something is wrong with the fetus or the fetal environment that prompts labor; very commonly, inadequate maternal nutrition is a major contributing factor. Thus, there is no assurance that preterm newborns have the same growth curve as those fetuses of the same gestational age who are still in utero; they may also be biologically different from fetuses who continue to term in other unidentified ways.

Myriad factors influence fetal growth in different populations. Ideally, each baby who may have a problem would be assessed by matching him to a large population of healthy infants who are of the same sex, race, ethnicity and genetic makeup and whose mothers were living in the same culture, environment and altitude. Most important, specifics regarding maternal nutrition are not factored into any of the existing growth curves. In addition, the statistical methods for establishing the data are poorly described, and almost all employ "smoothing" techniques to make the data more uniform. Many charts use data that includes babies who died during the neonatal period (first 28 days of life), which implies some intrinsic problem that prevented survival. For all these reasons, growth charts must be seen as generalizations only; as with any statistic, the findings on the chart should never supercede the actual condition of an individual baby (Sparks et al., 1998). Some of the best available charts are included at the end of this chapter.

Size-for-Dates Assessment

The normal baby is considered an appropriate size for his gestational age. His weight falls within the "average" part of the curve; this is considered to be between the 10th and 90th percentiles on a standard growth chart such as the graphs included at the end of this chapter. Size-for-dates criteria are summarized in the following chart; they are primarily classified by weight, unless otherwise noted.

SIZE CATEGORY AT BIRTH	RELATIONSHIP OF WEIGHT, HEAD CIRC AND LENGTH TO GESTATIONAL AGE
Extremely low birthweight (ELBW)	Less than 2 lb, 3.5 oz (1000 g), regardless of gestational age
Very low birthweight (VLBW)	Less than 3 lb 8 oz (1500 g), regardless of gestational age
Low birthweight (LBW)	Less than 5 lb 8 oz (2500 g), regardless of gestational age
Small for Gestational Age (SGA)	Below the 10th percentile for gestational age
Symmetric SGA growth	Weight, head circ and length are proportional, all falling below the 10th percentile
Asymmetric SGA growth	Weight below 10th percentile, head circ and length above 10th percentile
Intrauterine growth restriction (IUGR)	Weight, head circ and length may be above or below the 10th percentile, but the overall appearance of the baby indicates that the baby's weight is light for dates.
Symmetric IUGR growth	Growth is reduced, but is proportionate for all parameters.
Asymmetric IUGR growth	Low weight, short femur length and, in some cases, small abdominal circ
Appropriate for Gestational Age (AGA)	**Weight, head circ and length are proportionate, all falling between the 10th and 90th percentile for gestational age**
Large for Gestational age (LGA)	Weight above the 90th percentile for gestational age
Symmetric LGA growth	Weight, head circ and length proportional, all fall above 90th percentile (most likely a normal, healthy, big baby of a well-nourished mother)
Asymmetric LGA (macrosomic) growth	Weight above the 90th percentile, head circ and length below 90th percentile, or other types of asymmetric growth
High Birthweight	Over 4500g (9 lb 14.75 oz) regardless of gestational age

(Snow, 1998)

These graphs were derived from newborn populations born to mothers whose diets were not evaluated for excellence. Because many women have at least marginally inadequate nutrition and weight gain during pregnancy, the 10th percentile is probably too low to be considered truly normal. A baby whose weight falls in the 10th percentile at birth may be somewhat underweight and may have been bigger had her mother eaten better. Conversely, babies who weigh over 8 lb 13 oz (4000 g) can be perfectly healthy in women who eat well.

Babies who fall in the extremely low birthweight and very low birthweight categories are either quite preterm or IUGR. Although a baby may be born an appropriate size for her quite early gestation, her light weight and immature systems still place her at risk of problems in growing; her chances of coming through the neonatal period neurologically and otherwise intact are diminished (especially if her cord is clamped too quickly). In general, the smaller and earlier the baby, the poorer the prognosis for intact survival. Diminished growth can often be detected prenatally; in most cases, these mothers will have been evaluated prior to birth. If you are working far from medical facilities, it is possible that you will attend the birth of babies who are of extremely low to very low birthweight. Midwives in such circumstances must do the best they can to put together support for mothers and babies to maximize survival in such tiny infants. How to go about this is detailed in Volume III of this text.

The majority of homebirth midwives will only encounter infants who fall within the last five main categories. Infants are considered to be of low birthweight when they weigh less than 5 lb 8 oz (2500 g), regardless of their gestational age. The categories of small for gestational age (SGA), appropriate for gestational age (AGA), andlarge for gestational age (LGA) are based on percentile of growth for gestation utilizing standard growth charts. Asymmetric growth in any infant who is SGA or AGA may indicate intrauterine growth restriction (IUGR). Note that it is possible for a baby to be preterm, term or postterm and be either SGA, AGA, LGA or IUGR.

PRETERM				TERM				POSTTERM			
37 completed weeks gestation or less				37 to 42 completed weeks gestation				42+ completed weeks gestation			
SGA	IUGR	AGA	LGA	SGA	IUGR	AGA	LGA	SGA	IUGR	AGA	LGA

The pattern of growth combined with the gestational age for each baby helps determine what, if any, additional risks the baby may face beyond those intrinsic to preterm birth, a marginally nourished pregnancy or, at the other end of the spectrum, large size at birth (e.g., shoulder dystocia and associated birth trauma). However, keep in mind that these classifications only delineate risk rather than individual outcomes. The postbirth environment plays a major role in determining the response of a particular baby. For example, all babies, regardless of their size, will have the best chance of optimizing their potential from birth onward when they receive their placental transfusions and nurse exclusively.

The tables at the end of this chapter can be used to establish the proportions of the baby (use the ones by Miller, 1981, for babies born at term). Assign each of the three parameters of weight, length and head circumference to a category of SGA, AGA or LGA growth. In each instance, write in the actual measurement and the percentile into which the measurement falls. If all three fall in the same percentile, the baby is proportionately or symmetrically grown. If not, the baby is asymmetrically grown.

GESTATIONAL AGE OF BABY _______ WEEKS LMP			
PARAMETER	VALUES (TABLE USED_____________________)		
	MEASUREMENT	PERCENTILE	TYPE OF GROWTH
Weight			
Length			
Head circumference			

Characteristics and causes of small for gestational age (SGA) growth

A baby is considered to be small for gestational age when the birthweight dips below the 10th percentile on a standard growth chart. SGA babies may grow symmetrically or asymmetrically.

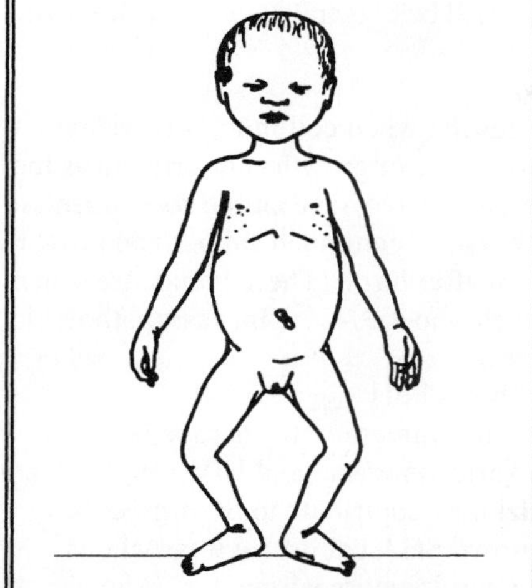

1. Normal 34 week preterm AGA baby

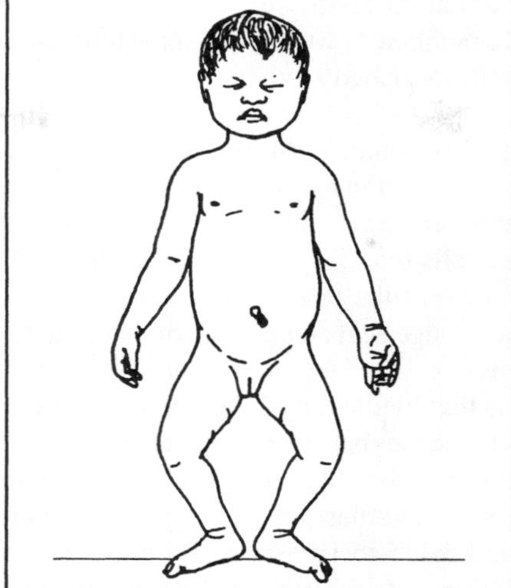

2. Symmetric SGA baby at term

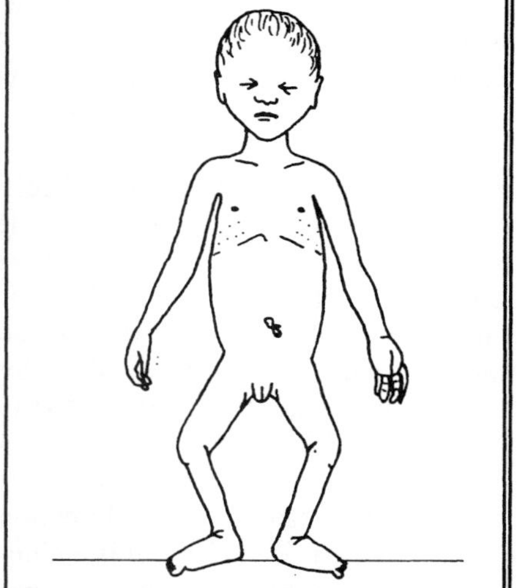

3. Asymmetric SGA baby at term

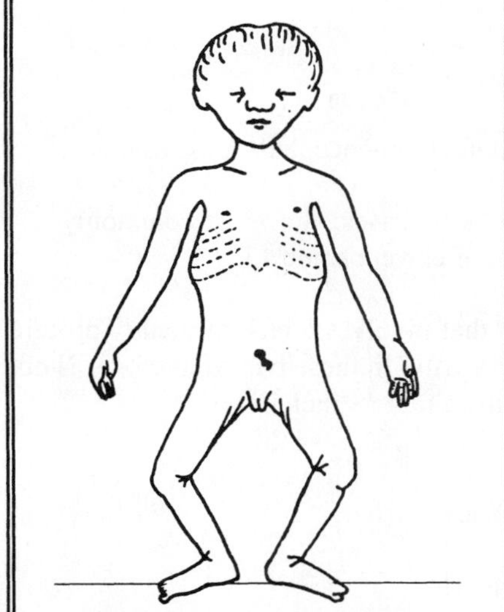

4. Symmetric IUGR baby at term

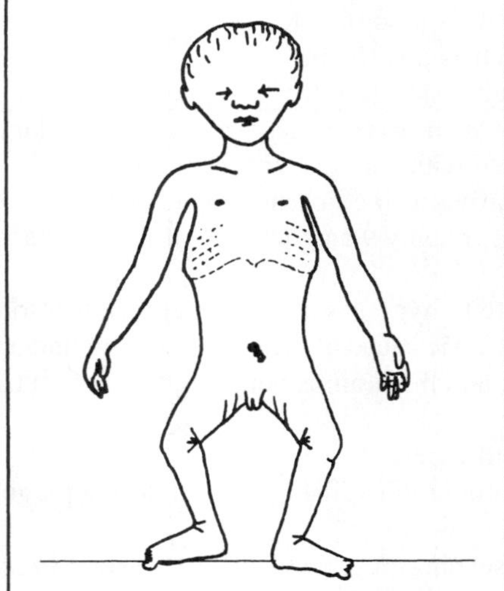

5. Asymmetric IUGR baby at term

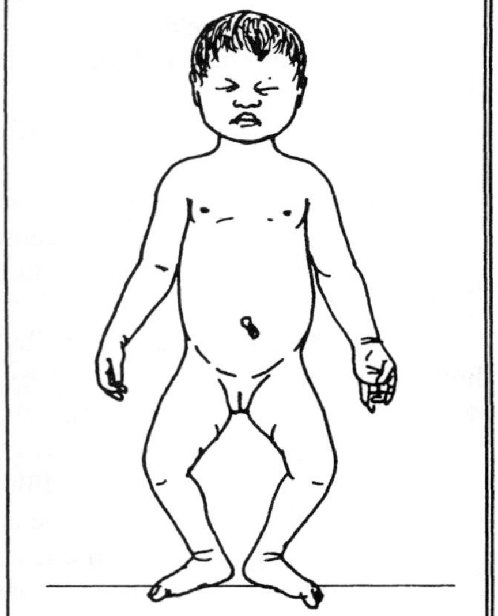

6. AGA baby at term

All babies are shown with extended limbs to better demonstrate their differences. Size parameters for 1, 2 and 6 are taken from the 50th percentile of the table from which they were derived. All others are estimates to show typical characteristics.

1. Weight 2160 (4 lb 12.2 oz), Length 45.3 cm, OFC 30.8 cm (Naeye & Dixon, 1978)
2. Weight 2890 (6 lb 5.8 oz.), Length 49.1, OFC 32.9 (Miller, 1981)
3. Weight 2495 (5 lb 8 oz), Length 49.1, OFC 32.9
4. Weight 2160 (4 lb 12.2 oz), Length 51.3 cm, OFC 34.5 cm (note sunken fontanelle)
5. Weight 1984 (4 lb 6 oz), Length 49 OFC 34 cm (femur length, abdominal circ. are also small for age; fontanelle sunken)
6. Weight 3430 (7 lb. 9 oz.), Length 51.3 cm, OFC 34.5 cm (Miller, 1981)

Symmetric SGA growth

Constitutional variation: These babies have length, weight and head circumference values that are proportionate; that is, they all fall below the 5th or the 10th percentile for their gestational age; which percentile varies among sources. The primary reason for symmetrical SGA growth is normal hereditary variation. Babies who are born to small, well-nourished mothers may be genetically predisposed to be smaller than average. Recall that the percentile ranking is just a statistical average. Just as there is a wide variation in "normal" labor, some of which will fall outside the "average," the same is true of some small babies. It is estimated that 80 to 85% of all symmetrically grown SGA babies are constitutionally small babies who are perfectly normal. Remember, however, that most term babies will be bigger than others in the same racial and ethnic population if born to well-nourished mothers.

Hypoplastic, proportionate growth: Proportionately diminished growth also results when cell mitosis (division) is disrupted or impaired during initial cell proliferation early in gestation. This early stage of growth is referred to as the **critical period** because it is when the organs are being formed, making the baby most susceptible to congenital malformations. The organs contain fewer cells than they normally would and the risk of continued suboptimal growth is high. Hypoplasia is irreversible, regardless of the provision of optimal nutrition after birth. These babies are seven times more likely to have a variety of major congenital anomalies compared to babies who are AGA. Intrinsic pathologic causes of symmetric SGA growth include:

- •Chronic nonbacterial fetal infections that begin early in pregnancy, especially syphilis
  - -Viral infections: The most evidence exists for a causal relationship for infection from rubella, cytomegalovirus and parvovirus, a possible relationship exists with varicella-zoster and HIV.
  - -Protozoan infections: Infection with toxoplasmosis or trypanosoma cruzi may contribute to SGA growth.
  - -Genetic disorders: It is estimated that 5 to 10% of all symmetrically grown SGA babies have associated genetic disorders; the correlation rises when the baby presents with neurologic impairment.
    - -The most common cause is triploidy (when there 3, rather than haploid [those in a sperm or egg] chromosomes: this results in death.)
    - -Single-gene defects
    - -Chromosomal disorders such as trisomies 13, 18 and 21
    - -Dysmorphic syndromes such as dwarfism
    - -Some inborn errors of metabolism
- •Congenital malformation anomalies such as renal agenesis, cardiovascular defects, anencephaly, gastroschisis, omphalocele and those associated with a single umbilical artery
- •Placental mosaicism may be causative in the absence of other risks in 6% of cases; the most commonly associated abnormalities include trisomy 9 and deletion of the short arm of chromosome 13.

Extrinsic factors may also contribute to hypoplasia. Maternal malnutrition that involves a lack of dietary protein throughout pregnancy is the primary extrinsic cause of proportional fetal undergrowth. In these babies, the liver is not affected any more than any other organ, and the brain is not spared. Other extrinsic factors include:

- •Inadequate maternal nutrition
- •Maternal malaria (in one-fifth of cases)
- •Conditions that decrease the amount of available oxygen during pregnancy, such as:
  - •Living at a high altitude
  - •Maternal pulmonary disease: chronic, severe asthma, cystic fibrosis, etc.
  - •Maternal cardiovascular disease or vascular abnormalities of the uterus
  - •Cigarette smoking, which can reduce birthweight by 135 to 300 g
  - •Chronic maternal hematological disorders such as anemia
- •Maternal genotypic disorders such as phenylketonuria (associated with IUGR and microcephalus)

Clinical signs and symptoms: Symmetrically small, term babies are miniature but normal babies, unless they have an obvious anomaly. They are normally filled out and plump, with limbs that are appropriately sized for their torso (unless they are small due to an abnormality of growth, such as dwarfism). Their heads do not appear large for their trunks. Their skin is normally thick, with the subcutaneous vascular pattern obscure or invisible, unlike infants of the same size who are AGA and therefore preterm. These babies are usually vigorous and less likely to be hypoglycemic or polycythemic than their asymmetrically grown counterparts. The primary risk in these infants is the increased likelihood of chronic infection or congenital anomaly (Korones, 1986).

Asymmetric (disproportionate), hypotropic SGA growth: Most SGA babies are asymmetrically grown, meaning that only one or two of the parameters of weight, length and head circumference fall within the 10th percentile for their gestational age. In most cases, the weight is reduced (below the 10th percentile) while the length is less affected and the head circumference is relatively normal for age. Shortened femurs may account for a slight reduction in length. Asymmetric growth reflects a developmental problem that occurred during the latter part of gestation after an initial period of normal growth. The total number of cells in affected organs is normal or nearly so, but organ size is diminished because the cells contain less than the normal amount of cytoplasm; thus hypertrophia has been disrupted, a process referred to as **hypotrophia**. This type of impairment is primarily due to extrinsic influences and is reversible to some extent. The cytoplasmic mass may approach normal with proper postnatal nutrition, and the resulting cellular enlargement will lead to normal organ size. Asymmetrically grown SGA babies look very much like IUGR babies. Extrinsic causes of asymmetric SGA growth include:

- Maternal alcohol intake of 1 to 2 drinks daily or maternal cocaine use; both can result in a reduction in birthweight and head circumference.
- High altitude (above 4500 m), which causes length to be slightly reduced (Mortola et al., 2000)
- Maternal hypo- or hyperthyroidism has no marked effect on fetal weight but may retard bone development and reduce protein synthesis in the fetal brain.
- Maternal chronic illness such as lupus, liver disorders or heart disease
- Advanced maternal diabetes involving generalized vascular damage and impairment of kidney function
- Complications of pregnancy (uterine and placental anomalies, polyhydramnios, toxemia, intrauterine infection)
- Multiple gestation with inadequate maternal nutrition or restricted intrauterine space (higher order multiples)
- Autosomal defects (especially trisomy 18–Edward's syndrome) have also been linked to growth restriction which develops after 26 weeks.

Impaired placental circulation during the third trimester of pregnancy due to late-onset maternal malnutrition produces asymmetric undergrowth in the fetus that has been misleadingly characterized as "brain-sparing." The belief that the brain is spared derives from the first studies of asymmetric growth, which were performed using animals. The overall birthweight of experimental rats was reduced by 20% when placental circulation was impaired throughout the third trimester; however, the weight of the liver was reduced by up to 50%. The adrenals were severely affected as well, while other organs were affected to a lesser extent, and the weight of the brain remained more or less normal. The difference between the weight of the brain and that of the liver was great due to the huge demand of the brain for glucose, which severely taxed the undernourished liver (Korones, 1986).

Clinical Differences between Hypoplastic Symmetric and Hypotrophic Asymmetric SGA Babies	
Hypoplastic, symmetric SGA Growth*	**Hypotrophic, asymmetric SGA Growth**
Universal, proportional reduction in size and weight; percentiles of head, length and weight are similar	Selective, disproportionate reduction in size and weight; percentiles of head and length above 10th percentile, with weight below the 10th percentile
Subcutaneous fat layer appropriate for weight; skin is normally taut, with normal horizontal creasing in the legs and elsewhere.	Subcutaneous fat reduced for size; skin is not filled out, and may be slightly loose; arm and leg creases run in a more longitudinal direction.
Congenital malformations 7 times more likely	Congenital malformation is infrequent.
Intrauterine, nonbacterial infection frequently found	Intrauterine, nonbacterial infection is rarely found.
Hematocrit usually normal	Hematocrit often elevated due to chronic hypoxia
Hypoglycemia and hypoproteinemia are uncommon.	Hypoglycemia and hypoproteinemia are common.

*Does not refer to constitutionally small but normal babies

In humans, research performed during the last quarter of the twentieth century found that asymmetric fetal growth is associated with a brain that is diminished in length, weight and size, although less so than when the baby has suffered from malnutrition throughout pregnancy. While head circumference may be above the 10th percentile, inadequate nourishment impairs brain development, with all parts of the brain feeling the lack, including the neurons, synapses, neurotransmitters and myelin. Malnutrition most severely affects the liver in humans, just as it does in rats and for the same reason. When the liver is undersized, the brain requires twice as much glucose as the liver can provide (Chamberlain, 1998). In humans, growth restriction due to malnutrition in later pregnancy results in diminished cytoplasmic mass in most organs, especially the liver and adrenals. Uteroplacental vascular insufficiency is the primary contributor to impaired fetal growth, reflecting an inadequately expanded blood volume in the mother and reduced nutrient delivery during this period of fetal weight gain. These babies may also experience chronic hypoglycemia long before birth, resulting in neurological damage before term.

Clinical signs, symptoms and problems associated with asymmetric SGA growth: IUGR babies who are not technically SGA (see below) and asymmetrically undergrown SGA babies present a similar, scrawny appearance. While the head appears large, the body appears long and thin in spite of its normal length, and the chest and abdominal circumferences are typically small in relationship to the baby's length. The skin is often pale, although the baby may be red due to polycythemia from prolonged hypoxia in utero. In extreme cases, the muscle mass and fat deposits over the buttocks, thighs and cheeks are poorly developed. Vernix is frequently abundant. Scalp hair is typically sparse; heavy hair growth is unusual in asymmetrically grown SGA babies. Skull sutures are often wide as a result of impaired bone growth. The anterior fontanelle, though large, is often soft and sunken, ruling out increased intracranial pressure as the cause. Ossification centers in the distal femur and proximal tibia may be absent in term SGA babies. Most asymmetrically grown SGA babies are more active than might be expected and have a vigorous cry. An alert, wide-eyed look is combined with tongue thrusting. This vigor is really irritative hyperactivity, and the tongue thrusting may indicate seizure activity in some babies. All of these are signs of chronic marginal hypoxia in utero. Many will begin to have seizures 6 to 18 hours later, especially those whose anterior fontanelle is firm due to edema from intrauterine hypoxia. However, when perinatal asphyxia has been more severe, the baby is usually flaccid and lethargic.

The primary problem that these babies face is hypoglycemia. The brain requires more glucose than any other organ, leaving little or no glycogen for the small liver to store. As a result, these babies are prone to hypoglycemia during the stress of labor and after birth. They also have a diminished fat layer. Both fatty acids and ketones are derived from broken-down fat deposits, which, when absent or scanty, cannot provide enough fuel in place of glucose. Some SGA babies do not have adequate levels of the enzymes required to activate glucose metabolism. This, plus a limited supply of protein, deprives the baby of another source of glucose. Hypoxia increases the body's demand for glucose, depleting what little glycogen the baby may have stored. The incidence of hypoglycemia may be as high as 40% among the most severely SGA babies and must be identified and treated promptly to avoid brain damage. Remember that hypoglycemia produces symptoms similar to those of hypoxia.

These babies are also prone to heat loss because they have little stored fat, although SGA babies born at term are more capable of responding to cold stress with increased heat production than equally weighted AGA babies who are preterm. Apparently, brown fat deposits are not as affected by maternal malnutrition. However, this benefit is obviated by the tendency of hypoxia as well as hypoglycemia to reduce any baby's ability to deal with cold.

Chronic intrauterine hypoxia may result in polycythemia as the baby's system tries to compensate for the lack of oxygen by producing more oxygen-carrying cells. While the baby may have a high hematocrit, allowing her to have her placental transfusion does not make this problem worse. It provides the benefits of continued oxygenation and nutrients found in whole blood during stabilization after birth and during infancy.

General concerns for all SGA babies: Unless constitutionally small, all SGA babies are at increased risk for many problems. They are poorly equipped to deal with perinatal asphyxia because of low glycogen stores; many have had chronic asphyxia during pregnancy. They may be hard to stabilize at birth, especially if labor has been at all difficult. They are also at more risk for meconium aspiration due to the increased possibility of asphyxia. All SGA babies should be monitored carefully for hypoglycemia at birth and encouraged to nurse right away. They often have suboptimal neurological responses and brain function as they mature.

Intrauterine growth restriction (formerly "growth retardation") (IUGR): The term "intrauterine growth restriction" is a designation often used synonymously with SGA. In fact, all SGA babies who are not constitutionally small can be properly described as having some form of growth restriction. IUGR babies may also experience either symmetric or asymmetric growth. Symmetrical IUGR generally results in an overall reduction in the parameters for weight, length and head circumference. Asymmetrical IUGR results in a low birth weight short femur length in some cases, and an abnormally small abdominal circumference (Anthony & Smith, 1999). However, while many IUGR babies are also SGA, this is not always the case, and a baby may be growth restricted yet not fall below the 10th percentile for any parameter. Thus, it is more precise to consider these babies in a different category, even though the differences between IUGR babies and those who experienced asymmetric SGA growth are often clinically vague. While IUGR babies are often malnourished, many factors can influence growth besides fetal nutrition. IUGR is best determined by comparing the newborn findings with the mother's medical and dietary history and the course of pregnancy. While the absolute definition of SGA may exclude some IUGR babies because they fall above the 10th percentile in weight, all IUGR babies are at some increased risk for postpartum complications.

To evaluate the SGA or IUGR newborn, first determine if the growth restriction is proportionate or disproportionate. Then, perform a complete physical exam with special regard to possible anomalies or dysmorphic features. If dysmorphic or multiple anomalies are noted, chromosomal studies are indicated. Review the pregnancy history to look for teratogenic exposure, infections, or other maternal illness. Maternal viral and antibody studies should be ordered as indicated. Uncontrolled maternal metabolic disorders should be ruled out, as they can wreak havoc with fetal growth as well.

Have infants with disproportionate IUGR evaluated for skeletal dysplasia or metabolic bone disease. For those with proportionate IUGR, consult a geneticist who may recognize one of the many associated dysmorphic syndromes. Submit the placenta for laboratory examination which may reveal confined placental mosaicism (where an abnormal cell line is confined to the placenta, a diagnosis of uncertain significance that may be associated with some cases of IUGR) or uniparental disomy (UPD). UPD occurs when both members of a pair of chromosomes are derived from a single parent; for example, the baby starts out with a trisomy defect (such as Down syndrome) and loses chromosome, to end up with two from the same parent. This is associated with a variety of syndromes (Korones, 1986; Sparks et al., 1999).

Appropriate for gestational age (AGA) growth

AGA babies fall in the midrange of size for weight, length and head circumference for most babies of the same gestational age. Technically, their measurements fall between the 10th and the 90th percentiles. Totally proportionate measurements would all fall within or nearly within the same percentile; for example, the baby's head, length and weight values might each fall in or near the 75th percentile. These babies are least likely to have problems of any kind. The exception is those infants who are technically AGA because their individual measurements are above the 10th percentile, but are actually IUGR due to inadequate maternal nutrition in the last trimester.

Large for gestational age (LGA) growth

As with SGA growth, LGA babies may grow either symmetrically or asymmetrically. **Macrosomia** means "big body"; technically, the term can be applied to all large babies. The use of this term is slowly falling out of favor because of its vagueness. Although some of the medical literature tends to lump all LGA babies into a pathological category, this generalization denies that healthy, bigger-than-average babies are often born to well-nourished women. Therefore, this textbook will confine the use of the term "macrosomia" to asymmetric LGA growth, as detailed below.

The cut-off for "high birthweight" has been variously set at values ranging from 4000 to 4500 g (8 lb 13 oz to 9 lb 14.75 oz), depending upon the source, with most using the 4000 g cut off. The 4000 g limit was chosen primarily because it is the size and weight at which the chances of birth trauma rise significantly among babies born in hospitals (where women are often drugged and cannot assume a variety of positions for pushing).

Symmetrical LGA growth: By and large, these are normal, big, healthy babies. About 50 to 60% of all LGA babies are large due to enhanced intrinsic growth. Their head, weight and length measurements are proportionate, all falling above the 90th percentile on a standard growth chart. Some of these babies are big because they are born to large parents and are constitutionally destined to be large adults; hereditary variation is the operative factor in their growth pattern. Others are large because maternal nutrition has been optimal, with fetal growth continuing right up to term. Well-nourished women often carry past their due date as well. This combination leads to a population of babies who are healthy in every way but larger than average. If born at or just past term, they are alert (but not hyperactive) and robust and have well-developed reflexes.

Asymmetrical LGA growth (macrosomia): A characteristic type of LGA growth occurs in babies of mothers who have poorly controlled or unrecognized diabetes. This is the most common cause of macrosomia, accounting for 35 to 40% of all large babies, who are sometimes referred to as "Infants of Diabetic Mothers" (IDM).

These infants are large with a disproportional growth ratio. Fetal growth parallels that of an AGA fetus during the first two trimesters, but the rate of abdominal growth begins to rise significantly after 24 weeks while head growth continues at a normal pace. Past the 28th week, skeletal growth, fat deposition and fluid retention begins to accelerate, and abnormal organ enlargement (excluding the kidneys and brain) occurs. At birth, the circumference of the trunk is large relative to the head; the chest circumference exceeds the head circumference in 80% of cases. The upper arms also contribute to a wider upper torso diameter and display deep skin folds. The abdominal circumference and thigh diameter also reflect soft-tissue mass that is usually significantly higher than average. These babies have head and femur measurements that vary in size and length but usually fall below the 90th percentile. Regardless of the baby's gestational age, those born to diabetic mothers are at increased risk for asymmetrical LGA growth (O'Leary, 1992). Not every feature of asymmetric growth is evident in every baby. These babies appear, fat, round and plethoric with a "tomato-face" and an obese body with tight, shiny skin, copious lanugo and often a generous covering of vernix. The placenta and umbilical cord are also usually enlarged. These babies are prone to a variety of problems, including birth injury, respiratory distress, polycythemia, hypoglycemia and transient hypertrophic cardiomyopathy.

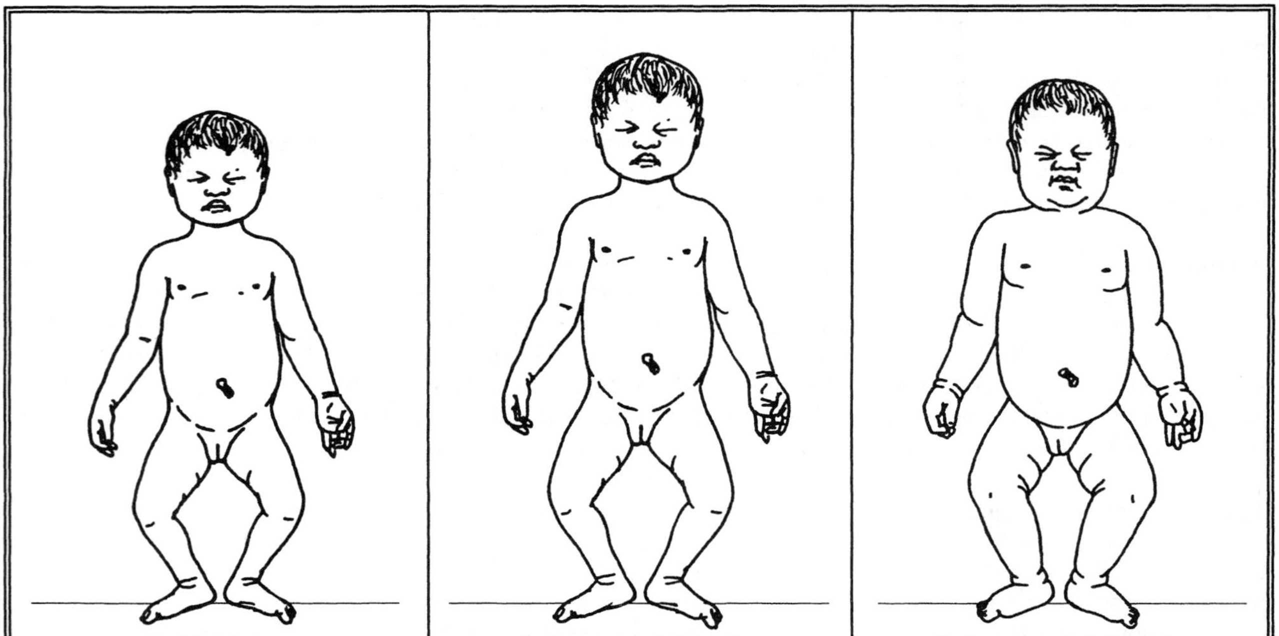

1. AGA baby — 2. Symmetric LGA baby — 3. Asymmetric LGA baby

Limbs are shown extended to better demonstrate the differences in size. Size parameters from the tables by Miller (1981).
1. Weight 3430 (7 lb. 9 oz), Length 51.3 cm, OFC 34.5 cm (50th percentile)
2. Weight 4030 (8 lb, 14.5 oz), Length 54.0 cm, OFC 36.2 cm (95th percentile)
3. Weight 4030 (8 lb, 14.5 oz), Length 52.0 cm, OFC 36.2 cm, Shoulder and abdominal circ. enlarged, femurs shortened.

This type of growth reflects the delivery of an abnormal nutrient balance to the baby from the mother, primarily comprised of excessive glucose but also including abnormal levels of growth factors, lipids and amino acids. High levels of glucose prompt the baby to produce more insulin, thus accelerating fuel use and growth. Chronic hyperinsulinemia causes the baby's islets of Langerhans in the pancreas to hypertrophy and leads to congenital hyperinsulinemia as the over-secretion continues. This is the most serious complication among these babies. It may occur even if the mother's diabetes is well-controlled (Johnston et al., 2003). Recurrent hypoglycemia presents in the first hours of life, which can lead to brain damage (Langer, 2000). Polycythemia is more common in these babies due to chronic intrauterine hypoxia.

Signs, symptoms and problems associated with asymmetric macrosomic growth in IDM: Many macrosomic babies of diabetic mothers die in the last six weeks of pregnancy because they have severe congenital defects or because they can no longer tolerate the abnormal nutrient supply coming from the mother. The baby who makes it through birth will be born fat and puffy, with a round, fat face and a weight that is often well above the 90th percentile for gestational age. The length and head appear relatively small because these measurements are not above the 90th percentile. Even though the baby is large, he can be quite preterm, so evaluate gestational age with care. Respiratory distress is common, with all the clinical features noted among other preterm babies. Polycythemia produces the characteristic tomato-red coloring and can lead to postnatal jaundice. Weight gain after birth is often slow as the baby adjusts to his intended genetic size.

The baby can become profoundly hypoglycemic after birth, the supply of glucose coming from the mother having been removed while the baby is still producing a high level of insulin. This is especially true during the first 6 hours of life. Hypoglycemia presents with jitteriness, cyanosis, lethargy, seizures, apnea, hypotonia and poor feeding, although many hypoglycemic babies are asymptomatic, at least at first. These babies should start nursing in the first hour of life to prevent a dangerous fall in blood sugar as the baby normalizes insulin production. Hypocalcemia often accompanies hypoglycemia during the first days of life because maternal diabetes causes immaturity of parathyroid function in the newborn; the symptoms are similar to those of hypoglycemia. Examine the baby carefully for traumatic birth injuries such as broken bones or nerve palsies if shoulder dystocia and subsequent manipulations took place at birth.

Macrosomic babies have a high incidence of congenital anomalies because of the teratogenic effects of abnormal maternal metabolism during early pregnancy. The incidence of major anomalies is about 6 to 9% overall but is disproportionately higher among babies of mothers whose diabetes was undetected or poorly controlled until pregnancy was well underway. The most common defects include cardiovascular (double the usual risk), central nervous system, and genitourinary anomalies as well as gastrointestinal and, more rarely, caudal regression syndrome, which involves severe defects of the pelvic bones and lower spine, including sacral agenesis (Johnston et al., 2003; O'Leary, 1992).

Macrosomia is also a feature of several congenital disorders that have a metabolic component including Beckwith-Wiedemann syndrome (presents with enlarged tongue, linear creases on the external ear lobes, and sometimes omphalocele), a variety of tumors (such as hemangiomata and Wilms, adrenocortical, or hepatic tumors), nesidioblastosis (a disorder of the pancreas, resulting in an infant with problems similar to those of IDM), Sotos syndrome (presents with a large, long head, and abnormal projection of the jaw with a narrow anterior mandible), Weaver syndrome (presents with accelerated skeletal growth, permanent flexion of both joints in one or more fingers, unusual facies, seizures and cerebral enlargement), Simpson-Golabi-Behmel syndrome (an X-linked dysplastic gigantism characterized by pre- and postnatal overgrowth, distinct, "coarse" facial appearance, dysplastic changes in several tissues, enlargement of the kidneys and tongue, rib and vertebral anomalies and hypoglycemia, as well as mild retardation in some cases. Polycythemia and respiratory distress are common at birth) (Langer, 2000).

Growth Charts

Georgieff (1995) lists five types of normative curves used to assess newborn nutritional status.

1. **Standard one-factor anthropometrics:** This is the most common set of measurements, including weight, length and occipitofrontal head circumference for gestational age, as described in this chapter.
2. **Specialty one-factor anthropometrics:** These give more information about body composition and include measurements such as midarm circumference and triceps skinfold thickness for gestational age.
3. **Calculated body-compartment anthropometrics:** These use a combination of specialty anthropometrics such as arm muscle area, arm fat area, and arm water area to further define body composition.
4. **Two-factor body-proportion assessments:** These assessments take advantage of the physiologic principles involved in the sparing of length at the expense of weight or occipitofrontal head circumference at the expense of peripheral muscles and fat during mild to moderate malnutrition. These include the ponderal index ([weight (grams) X 100/length (cm)]) and the midarm-circumference-to-head-circumference ratio.
5. **Biochemical assessments:** Lab tests of serum proteins with slow, medium and rapid turnover can provide insight into chronic, subacute and acute nutritional status changes, respectively, prior to birth.

All newborns should be evaluated with the standard one-factor anthropometric measurements. Only about 10% of these will require referral for further assessment. The most widely used one-factor growth charts come from a study done at the Colorado General Hospital in Denver in 1966 (Lubchenco et al., 1966). Although they are readily available in chart blanks printed by pharmaceutical companies, they are not the most accurate. This study excluded only infants with anomalies from its final data base (thus ignoring a number of variables that may have adversely influenced fetal growth). Thus, birthweights are rather light in this series, which is why these charts are not included here.

In 1996, a fetal growth curve was produced with data derived from national US birth statistics of singleton births. It was presented as a national reference tool in the February 1996 issue of OBSTETRICS AND GYNECOLOGY (Alexander et al., 1996). It attempted to address cases with implausible combinations of birthweight and gestational age and to smooth birthweights across gestational-age categories. There are several potential problems with the data that are described in the article. This table is included here for students for reference and comparison with the other tables that follow. This table is not recommended for use in newborn assessment, as its weight curve is low.

Assessing preterm infants: The tables from Naeye and Dixon (1978) attempted to better control for the timing of pregnancy, retained data only from those babies who survived the neonatal period and performed less smoothing of the data than some others. These tables are therefore recommended for use in babies born at 36 weeks or earlier.

Assessing term infants: The best charts available for babies born from 37 weeks to term are those by Miller (1981). They were derived from carefully controlled data that took into account 30 variables that may adversely impact fetal size and weight in order to arrive at the most normal standard possible. Miller analyzed populations of black as well as white infants and include data for both sexes. All of these charts are included. Because the normal fetal weight curve is higher in these tables, I recommend that you use these to assess your term babies.

Assessing postterm infants: McLean and associates (1991) did a careful study of babies born between 39 and 42.6 weeks gestation using due dates confirmed by ultrasound between 16 and 18 weeks gestation in conjunction with a known date for the first day of the last normal period. Conditions known to interfere with fetal growth were excluded. These tables are included after Miller's. Use them to compare findings when your babies are large or born past their due dates.

BIRTHWEIGHT (GRAMS) FOR GESTATIONAL AGE, BASED ON 1991 DATA FROM US RESIDENTS (ALEXANDER ET AL., 1996)						
GESTATIONAL AGE (WKS FROM LMP)	5TH PERCENTILE	10TH PERCENTILE		50TH PERCENTILE	90TH PERCENTILE	95TH PERCENTILE
	Smoothed data (♂♀)	Boys	Girls	Smoothed data (♂♀)		
23	385	446	426	582	882	1107
24	435	504	480	674	977	1223
25	480	570	535	779	1138	1397
26	529	644	592	899	1362	1640
27	591	728	662	1035	1635	1927
28	670	828	760	1196	1977	2237
29	772	956	889	1394	2361	2553
30	910	1117	1047	1637	2710	2847
31	1088	1308	1234	1918	2986	3108
32	1294	1521	1447	2203	3200	3338
33	1513	1751	1675	2458	3370	3536
34	1735	1985	1901	2667	3502	3697
35	1950	2205	2109	2831	3596	3812
36	2156	2407	2300	2974	3668	3888
37	**2357**	**2596**	**2484**	**3117**	**3755**	**3956**
38	**2543**	**2769**	**2657**	**3263**	**3867**	**4027**
39	**2685**	**2908**	**2796**	**3400**	**3980**	**4107**
40	**2761**	**2986**	**2872**	**3495**	**4060**	**4185**
41	**2777**	**3007**	**2891**	**3527**	**4094**	**4217**
42	**2764**	**2998**	**2884**	**3522**	**4098**	**4213**
43	2741	2977	2868	3505	4096	4178
44	2724	2963	2853	3491	4096	4122

These tables formulated by Naeye and Dixon (1978) are recommended for use when assessing babies born between 28 and 36 weeks of gestation.

Percentile	Body Length (Cm) in Newborns for Gestational Ages in Weeks from LMP								
	28	29	30	31	32	33	34	35	36
90th	39.8	40.7	41.9	43.4	44.4	46.0	47.8	49.4	50.8
75th	38.7	39.7	40.9	42.2	43.3	44.7	46.3	47.8	49.1
50th	38.0	39.0	40.3	41.4	42.5	43.9	45.3	46.7	48.0
25th	37.3	38.3	39.7	40.6	41.7	43.1	44.3	45.6	46.9
10th	36.2	37.3	38.7	39.4	40.6	41.8	42.8	44.0	45.2

Percentile	Occipitofrontal Circ. (Cm) in Newborns for Gestational Ages in Weeks from LMP								
	28	29	30	31	32	33	34	35	36
90th	27.6	28.4	29.3	30.1	30.6	31.4	32.2	33.0	34.0
75th	26.7	27.5	28.5	29.2	29.8	30.6	31.4	32.2	33.0
50th	26.0	26.9	27.9	28.6	29.3	30.1	30.8	31.6	32.4
25th	25.3	26.3	27.3	28.0	28.8	29.6	30.2	31.0	31.8
10th	24.4	25.4	26.5	27.1	28.0	28.8	29.4	30.2	30.8

Percentile	Weight (Grams) in Newborns for Gestational Ages in Weeks from LMP								
	28	29	30	31	32	33	34	35	36
90th	1363	1466	1648	1816	2004	2207	2529	2766	3121
75th	1245	1364	1524	1687	1863	2056	2308	2539	2822
50th	1165	1295	1440	1601	1769	1955	2160	2387	2621
25th	1085	1226	1356	1515	1675	1854	2012	2235	2420
10th	967	1124	1232	1386	1534	1703	1791	2008	2121

The following tables are those of Miller (1981), which are recommended for use with babies born at term.

Percentile	Crown-Heel Length (cm) in White Newborn Boys for Gestational Ages in Weeks from LMP					
	37	38	39	40	41	42-43
95th	52.0	53.0	54.0	54.5	55.0	55.3
90th	51.5	52.5	53.5	54.0	54.5	54.8
75th	50.5	51.5	52.5	53.0	53.5	54.0
50th	50.0	50.7	51.5	52.0	52.5	53.0
25th	49.0	49.7	50.5	51.0	51.5	52.0
10th	48.0	48.7	49.5	50.0	50.5	51.0
5th	47.5	48.2	49.0	49.5	50.0	50.5

Percentile	Occipitofrontal Circ. (cm) in White Newborn Boys for Gestational Ages in Weeks from LMP					
	37	38	39	40	41	42-43
95th	35.5	36.0	36.4	36.8	37.2	37.4
90th	35.2	35.6	35.9	36.3	36.7	37.2
75th	34.6	34.9	35.3	35.7	36.0	36.2
50th	34.0	34.3	34.6	34.9	35.2	35.5
25th	33.4	33.7	34.0	34.3	34.7	35.0
10th	32.8	33.2	33.5	33.8	34.2	34.5
5th	32.4	32.7	33.1	33.4	33.8	34.2

Percentile	Birthweight (grams) for Firstborn White Boys for Gestational Ages in Weeks from LMP					
	37	38	39	40	41	42-43
95th	3630	3820	3970	4100	4230	4340
90th	3500	3700	3860	4000	4130	4240
75th	3300	3480	3650	3780	3920	4030
50th	3100	3270	3430	3570	3700	3820
25th	2850	3000	3130	3260	3380	3490
10th	2700	2840	2960	3080	3180	3280
5th	2620	2760	2880	3000	3100	3200
Percentile	Birthweight (grams) for White Newborn Boys of Multiparas					
95th	3660	4000	4200	4390	4500	4600
90th	3470	3700	3900	4080	4240	4370
75th	3300	3500	3700	3870	4030	4150
50th	3100	3270	3440	3610	3750	3850
25th	2850	3020	3180	3340	3500	3620
10th	2710	2860	3020	3190	3340	3450
5th	2630	2780	2940	3080	3210	3320

Percentile	Crown-Heel Length (Cm) in White Newborn Girls for Gestational Ages in Wks from LMP (Miller, 1981)					
	37	38	39	40	41	42–43
95th	51.5	52.5	53.5	54.0	54.5	54.5
90th	51.0	52.0	53.0	53.5	54.0	54.0
75th	50.0	51.0	52.0	52.5	52.8	53.1
50th	49.0	50.0	50.7	51.3	51.7	52.0
25th	48.0	48.9	49.5	50.0	50.5	51.0
10th	47.5	48.5	49.0	49.5	50.0	50.5
5th	47.0	47.9	48.6	49.1	49.5	50.0

Percentile	Occipitofrontal Circ. (cm) in White Newborn Girls for Gestational Ages in wks from LMP					
	37	38	39	40	41	42-43
95th	35.0	35.5	35.9	36.2	36.5	36.8
90th	34.5	35.0	35.4	35.7	36.1	36.3
75th	33.9	34.3	34.7	35.1	35.5	35.8
50th	33.2	33.6	34.1	34.5	34.8	35.2
25th	32.5	32.9	33.4	33.8	34.2	34.5
10th	32.0	32.4	32.8	33.2	33.6	33.9
5th	31.8	32.2	32.6	32.9	33.3	33.6

Percentile	Birthweight (grams) in Firstborn White Newborn Girls for Gestational Ages in Weeks from LMP					
	37	38	39	40	41	42-43
95th	3440	3720	3900	4030	4120	4200
90th	3300	3600	3800	3920	4020	4100
75th	3170	3380	3570	3700	3820	3940
50th	3000	3150	3300	3430	3560	3660
25th	2790	2930	3070	3180	3290	3370
10th	2550	2720	3850	2970	3090	3170
5th	2460	2610	2760	2890	3010	3100
Percentile	Birthweight (grams) for White newborn Girls of Multiparas					
95th	3600	3860	4020	4140	4230	4310
90th	3500	3670	3840	3950	4070	4150
75th	3260	3480	3640	3750	3850	3950
50th	3000	3200	3340	3500	3620	3720
25th	2800	2950	3080	3230	3350	3450
10th	2670	2800	2930	3050	3160	3260
5th	2520	2670	2800	2920	3040	3150

Miller offers the only data on black newborns that I could find in the literature.

PERCENTILE	CROWN-HEEL LENGTH (CM) IN BLACK NEWBORN BOYS FOR GESTATIONAL AGES IN WEEKS FROM LMP (MILLER, 1981)					
	37	38	39	40	41	42-43
95th	51.5	52.5	53.5	54.5	54.5	54.5
90th	51.0	52.0	52.7	53.5	54.0	54.0
75th	50.5	51.5	52.0	52.5	53.0	53.0
50th	49.5	50.0	50.5	51.0	51.5	52.0
25th	48.5	49.0	49.5	50.0	50.5	51.0
10th	47.5	48.0	48.5	49.0	49.5	50.0
5th	47.0	47.5	48.0	48.5	49.0	49.5

PERCENTILE	OCCIPITOFRONTAL CIRC. (CM) IN BLACK NEWBORN BOYS FOR GESTATIONAL AGES IN WEEKS FROM LMP					
	37	38	39	40	41	42-43
95th	35.3	35.8	36.2	36.7	37.0	37.0
90th	35.0	35.5	35.9	36.3	36.7	36.8
75th	34.6	34.9	35.3	35.6	36.0	36.3
50th	33.6	34.0	34.4	34.7	35.1	35.5
25th	33.1	33.4	33.8	34.1	34.5	34.9
10th	32.4	32.8	33.1	33.4	33.8	34.1
5th	32.1	32.5	32.8	33.1	33.4	33.7

PERCENTILE	BIRTHWEIGHT (GRAMS) FOR BLACK NEWBORN BOYS FOR GESTATIONAL AGES IN WEEKS FROM LMP					
	37	38	39	40	41	42-43
95th	3440	3710	3970	4130	4290	4400
90th	3380	3620	3840	3970	4100	4150
75th	3300	3460	3620	3720	3820	3920
50th	3080	3180	3300	3400	3500	3600
25th	2830	2930	3030	3130	3220	3320
10th	2630	2730	2820	2900	2990	3080
5th	2540	2680	2720	2820	2950	3000

Percentile	Crown-Heel length (cm) in Black Newborn Girls for Gestational Ages in Weeks from LMP (Miller, 1981)					
	37	38	39	40	41	42-43
95th	51.0	51.7	52.5	53.3	54.0	54.0
90th	50.3	51.0	51.8	52.5	53.5	53.0
75th	49.5	50.5	51.0	51.5	52.0	52.5
50th	49.0	49.5	50.0	50.5	51.0	51.5
25th	48.0	48.5	49.0	49.5	50.0	50.5
10th	47.0	47.5	48.0	48.5	49.0	49.5
5th	46.5	47.0	47.5	48.0	48.5	49.0

Percentile	Occipitofrontal Circ. (cm) in Black Newborn Girls for Gestational Ages in Weeks from LMP					
	37	38	39	40	41	42-43
95th	35.0	35.1	35.6	35.9	36.2	36.5
90th	34.3	34.8	35.3	35.6	35.8	36.0
75th	34.1	34.3	34.6	34.8	35.1	35.3
50th	33.4	33.6	33.9	34.1	34.4	34.7
25th	32.7	33.0	33.2	33.5	33.7	34.0
10th	32.1	32.3	32.6	32.8	33.1	33.3
5th	31.7	32.0	32.2	32.5	32.8	33.0

Percentile	Birthweight (grams) for Black Newborn girls for Gestational Ages in Weeks from LMP					
	37	38	39	40	41	42-43
95th	3440	3650	3830	3970	4000	4150
90th	3320	3530	3730	3880	3980	4050
75th	3140	3320	3480	3600	3730	3850
50th	2930	3070	3220	3340	3460	3580
25th	2700	2830	2950	3080	3030	3320
10th	2530	2650	2770	2890	3010	3100
5th	2430	2540	2650	2770	2890	3010

Compare the values below with those on previous tables when your babies are large and born at term or later.

WEEKS + DAYS GESTATION AT BIRTH	BIRTH WEIGHT (GRAMS)	LENGTH (CM)	OCF HEAD CIRC. (CM)
Primiparous mothers			
39-39.6	2970-3764	48.55-52.65	33.32-34.88
40-40.6	3094-3900	49.04-53.36	33.72-36.18
41-41.6	3230-4020	49.65-53.75	34.14-36.46
42-42.6	3339-4131	49.43-54.37	34.4-36.6
Multiparous mothers			
39-39.6	3085-3597	48.66-53.14	33.46-36.34
40-40.6	3227-4015	49.13-53.67	33.73-36.47
41-41.6	3284-4204	49.62-54.18	34.27-36.53
42-42.6	3436-4282	49.84-54.96	34.39-37.01

(Based on McLean et al., 1991)

Assessing Babies Whose Mothers Experienced Pregnancy while Living at a High Altitude

At altitudes well above sea level, babies gestate in a thinner oxygen environment, which produces varying degrees of chronic hypoxia and therefore light-for-dates growth, with growth restriction beginning in the third trimester.

Moore (2003) states that weight reduction averages 100g per 3281 ft (1000 m) of elevation gain, although reductions become more evident at altitudes above 6562 ft (2000 m). Mortola and colleagues (2000) found that babies gestated at elevations below 6562 ft (2000 m) or at altitudes where the barometric pressure stays above about 590 mm Hg with an inspired oxygen partial pressure of above 114 mm Hg, show little variation from the birthweights of babies born at sea level.

Among people who have lived at the same altitude for many generations, the effect is less dramatic and their babies are larger than those who have not had the same degree of long-term adaptation. Among such populations, a 65 g drop in birth weight can be expected for those born at 6562 ft (2000 m), with further drops of 65 g for each additional 1640 ft (500 m) rise in elevation. A 105 g drop in birthweight may be expected for every additional 50 mm Hg drop in barometric pressure. Those gestated above 14,764 ft (4500 m) elevation also have a slight reduction in length (Motola et al., 2000).

ASSESSING THE NUTRITIONAL STATUS OF THE TERM NEWBORN WITH THE CANSCORE

Fetal malnutrition and the terms "small for gestational age" and "intrauterine growth restriction" are not equivalent conditions, and one may be present without the others. Malnutrition is a clinical diagnosis and can occur at almost any birthweight. In addition, those babies grouped into the IUGR or SGA category may or may not have suffered from fetal malnutrition because the range of causes of these growth abnormalities is wide. Fetal malnutrition affects body composition and interferes with brain development, with corresponding alterations in behavior. Its effect on humans remains vague partly because of the failure to distinguish SGA growth and malnutrition in newborns. Fetal malnutrition adversely impacts the central nervous system regardless of size at birth, and its short- and long-term effects are serious.

Fetal malnutrition is characterized by a reduction in or failure to acquire normal amounts of subcutaneous body fat and muscle. Weight, length and head circumference may, or may not, be affected. If the fetus fails to receive or utilize nutrients during the period of most rapid growth (20 to 36 weeks), the amounts of protein and fat synthesized are reduced, decreasing the body content of these nutrients. If the nutrient supply is acutely limited after 36 weeks, the fetus begins to break down and utilize previously deposited fat and protein. When this occurs, plasma amino acids and other nutrients may remain at normal to near-normal levels because the baby is catabolizing his own tissues. The clinical signs of malnutrition are partly affected by when it began during pregnancy.

ABNORMAL FINDINGS	PROBABLE TIMING OF ONSET OF MALNUTRITION AND COMMENTS
Length, head circ. and weight all significantly reduced	Began early second trimester
Length, head circ. less affected, but small with low weight (although may be above 10th percentile), with loss of subcutaneous tissues and muscle	Began early third trimester
Length, head circ. WNL, significantly reduced weight (may be above 10th percentile), obvious loss of subcutaneous tissues	Began after 36 weeks gestation due to insufficient or imbalanced nutrient supply

Clinical signs of specific types of malnutrition are included in the table below:

CLINICAL SIGN	NUTRIENT DEFICIENCY
Lethargy; muscle wasting	Protein, calorie
Pallor	Iron, copper, folate, Vitamin B_{12}
Edema; hair depigmentation	Protein, zinc
Dryness and ulceration of the cornea	Vitamin A
Inflammation of the corners of the mouth	Vitamin B_2
Swelling of the tongue	Niacin
Goiter (thyroid enlargement)	Iodine
Thickening around the hair follicles	Vitamin A
Inflamed skin on the arms and legs	Essential fatty acids
Dry, scaly skin	Zinc
Petechia and bruising	Vitamin C
Rachitic rosary (row of nobs where the ribs meet the rib cartilage on either side), bone thickening; craniotabes, frontal bossing	Vitamin D
Frail, thin, poorly mineralized bones	Calcium, phosphorus

The CANS (Clinical Assessment of Nutritional Status) scoring system was devised to differentiate malnourished newborns regardless of their weight, length and head circumference. The CANSCORE is used to assess the nutritional status of the term newborn of 37 completed postconceptual weeks, not preterm infants. The score is the sum of the nine parameters: hair, cheeks, chin and neck, arms, back and interior scapulae, buttocks, legs, chest, and the skin over the abdominal wall. Each of the assessments are rated on a scale of 1 (worst, most severe malnutrition) to 4 (most well nourished). A baby achieving a top score of 36 is healthy, plump and well nourished. Scores less than 24 indicate some degree of malnutrition with the lowest score, 9, indicating severe malnutrition in utero. The score can be done after birth to help determine the extent of intrauterine growth restriction or dysmaturity and to evaluate failure-to-thrive in the weeks after birth. The assessment is also used to further quantify growth in those babies who present at term with asymmetrically restricted growth.

<u>The CANSCORE assessments</u>

The malnourished baby appears emaciated to varying degrees. Any degree of malnutrition results in some reduction of the subcutaneous tissues and muscle, leaving a baby whose skin appears to be too large for the baby. To perform the CANS assessment, begin with the baby lying supine to evaluate the anterior features.

<u>Hair</u>: Run your fingers through the baby's hair. Assess the texture, amount, condition and manageability of the hair by lifting a hank of hair, looking at it and rubbing it between your fingers.

Scoring:
- 4: Large amount of smooth, silky, easily groomed hair
- 3: Thinner hair with some straight "staring" hair that sticks up or down
- 2: Very thin, straight, "staring" hair that does not respond to brushing and has depigmented areas
- 1: Very thin, straight hair which sticks out, with depigmented stripe (flag sign)

Straight and "staring" hair, which refers to dull, dry and inflexible (or wiry) strands, is a characteristic seen in severely marasmic babies. **Marasmus** is a form of emaciation due to prolonged protein and calorie deficiency. The flag sign describes bands of discoloration in the pigmentation of the hair. These may be reddish, blond, or gray depending on the genetic hair color. Such bands result from fluctuations in nutrition that are characteristic of the severe protein and calorie depletion seen in kwashiorkor.

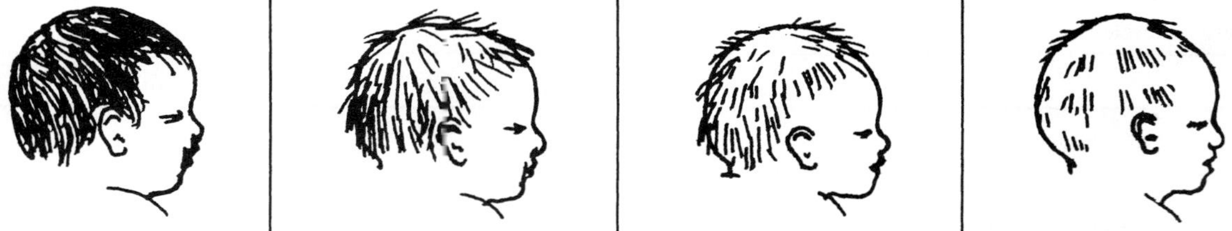

Score: 4 | Score: 3 | Score: 2 | Score: 1

In a study of the usefulness of the CANSCORE Score, Rao and colleagues (1999), found hair to be the least correlated of all the CANSCORE assessments with nutritional status. They recommended a modified score to exclude hair as a parameter, with a modified minimum normal score of 22 and a modified maximum optimal score of 32.

<u>Cheeks</u>: The cheeks are assessed by their appearance and, if necessary, by gentle palpation to determine the thickness of the fat layer.

Scoring:
- 4: Full buccal pads, round face
- 3: Face appears less full
- 2: Face thinner, with cheekbones more prominent
- 1: Significantly reduced buccal pads with a narrow, flat face

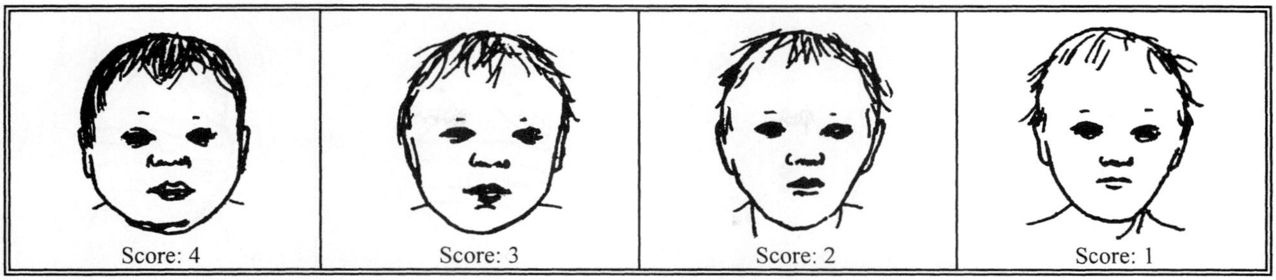

Chin and neck: The neck is assessed by appearance and palpation. Tip the head back to get a better view of the neck.

Scoring:
4: Double or triple fat folds under the chin, with the neck not evident
3: Single fat fold under chin with less fullness overall; neck somewhat evident
2: Minimal fat folds under chin; neck looks thinner with some wrinkling of the skin
1: No fat folds; loose, wrinkled skin very obvious, neck appears thin and scrawny

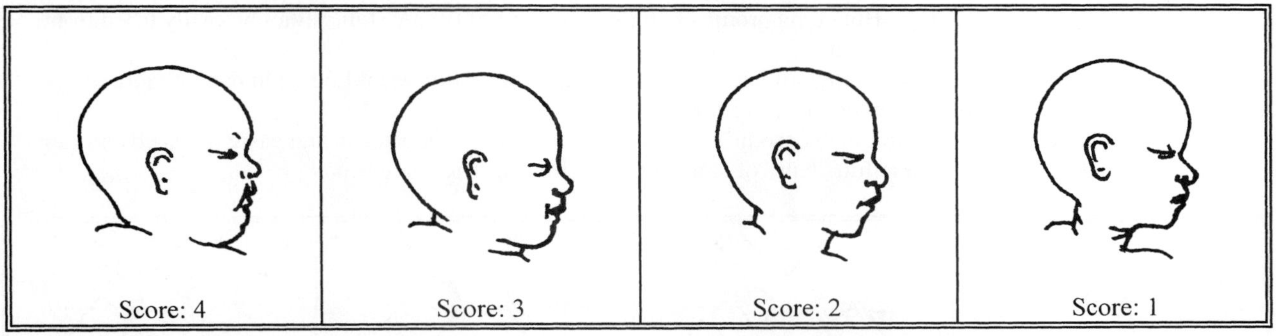

Chest: The chest is visually evaluated.

Scoring:
4: Full, round with no ribs visible
3: Ribs slightly visible
2: Ribs quite visible, with some loss of overlying fat layer
1: Progressively prominent ribs from the midline to the sides with obvious loss of intercostal tissue

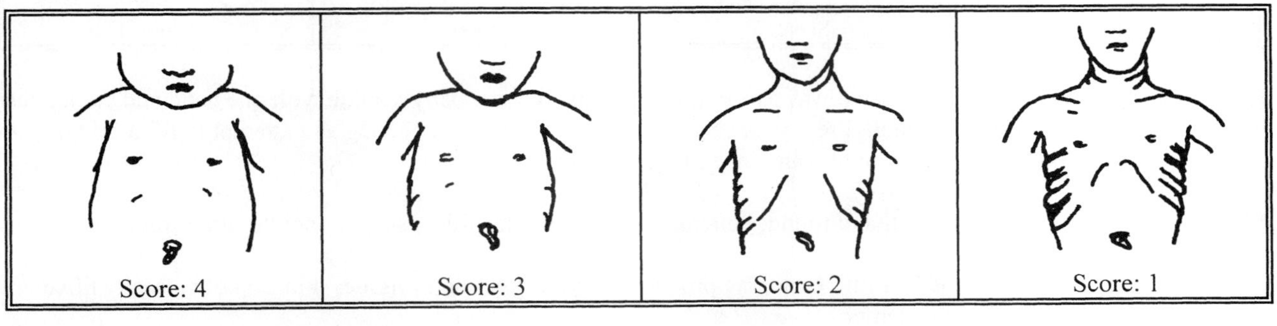

Abdomen: The abdomen is visually evaluated.

Scoring:
4: Full and round with no loose skin
3: Abdomen appears less full, with absent to very minimal wrinkling.
2: Abdomen is flat, with some wrinkling of the skin.
1: Distended or sunken with very loose skin that is wrinkled and easily lifted; accordion folding evident.

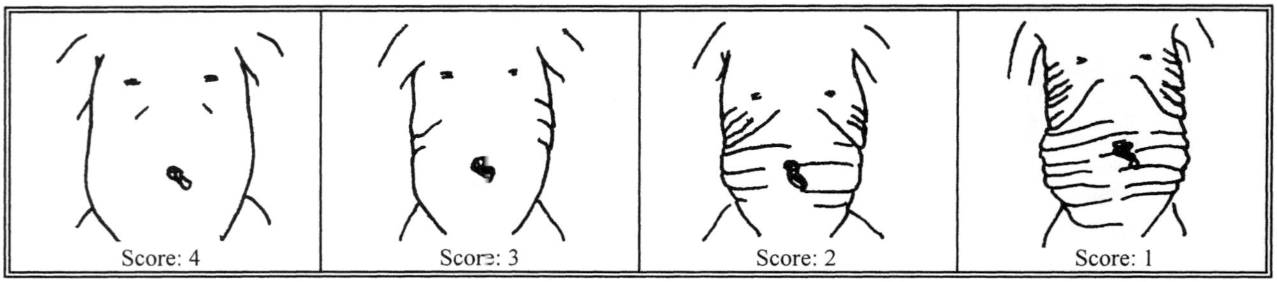

<u>Arms</u>: Grasp the baby's arm just below the elbow with one hand and encircle the wrist with the other or grasp the arm to either side of the elbow. Move your hands toward each other in an effort to bunch up the skin and underlying fat layer. Release the arm and attempt to lift the skin of the posterior upper arm above the elbow by pinching the skin with your thumbs and index fingers and pulling outward.

Scoring:

4: The arm is full and round. Bunching cannot produce accordion folds nor can folds be lifted from the elbow or triceps area.

3: The arm is less full. Bunching produces slight collection of tissue; skin cannot be easily lifted from the elbow or triceps area.

2: The arm looks thin. Bunching produces a moderate amount of wrinkling; skin can be more easily lifted from the elbow or triceps region.

1: Marked accordion folding is produced between your hands; skin is loose and easily grasped and can be pulled away in a thin "tent" of skin from the elbow or triceps region.

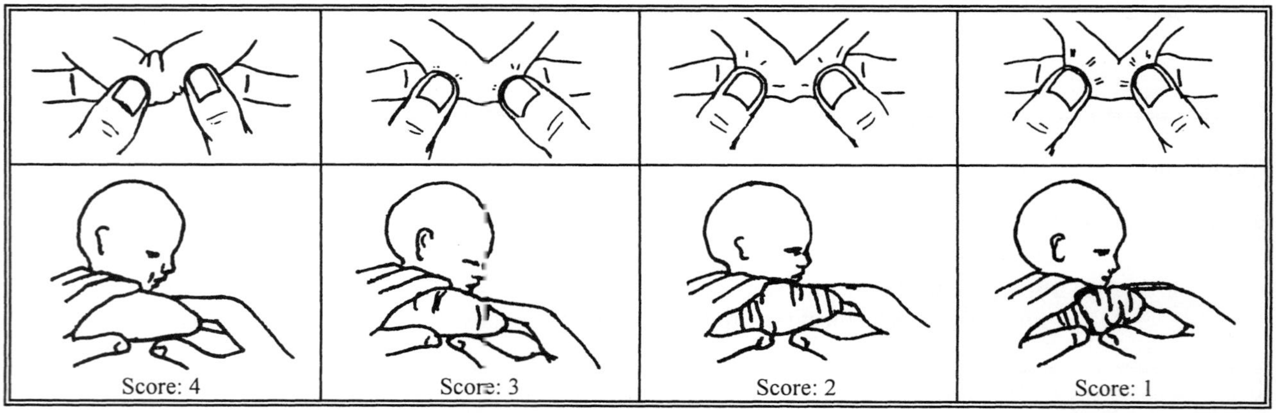

<u>Legs</u>: The legs are assessed in the same way as for the arms. Encircle the baby's ankle with one hand and the leg just below the knee with your other hand. Press your two hands together. Release the leg and attempt to lift a fold of skin over the anterior shin between your thumb and index fingers by pulling upward.

Scoring:

4: The lower leg is full and round; bunching cannot produce folds; skin cannot be lifted from the knee or femur.

3: The lower leg is less full; bunching produces slight collection of tissue; skin cannot be easily lifted from the knee or femur

2: The lower leg looks thin; bunching produces a moderate amount of wrinkling; skin can be more easily lifted from the knee and femur.

1: Marked accordion folding is produced between your hands; the skin overlying the knee or femur is loose and easily grasped and pulled away in a thin "tent."

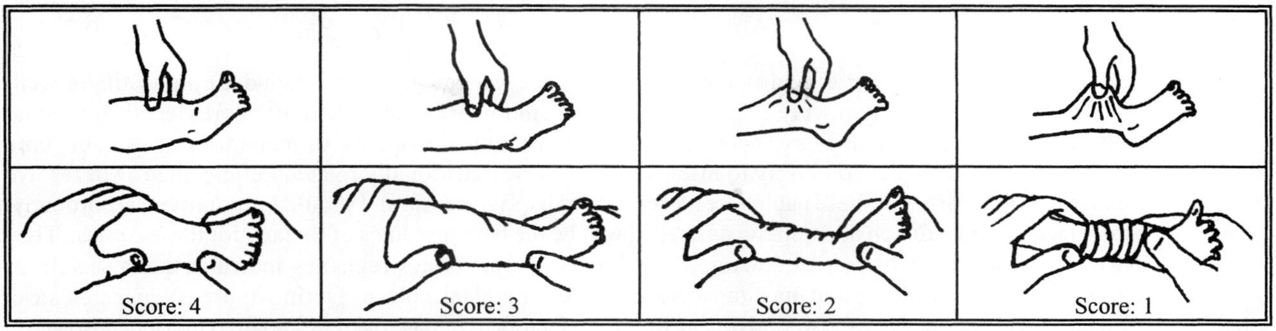

Back: Turn the baby over on her belly. Using your thumb and forefinger, attempt to grasp and lift a fold of skin between the scapulae.

Scoring:
4: Skin cannot be lifted between the scapulae.
3: Skin lifts slightly in a small fold; turgor is good.
2: Skin is moderately mobile and a moderately sized fold can be lifted easily.
1: Skin is loose and easily lifted in a deep, thin fold.

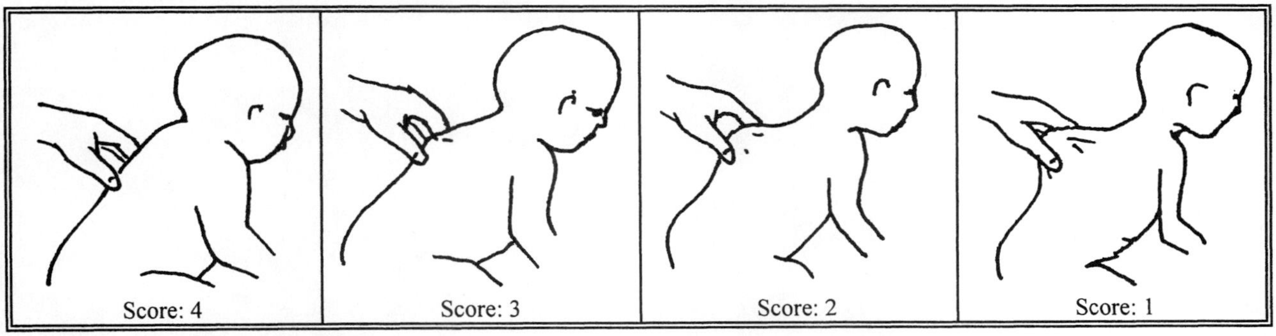

Buttocks: Lay the baby on his belly and look at the buttocks.

Scoring:
4: Full, round gluteal fat pads with filled out, chubby folds on the thighs leaving moderately deep creases.
3: Buttocks appear less full, with thinner folds and deeper creases at the upper thigh.
2: Sparse fat on the buttocks and thighs: buttocks are flat and sagging, with hips more apparent and wrinkling at the upper thigh.
1: Virtually no fat on the buttocks or thighs; skin of the buttocks and upper posterior thigh is loose, sagging and deeply wrinkled.

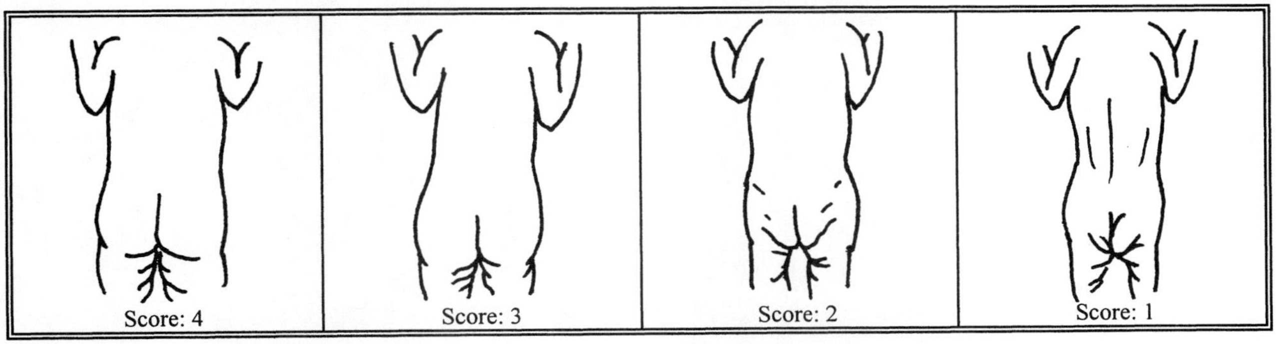

The Total Score

A “perfect” CANSCORE is 36 (or a modified score of 32, if the hair parameter is excluded), indicating a well-nourished, term newborn. The minimum score is 9, indicating severe intrauterine malnutrition. Scores less than or equal to 24 (or a modified score of 22 if hair is excluded) can be taken as clinical evidence of malnutrition. A poor score indicates a baby who should be watched closely to make sure that these nutritionally related deficits in growth resolve over the days and weeks postpartum. These babies are more prone to hypoglycemia and should be monitored accordingly. As always, a full placental transfusion and nursing as needed will be the best first lines of therapy for these babies. They are usually born quite hungry. A history of a malnourished baby in a previous pregnancy indicates that a search for possible underlying medical conditions that may impact fetal growth should take place. During future pregnancies, strict attention should be paid to excellence of maternal diet as well as to factors that may result in impaired nutrient absorption (Fletcher, 1998; Metcoff, 1994).

CANSCORE ASSESSMENT SHEET

Baby's name____________________ Date of birth__________ Weight:_______ Length_____ OCF circ.______ Sex: M F

Gestational age (wks)__________ Date of CANSCORE ________

CANS Nutritional Assessment Scoring

Hair	Cheeks	Chin/neck	Chest	Abdomen	Arms	Legs	Back	Buttocks

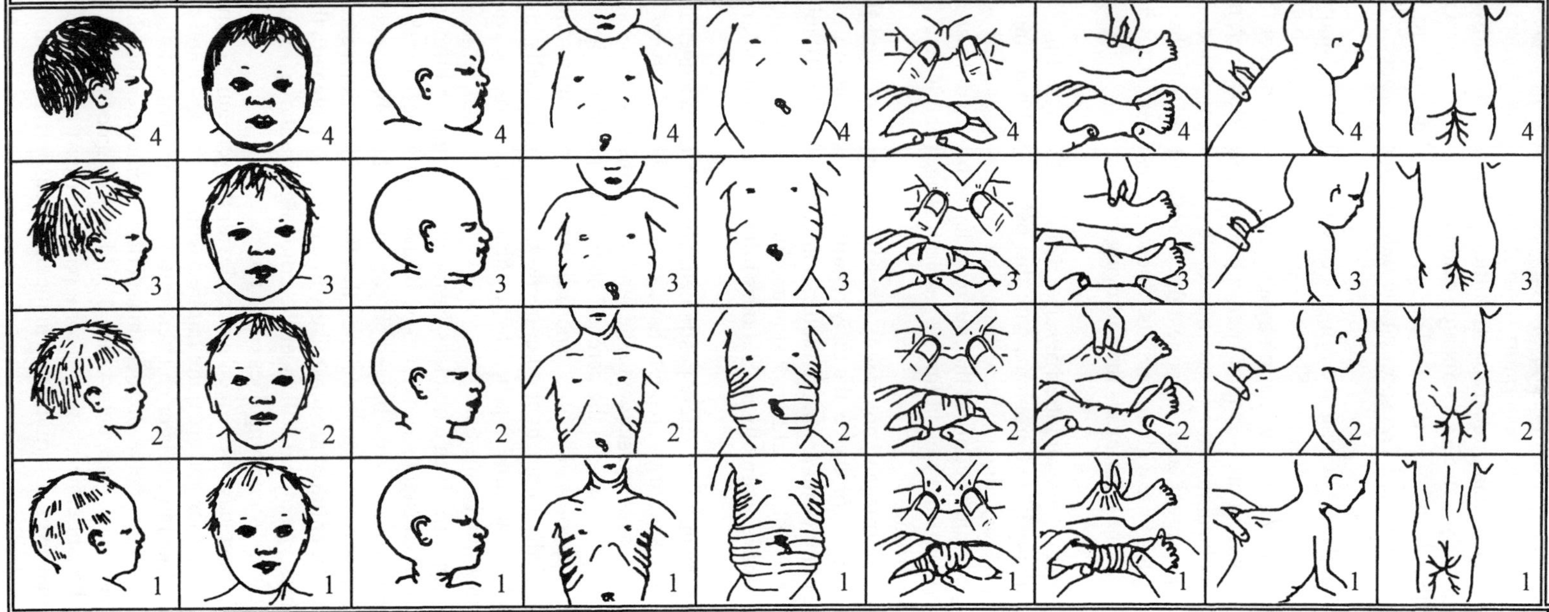

SCORE FOR EACH PARAMETER									TOTAL

INITIAL PHYSICAL ASSESSMENT OF THE NEWBORN

NOTE: This chapter assumes that the baby has appeared normal up until the time of the exam. Complications serious enough to cause acute respiratory distress, dramatically abnormal skin color, an inability to stabilize or the presence of gross anatomical abnormalities will prompt the midwife to support and transport the baby shortly after birth, in which case a screening exam would not be performed. Therefore, serious and obvious complications that tend to cause problems in the first hour of life are addressed in the part entitled "Assessing, Supporting and Transporting the Baby in Need of Specialized Care."

This text assumes that the midwife is the primary care provider for both the mother and the well infant at the time of birth and during the weeks that follow. She is therefore responsible for both examining the infant and considering whether her findings warrant further evaluation by a neonatal specialist. For this reason, detailed chapters on various aspects of newborn examination are included later in this section. However, not every baby will need, nor will every mother want, a full neonatal examination in the immediate postpartum period. The midwife may want to perform only a short initial newborn assessment, and postpone a full exam until the baby has had an opportunity to recover from the birth and spend uninterrupted time with his parents. Such an assessment is described in this chapter. A full examination can safely be delayed when the baby meets the following criteria:

- Both you and the parents have an intuitive sense that the baby is healthy.
- There have been no anticipated problems with this baby's health during this pregnancy based on maternal, sibling or family history, diagnostic tests or your prenatal findings.
- All histories and appearances confirm that the baby has achieved at least 37 completed weeks of gestation.
- The baby is a normal size and weight for her gestational age (not SGA, IUGR or asymmetrically grown) with no signs of malnutrition.
- Labor and birth were normal and not unduly stressful (vertex birth, well-flexed head, no fetal distress).
- All APGAR scores were 7 or above; the baby required no resuscitation.
- The baby has good color (with an oxygen saturation in the 90s after 10 minutes of age)
- The baby received a full placental transfusion and had a normal transition to extrauterine life.
- Baby appears and behaves normally in the hours following birth and after a basic assessment

For the full newborn exam to be safely postponed, you or a knowledgeable assistant should live close enough to return to the house quickly should the parents have concerns about the baby's well-being during the next 24 hours. Alternatively, you or an assistant can stay with the family until the first-day visit and the complete newborn exam have been performed. If you live hours from the parents' home, it is not wise to leave without performing a complete exam. If you do leave, make certain you will be able to perform a complete exam within or close to 24 hours after the birth (this means there are no other births imminent or other events that may potentially interfere with your ability to do so). If you have a very busy schedule at this time, it is best to go ahead and perform the complete exam before leaving the birth, to make sure it gets done in a timely manner.

While normal newborns are given a quick assessment at the time of birth in a hospital, it must be remembered that these babies are then under constant supervision by health practitioners for the next 24 to 48 hours. A more thorough exam is performed before the baby is discharged. If you attend a homebirth and then plan to leave after 3 to 4 hours, you and the parents must be satisfied that all is well and that the complete exam can reasonably be postponed until the first-day visit. Parents with older children are most likely to feel comfortable with this decision. The happy news is that the vast majority of the babies you attend will meet the criteria given above. Thus, the only real question is the parents' comfort and your proximity if something does come up.

If the criteria listed above have been met, proceed with the screening exam described below before you leave the house. This description assumes you are quite familiar with the purposes and procedures for the much more elaborate newborn examination outlined in the later chapters in this section. For details about how to perform any detail of this exam, refer to the relevant chapter elsewhere in this section. Remember that this exam serves as a screening exam *only* and *does not* include many basic parameters that should be evaluated shortly after birth. You can always choose to perform a more detailed exam either in full or for a particular part of the body depending upon what is found in the screening below. You may even determine that immediate transport is in order.

One of the primary things you are attempting to rule out is gross abnormalities. If any are found, you will want to be present with the parents when these are discovered so you can help them through their initial shock, as best you can, answering any questions and help decide about transport.

Basic newborn assessment

States of consciousness: The baby should be quiet and alert after birth and display normal transitions in consciousness for the entire postpartum stay.

Skin color and appearance: The baby should be a uniform, rosy pink (some bluing of the hands and feet may occur in the first hour or so). The skin should be free of all lesions except those that are clearly benign and that do not involve broken skin, such as peeling or milia. Blanch the skin and look for underlying yellowness (jaundice) or other abnormal coloring. Check the sclera for yellowing.

Cry: The baby should have a lusty, normally pitched, well-modulated, expressive cry.

Resting posture, limb movement and muscle tone: The baby should look and act appropriately for gestational age. Movement should be symmetrical and range of motion equal in all four limbs. Look for normal flexion and activity as the baby is handled after the birth. Check the baby's grasp by placing a finger in his palm. Check the suck by placing a gloved finger in the baby's mouth and rubbing the fingerpad against the hard palate; this should stimulate sucking. Observe the baby for normal Moro and startle responses while being handled.

Skeleton: Look for normal contours, posture and symmetry. Suspected skeletal malformations should be distinguished from postural deformations by passively moving the affected part to its normal position. If the limb can be passively moved to a normal position, deformation is more likely. Palpate the clavicles, humeri and femurs to rule out fractures or breaks; these may cause the baby to cry while being handled.

Body contours and proportions: Look for normal trunk size and limb length, normal head shape and size, symmetry of the chest wall and of the facial features and normal convexity of the abdomen.

Closed palate: Both visualize and palpate the palate while checking the baby's suck to ensure that the palate is complete and closed. A cleft palate may produce an inability to latch on well, with coughing, choking and respiratory distress when the baby tries to nurse. Discovery of a cleft palate requires a thorough exam followed by immediate consultation with a pediatrician, a lactation consultant who specializes in cleft palate, or both. Consider transport if other anomalies are found or suspected. Most babies with an isolated cleft lip do not require transport if they can nurse. If the defect is minor, a skilled lactation consultant may provide all the assistance that is required.

Genitalia: The genitals should appear normal in every respect, taking into account the gestational age of the infant. Palpate for the presence of testes in the scrotum and the absence of masses in the labia. Lift the penis and examine underneath. If there is any question *whatsoever* regarding the sex of the baby, transport is in order.

Gastrointestinal and abdominal exam: Check for normal abdominal contour, midline defects and peristaltic sounds. Note any difficulties with swallowing or the presence of excessive oral secretions.

Confirm normal elimination, anal patency and normal placement of the urethra and anus by observing the passage of urine and meconium whenever possible. The urinary stream should be continuous and moderately strong (and straight in boys).

Heart and lungs: Count both respirations and heart rate for one full minute. Listen to the lungs over the chest and back to determine if there are clear and equal breath sounds on both sides. Some crackly wet sounds are normal, but most of the lung field should sound clear. Auscultate the heart for normal heart sounds and the absence of murmurs.

Weight and measurements: Go ahead and weigh the baby now. This not only gives you a good baseline weight, but it is the one thing, other than sex, that everyone the parents contact about the birth will want to know. If the head is not moulded, you can also go ahead and get a head circumference, which is the most critical transverse body measurement.

Nursing: The baby should be able to latch on and suck normally without respiratory distress and while maintaining good color.

Upper and lower extremities: Observe the arms, legs, hands and feet in repose. Look for normal fisting and normal contour of the soles of the feet. Check for normally shaped limbs and normal creases and digits.

Umbilical cord vessels: If there are not three vessels in the cord, proceed with a full examination.

Skull, face, ears, eyes and mouth: Visually evaluate the presence of and normal shape and placement of the ears, eyes and mouth within a normal face. Abnormal facial characteristics are strongly associated with a variety of serious problems; if found, proceed with a full exam. Keep in mind that deformations from in utero positioning may mimic abnormal facial or other body features.

The back and spine: Even if everything looks great, always roll the baby over and check the back for open spinal defects by visualization and palpation. A spinal defect can be present in a baby who appears to be otherwise normal.

Spontaneously elicited reflexes: All reflexes that are stimulated by normal postpartum handling should appear normal for gestational age.

If all these evaluations are normal and remain consistently normal throughout the postpartum stay, you can postpone the full exam until the first-day visit.

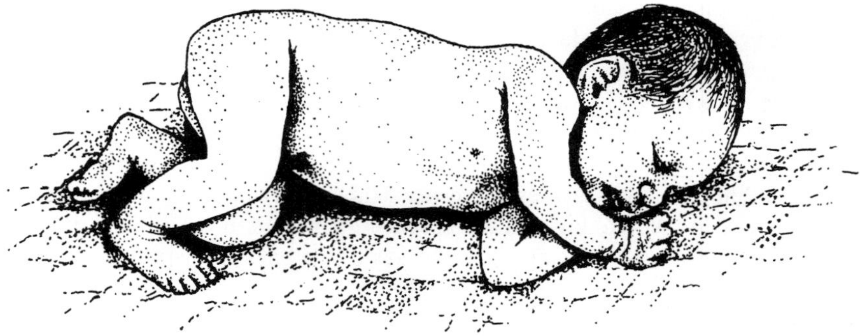

Complete Physical Examination of the Newborn

The Newborn Exam: An Overview

NOTE: This chapter assumes that the baby appears to be more or less normal at the time of the exam. Complications serious enough to cause acute respiratory distress, dramatically abnormal skin color, an inability to stabilize or remain stable or the presence of gross anatomical abnormalities will prompt the midwife to support and transport the baby shortly after birth, in which case a complete physical exam will not be performed. Therefore, while many subtle and more obvious signs of problems that require further evaluation are mentioned in this chapter, serious complications that tend to cause problems at or shortly after birth are addressed throughout the part entitled "Assessing, Supporting and Transporting the Baby in Need of Specialized Care."

Once mother and baby are ready, it is time to do the complete baby exam. Just as you perform a physical exam on the woman during prenatal care, you perform a screening exam on the baby, making it a very detailed one because it is the baby's first exam. You are looking to see how the baby is doing and what normal or possibly abnormal variations that require further evaluation may be present. Some of these abnormalities are mentioned in this chapter, but by no means are they all.

The student midwife often feels overwhelmed by the responsibility of newborn assessment. Many students have the impression that they need exposure to many abnormal situations in order to confidently assess the normal. This is definitely not true, especially when it comes to newborns. This is because newborns have not learned to mask or ignore physical signs and symptoms, as many adults have. Your familiarity with normal appearance and responses will become your best gauge of suspicious findings that need further investigation.

This does not mean, however, that you need only do a superficial exam. Attending births at home usually places the midwife in a more responsible role than a midwife working in the hospital (where input from the pediatric or neonatal medical staff is readily available and often unavoidable). Therefore, you need to perform a very thorough exam with an in-depth knowledge of normal parameters, the possible significance of abnormal findings, and supportive measures that might be needed prior to obtaining further evaluation or emergency transport. This does not mean, however, that you are expected to be able to accurately and precisely diagnose every newborn disorder. While some diagnoses are easily identified (such as an open spinal defect), many are subtle or complex, especially when genetic factors are involved. Not every possible problem is detectable at birth. You are only expected to be able to tell if something that is discovered needs further evaluation.

Remember that in medical settings, normal newborn responses are often altered significantly by interventions that occur both during and following birth. Even with comparatively benign hospital protocols, maternal drugs during labor, early cord clamping, separation of the baby from the mother to perform the baby exam, immediate administration of neonatal prophylactic medications and immediate weighing and drying are routine. At home, typically none of these interfering factors are present during the first hour or so. This gives you the opportunity to learn truly normal newborn responses. In doing so, you will develop a sensitive intuitive grasp of subtle variations that may indicate trouble.

Keep in mind that practitioners who have only had experience with hospital-born babies are likely to be unfamiliar with the subtleties of truly normal parameters. For instance, many years ago my midwifery partner (at the time still a student) brought a lethargic, inattentive newborn to a pediatrician for evaluation. He repeatedly asked if the mother hadn't merely received drugs during labor. She had not, but the physician obviously thought the baby's responses would have been in a normal range had that been the case. This baby turned out to be developmentally delayed. I have often heard doctors stress that a lack of interest in nursing and deep, prolonged sleeping is normal for newborns in the first three days of life. While this may be true for many traumatized hospital-born babies, it is not normal in untraumatized homeborn babies. Therefore I encourage you to learn from the healthy fully transfused homeborn babies you see, as they are the gold standard of normal.

The extent of your exam

The vast majority of the infants you examine will be normal. You may practice midwifery for an entire career and never encounter most of the anomalies mentioned in this chapter. As always, the intention is to give you more information than you would ever need, to cover unusual circumstances when they do arise and to facilitate being able to communicate enough detail to neonatal practitioners so that you sound like you know what you're talking about and how to make your findings meaningful. For those midwives working in regions where medical assistance is hard to access, the level of detail presented here may be even more important.

However, even in a more typical, urban homebirth practice, the midwife may not routinely recommend that parents take their newborn to a pediatrician in the days following birth. Being required to leave the house and go to a doctor's office full of sick kids a day or so after birth to have the newborn examined seems to defeat the idea of birthing at home. Therefore, you may choose to do a very complete exam yourself.

This chapter offers details pertaining to the more common congenital defects with an emphasis on those that can be recognized with an external exam. These associations are intended for students to use as they gain understanding of the range of variations and anomalies and how they are related. Those mentioned are not exhaustive and many syndromes are not explained here. Those that have major, obvious associated abnormalities are explained more thoroughly in the part entitled "Assessing, Supporting and Transporting the Baby in Need of Specialized Care." Volume III of this text also addresses some of these disorders. Do not casually suggest to the parents that a certain defect means that the baby has any particular diagnosis simply because it is mentioned in this text; such casual comments are only likely to cause great anxiety without being definitive. There are literally hundreds of disorders and syndromes, many of which have a number of features in common; they are definitely *not* all included.

With regard to any individual newborn exam, you are expected to use good judgement about how much detail is enough. For example, perhaps you are examining a boy's genitals and think his penis looks a bit small. You would want to actually measure to be sure; the inclusion of penile measurement in this chapter does not mean you would necessarily measure the penis of every baby boy. Likewise, not every type of evaluation is included in this chapter. For instance, a finding of disproportionate limb length is enough to decide that further evaluation is in order. You need not measure each individual bone; that will be done by a neonatal orthopedist when establishing a diagnosis.

<u>Variations and what they might mean</u>

Tappero and Honeyfield (2003) explain the meaning of neonatal variations well; the following discussion and the next on anomalies are both based on their excellent text. Each baby is an individual and carries with him traits from his family background, race and unique genetic makeup. The findings of your physical exam may be characterized as either normal, unusual or abnormal. Normal findings are, of course, expected; however, there is no one universal standard of normal but an accepted wide range of morphology or variation in physical structures. Gestational age has a significant influence upon what is considered normal. For example, fusion of the eyelids is normal at 24 weeks, as is full-body lanugo. However, both of these are considered abnormal at term. **Normal findings** include individual variations and family traits, which includes features that differ among races or ethnic groups. Unfortunately, many of the most utilized parameters have been established using Caucasian populations. **Familial traits** are unusual findings that may either be very subtle or very obvious and that persist throughout a family phenotype or genetic line. Such features may cause the child to have a subtly odd appearance with no evidence of outright abnormality. **Slight variations** that border on abnormal may not necessarily point to a problem but should not be dismissed. Some family traits may be more important, as is the case with extra digits. The ability to view each feature individually as well as to look at combined findings for any possible patterns will help in detecting both subtle and gross variations. Findings that go beyond the scope of individual variations enter the category of **anomaly**. Anomalies are classified by cause.

Deformation: A deformation is an alternation in the shape or structure of a previously normal part due to mechanical forces. This may occur when excessive pressure is applied to a limb for a prolonged period of time during gestation They are usually asymmetrical.

Malformation: Malformations arise from an abnormality that is present at the onset of development and results in imperfect formation. They may be intrinsic, resulting from a genetic error, or extrinsic, caused by exposure to agents coming from the outside, such as teratogens, infection or maternal metabolic disturbances. Seven and a half percent of malformations are associated with deformations.

Disruption: A disruption occurs when an extrinsic destructive agent interferes with tissues that were developing normally. It may be arise from vascular, infectious or mechanical causes. Common examples include damage or amputation resulting from the formation of amniotic bands and the limb damage caused by the drug thalidomide.

Dysplasia: An abnormal cellular organization of function that generally affects only a single type of tissue (such as cartilage anomalies that result in achondroplasia).

Anomalies are further classified as either minor or major. Minor anomalies are abnormal findings that will not cause any particular cosmetic challenges or functional impairment as the baby grows. They fall on the abnormal side of unusual, and many do not require any treatment. Most deformations fall in this category because they can be corrected with therapy or will resolve on their own. Minor anomalies occur primarily in the face, auricles, hair, hands and feet. The presence of two or more minor malformations are often associated with a more deeply seated major malformation.

Major anomalies are definite abnormalities that result in serious cosmetic or functional problems and that will require treatment. Malformations and disruptions usually result in major anomalies and are most likely to occur in regions of complex tissue development such as the face, hands or major organs.

Always keep in mind that some seemingly minor variations can be linked to serious genetic syndromes. In addition, those variations that may be insignificant to the health of the baby or that may be very familiar to you may be deeply distressing to the parents. Either way, the parents deserve the best explanation you can offer regarding the significance of any variations from perfect, without your resorting to an attempted diagnosis.

When a baby has or is suspected to have congenital anomalies

About 2% of all newborns have a significant malformation, which may range from relatively simple to very complex. The more simple the malformation, the later in fetal development the defect appears. Babies may present with one or more major congenital anomalies; however, there is usually only one, specific underlying cause, whether one or more organ systems are involved. A single anomaly–for example, a heart defect–suggests a primary defect of a single embryotic field. Multiple anomalies occur when two or more defects occur in different organ systems, such as the nervous and cardiovascular systems. Those infants with multiple anomalies often have a constellation of abnormal physical findings, each of which is nonspecific alone, but when found together form a recognizable pattern that can be confidently diagnosed by a practitioner familiar with the many variations of these relatively rare presentations. Such a pattern may be associated with a malformation sequence, association (complex) or syndrome, as described below:

Sequence: A sequence occurs when an underlying malformation or disruption that has an identified cause leads to a cascade of associated problems. One example is Potter sequence, where renal agenesis or amniotic leakage results in a lack of fetal urination and oligohydramnios, causing undue compression on the fetus and also leading to pulmonary hypoplasia.

Complex (association): A complex or association exists when several birth defects occur together (but less reliably so than in a syndrome) which may be related to a temporary intrauterine event. For example, when vertebral, anal, tracheoesophageal, renal and anomalies of the forearm occur together, VATER complex is present. When heart or other limb anomalies are also found, this is referred to as "VACTERL complex."

Syndrome: A syndrome is a group of signs and symptoms associated with any morbid process. Together, these signs and symptoms constitute the picture of a disease, for example, Down syndrome.

Cornelia Enning (2003) has found that the family cat can be a valuable member of the birth team when there is a question about the baby's health. She has the cat come in to examine the placenta. If the baby is healthy, the cat will try to eat the placenta; if not, the cat will walk away. It cannot hurt to perform a "cat scan" if you are concerned, although I would not advise taking the cat's assessment as the final word on the baby's condition.

Whenever a major anomaly is suspected, the baby should be transported for specialist evaluation, and the parents and siblings should be evaluated as well whenever a newborn anomaly is confirmed. The number of minor anomalies raises the chances of an associated major anomaly also being present.

MINOR ANOMALIES	CHANCE OF A MAJOR ANOMALY
None	1.4%
One	3%
Two	11%
Three	90% (most with multiple major anomalies)

(Marden, 1964)

The placenta should always be evaluated in the light of any abnormal findings in the newborn. For example, if a growth-restricted infant has a normally sized placenta, the growth restriction is more likely to be associated with congenital anomalies, whereas if the same baby has a small placenta, it is be more likely to be related to placental insufficiency.

The etiology of most congenital anomalies can be traced. A chromosomal abnormality can be found in 10% of all affected infants. In about 20%, the malformations are based on a single defective gene, with autosomal disorders predominating. Multifactorial inheritance accounts for 30%, which includes inherited as well as environmental influences. About 15% occur in babies of diabetic mothers or those exposed to a teratogen; in the remaining 35%, no cause can be identified. While chromosomal abnormalities are fairly common, occurring in about 1 in every 200 births, many of these babies appear normal. The categorization of a malformation as being the result of a single gene defect, chromosomal defect, multifactorial inheritance, or teratogenic exposure will help determine what types of tests and evaluations are relevant. In general, complete assessment of the cardiovascular system using two-dimensional echocardiography, ophthalmological exam, CT scan or ultrasound of the brain, renal ultrasound, spinal X-ray, photographs and chromosomal analysis are used to determine the nature and extent of the disorder. It is very important for the parents to have as clear an understanding as possible regarding the scope of the disorder, its etiology (including whether any chromosomal abnormality is present), the likely outcome of any proposed surgery, and the anticipated quality of life and mental capacity of the baby. They will also be concerned regarding the prospects of having a child with the same disorder in the future.

The most serious defects are often obvious at the time of birth, and transport is often advisable as soon as they are recognized. For the sake of consistency, some abnormalities are mentioned throughout this discussion; however, the major presenting signs and symptoms associated with immediately life-threatening newborn defects and information on how to support the baby until additional help is obtained are dealt with in the chapters in the part covering "Evaluating, Supporting and Transporting the Baby in Need of Specialized Care."

Preparing for the Newborn Exam

What the exam should include: (This explanation assumes a basic understanding of the "Basic Anatomy and Physiology for Midwives" section in Volume I, the section on newborn anatomy and physiology in Volume III and the chapters dealing with newborn anatomy and states of consciousness in this text. Study these before studying this chapter.)

The Complete Newborn Exam

General appearance and behavior: Posture, body proportions, muscle strength and tone, spontaneous movement, cry
Gestational age: See chapter entitled "Assessment of Gestational Age"
Size for date: See chapter entitled "Assessment of the Baby's Size and Its Relationship to Gestational Age."
Measurements: Weight; crown-heel length; head, chest and abdominal circumferences; body proportion; temperature
Excretory function: Timing, color, quantity, observation of normal passage of urine and meconium
Skin: Texture, color, opacity, turgor, bruises, edema, lesions, vernix, birthmarks, lanugo, peeling
Head: Moulding, presentation, fontanelles, caput, hair texture, skull firmness, sutures
Eyes: Spacing, conjunctivae, sclerae, corneae, red reflex, pupil reaction, hemorrhages
Ears: Shape, placement, cartilage
Nose: Discharge, patency, shape, flaring
Mouth & throat: Lips, teeth, mucous membranes, saliva, palate, cheeks, tongue, frenula
Neck: Position, masses, trachea, thyroid
Heart: Rate, sounds
Lungs: Respirations, breath sounds, inflation
Chest: Symmetry, breast cartilage, nipples
Arms: Range of motion, creases, radial and brachial pulses, clavicles
Hands: Size, shape, posture, creases, nails, fingers
Abdomen: Cord vessels, hernias, resonance on percussion, peristaltic sounds, masses, tenderness, liver, spleen, kidneys
Genitalia: Normal structure and appearance, orifices properly placed, testicles descended in males
Legs: Range of motion, assessing for hip dysplasia, creases, flexion, femoral pulses, inguinal area
Feet: Size, shape, posture, creases, toenails, toes, range of motion
Back & spine: Vertebral closure, scapulae, pilonidal dimple
Primitive reflexes: See subchapter entitled "Developmental Reflexes and Other Neuromotor Evaluations"

Perform your gestational age and size assessment before you begin this exam as that information is pertinent to what you will look for here. This discussion focuses on examination of the full-term infant, unless otherwise noted. For study purposes, it begins with the baby's head and moves down the anterior body, then the baby is turned to examine the back. Some practitioners, anticipating that the examination of the head will be more distressing to the baby, start with the chest and abdomen and then move to the extremities, back and head. You will find a flow that works for you and will learn to vary your approach for each baby, keeping in mind that a systematic exam minimizes the possibility of omissions and keeps random poking, prodding and repositioning of the baby to a minimum. It also helps you think through the exam as you inspect various organ systems. Even so, you will find yourself taking advantage of opportunities afforded by the infant as you become familiar with the exam. For example, should the baby yawn or cry, you can quickly do a visual inspection of the oral cavity.

Any physical examination entails some overlap of different systems; for example, pulmonary and cardiac function as well as thoracic skeletal structures are all examined when assessing the baby's chest. As you learn, the interrelationship between each component of the exam as well as your ability to evaluate multiple parameters at once will become second nature to you. During the newborn exam, you will move from making general observations to examining each newborn system for normalcy. Study all the chapters in this section of the book to get the most complete information about assessing newborn maturity and well-being.

Timing of the exam: The complete newborn exam can usually wait until the placenta is out, the mother has been checked for tears and had them repaired (if necessary), the mother and baby are out of the herbal bath (if they want one), nursing has commenced and the mother feels cleaned up and situated in bed. Ideally, the baby should have nursed well a half-hour to 1 hour prior to the exam and will neither be very sleepy nor hungry and irritated. However, if your initial observations of the baby cause you to suspect a problem, if the baby had difficulty establishing respirations, or if for any other reason the baby may be compromised yet no specific problem is evident, the newborn exam should be done as soon as possible to look for further signs of problems. Newborn transport may be in order and in some cases should not be unduly postponed.

Some midwives wait until the day after birth to perform a complete exam. The decision to delay the full exam may be appropriate if the baby was born in a birthing center or when there will be a knowledgeable person on hand at home throughout the night and when the baby seems perfectly normal. In this case, a preliminary assessment should be performed during the postpartum watch (see the preceding chapter for details). However, I personally prefer to do a full exam before completing immediate postpartum care. By doing so, the midwife as well as the parents are assured that all is well. Should something concerning be discovered, arrangements for follow-up consultation or transport can be made without delay, depending upon the findings and the circumstances.

Review the mother's medical history: Note any major systemic diseases, congenital defects, substance abuse or other health concerns in the family that may impact your findings during the baby exam. Review the mother's previous birth history and note the causes of any problems that siblings have had in the newborn period. For example, if the mother has a history of congenital heart disease, the baby has a 10 to 15% risk of also having a congenital heart problem (otherwise there is a 0.8 to 1% risk). Check the results of any prenatal tests that were done on the fetus.

Setting up for the baby exam: Ideally, the exam should be conducted on the bed beside the mother. The mother, her partner and other children, if present, should be able to watch the exam if they want to. As you go through each step, describe to the baby and parents what you are doing and why, and tell them of your findings.

The lighting should be adequate but indirect, so as not to hurt the baby's eyes. Indirect daylight is ideal, but if unavailable, use shaded incandescent lighting. Bright light may exaggerate the skin color, while florescent lights will make a normally perfused baby appear pale or slightly green.

The room should be quite warm, as you will need to uncover the baby during the exam. It is ideal to have the room warm enough so that the baby can be completely nude. This allows you to observe the baby better and look for symmetry from side to side. However, if the room cannot be made sufficiently warm, the baby should remain covered except for the area of the body you are examining. Even if the room is an ideal temperature, cover the baby back up if he seems distressed by being completely uncovered.

Place the nude baby on a clean receiving blanket or towel beside the mother. The baby can be nestled in a padded surface that allows her back to maintain the gentle convex curve familiar from her intrauterine stay. Placing the baby on a disposable Chux type pad or clean cloth diaper can minimize the mess if the baby has not yet urinated or passed meconium; the exam may stimulate elimination. The cord can still be intact.

An assistant can fill out the baby exam form, leaving your hands free to work with the baby. If no assistant is available, set your paperwork up on a TV table, book or chair seat so that you can easily move from examining the baby to taking notes. The following list includes all the equipment you may need to perform a complete exam:

- •Neonatal stethoscope
- •Flexible nonstretchy tape measure with inch and cm marks
- •25 in ruler with inch and cm markings to measure length
- •Small, clear plastic protractor
- •Goniometer
- •Small, bright flashlight
- •Newborn exam forms and pen
- •Tongue depressors
- •Infant reflex hammer
- •Adhesive tape
- •Ophthalmoscope
- •Exam gloves
- •Watch with a second hand
- •Baby scale (and sling, if needed)
- •Small, clear plastic ruler with cm and inch markings
- •Medium-sized, hand-held magnifying glass
- •Paper tape (IV tape)
- •Infant thermometer
- •Wood's lamp (not essential)

Gloves can worn if the baby is still wet with birth fluids, if the baby has any open skin lesions, and for examination of the oral cavity. If the herbal bath has been done, you may choose to eliminate gloves or only use them when palpating the oral cavity. Gloves not only protect you from oral fluids, but they protect the baby from contracting fungus or yeasts that may be on your fingers, even if your hands are clean. Nondisposable equipment can transmit infection, so be sure to wipe each item well with an antibacterial agent before using it on another baby.

The newborn exam form: You may choose to create your own form or use the one at the end of this chapter. Other sets of forms are available as well (see the last chapter in the text). The form included here is quite thorough, of a scope usually reserved for admission to an intensive care nursery. Although such a thorough form may seem like overkill, it is an invaluable tool when working with consulting physicians, and, for this reason alone, it is worth having. Aside from that, many midwives are often quite exhausted by the time the newborn exam rolls around. Having a thorough and detailed form to fill out helps avoid omitting parts of the exam; furthermore, the parents then have a very complete record for their newborn's future health care.

Relating to the baby

It must be remembered throughout the exam that huge transitional changes are in process for the baby as he adapts to life outside the womb. Every experience is new; contact with the air, breathing, nursing and direct encounters with others are chief among them. Slow, gentle handling of the baby, talking to the baby about what you are doing, and stopping to let the baby calm down or transition from one portion of the exam to the next will help the baby integrate the process. A "let's get this over with" approach and insensitive handling will usually lead to irritation and lack of cooperation on the baby's part. The baby exam is one of life's very first experiences; it should be performed consciously and with an attitude of respect. This may not be your first priority if you are very tired after a long birth. It is best to go wash your face, have a cup of tea and relax a little before you begin so you don't communicate lack of patience to the baby. Remember to breathe deeply into your belly. This will not only even out your emotional state, but will energize you and will help the baby remain calm as well.

If it is very late, you are very tired, there has been no evidence whatsoever that the baby is compromised in any way, and the baby's preliminary evaluation is normal (see previous chapter), you may postpone the baby exam until the next day's home visit. It's better to postpone it than to do an inadequate exam due to your exhaustion. However, if there is another midwife available who is less tired, she may perform the exam before you leave.

Newborn examination of____________________________

Mother______________________________ Examiners_______________ Birth Date ________/Time________ .m. Exam time________ .m.

NOTE: Checks or circles (Y N) may be placed to indicate findings which are within normal limits (WNL). Note other normal findings as appropriate. Unusual findings are to be circled, numbered and comments written in the section on the back of the page.

APGAR SCORES: 1 Min.____ Findings:____________________________ 5 min.____ Findings:____________________________

Est. gestational age____ weeks. SGA AGA LGA TEMPERATURES AFTER BIRTH: ____ at ____min./____ at ____min.

MEASUREMENTS: Weight___lbs.___oz./____gms. Length____in/___cm. Head____in/___cm. Chest____in/___cm. Abdomen____in/___cm.

GENERAL APPEARANCE: Proportion WNL ___ Muscle tone WNL___ Position of extremities___________ Activity WNL___ Cry WNL___

EXCRETORY FUNCTION: Passed meconium: before birth: passed urine/meconium while under midwife's observation after the birth.

SKIN: Texture___________ Color_______________ Opacity____________________ Turgor_____________________

Bruises___ Location____________________________________ Birth marks___ Location_______________ Type___________________

Edema___ Location____________________________________ Lanugo___ Location____

Milia___ Location____________________________________ Peeling___ Location____

Other lesions___ Location____

Vernix___ Color____________ Location____

HEAD: Moulding_______ Presentation_____ Fontanelles: Ant.____fingers Post.____fingers Caput________ Other ________

Hair texture___________ Skull firmness________________ Sutures_______________ Facial appearance WNL_______

EYES: Spacing WNL___ Conjunctiva healthy___ Sclerae WNL___ Cornea clear___ Red reflex: L___ R___ Pupil reaction: L___ R___

Hemorrhages: L___ R___ EARS: Shape L WNL___ R WNL___ Placement L WNL___ R WNL___ Cartilage L____ R____

MOUTH & THROAT: Lips WNL___ Teeth_____ Mucous membrane WNL___ Saliva WNL___ Palate WNL___ Tongue WNL___ Frenula WNL___

NECK: Position WNL___ Masses____________ Trachea WNL___ Thyroid WNL___ NOSE: Discharge WNL___ Patency WNL___
Shape WNL___ Flaring WNL___

HEART: Heart rate______/min. Sounds WNL___ LUNGS: Respirations_____/min. Clarity: L WNL___ R WNL___ Inflation L WNL____ R WNL____

CHEST: Symmetry WNL___ Breast cartilage_____mm. Nipples: WNL___ Clavicles: L________ R_________

ARMS: Range of motion: L WNL___ R WNL___ Creases match WNL___ Range of motion L___ R____ Radial pulses: L____ R____ Brachial pulses: L____ R____

HANDS: Fingers: L____ R____ Prints: L WNL___ R WNL___ Nails: L_______ R_______ Color of nail beds: L WNL___ R WNL___

ABDOMEN: Umbilicus: ___vessels Hernia____________ Percussion: Resonance WNL___ Peristaltic sds (X 4 quad.): WNL___

Superficial palpation: Masses_________ Tenderness___________ Deep palpation: Masses________ Tenderness____________

Kidneys palpated: L WNL___ R WNL___ Comments:____

GENITALIA: Female: Labia majora WNL___/minora WNL___ Clitoris WNL___ Urethra WNL___ Vaginal orifice WNL___ Discharge WNL___

Male: Scrotum______ Rugae_______ Penis WNL___ Urethra WNL___ Foreskin WNL___ Testes Descended: L___ R___

LEGS: Range of motion: L WNL___ R WNL___ Hip rotation: L WNL___ R WNL___ Creases match WNL___ Flexion: L WNL___ R WNL___

Femoral pulses: L___ R___ Inguinal area WNL___

FEET: Prints: L WNL___ R WNL___ Toenails: L______ R______ Color of nail beds: L WNL___ R WNL___ Toes: L WNL___ R WNL___

BACK & SPINE: Complete___ Closed___ Lesions___ Scapulae: L___ R___ Pilonidal dimple closed___ Anus patent___

REFLEXES: Moro WNL___ Grasp WNL___ Sucking WNL___ Rooting WNL___ Other____

NEWBORN PROPHYLAXIS: Vit. K Y N Reason___________ Type___________ Eye treatment Y N Reason___________ Type___________

NEWBORN EXAMINATION TECHNIQUES

(The chapter entitled "The Physical Examination of the Woman" in Volume I should also be reviewed. A complete description of taking the temperature and using the ophthalmoscope is included there.) The following section reviews skills which are particularly useful during the newborn exam and is based on Tappero and Honeyfield (2003), unless otherwise noted.

Skills

Observation: Quietly watching the baby without attempting any interaction is used throughout the exam; it is perhaps the most important and least interventive of all exam techniques. The way the baby moves, her facial expressions, her behavorial states (active, sleeping, waking, etc.), the skin color over the whole anatomy, symmetry of form and movement, and respiratory activities can all be observed quietly. Watching the baby for a while before proceeding with the exam can give you clues as to which areas may need to be examined first or which may require more careful attention.

Auscultation: This involves listening to body sounds either directly with the ear or with an infant stethoscope. The room should be quiet and the baby calm. Place the warmed head of the stethoscope firmly against the bare skin. Use the bell side to isolate sounds and the diaphragm to listen to diffuse sounds, such as lung sounds. Do not attempt to listen to a newborn through clothing, as sounds are hard to isolate in the small anatomy, and the friction of the head of the scope against the baby's clothes will confuse your findings.

Palpation: The fingertips, palms, sides of the hands and fingerpads of both hands are used to examine external structures (such as the skin), vibrations (such as pulses), and internal structures (such as abdominal organs). One or both hands can be used, depending upon the area to be examined. For example, a bimanual exam is helpful when palpating for kidney size and placement. Specifics regarding palpation will be found throughout the chapter.

Percussion: Percussion consists of striking or tapping a body part. This sends a vibration through the tissue, setting it into motion and eliciting vibrations or sounds that can be felt. These findings are assessed based on the quality and duration of any movement or sound produced. Percussion is not a technique commonly used on newborns because the results are very subjective. Hospitals routinely perform X-rays when gas entrapment or tumors are suspected.

Direct percussion involves firmly tapping the body surface to be assessed with the tip of the middle finger of the dominant hand. Indirect (mediate) percussion is more useful in newborn evaluation. It is performed by extending the middle finger of your nondominant hand and placing the first finger joint firmly against the part to be percussed. Take care to rest only the first joint of the finger on the baby, as contact between other parts of your hand and the baby's body may alter the findings. Cock the wrist of the other hand upward, with your middle finger partially flexed and poised to strike the distal joint of the finger in place for the exam. Strike the distal joint of the examining finger with the tip of the middle finger, using a quick, downward wrist motion. The bones of the joint of the examining finger will transfer vibrations to the underlying body part.

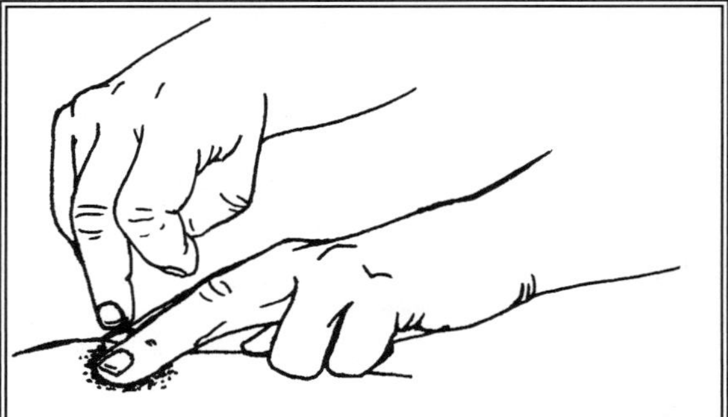

Finger posture during indirect percussion. Flex the non-dominant hand at the wrist and strike the examining finger.

Auscultatory percussion is helpful in outlining the margins of solid structures; it is particularly useful when examining the abdomen. The diaphragm of the stethoscope is placed over the presumed location of a solid mass or the lowermost right border of the liver or other solid organ. Scratch the skin lightly in a series of short motions, beginning a few centimeters beyond the anticipated border of the mass and away from the stethoscope, moving toward the stethoscope head. Listen to the character and pitch of the scratching sound. The point at which the sound changes in pitch is the margin of the mass. The entire outline of the heart, liver or spleen can be determined in this manner, even through the rib cage. Once the mass is identified, palpation can be used to locate the mass more accurately. This technique yields the same results as indirect percussion, but is easier and remains effective even when the abdomen is tense. (Fletcher, 1998)

Transillumination: Transillumination involves the use of a bright, cool light source to illuminate a body part. As light passes through the part, normal structure can be assessed. Transillumination is most commonly used to identify abnormal masses, empty spaces, and fluid- or air-filled spaces in the skull, chest, abdomen or scrotum of a newborn. Both solid and blood-filled masses will obscure the passage of light, while empty spaces or those filled with either clear fluid or air will allow more light to pass through (Donn & Kuhns, 1983).

Ideally, the lighted end of the instrument has a flexible black cuff that can seal firmly against the skin. If such a cuffed light source is unavailable, use a bright, small flashlight with a black rubber rim around the light end or any small bright light that has an end that will seal completely against the skin surface. Do not use a regular penlight, as it will not be sufficiently bright. Place the lighted end of the instrument in the finger of an exam glove or cover it tightly with new piece of plastic wrap secured with a rubber band to prevent contamination. Darken the room and allow a few minutes for your eyes to adjust. Hold the covered, lighted end against the body part (follow the specific instructions given throughout this chapter). Observe the area to see how much light penetrates the tissues. Around the lighted end, the light will extend into the tissues where it forms a pink halo or rim (corona). Measure the dimension of the corona, from the perimeter of the light source to the periphery of the halo, to determine if the finding is within normal limits. Normal findings are also assessed by observing the opposite side of the body to see how much light passes through a part or to visualize structures, as when the scrotum is transilluminated to determine if the testes are descended (Donn & Kuhns, 1983).

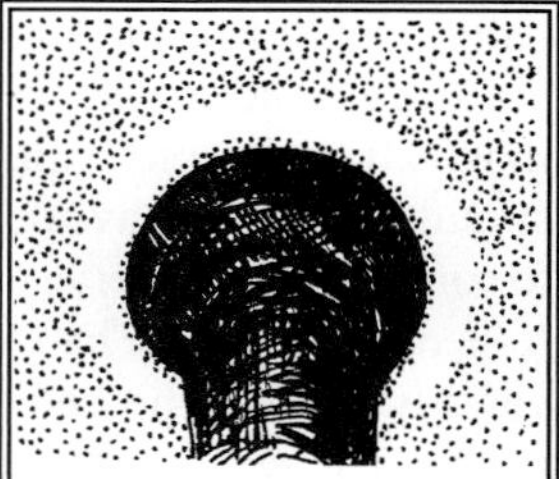

A corona during transillumination

Diascopy: A hand-held magnifying glass or blunt-edged, plain glass surface is used to check for color changes when examining the skin to distinguish vascular coloring from extravascular blood or pigment. Apply the surface of the glass flat against the skin firmly enough to induce blanching. Pressure decreases blood flow, causing vascular lesions and vasodilated areas to blanch, thus allowing better visualization of pigment; blood outside of vessels (such as that resulting from bruising or petechiae) will not blanch (Fletcher, 1998).

Measuring angles: A small clear plastic protractor is handy to measure angles, such as the angle of the ears. A protractor consists of a half-circle marked in 1° increments along its curved side. The long straight edge is held parallel with an established baseline. For example, to determine the angle of your fully extended thumb in relation to your hand, the long, straight edge of the protractor would be placed parallel with your index finger (the baseline) and the 90° line would be placed at the crotch of your thumb where it joins the hand. In most adults, the angle between the thumb and the index finger will actually be around 80° (measured at the pad of the thumb). In this text, a thick solid line will indicate the baseline, a large dot will indicate where to put the zero point of your measuring device and a finer line will be used to indicate the normal range for the angle in question. Another line will connect the baseline to the line showing the normal range. When relevant, an arrow will be used to indicate where to start the measurement in the illustrated part.

A clear plastic pocket goniometer with a 360° dial marked in 2 to 5° increments is the best tool to accurately measure anatomical angles as well as the limit of motion in the elbow, wrist, finger, knee and ankle joints. The device consists of two transparent plastic arms that rotate around a central axis. The baseline arm is marked in degrees, while the angle arm is marked with a straight line and an arrow. For most joints, the baseline or starting position is the extended, adult anatomic position. This position is described as zero. Fully extend the limb to be measured as well as the arms of the goniometer; then place the central axis of the goniometer over the center of the joint to be measured, with the 0° mark positioned away from the body (distally) and the baseline arm aligned with the center of the bone closest to the body (for example, the thigh or upper arm). Hold the baseline arm steady while moving the limb through its maximum range of motion, then hold it there. Align the angle arm of the goniometer with the axis of the extremity being held in place and determine the angle, measuring from the zero mark (Greene & Heckman, 1994).

Calculating a mean measurement: Whenever a measurement is difficult to obtain, a mean (average) of three readings can be taken as the assessment. This should be noted in the chart. Obtain the mean by taking three measurements, adding them together and dividing by three.

Comparison: Always compare paired anatomical features (e.g., hands, eyes, ears, nostrils) for symmetrical size, movement, contours, range of motion and other features.

OBSERVING THE INFANT AND EVALUATING POSTURE AND MUSCLE TONE

Observation

Unobtrusively observe the baby for normal appearance and behavior during the immediate postpartum period as the mother handles the baby and begins to nurse. You may already be alerted to anything unusual before it is time to do the baby exam. Place the baby on the bed beside the mother or on another padded exam surface on her back or side before you begin handling the baby for the exam. Do you have a general impression of a normal baby? The baby should stretch, move all extremities equally, open and close her hands, yawn with great expression, and root and start sucking when stimulated. If you have doubts about the general appearance of the baby, first look at the parents' features before jumping to conclusions. Observe the baby for normal breathing, skin color and body proportions (head size, length of limbs, torso-to-head ratio). Is the baby resting comfortably or is she distressed? Throughout the exam, you will be visually inspecting various parts of the body. For now you are getting an overall impression, which can tell you a lot about probable gestational age and the baby's neurological health. Severe conditions are often apparent on visual inspection alone.

State of consciousness

The baby's degree of alertness will affect how he responds to the exam and what you can determine as you proceed. It is best to examine the baby when he is in a quiet, awake and alert state. The baby is usually in such a state for the first one to three hours or so following an untraumatic birth. If you have missed the mark and the baby is already drifting off into his deep afterbirth sleep, you can still perform much of the exam, keeping in mind that some delayed neurological responses may be due to the sleepy state of the infant. It is quite normal for the baby to pass through several states of consciousness throughout the course of the exam. However, persistent irritability or lethargy is not normal. Do not confuse deep sleep with lethargy, which is a persistent impairment of consciousness resulting in reduced alertness and awareness. Lethargy is most commonly seen in babies who are either overheated or hypoglycemic and is caused by minimal brain dysfunction; if irresolvable, the baby should be transported (Fletcher, 1998; Tappero & Honeyfield, 2003).

Cry: Do not attempt to make the baby cry. However, should the baby cry at any time during the postpartum watch, be alert for the tone, intensity, volume, variability, pitch and duration of the sound. Pitch depends on the size of the baby. Preterm babies have higher-pitched, less resonant cries than do term babies. A term baby's normal cry is strong and loud and may be broken by gasps for air. Strong sustained crying may be accompanied by quivering of the lower jaw and, in extreme cases, temporary hoarseness. An inability to sustain a cry points to respiratory compromise. Likewise, abnormal irritability may exist if crying is excessive and the baby is inconsolable. While a baby is crying, note any skin color changes. Babies typically become redder while crying, indicating a healthy cardiovascular system. A baby that becomes pale or blue with exertion may have a heart condition. Take crying as an opportunity to quickly examine the interior of the mouth; also tune into what is happening when the baby is crying. Is the baby in pain? Did part of the exam elicit crying? These are clues to trauma or painful regions that require further investigation (Fletcher, 1998). Persistently high-pitched or weak cries are almost always abnormal.

TYPE OF CRY	MAY INDICATE
Hoarseness, weakness, very high or low pitched	Mild temporary hoarseness may occur after suctioning; these babies may refuse to nurse; it resolves quickly. More rarely, laryngeal or central nervous system abnormalities affect the size, shape or tension of the vocal cords. Also found in hypothyroidism and hypocalcemia.
Repetitive, inconsolable	Abnormal, may indicate physical or severe emotional pain
High pitched	Cerebral damage, metabolic abnormalities or drug withdrawal
Low, throaty	Congenital hypothyroidism
Stridor (harsh, creaking or crowing on inspiration)	May be due to partial vocal cord paralysis related to cervical nerve damage or partial webs, stenosis or malacia (softness) of the airway. If only one vocal cord is paralyzed, stridor will be worse when the baby lies on the back or unaffected side and improves when the paralyzed side is down. If continuous during both inspiration and expiration, it may be due to a relatively small larynx or delayed development of the cartilage of the tracheal rings.
Cat-like	Cri du chat syndrome (congenital abnormality)
Weak, poorly sustained	Airway obstruction, pulmonary pathology, premature, sick or cerebrally damaged infant

Note the shape of the baby's mouth as well as facial symmetry. Asymmetrical features during crying may be the only clue to a facial palsy. Unilateral facial palsy presents with impaired facial movement, drooping mouth and flattened nasolabial fold (space above the upper lip) on the affected side.

Posture

This refers to the arrangement of limbs, head and torso preferred by the undisturbed baby. It is determined by the strength of the flexor and extensor muscles and is clearly influenced by gestational age, with flexor tone becoming more dominant as the baby approaches term (Dubowitz & Dubowitz, 1977).

The normal term infant usually assumes a more or less symmetrical position when at rest. She lies with her neck slightly flexed or sometimes turned to one side, legs partially spread, hip joints partially flexed even when the legs are fully extended, and knees flexed, with all limbs held mostly off the mattress. The ankles are turned slightly, directing the feet toward the midline, with the soles facing each other at an angle. The feet are slightly plantar-flexed at rest. The upper legs are rotated outward, bringing the knees away from the midline, while the lower legs are rotated inward, bringing the feet toward the midline. The arms are partially spread and are flexed at the elbow. The hands may be loosely clenched with the fingers overlying the thumbs or the thumbs held alongside the fingers (Johnston, 1994).

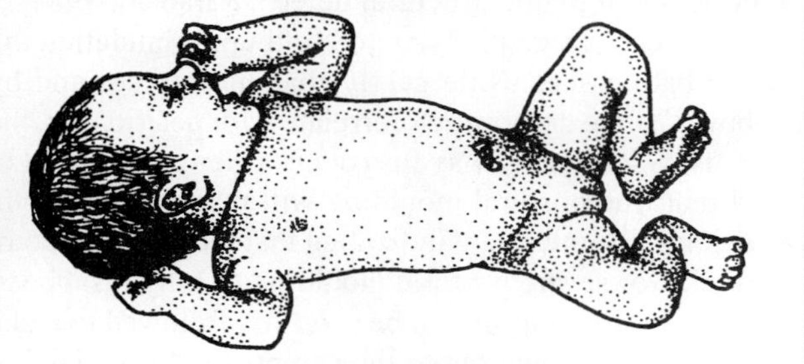

Term baby lying on her back

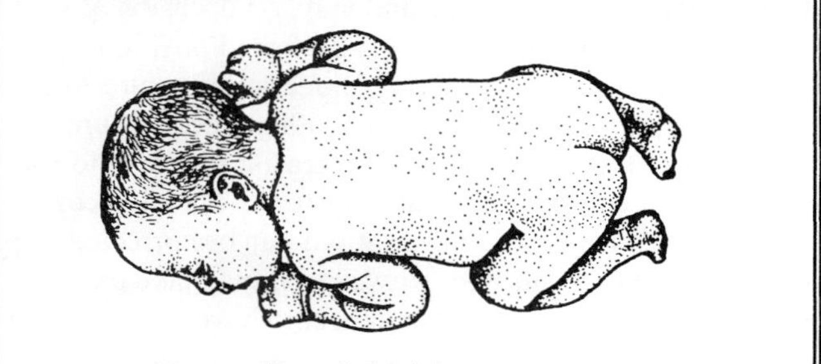

Term baby lying prone

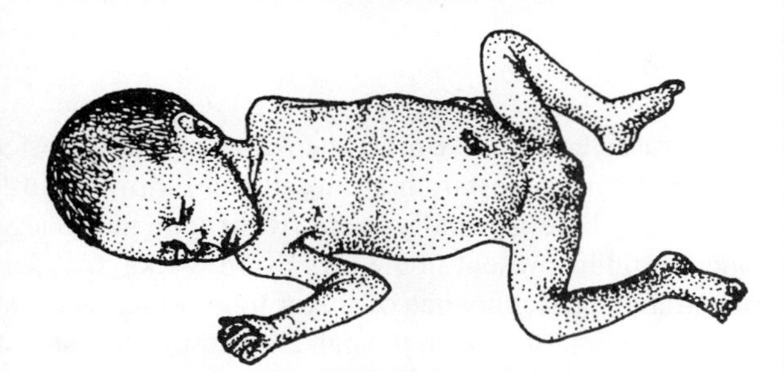

Preterm baby lying on her back

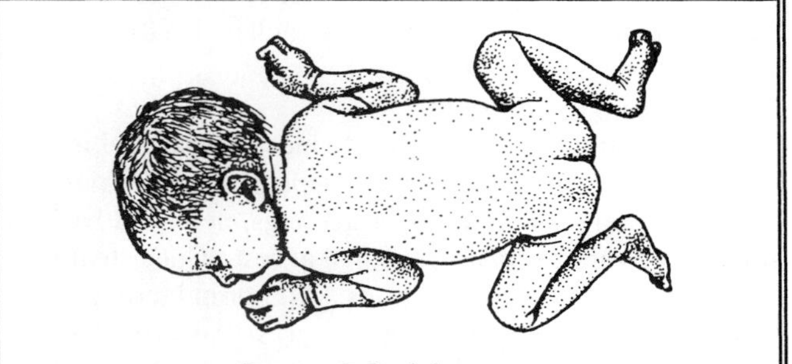

Preterm baby lying prone

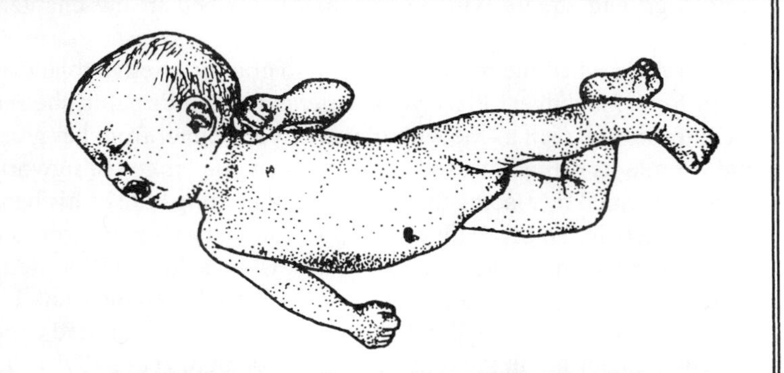

Opisthotonic posture in a newborn with hydrocephalus

The spine is a gentle convex curve from top to bottom. The legs are drawn up under the abdomen when the baby lies belly-down, the feet come to the midline under the buttocks (which raises the pelvis up), and the arms are held flexed and tucked up to the chest. Abnormal postures include persistent extension of the neck (opisthotonos) and obligate flexion of the thumb (Illingworth, 1987).

The legs assume a more splayed, frog-like posture if the baby is less than 36 weeks of gestation; there is little resting tone (this is abnormal in a term baby). This means the baby cannot hold the limbs up near the body, against gravity. Muscle tone is more lax and the arms are more extended out to either side at rest (Dubowitz & Dubowitz, 1977). Posture is further discussed in the chapters entitled "Assessment of Gestational Age" and "Evaluating the Newborn with Suspected Neurological Compromise."

Postural moulding or structural deformity? The preferred position and appearance of the limbs is often influenced by the position of the baby in utero, particularly when the intrauterine posture was extreme in any way. Frank breech position often results in flexed, abducted hips and extended knees; even a term breech baby may hold his legs in a splayed "frog leg" position for a few days following birth. The legs may also appear externally rotated and bowed, with feet that turn outward. Face presentation often causes the baby to rest with her head tipped far backward for the first few days. The neck can be compressed anteriorly, and the earlobes may be bent upward as well. The jaw or nose may also be displaced in a baby who descended in a pronounced asynclitic fashion. Compression of the chest or abdomen by the chin, an arm or a leg may give the appearance of a missing pectoris muscle or a scaphoid abdomen. These kinds of deformations can be extreme and may, on occasion, give the appearance of major structural defects (Graham, 1988).

Allow the baby to assume his preferred position of comfort, then encourage the baby to "fold up," simulating the intrauterine posture by applying moderate pressure to the relaxed baby's feet while gently shaking the legs and by directing the arms toward the body with gentle pressure on the elbows. If the deformities correlate with positioning, the "parts" will fit together, making the reason for the deformity obvious. Such a baby may fuss or cry when encouraged to assume a more normal postnatal posture. The chances are good that true postural moulding will resolve after birth. Furthermore, many postural variations can be corrected by passive joint manipulation, indicating that the bone structure itself is likely to be normal However, it may take days or even weeks for severe postural moulding to fully disappear. Any baby with deformities that appear to have been caused by in utero positioning should be carefully followed to make sure they spontaneously resolve. The specific areas of concern should be pointed out to the parents (and explained to the baby) so that they can also monitor resolution. These babies will greatly benefit from a craniosacral osteopathic or Network chiropractic adjustment (Fletcher, 1998).

Muscle strength and tone

Muscle strength correlates with muscle tone. Babies exhibit both passive and active tone, each of which can be tested separately and which may vary independently. Babies born prior to 32 weeks gestation are weak and limp with little flexor or extensor tone in the arms, legs, neck and back. By 32 weeks, there is usually some flexor tone in the legs, although the arms remain extended at rest. Consistent flexor tone should be present in the legs by 36 weeks, with less consistent flexor tone in the arms. All normal term babies demonstrate a predominance of flexor tone, which is to say they favor flexed over extended postures. Passive (phasic) tone is the amount of flexion the muscles retain when at rest. It is part of the deep tendon reflex response and is directly related to the baby's state of alertness and gestational age. It can be tested with the scarf sign and square window (already described in the chapter entitled "Assessment of Gestational Age."

Active (postural) tone is expressed when the muscles respond to gravity. Active tone can be tested by eliciting the palmar grasp reflex and the pull-to-sit maneuver. Place your finger in the baby's palm; she should grasp it and may pull back. The baby should resist extension as well as the withdrawal of your finger from her grasp as you gently straighten out her arm. The limb should resume its original flexed position when you let go (Illingworth, 1987).

The pull-to-sit maneuver is performed by placing the baby supine, holding both of his hands and slowly pulling him into a seated posture. The baby assists in the lift to the seated position by flexing his arms and maintaining his head in a nearly horizontal plane with his spine with no more than a 10° lag. Upon achieving a seated posture, the head remains erect for a second or two and then falls forward (3-second righting reflex). When the trunk is tilted forward, the baby's head should tip forward as well. Likewise, the baby should become erect when supported under the arms into a standing position if muscle tone and strength is normal in the trunk and legs (Scanlon, et al., 1979). The pull-to-sit maneuver is also covered in more detail in the subchapter entitled "Evaluating the Newborn with Suspected Neurological Compromise."

Muscle tone can be further evaluated in the awake baby by using the ventral suspension maneuver. Place your palm under the chest of a baby in the prone position and lift her up, tilting the body slightly to raise her head a bit higher than her pelvis. A healthy term baby can hold her head in line with her body for at least 3 seconds (or should, at a minimum, attempt to lift her head while suspended), with the back straight, hips slightly extended and arms and legs flexed, after which the torso will relax into a flexed posture, although the arms and legs will remain partly flexed (Illingworth, 1987).

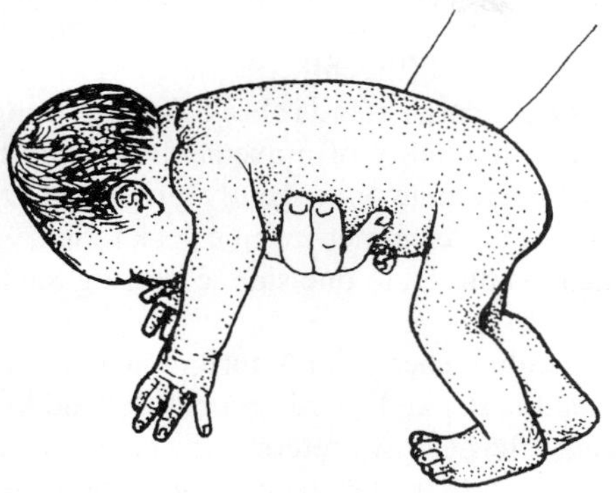

Ventral suspension with momentary head extension in a normal term baby

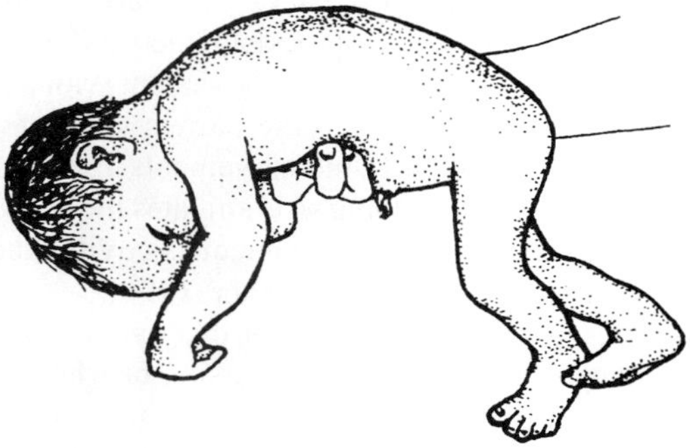

Ventral suspension in a normal term baby after head extension is relaxed.

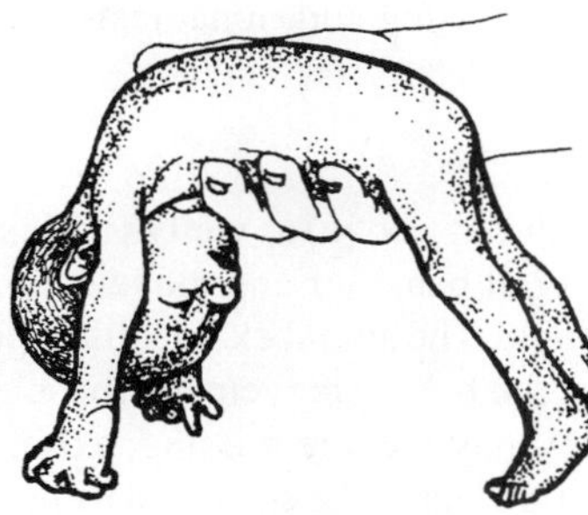

Ventral suspension in a normal preterm baby

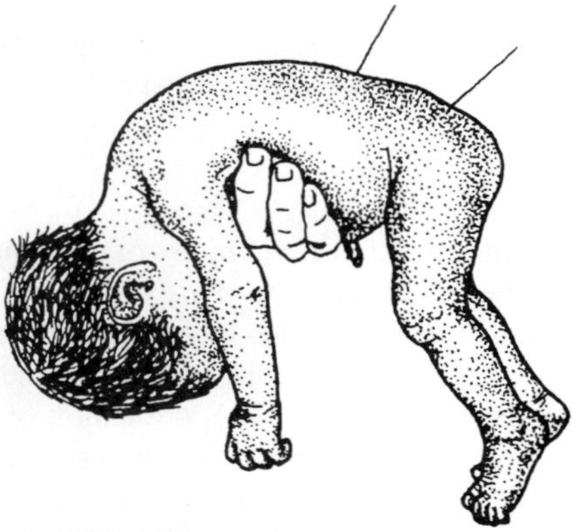

Ventral suspension in a flaccid, hypotonic term baby

Abnormal muscle tone in term babies may present as less flexor tone in the arms than in the legs. A generalized lack of tone or extreme hypertonus (pronounced flexion or stiffness of the extremities) are both abnormal and may reflect central nervous system damage, systemic disease or drug withdrawal. While increased flexor tone in the arms with increased extension of the legs is normal if the baby is crying, persistence of such posturing reflects central nervous system irritability, bleeding, or increased intracranial pressure. An increase in neck extensor tone over flexor tone (baby holds his head backward) is also seen in crying babies. Persistence may, however, indicate hypoxic-ischemic injury, meningitis or increased intracranial pressure. Unilateral lack of tone usually indicates nerve damage. Decreased activity or flaccidity may be associated with Down syndrome or heart defects. Swelling, asymmetry and signs of muscle wasting may indicate prenatal problems with muscle tone (Illingworth, 1987).

Spontaneous motor activity: The quality and quantity of spontaneous motor activity in an alert baby is particularly informative regarding overall well-being and as such is one of the most important general assessments that pertains to both regional and systemic health. Watch the baby before and after stimulation for movements in all the limbs. Normal limb movement alternates from side to side and between flexion and extension. It may appear random and uncoordinated from time to time but should be equal and symmetrical bilaterally. Slight intermittent tremors in the arms and legs are normal during the first 48 hours, especially when the baby is crying. Assess whether movement occurs with the limbs predominately extended or flexed (Prechtl, 1977).

The baby may display athetoid postures and movements, characterized by a succession of slow, writhing, involuntary movements of flexion, extension, pronation, and supination of the fingers and hands, and sometimes of the toes and feet. For example, some of the fingers may flex while the others are extended, the elbow may flex as the upper arm rotates, or the elbow may extend with rotation at the wrist. These changes should occur slowly. At term, expect to see occasional athetoid movements of the arms, forearms, hands and fingers, especially when the baby is lying quietly awake or is lightly sleeping. These movements are normal in babies but should not be continuous at term. More continuous athetoid movements are seen in preterm babies. They are infrequent or absent in depressed babies, may be exaggerated in babies who suffered asphyxia, and may be asymmetric if the baby is partially paralyzed (Prechtl, 1977).

Look for speed and intensity of movement with activity, and assess each parameter as absent, weak, strong or very strong, taking into consideration the baby's state of consciousness and the quality of movements. If you have any question about the quality of limb movements after observing the baby for a minute or so, gently guide the baby's head to center, facing forward. Doing so eliminates the confounding influence of the asymmetric tonic neck reflex, which can affect the resting posture and spontaneous activity when the baby's head is turned to one side; centering the head will help clarify what is happening (Fletcher, 1998).

Passive range of motion can be further evaluated by flexing and extending each joint in turn. The normally flexed hand should open when the baby is nursing or when the back of the hand is stroked. Preterm babies tend to lie more quietly even when alert; activity increases as the baby matures. Generally, the healthy preterm baby has a greater degree of waking activity than one who is unwell, although all preterm babies sleep more than do babies born at term. Abnormal activity includes stereotypic movements such as bicycling of the legs or arm waving, activity levels that do not match the degree of alertness, or unequal activity among the limbs in the absence of restraints (Fletcher, 1998).

Developmental reflexes: Volpe (1995) suggests using the Moro (see page 738), palmar grasp (see page 744), and asymmetric tonic neck response (see page 737) for all newborn examinations, using additional tests only if a problem is suspected.

Skeletal system

This assessment includes evaluation of the bones and joints (already discussed above) as well as their supporting and connecting tissues. Throughout your exam, you will be looking at the overall behavior and movement of the baby to detect any unusual findings. Also look for normal shape and size relationships. The spinal exam will be postponed until the end. Problems or defects of the muscles or skeletal structure will affect the baby's movement, muscle tone, posture of affected parts and, in some cases, the length of the limb or digit. Causes may include missing, extra, malformed or malfunctioning parts. A bone abnormality is suspected when an unusual posture cannot be corrected by passively moving the joints. Signs and symptoms pointing to infection, inadequate intrauterine nutrition and the like may also be noted during the skeletal exam (Scanlon et al., 1979).

On rare occasions, bones may break during birth. When this occurs, the attendant will often hear a snapping sound or may feel the bone give way as the baby emerges. If you hear a snap at the time of birth, which is most likely to occur during a breech delivery or shoulder dystocia, be alert for broken bones and dislocated joints during your exam, paying particular attention to the ball joints of the arms and legs. The most commonly broken bones are the clavicle, humerus and femur (in descending order of frequency). Suspect a break in any baby who fails to move one extremity as much as the others.

An otherwise normal baby may have missing parts, most frequently some portion of an extremity, due to the constriction or amputation of a limb by an amniotic band. A constriction band, an abrupt narrowing around the soft tissues of a limb, as though a tight rubber band had been there too long, may be present if constriction was not severe enough to result in complete amputation (Graham, 1988).

Jitteriness (tremor)

Jitteriness is a mild form of tetany that is normal in newborns. It is characterized by high-frequency (more than 6 times per second), low-amplitude (an arc of less than 3 cm) activity tremors that occur around a fixed point in one or more limbs or the jaw of a baby who is awake. Jitters often occur as the baby transitions from a sleeping to a waking state and may follow a startle reflex. They may present as an exaggerated or easily stimulated Moro reflex, may accompany an increase in muscle stretch reflexes, or may be prompted by external stimuli. Tremors should disappear when the baby enters a semidozing state. Normal jitteriness will also stop when the baby sucks, when the limb is grasped firmly and placed at rest or when the noncrying baby is otherwise soothed. Abnormal eye movements are never associated with normal jitteriness. If tremors are excessive and do not stop with sucking or resume when the sucking stimulus is removed, this may indicate hypoglycemia, hypocalcemia (rare in term newborns) or irritability associated with maternal drug intake (Fletcher, 1998).

In contrast, seizure activity presents with low-frequency (less than 6 times per second), high-amplitude (an arc over 3 cm) tremors, may include clonic movements. Clonus is a form of movement marked by a muscle contracting and relaxing in rapid succession. Seizure activity will not stop with sucking, soothing or steadying of the limbs and it is frequently accompanied by abnormal eye movements (Ahmann, 1996).

Jittering is most commonly seen in sleepy or active babies during or after crying. It is never observed in a normal baby who is deeply sleeping and, in awake babies, it is least common when they are in a quietly alert state. The incidence is slightly higher among smaller and shorter babies. Infants who are more jittery are harder to console during crying and less visually alert than other babies (Fletcher, 1998).

Mouth, body or urine odor

Fletcher (1998) notes that any discernable mouth odor in a newborn is so abnormal as to immediately raise suspicions of an oropharyngeal infection, gastroesophageal reflux or a metabolic disorder. However, be sure you are not picking up some weird odor from the home or the mother before you jump to any conclusions. Keep in mind that, without the presence of a gastrointestinal infection, reflux should not produce odor at birth because at that point the gut is still sterile. Babies of alcoholic mothers may have alcohol on their breath as they detox.

A distinctive body odor is also abnormal in the newborn. A foul odor or a sickeningly sweet odor may be due to an intrauterine infection. Distinctly scented urine is highly associated with a variety of metabolic disorders, depending upon the specific smell. However, a metabolic disorder is usually not obvious until the blood levels of the problematic substance have risen beyond the body's ability to cope with it.

Any baby with either a mouth or body odor should receive further evaluation without delay, and all feeding, except clear water, should be withheld until that time. Transport as soon as possible. If the parents have a history of unexplained death in other siblings, make sure they can detect the odor and ask if they ever detected this odor from their other children; this may give a clue as to a metabolic disorder.

Excretory function

Many babies pass meconium and urinate at the time of birth or shortly thereafter. Excretory function is covered in more detail in the chapter entitled "The Healthy, Full-Term Newborn in the First Hours of Life."

Assessing the Infant's Body Weight, Measurements, Proportions and Temperature

General body proportions offer many clues as to normal growth and development, especially of the skeleton and brain. The baby's head, chest and abdominal measurements can be taken as you move through the exam, which can end with the weight. For an explanation of the significance of body weight and proportion, see the chapter entitled "Assessment of the Baby's Size and Its Relationship to Gestational Age." As you examine the baby, keep in mind the various problems mentioned in that chapter that may be found whenever the baby is particularly large or small for dates. The following values are considered normal for term babies (37 to 40+ weeks) unless otherwise stated.

Weight

A hanging scale with 1 or 2 oz gradations is fairly accurate and easy to carry to homebirths. You will also need a cloth sling in which to place the baby; this should have large metal rings on either end to attach the sling to the scale. Line the sling with a fresh receiving blanket or clean Chux pad, plastic side down, to keep the sling sanitary for use with another baby. Then calibrate the scale to zero with the lined sling in place so that the weight of the sling (and protective liner) is not included in the overall reading. Now, spread the sling out on the mattress over which you will weigh the baby. Place the baby in the center of the sling, attach the rings on the sling to the hook on the scale, and have an assistant slip her hands under the sling to support the baby as you lift the scale until the sling is taut. Then have the assistant slowly remove her hands to allow a gentle shifting of weight from her hands to the sling, and note the weight. The term infant should weigh at least 5 lb 8 oz (2500 g). Small babies may be preterm or growth restricted. A very large baby (over 10 lb 8 oz or 4309 g) may result from excellent maternal diet or, in some cases, from undetected maternal diabetes. Should diabetes be the cause, the baby will have characteristic asymmetrical growth and is at higher risk for certain anomalies (see the chapter entitled "Assessment of the Baby's Size and Its Relationship to Gestational Age" for details).

Measurements

Head circumference: The newborn's head grows rapidly following birth. Establishing a baseline helps determine if continued growth and development of the brain are normal. The head should be measured at the level of the occipito-frontal circumference (OFC). To do so, place the measuring tape just above the eyebrow ridges in front and wrap it all the way around, level with the occipital eminence in back. Normally this measurement approximates two-thirds of the baby's total crown-heel length. The OFC measurement equals the infant's length in centimeters divided by 2 plus 10 cm, with a variation of 1.5 cm (OFC = [L ÷ 2] + 10 cm ± 1.5 cm) (Coen & Koffler, 1987).

The OFC is usually 2 cm larger than the chest circumference measured at the nipple line. A head circumference that varies more than 2 cm from the chest measurement calls for evaluation. The average head circumference in a full-term baby is 33 to 37 cm (13 to 14 5/8 in), with normal variations ranging from 31 to 38 cm (12.25 to 15 in). Moulding, caput formation or a cephalohematoma can falsely skew this measurement. A slightly large measurement may also reflect a normal genetic variation; look at the heads of parents and siblings before jumping to any conclusions. The father is usually the one to contribute a larger-than-average head. The OFC should always be within a normal range by several days after birth (Fletcher, 1998).

Chest circumference: The chest is not routinely measured. However, it is a good additional evaluation of normal body proportion, particularly if the baby is LGA. Measure horizontally around the upper body at the nipple line during expiration. If the level of the nipples is abnormal, measure from the intersection of the fourth intercostal space on the chest and a vertical line extended downward from the midclavicle (where the nipple should be). In term infants, the chest circumference ranges from 30 to 37 cm (11 7/8 to 14 in). The chest circumference is 1 to 2 cm less than that of the head at term; however the two measurements may be about the same in some babies for the first day or two following birth because of cranial moulding (Scanlon et al., 1979).

The more immature the baby, the greater the difference between the head and chest circumferences, with the chest being smaller. This difference is greatest at about 32 weeks gestation. Intrauterine growth restriction is suggested when the head circumference greatly exceeds that of the chest at term. Microcephaly is suspected when the head's circumference is less than that of the chest at term (Scanlon et al., 1979).

Abdominal circumference: The abdomen is not routinely measured, although this value may be informative if you suspect abdominal enlargement or if the baby is LGA. The normal abdominal circumference is 1 to 2 cm less than that of the head. It should be measured just above the umbilicus when the muscles are relaxed. Grasp the baby around the ankles, gently flex the legs at the hips, and lift the baby's bottom slightly off the bed to slip the tape measure into place. Cradle the flexed legs and knees in your hand to relax the abdomen while measuring. Abdominal circumference reflects liver growth and development, as well as whether there is gastrointestinal enlargement (Fletcher, 1998).

Recumbent crown-heel length: The baby's crown-heel length is the most difficult measurement to take because the baby tends to maintain a flexed posture. Since the baby cannot stand, a recumbent (lying down) length is the standard. Hospital practitioners typically stretch the baby out, pressing the knees down slightly to extend the legs, ideally lining up the head, trunk and lower limbs. This greatly distresses most babies as it forces his spine to straighten after so many months of being curled up in utero. An alternative method is to place a 25 in ruler beside the baby during the exam. When the baby stretches out naturally, an approximate measurement can be obtained. A less accurate method involves placing the baby on the examining surface, marking where the top of the vertex and the bottom of the feet are positioned at a time when the baby is fully extended, and then measuring between the marks. You can also hold the zero end of the tape at the heel, and stretch the tape out on the examining surface to the top of the head. Mark the tape with your finger and then read the measurement. Finally, the least accurate method is often the default option if the baby doesn't want to stretch out at all. Place the end of the tape on the crown of the vertex (just above the posterior fontanelle), then mold the length of the tape to the baby's body until you reach the plantar edge of the heel. This will give you an approximate length. If length seems abnormal, brace the top of the baby's head against a fixed vertical surface, stretch the baby's legs down and place the ruler along side the baby to get the most accurate assessment (Coen & Koffler, 1987).

The length for a full-term infant ranges from 47 to 55 cm (18.5 to 22 in). Abnormally short babies may be small for gestational age or earlier than you thought. Short length is also associated with a variety of growth and skeletal defects (Fletcher, 1998).

Crown-rump length: If you cannot measure the crown-heel length because the baby cannot or will not stretch out, the crown-rump length can be measured instead. This is the sitting height of the baby from the buttocks to the crown of the vertex and should approximately equal the baby's head circumference. It is measured by lying the infant supine and having an assistant flex the legs at the hips so the knees are sticking straight up. Measure from the top of the head to the level of the posterior undersurface of the thighs. This measurement ranges from 29.90 to 35.87 cm at term. The method of measurement should be noted in the chart (Coen & Koffler, 1987).

Body proportion

The relationship between extremity length and body length should be visually assessed. Determine the level of the fingertips in relation to the thighs when the arms are extended alongside the body. In the normal infant the fingertips fall below the hip joint in the midthigh region. When the upper extremities are short, they align with the hip joint or fall above this level, and when they are relatively long, they may reach to the knees. The head accounts for about one-fourth of the total body length at birth (Fletcher, 1998).

Body segment ratio: Fletcher (1998) is one of the few authors to describe neonatal ratios in detail. The body can be divided into upper and lower segments. The upper segment extends from the crown of the vertex to the pelvic (iliac) crest or pubic symphysis, depending on the reference. The lower segment is the distance from the top of the pelvic crest or symphysis to the bottom of the heel. Normal body proportion is illustrated in the drawing below as well as in most other drawings in this chapter.

The ratio of the upper body segment to the lower body segment should not exceed 1.7 to 1 at term. This means the measurement from the top of the head to the pelvic crest or symphysis should be just over one and two-thirds as long as the measurement from the pelvic crest or symphysis (pick one to use as your reference) to the heel.

To determine the upper-to-lower body segment ratio, start by measuring the distance from the upper border of the pelvic crest or middle of the pubis to the sole of the heel (this constitutes the lower segment). To obtain the length of the upper segment, subtract the length of the lower segment from the overall length from vertex to heel. A high ratio (greater than 1.7:1) suggests relative shortening of the extremities, and a low ratio (less than 1.7:1) implies either unusually long extremities or a foreshortened trunk. Upper and lower segment measurements should be taken and recorded if a discrepancy is suspected.

Body proportion measurements help to determine if a problem exists when a baby seems unusually short or otherwise disproportioned. Proportional growth restriction may be due to placental insufficiency. Disproportional growth in which the limbs are shortened and the trunk length is normal is associated with the chondrodysplasias (commonly referred to as "dwarf" or "midget" disorders).

Twenty-one different forms of skeletal dysplasia syndromes are recognizable at birth. The most common of all is thanatophoric dwarfism (1 in 6400 births), a lethal condition presenting with a small rib cage (leading to respiratory insufficiency and death), a relatively normal length torso and short limbs, flattened, U-shaped vertebrae, telephone receiver shaped femurs, macrocephaly and redundant skin folds giving the baby a pug-like appearance. An abnormally high ratio (in which the lower segment is too small), is associated with congenitally shortened legs, such as in achondroplasia, the most common viable skeletal dysplasia, occurring in 1 out of every 26,000 live births.

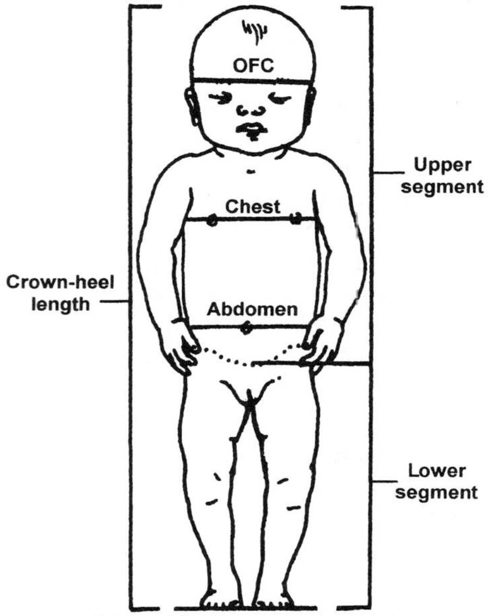

Normal body proportions and sites of transverse measurements

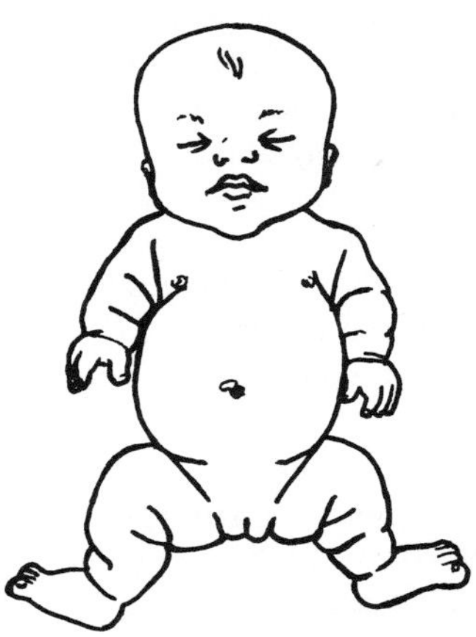

Body proportions of a newborn achondroplastic dwarf (short limbs, small thorax)

Temperature

The baby's temperature should be taken at least once during the postpartum stay. (For a more detailed description of how to take a temperature see the chapter in this text entitled "Parting Instructions for the Parents," and for a more complete discussion of body temperature and assessment, review the chapter entitled "The Physical Examination of the Woman" in Volume I of this text.) Either an axillary or rectal temperature are appropriate for newborn assessment. Do not attempt to use a tympanic thermometer on a newborn. If you choose to use an electronic thermometer, be sure it is accurate for both normal and abnormal readings. It is ideal to take the temperature using the infant thermometer the parents have purchased for the birth kit.

For an axillary reading, lay the baby on his side, lift his upper arm, gently remove any large accumulations of vernix and blot up any moisture (the skin does not have to be scrubbed clean). Place the tip of the thermometer in the pit of the arm. Lower the arm over the thermometer and place the forearm across the chest. Wait 5 minutes and read. Replace the thermometer for one more minute and read. Continue to do so until two consecutive readings are the same.

A rectal reading should not be done until after your examination of the anus and genitals or until the baby has passed meconium normally. Taking a rectal temperature may stimulate the passage of meconium, especially if no meconium has yet been passed, so be prepared by placing the baby on an absorbent underpad or diaper. The baby may either be lying on her belly or on one side. Gently flex the baby's legs, separate the buttocks, and insert the lubricated thermometer tip in the direction of the umbilicus to a depth of about ½ inch (1 cm). Do not force the tip in; inability to advance the tip may indicate that the baby has an imperforate anus. Steady the baby's legs, as necessary, to prevent injury or dislodgement of the tip. Wait two minutes and take the reading. Once finished, remove the thermometer, wipe off any secretions with tissue, using a rotating motion from where your fingers are holding the shaft to the bulb, and read.

Examining the Skin

The skin can tell you a great deal about the overall condition of the baby. The skin is the largest and most accessible of all the organs. Many serious disorders that affect the newborn cause skin alterations. The skin should be evaluated for overall color, opacity, hair distribution, staining, moisture, temperature and surface texture (smooth or parchment-like). The infant should be completely naked and warm while you are inspecting his skin so that all the skin can be observed and vascular events can be accurately interpreted.

Color, consistency and transparency of the skin change dramatically as the fetus matures. The less mature the infant, the more translucent, shiny, red and fragile the skin will be, with blood vessels more easily visible through the skin. This is more pronounced soon after birth, with prominent vessels seen over the abdomen. The skin of term infants is soft, velvety smooth and opaque, with only a few of the largest blood vessels visible through the tissue. Postterm or dysmature babies have skin that feels drier and may be peeling (Dubowitz & Dubowitz, 1977).

Any changes or unusual findings need to be described as accurately as possible. While any baby with suspicious or unidentifiable findings should be seen by a physician, your careful record of what was found at birth can help determine if it was actually present at birth and whether it is increasing or decreasing in size.

Palpation is used throughout the exam, as appropriate to the size or extent of any lesions or other variations, unless the lesion is open. Gently squeeze around the edges of a lesion to assess depth. If a cyst is suspected, transilluminate the lesion to look for differences in tissue density compared with the surrounding area. Rub a closed lesion to look for smooth-muscle contraction, vasodilation or constriction. If the lesion appears to be highly vascular, palpate for pulsation and thrills. Take a close-up photograph of any suspicious findings to show to the consulting physician (Bates, 1991).

Color

Skin color is an excellent indication of overall health. Color is best observed when the infant is quiet or sleeping in a thermoneutral environment under natural daylight and lying on a neutrally colored surface. The use of natural or incandescent lighting and a white background are especially important when the skin color is thought to be abnormal. Although skin color is partly determined by gestational age and racial background, the predominant color of the newborn who has received an optimal placental transfusion is a rosy pink, regardless of race. Very dark-skinned infants will be a rosy pink-brown and Hispanic and Asian babies may have a slight olive or yellowish undertone, but the pink will predominate in the immediate postpartum hours. Crying babies generally become more pink and babies with a thick fat layer are somewhat less pink. Gestational age also influences the depth of normal color; very early babies present with dark red skin; term babies with a medium rose pink; postdates babies are somewhat lighter, but the "pale pink" color often described as normal in postterm babies is more a product of a thicker skin layer combined with the effects of early cord clamping than it is of maturity alone (Fletcher, 1998).

A rundown of skin color variations and what they signify follows. Any suspected abnormal variations may clear up when the baby is returned to a quiet state in a thermoneutral environment, so these factors should always be attended to before a decision is made regarding the appropriate course of action. Variations indicative of a problem may be harder to detect in babies-of-color; check the tongue, mucous membranes, gums and nail beds if you are in doubt about skin tone.

Centrally pink with pink lips, blue hands and feet (acrocyanosis): This uneven coloration is commonly seen in babies less than three days old and is usually indicative of vasomotor instability secondary to chilling. The baby does not have to be very chilled for this to develop. Acrocyanosis may last as long as 48 hours; circumoral cyanosis (see below) may normally be present for 12 to 24 hours. Acrocyanosis occurs in the presence of low cardiac output when the oxygen saturation of arterial blood is within normal limits. A low cardiac output (which can be caused by clamping the cord too soon) causes the hemoglobin level in the arterial and venous bloodstreams to vary more than usual, resulting in an increased amount of reduced hemoglobin in the capillaries (Hernandez & Hernandez in Thureen, 1999).

The presence of numerous petechiae on the face or head can give the appearance of cyanosis. A magnifying glass can be used to identify the petechiae and determine the underlying skin tone. The local nature of this finding distinguishes it from true cyanosis.

Blue ring around the mouth (circumoral cyanosis): Even though cyanosis of the surrounding skin and mucous membranes of the mouth can be normal during crying, it is more worrisome than acrocyanosis. Circumoral cyanosis that persists requires further evaluation. Problems with the cardiovascular and pulmonary systems as well intracranial pathology could be causative. Circumoral cyanosis is often seen with cyanotic heart defects.

Blue all over (central cyanosis): This refers to a bluish or dusky blue-gray skin tone that involves the torso, limbs, lips, tongue, earlobes, nail beds and, in boys, the scrotum. In dark-skinned infants, check the lightest areas (palms, soles, and nail beds as well as mucous membranes), to evaluate color. Blueness of the mucous membranes, lips, nail beds and tongue often indicates that unsaturated hemoglobin exceeds 3 gm/dl (1.86 mmol/l). Record the effect of crying and activity on the depth and areas of cyanosis. Although concerning, central cyanosis alone does not always indicate impaired oxygen saturation. After 10 minutes of age, an oximeter reading of 89-100% is desirable in the first 24 hours.

Central cyanosis may result from lung disease, sepsis, persistent pulmonary hypertension or neurological disease. It is one of the two best indicators of congenital heart disease, the other being respiratory difficulty. Cardiac causes are likely if there is no improvement at all or if there is only a temporary rise in O_2 saturation with the administration of blow-by oxygen or if cyanosis increases with crying. Central cyanosis that does not resolve requires prompt investigation.

Differential cyanosis: Differential cyanosis, as described by Fletcher (1998), occurs when there is either a visible color difference in different body regions. It is usually related to varying oxygen saturation levels between the upper and lower portions of the body. Deoxygenated blood is perfusing the blue region of the body while well saturated blood is perfusing the pink area.

Harlequin color change: Low-birthweight babies are particularly prone to a primarily benign phenomenon called "harlequin color change." This presents as a clear line of demarcation that divides the body into an area of redness and an area of paleness. It most commonly presents when the baby is lying on her side, when the dependent side of the body becomes reddened with a sharp head-to-toe border between the lowermost and uppermost side, which now appears pale. If the baby lays on her other side, the pattern reverses (sometimes the division of color appears in other configurations, but its main feature is that it is transient). It lasts from a few seconds to 20 minutes and resolves if the baby is positioned on her back or belly. This is said to occur in both well and sick babies and is assumed to be due to immature vasomotor control and is rarely seen after the first 10 days of life. I postulate that it may be related to early cord clamping. Harlequin color change may be benign; however, in some babies it indicates that shunting of blood is occurring across fetal circulatory pathways, which can be due to sepsis or persistent pulmonary hypertension.

Pink upper body with blue lower body: This occurs when blood shunts from the pulmonary artery to the aorta (right to left) at the level of the ductus arteriosus and may occur during early transitional circulatory changes, especially if the cord is clamped too early. It is also associated with obstructive lesions of the left side of the heart or persistent pulmonary hypertension, which requires transport.

Blue upper body with pink lower body: This reverse differential cyanosis occurs only in the presence of dextrotransposition of the great arteries in combination with either pulmonary hypertension or coarctation or interruption of the aorta. Oxygenated blood from the left ventricle enters the pulmonary artery and is shunted right to left, causing oxygenated blood to travel to the lower body and deoxygenated blood to enter the aorta. This cyanosis is persistent and requires transport. (See the subchapter entitled "Cyanosis, Rapid Breathing, Congestive Heart Failure, Shock or Arrhythmia: Detecting Heart Defects at Birth.")

Mottling (cutis marmorata): This transient lacy or marbling pattern of dilated veins is a vasomotor response to cold stress or chronic exposure to radiant heat, overstimulation, hypovolemia or sepsis. It vanishes when a normal baby is warmed but may persist in the presence of many genetic disorders (notably trisomies 18 and 21), in preterm babies and in those with hypothyroidism. Pallor seen with mottling of the skin may indicate shunting of blood away from the skin to more vital organs; mottling is also seen in cardiogenic shock. Persistent, extreme or unusual mottling or mottling that is regional or unilateral may also be seen with sepsis or with a few rare vascular malformations. These findings are alarming and require transport.

Boiled lobster look (erythematous flush): Some normal babies may display a generalized bright red flushing over the entire body and limbs at some point during the first 8 to 24 hours of life, after which they return to their normal rosy pink color. This often occurs with the first bath. This reassuring sign will not occur in babies with cyanotic heart disease.

Diffuse redness: Generalized cutaneous dilation It is common in babies less than 12 hours old but unusual thereafter.

Red palms, soles, ear lobes and mucous membranes: Exceptional ruddiness in these areas may be due to the excessive use of supplemental oxygen or a high hematocrit.

<u>Purplish, tomato, or deep rosy red (plethora)</u>: Plethora refers to an overfullness of blood vessels or of the total quantity of any other type of bodily fluid. This coloration may be seen in overoxygenated or overheated babies. Eliminate these factors and see if the baby's color changes. True plethora will persist as a dark ruddy red that is prominent in the mucous membranes and less so on the palms and soles. This skin tone may also result from a combination of saturated and unsaturated hemoglobin. The baby is likely to be polycythemic, which suggests the presence of cardiopulmonary or neurological problems, as well as chronic hypoxia in utero. This baby is more susceptible to jaundice, even if he is not technically polycythemic. This purple tint must not be confused with cyanosis, although the polycythemic baby can become cyanotic because of the presence of reduced hemoglobin in the capillaries.

<u>Pale, washed out or white all over (pallor)</u>: When pallor is present, the baby is whitish or pale pink as opposed to blue. Note the distribution over the body. When generalized pallor due to peripheral vasoconstriction is present (producing blue extremities and cool skin), acute heart failure, hypovolemia, birth asphyxia and shock are chief concerns. Pallor may be masked by the presence of other discoloration such as cyanosis or jaundice. Pallor with mottling is alarming and requires prompt investigation (see "Mottling," above).

<u>Slate gray</u>: This is due to the presence of methemoglobin (abnormal hemoglobin) or to profound peripheral vascular constriction or collapse and cyanosis, often secondary to hypovolemia. This baby is likely to require volume expansion; see the subchapter entitled "Evaluating and Assisting the Infant in Need of Resuscitation." Transport the baby right away if it does not resolve with resuscitative efforts.

<u>Green-gold to dull green to dull brown (meconium staining)</u>: The skin, finger- and toenails, body creases of the arms, legs and buttocks, umbilical cord and vernix should be inspected for meconium staining.

Region Exposed	Degree of Staining	Time since Meconium Was Passed
Vernix	Yellow	12 to 14 hours
Fingernails	Yellow	4 to 6 hours
Placental surface	Proportional to the length of exposure and concentration of meconium in the fluid	Surface stains appear within 1 hour
Placental macrophages*	Depends on length of exposure	Always detectable by 3 hours
Umbilical cord	Visible (5% concentration in amniotic fluid)	1 hour
	Visible (10% concentration in amniotic fluid)	15 minutes
Pulmonary macrophages*	Visible	Indicates prenatal aspiration

*Stained white blood cells found on microscopic exam

Use the preceding chart to determine approximately how long meconium was in the fluid before birth. A placenta, cord and membranes that have been standing at room temperature for many hours will appear more severely stained than they actually were in utero because the pigments will have had more time to absorb into the tissues.

<u>Greenish yellow</u>: This indicates an elevation of conjugated (direct) bilirubin, usually in the range of 3 to 5 mg/dl (51.3 - 85.5 μmol/l). Babies with this type of jaundice should also be evaluated soon after birth. This should not to be confused with meconium staining of the skin. The two can be distinguished by blanching: if the baby is jaundiced the blanched area will remain jaundiced, if not, it will turn white. Also, if the amniotic fluid is not clear and you are in doubt, check the base of the cord and the nails for a green or brown tinge, indicating meconium staining.

<u>Yellow to lemon or orange tone</u>: Yellow jaundice indicates elevated blood concentrations of unconjugated (indirect) bilirubin. This is pathological when present at birth, is often related to blood group incompatibility or infection and requires prompt investigation. Jaundice is not to be confused with meconium staining of the skin (see above). Jaundice progresses from the head down. As bilirubin rises, the yellow hue deepens and extends down the body, eventually reaching the soles of the feet. The "rule of threes" can be used to estimate the degree of jaundice.

BODY REGION	BILIRUBIN LEVEL
Head only	3 mg/dl (51.3 μmol/l)
Head and upper trunk	6 mg/dl (102.6 μmol/l)
Head and entire trunk	9 mg/dl (153.9 μmol/l)
Head, trunk and upper abdomen to umbilicus	12 mg/dl (205.2 μmol/l)
Head, trunk and entire abdomen	15 mg/dl (256.5 μmol/l) or more
To soles of feet	18 mg/dl (307.8 μmol/l) or more

Muddy green: In dark-skinned or cyanotic infants, jaundice causes the skin to appear muddy green.

Other common, often normal, dermatological findings

Lanugo: A fine, soft, downy body hair, called "lanugo," appears at 20 weeks gestation. It first covers the body extensively, then begins to fall out as the baby matures. Much of this hair is gone by term; however many babies have a fine, peach-fuzz-textured hair on their back, shoulders, upper arms and along the hair line. This hair is usually pale in light-skinned babies, but it may be brown or black in dark-skinned babies. Normal Hispanic babies may have fairly abundant hair on the forehead and body, while babies of African descent usually have less than average.

Vernix caseosa: In Latin, *vernix caseosa* means "cheesy varnish." The baby may have this cream-cheese-like, greasy, waxy white or pale yellowish material anywhere on the body. Vernix may be stained green if meconium was in the amniotic fluid. Vernix production increases early in the third trimester. Production starts to drop off at about 37 weeks, with term babies having vernix only in their creases and hair. Postterm babies have little remaining. Vernix protects the baby's delicate skin before and after birth. Do not remove it, except as necessary to perform the exam.

Lymph nodes: The lymph nodes can be felt in over one-third of all newborns, usually in the inguinal area, regardless of the baby's history. They range from 3 to 12 ml in diameter and tend to remain enlarged for a while after birth.

Body fat: The subcutaneous tissue of the term infant contains abundant fat cells, making the well-nourished term baby appear round, plump and filled out. The underlying dermis should be palpated for consistency. If subcutaneous fat is absent or lacking, you will find thin, loose or hanging folds of skin that may appear wrinkled on parts of the body or all over the body, giving the impression that the skin is too big for the baby; in this case, you can assume there is little fatty tissue elsewhere in the body.

Subcutaneous fat necrosis (pseudosclerema) is a sharply demarcated, localized area of firmness (induration) of varying size usually found on the back and occasionally over the face or thighs, although it may occur anywhere. The overlying skin may appear blotchy and red. The lesion is fixed to the overlying skin, to the point that lifting a skin fold is impossible. It may develop as a result of localized pressure although often no reason can be found. It will gradually resolve over the days or weeks, occasionally persisting into the first year of life.

Checking motility and turgor: "Motility" refers to how much the skin can move over the underlying surface. "Turgor" means fullness and represents the natural rebound elasticity of the skin. These qualities should be assessed on the anterior abdomen, anterior thigh and the posterior arm, although the abdomen gives the most reliable information on early or small babies. Place your fingers at least 1 in (2.25 cm) apart, then use the pad of your thumb and index finger to gently grasp and lift a good-sized fold of skin away from the surface. Roll the skin fold gently between your fingers to assess the consistency, the amount of subcutaneous tissue and the degree of hydration. Then release it. The ease with which it lifts indicates the mobility of the skin. Upon release, the ease with which the skin returns to its original position reflects normal turgor and elasticity: it should return immediately. If the skin "tents" (that is, it remains pinched up for a varying length of time after release) or if it wrinkles during or after release, dehydration, a lack of subcutaneous fat, weight loss or all three could be causative as could a hyperelastic disorder such as Ehlers-Danlos syndrome. Preterm and dysmature infants who suffered late nutritional deprivation in utero lack subcutaneous fat and have loose skin with sluggish turgor. Thin, tight skin overlying joints is seen with early onset lack of mobility due to neurologic impairment (Fletcher, 1998).

Muscle mass: Newborn musculature is not as defined as in an adult. It normally feels doughy. Poorly developed or wasted muscles feel thin and fibrous. Muscles that are clearly defined may be hypertonic or contracted and fibrotic.

Edema: Check for swelling over anterior shins, tops of the feet, lower back, scapulae and sacrum by pressing a fingerpad firmly into the skin. Mild to moderate localized swelling or bruising is normal if it can be explained by the circumstances of the birth, such as when it is secondary to tissue trauma due to pressure on the presenting part. Mild puffiness of the eyelids, hands, feet, lower legs, pubis and sacrum, even to the point of pitting, may be present in some normal babies; this should disappear by the second to third day of life. More extreme generalized peripheral swelling or pitting edema results in stretching of the skin, causing it to appear shiny, with a loss of skin creases and folds. Such edema shifts with position changes. It may be related to disorders of fluid balance or metabolism, especially in dependent areas of the body (these areas are the buttocks, back and occiput when supine). **Lymphedema** is characterized by puckering as it forms clefts between regions with accentuation of skin creases; it also has some degree of pitting. The baby should be evaluated promptly if edema is generalized, pronounced and regionalized, or inexplicable. Isolated regions of peripheral edema (such as one swollen leg or swelling of the tops of the hands and feet) is a sign of Turner syndrome in full-term girls; this disorder is associated with a high incidence of coarctation of the aorta, a heart defect. Swelling of the tops of the feet and hands is seen in almost all preterm babies of less than 2000 g (4 lb 6.5 oz).

Loose (redundant) skin: Loose skin is generally indicative of a problem and may have several origins. Distension can produce loose skin due to pressure from within from an unusual force that has regressed (such as lymphatic swelling or edema), compression by an external force (such as the loose facial skin associated with oligohydramnios) or malformation with overgrowth of normal forces (such as in cutis laxa) or of unknown or idiopathic cause (as occurs in achondroplasia).

Skin temperature: Assess the skin temperature in several body regions by applying the back of your hand to the skin surface. The hands and feet may normally be cooler on palpation than the rest of the body during the first few hours of life. However, a repeated finding of coolness in the extremities, despite normal environmental and core temperatures, is abnormal. Be especially attentive to lesions and areas that appear red, hardened or pale, and compare their temperature with an adjacent region that appears normal.

Sweating: Sweating is usually not seen in the normal newborn. However, in large infants, some sweating may occur in otherwise normal babies. This manifests as beads of perspiration on the forehead or the palms after birth fluids in the hair have dried. Generalized sweating in the presence of a normal environmental temperature may be due to drug withdrawal or, rarely, congestive heart failure.

Dimpling: Dimples develop anywhere the skin is relatively tightly fixed to the deeper tissues and the underlying bony prominences. They may be a familial trait or may signal an underlying defect or bony prominence. The presence of a skin dimple, whether pigmented or not, is normal if it is located over a joint, commonly appearing over the knees, the side of the elbow, the acromion process of the shoulder and the lumbosacral area. Mild dimpling may occur over the bony prominences as the result of intrauterine pressure. Dimples may be related to postural deformities that later resolve. Dimpling over the lower sacrum is a pilonidal dimple, discussed later in this chapter under examination of the spine.

Dimples found in an area that is between two joints (such as along a long bone) are considered pathologic until proven otherwise. Abnormal dimpling may occur anywhere there has been closer than usual proximity between the skin and underlying bone structure during fetal life, resulting in the development of deficient subcutaneous tissue at that site and usually arising from intrauterine pressure resulting in lack of movement. There may also be breakdown of tissue with ulceration. Further evaluation is warranted when dimpling is deep, in an unusual location, apparently unrelated to intrauterine posture, or persistent when assumed to be related to intrauterine posture.

Normal pigmentation variations in infants-of-color: Regular transverse folding creases (not wrinkling) across the lower abdomen may be present, giving the trunk a gridiron appearance. Compared to Caucasian babies, this finding is most prominent in dysmature black infants, although pinkish creases may be noted in dysmature Caucasian infants as well. The areola, nail beds, linea negra (line of increased pigmentation extending from the umbilicus to the genitalia), and genitals (especially the scrotum) may be much darker (ranging to near black) than the surrounding tissues. Regions of the skin that were protected by flexion in utero, such as the inner thighs, may be more lightly pigmented than surrounding areas. Babies-of-color tend to be lightly pigmented at birth. African American mothers report that the color of the upper auricle of the infant's ear indicates the mature skin tone (Fletcher, 1998).

Lesions

Unpigmented, nonvascular lesions: At term, newborn skin is velvety smooth and normally free of lesions, although a little superficial peeling may occur as the skin dries. A lesion includes any area of altered skin texture or appearance. Irregularities of the skin should be noted as to location, color, texture, depth, consistency (hard or soft), size, shape, if the legion is singular or in clusters (scattered, patches, etc.), temperature, and any other distinguishing characteristics. As in the adult, the presentation of skin lesions is highly variable. Pay close attention to any irregularities in the surface of the skin or to a regionally hyper- or hypopigmented area. Blanch the skin over the lesion by pressing a magnifying glass or other flat clear object over the area to further examine suspicious skin lesions. This empties underlying blood vessels but will not alter the appearance of bruises or pigmented lesions. A number of skin lesions may be present, most of which are totally benign and disappear in the days, weeks or months following birth. Fletcher (1998) offers this basic vocabulary to describe lesions:

CHARACTERISTIC	DEFINITION AND IMPLICATIONS
Abrasion (scrape) and laceration (cut)	Injuries may be related to attempts to free the shoulders, a tight cord, or any difficult delivery. They usually result from scraping with a fingernail or instrument. Babies may also scratch themselves in utero.
Bruise (ecchymosis)	A subepidermal hemorrhage may develop in areas traumatized during birth such as the buttocks in a breech, face in a face presentation, or arms and shoulder areas after a shoulder dystocia.
Bulla	A blister >1 cm in diameter that may be tense and full or flaccid. Any baby with a bulla requires further evaluation; it may be infectious.
Erythema	A reddened area that blanches with pressure
Induration	A loss of softness of the dermis or its underlying subcutaneous tissue. May indicate infection, obstruction or tumor. May cause the overlying skin to appear taut and shiny.
Lesion	Any region of tissue that is different or altered
Macule	A flat lesion less than 1 cm in diameter that differs in color from the surrounding skin. Freckles are one example. They may be hypo- or hyperpigmented.
Nodule	A papule greater than 1 cm in diameter. Blue-toned subcutaneous nodules may be present causing the baby to look like a blueberry muffin. They are associated with either metastatic neuroblastoma or dermo-erythropoiesis due to intrauterine viral infection with rubella or cytomegalovirus.
Plaque	A raised legion whose width is greater than the degree of elevation. They can arise directly from the skin, or be formed by a group of papules. These vary in size from 1 cm to very large, covering most of the body. Note surface texture (smooth or rough, taut, hard, etc).
Papule	An elevated, palpable, solid, distinct lesion <1 cm in diameter. Note distribution, color, consistency and texture.
Patch	A macule > 1 cm in diameter
Petechia	A pinpoint subepidermal hemorrhage that does not blanch with pressure. Multiple lesions are often found on the faces of babies who experienced rapid descent during pushing, who had a tightly wrapped cord or who had cranial congestion during birth (i.e., shoulder dystocia). More likely to be associated with thrombocytopenia (low platelets) or congenital infection if found on the torso or if they increase in number or size; the baby requires careful evaluation. Petechiae normally fade in the days after birth.
Pustule	A small vesicle that contains pus
Scale	A peeling up of dead or dying fragments of skin. May result from excess skin cells. The most serious associated condition is ichthyosis, an often severe skin disorder causing cracking and peeling. Note if the scales are coarse, fine, greasy, silvery, white or yellow, peripheral, or associated with another lesion or adherent to it.
Vesicle	A blister <1 cm in diameter
Wheal	A circumscribed papule or irregular plaque of edema, appearing as slightly reddened, often changing in size and shape and extending to adjacent areas, and usually accompanied by intense itching; produced by stroking or by exposure to allergenic substances (Darier sign). It is very transient.

Sucking blisters or sores: Large or small blisters may develop on the baby's lips, fingers, hands or wrists as a result of sucking in utero. They may be intact or ruptured. They require no treatment other than being kept clean, although they will not heal if the baby continues to suck there.

Blisters, fragile skin: Some babies are born with localized blisters that heal rapidly and do not spread. This can be a normal variation, but infection should be ruled out. Epidermolysis bullosa is an inherited skin disorder that causes localized tearing and separation of the skin due to inadequate tissue bonding, resulting in blistering with rupture, revealing red underlying tissue (Nikolsky's sign). This may occur with minimal friction, such as rubbing the skin. It commonly affects the extensor surfaces of the limbs and the feet, as they are so active in utero. Depending upon the type, the wounds may resemble second-degree burns or common ruptured blisters; one type produces atrophic changes in affected limbs. The baby is at risk for fluid and electrolyte loss as well as infection if the lesions are large.

Erythema toxicum: This very common, benign, newborn rash that usually appears between 24 to 48 hours of life, although on very rare occasions it is present at birth or develops in the hours following birth. It presents as small irregular reddened macules or patches with a central papule or vesicle that is yellow or white (depending upon the baby's serum bilirubin level) that may or may not be red at its base. If seen at birth, the vesicles should be white in normal, unjaundiced infants. Lesions can appear anywhere on the body except the palms and soles and are most commonly seen on the face, trunk or limbs. This rash can appear and disappear and then reappear minutes later elsewhere on the body. It must be distinguished from infectious lesions. Especially if the mother's history raises concerns of infection, a diagnosis can be made by doing a microscopic examination of the exudate from a lesion.

Round or oval patches with moist, whitish yellow surfaces that may rupture to reveal underlying shiny red tissue with ulceration should be assumed to be syphilitic until proven otherwise; if they are, the secretions are highly infectious.

Milia (whiteheads): Milia are tiny vernix-filled epidermal cysts in sebaceous follicles, appearing at birth as discrete, pinhead-sized yellow to pearly white papules of vernix that disappear in the first weeks of life. They are usually localized to the nose, forehead and cheeks. They can be felt with the finger and are benign. They are seen in 66% of Caucasian infants and less commonly in black ones.

Miliaria: Miliaria may develop during the first 12 hours of life in a warm, humid environment. They are tiny eruptions of minute vesicles and papules due to retention of fluid at the orifices of sweat glands commonly appearing on the forehead, scalp and skin folds. Superficial lesions appear as thin-walled groups of vesicopapules (miliaria crystallina). "Pustularis" refers to cloudy vesicles without inflammation. If the glandular obstruction is deeper, the lesions appear in groups of red papules (miliaria rubra). Miliaria often clear within the first few days to 1 week if the infant is not overheated and are benign.

Pustular melanosis: These benign lesions may be confused with milia. They begin as small (2 mm) fragile vesicopustules usually on the forehead, neck and submental area, although they may appear on the palms and soles or elsewhere. The intact vesicle ruptures, leaving a whitish scaly halo at the base with no redness. The base is more pigmented than surrounding skin in babies-of-color. They may be present at birth and occur more frequently in African American babies than in Caucasian ones.

Sebaceous gland hyperplasia: Tiny white or yellow legions at the opening of each pilosebaceous follicle, commonly seen on the nose, upper lip and cheeks. They get smaller and disappear in first weeks of life and are benign.

Pinched-up skin folds: On rare occasions, intrauterine positioning produces a fold of skin that may be hard and fibrotic and therefore does not resolve even though the region is no longer under pressure. It can be massaged regularly with castor oil or evening primrose oil to help the tissues relax.

Skin tags: A baby may be born with a vestigial tail at the base of the spine where the pilonidal dimple would be. The tail consists of soft tissue or contains a tiny bone. Skin tags may also appear between the ear and mouth, as bridges of skin from the chin to the neck or elsewhere, or as redundant skin that forms as a result of intrauterine positioning (for example, flexion of the head on one shoulder in utero may make the skin on that side form more tightly, creating a web when the baby's neck is straightened). Midline tags found anywhere from the back of the neck to the tip of the spine warrant evaluation of the neural axis. Any tag should be examined carefully to rule out underlying sinuses or drainage of fluid. Babies with skin tags should be evaluated by a specialist soon after birth to rule out other anomalies.

Dermoid cysts: These cysts contain ectodermal structures and may present as smooth, round elevations of the skin that can rupture during birth. They often develop along the lines of tissue fusion on the head, especially around the eyes and nose, giving a dramatic appearance. The cysts can be attached to underlying structures; this possibility should be excluded before removal by a neonatal surgeon.

Peeling (desquamation): Exposure of the skin to air results in drying at all gestational ages. Slight peeling is often noted over the palms and soles and in the groin. Extensive peeling indicates that the baby has been without protective vernix for some time. Some congenital skin disorders involve rapid drying after birth, leading to extensive peeling and cracking of large areas of very dry, scaly skin. These babies are prone to injury and infection and should be transported for evaluation as soon as possible.

Note that tense shiny skin with peeling or blisters filled with bloody secretions with underlying redness and ulceration of ruptured blisters should be assumed to be syphilitic until proven otherwise, especially when the lesions are limited to the palms and soles of the feet. If syphilitic, the secretions are highly infectious.

Absence of skin: Referred to as **cutis aplasia** or **cutis congenita**, this congenital abnormality involves regions in which some or all layers of the skin and sometimes underlying tissue have not developed, leaving an area that appears hairless, ulcerated or scarred. It most commonly appears as a sharply defined, hairless, round, 2 to 3 cm lesion on the scalp, most frequently over a parietal bone or near the sagittal suture. Rarely, these lesions will be found in other areas of the body as well. Cutis aplasia may be an isolated finding secondary to a familial trait or mechanical pressure during pregnancy but can also be associated with midline spinal defects if found along the midline of the lumbosacral region or with genetic disorders, notably trisomy 13. Aplasia may also result from exposure to embolic microthrombi from the placenta or a fetus papyraceus. The area should be kept clean and dry, and the baby should receive further evaluation. Most such lesions will heal over in time, although large ones may require skin grafting (Coen & Koffler, 1987).

Evidence of infection: Any baby born with skin lesions that present as vesicles, open or crusted sores, tense or flaccid blisters, pustules, erosions (areas where the skin has worn away), scars or missing skin may be suffering from any number of infections acquired during pregnancy. Many of these skin conditions are also associated with noninfectious genetic syndromes or conditions, such as an antibody-mediated reaction to maternal lupus. The maternal history should be reviewed, the lesions should be considered infectious until proven otherwise and a culture swab can be taken from any fresh exudate as soon as the lesions are recognized. Further evaluation may be called for as soon as possible, depending upon the overall history, the appearance and distribution of the lesions, and whether they appear to be one of the lesions already described in this chapter.

Vascular lesions: The gamut of vascular lesions are commonly referred to as "birthmarks." The formal term, **hemangioma** (angiomatous nevus), refers to an overgrowth of blood vessels (typically capillaries) that forms a tumor that increases the size and number of endothelial cells, resulting in a lesion that grows faster than the rest of the body during infancy, followed by reduction in size or total disappearance. Most of these do not require treatment. Hemangiomas occur in about 10% of all white infants during the first year of life. Premature babies of all races have a higher incidence and larger numbers of hemangiomas than term infants; most of these begin to disappear during the first year as well. Although three term girl babies have a hemangioma for every boy, the incidence is roughly equal in the preterm population. The more hemangiomas a term baby has, the greater the likelihood of internal involvement (Low, 1994).

Most hemangiomas are not obvious at birth; only 2% of affected full-term newborns have a visible lesion presenting as a

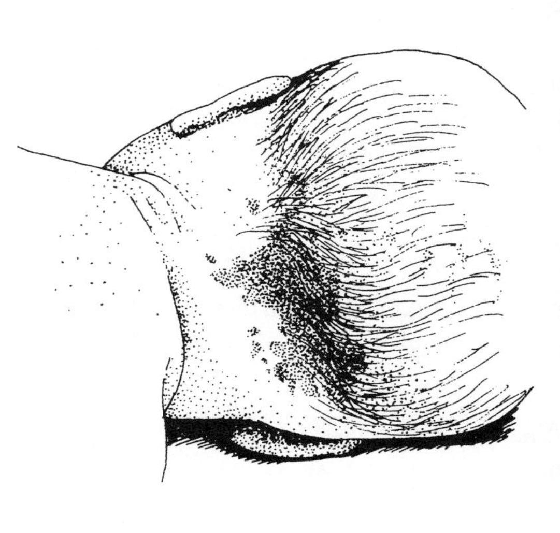
"Stork bite" on the nape of the neck

flat, bright pink red macule that may be distinguished from a bruise because it blanches with pressure. Stroking the lesion causes blanching around its edges and deepening of the color in the center due to blood vessel dilation. The site of a future hemangioma may also present at birth as a diffuse reddish lesion (telangiectasia) or a localized patch of pallor (herald spot). Fine, threadlike blood vessels within its boundaries may be a precursor to the development of a strawberry hemangioma. On rare occasions, hemangiomas that manifest prenatally significantly interfere with normal development of the underlying bones and other structures. This is a prominent feature of Klippel-Trenaunay syndrome (Low, 1994).

In contrast to hemangiomas, vascular malformations consist of abnormalities of vessel development. They are subcategorized by their predominant channel type (capillary, venous, arterial, lymphatic or combination). They grow at the same rate as the baby and show no sexual preference. Although some may reduce in size if the vessels supplying them become occluded, they do not recede by involution. Vascular malformations are always present at birth, although many are not clinically evident on initial exam because they tend to be faint. A notable exception is stork bites (salmon patch), which are commonly found at birth. Stork bites and port-wine stain lesions are categorized as vascular stains (telangiectatic nevi), a form of vascular malformation. The following table describes the most common hemangiomas and vascular malformations (Fishman & Mulliken, 1993).

TYPE	TYPICAL LOCATION AND INCIDENCE	APPEARANCE
Flat macular (nevus simplex, telangiectasia, salmon patch; stork bites; beak marks)	Nape of neck, eyelids, bridge of nose, upper lip. Seen in 50% of newborns.	Splotches of salmon-pink to red color with indistinct borders; blanch with pressure and darken with crying; disappear by two years of age, although those on the nape of the neck may persist. They may brighten when the baby is hot, after a bath or with crying.
Nevus flammeus (port-wine stain) Capillary vascular malformation	Anywhere on the body. Seen in 3 of every 1000 newborns.	Sharply delineated, flat splotch of color which presents at birth as a pale pink legion that blanches only slightly or not at all with pressure. Usually unilateral, but may occasionally cross the midline. May accompany eye disorders, Sturge-Weber syndrome or angiomatous malformation of the brain if found in the trigeminal area (eyes, nose and jaw). Lumbosacral legions may be associated with spinal disorders.
Nevus anemicus	Often a precursor to a strawberry hemangioma	Nevus is pale with prominent capillaries or has a red speckled appearance and is surrounded by an area of localized pallor.
Strawberry hemangioma (nevus vasculosus)	Anywhere on the body. 75% appear on the head. May also occur in the throat, resulting in airway obstruction.	Only 30% of affected babies have visible lesions, appearing as a flat, bright pink macule that reveals some underlying pigmentation with pressure.
Cavernous venous malformation		Deeper cavernous form occurs beneath the skin surface. Presents as a soft, compressible swelling that usually causes the overlying skin to appear reddish blue; may have its edges obscured by overlying skin. Tends to be small and not very prominent at birth. Most regress in size at least partially; those that persist may require surgical removal.

Types of lesions can often be distinguished by changes noted during both stroking and blanching. Areas appearing more pink than the surrounding tissues should be rubbed to increase blood flow. Note whether a magnifying glass pressed against the area causes the lesion to blend into the surrounding blanched skin (Fletcher, 1998). Because lesions in this broad category create problems beginning in the weeks following birth, more details will be found in Volume III.

Lesions involving pigmentation or discoloration that suggests pigmentation: The following lesions are commonly referred to as "birthmarks" but are caused by variations in pigmentation. These descriptions are based on Fletcher (1993), unless otherwise indicated.

Mongolian spots: These common, usually benign lesions result from a variation in pigmentation where melanin-producing cells infiltrate the dermis rather than the epidermis. They are usually associated with dark-skinned infants occurring in 80% of African American, Hispanic, Native American, East Indian and Asian babies but in less than 10% of Caucasian babies. They present as dark blue-gray to dark blue hyperpigmented macules that may resemble and must be distinguished from bruising. They are never raised and are not palpable, as are blue nevi. They appear most commonly over the sacrum, posterior thighs, legs, back and shoulders and less so on the abdomen to either side of the umbilicus, tending to occur on the outer surfaces of the body when the infant assumes her fetal position. Mongolian spots sometimes persist into early childhood but usually fade sooner (Johnston, 1994).

Mongolian spots or a variant ("nevus of Ito," which is usually a singular lesion) may also appear above the clavicles, on the upper arms or in the scapular regions. Isolated nevi of Ito may also occur with a nevus of Ota, which covers the trigeminal region of the face, often involving the eyes, nose and jaw. At times this results in damage to the eye and requires ophthalmologic screening. Both variants are darker than typical Mongolian spots and have more defined borders. These variants do not fade and may rarely become cancerous, especially in Caucasian babies (Fletcher, 1998).

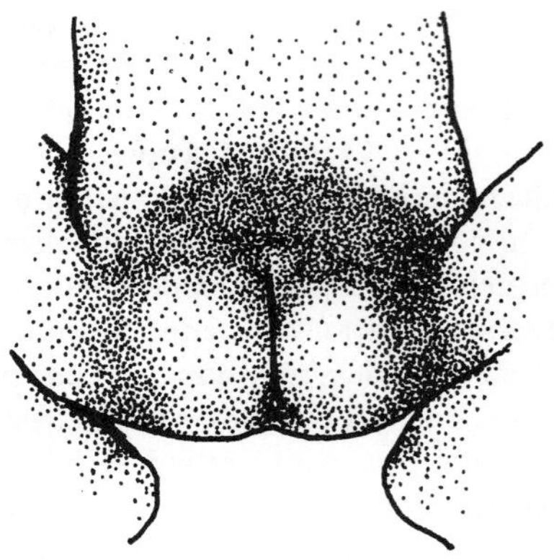

Mongolian spots

Lentigines: These are smooth, freckle-like pigmented macules. They present in a scattered pattern and disappear by 6 to 8 weeks.

Café-au-lait patches: These brown, tan or black macules or patches are areas of darker pigmentation producing a freckle-like spot that is not raised or textured and is usually less than 3 cm in diameter. They occur in 15% of black babies (120/1000 live births) but are only occasionally seen in Caucasians (3/1000 live births). Small spots are not significant; however, large spots that exceed 1.5 cm in diameter, spots found under the arms, or clusters of more than 5 or 6 patches may indicate an underlying neurofibromatosis lesion and require follow-up evaluation. Ask the parents if they or any family members have similar lesions (Scanlon, et al., 1979).

Mastocytosis (urticaria pigmentosa): These result from an excess of mast cells in the superficial dermis, usually producing a chronic eruption characterized by flat or slightly elevated reddish to tan or brownish papules that produce wheals when stroked. Less commonly, it can present as a nasty looking bullous swelling. Mild forms may or may not be localized and usually resolve spontaneously. The systemic form presents as a generalized body rash with liver and spleen enlargement and bone involvement.

Diffuse hyperpigmentation: This occurs in the presence of scattered melanocytes (skin pigment cells) and is unusual. It presents as scattered areas of pigmentation. A benign form occurs exclusively in babies of African descent, presenting as irregular patches and streaks of deeply pigmented lesions. However, hyperpigmentation may be associated with intersex disorders, adrenal insufficiency, and some other metabolic disorders. The baby should be evaluated right away.

Incontinentia pigmenta (Bloch-Sulzberger syndrome): This rare disorder is characterized by hyperpigmented lesions in linear, zebra stripe, and other unusual configurations. It is occasionally accompanied by other developmental anomalies of the eyes, teeth, nails, skeleton, and heart. The dermatologic features involve four stages; stage 1 is characterized by erythema, vesicles, and pustules and is the only stage that may be present at birth. A variant, hypomelanosis of Ito (incontinentia pigmenti achromians) is associated with many forms of mosaicism; it is characterized by unilateral or bilateral hypopigmented macules in whorls, streaks, and patches in a "marble cake" pattern that may be patchy and localized. These are often most obvious on the front of the body and flexor surface of the limbs. It is variably associated with epidermal nevi and alopecia, as well as ocular, skeletal and neural abnormalities.

Hypopigmentation: Pigmentation may be somewhat irregular at the time of birth. Therefore, any areas that appear to be poorly pigmented should be monitored over the first few weeks of life to see if they fill in with normal coloration. Areas of true hypopigmentation may be the earliest and often the only early sign of tuberous sclerosis, a progressive degenerative neurologic disease. These lesions are typically shaped like an ash leaf (a single-lobed leaf, pointed at one end and rounded at the other, shaped like an elongated teardrop with jagged edges), 1 cm across or less. One or more lesions may be found on the buttocks, hips and trunk. Their appearance becomes more pronounced when examined under an ultraviolet light source (such as a Woods' lamp). Shagreen patches may also be found on the sides of the abdomen and the back. These are irregularly outlined areas a few centimeters across consisting of slightly thickened, firm, yellow skin with a finely textured surface resembling an orange skin and are also associated with tuberous sclerosis.

Albinism: Albinism is characterized by varying degrees of reduced pigmentation in the skin, hair and irises, as well as by photosensitivity. The baby shows markedly reduced pigmentation, yellow or white hair, pink pupils, blue or pink irises and photophobia with photosensitivity. Nystagmus with reduced vision is also common. Piebaldism or partial albinism is characterized by off-white macules on the scalp, widow's peak and forehead that may extend to the base of the nose, chin, trunk and limbs. An isolated white forelock may be the only manifestation. In true piebaldism, the light areas contain normally pigmented islands 1 to 5 cm across, distinguishing it from vitiligo, nevus anemicus, Addison disease and the ash leaf-spots of tuberous sclerosis.

Hamartomas (epidermal nevi): As described by Coen and Koffler (1987), hamartomas of the skin are composed of epidermal tissue and its appendages. In general, hamartomas are focal malformations that resemble tumors both grossly and microscopically. They result from faulty development of the skin and are composed of either an abnormal mixture of tissue elements or an abnormal proportion of a single element that is normally present in that region. They develop and grow at virtually the same rate as normal components and are not likely to result in compression of adjacent tissue (in contrast to a neoplasm). Two varieties are present in newborns:

Verrucous (verrucosus) nevus: These fleshy, yellowish-brown or grayish nevi may be warty, granular, rough or smooth oval or linear plaques. If extensive, they can be associated with developmental defects of the skin and eyes. This baby should have further evaluation.

Sebaceous nevus (of Jadassohn): This common nevus is present at birth in 0.3% of all babies. It often appears first as a bald spot in the scalp with or without a few hair follicles; very rarely, it appears in multiple sites. Nevi vary from 1 to 10 cm in diameter and may be round, oval or linear. They develop a slightly raised, finely pebbled, rough, waxy, hairless surface ranging in color from pink to yellow to orange, orange-brown (some have a very fine cauliflower-like appearance) with an oily, waxy or velvety texture. They can continue to grow and will generally transform into basal cell carcinoma by puberty. It should be removed before adolescence. Sebaceous nevi that occur in a linear pattern are rare and are associated with a complex of severe malformations including leptomeningeal hemangiomas, cystic adenoma of the liver, horseshoe kidney, patent ductus arteriosus and conjunctiva lipodermoids. Yellowness increases if the baby is jaundiced. A long list of lesions mimic sebaceous nevi, so further evaluation is in order.

Fletcher (1998) notes a variety of other epidermal nevi, commonly referred to as "moles," and classified according to their predominant cell type. Many, but not all, are pigmented. Some nevi are associated with multisystem defects or syndromes, many of which involve the skeleton or central nervous system.

Junction nevus: These slightly raised pigmented lesions range from brown to black in color and are usually less than 1 cm in diameter. They are seen in up to 15% of black babies and 1 to 2% of all neonates and are usually benign. In large numbers, they may be associated with syndromes such as tuberous sclerosis, xeroderma pigmentosus and generalized neurofibromatosis (Scanlon et al., 1979).

Congenital melanocytic nevus: These vascular lesions are rare, occurring in fewer than 1 in 20,000 babies and more frequently in girls than in boys. These nevi appear over the posterior trunk with irregular topography and may include coarse hair, irregular pigmentation and tumor nodules. Cranial or midline posterior lesions are associated with neurological involvement. These lesions are difficult to distinguish from others at birth; they should be watched and evaluated by a dermatologist.

Congenital pilar (smooth-muscle nevus): This rare nevus consists of smooth-muscle bundles in the dermis. It is studded with fine hairs that may or may not be slightly pigmented, with the hair being the notable feature. It occurs in 1 out of every 2600 babies and is slightly more common in boys than in girls. It is usually found adjacent to the midline in the lumbosacral area, presenting as an oval plaque 2 to 4 cm in length. The lesion feels superficial but firm. Stroking it causes the skin to wrinkle and the hair to stand up; but there is no blistering or wheal formation with rubbing. These lesions are benign.

Giant pigmented nevus: This compound nevus presents an extensive, sharply outlined, highly pigmented lesion that covers a large area of the body, often the entire back of an extremity. It has a nodular or raised surface with fleshy features and a somewhat leathery texture, and may include dark coarse hairs. There may be skin breakdown and ulceration over the lesion at birth.

Nevus unius lateris: These lesions appear as warty, flesh-colored or yellow orange ridges or raised areas. They are often extensive and may be arranged in elaborate, continuous or interrupted pattern such as a line or spiral over multiple sites. There may be pigmented nevus on the limbs. Sebaceous glands overlying these lesions may become enlarged when the scalp, face or neck are involved; when this occurs, eye, skeletal, pigmentary and central nervous system defects are likely.

Dermal signs in the newborn reflecting autoimmune disease in the mother: Edematous lesions of varying size may present in babies born to mothers with a history of lupus, rheumatoid disease or other autoimmune disease. They may be round violet lesions or red edematous lesions of varying size that are partly ring-shaped, fading in the center and spreading on the edges. They commonly appear on the head, neck or extensor surfaces of the arms but may occur less frequently in other areas. Most of these babies will be otherwise normal, although two-thirds may show laboratory abnormalities at birth.

Transillumination of Skin Lesions

Lesions of the extremities can be further examined using a light source. Place the probe tip on the body surface posterior to or oblique to the lesion or against the palm of the hand or sole of the foot when the lesion is on an extremity. Cystic and fat-filled lesions will both transilluminate nicely. Lesions over joints do not transilluminate well because of the density of tissues in these areas. When hypervascularity is present, the extra vessels can be easily seen (which may sometimes indicate malignancy) (Fletcher, 1998).

Further evaluation of unusual lesions

There are literally dozens of different types and subtypes of neonatal dermatologic lesions. The above descriptions include many of the more common and a few of the more rare but serious lesions that may be present at birth. It does not represent an exhaustive description of them all. Any unusual skin lesions should be further evaluated by a pediatric dermatologist whenever you are uncertain as to their significance.

EXAMINING THE HEAD AND NECK

The head and neck region merit careful attention. Ninety percent of all congenital anomalies that are visible at birth occur here, although facial features considered diagnostic of a number of conditions are not always obvious at birth. In such cases, growth will reveal these abnormalities and, in some cases, birth-related changes will resolve otherwise suspicious features. The normal shape of the skull is reviewed in detail in the chapter entitled "Features of Fetal Anatomy Pertinent to the Birth Process." Ridges, narrowing of the midline, bossing or protrusion of the forehead, small jaw, elongation of the entire skull, shallow eye sockets, and a depressed nasal bridge are associated with a variety of congenital disorders. Unusual features in the midline of the face or vertex, even if minor, may be indicative of significant associated disorders. The content of this chapter is based on Thureen and colleagues (1999), unless otherwise noted.

Examining the Head

The appearance of the newborn's head and face give clues about brain development as well as fetal position and engagement. Look for symmetry, size, shape and relationship of all the features to each other as well as how the baby holds his head and moves his face. The baby's head has been subjected to pressures for many hours if the baby was born cephalic and to sudden pressure changes if born breech; it should be carefully and gently handled.

Hair

Note the quantity, length, continuity, texture and color of the hair. Preterm newborn scalp hair is fuzzy with ends that tend to clump. By term, the strands are distinct, thicker and silky. The quantity varies with gestational age, race and maternal nutrition. Term infants will have more hair than preterm babies. Hispanic infants and other babies-of-color tend to have more abundant scalp hair at birth than do Caucasian babies.

Hair color should be racially concordant with that of the parents. The color of the hair may be uniform or a salt-and-pepper mix of light and dark that is uniformly distributed. Random patches of white are a normal familial variation, but a white forelock with other pigment defects and anomalies is associated with deafness and retardation. Reddish or blonde hair in a baby from dark-haired parents (especially in families-of-color) suggests a degree of albinism, but always check with the parents to find out if light to dark hair color changes with maturation are a family trait. (The baby could also have another father!)

The hair line can vary among normal infants but should be fairly uniform and racially concordant. The hairline above the forehead may vary widely. Normal hirsute babies (those with excessive body hair) may have fine hair that extends down the forehead and over the face, arms and torso. Hirsutism can be normal as long as the eyebrows are not continuous across the brow (seen in Cornelia de Lange syndrome). The posterior hairline is more consistent in its formation. The presence of hair roots well below the neck creases or along the side of the baby's neck (below the level of the lower tip of the ear lobes) is associated with syndromes involving a short or webbed neck, such as Turner and Noonan syndromes. A trident posterior hairline (with a central point and points on either side) is also seen with Turner syndrome.

The hair typically has an unruly appearance at birth; however, it should be manageable after it is dried. It is unruly if it stands straight up over the top of the head from the posterior parietal whorl toward the frontal hairline despite attempts at grooming. It is also uncommon for the hair to be strongly upswept at the neck or forehead at birth. Extreme unruliness with multiple directions of growth, especially when found with unusual facies, microcephaly or in SGA age infants may be associated with poor brain development and is characteristic of a number of genetic disorders.

An absence of hair from a normal location is not unusual in newborns, because newborn hair grows in synchronized waves; however, some downy hair is almost always present. Friction in utero from head movement may produce hair loss at the back of the head that resolves once the baby is able to move at will. Alopecia (complete lack of hair) occurs in several syndromes (ectodermal dysplasias where the hair is sparse over the scalp, eyebrows and eyelashes; progeria; Hallermann-Streiff syndrome and cartilage-hair hypoplasia).

A baby who appears to have an unusual quantity of hair or kinky, brittle or abnormally textured hair may also have poor brain development, especially if the baby has other signs of problems such as a small skull, being small for gestational age, or having unusual facial features. These associations occur in a wide variety of genetic disorders. Most abnormal hair textures are not apparent in the newborn at birth.

Hair Texture	Possible Associated Problems
Kinky	Menkes syndrome
Coarse	Mucopolysaccharidoses (metabolic disorders)
Sparse	Ectodermal dysplasias
Hypopigmented	Albinism (for example, reddish or blonde hair with parents-of-color)
White forelock	May be associated with Waardenburg syndrome when seen with other pigment defects in the eyes or skin

The direction of growth, position and number of hair whorls should also be assessed by smoothing the hair out and noting the direction of growth over the entire scalp. This will be easiest to do after the baby's hair has been rinsed of any birth fluids and is completely dry (for example, after the herbal bath). The direction of growth is normally consistent except for the hair whorl. Ninety-five percent of all babies have a single, off-center, variably positioned whorl (spiral) of hair located over one of the parietal regions, regardless of race. The whorl is located 1 to 2 cm anterior to the posterior fontanelle in 56% of babies; 55% are to the left, 30% are right-sided and 15% are midline. The hair grows in a clockwise spiral 80% of the time. Note that 90% of normal black infants with short, curly hair tend not to have a hair whorl. About 5% of normal babies have two whorls. If there are more than two whorls, or if the whorl is found in the midline, over the frontal bone or behind the posterior fontanelle, the underlying brain may be abnormal.

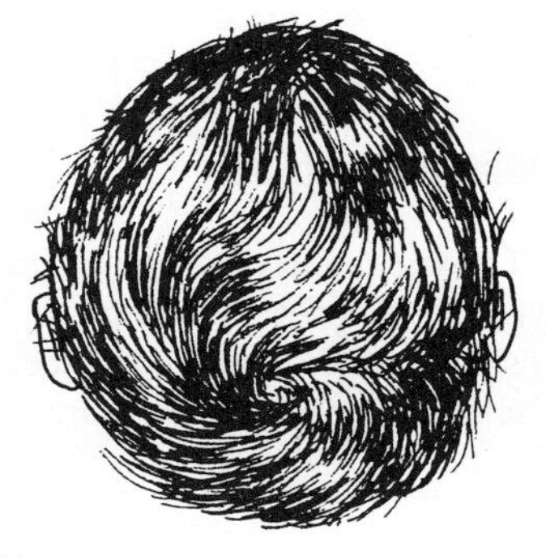

Typical clockwise hair whorl viewed from above and behind.

Scalp: Examine the scalp for uniform, normal development, texture and thickness. Look carefully through thick hair and vernix. Lesions of the scalp may be caused by localized trauma during birth (for example, if the membranes were ruptured with an instrument). Check for coarse furrowing that looks similar to the folds of the brain; this most commonly presents on the scalp and neck, and may be seen with some genetic disorders. Congenital lesions or defects such as sores or raw or bald areas are also associated with a variety of congenital defects, particularly trisomy 13. Localized absence of the skin may appear as single or multiple lesions to either side of the midline. Dilated scalp veins indicate long-standing intracranial pressure.

Examining the skull

Look at the head from the front, back, top and each side to get an overall feel for its shape. Assess the size of the head in relationship to the rest of the body, keeping in mind that the head is relatively large at birth, comprising one-fourth of the total body length.

Look for any flattening, depressions, abnormally prominent areas or areas of apparent decrease in volume. Compare the shape from diagonally opposite corners and from above. Keep in mind that a caput or hematoma may temporarily cause a marked oblique distortion; a true oblique distortion of the skull shape is termed **plagiocephaly**. This gives the entire skull an asymmetrical appearance of flattening with fullness over the diagonally opposite corner, especially when viewed from above. Parietal flattening with diagonal fullness causes the face to be asymmetrical.

Look at the overall contour of the baby's head to get an idea of the position the baby assumed as the head came down the birth canal. (Moulding is covered in detail at the beginning of this volume and will be further addressed in Volume III.) Compare your findings to the drawings of the various types of moulding associated with the different presentations. This will allow you to double-check your assessment of fetal presentation during labor. Note whether moulding is absent or seems excessive. Moulding of the head due to fetal positioning may also result in temporary facial asymmetry, therefore any abnormal findings that appear to be caused by moulding should be carefully reassessed at each home visit in the days following birth. Although most types of moulding are not considered damaging in the medical model, be alert for moulding that does not resolve as well as pathologic conditions that inhibit normal moulding, such as premature fusion of one or more suture lines or macrocephaly when the baby has not been born head first or descent was much delayed.

Suture lines: If there are no mismatched or overlapped edges, the borders of the sutures should be firm but give slightly with gentle pressure. Normally the edges of sutures are flush and slightly mobile. Up to 1 cm of separation may exist between the sutures, but this is unusual in normal term babies. Preterm infants will have wider and more flexible sutures than a full-term baby.

To evaluate the amount of moulding that took place during labor and to determine whether premature fusion of the sutures has occurred, palpate along the frontal, sagittal, coronal and lambdoidal suture lines. Attempt to determine if they are fused. Some of these sutures may be mismatched or overlapped immediately after birth, especially if moulding has been extreme. Commonly, the edges of the lambdoidal suture are staggered due to occipital molding: the edge of one bone can be felt above the other, with the higher edge forming a cliff over the other. Normally the coronal suture is barely felt from the edges of the anterior fontanelle down half the length of the side of the head with no gap noted. A small gap between the frontal bones at the metopic suture is frequently noted. The posterior angle of the anterior fontanelle may be elevated due to moulding of the frontal bones. If you do not note a clear separation, place the thumbs on the bones on either side of each suture line and alternately press down with one thumb and then the other. If moulding is palpable, repeat this exam during a postpartum visit after moulding resolves. If there is no moulding, you should still be able to detect a tiny membranous gap between the bones. Widened suture lines with a normally sized anterior fontanelle may be due to abnormal ossification secondary to intrauterine growth restriction. Wider separation or a bulging fontanelle should alert you to the possibility of increased intracranial pressure. Any suture, especially the frontal, may be normally widened without increased intracranial pressure. However, a wide lambdoidal or squamous suture is strongly associated with increased intracranial pressure. Bones between the sutures or in the fontanelles may be hard to detect without an X-ray, but if you suspect their presence in association with widely spaced sutures and fontanelles, check carefully to see if the clavicles are normal; if not, clidocranial dysplasia is likely.

The most common causes of an abnormal skull shape are either a caput or hematoma (discussed later). More rarely, premature closure of one or more of the cranial sutures, known as **craniosynostosis**, occurs with an overall incidence of 1 in every 2000 to 2500 births. This defect has many presentations, as described in the chart on the next page; the incidences mentioned in the first column refer to the percentages of that type of craniosynostosis within the overall population of affected babies. When craniosynostosis is present, the sutures may feel at first as though they are overriding, but on closer inspection it becomes apparent that the edges are rigid and immobile, more like a mountain range that peaks over the suture line than a cliff, in which one edge is elevated above the other. The edges do not move when alternately pressed. Premature closure of one or more sutures is a serious problem, which inhibits growth of the skull and brain perpendicular to the line of fusion. It is accompanied by compensated growth in unrestricted regions. This distorts the shape of the head in characteristic ways, depending upon which sutures are involved. The baby should be evaluated without delay whenever fusion is suspected along a suture line. Some forms of this defect require immediate surgery while others will only require cosmetic surgery later.

Fusion may result from a variety of causes, although many cases have no identifiable cause. The small, normally shaped head with fused sutures results from abnormal brain growth. Craniosynostosis may also be associated with a metabolic disease such as rickets, hyperthyroidism, prolonged constraint of the fetal head in utero, and certain genetic disorders, or it may be a primary congenital defect of skull growth. Numerous problems may arise including impairment of brain and nervous system function and growth, elevation of intracranial pressure, impaired blood flow to the brain and mental retardation, although a surprising number of these children have normal intelligence. Vision and hearing impairment as well as airway obstruction may occur. Even when the child is not mentally delayed, learning difficulties may be present (Graham, 1988).

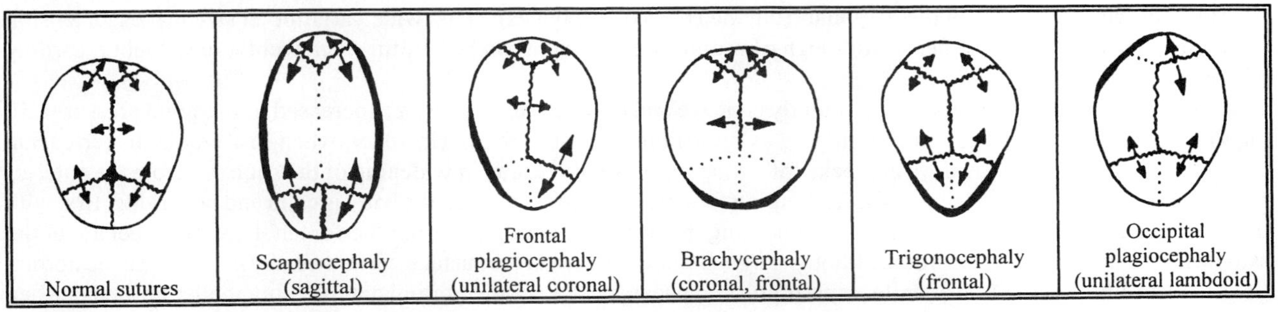

These drawings show the most common configurations of fusion from an overhead view, which sutures are involved in each (shown as dotted lines and listed in parentheses), and the abnormal shape such fusion produces (note that the abnormal shape may not be marked at birth). Normal sutures are shown as solid, serrated lines. The thicken black outlines, when shown, indicate areas of marked flattening as the deformity becomes more severe. The arrows indicate the directions in which the skull can grow. More complex distortions of shape occur when multiple sutures are involved.

SHAPE/INCIDENCE	CHANGES IN THE SKULL SHAPE	FUSED SUTURES	COMMENTS AND ASSOCIATIONS
Scaphocephaly (dolichocephaly), 40-50% (80% boys)	Elongated AP axis	Sagittal	Sagittal suture feels like bony keel
Frontal plagiocephaly, 20–25% (more frequent in girls)	Face asymmetrical, with flattening over one side of forehead; elevation and recession of eyebrow and orbital border with one prominent eye; bulge in the opposite parietal vault.	One coronal and sphenofrontal	Saethre-Chotzen syndrome
Brachycephaly, 12%	Widened skull with short AP diameter	Bilateral coronal	Apert, Antley-Bixler and Pfeiffer syndromes
Turricephaly (acrocephaly), 5–10%	Broad, tower shape with no anterior fontanelle	Bilateral coronal, sphenofrontal and frontoethmoidal	Crouzon (common) and Apert syndromes (less common; anomalies of skull base)
Occipital plagiocephaly, 2–10%	Flattening over occiput with prominent forehead but little facial deformation; ear sometimes prominent	Single lambdoid	Similar findings in postural deformations with preterm babies, torticollis, spinal tumors, cervico-occipital defects. Usually does not require surgery.
Trigonocephaly, 5% (more frequent in boys)	Triangular, prow-like forehead. Fusion of frontal suture with central ridge down the forehead.	Frontal	Bilateral frontal lobe dysplasia presents a similar appearance but no forehead ridge. Opitz syndrome.
Oxycephaly, rare	Cone-shaped with forehead sloped to bony elevation at bregma	Multiple	
Triphyllocephaly (Kleeblattschädel), rare	Cloverleaf with bilateral temporal bulges, narrowing at level of forehead and central bregmatic bulge	Multiple	
Pachycephaly, rare	Back of head flattened, skull widened, short AP diameter	Bilateral lambdoid	

(Adapted from Simpson, 1986)

Fontanelles: Usually six fontanelles can be identified at birth (two mastoid, two sphenoid, the anterior, and the posterior), although less commonly a seventh (the sagittal) is noted. The anterior and the posterior are the most clinically significant. The anterior fontanelle is easily identified as a soft, diamond-shaped area at the junction of the coronal and sagittal sutures that remains flat when the quiet infant is supine or held upright.

The size of the anterior fontanelle is widely variable. It may be barely palpable or may measure up to 5 × 4 cm at its widest points (measured on the diagonal from the edges of the bones). This wide variation in size makes its tension more informative than its size per se, although a baseline measurement can be helpful whenever there is doubt regarding whether the opening is normal.

Normally, the anterior fontanelle is slightly concave and may be seen to pulsate. Increased intracranial pressure will manifest as tension that progresses to bulging as intracranial pressure rises. However, when intracranial hypertension is present, head growth in the days or weeks following birth usually results in widening of the sutures before the anterior fontanelle begins to bulge. If you suspect a bulging fontanelle, reassess it when the baby is calm and not crying, first with the baby in a supine position and then while holding the baby in a sitting position; the fontanelle should feel about the same with the baby in either position, although *slightly* more fullness in the surface when the baby is sitting can be normal (it should still be soft). Occasionally arterial pulsations can be seen in the normal anterior fontanelle; however, when this occurs, an overfull fontanelle or increased arterial pressure must also be considered. A sunken fontanelle is a late sign of severe dehydration.

The posterior fontanelle is smaller, triangularly shaped and bordered by the sagittal and lambdoidal sutures. It is often patent at birth, although in some babies it closes during the last two months of gestation. It is measured by extending a line from its anterior corner (at the posterior end of the sagittal suture) to the midpoint of a line connecting the two posterolateral corners created by the occipital bone. If the sagittal suture is wide, establishing the anterior corner is difficult. Only 3% of all term babies have a posterior fontanelle that exceeds 2 cm and it is usually much smaller.

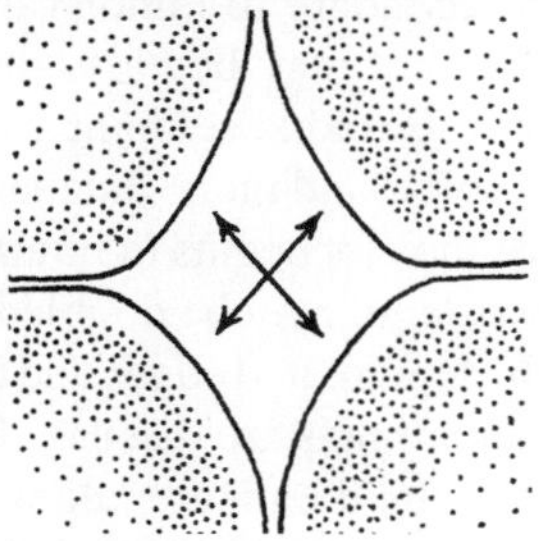

Measuring the anterior fontanelle

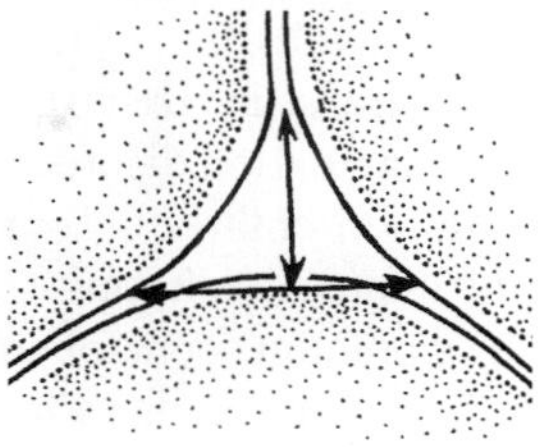

Measuring the posterior fontanelle

A sagittal fontanelle is sometimes found along the sagittal suture, halfway between the anterior and posterior fontanelles. This developmental feature persists to term in about 5% of all babies. It can be a normal variant but is also associated with Down syndrome and congenital hypothyroidism.

Rarely, one or both parietal bones have a palpable parietal foramen. This presents as a depression over the parietal area, ranging in diameter from 1 mm (the normal size) to 3 cm (very large and *very* rare). Large foramina present similarly to fontanelles and, like fontanelles, may pulse or bulge. Unlike fontanelles, they do not intersect suture lines. They interrupt the contour of the otherwise dome-shaped parietal bone when the head is viewed from the correct angle. They are generally harmless and may appear in otherwise normal infants; they usually close as the baby matures (Rudolph, 1997).

The squamosal sutures curve over and above the ears, separating each parietal bone from each temporal bone. The sphenoid fontanelle is at the anterior end, and the mastoid fontanelle at the posterior end, of this suture. These fontanelles are usually only obvious at term in the presence of increased intracranial pressure, as in hydrocephalus. They may be more easily palpated in preterm infants.

Skull firmness: Hand in hand with checking the sutures is an assessment of skull firmness. Normally, the skull at term is firm enough to retain its shape during normal descent and birth. Be alert for depressions or irregularity that suggest a fracture (follow up with referral for X-rays). Soft areas of bone (craniotabes) may also be present anywhere over the skull but are most common in the parietal bones near the sagittal suture. Pressing on the bone causes a give-and-return sensation similar to that elicited by pressing on an empty aluminum soft-drink can or ping-pong ball. Such areas are usually not significant but may be associated with preterm birth as well as with prolonged pressure on the head of a baby who has been engaged in a vertex presentation for at least five weeks; they are, at times, associated with pressure from the uterine fundus on the fetal head in a breech presentation or hydrocephalus. Prolonged intrauterine pressure can interfere with proper bone mineralization. Pathologic craniotabes occur in syphilis but are usually not apparent at birth (Graham, 1988).

Cranial swellings: Pape and Wigglesworth (1979) offer excellent descriptions of the three most common cranial injuries. Either a caput or a hematoma can influence the shape of the skull as well as the way it feels on palpation. Any baby with one of these lesions should receive homeopathic arnica after birth (30C or 200C).

Caput succedaneum: Caputs are the most common type of scalp swelling. Pressure on the presenting part restricts venous and lymphatic return resulting in a diffuse subcutaneous hemorrhagic edema over the leading area of the presenting part producing a thick, boggy scalp. Caput formation is highly associated with continued labor (usually of at least several hours duration or with a long pushing phase) in the presence of ruptured membranes. They rarely (if ever) form in the presence of intact membranes. It will feel nonfluctuant (not boggy), somewhat firm and spongy, will pit on pressure and will obscure palpation of the underlying skull bones and sutures. Superficial bruising can cause it to mimic a hematoma. A caput may overlie suture lines or fontanelles; which differentiates it from a cephalohematoma. Although the much more serious subgaleal hematoma may also overlie suture lines, a caput is most pronounced at birth, does not enlarge more after birth, is confined to the region of the presenting part that received the most direct pressure during descent and gradually resolves during the first hours or day of life. A caput usually develops on the head, but similar swellings may develop on any other presenting part of the baby that received prolonged, direct pressure during descent.

Cephalohematoma: This consists of a collection of blood that forms secondary to minor vascular trauma occurring between the periosteum and the skull. It is often not apparent at birth but may begin to develop during the hours following birth and continue to increase in size up to three days postpartum. Rapid development of any type of hematoma suggests extensive trauma or a coagulation disorder. A hematoma feels softer and more fluctuant than a caput, does not pit as much and feels more doughy after three or four days as the center of the clot begins to liquify. There may be a ridge mimicking an underlying bony depression because the edges of the periosteum may be doubled slightly under pressure at the border of the hematoma. Common cephalohematomas have clearly demarcated edges and do not cross suture lines. There may be pitting edema if a caput overlies a hematoma. Cephalohematomas are discussed further in Volume III.

Extradural hemorrhage occurs with bleeding between the bone and the dura mater along the inner surface of the skull. It is nearly always associated with skull fracture and is usually accompanied by an overlying cephalohematoma. Skull fracture is associated with a hematoma in 5 to 10% of all cases, probably more with instrumental deliveries.

Subgaleal (subaponeurotic) hematoma: This rare and serious form of hematoma is almost exclusively associated with instrumental deliveries, although it may occur even more rarely with precipitous birth. Bleeding develops beneath the thin, tendonous epicranial aponeurosis, which attaches the frontal and occipital portions of the occipitofrontal muscle. Unlike a cephalohematoma, a subgaleal hematoma occurs in a layer of the scalp that has poorly defined borders, thus bleeding can extend into the neck or forehead area and may cause the ear on the affected side to protrude. The swelling may feel firm or fluctuant and can cross suture lines. It will typically pit with pressure, although less so than a typical caput, and may produce a fine grating sensation (crepitance) on palpation, especially near the borders as minerals have time to precipitate out of the blood. It may also form what looks like a swollen bruise localized over the upper eyelids, jaw and nape of the neck. Small lesions are the rule, although large amounts of blood can accumulate and compromise the circulating blood volume. If you suspect a subgaleal hematoma, watch carefully to make sure it is not enlarging. If it is, the baby should be transported for monitoring of blood pressure and hematocrit and may need a transfusion.

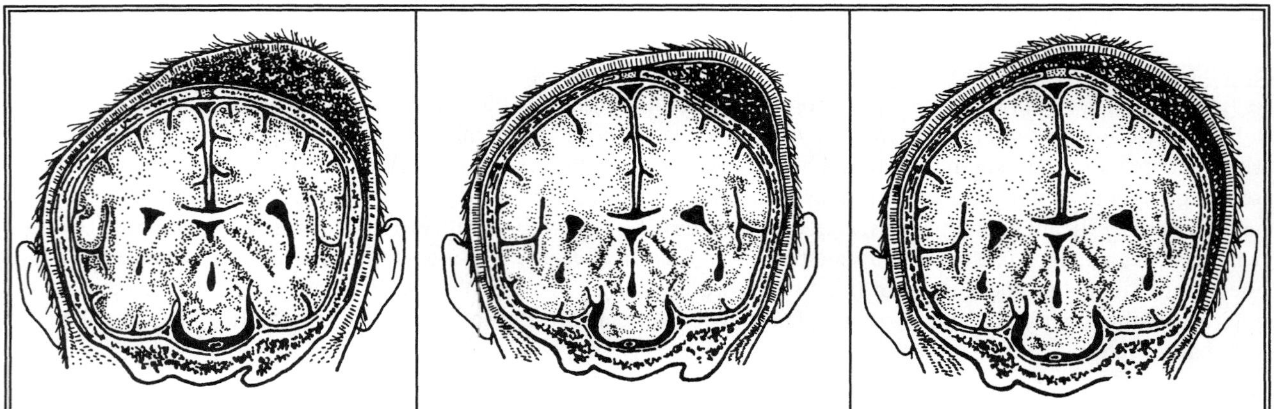

Caput succedaneum | Cephalohematoma | Subgaleal hematoma

(These babies ears appear to be misaligned due to normal moulding.)

<u>**Other cranial defects**</u>: Fletcher (1998) discusses other, more obvious pathological findings of the cranium, all of which result from abnormalities of the vault.

Defects involving incomplete closure of the skull: These include anencephaly (exposed brain tissue with an open skull), encephalocele (herniation of the brain and meninges through a defect in the skull) and cranial meningocele (defective bone allowing an outpouching of spinal fluid-filled meninges). Because these defects present dramatically, they are covered in more detail in the subchapter entitled "Externalized Organs and Neural Tube Defects."

Hydrocephalus and related defects: This group of defects involves an increase in spinal-fluid pressure within the ventricles of the brain, often with decreased or absent brain growth and sometimes with severe malformations of the face. It has an incidence of 5 to 25 per 10,000 total births. When noticeable at birth, you will find wide sutures (particularly the lambdoidal and squamous sutures) and fontanelles, increased head circumference, perhaps a bulging forehead, and if pronounced enough, positive transillumination. A baby whose head circumference is greater than the 90th percentile for gestational age and whose weight and height are below the 90th percentile may have hydrocephaly, macrocephaly or hydranencephaly. (See the chapter entitled "Assessment of the Baby's Size and Its Relationship to Gestational Age.") The vault of the skull may also appear globular. These babies should be transported for evaluation by a neonatologist without undue delay. Sometimes these growth discrepancies are not obvious at birth. Postnatal growth charts will be discussed in Volume III of this textbook.

Microcephaly: This occurs when the cranial vault is abnormally small (two standard deviations below the normal percentile for gestational age with the weight and length closer to average) and usually indicates underdevelopment of the brain with or without premature fusion of sutures. It may occur secondary to infection, chromosomal abnormality, or maternal drug or alcohol use. The head may also appear microcephalic if a baby has extensive cone-shaped moulding.

Specific examination technique: These techniques are rarely needed, but all are noninvasive and easy to perform if there is a question about your findings.

Auscultation: Flow disturbances through vessels may cause vascular wall vibrations, called **bruits**, which sound like systolic murmurs. Listening through the skull for bruits is not normally a part of the newborn exam but may be valuable when arteriovenous defects or an aneurysm is suspected. Listen to the skull through the bell of a stethoscope placed over the temporal, frontal and occipital areas. These harsh, intermittent swishing sounds may also be heard in Sturge-Weber syndrome, which is usually associated with a facial hemangioma.

Percussion: Tap over the parietal bones on each side. This should produce a "cracked pot" sound (Macewen's sign) in normal babies prior to closure of the sutures (Coen & Koffler, 1987).

Transillumination of the skull: As Donn and Kuhns discuss (1983), transillumination may prove informative if the head is oddly misshapen, larger or smaller than normal; if the sutures appear abnormal; if other findings suggest brain abnormalities or if the baby exhibits abnormal neurological signs. Place a light source firmly against the skull, first over the anterior fontanelle, then over each parietal bone and finally over the occiput. Various factors affect the normal transmission of light. The presence of a thick scalp or thick subcutaneous fat layer, darker color or density of the skin or hair, or a collection of blood (as with a hematoma) all diminish light transmission. Skull thickness also effects transillumination; no light will pass through a bone thicker than 2.5 mm. The skull of a normal term baby is less than 2.5 mm thick. Conversely any collection of clear fluid from a caput, generalized edema or ventricular enlargement may increase transmission.

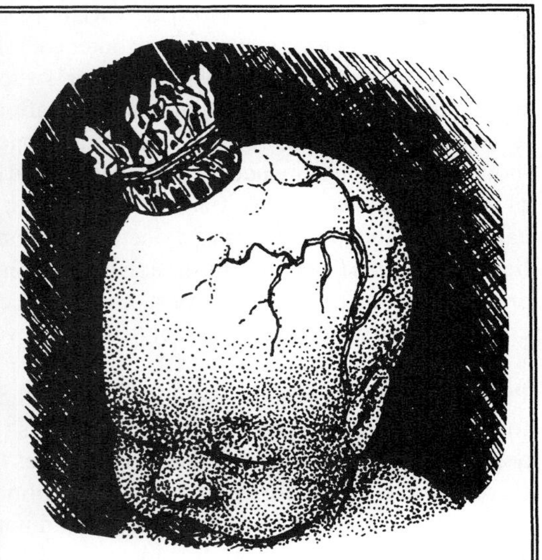

Abnormally bright transillumination of the skull suggesting a lack of brain development.

When the light is placed over solid bone in babies 37 to 42 weeks gestation, the frontal region often illuminates most brightly (2.2 to 4.9 cm corona); followed closely by the parietal regions (2 to 4.9 corona); generally speaking, the occiput admits less light (0.7 cm to 3.9 cm corona), but it is more variable (Vyhmeister et al., 1977). Fletcher (1998) gives more standardized values. She says the rim of light over the frontal or parietal area will be about 2 cm with a 1 cm halo over the occipital area. The entire forehead may light up in the presence of a normal brain. There is a normal increase in glow over sutures, fontanelles and craniotabes. Rim diameters are somewhat smaller in normal babies-of-color because of their pigmentation. A rim of more than 2 cm suggests increased fluid or decreased brain tissue in the cranium.

A larger corona is widely held to be normal in preterm infants. However, Swick and colleagues (1976) and Volpe (1995) state that, in fact, the corona in a normal preterm infant is often smaller than in term babies and enhanced as term approaches. Light transmission is greatly increased in the presence of increased amounts of fluid in the subarachnoid, subdural and ventricular spaces. Brighter than normal transillumination may therefore signify hydrocephalus, hydranencephaly (absence of the cerebral hemispheres of the brain), porencephaly (cysts of the brain) or extreme thinning of the cranial bones, although a false positive result may occur if the baby has a large caput or other forms of scalp edema, both of which diffuse light across the region being examined.

It should be noted that transillumination of the skull is a screening assessment only, as it can only detect large fluid accumulations or large empty areas; more precise techniques are required to rule out brain disorders.

Face and ears

Examine the face by viewing it from the front, in profile from each side, from above, and in its relationship to the rest of the skull. Divide the face in half; focus on one side, then the other, from the front and from above. Look for symmetry, shape, size and the relationship of all the facial features in repose as well as during movement. The space between the eyes and the lower forehead is richly supplied with blood vessels. Prominent redness may be present; the junction of the brows is also a common site for stork bite birthmarks.

The normal newborn face can be roughly divided into horizontal thirds, with the top third consisting of the forehead, the middle third the eyes and nose, and the lower third the mouth and chin. Symmetry of facial muscle strength and tone are noted with the baby at rest as well as when she is yawning or crying. Look for signs of distress and jitteriness of the jaw. Notice if the size of the head, especially the vault, is proportionate to the size of the face, even if the circumference of the head was normal.

Ears: Fletcher (1998) gives a detailed description of the ear exam. First, get an overall impression of the ears, observing for shape, size, symmetry and their relationship to the facial features. View the ears from above, from behind and in front of the head with your eyes level with the infant's. Viewing the head from the front, assess the vertical and lateral position of the ears by comparing the position of the tragi (tab of cartilage in front of each ear canal) and the linear distance between the tragi with the midline of the face. If the shape of the head is obliquely distorted when viewed from above, lateral positioning may be distorted, with one ear appearing more anterior than the other. From the sides, assess the horizontal position of the ears in relationship to the eyes; the point at which the top of the ear cartilage attaches to the head should be at the level of the inner canthi of the eyes (more about this assessment is included later in this section)

Normal ears are subject to wide variations in position, size, and structure and are almost as unique as fingerprints. In a term infant, the auricle (pinna or outer ear) should be well formed and curled along the edge or helix (the border that extends from above the earlobe to the ear's superior attachment point). The cartilage should spring back easily when folded and released. Preterm infants have softer cartilage, which recoils more slowly after folding. Often the right ear is larger than the left. Normal ears may appear temporarily asymmetrical at birth due to intrauterine pressure or moulding. Ears that are poorly formed, irregularly shaped, asymmetrical or extreme in size or that are attached to the side of the head in an unusual way are associated with a wide variety of genetic syndromes, hearing impairment or both. Hairy ears may be found in babies of diabetic mothers. Downward folding along the curve of the helix is called "lop ear" (to be distinguished from a malformation due to prenatal positioning). It is associated with weak superior auricular muscles, anencephaly, microencephaly vera, and severe congenital neuromotor disorders and fragile-X syndrome. A transverse crease in the earlobe is also associated with several disorders.

Palpation and inspection: Visually examine the preauricular region (the area over, in front of and adjacent to the tragus) for skin tags, fleshy appendages, and pits. Pits (usually pinpoint indentations) are commonly found on the helix or just anterior to the point at which the helix attaches to the head or in front of the auricle but may be found almost anywhere on the auricle. A preauricular pit may be a blind pocket or may communicate with the internal ear or brain, leaving the infant vulnerable to infections. A pit should never be probed to determine if it is blind. Rather, spread the skin to the sides and use a magnifying glass to see if a bottom to the pit can be found. A pit that is truly blind poses no problem unless it fills with debris and becomes infected. Tags and pits may be associated with kidney disorders or hearing loss. Rarely, multiple skin tags extend in a line to the mouth; these may reflect other craniofacial defects. Palpate the auricle and around the ear for any hardened areas, swelling, masses or tenderness. A Darwin tubercle is a small fleshy nodule on the upper helix; it is a normal variation (Fletcher, 1998).

Ear canal: The newborn ear canal is extremely short, small, sensitive and likely to be filled with vernix and amniotic debris. All this makes otoscope examination of the newborn ear canal difficult or impossible right after birth. Inspect the canal with a penlight to assess presence, size, angle and patency, as far as it is possible to do so. Bleeding from the ear canal is associated with basilar skull fracture. Be sure this isn't maternal blood from the birth by gently cleaning the blood away from the outer canal with a moistened cotton swab to see if you can tell if it is coming from within the ear (do not push the swab down into the ear canal; this could be especially dangerous if a fracture is present).

Infant hearing may be assessed during the course of your immediate postpartum watch. The infant with normal hearing will startle, cry, alert or turn his gaze toward a loud noise or his mother's voice. Infants are especially responsive to high pitched vocalizations. Hearing assessment must be done carefully, since other stimuli may cause the baby to behave as if he can hear when, in fact, he cannot. Be sure to eliminate drafts, lights, sound vibrations and extraneous motions that may attract the baby's sight, and perform the test only when the baby is quietly alert. All babies, especially those with small or misshapen ears, should be assessed for hearing loss at a later date (Tappero & Honeyfield, 2003).

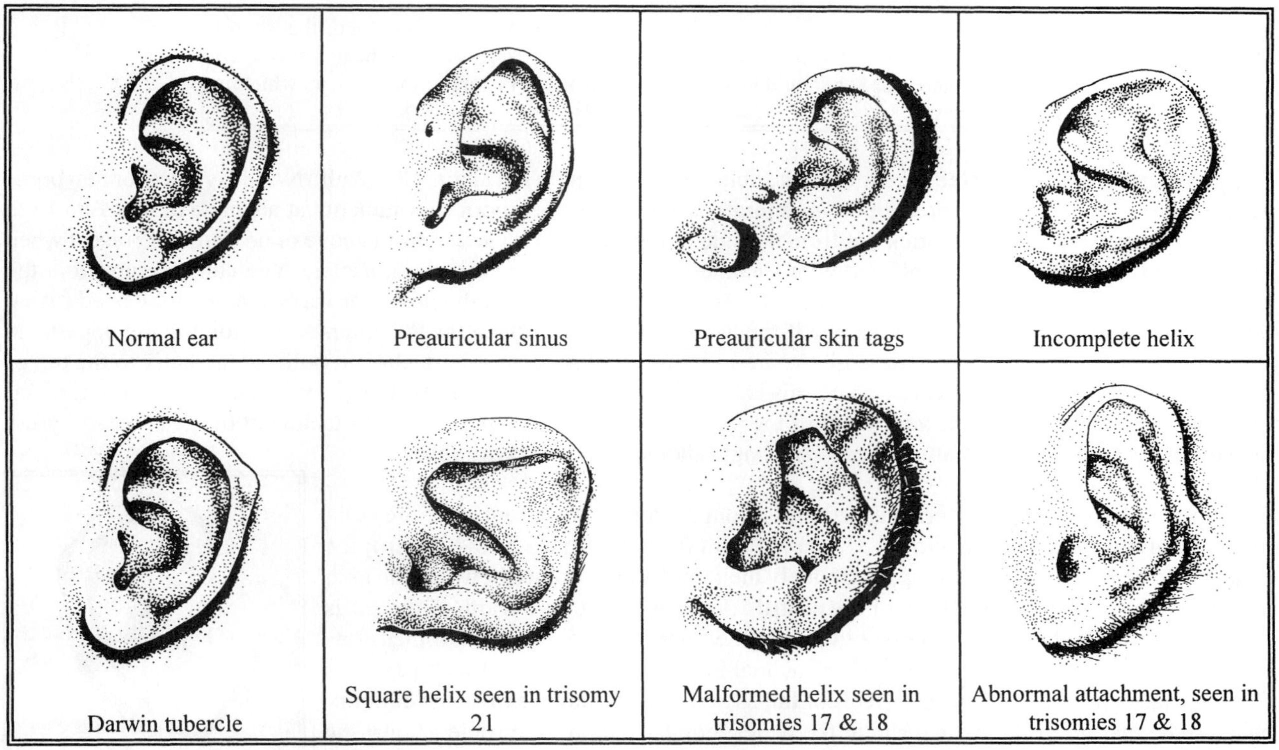

Normal ear | Preauricular sinus | Preauricular skin tags | Incomplete helix

Darwin tubercle | Square helix seen in trisomy 21 | Malformed helix seen in trisomies 17 & 18 | Abnormal attachment, seen in trisomies 17 & 18

Ear rotation: The longitudinal axis of the ear is normally rotated backward about 17 to 22° (range is 10 to 30°) in relationship to the vertical axis of the skull. An angle greater than 22° indicates posterior rotation. Moulding may cause the ears to appear more posteriorly rotated than they are. If the ears seem abnormal in any way, assess ear rotation by measuring the angle between the longitudinal axis of the ear and the vertical axis of the head.

Vertical axis of the head: First, establish a horizontal plane by extending a line connecting the inner canthi of the eyes around the head posteriorly to the occiput. This can be more easily done by using a clear plastic flexible ruler and bending it around the side of the head. The vertical axis of the head, the baseline, is perpendicular to this line. When moulding is present, a good estimate of the vertical axis of the head can be obtained by extending a vertical line that follows the coronal suture straight down.

Longitudinal axis of the ear: This is the straight line that passes from the top border of the helix to the lowermost border of the earlobe.

Align the straight edge of your protractor with the vertical axis of the head, with the curved edge to the back of the head. Keeping the protractor vertical, place the zero line along the straight edge over the lowermost tip of the earlobe. Extend a line from this point to the upper attachment of the ear and read the angle.

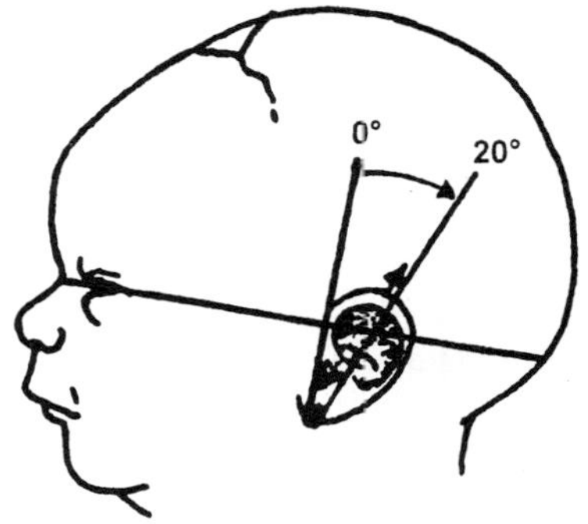

Ear rotation: arrow between the angle range indicates where this ear should be measured, which is about 19.5°

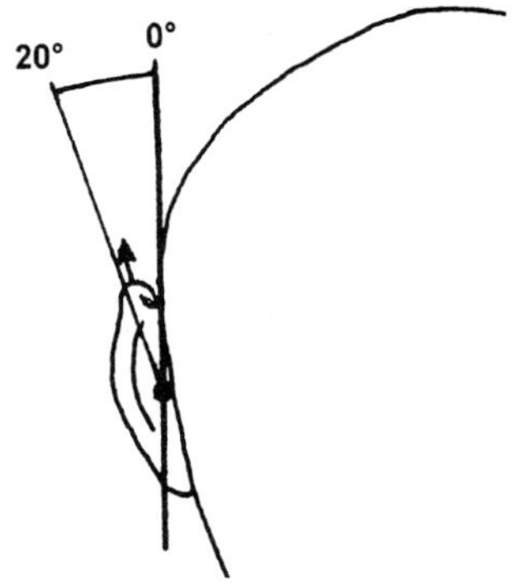

Ear protrusion from behind: this shows the 20° arc; arrow indicates where to measure the angle for this ear: which is about 17°

Ear protrusion: The upper free border of the auricle is normally quite flat against the skull. Normal values for newborns have not been formally established, but it is generally accepted that newborn ears stick out at an angle of less than 15 to 20°. Prominent ears (those that stick out from the side of the head when viewed from above or behind) are present when this angle exceeds 20° and is associated with weakness of the posterior auricular muscles. You can measure from the back of the baby's head by lining up the straight edge of a protractor with the posterior vertical axis of the head (using the sagittal suture to create a reference line if the head is moulded). Place the 90° intersection point at the uppermost attachment point of the helix and measure the angle from the most posterior attachment point of the helix to the top of the free border of the helix. A variation on this is to look down on the head from above. Hold the protractor horizontal to the top of the head, place the zero point of the protractor above the upper point of attachment of the helix and press the straight edge against the baby's head. The angle should now be easy to read.

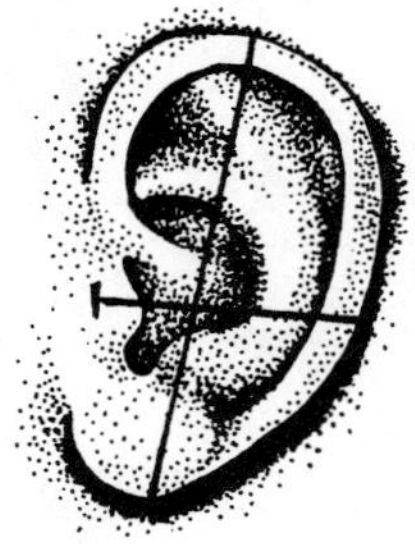

Where to measure ear size.

Ear size: The length of the external ear extends from the top of the outer rim of the helix to the tip of the ear lobe. It averages 3.75 cm at term (ranging from 3.5 to 4.25 cm); the ears should be symmetrical. It is approximately the same as the distance between the arch of the eyebrow and the lateral base of the nostril. At birth, the normal width of the ear is about two-thirds its length. Measure both ears in their horizontal and vertical dimensions if they appear to be too large, too small or unequal in size. The horizontal width extends from the anterior base of the tragus (feel for the edge of the cartilage) across the auditory canal to the margin of the helical rim at the widest point. Flatten the auricle against the head before measuring if it protrudes or is cupped (found with weakness in all three external auricular muscles). If the rim is unfolded because of intrauterine pressure, form the natural curve at the rim and measure from its border. A cup ear is generally smaller than average and appears to be gathered up around the border of the helix as though a draw string were in the edge, causing the entire pinna to be cupped; this baby should be evaluated for genetic disorders and hearing.

Ear position: This refers to the placement of the ears on the side of the head. Asymmetrical moulding can cause one ear to appear more anteriorly placed than its mate. Low-set ears are associated with a variety of congenital defects. To assess the baby for low-set ears, examine the ears from the front, with the baby's head held erect in the midline with her eyes facing forward. Assess ear symmetry in the vertical position by comparing the position of the tragi.

Using a clear, flexible plastic ruler or one arm of a gyrometer (use the edge of a strip of paper if you have nothing else), line up the inner canthi of the eyes to establish a horizontal baseline and extend the line posteriorly toward the ear by bending your measuring device to follow around the side of the head. The uppermost attachment point of the auricle should be at or above that line, with between 10 to 30% of the unattached auricle projecting above this level as well.

Assessment of ear position is tricky, and minor departures from appropriate technique can result in major errors. Assessing the height of each ear in relationship to the inner corners (canthi) of the eyes helps prevent an inaccurate measurement. If the outer canthi are used as landmarks but are slanted upward, for example, the ears may appear to be low-set when they are not. Likewise, a downward slant to the eyes may lead to the false impression that the ears are normally placed when they are not. When the attachment of the external ears is posteriorly rotated, this can create the illusion that the ears are low-set when they actually are not. The ears may also appear low-set if the head is extended. The relation of the vertex to the chin and shoulder in the newborn can also result in a misdiagnosis of low-set ears when examined from the side. The ears may also appear to be low-set if the head is an unusual size or shape, if the helix is poorly formed, if the baby's jaw or nose is quite small, if the midfacial structures are poorly developed, if the eyebrows are positioned too high or if the forehead is high. If the ear positioning is slightly off and the head is quite moulded, reassess their position at a postpartum visit after the moulding has resolved.

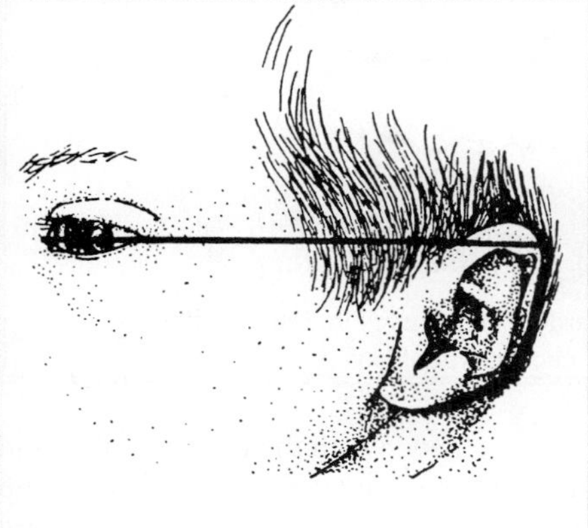
Normally placed ear

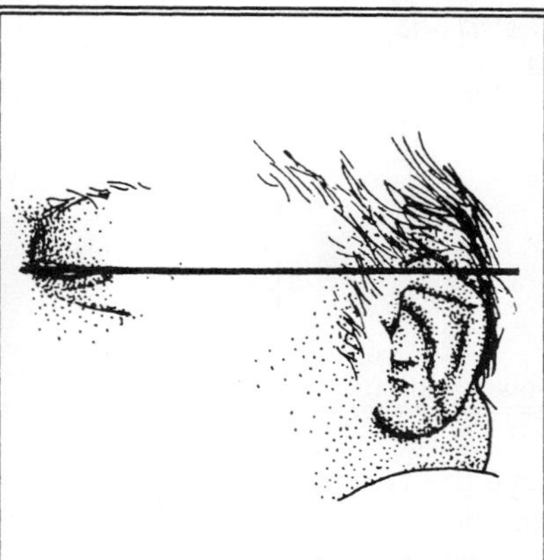
This ear appears low-set because the helix is twisted.

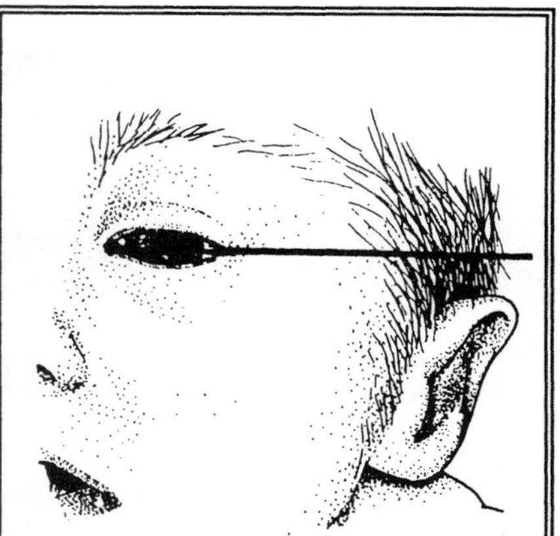
Truly low-set ear

Eyes: Observe the placement of the eyes in the face. Are they deeply set or prominent? Does the eye seem too large or too small for its socket (orbit)? Exophthalmos (protrusion of the eyeball, sometimes with lid retraction) is seen with some craniofacial deformities involving shallow orbits, hyperthyroidism and congenital glaucoma. Marked moulding with depression of the forehead can make the eyes appear to protrude, unless their position in relation to the cheekbones is considered. If the size of the eyes is unequal, try to determine which eye is most normal. Any distinct variations from normal in the relationship of the eyes to the face should lead to a careful search for other problems. For example, abnormal placement or small eye openings should alert you to the possibility of a syndrome or chromosomal abnormality. The corners of the mouth are usually aligned vertically with the inner border of the irises (Scanlon et al., 1979).

Many of the following assessments are best performed when the baby's eyes are open. Talk to the baby and divert hin with bright lights. This may be sufficient to encourage opening of the eyes. If not, hold the baby upright at eye level by supporting him under the arms and behind his head and gently rock his entire body toward and away from you. This triggers the vestibular (also know as the vertical doll's eye) reflex, which should cause him to open his eyes at least for a moment or two. If this doesn't work, look straight down into the supine baby's face while he is awake and alert. The eyes should move symmetrically and the baby should be able to focus on your face for at least a moment or two. A fixed squint or persistent nystagmus (involuntary rhythmic oscillation of the eyeballs, either pendular or with a slow-and-fast component) is always abnormal and requires follow-up (Tappero & Honeyfield, 2003).

Eyebrows and lashes: The eyebrows normally extend above the eye in a curve approximately the length of the palpebral fissure. They do not meet over the nose or flare in the midline, nor should the arch be noticeably elevated. The eyebrows are not always distinct in babies and may be sparse, especially in infants who are early or light skinned. Babies with dark facial hair may appear to have heavy eyebrows. Normal eyelashes are soft, sparse and continuously distributed across the eyelid in a single layer, with a slight upward curve. They may also be lightly pigmented. Eyebrows that meet at the glabella and abnormally long or tangled eyelashes are associated with some congenital syndromes, most notably Cornelia de Lange syndrome (Fletcher, 1998).

Slant of the eyes: Note the slant of the palpebral fissure (eye opening). The horizontal positioning of the eye fissures in the face reflects midface formation and is primarily related to race. Wait until the baby has her eyes open, is relaxed and is not crying, then draw a horizontal baseline from one inner canthus to the other and extend it horizontally to the sides of the head. Hold a clear protractor up to the baby's face, aligning the zero line with the inner canthi. (There is a more accurate but complex way to establish a baseline; this will do for screening.) Draw another line connecting the inner and outer canthi of each eye. If the inner-outer canthus line is oblique, with its outer end more than 2 mm higher than the outer end of the baseline, the slant is upward. The upper range of normal for an upward slant is less than 7°. If the canthus line falls more than 2 mm below the baseline, the slant is downward. Unequal or pronounced slanting is typically associated with a variety of syndromes, especially if the slant is below the horizontal. Be sure the eyes are open, as the degree of slant can change significantly if the eyes are closed (Fletcher, 1998).

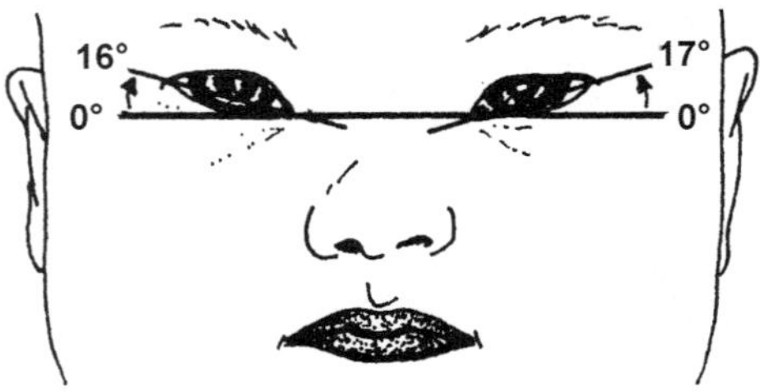

Upwardly slanted eyes in a baby with Down syndrome

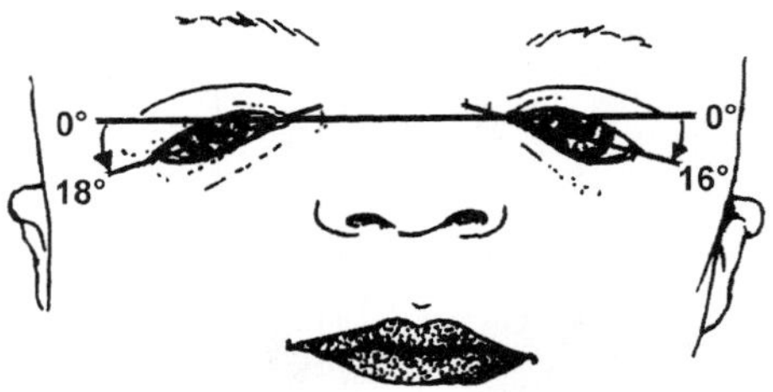

Downwardly slanted eyes in a baby with Treacher-Collins syndrome

Palpebral fissure length: This is measured from the inner to the outer canthus of each eye when the eyes are open and the baby is calm. There is wide racial variation (see chart below). The length for each eye may normally differ by up to 1 mm, but the normal width roughly equals the distance between the inner canthi. Short palpebral fissures are associated with many disorders, one of the most common being fetal alcohol syndrome (Fletcher, 1998).

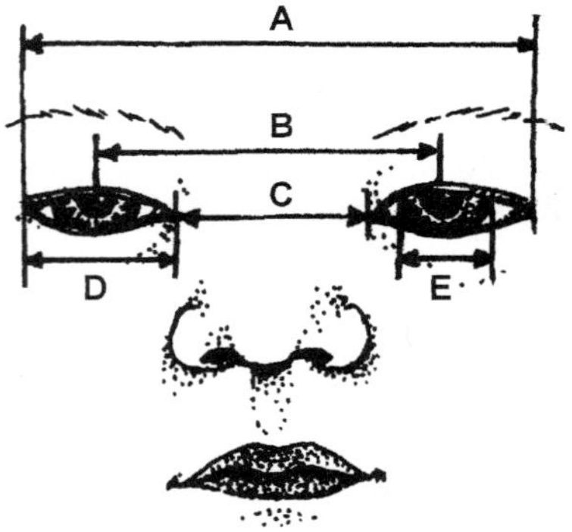

Eye Measurement	Normal Values at Term
A. Outer canthal distance	Palpebral fissure × 3
B. Interpupillary distance	33 to 46 mm
C. Inner canthal distance	16 to 24 mm
Anteroposterior diameter of orbit	16.5 to 17 mm
Palpebral area (eye open)	18 × 12 mm
D. Palpebral fissure length:	
African	17.8 to 22.2 mm
Asian	17.7 to 21.1 mm
Caucasian	17.2 to 19.8 mm
Hispanic	17.5 to 21.5 mm
E. Cornea (iris) diameter	9.5 to 10.5 mm
Eye slant: Upward	< 7°
Eye slant: Downward	None to < 2 mm
Undilated pupil diameter	1.8 to 4 mm
Dilated pupil diameter	5.4 mm

Vision: A newborn with normal vision will follow with his eyes and attend visually to things that are of interest, such as his mother's face. The newborn focus distance is about 7.5 in (19 cm) or about the distance from the eye to the breast. Assessing vision is done most easily with a quiet, alert baby, but a startle response to a bright light flash through closed eyelids even with the baby asleep indicates intact optic pathways.

Eyelids: Visually inspect the eyelids while the baby is quiet and alert, looking for ptosis (drooping of upper lid), edema (common after birth) or signs of trauma, such as bruising. The border of the upper lid should form an arch above the midpoint of the pupil when the eyes are open in a neutral position. Inspect the edges of the lids; they should be smooth with no clefting. Stork bite vascular stains are frequently found over the eyelid and are benign. Malformation of the eyelids is rare, but coloboma, a defect in closure of a portion of the lid or eye, is sometimes seen, presenting as a "bite" out of the margin of the lid. Rarely, the border of one or both lids may be flipped back on itself (ectropion), revealing the conjunctiva and presenting an alarming appearance with a oval, red-orange-colored membranous pouch of tissue occluding the eye. This should be evaluated by an neonatal specialist, but if this is all it is, it is usually easy to correct. An orbital encephalocele can present a similar appearance and must be ruled out (Fletcher, 1998).

More frequently, eye anomalies include an oddly shaped pupil or partial or complete fusion of an otherwise normal eyelid opening. To check for this, see if you can get the baby to open her eyes. If not, place a fingerpad above and below the lids and gently try to part them, looking for separation of the fissure. Do not try to pry them apart.

There is no significant amount of tear formation until the baby is 2 to 3 months old. Tearing that is not an immediate response to a chemical irritant (such as silver nitrate) is abnormal and may be due to excess tear production or the inability to clear the tears. Disorders of the nasolacrimal drainage system are likely causes (particularly blockage), but possible infection or glaucoma must also be considered. Excess tearing presents with a moist eye or matting after sleep.

The nasolacrimal glands have ducts that should be visible near the inner corners of the upper and lower lids. Placing the tip of your fingerpad adjacent to the inner canthus on one side, gently press inside the bridge of the nose. First, stroke upward to remove stagnant material; then stroke downward over the same area with firm pressure, stopping at the nasal bone. These ducts are often not fully patent until 5 to 7 months of age, and purulent or mucoid drainage is common. If material is expelled, an obstruction probably exists in the nasal communication of this drainage system, and the massage should be continued postpartum (Scanlon et al., 1979).

Palpate the upper lid to assess the size of the orbits as well as for swelling or masses while the eyes are closed. A blue gray cystic swelling about 1 cm in diameter may form just beneath the inner canthus if the nasolacrimal ducts are quite obstructed. In the uncommon event that the swollen nasolacrimal gland is prolapsed inside the nasal passage, it may cause respiratory distress. Nothing may be visible outside the nose, but the swelling will be apparent if the inside of the nostril is checked at the level of the internal duct on the outermost turbinate.

Another lacrimal gland is located along the outer half of the upper lid. Swelling between the inner corner of the eye and the bridge of the nose (dacryocystocele) results if one or both of its ducts are obstructed. This may sometimes be mistaken for a hemangioma. It usually occurs on only one side, most often in girls. However, more rarely it may be mimicking a more serious condition. Large lesions, midline lesions and others that present with an unusual location or appearance, or those presenting in a baby with any unusual facial features, should be evaluated to rule out brain involvement. Differentiation of such lesions is outlined in the following chart (Fletcher, 1998).

Cause of Swelling	Color of Skin Overlying the Swelling	Palpation	Transilluminates?
Obstructed lacrimal gland	Blue gray to purplish	Tense, firm	Yes
Encephalocele	Blue or gray	Soft, may have a pulse	Yes, if fluid-filled only
Hemangioma	Violet	Compressible	No

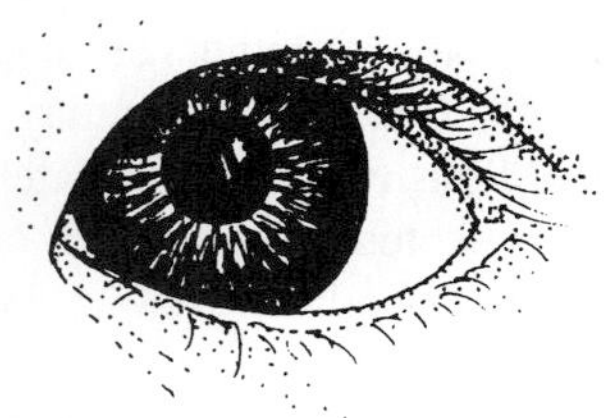

Epicanthal fold of upper lid over inner canthus

Epicanthal folds: An epicanthal fold is a crescent-shaped fold of skin that runs vertically between the eyelids over the inner canthus and the lacrimal caruncle. The fold can be most prominent in the upper eyelid, lower eyelid or equally distributed between the upper and lower lids. It can begin at the eyebrow, at the skin of the upper lid or at the tarsal (eyelid) fold. These folds result from flattening of the bridge of the nose and may resolve if the nose becomes more prominent with growth. They are normal in Asian infants. Epicanthal folds accompanying a Mongolian slant are associated with Down syndrome. Epicanthal folds that cover the inner canthi can interfere with the assessment of eye spacing because they prevent visualization of the inner canthi, thus causing the eyes to appear widely set when they are not. Likewise, the presence of epicanthal folds can cause closely spaced eyes to appear normally spaced. Unilateral folding may occur when the shape of the head is obliquely distorted, although it does not necessarily indicate the side of the skull that is flattened.

Conjunctivae: The mucous membranes lining the inner surface of the eyelids, the conjunctivae, may appear highly vascular and swollen in the first days of life. In general, however, they should be deep pink and healthy, with no discharge, jaundice or prominent hemorrhages. Infectious conjunctivitis is rarely noted at birth; when it is, it presents with a purulent discharge that can be cultured (Scanlon et al., 1979).

Sclerae (whites of the eyes): The sclera should be white to bluish white. A yellow tinge indicates an elevated bilirubin level. A distinctly blue coloration, indicating the sclerae are thin, is seen with preterm babies and with connective tissue disorders such as cutis laxa and osteogenesis imperfecta, a severe skeletal disorder. The sclerae should not be persistently visible above the irises. Called the "sunset sign," this is often due to intracranial pressure from hydrocephalus producing lid retraction and a downward gaze. Unusually large eye orbs can be caused by congenital glaucoma.

The eyes may be bloodshot due to pressure from birth, and hemorrhages may also commonly occur around the iris after normal birth. Conjunctival or subconjunctival hemorrhage results from rupture of a capillary of the mucous membrane that lines the eyelids and bleeds over into the eyeball. This is seen as a bright red, often crescent-shaped area on the white of the eye near the iris and usually disappears within a week to ten days. Note that any hemorrhaging of the eyes, including any apparently benign bruises near the eye, may on rare occasions be associated with bleeding inside the orbit, which can lead to blindness. Advise parents to have the baby seen by a pediatric ophthalmologist at two months of age to rule this out. An appointment should be scheduled as soon as possible to ensure that the baby will be seen at the appropriate time. Vitamin K should be given to such babies (Scanlon et al., 1979).

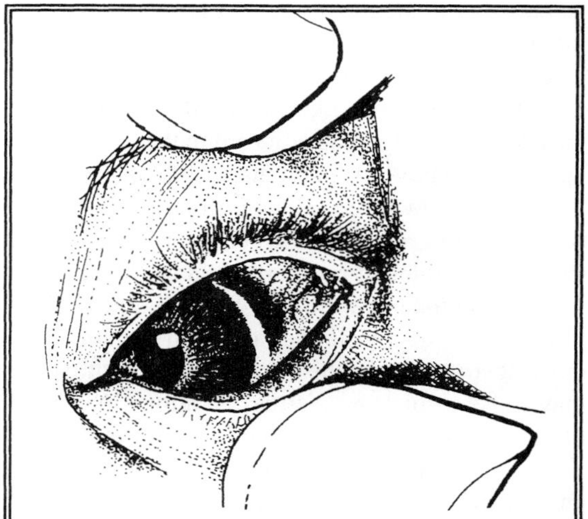

Opening the eye to reveal a typical crescent-shaped scleral hemorrhage at the outer border of the iris.

Eye spacing: Eye spacing is another important consideration. The distance between the outer canthi should be divisible into equal thirds, with one normal palpebral fissure length fitting between the inner canthi. This method of measuring works if the canthi are not deviated downward and there are no epicanthal folds. If you have questions regarding eye spacing, assessment should be done by measuring the interpupillary distance. Hypertelorism (wide spacing of the eyes) occurs when the interpupillary distance is increased and is a common finding in many congenital syndromes. The eyes may only appear to be widely spaced if the inner canthi are laterally displaced or if epicanthic folds are present. In this case, a normal interpupillary distance will be found (telecanthus). In hypotelorism, the interpupillary distance is decreased; this is seen exclusively in infants with trisomy 13 or holoprosencephaly.

Eye movement: Watch the baby to see how and if he uses his eyes when he is definitely awake and alert. Normal eye movement depends on normally developed ocular muscles and is generally prompted by the ability to see. At birth, the baby usually maintains a horizontal visual field (looking straight ahead) with rotation to the left or right. The eyes move in conjugate (that is, together) in a coordinated fashion. Vertical gaze movements do not appear until 4 to 6 weeks of age in term babies. Limited motion may be related to a palsy of some sort (Fletcher, 1998).

Corneal light reflex: Stimulate simultaneous fixation of the baby's vision on a penlight; note the location of the reflected light on each cornea. If the reflections are in the same place on each cornea, the vision is conjugate and there should be no dislocation of the lens. While a positive test is reassuring at birth, lack of this response may be normal up to 8 weeks of age.

Fixing and maintaining a gaze: Hold the baby out about a foot from you so his eyes are level with your gaze. If the baby continues to look at you after blinking, he is maintaining his gaze. Observe to see if he turns his gaze toward a light source such as a window.

Doll's-eye maneuver: The "doll's-eye maneuver" consists of fixing the position of the head in the midline and then gently rotating the baby from side to side and watching to see if the eyes deviate away from the direction of rotation (i.e., if the head is turned to the right, the eyes should track to the left). If the eyes remain fixed or move in the same direction as the head, brain or nerve dysfunction may be present.

Strabismus occurs due to muscular incoordination and gives the appearance of crossed eyes. Symmetrical eye movement in the newborn is intermittent; therefore, a cross-eyed appearance that comes and goes is commonly noted. Pseudostrabismus, appears when the eyes are at rest, is associated with a flat nasal bridge or epicanthal folds and usually resolves by 1 year of age. Most other abnormal eye movements are highly associated with a number of serious neurologic disorders and are unlikely to appear without other signs of central nervous system compromise. Any abnormality of the eyes should be evaluated by an eye specialist in the day or two following birth, as uncorrected eye disorders can have a profound affect of the development of normal sight (Fletcher, 1998). (Abnormal eye movements are discussed further in the subchapter entitled "Evaluating the Newborn with Suspected Neurological Compromise.")

Irises, pupils, corneae and funduses: The iris may be dark gray, blue, or brown. A red iris lacks pigmentation, the color being due to underlying blood vessels. This may be seen in albino babies (along with abnormally light hair, if the family is dark skinned) or in a form of albinism that is limited to the eyes. A baby whose irises are different colors or with more than one color in the same eye (heterochromia) may later develop a renal neoplasia. Brushfield spots, white streaks and spots scattered throughout the iris, may be a normal variant, although they are also associated with Down syndrome.

The iris should form a complete, uniform ring around a centrally located, round, black pupil. A coloboma is any cleft-shaped fissure in the eye area. An irregularly shaped iris or pupil is frequently associated with abnormalities of other organ systems, although if limited to the iris, it is not associated with visual difficulty (Fletcher, 1998).

Although the newborn reaction to light is relatively immature, the pupils should be equal in size and react identically to light. Note that the pupillary light reflex is entirely subcortical and its presence does not rule out blindness. Check pupillary response by darkening the room and bringing a bright, focused light source into the baby's peripheral vision (from the side). If there is no response and the pupils are naturally dilated, use a brighter light and repeat the test. Repeat a third time to confirm that any change in pupil size is in response to light and not merely random. A small pupil in one eye and a droopy upper lid (ptosis) suggest a lesion of the cervical sympathetic nerves. If this is the cause, the baby will not sweat on that side of the face. A gray or white pupil or lack of a red reflex (see below) may indicate that cataracts are present, although cataracts, unless they are well developed, can be difficult to identify without an ophthalmoscope (and lots of experience). Use an ophthalmoscope lens with the diopter set at +1 to inspect for cataracts by holding the otoscope light 6 to 8 in from the eye. A normal optical lens transmits a clear red color back to the examiner: this is the red retinal reflex. When cataracts are present, the red reflex is interrupted by black opaque areas. Some cataracts present with an amber discoloration of the lens, which may be present at birth in babies with galactosemia. Note that the pupil size determines the amount of the lens you can examine. Therefore, without the use of a dilating medication in the baby's eyes, you may not be able to fully confirm the presence or absence of cataracts with this exam (Scanlon et al., 1979).

The cornea is inspected for clarity using a pinpoint source of bright light, such as an otoscope. Cast the light at an oblique angle across the eye from the temporal side. The normal cornea is smooth, shiny and glossy, although all babies may display a slight haziness for the first few days of life. Note any asymmetric, irregular or dense cloudiness. Measure the cornea if there is excessive tearing or photophobia in the absence of conjunctivitis. A corneal diameter of 12 to 13 mm raises the possibility of congenital glaucoma (Scanlon et al., 1979).

Ophthalmic exam: Try to perform a quick ophthalmic exam. Adjust the ophthalmoscope to obtain a round, white beam of light. Direct the light into the baby's pupil from a distance of about 6 inches to assess equality of size, pupillary reflex (contraction with bright light) and red retinal reflex. The pupils should be equal and reactive to light. If the baby resists this exam, it can wait until a day or two after birth or until the baby is seen by a pediatrician. A complete ophthalmic exam requires dilation of the pupils and should be performed by a eye specialist. It is not required unless eye abnormalities are suspected (Scanlon et al., 1979).

The fundus is best examined through a dilated pupil. However, you may be able to assess the retina without dilation if you are skilled and the baby is unusually cooperative. Dim the room lights to maximally dilate the pupil. This will also encourage the baby to keep her eyes open. Adjust the ophthalmoscope diopter lens between +1 and +3. Direct the light through the pupil. Bright light elicits a clear orange-red color when it hits the retina; this is somewhat paler in babies-of-color. The retina should look transparent and glistening with no demarcated pigmented or depigmented areas, and should appear decreasingly vascular as the temporal periphery is approached. The blood vessels should not be twisted or appear connected. The neonatal fundus appears flat and is usually reddish pink; however, it may also have a pale greyish tinge and appear relatively streaky, especially under the edges. The optic nerve may appear pale, but its margins should be sharp. The macula is often indistinct if the baby is preterm, but the full-term macula is reddish brown. It is located 1.5 disc diameters to the temporal side of the disc. About 3% of term infants have remnants of the hyaloid artery; these appear as thin strands extending from the retina to the lens. Isolated retinal hemorrhages are commonly seen in full-term babies and are not significant (Scanlon et al., 1979).

Any suspected or identified abnormalities of the lens, fundus or cornea should be considered an optic emergency. Although the baby need not be taken immediately to the hospital for this reason alone, plans should immediately be put in place for an eye exam by an neonatal ophthalmologist in the first day to two of life. If correctable problems are not dealt with in the first 6 weeks, blindness can result.

Nose: Observe the nose for placement, number of nostrils, fistulae, swellings and deviations from the midline. The newborn's nose is normally symmetrical and relatively flat in comparison to older children. Abnormal findings include small or otherwise unusual nares, extreme thinness or a flat, wide or pronounced bridge, any of which may be associated with a variety of congential syndromes.

Normal respiratory variations: There is often no visible movement of the nose with normal breathing. However, slight movement around the openings of the nostrils may be seen in normal newborns without additional signs of respiratory distress for the first few days of life; be sure the baby is warm and monitor to see if this minor flaring resolves or if other signs of distress become apparent. If such slight flaring persists and does not increase and no other signs of distress are found, this is a normal variation. Intermittent occasional sneezing is also common and normal. It is often because of slight swelling of the nasal passages in the first few days of life. Stuffiness may occur as the baby discharges mucus from birth, which may lead to snorting, flaring and fussing or crying if the nasal passages are obstructed. Colostrum will help the baby bring up and get rid of mucus in the respiratory passages. Normal nasal secretions are clear and minimal. Persistent nasal stuffiness is associated with maternal drug use. "Snuffles," which presents as a copious mucopurulent or bloody discharge, is associated with congenital syphilis and is highly infectious.

Patency of nostrils: Nasal patency is assessed by observing the baby's breathing. Infants are preferential nose breathers, primarily because their relatively large tongues touch their palates when at rest, making mouth breathing difficult. Therefore, blockage of both nostrils for any reason may result in cyanosis at rest and improved color during crying or mouth breathing. Obstruction may also be due to the presence of swelling, a mass or secretions. It is possible for one or both nostrils to be blocked completely or to have a degree of stenosis (narrowing). When an obstruction is suspected, there are a number of techniques that can be used to assess both the presence and degree of blockage. You can hold a cold metal spoon or safety-edge mirror beneath the nostrils and look for two areas of mist formation, indicative of air movement. The relative size of each area of mist will help determine if air passage is equal on both sides. You may also hold a string in front of each nostril to try and see air movement. Alternatively, you can use your fingerpad to press against the side of one nostril to see if the baby can continue to breathe out of the uncompressed side or if he must open his mouth to breathe. Then, apply pressure to the other nostril. You can also use the bell of an infant stethoscope to listen over each nostril to detect poor air flow or any other respiratory sounds. Stenosis of the nostril produces a high-pitched or whistling sound. As a last resort, a soft #5 French catheter can be passed through both nostrils to assess patency by first lifting the tip of the nose and then directing the tip of the tube toward the occiput. However, this may further irritate the sensitive lining of the nose and thus increase breathing difficulty.

External features: The surface of the nose should be inspected for normal contours. Abnormalities may include underdevelopment of the nares, or extreme thinness, depression, widening or prominence of the nasal bridge, all of which are associated with a variety of congential syndromes.

Nares: Lift the tip of the nose to visually examine the septum, the nasal membranes and the turbinates. The nasal mucosa should be pink and moist, without pallor, cyanosis or other discoloration. Normal secretions are thin, clear and scanty.

Nasal base: The base of the nose (the area between the inner canthi of the eyes) should be measured. The normal value in term infants is 2.5 cm or less or the length of one palpebral fissure (Fletcher, 1998).

Nasal length: Length is assessed by measuring in the midline from the deepest depression at the root of the nose between the eyebrows to the deepest concavity at the base of the columella; the range at term is from 20 to 32 mm (see next page for an illustration of nasal measurements) (Fletcher, 1998).

Interalar distance: The width of the nose is usually assessed visually in relationship to other facial features. It is measured from the widest side of one alar to the widest side of the other. The width varies by race, ranging from 18 to 24 mm (Fletcher, 1998).

Columella (kau-loo-MEL-ah) length: The columella is the fleshy, skin-covered lower border of the nasal septum that projects out at a 90° angle above the philtrum at the base of the nose. It is visually assessed. Measuring is done along the bottom from its attachment point above the philtrum to the level of the anterior border of each nostril. If it is curved, the tape is moulded along its length to include the curved portion. Length is related to birthweight and gestational age but will be decreased in conditions involving severe hypoplasia of the midline of the face. Normal values have not been established for newborns, so you must evaluate its size in relationship to other facial features (Fletcher, 1998).

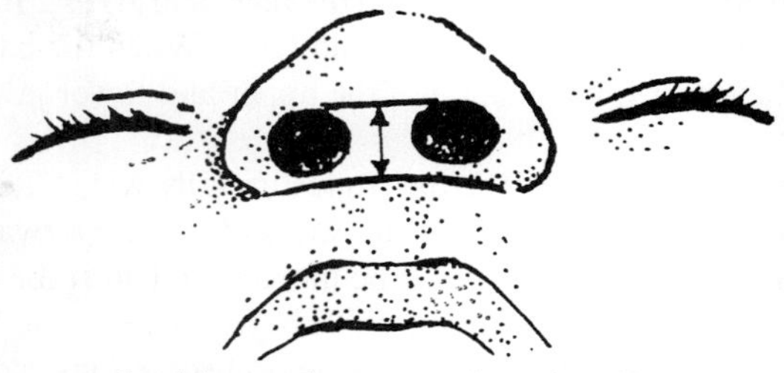
Looking up the nose at the columella

Nasal deformities: Nasal deformation is addressed by Graham (1988) and is common in newborns at birth and usually resolves along with other forms of moulding. Congenital hypoplasia (underdevelopment) may be present if the nares are asymmetrical or extremely flat. Deviation of the nasal septum, tip of the nose or the alar to one side may be a temporary result of prenatal positioning or may be caused by a dislocated septum. Nasal "fractures" are usually dislocations of the cartilaginous portion of the nose, causing it to be flattened or displaced, often without swelling or bleeding. A dislocated nose cannot be easily moulded into a normal shape with the fingers. Obstruction of respiration with distress is common. Cranial adjustment should be the first type of therapy sought for these babies. Graham (1988) describes two ways to assess for dislocation:

1. Compress the tip of the nose. If the septum is dislocated, this maneuver will deviate the base further from the midline (a normal septum will curve laterally into the nostril opening but will not move at the base).
2. Push the tip of the nose toward the midline. If the septum does not easily return to upright and the nostril openings remain asymmetrical, the septum is dislocated and will require treatment.

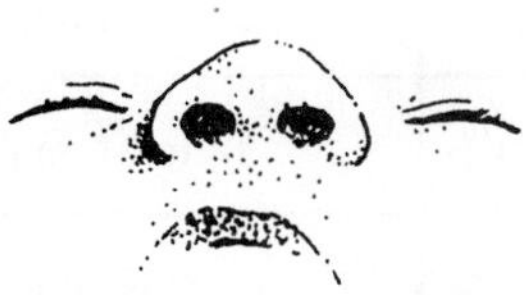
Normal nose

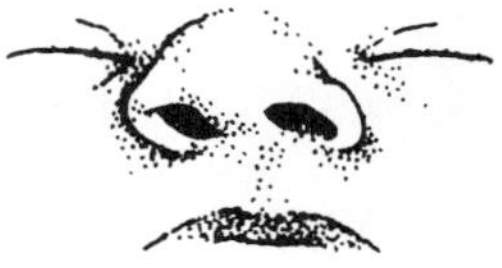
Septum deviated to the right and asymmetrical nostrils

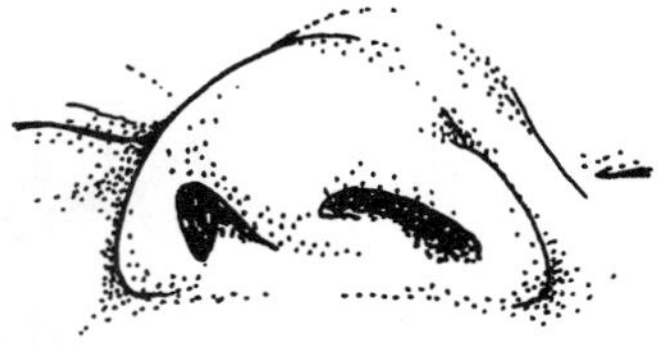
Septum deviated to the right.

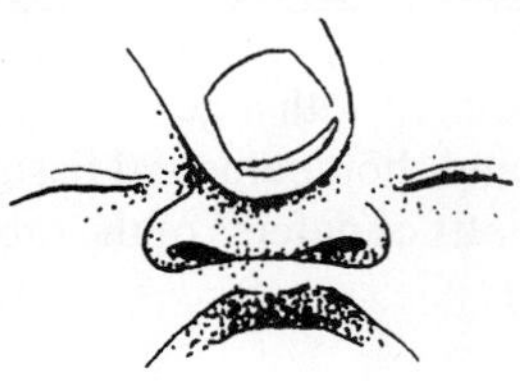
Pushing down on the tip of a normal nose causes the septum to flatten.

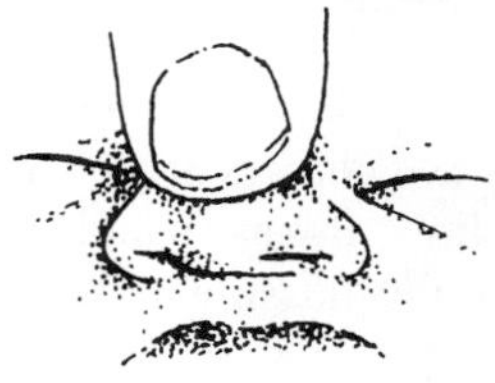
Pushing down on the tip does not correct the asymmetry

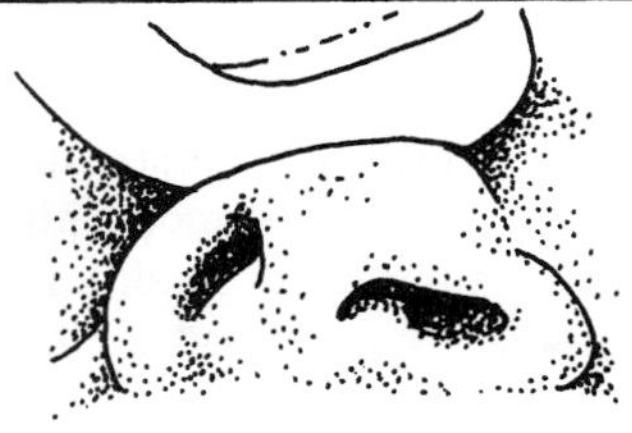
When the tip is pushed toward the midline, the asymmetry persists.

When released, the deviated septum will not return to normal. A dislocation may resolve by itself in the first 72 hours as other moulding dissipates. The cartilage can also be repositioned at the third day visit if this does not occur. Midline craniofacial defects often involve flattening or poor development of the nose, which, when severe enough, will result in upper airway obstruction.

Mouth: Examination of the mouth consists of close inspection and palpation of the lips, nasolabial fold and philtrum, frenula, gums, tongue, palate, oropharynx and jaw. Observe the shape of the mouth, lips and face when the baby is crying, or otherwise moving the face, and at rest. Assess the size and shape of each individual feature as well as how each relates to the entire mouth and face. When the baby is crying or yawning, look for symmetry of structures (especially the lower lip, the angle of the upper and lower jaws relative to each other, and the tongue).

Oral secretions: The mouth is normally wet. Clear to frothy white secretions are usually present in moderation during the minutes after birth as the baby clears her airways. Some babies have scanty secretions during the first few hours of life. Secretions may also be more abundant if the baby has swallowed a lot of fluids during birth and there is therefore a lot of fluid in the stomach. They may be stained with swallowed meconium or, rarely, maternal blood.

However, as a rule, notable oral secretions are not normal beyond the first few hours of life. They should never be constant and copious beyond the first few minutes of life. Some defects, such as esophageal atresia, result in the production of excessive amounts of white foamy mucus that does not diminish over time. Abnormal drooling is most commonly associated with upper gastrointestinal obstruction. More rarely, consistent drooling may be due to an isolated neuromuscular swallowing disorder, which is also associated with abnormal cranial nerve function.

To further evaluate the cause of drooling, insert a soft catheter into the mouth to the stomach. If you cannot confirm that it has reached the stomach (listen over the stomach with a stethoscope while air is forced into the tube with a syringe), an obstruction is likely. Esophageal atresia, which occurs by itself in only 10% of all affected babies, is most often found with a tracheoesophageal fistula (85% of cases). When a baby presents with copious and persistent drooling, assume there is an esophageal defect and withhold oral feedings until this can be ruled out. Transport soon after birth.

Fletcher (1998) points out that the production of very small bubbles of saliva that last only a second or two may be a tip-off that the baby has an immature level of surfactant, whereas long-lasting bubbles offer reassurance that the baby's surfactant levels are normal.

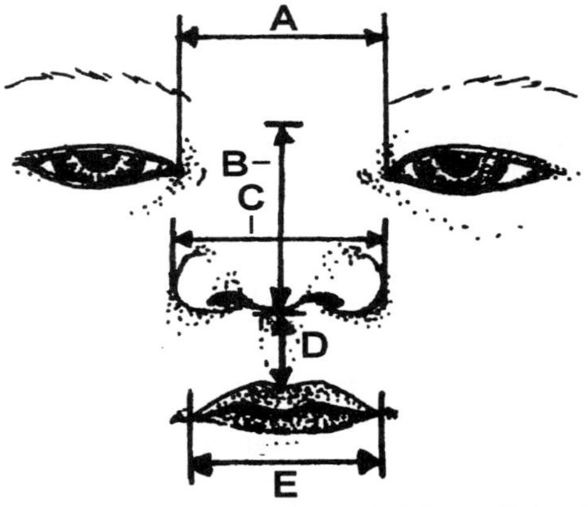

NOSE AND MOUTH MEASUREMENTS	NORMAL DIMENSIONS AT TERM
A. Width–nasal base	One palpebral fissure length (averages 25 mm)
B. Nasal length	20 to 32 mm
C. Interalar distance	18 to 24 mm
D. Mouth width	averages 20 mm
E. Philtrum length	8 to 13 mm

Size: Abnormal shape or size of the mouth opening, lips, philtrum or jaw may be associated with a genetic syndrome. A thin upper lip with a smooth philtrum, downturned corners of the mouth (fish mouth) and short palpebral fissures may be seen in fetal alcohol syndrome. A thin upper lip is also associated with submucous clefts or defects of the orbicularis oris muscle, a type of oral sphincter, often called the "kissing muscle" (Fletcher, 1998).

Shape: To evaluate the shape of the mouth, assess how well the lower jaw fits in relation to the upper jaw. It should open at equal angles on both sides. The shape of the mouth is influenced by fetal positioning, which may produce asymmetry at the angle of the jaw. Unequal opening of the mouth is also seen when a depressor anguli oris muscle is absent. These muscles are found at the lower corners of the mouth on either side. When absent, it mimics the appearance of a facial palsy except that the upper lip and the nasolabial fold appear normal, and there will be no difficulty with sucking. The angle of the lower lip feels thinner than normal on the side where the muscle is absent. If the face becomes asymmetrical with crying, the baby may have a facial nerve paralysis; this may not be detectable when she is calm. Such a palsy can cause the mouth to pull to the undamaged side during crying, asymmetry of the nasolabial folds, an inability to close the eye on the affected side and problems with sucking. A short philtrum, wide upper lip, and thick lower lip combine to create a carp-like mouth, a feature of several disorders.

Width (intercommisural distance): The width of the mouth from corner to corner averages 2 cm. The corners of the mouth at rest generally align with the nasal margin of the iris, which is assessed by dropping a line straight down from the inner edge of the baby's iris to the corner of the mouth on each side (Fletcher, 1998). A small mouth opening (microstomia) is associated with some trisomies, most frequently 18 and 21, and defects involving a small jaw. A large mouth (macrostomia) results when the oral opening fails to fuse properly during development; it may cause drooling and problems with nursing. It may be associated with poor development of the maxilla, mandible, and ear structures and is seen with Beta-d-glucuronidase deficiency (mucopolysaccharidase), a metabolic disorder (Scanlon et al., 1979).

Philtrum: The philtrum is the wide vertical groove spanning the midline nasolabial fold (space above the upper lip) and forms the cupid's bow at its base. Its length is measured from the base of the lower border of the nasal septum to the top of the border of the lip in the midline when the infant is quiet and not sucking. At term, it ranges from 8 to 13 mm. A long philtrum is often seen with a short nose; conversely, a short philtrum is often found with a long nose. The absence of a philtrum is seen with some disorders; poor development often occurs with fetal alcohol syndrome (Fletcher, 1998).

Lips: Assess the lips for shape, size and thickness, including the nasolabial fold (the space between the upper lip and the base of the nose). The lips are normally closed when the mouth is at rest. The upper and lower lips should be roughly the same size. A central calloused swelling in the midline, usually of the upper lip, is a sucking blister, sometimes present at birth. Shallow pits may develop in the corners of the mouth, but when otherwise located may be a sinus tract or subepithelial cleft. The lips and mucous membranes of a healthy infant are deep pink and free of lesions. Mild cyanosis around the mouth can be normal in the first hours of life, but this also occurs when the baby is chilled; make sure he is warm. Very rarely, one or a pair of fistulas are present on the lower lip in the midline, with tiny nipple-like protrusions. These occur more often in girls than in boys and can be associated with a cleft lip or palate.

The width and thickness of the lips are related to race, but extreme thickness is unusual in the newborn. Swelling without associated birth trauma often accompanies masses, commonly hemangioma or lymphangioma. Much more rarely, it results from the doubling of lip tissue during development. A double lip, occurring once in every 200 to 480 babies, exists when a transverse furrow forms in the lower lip during smiling, giving the appearance of two vermilion borders. Masses of tissue on either side of the midline create a dent in the center.

A cleft is a separation or space between parts that are normally joined, thus interrupting the continuity of the structure. Cleft or "split" lip usually develops as a notch or open vertical cleavage on one or both sides of the upper lip extending up from the peak of the cupid's bow along the philtrum ridge to the midpoint of the nasal opening. It may only involve part of the lip or extend completely into the nostril or through the upper jaw. More severe lip clefting is usually seen with cleft palate and may be a clue to midline central nervous system defects. When a cleft lip is found, examine the baby's lower lip and those of both parents for lip pits. Van der Woude syndrome is a genetic defect in which a parent may only have lip pits, but a child may have full expression with clefts of the lip or palate or both. Rarely (in less than 1% of cases), clefting occurs in the midline, which may extend from the center of the anterior gum and cupid's bow to the nose. Major forms of midline cleft lip are associated with widely spaced eyes and midline cerebral malformations, as well as other structural and some major chromosomal anomalies.

Jaws: The normal newborn mandible is slightly recessed, which helps the baby latch on and nurse. Sometimes what appears to be a small jaw is because of intrauterine moulding; this will self-correct or can be treated by a craniosacral therapist after birth. However, underdevelopment, or micrognathia, is a fairly frequent oral abnormality. Proper oral development requires tongue movement against an intact hard palate; when this does not occur, the lower jaw recedes. A small lower jaw leaves less room in the oral cavity, displacing the tongue backward into the pharynx, which causes the tongue to appear enlarged. Micrognathia can occur by itself but is usually associated with other problems, notably Pierre Robin syndrome (referred to as a sequence in some texts), which is also associated with a high-arched or cleft palate. The maxillary area may also be flattened in fetal alcohol syndrome.

Internal inspection: It is easiest to see inside the mouth when the baby is yawning or crying. If the baby is calm, press down gently on the chin to open the mouth. Hold the baby's head in the midline during your visual inspection to avoid misinterpreting an angled view for asymmetry. Inspect the gums and buccal mucosa (inside walls of the cheeks) for normal color, lesions and any structural abnormality.

Tongue: The newborn tongue is fairly smooth on all its surfaces. All the taste buds are present, but fewer of them are well developed in comparison to an adult. A whitish coating may be present if the baby has just nursed. Babies-of-color have a white coating more consistently. Note the size of the tongue, which should fit nicely inside the mouth when the baby is resting. Watch for symmetrical movement as well as protrusion forward and other general movements. Deviation to one side occurs with lower cranial nerve palsy.

The normal newborn tongue appears large, but true macroglossia is uncommon. If found, it may be congenital or may be acquired by overdevelopment of the tongue muscles. The tongue may appear to be enlarged when localized masses or cysts are present beneath it. This could be due to several types of cysts, tumors or obstruction of glandular ducts, and requires further evaluation. Congenital enlargement is found with Beckwith syndrome, Pompe disease, Down syndrome, hypothyroidism, mucopolysaccharidosis and several other disorders. A large tongue may block the airway. Underdevelopment or absence of the tongue is rare and almost always found with other anomalies.

Frenula: Look for a narrow, vertical membrane attaching the midline of the underside of the tongue to the floor of the mouth. It usually extends halfway between the root of the tongue and the tip, although its placement is widely variable. It may be thick or extend to the tip (tongue tie), but the tongue should still be mobile enough for the baby to suck. True limitation of movement sufficient to impair sucking or speech is uncommon. As long as the baby can stick his tongue out beyond his lips, no intervention is necessary, as the tongue will grow more rapidly than the frenulum and soon become freely mobile. If the frenulum does reach the tip of the tongue, it may be thick and produce a groove in the tip of the tongue, limiting movement and protrusion. The idea that cutting a tight frenulum is not necessary evolved in an era of bottle feeding. However, for some babies, nursing at the breast is so painful that they may refuse to suck at all. In such cases, cutting the tip of the frenulum may preserve the nursing relationship (Schlinger, 2003). Two more midline labial frenula may be found between the top lip and the gum and between the bottom lip and the adjacent gum. A thick frenulum of the upper lip is sometimes associated with dental or tongue abnormalities. Multiple or enlarged frenula are not normal and suggest the presence of a multisystem syndrome, especially one involving the skeletal system.

Gums: The newborn gums are smooth with a 1 mm serrated fringe of tissue firmly attached to the edges along either side. Look and palpate for teeth and Epstein's pearls (described later in this section). Check to see that the inner surface of the cheeks and lips are separate from the gums. The frenulum may extend from the superior midline of the inner, upper lip up and over the midline of the gum, creating a deep notch in the center of the gumline. Large gums with pronounced fringing along the top are seen in several disorders.

Teeth: Teeth are present in about 1 in every 2000 newborns. They usually appear at the position of the lower incisors and may either be supernumerary (extra or natal teeth) or prematurely erupted baby teeth; an X-ray can determine which. Palpate any cysts in the midline of the upper or lower jaw as these may contain partially erupted teeth (eruption cysts). These teeth usually erupt in the days following birth. Natal or supernumerary teeth most commonly appear in the lower jaw but may appear in the upper, especially in association with cleft lip or palate. These teeth are usually soft with no enamel and are poorly attached to the gum. They should either be watched closely to see when they fall out or be removed as soon as possible to prevent choking. Teeth that are firmly rooted or not completely erupted should be left alone. Teeth may interfere with nursing and lead to lacerations of the tongue or lip (not to mention mother's nipple!). Consultation with a pediatric dentist is advised (Scanlon et al., 1979).

Palate: The newborn palate is normally round and smooth with a small midline ridge (like a backbone). Visualize it with the help of a flashlight to detect pinhole defects. It should be complete and closed all the way back to the uvula, which usually appears as a single, midline, drop-shaped structure hanging from the posterior soft palate. A split or bifid uvula is found in 2% of the US population and is the most minor type of clefting defect. A narrow palate or one with a high arch may indicate lack of normal tongue motion against it. Also check for elevation and integrity of the soft palate when the mouth is spontaneously opened. To see what this should look like, say "ahhh' as you look inside your own mouth in a mirror. (Also palpate your soft palate with your finger while saying "ahhh.")

Cleft palate: An otherwise normal infant may have a cleft lip and palate, which occurs in 1 out of every

750 live births, with 60% occurring in boys. The incidence of isolated cleft palate that is unrelated to a syndrome is 1 in every 2000 births. Clefting of the palate can involve one or both sides or may occur in the midline only. Cleft palate that occurs with a cleft lip usually presents as a long, narrow opening. Isolated clefts of the palate appear as U- or V-shaped defects. U-shaped clefts occur when the tongue is displaced posteriorly between the "shelves" of the developing palate and are associated with other anomalies, such as a small jaw. V-shaped clefts are due to interference with fusion of the palate during development (Biavati, 2002).

Submucous clefting of the hard palate: Submucous clefting of the hard or soft palate occurs once in every 1200 to 2000 live births. The hard palate appears to be structurally intact, but there is a bony defect indicated by a central, palpable bony notch in the posterior hard palate. The bony notch can be seen or felt where normally the posterior nasal spine is found along the posterior border of the hard palate. Submucous clefting of the hard palate is not functionally significant (Biavati, 2002).

Submucous clefts of the soft palate: In some cases a split, or bifid, uvula is associated with a submucous cleft of the soft palate. This muscular defect is often functionally significant and may result in feeding and choking problems. This cleft is seen as a bluish line through the length of the soft palate, reflecting defects in the musculature. The levator palatini muscles in these cases are often found to be inserted into the hard palate instead of interlocking to form the normal levator palantini sling. This condition foreshortens the functional soft palate and creates a more complex defect. Normally, the levator palatini muscles elevate the posterior part of the soft palate, the velum, and pull it slightly backward, effectively separating the nasal from the oral pharynx. Submucous clefts of the hard and soft palate often occur together (Biavati, 2002).

Posterior pharynx: The newborn oropharynx is not usually the site of abnormalities and is not routinely examined except by visual inspection while the baby yawns or cries. At this time, look for healthy mucosa and symmetrical features; try to rule out tumors and obvious anomalies (Scanlon et al., 1979).

Palpation: Palpate the interior of the mouth using a gloved finger to check the texture, consistency and continuity of the lips, the cheek pads and the tongue. Be alert for thickening, indicating a tumor, or thinning, which may indicate a missing muscle. Push the cheek walls away from the gums, lift the tongue up, push it down and to each side to visualize all sides (you only need to do this if the baby has not moved her tongue around for you).

Check the palate for closure and uniform firmness by pressing with the pad of your index finger along the center from the front of the mouth to the back along the entire length, and for fistulas or thinning, which may indicate a submucous cleft. The parotid ducts may be seen or palpated bilaterally in the upper, posterior buccal mucosa near the gum line and just in front of the tiny web of tissue that forms in the joint of the jaws when the mouth is widely opened. (To practice, check your own mouth to locate these landmarks.) If you can't find these ducts, confirming normal size of the glands with your digital exam is sufficient.

Mouth lesions: Several types of benign cysts may be present in the mouth at birth. The first four will usually disappear within a few weeks.

Bohn's nodules: These are essentially milia of the mouth. These epithelial inclusion cysts develop on the buccal or alveolar surface of the gums and appear as firm, white, irregularly shaped papules either singly or in small groups.

Epstein's pearls: These small white pockets of epithelial cells are often found on the gums or on either side of the ridge that runs down the midline of the upper palate. Cysts that appear on the alveolar ridge of the gums are the same types of lesions but tend to be flat and white.

Sublingual cyst: Small, bluish white, fluctuant, transparent swellings of variable size are sometimes found on the floor of the mouth. These benign mucous-gland retention cysts rarely require any intervention but may rupture during vigorous nursing.

Mucocele: These collections of mucus surrounded by connective tissue appear as glistening clusters of red bumps, usually inside the lower lip. They are harmless but must be distinguished from herpetic lesions.

Epulis: This firm mass looks like the surrounding oral mucosa. It protrudes from the mouth and may be pediculated. It usually occurs in the cavity formed by the gum and the upper jaw bone. These lesions vary widely in size; large tumors may cause respiratory distress and should be removed.

Alveolar lymphangiomas: Singular, firm, bluish cysts of the alveolar ridge that range from 3 mm to 1 cm in diameter are reported in less than 4% of black babies at birth; the incidence is even less common in white infants. More than one may be present but never more than one in each of the four lateral quadrants of the oral cavity. They will slowly regress or become more fibrous; they do not contain teeth.

Teratoma: Very rarely, teratomas may develop in the oral cavity, on the tongue, in the posterior mouth, in the nasopharynx or in other locations. They may be friable and bleed easily; if sufficiently large, they can block the airway (Fletcher, 1998).

Oral encephalocele: As a midline defect of closure in the skull, on rare occasions an encephalocele may protrude from the mouth. It may contain brain tissue and could block the airway. Rupture of such a lesion can be dangerous. Encephaloceles are fluctuant and may pulsate. If you suspect this, get the baby evaluated right away (Fletcher, 1998).

The Neck

The resting posture of the baby's head is often consistent with in utero positioning, especially if it was exaggerated, as in a face presentation. Positioning should normalize in the days following birth. In all other cases, there should be little visible space between the cervical spine and the mattress when the baby is resting on his back.

Length

Newborns have short, thick necks that should be fully mobile and display multiple horizontal skin folds. Unusual shortness may be associated with a syndrome. Several defects involve either a reduction in the number or fusion of two or more cervical vertebrae or of the basioccipital bones and the atlas; these result in a short neck with limited motion in all directions and asymmetry in rotation and lateral flexion.

Shape and symmetry

To observe the shape and symmetry of the neck, support the infant beneath the shoulders and gently allow the head to tilt back. When the exam is done shortly after birth, asymmetry of midline features is most likely a result of positioning in utero. To assess the sides of the neck, stroke the baby's cheek to elicit the rooting reflex. The baby should turn his head to the stimulated side, which will facilitate your exam of the opposite side of his neck. Palpate the neck on all sides. Anteriorly, you are assessing the thyroid gland and the position of the larynx and trachea, which should be in the midline. Locate the carotid and jugular pulses on either side. The connecting bridge between the lobes of the thyroid (the isthmus) is just palpable in the sternal notch and may be felt as a smooth, soft rim of tissue crossing the midline. The thyroid gland is not usually felt unless enlarged, which is quite unusual in newborns but should be looked for if the family has a history of thyroid problems (Fletcher, 1998).

The neck is palpated posteriorly along the cervical spine and laterally over the sternomastoid and trapezius muscles. Lumps overlying or misplacement of any of these structures should alert you to the possibility of an underlying mass. Fibrous sternomastoid muscle tumors are often mistaken for hematomas and may be associated with facial asymmetry and a head tilt due to a shortened, hypotrophic (poorly developed) sternomastoid muscle. A mass in the upper neck may be a thyroglossal duct or branchial cleft cyst. Cystic hygroma is the most common neck mass and is caused by the development of trapped lymph channels, which dilate into large cysts. They are soft, fluctuant and usually located on the sides of the neck or over the clavicle. They can range in size from a few centimeters across to massive and may put pressure on the airway, interfering with breathing or nursing. Very small cysts may resolve on their own, but many will require surgical attention. A cyst can be distinguished from a tumor by transillumination, but any positive findings require further evaluation. Look for clefts, indentations, fistulas or open sinus tracts as you examine the neck and shoulder area. Thyroglossal duct cysts are only rarely present at birth. They are small, rounded and firm, and are distinguished from subcutaneous lesions by their movement during swallowing (Scanlon et al., 1979)

Also check for excess skin along the sides of the neck (webbing) that presents as flaps or folds of tissue or a pouch of extra skin extending from the backsides of the neck down to the midshoulder. They may be associated with a congenital disorder such as Turner, Down or Noonan syndromes (Scanlon et al., 1979).

Muscle tone

The neck is normally flexed and the muscles relaxed, regardless of gestation. Although a prominent occiput may interfere with an accurate assessment, compare your findings with other signs of muscle tension, such as a change in tone with repeated forward flexion of the head, and the amount of head control the baby displays when brought into an upright position. Nuchal hypertonicity prevents the neck from lying nearly flat (leaving an obvious space under the neck), a resting position of the head that tends toward lateral rotation with posterior extension or opisthotonus (extreme, rigid extension of the entire body).

Movement: The neck can rotate 80° (turning the neck to the shoulder on each side) in the term newborn. Rotational distance is slightly more when the baby is early. The head overrotates when there is weakness of cranial nerve XII or when muscle tone is reduced. The term baby has a 40° range of lateral flexion on either side (with the head centered in the midline, tilt the ear toward the shoulder on either side). Anteriorly, the baby should be able to touch or nearly touch her chin to her chest. On extension, the occiput should touch or nearly touch the back of the neck; normally the neck can extend 45°. Asymmetrical range of motion during lateral flexion or a limited range of motion should be reassessed at the third day visit. If not resolved, the baby should be evaluated by a specialist (Fletcher, 1998).

Torticollis involves unilateral shortening of the midportion of one sternomastoid muscle when the head is held in a cocked position for a prolonged period during gestation. It prevents the head from rotating fully in the direction opposite the lesion, and the head tilts to the shortened side. Fronto-occipital plagiocephaly may result in a unilateral epicanthal fold or asymmetry of the ears and is often seen with torticollis. Torticollis is not often obvious at birth (Graham, 1988).

EXAMINING THE CHEST, LUNGS AND HEART

Respiratory Assessment

Checking pulmonary function is a very important part of the exam. Observe the chest for respiratory movements, symmetry, and signs of effortful breathing, such as intercostal retractions. Remember that the baby's color, muscle tone and activity level are dependent upon and indicative of adequate oxygenation. All babies are born as diaphragmatic (or paradoxical) breathers. The baby's lower ribs will dip very slightly as the belly rises with inspiration; the belly will fall with expiration, with the umbilicus moving downward slightly. The upper chest will move less, but will rise and fall in concert with the belly. This pattern is often more apparent when the baby is asleep, and less so when she is stressed, frightened or angry. Under abnormal circumstances, the baby will use more accessory abdominal muscles to breathe. This is known is known as "seesaw breathing" because the abdomen and chest move asynchronously up and down. Also look for a slight lag in chest expansion on inspiration, which is a minor form of seesaw breathing (Scanlon et al., 1979).

Chest movement

Watch for asymmetric chest movement where one side of the chest rises more than the other during inhalation or exhalation. Under- or overexpansion should be easy to recognize if you stand at the foot of the baby and look at the width of the chest in profile. Also look for excessive expansion of the entire chest wall, which can occur when a baby is frightened or when he is trying to compensate for an inability to inflate the lungs because of poor perfusion or a mechanical difficulty, such as meconium aspiration. Asymmetric chest expansion is seen with pneumothorax and sometimes with diaphragmatic hernia. Consistent asymmetry is more rarely indicative of a heart disorder.

Counting respirations

Normal pulmonary findings vary widely and are dependent upon gestational age, ambient temperature, time since birth, the baby's state of consciousness, feeding, any maternal drug intake, the level of disturbance and the amount of placental transfusion the baby received. The baby's state of wakefulness significantly influences the breathing pattern as well. Deep sleep is associated with fairly regular respirations while awake states with accompanying movement, sucking and crying are typified by a grossly irregular respiratory pattern, including breaths of varying depths interspersed with brief periods of apnea that last 10 seconds or less. Skin color provides information about oxygenation as well and has been covered in the subchapter entitled "Examining the Skin."

RANGE OF RESPIRATORY RATES AT VARIOUS AGES AFTER BIRTH IN EARLY AND IMMEDIATELY CLAMPED INFANTS

GROUP	5 MIN	10 MIN	15 MIN	30 MIN	45 MIN	1 HR	2 HR	3 HR	4 HR	5HR	6 HR	24 HR
Early clamped	53.5-60.5	57.3-62.7	56.1-61.9	52.5-57.5	55.1-60.9	56-62	50.5-53.5	48.6-53.4	42.3-45.7	42-46	45.9-52.1	45.2-48.8
Immediate clamped	49.4-54.6	48.2-53.8	53.3-58.7	52.8-57.2	50.1-53.9	46.3-49.8	41-45	41.1 44.9	38.9-43.1	36.8-43.2	36.9-43.1	41.9-46.1

(Data from 50 babies born between 38 and 42 weeks gestation, averaging 3410 grams split evenly into two groups. Early clamping [called "late clamping" in this study], occurred after pulsing had ceased in the midcord, an average of 3 min, 54 sec after birth; during this time the baby was held 10 cm below the introitus. Immediate clamping [called "early clamping" in this study], occurred an average of 7.6 sec after birth. Adapted from Oh et al., 1966.)

Count the respirations while the baby is quiet, undisturbed and not overly warm or chilled. The requirement of no disturbance means that counting respirations may be the first thing you do when examining the baby because as soon as the baby is touched, the respiratory rate and depth change. Assessment can be done by watching the baby breathe; however, because newborn breathing is irregular in volume and rhythm, listening with a stethoscope will give more accurate information. Be sure the diaphragm of the stethoscope is turned to the listening position and then hold the head of the scope in your hand or under your arm to warm it before applying it to the right chest wall. Listening here will help minimize heart sounds from obscuring breath sounds. First, just focus on counting respirations, as trying to also move around to listen for proper inflation will prevent an accurate count (Fletcher, 1998).

Because newborns breathe irregularly, it is important to count breaths for at least one full minute. There is considerable variability in the normal respiratory rate, but it averages about 50 respirations per minute (rpm) in babies who have experienced physiologic cord closure. Irregularity will be more pronounced in preterm infants; they are also more likely to have periodic breathing episodes during which the baby breathes, sometimes vigorously in a "respiratory burst," for 10 to 18 seconds (during which the rate may rise as high as 50 to 60 rpm) and then lapses into pauses for at least 3 seconds and sometimes as long as 10. These brief periods are usually associated with startles, movement, defecation or swallowing during feeding and are not associated with bradycardia (<100 bpm). Periodic breathing will persist for a few days in term infants and until close to the due date in preterm infants. It may also be seen more commonly in normal babies born at higher altitudes.

A lapse of more than 10 (at the most, 20) seconds between one inspiration and the next expiration accompanied by bradycardia (lowered heart rate to <100 bpm) or color changes indicates apnea. Periodic breathing (i.e., pauses of shorter duration) that occurs in the presence of low oxygen saturation or bradycardia is also considered apnea. Apnea is associated with preterm delivery and is outgrown as the baby approaches term. Prolonged apneic spells in the term or nearly term infant, however, are usually abnormal, imply a cardiovascular response to asphyxia and may be ominous. They can also be associated with underlying illness (sepsis, hypoglycemia, or central nervous system insult) or may be secondary to maternal drug ingestion (Fletcher, 1998).

The baby who is too hot or too cold will usually have a higher respiratory rate (tachypnea) but occasionally may have a low respiratory rate (bradypnea). Respiratory rates in normal newborns do vary. Transient tachypnea of the newborn is the most common benign newborn respiratory variation (it is further discussed in the chapter entitled "Evaluating the Apparently Normal Baby Who Develops Respiratory Distress"). However, persistent tachypnea with rates over 60 breaths per minute may also indicate a problem such as respiratory distress syndrome, meconium aspiration, pneumonia, hyper- or hypothermia, or pain. Very low respiratory rates are seen with central nervous system depression, which may be due to maternal drug intake, asphyxia or birth injury. Persistently shallow respirations with minimal chest movement may be associated with overall central nervous system depression. Signs of respiratory distress–such as grunting, flaring, retractions, tachypnea, and crackles–may also be signs of immature lungs or congestive heart failure, as well as other anomalies. Irregularity of the contour of the chest wall with labored breathing may indicate a pneumothorax (a hole in the lungs that allows air to become trapped between the lung and chest cavity). However, it can also be seen with disorders of the diaphragm or hypoplastic muscles (Scanlon et al., 1979).

Listen to the lungs

To auscultate breath sounds, use the bell side of a warmed neonatal stethoscope. Breath sounds are more pronounced in babies than in adults because infants have less padding to muffle the sounds, bringing the stethoscope head closer to the origin of the sounds and causing them to be louder, harsher, less subtle and more difficult to isolate than when the anatomy is larger. Sounds will often be diminished on the side of the chest opposite the direction in which the head is turned, therefore try to listen with the head in the midline, facing forward. Crying usually enhances auscultation as it produces deep breath sounds on inspiration. However, should the baby continue to cry during exhalation, auscultation will not be so enhanced. Sounds are rarely completely absent, even when severe problems exist, because the rib cage is small and sounds are easily transmitted. Begin listening at the top of the chest and move systematically over the anterior chest wall in all four quadrants and under the arms, taking into account the interference from cardiac activity (Tappero & Honeyfield, 2003). Listen systematically in the following the order in each of the columns below.

ANTERIOR CHEST	POSTERIOR CHEST
Right upper chest above the nipple Right midchest in the center of the triangle formed by the nipple, sternum and xiphoid Right lower chest under the arm Left upper chest but not directly over the heart Left lower chest under the arm	Above the midpoint of the scapula on either side Below the midpoint of the scapula on either side Below the tip of the scapula on either side (Listening through the back may be postponed until the spine is being examined.)

If there is a question about the baby's respiratory rate, evaluate the environment, anything else that might be affecting respirations (such as the baby's position, nasal obstruction, etc.) and whether the baby can breathe and nurse at the same time. Make periodic assessments or watch constantly (depending upon the apparent degree of distress) to decide if the abnormal rate persists or if the breathing pattern normalizes. If not, further observation or evaluation may be necessary, depending upon all the findings involved. More about assessing newborn respiratory variations can be found in the chapter entitled "Evaluating the Apparently Normal Baby Who Develops Respiratory Distress."

Compare sounds on each side of the chest. Normal breathing sounds like what you would hear if you lightly brushed your fingerpad over the diaphragm when listening through the stethoscope. You are listening for pitch, intensity and duration of the sounds. Breath sounds may be decreased or distant for a number of reasons but are seldom absent, even over areas of lung collapse (atelectasis) or pneumothorax. Any area of distant, absent or extremely noisy sounds should be transilluminated. Absence of sound indicates a region of lung that has not yet expanded or that has totally collapsed.

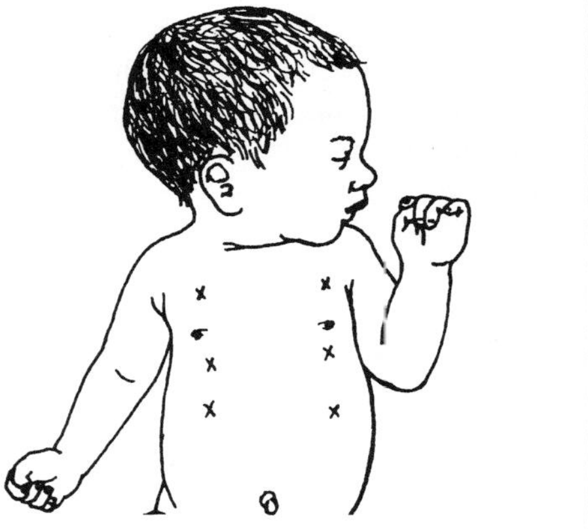
Where to listen on the anterior chest

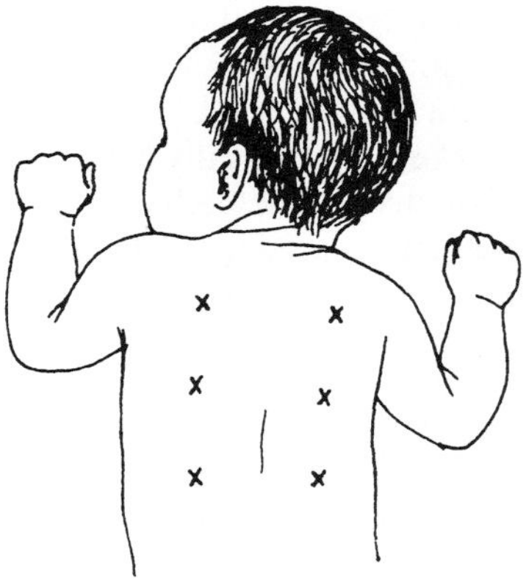
Where to listen on the posterior chest

Normal Lung Sounds	Characteristics and Clinical Implications
Vesicular	Soft to medium sound, pitch lower than other normal sounds, dominant on inspiration. Expiration soft, short, low pitched. Normally heard over the entire chest except over the trachea and upper sternum.
Bronchovesicular	Inspiratory and expiratory sounds are equal in quality, intensity, pitch and duration. Medium volume and pitch. Heard over the upper sternum and between the scapulae.
Bronchial	Loudest of all normal breath sounds, high pitched, dominant on expiration, but seldom auscultated in newborns, located in the anterior trachea.

(Bates, 1991)

In adults, "adventitious" (accidental) lung sounds are abnormal. Adventitious lung sounds in newborns, commonly called "junky sounds" in midwifery vernacular, may indicate a problem but are most often due to unabsorbed fetal lung fluid. When present, these sounds are heard right after birth and become increasingly less obvious by the time of the baby exam. Persistent crackles are abnormal. Frequently, you may think you hear fluid or mucus in the lungs when in fact the sounds are originating in the upper airway; this is especially true if the baby sounds like she is wheezing. To differentiate the two, start by placing the head of the stethoscope on the sternum and listen at intervals as you move up toward the neck. If the sounds are more pronounced as you do so, they are coming from the upper airway and are not so concerning, unless significant mucus blockage, structural blockage, meconium aspiration or sepsis is suspected. Listening over the nose can help tell these sounds apart as well. Nursing should help clear normal fluids and mucus. (Tappero & Honeyfield, 2003; Fletcher, 1998).

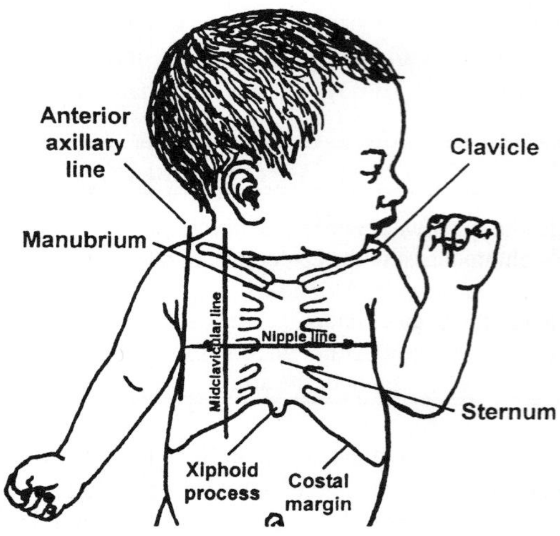

Reference lines and other landmarks of the chest.

Bubbling gastrointestinal sounds may be heard through the lower chest even when the esophagus and stomach are normally located but can also be a tip-off to a diaphragmatic defect that has allowed loops of bowel to enter the chest cavity. Adventitious sounds that not due to lung fluids from birth *are* abnormal in newborns. If you are having trouble differentiating where sounds are coming from, try gently suctioning the nose with a bulb syringe and then check again.

Abnormal Lung sounds	Characteristics and Clinical Implications
Crackles (formerly rales)	Isolated, noncontinuous, brief popping or bubbling sounds; the sound of wet alveoli popping open
Fine crackles	Intermittent sounds of short duration like rubbing strands of hair together in your fingertips. Originate in the alveoli, usually heard at the end of an inspiration. May simply represent fluid resolution from the lungs but are also found with RDS and bronchopulmonary dysplasia.
Medium crackles	Intermittent sounds like a carbonated drink and occur when air passes through sticky surfaces as the alveoli pop open. This occurs in pneumonia, lung congestion, or transient tachypnea.
Coarse crackles	Intermittent low-pitched, loud and long-lasting bubbling during inspiration, like Rice Crispies in milk. Not resolved by coughing.
Rhonchi	Continuous, low-pitched, coarse, snoring sound occurring at any point during breathing associated with secretions or foreign material in large airways. Coughing may eliminate sound. Uncommon in neonates.
Wheezing	Palpable and audible vibrations (squeaky, high-pitched rhonchi) caused by air rushing through a narrowed segment of the airway, which in infancy may be caused by slight swelling, structural defects, spasm or the presence of mucus. May be heard at any point during breathing, although often loudest during exhalation. Rare in babies.
Pleural friction rubs	A dry rubbing or grating sound associated with inflammation of the pleural membrane, heard at any point during breathing and loudest over lower lateral anterior chest. To mimic sound, hold cupped hand over your ear and rub a finger over the cupped hand.
Stridor	High-pitched, hoarse sound from the larynx or upper airways heard at any point during respiration. Found when the airway is partially blocked.
Bowel sounds	Distant bowel sounds may be referred from the abdomen. If loud or persistent, rule out diaphragmatic hernia.

(Adapted from Thompson et al., 1989)

Chest Contour, Structure and Features

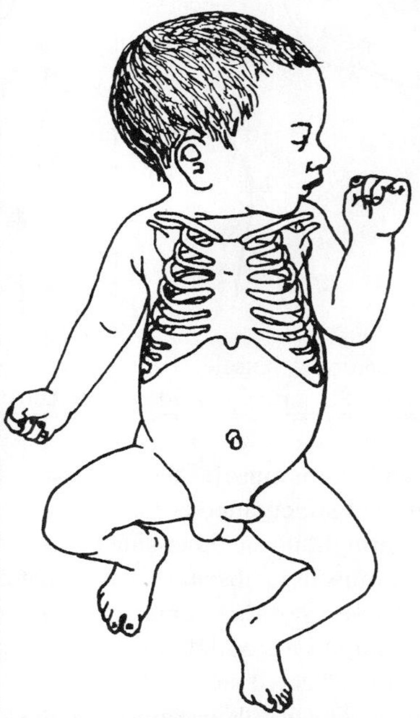
Normal bone structure of the chest

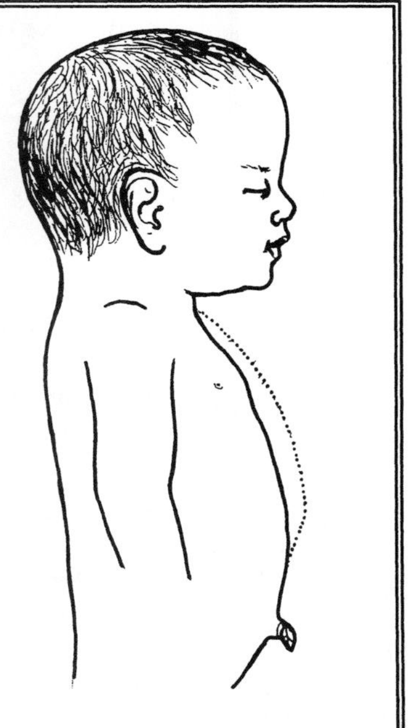
Dotted line shows the typical contour of a barrel chest

After observing for and listening to breathing, you should examine the chest structure. The bone structure should be smooth, symmetrical and round both in general and during breathing. The rib cage should be slightly wider than it is deep. The ribs are more horizontal than in adults. The normal newborn chest is narrower at the top and flares at the bottom so that the overall shape is a gently sloped elliptical cone. Palpate the chest gently to detect any irregularities of contour or structure that are not visually apparent. Check the sternum and ribs for asymmetry in their contour or number. The xiphoid process presents as a small, sharp cartilaginous mass at the base of the sternum. The tip of the xiphoid often protrudes anteriorly and may pivot backward with slight pressure. Any bulges, masses, areas appearing to lack musculature or overdeveloped regions should be noted. Lumps or masses may be associated with a fractured bone. Crepitance, a bubbly popping or crackling feeling, is noted when air is trapped subcutaneously and is often associated with pneumothorax. Place both hands on the chest and feel for transmitted vibrations or rattling (Scanlon et al., 1979).

A barrel chest is characterized by an increased anteroposterior diameter, making the chest fuller and rounder than usual. It may be hard to recognize as the newborn chest is rounded to begin with. It is seen with transient tachypnea of the newborn, meconium aspiration, hyperinflation, air trapped in the pleural space, cardiac enlargement or gastrointestinal tract and diaphragmatic hernia, although most such changes are associated with abdominal enlargement. Sternal bulging may also occur because of underlying masses or trapped air. This also results in distant heart sounds and a decrease in precordial impulse on palpation (see the section on examining the heart for more information). A "dog chest," which is narrow on both sides of the rib cage, may develop in the presence of lung hypoplasia; these babies will present with intractable respiratory distress. If in doubt about a finding, view the chest from all angles to get a better sense of what you are seeing. A small chest is associated with many severe skeletal disorders. In most such cases, the abdomen appears large and distended relative to the chest size (Fletcher, 1998).

Two other types of chest deformities may present at birth but usually do not become pronounced until later in childhood. Funnel chest or pectus excavatum (1/300 to 400 live births), is present when the region of the xiphoid and lower rib cage is markedly angled inward due to overgrowth of lower costal margin, giving the lower chest a caved-in appearance, usually more on the right, which can displace the heart. It is associated with musculoskeletal deformities. It may cause respiratory distress but is usually asymptomatic in infancy. Pectus carinatum, or pigeon chest, causes the chest wall to protrude; one variant is associated with cardiovascular defects (Tappero & Honeyfield, 2003).

Symmetry

The chest should appear symmetrical during all phases of respiration. A number of things can cause asymmetry, ranging from external forces of compression brought to bear during late gestation (compression may occur due to pressure from a maternal fibroid, a twin, arm position, uterine shape or severe oligohydramnios) to space-occupying conditions such as pneumothorax, masses, cardiac enlargement or overdistended lobes of the lung. Unilateral rib fractures are usually associated with disorders of bone strength; however, prolonged compression of a portion of the chest wall during gestation can cause that side of the chest to be more caved in, mimicking rib fractures. Missing ribs or cartilage or the presence of a tumor may also result in asymmetry.

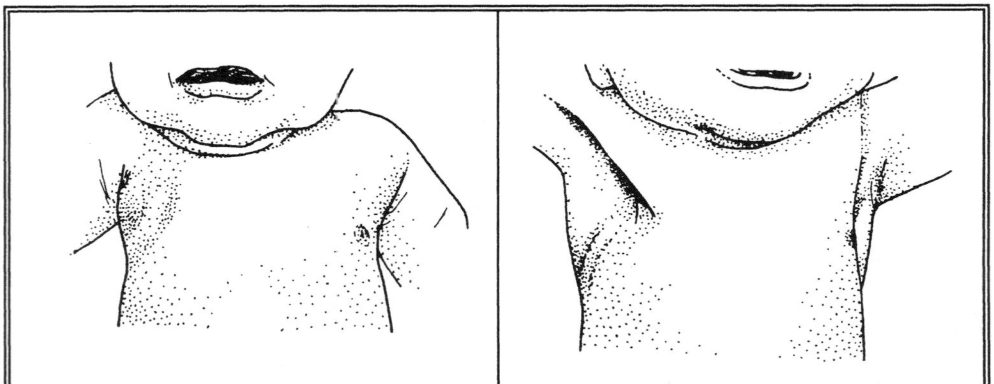

Aplasia of the right pectoralis muscle; note missing nipple (compare with normal left side)

Arms extended, revealing a fold of skin over the defect and normal appearance of left side.

Aplasia of the pectoralis major and minor muscles will cause the chest to be concave above the breast and the anterior axillary fold to be absent with minimal subcutaneous fat, resulting in asymmetry of the upper thorax. To check the axillary folds, raise the baby's arms straight up to either side of the head and look at the folds created in front of the arm pit; they will be asymmetrical if the muscle is absent or hypoplastic. There may be normal underlying ribs or severe underdevelopment. If there are subtle signs of this abnormality, raise the forearms so that the humeri are parallel with the shoulder. This should produce an obvious unilateral fold of skin that runs at a diagonal angle from the arm to the chest wall in front of the armpit on the affected side. Absence of the pectoralis muscles does not produce respiratory distress or limitation of arm movement. The breast and nipple on the affected side may be displaced upward, hypoplastic or absent, which suggests Poland syndrome. Associated hand defects such as fused or stubby fingers or mitten or claw-like hands are seen with Poland syndrome (Fletcher, 1998).

Disorders of the diaphragm, such as complete absence or paralysis, may also lead to chest asymmetry. A number of signs will be evident when the baby is breathing spontaneously and sufficiently deeply. The side on which the diaphragm functions normally presents the expected minimal subcostal retractions when the baby inhales. Although the affected side shows no subcostal retractions, it collapses more than normal and the ribs flare up and out. The umbilicus moves upward and toward the affected side; this is called the "belly dancer's sign." It is best noted by holding a ruler just over or under the level of the umbilicus at full expiration and watching for a shift with each inhalation. Unilateral paralysis is usually associated with brachial or spinal injuries. Bilateral paralysis is rare but causes respiratory failure at the time of birth. It may be associated with injury but can be because of congenital absence of the phrenic nerves as well.

Incomplete closure or total absence of the diaphragm results in diaphragmatic hernia, whereby some or most of the abdominal organs migrate to the lung field during gestation. This leads to progressive respiratory distress, the severity of which depends upon the degree to which the pulmonary space is encroached upon by misplaced organs. (Diaphragmatic hernia is discussed in more detail in the subchapter entitled "Complicated Respiratory Distress.")

Percussion

Although chest percussion is not usually included as part of this exam, it can be used by the skilled practitioner to distinguish between air and fluid in the chest cavity. A good way to become skilled at detecting this problem (as with many others) is to become expert at recognizing normalcy. Use the two-finger technique for this exam. Place one finger firmly against the chest wall and tap that finger firmly with the index finger of the other hand. There should be uniform and hyperresonant (low-pitched and prominent) sounds throughout the chest cavity. A change in resonance indicates a change in the consistency of the underlying tissue. The area of cardiac dullness can be mapped out with your fingers. An alternate technique uses the diaphragm of the stethoscope placed over an area of high tissue density such as a suspected collapsed lung; the chest is lightly scratched and a change in pitch is listened for as the scratching is moved closer to the stethoscope head. The pitch of the scratching sound should become higher and sound closer when it is done over dense structures; however, the presence of the liver or heart may obscure findings during this exam (Bates, 1991).

Transillumination of the chest wall

Transillumination can help identify abnormalities that may be due to trapped air from a thoracic air leak, such as a pneumothorax. With the baby supine, place the light source above one nipple, starting on the side believed to be unaffected; normally a 2 to 3 cm corona should extend around the end of the flashlight (less if the room is not completely dark). The light will shine brightly through any trapped air, extending the corona. Continue the examination, placing the light source below the nipples, on the sternal border and in the axillae and costal regions on either side to compare the amount of light that can penetrate different regions of the chest wall. Pay particular attention when comparing upper and lower and right and left sides of the chest. An air pocket will cause the region of chest in which it is trapped to brightly illuminate, the classic "Chinese lantern sign." The glow in an air pocket will take the shape of the space it occupies and change shape as the heart beats and the baby breathes. Air will also tend to seek the most anterior surface of the baby's body and therefore moves up if the baby's position is changed. Subcutaneous swelling or air may produce a false positive finding. Chest wall edema or dark skin may also interfere with a positive finding (Donn & Kuhns, 1983).

Nipples and breast buds

Examine the nipples and breast buds for placement, location, spacing, number, pigmentation, cracks and discharge.

Size: Size varies according to the infant's size and maturity. Normally, the areolae of term infants are elevated, more darkly pigmented than the rest of the skin, and stippled or textured. Palpate gently with a fingerpad to detect 0.75 to 1 cm of palpable breast bud tissue directly beneath. At least one bud should be over 1 cm in diameter. Areolae range in size from 6.5 to 10.5 mm, although girls tend to have slightly larger nipples than boys. Preterm infants will have smaller or absent breast buds; the areolae will be smaller as well (Johnston, 1994).

Spacing and location: The distance from the outside edge of one areola to the outside edge of the other should be less than .28 (a little more than one-quarter) of the chest circumference. Widely spaced nipples are associated with some genetic syndromes but may also appear in normal infants. The nipples usually overlie the fourth intercostal space but may be found anywhere along the milk line, which extends from the axilla to the pubic bone (Rudolph, 1997, Vol 4).

Extra nipples: Supernumerary nipples are a relatively common finding, especially in babies-of-color, and often appear as raised or pigmented areas 5 to 6 cm below the normal nipple. They may also be located anywhere along a vertical line drawn from the midaxilla to the midclavicular axis down through the true nipple toward the inguinal canal and middle thigh. (The nipple line is illustrated in the anatomy section in Volume I of this text.) These nipples may be very tiny and have no external resemblance to breast tissue, appearing as only shallow dimples along the mammary line, as oval pigmented spots less than half the size of the normal nipple or as another fully developed nipple. Usually only one or two extra nipples are found below the true nipples (Thureen et al., 1999).

Absence of nipples (athelia): Poland syndrome presents with an absence of the nipple on one side; some ectodermal dysplasia disorders have bilateral athelia as a feature. This is otherwise a rare finding (Fletcher, 1998).

Breast variations:

Extra breasts: These are rare and are distinguished from an extra nipple alone by the presence of an underlying breast bud. Most supernumerary nipples do not contain glandular tissue. Supernumerary breast tissue may develop under the arms with no accompanying nipple. This tissue may swell and become tense in the neonatal period, are event that heralds similar changes at puberty and during breastfeeding in girls. Removal during childhood may therefore be desirable. Extra nipples may be associated with congenital abnormalities in Caucasian babies (Fletcher, 1998).

Amastia: Complete absence of the breasts with no signs of a nipple, areola or breast bud is rare. The entire milk line should be palpated carefully to confirm this finding (Fletcher, 1998).

Heart

Note the baby's behavior, breathing patterns, color and activity throughout the exam. All of these are valuable clues to the health of the cardiovascular system. Adaptation of the newborn heart and lungs to breathing occurs over the first weeks of life, making early assessment challenging. Ideally, cardiac function is to be assessed shortly after birth, again within the first six hours, again at the end of the first and the third day of life and at regular intervals thereafter.

Skin color

(See the subchapter entitled "Examining the Skin" for more detailed information about skin color.) Normal babies become red when crying or exerting themselves, which reflects cardiovascular health. A baby who cannot tolerate exertion will become blue or pale. Cyanosis in the hands and feet or cyanosis confined to the face and scalp are normal during the first few hours of life. If other evidence of cyanosis is present, its distribution over the body, its depth, the effect of crying on cyanosis, as well as the time it takes for the baby to recover to a normal rose pink should be recorded. Cyanosis of the mucous membranes during crying in the first hours after birth is often normal but needs reevaluation. Extrapulmonary shunting is facilitated by temporarily increasing intrapulmonary pressure; this occurs when the baby forces expiration, as when he cries. It is important to remember that differential diagnosis of cyanosis is not confined to examining the cardiovascular system because pulmonary or intracranial pathology could be involved. Whenever there is a question about the color of the baby, examine him against a white background under natural or incandescent light (Scanlon et al., 1979).

Likewise, the distribution pattern of any pallor should also be noted. Generalized pallor, peripheral vasoconstriction, acute cardiac failure and a lack of adequate circulating hemoglobin (anemia) are prominent concerns. Pallor can be disguised by the presence of other skin coloring, such as jaundice or cyanosis (Scanlon et al., 1979).

The depth of pinkness should be assessed. While this is usually reflective of skin opacity and pigmentation, some qualitative assessment of circulating blood volume can be inferred from the intensity of the pink color. Purplish coloration may result form a combination of saturated and unsaturated hemoglobin. This is seen in plethora (hypervolemia), a condition sometimes associated with both cardiopulmonary and neurological findings.

Capillary refill time: Conditions that compromise the circulation, such as hypovolemia, persistent peripheral vasoconstriction, sepsis or heart defects, may prolong capillary refilling time. Assess this by pressing your fingerpad firmly against the baby's sternum, sole of the foot or palm for one second. Release the pressure and note how long it takes for the color to return to normal; this should be 2 seconds or less. Two to three seconds is delayed, and longer than 3 seconds calls for evaluation. Check variations between central and peripheral filling times by checking one central area, such as the chest or abdomen, and one peripheral area, such as the shin or the back of the hand, and note any differences. If you are unsure, compare with your own refill time (assuming your circulation is normal) (Thureen et al., 1999).

Peripheral pulses

Tappero and Honeyfield (2003) describe how to examine the peripheral pulses, the strength and character of which offer indirect information about cardiac output. The baby's postnatal age is important, as hyperdynamic pulses are usually found in the first several hours of life, but by the second or third day, they are uncommon and often pathological. The axillary, palmar, brachial, radial, femoral, popliteal, posterior tibial, and dorsalis pedis pulses may be palpated. The dorsalis pedis pulse is not often detectable in newborns.

Use the pads of your index fingers to palpate pulses when the baby is lying quietly. Although you may be tempted to use your thumbs, the pulse in your thumb pads may confuse your findings. Pulse assessment is described below in a systematic fashion; however, you may find you need to check various pulses at different times throughout the exam according to the baby's level of calmness and cooperation. Palpate the pulses on each side simultaneously to see if they are present and equal bilaterally. The presence or absence of the pulse, its amplitude (magnitude or volume) and symmetry should be noted. The amplitude and character of a pulse's rise and fall are the two most important findings in newborn pulse assessment.

Note the rate, any irregularities in rhythm or skipped beats, and any difference between the pulse and the heart rate counted simultaneously by auscultation (a frequent finding with ectopic rhythms) when assessing the character of each pulse. Bounding pulses, especially femoral pulses, are usually associated with heart defects such as patent ductus arteriosus and other aortic-run-off lesions. Preterm babies normally have prominent peripheral pulses, but strong palmar or digital pulses may also be associated with patent ductus arteriosus. Weak or absent pulses occur secondary to low cardiac output regardless of the exact cause but are often associated with left-sided obstructive cardiac lesions. Amplitude is assessed on the following scale:

GRADE	DESCRIPTION OF AMPLITUDE OF PULSE
0	Not felt
+1	Hard to find, weak or thready, and easily occluded with finger pressure
+2	Hard to find, may be occluded with finger pressure
+3	Easy to find and not easily occluded with finger pressure (normal)
+4	Strong, bounding, finger pressure does not occlude pulse

The drawing and chart on the next page show the locations of the pulses that can be assessed. For a basic exam, start by assessing the brachial pulses and comparing their timing and intensity. Next, simultaneously palpate the femoral pulses, which are located on the lateral side of the femoral triangle just below the inguinal ligament. First, place the baby in a relaxed supine position with her hips slightly abducted and flexed. Stand at the foot of the baby, hold your index fingers along the long axis of her femurs with your fingerpads resting just below the inguinal creases, and feel for the pulses with a light touch. If you cannot find them, move your fingerpads a few millimeters up toward the abdomen. It is easier to feel the pulses when your fingers lie parallel with the artery rather than across it. Keeping your fingerpads flat, palpate the femoral triangle. You may be able to detect a soft mass 3 to 5 mm long, which is a lymph node that overlies the pulse. When the node is felt superficially, advancing your finger toward the abdomen slightly usually leads right to the pulse.

Individually compare each femoral pulse to each contralateral brachial pulse using simultaneous palpation. Use your right hand to feel for the left femoral pulse and your left hand to find the right brachial pulse, then reverse your hands. The brachial and femoral pulses should be equal in intensity and timing. Weak or absent femoral pulses or a significant difference between the brachial and femoral pulses, such as a lag between them, as well as decreased femoral pulse intensity–especially when compared to the right brachial pulse–are abnormal and may indicate decreased aortic blood flow. Absent femoral pulses suggest an arterial obstruction or shock. Pulse irregularities are seen in several heart defects (coarctation of the aorta, aortic stenosis, patent ductus arteriosus and hypoplastic left heart syndrome). The femoral pulses can be hard to find and are often subtle during the first days of life. Their assessment is an important part of the exam. With patience the pulses can usually be felt, so don't rush through it. If you are unsure, you haven't found them. When the brachial or femoral pulses are abnormal, palpate the other pulses as well.

Whenever there is a decrease in palpable pressure in any of the pulses, palpate the carotid pulses as well. If there is any question about whether the pulses are bounding, elevate an arm above the head and observe the axilla for visible arterial pulsations, which are seen with palpable bounding.

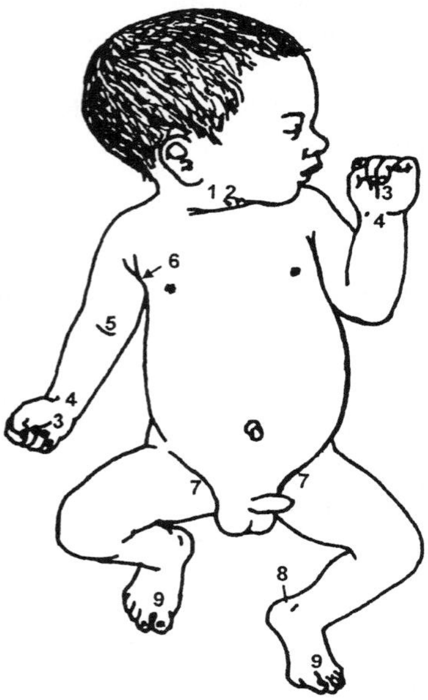

PULSE	WHERE TO PALPATE
1) Jugular vein	Observe the lower portion of the neck under the posterior corner of the jaw with the head turned away from the side being examined (posterior to and parallel with the carotid artery)
2) Carotid	Place finger pad on the anterior midline of the neck just under the chin and slide it to the side until you feel a pulse under the jaw line.
3) Palmar	Found in the lower half of the palm in the midline
4) Radial	Radial flexor surface of wrist just medial to the distal end of the radius
5) Brachial	In and above the groove of the elbow, medial to the biceps muscle and tendon
6) Axillary	In center of the armpit
7) Femoral	Below inguinal ligament, an equal distance between pubic tubercle and anterior superior iliac spine
8) Posterior tibial	Just behind and slightly below the medial malleolus (inner ankle)
9) Dorsalis pedis	Follow an imaginary line extending from the groove between the first and second toes onto the surface of the foot until the pulse is found just above this groove.

The pulse in the jugular vein can sometimes be visualized as it reverberates through surrounding soft tissues. To look for this, lie the baby supine and turn his head to face the side opposite the pulse to be examined. The atrial and ventricular waves of the external jugular pulse can be seen in the lower half of the neck in the sleeping newborn. An alternate technique is to raise the baby's upper body between 15 and 30°, shine a flashlight across the neck at an oblique angle and see if the pulse becomes visible. Unilateral distention may be due to either a structural obstruction or positional compression. The level on the neck at which the pulse can be seen may move down slightly on inspiration. The atrial wave is produced by atrial contraction at the end of diastole. The ventricular wave reflects the end of ventricular systole and gradual right atrial filling from systemic return. A prominent jugular venous pulse is often seen in the first few hours after birth, particularly in babies who received their full placental transfusion. The internal jugular pulse may also be visible in the suprasternal notch, between the attachments of the sternomastoid muscle on the sternum and clavicle or just behind the sternomastoid muscle. The jugular pulse can be distinguished from that of the nearby carotid artery because the carotid pulse is always palpable, is more vigorous, cannot be occluded with finger pressure, is not altered by position changes and has a level of pulsation that is not affected by inspiration. The speed of the heart rate makes counting pulses difficult. When venous pulsations can be distinguished from arterial, they may indicate an increase in the venous volume or obstruction to emptying the right atrium. If there is right arterial obstruction, liver pulsations may be palpated. The pulses of the neck are not usually assessed if the baby seems otherwise normal (Scanlon et al., 1979).

<u>Chest wall overlying the heart</u>

The heart lies in the midline of the chest in the newborn, extending from the level of the 3rd rib down to the 6th, and over to the left midclavicular line. Observe the chest wall overlying the heart. This area, the precordium, may have a visible pulse in the first few hours of life in the term baby; however, if this persists it usually indicates heart disorders involving increased ventricular volume. A prominent pulse in the epigastric area (just below the sternum) indicates that the heart is probably quite enlarged. Finding the point of maximum impulse and the apical impulse help to confirm that the heart is of a proper size and in its normal location (Thureen et al., 1999).

Point of maximum impulse (PMI): Lay your warmed, open palm over the upper chest to get a feel for heart activity. Then palpate the chest wall with the pad of your index finger to locate the point of maximal impulse, which is the area where the contraction of the heart can be most easily felt and is usually strongest; it should be located slightly to the left of center over the fifth intercostal space at the lower border of the sternum or even below the sternum. If not found there, palpate the right side of the sternum as well. Palpate across the entire chest when feeling for the PMI because it can be shifted by a congenital or acquired misplacement of the heart, from defects such as diaphragmatic hernia or from an injury such as pneumothorax. If you are in doubt whether the PMI is normally placed, attach a small piece of paper tape over the spot where you find the PMI to help with repeat comparison. Also record its location by drawing it in your chart. Closure of the pulmonary valve may be felt over the second intercostal space to the left of the sternum in some normal newborns, especially if there is little subcutaneous tissue (preterm babies are the most likely candidates). Now palpate the precordium with the portion of your palm at the base of your fingers. A heave (or lift) at a point of maximum impulse that is slow to rise and diffuse may be associated with ventricular dilation or volume overload. A sharp, well-localized PMI is called a "tap" and is associated with cardiac pressure overload or enlargement. Thrills are palpable low-frequency murmurs that feel very much like those of a purring cat. All these findings may be normal in the first few hours after birth, but should disappear after several hours. These findings may be related to the anterior placement and prominence of the right ventricle in full-term newborns. However, such findings are uncommon in older newborns and usually indicate a cardiac defect (Scanlon et al., 1979; Tappero & Honeyfield, 2003).

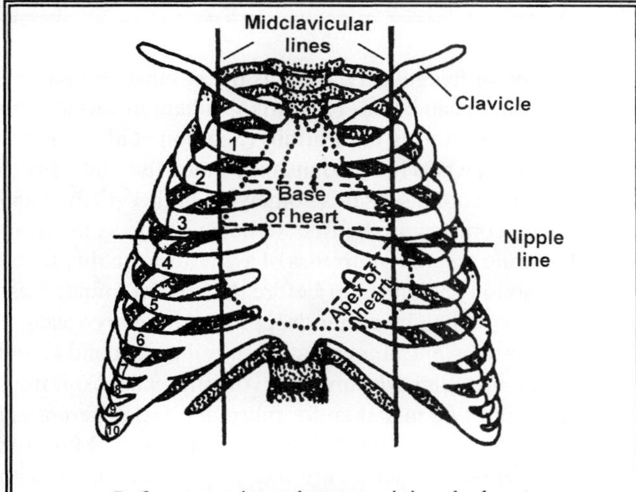

Reference points when examining the heart

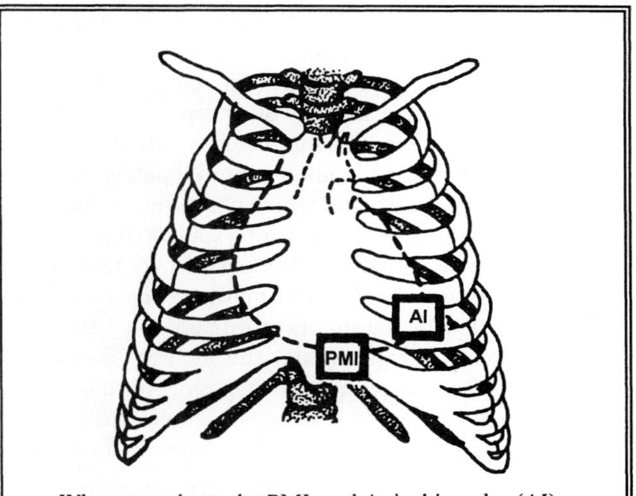

Where to palpate the PMI and Apical impulse (AI)

Apical impulse: The apical impulse (forward movement of the left ventricle during contraction) and the PMI impulse may be in the same location. However, it is normal for the PMI to be found farther to the center, even below the left sternal border, during the first hours or days after birth, indicating normal right ventricular activity with the apical impulse located in the 4th or 5th intercostal space. The locations of the PMI and the apical impulses are usually found in the fourth or fifth intercostal space after the first few hours of life, either at or to the left of the midclavicular line. An apical impulse that is misplaced downward to the left or that feels sharp may indicate problems such as high cardiac output or enlargement of the left ventricle. Both the PMI and the apical impulse can be displaced in dextrocardia (when the position of the heart is reversed), in tension pneumothorax and in diaphragmatic hernia. The nuances of evaluating the heart will become clearer to you with experience and with learning what is normal for most babies (Scanlon, et al., 1979).

Heart sounds: The heart rate and sounds should be evaluated next, as described by Tappero and Honeyfield (2003). As with other findings, the heart rate is influenced by gestational age, postnatal age, sleep-wake state, feeding and physical environment. Place the bell of a warmed stethoscope over the center of the left wall of the chest and count for one full minute to allow for normal variability. A full-term neonatal heart rate at rest should be 80 to 160 beats per minute. The heart rate may be in a high normal range at birth and drop to the midrange by 3 hours of age (103 bpm), where it plateaus until the end of the first 24 hours. Deeply sleeping, healthy babies may have a heart rate as low as 70 bpm. Are the sounds clear, strong, distant, crisp or weak, harsh or muffled? Next, move the diaphragm over the chest,

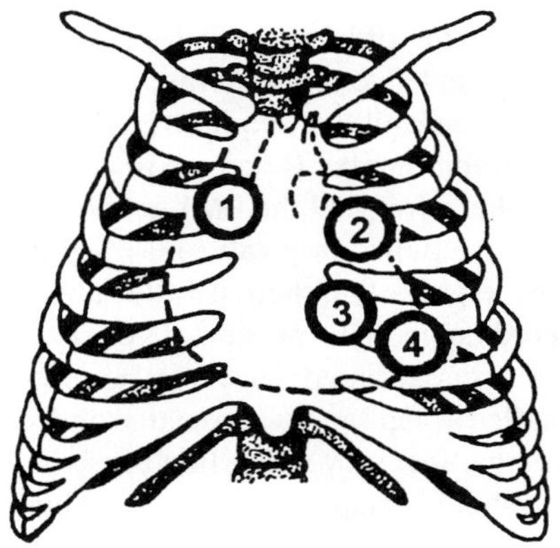

Auscultatory regions of the heart: (1) Aortic; (2) Pulmonary (3) Tricuspid (4) Mitral (apical)

noting how far from the PMI the heart sounds can still be heard.

Sinus bradycardia, or a heart rate less than normal for age (usually less than 80 bpm), may also be seen in normal babies. Stimuli such as yawning or urinating, may result in vagal stimulation and produce bradycardia. Episodes of bradycardia may be as frequent as once per hour in up to 30% of normal newborns, with even more frequency in preterm infants.

Sinus tachycardia is defined as a heart rate that is higher than normal for age (usually 180 to 200 bpm). It is the most common form of rapid heart rate in the newborn and can occur with any stimulus that causes increased demands on the heart, such as crying, feeding, fever or activity. The heart rate should return to baseline once the stimulus is removed. As with the fetus, heart rate variability is seen as a healthy response to stimuli; lack of responsiveness (a fixed heart rate) is clearly abnormal. Persistently high heart rates greater than 200 bpm result in decreased cardiac output and constitute a medical emergency requiring immediate transport.

Also note the rhythm of the heart rate. It may be hard to detect abnormal rhythms because of the fast pace of the newborn heart rate. Any unusual rhythm should be further assessed for the type of irregularity, such as the number and pattern (if any) of missed beats, and any other repetitive sounds. Sinus arrhythmia can occur, resulting in a benign variation in the heart rate with breathing (an increase during inspiration and a decrease during expiration) (Scanlon et al., 1979).

The newborn heart sounds are approximately equal in intensity, and the two heart sounds are much the same due to the rapidity of the heart rate, with a characteristic tock-tick sound. The second sound is somewhat higher pitched and sharper than the first. Extra swishing sounds (murmurs) and clicks are common in the first 48 hours of life as the heart undergoes its transformations. Sixty percent of these will be mild systolic ejection murmurs of a vibrating quality in the 2nd left intercostal space. Systolic murmurs occur after the first heart sound and end at or before the second sound. Less frequently, a systolic murmur is heard between 4 and 6 hours of age, explained by either dropping pulmonary vascular resistance, changing flow through the ductus arteriosus or both. Continuous murmurs persist beyond the second sound into diastole. Remember that these types of murmurs are more common in babies who are hypovolemic. The respiratory rate can match the heart rate in newborns, so breath sounds can sometimes be mistaken for murmurs. To differentiate suspicious sounds, pinch off the baby's nose for a second or two and listen to see if the "murmur" disappears. Murmurs that persist beyond the first 12 hours are less frequent and require evaluation. These are likely to be associated with structural defects, even though they may not compromise the baby. As a rule, innocent murmurs will change in intensity and quality when the baby changes position and are usually not associated with additional signs or symptoms of cardiac problems. Also look at the overall well-being of the baby to ascertain if what you are hearing warrants immediate referral. Reassessing the peripheral pulses may also offer clues. Recordings of normal and abnormal heart sounds are available through medical publishers. There is no substitute for hearing what you are listening for. Any unusual heart sounds that persist beyond 48 hours should be further evaluated, regardless of how normal the baby appears to be.

If the heart sounds are strangely distant or nearly inaudible, further evaluate perfusion by checking the femoral pulses. If the pulses are normal, the faint sound may be due to a pneumothorax, while poor pulses suggest shock or cardiac pump disorders.

Locating the borders of the heart: If you suspect cardiac enlargement, the borders of the heart can be mapped using the scratch technique. The normal neonatal heart is relatively narrow, with little heart identifiable on either side of the sternum. Place the diaphragm of a stethoscope over the sternum at the third or fourth interspace. Listen while you scratch the surface of the chest gently, starting laterally and moving closer to the sternum along an intercostal space until the pitch of the sound changes. Repeat over each intercostal space on either side of the chest until the entire border in outlined.

Determining Blood Pressure in the Newborn

Infant blood pressure is not normally assessed by midwives, even in an exam of this depth. If all other findings are normal, the baby's blood pressure is likely to be normal as well. Newborn blood pressure measurement is tricky at best, and there are inherent problems with obtaining the blood pressure in newborns using the same techniques that are used in older children and adults; it is almost impossible to auscultate a pulse while the baby is moving or crying, and irregularities of respiration, as well as activity, influence the findings. Blood pressure is therefore indirectly assessed by evaluating the peripheral pulses. The baby should be evaluated further by a clinician knowledgeable about cardiovascular defects whenever any abnormalities of the peripheral pulses are noted.

All that said, newborn blood pressure measurement can offer vital information when evaluating a baby suspected of having coarctation of the aorta, kidney defects, or a metabolic disturbance such as hypoglycemia, as well as a baby born to a toxemic or diabetic mother. Therefore, though you may never find the need to check the blood pressure of a neonate, for the sake of completeness, two very low-tech methods are included here. This section is based on the work or Kitterman and colleagues (1969), Goldring and Wohltmann (1952) and Oh and associates (1966).

Equipment: A properly sized neonatal cuff is essential for an accurate reading. Too small a cuff results in a falsely high reading, while too large a cuff will give a falsely low reading. The width of the cuff should be to 25% wider than the diameter of the limb at the level at which the pressure is to be measured (upper arm, thigh, wrist or above the ankle). It should also cover about two-thirds of the arm or leg or the wrist or ankle when in place. (The use of limb length alone to determine the size of the cuff disregards the larger limb diameter of LGA babies and may result in an inaccurately elevated reading.) The bladder should encircle the entire limb without overlapping. A 2.5 cm wide cuff is usually adequate for assessing the pressure at the wrist or ankle in most term babies, while a 4 cm cuff is appropriate for upper arm measurements in most term babies.

Flush method (Goldring & Wohltmann, 1952): This is a fairly accurate, though not precise, method that is practical for use with a newborn. Do your best to ensure a quiet, cooperative baby. Consider taking the pressure while the baby is nursing or drowsy. It is important to have good lighting so that you can clearly see the color return.

1. Place the cuff around the baby's ankle or the wrist as you would on the upper arm in an adult, closing it snugly and smoothly around the limb.
2. Wrap a length of elastic support bandage around the entire exposed hand or foot that is below the cuff, beginning with the fingers or toes and working upward, blanching the skin by pressing the blood up and out of the extremity.
3. Inflate the cuff to a pressure slightly above the suspected systolic pressure.
4. Remove the bandage.
5. Reduce the pressure in the cuff slowly, no faster than 6 to 7 mm per second. An approximate mean blood pressure is the reading at which blood reenters the foot or hand, causing a sudden flush.
6. Repeat until you obtain two consistent readings.

Palpation method: If the infant will cooperate, systolic blood pressure can approximated with palpation.

1. Apply the cuff in the usual manner (as above). (Do not wrap the limb with a support bandage.)
2. Find the pulse distal to (below) the cuff (brachial, radial, or tibial pulse).
3. Pump up the bladder and slowly release the pressure while feeling for the pulse.
4. The approximate systolic blood pressure is obtained by noting the gauge reading corresponding to the reappearance of the pulse during deflation.

Normal values depend on many variables, such as activity, body weight and temperature, posture, gestational age, postnatal age, type of birth, the amount of placental transfusion and asphyxia. Readings taken when the limb is positioned below the level of the heart may be elevated, but only very slightly. Pressures taken in the legs are just about equal to or are one standard deviation above (6 to 9 mm Hg more than) those obtained in the arm (the reverse is true in obstructive lesions of the aorta). Awake infants also have pressures averaging 6 to 10 mm Hg higher than those who are sleeping. Supine positioning raises the blood pressure slightly over readings obtained when the baby is prone. Cuff inflation can trigger a startle response, which will also raise the reading. Expect a rise during nursing, when the baby is upright and sucking, as well as when she is irritated or crying. Values in preterm infants are proportional to their age and size. Babies suspected of having a problem will be evaluated using a more precise Doppler technique once they have been transported.

At any age, a hallmark of normal blood pressure is variability, so having the baby quiet and comfortable is important. Average blood pressure is more informative than an isolated reading. A better gauge of normal values can be obtained when the baby is left quiet and undisturbed for 90 minutes prior to the evaluation. For serial readings, the baby should be in the same state from one to the next with several readings taken over a period of 5 to 10 minutes. For example, if the only way to obtain a reading is during nursing, make sure to obtain each reading during nursing for comparison. Three separate readings recorded at 2 min intervals on a quiet baby can be averaged to estimate blood pressure.

Normal term babies who have received a full placental transfusion have higher average systolic blood pressures during the first three hours after birth and again at 24 hours than those who have not. Normal variations include a relative drop during the first three to four hours of life as fluid shifts occur in and out of the vascular space. The systolic pressure reaches its nadir at three to four hours and then slowly returns to its birth level by 4 to 6 days of age. Blood pressure tends to be less variable in babies whose cords are clamped too soon because they must mobilize fluid from the extravascular spaces in order to maintain their already low blood pressure.

Hypertension during the first six weeks of life is defined as any reading greater than 90/65 at term and over 80/45 for preterm infants. Hypertension may result from congestive heart failure, vascular and other types of kidney defects, disorders involving the aorta, increased intracranial pressure, certain tumors, cocaine intoxication and disorders of the endocrine system, such as adrenogenital syndrome. **Hypotension** is defined as a systolic reading less than 50 mm Hg for term babies (or those over 3000 g) and less than 40 mm Hg for those weighing 1000 grams or less. Hypotension primarily results from low blood volume and other causes of shock. Respiratory distress is associated with a low to normal pressure. A **mean arterial pressure** falls roughly between the systolic and diastolic readings. Mean pressure averages 43 to 51 mm Hg in term infants and 35 to 40 mm Hg in preterm babies. **Pulse pressure** is the actual numerical difference between the diastolic and systolic readings, averaging 25 to 30 mm Hg in term babies and 15 to 25 mm Hg in preterm babies. Narrow pulse pressures are seen in babies with low blood volume, heart failure, peripheral vaso-constriction or generalized vascular collapse. The values below are for babies whose cords were clamped shortly after birth. Compare them with the values in the next table, which shows readings for babies whose cords were clamped at different times after birth.

BIRTH-WEIGHT	BLOOD PRESSURE READING	HOURS FOLLOWING BIRTH											
		1	2	3	4	5	6	7	8	9	10	11	12
1001 to 2000 g	Systolic	49	49	51	52	53	52	52	52	51	51	49	50
	Diastolic	26	27	28	29	31	31	31	31	31	30	29	30
	Mean	35	36	37	39	40	40	39	39	38	37	37	38
2001 to 3000 g	Systolic	59	57	60	60	61	58	64	60	63	61	60	59
	Diastolic	32	32	32	32	33	34	37	34	38	35	35	35
	Mean	43	41	43	43	44	43	45	43	44	44	43	42
>3000 g	Systolic	70	67	65	65	66	66	67	67	68	70	66	66
	Diastolic	44	41	39	41	40	41	41	41	44	43	41	41
	Mean	53	51	50	50	51	50	50	51	53	54	51	50

(Kitterman et al., 1969)

RANGE OF SYSTOLIC PRESSURES AT VARIOUS AGES AFTER BIRTH IN EARLY AND IMMEDIATELY CLAMPED INFANTS												
GROUP	5 MIN	10 MIN	15 MIN	30 MIN	45 MIN	1 HR	2 HR	3 HR	4 HR	5HR	6 HR	24 HR
Early clamped	78.1-81.9	72.6-75.4	74.9-77.1	69.4-72.6	71.6-74.4	70.5-73.5	65.7-68.3	66.3-69.7	63.5-68.5	62.4-67.6	61.1-64.9	71-75
Immediate clamping	59.2-62.8	59.4-62.6	62.7-65.3	61.6-64.4	65.7-68.3	63.8-66.2	59.7-62.3	61.5-64.5	62.8-67.2	64.6-69.4	61.6-68.4	65.7-68.3

(Data from 50 babies born between 38 and 42 weeks gestation, averaging 3410 grams split evenly into two groups. Early clamping [called "late clamping" in this study], occurred after pulsing had ceased in the midcord, an average of 3 min, 54 sec after birth; during this time the baby was held 10 cm below the introitus. Immediate clamping [called "early clamping" in this study] occurred an average of 7.6 sec after birth. Adapted from Oh et al., 1966.)

Examining the Arms, Clavicles and Hands

Examination of the upper extremities includes the bones and tissues of the shoulder girdle, clavicle, humerus, elbow, forearm, wrists and hands. Observe the baby for symmetrical upper extremity activity and normal range of motion. Normally, the term infant holds his arms in some flexion with the hands varying between clenched and partially open. Asymmetry of motion may indicate weakness, paralysis, fractures or infection. Inability to move an arm may reflect spinal cord injury or brachial plexus palsy. The overall incidence of upper limb malformations is estimated at 1 in 626 live births, with only 10% of these requiring surgical treatment.

Examining the Arms

Arm contour, structure and length

Hold the baby's arms to the sides of her torso to assess their length and contour whether the creases (skin folds) match. Look for smooth, matching contours on each arm. The limbs should be plump but not swollen. The fingertips should reach to the upper thigh and be parallel from side to side, and the elbows should be in the same horizontal plane and the same height from the shoulder. If the arms appear asymmetrical, bend the elbow 90°, if the wrists are the same height, the discrepancy is in one forearm. Compare the circumferences of the arms by encircling the widest area with your thumb and forefinger as you palpate for muscle mass. If you detect asymmetry, measure the circumference at the same distance from a chosen landmark. If one side appears enlarged or too small, palpate for abnormalities as already outlined in the "skin" section. If any of these findings are off, a congenital absence or shortening of a bone, a break, or a dislocation could be causative. Breakage of the humerus is the second most common birth-related fracture, the clavicle being first (Fletcher, 1998).

The elbow, forearm and wrist should be examined for position, shape, size and number of bones and for joint motion. Wrist flexion varies with gestational age, with greater wrist flexion seen in full-term babies. Radial nerve palsy presents with the hand dropped forward in a "limp wrist" posture, although the bone structure is normal. This probably results from compression of a nerve due to intrauterine posture. Postural deformity or hypotonia can mimic wrist drop. To distinguish them, see if the baby can voluntarily straighten his wrist. If so, the nerves are okay (Scanlon et al., 1979).

Absence of either the radius or ulna may be noted and is often found with other congenital anomalies. Complete absence of the radius (1 in 100,000 births) is easily recognized because the outer border of the hand and wrist are severely bowed and are held at a 90° angle to a shortened forearm. The thumb is often absent or hypoplastic and the elbow has limited movement. This defect requires consultation with a pediatric hand surgeon and may be associated with several disorders. Absence of the ulna will produce an unusually thin forearm that does not exhibit a full range of motion. A defective radius causes the hand to be bent at an odd angle at the wrist (Scanlon et al., 1979).

Examining the Anterior Shoulders and Clavicles

Observe the clavicles for irregular contour, shortening or incurving of the shoulder region on one side, or tenderness on palpation. Stand at the foot of the baby and evaluate the clavicles for symmetry. Palpate to determine if they can be outlined easily. Press your fingerpads the length of each clavicle, feeling for abnormal movement along the bone, crepitation (grating sensation), tenderness or swelling (which may be a hematoma or a misplaced, broken end). The ends of a broken bone will be mobile beneath your fingers. Although it rarely occurs in homebirths, a broken clavicle is one of the most common birth injuries and is more likely to occur with a difficult shoulder birth. A hematoma may form at the site of a break, and the baby may react to pain during the exam. Bruising may be evident over the area as well (Scanlon et al., 1979).

Further assess the clavicles by palpating each along its entire length while simultaneously moving the arm on the same side through a passive range of motion, a process that may reveal a break. More rarely, pseudoarthrosis of the clavicle occurs, resulting in a false joint usually in the mid-third of the bone, that presents as a lump, usually on the right, that may be confused with a fracture. The affected shoulder droops lower and more forward and is nearer the midline than usual, although these signs become more marked with age. There is a variable degree of painless motion at this false joint, but seldom any functional problems (Fletcher, 1998).

The clavicles may be incompletely formed or missing. Marked passive abduction of one or both shoulders toward the midline may also reveal the absence of clavicles. To assess for this, grasp both of the baby's arms with one hand while you stabilize the baby with the other. Bring the arms toward the midline and compress the upper arms as if to bring the shoulders together. If the shoulders almost meet, or if one flexes more toward the midline than the other, absence of one or both clavicles (cleidocranial dysostosis) is likely on the squashed-in side. This inherited disorder of bone formation affects the skull, clavicle and sometimes pubic bone development, although treatment is not usually needed (Tappero & Honeyfield, 2003).

Examining the Hands and Fingers

General observations of the hand

Each hand is examined for shape, size and posture when opened and closed in a fist. The incidence of some type of hand deformity occurs in 1 out of every 626 live-born babies. The hand maintains a fairly constant proportion throughout life. The distance from the tip of the middle-finger to its base where it joins the palm is 5.5 to 8 cm in full-term infants. The ratio of middle finger length to total hand length is usually 0.38 to 0.48:1 in newborns (meaning that the length of the middle finger should be just over ⅓ to just under ½ as long as the total hand length). The thumb's tip should reach just beyond the base of the index finger. The tip of the little finger should extend to the distal (outermost) flexion crease of the ring finger.

The term baby normally holds his hand in a fist, with the thumb overlapping the index finger. Abnormal postures include tight fisting with the thumb tucked in, which is rarely normal or transient and may be a precursor to spasticity (Hill, 1998).

Creases of the palms and soles

The location of these creases is determined by the attachment of the skin to underlying structures between the 7th and 14th weeks of gestation. Well-developed creases are a product of maturity, as the fetus at term is in a cramped environment. Unusually severe uterine space limitations associated with multiple gestation, oligohydramnios, hypotonia or uterine anomalies may inhibit or prevent normal fetal activity and therefore interfere with normal crease development. Extreme creasing for a given gestation or in unusual places suggests that the limb may have been abnormally folded or restrained. An absence of creasing indicates a lack of normal movement from the first trimester on and requires further evaluation (Davies, 1968).

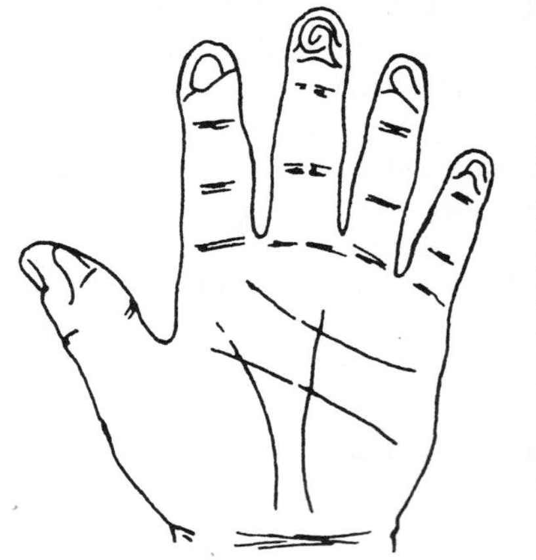
Normal hand proportion, creases and fingerprint distribution

The study of crease patterns and ridges on the palms and soles of the feet is called **dermatoglyphics**. There are two general categories of crease alterations. Specific, characteristically aberrant patterns of creases and other anomalies of the hands occur with unusual frequency in specific syndromes. Such alterations are seldom indicative of a particular condition, but when considered with the total constellation of any other defects may enhance the specialist's ability to arrive at a specific diagnosis. Secondly, the distribution of a particular pattern of fingerprint can be associated with certain syndromes (fingerprints are described on the next page). For example, ulnar loops may appear on all the fingers in Down syndrome. Crease patterns may also be altered by nongenetic effects, including fetal alcohol syndrome, intrauterine infection, chronic intrauterine pressure or hypotonia, to name a few (Davies, 1968). Any unusual crease patterns should be pointed out during a pediatric evaluation.

Palmar creases: Examine the palmar creases. Normally there are three prominent creases at birth: two transverse creases and a thenar crease, which forms a semicircle curving around the large palmar pad at the base of the thumb. The distal transverse crease (nearest the fingers) extends from the ulnar edge of the palm to below the base of the index and middle fingers. The proximal transverse crease (nearest the wrist) extends from the inside of the palm to the oblong palmar pad on the outer border of the hand, under the little finger (Davies, 1968).

The transverse creases have received the most attention in genetic studies. A **simian crease** presents as a single, prominent transverse crease across the upper third of the palm. It is associated with Down and other syndromes, although 4% of genetically normal persons have a simian crease on one hand and 1% have one on both (twice as often in males).

A single transverse crease reflects a shortened palm. Down syndrome in more likely when short fingers, an incurved little finger, a low-set thumb and a Simian crease are seen in combination (Fletcher, 1998).

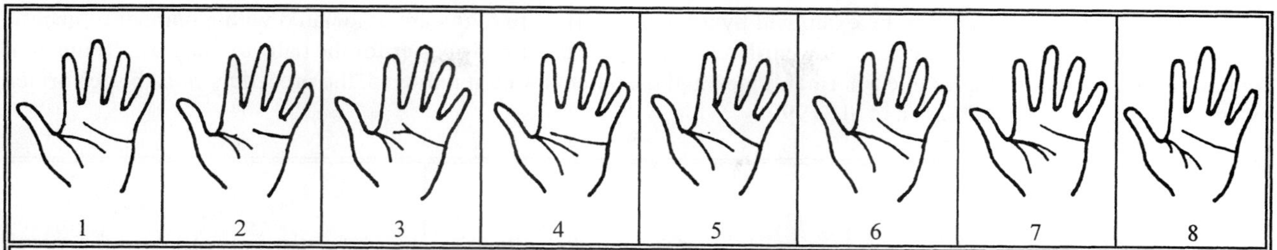

Normal Variations in Palmar Creases (1 is found in 94% of normal individuals;
2-5 show variants of the distal transverse crease; 6-8 show variants of the proximal transverse crease)

(Schmidt & Nitowsky, 1977)

A **Sydney line** consists of a proximal transverse crease that spans the width of the palm (as does the single simian crease). However, in a Sydney line, a distal transverse crease that terminates between the middle and index fingers is also present. These two lines are often bridged by another diagonal crease. A Sydney line is found in 6.6% of normal infants. There have been attempts to establish a link between a Sydney line and some syndromes, as it was originally noted in association with congenital rubella. It is frequently seen in babies who later have learning difficulties, delayed development and minor behavioral problems. Some consider it a variant of a simian crease.

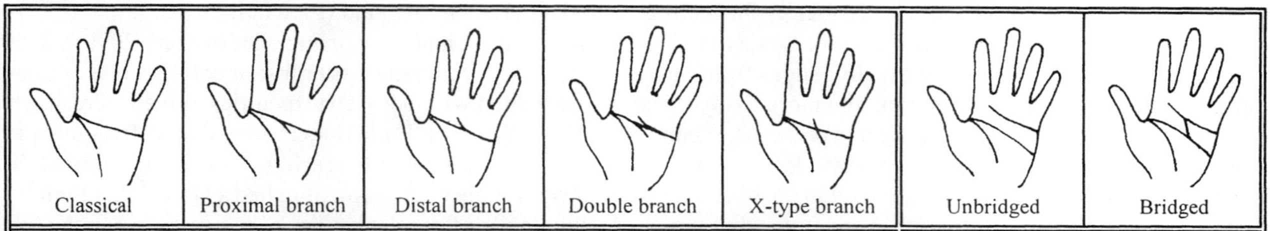

Major Variants of the Simian Crease | Sydney Line

(Adapted from Hook et al., 1974)

A Sydney line is not always permanent; it sometimes appears later in childhood, and sometimes it is present at birth but absent 10 to 14 months later among normal children. Its disappearance may be related to growth of the palm, with relative shortening of the proximal palmar crease (so it no longer spans the hand). It may also result from the clenched posture of the fetal hand.

There are a large variety of other abnormal palmar crease patterns including complex creasing, where a simian crease is joined by two other deep creases to form a triangle in the center of the palm. Broken or shortened creases are also among these widely disparate types.

Fingers

The fingers are assessed for number of digits, shape, length, contour, spacing, bending, curvature, posture at rest and sounds on joint motion. Dermoid cysts may appear on the fingers as round, skin-covered masses and transilluminate well. Look for overlapping and separate each finger to assess for webbing. Curvatures of the fifth (little) finger less than 10 to 15° are normal. The creases of the little finger should be parallel. Macrodactyly, an enlarged finger or toe, can be normal, but is also associated with neurofibromatosis. Isolated flexion of the index finger is seen in normal crying babies but when persistent may indicate focal cerebral injury (Hill, 1998). Overlapping of the second and third fingers is seen with trisomy 18 (Scanlon et al., 1979; Rudolph, 1997).

Palpate each finger to confirm the presence of three phalanges. There should be two parallel creases on each finger, dividing the length roughly into thirds. Absence of one crease indicates a shortened digit. Shortening of the midphalanx results in nonparallel creases indicating a radial deviation (the finger is twisted). Shortening of any of the metacarpal bones results in a short knuckle and is seen with Turner syndrome and pseudohypoparathyroidism (Fletcher, 1998).

An extra digit (polydactyly) may present as an entire extra finger with bones or a small stub of tissue with no bones. It is more commonly seen in babies of African descent, and there is often a familial tendency. An appendage that is small and is only attached by a fleshy pedicle with no attached bones may be tied off at its base with wide dental floss; however, this should wait until the baby can be examined by a specialist as extra digits are associated with a number of genetic syndromes. Waiting at least a few days after birth may also make the trauma easier for the baby to integrate. If the digit contains an attached bone, more like a normal finger, and the parents want it removed, the procedure must be performed by an orthopedic surgeon (Thureen et al., 1999).

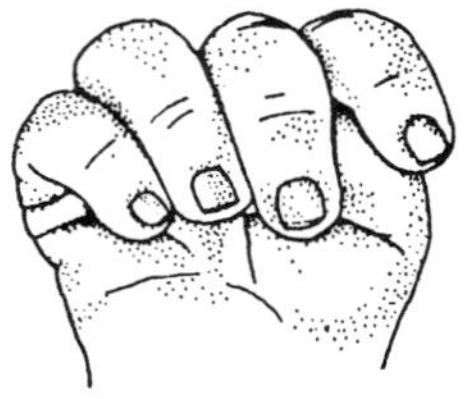
Normal grasp at term

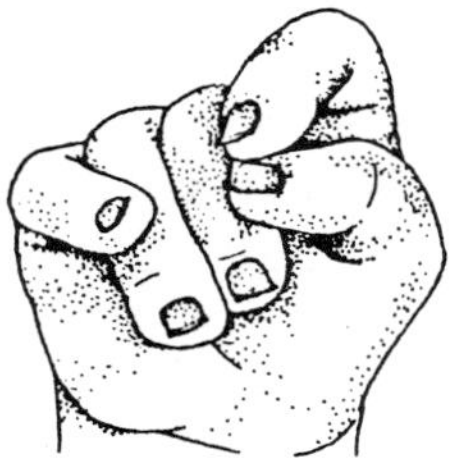
The grasp is similar in trisomy 13, 18, Smith-Lemli-Opitz and Pena-Shokeir syndromes

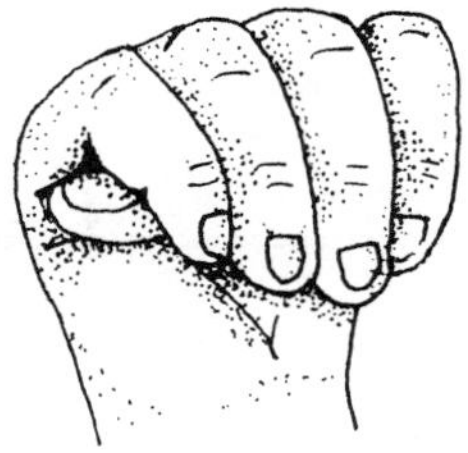
In Marfan syndrome, the fingers are long and thumb often extends beyond the little finger.

Extra digits that are placed slightly back from the attachment of the little finger or on the outer edge of the hand are usually familial. Those that develop on the inner edge of the hand (thumb side) may be associated with hematologic and heart defects; these babies should be further evaluated regardless of racial background (Fletcher, 1998).

Syndactyly, or webbing of the fingers or toes, is a common congenital anomaly, occurring once in every 2000 to 2500 live births. It is often familial. Severity ranges from minimal bridging to complete tissue fusion between one or more digits. The more severe the webbing, the more likely it is to be associated with bony abnormalities as well. Treatment depends on the extent of the webbing and presence of bone anomalies. When multiple fingers are webbed, function may depend on early correction, so the baby can learn to use her fingers. The thumb should reach just beyond the base of the index finger. A forward-placed thumb, with the long axis at a near right angle to the palm, is called a "hitchhiker thumb"; it presents when the first metacarpal bone is poorly formed. A "floating" or floppy thumb may also result when the first metacarpal bone is poorly formed or absent. When the thenar muscle is poorly formed, the thumb is retroflexed (pushed back). A low-set thumb is seen with Down syndrome. Duplication of the thumb occurs once in every 100,000 births, is usually unilateral, and is more common in males, especially among Caucasians and Asians (Fletcher, 1998).

Fingerprints: There are three basic, normal configurations that the fingerprints may assume; the whorl, the loop and the arch. Which pattern develops is thought to depend upon slight variations of positioning of the finger-pads during early fetal development. The loop is further designated as ulnar (toward the little finger) or radial (toward the thumb), depending upon the side of the hand to which it opens. Commonly the thumb sports a whorl, the index finger a radial loop, the middle finger an ulnar loop, the fourth finger a whorl and the little finger an ulnar loop. Many syndromes are associated with a particular distribution of these patterns on the fingerpads (Preus & Fraser, 1972).

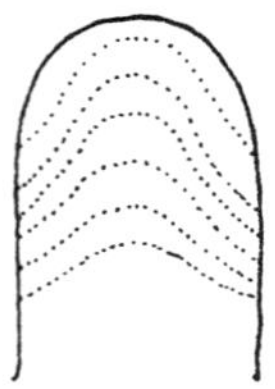
Simple arch

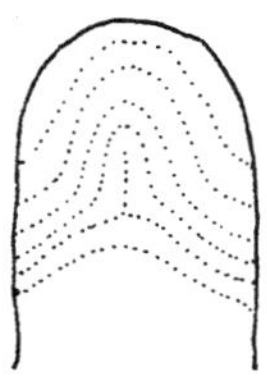
Tented arch

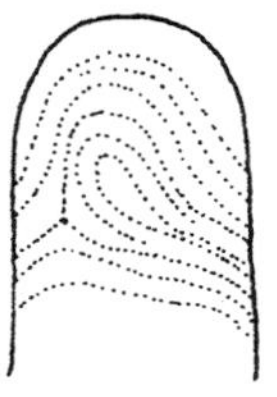
Ulnar loop

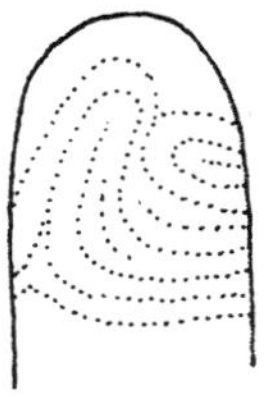
Double-looped whorl

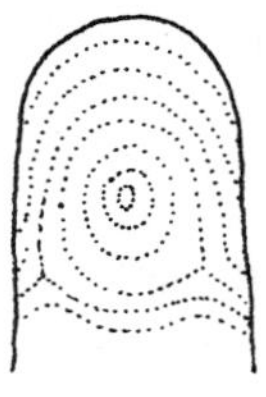
Circular whorl

Fingernails: The nails should be examined for normal placement, growth, underlying color and smoothness. Nails reach the fingertips by 32 weeks and in full-term babies usually extend beyond the nailbed. They are thin, easily bent or torn, soft and smooth without pits or ridges. They may appear cupped or bent. The most frequent abnormality involves poor growth (with surrounding cuticle flush with the nail surface). Note that edema will override the edges of the nails, making them appear hypoplastic. Spoon-shaped, dysplastic or absent nails are seen with systemic disorders such as fetal alcohol syndrome or maternal ingestion of anticonvulsant drugs, although some normal babies have spoon-shaped nails that straighten out during infancy. While trauma or infection may cause nails to appear abnormal, most defects or missing nails are due to congenital disorders and may be associated with absent patellae (kneecaps), as well as renal and iliac bone anomalies (e.g., osteo-onychia dysplasia). Underdevelopment, as seen in fetal hydantoin syndrome, may be a mild form of limb reduction. Overgrowth of the nails is rare in newborns but occurs in diseases such as congenital hemihypertrophy or familial onychogryposis. The nails may be stained from passage of meconium in utero or the beds may be bluish in the presence of acrocyanosis. Small mucinous pseudocysts may appear near the nail. Transillumination with the probe pressed against the pad of the finger and the light directed to the nail reveals a mass that, being mucus filled, admits light (Fletcher, 1998; Donn & Kuhns, 1987).

Assessing the Movement of Major Joints in the Shoulders, Arms and Hands

Performing range of motion assessments

With the exception of Fletcher (1998), neonatal range of motion assessment is not described in the general neonatal literature; therefore, it is included here. You will be evaluating spontaneous range of motion during the course of your postpartum stay. Most of the time, it is obvious that everything is fine; there is no need to subject obviously normal babies to a battery of range of motion tests. However, if there is a question about a limb, because either structure or function seems amiss, you can select the appropriate assessments from the descriptions below to further evaluate the limb.

Range of Motion in the Arms and Hands

Joint or Bones	Flexion	Extension	Abduction	External Rotation	Internal Rotation
Shoulder	Close to 180°	≥ 25°	Close to 180°	≥ 45°	≥ 80°
Elbow	145°	165 to 170°			
Forearm				Supination* ≥ 80°	Pronation* ≥ 80°
Wrist	75 to 80°	65 to 75°			
Digits	Able to clench	Full extension			
Knuckle joint (Metacarpal-phalangeal)	90°	0°			
Finger joints (Interphalangeal)	Normal clenching	0°– 5° to 15°			

*These maneuvers are performed with the upper arm held immobile and the elbow bent to a 90° angle (Scanlon et al., 1979).

Calming the baby during assessment: It is essential for the baby to be relaxed during any range of motion tests. Wait for the baby to be calm and make sure he is warm. Explain what you are doing. Go slowly. Have an assistant offer the baby a finger to suck. Work with the baby's spontaneous movements. If the baby becomes agitated, stop and allow him to settle before you continue or proceed with another portion of the exam, and come back to the problematic assessment later. Be aware that lack of cooperation may also indicate pain or a limited range of motion in that region.

Establishing a baseline: A baseline from which to measure must be established for each assessment so that an angle can be determined. The baseline should be lined up with the zero line of your protractor. One end of the baseline is designated as the zero point and, when referred to, is the point from which to begin the arc of movement. In most cases, a motion line is drawn perpendicular to the baseline, depending upon the measurement to be obtained. To obtain the arc of rotation, an angle is assessed when the limb reaches its limit of motion. Assessment includes evaluating the limb and joint for normal strength and tone as well as spasticity or flaccidity (Greene & Heckman, 1993).

Understanding flexion contracture: The larger newborn joints normally have a degree of flexion contracture. This means, for example, that the baby cannot completely straighten her arm at the elbow to a full 180° until a few weeks after birth. Any tests evaluating limb extension will result in the baby resisting full extension. Testing the baby when she is very relaxed and almost drowsy may help. Note that abnormal flexion contracture, from such problems as fusing at the elbow (synostosis), is easily recognized by a lack or obvious limitation of range of motion during spontaneous motion and smaller anatomy on the affected side (Herring, 2002).

Range of shoulder motion

The shoulder has the greatest range of motion of any joint in the body, allowing it to assume many positions and planes of motion, which also makes it vulnerable to injury.

Flexion (vertical or forward elevation) and extension of the shoulder: Begin with the baby supine with her arm lying alongside the torso. Draw a head-to-foot baseline straight through the head and torso, centered through the shoulder joint. Keeping the arm straight, with the palm toward the midline, raise the entire arm up above the body to a 90° angle (the arm forms the motion line), and then move it upward in an arc and then to the side of the baby's head (like raising your hand in school). Flexion of the humerus or forward elevation of the scapula off the mattress during this maneuver indicates the maximum upward range of arm motion (Fletcher, 1998; Herring, 2002).

Extension of the shoulder, which is sometimes referred to as "posterior elevation," is motion in the opposite direction from forward elevation. To assess this, position the baby on her back so that one arm can be rotated down off the edge of the examining surface. From the resting position alongside the torso, the arm is kept straight, with the palm facing the body, and posteriorly elevated or extended backward from the neutral position. In other words, it drops off the side of the mattress as far as it can comfortably go. Maximum posterior extension requires some internal rotation (see the illustration below). Do not expect the arm to fall freely off the edge in a term newborn, as the natural tendency to stay flexed will override gravity; if it does drop off, suspect preterm birth or hypotonia (Fletcher, 1998).

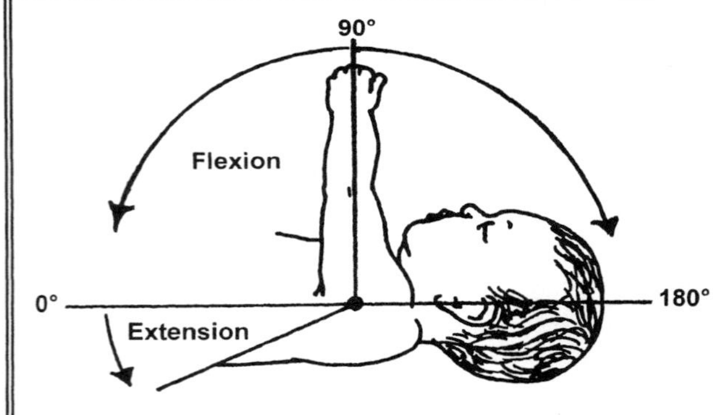

Flexion and extension of the shoulder

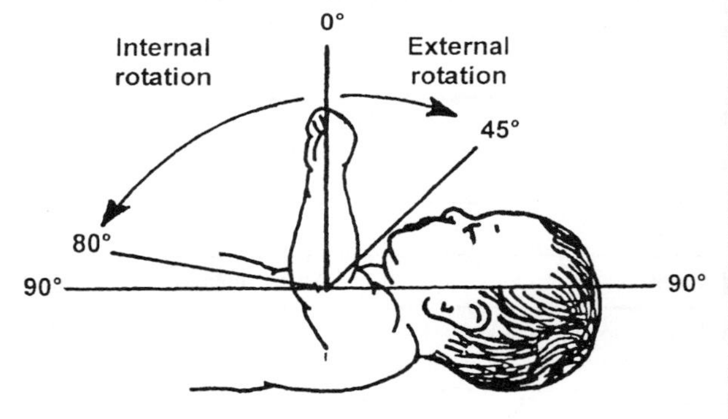

External and internal rotation of the shoulder

External and internal rotation of the shoulder: Begin with the baby supine and the upper arm extended straight out to the side in a "T" position–that is to say, abducted 90°–and aligned with the plane of the scapulae (this will raise the arm up off the mattress slightly, as illustrated). Flex the elbow 90° so that the forearm is perpendicular to the mattress with the palm directed toward the feet. Establish a vertical baseline straight down through the forearm and a head-to-foot motion line running through the ear. External rotation is assessed as the number of degrees the forearm moves away from the perpendicular as it is moved in an arc toward the head. Internal rotation is the number of degrees the forearm moves away from perpendicular as it is moved in an arc toward the feet (the palm moves down to rest on the mattress) (Greene & Heckman, 1993).

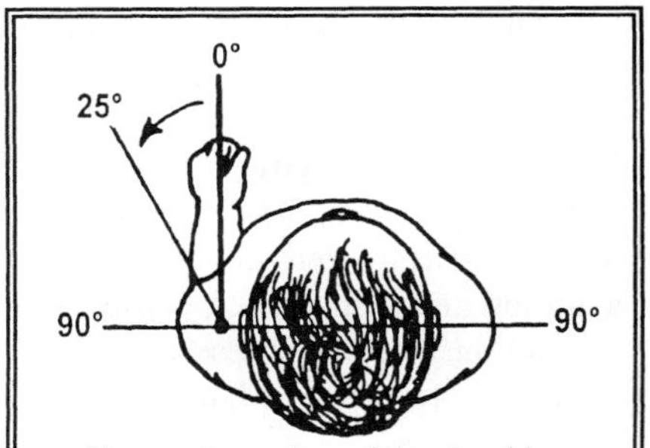

External rotation of the shoulder

External rotation of the shoulder: The arm is held to the supine infant's side with the upper arm held comfortably against the side of the chest. Flex the elbow 90° to bring the forearm straight up in the air. The baseline is drawn straight down through the forearm. A horizontal 90° line is centered through the ears from side to side. The degree of external rotation is determined by the number of degrees the forearm can move to the side, away from the midline. The presence of the trunk prevents the estimation of internal rotation from this position (Herring, 2002).

Neutral abduction of the shoulder: Begin with the baby supine and the arm extended alongside the torso. The baseline is designated by the starting position of the arm. The 180° point is on the opposite end of this line. A motion line is extended at a 90° angle from the center of the baseline, level with the shoulder. Keeping the arm parallel with the mattress and in the same plane as the ear, move the arm out to the side and up by the head in an arc (Herring, 2002).

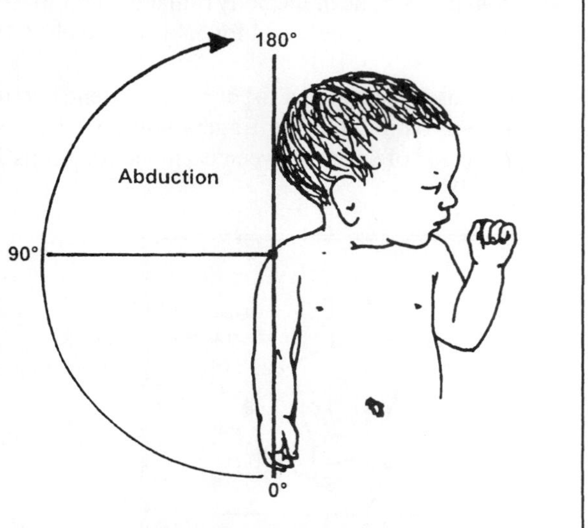

Neutral abduction of shoulder

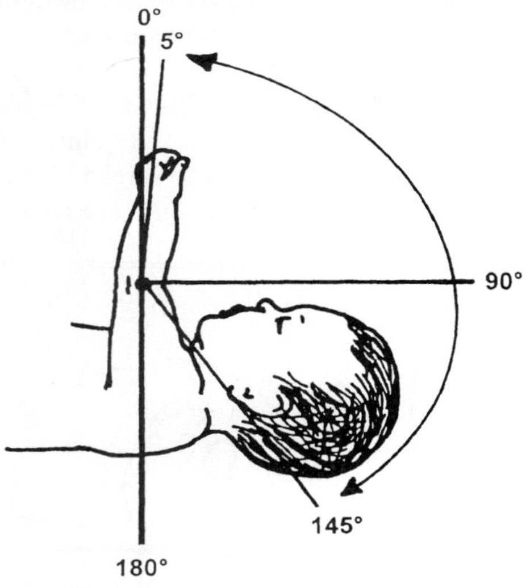

Range of motion in the elbow joint

(after Fletcher, 1998)

Range of elbow flexion and extension

Begin with the baby supine. Extend the arm straight up in the air, palm toward the head. Bend the forearm toward the head as far as it will go. Bending the forearm backward from the elbow (hyperextension) is not possible in the newborn because of flexion contracture in the joint (Greene & Heckman, 1993).

Range of forearm and hand motion

Forearm rotation: Begin with the baby supine and the arm to the baby's side. Flex the forearm 90° at the elbow with the palm facing the baby's midline (thumb toward the head). A line drawn across the base of the fingers establishes the baseline. Hold the upper arm in place with one hand while rotating the forearm with the other to move the baby's hand. **Supination** occurs as the thumb moves laterally as the palm turns in the direction of the head. **Pronation** occurs when the forearm rotates to move the hand in the opposite direction, bringing the thumb toward the midline and the palm toward the feet. While the hand motions are the easiest to describe for this maneuver, remember that you are checking for normal motion of the forearm, as abnormalities will otherwise be missed. Synostosis (fusion) of the radius or ulna will either impair or prevent supination and pronation of the forearm (Greene & Heckman, 1993).

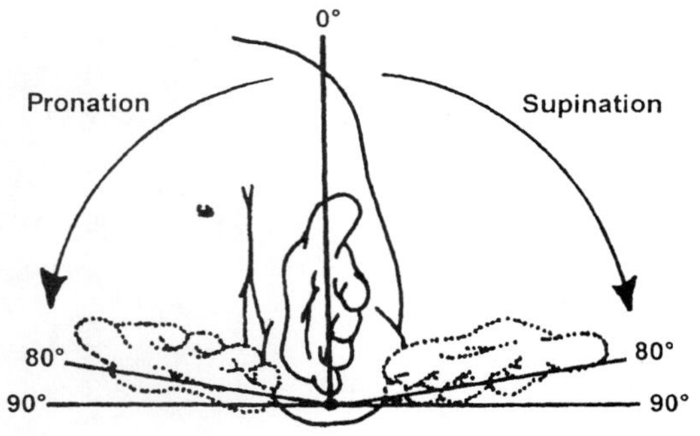

Rotation, supination and pronation of the forearm

Range of wrist motion: Begin with the baby lying supine and the forearm prone (thumb on top, palm toward the thigh); the fingers and wrist are held straight in line with the forearm. A baseline is drawn straight down along the back of the third finger and the outer border of the forearm. Extension is assessed by how far the back of the hand can bend toward the outer forearm. Flexion is described by how far forward the palmar side of the hand can bend toward the inner forearm.

Next, begin with the baby supine and the forearm in pronation, that is, the inside of the forearm and the palm rest on the mattress, with the wrist in a neutral position and the fingers in a straight line with the forearm. A baseline is drawn through the third finger and center of the wrist. A 90° line is drawn across the wrist, level at the base of the thumb. Move the entire hand at the wrist side to side in a waving motion, first moving the thumb side toward the midline of the body (radial deviation) and then moving the other side of the hand away from the midline of the body (ulnar deviation). Radial deviation averages 20° and ulnar deviation averages 55° in adults (no values could be found for babies) (Fletcher, 1998).

Range of hand and finger motion: The baby should be able to fully close his hand in a fist and fully extend his fingers straight out from the palm. The knuckle joints should flex 90° during fisting, but the fingers will not hyperextend backward. The baby should be able to spread his fingers, leaving 10 to 15° of space between each one (this constitutes lateral extension of the fingers in relation to each other) (Fletcher, 1998).

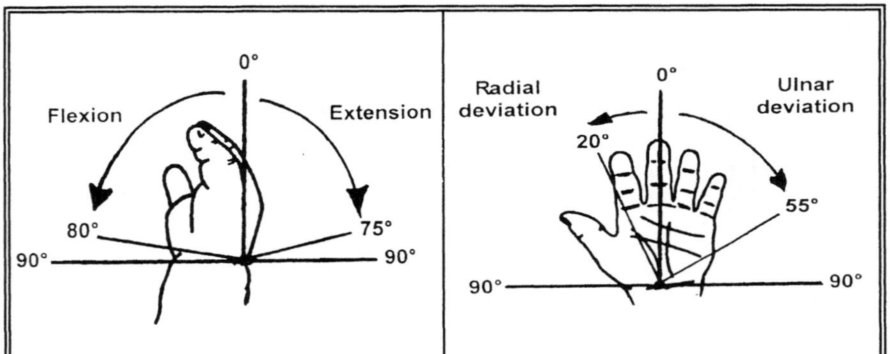

Flexion and extension of the wrist | Radial and ulnar deviation of the hand

(after Fletcher, 1998)

EXAMINING THE ABDOMEN AND GROIN

Examining the Abdomen

The abdominal exam is based on the work of Scanlon and associates (1979), unless otherwise noted.

Visual inspection

The normal newborn abdomen is slightly rounded or protuberant, soft and symmetrical, and moves synchronously with the chest as the baby breathes. The skin overlying the abdomen of a term newborn is thick and smooth, with only a few large blood vessels visible. These veins should not appear distended (swollen and elevated), although it is not abnormal for the veins of the upper abdomen to appear dilated and darker. A preterm baby may appear slightly potbellied due to immature muscular tone, with more translucent skin and more visible veins.

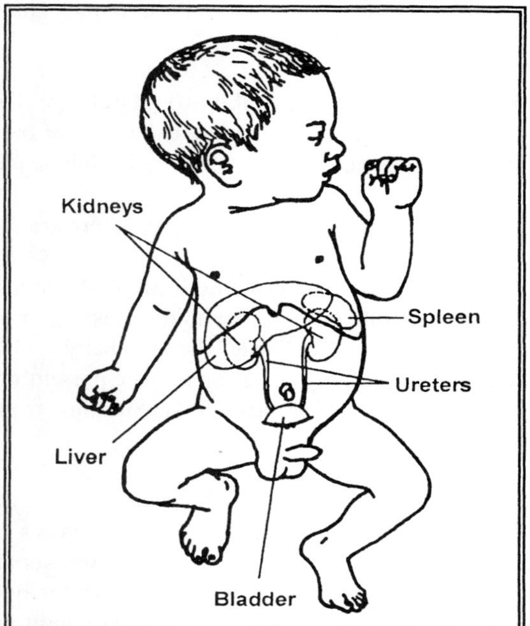

The normal abdomen at 2 hours of age showing the location of organs to be examined (excluding GI tract).

Intermittent peristaltic movement may be visible through the abdominal wall in some infants after the first hour of life, especially after the baby has swallowed some air. They present as subtle wave motions. It is also very common to see multiple loops of bowel through the abdominal wall in the first hour of life, especially in babies with little subcutaneous fat, such as early infants, IUGR babies or those with lowered abdominal muscle tone. (The same phenomenon may occur, but is less visibly apparent, in babies born closer to term who have a normal fat layer.) Peristaltic waves are seen to carry air along the loops and should become invisible after the first hour (Fletcher, 1998).

Upper abdominal distension that may be asymmetrical is commonly seen after nursing, when the stomach is full, or after crying (due to swallowed air). Persistent asymmetry of the abdominal wall may be due to a mass, organ enlargement, or intestinal obstruction, while concavity can be associated with diaphragmatic hernia (especially with accompanying respiratory distress) or extreme malnutrition.

A flat, flabby abdomen with loose folds of skin indicates weight loss or decreased muscle tone, which may be induced by maternal drug intake or neurological depression. More rarely, congenital absence of the muscles may be the cause of a lax, baggy abdominal wall, as in prune belly syndrome, which causes the abdominal contents to be outlined by the overlying skin and the sides of the belly to appear widened without an increase in the anteroposterior diameter. This syndrome is usually seen in males and is often associated with urinary tract abnormalities.

While the normal newborn abdomen appears full and rounded once the baby has swallowed some air, marked distention is a reliable but nonspecific indication of a disease or defect. It may be associated with gastrointestinal obstruction, ascites (fluid build-up), infection, masses or enlargement of abdominal organs. Fullness above the level of the umbilicus is increased with duodenal atresia, gastric distention or liver enlargement. Fullness is increased below the umbilicus with distention of the urinary bladder. An abdomen that is very distended will be tense and may be shiny. Serial measurements of the abdominal girth will detect more subtle changes over time.

Persistent, localized enlargement suggests a tumor or other mass. Its location can be suggestive of the source; for example, localized bulging along one or both sides of the lower abdomen suggests enlarged kidneys. The presence of persistent visible peristalsis in a distended abdomen alerts the observer to a possible obstruction and may indicate its location. Persistent peristaltic waves with visibly distended loops of bowel in the same area, especially if located in an upper quadrant, raise the suspicion of a bowel obstruction. Visible upper left quadrant distension and peristalsis suggests pyloric obstruction. An obstructed duodenum is the likely cause when two distinct "bubbles" persist in the bowel loops beyond the first hour, particularly when the rest of the abdomen is relatively less distended; about one-third of these babies will also have Down syndrome. Obstruction is especially likely if the baby is also vomiting. Distention may also occur due to either enlargement of a solid abdominal organ or to infection.

Seesaw breathing (the chest rises as the belly falls during inspiration and the chest falls as the belly rises during expiration) suggests respiratory distress, central nervous system disease, or peritoneal irritation.

Localized edema or discoloration of the abdomen are both abnormal, in most cases indicating intraperitoneal disease. Rarely, bruising results from internal leaking of an umbilical vessel at the base of the cord. Edema at the base of the cord results from urine leakage from a patent urachus (embryological communication between the urinary bladder and umbilicus). In either case, these findings are localized to the abdominal wall below the umbilicus. Abnormal abdominal findings are discussed more fully in the subchapter entitled "Abdominal Distension and Vomiting at Birth: Detecting Gastrointestinal Anomalies."

Serious visible, midline abdominal defects: There are three varieties of serious midline defects of the abdominal wall: omphalocele, gastroschisis and exstrophy of the bladder. The recognition, support and transport of the newborn with these obvious defects is covered in the subchapter entitled "Externalized Organs and Neural Tube Defects."

Checking for abdominal hernias: There are several types of minor abdominal variations that may be present at birth.

Diastasis recti: This is a mild form of herniation that occurs due to the nonunion of the two rectus muscles that extend from the umbilicus to the xiphoid. Diastasis presents as a gap between the rectus muscles, forming a palpable midline depression up to 1 cm wide when the baby is at rest, with visible bulging along this gap when the baby strains or cries. Varying degrees of separation may be present in normal babies, and the gap tends to close as the baby becomes active in the first weeks after birth. Be sure nothing from within protrudes through this gap (which would classify it as a hernia) by palpating along its length.

Umbilical hernia: The newborn umbilicus is normally protuberant with redundant skin and gives no indication of its appearance in adulthood. Umbilical hernia is a common defect in which the abdominal muscles fail to close around the umbilicus. Intestines protrude into the weaker area, causing the base to feel solid on palpation. These hernias usually present with a diameter less than 4 cm and may protrude 3 to 4 inches from the abdominal wall when intra-abdominal pressure rises. They are especially common among preterm babies as well as male African American infants. If sufficiently large, a small loop of intestine may protrude through the defect, although incarceration is rare; the loop can usually move in and out of the defect and thus poses no immediate problem. These hernias occur when the otherwise normal umbilical ring fails to contract as it should between the 8th and 10th week of gestation. Babies with hypothyroidism usually have umbilical hernias. Palpate the area below and around the umbilicus to confirm that abdominal contents are not distending the area in the gap between the muscles. A large hernia or one that strangles abdominal contents requires surgical intervention.

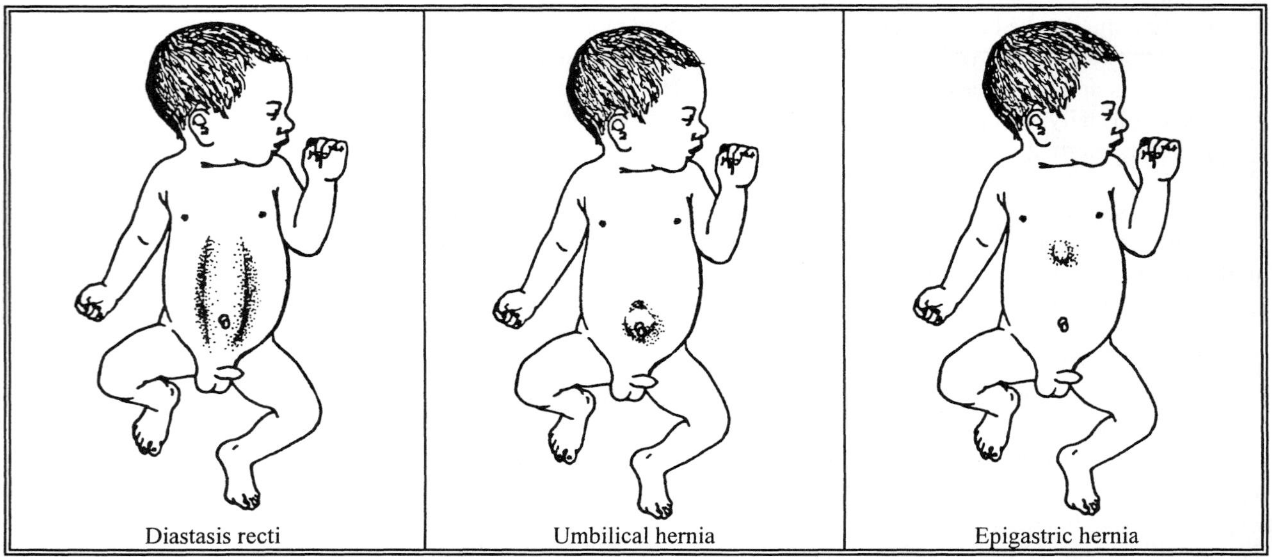

Diastasis recti	Umbilical hernia	Epigastric hernia

Epigastric hernia: An epigastric hernia is a bigger problem. Here, a small, irreducible, fatty protrusion escapes through a rectus muscle defect located anywhere along the midline from above the umbilicus to the lower end of the xiphoid. Palpation may be painful to the baby and surgical correction may be required.

Parietal (Richter) hernia: This rare hernia resembles an epigastric hernia as it also presents between the umbilicus and the xiphoid. It occurs when a portion of the wall of the intestine protrudes (Clark, 2000).

Umbilical cord: The insertion point for the umbilical cord is located midway between the xiphoid and the pubic bone in the center of the abdomen (or 1.5 cm below the midpoint between the crown and the heel) (Crelin, 1973). The circumference of the base averages 7/8 in (2 cm). Some umbilici have a cutaneous, or skin-covered, portion (umbilicus cutis) of varying length that extends from the abdomen until the tissue transitions into the cord proper. The skin on the top side ranges from 7.96 to 15.12 mm while the skin on the underside ranges from 5.82 to 11.6 mm. This is more common in African American babies and, when long enough, heals to form a true "outie" belly button or "skin navel." Umbilicus cutis is not a variation of an umbilical hernia, is soft at the base and cannot be reduced. Excessive length of this skin is seen with Rieger's syndrome. More commonly, the translucent cord terminates at the abdomen (umbilicus amnioticus). The cord should be limp, pearly white and empty of blood if the baby has received a full placental transfusion (Hoekelman, 1991).

If the cord has been cut, the end is typically moist and slightly gooey from the presence of Wharton's jelly. However, the presence of either edema or clear fluid (less commonly, meconium) that oozes from the base of the cord is abnormal. A constant trickle of fluid or moistness is found with a patent urachus. Fluid or meconium may be seen in the very rare event that the vitellointestinal duct, which leaves a communicating tract between the ileum and the umbilicus, is patent. Frank fecal drainage is associated with a fistula into the colon. Any of these defects require transport for surgery as bowel obstruction may result from intestinal kinking or prolapse around the duct. Any drainage other than a tiny amount of residual blood issuing from the cord vessels themselves should be further evaluated by a physician.

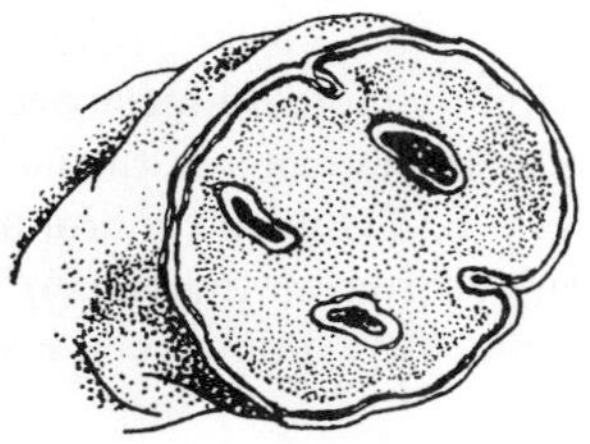

The umbilical stump showing the stumps of the two flattened, collapsed veins and muscular artery

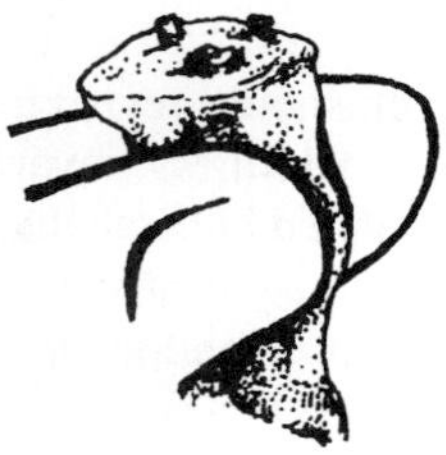

Squeezing the end causes the arteries to protrude and the vein to pout

The umbilical vessels: If the cord has been cut, check the end to determine the number of vessels by grasping the cord stump just below the end between your thumb and forefinger and looking straight down on the cut end. Squeeze the stump between your fingers. This will cause the artery stumps to pucker upward and the opening of the vein to pout, making them all easier to see. A bit of blood may ooze from the open ends of the vessels as you do this; if so, use a gauze pad to pat it dry. The blood helps make the vessels more obvious. There should be two arteries and one vein. The arteries, two little tubes that project upward, have thick, muscular walls. The larger vein has thin, floppy walls and usually exits the abdomen at the 12 o'clock point (keep in mind that the cord tends to spiral; this may displace the vessels if the cord stump is long). If you are unsure that three vessels are present, use your fingers to milk a bit of blood to the ends from further down the cord. Evaluate the cord near the baby's end, in the center and near the placenta to be sure of the number of vessels (for more details about evaluating the number of vessels, extra vessels and missing vessels, see the chapter entitled "Examination of the Placenta"). If you only find two vessels, the baby should receive further evaluation. About 1 out of every 200 babies lacks one of the cord arteries; out of these, about 15 to 20% will have associated cardiovascular or renal anomalies.

If the parents have chosen Lotus birthing, transilluminate the cord in the three places mentioned above to determine the number of vessels. It would only be necessary to discuss cutting the cord for further examination if you were unsure of the number of vessels. To assist in further examination, a cord left intact can also be rehydrated once it falls off.

Cord thickness: Blood flow is the primary determinant of thickness when the vessels are fully engorged. As blood flow diminishes and ceases, the amount of Wharton's jelly, which forms a protective layer around the vessels, becomes the primary determinant of cord thickness. Larger infants tend to have thick, gelatinous cords, while a small, thin cord is often associated with intrauterine growth restriction. Note that congenital syphilis may also result in a very thick umbilical cord. If the base of the cord is broad or remains fluctuant once pulsations have stopped, it may indicate the presence of a small omphalocele, with a portion of the abdominal contents herniated within it; in this case, the cord base may merely appear enlarged or edematous.

Auscultation of the abdomen

Next, with the diaphragm of the infant stethoscope, listen to the baby's belly in all four quadrants of the abdomen. It is common to hear referred breath sounds in the upper abdomen. Normal bowel activity produces intermittent metallic, tinkling sounds that are usually heard every 15 to 20 seconds between feedings. These may become audible within the first 15 minutes after birth, as the baby begins to breathe and swallow air. The normal movement of air through the gastrointestinal tract follows a well-defined pattern. It is found in the stomach shortly after birth, in the proximal bowel by 1 hour, in the distal small bowel by 3 hours and in the distal colon as early as 3 to 4 hours after birth. Progressive air accumulation occurs within the first 4 to 8 hours in both the small and large intestines, and after 8 hours, air predominantly accumulates in the small intestines. Early nursing may alter this sequence, with small bowel air diminishing and colonic air becoming more prominent (Evans, 1951; Wasch & Marck, 1948).

Normal bowel function is reflected by sounds that intensify immediately after a feeding and diminish prior to the next feeding. Peristaltic sounds that are either consistently absent or overabundant suggest an obstruction or hypermotility of the gastrointestinal tract. Bruits are harsh, intermittent swishing sounds similar to a systolic heart murmur; they are heard with dilated, tortuous or constricted vessels. If you think you hear an abdominal bruit, change the baby's position to see if the sound continues. If it does, renal artery stenosis, an abnormality of the umbilical vein or the hepatic vessels or a hemangioma of the liver are all possible associated factors. Auscultate over the kidneys. If a bruit is heard there, renal artery stenosis is likely.

Abdominal percussion

Percussion of the abdomen should reveal uniform dullness, with slightly more dullness over dense organs such as the liver and spleen. Pronounced dullness may indicate enlarged organs, a tumor or an intestinal obstruction. Dull sounds that shift as the baby is repositioned indicate that the abdomen contains fluid. Tympanic or drum-like sounds are normal when found below the border of the left rib cage but suggest air-filled regions from air trapped in the gastrointestinal tract when they are found over the central abdomen. These variations are subtle. Any pronounced irregularity of sound over the abdomen is abnormal.

Abdominal palpation

Palpate the quiet supine baby's belly with warm hands. (A crying or struggling baby will have tense abdominal muscles.) In the first 24 hours, the baby's belly may be distended with meconium, which can also render palpation somewhat difficult. Babies tolerate palpation best when the organs are brought to the examining hand, rather than probed by the fingertips pushing into the abdomen. If you are right-handed, stand to the baby's right; if you are left-handed, stand to the baby's left. Use your nondominant hand to help relax the abdominal muscles by flexing the baby's knees and hips or by grasping the ankles and lifting the baby's bottom off the mattress slightly. Keep your dominant hand flat and use the fingerpads rather than the tips to palpate the entire abdominal region for masses. Begin below the umbilicus on both sides and move up toward the diaphragm. Holding the fingers together, use the pads to press in shallow, smooth, gentle, rocking movements and then repeat, pressing deeper into the tissue. Do not use rough, poking or abrupt movements. Watch the baby for signs of distress during this exam, including crying, grimacing, drawing up of the legs or contraction of the abdominal muscles. When reaching for organs or masses, press more deeply as the baby exhales and the abdomen recedes. If the organs are difficult to find with the baby supine, try turning the baby over, which allows the organs to fall toward your hands, and reach your fingers under either side of the abdomen to palpate from beneath.

Consistency: The overall consistency of the abdomen on superficial palpation should be about the same throughout the belly. Tension or rigidity suggests peritoneal irritation or distention. When you are just learning, note that a baby who has not passed meconium will have a more firm and full-feeling belly than one who has. Flaccid tone suggests neuromuscular disease or exposure to drugs causing neonatal depression. The meconium-filled descending colon, which may be easily felt in the lower left quadrant, has a pliable sausage shape but will not be very distinct nor remarkably firmer than the surrounding region.

Rarely, a portion of the bowel channel slips into another (causing a folding inward and doubling of the walls, similar to folding a cuff on a sock). This is called **intussusception** and presents a sausage-like mass in the right or left upper quadrant. Although pyloric stenosis rarely presents at birth, an oval mass about the size of an olive between the umbilicus and the right lower costal margin is palpable in most infants that will later manifest pyloric stenosis. This mass is most easily found after feeding or vomiting. Solid or fluctuant (cystic) masses may be located in the urinary tract, especially the kidneys, or on the ovaries in a girl. Note that an enlarged ureter may be mistaken for a large loop of bowel on deep palpation. It would be found to one side the spine but be less mobile than a loop of bowel.

Palpating the liver: Normally, the lower border of the liver is felt about 1 to 3 cm below the margin of the rib cage at the midclavicular line; the border is followed across the upper abdomen as it slopes upward toward the midleft costal margin. At term, the normal liver is 5.1 to 6.7 cm high at the midclavicular line. The height of the liver can also be determined by percussing the upper and lower margins. The body of the liver is smooth and firm, with a soft but well-defined border. A very hard or nodular surface is not normal. A full or overly firm edge may be associated with a markedly increased total blood volume as well as elevated extramedullary hematopoiesis, chronic infection, an infiltrative process and sometimes congestive heart failure.

Palpate the liver to define its margins, size and location of the lobes. To do so, place the pad of your thumb or index finger in the lower right quadrant of the abdomen just above the groin in the midclavicular line parallel to the edge of the rib cage. Using a gentle compressing motion. Too firm a touch may cause you to miss the soft edge. Gradually move the finger upward until the edge of the liver slips below it. You should feel a resistance that falls away as your fingers pass over the edge, which should be soft but distinct. Another technique calls for standing at the head of the baby, reaching down to the midabdomen on the right with the fingertips toward the groin. Using a gentle compressing and rocking motion, move upward until the lower margin of the liver is identified. Liver enlargement cannot be accurately assessed by finding the lower border alone, because it does not distinguish displacement downward from a variety of causes. To find the upper border of the liver, place the diaphragm of an infant stethoscope over the liver and scratch the skin lightly with a finger, starting at a point above where you think the upper edge of the liver is. Move the scratching downward until there is a definite increase in the intensity of the sound, indicating the location of the liver's edge. If the upper margin is at or near the fifth intercostal space in the midclavicular line, palpation of the lower edge is a reliable index of actual liver enlargement. If the upper margin is lower than the fifth intercostal space, intrathoracic pathology may be displacing the liver downward due to such conditions as deformities of the thorax, space-occupying lesions such as pleural effusion, pneumothorax, or abscess, as well as relaxation of the abdominal muscles caused by hypotonia or a congenital defect of the abdominal wall.

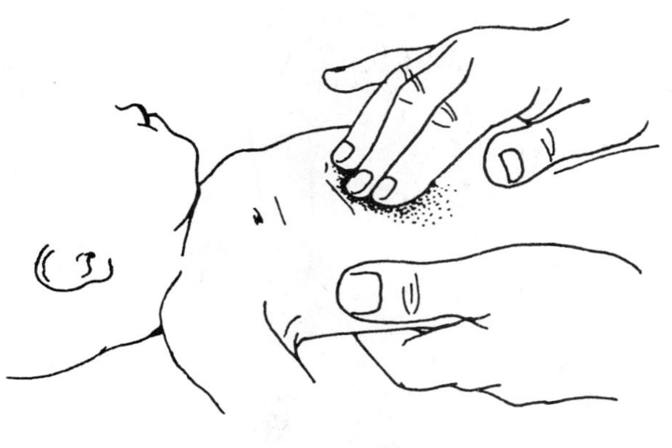

Liver palpation: moving up to the margin from below

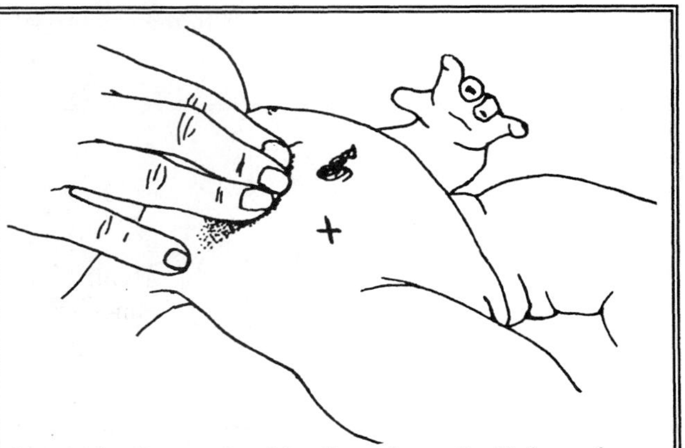

Liver palpation: approaching from above, the X shows the level at which palpation should begin.

As you palpate the liver and spleen, remember that traumatic or aggressive handling of the baby at birth or during resuscitation can lead to rupture, although if the liver *is* ruptured, the baby will appear normal for the first 24 to 48 hours thereafter. A mass in the liver region may be felt, with abdominal distention following as blood fills the peritoneal cavity.

Feel for liver pulsations with your index and long fingers, taking care to differentiate pulsations from movement due to rapid breathing. Pulsations are highly abnormal and indicate cardiac defects. A liver that has a rounded, full or firm edge or one that extends more than 3 cm below the right costal margin or that is soft and large with a poorly defined border suggests congestion, an early sign of congestive heart failure. The liver can be thought of as a venous pressure bag; it is a sensitive indicator of elevated right atrial pressure, which is indicated when pulsations can be felt in the liver. Enlargement may also be present with perinatal infection, blood group incompatibilities, tumor or cyst formation, or hemangioma. Note that a hyperexpanded chest will cause the lower border to be displaced downward, giving the impression that a normal liver is enlarged.

Palpating the spleen: Use the same maneuvers described above on the left side of the baby's abdomen, beginning at the level of the umbilicus, to examine the spleen, which is usually not palpable. With sufficient skill, the tip may just be felt on deep palpation 1 to 2 cm below the left costal margin in 10 to 20% of all normal babies. A spleen tip felt 1 cm or more below the left costal margin may indicate a disorder wherein an enlarged liver is misplacing the spleen. Chest hyperexpansion can also displace the spleen downward, causing it to be more easily palpable, although the normal spleen is small. Spleen enlargement is seen with infection and extramedullary hematopoiesis.

Palpating the kidneys: Attempt to palpate the kidneys, although this is usually not an easy exam. They are most easily found in the first day or two of life, before the bowel has become distended. Ideally, the kidneys are palpated at birth, before the abdomen has had a chance to fill with air. The newborn kidneys are typically 4 to 5 cm long, 2 to 2.5 cm wide and 1.2 to 1.5 cm deep to the surface of the abdomen and feels like a stuffed, medium-sized olive under four or five blankets. The left kidney is more easily palpated than the right, unless the descending colon is filled with meconium. The right kidney is slightly lower in the posterior abdomen, but the liver partially overlies it, which often prevents palpation, although its lower pole can sometimes be located with patience. Both kidneys are more difficult to locate in an irritable crying infant because of abdominal tension as well as limb movement. However, if the abdomen is quite relaxed, lobulations of the kidneys may sometimes be identified. Note that kidneys that are easily felt are most likely enlarged.

Because palpating the kidneys is distressing to most babies, this assessment can wait until you are almost done with your exam. There are two examination techniques that can be used to find the kidneys. With either of these, flexing the hip on the side to be examined will relax the abdominal muscles and make the exam easier.

1. The baby should be supine. Stand at the baby's feet. Place the fingers of each hand on either side of the baby under the baby's back, with the index fingers at the level of the lowest costovertebral angle on either side of the spine. The thumbs are parallel with the umbilicus. Examine one side at a time. Gently compress the thumb into the abdomen while lifting up with your finger as if to cause them to meet. While maintaining the pressure, gently move your thumb up and down from the midline and to the side to palpate the kidney region. Deep palpation with a smooth, firm pressure is used.

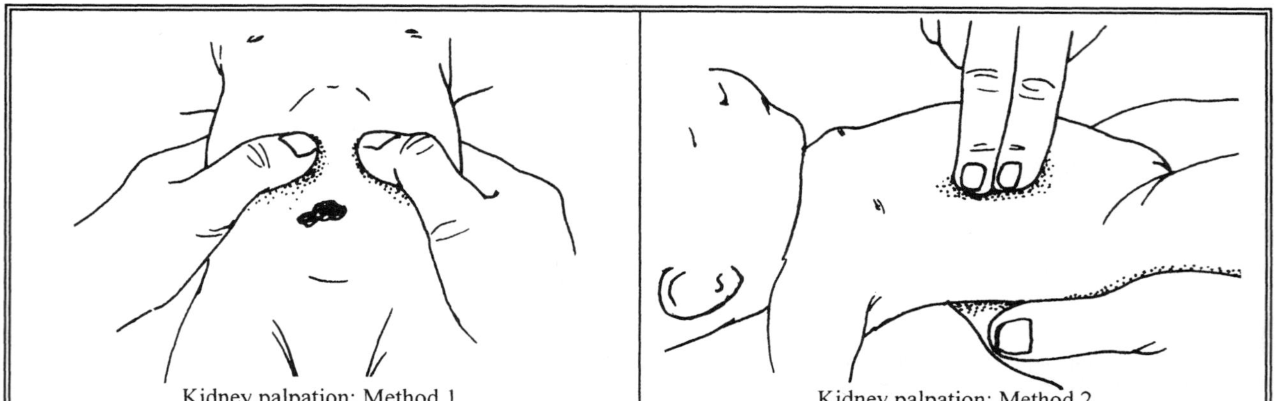

Kidney palpation: Method 1

Kidney palpation: Method 2

2. Another method is to place the baby supine and stand to the baby's left to palpate the right kidney. Place your left hand

under the right side of the baby's lower back, with the third finger in the lowermost costovertebral angle and lift upward. Use the index and third finger pads of your right hand anteriorly to press downward over the region of the left kidney to trap it between your fingers. Stand on the opposite side of the baby and reverse hand maneuvers to examine the right kidney. While the upper end of the right kidney is often not felt (it may be noted if enlarged), the lower portion may be found with careful examination as you become more skilled. If that technique doesn't work, try placing your left hand flat between the baby's right rib cage and the pelvis and palpate from the pelvic brim upward with your other hand (Ziai et al., 1984). You may detect abnormal kidneys, bladder or other masses with this technique.

The lower end of a normal newborn kidney has about the consistency and texture of a large grape that slips between your fingers. While fetal lobulation is occasionally noted, the texture should be smooth and firm, not depressible or too irregular; truly lumpy or enlarged kidneys are reasons for concern. To detect abnormal placement or orientation, palpate along either side of the lumbar vertebral column and the upper quadrant of the abdomen as you compress from the sides, allowing the contents to slip under your fingers. If the lower pole of the kidneys are close to the midline, horseshoe kidneys may be present.

Palpating the bladder: The newborn bladder is narrower and located higher in the abdomen, 1 to 4 cm above the symphysis pubis, than in older children. Distention is a normal finding immediately after birth and before the first urination or an hour after feeding. Newborns should void within the first 24 hours after birth. A frequently or continuously full bladder is a sign of central nervous system defects or urethral obstruction.

The bladder is best examined with palpation and percussion. Start by sliding the fingers downward from the umbilicus to detect a swelling in the midline above the pubic bone. The full bladder can be found with percussion before the first urination and then about an hour after nursing (Scanlon et al., 1979).

Palpating for the ureters: Normally the ureters cannot be felt in either sex upon abdominal palpation. Enlarged or distended ureters feel like soft, rounded, compressible masses located in the intra-abdominal area and may be mistaken for loops of bowel, although they are less mobile. Palpable ureters suggest an obstructed urinary tract.

Transillumination of the abdomen

As described by Donn and Kuhns (1983), when suspicious findings are detected, transillumination can be used to further evaluate the abdomen for solid masses or for trapped air or fluid. Fluid- or gas-filled masses can be illuminated when the abdominal wall is thin and lightly pigmented, allowing you to outline their position and size. Meconium-filled bowel loops will not transilluminate; however, an air-filled stomach or bowel, fluid-logged hydronephrotic kidneys, or a distended bladder will. Clear fluid within the peritoneal space (ascites) produces a uniform glow over the anterior abdominal wall when the probe tip is placed against the anterior abdomen. A feature that lights up and shifts when the baby is moved around suggests free air (pneumoperitoneum), which is usually a result of gastric perforation, producing a bright area of abnormal transillumination in the anterior abdomen. Place the tip of the probe in the upper abdomen to the left of center; push it deep and look at the abdomen from the right to visualize the falciform ligament (which longitudinally divides the primary lobes of the liver). Seeing the ligament is helpful in determining that the abnormal findings are due to air rather than loops of bowel. The anterior edge of the liver can sometimes be seen outlined by air; however, air accumulates in front of the liver and tends to push both it and the spleen posteriorly. The liver is more visible in ascites because fluid surrounds the liver and spleen but does not displace them backward.

The liver can be visualized by placing the light source beneath the liver's edge just below the right costal margin. Bowel loops beneath the liver's border transilluminate and allow detection of the opaque edge. The spleen can be seen along the large curve of the stomach when the stomach is filled with gas, and the probe is placed in the upper left quadrant. The liver and sometimes the gall bladder can also be detected when there is fluid in the abdomen. The spleen can be found floating in the fluid as well.

Transillumination of the kidney region begins with placing the baby on her side, legs flexed. The uppermost side of the abdomen is then examined by placing the tip of the flashlight (with the cuff, if any, removed) deep into the upper abdominal quadrant. The light source is then redirected like an examining finger, applying soft, gentle pressure until the probe tip is in the region of the kidney. Bowel loops will tend to be displaced away from the probe tip. However, if the kidney is absent, bowel loops can occupy the renal space and simulate a hydronephrotic kidney (a condition of swelling that, when marked, renders the kidney outline invisible). Once the probe is believed to be in place, look at the costovertebral angle on the back of the baby and attempt to see if an abnormal area of transillumination exists, which suggests a cystic or obstructive lesion of the kidney. Occasionally, a normal kidney outline can be seen when there is sufficient air in the surrounding bowel anterior to the kidney. Most of the time, however, the kidneys cannot be seen when they are normal. A dilated ureter can sometimes be seen in the anterior inferior abdomen when the light is placed anteriorly on the abdomen; however, loops of bowel filled with air or fluid may stimulate a dilated ureter.

A full bladder can be easily identified when the cuffed probe tip is placed in the suprapubic region on either side of the rectus muscle and directed toward the midline.

Examining the Groin

The groin is longitudinal region of the lower abdomen along the anterior crease of each thigh, where the legs join the body. It should be observed when the baby is quiet. Here, on either side, lie the inguinal canals. Each canal is a tube that begins at an internal ring about midway between the hip and the symphysis and exits via an external ring that opens at the top of the scrotum in a boy and the top of the labial mound in a girl. This area should be flat, although some babies have a prominent pubic mound, which is symmetrically soft. Visible femoral pulses are sometimes evident. The femoral triangle's base runs along the inguinal canal and extends to a point in the midline of the thigh, terminating about half-way to the knee. This area is visualized and palpated for the presence of bulges, masses and pulses. The mnemonic "NAVEL" can be used to help remember what you are looking for: nerve, artery, vein, empty space and lymph nodes. (Note that the examination of the groin overlaps with the genital exam.)

Swellings

All swellings in or near the groin are abnormal. Any swelling in the crease is most likely a herniated part that is lying in the canal, and any swelling beyond the crease is most commonly a herniated part that has passed down through the external ring into the genitals. If the part is still in the canal, place your fingertip at the external opening to see if you can feel anything descending further down the canal. You are less likely to detect a hernia if the baby is quiet and relaxed; many are only obvious when the baby is crying or straining. Use a stethoscope to listen over the herniated bulge. Bowel sounds may be heard if loops of intestine are involved. Bleeding may also lead to swelling, which is usually associated with testicular trauma during the birth.

An incomplete hernia produces a soft swelling just above the crease of the leg. The swelling may extend down into the scrotum to the side of the penis. The bulge may only be apparent during straining or crying, characterizing it as a reducible hernia. The parents may notice a hernia appearing intermittently after birth, and any such reports should prompt a careful examination. An increase in intra-abdominal tension may cause the hernia to descend. To produce straining, have an assistant hold the baby's arms over his head and press the knees into extension while you watch and feel the groin on both sides; the bulge may appear only briefly or not at all. If the baby has a normal but prominent pubic mound, it may confuse your findings. The normal pubic mound is in the midline and symmetrically rounded and soft. A hernia will be off the midline and located above and to the side of the symphysis; it is also softer.

Indirect inguinal hernia: An indirect inguinal hernia is so named because the prolapse occurs through the inguinal canal but is contained in a pouch of peritoneum. It is the most common surgical problem in the newborn. An indirect hernia results from persistent patency of the processus vaginalis, an embryonic structure that appears during the third month of gestation as an outpouching of the peritoneum at the internal inguinal ring. In boys at about 28 weeks, it attaches to the testicle during its descent through the inguinal canal into the scrotum. The upper end of the processus vaginalis normally fuses, closing off its entrance to the peritoneal cavity in both sexes during the last few weeks of gestation. The portion attached to the testes forms the tunica vaginalis. In boys, persistent patency is known as a patent processus vaginalis; in girls, it is known as the canal of Nuck. It is still patent at birth in 1 to 5% of all babies, with a 10% incidence in preterm babies (35% of these occur in babies less than 28 weeks of gestation). These hernias are 4 to 10 times more common in boys than in girls. The reported incidence of inguinal hernia ranges from 0.8 to 4.4% in children, of which 98.6% are indirect, 1.2% are direct and 0.2% are femoral (Fletcher, 1998).

The opening at the inguinal ring may allow abdominal contents to descend into the pouch formed by the patent processus vaginalis. This prolapse can descend as far as the scrotum in boys. The right side is involved about twice as often as the left, although bilateral hernias are commonly found later when a left-sided hernia is obvious at birth. If the opening is small, only fluid will descend, resulting in a hydrocele in either sex, but most commonly in boys. A larger opening allows a loop of small intestine to descend as well (an indirect congenital inguinal hernia is always accompanied by some degree of hydrocele). The testis or lymph nodes present as abnormal groin swellings. In preterm boys, the testes may not be fixed in the scrotum and can be repositioned into the inguinal canal. Inguinal lymph nodes seldom swell to the size of an inguinal hernia and are positioned below the inguinal crease, where they mimic a femoral hernia (Fletcher, 1998). In boys, an inguinal hernia can be differentiated from a hydrocele or a hematocele because the spermatic cord cannot be felt to overlie the hernia, whereas in the other two conditions it is palpable.

Indirect inguinal hernias are uncommon in girls but feel exactly the same as in a boy. They may be located in the labia majora, where they form a pronounced bulge over the mound of Venus on one or both sides. Egg tube or ovary prolapse into the labia majora may occasionally occur in girls. The ovary is felt as a small, movable marble in the inguinal canal that is similar to a swollen lymph node. However, the presence of a groin swelling in a girl may also be an abnormal gonad; genotyping to confirm the genetic sex is mandatory before the hernia is explored (Fletcher, 1998).

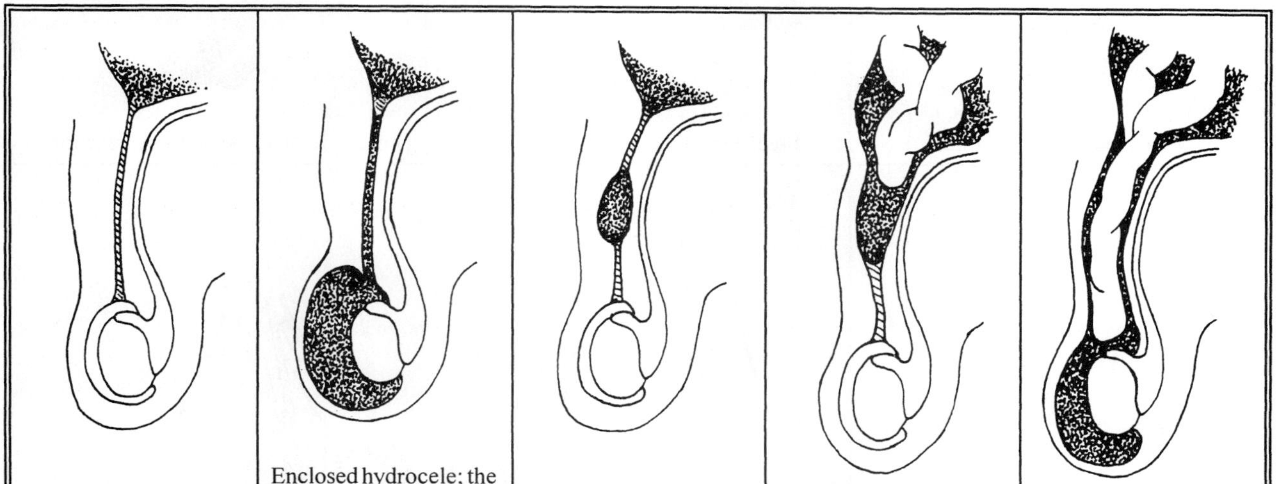

Lateral view of left groin in a normal boy	Enclosed hydrocele; the processus vaginalis is fused superiorly.	Hydrocele of the processus vaginalis	Incomplete indirect hernia	Complete indirect hernia

Direct inguinal hernia: Far less commonly seen in the neonate, a direct hernia is a defect in the musculature of the abdominal wall that occurs between the deep epigastric artery and the lower edge of one of the rectus abdominal muscles. Such a defect allows loops of intestines or fluid to prolapse into the area immediately above and anterior to the lower end of the inguinal canal. The hernia bulges outward, pushing the side of the examining finger forward when the baby strains. It rarely descends as far as the scrotum. An extremely large direct inguinal hernia presses against the lower end of the inguinal canal where it can strain the attachment of the rectus muscle.

Femoral hernia: The femoral canal is a funnel-shaped passage, located about one-quarter of the way between the pubic bone and the hip, that allows passage of lymphatics to the upper leg. A femoral hernia passes under the inguinal ligament, through the femoral canal and exits at the external ring, which is the lower opening of the femoral canal. The femoral ring is normally closed only by a septum of modified extraperitoneal tissue and is therefore a weak spot. When a loop of intestines bulges into the femoral canal, a sac of peritoneum is pushed ahead of it. The loop descends through the femoral ring, where it is prevented from descending further due to the narrowing of the femoral sheath. It is then pushed forward, upward and somewhat laterally toward the inguinal ligament. Once it reaches the loose connective tissue of the inguinal ligament, it enlarges. Attempts at reduction should follow this path in reverse. The hernia may present beside and medial to the femoral artery producing a small round bulge that is often difficult to distinguish from a lymph node. It may also present along the inguinal ligament, adjacent to the genitals. The femoral ring is wider at the top and larger in females, hence the higher prevalence of femoral hernias in girls. This type of hernia can also occur in boys, but the anatomy is such that it never descends into the scrotum. Overall, this is the least common type of hernia in newborns (Fletcher, 1998).

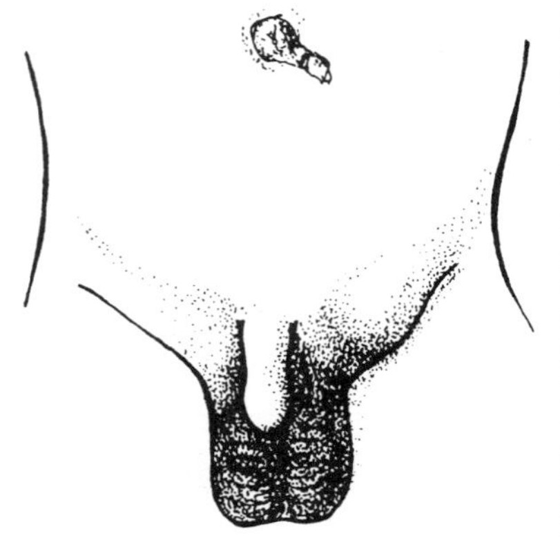

Indirect hernia that has not descended into the scrotum

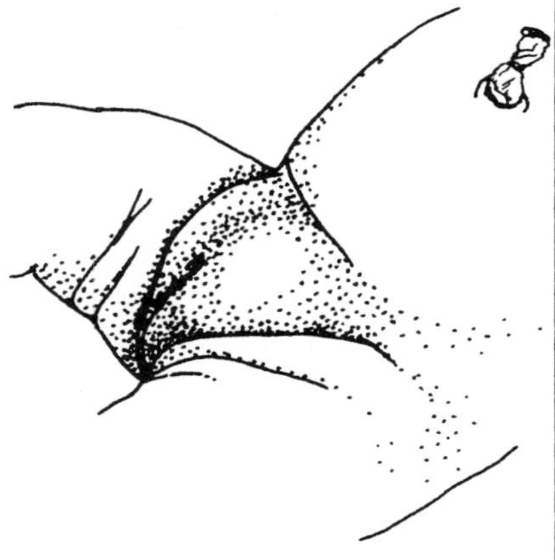

Indirect hernia on her left side in a girl

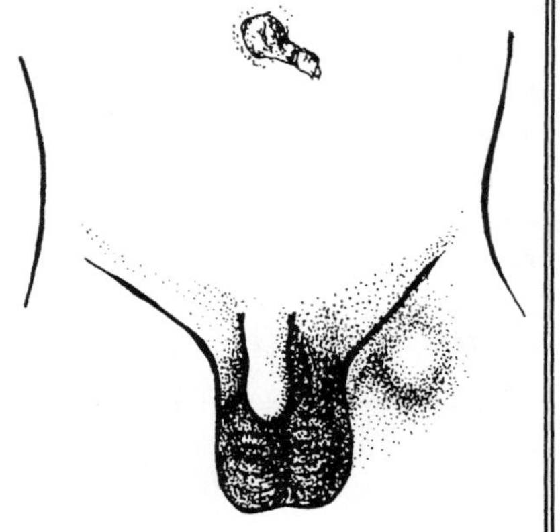

Femoral hernia (looks the same in girls)

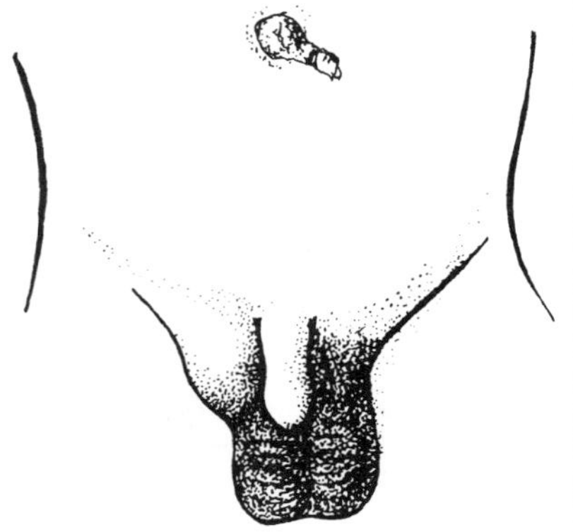

Direct hernia

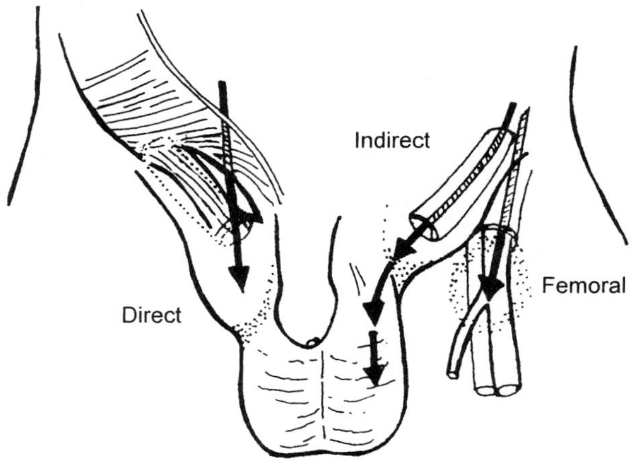

Pathways of indirect, direct and femoral hernias

Interstitial hernia: This rare defect may appear by itself or in conjunction with an inguinal or femoral hernia. It usually protrudes between the internal and external oblique muscles. It is more common in males and is associated with abnormal testicular descent. It presents as an ill-defined swelling extending upward and laterally from the level of the internal inguinal ring toward the hip. It may become incarcerated and be confused with torsion of the undescended testicle. If suspected, the baby should be evaluated further by a pediatrician (Johnstone, 1994).

Reducing a hernia: If an inguinal hernia is found, gently try to return it to its proper position. Sometimes, simply elevating the baby into a steep Trendelenburg position will cause it to retract as a result of tension on the mesentery. If not, try manual reduction. If the hernia is on the baby's right, form an inverted "V" (or wide "pinch") with the tips of the thumb and index finger of your left hand at the level of the external inguinal ring, which is found at the top of the inguinal crease, and apply gentle downward pressure to prevent superficial reduction of the prolapse. With your right hand, position your fingers on the scrotum (or labia) below the prolapsed part. Use a gently pinching and pushing motion with upward pressure *below* the prolapse to push the protruding parts directly back toward the opening. The contents may slip back into the abdomen with a characteristic gurgling sound if air has had time to traverse the bowel to reach this level. If the hernia is on the baby's left, reverse your hand maneuvers (Johnstone, 1994).

When reduced and empty, the open canal may feel like a thickened cord. With experience, you may be able to feel the slippery inner surface of the canal as the two sides are rubbed against each other, the "silk-glove sign," although this is often hard to detect in newborns Replacement will not be possible if the baby is tense and should be stopped if it seems to cause pain. If you cannot replace the parts or it is very difficult to do so, the herniated organs are said to be "irreducible" and are more susceptible to strangulation; surgery is indicated. A hydrocele of the cord may mimic an incarcerated hernia; distinguishing the two is covered under "Scrotum" in the subchapter entitled "Examining the Genitalia, Perineum and Anus," which follows. Any baby found to have a hernia on one side should be carefully examined on the other (Johnstone, 1994).

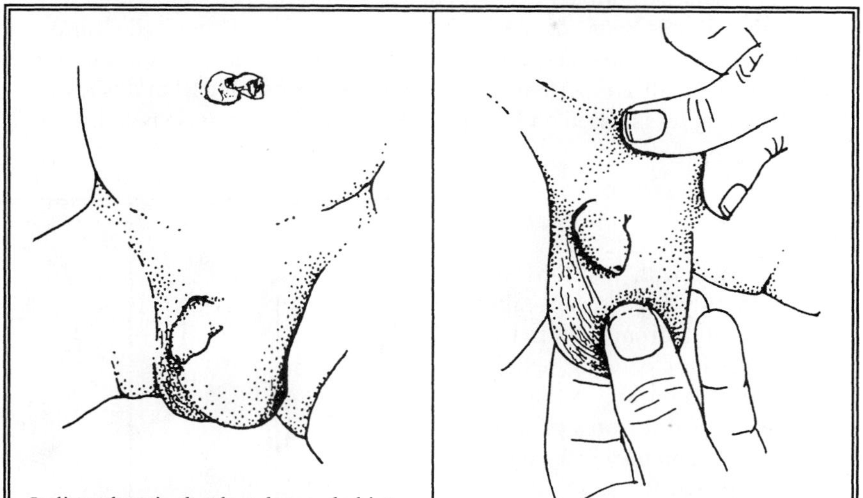

Indirect hernia that has descended into the scrotum

Reducing the hernia

EXAMINING THE GENITALIA, PERINEUM AND ANUS

Examination of the genitals includes visualization and palpation and sometimes auscultation, percussion, measurement and transillumination. You are looking for normal formation of the genitals and unequivocal evidence of the sex of the infant. Be sure of the gestational age of the baby and be familiar with the normal variations that occur in the genitals as the baby matures, otherwise normal features of maturation may be mistakenly interpreted as atypical. Note that the term "ambiguous genitalia" has been replaced with the term "atypical genitalia" in deference to the vocal movement of intersex adults who have suffered at the hands of a medical profession that has tried to fit them into either the "boy" or the "girl" box. More about this important topic is addressed in Volume III of this text and in a recent edition of my DIAGNOSTIC TESTS. This chapter is based on Fletcher (1998), unless otherwise noted.

Female Genitalia

Position the baby on her back with her hips fully abducted and her knees flexed to fully expose the genitals. Inspect and gently palpate the genitals from front to back, examining the labia, clitoris, urethral opening, external vault of the yoni and perineum. You are noting size, location and the relation of the external features to the rest of the baby's anatomy. Your inspection may be hampered by the presence of vernix in the genital folds; however, do not attempt to remove all of it. Try instead to work around it and remove only enough to complete your exam. Be alert for any unusual findings, even one of any of the abnormalities presented in this discussion is suspicious; the presence of two or more greatly increases the probability of an intersex condition.

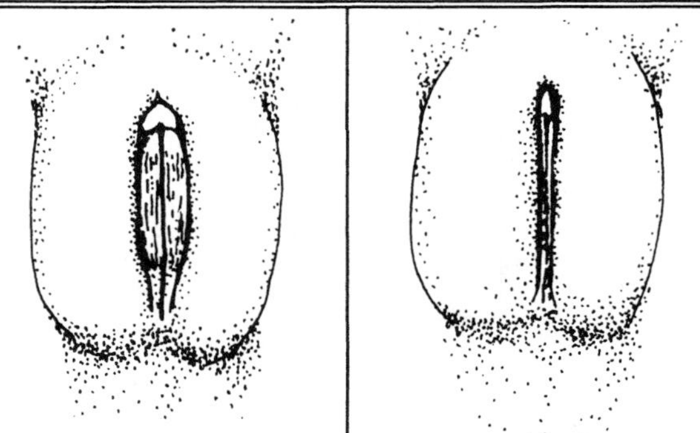

Normal female genitals at 37 weeks | Normal female genitals at term

Labia

The labia majora of the term infant are large and usually completely or almost completely cover the clitoris and labia minora. In an early baby, the labia minora are larger, the labia majora are more separated and proportionally smaller, and the clitoris appears more prominent. Most of the fat in the labia majora is laid down near term.

The labia minora and majora are usually edematous at birth and should be smooth, with only tiny scattered wrinkles as the skin dries. These may be more pronounced if the baby has lost weight in utero; however, there should be no true rugae. Pigmentation along the edges of the labia minora is normal in babies, regardless of gestational age, and is more pronounced in babies-of-color. Gently part the labia majora and the labia minora to rule out fusion along their edges. Masculinization results in posterior fusion of the labioscrotal folds with or without enlargement of the clitoris.

While the normal labia majora can be quite plump, bulging is not normal. Gently palpate the labia and inguinal region to rule out any masses. A mass may indicate a hernia or may be a gonad that has descended; it could be a normal, herniated ovary, but this is rare. It is more likely to indicate an intersex state. The baby should be evaluated without undue delay.

On occasion, benign vesicles similar to milia may be found grouped around the genitalia. Like milia, they should not be red at the base. They may range in diameter from 0.5 to 1 cm. These often rupture in the days following birth.

Bruising and edema may be present when a baby has been born in a frank breech position. Watch for excoriation (peeling and breaking of the skin) of the edematous areas over the next few days.

Clitoris

The clitoris is found in the triangular point of the cleft between the labia minora. Its full size is achieved by 27 weeks gestation. By term, it is usually covered by the labia majora, but in preterm girls, it is exposed and may appear prominent. Enlargement of the clitoris at birth is usually due to edema. True enlargement suggests pseudohermaphroditism and is associated with adrenal hyperplasia, which affects 1 in every 14,000 live births. Underdevelopment is associated with syndromes that cause hypogonadism and microgenitalia in males, such as Prader-Willi syndrome, and with growth hormone deficiency. The clitoris can be measured whenever there is doubt about its size. Gently and firmly press the shaft between your thumb and forefinger to exclude excess skin from the measurement, allowing the width of the corpora cavernosa to be assessed. Use a small ruler to measure the width of the shaft; this normally ranges from 2 to 6 mm, averaging 3.22 mm in the term newborn. Width and length are roughly the same, and width is easier to measure than length.

Urethral meatus

The urethral meatus is located directly beneath the clitoris. It can be very hard to see, but should be visualized to confirm its normal placement. Place your gloved thumbs and index fingers on the labia majora and gently press down and to either side to spread the labia apart. Alternatively, gently "pinch" each labia, then pull them forward and spread them to either side slightly. Either of these techniques should render the meatus visible.

Misplacement of the meatus may occur in both sexes. If the meatus is placed near or inside the yoni (female hypospadias, which occurs in 1 of every 500,000 female births), it is associated with other genitourinary anomalies (Smith, 2004).

Female epispadias presents with anterior displacement of the meatus above or through an enlarged clitoris, which usually also involves an accompanying split down the midline of clitoris, separated labia and a flattened mons. In its mildest form, the urethra may only form a pouch. Intermediate forms present a dorsal separation of most of the urethra. Most severely, the cleft extends to involve the external sphincter of the urethra, resulting in incontinence. This is also quite rare, affecting 1 baby in every 100,000 live births with 5 boys affected for every girl (Medcylopaedia, 2004). In either case, the baby requires further evaluation.

The normal urine stream is emitted in a steady flow and does not dribble or markedly project. An ectopic ureter is located to the side of the normal urethra and will result in constant drainage of urine. Prolapse of the urethra appears as a red, lobulated (raspberry-like), mass of mucous membrane extruded from the urethra; neural tube defects should be ruled out. Another variation that may be found in some normal babies is periurethral bands; these symmetrical bands originate to either side of the urethra and are connected to the wall of the vestibule (the region between the labia minora).

Yoni

The opening of the yoni is normally visible upon spreading the lower labia majora. It should be pink and glistening, and normally appears as a 3 to 4 mm slit or star-shaped opening with crinkled, heaped-up mucosa around the orifice. Patency is implied if a creamy white mucoid secretion fills the opening (this may be slightly blood tinged due to the influence of maternal hormones). About 25% of all normal girls have a midline white streak or spots in the area between the fourchette and the posterior hymenal border. This is known as **linear vestibularis** and occurs due to avascularity or a posterior fourchette raphe (line of union between symmetrical structures). It is best observed with the labia fully parted.

Fecal discharge from the yoni indicates the presence of a fistula between the rectum and the yoni. Genital prolapse through the hymenal ring presents as a pink mass at the introitus. This is usually associated with congenital spinal defects or neuromuscular disorders. An intersex condition or adrenogenital syndrome both can produce a double-orifice perineum with an anterior urogenital opening and a normally positioned anus. Complete agenesis of the yoni occurs in only 1 out of every 4000 to 5000 live births; these babies usually have a normal female karyotype. Duplication of the yoni, uterus, cervix or some combination thereof may also occur in genetically normal females.

Hymen: Newborns often have large, lax hymens that are widely variable in shape and appearance. The edge may be smooth and rounded, crescent shaped, or frilly. The hymenal opening may be centered, positioned slightly above center or slightly off to one side. Tags of glistening mucosal tissue may extend from 1 to 15 mm beyond the rim of the hymen; these generally disappear in a few weeks.

Up to 14% of all newborn girls have a degree of imperforate hymen. A completely imperforate hymen occurs in 1 out of every 2000 girls. This may or may not be obvious at birth; if it is, it will present as a pale pink to whitish bubble-like mass protruding from the introitus. It may rupture on its own; if not, it should be opened by a physician so that normal yoni discharges can escape. Genital tract obstruction can be due to a partial or completely intact hymen, hymenal bands, a membrane that spans the yoni or yoni atresia. **Hydrometrocolpos** occurs when secretions accumulate in the yoni and uterus because of excessive intrauterine hormonal stimulation coupled with obstruction. If secretion build-up is limited to the yoni, the condition is termed **hydrocolpos**. A uterus that is enlarged from backed-up secretions presents as an abdominal mass; it may obstruct bowel function or urination and may even produce edema of the lymph nodes in the lower extremities with impaired venous return. An enlarged greater vestibular (Bartholin) gland may appear to be an imperforate hymen with discharge backed up behind it.

Perineum

The perineum should be smooth, with no pockets or fistulas. Incomplete fusion of the perineum from the posterior fourchette to the anus is a benign variation not to be confused with injury. Openings or dimpling in the perineum may be seen with intersex conditions.

The perineum is also inspected for normal location of the anus and the presence of any rectal fistulas. The number of genital orifices should be counted. An abnormally placed anus may be located anywhere along the perineum as well as in the opening between the fourchette and hymen (it may appear to be the normal opening of the yoni), within the yoni above the hymen, or on the dry perineal skin. Bulging of the perineum, with or without accompanying lower abdominal enlargement, may be due to build-up of fluid behind a transverse yoni septum (hydometrocolpos).

Uterus

It is assumed that a normal uterus is present when the external genitalia appear completely normal. The uterus averages 7/8 in (2 cm) in length at term. While a rectal exam using the little finger is described in the literature to examine the newborn uterus, this is no doubt a painful and traumatic exam for the baby. Furthermore, the newborn rectal and anal mucosa are very fragile and prone to laceration, compounding the baby's discomfort and possibly resulting in long-term emotional damage. Ultrasound may be used to determine if a uterus is present in a baby whose genitals are not clearly female. However, this, too, is problematic as it exposes her eggs to ultrasound, an unproven technology. Any question regarding the presence of a uterus in a baby presumed to be a girl should be left to the experts.

Findings That Constitute a Normal Genital Exam in a Girl*
•Opening of the yoni is fully visible as a 3 to 4 mm slit or star-shaped orifice with crinkled, heaped-up mucosa. •The lowermost borders of the labia are completely separate (not fused). •Clitoris is 2 to 6 mm wide. •No masses (which might be gonads) are palpated in the labia majora or inguinal region. •The distance between the anus and the fourchette is within normal limits (about 1 cm at term).

*The only exception to this rule is babies with androgen insensitivity syndrome (AIS), who have normal female genitalia externally but who are genetically male with fully developed, undescended testes. If not detected before puberty, this condition is often discovered when the adolescent is evaluated for primary amenorrhea.

Congenital adrenal hyperplasia and virilization of the female genitals

Virilization of the external genitalia is the primary presenting sign of congenital adrenal hyperplasia due to 21-hydroxylase enzyme deficiency in females, the most common case of atypical genitalia in the newborn, occurring in 1 out of every 14,000 live births. The severity varies from mild with an isolated enlarged clitoris or labial fusion to complete labial fusion with scrotalization of the labia majora, a large clitoris and a penile urethra. Typically, the baby has a large clitoris, a single perineal opening for the yoni and bladder and fused labia that have rugose, pigmented skin. The fused labia may obscure a urogenital sinus into which the urethra and yoni open. The baby may appear to be male with bilaterally undescended testes and severe hypospadias. Three-quarters of these babies have the life-threatening, salt-losing form of this defect (see the section on "When the genitals appear atypical" at the end of this subchapter for more details.)

Male genitalia

The glans and shaft of the penis, urethral opening, prepuce (foreskin), scrotum and perineum are examined for size, position and deformity.

Examining the penis

Penial shaft: The penis is assessed for size, downward or upward curvature, rotational deformity and length. A number of normal variations may be found. The length of the shaft is usually lined up in the midline but may be slightly deviated to the left or right. A line of tissue closure, the median raphe, is found on the underside of the shaft, and extends over the midline of the scrotum to the anus in many babies. (A raphe is the line of union between two structures; this one appears as a longitudinal ridge of tissue down the underside of the penis.) Mild to pronounced rotational deformity or torsion (twisting or deviation from the midline) of the median raphe or the entire penile shaft may also occur in some babies. While this can be a normal variation, it can also be associated with hypospadias (described later) or deviation of the meatus.

Large babies may have a pad of fat over the pubic bone that obscures visualization, creating the appearance of a short retracted penis; pressing down on the pad will usually reveal a normal penis. Make a visual assessment. A penis that looks retracted should be lifted carefully to compare the top and bottom lengths; a short underside indicates a high scrotal insertion and a greater chance of problems if the parents choose circumcision.

A **webbed penis** has deficient ventral shaft skin that is buried in the scrotum or tethered to it by a fold or web of skin. The urethra and erectile bodies are usually normal. Webbing commonly occurs with hypospadias, chordee or micropenis.

Ventral bowing of the penile shaft is called **chordee** and is often associated with hypospadias. Chordee restricts the full erection of the penis, producing a downward and inward curve. Chordee is exceptionally rare in the uncircumcised, otherwise normal penis. Intermittent erection is a common and normal occurrence in the newborn.

Constant erection, or **priapism**, is abnormal and may be associated with a spinal cord defect. Webbing occurs when the scrotal skin extends onto the underside of the penial shaft, causing the penis to appear short; the testes may drop down into the scrotal sac level with the glans; the urethra and scrotum are otherwise normal.

Rarely (1 in 10 to 30 million boys), the penis is completely absent in the presence of an otherwise normal scrotum, with the urethra exiting on the perineum. Penile duplication is also rare.

Measuring the penis: Measure the penis only if you suspect the size to be abnormal. Use a small, rigid ruler, or better, mark measurements on a tongue depressor; as its rounded end will be more comfortable for the baby. A piece of opaque tape wrapped around the end of a rounded spoon handle could also be marked and used as a makeshift ruler.

Penile length is measured by stretching the shaft to its full length first. Grasp the penis just beneath the glans with your thumb and forefinger and gently extend it. Use your other hand to press the ruler against the pubic ramus, depressing the fat pad as much as possible. Measure to the tip of the glans only, not the end of the loose foreskin. The tip of the glans can be easily felt through the unretracted foreskin, do not attempt to push the foreskin back for this measurement. The width is measured at the midshaft of the gently stretched penis. The term infant's stretched penis length normally ranges from 3 to 3.5 cm, with findings less than 2.5 cm being abnormally short. The average penile width is 0.9 to 1.5 cm. If the dimensions of the penis are less than 1.5×0.7, the baby should be evaluated further.

Micropenis (or penile hypoplasia) is present when the urethra is both normally formed and placed but either the stretched length of the penis is less than 2.5 cm at term or the penile corpora cavernosa are absent or severely deficient, resulting in an abnormally thin penis (excluding atypical genitalia or the penis with hypospadias or chordee). Micropenis is associated with cryptorchidism, persistent jaundice and cleft lip or palate, and strongly suggests congenital hypopituitarism. It is found in more than 30 clinical syndromes; however, it is not associated with atypical genitalia. Most commonly, it results from hypogonadism and responds well to testosterone therapy. Intersex conditions of the male genitalia center on the incomplete formation of or defects of the penis rather than hypoplasia per se.

Foreskin: The normal foreskin usually covers the entire glans, is quite tight and is usually not retractable in newborns. *NEVER attempt to forcefully retract the foreskin to visualize the glans.* The newborn foreskin is attached to the glans by a number of adhesions, which will stretch and break as the child matures. Premature rupture of these adhesions may lead to bleeding, swelling, pain, infection, and an inability to return the foreskin to its unretracted position. A benign squamous-cell inclusion cyst, also called a **urethral retention cyst** (a form of Epstein's pearl) may be present as a little whitish or yellowish pimple on the foreskin or the tip of the glans. The foreskin is partially absent in 10% of otherwise normal boys, however it should raise your suspicion of hypospadias, which is often accompanied by partial absence of the foreskin.

Glans: In the normal penis, the glans cannot be directly examined because the foreskin tightly overlies it. The blunt-tipped cone of the glans can be gently palpated and sometimes visualized through the foreskin. It can be inferred that the glans is normal when the foreskin is normal. In rare cases, when the foreskin can be retracted enough to expose the glans, the glans normally appears cherry red with an exquisitely smooth surface. The glans is also exposed when the baby has hypospadias and is often heart shaped and may be deeply cleft, depending upon the location of the urethra. Numerous other anomalies of glans formation are possible, usually involving anomalies of the foreskin as well.

Urethral meatus: Some foreskins will naturally retract enough to allow visualization of the meatus. To determine if this is the case, hold the penis upright with one hand and grasp the penis on either side of the glans with the thumb and forefinger of your other hand. *Slowly and very gently* move the foreskin downward *only as far as it will go easily.* You are taking advantage of the foreskin's natural range of looseness, not forcing it back. This may move it just enough to expose the urethral opening, or meatus. This should be a very small (1.8 to 3.4 mm) vertical slit in the upper center of the glans. A round, rigid meatus suggests stenosis. It can be inferred that the urethral opening is normal and correctly placed at the tip of the glans when the foreskin is fully developed and covers the tip of an otherwise normal glans. Visualization to confirm this is not required.

If the anterior portion of the foreskin is not fully formed, locate the urethral opening by gently pulling outward on the anterior skin just enough to take up any slack. This may reveal a functioning meatus that is further down the shaft, to be distinguished from a commonly present blind pit that develops closer to the tip of the penis.

A relatively common abnormality involves misplacement of the meatus and associated problems. A urethral opening on the ventral surface (underside) of the penis is called **hypospadias**. A urethra which opens on the dorsal (top) side of the penis is defined as **epispadias**; this rare but severe defect is associated with urinary incontinence and some degree of dorsal chordee. The varieties of each of these defects are described in the table below.

DEFECT	AS SEEN IN MALE HYPOSPADIAS (1 IN 250 TO 300 LIVE BIRTHS)	AS SEEN IN MALE EPISPADIAS (1 IN 100,000 LIVE MALE BIRTHS)
Associated findings	Abnormal foreskin, penile torsion or chordee; 30% of those who also have an undescended testes have an intersex condition.	Extrophy of the bladder, short penis
Glanular	The meatus is located on the underside of the penis at the base of the glans; requires no treatment unless the meatus is so small that the flow of urine is restricted.	The glans appears split open at the end, with the meatus located on top of the glans.
Distal or midshaft	The meatus is located on the underside of the shaft, between the glans and the scrotum; chordee, a flattened glans, and absent ventral foreskin are common associated defects.	The meatus is located along the top the shaft, which appears split open to the level of the meatus.
Penoscrotal (penopubic)	The meatus is located ventrally where the base of the penis meets the scrotum.	The entire penile shaft is split with meatus located directly below the symphysis pubis (not on the shaft at all); almost always associated with extrophy of the bladder.
Perineal	The meatus is located ventrally at the base of the scrotum where it meets the perineum, the scrotum may be bifid (divided), and the penis, small with a large meatus, may be bent so that the glans is attached to the perineum. The testes are usually undescended. Intersex conditions are associated with this type of hypospadias.	Not applicable

Malposition of the urethra is often associated with a malformed foreskin and glans. Meatal atresia (closed meatus) may be missed due to its small size but will result in failure to void and a distended bladder. Babies with any type of penile defect should not be circumcised.

The normal urine stream is expelled straight from the tip of the penis in a moderately strong, steady projection. If you have the opportunity, observe the baby from the side while he is urinating. In a penis that otherwise appears normal, urine streaming from the abdomen or the perineum may be the result of a fistula. A deviated or weak stream is associated with stenosis of the meatus or other urinary tract malformation as is an unusually powerful but fine stream. There should be no ballooning of the foreskin prior to urinating, nor should this occur during urination. A rectal fistula into the urinary tract results in meconium-stained urine.

Examining the scrotum

Assess the scrotum for rugation (closely and uniformly distributed, distinct, mostly horizontal wrinkles), color, size and bulges along either side. The term infant has fully developed rugae with brownish pigmentation, which may normally range from pinkish brown in Caucasian infants to almost black in some infants-of-color. Well-formed rugae and a pendulous scrotum are good indications that the testes are or have been descended (but may be currently retracted), however, this cannot be taken as a guarantee. Preterm babies have few or no rugae, which first appear at about 36 to 37 weeks gestation and cover the entire sac by 40 weeks gestation. The scrotum becomes more pendulous as gestational age advances. Bruising and swelling of the scrotum commonly occur with frank breech presentation.

The contour and size of the scrotal sac varies among normal infants. The scrotal sac's attachment to the body is its smallest diameter and the sac is widest at its far end. The skin may be tight and firm and the sac small, or the skin may be loose and hanging.

An unusually large or stretched sac suggests that a mass, hydrocele (accumulation of fluid) or herniation of bowel is present. A hydrocele occurs with incomplete closure of an embryonic channel that allows peritoneal fluid to enter the sac. This fluid may be trapped anywhere along the spermatic cord, where it forms an encysted hydrocele, most frequently surrounding the testicle as a soft fluid-filled oval or round sac that results in enlargement of the scrotum. The testes is not palpable as a result. The borders of the hydrocele are well defined. If it communicates with the inguinal canal, the canal may appear enlarged. When the hydrocele is moved into the scrotum, away from the groin, the groin appears normal and not swollen, distinguishing it from a hernia. Only very rarely does a hydrocele develop into a hernia. Treatment may be required if the hydrocele is extremely large and noncommunicating. Scrotal hydroceles transilluminate well, a technique discussed later in this section. A scrotal hematoma will not transilluminate and may cause difficulty with urination, but this should clear up within a few days. Give the baby homeopathic arnica to speed resolution.

A hydrocele of the spermatic cord, often found with an inguinal hernia, is not as likely to transilluminate as is one in the scrotum, but it is easily palpated. Note that a hydrocele of the cord may be relatively fixed because the fluid it contains cannot be compressed back into the abdomen, thus mimicking an incarcerated inguinal hernia. There are three things that distinguish the two. The upper border of an incarcerated portion of intestines is fixed to the border of the inguinal ring, while the upper border of most hydroceles can be moved away from the inguinal ring. Manipulating the upper border of an incarcerated hernia causes pain, while a hydrocele is painless on manipulation. Finally, a finger in the baby's rectum may be able to palpate the internal ring allowing the examiner to identify the presence of a descended loop of bowel (it is not recommended that a rectal exam be done at home). Most hydroceles resolve rapidly on their own.

Anomalies of the scrotum include bifid and triple sacs where there are two or three distinct pouches.

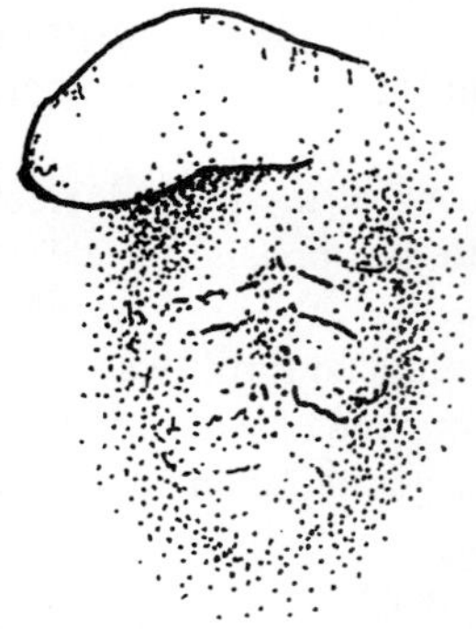

Normal male genitalia prior to term (testes undescended)

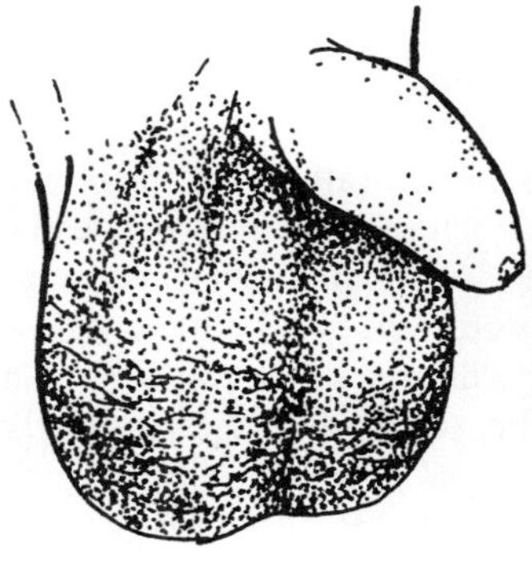

Normal male genitalia at term (both testes descended)

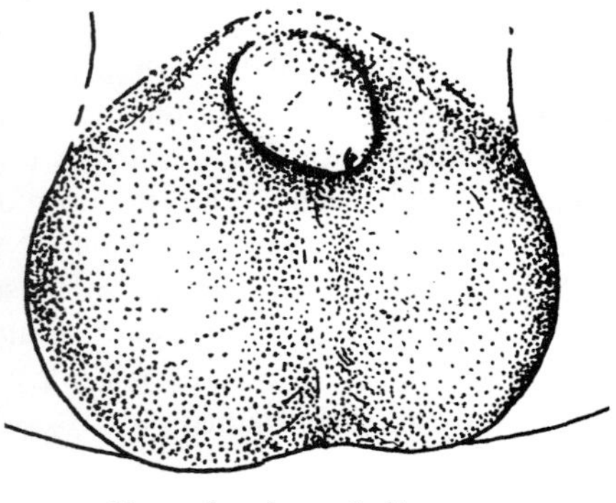

Normal male genitalia at term (bilateral hydrocele)

Testes: Regardless of the appearance of the scrotum, palpate the scrotal sac for the presence of two testes. The term newborn's testes range from 1.4 to 1.6 cm in length and are considered abnormally small if they are less than 8 mm in their longest diameter. Descent into the inguinal canal begins at about 28 to 30 weeks gestation. By 36 weeks, the testes are at the neck of the scrotum; by 37 weeks, they are high in the scrotal sac. At least one testicle will have descended below the inguinal canal by term in 96.6% of all male babies. Bilateral undescended testes present in 10% of all males at birth, and 3 to 5% are missing a testis altogether.

The newborn testes feel like small, slightly indentable, very slippery, ovoid grapes within the scrotal sac. They are small within the relatively large cavity of the term scrotum and can easily elude your exam. Furthermore, the newborn inguinal canal is open and the testes can slip up inside, out of your reach, as you try to palpate them. Touching and cold air both can prompt the cremasteric reflex, which results in the abrupt retraction of the testes up into the inguinal canal, although this reflex is weak in the first two days of life. Nevertheless, be sure your hands are warm before you proceed.

To begin your exam, use the thumb and forefinger of each hand on either side of the scrotum to palpate for both testes simultaneously. Place your index fingers under the scrotal sac and your thumbs on top. Start where the scrotum joins the body and gently compress your fingers together in a pinching motion, continuing to palpate in a downward direction until you find both testes. If both are descended, you should be able to easily identify each one. Bilateral palpation helps eliminate the chance that you will identify the same testis twice (Schlinger, 2003). The finding of normal descended testes rules out the possibility of congenital adrenal hyperplasia.

If the testes cannot be located with this technique, if they appear not to be descended or if you are otherwise unsure of your findings, proceed as follows. First block the "escape route" of the lower opening of the inguinal canal. Before you touch the scrotum, slide your index finger down the groin on one side toward the midline along the inguinal ligament, moving down along the canal toward the top of the scrotum and apply gentle pressure. Now, with the other hand, palpate using the thumb, index and middle fingers, starting where the scrotum joins the body. Move your fingers downward with a gentle pinching motion to locate the testis, which should slip between your fingers. Reverse your hands and palpate for the other testis. Be sure you are feeling two separate testes and not just the same one over again. If you think you have identified both testes, attempt to reconfirm your findings using bilateral palpation.

Undescended or small testes may be even harder to identify. Assessment is easier if you use soap or oil on your finger to reduce friction. With the baby lying supine, apply gentle pressure on the abdomen just to the inside of the iliac crest at the level of the internal inguinal ring. Glide two or three fingers along the inguinal crease toward the scrotum, using gentle to firm pressure and repeating several times if necessary. As you do so, palpate the side of the scrotum toward which you are stroking with the other hand. The testis will pop out of the canal into your fingers. Be careful to reach up, through the scrotum toward the testis to find it, rather than forcing it down toward your fingers. This will prevent mistaking a low but undescended testes from one that is descended. Note its location at the internal or external inguinal rings, the scrotal inlet or as ectopic if outside the normal path of descent.

Cryptorchidism occurs when one or both testes are not completely descended into the scrotum, a condition often accompanied by an inguinal hernia. This most commonly occurs on the right. An undescended testis can identified at times by sitting the baby in a frog-leg position (supine with soles of feet together and knees apart to expose the perineum), which may cause the testis to descend into the lower inguinal or scrotal region. This is especially likely if the baby cries or strains, which increases intra-abdominal pressure. Often, only one testis is descended, more often the left. If you cannot identify both testes, place the baby frog-legged (as above) and gently probe upward into the inguinal canal on the questionable side to see if the testis is on the way down. The finding of a small, very slightly mobile mass affirms that all is likely to be well and that it should descend. About 50% of full-term babies with a normal undescended testis at birth will experience testicular descent by six weeks of age.

If you still cannot find it, palpate the abdominal wall, upper thigh, perineum and base of the penis for ectopic placement. Exceedingly rare is the form of ectopic testes in which one testis descends into the opposite scrotal pouch, resulting in a finding of two testes on the same side, usually with an accompanying hernia.

Progressive tissue damage, an increased risk of cancer of both the testes, torsion and reduced fertility are possible complications if the testis has not descended by the age of 6 months. Treatment is recommended within the first 18 months of life. If one or both testes cannot be identified in the presence of significant genital anomaly, extensive evaluation is called for immediately.

The presence of two testes almost always confirms that the baby is genetically male, as a normal ovary virtually never descends. Therefore, a palpable gonad is usually a testis. If only one is palpable, that is probably a testis on that side; however, there could be a normal testis, a streak gonad or an abdominal ovary on the other. Magnetic resonance imaging is used to look for intra-abdominal testes if one or both cannot be felt. Hermaphroditism is suspected when only one testis is found. Complete absence of both testes in an infant that otherwise appears male is associated with female pseudohermaphroditism; the baby should be transported for immediate assessment for adrenal hyperplasia.

Unless the baby was born breech and has bruised genitals, discoloration suggests testicular torsion or a hematoma. Either of these complications require transport. Torsion of the testis occurs when the entire testis and its attachments are twisted in the lax scrotal sac, inguinal canal or abdomen. This can occur in utero, presenting at birth as a nontender or mildly tender, slightly enlarged, hard mass. The affected side may be shorter due to spasm of the spermatic cord. In most cases, the overlying scrotum looks normal early on, although rarely it is accompanied by reddish to bluish coloring of the scrotal skin. Torsion in an undescended testis is hard to identify. The baby is often pain-free or may exhibit only intermittent pain with irritability. The combination of an abdominal mass, irritability and an undescended testis should lead you to suspect testicular torsion. Most of the time, the twisted testis must be removed surgically to prevent malignancy.

The epididymis is felt as a vertical ridge of soft, nodular tissue closely attached behind and to the outer side of each testis. The vas deferens is a hard, distinct cord. Other, less distinct cord-like parts are nerves, arteries and fibers of cremasteric muscle. A mass on the epididymis suggests a spermatocele or retention cyst. A palpable sausage-shaped smooth bulge above the testis is likely to be a hydrocele of the vas deferens. A hematoma of the vas deferens feels boggy and is usually associated with a breech delivery.

Besides a hydrocele or hernia, other masses may be palpated in the scrotal sac while you are attempting to locate the testes. A **hematocele** is an accumulation of blood that occurs with trauma to the scrotum. A **varicocele** is a varicose vein of the scrotum, causing the scrotum to feel like a bag of worms. Varicocele occurs most often on the left side and suggests vascular obstruction above the scrotal sac.

Transillumination of the scrotum: Whenever your are unsure about your findings regarding the scrotum, you can transilluminate the sac. Transillumination may help in identifying an otherwise elusive testicle, varicocele, fluid in the form of a scrotal hydrocele, blood, a twisted testicle or loops of bowel that have herniated into the scrotum. Hold the light source directly against the scrotum and look at the scrotum from the opposite side. The normal scrotum admits light uniformly except for the two tiny testicles near where the sac joins the body. A hernia is present when loops of bowel are clearly visible. Masses filled with clear fluid, such as a hydrocele or a cyst, appear translucent, while those that are blood-filled or solid, such as a swollen twisted testicle, do not admit light. While intestines are usually opaque on transillumination, note that thin-walled bowel (which may accompany a hydrocele) may transilluminate at times as well. (Donn & Kuhns, 1983)

Perineum

The perineum should be carefully examined to locate any abnormal communication with the bowel. When present, this track can be filled with air, white epithelial pearls or meconium. It may be located anywhere from the normal anal site to the tip of the penis. When a fistula is present, the perineum may look flat with bulging during crying, or more normal with a deep intragluteal groove and anal dimple.

FINDINGS THAT CONSTITUTE A NORMAL GENITAL EXAM IN A BOY
•The urethra is located at the tip of the glans (may be inferred by the presence of a fully developed foreskin). •The penis is a normal length when stretched (2.5 to 5 cm) and diameter (0.9 to 1.3 cm). •Bilateral testes of normal size (8 to 14 mm) are located in the scrotal sac.

Congenital adrenal hyperplasia in males

Affected boys generally present with normal external genitalia. Details regarding signs and symptoms will appear in Volume III of this text and in a recent edition of my DIAGNOSTIC TESTS.

Examining the Anus

The structure of the anus is the same in both sexes. Part the buttocks to see if the anus is properly placed and apparently patent. The normal anus has a longitudinally-oriented puckered, oval "mouth," the orifice of which forms a small slit best visualized when the buttocks are held open to either side, although this oval appearance may not always be obvious at birth, in which case the opening will look like a large, puckered dot. Lack of puckering suggests that the opening is a fistula and that the anal sphincter is not encircling the opening. The orifice should also contract when gently touched. If the baby has not passed meconium, look carefully, as the normally deeper pigmentation in the region can make an imperforate anus (1 in 5000 to 20,000 live births) easy to miss, especially if a nearby fistula exists that allows meconium to escape. Small skin tags in the anal opening are usually normal variations.

Measuring normal anal placement

To measure for the normal placement of the anus, first tear off a strip of paper IV or cloth adhesive tape and fold it in half lengthwise (masking tape can be used if that is all that is available). This will provide a soft, pliable measuring device that will not produce a paper cut; it is held just off center so you can see the anal orifice as you measure. Alternatively, place a piece of clear adhesive tape lengthwise over the area to be examined, centered over the anus (this method is further described below). This makes it easier to take your measurements without worrying about moving your measuring device. Make sure the baby is relaxed; cradle the legs in an unforced frog position by first flexing the knees and hips and bringing the soles of the feet together; then rest the lower legs and feet on the pubic bone. This relaxes the perineum. The baby should not be pushing and struggling; as this will increase intra-abdominal pressure and cause perineal bulging, which will distort measurements. This ratios described below do not change with maturation.

Perineal length and anal placement in boys: In boys, the anus is normally located just below the midpoint between the tip of the coccyx and the scrotal-perineal junction on the underside of the scrotum (the horizontal boundary where the scrotal skin stops and the perineum starts). The scrotum will have to be lifted toward the abdomen to reveal this area. Anterior displacement falls above the normal location and is rare in boys.

To measure exactly, lay the tape lengthwise on the midline of the perineum by lifting the scrotum and placing one end of the tape level with the scrotal-perineal junction. Smooth the tape over the midline of the perineum, crossing over the center of the anus to the tip of the coccyx (palpate in the midline just below the anus to locate it). Mark the midpont of the anal opening, the tip of the coccyx and the end that was level with the scrotal-perineal junction on the tape. Stick the tape to white paper and overlay it with a clear centimeter ruler. Use the parameters developed by Reisner and associates (1984):

Scrotum-coccyx (SC) length: The distance between the scrotal-perineal junction and the tip of the coccyx.

Scrotum-anus (SA) length: The distance from the center of the anus to the scrotal-perineal junction.

Anal placement: Normally, the upper segment (the distance from the scrotum to the anus) is just a bit under three-fifths of the total distance from the scrotum to the coccyx (0.58) with a normal range of 0.52 to 0.64. A distance of less than 0.46 (or less than half) constitutes anterior anal placement.

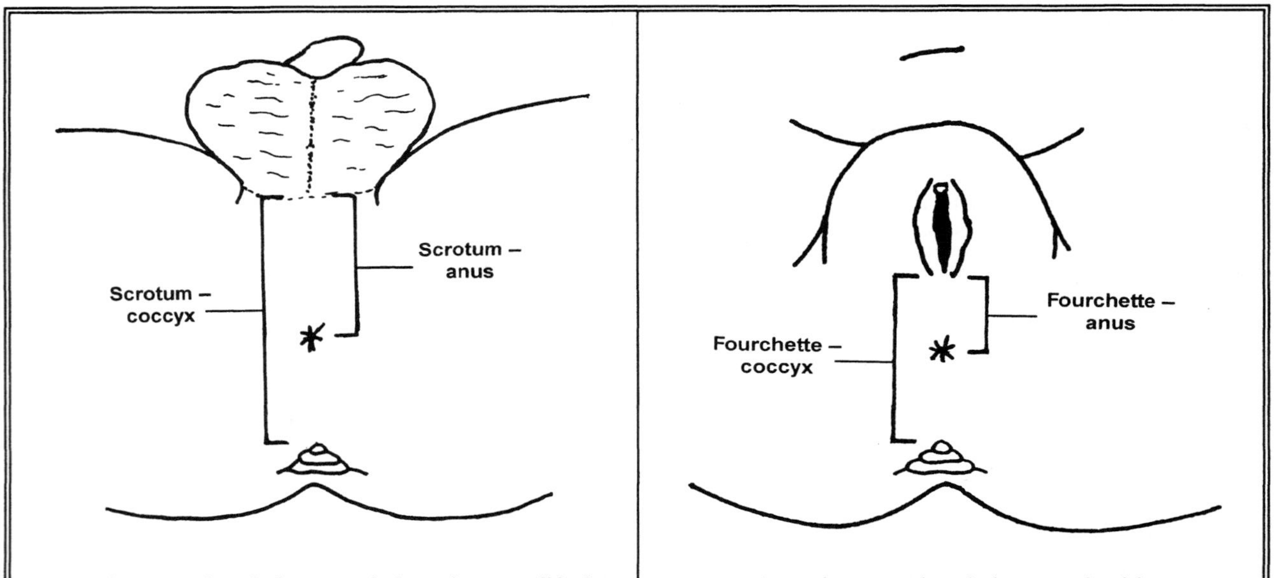

Assessing normal anal placement in boys (scrotum lifted) | Assessing normal anal placement in girls

(Anatomy proportionately enlarged to more easily demonstrate how to measure)

Perineal length and anal placement in girls: There should be roughly 1 cm (± 3.5 mm) of space between the posterior border of the yoni orifice and the center of the anal opening in the term infant (Callegari et al., 1987). According to Reisner and colleagues (1984), the anus is normally placed slightly anterior to the midpoint between the fourchette and the coccyx in girls (i.e., closer to the genitalia). Anterior displacement in girls falls about a third of the way between the posterior fourchette and the coccyx. When there is a question about masculinization (labioscrotal fusion), anal placement can be assessed by placing the upper end of a piece of clear adhesive tape level with the lower border of the fourchette (where the labia minora meet at the base of the yoni orifice); smooth the tape over the midline of the perineum and the center of the anal opening to the tip of the coccyx (Genc et al., 2002). Mark the tip of the coccyx and the center of the anus and the end that was level with the fourchette. Carefully remove the tape and stick it to a piece of white paper, overlie it with a clear plastic centimeter ruler. Use the parameters developed by Reisner's team:

Fourchette-coccyx (FC) length: The distance between the fourchette (the midpoint of the lowermost labia minora at the junction of the perineum and yoni mucosa) and the tip of the coccyx.

Fourchette-anus (FA) length: The distance between the fourchette and the center of the anal opening.

Anal placement: Normally, the upper segment (AF) is just a bit over two-fifths of the total distance from the fourchette to the coccyx (that is, 0.44) with a normal range of 0.39 to 0.49. A distance of less than 0.34 (slightly more than a third) constitutes anterior anal placement.

Another way to assess anal placement in girls is by measuring as follows (Callegari et al., 1987):
Anus-Fourchette (AF): Measure from the center of the anus to the fourchette (as above).
Fourchette-Clitoris (FC): Measure from the fourchette to the external, uppermost base of the clitoris, at the superior junction of the labia minora.
Anus-Clitoris (AC): Measure from the center of the anus to the base of the clitoris.

In normal female babies, the lower segment (AF) should be at least one-third the total distance from the anus to the clitoris.

If the anus is misplaced, the skin overlying the sphincter is often slightly depressed. Stimulation along the perineum with a cotton swab may result in contraction of the sphincter (the anal "wink"), thus identifying its location. Anterior displacement of the anus may be associated with chronic constipation in both sexes. Anal anomalies or displacement also alert you to the increased possibility of a spinal defect or sacral agenesis (see details in the part of this chapter covering the examination of the back and spine). Spinal anomalies are present in 30% of these babies. More about evaluating anal defects can be found in the subchapter entitled "Abdominal Mass, Single Umbilical Artery, Edema, Atypical Genitalia: Detecting Kidney and Genitourinary Tract Disorders."

Normal diameter

Anal diameter steadily enlarges as the baby gains weight. Normal anal diameter is assessed when it is dilated to its maximum size and is calculated in mm as follows: 7 + (1.3 × weight in kilograms [weight in pd ÷ 2.2]). In the study by El Haddad and Corkery (1985) normal values were obtained by inserting Hegar uterine sounds into the anuses of newborns in seven weight groups. The normal anal diameter was taken as the size at which the dilator filled the canal comfortably with blanching of the edges of the orifice. Do not attempt to assess the diameter of the anus by inserting anything into it. The values in the following table are given for reference only.

Birthweight		Average Dilated Anal Diameter
5 lb 8 oz to 6 lb 9.5 oz	2.5 to 3 kg	11.7 mm
6 lb 9.5 oz to 7 lb 11.5 oz	3 to 3.5 kg	12.3 mm
7 lb 11.5 oz to 8 lb 13.5 oz	3.5 to 4 kg	12.6 mm
8 lb 13.5 oz to 9 lb 14.5 oz	4 to 4.5 kg	12.8 mm

Meconium passage

Passage of meconium may occur through a misplaced opening in the yoni (girls), the urethra or bladder (boys), or even the umbilicus, so check to be sure the placement of the anus is anatomically correct, even if meconium has been passed. This is facilitated by observing the infant passing meconium exclusively through the anal orifice. Babies should pass a large volume of meconium when they defecate: beware of those who pass quarter- or silver-dollar-sized blobs through an otherwise apparently normal anal opening, as they are more likely to have stenosis. A large fistula can be mistaken for a normal anal opening but is usually anterior or posterior to the normal location of the anus. If no meconium has been passed and there is a depression or orifice at the anal opening, insertion of a well-lubricated soft catheter will help determine if the anus is truly patent. This must be done gently, as you do not want to perforate a membrane if the anus is not patent. To do so, direct the tip of the catheter toward the baby's umbilicus and insert it slowly and gently to a depth not to exceed 2 cm. This is rarely necessary as most babies will be happy to pass meconium for you. A variety of anal anomalies can occur, causing anything from an obviously imperforate anus with a membranous covering flush with the skin surface to a blind pouch where the rectal canal should be. Any question regarding anal patency requires immediate withholding of oral intake, transport and evaluation.

Examining sphincter tone

Depending upon your observations, you may want to discuss an anal examination to rule out anal stenosis with the parents. Most midwives do not perform an internal exam, but knowing ways to assess stenosis may be important if a baby starts to have problems later on; an examination of the newborn may be warranted. If the parents or any siblings have had a history of anal problems, constipation, withholding of stool or pencil-thin stools, an examination of the newborn is warranted. When present, anal stenosis is a major impairment to the development of normal stool habits in childhood. That an infant thermometer can be inserted with ease does not rule out stenosis because the diameter of the thermometer is not large enough to reveal a problem. The apparent size of the anal orifice is unrelated to the presence of stenosis. Infants with stenosis may be able to pass meconium without apparent difficulty because meconium is normally quite soft.

Cotton-swab method: The least invasive way to obtain more information about sphincter tone is suggested by Joe Gilhooly (2003), a neonatologist in Portland, OR. He uses the soft end of a cotton swab to gently insert into the anus just deeply enough to assess sphincter tone by moving the end side to side to press against the muscle. The only way to know if there is a problem would be to examine normal babies to get a feel for normal resistance to this kind of pressure.

Digital exam: Note: digital exam is invasive and potentially harmful and is *not* recommended unless you are the primary care provider far from a pediatric consult the swab technique is inconclusive and you still suspect a problem. Digital exam risks tearing the extremely delicate mucus membranes of the anus and internal tissues. If you are in a position where you feel it is warranted, the tip of the little finger is an ideal anal probe because it can be used to assess the diameter and the elasticity of the sphincter. First, explain to the baby and parents what you plan to do and why. Measure the diameter of your fingertip and trim your nail short. Flex the baby's legs up against his abdomen into a open knee-chest position and explain to the baby what you are doing and why. Have someone offer the baby a finger to suck. Wear a well-fitting glove and lubricate your fingertip and the external anus liberally. Ask the baby to relax and continue to talk to him as you very gradually introduce your finger into the anal opening by placing the pad of your finger against it and applying gentle, continuous pressure until the sphincter relaxes and allows you to insert your fingertip. Insert your finger only far enough to feel that the tip is just beyond the ring of muscle. Note resistance and external diameter, then remove your finger very gradually. A stenotic sphincter is tight and inelastic, even when the baby is otherwise relaxed. The one advantage of this technique over the swab method is that a truly stenotic sphincter should leave an indentation around your fingertip. With gentleness and patience, most babies can be examined without evidence of discomfort.

Anal prolapse

On rare occasions, the anus may be prolapsed to varying degrees, presenting a bumpy red mass of mucous membrane; prolapse is usually associated with other disorders, particularly spinal defects and cystic fibrosis.

Pubic hair

Newborns generally lack genital hair. Its presence may or may not indicate increased androgen levels and requires follow-up.

When the Genitals Appear Atypical

Be on the lookout for the findings in the following table.

The Primary Characteristics of Atypical Genitalia	
When the genitalia appear more male you may find	**When the genitalia appear more female you may find**
Micropenis More severe forms of hypospadias Undetectable or small gonads Inguinal mass (may be the uterus or an egg tube)	Enlarged clitoris at term Posterior fusion of the labia Palpable mass in the labial or inguinal area (may be a testis)

More congenital malformations occur in the genitourinary system than any other, and the range of variation in how they can present is simply enormous. Because such defects can manifest in very subtle ways, it is frequently the case that babies with atypical genitalia are labeled as one sex by the parents and care providers at birth, and later it is discovered that the sex of the baby is in question. An abnormality of two or more of the following physical characteristics is highly associated with sex-linked disorders: the size of the penis or clitoris, the location of the urethra, improper fusion of the labioscrotal folds, and abnormalities of the location or size of the gonads (testes or ovaries). Even though the clitoris may be enlarged in both width and length, it is still not possible to tell if it is a masculinized clitoris or a severely feminized penis by examination alone, even if apparent scrotal masses or a yoni opening are present. Whenever an intersex condition is suspected, if there are abnormal openings in the perineum, or if the testes cannot be palpated in a baby presumed to be male, the abdomen and groin must be carefully reexamined for masses.

Gender will undoubtedly be assigned by the parents following a cursory visual inspection at the time of birth unless the genitals are very unusual. Never officially assign gender during the newborn exam without first palpating for testes. Palpate the labia for testes in a baby you believe to the female; if masses are found, the sex of the baby is uncertain. If no testes are found in the scrotum or inguinal canal in a baby presumed to be male or if, in spite of these evaluations, you are still unsure, do not formally assign gender until a more complete evaluation can be performed.

Regardless of the circumstances and the particular desires of the parents, this is a complex situation and must be handled with care, for the sake of the baby's future self-esteem as well as the parents' attitudes toward the baby. (For example, was either parent quite attached to the baby being a particular sex, and was it assumed at birth that the baby *was* the desired sex?) Once you or the parents realize that there is a question as to the baby's genetic sex, be sure not to compound the problem by guessing. When the genitalia have subtly unusual features, it is best to tell the parents that there are variations of the genitals that require further assessment. If the genitals are frankly atypical, tell them the truth. Explain that the baby's genitals are atypical and that further examination and testing will be required to determine the baby's genetic sex. Tell the baby and the parents how beautiful the baby is and that the baby needs their unconditional love in infancy, regardless of sex. As always, your attitude can help set the tone for the parents' acceptance or difficulty in dealing with such a crisis.

The mainstream medical practitioners the parents encounter are likely to foster any fears they may already have and encourage them to surgically alter the baby to match the genetic sex or reconstruct the genitals to match the sex that will give the most "cosmetically normal" result, regardless of genetics. While the wisdom of this approach is starting to be questioned, it is up to you to make sure parents understand the serious psychological ramifications of forcing a child into an assigned sex role. Without a clear medical indication, there is no need whatsoever for the baby to undergo surgery. Advise the parents not to allow the medical staff to rush them into a particular decision without first thoroughly researching the proposed treatments versus the ramifications of no surgery at all. An excellent place to start is the website www.isna.org.

The cultural, medical and social aspects of supporting parents to make reasonable choices for their newborn with an intersex condition are further discussed in Volume III of this text. See the most recent edition of my DIAGNOSTIC TESTS for more details about testing to diagnose intersex conditions.

Associated disorders: All babies who are suspected of having an intersex condition must be transported for evaluation within an hour or so after birth because a major associated problem is salt-losing adrenal hyperplasia. Depending upon the severity of the condition, it can produce severe electrolyte imbalance leading to vomiting, dehydration and metabolic derangement resulting in complete physiologic collapse, usually within 7 to 28 days after birth. Detecting adrenal hyperplasia requires laboratory assessment of adrenal and pituitary function.

Other babies lack any atypical genital characteristics but have other findings that may lead to the diagnosis of an intersex condition. Examples include signs of Turner syndrome, dwarfism with bowing and angulation of the lower limbs, flat face and shortened vertebrae, hyperpigmentation, and sodium wasting or failure-to-thrive in males with congenital adrenal hyperplasia. Intersex babies whose external genitals appear normal may have certain associated metabolic disorders that can be life-threatening.

Examining the Legs, Knees, Hips, Ankles and Feet

This part of the exam should include evaluation of the hips, femurs, tibias and fibulas and is based on Fletcher (1998), unless otherwise noted.

Examining the Legs

Visual inspection

The term newborn holds her flexed legs spread to a varying degree when at rest on her back, with the thighs rotated externally, knees apart, and lower legs rotated internally with the feet held at a toed-in angle, resting on the heel. However, bowing in an anterior direction is abnormal, indicating the presence of sclerotic or dysplastic bone (Scanlon et al., 1979). Both the hips and the knees are held in 15 to 20° of flexion. Compare knee height with the legs extended. Compare the circumferences of the legs by encircling the widest area with two fingers as you palpate for muscle mass. If you defect asymmetry, measure the circumference at the same distance from a chosen landmark. If one side appears enlarged or too small, palpate for abnormalities, note irregularities of contour or horizontal thigh creases, check for other abnormalities as already outlined in the "skin" section. If any of these findings are off, soft tissue hypoplasia, a congenital absence or shortening of a bone, a break, or a dislocation could be causative. Adduction of a thigh at rest is also associated with hip dislocation. Note, however, that asymmetrical posture or hyperflexion is often seen with babies who were born breech as well as in those who have hip dysplasia. Gentle pressure against the soles of the feet with slight shaking often encourages the baby to curl up into her fetal position, which will allow better appreciation of her preferred position of rest after birth. Look for webbing of the skin behind the knees, spanning the posterior thigh to the upper calf, which may contain the sciatic nerve, a finding associated with popliteal web syndrome. This is often accompanied by clubbed feet, lip pits, cleft palate and lip, genital anomalies and a band connecting the gums.

Palpation

Palpate the legs to make sure the femur, tibia and fibula are all present. When the tibia is absent (1 in 1,000,000 live births), the position of the foot may be normal or it may be bent toward the midline (varus position) with mild to extreme shortening of the lower leg; the knee is unstable and has a flexion contracture, causing it not to straighten even as much as a newborn's leg normally would (Scanlon, et al., 1979). Absence of the fibula is more common; the involved leg is shortened with bowing of the tibia anteriorly and to the midline. There is often an associated pronounced foot deformity, causing the foot to turn away from the midline (valgus position). Related deformities are likely to be less severe when only a portion of one of these bones is missing. If bone hypoplasia is suspected, consult a pediatric orthopedist soon after birth.

Fractures or hip dislocation may result from a traumatic birth, particularly if the baby was breech. Further evaluation is needed if you find irregularities in the contour of the legs, crepitance on palpation (a grating sound or vibration) or masses, which may be due to hematoma formation or a displaced break. Although breakage of the femur rarely occurs, bruising is more common and will cause the baby pain, resulting in little spontaneous movement of the leg.

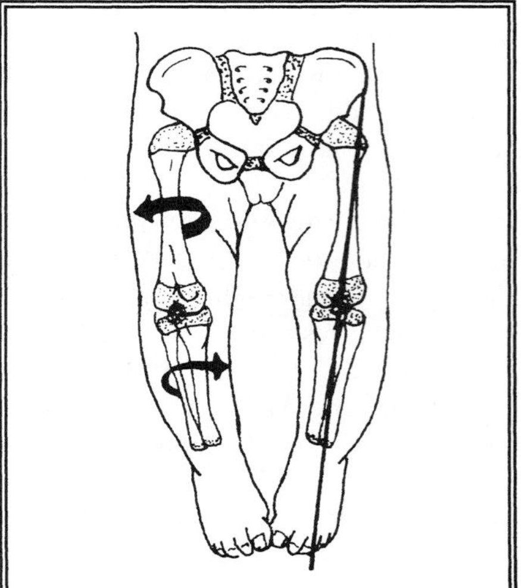

Normal internal torsion occurs when the femur rotates outward and the tibia rotates inward. To check the type of torsion: draw a line from the antero-posterior iliac spine through the mid-patella, then straight down to the foot.

Estimating tibial torsion

At least half of all infants present with a degree of torsion of the femurs, tibias, or feet, making physiological bowing of the legs a common finding in the newborn. It occurs when external femoral torsion causes the knees to be angled away from the midline in conjunction with internal tibial torsion, which rotates the feet toward the midline, causing the feet to appear pigeon-toed (toes turned inward). Such bowing occurs due to fetal positioning resulting in rotational contractures at the hip and knee. In postural deformity, the leg can be manually straightened (Staheli, 1986).

Screening for the type of torsion: With the baby supine and the legs extended, establish a horizontal baseline connecting the anteroposterior iliac spine with the middle of the knee. Continue this line straight down to the foot. If the line falls inside of (medial to) the big toe, external tibial torsion is present. If the line falls inside the second toe, a small degree of internal tibial torsion, or a varus curvature, is present (Tappero & Honeyfield, 1993). If the line falls past the second toe (even more toward the side), the tibial torsion is more extreme, depending upon the location of the line. While this test can be done in newborns, the thigh-foot angle is easier.

Thigh-foot angle: Lie the baby on her belly. Flex the knees to 90° so that the feet stick straight up. Stand over the baby and look straight down at the soles and posterior thighs. From this vantage point, it will be apparent if the tibias lean inward or away from midline.

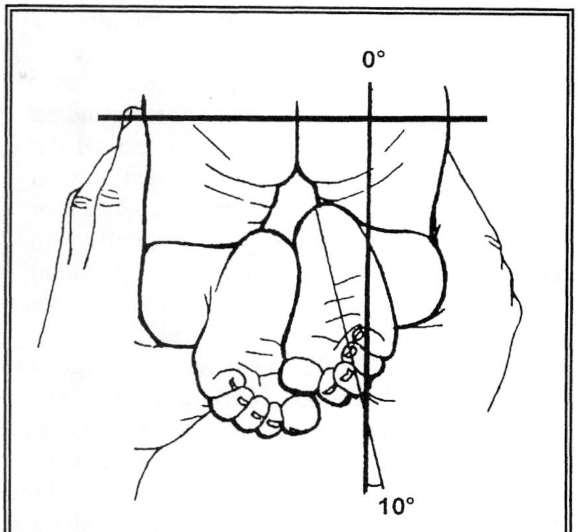

With the baby prone and lower legs held straight up, internal tibial torsion is readily apparent. Lines on sole and thigh allow an angle to be measured; in this case it is 10°.

The degree of internal tibial torsion in normal newborns ranges from zero to 20°. This is measured by extending a baseline through the posterior center of the thigh and an angle line from the center of the heel through the third toe. The angle is measured at the intersection of these lines. Normal internal torsion gradually changes to external tibial torsion by childhood. Lateral tibial bowing without significant shortening of the extremity is considered normal in the newborn, while anterior bowing is an abnormal finding, requiring an orthopedic consultation. The tibia may be bowed between its middle and lower third. Bowing may be anterior or posterior and to the side. Posterolateral bowing is usually an isolated finding and typically occurs on only one side; it may be associated with intrauterine posture and often resolves on its own. Simple anterolateral bowing in the midshaft of the tibia is usually associated with a bowed fibula at the same level and may also resolve on its own. A cystic form (with a cyst at the junction of the middle and distal thirds) and the pseudoarthrosis form (with an hourglass constriction) both increase the risk of fracture and require orthopedic evaluation shortly after birth. Seventy percent of those with the pseudoarthrosis form will eventually be diagnosed with neurofibromatosis (Staheli, 1986).

Knees: The newborn knees are usually outwardly bowed (genu varum) to about 10°. The patellae (kneecaps) are very small and flat, with a dent below where they will eventually develop; this finding is accentuated when the knee is flexed. On the rare occasions when the quadriceps muscle is deficient, weakness of the knee extensors results in knee flexion deformity with absence of the patella. Rarely a patella can also be dislocated at birth, presenting with flexion of the knee and excessive lateral rotation of the tibia, causing the lower leg to stick out to the side. On palpation, the patella can be felt lying alongside the knee above the head of the fibula, where it is fixed; the quadriceps muscle is also displaced and rotated to the side, pulling the tibia out and to the side.

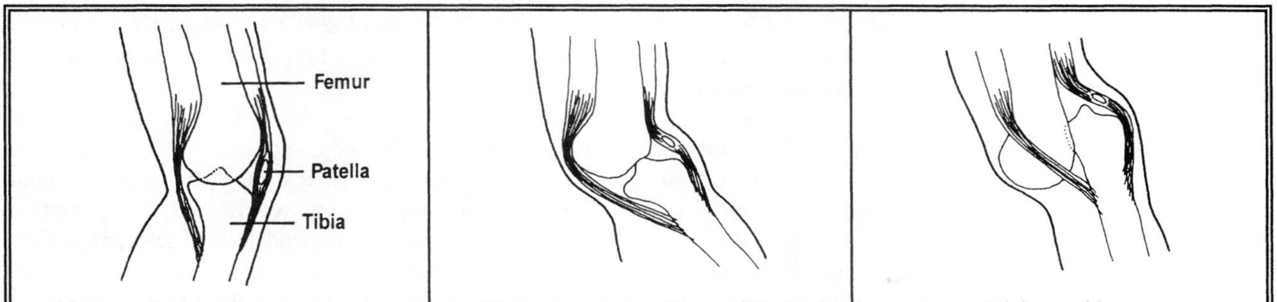

Normal knee | Hyperextended, subluxated knee | Dislocated knee

Range of motion: Establish a horizontal baseline extending from the center of the hip to the knee. To assess flexion with the baby on her belly, bend the leg at the knee to bring the foot straight up in the air, and then gently bend the calf further back toward the posterior thigh. To assess this with the baby supine, lift the entire leg off the mattress and bend the leg at the knee (illustrated). The leg can usually be flexed at the knee between 120 and 151°. Limitation of flexion may be more a product of a fat thigh and calf rather than a problem with the joint (Broughton et al., 1993).

Full extension of the newborn knee usually reaches its limit between 165° and 170° (with the zero point of the baseline starting at the hip [see drawing, next page]), preventing the leg from fully straightening and representing a flexion contracture of 15 to 20°. This is such a normal finding in newborns that the ability to fully extend the knee raises the likelihood of hip dislocation. On the other hand, a tight popliteal angle (tighter than the rest of the tone in the leg) is associated with intracranial hemorrhage; asymmetric popliteal angles in babies of 40 weeks gestation or older reflects hypertonia or unilateral paralysis (hemiplegia) (Hill, 1998). Hyperextension (genu recurvatum) or backward bending at the knee occurs when the proximal surface of the tibia and the distal surface of the femur are still in contact; it is seen most often in girl babies born in a frank breech position. The leg does not remain straight with extension but bends further backward at the knee, bringing the foot over the thigh well past 0° (straight) to between 10 to 15°. Congenital dislocation is much more rare. A dislocated knee can be hyperextended but will not flex beyond neutral (leg straight), and the tibia will be anteriorly displaced on palpation. There may be horizontal creases over the anterior knee. Dislocation is also seen with oligohydramnios, sacral agenesis or absence of the quadriceps muscle. When dislocation of the knee occurs, it is usually present in both legs. An orthopedist should be consulted shortly after birth, although this condition usually requires no special treatment (Broughton et al., 1993).

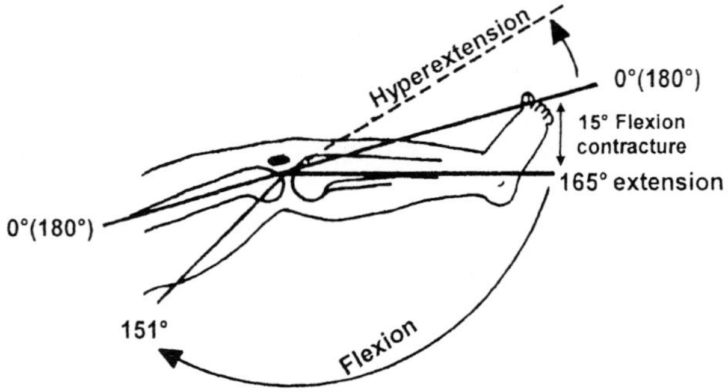

Range of motion at the knee

Hips

Even if no other joints are formally evaluated, the stability of the hip joints should always be carefully assessed to rule out developmental dysplasia of the hip (DDH). This is a very important exam. Hip problems are usually easily resolved in the newborn period. When they are not, disabling complications requiring prolonged corrective therapy can result. Some 2.5 to 6.5 infants per 1000 live births develop hip problems, and a significant portion of these are not detectable at birth, therefore routine examination is recommended for the first year of life at well-baby visits. There are three different degrees of hip dysplasia, as described by Tachdjian (1997):

Fully dislocated hip: The femoral head is completely out of the acetabulum. The dislocation may be temporarily corrected by simple flexion and abduction of the hips with a definite "clunk of entry," or it may be uncorrectable.

Dislocatable hip: The femoral head is still located in the acetabulum but can easily be displaced by adduction and extension of the hip. This produces a distinct "clunk of exit."

Subluxatable hip: The femoral head can be partially, but not completely, displaced out of the acetabulum, rendering the joint unstable. The subluxatable hip produces a giving sensation but no clunk. It may be loose and easily corrected or rigid and uncorrectable.

Babies who presented breech, especially frank breech, are at high risk for hip dysplasia, with some 30 to 50% of these children being affected. Other associated factors include family history (including Native American, Northern Italian or Yugoslavian descent), oligohydramnios, intrauterine crowding in multiple gestation, severe hypotonia, bilateral deformations of the ankle and foot (varieties of talipes), severe contracture of the joints, and female sex (particularly when she is the firstborn), with six to eight girls being affected for every boy. Other skeletal anomalies, spinal defects and chromosomal disorders may also be involved. Be especially alert for hip dysplasia if the baby has any foot deformities, torticollis, plagiocephaly or extensive contracture of the knee. Conversely, some otherwise normal babies may have hip dysplasia. The left hip is involved 60% of the time and the right hip only 20%; both hips are involved in 20% of cases. When both hips are affected, the left is usually more severely affected than the right; a result of the tendency of babies to position their backs to the mother's left in utero (Illingworth, 1987). Note that hip dislocation is painless in infants, although the exam may make many babies cry from anger. True pain is likely to be found with a bone fracture.

There are several observations and maneuvers used to assess hip dysplasia that should be performed on every baby. The Barlow and Ortolani rotation maneuvers should be performed even if all preliminary assessments are normal. Hip subluxation or dislocation is still a possibility even if the baby seems to move his legs normally. A dislocation can also be present when all these screens are negative, as some of these signs do not appear until the baby starts to bear weight on her legs. While just about every possible assessment is described in the pages that follow, some of them overlap, and every single assessment need not be performed in every baby. They are all described here to make sure that you understand the range of tests that can be performed and that you fully appreciate the combined assessments entailed in the Barlow and Ortolani maneuvers. The items marked with an asterisk should be performed individually on every baby.

*Movement
*Symmetrical length and creases of the legs
•Knee height
*Hip flexion
Hip extension
Hip abduction in flexion and extension
Hip adductor angles
Hip adduction
Extension limitation for flexion contracture
Assessment for telescoping
Barlow hip dislocation maneuver
*Ortolani hip relocation maneuver
*Tibial torsion

If limb movement is normal and length, knee height and thigh creases are symmetrical, the midwife should carefully perform the Barlow and Ortolani maneuvers. (These maneuvers are often referred to together as simply the Ortolani maneuver.) The angle of hip abduction can be assessed simultaneously. The Barlow and Ortolani maneuvers combine many different assessments of hip flexion, abduction in flexion and adduction in flexion. The midwife should have a thorough understanding of the individual components of the maneuvers, studying the separate descriptions for hip flexion, hip extension, hip abduction in flexion and extension, angle of abduction and hip adduction before proceeding to study the maneuvers themselves. Complete knowledge of each component allows the midwife to go back to a particular assessment whenever an abnormality is detected, providing a good foundation in what the problem may be and how to assess it more specifically. For example, if a joint seems loose but cannot be dislocated, assessment for telescoping would be appropriate.

Normal ranges of movement in the lower limbs are summarized in the following chart. Note that the knees are evaluated using many of the same assessments as for the hips.

Hip Joint	Flexion	Flexion Contracture	Extension	Abduction	Adduction	Internal Rotation*	External Rotation*
Girls	160°	average 19°	average 40°	55–103°	0– 30°	30–90°	40–100°
Boys	160°	average 21°	average 40°	50–100°	0–30°	30–90°	40–95°

*Values are the same for both prone and supine assessment. (Schwarze & Denton, 1993)

A baseline from which to measure must be established for many of the range-of-motion assessments so that an angle can be determined. One end of this line is designated with a zero and is where the arc of movement begins. The zero line of your protractor or goniometer is aligned with the baseline. In most cases, a motion line is drawn perpendicular to the baseline, depending upon the measurement to be obtained. An angle is assessed when the limb reaches its limit of motion, which gives the arc of movement. Evaluation includes assessing the limb and joint for normal strength and tone as well as spasticity or flaccidity.

Sounds during assessment: Note that with any of the following maneuvers, short, high-pitched clicks, a dry crunch or a snap may be heard or felt. These sounds are not associated with hip pathology and are usually due to movement of the tendons, ligaments, or fluid in the hip joint (they are the same sounds heard when one cracks his knuckles). The sound you are looking for is a heavier, thunk or clunk accompanied by a palpable and visible jolt which can sometimes been seen from a distance as the head of the femur moves forward and drops into the acetabulum (Hensinger, 1979).

Preliminary assessments:

***Movement:** First, observe the baby while he is lying calmly on his back and moving his legs. Look for equality of movement as the baby spontaneously moves his legs to the side (abduction) and extends his legs. In some babies, spontaneous movement is more effective at dislocating the hip than any of the following assessments. This may be noted as a jerking of the leg with flexion and extension, as the femoral head moves in and out of the socket.

***Symmetrical length and creases of legs:** Lay the baby supine, allow the baby to separate his legs naturally. Grasp the legs and extend them as straight as possible, holding them just below the knees. Look at the horizontal skin folds on the anterior thighs. Assess the legs for equal length and note whether the knees are parallel. Then grasp the baby's ankles in one hand and hold the legs together straight up in the air at a 90° angle to the torso. Look to see if the legs are still equal in length and look at the underside of the knees to see if they are still level with each other. Assess the symmetry of creases on the posterior thighs and behind the knees. (The posterior assessment can also be made with the baby lying on her belly and the legs held straight.) Tightly spaced or bunched creases that are noted in any of these positions and that are persistent suggest dislocation on that side.

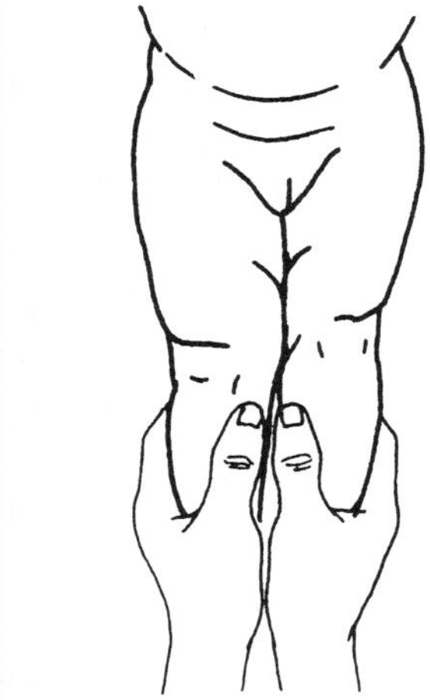

Checking for leg length and creases, legs extended (left leg is short)

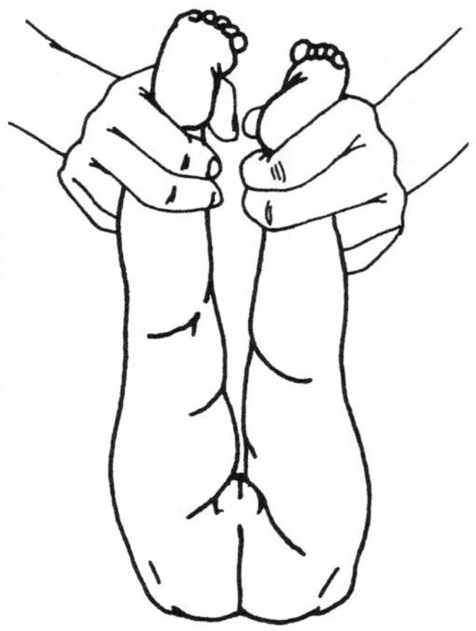

Checking creases, legs held up (left leg is short)

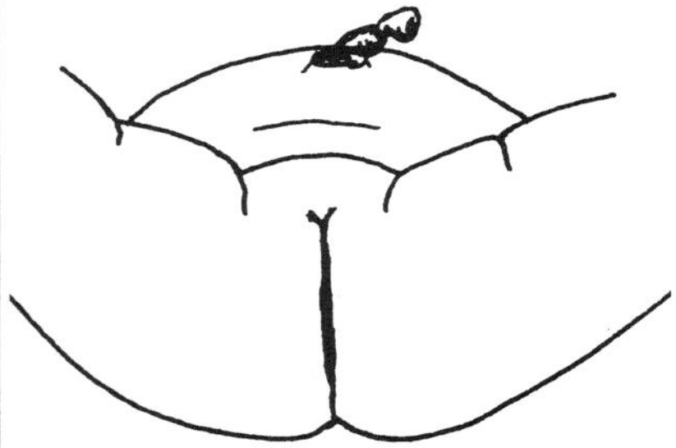

Normal inguinal creases

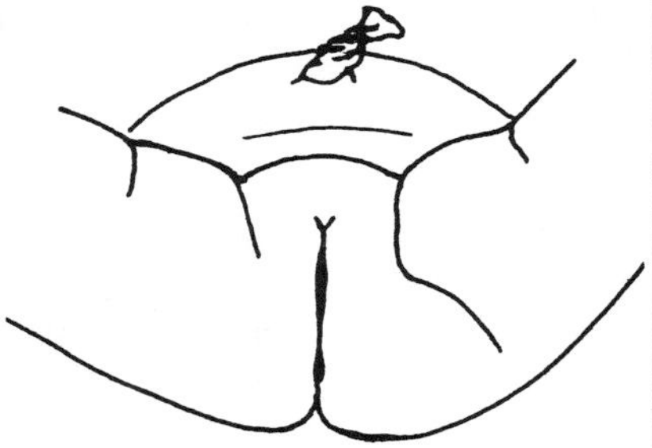

Asymmetrical–dislocation of left hip

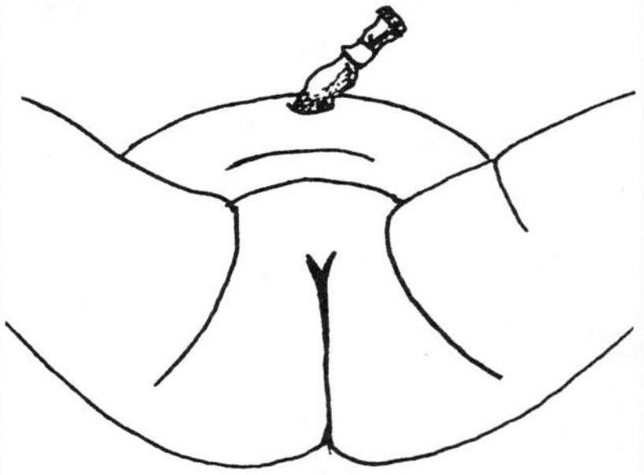

Bilateral dislocation

Note that slightly asymmetrical creases that are otherwise normally spaced can occur in normal babies in all these locations just from soft-tissue positioning. When this is suspected, relax the legs and recheck the creases a few times to see if the apparent asymmetry resolves. Asymmetry of the creases with equal leg length is unlikely to reflect a problem. Asymmetry can also present in some babies who have defects other than hip dysplasia. For example, they may be seen with pelvic obliquity with abduction contracture of one hip and sometimes with varying degrees of adduction contraction of the opposite hip. The adducted hip may be dysplastic (abnormally formed) (Tachdjian, 1997).

Next, lower the legs, spread them part way and look at the inguinal creases (where the thighs join the torso). Normally, the inguinal folds are symmetric and stop about one-third of the way around the joint. The inguinal folds will not be symmetric when the femoral head is dislocated toward the back and displaced upward; the folds on the affected side will extend down and around the joint to the anus. When both hips are dislocated, the creases may be symmetric but will extend around the joint beyond the level of the anus (Tachdjian, 1997).

***Knee height (Allis' sign):** Compare the height of the knees. The length of the femur as well as hip dislocation can be assessed by using this technique. With the baby on his back, place his feet flat on the mattress, then align and flex the legs so that both knees are pointing straight up. Make sure that the tips of the big toes are lined up in the same horizontal plane and that the hips are symmetrical. (When one hip is tilted into abduction, the other leg becomes adducted and appears shorter.) Now arrange yourself at the foot of the baby, your eyes level with the baby's feet. Observe the height of the knees; it will be obvious if one knee is higher than the other. A discrepancy in knee height suggests that one hip is dislocated or that the femur on the low side is shortened (Galeazzi's sign); the tibia could also be shortened with this finding. Apparent shortening of the femur is usually not seen in newborns unless the dislocation occurred in utero (Tachdjian, 1997).

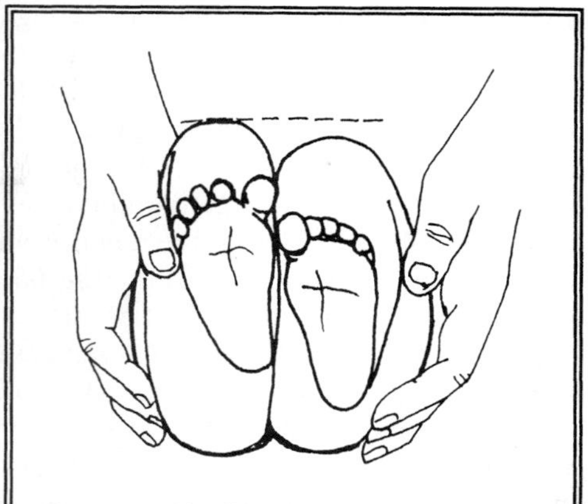

Checking knee height

Palpating the hip joint: Before you move on to rotational maneuvers, palpate the groin for the femoral head and note its relationship to the acetabulum. It should be well seated in the acetabulum. You should not be able to feel the ball of the femur.

Hip flexion: Start with the supine baby's legs as fully extended as possible against the mattress. Raise the legs, allow flexion at the hips and knees and see how far the knees can move directly up and over the torso in an arc toward the head (that is, move the legs into a knee-chest position). Using a horizontal line drawn through the length of the body as the baseline, find the angle between it and a line drawn straight through the knee and thigh. Maximum flexion occurs at the point just before the pelvis begins to lift off the mattress. A full range of motion is about 160°; however, hip flexion may be limited by a protuberant abdomen and a fat thigh rather than a problem with the hip joint. Extreme flexion renders an unstable hip more stable because it brings the femoral head closest to the acetabulum with the least strain on the joint.

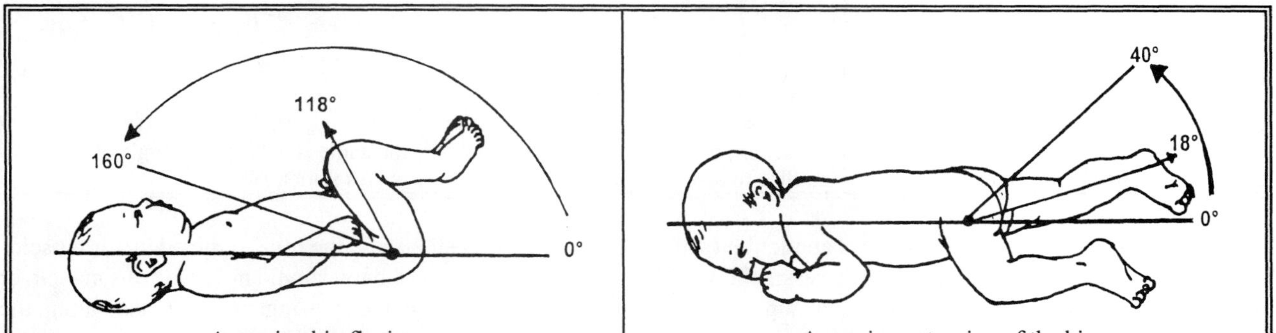

Assessing hip flexion

Assessing extension of the hip

Hip extension: This is the motion made when a person stands and swings a straightened leg out behind him. Extension of the hip increases any existing instability. For a newborn, begin with the baby lying on her belly. Use a horizontal line drawn through the length of the body as the baseline. The legs should be as straight and as flat against the mattress as is possible, although a true starting position is not achievable until the baby is several weeks old. Hold one leg as straight as possible and gently lift it directly off the mattress. A line drawn straight through the raised leg is used to get an angle with the baseline. The angle on each side should be equal. If you believe a hip to be dislocated, you can further assess the baby by turning her over on her back and placing that leg so that it hangs off the side of the mattress. When the hip is dislocated, it will easily hyperextend at the hip and, in many cases, at the knee as well (Tachdjian, 1997). As you extend the leg, palpate to notice what happens to the femoral head. If it is dislocated, a depression will develop in the groin where the femoral head should be normally located (Chung, 1981).

Abduction of the hip: Spontaneous abduction (separation of the thighs) of the affected side is limited in true dislocation; difficulty in abducting either hip to 80° should always raise suspicion of congenital dislocation. There are two ways to assess hip abduction. Wait for the baby to be resting quietly on his back before performing the following assessments.

Abduction in flexion: Starting with the legs in a flexed posture is the preferred way to assess abduction in the newborn because of the natural flexion contracture that is present. A relaxed baby should be able to have her flexed leg gently abducted from the hip through an arc of 80 to 90°. The baseline runs down through the center of the hip joint to the mattress. Gently grasp one leg, flex it at the hip and knee, and spread the leg over to the side until the lateral border (outside) of the thigh is almost flat on the mattress. A distinct restriction of this movement usually indicates an established congenital dislocation, although bilateral restriction could also be due to increased muscle tone or spasm, coxa vara (where the ball joint of the femur is angled to the side more than usual) or merely normal variation. Maximum abduction is achieved when the opposite side of the pelvis starts to tilt, which can be detected by stabilizing the opposite hip with one hand placed on top of it while moving the opposite leg. An angle is obtained by comparing the baseline with a line extended from the knee to the center of the hip joint. Dislocation reveals a palpable depression just to the outside of the ischial tuberosity if the femoral head is dislocated (Chung, 1981).

Abduction in extension: Straighten both legs as much as possible into a neutral position. A baseline is established with a horizontal line across the hips and then extending a perpendicular line straight down from the first. Abduction is assessed by keeping the leg as straight as possible and moving the entire leg away from the midline (spreading one leg outward with the knees more or less straight).

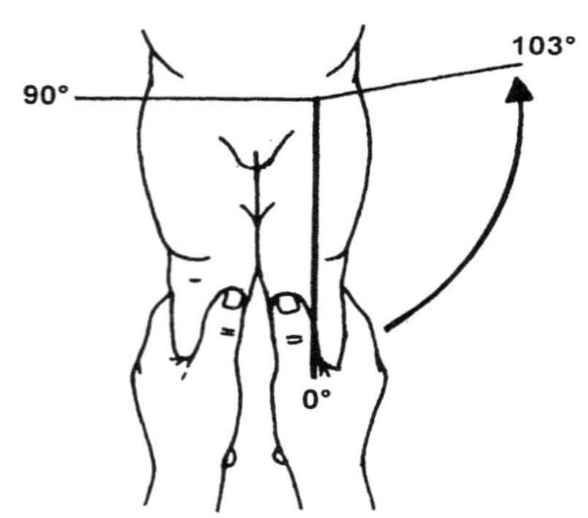

Abduction in extension

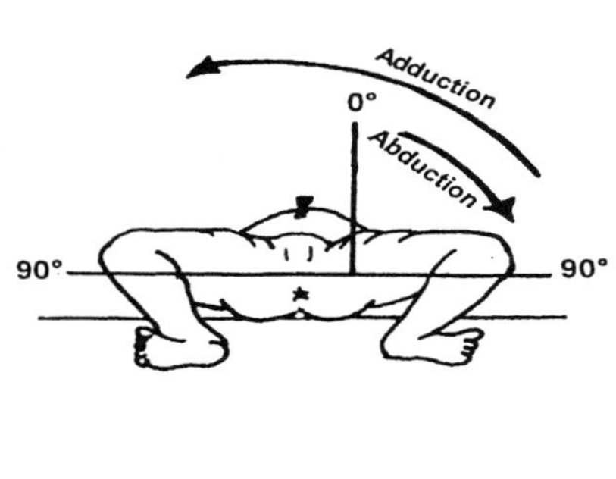

Abduction/adduction in flexion (move knee away from baseline to assess abduction; move it past the abdominal midline to assess adduction)

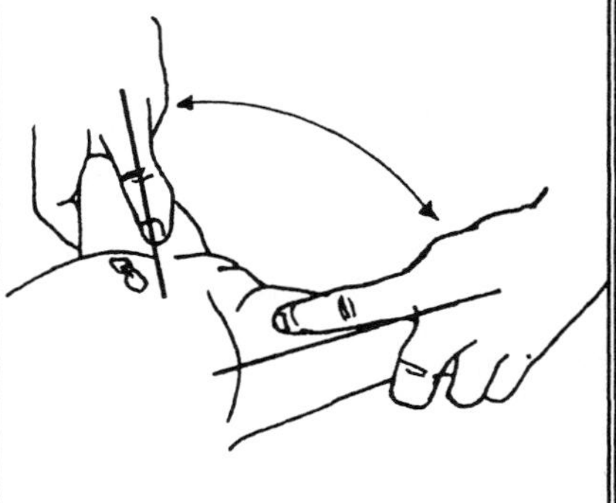

Checking adductor angles (in this case, the angle is 90°, but the angle of view makes it look larger)

****Adductor angles:*** This maneuver uses abduction (separation of the thighs) to assess the tone in the adductor muscles of the hip and can be performed during assessment of abduction in extension. The baby should not resist this maneuver for it to be truly informative. Lie the infant supine, and extend the legs by placing the forefinger of each hand along the inner thighs and gently separating them as far apart as possible. A baseline is established with a horizontal line through the baby's midline to the center of the crotch. Measure the angle formed by the legs, with a line that extends from each knee to the baseline. Assess any asymmetry in how far the legs can be spread. Abnormal hip development results in asymmetry in the angles; abnormal adductor tone can lead to hip dislocation. The angle ranges from 40 to 80° with equal abduction on both sides. The baby can spread his legs further apart as term approaches, but the angle should be no greater than 90°.

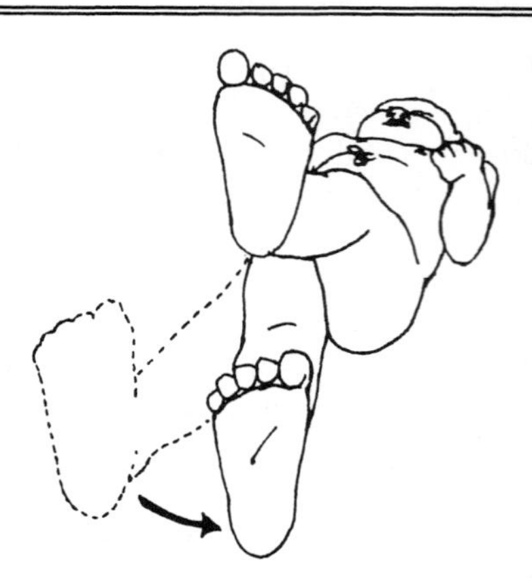

Method 2: Adduction of the extended hip

Adduction of the hip: Begin with the baby supine. Establish a baseline as for abduction in extension, (see above). The maximum range of adduction is 30° past the baseline and should be equal on both sides. This assessment can be performed in two ways:

- Method 1. Beginning with the legs straight in the neutral position, lift one leg over the other toward and past the midline as far as possible.
- Method 2. Beginning with the legs as straight as possible, lift one leg and pass the leg to be examined under it.

Hip rotation, hips extended, knee flexed: Begin with the baby on his belly with one knee flexed. The baseline is established with a vertical line drawn through the center of the top of the knee, passing between the big toe and the second toe to the mattress. Grasp the foot and, keeping the knee in line with the trunk and flexed at a 90° angle, rotate the leg so that the foot is moved away from the midline, which will result in internal rotation of the hip joint. Then return to the start position and move the foot toward and past the midline of the back as far as it will go, which will cause the hip joint to rotate externally. With both maneuvers, maximum rotation of the hip joint is achieved when one side of the pelvis begins to lift off the mattress. Rotation in each direction should be symmetrical in both hips.

Once you have assessed both legs, you can stabilize the pelvis with one hand while reassessing each leg individually, if indicated. Watch for unusual bulging at the hip, indicating abnormal movement of the femoral head.

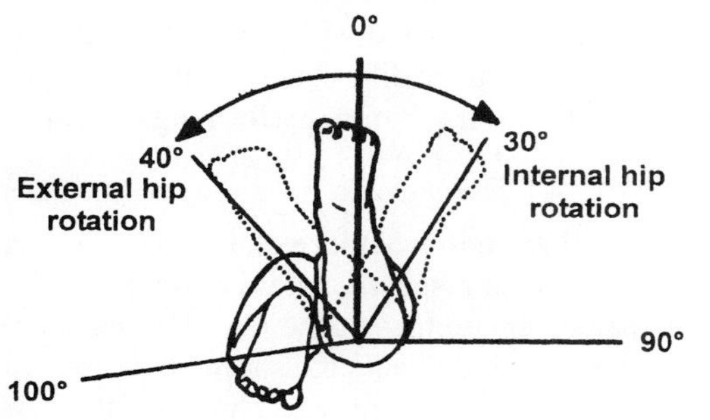

Hip rotation with the hip extended, knee flexed

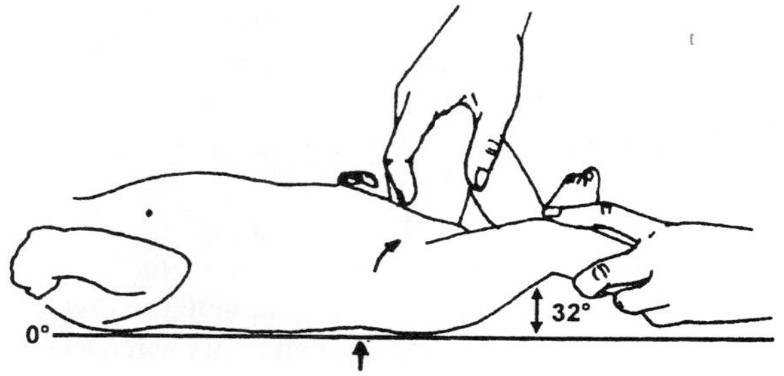

Thomas test: straight arrows indicates where the spine will begin to lift as hip rotates (curved arrow), When it does, measure the angle under the thigh: in this case 32°

Flexion contracture (extension limitation, Thomas test): The number of degrees that the extended thigh lacks from going to complete 0° extension is the degree of extension limitation, more commonly known as "flexion contracture," present in that hip. When the hip is dislocated, the hip and knee can often be fully extended. This kind of laxity is a very reliable indication that dislocation is present. Conversely, an immobile, dislocated hip may present with less than normal extension. The Thomas test can be used to assess flexion contracture whenever dislocation is suspected (Chung, 1981).

To perform this test, the baby needs to be quiet and cooperative. Lie her supine with her legs level and square to her trunk so that a line drawn between the superior iliac spines is perpendicular to the axis of her spine. Fully flex both hips. Stabilize the pelvis and prevent pelvic motion on the side not being examined by holding that leg flexed enough to flatten the lumbar spine. Use your other hand to extend the other left leg straight down in a "standing" position until that hip rises off the mattress (that is, the pelvis starts to tilt also signaled by the lumbar area starting to arch), indicating the leg's limit of motion. Flexion contracture, which is normal in newborns, exists when the leg cannot be extended to a completely straight position. Measure the angle between the thigh and the horizontal plane of the examining surface, which indicates the degree of flexion contracture. Normally this is 25 to 30°, but it may range up to 45° in normal infants. Reverse your hand maneuvers and examine the right leg. If there is an inequality in the angles or if one angle exceeds 30°, the increased contracture may be in either the hip or the knee. If there is asymmetrical extension, the hip that can extend the farthest may be dislocated or unstable (Chung, 1981).

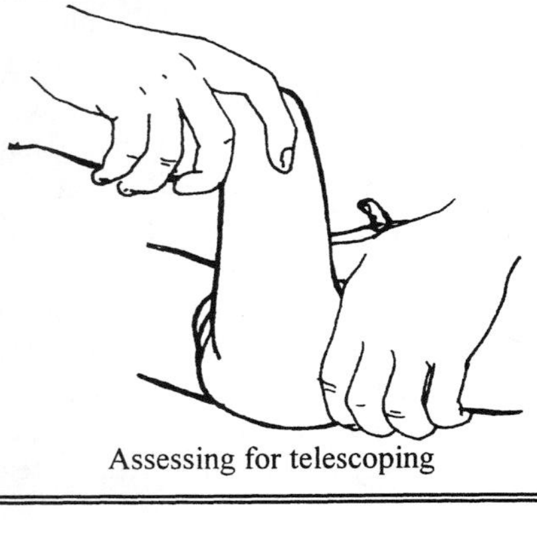

Assessing for telescoping

Telescoping (Dupuytren sign): The normal hip joint feels firm and stable in both adduction and abduction. Laxity of the supporting ligaments results in free movement known as **telescoping**. Lie the infant supine. Use the hand on the same side to be examined to brace the hip against the mattress by encircling the anterior hip joint with the thumb and forefinger and bracing the pelvis on that side with the palm. Use the other hand to flex that hip to 90°, extend the knee and pull the leg upward so as to lift the head of the femur out of the hip socket. Lower the leg back toward the mattress, extend it and pull straight down in relationship to the hip. Reverse your hand maneuvers and repeat on the other leg. Lots of free movement at the hip joint indicates that the joint is unstable. It is always abnormal for a hip to be dislocated before any pressure is applied (Chung, 1981).

Combined maneuvers to evaluate hip dislocation and relocation: After performing the appropriate screening maneuvers, you should have some idea if the hips appear to be normal or if a problem is suspected. The next maneuvers are designed to reveal or confirm a dislocated hip. If the hip joints are normal, they should remain stable throughout these assessments. Both tests should be negative. In most cases, a dislocation is posterior, meaning the head of the femur moves to the rear. Proceed according to your findings thus far.

If the legs appear symmetrical: If both legs appear symmetrical, are the same length and have equal angles of abduction, or if the baby rests with his legs spread (abducted, which is not normal in a term baby and may indicate lax connective tissue), perform the Barlow maneuver before you do the Ortolani maneuver.

If the legs appear asymmetrical: If asymmetry of length, knees or creases is found with any of the preceding assessments, the shorter side, with the bunched-up creases, is most likely to be dislocated. With any of these findings, perform the Ortolani maneuver first, beginning with the shorter leg, before performing the Barlow maneuver.

Which maneuver you start with may be different for each leg, depending upon whether you believe it is currently dislocated. Since these maneuvers are intended to dislocate and relocate the hip respectively, it is common practice to perform both maneuvers on one leg and then switch to perform both maneuvers on the second leg. This ensures that a dislocated hip is not left that way for a period of time while the other leg is examined, reducing strain on the tendons and ligaments as well as minimizing discomfort for the baby. Note that both of these signs cannot be elicited in the same hip. *Either* the femoral head is located in the acetabulum and can be temporarily displaced (Barlow's sign) *or* it is already out of the its socket and can be temporarily replaced during the exam (Ortolani's sign) (Tachdjian, 2002).

Several different ways of performing both the Barlow and Ortolani techniques are presented. While different methods may be confusing for the novice, they are all included to give the student a variety of approaches; no doubt some of the nuances of technique may come in handy during individual assessments. I recommend getting a more or less term-sized doll with flexible cloth legs so you can practice the maneuvers as you study. This will help clarify the relative merits of each approach. Be gentle, using firm but not excessive pressure; you do not want to damage an unstable joint. The baby must be relaxed for the maneuvers to be informative as a kicking, crying baby will tighten her adductor and hamstring muscles, leading to a false result.

Barlow hip dislocation maneuver: The Barlow maneuver screens for an unstable, dislocatable hip. A dislocatable hip is currently in its socket but the connective tissue is lax, allowing the femoral head to become partially displaced. When the hip is flexed and the thigh is brought into an adducted position, the dislocatable femoral head will either fall out and to the rear of the acetabulum or can be gently pushed posteriorly out of the socket. While a positive Barlow test by itself does not necessarily diagnose a problem hip, babies with positive tests should be referred for further evaluation for this possibility.

Use your left hand to examine the baby's right leg and your right hand to examine the left leg. To examine the right leg, flex the shin toward the thigh at the knee by placing the crotch of your left thumb and forefinger over the shin, just below the knee. Apply your thumbpad to the inner side of the thigh just below the knee, which is bent at about a 30° angle (do not dig your thumb into the femoral triangle; this will be painful to the baby). Stretch your index and ring fingers along the length of the outer femur, with your ring finger over the outer side of the hip joint (greater trochanter) as illustrated. Your last two fingers may either pass under the knee to grasp the upper calf from the outside or extend along the outer thigh (depending on the size of your hands and the size of the baby). The leg should now be held with the hip at 45° of flexion and 5 to 10° of adduction, which is an unstable position.

Use your other hand to stabilize the opposite leg under the upper thigh, with your thumb braced against the lateral pubic bone in front, the crotch of your index finger and thumb around the side of the thigh, your index and ring fingers extended along the flank and palm adjacent to the thigh on that side, applying equal pressure to steady the pelvis. This is a particularly helpful grip if the pelvis proves difficult to stabilize, although the hand can be placed on the left leg in exactly the same manner as the examining hand. This stabilizing hand prevents the unexamined side of the pelvis from moving when you apply downward pressure to steady it and keep the lower back straight while holding the leg at 90° of flexion and 45° of abduction unless otherwise recommended below.

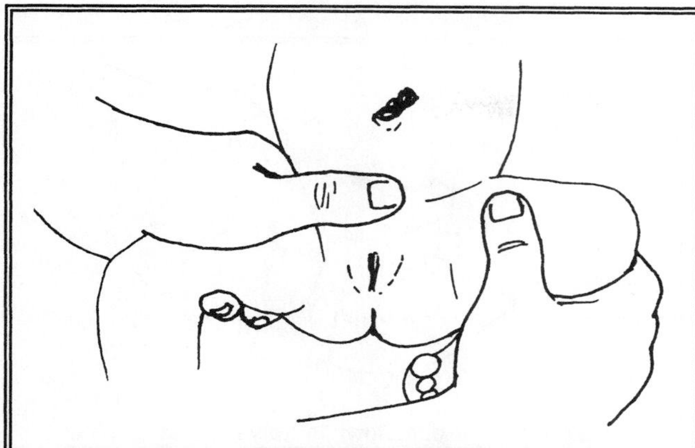

Hand positions with left hand stabilizing the pelvis

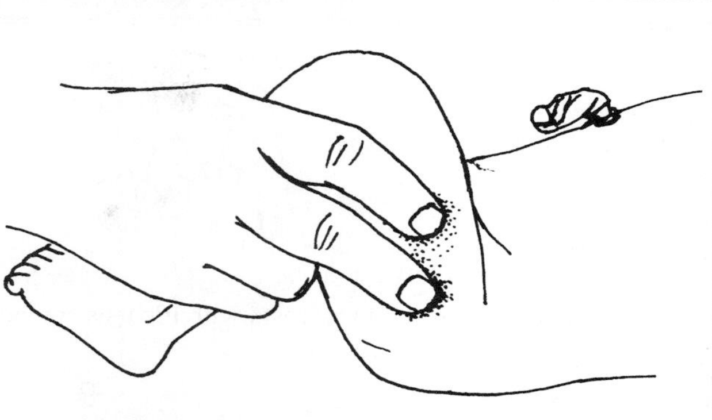

Side view of the right hand, showing fingers stretched along the outer thigh

There are basically two different ways of performing the Barlow maneuver described in the literature. Start with your hands positioned as above, using the first method, as it is more gentle and usually sufficient. If you are having trouble determining if the test is positive, further adduct the leg, as that will render the hip even more unstable.

Barlow, method 1: As you adduct the thigh at least 20° toward and past the midline of the baby's belly, use your thumb to apply pressure backward and outward against the inner thigh and the rest of your hand to assist in applying pressure to the knee in an outward (from the midline) angle toward the mattress in an effort to dislocate the hip. Normally, no movement is felt. If the joint is lax, you will feel for movement of the femur to the side against some resistance as it slips out over the posterior rim of the acetabulum and pops out; if this happens, the knee heights should now be asymmetrical, with the shorter leg dislocated (a positive Allis' sign) (Fletcher, 1998; Hensinger, 1979). The femoral head may or may not immediately relocate back into the socket when pressure is released.

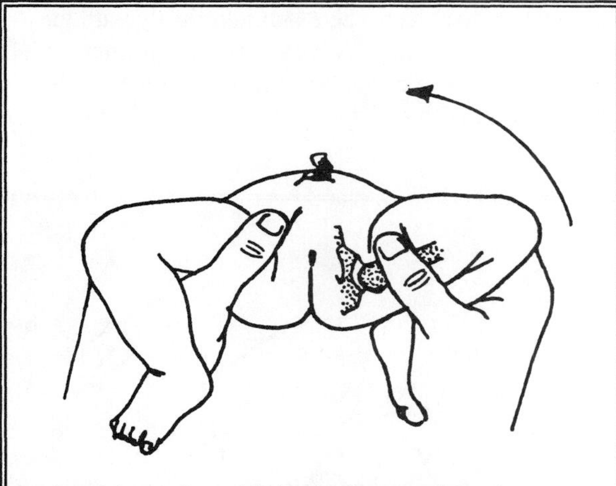

Barlow (1): starting with the thighs spread, begin to move the leg to be examined toward the midline

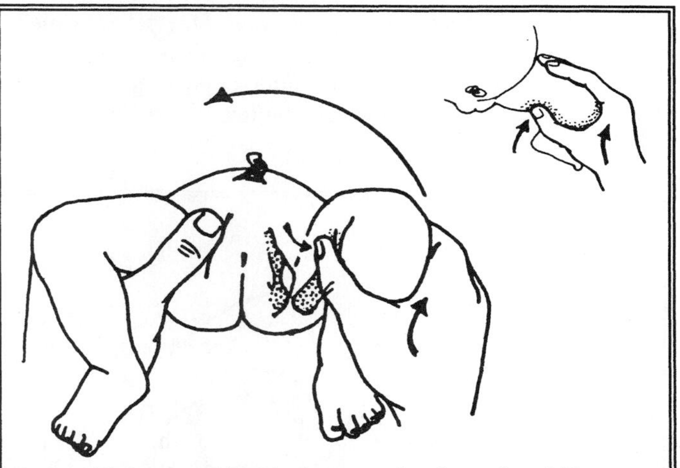

Barlow (1): as you adduct the leg toward and past the midline, press with your thumb and hand to try and dislocate the hip

(after Fletcher, 1998)

Barlow, method 2: This approach involves telescoping the femur. Brace one side of the pelvis. To examine the other side, grasp that lower leg and knee and pull straight up on the femur. This should lift a loose femur head out of the socket. While the leg is still under tension, you can use your thumb to push the femur outward (away from the midline) and backward to complete the dislocation if necessary. Upon dislocation the knees should now be at different heights, with the dislocated leg being shortened. Now push straight down on the leg, which should yield a noticeable clunk as the dislocated femoral head knocks against the outer edge of the acetabulum (Graham, 1988).

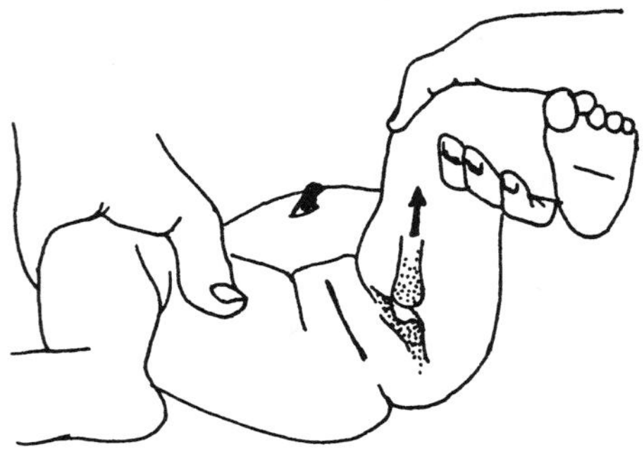

Barlow (2): Pulling up on the femur to take it out of the socket

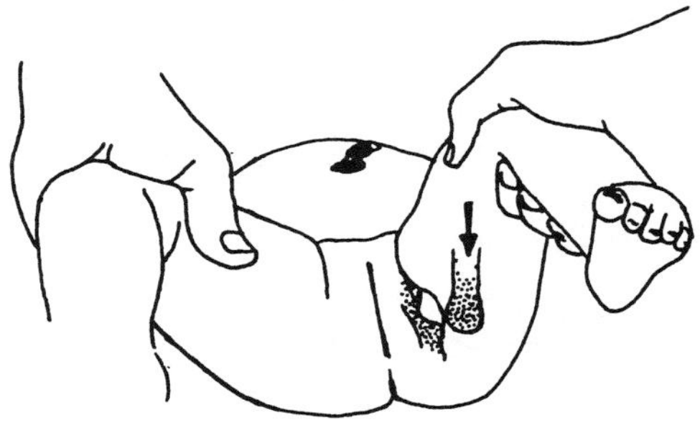

Barlow (2): pushing down to fully dislocate the hip

(after Graham, 1988)

If the Barlow test is normal on one leg and you believe the other leg is also normal, perform the Barlow maneuver on the other side now by reversing your hand maneuvers. If the ball of the femur moves to the edge but not out of the socket, it is subluxable. If the femoral head appears to have come out of its socket or if you have completed the Barlow maneuver on both legs, proceed with the Ortolani maneuver.

Ortolani hip relocation (reduction) maneuver: The Ortolani maneuver is a very reliable screening tool for evaluating the presence of a currently dislocated hip. This maneuver is intended to reposition the head of the femur into the acetabulum, thus reversing the effect of a positive Barlow test. The baby should be relaxed and lying supine on a firm surface. The hand positions are the same as for the Barlow test unless otherwise noted. Some have erroneously stated that this maneuver is used to demonstrate that the hip can be fully abducted. However, most dislocated hips will permit full abduction without relocation of the ball within the socket at birth; thus the finger pressure techniques are important to an accurate test. There are three slightly different ways of performing the Ortolani maneuver described in the literature.

Ortolani, method 1: Brace one side of the pelvis while holding the (other) leg to be examined firmly with the knee straight up. Abduct the leg (move it laterally, away from the midline). Now use your ring finger to apply light pressure to the outer, upper thigh in an upward and midline direction, thus lifting and pushing the femoral head into the acetabulum. A positive test is felt as a clunk with a visible jerk as the femoral head is replaced in its socket (Fletcher, 1998).

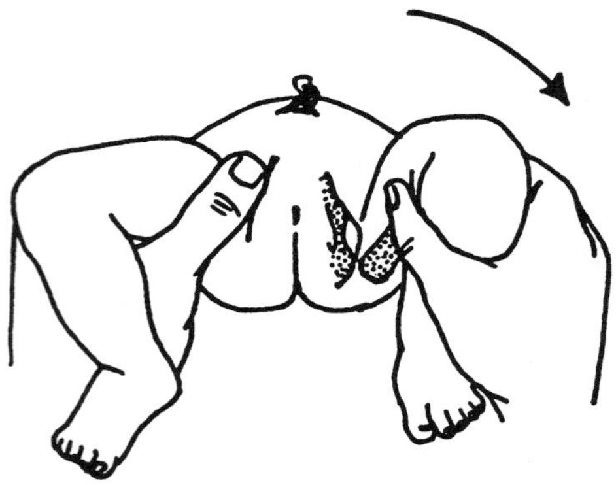

Ortolani (1): Bracing the right hip and beginning abduction of the left hip.

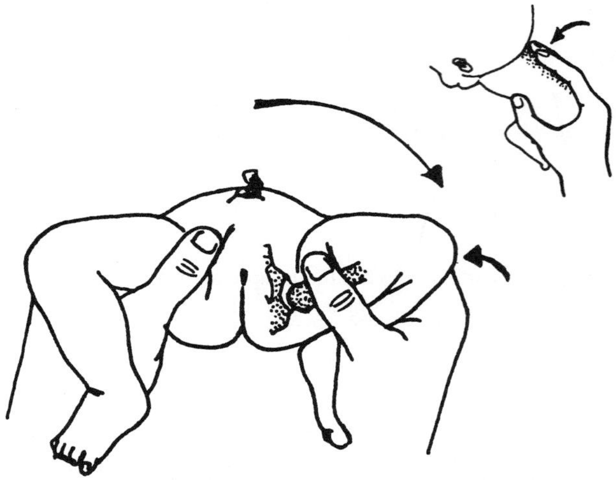

Ortolani (1): Pushing from behind to relocate the left hip

(After Fletcher, 1998)

Ortolani, method 2: Brace one side of the pelvis as you grasp the (other) lower leg and knee and raise the knee straight up. Now, push straight down on the femur. This should further dislocate a dislocated hip. Now, abduct the leg (move it laterally, away from the midline); this will cause the head of the femur to pivot inward. Simultaneously apply pressure to the outside of the thigh in an upward direction with your index finger. This should produce a noticeable clunk as the dislocated femoral head is pushed over the rim of the acetabulum and into the socket (Graham, 1988).

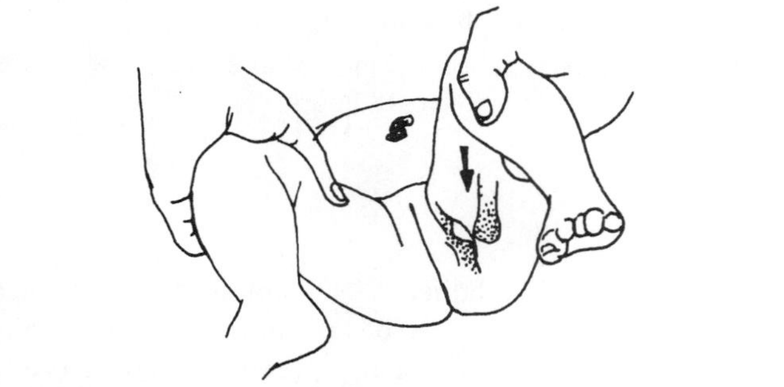

Ortolani (2): After pulling up on the leg, push straight down to fully dislocate the hip.

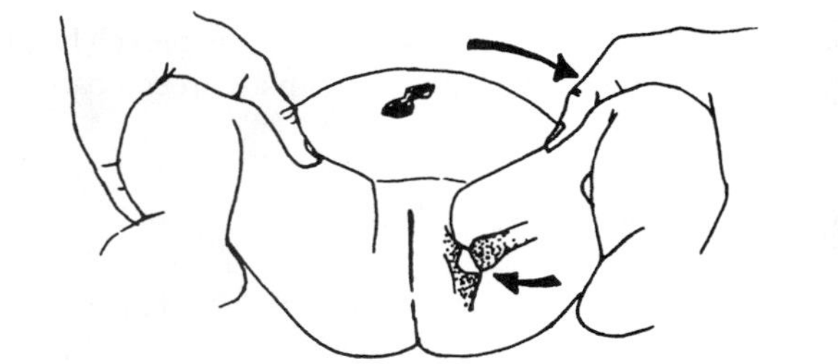

Ortolani (2): Rotating hip while pushing with fingers toward the midline.

(after Graham, 1988)

Ortolani, method 3: The hand positioning for this, the gentlest method, differs from that described above. With the baby supine, place your palms over the knees bringing them together in the midline. Extend your fingers down the outside of each thigh toward the hip joints, placing the index fingers over the greater trochanter of each femur and the thumbs over the lesser trochanter of each femur (that is, as near to the hip joint as possible). Simultaneously spread both legs slowly until the outer side of the knees touch the examining surface. A positive test produces a clunk as the dislocated femoral head, which lies posterior to the acetabulum and enters the socket at some point during the 90° arc of movement. Since this method tests both legs at once, it allows ready comparison of mobility and range of motion. If a problem is suspected, retest that leg using one of the two methods for the Barlow maneuver described above (Hoekelman, 1991).

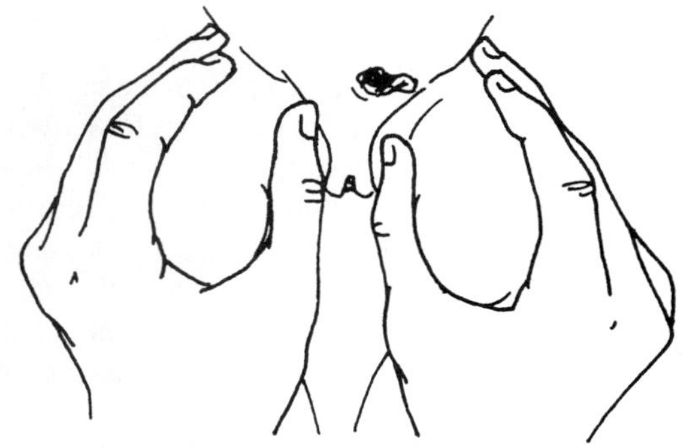

Ortolani (3): Both hands positioned to begin exam

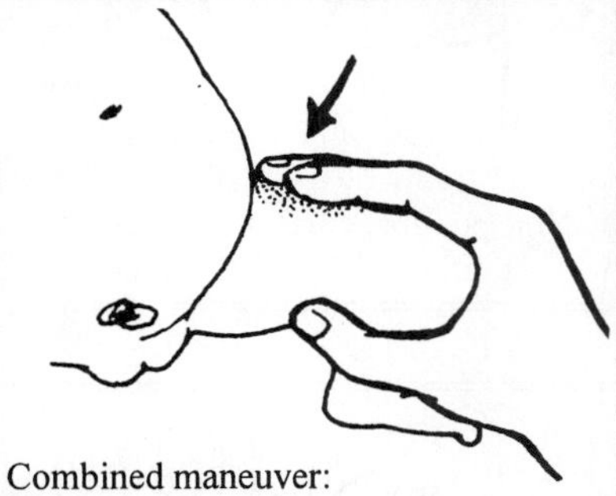

Combined maneuver: Pushing toward the symphysis

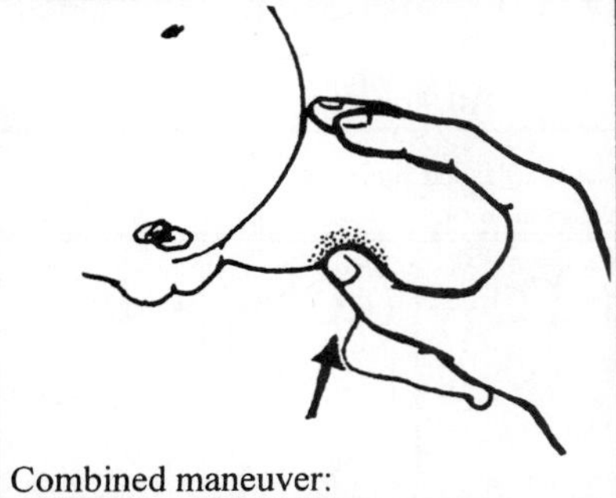

Combined maneuver: Pushing toward the mattress

<u>**Combined Barlow-Ortolani maneuver:**</u> This method combines techniques already described for both maneuvers. Place your hands as described for Ortolani, method 3. Starting with the legs flexed at a 90° angle to the torso and the knees straight up, spread both legs until each is at about a 70° angle in relation to the baby's midline, an extremely unstable angle if hip joint laxity is present. Each leg is then assessed individually. Starting with one leg only, use

your middle finger to exert pressure against the outer thigh, at an upward and inward angle (i.e., away from the mattress) as if to push the trochanter toward the symphysis. Normally no movement occurs. If the hip is dislocated, the greater trochanter and head of the femur can be felt to move toward the midline as it slips back into its socket. Keeping the leg spread to 70°, use your thumb, which is applied over the upper, inner thigh, to exert pressure toward the mattress. If the hip sits loosely in its socket and can be dislocated, it should slip out of the acetabulum and return immediately once pressure is released. Examine the other leg in the same manner (Illingworth, 1975).

Both the Barlow and Ortolani maneuvers will be negative if a hip is dislocated and cannot be relocated. In these cases, leg length and range of motion may or may not show a problem. Conversely, normal hip joints may be unstable on the first day of life, especially following breech birth. Many of these hips will become more stable within a few days; therefore, if there is any doubt and in all breech babies, reexamine the hips after 24 to 48 hours.

Examining the Ankles and Feet

The examination of the ankles and feet is based on the excellent work of Tachdjian (1997), unless otherwise noted. The ankles and feet are assessed at rest and when in active motion. The forefeet tend to be toed-in with the soles facing each other in a posture of slight plantar flexion; however, the posture of a normal foot can vary considerably according to intrauterine positioning. The plantar arch in most newborns is filled with a pad of fat, resulting in "flat" feet. This will gradually disappear during the first year of life. Passive motion of the ankle is dependent upon fetal positioning at birth. Stimulate active motion by stroking the sides, top and bottom of each foot and observe how the foot moves. A number of different foot deformities may occur. In all cases, if the foot can be passively repositioned to a normal posture, the cause is intrauterine positioning and the deformity should resolve on its own. If the foot is rigid and cannot be manipulated into a normal posture, the baby should be evaluated by an orthopedist or osteopath.

Plantar creases

(See the section on palmar creases in the subchapter entitled "Examining the Arms, Clavicles and Hands" for general information about creases.) The plantar creases have received far less attention than those of the palm, partly because they fade or disappear in early infancy. There is an wide range of normal variation, with slight differences between sides and sexes. The anterior sole is focused upon, which has 9 major creases, although the number which appear in normal individuals varies widely. Because foot creases are less familiar and the variations more complex than in the palm, creases, numbered according to Hauser and colleagues, are shown to the right. There is little information on abnormal plantar creases; an exception is the arch fibular S crease, which is associated with trisomy 13 (Hauser et al., 1983; Hiroshi & Kadowaki, 1975).

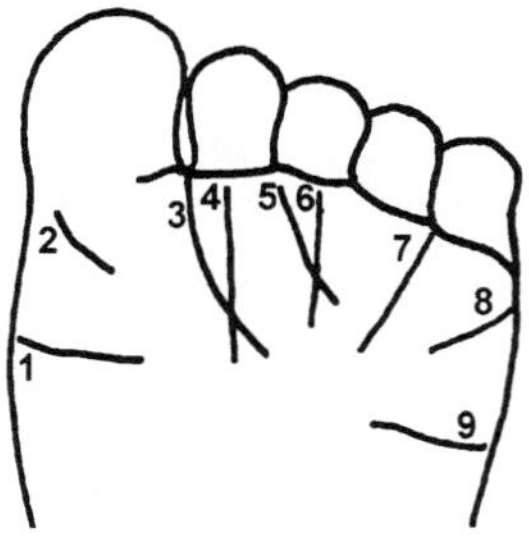

Nine possible creases in the anterior portion of the newborn foot

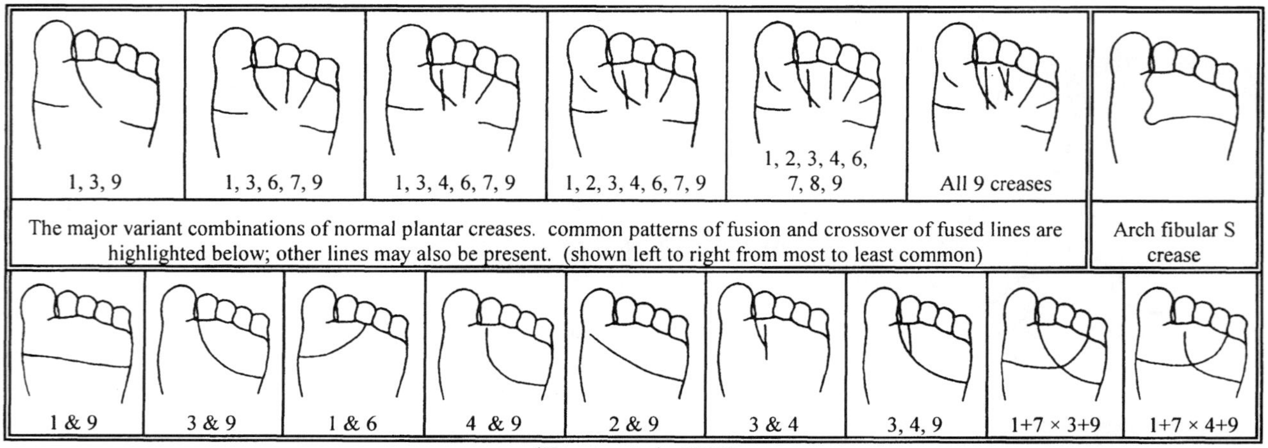

(Hauser, et al., 1983)

Toes

Look over the toes for number, size, spacing, fusion or webbing. Curving that does not exceed 8° is normal. Overlapping of toes in babies is usually hereditary; correction is often accomplished by stabilizing the toes in the correct position with adhesive tape for about six weeks. Dorsiflexion of the big toe (i.e., a spontaneous Babinski reflex), is often noted in normal crying babies, but when persistent may reflect an upper motor neuron lesion on the contralateral side (Hill, 1998). Slight webbing (syndactyly) of the 2nd and 3rd toes is a common minor congenital anomaly that is not particularly significant. Assess the toenails for presence, size, firmness, length and any irregularities. The growth of the toenails lags behind the fingernails, reaching the tips of the toes by 36 weeks. Because of this, hypoplastic toenails are often temporary variations in babies. Edema that raises the surrounding cuticle can mimic hypoplasia. However, as with fingers, poorly formed nails and extra digits are often associated with genetic syndromes. For this reason, extra digits should not be removed until the baby can be examined by a specialist.

Attention to the toe prints is usually limited to the big toe, which normally displays one of the three basic patterns seen on the fingers–the arch, loop or whorl–oriented toward either the tibial or fibular side of the foot. A tibially-oriented arch is associated with Down syndrome (Shiono & Kadowaki, 1975).

Assessing normal structure and function of the ankles and feet

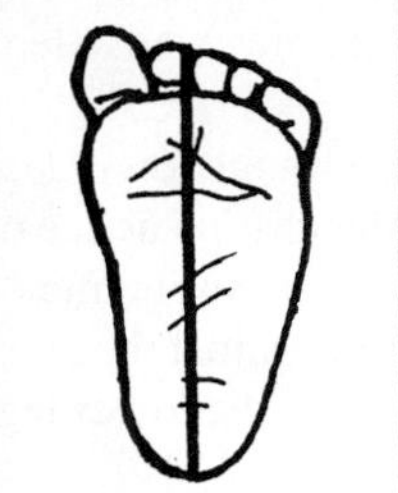

Heel bisection

Heel bisection: To begin your assessment of normal foot formation, check the position of the forefoot in relation to the hindfoot. First, locate the center of the posterior border of the heel. Extend a vertical line up the sole of the foot from the center of the heel toward the toes. Note where the line intersects the toes. Normally it passes between the 2nd and the 3rd toe, with a range of bisection from the interspace between the 1st and 2nd toe to the interspace between the 3rd and 4th toe. Findings outside this range are associated with abnormal bending of the foot.

Another way to gauge this is to draw a parallel line straight through the ankle eminences. In a normal foot, this line forms an 85° angle to a vertical baseline drawn through the sole when the foot is held straight. It is easier, however, to establish a vertical line through the sole as described above.

If bisection suggests deformity, draw a line across the top of the foot at the junctions of the tarsal and metatarsal bones, located just in front of the point where the foot joins the leg (the tarsal-metatarsal line). The portion of the foot in front of this line is the **forefoot**, the portion behind is the **hindfoot**. The portion in the region of the line is the **midfoot**. In the newborn, the ossification centers of the calcaneus (heel), talus and cuboid (ankle), metatarsals (midfoot) and phalanges (toe bones) are usually present. However, much of the bone structure is still cartilaginous at term, making the foot especially vulnerable to deformity. A variety of positioning malformations that can cause the foot to be turned either in or out and that may simulate a club foot (talipes equinovarus) can be identified with this simple division of the foot. Clubfoot, if present, reflects a structural abnormality.

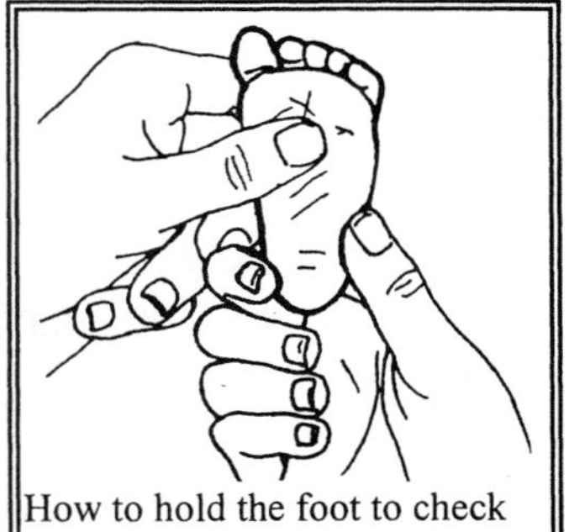

How to hold the foot to check for postural deformity.

Distinguishing postural from structural deformity: Deformities that are due to in utero positioning allow the joints to remain flexible because there is no bone involvement, while those that are structural render the foot inflexible because bones are deformed. To distinguish a positional deformity from a structural defect, first scratch or stroke the outer edge of the affected foot to see if the baby will move it into a normal position. If not, grasp the base of the heel with one hand while using your other to bend the forefoot side to side: if it can be manually abducted beyond neutral, no correction is necessary. If it will not abduct beyond neutral or if it cannot be corrected into a neutral position, the deformity is fixed. Passively position the foot in the midline and dorsiflex it (push the sole up toward the shin). A structurally abnormal foot and ankle will not have a full range of motion and will resist one or both of these movements.

Test the range of abduction next. Hold the foot by the heel so you can see the sole; use your other hand to press against the pad below the big toe. Positional deformity allows the foot to be easily abducted past the midline, with the foot usually assuming a neutral position or twisting toward the midline at rest (varus position). With structural deformities, the arch of the foot appears high; there is often a crease in the middle of the arch toward the midline, and the forefoot cannot be abducted past the midline (the normal anatomical position of the mature foot). If severe, the heel is twisted away from the midline (valgus position).

Range-of-motion assessments of the ankle and foot: The following assessments can be performed whenever there is a question about positional versus structural defects. Normal values for range of motion are charted below. While the motions of inversion and eversion may be tested independently from those of abduction and adduction, normal movement of the foot combines inversion with adduction (supination) and eversion with abduction (pronation), thus independent assessment of each motion is extremely difficult.

Joint or Bones	Flexion	Abduction	Adduction
Ankle: Dorsiflexion Plantar flexion	36 to 71.7° 10 to 41.7° (>10° from normal resting position)		
Forefoot		≥10° to 15°	≥10° to 15°
Hindfoot (heel)		Valgus 5–10°	Varus 5–10°

(**Valgus** refers to the foot turning away from the midline. **Varus** means the foot turning toward the midline.) (Scanlon et al., 1979)

Ankle flexion: This angle decreases as term approaches and uterine space diminishes, so that by term the top of the foot can be pushed against the leg. Any factors that further restrict intrauterine space, such as oligohydramnios or multiple gestation, may result in an angle that is decreased beyond that which is expected for gestational age. In most babies, dorsiflexion is up to twice as great as plantar flexion. The values in the table above were obtained in babies whose legs were flexed at the hip and knee during assessment.

Begin with the baby supine and the knee flexed to relax the heel, with the foot at its natural angle with the lower leg, noting that the entire newborn foot rests at a slightly plantar-flexed posture. (Flexing the leg eliminates the influence of muscle tone when assessing mobility.) A baseline is established parallel with the bottom of the foot. The angle line of 90° is centered through the lower leg, extending to the center of the heel. Dorsiflex the foot by pushing against the sole, bringing the top of the foot as close as possible to the shin; at term, the foot should dorsiflex fully against the lower leg.

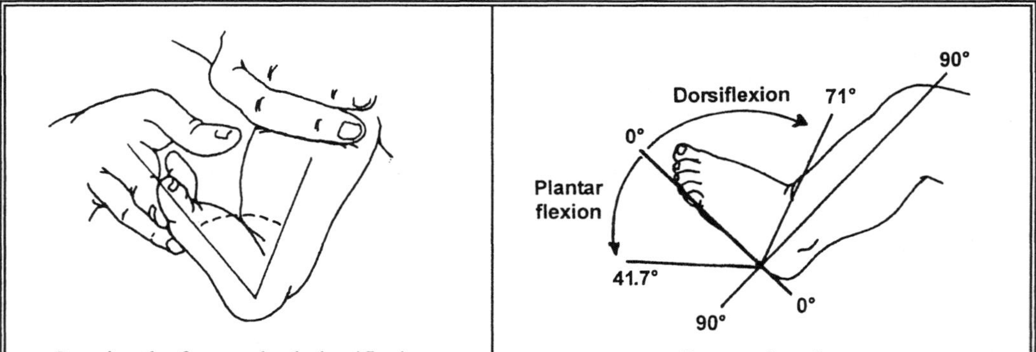

Pressing the foot to check dorsiflexion — Range of motion

To test this joint further, slowly apply moderate pressure to the sole of the foot until the smallest possible angle is achieved. Release, then reapply pressure quickly and suddenly. The range of motion elicited by both maneuvers should be the same. A difference of more than 10° suggests an abnormally exaggerated stretch reflex.

Ankle extension (plantar flexion) is assessed by pushing down on the top of the foot to bring the sole as close to the mattress as possible (pointing the toes downward like a ballerina's).

Note: When dorsiflexion is evaluated to test for either gestational age or motor tone, the leg should be fully extended so that the gastrocnemius and soleus muscles of the leg are involved in the motion. Extending the leg also tests muscle groups across the knee and ankle joints. If there is decreased dorsiflexion when the leg is held straight, flex the knee and recheck. Improvement indicates a tightened Achilles tendon, while continued decreased dorsiflexion suggests congenital inflexibility of the talar joint.

Heel mobility (subtalar motion, both inversion and eversion): Begin with the baby lying on his back. Draw a horizontal baseline beneath the toe pads. Grasp the heel with one hand and steady the leg with the other. Now pivot the foot obliquely at the ankle joint to direct the sole toward the midline. The degree of inversion is measured by how much the heel bone tilts inward in relation to the baseline. Move the heel away from the midline to check the rate of eversion. The degree of motion is measured by how much the plantar surface of the foot tilts away from the baseline. Fixed deformities of the foot will limit or prevent normal flexibility.

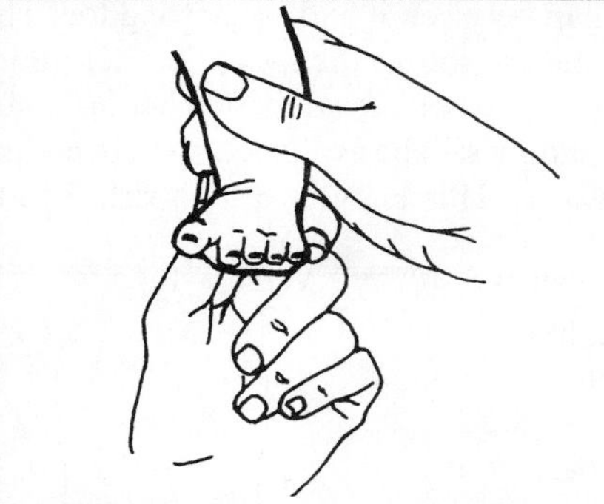
Holding the foot to check subtalar motion

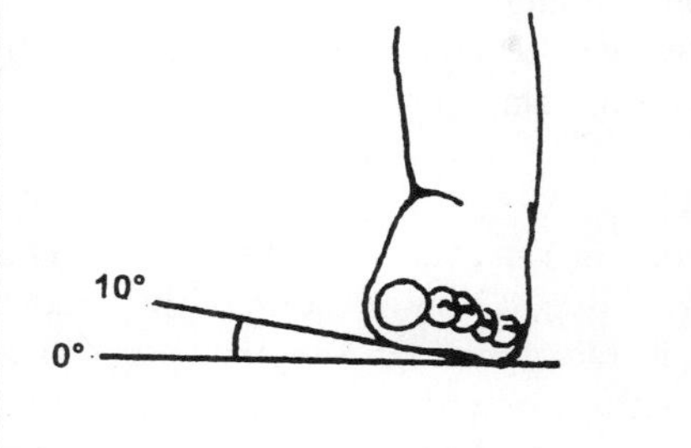

Inversion of the heel

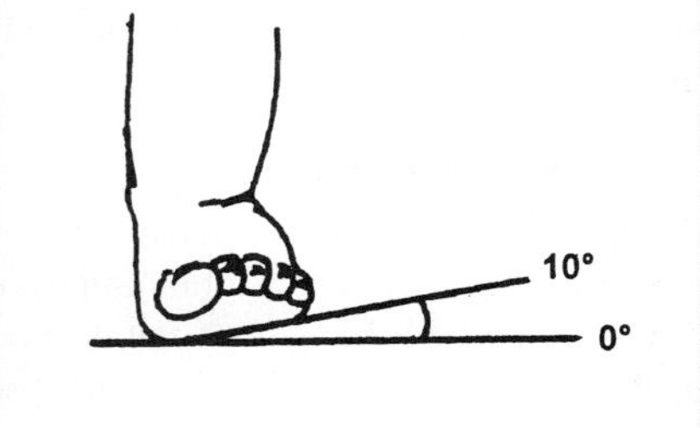

Eversion of the heel

Forefoot motion (abduction and adduction): The movements of the forefoot take place primarily at the midtarsal joint. To assess forefoot motion, grasp the heel with one hand to stabilize the foot in the neutral position, while grasping the forefoot with the other hand. Pivot the forefoot toward the midline (adduction) and away from the midline (abduction). This should be easy if there is no structural deformity. If there is, the foot will be rigid or the range of motion limited.

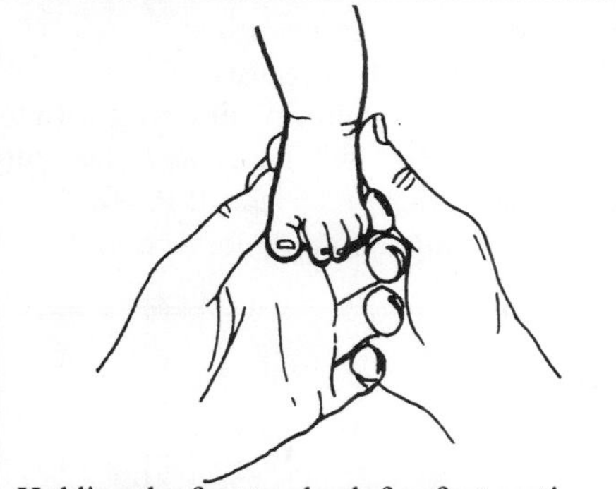
Holding the foot to check forefoot motion

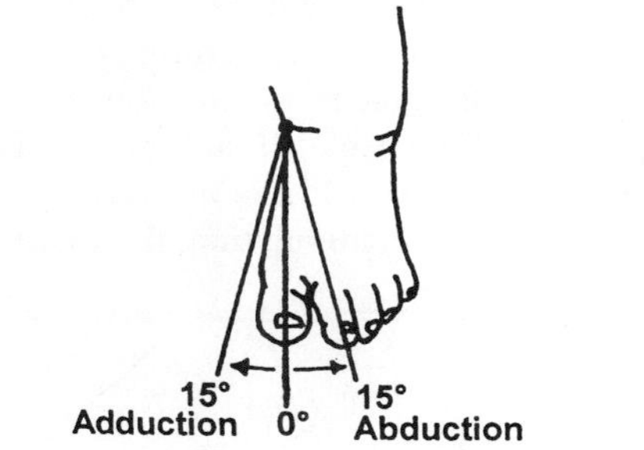

Range of motion (entire foot moves)

<u>Foot deformities</u>

<u>Turning inward of the foot</u>: The primary foot deformities that involve the foot turning inward are described below.

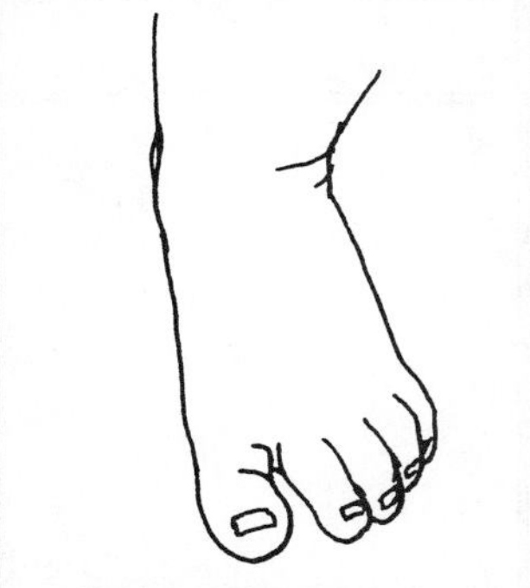
Normal foot posture

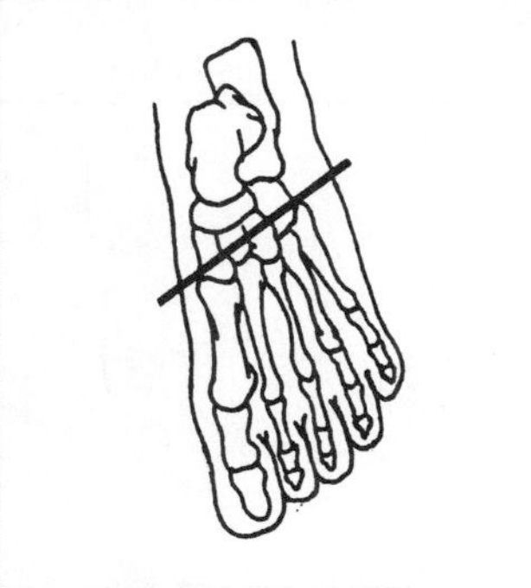
Tarsal-metatarsal line

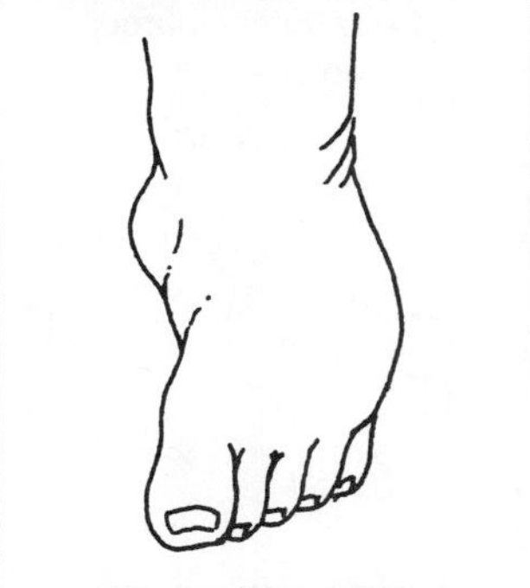
Postural pes varus

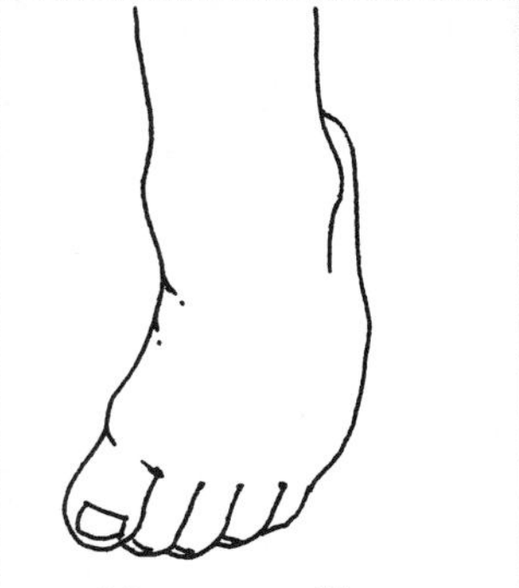
Metatarsus adductus

Postural pes varus: The forefoot points to the midline and the back of the foot is inverted as well, causing the entire foot to appear bent at the tarsal-metatarsal line.

Metatarsus adductus or adduction of the forefoot (toeing-in): This postural deformity occurs when the anterior portion of the foot is turned so that the toes are directed toward the midline, causing the inside border of the foot to form a "C"shape. The big toe points inward more than the rest, resulting in a wide gap between it and the second toe. The posterior portion of the foot is normally positioned, and there is no crease on the medial sole of the foot. This deformity can be corrected by passive manipulation. Spontaneous correction occurs by age two when the adduction begins distal to the tarsal-metatarsal line (that is, on the toe side of the line), although the baby should still be evaluated by a specialist. In metatarsus primus varus, only the first metatarsal and the big toe point inward. This baby is at high risk for hip dysplasia.

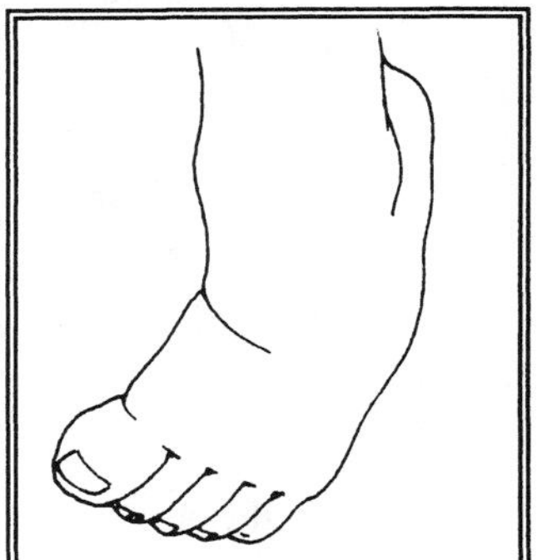

Metatarsus varus

Congenital metatarsus varus: This occurs in 1 in every 1000 live births. The anterior portion of the foot is turned in and inverted due to a subluxation of the tarsometatarsal joints. A crease is present on the middle, inside of the foot, wrapping part way up the top of the foot from the sole. It is a rigid deformity and cannot be corrected by passive manipulation.

Postural clubfoot: The entire foot is pointed downward and is longitudinally rotated inward at the ankle; both ends of the foot are bent inward, toward each other. It is correctable by passive manipulation.

Congenital clubfoot (talipes equinovarus): So called because the foot looks like a golf club, this complex foot deformity is obvious at birth, with males affected twice as often as females. It occurs in 1 in 1000 live births and involves three specific deformities: adduction (varus angulation) of the forefoot, turning inward toward the midline; varus angulation of the ankle so that the foot is turned on its side and the sole is directed toward the midline; and equinus positioning with the toes down and the heel up, rendering the side of the heel difficult to feel. The big toe is relatively shortened, the lateral border of the foot is convex and the inner border is concave with a furrow on the inside, plantar surface of the foot. A deep crease appears on the posterior ankle joint. On manipulation, the foot is rigid and range of ankle joint motion is limited.

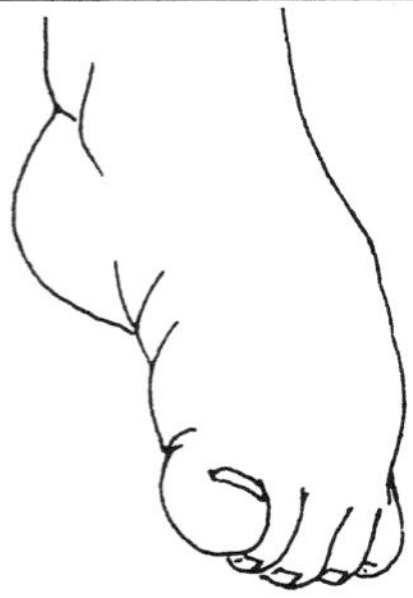

Postural clubfoot

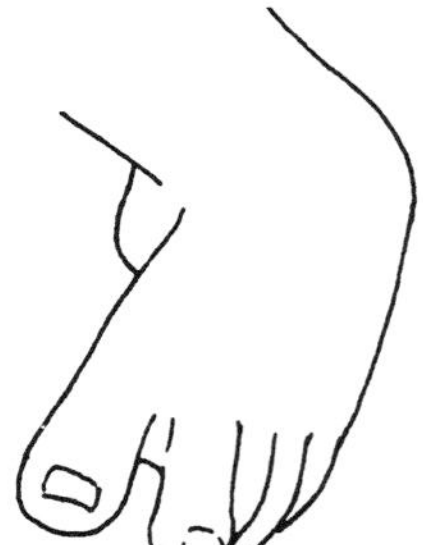

Congenital clubfoot: anterior view

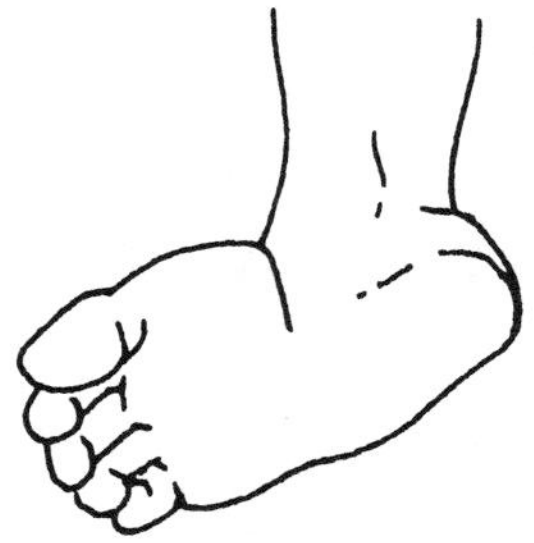

Clubfoot: medial view

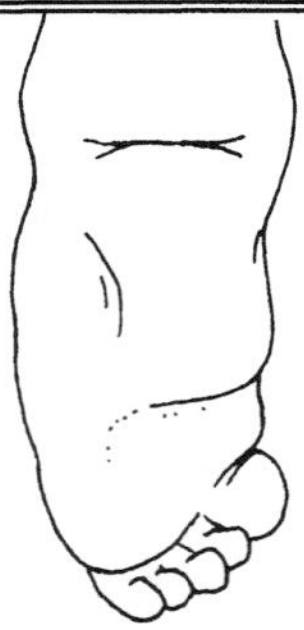

Clubfoot: posterior view

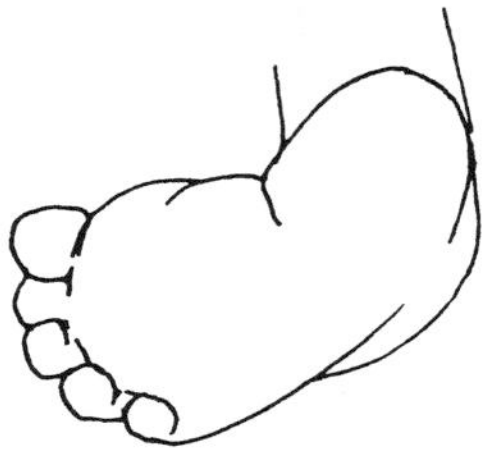

Clubfoot: inferior view

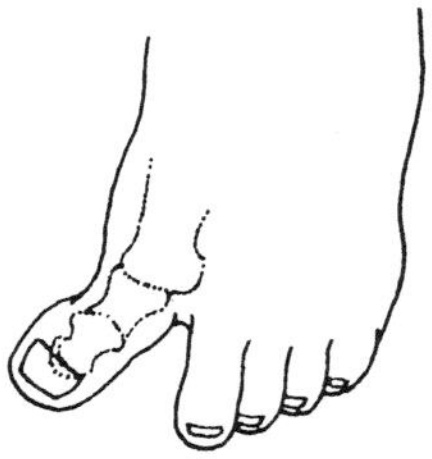

Hallux varus

If only one foot is affected, it is usually smaller than the other, with thickened and contracted ankle and foot joints, which impair movement. Whether one or both feet are affected, an orthopedist should be consulted as soon as possible, as treatment often begins just after birth. Clubbed feet may be associated with neurologic problems in some babies; they may also be found with hip dislocation and contracture of other joints (arthrogryposis).

Hallux varus: The big toe points inward at the second (metatarsophalangeal) joint and the first metatarsal is usually short. In some cases, all the metatarsals point toward the midline. This deformity is rigid and cannot be corrected with passive manipulation.

Outward turning of the foot: The primary foot deformities that involve the foot turning outward include those described below.

Talipes calcaneovalgus: This is the most common postural deformity of the foot, occurring in up to 30 to 50% of all live births. It presents with extreme dorsiflexion of the foot when at rest, with piloting of the foot outward at the ankle joint. Hip dysplasia is a common associated finding. Also check carefully for spinal defects. Talipes calcaneovalgus may be associated with lower nerve dysfunction, therefore assess the calves to rule out muscle atrophy, and evaluate motor function of the plantar flexors to see if the baby can point her toes downward. Assess the cremasteric reflex in boys, and in both sexes, assess the presence of the superficial abdominal umbilical reflex by stimulating the abdomen and watching for motion of the umbilicus. Assess the Babinski response and rule out angular deformities of the tibia. (A posterior dimple of the lower leg suggests tibial defects.) Posterior inward angulation of the tibia and fibula are often associated with a moderate or severe deformity of the heel bone of the foot.

Postural pes valgus: The midfoot and forefoot are turned outward. The forefoot is rotated outward on its longitudinal axis at the ankle joint, with a varying amount of outward rotation of the hindfoot. The ankle is pointed downward and oblique to varying degrees. This deformity is flexible; when the ankle joint is plantar flexed, the normal posture of the foot can be restored. It must be distinguished at birth from two similar deformities, the first being tarsal coalition, in which the entire deformity is fixed. Check the range of eversion and inversion of the heel with the ankle in a neutral, dorsiflexed position. (Do not confuse range of ankle motion with that occurring in the heel.) The other condition is congenital convex pes valgus, in which the posture of the ankle joint and heel is misdirected and fixed toward the back and side. When the ankle is plantar flexed and the forefoot inverted, the vertical position of the ankle is not restored to normal.

Congenital convex pes valgus (vertical talus), congenital: Commonly referred to as a "rocker-bottom foot," this rare rigid deformity causes the ankle to be fixed in 90° of flexion with the head of the talus (ankle) projecting into the plantar surface of the foot. The incidence is 1 in 10,000 births. The sole is convex, the heel is drawn up and the forefoot and midfoot are turned up and outward. This condition may occur as an isolated deformity, but it is often associated with neuromuscular disorders, including a variety of spinal defects, dislocation of the hip or knee, and other deformities of the opposite foot.

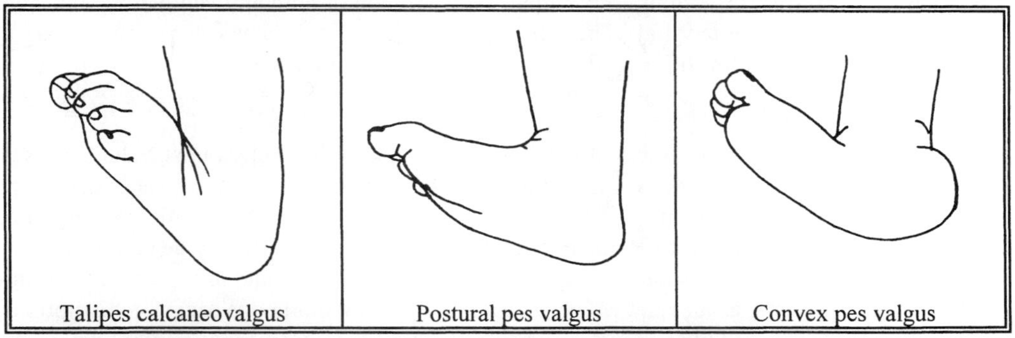

EXAMINING THE BACK, SPINE SCAPULAE AND BUTTOCKS

Turn the baby over to examine the back, spine and scapulae. The baby should spontaneously turn his head to the side to breathe more easily when he is lying prone. First allow the baby to adjust to being on his belly, then, if you have not already done so, you can assess posterior lung sounds before proceeding with the examination of the spine. This chapter is based on Tappero and Honeyfield (2003), unless otherwise noted.

Spinal movement and curvature

The normal convex curvature of the newborn spine can be appreciated when the baby is supported in a sitting position or lying on her side with the back slightly curled forward. Extension and lateral flexion of the spine can be observed during passive flexion. Movements should be smooth and rhythmic; the back should have smooth contours, with no muscle spasm. Lateral flexion may be somewhat asymmetric as a result of in utero positioning.

A side-lying baby may appear to have a curvature. Thus, any lateral curvature of the spine is first assessed with the infant resting comfortably on her belly. The normal newborn is gently kyphotic; that is, the spine curves from top to bottom in a gentle "C" shape with the convex curve to the back. Lordosis of the neck and lower back develop as the child matures. Palpate along the length of the spine, noting any scoliosis (curving to the side and with abnormal rotation), lordosis (anteriorly convex curving) or an unusual degree of kyphosis (excessive posteriorly convex curving). Lateral curving may be a product of in utero positioning and will require follow-up assessment in the days after birth. Abnormalities of the vertebrae are often not identified during palpation. To differentiate a structural curvature (such as scoliosis) from a positional one, hold the baby upright while supporting her under her arms with your hands. Any structural curvature should then be obvious, since positional curvatures will straighten out with this maneuver.

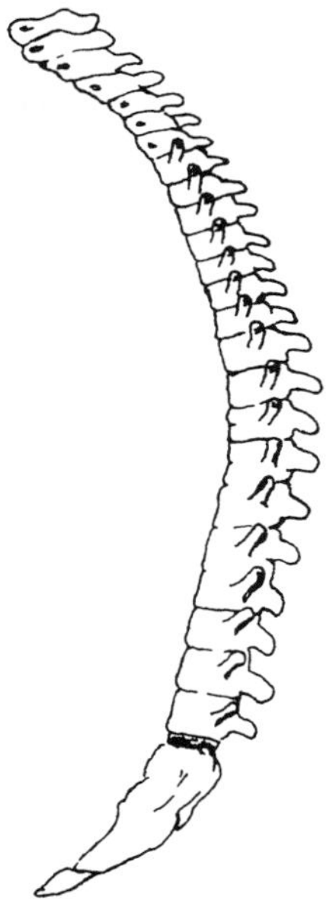

Newborn spinal curvature

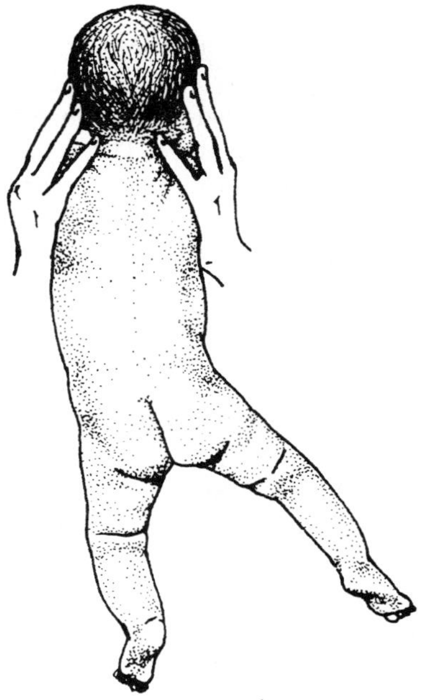

Suspending this baby reveals a true scoliosis of the lumbar spine.

(Left box after Alexander & Brown, 1979
right box after Milner & Herber, 1984)

Any abnormal findings will require further assessment. Scoliosis is a rare disorder usually associated with structural abnormality resulting from a failure of vertebral formation, segmentation or both anywhere along the spine. It is more common in female infants and may be familial. These babies should also be evaluated for genitourinary abnormalities such as Klippel-Feil and Sprengel deformities, which are often associated findings.

Spinal closure

Fusion of the spinal bones should be assessed with the baby lying on his belly or with the baby suspended by a supporting hand under his chest. First, look over the spine from the gluteal crease to the base of the occiput. Note any skin disruption, tufts of hair, soft or cystic masses, birthmarks, dimples, sinus tracts (pinhole openings along the spine) or moisture around an otherwise dry dimple. Remember that a stork bite birthmark may be at the nape of the neck, but is not indicative of a problem. Neural tube defects may be small but are always found in or very near the midline. While a neural tube defect usually presents as an open lesion protruding into a membranous sac, skin disruption is not always present. Therefore any soft mass noted over or just to the side of the midline means that a spinal defect should be ruled out by a specialist.

A closed dimple, which is usually harmless, must be distinguished from a sinus tract. A dimple is often noted just above the anus and is usually a blind indentation. A dermal sinus can be found anywhere along the midline of the spine but is most commonly found in the lumbar region. If it is a sinus, a "bottom" or blind end usually cannot be found. *Never probe a dimple to try and determine if it is closed.* A sinus may be associated with a defect in the underlying vertebra and extend directly to the spinal cord. To try and see the bottom of it, spread the tissue apart using fingers on either side, using a magnifying glass if necessary. A closed sinus can terminate in subcutaneous tissue (the bottom would look raw), a cyst, or a fibrous band. Muscular impairment or paralysis below the level of the defect strongly increases the chances that a spinal defect is present. Any suspicious signs may indicate a congenital spinal or neurological anomaly and call for further evaluation. A palpable, mobile mass frequently turns out to be a lipoma, a fatty tumor that is covered with normal skin. A sacrococcygeal teratoma is a type of neonatal tumor that can reach huge proportions and that is usually benign at birth but may become malignant if not removed. It tends to be a fixed mass and will usually be located just off to the side of the midline in the region of the coccyx; only rarely is there spinal involvement. Removal can result in neurological or muscular impairment if the tumor is quite large.

Next, use the pads of two fingers to palpate over and to the side of each vertebra down the entire length of the spine to check for the presence of dorsal spinal processes (extra lumps), absence of bone (gaps where there should be bones), or subtle indentations and to further assess any abnormal curvature. To avoid damaging nerves or rupturing a swelling, do not palpate any obvious lesions. Any suspicious findings should be reevaluated while you are holding the baby suspended prone in one hand to open the posterior spaces between the vertebrae, which helps in further assessing the region in question.

Buttocks and sacrum

Palpate to identify the tip of the coccyx and note whether the buttocks are normally rounded with a normal gluteal cleft. Flat buttocks with little or no gluteal cleft suggests sacral agenesis, which may be subtotal or total. A minimum of three sacral segments are required for normal continence. Sacral agenesis is associated with rectoanal anomalies.

The pilonidal region: This is where the distal end of the neural tube attaches to the coccyx. It is also the location of the embryonic tail, which has usually disappeared by birth but in rare cases may persist as a fleshy appendage that may or may not contain tiny bones. Check in the area overlying the coccyx for a pilonidal dimple or sinus. Usually, the loss of the tail leaves a blind depression and does not cause problems. However, occasionally there will be an open tract in this area; suspect this if the bottom of a dimple is not visible or there is moisture around an otherwise dry lesion. During gestation, the neural tube remains open at its upper (caudal) end until closure occurs with the fusion of the ectodermal layer of skin in the midline. The distal end of the tube becomes a delicate fiber that remains attached in the region of the coccyx. A midline depression in this area may indicate the point of attachment. Failure of closure leads to the formation of a sinus tract opening to the exterior. Babies with such a sinus need further evaluation. Sometimes infections or cysts develop in the area and must be removed. Open defects may also be associated with spinal anomalies.

Transillumination of the spine: Confine your use of transillumination to skin-covered defects, if you use it at all; extreme care must be taken not to rupture a lesion during your exam. Fluid-filled spinal defects transilluminate very well. Nerve roots can sometimes be seen floating in a meningomyelocele. Lipomas do not transilluminate as well, as fatty regions admit less light than fluid-filled ones. Sacrococcygeal teratomas can be evaluated using transillumination, which can identify whether a mass is cystic, solid or a combination. The size and extent of a tumor that is largely cystic can also be evaluated in the same manner. Place the tip of the probe on the teratoma; a glow within the pelvis can be seen if the tumor extends into the pelvis (Donn & Kuhns, 1983).

Scapulae

Note the position of each scapula; a winged (elevation of the outer edge) scapula is abnormal. This disorder, known as Sprengel deformity, may be seen on one or both sides; the unilateral variety is easier to spot. The scapula may also be somewhat hypoplastic and malrotated, with palpation revealing that the vertical border is higher and more horizontal than normal. There will be some accompanying limitation of shoulder abduction and flexion. Sprengel deformity is often found in babies with spinal and kidney problems as well as those with Klippel-Feil syndrome.

When You Suspect a Problem during the Newborn Exam

Any unusual findings that may change (such as lesions) can be photographed for your record and to show the physician when the baby is evaluated. Unusual crease patterns of the palms and especially the plantar surfaces (because they start to change in early infancy) should also be photographed, making sure that the crease pattern is clear.

Communicating with the parents and transmitting information in a sensitive fashion is a delicate art. Remember that words and impressions imparted in the immediate postpartum period can have long-term impact on the parents' attitudes and relationship with their baby. If you detect something unusual, you should communicate this in as positive a way as possible, avoiding loaded phrases such as "Your baby seems to have deformed ears." While the term "deformity" has been used appropriately throughout this chapter and often applies to temporary postural moulding due to in utero positioning, it is a frightening term for parents to hear. Instead, you might say "The shape of your baby's ears is a little unusual. I think we should have your pediatrician take a look." It is very important to differentiate findings that constitute temporary postural moulding from structural defects. In either case, do not go on and on about strange findings in the baby. Help the parents affirm what is normal and beautiful about their baby. This is not to say that you should withhold information, just that focusing on the things that are different will not help the parents bond with their baby, which will be *more* important with a baby who has unique physical features or is actually compromised. At the same time, you don't want to downplay potentially serious findings and especially don't want to minimize things to the point where the parents postpone further evaluation, when it is appropriate.

While you may suspect a problem, in many (if not most) cases you will not be in a position to make a diagnosis. Depending upon what the problem appears to be, immediate transport or referral for a physician's exam in the first hours or days after birth may be appropriate. It will be necessary to describe to the parents specifically what you are seeing that is cause for concern and to tell them what you suspect in general terms (such as "This finding is sometimes associated with other organic problems that would require assessment right away"). Be very clear that you are in no position to make a diagnosis and that there are other practitioners whose knowledge and experience will allow them to do so. This is especially important if the baby's problems are not that obvious and the parents do not want to transport, but you feel it may be necessary because of possible underlying defects or impending associated complications.

Be sure the parents understand that the baby who requires more evaluation than you can provide will usually need to see an expert in neonatal care; in most cases, simply another opinion will not be adequate. Private pediatricians may not see babies until they are at least two weeks old. Family practice doctors are often even less familiar with the immediate newborn period. Therefore, consultation with a neonatal specialist is strongly recommended. Consult a clinical genetic specialist if multiple anomalies are present or you suspect a problem of genetic origin; they can be accessed through the neonatology department of a hospital that provides advanced intensive newborn care (i.e., a Level-III hospital). You want someone who knows *more* than you do, not less! Stay with the parents throughout the decision-making process about whom to contact; act as a liaison whenever possible to make sure all pertinent records and information are provided. If the parents so desire, you or someone in your practice whom they know well should be available to accompany them to follow-up appointments. If not, be sure to stay in close touch with them over the days and weeks following birth and visit the hospital frequently, should the baby require admission. Be sure to let the parents know that you are available to provide postpartum care to the mother as you normally would.

Reflexes and Neuromotor Responses in the Newborn: An Overview

Neuromotor responses and reflexes are distributed throughout this volume, as noted in the chart below:

Newborn Reflexes and Neuromotor Responses

General reflexes	Tests of passive muscle tone	Tests of active muscle tone	Additional reflexes
•Asymmetrical tonic neck‡ Athetoid movements* ✛Cold crying✦ Jitteriness*> •Moro‡ Motor activity*> Posture†*> •Startle‡ **Oral-motor** •Babkin‡ •Biting‡ •Gag‡ ✛Lip❖ •Palmomental‡ •Rooting‡ •Sucking‡ •Suck-swallow‡ •Tongue thrust‡ **Respiratory** ■ Carotid body ■ Distal esophageal ■ Laryngeal chemoreflex ■ Laryngeal protective ■ Lung inflation/deflation	**Upper body** Forearm recoil†* Lateral rotation of head* •Perez‡ Scarf sign† Square window† ✛Trunk incurvation‡ Ventral suspension*> •Vollmer‡ **Lower body** Adductor angles* Dorsiflexion of the foot* Flapping of hands and feet> Heel to ear† Leg recoil‡ Leg traction‡ Popliteal angle†	**Upper body** Arm release to prone position‡ •✛Palmar grasp*‡ Pull-to-sit*> **Axial (midline)** Held sit‡ Neck extensors‡ Neck flexors‡ **Lower body** •Automatic walking‡ ✛Crossed extension‡ ✛Magnet response‡ ✛Placing reaction‡ •✛Plantar grasp‡ Supporting reaction‡	**Deep Tendon** Adductor & crossed adductor☆ Ankle clonus☆ Brachioradial☆ Biceps☆ Deltoid☆ Finger flexors☆ Jaw jerk (masseter)☆ Knee jerk☆ Pectoral☆ Triceps☆ **Other skin reflexes** ✛Abdominal reflex‡ ✛Anal wink‡ ✛Babinski‡ ✛Chaddock ✛Cremaster reflex‡ **Optical reflexes** Acoustic blink❖ Corneal❖ Corneal light* Doll's eye❖ Glabella❖ Optical blink*❖ Photic sneeze❖ Pupillary*❖ Rotation❖ Vestibular*

•Developmental (primitive or primary) reflexes, which normally disappear as the baby matures.
✛Skin reflexes (also known as skin-muscle reflexes).
✦See the chapter entitled "The Baby's Journey through Labor to Birth."
†See the subchapter entitled "Evaluating the Arms, Clavicles and Hands."
*See the subchapter entitled "Observing the Infant and Evaluating Posture and Muscle Tone."
>See chapter entitled "Evaluating the Newborn with Suspected Neurological Compromise."
‡See subchapter entitled "Developmental Reflexes and Other Neuromotor Evaluations."
☆See subchapter entitled "Deep Tendon Reflexes."
❖See subchapter entitled "Assessment of Cranial Nerve Function."
■See chapter entitled "Autonomic Neuromuscular Reflexes and the Baby's Response to Resuscitation."

Volpe (1995) suggests using the Moro, palmar grasp and asymmetric tonic neck response for all newborn examinations and using additional tests only if a problem is suspected.

Developmental Reflexes and Other Neuromotor Evaluations

Fletcher's book Physical Diagnosis in Neonatology (1998) describes a total of 67 newborn reflexes, some of which are more informative than others. This text discusses many but not all of these, focusing on a wide representative sample to provide in-depth learning and screening tools. Many of these reflexes can be observed or will be spontaneously elicited during the types of activities and handling that typically occur during the early postpartum hours. A midwife who is familiar with these responses will recognize them when they occur and will not need to formally elicit most of them to satisfy herself that they are present.

Reflexes are divided into passive and active responses. A passive response occurs when the examiner positions or moves the baby's body in such a way as to elicit the reflex. A response is considered active when the baby assumes the position or reacts spontaneously. Any reflex responses that you observe may be considered the summation of automatic body responses to a stimulus, the responses being mediated only by the nervous system. The primitive reflexes have been divided by Capute (1986) into three main categories:

Primitive reflexes I: These reflexes appear and then disappear during gestation, usually extinguishing before the 20th week, and are not present at birth.

Primitive reflexes II: These reflexes appear during intrauterine life as the fetus matures, are present at birth, and disappear or change into their mature form, usually by 6 months of age.

Primitive reflexes III: These reflexes appear during early infancy after type II reflexes have become suppressed. They include postural reactions such as righting and equilibrium reactions, which present just before voluntary motor activity begins.

Type II reflexes are addressed in this volume. In general, normal newborn reflexes are a reliable indication of an intact spinal cord and brain stem because these structures are fairly well developed at birth. This makes them valuable in assessing maturity. However, they do not depend on higher brain function, as they do not require functional brain activity above the diencephalon. Therefore these reflexes may be normal in the presence of serious brain damage; at the same time, absence of these reflexes at birth strongly suggests a malfunction of the central nervous system beneath the cortical level. Most of these primitive reflexes will disappear as the higher brain functions mature after birth, and the cerebral cortex begins to exert control over the brain stem and spinal cord. Other than the specific exceptions described in this chapter, the most important considerations are the symmetry, tone and strength of the baby's reflexive responses of the limbs and trunk. The behavioral state of the baby greatly impacts how she will respond to these maneuvers; when relevant, the ideal state is noted (see the chapter entitled "States of Newborn Consciousness and Behavior").

This subchapter includes both primitive reflexes as well as a few miscellaneous neuromotor evaluations that are not strictly primitive reflexes but that do change with advancing gestation. The classification of each reflex is clearly indicated in the charts that follow.

Should you decide to formally elicit one or more reflexes, note the relative ease or difficulty of elicitation. Ideally, a formal evaluation, if deemed necessary, is postponed until the baby is at least three days old to eliminate birth-related influences and to give the baby the opportunity to stretch out from his constantly flexed fetal position. Any abnormal assessments noted after birth should be rechecked during the first two postpartum visits.

General reflex-related activities such as posture, spontaneous motor activity, athetoid postures and movements, and jitteriness and are covered in the subchapter entitled "Observing the Infant and Evaluating Posture and Muscle Tone."

Primitive Reflexes

Flexor habitus

In order to appreciate the progression of reflexive response in the newborn, it is important to understand the concept of flexor habitus. In plain English, this simply means that the term newborn's joints, muscles and ligaments have become accustomed to a flexed posture during late gestation, a tendency that persists for the first 2 to 3 months of life. It is not known whether flexor habitus is the result of the tonic labyrinthine flexor reflex or simply due to the contour of the uterus. However, it seems reasonable that the term baby would have reflexes that encourage a flexed posture, since it is the ideal attitude to both accommodate a tight space in late gestation and the dilation phase of labor. Flexor habitus results in the flexor portion of reflex responses being somewhat stronger than the extensor responses, a tendency which becomes increasingly pronounced as the fetus nears term (Capute, 1986).

Tonic labyrinthine reflex, supine (TLS) or prone (TLP)

Neck extension produces shoulder retraction, secondary flexion of the arms and extension of the legs. Neck flexion produces total flexion habitus, the typical fetal position. Clinically the extended version of this reflex is referred to as "opisthotonic posturing" or "decorticate rigidity," and is seen as an obligatory response following head trauma or cerebrospinal infection at any age (Capute, 1986).

Asymmetrical tonic neck (fencing) reflex (ATNR)

This is perhaps the most important of all primitive reflexes. Normal infants exhibit an asymmetrical response in their extremities when their head is turned far to one side. The baby should extend her limbs on the side to which the face is turned while flexing the limbs on the other side. This reflex can be noted in babies lying either on their stomach or their back, but is most often tested with the baby supine. It is spontaneously elicited during both land and waterbirth (when the water is not too warm), when the baby actively participates in his birth (note that it is a motion similar to swimming). Forty-four percent of all babies have a spontaneous, complete ATNR. Preterm babies may lie at rest in this asymmetrical posture whether they are placed on their back or their belly for extended periods. This reflex appears by 35 weeks; after 36 weeks, the flexor tone becomes dominant and the reflex is present but less obvious.

Type and duration	Developmental reflex. Generally starts to diminish by 4 months of age and disappears by 6 months.
Behavioral state	Lightly sleeping or dozing. Do not attempt it if the baby is sleeping deeply or crying.
Elicitation of reflex	Start with the baby resting on her back. Turn her head to one side without flexing it. The limbs on the side to which the face is turned should extend and the limbs on the other side should flex.
Normal response	The baby extends her chin and tips her occiput back (in a modified brow presentation). The arm (and sometimes the leg) on the side of the face will become rigid and extend; the arm and (sometimes the leg) on the side of the occiput will flex. The grasp reflex is more easily elicited on the side to which the occiput is turned. The response is stronger in the legs of preterm babies. Response time varies from 1 to 7 seconds, with resistance demonstrated by 15 seconds of holding the head in most babies. The baby will spontaneously move out of the posture after a few seconds or lessen the degree of either flexion or extension. Response may be absent or incomplete immediately after birth. The responses of the lower limbs are more constant than those of the upper limbs, especially in preterm babies. Types of normal variations in passive response that are typically noted include: Complete (50%): Both chin-side extremities extend and both occiput-side extremities flex. Leg ATNR (25%): Chin-side leg extends; occiput-side arm flexes. Arm ATNR (4%): Chin-side arm extends; occiput-side leg flexes. Unidirectional (15%): Reflex occurs only when the head is turned to one side but not the other.
Abnormal response	Sustained or exaggerated response in which the baby cannot change positions when the head is held for 15 seconds or after the head is released. Consistent failure to move an extremity. The reflex is obligatory when the baby cannot change position while the head is rotated. This should not occur every time the reflex is evoked. In pathologic conditions, such as cerebral palsy, the ATNR persists and may increase. Increased extensor tone on the face side and increased flexor tone of the occiput side may be the only findings when the positive response is weak. Persistence after 6 months of age may indicate neurological injury.

Variation in this response is always abnormal. To assess for it, lift the baby under the arms so she is facing you. An abnormal response is present if the baby holds her head tipped back (extended) in the midline with her arms rigidly extended to either side with the fists clenched.

Moro reflex

The Moro reflex first appears at 28 to 32 weeks and is well established by 37 weeks gestation. It is one of the most interesting of the primitive reflexes. It is thought to be an evolutionary remnant that relates to the way that our foremothers carried their infants. Primates carry their babies in front, and the young typically wrap their arms and legs around their mother. With movement, the baby's limbs extend and tighten to hold on.

As this vestibular reflex simulates falling, it is, no doubt, frightening to the baby. It should be explained to the baby prior to proceeding. The elicitation of this reflex should be done last, as the baby is likely to start crying.

It is important to control the positions of the baby's head and body when using any of the elicitation techniques described below to ensure that the baby has a symmetrical response. The limbs cannot be restrained. A partial Moro reflex may also be elicited when a normal term newborn is exposed to sudden movements or a loud noise. The baby abducts and flexes her limbs and may start crying.

Type and duration	Developmental reflex. Starts to fade at 4 months and normally disappears at 6 months.
Behavioral state	Drowsy or quiet and alert.
Elicitation of reflex	**Method 1 (traction and release):** With baby supine, pull on both arms to raise the shoulders a few centimeters above the mattress (just enough to create a space between the mattress and the baby's neck). Release the arms to allow the baby to fall back to the mattress. Repeat until the response disappears. Although the upper limbs are starting from a more extended position than in methods 2 and 3 below, this method allows you to combine tests for Moro, palmar grasp and arm traction, and is suitable for most screening exams. If there is any doubt regarding response, proceed with method 2, 3 or 4.
	Method 2 ("drop" the baby): Hold the baby in your hands above the mattress by supporting the trunk with one open palm and the head with the other. Rapidly lower both hands 10 to 20 cm without flexing the baby's neck. Do not tilt the baby during the "drop." Repeat until the reflex disappears.
	Method 3 (head-bang): Lie the baby supine in a symmetrically midline posture. Slap the flat of your hands down sharply on the mattress on either side of the baby (or jerk the end of the mattress sharply). Repeat until the reflex disappears. Part of the response to the noise from hitting the bed may be a startle to sound. This or method 4 should be used if this evaluation is felt to be absolutely necessary in ill babies or those with spinal cord injuries.
	Method 4: Space your index finger and thumb widely apart and pinch the baby's epigastric area (the soft tissue just below the sternum). Gently tapping the abdomen sometimes works as well.
Normal Moro response	Any of the above maneuvers should cause the baby to suddenly extend his spine and symmetrically extend his arms from the elbows, open his hands completely and spread his fingers. The baby's thumbs and forefingers may open fully during arm extension and then form a "C," while the rest of the fingers remain extended before curling. The legs may simultaneously extend as well, but not in as uniform and stylized a manner as the arms. This is followed by adduction of both arms at the shoulders and the elbows, bringing them together in a wide, embracing motion, with curling of the fingers. If the legs extended, they will flex as well, but not in as uniform and stylized manner as the arms. The baby then resumes a relaxed, flexed posture. At the end, the baby cries or grimaces. In term babies, the response should diminish after 3 tries; premature babies require more attempts to get a complete response and should extinguish after 10 attempts. In preterm infants, the limbs tend to fall backward during the adduction phase due to muscular weakness.
Abnormal response	Lack of response may be associated with normal newborn sleep as well as neurological disorders or deafness, although use of the reflex to evaluate hearing is often less effective in the first 24 to 36 hours of life. Hypertonicity decreases the response because the increased muscle tone prevents full range of motion; the limbs may move only partially at the height of the reflex, the hands may fail to open, or there may be no response because the limbs are tightly flexed. Hypotonia or flaccid paralysis also impairs the response. Asymmetrical response is seen with peripheral nerve injury.

Lesny (1967) found that elicitation of the Moro reflex by method 4 was the most sensitive of all because the Moro could be elicited in some babies he studied by this method alone. This suggests that an absence of response to method 4 is a serious sign of compromise.

An asymmetric Moro response in the extremities suggests possible brain injury on one side (hemiparesis). A lack of response in both legs (paraparesis) suggests a problem in the lower spinal cord or a congenital hip dislocation. If one arm fails to respond, the baby may have a fractured clavicle or humerus or may have sustained injury to the brachial plexus. Asymmetry of response in the arms is also associated with craniosacral disruption at the lower neck or upper thoracic area. Inability to elicit the Moro reflex and the Perez reflex (described at the end of this chapter) indicates a serious problem with the cerebrum or the cervical spinal region, or severe, generalized muscle disease (myopathy) (Upledger, 1996).

Failure of the repeated reflex to fully disappear indicates lack of cortical inhibition and is often a primary indication of poor cerebral function above the level of the brain stem or of cortical irritability in the early newborn period. Repeated trials in normal infants lead to absence of the motor reflex and anger.

Startle reflex

The startle reflex is a mass myoclonic reflex. It is similar to but differs from the Moro response in that the complete sequence of reflexes demonstrated in a Moro are not seen. The Moro is likely to stimulate a startle as part of the entire response. Some authorities consider the Moro reflex and the startle to be the same response, or consider the Moro to be a form of startle, and find that the techniques used to stimulate the Moro are likely to produce a startle. However, less marked startles are seen more frequently than the complete Moro response.

Type and duration	Developmental reflex. Present throughout life.
Behavioral state	Any except but deep sleep. Response may be absent or diminished during sleep.
Elicitation of reflex	Noise and spontaneous movement in the course of care. Alternatively, place the baby supine with the limbs in natural extension. Make a sudden, loud noise or tap on the baby's sternum.
Normal response	Flexion of all extremities while the hands remain closed, with a total body reaction; may elicit crying. Repeated stimulation causes the term baby to inhibit and react less intensely until he completely ignores the stimulus or becomes angry and starts crying.
Abnormal response	Markedly exaggerated or easily elicited response; failure to habituate to repeated tests; frequent spontaneous startles without external stimulation; initiation of mass, exaggerated or easily elicited response; absence of the reflex may indicate neurologic deficit or deafness.

An increased startle reflex is sometimes noted in hypertonic infants.

Infantile Oral-Motor Reflexes

These reflexes are related to the baby's innate ability to nurse. This section relies heavily on Walter (1994).

Palmomental reflex

This reflex is not as immediately obvious as some of the others described here but can be easily elicited in preterm and term babies.

Type and duration	Developmental reflex. Can persist into adulthood.
Behavioral state	Drowsy or quiet and alert
Elicitation of reflex	Stroke the palm of the hand.
Normal response	Elicits wrinkling of the skin overlying the chin
Abnormal response	Absent, weak, or asymmetrical

Rooting reflex

Rooting describes the newborn's instinctive search for the mother's nipple that occurs when the lips (and often the cheek) are touched, simulating the touch of the breast as the mother holds the baby. This reflex appears at 28 weeks and becomes well established between 32 and 34 weeks.

Absence of this reflex suggests a decreased level of awareness. A normal sleeping baby may have a negative response; however, decreased awareness is often associated with serious central nervous system disorders, development impairment or with more localized problems involving the medulla oblongata. Medullary problems may be referred to as "bulbar disease" because the medulla oblongata is often characterized as a bulb. The rooting reflex may be suppressed by the residual effects of maternal sedation during labor.

Type and duration	Developmental reflex. Disappears by 3 to 4 months of age but may be present longer during sleep.
Behavioral state	Drowsy or quiet, and alert
Elicitation of reflex	Lie the baby supine with the head centered; hold the baby's hands against her upper chest. Touch either corner of the baby's mouth or first her upper, then her lower lip at the corner of her mouth with a finger or the mother's nipple. The baby should lower her lower lip, open her mouth wide, move her tongue toward the stimulation and turn her head to that side. Variants of this reflex include moving a finger along the baby's upper lip or nasolabial fold; this should cause the baby to flex his head backward. Moving the finger to the side should cause the head to turn to follow it. Stroking the middle of the lower lip causes the lip to be lowered, the tongue to move toward it and the chin to drop. Moving the finger toward the chin causes the jaw to drop and the neck to flex.
Normal response	Stimulation of the upper lip causes the baby to turn her head and open her mouth as if to catch the stimulus. With stimulation of the lower lip, the mouth opens and the jaw drops. The baby tries to suck the finger. Normally the baby turns her head fully to the side of stimulation and grasps with the lips. The baby may turn away from stimulation if she has just nursed.
Abnormal response	Early babies, those with neurologic disorders or injuries, or central nervous system depression (e.g., from maternal drugs) may have little or no response to stimulus. Asymmetry is also abnormal.

Sucking

Newborn sucking differs from that of the older child or adult and is uniquely suited to express milk from the breasts. The baby will instinctively suck on an object placed far enough back into the mouth and pressed against the hard palate. Sucking is first noted at 28 weeks and is well established between 32 and 34 weeks. Sucking can be evaluated as in the description of the suck-swallow reflex on the next page, but it is easier to tell if the baby is moving his tongue correctly when it is evaluated independently, as described here. Show the parents how to insert their finger to check for the character and strength of the baby's suck before you leave.

Type and duration	Developmental reflex. Neonatal sucking disappears by 3 to 4 months of age unless nursing is continuous, in which case the baby will suck at this breast in this manner until weaned.
Behavioral state	Drowsy or quiet and alert
Elicitation of reflex	Insert your index finger into the baby's mouth until the tip is level with the margin of the hard and soft palate. Stroke the roof of the mouth with the fingerpad. The baby initiates strong coordinated sucking as the flat of the tongue presses the finger against the hard palate and moves rhythmically along the length of the finger in an anteroposterior stripping motion. The tongue then thrusts forward to repeat the stripping action. This tongue action is exactly what is needed for the baby to strip milk from the ducts in the mother's breasts. Rooting and sucking reflexes are closely related.
Normal response	The response is strong and coordinated in babies born at term.
Abnormal response	Tonic biting or up and down motion of the lower jaw with no tongue movement to strip and propel the fluid. Early babies, those with neurologic disorders or injuries, or central nervous system depression (e.g., from maternal drugs), may have little or no response to stimulus.

Suck-swallow

Swallowing will be elicited when sufficient fluids are in the baby's mouth, but do not give the baby any liquids to try and induce swallowing, instead observe the baby at the breast. Normal rooting, sucking and swallowing reflexes are associated with intact, normally functioning cranial nerves V, VII, IX, X and XII.

Type and duration	Developmental reflex. The swallowing reflex never disappears but changes around 6 months to a pattern of mature adult suck-swallow.
Behavioral state	Drowsy or quiet and alert
Elicitation of reflex	**Observation:** Look at the throat for signs of swallowing in coordination with sucking during nursing. It may take a while as the mother does not have a great quantity of colostrum at the time of birth. **Manual:** Stroke anterior third of the tongue or the center of the lips to elicit suck-swallow movements.
Normal response	The response is strong and coordinated in babies born at term.
Abnormal response	Babies who gag, cough or regurgitate fluid repeatedly may also have cyanosis associated with prematurity, or neurological injury or defects.

Biting

This reflex may be noted while evaluating the baby's sucking response or it may be elicited independently.

Type and duration	Developmental reflex. Disappears by 6 months of age.
Behavioral state	Drowsy or quiet and alert
Elicitation of reflex	Stroke the gum
Normal response	Elicits rhythmic vertical biting motion of the jaw
Abnormal response	Weak, absent or asymmetrical

Extrusion (tongue thrust)

The tongue thrust is part of the infant's suckle-swallow movement in which the tongue is placed in position on the midline, anterior alveolar ridges during the initial stage of swallowing, sometimes resulting in an open biting motion. This action results in the tongue pushing forward slightly past the lips.

Type and duration	Developmental reflex. Normal extrusion disappears by 6 months of age.
Behavioral state	Drowsy or quietly alert
Elicitation of reflex	The baby pushes her tongue outward when the tongue tip is touched with a finger or nipple.
Normal response	The response is strong and coordinated in babies born at term.
Abnormal response	Babies who have central nervous system abnormalities, including seizures, may continuously extrude their tongue or may display repetitive tongue thrusting. An attitude of persistent tongue thrust may be present in babies who have genetic defects, notably Down syndrome.

Gag

An intact gag reflex prevents the baby from choking while nursing.

Type and duration	Developmental reflex. Sensitivity shifts to the back quarter of the tongue and pharyngeal in adults.
Behavioral state	Drowsy or quietly alert
Elicitation of reflex	Stimulate the posterior three-fourths of the tongue and the pharyngeal wall
Normal response	Elicits constriction and elevation of the pharynx
Abnormal response	Ineffective, weak, absent or asymmetrical

Babkin

As with the palmomental reflex, stimulation of the baby's palm should elicit an oral-motor response.

Type and duration	Developmental reflex. Disappears around 3 to 4 months of age.
Behavioral state	Drowsy or quiet and alert
Elicitation of reflex	Stroke the palm of the hand
Normal response	Elicits mouth opening, eye closing, head moving forward and to the midline
Abnormal response	Weak, absent, asymmetrical or persistent

Neuromotor Reflexes That Evaluate Passive Muscle Tone in the Upper Body

Ventral suspension

Various responses to ventral suspension are also discussed and illustrated in the subchapter entitled "Observing the Infant and Evaluating Posture and Muscle Tone."

Type and duration	Developmental reflex. Disappears at 4 months of age.
Behavioral state	Awake
Elicitation of reflex	Hold the baby under the chest so he is prone, suspend him so the head is slightly higher than the pelvis and note the posture of the head, trunk and limbs.
Normal response	Attempts to extend head and trunk and flex limbs, with increasingly strong limb flexion with maturity. If there is no spontaneous lifting of the head, stimulate by stroking firmly to the side of the upper spine. If still no lifting occurs, stroke up and down beside the spine.
Abnormal response	None, flaccidity, asymmetry with flaccidity on one side, in one limb or in the upper or lower extremities only with a strong response in the opposite set of extremities. A pronounced response in neck and trunk extension, especially with failure to drop the head when held in a sitting position, suggests abnormally increased extensor tone.

Perez reflex

The Perez reflex, along with the Moro reflex, is a summation response that demonstrates normal development and control by the subcortical brain. The cortex will usually obliterate these reflexes by 3 to 4 months as the brain matures.

Serious neurologic malfunction should be suspected if both the Moro and Perez reflexes are absent. Abnormal cortex development is likely if the Moro and Perez reflexes persist beyond four months. If they persist past 6 months, the chances of this are increased even more.

Type and duration	Developmental reflex. Diminishes starting at 4 months and disappears by 6 months.
Behavioral state	Drowsy or quiet and alert
Elicitation of reflex	Hold the baby face down with one palm and forearm under the baby's torso so that the body and limbs are suspended over an absorbent surface. Move your other thumb up the spine beginning at the sacrum and exerting firm pressure on each spinous process as you do so.
Normal response	Backward bending of the head and spine, flexion of the arms and legs (knees toward the chest), crying and emptying of the bladder. (More pronounced response from the upper extremities may occur with an upward stroke along the spine.)
Abnormal response	Marked extension of pelvis and neck. Absent, weak or asymmetrical response; failure to lift head.

Vollmer reflex

This is similar to the Perez reflex and likewise reflects normal subcortical development.

Type and duration	Developmental reflex. Disappears around 3 months of age.
Behavioral state	Drowsy or quiet and alert, not crying
Elicitation of reflex	Holding the baby by a hand under the chest, suspend her and firmly stroke down the spine.
Normal response	Similar to the Perez response but tends to stimulate more response in the lower trunk with flexion of the legs and extension of the lower back
Abnormal response	Absent, weak, exaggerated or asymmetrical response or persistence after 3 months

Trunk incurvation (Galant's reflex)

This is a type of skin reflex. A normal trunk incurvation reflex is present when the spinal cord is healthy and normally formed. This assessment roughly evaluates the segmental integrity of the spinal nerves from T-2 to S-1. It appears at 28 weeks and is well established by 40 weeks gestation.

Type and duration	Developmental skin reflex. Disappears at 4 months of age.
Behavioral state	Any state but sleeping or crying
Elicitation of reflex	Start with the baby lying face down on a mattress. The test may be performed with the baby lying prone, or you can insert one open palm under the baby's midtorso and lift him so that his limbs are suspended. Using a finger from the other hand, apply pressure as you draw a line down the length of the back about an inch to one side of the spine.
Normal response	The normal newborn flexes his spine and pelvis in the direction of the stimulated side (if you draw a line on the baby's left, the torso should flex to his left in a "C" curve). A similar response occurs by running a finger in the paravertebral region from the infant's buttock up to the base of the neck to stimulate the paravertebral muscles on one side and then the other. Response varies, but should be present in all babies. Is should be apparent by 5 to 6 days if not seen in the first days of life.
Abnormal response	No response is associated with a complete transverse lesion of the spinal cord or CNS depression. Exaggerated response is a rapid and sustained swing to one side with minimal stimulus. Asymmetry seen with sensory or motor deficit problems involving the spinal cord.

The organization of the remainder of the chapter and much of its content follows Fletcher (1998).

Neuromotor Reflexes That Test Active Muscle Tone in the Upper Body

Arm traction (pull-to-sit)

This can be done after eliciting the palmar grasp.

Type of response	Neuromotor reaction reflecting gestational maturity, becomes stronger as gestational age advances
Behavioral state	Awake
Elicitation of reflex	With the baby supine, grasp the hands and pull the baby up and forward to stimulate flexion of the arms and neck.
Normal response	The baby should pull with his arms while keeping his head aligned with the spine. The legs should flex for a few seconds. Preterm babies will pull less and have less head control.
Abnormal response	Absent, weak or asymmetric effort in the arms or head lag without being able to lift the head in line with the spine in a term baby.

Palmar grasp

Normal infantile hand reflexes reflect that the volar branches of the ulnar and median nerves are intact and that the flexor digitorum muscles are working properly, assuming there is no Erb's, Klumpke's or mixed palsies originating from damage to the brachial plexus. The strength and duration of this reflex are related to gestational age, although preterm babies often have remarkably strong grips.

The grasp reflex remains intact in the presence of a brachial plexus palsy, but the Moro reflex will be absent on the affected side. Persistence of the palmar grasp past 4 months of age may be associated with cerebral dysfunction.

Type and duration	Developmental skin reflex. Strongest at term, weakens by 2 months and disappears by 4 months.
Behavioral state	Optimal when baby is drowsy or quietly alert; do not perform if the baby is sleeping or crying.
Elicitation of reflex	Lie infant supine with head centered and arms semiflexed. Without touching the back of the hand, place your finger across the newborn's palm, approaching from the outer edge, and apply slight pressure. Test both hands simultaneously. If the fist is tightly clinched, stimulate opening by stroking along the side of the hand opposite the thumb or the back of the hand and look for uncurling of the fingers. Firmly touching the back of the hand may also stimulate opening the fingers. Allow the baby to suck on your finger to facilitate a grasp if the first test is poor.
Normal response	The baby should use all her fingers to respond with a strong grasp that is sustained for several seconds and then relaxes. The baby should tighten her grip when you attempt to withdraw your finger; this may be of sufficient strength to suspend the baby for a moment. Make sure the baby is positioned perfectly symmetrically before deciding that the grip is asymmetrical between hands. If the head is not midline, the grasp will be stronger on the side to which the occiput is directed.
Abnormal response	Asymmetry of intensity may indicate a peripheral nerve weakness. A weak or absent grasp is strongly associated with neurological or muscle disorders or injury. Persistence beyond a few seconds or clenching to the point of blanching is also abnormal, as is bilateral weakness with a short attempt at grasping despite stimulation.

Arm release to prone position

Type of response	Neuromotor reaction reflecting gestational maturity, becoming stronger as term approaches
Behavioral state	Awake or light sleep
Elicitation of reflex	Lie the baby on her belly with her head centered and arms extended next to the trunk so the palms face up. Note the time it takes and the extent to which the baby brings her arms forward.
Normal response	At term, the baby should bring her arms near her face rapidly. Response depends on maturity, although healthy preterm babies should be able to bring each arm to the same level.
Abnormal response	No effort or inability to raise either wrist to nipple level. Asymmetry may indicate partial paralysis in an upper segment of the spine.

Axial Reflexes

Although the newborn cannot normally hold his head erect for extended periods, contraction of the neck muscles should be evident. The assessments below demonstrate strength of flexion and extension of the infant's neck.

Flexor muscles of the neck

Type of response	Active neuromuscular tone and strength of the flexor muscles; strengthens as gestation advances.
Behavioral state	Awake, not crying
Elicitation of reflex	With the baby supine, grasp the shoulders with both hands and slowly raise the baby into a sitting position, allowing time for the baby to flex the neck muscles and assist.
Normal response	Active contraction of the neck muscles causes the head to come forward before the trunk is completely upright. The head is aligned with the spine for a second or two with the trunk curled slightly forward, the head then falls onto the chest. At term, there is full flexion while raising the head, after which the head is held upright for more than a few seconds until the trunk is tilted past vertical. Preterm infants show little effort before 34 weeks.
Abnormal response	Absent or weak flexion indicates specific flexor weakness, general hypotonia or central nervous system depression. More competent head control for gestational age, failure of the head to fall forward or falling only when the trunk is very tilted indicates abnormally increased extensor tone.

Extensor muscles of the neck

Type of response	Assesses active tone, strength and neuromuscular integrity of the extensor muscles, becomes stronger with advancing gestation
Behavioral state	Awake
Elicitation of reflex	Support the baby by the shoulders with both hands, allowing him to lean forward in a sitting position so the head is flexed onto the chest. Wait at least 30 seconds to allow the baby to lift his head, then move the baby backward to stimulate an active lifting of the head.
Normal response	A term baby tilted back and forth in a vertical plane in a sitting position should alternately and symmetrically flex and extend his neck to try and keep his head upright. The neck extensors develop earlier than do the flexors, so some response should be noted by 32 weeks.
Abnormal response	Absent or minimal effort, very brisk or strong response for age, especially with an imbalance between the extensor and flexor muscle groups and failure of the head to drop onto the chest

Held sit

Type of response	Active muscle tone in the neck and extensor muscles of the back; strengthens as gestation advances.
Behavioral state	Alert
Elicitation of reflex	Support the baby by the shoulders in a sitting position with both hands. Note the length of time the head is held in an upright position. If the head is maintained upright for more than 10 seconds, determine the level of the lumbar vertebra from which the back bends.
Normal response	A term baby should hold her head up for more than 10 seconds; this may be encouraged by visual fixation at her eye level. The curve of her back should be rounded and anteriorly concave. The stronger the back extensors, the lower the level of back curve.
Abnormal response	Failure to lift the head or inability to keep it upright for more than 3 seconds

Neuromotor Reflexes That Assess Passive Muscle Tone in the Lower Body

Leg recoil

Type of response	Tests passive muscle tone in the legs; becomes stronger with advancing gestation.
Behavioral state	Ideally, the baby is awake and fully relaxed
Elicitation of reflex	With the baby supine, hold both ankles and fully flex the legs for about 5 seconds, then fully extend the legs level with the table. Hold them in place for 2 seconds and then release.
Normal response	The term baby should completely flex the hips and knees immediately upon release. The intensity of the response increases with gestational age. Babies born breech may resist extension but should demonstrate symmetrical recoil from the point of maximum extension unless they were in a hyperextended breech position in utero.
Abnormal response	Asymmetry; decreased intensity or delayed reaction outside the range expected for gestational age

Leg traction

This examination tests the strength of the lower legs.

Type of response	Tests passive tone and strength of the lower legs; becomes stronger with advancing gestation
Behavioral state	Ideally, the baby is awake and fully relaxed
Elicitation of reflex	With the baby supine, grasp both legs near the ankles and pull up until the pelvis is lifted 2 to 5 cm off the mattress (as though changing a diaper). Note both the resistance of the legs to the pull and the popliteal angle.
Normal response	Flexion of both knees to an angle less than 100° with a strong resistance to the pull.
Abnormal response	Absent, weak or asymmetrical response

Neuromotor Reflexes That Evaluate Active Tone in the Lower Body

Withdrawal reflex

Type and duration	Developmental reflex that also tests active muscle tone. Disappears by 1 to 2 months of age.
Behavioral state	Best when the baby is quiet and alert
Elicitation of reflex	Starting with the baby supine with the lower limbs in the midline in natural extension, stroke, apply a pinprick or other noxious stimulus such as an ice cube to the sole of one foot.
Normal response	Withdrawal of the limb from the stimulus by dorsiflexing the ankle and flexing the hip and knee.
Abnormal response	Weak or absent with meningomyelocele or flaccid paralysis. Abnormal persistence may be due to spasticity of the lower limbs as in cerebral palsy.

Crossed extension

A normal crossed-extension reflex is associated with the intact functioning of spinal nerves L4 through S1.

Type of response	Developmental reflex that also assesses active muscle tone. Disappears by 6 months of age.
Behavioral state	Best when the baby is quiet and alert but can be performed during light sleep
Elicitation of reflex	Starting with the baby in a supine position, gently pull one leg straight out to full extension; press the knee down and stimulate the sole of that foot.
Normal response	The baby's opposite leg should flex, then extend and adduct rapidly; the toes may fan out, as if he is trying to kick away the stimulus to the other foot. The response should be strong if limb strength is normal in both extension and flexion. Flexion and extension are present regardless of gestational age, but adduction of the foot may not be fully present until term.
Abnormal response	Asymmetry. Little or no response is seen with peripheral nerve injury or fracture of a long leg bone. Persistence of strong response after 44 weeks of corrected gestational age.

Placing response (lower extremities)

This reflex should be present during the first day of life. Its absence within the first week or so suggests lower extremity motor dysfunction.

Type and duration	Developmental skin reflex that is part of the automatic walking reflex, tests active muscle tone. Its duration is not mentioned in the literature.
Behavioral state	Awake
Elicitation of reflex	Hold baby upright in a standing position with both hands under the arms and around the chest. Support the back of the head with your thumbs and the jaw with your index fingers. Lightly bring the top of the baby's foot or the anterior shin in contact with the edge of a table or mattress and lift her to draw her foot against the edge
Normal response	Flexing of the leg enough to bring the foot up and place it on the surface.
Abnormal response	Asymmetrical, absent or weak response with minimal movement of the leg or marked extension after initial stimulus.

Positive support response (redressement de tronc; leg-straightening reflex)

Type and duration	Developmental reflex. Disappears by 4 months of age.
Behavioral state	Best when the baby is quiet and alert
Elicitation of reflex	Hold the baby upright in a standing position facing away from you, with both of your hands under the arms and around the chest; support the chin with your fingers so the head is in a neutral upright position. Press the soles of the feet to the mattress several times.
Normal response	The lower limbs and trunk extend; the legs thus act as support for weightbearing for a few seconds. The baby then relaxes by taking a few walking steps or by flexing both hips. The knees may remain slightly flexed as long as there is some attempt to straighten the legs and bear weight.
Abnormal response	Arching of the back with hyperextension of the legs seen with marked hypertonia of the posterior muscles. Absence of any extension at the hips or legs, or asymmetry. Persistence prevents reciprocal leg movement required for walking.

This reflex is elicited during automatic walking (stepping) and tests active muscle tone. It can be used to understand the stages through which a primitive reflex passes as the baby moves out of flexor habitus. During the flexor phase of early infancy, it can be difficult to elicit momentary extension of the legs followed by flexion when the baby is suspended by the axilla and his big toe touches the surface. A more mature response evolves by the second month of life, evidenced by full extension of the legs with support. A hypotonic baby will "sit in air" with no support response.

Stepping (automatic walking)

This reflex evaluates the strength and active muscle tone of the lower limbs. It first appears at 35 to 36 weeks, and should be readily elicited after 37 weeks. This response must disappear before voluntary walking can begin.

Type and duration	Developmental reflex. Increases after the first few 2 or 3 days of life, then diminishes by the end of the first month after term. Disappears by 3 to 4 months of age.
Behavioral state	Quiet and alert
Elicitation of reflex	Hold the baby upright with both hands under the arms around the chest, and support the chin. The feet are allowed to touch the mattress, and the baby is tilted forward slightly. First, observe for a support response, where the baby tries to support her weight rather than stepping. If necessary, shift the baby's weight from one side to the other to facilitate alternate weight bearing on the legs. Extend the neck slightly if there is no initial response by pushing up on the chin.
Normal response	The baby should take at least three steps by flexing her hips and knees on both sides. The response should be rhythmic and coordinated, needing only forward movement for stimulus. Babies born breech may not be able to fully extend their legs as required for the first few days.
Abnormal response	Asymmetrical flexion or a hyperactive response wherein the baby displays extreme flexion or extension. Absent or weak response is seen with flaccid paralysis.

Plantar grasp

This is reflex is similar to the palmar grasp and tests active muscle tone in the toes.

Type of response	Developmental skin reflex. Disappears by 8 to 9 months, usually as a predictable prelude to walking. A delay in disappearance may indicate abnormally increased motor tone.
Behavioral state	Awake, otherwise not important to the test
Elicitation of reflex	Lie the baby supine. Lightly press your thumbpad against the ball of the baby's foot under the four smaller toes close to the toe joints. Do not touch the top of the foot and take care to apply firm pressure rather than a tickling touch.
Normal response	The toes should flex forward over your finger in a strong, sustained, grasping motion that gradually relaxes. The response should be equal in both feet.
Abnormal response	Reflex is absent or asymmetrical in defects of the lower spinal cord with flaccid paralysis. Delayed relaxation suggests generalized hyperirritable or hypertonic state.

Additional Neuromotor Assessments

Babinski reflex

Also called the "plantar response," this reflex first appears at 34 to 36 weeks and is well established by 38 weeks. Several other neonatal reflexes tend to be simultaneously stimulated by this reflex, which may confuse the findings. Nociceptive withdrawal (response to a painful stimulus) produces extension of the toes with flexion of the hip, knee and ankle.

This response involves at least four competing reflexes leading to movement of the toes. Two of these result in extension: the nociceptive withdrawal, which is often accompanied by simultaneous flexion of the hip, knee and ankle, and contact avoidance, which is best elicited by stroking the top of the foot (which may occur inadvertently when the foot is held to elicit the plantar response). The two responses that promote flexion include the plantar grasp and the positive supporting reaction, both of which are elicited by applying pressure to the sole of the foot. While the plantar response is usually said to be an extensor reaction, extension is related to the way in which the response is elicited. Flexion is more likely to occur when a thumbnail is dragged along the outer side of the sole. When a sharper object such as a pin or a pinprick is used, most babies will have an extensor response.

Type and duration	Developmental skin reflex. No change during the neonatal period, disappears by 12 months of age.
Behavioral state	Quietly alert
Elicitation of reflex	The legs should be semiflexed. Use a thumbnail to scratch the sole of the foot along the outside edge from the toes to the heel. (Be sure not to stimulate the plantar grasp by touching the sole of the foot.)
Normal response	The big toe should extend backward (dorsal flexion), with fanning of the other toes a far less consistent response, or the big toe may curl forward in a grasp-like motion. Should be symmetrical in both feet.
Abnormal response	Absent or weak with minimal spread of toes; asymmetrical response; strong, obligatory response with no relaxation afterward; may be absent in severely depressed or brain-damaged babies.

Chaddock maneuver: A plantar response can also be elicited by stroking below the outer ankle. This avoids the plantar surface of the foot altogether, and the confounding effect of other responses is eliminated. The big toe should flex toward the sole of the foot (Ziai et al., 1984).

Lateral abdominal reflex

This assessment tests the integrity of the cutaneous branches of the intercostal nerve and the connections to T7 through T12.

Type and duration	Developmental skin reflex. The timing of disappearance varies. Always present in the first 10 days of life at term but may be weaker during the first two days.
Behavioral state	Not important but exclude all states in which the abdominal muscles are contracted.
Elicitation of reflex	The baby should be supine. Use a rough blunt object to lightly scratch the surface of the skin in all four abdominal quadrants, in line with the axilla.
Normal response	Quick contraction of the abdominal muscles in the stimulated area, with trunk incurvation and slight hip flexion. Strong muscle contraction only or slight muscle contraction.
Abnormal response	Asymmetry of response is abnormal, but a total lack of these reflexes may be within normal limits.

Cremaster reflex

This reflex may or may not be present, but the response should be equal on both sides.

Type and duration	Developmental skin reflex. The timing of disappearance varies. Always present in the first 10 days of life but may be weaker in the first two days.
Behavioral state	Not important
Elicitation of reflex	Scratch the skin gently on the inner thigh.
Normal response	**Male:** The testis on the stimulated side should retract. The response may take place on both sides and may happen even if the testes are not fully descended.
	Female: The skin overlying the vulva on the stimulated side may blanch, but not reliably.
Abnormal response	Absent in spinal cord lesions at segments L1 and L2; may not appear in some normal babies up to 3 months of age

Anal wink

The presence of this reflex reflects the integrity of dorsal branches of the sacral spinal segment at S4 and S5.

Type of response	Developmental skin reflex. The timing of disappearance varies.
Behavioral state	Not important, but the lower limbs must be relaxed.
Elicitation of reflex	Brush the tip of a cotton swab to the side of the anal opening.
Normal response	A quick muscular contraction of the sphincter, that looks like a wink, indicates intact spinal nerves at S4 and S5.
Abnormal response	None or weak

DEEP TENDON REFLEXES

This chapter is based on Fletcher (1998), unless otherwise noted. The deep tendon reflexes are not routinely assessed but are included for completeness and reference should the need arise. These are spinal reflexes that involve peripheral sensory, motor and proprioceptive nerve fibers. Normal reflexes depend upon intact sensory or afferent nerve fibers, functional synapses in the spinal cord, intact motor or efferent nerve fibers, functional neuromotor junctions and competent muscle fibers. They can be assessed by using an infant reflex hammer or your two hands. Place one fingerpad over the structure to be tested and strike the fingerpad with your other index finger or the hammer, or flex the joint gently while supporting the limb with the same hand and use the middle finger of the other hand to tap the tendon. The direct strike of a fingertip can be used in place of the hammer for some assessments. Gestational age affects the ease with which a reflex can be tested, with more reliable response in babies who have reached at least 33 weeks gestation. The spinal reflex mechanisms upon which deep tendon reflexes depend are variable during infancy because the corticospinal pathways are not fully developed in the newborn. Their exaggerated presence or absence is of little significance during a single examination. Therefore, whenever the deep tendon reflexes are evaluated in a baby, they are performed to establish a baseline, as changes in response can be important over time.

Testing should be performed with the quiet, awake baby lying supine, with the head facing forward and centered on the shoulders; otherwise, the asymmetric tonic neck reflex may be invoked, which tends to increase tone and reflexes on the side to which the head is turned. The normally flexed position of a baby's arms at term makes the reflexes in the upper extremities, especially the triceps reflex, difficult to elicit. Because of this, it is common to find that the reflexes in the lower extremities are more brisk than those in the upper. Do not attempt to test crying babies. The limb can be gently shaken to facilitate relaxation. As with adults, distracting techniques may help the baby relax more fully. In babies, visual engagement or oral diversion with a pacifier or finger can help, especially if the baby is crying. Tendon reflexes are more brisk in newborns than in most older children and adults and are influenced by the baby's state of consciousness. There may be markedly different briskness noted when reflex testing is repeated later on the same infant. It is impossible to elicit any deep tendon reflexes in about 10% of normal newborns.

The speed, strength, amplitude (or range of movement) and duration of muscle contraction should all be noted. However, reflexes can be difficult to elicit in some normal babies, and the significance of increased response may be less important than if the reflexes are asymmetrical, therefore always test both sides. Each response should be graded according to the scale in the table below.

SCORING	PARAMETERS
0	No response
± or trace	Very faint, visible or palpable contraction without movement
1+	Hypoactive
2+	Normal
3+	Hyperactive
4+	Hyperactive and reduplicated, with clonus or strong overflow, especially to surrounding muscles. Sustained clonus, characterized by more than 8 to 10 beats when the reflex is elicited, is never normal.

Note: The spinal and cranial nerve (CN) levels in bold indicate the primary nerve supplying the muscle. The reflexes marked with an asterisk indicate those most frequently tested.

Jaw jerk (masseter) reflex

This reflex depends upon intact trigeminal and facial nerves and tests **CN V** and VII.

Elicitation: Place the tip of the index finger of your nondominant hand on the baby's chin well below the lips with the mouth slightly opened. Sharply tap your fingertip with the other index finger or a reflex hammer.

Response: This should prompt contraction of the masseter muscle, which elevates the chin. An absent or weak response after the first two days suggests a brain stem lesion or damage of the fifth cranial nerve.

Deltoid muscle

The deltoid muscle is supplied by the axillary nerves, whose roots enter at **C5** and C6.

Elicitation: Gently press the shoulder back away from the midline with the flat of your finger; your fingertip should lie on the outer side of the baby's arm. Tap the side of the humerus at the junction of the upper and middle third of the arm where the deltoid muscle inserts.

Response: The arm should raise.

Pectoral muscle

This reflex requires intact innervation of the pectoralis major muscle by the medial and lateral pectoral nerves, which insert at C5 and **C6** and move the inside head of the clavicle. It also involves movement of the sternocostal end of the clavicle, supplied by C7, **C8** and T1.

Elicitation: Support the supine baby's shoulder toward the midline slightly by placing a small hand towel behind the shoulder or having an assistant support the shoulder to be examined. Place the flat of your index finger pointing either toward the baby's feet or toward the head on the front of the chest just above the armpit with the finger directed firmly against the pectoralis major muscle. Tap your index finger with the tip of the other or with the hammer.

Response: The arm should move toward the midline and rotate inward slightly as the clavicular fibers flex the arm.

***Biceps reflex**

This reflex relies on an intact musculocutaneous nerve, which is attached to C5 and **C6** of the spinal cord.

Elicitation: Hold the baby's arm with the elbow partially flexed and the palm facing downward. Place your index finger over the insertion of the biceps tendon, that is, in the midline just above the bend of the arm. Tap your finger with the tip of the reflex hammer (you are stimulating the superomedial aspect of the antecubital fossa on the biceps tendon).

Response: This should produce flexion of the forearm and contraction of the biceps muscle. At times, associated supination occurs, with rotation of the forearm so that the palm faces upward when the arm is flexed at the elbow.

Triceps muscle

This reflex tests the triceps muscle, supplied by the portion of the radial nerve that inserts at C6, **C7** and **C8**.

Elicitation: Place your fingerpad over the triceps tendon above the olecranon (the "funny bone" in the elbow), then tap it. Another way to perform this test is to flex the arm at the elbow, pull the forearm across the chest with the baby's palm facing the chest, and use a direct tap from directly behind the elbow.

Response: The forearm should extend with contraction of the triceps muscle.

Brachioradialis (supinator) muscle reflex

This reflex requires normal innervation of the brachioradialis muscle by the portion of the radial nerve that is rooted at C5, **C6** and C7.

Elicitation: Position the baby's arm with the elbow partly flexed and the forearm turned so that the palm is about three-quarters of the way toward the body. Use a fingertip or the flat side of the hammer to strike directly over the side of the outer third of the arm just above the wrist.

Response: The forearm should flex and supinate (rotation of the forearm so that the palm faces upward).

Finger flexors

This reflex tests the flexor digitorum superficialis and profundus muscles, innervated by the median and medial part of the ulnar nerve, which is rooted at **C8** and T1.

Elicitation: Lay your index finger horizontally across the base of the baby's fingers to elicit a partial grasp. Then tap your index finger.

Response: Flexion of finger joints.

<u>*Knee jerk (patellar) reflex</u>

This reflex is the one most easily elicited in newborns and the one most reliably present at birth. It requires a normal nerve supply to the quadriceps femoris muscle via the femoral nerve and tests spinal nerves entering at L2, **L3** and **L4**.

Elicitation: Stand to the baby's side. Lay the baby supine and center his head in the midline. Support the leg to be tested with your nondominant hand. Strike across the patellar tendon just below the knee in the crease or just above the patella on the quadriceps tendon. The area of stimulation is often wider than in older persons.

Response: This should produce extension of the lower leg at the knee with visible contraction of the quadriceps muscle in the thigh. There is often an associated movement of the opposite leg toward the midline. If the knee jerk is not elicited, the adduction of the opposite leg may occur by itself. The knee jerk may be absent in a severely shocked baby.

<u>*Thigh adductor and crossed adductor muscle reflexes</u>

This assesses intact innervation of the adductor muscles of the hip, which are supplied by the obturator nerve, which is linked to L2, **L3** and **L4**.

Elicitation: Spread the thighs slightly. Reaching down from the baby's head, place your index finger diagonally across the inside of the knee, with your little finger on the opposite leg to maintain a 45 to 60° angle of the index finger. Tap your index finger.

Response: The stimulated thigh should rotate toward the midline at the hip.

<u>Ankle jerk (Achilles) reflex</u>

This tests the gastrocnemius and soleus muscles, which are innervated by the tibial nerve, which is linked to L5, **S1** and S2.

Elicitation: With the infant supine, hold the leg in a flexed position with the foot partially dorsiflexed (bent back toward the shin). Tap horizontally across the back of the baby's foot where the Achilles tendon inserts above the heel.

Response: This produces plantar flexion of the foot at the ankle (foot jerks away from the shin; there may be several repetitive beats). Sustained clonus, with more than 8 or 10 repetitions, may indicate cervical irritation. However, bilateral clonus of 5 to 10 beats may be a normal finding, especially in babies who are crying, hungry or jittery. This is particularly true if the clonus is unaccompanied by other signs of upper motor neuron dysfunction.

ASSESSMENT OF CRANIAL NERVE FUNCTION

This chapter describes some basic newborn responses that reflect cranial nerve function and how they may be elicited. In the vast majority of cases, there will be no need to perform formal cranial nerve assessments, as the baby's normal responses will be self-evident. Many of the examinations discussed below have already been addressed in the previous chapters. Those findings most pertinent to neurological assessment are repeated here for clarity of presentation. My discussion is based on the writings of Fletcher (1998), Scanlon and colleagues (1979) and Simpson and Creeham (2001).

Birth Trauma

Evidence of birth trauma may include bruising, broken bones, cephalohematomas, a depressed area of the skull, forceps marks, lacerations, abrasions, petechiae and localized swelling. Any of these, especially if on the face or limbs, could be associated with underlying nerve damage that would be reflected in abnormal spontaneous movement or asymmetrical movement. Lack of movement in an arm may indicate Erb palsy (damage to the upper spinal roots C5 and C6), Klumpke palsy (damage to the lower spinal roots C8 and T1), or both. Facial asymmetry or lack of expression is seen in infants with facial weakness due to Bell's palsy.

Evaluating the Cranial Nerves (CN) for Intact Functioning

Below are screening protocols for assessing the normal function of each cranial nerve. The nerves listed on the left are not all in numerical order but are ordered according to the relevant evaluation as you move down the baby's body.

CN I (olfactory): CN I is rarely assessed at birth because problems with the sense of smell are rarely associated with neonatal neurologic disease and babies rapidly habituate to smells. However, babies respond to strong scents and the smell of their mother by grimacing, widening the eyes, sniffing, startling or changing their heart rate. Oil of cloves or peppermint or smelling salts can be passed under the baby's nose to elicit a response. Do not apply these substances to the baby.

CN II (optic): At term, the alert baby's eyes will follow faces or brightly colored objects, and she will blink in response to light. Bright lights in the room will alter this response, so dim the room lights before assessment. The visual field can be assessed by shining a penlight at the periphery of the baby's vision. Pupil constriction or response (also discussed under CN III) is an indication that the eyes are registering light. Constriction should be bilaterally equal. Pupil constriction tests the retina, optic nerve and the third cranial nerve. Note that if the room is too bright, the baby too deeply asleep, or the baby's other senses are overstimulated, tests of the optic nerve will be unreliable.

Wandering nystagmus (involuntary rhythmic oscillation of the eyeballs, either pendular or with a slow-and-fast component) may be transiently present but should not be persistent. Sometimes nystagmus occurs in the direction opposite the visual stimulus. If it occurs with limb tremors, seizure activity must be ruled out. (If the tremors subside when the affected limb is held, the baby is not seizing.)

Optokinetic (coordinated) eye movement can be elicited after nystagmus (or in its absence) when the baby is awake. This test of cortical vision requires clear corneas and lenses plus a normal retinal and optic nerve. Hold the baby 12 to 18 inches from you so that you are in his line of vision, with his eyes in the same horizontal plane as your own. If the baby fixes his eyes on yours, hold him still and move your face from side to side slowly, watching his gaze to see if he follows yours. The eyes should follow the direction of horizontal movement over an arc of 30 to 60° at term; most normal 32-week babies can fix on an object briefly. Sometimes nystagmus occurs in the opposite direction of motion.

Optical blink reflex: If the baby will not fix on you, use a light source of increasing intensity until a blink reflex is elicited. In a dimly lit room, with a baby who is either lightly sleeping or awake but not crying, shine a bright light suddenly in the eyes about 12 to 18 inches from the face. This should produce quick closure of the eyes; there may be a slight backward tilt of the head as well. This reaction depends on adequate clearing of the cornea and vitreous body after about 28 weeks gestation.

A lack of reaction occurs when there is impaired perception of light, which may be due to a cataract or cortical blindness. A startle that occurs with the blink reflex may reflect hyperirritability.

Photic sneeze reflex: Shining a bright light in the eyes causes reflexive sneezing, which confirms visual perception of light, although its absence is not abnormal. There may be a familial tendency.

CN III (oculomotor): Pupillary constriction in response to light is controlled by CN III and should first appear between 28 and 30 weeks of gestation. It depends upon an intact cranial nerve as well as clarity of the ocular tissues sufficient to allow light to reach the optic nerve; therefore, it is not always present prior to 35 weeks of gestation.

Pupillary response: Use your hands over the infant's eyes to shield them from ambient light and to encourage the baby to open her eyes. Move your hand and watch the reaction as the shadow moves off the eyes. If there is no reaction, use a stronger light source and bring it from the side to focus on a pupil; observe for constriction of both pupils. Avoid shining the light directly in the baby's eyes, which will elicit the blink reflex and prevent your observation of the pupils.

CN III (oculomotor), CN IV (trochlear), and CN VI (abducent): These nerves supply the pupils and the muscles around the eyes. First observe the spontaneous movements of the eyes and evaluate their shape and symmetry. Do not attempt to force the baby's eyes open. Also note that ocular alignment is normally poor in newborns.

Rotation test: This test requires an awake, strong term baby. Hold him upright under his arms, facing you with your hands around his chest. Rotate his entire torso slowly to about 90°; first in one direction, then in the other. Do not restrain the head on the first try. The head should turn toward the direction of rotation.

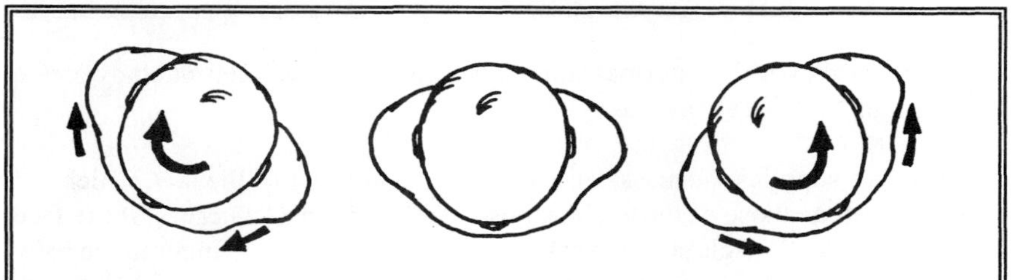

Rotation test: when the torso is rotated and the head is free to move, the head follows the direction of rotation

On the second try, support the head so that the baby cannot turn his head from a neutral (facing forward) position and rotate the torso as above. When head and body turn in unison, his eyes should follow in the direction of rotation, and the gaze should return to the midline when rotation stops. There may be brief saccadic movements of both eyes (this occurs when the eyes fix, then jerk to the next focus point and fix again in a series of rapid start-and-stop movements). There should be no sustained nystagmus. This response will be absent or variable in babies who have lesions that interfere with vestibular response. Absence in one direction only with a normal opposite response may be due to an abnormal CN VI. Elicitation of an accompanying startle (mass reflex) or a lack of return of the focus to midline after rotation ceases is also abnormal.

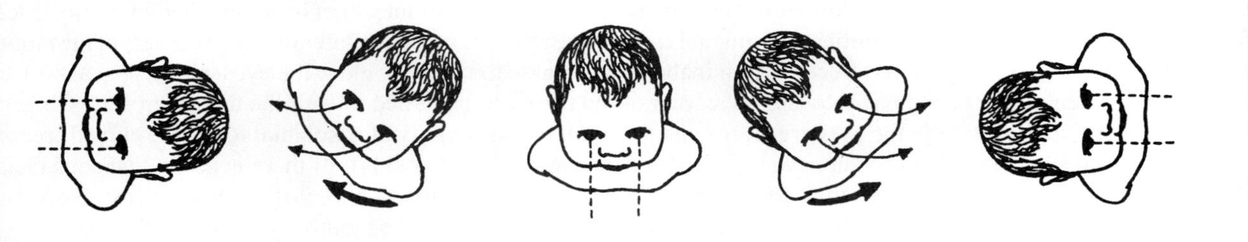

Rotation test: when the torso and head are rotated together, the eyes follow the direction of rotation. When rotation stops, the gaze returns to midline.

Doll's eye maneuver: This test assesses CN II, IV and VI. The baby should be awake and not crying. The eyes should not be focused in the midline. The lids may be open. Hold the baby so she faces you. The lateral doll's eye maneuver is elicited by turning only the baby's head slowly from side to side while observing for the direction of eye movement. Hold the head in each position for several seconds. The eyes should move in the opposite direction of rotation. If the baby is tilted forward, the eyes should roll upward. If the eyes remain fixed or move in the same direction as the head, brainstem or oculomotor nerve damage may have occurred. A normal response to the doll's-eye maneuver indicates an intact vestibular nerve.

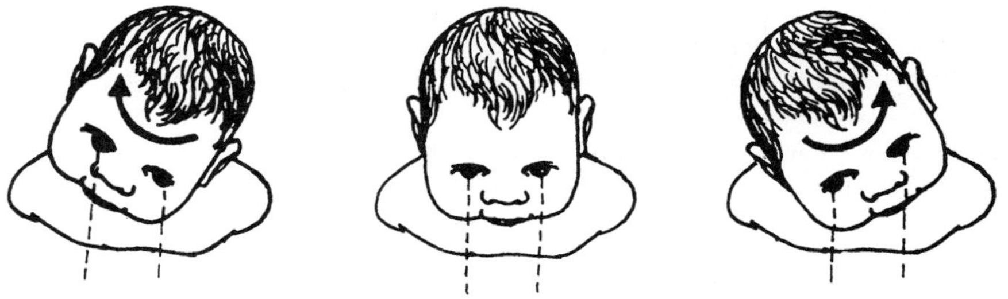

Doll's eye maneuver: the eyes are "left behind" when the torso remains stationary and only the head is turned

Persistent strabismus (crossed eyes) is abnormal, although occasional asymmetrical movements are seen, especially in babies who are sleeping lightly or barely awake.

CN V (trigeminal): This nerve supplies the masseter and pterygoid muscles of the jaw, which are involved in the jaw-closing phase of sucking, as well as those of the eyelids, nose and other sensory nerves of the face. The rooting reflex tests the sensory pathways of CN V. Muscle strength can be assessed by placing a finger in the baby's mouth and feeling the force of his bite. These assessments are most accurate when performed on a hungry baby.

Rooting reflex: The rooting reflex, induced by stroking to the side of the lips, should cause the baby to open her mouth and turn toward the stimulus. If not, a light pinprick can be used to elicit a grimace.

Corneal reflex (lid reflex): The eyes must be open. Barely touch the cornea with a sterile thread of cotton, which should cause the eye to close immediately.

Jaw jerk reflex: When the baby's mouth is slightly open, place the pad of one index finger on the baby's chin well below the lips. Tap this forefinger sharply with the other. This should cause the mouth to close. It is easier to feel the jaw movement than it is to see it. An absent or weak response after the first 2 days suggests a brain stem lesion or damage to CN V.

CN VII (facial motor), assessing: This nerve governs facial expression. An intact nerve is indicated by symmetrical facial movements during crying or smiling. Nasolabial creases are normally present bilaterally. The corners of the mouth should not droop. Severe injury is reflected by an inability to wrinkle the brow or close the eyes with crying as well as obvious facial weakness. Facial palsy causes the corner of the mouth to be pulled toward the uninjured side. Observe the resting infant for how tightly the eyes are closed and the fullness and equality of nasolabial folds (the curved creases that extend from above the ala of the nose to the corner of the mouth on either side). If there is no spontaneous facial movement, stimulate a response and look for symmetrical opening of the mouth and closing of the eyes. Note that absence of the depressor anguli oris muscle may cause incomplete opening of the mouth on the affected side.

Lip reflex: Tap sharply near the corner of the mouth with a fingertip. This should prompt contraction of the orbicularis oris muscle, causing the lips to protrude. Only a light touch is needed in a baby who is sleeping lightly, although the reflex may be absent if the baby is sleeping deeply. This response should decrease with repetition.

Glabella reflex: Hold the baby's head firmly with one hand while sharply tapping the center of the forehead just above the nose with your other index finger. This should produce tighter closing of the eyes and wrinkling of the brow. An abnormal response would be asymmetrical, absent or extremely pronounced with sustained closure lasting more than one second or resulting in a generalized startle response.

CN VIII (auditory): The intactness of CN VIII is grossly assessed when the baby moves in the direction of sound or quiets to voices. Tests for hearing must take place with little or no background noise when the baby is either lightly sleeping or quietly alert. If the room is too noisy, this assessment will be useless. Normal babies habituate to sounds quickly, so the same type of sound can be used to test hearing only once or twice. Use sounds such as a single tone, clicker toy, bell, wrinkled paper or rattle. The sound source should be held about one foot out on either side of the baby. The baby may blink, change his sucking pattern, startle or alert to the sound. The baby may also become quiet or alter his breathing pattern when talked to. It can be very difficult to distinguish unilateral hearing impairment. A positive Moro reflex also includes a vestibularly mediated response to head drop.

Acoustic blink reflex: The baby has a pronounced blink upon hearing the sound; this decreases after several repetitions. Abnormal responses would be none, persistent blinking with repeated tests or elicitation of a startle reflex (mass response). Mass response, difficulty habituating or complete shutdown may be seen in normal but immature babies.

CN IX (glossopharyngeal): Evaluate by inspecting the tongue for normal movement during sucking and in general as well as when eliciting a gag reflex. The gag reflex should be strong, and the uvula should not deviate to one side while the baby is gagging. This reflex can be affected by an irritated throat (which may result from suctioning).

CN VII & IX (taste): The newborn can discriminate tastes and will tell you if she likes them or not by facial expression, grimacing, rate of sucking or changes in heart rate. Touching the tongue with a cotton swab dipped in safe but strong flavors (such as glucose, white vinegar, lemon juice or salt solution) can demonstrate this ability. Do not use honey, as it may contain botulism spores. Babies habituate to tastes rapidly.

CN X (vagus): This nerve supplies the soft palate, pharynx and larynx in the head and neck. Evaluate the baby by listening to his cry and assessing the presence of any hoarseness, stridor or loss of the voice (aphonia), any of which may indicate injury to this nerve.

CN XI (accessory): This nerve supplies the sternocleidomastoid and trapezius muscles. Impairment of flexion and rotation of the head is difficult to detect in the newborn period. Look for notably asymmetric head control (although this is most likely due to shortening of the neck muscles on one side rather than dysfunction of CN XI). Assess head control by placing the baby on her back and turning her head to one side; the baby should attempt to bring her head back to the midline. The height of the shoulders should also be symmetrical. Also palpate the length of the muscles on both sides of the neck and check for symmetry and definition of outline.

CN XII (hypoglossal): This nerve supplies the tongue, so it governs coordination of the suck and swallow reflexes. It is evaluated by assessing both the strength of the tongue during sucking and the baby's ability to swallow and gag. The tongue should remain in the midline when the mouth is open. The integrity of the nerve can also be assessed by pinching off the nostrils, which should produce a reflex opening of the mouth and a raising of the tip of the tongue. The tip of the tongue will deviate toward the affected side if there is partial paralysis of the nerve. Enlargement of the tongue can adversely affect the reliability of your results.

References and Further Reading on Evaluating Newborn Well-being

References used in multiple chapters

Fletcher MA. Physical Diagnosis in Neonatology, Lippincott-Raven, Philadelphia PA, 1998.

Fletcher MA. Chapter 19: "Physical assessment and classification," in Avery G, et al., eds. Neonatology: Pathophysiology and Management of the Newborn, 5th ed. Lippincott, Williams & Wilkins, Philadelphia PA, 1999.

Hill A. "Chapter 194: Development of tone and reflexes in the fetus and newborn," in Polin R, Fox W, eds. Fetal and Neonatal Physiology, Vol 2, 2nd ed., WB Saunders, Philadelphia PA, 1998.

Illingworth R. The Development of the Infant and Young Child: Normal and Abnormal, 4th ed. E & S Livingstone, Ltd, Edinburgh UK, 1970.

Illingworth R. The Development of the Infant and Young Child: Normal and Abnormal, 6th ed. Churchill Livingstone, Edinburgh UK, 1975.

Illingworth R. The Development of the Infant and Young Child: Normal and Abnormal, 9th ed. Churchill Livingstone, Edinburgh UK, 1987.

Johnston P, et al. The Newborn Child, 9th ed. Churchill Livingstone, Edinburgh UK, 2003.

Mead-Johnson Co. A Clinical Review of Concepts and Characteristics in Infant Development. Mead-Johnson & Co., Evansville IN, 1974.

O'Doherty N. Neurological Examination of the Newborn: A Routine for All, MTP Press, Lancaster UK,1986.

Polin R, Spitzer A, eds. Fetal and Neonatal Secrets, Hanley & Belfus, Inc, Philadelphia PA, 2001.

Prechtl H. The Neurological Examination of the Full Term Newborn Infant, 2nd ed. Clin Dev Med, Vol. 63. JB Lippincott, Philadelphia PA, 1977.

Scanlon, J, et al. A System of Newborn Physical Examination. University Park Press, Baltimore MD, 1979.

Swaiman K. Chapter 4: "Neurologic examination of the term and preterm infant," in Swaiman K, Ashwal S, eds. Pediatric Neurology: Principles and Practice, 3rd ed., Vol. 1. Mosby, St Louis MO, 1999.

Thureen P, et al. Assessment and Care of the Well Newborn. WB Saunders Co, Philadelphia PA, 1999.

Vlach V. "Evolution of skin reflexes in the first years of life," Dev Med Child Neuro, 31(2);196-205, Apr,1989.

Volpe J. Neurology of the Newborn, 3rd ed. WB Saunders, Philadelphia PA, 1995.

Volpe J. Chapter 3: "Neurological examination: normal and abnormal features," in Volpe J. Neurology of the Newborn, 4th ed. WB Saunders, Philadelphia PA, 2001.

Ziai M, et al., Assessment of the Newborn: A Guide for the Practitioner, 1st ed. Little, Brown and Co, Boston MA, 1984.

The Healthy Newborn in the First Hours of Life

Ariel I, et al. "Nesidiodysplasia–a histologic entity?" Hum Pathol.19(10);1215-1218, Oct, 1988.

Enning C. "Birth on demand," all day workshop on waterbirth, Midwifery Today conf., Springfield OR, Mar, 2003.

Gruener JS. "Fetal and neonatal heart rates observed during involuntary expulsive efforts in the second stage of labor." Unpublished master's thesis. Graduate College of the U of IL, at the Medical Center, Dept. of Nursing Sci., Chicago IL, 1982.

Karlberg P, et al. "Respiratory studies in newborn infants, II, Pulmonary ventilation and mechanics of breathing in the first minutes of life, including the onset of respiration," Acta Pediatr, 51;121-136, March, 1962.

Mercer J. "Current best evidence: A review of the literature on umbilical cord clamping," J Midwif Women's Health, 46(6);402-414, Nov-Dec, 2001.

Oh W, et al. "The effects of placental transfusion on respiratory mechanics of normal term newborn infants," Pediatr, 40(1);6-12, July, 1967.

World Health Org. Thermal Protection of the Newborn: A Practical Guide, Safe Motherhood, Geneva Switzerland, 1997.

Yao AC, et al. "Expiratory grunting in the late clamped normal neonate," Pediatr, 48(6);865-870, Dec, 1971.

The APGAR Score

ACOG. "Fetal and neonatal neurologic injury," ACOG Technical Bulletin, 163, Washington DC, 1992.

ACOG. "Inappropriate use of the terms fetal distress and birth asphyxia," ACOG Committee Opinion 197,Washington DC, 1998.

ACOG. "Use and Abuse of the Apgar Score," ACOG Technical Bulletin 174:Washington DC, July, 1996.

ACOG. "Utility of umbilical cord blood acid-base assessment." ACOG Committee Opinion 138, Washington DC, 1994.

Apgar V. "A proposal for a new method of evaluation of the newborn infant," Curr Res Anesth Analg, 32(4);260-267, July-Aug, 1953.

Apgar V, James LS. "Further observations on the newborn scoring system," Am J Dis Child, 104;419-428, Oct, 1962.

Blair E, Stanley FJ. "Intrapartum asphyxia: a rare cause of cerebral palsy," J Pediatr, 112(4);515-519, Apr, 1988.

Dennis J, et al. "Acid-base status at birth and neurodevelopmental outcome at four and one-half years,"Am Col Obstet Gynecol, 161(1);213-220, July, 1989.

Drage JS, et al. "The Apgar score as an index of neonatal mortality, A report from the Collaborative Study of Cerebral Palsy," Obstet Gynecol, 24;222-230, Aug, 1964.

Ekert P, et al. "Dexamethasone prevents apoptosis in a neonatal rat model of hypoxic-ischemic encephalopathy (HIE) by a reactive oxygen species-independent mechanism," BRAIN RES, 747(1);9-17, Jan,1997.

Fee S, et al. "Severe acidosis and subsequent neurologic status," AM J OBSTET GYNECOL, 162(3);802-806, Mar, 1990.

Graves B. "Challenges of neonatal resuscitation for nurse-midwives," JNM, 33(5);217-224, Sept-Oct, 1988.

Jain L, et al. "Cardiopulmonary resuscitation of apparently stillborn infants: survival and long-term outcome." J PEDIATR, 118(5);778-782, May, 1991.

Levinson G, et al. Chapter 37: "Evaluation of the neonate," in Hughes S, et al., eds. SHNIDER AND LEVINSON'S ANESTHESIA FOR OBSTETRICS, 4th ed. Lippincott, Williams & Wilkins, Philadelphia PA, 2001.

Morley G, Ob-Gyn. "How the cord clamp injures your baby's brain," www.cordclamping.com, Feb 26, 2002.

Nelson KB, Ellenberg JH. "Apgar scores as predictors of chronic neurologic disability," PEDIATRICS, 68(1);36-44, July, 1981.

Nelson KB, Ellenberg JH. "Antecedents of cerebral palsy, Multivariate analysis of risk," N ENGL J MED, 315(2);81-86, July, 1986.

Nelson KB. "Perspective on the role of perinatal asphyxia in neurologic outcome: its role in developmental deficits in children," CAN MED ASSOC J, 141(S);3-10, 1989.

Ruth VJ, Raivio KO. "Perinatal brain damage: predictive value of metabolic acidosis and the Apgar score," BMJ, 297(6640);24-27, July 2, 1988.

Sniderman S, et al. Chapter 38: "Resuscitation of the newborn," in Hughes, S, et al., eds. SHNIDER AND LEVINSON'S ANESTHESIA FOR OBSTETRICS, 4th ed. Lippincott, Williams & Wilkins, Philadelphia PA, 2002.

Stanley FJ. "Cerebral palsy trends, Implications for perinatal care," ACTA OBSTET GYNECOL SCAND, 73(1);5-9, Jan, 1994.

STATES OF NEWBORN CONSCIOUSNESS OR BEHAVIOR

Brazelton TB. NEONATAL BEHAVORIAL ASSESSMENT SCALE, 1st ed., Clin Dev Med, Vol. 50. Spastics International Medical Publications with JB Lippincott, London UK, 1973.

Brazelton TB. Chapter 20: "Behavioral competence," in Avery G, et al., eds. NEONATOLOGY: PATHOPHYSIOLOGY AND MANAGEMENT OF THE NEWBORN, 5th ed. Lippincott, Williams & Wilkins, Philadelphia PA, 1999.

Pearson J. "Crying and calming: important information and effective techniques to teach parents of full-term newborns,"MOTHER BABY J, 4(5);39-42, 1999.

ASSESSMENT OF GESTATIONAL AGE

Ballard J, et al. "A simplified score for assessment of fetal maturation of newly born infants," J PEDIATR, 95(5, Pt 1);769-774, 1979.

Ballard JL, et al. "New Ballard Score, expanded to include extremely premature infants," J PEDIATR 119(3):417-423, Sept,1991.

Chow M, et al. HANDBOOK OF PEDIATRIC PRIMARY CARE. John Wiley and Sons, New York NY, 1979.

Dodd V. "Gestational Age Assessment."NEONATAL NETWORK, 15(1):27-36, Feb, 1996.

Donovan E. "Inaccuracy of Ballard scores before 28 week's gestation," J PEDIATR, 135(2, Pt. 1);147-152, Aug, 1999.

Dubowitz L, et al. "Clinical assessment of gestational age in the newborn infant," J PEDIATR, 77(1);1-10, July, 1970.

Dubowitz L, Dubowitz V. GESTATIONAL AGE OF THE NEWBORN: A CLINICAL MANUAL. Addison-Wesley, Reading MA, 1977.

Rudolph A. ATLAS OF THE NEWBORN, VOL. 1: NEONATAL AND PERINATAL MEDICINE. BC Decker, Inc, Hamilton, Ont, Canada, 1997.

Schlinger H. Editing notes, 2003.

Sola A, Chow I. "The coming of (gestational) age for preterm infants," J PEDIATR, 135(2, Pt 1);137-139, Aug, 1999.

Sullivan R, Schreinder R. "Determining A Newborn's Gestational Age," MCN AMER J MAT CHILD NURS, 4(1);38-45, Jan-Feb, 1979.

ASSESSMENT AND RELEVANCE OF THE BABY'S SIZE IN RELATIONSHIP TO GESTATIONAL AGE

Alexander G, et al. "A United States national reference for fetal growth," OBSTET GYNECOL, 87(2);163-168, Feb, 1996.

Anthony J, Smith P. "Intrauterine growth restriction," in Jaffe R, Bui, TH. TEXTBOOK OF FETAL ULTRASOUND, Parthenon Pub, New York, NY, 1999.

Chamberlain D. THE MIND OF YOUR NEWBORN BABY. North Atlantic Books, Berkeley CA, 1998.

Fox H. PATHOLOGY OF THE PLACENTA, 2nd ed. WB Saunders Co, Ltd, London UK, 1997.

Georgieff MK. "Assessment of large and small for gestational age newborn infants using growth curves," PEDIATR ANN, 24(11);599-607, Nov, 1995.

Girling J, Dornhorst A. "Chapter 65: Pregnancy and diabetes mellitus," in Pickup J & Williams G, eds. TEXTBOOK OF DIABETES 2: VOL 2, 3rd ed, Blackwell Science, Malden MA, 2003.

Korones S. HIGH-RISK NEWBORN INFANTS: THE BASIS OF INTENSIVE NURSING CARE, 4th ed. CV Mosby, St. Louis MO, 1986.

Langer O, "Fetal macrosomia: etiologic factors," CLIN OBSTET GYNECOL, 43(2);283-297, June, 2000.

Lubchenco L, et al. "Intrauterine growth in length and head circumference as estimated from live births at gestational ages from 26 to 42 weeks," PEDIATRICS, 37(3);403-408, Mar, 1966.

McLean F, et al. "Postterm infants: too big or too small?" AM J OBSTET GYNECOL, 164(2);619-624, Feb, 1991.

Miller H. "Intrauterine growth retardation, An unmet challenge," AM J DIS CHILD, 135(10);944-948, Oct, 1981.

Moore, L. "Fetal growth restriction and maternal oxygen transport during high altitude pregnancy," HIGH ALTITUDE MED BIO, 4(2); 141-155, 2003.

Mortola JP, et al. "Birth weight and altitude: a study in Peruvian communities," J PEDIATR, 136(3);324-329, Mar, 2000.
Naeye R, Dixon J. "Distortions in fetal growth standards," PEDIATR RES 12(10);987-991, Oct, 1978.
O'Leary J. SHOULDER DYSTOCIA AND BIRTH INJURY, McGraw-Hill, New York NY, 1992.
Snow C. INFANT DEVELOPMENT, 2nd ed. Prentice Hall, Upper Saddle River NJ, 1998.
Sparks J, et al. Chapter 26: "Intrauterine growth and nutrition," in Polin R, Fox W, eds. FETAL AND NEONATAL PHYSIOLOGY, 2nd ed., VOL. 1., WB Saunders Co, Philadelphia PA, 1999.

ASSESSING THE NUTRITIONAL STATUS OF THE TERM NEWBORN

Metcoff J. "Clinical assessment of nutritional status at birth, Fetal malnutrition and SGA are not synonymous," PEDIATR CLIN NO AM, 41(5);875-891, Oct, 1994.
Rao M, et al. "Suitability of CANSCORE for assessment of the nutritional status of newborns," INDIAN J PEDIATR, 66(4);483-492, July-Aug, 1999.

REFERENCES USED IN THE CHAPTER ENTITLED "PRELIMINARY PHYSICAL ASSESSMENT OF THE NEWBORN" and all the subchapters under "THE COMPLETE PHYSICAL EXAMINATION OF THE NEWBORN"

Ahmann E. HOME CARE FOR THE HIGH-RISK INFANT: A FAMILY CENTERED APPROACH, 2nd ed, Aspen, Gaithersburg, MD,1996.
Alexander M, Brown M. PEDIATRIC HISTORY TAKING AND PHYSICAL DIAGNOSIS FOR NURSES, 2nd ed. Mosby, St Louis MO, 1979.
Asher M. "Screening for congenital dislocation of the hip, scoliosis, and other abnormalities affecting the musculoskeletal system," PEDIATR CLIN NO AMER, 33(6);1335-1353, Dec, 1986.
Avery G, et al., eds. NEONATOLOGY: PATHOPHYSIOLOGY AND MANAGEMENT OF THE NEWBORN, 5th ed. Lippincott, Williams & Wilkins, Philadelphia PA, 1999.
Bates B. A GUIDE TO PHYSICAL EXAMINATION AND HISTORY TAKING, 5th ed. JB Lippincott, Philadelphia PA, 1991.
Berger A, et al. "Changes in the Sydney line during the first year of life," DEV MED CHILD NEUROL, 25(4);490-492, Aug 1983.
Biavati M. "Cleft palate," E-MEDICINE.COM, web article, updated, May 15, 2002.
Broughton N, et al. "Range of knee motion in normal neonates," J PEDIATR ORTHOPED, 13(2);263-264, Mar-Apr,1993.
Callegari C, et al. "Anogenital ratio: measure of fetal virilization in premature and full-term newborn infants," J PEDIATR, 111(2)24-243, Aug, 1987.
Chasler C. ATLAS OF ROENTGEN ANATOMY OF THE NEWBORN AND INFANT SKULL, Warren H Green, Inc, St. Louis MO, 1972.
Chung S. HIP DISORDERS IN INFANTS AND CHILDREN, Lea & Febiger, Philadelphia, PA, 1981.
Clark D. ATLAS OF NEONATOLOGY: A COMPANION TO AVERY'S DISEASES OF THE NEWBORN, WB Saunders Co, Philadelphia PA, 2000.
Coen R, Koffler H. PRIMARY CARE OF THE NEWBORN. Little, Brown and Co, Boston MA, 1987.
Crelin e. FUNCTIONAL ANATOMY OF THE NEWBORN. Yale U Press, New Haven ST, 1973.
Davies P. "Dermatoglyphics and palmar creases," NURS TIMES, 64(30);994-996, July 26, 1968.
Donn S, Kuhns S. PEDIATRIC TRANSILLUMINATION. Year Book Medical, Chicago IL, 1983.
Dunne K, Clarren S. "The origin of prenatal and postnatal deformities," PEDIATR CLIN NO AMER, 33(6);1277-1297, Dec, 1986.
El Haddad M, Corkery J. "The anus in the newborn," PEDIATR, 76(6)927-928, Dec, 1985.
Enning C. "Birth on demand," all day workshop on waterbirth, MIDWIFERY TODAY conf., Springfield OR, Mar, 2003.
Evans C. "Atresias of the gastrointestinal tract," INTERNAT ABSTRACTS IN SURGERY, 92;1, 1951.
Fishman S, Mulliken J. "Hemangiomas and vascular malformations of infancy and childhood," PEDIATR CLIN NO AMER, 40(6);1177-1200, Dec 1993.
Genc A, et al. "Evaluation of the location of the anus by a modified technique in the neonate," J PEDIATR SURG, 37(1);80-82, Jan 2002.
Gilhooly J. Personal e-mail communication, March 2003.
Goldbloom R, ed. PEDIATRIC CLINICAL SKILLS. Churchill Livingstone, New York NY, 1992.
Goldring D, Wohltmann H. "Flush method for blood pressure determination in newborn infants," J PEDIATR, 40(3);285-289, 1952.
Graham J. SMITH'S RECOGNIZABLE PATTERNS OF HUMAN DEFORMATION, 2nd ed. WB Saunders Co, Philadelphia PA, 1988.
Greene W, Heckman J, eds. THE CLINICAL MEASUREMENT OF JOINT MOTION. Amer Acad of Orthopaedic Surg, Rosemont IL, 1994.
Hauser G, et al. "On the variablity of "flexion creases" in the distal plantar areas of newborns," AM J PHYSICAL ANTROPOL, 60(1);29-37, Jan 1983.
Hensinger R. "Congenital dislocation of the hip," CLINICAL SYMPOSIA, 31(1), CIBA Pharmaceutical, Summit NJ, 1979.
Hensinger R, Jones E. "Developmental orthopedics, I: the lower limb," DEVELOP MED CHILD NEUROL, 24(1);95-116, 1992.
Herring J. Chapter 3: "The orthopaedic examination: a comprehensive overview," in Herring J, ed. TACHDJIAN'S PEDIATRIC ORTHOPAEDICS, 3rd ed. VOL. I. WB Saunders, Philadelphia PA, 2002.
Hoekelman R. "Chapter 19: The Physical Assessment of Infants and Children," in Bates B. A GUIDE TO PHYSICAL EXAMINATION AND HISTORY TAKING, 5th ed. JB Lippincott, Philadelphia PA, 1991.
Hook E, et al. "The human simian crease and its variants: a model for investigation of serious congenital malformation," in Bergsman D, ed. MALFORMATION SYNDROMES, Birth Defects Original Article Series, 10(7);7-16, 1974.
Johnston P. VULLIAMY'S THE NEWBORN CHILD, 7th ed. Churchill Livingstone, Edinburgh UK,1994.

Johnstone J. Chapter 26: "Hernia in the neonate," in Freeman N, et al., eds. SURGERY OF THE NEWBORN. Churchill Livingstone, Edinburgh UK, 1994.

Jones K. SMITH'S RECOGNIZABLE PATTERNS OF HUMAN MALFORMATION, 5th ed. WB Saunders Co, Philadelphia PA, 1997.

Kitterman J, et al. "Aortic blood pressure in normal newborn infants during the first 12 hours of life," PEDIATR, 44(6);959-968, 1969.

Korones S. HIGH-RISK NEWBORN INFANTS: THE BASIS OF INTENSIVE NURSING CARE, 4th ed, CV Mosby, St. Louis MO, 1986.

Lajeunie E, et al. "Genetic study of scaphocephaly," AM J MED GENET, 62(3);282-285, Mar, 1996.

Low D. "Haemangiomas and vascular malformations," SEM PEDIATR SURG, 3(2);40-81, May, 1994.

Marden PM, et al. "Congenital anomalies in the newborn infant, including minor variations." J PEDIATR, 64;357-371, Mar, 1964.

Marieb C. HUMAN ANATOMY AND PHYSIOLOGY, 4th ed., Benjamin/Cummings, Menlo Park CA, 1998.

Mead-Johnson Co. VARIATIONS AND MINOR DEPARTURES IN INFANTS. Mead-Johnson & Co, Evansville IN, 1978.

Medcyclopaedia. "Epispadia," www.amershamhealth.com/medcyclopaedia/Volume%201V%202/EPISPADIA.asp, accessed Feb 2004.

Milner R, Herber S. COLOR ATLAS OF THE NEWBORN. Medical Economics, Oradell NJ, 1984.

O'Doherty N. ATLAS OF THE NEWBORN, 2nd ed. MTP Press, Boston MA, 1985.

Oh W, et al. "The circulatory and respiratory adaptation to early and late cord clamping in newborn infants," ACTA PAEDIATR SCAND, 55(1);17-25, Jan, 1966.

Pape K, Wigglesworth J. "Haemorrhage, ischaemia and the perinatal brain," CLIN DEV MED, (69/70), JB Lippincott, Philadelphia, PA 1979.

Preus M, Fraser F. "Dermatoglyphics and syndromes," AMER J DIS CHILD 124(6); 933-943, Dec 1972.

Reisner S, et al. "Determination of anterior displacement of the anus in newborn infants and children," PEDIATR, 73(2);216-217, Feb, 1984.

Rudolph A. ATLAS OF THE NEWBORN VOLS. 1-5. BC Decker, Inc, Hamilton, Ont, Canada, 1997.

Scammon R. Chapter 3: "A summary of the anatomy of the infant and child," in Abt I, ed. PEDIATRICS, VOL. 1. WB Saunders Co, Philadelphia PA, 1923.

Schlinger H, CPM, CNM. Editing notes, 2003.

Schmidt H, Nitowsky H. "Palmar crease variants and their clinical significance: a study of newborns at risk," PEDIATR RES, 11(2);103-108, 1977.

Schwarze D, Denton J. "Normal values of neonatal lower limbs: an evaluation of 1,000 neonates," J PEDIATR ORTHOPAEDICS, 13(6);758-760, Nov-Dec, 1993.

Seidel H, et al., eds. PRIMARY CARE OF THE NEWBORN, 3rd ed. Mosby, St. Louis MO, 2001.

Shiono H, Kadowaski J, "Dermatoglyphics of congenital abnormalities without chromosomal aberrations: a review of the clinical applications," CLIN PEDIATR, 14(11);1003-1013, Nov 1975.

Simpson K, Creehan P. PERINATAL NURSING, 2nd ed. Lippincott Williams & Wilkins, Philadelphia PA, 2001.

Simpson P. "Craniosynostosis," p. 327, in Hoffman H, Epstein F, eds. DISORDERS OF THE DEVELOPING NERVOUS SYSTEM: DIAGNOSIS AND TREATMENT, VOL. I. Blackwell Science, Oxford UK, 1986.

Smith J. "Hypospadias and epispadias," www.chclibrary.org, Thomson Corp, accessed Feb 10, 2004.

Staheli L. "Torsional deformity," PEDIAT CLIN NO AM, 33(6);1373-1383, Dec, 1986.

Swick H, et al. "Transillumination of the skull in premature infants," PEDIATR, 58(5);656-664, Nov, 1976.

Tachdjian M. CLINICAL PEDIATRIC ORTHOPEDICS. Appleton & Lange, Stamford CT, 1997.

Tappero E, Honeyfield ME. PHYSICAL ASSESSMENT OF THE NEWBORN: A COMPREHENSIVE APPROACH TO THE ART OF PHYSICAL EXAMINATION." NICU Ink, Petaluma CA, 2003.

Thompson JM, et al., eds. MOSBY'S MANUAL OF CLINICAL NURSING, 2nd ed. Mosby-Year Book, St. Louis MO, 1989.

Turner T, et al. CRAIG'S CARE OF THE NEWLY BORN INFANT, 8th ed. Churchill Livingstone, Edinburgh UK, 1988.

Vyhmeister H, et al. "Cranial transillumination norms of the premature infant," J PEDIATR, 91(6);980-982, Dec, 1977.

Wasch M, Marck A. "The radiographic appearance of the gastrointestinal tract during the first day of life," J PEDIATR, 32;479, 1948.

Waugh K, et al. "Measurement of selected hip, knee, and ankle joint motions in newborns," PHYSICAL THERAPY, 63(10);1616-1621, Oct, 1983.

Wilkins K. "Bowlegs," PEDIAT CLIN NO AM, 33(6);1429-1438, Dec, 1986.

REFERENCES USED IN MULTIPLE CHAPTERS ADDRESSING NEONATAL REFLEXES AND OTHER NEUROMOTOR RESPONSES

Capute A. "Early neuromotor reflexes in infancy," PEDIATR ANNALS, 15(3);217-218, 221-223, 226, Mar, 1986.

Goldbloom R, ed. PEDIATRIC CLINICAL SKILLS. Churchill Livingstone, New York NY, 1992.

Lesny I. "A more sensitive way of eliciting the Moro response by pinching the epigastrium," DEV MED CHILD NEUROL, 9(2); 212-215, Apr, 1967.

Simpson K, Creehan P. PERINATAL NURSING, 2nd ed. Lippincott Williams & Wilkins, Philadelphia PA, 2001.

Upledger J. A BRAIN IS BORN: EXPLORING THE BIRTH AND DEVELOPMENT OF THE CENTRAL NERVOUS SYSTEM. North Atlantic Books, Berkeley CA, 1996.

Walter RS. "Issues surrounding the development of feeding and swallowing," in Tuchman DN, Walter RS, eds. DISORDERS OF FEEDING AND SWALLOWING IN INFANTS AND CHILDREN. Singular Pub Group, San Diego CA, 1994.

Care of the Mother and Baby during the Hours Following the Birth of the Placenta

The Postpartum Watch: An Overview

The midwife's job is not done once the baby and placenta are born and the mother is stable. It is important to remain for a few hours afterward to make sure that things are going smoothly before you take your leave.

How Long Should You Stay after the Birth?

This will vary from case to case. It will primarily depend upon the condition of the mother and baby, and any manifest problems that need watching as well as any potential problems that are likely to arise for this birthing pair. In most situations, you will want to stay a minimum of three or four hours. However, in some cases you may wish to stay longer, while in still others you may be able to leave at the two-hour mark. Take into account:

Maternal considerations:

- Length of labor and degree of maternal exhaustion (if relevant)
- Need for perineal repair
- Need for postpartum transport (perhaps you have returned home after birth in the hospital)
- Overall blood loss before, during and immediately after the birth of the placenta
- Postpartum blood loss since the placenta was born
- Evidence of possible problems, such as a hematoma
- Ability to urinate spontaneously
- Vital signs
- Mother's assessment of her own condition and well-being
- Ability to ambulate confidently without feeling faint
- Number of support people on hand or available to help her

Newborn considerations:

- APGAR scores and condition immediately following birth
- Overall condition and responsiveness of baby, including vital signs
- The need for resuscitation
- Your findings during the baby examination (was a complete physical exam deemed necessary?)
- Trauma or suspected injury incurred during the birth process
- Suspected or obvious birth anomalies
- Gestational age
- Growth and size assessment
- Response to nursing

You should stay until any questions about the condition of the mother or baby are resolved or until you are confident that the parents understand what to look for and will call you if the issues in question do not resolve. This may entail having at least one midwife or an apprentice with enough experience to monitor the situation stay the night. Do not leave an unprepared apprentice to monitor a questionable situation; it defeats the purpose and may endanger the mother or baby. Alternatively, if the circumstances are potentially serious, you should accompany the parents for a postpartum transport.

You or your midwifery associates may attend to cleaning up, but your clinical evaluation of both mother and baby and assisting the mother in getting started with caring for the baby should be your first priority. When more than one midwife is present, your roles may have been decided prior to birth; each midwife can continue to monitor the mother or baby as she has been during the labor; or you can alternate checks. If all of you are very tired, once the mother and baby are stable and basic cleanup is complete, one of you can monitor both mother and baby while the others rest. It is best not to send everyone home shortly after birth, as there is a lot to be done. This is especially true if all of you are tired; the burden may unfairly fall on only one of you to safeguard the mother and baby.

Immediate Tasks

Being there for the family

First and foremost, honor the rhythm of the family you are attending by respecting their pace with integrating the immediate experience of the birth. This is especially important for the mother-baby pair as they come down from their birth-hormone high. Your need to examine the mother and baby and clean things up should never take precedence, unless you truly feel you need to investigate something immediately for the sake of their safety and well-being.

Finishing up your record-keeping

Review the chart once the birth is essentially over; make sure each entry is dated, timed and initialed; complete the statistics form; and finish recording any events that require an unusual amount of description. It is always best to complete the chart before leaving the house, when the events are freshest in your mind. Be sure your partners have reviewed the chart and completed their notes before they leave as well. The statistics form can be completed by an apprentice with your help; this is a good way to review the birth.

Cleaning up and packing

Clean and straighten up after the birth. Tasks that can be assigned to visiting friends and relatives include such things as returning furniture to its original location (unless this involves movement of furniture in and out of the mother and baby's room), cleaning the kitchen, preparing food to feed to the new family, changing the labor bed, doing laundry and caring for older siblings.

Meanwhile, the midwives can assist with the herbal bath, clean and possibly even sterilize equipment, and reorganize birth and prenatal bags. Make a list of items you used that need to be replenished. Leave accessible those items that may still be needed, such as antihemorrhagic agents, resuscitation equipment and oxygen, bulb syringes and mucus-trap suction devices.

Record-keeping during the postpartum watch

The next page shows a sample form for monitoring the condition of the mother and baby after birth. This should be filled out for as long as regular checks are performed after birth and filed in the chart. Be sure that each attendant initials her notes in the comments section at the end of the form.

Below is a form to record your findings during the placental exam:

PLACENTAL EXAMINATION: Examined by____________________________ at ____ m.

Separation gush at ___ .m. Placenta delivered at ___ .m., ________min.: Schultz Duncan

CORD: Length_ ___in. No. of vessels___ Knots__________ Size___________ Point of attachment___________________

PLACENTA: Weight_____Lbs._____oz Type:______________Staining_________ (Illustrate unusual features below)

Infarcts________________________

Calcifications__________________

Cotyledons____________________

General condition:

healthy postdue friable

poor fair good excellent

Unusual findings/abnormalities:____

MEMBRANES: Chorion intact____ Amnion intact____ Comments______________________________________

AMNIOTIC FLUID: Color: clear stained (lt/med/dark) Amount: normal large scant none Odor: normal foul

Comments:____

____

IMMEDIATE POSTPARTUM RECORD

Date ______________ Monitoring by ______________________ Initial blood loss: _____ measured. Care ended at ______ .m. on ________

	MOTHER ________________						BABY ____________					
Time	Clean pad	Fundus	Lochia	Vitals	Food Drink	Void	Color	Cord	Vitals	Alertness	Nursing	Comments/initials

Caring for the Mother in the First Hours after Birth

Maternal condition after birth

Reassess the mother's overall condition after the placenta is out and before she gets up for the first time to take an herbal bath or go to the toilet. Blood pressure and pulse should be assessed and respirations observed as indicated. These evaluations are especially important if the mother is exhausted, bleeding has been excessive or any vital signs have been abnormal during labor. Respirations should be counted if they appear abnormal. The acute onset of abnormal respiration should alert you to the possibility, albeit very rare, of amniotic fluid embolism. If the mother is at increased risk for infection, her temperature should be checked after at least 45 minutes have passed after the birth. If it is not within normal limits, infection should be suspected. It is especially important to check her temperature if the membranes were ruptured for some time prior to birth or if the risk of infection is elevated for some other reason (such as manual entry into the uterus). Any variations in vital signs should alert you to the possibility of an underlying problem, such as hemorrhage, that may be concealed.

You probably don't need to check the blood pressure during the first hours following birth if everything has been fine, bleeding is well under control and all is well. However, if there is excessive bleeding, if the woman feels lightheaded or "funny," if the placenta took a while to deliver or if you are otherwise concerned, then, by all means, check the blood pressure and pulse as often as indicated.

Preliminary clean up

Be sure to remove all bloody underpads from the bed. This will help you monitor postpartum bleeding and assess how much blood the mother has lost so far. Arrange the bed so that the mother is comfortable. Use a washcloth and plain warm water to clean the mother's legs, genitals and perineal area (soap will only need to be rinsed off and is usually unnecessary). Use a clean cloth for the anal area and clean up any fecal matter; take care to do those last. If fecal matter has soiled the perineum, mild soap and water can be used to cleanse the area, but it will have to be rinsed throughly. Alternatively, wipe off any debris and lavage the perineum with an antiseptic solution.

Examining the mother for birth-related tissue damage

Arrange the mother for perineal examination: The woman will need to be positioned so that you can check for tears. Move her bottom to the edge of the bed and prop her feet on chairs to either side, then sit between her legs. She may or may not wish to hold the baby during the examination.

Check for tears: Check the mother for any damage to her yoni, cervix, perineum, anal sphincter, labia, periurethral region and surrounding tissues. If damage is found, assess the need for repair and whether you are qualified to perform the repair. If not, the mother should be transported, with the goal of having the repair completed within six hours of the birth. (See my text HEALING PASSAGE for complete details regarding examination for damage following birth.)

If repair is needed: If you can perform the repair, it should be done soon after the birth. If it is not, swelling will increase. The repair will also be more painful because the natural "anesthetic" from the pressure of birth will have worn off. (See the text HEALING PASSAGE for complete details regarding repair of the perineum.) The mother can decide if she wants to hold the baby during the repair. Some women find it a welcome distraction while others prefer that their partner hold the baby. A support person should be face to face with the mother during the repair.

If repair is not necessary or when it is complete: Arrange the mother so that she is comfortable. Place an absorbant pad under her bottom, place a maternity sanitary pad against her vulva and give her the baby. Allow the mother and her partner quiet time together, but do not leave them completely alone. At least one midwife should remain in the room to discreetly observe the mother and perform periodic checks to assess whether the uterus is remaining contracted.

Checking the uterus and evaluating postpartum blood loss

Begin postpartum uterine checks: The uterus should be checked periodically to make sure it is contracted. Once the placenta has been born, the fundus should be firm and about the size of a grapefruit, positioned above the pubic bone, but below the navel. If it is not, cup your palm over and around the fundus and gently rock the uterus until a contraction begins.

The fundus can also be pressed downward to expel any clots or bleeding that may have collected in the os since the last check. While vigorous massage and brute force should be avoided, enough pressure and firmness should be used to release any retained clots or blood. Too much massage of the uterus can exhaust the myometrium, break up clots that are trying to form over the placental site, and may lead to more bleeding; however, if bleeding is occurring, clots must be expelled. Not to do so is to invite ballooning of the uterus, which prevents it from closing down and results in more bleeding.

Little or no blood loss will be noted if clots are plugging up the cervix, but the woman may feel queasy and just "not right." When checking, always note the size of the uterus as well as what comes out. Enlargement or rising of the fundus between checks points to concealed blood loss. In addition, note whether pressing on the uterus is painful for the mother. Ironically, the mother who most fervently tries to stop you from pressing on her uterus is invariably the one who most needs clots expelled (Schlinger, 2003).

At the same time that the fundus is pressed, look at the sanitary pad or underpad to check for the discharge of lochia by observing the introitus to see how much, if any, blood is expelled. This is a dark red discharge of liquid blood, clots, decidual debris and sometimes minute fragments of membrane and placental tissue. Any discharge that appears to contain tissue should be further examined by placing it in a clear glass of tepid water. Blood clots may have strings of fibrin in them, which causes them to appear to be tissue fragments, but any fragment that can be dissolved completely by gently working it with your fingers is a blood clot. Any tissue or membrane fragment remaining should be compared to any suspicious ragged areas found on the placenta during its exam.

Assessing postpartum blood loss: While this assessment is of vital importance to maternal well-being, the literature is virtually silent on it, save for a very few articles that have appeared in nursing journals. Jacobson (1985) is the only author who has attempted to develop a standard to assess postpartum fluid blood loss (see the illustrations on the next page).

Normally, the discharge that occurs after the initial postplacental separation bleeding has ceased is a progressively diminishing flow. Normal blood loss during the next two to three hours postpartum consists of a dark, sporadic flow that should not exceed that of a heavy menstrual period and is often much lighter. The blood should be medium to dark red transitioning to dark pink. It should feel thick and substantial, similar to mucus. Constant or bright-red or more fluid bleeding calls for ruling out missed perineal or cervical damage and could be from the placental site as well. Bright orange-red blood is probably from a torn artery, which may or may not spurt when disrupted during an exam. A constant, watery reddish to dark pink trickle suggests bleeding from behind clots lodged in the cervix. It could also be caused by a depletion of clotting factors, which is usually only seen when intrapartal or postpartal bleeding has been prolonged and severe; in this case any open site will ooze blood.

Small clots may be expelled with fundal checks. After the first hour, normal blood loss may contain clots that would fit in a rounded tablespoon and may be as large as a lemon; often they are smaller. Numerous tablespoon-sized clots with each check are cause for concern; one such clot and one or two smaller ones are more normal. Herbal tinctures such as white oak bark can be given to help normalize this type of bleeding. When a woman changes position or arises, it is common for any lochia pooled in the yoni to be discharged all at once, but this usually consists of only a tablespoon or two of blood and should not continue as a constant flow. Discharge of pooled blood is especially likely to occur if a woman has had little or no visible blood loss for the 30 to 45 minutes prior to arising.

Generally speaking, it is considered excessive for the woman to soak more than one maternity-sized sanitary pad every 15 minutes during the first hour after birth. (This is a medical standard and, is in fact, an outside limit of normal.) A more common finding is soaking 1.5 pads during the first hour, with a maximum of three pads used in the first two hours. A "soaked" pad contains about 100 ml (3.33 oz) of blood and is fully saturated in the center of the pad, which was directly covering the introitus. Record each change of pad, the characteristics of the blood loss and any clots that are passed.

The amount of blood loss the mother experiences after the birth should be judged in relationship to the amount she lost before, during and after the birth of the placenta. If she lost very little at that time, the chances of her having heavy lochial bleeding after the birth are much less. However, she can probably tolerate somewhat heavier bleeding by virtue of the minimal loss she had with the placenta. Regardless of how little was lost during the birth of the placenta, the norm is for the lochial flow to progressively diminish; therefore, investigate the source of any heavy or increased bleeding. Conversely, a woman whose blood loss was heavy after birth can ill afford to lose much more during the hours postpartum. If such a woman has heavy lochial bleeding, herbal tinctures should be freely given by diluting dropperfuls of tincture in a little hot water or ginger tea and having her take them at 15 to 30 minute intervals. She should hold the solution in her mouth for quick absorption.

Be sure to look at the underpad below the mother to determine if additional blood loss has pooled beneath her between checks. If the underpad is wet with blood, change it. Have the mother roll to her side enough for you to remove the pad from behind. Take this opportunity to look for additional blood that may have pooled on or beyond the edges of the underpad and check to see if her clothing, if she is wearing any, or the bedding is also bloody. Check her back and thighs to see how far up any pooled blood has extended. If blood loss has been missed or seems excessive, monitor the mother more closely. If necessary, sit beside the woman, keeping one hand on the fundus and an eye on the introitus, to determine whether bleeding is continuing.

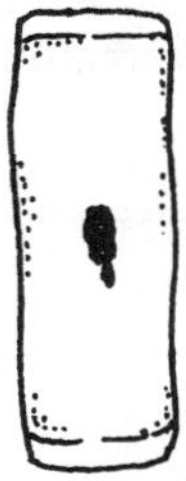	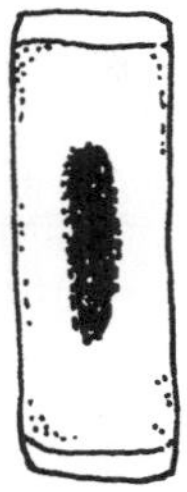	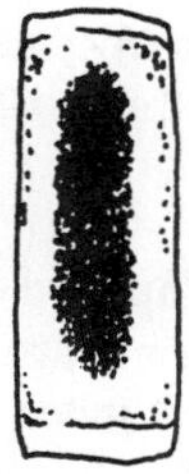	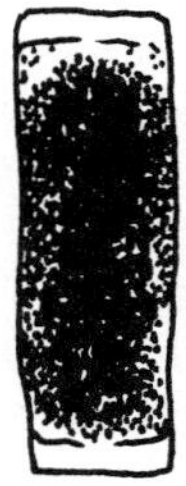
Scant: Less than 1" stain on pad, or staining only with wiping	**Light:** Less than 4" stain on pad	**Moderate:** Less than 6" stain on pad	**Heavy:** Pad fully saturated within one hour

<u>How often should uterine checks take place</u>? Once the placenta has been born, the uterus should be checked *at least* every 15 minutes during the first two hours after birth. Some midwives check the fundus every 5 minutes during the first hour, every 10 minutes during the second hour, every 15 minutes during the third hour and every 30 minutes during the fourth hour. This takes into account the probability that excessive bleeding is most likely to occur in the minutes immediately following birth. The risk is proportionately less as time goes by. A normal lochial flow should be established by the end of the fourth hour, and, as a rule, further frequent checks are no longer needed.

Of course, common sense is called for here. If the mother bled excessively to begin with, more frequent checks are in order to make sure the uterus is not becoming atonic and to minimize further blood loss in an already compromised situation. When excessive or constant bleeding is discovered upon exam, subsequent exams should be spaced more closely until the bleeding is under control. On the other hand, if the mother is stable and has lost very little blood with the birth of the placenta, and her uterus is staying firm with little or no additional loss at each check, it is reasonable to reexamine her less frequently.

<u>Checking the os for clots</u>: A woman who drifts in and out of a state approaching shock should be assumed to be losing blood until this is ruled out. Quickly place a clean placenta pan under her bottom. Don a sterile glove and perform an internal exam. Place your other palm over the fundus abdominally while you reach for the os and feel for clots. The os will be large, soft and floppy. Clots will feel like warm soft masses of gelatin. Use two fingers to gently scoop clots out of the os. Apply fundal pressure. You may be rewarded with a gush of backlogged blood from the uterus. Emptying the full uterus in this fashion will usually result in the mother feeling much better very quickly. Stay with her as you continue to monitor the fundus with one hand and help remove any additional clots with the other. The fundus should be firm and contracted before you quit.

<u>Checking for blood loss due to unrecognized tissue damage</u>: Bleeding from tissue damage usually begins during the birth and continues even though the uterus is well contracted. On rare occasions, you may discover that some sort of damage that is continuing to bleed has been missed. For example, a blood vessel may have clotted over and something (such as getting the mother up) dislodged the clot, causing bleeding to resume. A torn cervix can produce a continuous heavy discharge of blood but often produces sporadic bleeding when the mother stands or walks. Bleeding sites must be repaired or transported for repair. If the mother is to be transported, apply pressure to the site if possible, and take her in as soon as you can. (See the chapter entitled "Postpartum Hemorrhage: An Overview" for more details on the causes of bleeding after birth.)

When to give oxytocics: If the uterus is not clamping down as it should, have an assistant give the mother something to cause the uterus to contract. It is imperative that the action of any herbs given will produce uterine contractions because that is the only thing that will really stop uterine bleeding. Shepherd's purse and white oak bark may be helpful if the bleeding is coming for somewhere other than the uterus (shepherd's purse can also produce large, retained uterine clots, so be judicious in its use). If herbs and other nonallopathic modalities fail to control the bleeding, give oxytocin or Methergine IM. Methergine tablets are another option at this point.

Maternal vital signs

The mother's blood pressure, pulse and respiratory rate all gradually return to prelabor levels during the first hour after birth. Her temperature may continue to remain slightly elevated up to 2°F (1.1°C) over her prelabor normal, but is should never rise above 100.4°F (38°C). Any nausea and vomiting that occurred during labor should have subsided. Thirst followed by hunger is the norm (Varney, 1997).

Monitor the bladder

A full bladder can displace the uterus upward toward the umbilicus. The bladder may be hypotonic after birth because of the pressure and compression it underwent as the baby descended, especially if the woman has labored with a full bladder (it is less likely to occur if the bladder stayed empty during labor). This can lead to urinary retention of which the mother is unaware. In most cases, the sensation of fullness comes back within the first few hours of birth (Varney, 1997). However, in the meantime, a full bladder can cause painful postpartum cramping as the uterus tries to work against the pressure, and the lower segment is stretched. It can also contribute to additional bleeding, as the uterus cannot effectively clamp down when it is displaced. The mother should be assisted to urinate either into a placenta pan, a bed pan, a towel or on the toilet. If she cannot urinate spontaneously, she should be catheterized.

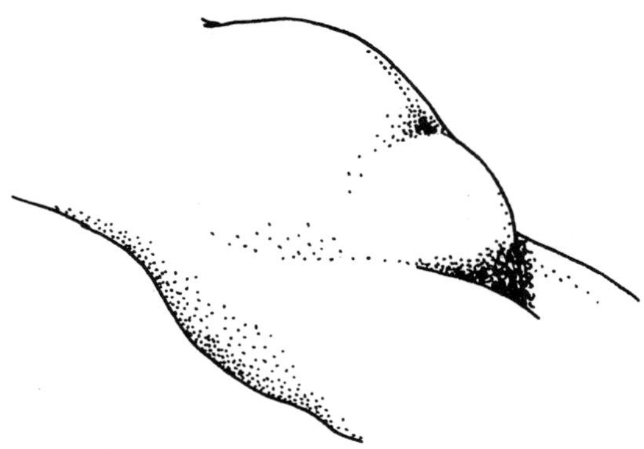

A full bladder displacing the uterus upward

Food and liquids for the mother

The mother may express that she is hungry and should be encouraged to eat whatever she wants within the first two or three hours after birth. Very often, support people are happy to prepare a meal for her. Eating and hydration will revive her if the labor has been long and tiring, will draw blood to her digestive tract (and away from the uterus), raise her blood sugar and will help ground her after the expansive experience of labor. All this paves the way for her to be able to get up for the first time without problems.

Getting the mother up during the first hours postpartum

It is important to have someone stay with the mother *at all times* during the immediate postpartum watch to make sure that she can walk and care for herself without becoming unsteady on her feet or fainting. This is important even if the mother has had a perfectly wonderful birth with minimal blood loss. Women are in an altered state, and coming down from the birth does not happen all at once. In addition, they often do not realize how tired they are until they get up. Some women will respond more severely than others to a moderate blood loss. Also, if a woman is getting up to urinate because her uterus is high and crampy, it is possible that she has retained blood in the uterine cavity; arising can easily result in lightheadedness, fainting or shock.

To get the mother up, first have her sit up in bed for a minute or so. Ask her how she is feeling. If she feels fine, help her to swing her legs gently over to the side of the bed and have her sit on the edge of the bed for a few minutes more. Ask her how she is feeling. Only if she reports that she feels fine, have her put her feet on the floor and slowly rise to standing. A support person, preferably someone big enough to actually catch her should she fall or faint, should be at her elbow. She should then be escorted to the toilet or shower, and the support person should remain near her side the entire time. If she is quite tired or has lost a fair amount of blood, have her get up and then lie back down; then after resting she can arise again to bathe or shower if she still feels up to it.

Do not leave a woman alone, especially not in the bathroom, where collapse will result in falling on a cold, often tiled, floor. If she requests privacy, have someone stand by the cracked door and ask her how she is doing every few minutes. This is particularly important during a shower as the combination of heat, even minimal blood loss and exhaustion can cause a woman to suddenly faint even if she has previously felt fine. Her partner can join her in the shower, to monitor her and catch her if she falls, although the partner frequently wishes to stay with the baby during this time.

If the mother feels faint on arising: Have the mother who feels lightheaded or faint lie back down immediately. Reassess her fundus and her blood loss. Sometimes getting up will result in a flood of blood from the uterus. If this does not occur, there could be unseen blood loss blocked by clots at the os. The mother who moves from bed and is seemingly fine and then feels faint or actually passes out can be gently eased down onto the floor. There you can examine her vital signs, check her for bleeding, hold a bottle of smelling salts under her nose and help revive her. A whiff or two of oxygen by mask is likely to help bring her around as well. If the mother has felt faint and her only goal was the toilet, have her return to bed and urinate in a bedpan or a towel while she regains her equilibrium in a horizontal position.

Comfort measures

Heat and the postpartum period: According to Chinese medicine, birth causes a rapid reduction of internal heat in the mother's system. Women are usually warm during pregnancy as a result of increased metabolism (i.e., internal heat). After birth, women frequently shake as if they have chills. The Chinese explain that this is due to the *ming men* (life gate fire) being opened by the birth.

The Chinese consider the *ming men* to be the basis of all strength. This energy center is located between the kidneys; it extends down the lower back and the abdomen, and from two finger-breadths below the navel to the pubic bone. The kidney energy governs sexuality, reproduction, growth and decline. The gate of life opens to allow passage of the baby and, with proper postpartum care, closes again, contributing to stronger lower back and kidney Qi.

Postpartum shivering is symptomatic of the internal heat loss that has taken place. The Chinese feel that applying cold encourages this internal cold and may create long-term complications such as weakening the back or kidneys. Therefore, ice should be used only in the most extreme cases of swelling or hematoma formation. Otherwise, heat-producing fluids (such as ginger tea), warm packs applied to the perineum and ensuring that both mother and baby are warm will help to balance out the rapid heat loss that follows birth (Lang, 1985).

Warm packs and dry heat: Warm (tepid) herbal packs on the perineum help stimulate circulation. This will carry away local anesthetics and edema, as well as promote oxygenation of the area and enhance healing. Hot packs should not be used at this time. Some women enjoy drying their stitches with a hair dryer or exposing them to a high-wattage light bulb for a few minutes after their bath. (Infrared heat lamps should be used with great care. A sunburned perineum will not feel better!)

Ice packs: The perineal area can benefit from the application of ice when swelling is extreme. Ice packs can be made by liberally dribbling comfrey leaf infusion on maternity napkins that have been cut in half. Freeze several for use after birth. (Soaking rather than dribbling creates large ice chunks, which will be unpleasant for most women). A quick ice pack can be made by filling a sterile glove with crushed ice and tying off the end. Ice should not be applied for longer than 24 hours except in the event of an enlarging hematoma.

Hot ginger tea (1 tsp powdered or fresh grated ginger to a cup of water) and warm blankets can be used to help offset the chilling effect of the ice. Homeopathic arnica taken orally can be used instead of, or in addition to, ice. It does not expose the mother to the internal chilling that ice promotes.

Arrange for lab work to be performed

If the mother is Rh_0D negative, you will need to make sure her and her baby's blood samples get to the lab in a timely fashion. Make sure all tubes and forms are filled out accurately and completely to avoid having to get another specimen.

Afterbirth Pains

The uterus continues to rhythmically contract after every birth as it closes down the site of placental attachment. This prevents bleeding, helps to regenerate the placental site as it returns to its nonpregnant state and restores the tone and size of the uterine muscle. Afterbirth cramps tend to become more severe in all women when they breastfeed. These contractions are often most painful in women who have had previous babies, usually becoming more severe with each subsequent birth. In fact, some multiparous women dread these afterbirth pains and feel they are the worst part of having a baby. Some women have severe pains that begin in the immediate postpartum period and may last anywhere from 24 to 48 hours.

Increasing parity tends to be associated with stronger afterbirth pains because each pregnancy results in additional stretching of the uterus and a slight corresponding decrease in uterine muscle tone. During the postpartum period, this leads to an exaggerated relaxation phase, which causes the uterus to tighten up more firmly with each postpartal contraction. In contrast, the firm, well-toned uterus of the first-time mother tends to remain more or less contracted without much intermittent relaxation. Oxytocin is released during nursing, causing the uterus to contract even more, regardless of parity. Because of the overstretching involved, contractions are also more noticeable after a pregnancy that involved polyhydramnios or extreme enlargement from a multiple gestation.

Normal afterbirth pains are relieved or at least made much more tolerable if the uterus can remain well contracted at all times; that way, it doesn't have to work so hard to achieve a state of contraction. An important contributory element in this is keeping the bladder empty. A full bladder displaces the uterus upward. This stretches the cervical canal and results in inefficient uterine contractions with more relaxation between. Sometimes afterbirth pains are completely relieved when the woman urinates, especially if she has had only one or two babies.

If emptying the bladder does not provide relief, the woman can apply hot compresses to her lower abdomen, either in the form of a hot water bottle or a heating pad. This is soothing to many women. A heating pad should not be left in place if the woman falls asleep. Varney (1997) recommends that the woman lie face down, either flat or with a pillow under her lower abdomen. The counterpressure upon the uterus provides constant stimulation and will eliminate afterpains after about 5 minutes, during which time the cramps may be severe. Breastfeeding will require the woman to assume another position, so applying a weight (such as a hot water bottle) above her pubic bone may provide some measure of counterpressure but is probably not as efficient as lying prone.

CARE OF THE BABY AFTER THE BIRTH

The following things should be periodically assessed during the hours postpartum.

Nursing

The initiation of successful latch-on and sucking is a top priority during the initial postpartum period. Ideally, a normal, healthy baby will latch on during the first two hours of life before falling into a deep, postbirth sleep this early nursing greatly assists with nursing continuing to go smoothly in the days after birth. Provide the mother with appropriate information and hands-on assistance if difficulty is noted. The baby who refuses to latch on and nurse in a certain position, or favors one breast over the other, may have pain related to unresolved cranial moulding or birth position. Assist the mother to accommodate the baby for now and suggest that the baby be seen by a craniosacral practitioner as soon as is practical. Hopefully, a practitioner in your area will make house calls for newborn patients. The mother can also assist with the resolution of moulding by using the energy technique described in Volume III of this text. In the meantime, suggest a nursing position that provides the maximum maternal control over breast positioning.

Vital signs (temperature, pulse and respirations)

The baby's temperature should be assessed by noting skin temperature with the back of your hand, as well as observing skin color. If the baby seems cold, wrap him in one additional blanket, put a stocking cap on his head, booties on his feet and warm the room. Sometimes taking the temperature is appropriate; obtain an axillary temperature and record the results. Retake the temperature once any chilling or overheating has been corrected. Show the parents how to assess the temperature and help them read the thermometer if they are unfamiliar with the procedure.

The baby's heart rate should be checked periodically, especially if it was unusually fast or slow after the birth. The baby can remain in the mother's arms while this is done. Be sure to auscultate the heart rate over the bare chest. Respirations should also be assessed periodically for rate, effort and grunting. Reappearance of any sign of respiratory distress that has previously disappeared should be considered an indication of a potentially serious problem. Seek pediatric consultation or consider transport. See the subchapter entitled "Evaluating the Apparently Normal Baby Who Develops Respiratory Distress" for more information.

State of consciousness

The baby should remain awake and aware for approximately two hours or so after birth (give or take 30 min). Reassess the respirations, muscle tone and responsiveness of any baby who appears to be going to sleep sooner than this after birth. During this initial period of wakefulness, the baby should nurse well at both breasts for several minutes at least and then drift off into a very deep postbirth sleep of several hours. After this, the baby should wake again and nurse every two to three hours for the next few weeks, day and night.

Skin color

Watch the baby's color throughout the postpartum stay. Be especially alert to color changes for the worse, which are associated with exertion and may indicate a heart or respiratory problem.

Elimination

Urination: Ninety-four percent of all babies whose urinary tract is functioning normally will void within 24 hours, many in the process of birth or soon thereafter, in which case urination is often easy to observe. Urine should flow in a stream; this will be easy to see in boys. Urine that only trickles out, especially in large quantities, may be cause for concern regarding a defective urethra. After the baby has voided initially, the next urinations will usually be light and odorless and therefore easy to miss. This is even more true if highly absorbent disposable diapers are used. Therefore, the use of cloth diapers is especially important during the initial postpartum hours or until you (or the parents in your absence) are satisfied that the baby has voided. Passage of clear or very pale urine shortly after birth and continuing at frequent intervals is the norm in babies who have received their full cord transfusion. (See Volume III for ways to facilitate elimination if none has occurred by the first-day visit postpartum.)

Meconium: Ninety-nine percent of all infants whose gastrointestinal tract is functioning normally have passed meconium by 48 hours; any further delay suggests functional or organic bowel obstruction. Passage of meconium per rectum prior to birth counts; be sure, however, that the baby has not vomited meconium due to a gastrointestinal obstruction.

Normal meconium passage begins with the release of a small amount of colorless or whitish mucus from the lower rectum, although this mucus is easy to miss. Occasionally, the mucus becomes dehydrated enough to be firm and formed, in which case it is called a “meconium plug.” After passing mucus or this plug, the baby’s anus pushes outward slightly, opens, and a large flow of soft, thick, semiformed stool is expelled. It usually has a uniform consistency similar to that of artist’s paint as it is squeezed from a tube; that is, it comes out in a soft column and puddles into a blob. Its normal consistency can vary, however, and may be slightly less formed. Its color ranges from deep, dark green-black (the most common) to mustard-brown. Normal meconium is odorless because it is sterile. Any odor may indicate an infection.

If you are concerned about drug use in the mother, collect a sample of the first meconium for drug screening. You should discuss your concerns with the parents and reiterate the negative repercussions for both mother and baby and the possibility of the baby having to suffer withdrawal symptoms.

Meconium is very sticky and stains everything it touches. Oil the baby’s bottom, genitals and upper thighs generously with olive oil after each diaper change to keep meconium from sticking to the skin. The mother can use old cotton diapers, which can be thrown out rather than washed, or a “natural” version of a disposable diaper until the stools have transitioned to those of a normal breastfed baby.

Heading off jaundice: The bile from retained meconium can be reabsorbed through the intestinal walls, increasing the likelihood that the baby will jaundice if meconium passage is delayed. Because of this, some midwives use gentle means to encourage the passage of meconium soon after birth, such as massaging the baby’s abdomen with olive oil in a circular pattern, moving up the right side of the belly, across under the rib cage and down the left side of the belly several times. The baby’s thighs are then gently flexed up on her belly; this will often prompt baby to expel meconium. Taking rectal temperature is another activity that may prompt the passage of meconium.

Cord care

If the cord has been cut, each time you check the baby for any other reason, examine the cord stump to make sure it is not oozing blood. Oozing is very uncommon for a cord that has been allowed to completely cease pulsing at the base of the umbilicus prior to being cut, although a tiny bit of blood can sometimes leak out, especially after a warm herbal bath. This is usually residual blood from a tiny semicoagulated clot in a cord vessel and is not a cause for concern. However, immediately clamp any cord that begins to bleed. Frank seepage of blood suggests a coagulation disorder. If the cord is left uncut, abnormal bleeding would be observed as blood begins to fill the umbilical vein.

Newborn prophylactic medications and screening tests

In the medical model of care, the newborn is routinely given the following medications during after birth:

- Eye prophylaxis to prevent ophthalmic gonorrhea or chlamydia infection. This is usually administered in the form of a petroleum-based ophthalmologic ointment containing an antibiotic such as erythromycin.
- Vitamin K administration to prevent hemorrhagic disease of the newborn. The dose can be given orally or by intramuscular injection in a neonatal concentration.
- Hepatitis B vaccine for babies exposed to hepatitis B via maternal blood contamination during the birth process.

When parents choose one or more of these, midwives usually postpone administration until the second or third hour of life to allow the baby a chance to orient herself to the world. (The exception is a known maternal infection that may lead to an eye infection in the newborn; in this case, ocular prophylaxis will be most effective if used shortly after birth.) Record the time it was given and the type of medication used. The ease with which parents can decline one or more of these treatments varies from region to region. In most places, parents can sign informed consent agreements to waive treatment, regardless of health department requirements. Refusal should be based upon a careful consideration of the pros and cons of both accepting or rejecting treatment, as well as the overall circumstances. These factors should have been reviewed prenatally and can be reviewed again after the birth. The waiver can be given to the parents to read prior to birth but should not be signed until the birth is over and the condition of the baby is known. Once signed, the waiver should be placed in the chart. (For a full, up-to-date discussion of the indications, theories, risks, benefits, and administration of neonatal prophylactic medications see the most recent edition of my DIAGNOSTIC TESTS.)

Newborn screening for a variety of metabolic disorders is available throughout the United States. Some tests can pick up problems at the time of birth by testing cord blood. These include hypothyroidism, biotinidase deficiency and galactosemia. It is therefore recommended that the first sample be obtained within the first 48 hours and the second between 5 and 14 days after birth. These tests are discussed in my DIAGNOSTIC TESTS and also in Volume III of this text.

THE HERBAL BATH

The mother and baby can get into an herbal bath together once they are both stable. The bath helps to soothe, heal and cleanse the yoni area, as well as to dry and heal the baby's cord. Soap should not be used while the baby is in the tub. The water can be drained and someone can hold the baby while the mother takes a shower with soap once she has finished with the herbal bath.

Prepare the tub by scrubbing it with an abrasive cleanser. Rinse thoroughly; check for dirt and grit; wipe, rinse or clean again. Spray generously with an antibacterial agent such as Seventh Generation Kitchen Cleaner wipe, and then rinse once more. Fill with temperate water (no more than 92 to 94° F [33.5 to 34.7° C]).

Yourbirthherbs.com formulates prepackaged herbal baths that are easy to have your parents order prenatally. Alternatively, a bath may also be made using garlic, sea salt and one or more of the following dry herbs:

•Comfrey leaf (*Symphytum officinale*)–promotes cell growth and healing
•Rosemary leaf (*Rosmarinus officinalis*)–antiseptic and reduces swelling (found in most kitchens)
•Uva ursi leaf (*Arctostaphylos uva-ursi*)–heals the urinary tract
•Shepherd's purse (*Capsella bursapastoris*)–promotes clotting

The dry herbs (or any combination of healing herbs you concoct) should be steeped (not boiled or simmered) from the onset of labor until the mother and baby are ready for their bath. Boil a large pot of water; remove the boiling water from the heat and then add a half ounce of each herb. Let it sit for the duration of labor. This makes a medicinal strength infusion for use after birth. Now take a whole bulb of fresh garlic *(Allium sativum*, used for its antiseptic properties) and peel it enough to remove the outer "paper" membranes (no need to peel every single clove). Whiz in a blender or food processor with enough water to process. This antiseptic mash can now be added or placed in the colander before the infusion is strained.

When bath time is near, fill the tub, then strain the herbal infusion through a colander lined with an old T-shirt, diaper or a couple of layers of cheesecloth. Do not make the mistake of dumping the herbs directly into the tub, as this will clog the plumbing. Add ½ cup of sea salt directly to the water, then strain the herbal infusion directly into the tub. Tie the remaining herbs up in the cloth to make a big tea bag and throw it into the tub as well.

You might want to check to be sure all is going well with preparations. One mother found herself soaking in collard green liquor (the father had inadvertently dumped the infusion). Another father carefully disposed of the infusion and saved the herbs. An occasional friend or relative, overwhelmed with the birth experience, has attempted to steep prepackaged herbs without first removing them from the plastic bag. Be sure postpartum helpers know how to prepare the bath.

USES FOR THE PLACENTA

The word "placenta" comes from the Latin word for "cake" via an obsolete English term, "placent," which also means "a flat, round cake." This word is also common to French, Spanish and Italian. German has two words for placenta, *mutterkuchen* (literally, "mother cake") and *fruchtkuchen* ("fruit cake"). Western birthday celebrations include cakes; traditionally, this was a rich fruit cake with nuts and dried fruits. Candles were incorporated to represent the years of life. Could the cake and candles be symbolic of the placenta and cord at birth?

The placenta contains female hormones as well as concentrated nutrients, making it an ideal medicinal and nourishing substance for those women who can get past cultural taboos to the contrary. Throughout history, human cultures in many parts of the world have used the placenta and cord for various purposes, most of them medicinal (Ober, 1979).

Antihemorrhagic properties

Midwives sometimes use one or two tablespoons of raw cotyledon tissue to slow or stop bleeding. After a quick examination, tissue from the parenchyma can be removed and given to the mother to chew. She should then hold it between her cheek and gum, allowing direct absorption of the hormones through the mucous membranes. Other midwives put the tissue in a blender with tomato juice first. The benefit of this practice is explained to the mother prior to labor; some women will feel quite amenable to consuming some or all of the placenta for this purpose. While this practice does disrupt the placenta for those planning Lotus birth, at least the placenta is being incorporated back into the mother-baby duo. Be sure to explain to the Lotus-birth baby what you are doing and why.

Placental keepsakes

You can create a keepsake by separating the entire cord from the placenta after the exam (or even after the cord falls away naturally in a Lotus birth). If the cord is fresh, rinse it and then arrange it in a spiral shape on a dinner plate to dry, or place it in a very slow oven or a dehydrator. (If the cord is dry, rehydrate it in water, then proceed as above.) If the cord had a true knot, preserve the cord with the knot intact. The parents may also wish to preserve the membranes, especially if the baby was born in the caul. To do so, rinse them throughly and spread them out to dry. Sometimes a Native American dream catcher is made with the membranes. The parenchyma can be used to fertilize a special tree planted in the baby's honor.

Placental prints: Art prints can be made with the fetal side of the placenta and cord either by the midwives or family after the birth or the following day. This would be a great project for older siblings. You will need white watercolor paper no smaller than 11 × 14 in on a tablet that is not spiral bound. Colored or patterned papers tend to obscure detail and are therefore less desirable. Stamp pads in a variety of colors can be used to apply ink to the placenta. Darker colors tend to work better than light, picking up more detail. Paint is another possibility. Watercolors or tempera paints may work. If the placenta is to be consumed, be sure the paints are nontoxic and washed off immediately after the printing is done. Set up on a large table or the floor by spreading newspapers down to minimize the mess. To prepare the paper, either leave it in the pad or tear off a piece and attach it with masking tape to a thick piece of cardboard (check at the art supply store for possibilities).

If a print from the maternal side is desired, place the placenta parenchyma up (no ink necessary). A tree of life print can be made from the fetal side of the placenta by washing it off, blotting it dry with paper towels and then blotting all over the surface of the placenta and cord with the ink pad or pads. Now, either bring the placenta to the paper (kind of tricky, but you get better cord prints) or the paper to the placenta. To bring the placenta to the paper, have an assistant hold the paper for you while you work your open hand in under the edge, lift the entire placenta and press it against the paper. Flip placenta and paper over like a pancake and press the cord to the paper, then lift the placenta away. Or, arrange the placenta as desired, hold the paper above it and lower the entire piece of paper over it. Apply gentle but firm pressure against the board to make the print, peeking under to make sure the cord was printed as well. Then lift the paper and board directly up and away from the placenta. Plan to make several prints (Forester, 2002).

Eating the placenta (placentophagy)

The parenchyma consists of a tender meat that tastes like organ meat, such as kidney or liver, but is sweeter and milder than either (it actually tastes more like calf's brains). Some women want to eat their placenta after the birth. Although higher primates (chimpanzees and gorillas) do not always eat their placentas, lower primates and omnivorous animals usually do. Women who eat their placenta report feelings of well-being and strength as a result. The practice is also said to minimize postpartum depression, as well as act as a powerful restorative (Field, 1988). Placenta is the only meat that is a by-product of life, not death. Squeamish meat-eaters and vegetarians alike should keep this in mind. Sometimes all who are present partake of this special meal; a literal sharing of the body and blood of the mother and baby in a communion honoring the holy sacrament of physical incarnation. If this is to be done, most of the stew should be set aside for the mother and the rest heated to at least 320° F (160° C) and cooked for a minimum of one hour to kill any pathologic organisms unless the mother is known to be free of all blood borne infections and the entire company feels comfortable with less cooking.

Any recipe that calls for kidney or liver can be used to prepare placenta. Cooking temperatures should not exceed 212°F (100°C), since the steroid hormones it contains are unstable at higher temperatures. Here is one highly recommended recipe from Shaheeda Pierce, a midwife in Washington State (1999):

1 freshly birthed placenta (thoroughly examined before use)
1 bottle of red wine, preferably organic
½ cup olive oil
¼ cup lime juice
2 cloves of garlic
1 medium onion
3 potatoes
fresh or dried herbs such as rosemary, tarragon, ginger, thyme, bay leaf, parsley, basil, etc., to taste
One or more additional vegetables such as squash, kale, collard greens or carrots
Seasonings: salt, pepper, tamari, etc, to taste
Cornstarch or arrowroot

Preparing the placenta: The cook should wear gloves when handling the raw placenta. Wash the placenta to remove any clots and excess blood. Then use sharp scissors to slice off the umbilical cord and membranes

Marinating the placenta: Place the placenta in a large container with a tight-fitting lid. Add most or all of the wine, half the olive oil and all of the lime juice. Cover and place in the refrigerator for one to three hours or up to three days. If you plan to marinate the placenta for just an hour or so, first remove the cotyledons from the membranes by cutting them away from the basal plate with a sharp knife. Discard any portions that are very calcified. If the placenta is to be marinated from 1 to 3 days, don't bother skinning the membranes, because the marinade will soften everything.

Cooking the placenta: After marinating, cut the placenta into bite-sized chunks and brown it in olive oil, preferably in a cast iron skillet (which will add iron). Cook about 6 minutes, stirring occasionally. As the placenta is browning, chop the onion and garlic and add them to the pan. Add herbs of your choice.

Cut the potatoes into bite-sized pieces. Then cook them in water in another pan until almost done. Cut up any additional vegetables and add them to the water. When done, add the strained vegetable mixture to the pan with the placenta. Cook for a few minutes on low heat. If desired, add some of the marinade or make a gravy.

Gravy: Combine the olive oil and marinade in a small saucepan. Dissolve 2 tablespoons cornstarch or arrowroot in a little cold water, stirring until smooth. Add to the marinade and oil, and stir over medium heat until thickened. Season to taste. Serve hot over the placenta or a grain such as brown rice.

Preparing restorative remedies from the placenta

Chinese restorative formula: The medicinal properties of the placenta can be preserved for later use by the mother. Use the following recipe, which comes from Raven Lang, a midwife of many years and now a Chinese medical doctor in California (Hobbs, 1999). Use the preparation as a general restorative for the first two weeks after the birth. Save the rest for the mother to take if she later becomes ill with a cold or the flu.

1 placenta	Vegetable steamer
½ lemon	Oven or dehydrator
1 hot pepper	Electric food grinder
fresh ginger	Sharp knife

1. Wash excess blood from the placenta.
2. Milk out any excess blood from the cord.
3. Place the placenta, membranes and cord in a steamer with a hot pepper of your choice, half a fresh lemon (preferably organic) and several generous slices of fresh ginger.
4. Steam for 15 minutes; turn over and steam another 15 minutes or until no juice comes out when pricked with a fork.
5. Slice into ⅛ inch slices and place on a baking sheet.
6. Put in a very slow 100 to 150°F (38 to 65°C) oven for many hours or overnight until the slices are completely dry and break easily. A food dehydrator also works well for this purpose.
7. The dehydrated placenta can now be stored by either freezing or placing it in capsules.

    To freeze the dried strips: Wrap them tightly in plastic wrap and then place in resealable plastic freezer bags. Press as much air out of the bag as possible, date and label and place in the freezer. To use, break off a small piece and place in a cup. Pour hot but not boiling water over it, stir and drink.

    To make capsules: Grind the slices in a clean coffee grinder or a food processor, using the metal blade. Place the powder in 00 gelatin capsules. The mother should take 2 capsules, 3 times a day for the first two weeks after the birth.

The placenta can also be prepared by simply slicing, drying, powdering and capping it as above, but without the herbs. This is called Ze He Qi (Bastien, 2004)

Tincture of placenta: A simple tincture of placenta can be made by rinsing and cutting the placenta into pieces, placing them in a jar and filling the jar to the brim with 100 proof vodka or grain alcohol. Close tightly. Allow this to steep in a cool, dark place for six weeks, gently rotating the jar from top to bottom every few days. When done, strain and decant the tincture into a dark, tightly lidded glass container.

A more elaborate recipe comes from Doña Irena Sotelo (2001), a renowned traditional Mexican midwife and healer. For her tinctures, she uses the placenta of a very healthy, first-time mother who has had no problems during her pregnancy and who has never taken artificial hormones (such as contraceptive pills) and whose lab results have all been normal. Once the cord is cut and the placenta has been examined:

1. Remove all membranes.
2. Wash the placenta with clear water.
3. Weigh the placenta. If it weighs one pound or more, cut it in half.
4. Place each piece of placenta in 1 pint of water in a wide-mouthed, lidded glass jar and freeze overnight. Be sure there is expansion space in the top of the jar or it will burst.
5. The next morning, place all the frozen placenta including the frozen water into a blender or food processor fitted with a metal blade and blend thoroughly.
6. Add half a liter of sugar-cane alcohol (this is similar to grain alcohol and is often available in Mexican markets).
7. Strain through a fine cloth.
8. To the strained liquid add five times as much sugar-cane alcohol (e.g., if you have 1 cup of tincture, add 5 cups of alcohol).
9. Decant into a dark glass container and cap tightly.

Tincture of placenta can be given to any woman who needs the hormonal boost it provides. Heavy or prolonged postpartum lochia can be treated by giving 5 to 10 drops three times daily in a little water for up to two months. When prolonged use is necessary, the woman should take the drops for 21 days, take a 9 day break and resume. It is also helpful in preventing postpartum depression. Placenta cream (described below) can be used as an alternative to taking tincture.

Placenta cream: Sotelo adds the tincture described above (the elaborate recipe) to any good-quality, thick body cream, preferably one that does not contain petroleum products such as mineral oil. Use 2.2 lbs (1 kg) cream to 4.5 oz (125 ml) of tincture. Mix with a spoon or whisk for about one hour and let the mixture rest overnight. It can be rubbed under the breasts and lower abdomen once at night for up to 21 days, with a 9 day break before beginning again.

Cornelia's placenta remedies: Cornelia Enning (2003) shares these thoughts regarding her version of a placenta remedy. She finds that the functioning of the maternal glands affects the chemical composition of the placenta. A good placenta for this purpose is one from a mother with a good thyroid balance, clear skin and a healthy baby. Therefore, do not make a remedy from the placenta if there is a history of placental bleeding, varicosities, preeclampsia, use of intoxicants or drugs, infections or early labor. Each remedy is made from a powdered preparation of placenta and is intended for the sole use of that mother.

Placenta powder: First, powder the placenta using a healthy human or animal placenta, as follows:
1. Pasteurize the placenta for 1 hour at 158°F (70°C). Then reduce the temperature to warm and open the oven door for the next 30 hours to dehydrate it. Alternatively, place it in a dehydrator after the first hour.
2. Grind the completely dried placenta in a clean, manually operated coffee mill and then grind further with a mortar and pestle.

The powder may be either black, yellow or red and should smell good to the mother.

Placenta ghee: Clarify 4 oz (a quarter pound) of butter. To do so, place the butter in an enamel or stainless-steel saucepan and heat it until the solids separate and sink to the bottom of the pan. Carefully use a turkey baster to draw off the clear oil on top, then discard the milk solids. Add 1 to 2 tsp of powdered placenta (use 1.5 tsp if the salve is to be used on the baby). This salve is great for acute skin problems including varicosities and even skin cancer, but it should not be used prophylactically (those with skin cancer should seek the advice of a medical professional as well). This will keep unrefrigerated for three weeks.

Placenta drinks: The placenta contains lots of B vitamins, can enhance milk production, may help stop preterm labor and may treat infertility. It can be used to make a drink or extract.

Mother's Milk Bavarian Drink

1 bottle of beer with a high hops content
1 bottle of good-quality malt beer
1 tsp placenta powder
1 16 oz glass (half-liter)

Place 1 tsp of placenta powder in the tankard. Add the first beer (the one with a high hops content), and then add malt beer until the glass is half-full. It will froth, filling the rest of the tankard. This drink is good for treating depression, to increase milk production and to fortify thin women.

Mother's Milk Vineyard Drink

1 pinch of placenta powder
1 glass of champagne

Add a pinch of placenta powder to a champagne glass, and then fill the glass two-thirds full with champagne. The drink will sparkle. This is indicated to bring on early milk production. If this drink is taken two hours after a waterbirth, it will bring the mature milk after five hours. Early onset of mature milk production can be important for large babies, for particularly small babies, in cases of multiple birth and in cases of maternal gallbladder problems.

Caring for the Lotus Placenta

After the baby's placenta is born and has been examined, place it in a bowl near the baby. After the pulse has disappeared at the baby's umbilical base and the herbal bath is finished, the placenta can be gently washed with plain water and patted dry with paper towels or old cloth towels. Place it in a colander set over a large bowl to dry from all sides. This works especially well if the family lives in a dry climate. Once the placental exam is complete, the Lotus placenta can also be coated with herbs. While some midwifery literature has talked of using salt to preserve Lotus placentas, salt draws fluid to the surface and tends to make the placenta sticky and messy. Herbs work much better for this purpose.

The single best herb to use is rosemary with the leaves finely powdered. Both sides should be thoroughly coated with rosemary after the placenta is partially dried (a few hours after birth). Make sure the powder gets between the septa of the cotyledons. Rosemary's strong, clean smell and antiseptic properties make it an ideal herb for this purpose. Powered turmeric is also an excellent herb for this purpose and is also widely available as a bulk kitchen herb. When using a powdered herb, take care not to create a big dust storm as you apply it, as breathing the dust will not be helpful to anyone, especially the baby. It is not toxic but could cause respiratory symptoms, just like breathing any other dust. To avoid airborne dust, take it outside and put the powder in a large bowl. Bring it back inside and carefully place the placenta on the powder, and then use a spoon or your gloved fingers to work the powder into the parenchyma. Once the rosemary has been applied, the placenta can then either be returned to the colander unwrapped for continued drying or it can be wrapped in any absorbant, waterproof material. Robin Lim, a CPM from Idaho, says she has wonderful results with using disposable diapers (as much as we both hate them) to wrap Lotus placentas. The diaper draws the fluids out of the placenta, makes it much easier to deal with in the days after birth, and can be changed as frequently as necessary. (I wonder if disposable diaper producers would like to do a few commercials featuring babies wearing cloth diapers while their intact placentas wear disposables?) However, be aware that most brands of disposable diapers contain a lot of chemicals; if the parents are being so organic as to leave the cord intact, they may wish to purchase a pile of new, thin kitchen towels or an ecological brand of disposable diapers to use for this purpose. If cloth is used, a Chux pad can then be wrapped around the cloth-wrapped placenta, or the wrapped placenta can be contained in any suitably sized plastic bag. Be aware, however, that keeping it in plastic will tend to keep it moist, whereas exposing it to air will help it to dry and shrink and smell less potent.

PARTING INSTRUCTIONS FOR THE PARENTS

You are satisfied that the mother's and baby's transitions are coming along smoothly and the initial three to four hours after birth have passed without major concerns. The house is more or less in order; your bags are reassembled and packed. The family members are probably ready to have some time completely to themselves, or they may want to go to sleep. Before you go, however, you need to give the parents parting instructions, including when to call you regarding concerns. Both parents will likely be in an altered state of consciousness, from exhaustion as well as elation. Therefore, it is important to give your instructions orally and in writing to both of them. Your instructions should be comprehensive enough to cover the basic information the parents will need for the next few days. Do not expect all your instructions to sink in at this point, many will have to be reviewed at the 24 hr visit as well.

In addition, you will want to provide the parents with more extensive information to carry them through the first 6 weeks after the birth. This can be given at the day-3 postpartum visit or in one comprehensive handout that you give them before you leave the birth. Most of the topics introduced below are covered in detail in Volume III of this text or in my other texts.

If the cord has been cut, left long and is not clamped, you will want to leave a clamp with the parents and instruct them how to use it. It is very unlikely that it will ooze even a drop of blood, but it will make them feel secure, knowing they can clamp it if need be.

For the Parents

From here to the end of the chapter, "you" refers to one or both of the parents.

Dealing with family and friends

When you give birth at home, family and friends view you as more accessible and may unintentionally wear you out with visits. Set up your phone answering system to let people know a good time to call. You can say something like "Our beautiful baby boy, Andrew, was born at home at 6 am yesterday. We are delighted. We are resting and having plenty of family time. Our midwives told us to tell you that if you wish to support us during the next few weeks, we would love for you to bring a hot meal, take our other kids for an outing or do a load of laundry, and we are open to suggestions if you remember something you wish had been done for you when you gave birth. We will return your call, let you know a good time to visit and find out if you can help us preserve the sanctity of these precious first days and weeks with your support. Leave your message after the tone and thanks for calling."

This way, you lay the heavy rap on the midwives and right off the bat send a clear message regarding what will truly be supportive to you as a family.

Baby care instructions

- Nurse whenever your baby wants to or every 2 to 3 hours; never go longer than four hours, regardless of the time of day. The hotter the temperature outside, the more critical it is to follow this schedule for the first four to six weeks. Babies can quickly become seriously dehydrated or hypoglycemic. Frequent nursing will prompt the baby to want to wake up on her own and nurse more. Infrequent nursing will often result in a sleepy baby who falls into a hypoglycemic state from which it is hard to be roused.
- The baby should not become overheated or chilled. Babies can easily become overheated from too much clothing or chilled from too little. If, after correcting any possible environmental factors, the baby's temperature seems abnormal in either direction, take an axillary or rectal temperature and call immediately if it is abnormal. The baby's axillary temperature should be between 96.6 and 98.6°F (35 to 37°C). The baby's rectal temperature should be between 98.6 and 100.6°F (36 to 38°C). See "Taking a temperature" at the end of this sheet, if you have any questions about how to do this.
- The baby should pass stool within 48 hours and urinate within 24 hours of birth (if not already noted during the immediate postpartum hours). Babies whose cords are left intact for many minutes or hours after birth tend to urinate frequently.
- Watch for skin rashes and report any red patches, pimples or red bumps right away.
- If the cord has been cut, the stump can be cleaned thoroughly with a Q-tip moistened with either peroxide, echinacea tincture, plain grain alcohol or a strong sterile saline solution (½ tsp salt per cup of water) after

each diaper change. Do not use rubbing alcohol as it is toxic and too irritating. For the first 24 hours, the cord will be cold and clammy but empty of blood. Over the first 36 to 48 hours, it will become dry and brownish or even blackish. Most of the cord will become brittle, with the base a dirty white color before it falls off. The base will be slightly moist and flexible and then become very narrow until it hangs on only by a thread; this thread is often the umbilical vein, so do not pull on it. If the length of the cord becomes moist after it has begun to dry, dry it lightly from a distance with a hair dryer set on low. Call at once if you notice any swelling of the cord stump, constant wetness or slight leakage of fluid, blood or meconium from the base.

•Diapers should be folded so that the umbilicus and cord are exposed.

•A cord that has been cut long after all pulsing has ceased at the navel and not clamped, should not bleed from the end. If it should start bleeding, clamp or band it; then call the midwives immediately.

•If you are doing a Lotus birth, and live in a dry climate, pack the placenta with rosemary or turmeric or both and place it in a colander beside the baby to dry. If you are not in a desert area, pack it with herbs and place it in either a disposable diaper or a cloth diaper wrapped in a disposable underpad. Change the diaper when you change the baby so that can continue to absorb moisture.

•If you have a boy, *do not* attempt to forcefully retract the foreskin. It is held in place by adhesions that will tear if you do so.

•If blocked tear ducts were detected during the newborn exam, to help open the tear ducts, gently press inside the bridge of the nose, placing the tip of your fingerpad adjacent to the inner corner of the eye on one side. First stroke upward to remove stagnant material, then stroke with firm pressure downward parallel to the nose, stopping at the nostril. Mucoid material may be expelled in the corner of the eye. This should be done using three to four strokes at a time, several times a day.

•Preferably, sleep with the baby. If this is not possible, sleep with the baby beside your bed.

•If the baby's skin starts to appear yellow (jaundiced) within the first 24 hours, call us.

•If the baby starts "acting funny," is extremely lethargic or very irritable for no obvious reason, and especially if this behavior persists regardless of what you do, something may be seriously wrong. Call immediately.

•Call us immediately, day or night, if you have questions or other concerns.

Mother care instructions

Nursing and breast care:

•Do not wash your nipples with soap and do not wash them at all prior to nursing.

•During the first 36 to 48 hours, the breasts produce colostrum, the perfect food for the newborn. Most women only produce a relatively small amount of this rich premilk. This is all your baby needs. Do not offer the baby water or any other fluids.

•Colostrum will begin to transition into breast milk after the first couple of days. Breast milk is thinner, may have a bluish white cast, and is much more plentiful. As this occurs, your breasts will feel full and tender and may feel hard and warm. Frequent nursing will help ease this fullness until the milk supply is established and stabilizes. Warm compresses or freshly steamed whole cabbage leaves can be applied to the breasts to ease engorgement. If your breasts are increasingly or persistently hard and tender, if they become painful, red and swollen or if they develop localized areas of redness, swelling or palpable lumps, call immediately.

•Using the following basic principles, experiment with different nursing positions:

1. Position the baby belly to belly, his hips flexed, mouth and nose facing nipple with no blankets in between.
2. Place the baby's arm under your arm. Encourage him to open his mouth wide and aim your nipple at the roof of his mouth. Use your hand to support his upper back and neck, not his head.
3. Be sure the baby has at least a half-inch of your areola in his mouth and is not sucking on the tip.
4. Be sure baby's lower lip is not curled under.

•Breast and nipple tenderness:

-If your nipples are beginning to get sore and the baby is finished nursing for nourishment, give the baby a clean finger (clean under the nail as well) for comfort.

-Apply Vitamin E from capsules or Lansinoh Lanolin® salve to nipples after each feeding.

-Dry your nipples gently (at a distance) with a light bulb after feeding.

-Change nursing positions often.

-Expose nipples to air as much as is practical.

-Check the baby's mouth for thrush; if you find whitish patches that won't rub off, call immediately.

-Know it will get better; the first week is the hardest.

Caring for your uterus

•Check your uterus for position and firmness regularly (but do not wake up just to do this). It should feel about the size of a grapefruit and be no higher than your navel.

•To keep your uterus clamped down and firm:

-Empty your bladder frequently.

-Nurse your baby as she desires or at least every 2 to 4 hours. This stimulates the production of oxytocin, the hormone that causes your uterus to contract.

-If your uterus feels soft or mushy, gently massage (stimulate) it by placing your hand over the top and rocking it gently until it firms up. Vigorous massage is not necessary and may break up clots over the placental site. Your uterus should not feel sore and should feel increasingly less tired as the hours go by. If you find that you cannot tolerate touching your uterus or that your uterus is becoming increasingly painful or sensitive, you may have an infection. Call immediately!

•Passage of small clots and small gushes that occur upon arising from a reclining position are normal during the first 12 to 24 hours.

•Your bleeding is coming from the placental implantation site and should taper off gradually as the hours and days pass and the endometrial lining regenerates. This bleeding, called lochia, transitions from dark red to pinkish brown and finally to a creamy color before it disappears. Normal, healthy lochia smells like strongly scented menstrual blood. It should not smell foul or like rotten meat; if it does, call immediately.

•Take 800 IU Vitamin E daily; increase to 2000 IU with increased bleeding or activity. Vitamin E causes the lochial discharge to taper off much faster than is ordinarily expected because it speeds the regeneration of the placental site. Vitamin C with bioflavonoids (500 mg) will also help regenerate the placental site and can be taken as well. If you have bled excessively after the birth, an assimilable form of iron should be taken to help rebuild your red blood cells.

•Watch for excessive bleeding.

-If you soak more than two super-sized napkins in one hour, call immediately.

-If you pass a clot larger than a lemon, call immediately.

-If blood starts to pour out continuously and is not containable, go to the hospital immediately and have someone call us to let us know to meet you there.

•Avoid substances that promote blood flow, such as aspirin or other medications that contain acetylsalicylic acid, alcoholic beverages or herbal products containing willow bark or red clover.

Afterbirth pains

•Your uterus contracts as it works to close down the placental site. These contractions feel different to different women and tend to be stronger the more babies you have had. Nursing will also increase the frequency and intensity of afterbirth pains. To take the edge off these cramps, try the following:

-Apply a wrapped hot water bottle or a heating pad to your lower abdomen. Either must be removed and the pad turned off before you fall asleep, so it is a good idea to tell someone else you are using a pad to help you remember or so he can turn it off for you in case you don't.

-Take extra supplemental calcium or eat additional dairy products such as yogurt.

-Take an herbal tincture or homeopathic remedy indicated for easing afterbirth pain. If you are really miserable, you can take acetaminophen; again, *do not* take any products containing acetylsalicylic acid.

-Lie on your belly with a pillow under your lower abdomen to create pressure against your uterus. The frequency and intensity of your afterbirth pains may increase for the first 5 minutes, after which you should experience complete relief. You cannot breastfeed in this position, but a break from nursing also helps, because nursing stimulates the uterus to contract.

Bathing and personal hygiene

•Change your sanitary pad with every bathroom visit. Do not use tampons or other internal menstrual collection devices. Do not douche. Rinse your perineum each time you use the toilet. This can be done with a bidet, a mobile shower spray head, or a peri-bottle filled with clean water to which a dropperful of calendula tincture has been added. Rinse and pat dry from front to back.

- Take an herbal bath once or twice a day until all your herbal bath packs are gone. This is helpful for sutures as well as healing to the entire reproductive tract. If you have stitches or an unrepaired tear, limit your baths to once or twice a day; more can waterlog the area and prolong healing. Shower for all other bathing requirements.

Diet, rest and exercise

- Eat well, with even more protein than during pregnancy.
- Eat foods you know to be agreeable and nonconstipating for you. Prunes and prune juice can provide natural laxative effects, but some babies get gassy when their mothers eat prunes. Black cherries and black cherry juice are also good for this purpose, and babies tolerate them better.
- Drink lots of clear fluids; at least a half-gallon daily. When you nurse, have a large glass of water or clear fluid to sip. Avoid caffeinated, carbonated and sugared beverages, all of which may seriously disrupt your sleep and your baby's.
- Whatever you eat will get to the baby. If the baby starts having digestive distress, think about what you ate in the previous few hours or the day before. Caffeine, chocolate and certain spices and additives may negatively impact the baby's behavior or sleep pattern.
- Rest a lot; a minimum of a two-week break is recommended. You should rest in bed or on the couch for the first few days and avoid climbing stairs if you have stitches or an unrepaired tear. If the weather is mild and there is a safe and protected outside area for you and the baby to enjoy, do so. Otherwise, stay inside for the first two weeks or so.
- When you do get up, have someone with you for the first 12 to 24 hours to make sure you do not become dizzy or feel faint. If pronounced or persistent faintness or dizziness does occur, call immediately.
- Walk the length and breadth of your house twice daily to help circulate blood to your lower extremities. This is especially important if you have varicose veins in your legs or vulva. You do not have to behave like an invalid; just take it easy.
- During the first two weeks, your primary task should be taking care of the baby and your own personal needs. Let others take care of you, your other children and household responsibilities.
- Do not lift anything heavier than the baby for the first three weeks. If you have a history of any type of pelvic prolapse (or a family history of prolapse), do not lift anything heavier than the baby for 4 to 6 weeks.
- Your activity level will directly impact how much and how long you bleed after the birth. If you notice an increase in your flow, or a change from brownish to bright red bleeding, you are probably doing too much. Decrease your activity, increase your Vitamin E dosage and call us.
- Regular exercise can resume when your lochia stops flowing and you feel ready. Begin with stretches and short walks. Avoid heavy aerobics and jarring exercise such as jogging or running for the first 6 weeks.
- Perineal strengthening exercises (Kegels) can resume immediately and will help speed healing to the area.

If you have stitches or an unsutured tear

- Be careful not to put undue stress or strain on sutures by avoiding climbing stairs. Also don't swing your legs widely when entering or exiting a car, avoid tailor-sitting and do not lift anything heavier than the baby.
- Wear sanitary pads and underwear as little as possible, especially if you have unsutured labial damage. Instead, rest on extra plastic-backed underpads from your birth kit.
- After using the toilet, rinse your perineum with normal saline solution (¼ tsp to 1 cup water) or an herbal solution, such as rosemary infusion (made by using 1 oz or dried leaves, pour 1 quart of boiling water over leaves and allow to steep overnight). If you have a movable shower head, you can use that as well.
- If desired, dry your stitches gently with a light bulb or a hair dryer set on warm; do not use a high-intensity infrared lamp.
- Call immediately, day or night, if there are questions or concerns.

Resumption of sexual activities

- It is best to postpone all penetration until the cervix is fully closed. Closure is usually indicated by a complete absence of tinted discharge for at least 5 days.
- If you have sutures or tears that were not sutured, it is best to postpone for 6 weeks any activities that may disrupt healing.

•To resume penetration, go slowly and gently; a water-based lubricant may be helpful.
•Ovulation will occur prior to your first regular period for 80% of all women.
•If you provide all your baby's nourishment (no supplemental feedings), have no return of your menses and your baby is less than 6 months old, the chances of getting pregnant are less than 1%, but only if all these criteria are met fully. If not, conception can occur as soon as three weeks postpartum!
•Barrier methods of contraception, such as a diaphragm, can be used once healing is complete. Hormonally based methods should not be used. If you have questions regarding suitable contraception during nursing, please ask.

Call immediately if you have any of the following signs of infection, concealed bleeding, or inflammation:
•A fever. (Your temperature should not exceed 100.6°F [38.1°C]).
•Foul-smelling discharge
•Uterine tenderness (It may feel vaguely sore, like muscle soreness after exercise for the first day or so, but if you cannot tolerate any external pressure or if your uterus is becoming increasingly sensitive to touch, this is an abnormal sign associated with infection.)
•Leg or calf pain with tenderness; localized hot spots, redness or swelling, with or without visible varicose veins
•A sick, flu-like feeling, with or without chills or fever
•Pronounced or persistent dizziness or faintness
•Increasing and continuous bleeding; passage of more than one large clot (lemon sized or larger)
•Family members notice a change in mother's level of consciousness or behavior that is concerning

Taking temperatures
The basics:
To shake down a glass thermometer: Hold the thermometer firmly in your hand with the colored end pointing down. Shake it using a fast, snapping motion until the colored column reads 95°F (35°C) or below. This can be done after each reading.

To read a glass thermometer: Hold the thermometer by the end that isn't colored. Place it horizontally at eye level and rotate it slowly in good light until the colored column becomes visible and the degree markings face you. Note the mark above where the colored column ends.

Fahrenheit: Each long line indicates one degree of elevation in temperature. Only every other degree is marked with a number. Each short line indicates 2/10 of a degree. The average normal temperature is indicated by an arrow below the line. If the colored column is between two marks on the glass, assess it as the higher reading.

Celsius: Each long line indicates one degree in temperature. The lines between the long ones each indicate 1/10 of a degree. These alternate between short- and medium-length lines to make it easier to read. The average normal temperature is indicated by an arrow below the line.

Taking baby's temperature: Take the baby's axillary or rectal temperature if you suspect that the baby is feverish or too cold. Nursing, hot or cold baths, environmental overheating or chilling, or vigorous activity can temporarily alter the temperature. Wait at least 15 minutes after the baby has experienced any of these before assessing the temperature.

To check the axillary temperature: The axillary route is much preferred as it is safer than the rectal route. Dry the thermometer and the armpit. To use a glass thermometer, place the colored thermometer tip into the deepest center of the armpit, lower the arm over the thermometer and hold it in place along the baby's side for 5 minutes, remove and read. Reinsert the thermometer for another minute and read again. If the temperature is continuing to change, repeat the readings until it stabilizes. Write down the time, date and reading on a note pad. If you are using a digital thermometer, place the tip as described and follow package instructions regarding the length of time to leave it in place. Record the date, time and reading.

To check the temperature rectally: Lay the baby on the bed. Sit beside the baby and roll her to her side, away from you (so her back is to you). Flex her legs. Lubricate the thermometer tip with oil or a water-based lubricant. Lift the top buttock and insert the tip into the anal passage, pointing the tip toward the umbilicus. For a glass thermometer, leave it there 3 to 4 minutes, remove and read. If you are using a digital thermometer, place the tip as described and follow package instructions regarding the length of time to leave it in place.

Taking mother's temperature: Take your oral temperature once daily. Take your temperature twice daily if your membranes were ruptured more than 12 hours prior to the birth. Also take it if you begin to feel feverish. Eating, drinking, smoking, hot or cold baths, or exercise can temporarily alter the temperature; wait at least 15 minutes after any of these activities before assessing the temperature.

To take an oral temperature: Place the colored tip of an oral thermometer just to the side of your frenulum, as deeply as possible under your tongue. Relax your tongue over the thermometer, close your mouth and do not talk until it is removed. Wait 2 to 4 minutes, remove and read. If you are using a digital thermometer, place the tip as described and follow package instructions regarding the length of time to leave it in place.

TAKING YOUR LEAVE

Sit by the bed and ask the parents if they have any last-minute questions before you leave the house. Recheck anything that has been concerning during your postpartum watch and confirm that the problem has resolved or that the parents are well informed about calling you should it not continue to resolve once you leave. Let them know when you expect to return to perform the first home visit, which is ideally scheduled between 24 to 36 hours after the birth. When it actually will occur will depend upon the time of day the birth occurred, the travel time to the home and your schedule. If you will not be making the visit yourself, make sure the parents know who will be coming (presumably another assistant who also attended the birth with you).

Now your bags are packed and you are ready to slip out the door, leaving a contented family to bask in the glow of an extraordinary event that is as old and as sacred and as commonplace as human life on earth. As you go home, to your office, or to do errands or to your own little ones, you will reflect on the miracle you have just witnessed and the special intimacy that is part and parcel of the calling to homebirth midwifery and the privilege of being a handmaiden of the universal life force.

References and Further Reading on Care of the Mother and Baby during the Hours following the Birth of the Placenta

Caring for the Mother in the First Hours after Birth

Jacobson H. "A standard for assessing lochia volume," MCN Am J Matern Child Nurse, 10(3);174-175, May/June 1985.

Lang R. Mother Roasting: The use of Traditional Chinese Medicine in Postpartum Care, privately published, Sept 16, 1985.

Long P. "Management of the third stage of labor: a review," J Nurse-Midwifery, 36(4);240-244, July/Aug, 1991.

Schlinger H. Editing notes, 2003.

Varney H. Varney's Midwifery, 3rd ed. Jones and Bartlett Pub, Boston MA, 1997.

Afterbirth Pains

Varney H. Varney's Midwifery, 3rd ed. Jones and Bartlett Pub, Boston MA, 1997.

Uses for the Placenta

Bastien A. "Placental rituals, placental medicine," Midwifery Today, (71);54-55, Autumn 2004.

Enning C. "Birth on Demand," all day workshop on waterbirth, Midwifery Today conf., Springfield OR, March, 2003.

Enning C. Placenta Remedies. English edition, Forthcoming.

Field M. "Placentophagy (eating the placenta)," Childbirth Alternatives Qtrly, IX(3);6, Spring, 1988.

Forester E. "A treasured keepsake: placenta prints," Midwifery Today, (62);30-31, Summer, 2002.

Hobbs V. Personal communication, medicinal use of the placenta, 1999.

Janszen K. "Meat of Life," Sci Digest, 88(6);78-81, 122, Nov-Dec, 1980.

Ober W. "Notes on placentophagy," NY Acad Med, 55(6);591-599, June, 1979.

Pierce S. Personal communication, 1999.

Sotelo I. "Practices of Traditional Midwifery in Mexico," 5-day midwifery intensive, Midwifery Today workshop, Aug 27-31, 2001.

Caring for the Lotus Placenta

Baker J. Lotus Birth Information Pack, privately printed, bound handout, 1999?

Rachana S. Lotus Birth. Greemwood Press, Steels Creek, Victoria Australia, 2000.

WHEN LABOR AND BIRTH DEMAND SPECIFIC MIDWIFERY SKILLS

Remedies, Skills and Equipment for Complex Labor Situations

Useful Remedies

Naturopathic Remedies

Western Herbs

Throughout my textbooks, you will find mention of numerous herbs for treating conditions during pregnancy, labor and postpartum. Here are some basic, widely used remedies that most midwives who use herbs would want to have on hand at a birth, along with their commonly accepted uses. There are, however, many more herbs that can be used during labor and birth, but it is beyond the scope of this text to list them all. This list gives you a good basic apothecary. These herbs are all prepared as alcohol-based tinctures from the parts of the fresh plant mentioned unless otherwise noted. Full instructions regarding the preparation of herbal medicines can be found in the appendix of DIAGNOSTIC TESTS.

Angelica root *(Angelica archangelica, A. sylvestris, A. Atropurpurea)*: This helps with placental detachment after birth. In doses of 30 to 50 drops of tincture under the tongue, it can work in 5 minutes. If necessary, it can be repeated after 15 minutes. Some may be sensitive to the its effects, with fresh root preparations causing more reactions than dried.

Basil leaf (*Ocimum basilicum*): The infusion can be used to stimulate the uterus after birth to help deliver the placenta.

Bayberry bark (*Myrica cerifera)*: Highly astringent, this is used to help stop postpartum uterine bleeding.

Bethroot or birthroot (*Trillium pendulum*): The white-flower variety was preferred by Native American midwives as a uterine stimulant to augment labor and control postpartum bleeding. Chewing raw root may work quickly but tastes acrid, causing profuse salivation and watering of the eyes. Use ¼ to ½ tsp of tincture and repeat twice at 30 min intervals.

Black cohosh (*Cimicifuga racemosa*): This herb stimulates and enhances the action of blue cohosh, with which it is often used in combination. It helps produce coordinated and effective contractions. It is also good in combination with blue cohosh as a priming tincture to prepare for induction. The use of 10 drops of tincture under the tongue every hour helps to ripen the cervix.

Blue cohosh (*Caulophyllum thalictroides*): This uterine contractant is best used in small amounts prior to labor to prime the uterus in preparation for induction. It stimulates the production of oxytocin, helps the uterus begin contracting and increases the force of contractions. Although widely used to augment contractions once labor begins, cotton root bark is a better herb with fewer side-effects. Blue cohosh causes nausea in many women, has been associated with an elevated fetal heart rate in labor, is toxic to the liver and kidneys in very large doses and is contraindicated if the woman has low blood pressure.

Catnip leaf (*Nepeta cataria*): This very safe sedative and calmative can be used on babies and laboring mothers; the infusion can be used to release the placenta after the birth and to ease afterbirth pains.

Cinnamon bark (*Cinnamomum zeylanicum*): A strong infusion assists placental detachment postpartum.

Cotton root bark (*Gossypium herbaceum*): The best all-around herb for labor induction. It can be used in a tincture or as an infusion. Since this is the root of the cotton plant from which fabric is made and most cotton is heavily sprayed with pesticides, it is imperative to get cotton root bark from an organic source.

Don quai (*Angelica sinensis*): An infusion can be used to stimulate the uterus after birth and help deliver the placenta.

Gelsemium root or yellow jasmine root (*Gelsemium nitidum*): This potent herb can be used orally to soften a rigid cervix, but it must be used very carefully as it is a respiratory paralytic. (Safe use is described in the chapter entitled "Cervical and Other Soft-Tissue Problems during Labor.")

Ginger root (cultivated form: *Zingiber officinalis,* wild form: *Asarum canadense*): Small quantities of ginger will potentize the effects of other herbs when combined with them; it is also an antinauseant and a stimulant that can help with fatigue in labor. To make a tea, use 1 oz of grated fresh root, ¼ oz shredded dry root, or ½ to 1 tsp of powder and steep for 5 to 30 minutes. The tea can be sipped throughout labor to maintain energy. To increase energy, give a full cup as often as every 30 minutes, or give 15 to 20 drops of tincture in a cup of hot water. Stimulate perfusion in the perineum by slicing fresh root into hot water for perineal compresses during pushing. Wild ginger helps the woman open to birthing energy. Brew a teaspoonful of dried root in 1 cup of water for 5 to 15 minutes or use 3 drops of the tincture under the tongue and repeat no more than 3 times. Both wild and cultivated ginger stimulate circulation to the uterus; however, internal use within an hour of birth should be avoided to decrease the risk of postpartum hemorrhage.

Ground ivy leaf (*Glechoma hederacea*): Fifty drops of tincture assists in releasing the placenta after birth and clamping down the uterus. It can be repeated in 2 to 5 minutes, if indicated.

Hops flower (*Humulus lupulus*): A sedative very safe for mother and baby.

Lady's mantle (*Alchemilla vulgaris*): A blood coagulant for postpartum hemorrhage; give 20 to 30 drops of tincture. Use in combination with uterine contractant herbs such as witch hazel, blue cohosh and cotton root bark to stop bleeding and contract the uterus. Combine 10 drops of one of these oxytocic herbs with 20 of lady's mantle.

Life root (*Senecio aureus*): This can be used to augment established labor. A tincture made from fresh flowering plants can be given in 10 to 15 drop doses, diluted in warm water, and repeated several times on the half-hour.

Lobelia (*Lobelia inflata*): A sedative and powerful relaxant. It can relax all voluntary muscles and is excellent for relaxing the cervix if the tincture is given in a sufficiently large dose. Try 60 to 150 drops of tincture of fresh plant material (leaf, flower and seed) in a small amount of water. An effective dose produces tingling in the extremities, flushing, and a rubbery sensation in the face. An inadequate dose is stimulating, resulting in heightened nervous energy and talkativeness. Small, repeated doses of 3 to 5 drops of tincture under the tongue is specific for shock. Note that lobelia is considered dangerous as it can cause nausea, burning in the throat and other side-effects. It may also lower blood pressure.

Motherwort (*Leonurus cardiaca*): A calmative good for restlessness in early labor and for preventing postpartum hemorrhage; use 10 drop doses of the tincture. It is also good for shock, which it eases as it centers the mother and strengthens the heart. Give one 10 drop dose under the tongue.

Passion flower (*Passiflora incarnata*): Use 15 drops of the tincture as a dose to bring down high blood pressure. Once pressure returns to normal, continue to take it.

Shepherd's purse (*Capsella bursa-pastoris*): This promotes clotting in doses of 20 to 40 drops of tincture and is said to stop a postpartum hemorrhage rapidly. Although it is a vasoconstrictor and said to promote uterine contraction, in my experience shepherd's purse used alone causes huge clots to form in the uterus. For this reason, it should never be used prophylactically to prevent hemorrhage. I recommend using it in combination with a uterine contractant herb. It should be prepared from the fresh whole plant in flower, as it loses potency rapidly after drying.

Skullcap (*Scutellaria tateriflora*): A very safe sedative, the tincture is good for all tension-related concerns and reduces anxiety. The infusion is useful in reducing hypertension.

St. John's wort flower (*Hypericum perforatum*): The tincture can be used internally for nerve pain, especially sciatic pain, and the oil is used externally for muscle pain and spasm.

White oak bark (*Quercus alba*): An astringent, the tincture can be given for postpartum bleeding. The infusion can be used as a compress for hemorrhoids or varicosities. It is healing and antiseptic.

Witch hazel bark (*Hamamelis virginiana*): An astringent and a powerful, rapidly acting hemostatic, this herb is good for controlling bleeding prior to the birth of the placenta because it does not close down the os. Use a dose of 10 to 20 drops of tincture. It is also good for persistent, excessive postpartum lochia but does not assist in contracting the uterus.

Cayenne and uterine bleeding:

Cayenne (*Capsicum minimum*) is a powerful equalizer of the circulation and works well to control bleeding that results from injury. However, it will only stop a uterine hemorrhage temporarily; then bleeding will resume. This is because uterine bleeding is due to atonicity of the myometrium, which cayenne does not correct. Cayenne should not be used to stay uterine bleeding and may aggravate uterine bleeding if it is used to stop bleeding from other sources, such as a perineal laceration. It should not be used after labor.

Combination herbal tinctures

Labor tincture: 1 part black cohosh, 1 part blue cohosh, ½ part ginger root, ½ part birth root. Make a combination tincture from the dried plant materials or give a combination dose using each of these herbs (for example, 10 drops each of blue and black cohosh combined with 5 drops each of ginger and birth root). Give twenty drops of the combined tinctures under the tongue in a single dose. While called "Labor tincture," this is best used to prime the uterus in the days before labor begins or as a preliminary to induction.

Antihemorrhage tincture 1: Use 1 part each blue cohosh, shepherd's purse and motherwort tinctures in combination in dropperful doses under the tongue and repeat as necessary for postpartum bleeding.

Antihemorrhage tincture 2: As an alternative to the above tincture, you can use 1 part each of dried blue cohosh root and dried witch hazel bark to ½ part dried valerian (*Valeriana officinalis*) or lady slipper root (*Cypripedium pubescens*). The valerian or lady slipper prevents spasms and eases pain and tension. Use two dropperfuls or 50 drops of the combination remedy under the tongue; repeat one minute later and again in 10 minutes if necessary.

(The section on herbs written with extensive reference to Susan Weed's wonderful book WISE WOMAN HERBAL FOR THE CHILDBEARING YEAR [Weed, 1985]. This book is a must for all midwives.)

Flower essence remedies

Although the Bach remedies are the most well known of the flower essences, there are several different lines of flower remedies available today. Flower remedies are similar to homeopathic remedies in that they contain a minute amount of the remedial substance. They are prepared from the fresh flowers of each plant, which are used to create a mother tincture that is then diluted to create the stock remedies. Stock remedies can be added by the drop to water or juice or taken directly from the bottle. Flower essences are designed to balance the emotional body. They should not be confused with aromatherapy preparations. They contain no oil and have no specific scent. They are easily prescribed based on the presenting emotions of the moment. They are totally safe and will not interfere with any other treatment that is being given concurrently.

Flower essences can be administered in 4 drop doses as frequently as the condition warrants. Increasing the amount per dose does not increase their effectiveness; as with other homeopathic remedies, the best results will be obtained by repeating the dose frequently to treat acute symptoms. The remedy may be diluted in water, given directly from the dropper under the tongue, applied directly to the skin, or diluted in bath water. It can also be aerosolized by diluting several doses in a spray bottle and spraying the person periodically. Skin application can be done by direct spray from the bottle, by pouring the diluted remedy over the woman and massaging or by spraying it on and rubbing it in.

Any flower remedy that matches the mother's emotional state may prove helpful in labor. However, there are some that come highly recommended by Kate O'Reilly, a flower essence practitioner from Oregon.

Cauliflower (Perelandra Essences): Use at the time of birth on the baby's forehead. This helps the new baby make a smooth transition into this world.

Cowkicks (Living Essences): Use for the woman who has run out of steam during labor. This essence is excellent for recharging one's batteries.

Dampiera (Living Essences): Use at crowning to open the perineum, prevent tearing and allow the woman to let go.

Green bells of Ireland (Alaskan Flower Essences): Helps newborn children connect to the earth's vibration so they can more easily make the transition from the spiritual world to the physical world.

Grove sandwort (Alaskan Flower Essences): Strengthens the feminine connection to the earth and enables the mother to receive nurturing energy from the earth before and after the birth. It has a stabilizing and centering effect.

Honeysuckle (Healing Herbs): Assists the mother in letting go of the past and of any past issues that may come up during labor. For example, it could be used for a woman who anticipated a labor very unlike the one she is having, and for each parent if faced with the birth of a baby with trauma or defects.

Impatiens (Healing Herbs and Bach): Use for impatience. It may also help the mother and her baby be more tolerant of early labor.

Kapok bush (Australian Bush Flower Essences): Use during the middle stages of labor when the mother feels like giving up.

Ladies's tresses (Alaskan Flower Essences): Useful when something has happened that keeps the body and soul from uniting at birth. Use it for premature birth and maternal shock. It is useful for birth trauma at any point in life.

Macrozamia (Living Essences): The queen of essences in birth, it brings on contractions, allows vulnerability, and gets a woman in touch with her primordial self.

Mariposa lily (FES–Flower Essence Services): This flower is called the "Madonna of the rocks" and brings nurturing and warmth to the young soul who has not been able to receive proper mothering due to disrupted bonding with the mother because of trauma, separation or neglect.

Menzies banksia (Living Essences): Use for pain and for when the woman feels there will be no end to pain.

Pear (Master's Flower Essences): Use for traumas, difficult births, accidents, minor injuries, pain, and hurt feelings.

Pink trumpet (Living Essences): For keeping focused on one's goal. Give to the laboring woman who feels that she would prefer to be somewhere else–any other place where there is less discomfort and trauma.

Sticky geranium (Alaskan Flower Essences): Good for getting the energy unstuck. Midwives use it to help mothers move to the next stage of labor.

Shooting star (Alaskan Flower Essences): Used for alienation, this remedy helps the soul take hold of the physical body and incarnate. Use it for premature babies, those who are having trouble stabilizing after birth and women who are always in a hurry to "go home."

Sweet potato (Starmen of Kauai): For fetal trauma and distress; for example, to correct a worrisome fetal heart rate pattern. It can be applied externally over the baby and massaged directly onto the mother's belly.

Combination flower remedies to have on hand: Note that some manufacturers do not reveal the contents of their formulas. Those that are available are given below.

Rescue Remedy (Bach): If you carry only one flower remedy, that one should be Rescue Remedy from the Bach Flower remedy line. This is a combination of five remedies intended to be given during or after any kind of crisis. It can be used freely on mother, baby and support people when things get tough in labor, during birth or thereafter. It contains the following remedies:

Cherry plum–desperation and fear of losing control
Clematis–for the bemused, faraway, out-of-the-body feeling that often precedes fainting or loss of consciousness and that often accompanies shock
Impatiens–for mental stress, tension, irritation, impatience and intolerance
Rock rose–for terror, panic and deep fears
Star of Bethlehem–shock and want of comfort and reassurance

Emergency Essence (Australian Bush Flower Essences): For the mother and partner during the birth process, this essence helps the mother to center herself and help her partner to remain calm. It contains the following essences:

Fringed violet–for distress
Spider flower–for terror
Sundew–for lack of focus and indecisiveness
Waratah flower essence–for inability to respond to a crisis
Crowea–for worrying and a sense of being "not quite right"

First-aid formulas (Five Flower, Bush Emergency, Wildflower Relief, Terra, Soul Support): A variety of other formulas can be used when labor or birth is difficult. Soul Support contains the following essences:

Cattail pollen–for gaining inner support
Chalice well–water from the well at Glastonbury, England, for when support is needed
Cotton grass–helps to release physical trauma
Fireweed flower essence–for grounding and to heal from shock
Labrador tea–for centering and rebalancing the body after extreme trauma or distress
Malachite (a mineral)–for grounding and aligning all aspects of the body
River beauty–for emotional recovery, reorientation and regeneration
White fireweed–for calming the emotional body after shock

New Mother's Formula (Flower Essences of Fox Mountain): This is used to help the bonding process between the mother and her baby. This formula contains angelica, borage (for courage), houseleek, lemon lily and trout lily.

RQ7 (Korte PHI Mother Earth Essences): This remedy contains all the flower essences listed for Bach Rescue Remedy plus lotus (for high spiritual connection) and self-heal flowers (for activating the body's natural healing process).

Aromatherapy

Smell is the oldest of our senses, and odors have profound physiological and emotional effects, acting directly on the limbic region of the brain. Aromatherapy is the therapeutic use of pure essential oils for their health promoting properties. Here is a small repertory of oils from a study done by Burns and Blamey (1994) you may want to start with:

ESSENTIAL OIL	THERAPEUTIC PROPERTIES
Chamomile	Anti-inflammatory; soothing
Clary sage	Reduces stress and tension; enhances contractions; antispasmodic; estrogen-like in effect
Eucalyptus	Cooling; refreshing; nasal decongestant; antiseptic
Frankincense	Useful for hyperventilation; slows and deepens breathing; calms anxiety; helpful for asthma
Jasmine	Antidepressant; relaxant
Lavender	Calming; sedating; relaxing; antiseptic; can quieten and strengthen contractions
Lemon & Mandarin	Refreshing; uplifting emotionally; cooling; often mixed with other oils to enhance their effect
Peppermint	Cooling; refreshing; useful for nausea and vomiting
Rose	Antidepressant; calming

Oils can be administered in various ways. A solution can be prepared using 100 ml of tap water with 2 drops of oil to mist over the face or spray on a face cloth or pillow. Four to 6 drops of oil can be added to a bath or 2 to 3 drops can be added to a footbath. A drop of oil can be applied to an absorbent card for inhaling, or 2 drops of oil can be added to 50 ml of carrier oil for massage (Burns & Blamey, 1994).

Whenever an essential oil is mentioned in this text, you should assume it must be of the purest medical-grade quality. Essential oils are potent and therefore rarely used in undiluted form. A carrier oil is one of several neutral oils into which essential oils can be diluted. Good carrier oils include sweet almond (*Prunus amygdalis*), apricot kernel (*Prunus armeniacea*), grapeseed (*Vitis ninferi*), sesame seed (*Sesamum indicum*), borage (*Borago officinalis*) and evening primrose (*Oenothera biennis*). Mineral oil should never be used as a carrier oil, and peanut oil should not be used as a carrier oil during pregnancy.

Aromatherapy is potent medicine and requires a great deal of background knowledge to be used safely. Always inform the woman that you intend to use essential oils and rule out any allergies before doing so. Essential oils of any kind are very potent and can carry both therapeutic and toxic effects. There will be a few specific suggestions regarding the use of aromatherapy throughout this book; do not assume you can use the suggested oil during pregnancy or for some other purpose unless this is clearly stated here or elsewhere. Midwives interested in using aromatherapy extensively are strongly encouraged to seek professional training at a qualified school. See the last chapter for suggestions.

Essential oils are extremely volatile and prone to lose their potency when exposed to light, air and high temperatures. They are expensive and must be purchased in small quantities and handled with great care to preserve their medicinal properties. All essential oils should be carefully stored in dark bottles, away from light and kept safely out of the reach of children. Small quantities of diluted oils can be prepared for use at births, keeping the rest of the pure oils in a dark, cool place at home. To maintain their highest potency, mixed oils should be kept in a separate, airtight bag or container that is placed in a dark place at home between births where it can be easily grabbed on the way out the door. Essential oils should be stored separately from homeopathic remedies and flower essences. The intense smell of the oils could neutralize your homeopathic remedies.

Books on complementary modalities

THE ALEXANDER TECHNIQUE BIRTH BOOK: A GUIDE TO BETTER PREGNANCY, NATURAL BIRTH AND PARENTHOOD by Ilana Machover, Angela Drake and Jonathan Drake, Sterling Pub Co, New York NY, 1993. The Alexander technique is a method of teaching people how to become more aware of and eliminate ways they abuse their body to balance physical and emotional disorders.

AROMATHERAPY FOR PREGNANCY AND CHILDBIRTH by Margaret Fawcett, Element Books Ltd, Shaftsbury, Dorset UK, 1993. This book is aimed at childbearing women, so it is simply written and not very in-depth. It offers basic information about the use of aromatherapy along with much adjunctive advice about general pregnancy and birth care.

Complementary Therapies for Pregnancy and Childbirth, 2nd ed., edited by Denise Tiran and Sue Mack, Baillière Tindall, Edinburgh, UK, 2000. This book introduces a wide range of modalities as they pertain to midwifery practice, including homeopathy, osteopathy, chiropractic, acupuncture, herbal medicine, massage, aromatherapy, reflexology, shiatsu, hypnosis, hydrotherapy, flower remedies and the Alexander technique. It would be an excellent book with which to begin more in-depth study.

Homeopathic Remedies

Basic homeopathic principles are explained in Volume I in the chapter entitled "Health Care Modalities." Homeopathic remedies can be very useful during labor. When the right remedy is chosen, it can work miraculously to alter imbalanced energy on a physical and nonphysical level. The key to the effective use of homeopathy is an in-depth knowledge of a range of remedies coupled with acute observational skills so that the condition of the patient can be matched to the remedy picture. Therefore accurate and quick homeopathic prescribing requires a broad knowledge base of many remedies, and there is no substitute for a natural talent for this type of therapy.

One of the most frustrating things about trying to learn homeopathy is having too few remedies at your disposal, as often the symptom picture will suggest the use of a remedy that you do not have. Therefore, I highly recommend finding one book that seems easy to understand and obtaining at least one potency of all the remedies it lists: 30C is a good, all-purpose potency. As you become more skilled, you may increase your pharmacy to include 200C potencies of the most used remedies. Affix a round stick-on label to the top of each remedy with the name and potency of each one. Arrange the tubes in alphabetical order in a box. Use strips of thin cardboard to separate the rows of remedies so you can remove one or more without all of them getting mixed up. This is the most space-efficient way to carry a number of remedies. One text and a full pharmacy of remedies that it covers gives you a good starting point for prescribing and really learning about homeopathy. I suggest you look over the following books to see which one speaks to you:

Guide to Homeopathic Remedies for the Birth Bag, 3rd ed., by Patty Brennan, 1997, Trusting Nature, 128 N. Seventh, Ann Arbor, MI, 48103, 313-663-1523. This book, in my opinion, offers the best and clearest explanation for beginners.

Herbals and Homeopathics for Women and Newborns by Lisa Goldstein, Midwifery in the Mountains, Inc, 239 Gravy Hill, Burnsville, NC 28714-7573. This combination text offers a wealth of detailed information on the use of herbs, aromatherapy and homeopathics. The writing style is easy to access and she answers lots of questions.

The Homeopathic Childbirth Manual: A Practical Guide for Labor, Birth, and the Immediate Postpartum Period, 2nd ed., by Betty Idarius, 1999, Idarius Press, PO Box 388, Talmage CA, 95481, 707-463-3739.

Homeopathy for Birthing: A Simplified Guide for Mothers, Midwives and Other Health Care Professionals, 2nd ed., by Jana Shiloh, 1990, Rocky Mountain Homeopathics. While this book mentions only 30 remedies, the fewest of all of these references, it is not as easy to use. It does, however, have some interesting additional concepts that will prove useful as you learn more. Therefore it can be considered an adjunct reference once you have mastered the basics.

Homeopathy for the Modern Pregnant Woman and Her Infant: A Therapeutic Practice Guidebook for Midwives, Physicians and Practitioners by Sandra J. Perko, 1997, Benchmark Homeopathic Publications, 13526 George Rd, Ste 101, San Antonio, TX 78230-3002. This is by far the most advanced presentation of obstetric homeopathy in this list.

Homeopathic remedies, like flower essences, are prescribed according to the manifest symptoms of the affected individual (*not* the Western diagnosis). Unlike flower remedies, which focus on emotional states, each homeopathic remedy has indications for conditions ranging from the mental state to every organ system in the body. Therefore, it is not appropriate to give a this-for-that list of remedies, as one can with just about any other therapeutic agent. There are, however, a few remedies that are so strongly associated with just one or two symptoms that they can be used when the practitioner has little additional knowledge of the remedy pictures of a variety of remedies. These remedies fall in the category formerly known as polycrests, a class of about 100 remedies whose effects are most well known. Most of the remedies in the first book listed above fall in this category. Some are so strongly linked to general symptoms that they can be recommended almost like allopathic medicines. Good examples include arnica for bruising and swelling, bellis perennis for deep-tissue trauma that does not respond to arnica, belladonna for sudden conditions producing bright red symptoms that are worse with the slightest motion, and carbo veg for someone who looks dead or nearly so.

TRADITIONAL CHINESE MEDICINE

The basic principles of Chinese medicine are reviewed in Volume I in the chapter entitled "Health Care Modalities."

Patent Remedies

Patent Chinese remedies are prepared in tablet or liquid form, making them easy to obtain, carry and administer.

Safety issues

There has been concern among Chinese herbalists about the safety of patent remedies because of contamination with heavy metals such as lead, mercury or arsenic, the substitution of plant species with potentially harmful plants and the adulteration of formulas with Western drugs. Recent and extensive lab analysis of patent remedies has shown that blanket rejection of any patent remedy is unwarranted. While contamination is documented, the contamination is limited to certain factories and certain preparations. A great deal of industry pressure, particularly from the United States, Australia and Taiwan, for all factories to follow Good Manufacturing Practice (GMP) standards has developed to address this problem. It is important for practitioners to be aware of the issue and assure that any preparation they suggest or provide be prepared using proper standards and be tested to confirm they are free of contaminants. The remedies described below have all met these standards or have shown in laboratory testing that they do not contain pharmaceutical, pesticide or heavy-metal contaminants. If you are unsure, check with a local practitioner of Chinese medicine or call the pharmacy at a Chinese medical school.

Yunnan Paiyao (Yun Nan Bai Yao)

Also called "Yunnan White Medicine," this remedy is produced at the Yunnan Pai Yao Factory, in Kunming [Yunnan] China. This secret formula, passed down through a family in China, is an excellent remedy for postpartum bleeding. Some authorities warn never to use it while the baby is still inside, as it can seriously reduce the blood flow to the uterus. Yunnan Paiyao is supplied in a 4 g bottle of powdered herb or in packets of 16, 0.25 g capsules, the capsules being the most commonly found. A small red pill which is for torrential bleeding (such as from a gunshot wound), is include in the package and may be used for a gushing postpartum hemorrhage. The exact ingredients of this pill are undivulged but are described as herbs known to treat shock and restore consciousness.

The powdered form is preferable to the capsules for use in labor because you do not have to get the capsules out of the blister pack, and the herbs absorb more quickly when mixed in hot water. The bottle will have a little rubber stopper with a hollow neck. The small red pill mentioned above is wrapped in cotton and stuffed into the stopper neck. Be sure it doesn't fall out or get mixed into your dose when you pour out the powder. Use one-third of a vial (1.33 g) for each dose, mixed thoroughly into ¼ cup of hot water and have the mother drink it through a straw (this helps bypass the tongue, as the herbs are strongly flavored). If it is going to work, it works within 5 minutes at the most. A second dose is only rarely needed but can be given if bleeding has slowed but not stopped; the timing of the second dose is judged by the amount of bleeding. If you only have access to the capsules, pop them out of the blister pack and store them in a well-marked, dated, pill bottle. To mix one dose, open five 0.25 g capsules and pour the powder into hot water. The woman should not eat any broad beans, fish, or cold or sour foods during the 24 hours following administration (Edmonds, 2003)

The active ingredient in Yunnan Paiyao is an herb called *Panax notoginseng* or *Panax pseudoginseng* (San Qi). It is of the same genus as Chinese ginseng (*Panax ginseng*) but is a different species and should not be confused with American ginseng. Notoginseng, also known as pseudoginseng, has been shown to shorten thrombin time, thus the probable mechanism of action is in aiding blood clotting. An alternative to the brand from China, in a powdered raw form, is a product from Herbal Times Brand called Pseudoginseng Capsules.

Astragalus

Many companies provide an extract of the herb *Astragalus membranaceus* (Huang Qi) in small glass vials with honey. They often come ten glass vials to a box, including small straws to sip the remedy. The Plum Flower Brand Imperial Astragali Extract meets Australian GMP standards. An entire vial can be given to a woman to enhance energy, prevent fatigue, or to facilitate progress during a prolonged labor particularly when exhaustion is a factor that needs to be addressed or prevented. The liquid extract with honey is the most desired way to administer small, potent doses to a laboring woman whose digestion might not tolerate the taste or amount of decoction that would have to be administered to produce the same effect.

A laboring woman can drink a vial every hour or more often if her digestion will tolerate it. Astragalus is known as a "Qi tonifier," meaning that it confers energy, restores normal functioning, and enhances immune function. Its effects are wide ranging, and it is one of the safest herbs of this kind. Astragalus increases metabolic function, raising the energy level immediately. Its use is preferred over the use of similar extracts of ginseng root. Ginseng root has comparable effects on the metabolism when taken long-term, suggesting that it takes some time for ginseng to reach its optimal potential in this regard.

Panax ginseng (ren shen) or Chinese ginseng

This is a very powerful warming herb and is excellent for restoring the body's ability to hold blood. Ginseng can be carried as a root to make a decoction for every woman to drink immediately postpartum as a restorative or as a first-line remedy in case of postpartum hemorrhage. A decoction produces the strongest restorative to uterine function in case of hemorrhage from uterine atony. Gently simmer fifteen grams of ginseng root at a low boil in 2 to 3 cups of water for 90 minutes. Add water if needed. Start making the decoction as soon as active labor is well established, and then administer as much as a cup immediately after the baby is born.

When purchasing ginseng, it is important to ask the supplier if the ginseng has been tested for pesticides and fungicides. Purchase only ginseng that has been so tested. The form to purchase is Chinese (or "red") ginseng. American ginseng does not have the same properties.

Sorting through indications for Chinese herbs

The use of Chinese ginseng, rather than astragalus, for postpartum hemorrhage illustrates the difficulty in fully translating the actions and indications set forth in Chinese herbology into English. While astragalus confers energy immediately, ginseng is a more powerful restorative. A more powerful yang tonifier, such as ginseng, is indicated in the case of an extremely yin condition such as hemorrhage, either to treat it or prevent it, as it is the restoration of uterine contractility, a yang response, that is desired. When labor is prolonged, however, the use of an energy sustainer is required. In dysfunctional labor, when contractions have ceased or become weak, a decoction of ginseng is an appropriate remedy, if the taste can be tolerated. When the concern is exhaustion related to the length of labor rather than the strength of contractions, astragalus is more appropriate.

Acupressure and Acupuncture in Midwifery

Acupuncture involves inserting very fine needles into acupuncture points, or specific locations along meridians or energy channels in the body. There is a great deal of controversy about midwives needling acupuncture points, and in some states the use of acupuncture without a degree in Chinese medicine is illegal. Just as midwives have lobbied to use selected pharmaceuticals (such as oxytocin), we can lobby to be allowed to use a limited repertoire of acupuncture techniques during labor. If your legal situation does not allow you to use needles, keep in mind that any point that can be needled can also be stimulated with finger pressure, which, in some cases, is even more effective (Lowe, 2003).

Acupuncture equipment

Acupuncture needles: Acupuncture needles can be a valuable addition to the birth bag, although they will receive very limited use unless you are a practitioner of Chinese medicine. These specialized needles are single-use, sterile and disposable. They come in a wide variety of lengths and gauges. For use in neonatal resuscitation, 36 gauge (0.20 mm), which is the width of the needle, and 25 mm (1 in) length is sufficient. Purchase acupuncture needles that are packaged with a guide tube. The guide tube is slightly shorter than the needle and greatly helps with placement as well as regulating the depth of penetration during insertion.

Ear press needles: Ear press needles are tiny, short needles that can be used in place of finger pressure to stimulate a point without inserting a longer, deeper needle. They can be taped in place with IV paper tape or a similar product. Beccaria seeds are also used for this purpose and do not involve penetrating the skin.

Lancets: Standard blood lancets can be used to stimulate an acupuncture point to stop postpartum hemorrhage. (This is described in the chapter entitled "Immediate Postpartum Hemorrhage.")

General tips on inserting needles: The needle is attached to the guide tube by a plastic bridge or small plastic tab inserted in the top of the tube. Before use, twist the needle in the tube to break the plastic attachment or remove the colored plastic tab. Once you do this, you will have to hold the top of the needle together with the guide tube between your thumb and index finger or the needle will fall out. Place the needle and guide tube perpendicular to the insertion point, release the top of the tub and abruptly tap the top of the needle; this will result in the tip quickly penetrating the skin. The guide tube can then be lifted off the shaft and the needle inserted more deeply, or the point can be stimulated by twisting the needle with small movements only. It is a lot easier to do than to describe. Practice on an arm or leg of a willing volunteer before you have to insert a needle in an emergency.

Acupressure

Once the relevant point is located, apply firm, even pressure directly down into the point with your thumbs, index fingers, knuckles or elbows or an object with a small, blunt end such as the end of a wooden kitchen utensil. When using a finger, the force should be directed from your shoulder down your arm and through your finger, rather than from the finger alone, or you will quickly become tired. Aside from this adverse side-effect, acupressure can be surprisingly effective without the need to insert (or purchase) needles. Seabands™ (available at many pharmacies and health food stores) are elastic bands with a rounded button on one side that are used to apply pressure to a point wherever the bands can be placed. Seabands™ are designed to stimulate points at the wrist. Similar bands could be made to stimulate points on the leg, ankle or bottom of the foot.

Nomenclature variations

There are a few terminology variations among schools of Chinese medical training in the United States and Europe. For example, a five-element acupuncturist would label "Colon 4 " what Traditional Chinese Medicine practitioners would call "Large Intestine 4." There may also be slight variations in other names, depending upon the source. This could be confusing when cross-referencing sources, so it is something to be aware of. Also, British training programs use slightly different English names for meridians, but the energetics of the points are the same.

Locating the points

The Chinese system of point location uses individual body measurements with the finger length of the person as the criterion. These lengths are called cun, which is about an individual inch. These methods (also referred to as "identical measuring methods") are simple to determine but not quite as accurate as proportional measurement, which is a more precise technique. If your body build and that of the woman is similar, you can use your own fingers as a guide. If not, first find the woman's cun by taking the following measurements.

Measure her middle finger: Measure the distance between the two creases of the joints of the distal and middle phalanges of the middle finger (the middle section) as one cun.

Measure her thumb's width: The width of the first joint of the thumb is taken as one cun. Average this measurement with that of the first, to arrive at one average cun.

Measure her fingers together (excluding the thumb): Measure the breadth of the four fingers held straight out and together at the level of the second joint of the middle finger. This equals three cun.

Recognizing the point: This depends upon the surrounding anatomy. The point itself generally feels subtly different (often softer or indented) than the region around it and is often tender to pressure. When the point is stimulated, the response of the Qi can often be detected by a change in the way the point feels. How this manifests is unique to each individual and may vary from point to point. There may also be a communicating sensation that runs along the entire meridian when a point is stimulated. This is often described as a subtle vibration, flow of energy or electric zapping sensation by the person being treated and can sometimes be felt by the person providing the treatment as well.

The following chart will detail the relevant facts regarding the 15 points mentioned in this text. For ease of study and comparison, they are all listed in anatomical order from head to toe. These points can be stimulated with finger pressure or needles. The use of these points will be further discussed throughout the text; however, the details regarding how to locate each one will not be repeated.

Note that most of the following points should not be used during pregnancy prior to term, as they may induce premature labor or have other undesirable effects.

Anatomical Location of Point	Descriptive Location	Actions and Notes
Points located on the head, shoulders, arms and hands		
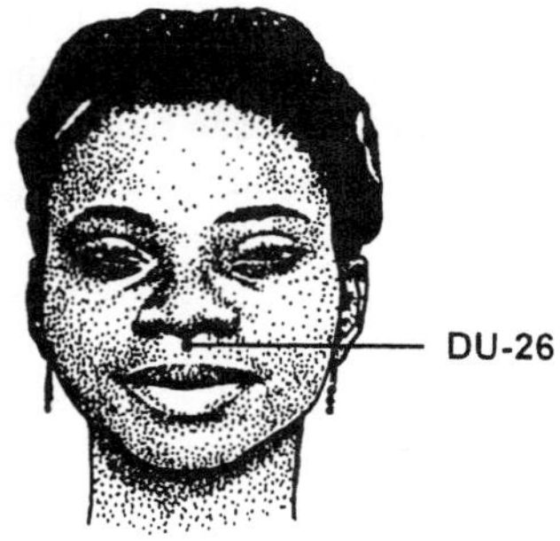	Renzhong (Man's Middle) Governing vessel (DU or GV) 26 Above the upper lip on the midline at the junction of the upper third and lower two-thirds of the philtrum (i.e., two-thirds of the way above the upper lip)	Restores consciousness, calms spirit. Resuscitation point, can revive a woman who has fainted or is shocky, fearful or hypertensive. Assists in reviving a baby who is not breathing.
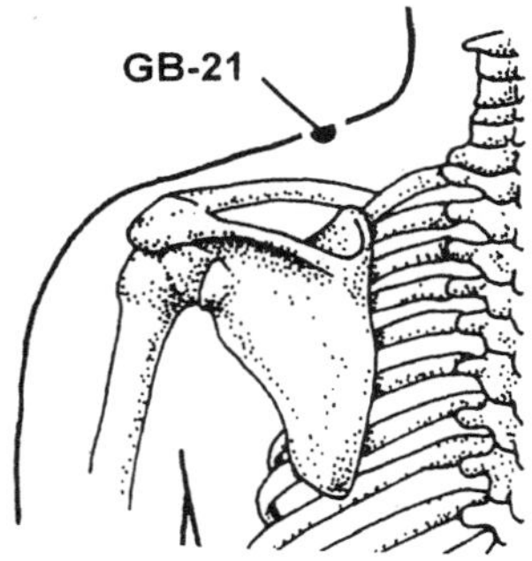	Jianjing (Shoulder Well) Gall Bladder (GB) 21 Draw a line from the center of the 7th cervical vertebra (uppermost prominence on the back of the neck when head is bent forward, moves slightly with turning the head) and the top of the shoulder bone (acromion process). GB-21 is midway between these points.	Descends Qi to strengthen labor and pushing contractions. Helps center a woman who is afraid, anxious or who is disassociating from her present reality (may be helpful in a history of sexual abuse). Relaxes the shoulders and relieves excessive labor pain. Helps descend the baby during labor and the placenta after birth. *Do not use this point prior to term.*
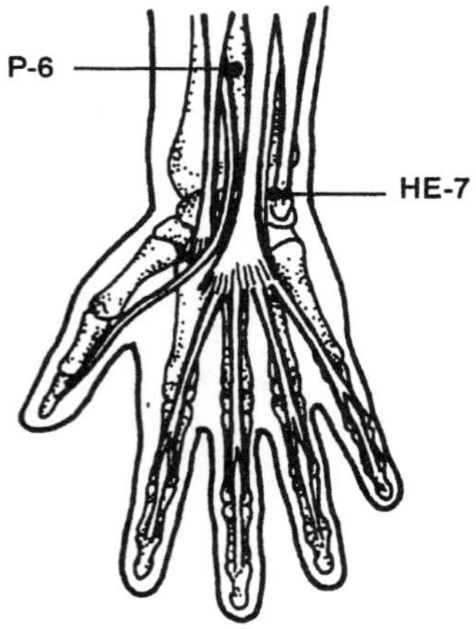	Neiguan (Inner Pass) Pericardium (P or Pc) 6 On the palmar surface of the hand, 3 of the woman's finger-widths above the transverse crease of the inner wrist, between the palmaris longus and flexor carpi radialis tendons.	Relieves nausea and vomiting; Sea Bands™ wrist bands can be used to stimulate these points as well as acupressure.
	Shenmen (Spirit Gate) Heart (HE) 7 On the palmar surface of the wrist joint, below the heel of the hand on the radial (little finger) side, in the depression on the inner border of the pisiform bone.	Calms the spirit; regulates and tonifies the heart; relieves symptoms of shock such as restlessness, disorientation, agitation, fright, difficulty breathing, shortness of breath and shivering.
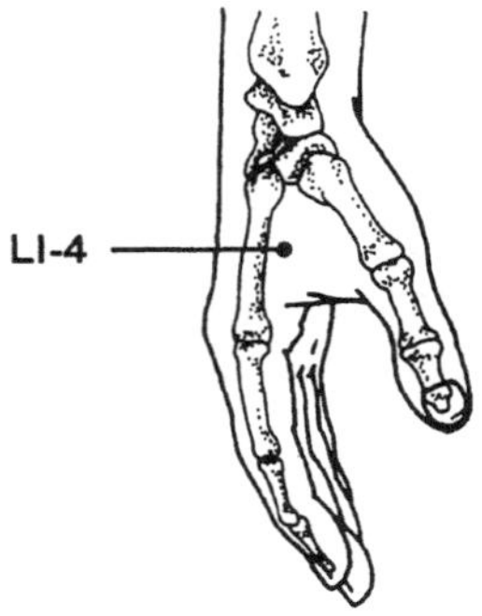	Hegu (Joining Valley) Large Intestine (LI) 4 or Colon (Co) 4 Point located between the first and second metacarpal bones in the pad above the crotch of the thumb and forefinger.	Increases frequency and intensity of contractions while decreasing sensations of pain. Best point to use to assist with pushing. Descends the baby during labor and the placenta after birth. Traditionally used with Sp-6. *Do not use this point prior to term.*

Anatomical Location of Point	Descriptive Location	Actions and Notes
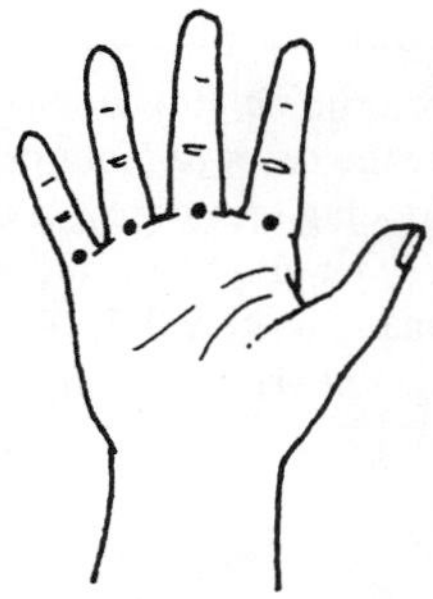	Hand points Referred to as "extra points" these are located in the crease formed where the fingers join the palm.	Stimulation helps release endorphins and therefore assists with pain management.
Points located on the abdomen and in the pelvic region		
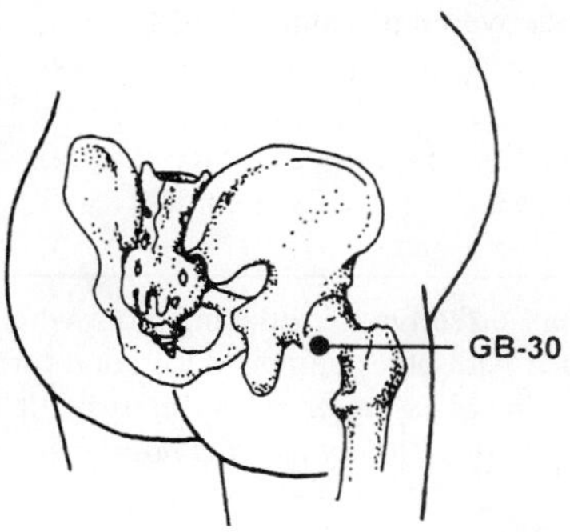	Huantiao (Jumping Circle) Gall Bladder (GB) 30 Draw a horizontal line from the top of the gluteal crease along the side of the body below the iliac crest; press along this line until you hit a tender point overlying the posterolateral region over the ball joint of the femur.	Used to help loosen up pelvic energy to encourage labor.
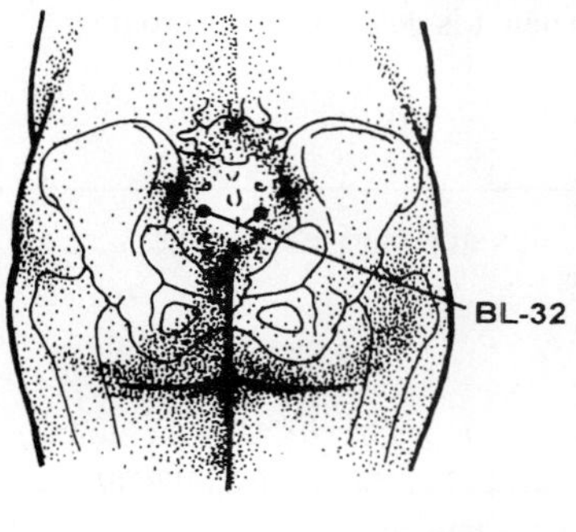	Ciliau (Second Crevice) Urinary Bladder (BL) 32 Centered between the inferior margin of upper sacral dimple of the rhomboid of Venus and the spine on either side of the rhomboid of Venus, overlying the second sacral foramen. (Or one of the person's index finger-widths above the top of the gluteal crease and one of her thumb-widths lateral to the outer border of the spinal vertebrae).	For delayed labor, affects the uterus, enhances dilation as well as relieving or preventing radiating pain in the sacrum and lower back. Can be stimulated with pressure, needles or sterile water injections. See the chapter entitled "Sterile Water Injections for the Relief of Excessive, Localized Pain."
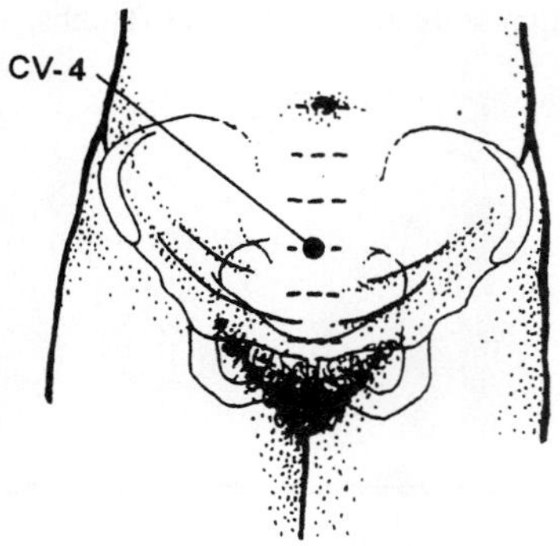	Guanyuan (Gate of Origin) Conception vessel (CVor REN) 4 Midline of lower abdomen, 3 cun below the navel and 2 cun above the symphysis.	Regulates the uterus and moves the blood; use for retention of urine, retained placenta, abdominal pain after birth. *Do not use this point prior to term.*

Anatomical Location of Point	Descriptive Location	Actions and Notes
Points located on the lower leg and foot		
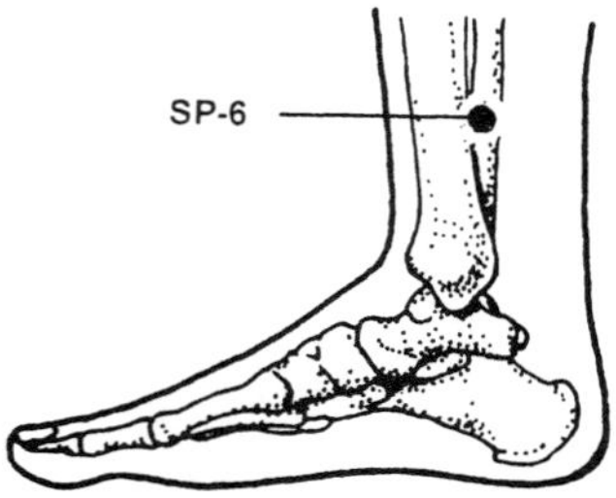	Sanyinjiao (Three Yin Intersection) Spleen (SP) 6 On the inner surface of the leg, 4 cun above the tip of the little prominence behind the inner, upper ankle.	Good for priming the uterus, may stimulate the onset of labor or enhance labor-inducing techniques, use for difficult labor and to assist dilation. Traditionally used with LI-4. *Do not use this point prior to term.*
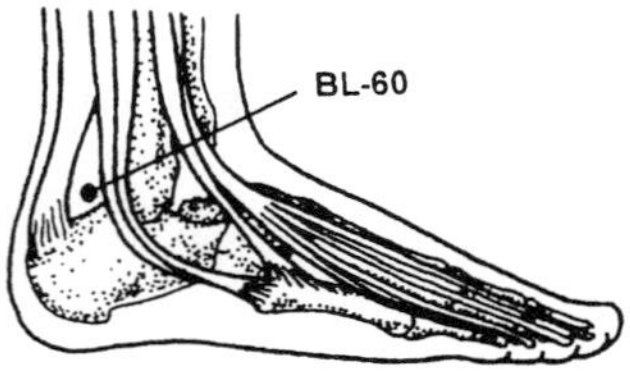	Kunlun (Kunlun Mountain) Urinary Bladder (BL) 60 On the outer side of the ankle in the depression between the prominence of the ankle and the Achilles tendon.	Helps downward movement: used for undetached placenta or retained but undelivered placenta
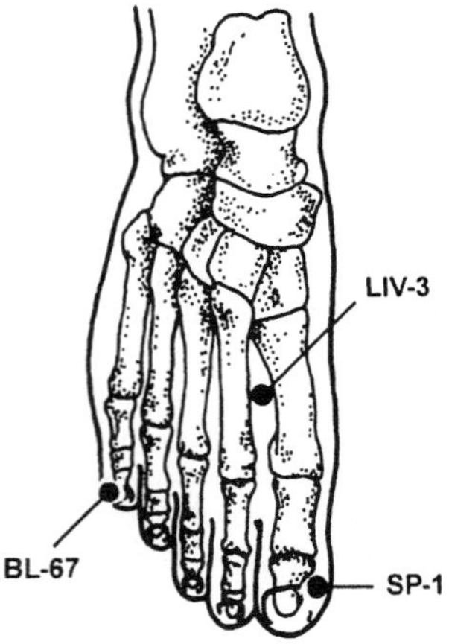	Taichong (Great Rushing) Liver (LIV) 3 Between the big toe and the next toe on the top of the foot in the depression below the junction of the 1st and 2nd metatarsal bones.	Very effective for inducing labor when used with other points. Also good for uterine bleeding or prolapse; difficult urination. *Do not use this point prior to term.*
	Zhiyin (Reaching Yin) Urinary Bladder (BL) 67 Lower outer corner of small toe at the base of the nail on either side.	Useful for correcting the fetal position when it is delaying labor progress
	Yinbai (Hidden White) Spleen (SP) 1 Near base of big toenail at the medial corner of the nailbed, 1/10 of an inch medial and proximal to the nail root.	Helps stop uterine bleeding.
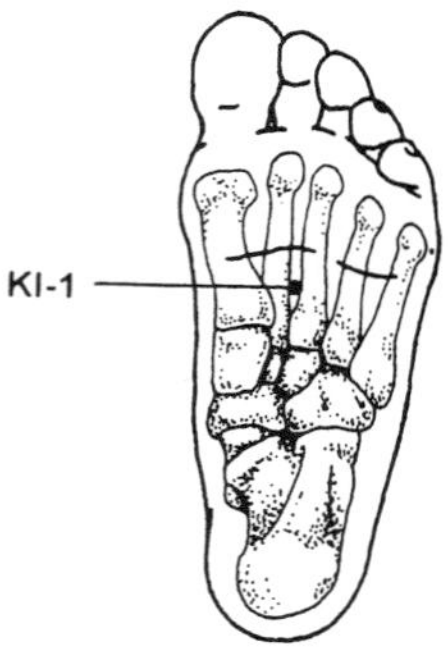	Yongquan (Gushing Spring) Kidney (KI) 1 On the sole of the foot, between the 2nd and 3rd metatarsal bones, about ⅓ the distance between the base of the second toe and the heel. Plantar flex the toes (toward the sole of the foot). Point lies in the central depression.	Helps with perineal relaxation during pushing. Resuscitation point for use with nonbreathing newborns (Hobbs, 2002).

Books and Readings on Chinese Medicine

ACUPUNCTURE IN MIDWIFERY by Sharon Yelland, Books for Midwives Press, Hale, Cheshire, UK, 1996. Its disappointingly general but a good introduction to what acupuncture can do for pregnancy and laboring women.

ACUPUNCTURE IN PREGNANCY AND CHILDBIRTH by Zita West, Churchill Livingstone, Edinburgh, UK, 2000. This book is aimed at acupuncturists who wish to know more about the application of acupuncture in maternity care but is written clearly enough that one need not be trained in Chinese medicine to gain a lot from studying it.

A MANUAL OF ACUPUNCTURE by Peter Deadman and Mazin Al-Khafaji. The point bible with complete, well-written descriptions of every point and meridian. This text is technical but still accessible for those with a basic understanding of Chinese medical theory.

NATURAL PAIN RELIEF TECHNIQUES FOR CHILDBIRTH USING ACUPRESSURE: PROMOTING A NATURAL LABOUR AND PARTNER INVOLVEMENT by Debra Betts. Debra is a New Zealand acupuncturist who has very generously explained how to use a variety of acupuncture points in late pregnancy and labor. This practical and succinct manual is designed for couples and is available free on the Web. The following link takes you to her homepage: http://home.clear.net.nz/pages/debra_betts/. Look to the left and click on "download booklet" to view and print this manuscript (you will need Adobe Acrobat Reader). It prints out in booklet form and is easy to place in a folder and carry in your birth bag. You can start with no background in Chinese theory and still make good use of all of Debra's manuals. They are the best place to start if you want to use Chinese medicine right away.

INFORMATION FOR MIDWIVES by Debra Betts. This is the midwifery-level version of the information included in the manual for parents. It can be downloaded from http://home.clear.net.nz/pages/debra_betts/Info4Midwives.

INFORMATION FOR ACUPUNCTURISTS by Debra Betts can be downloaded at http://home.clear.net.nz/pages/debra_betts/Info4Acupuncturists.htm. This is aimed at acupuncturists but also has interesting tidbits of information that are not included in the other manuals and is very accessible reading for those who are not acupuncturists.

OBSTETRICS AND GYNECOLOGY IN CHINESE MEDICINE by Giovanni Maciocia, Churchill Livingstone, New York, NY, 1998. This is a highly technical textbook aimed at Chinese practitioners. Comprehension requires a thorough background in Chinese theory.

(Thanks to Valerie Hobbs LAc, Dean of the Denver School of Chinese Medicine, long-time midwife and old friend and to Catherine Lowe, CNM, LAc, for much of the content of this chapter on Chinese medicine. Also with reference to Betts, 2002; Deadman & Al-Khafaji, 1998; Maciocia, 1989 & 1998; Rizack & Trinidad, 1992; Yelland, 1996; West, 2001; Wolfe, 1993.)

ALLOPATHIC PHARMACOLOGIC AGENTS FOR TREATING UTERINE ATONY

Many midwives are familiar with a variety of complementary therapies that are often successful at arresting hemorrhage. Most midwives also carry one or more antihemorrhagic drugs to use in the event that other therapies are ineffective. The knowledge base needed to administer these drugs is included in this chapter. The chapters dealing with the birth of the placenta and postpartum hemorrhage will also indicate when they should be used. An oxytocic is defined as anything that hastens childbirth; therefore all the drugs mentioned in this chapter can be broadly classified as such. Today, there are three basic types of antihemorrhagic drugs available: oxytocin, ergot derivatives and prostaglandins.

Some of these drugs are among just over a dozen that have been approved for use in obstetric care. None of the approved drugs have been proven safe for fetal exposure. There are no adequate, well-controlled studies to determine the long-term effects of any of these drugs on pregnant women or on the neurologic, as well as the general, development of offspring exposed in utero or during lactation (Haire, 2004a). The manufacturers have removed the FDA approved labeling for more than half of these drugs from the PHYSICIAN'S DESK REFERENCE (PDR) (Haire, 2004a). Listing in the PDA costs money and manufacturers frequently remove labeling for drugs whose patents have expired and fund the listing of newer drugs that are still under patent, and therefore make the most money (Pozner, 2004).

Oxytocin (generic form [American Pharmaceutical Partners]), Pitocin [Monarch Pharmaceuticals], Syntocinon [Wyeth-Ayerst Pharmaceuticals])

Before the advent of prostaglandins, ergot, then quinine and later oxytocin were the only drugs used to induce or augment labor. Among these agents, oxytocin is still used to augment labor and remains the most commonly used drug in the treatment of postpartum hemorrhage. Oxytocin is a polypeptide consisting of nine amino acids and is one of two neurohormones released by the posterior pituitary gland. Natural secretion is enhanced by an increase in plasma osmolarity and suppressed by alcohol consumption, hence the observation that alcohol given to the mother may, at times, stop premature labor. The uterine muscle becomes increasingly sensitive to the effects of oxytocin as term approaches and the number of uterine oxytocin receptors rises. Oxytocin is an agonist, that is, it works by linking with these receptor sites on the uterine muscle. Oxytocin stimulates uterine contractions during pushing and placental delivery, and administering it during labor apparently augments contractions, although exactly how this occurs is not fully understood. It also appears to increase local prostaglandin production. It has a potent action on the breast, stimulating milk letdown. Oxytocin is released in women and men during stress and sexual activity; Michel Odent calls it the "love hormone." It is inexpensive and generally effective as an antihemorrhagic agent with a long history of use and a good safety record when used appropriately.

Oxytocin is one of the drugs that have been approved for use in obstetric care. Oxytocin is approved for use in the medically indicated induction and augmentation of labor (i.e., not elective). The FDA approved labeling for all three products listed above has been removed from the PDR (Haire, 2004a).

Packaging and strength

Oxytocin is supplied in individual-use ampules, single- and multi-use vials, and prefilled syringes. The strength of oxytocin is expressed in United States Pharmacopeia units, also known as USP. In the United States, each unit equals about 2 µg of pure hormone. The amount of drug in each milliliter of solution varies according to the country in which it is sold and may be in either 5 or 10 units/ml increments. Pitocin (Monarch) contains 0.5% chlorbutanol, a chloroform derivative, as a preservative and may contain up to 25% of total impurities. Check package inserts for other products for preservative information.

In the United States, it is usually sold as a generic drug by its chemical name oxytocin or under the brand name Pitocin (often referred to as "Pit") and Syntocinon. It typically comes in individual ampules containing 10 units each.

Syntocinon is the most commonly used synthetic oxytocin in Europe and England. It is available in individual 1 ml ampules containing either 3 or 5 units of oxytocin each, and in 1 or 2 ml ampules containing 10 units of oxytocin each.

Metabolism

Oxytocin is quickly taken up from the plasma and metabolized in the liver by the enzyme oxytocinase. The plasma half-life of oxytocin ranges from 1 to 6 minutes; the half-life shortens as pregnancy advances. Half-life is the length of time it takes the body to eliminate half of a substance through metabolism and excretion. When oxytocin is given IV, the effect lasts approximately 1 hour; the effect of an intramuscular injection lasts 2 to 3 hours.

Action and effects

Oxytocin links to receptor sites on the uterine muscle. It stimulates rhythmic contractions of the uterus, increases the frequency of existing contractions and raises the tone of the uterine muscle. Oxytocin is capable of eliciting graduated increases in uterine muscle activity, resulting in a moderate increase in the rate and force of spontaneous motor activity. If oxytocin is used in excess or if women are hypersensitive to its effects, it can produce sustained (tetanic) contractions.

When compared to vasopressin (the other hormone produced by the posterior pituitary gland), oxytocin appears to produce a much weaker constrictive effect on the vasculature of the mesentery, stomach, pancreas and intestines, kidneys and skeletal muscle as well as the carotid and hepatic arteries. However, as tone increases, the stage is set for relaxation of the vessels of the mesentery, stomach, pancreas and intestines and skeletal muscle arteries in particular, accounting for the hypotension and increased diuresis that can be induced when high dosages are given IV (Altura & Altura, 1984).

With respect to the vasculature in the placenta and umbilical cord, oxytocin appears to have a more potent constricting effect, even at levels know to be present in term pregnancy. This suggests oxytocin may play a role in the closure of the umbilical vessels after birth (Altura & Altura, 1984).

Stability and storage

Oxytocin is remarkably stable at all temperatures, even if exposed to light. It should be clear, colorless and free of particulate matter. Glass ampules completely seal out air and preserve sterility, making them the best choice for the longest preservation of any drug. However, it is wise to replace ampules by their expiration date, since you want the oxytocin to work reliably when you do choose to use it. Plastic, rubber-topped vials are more prone to air entry and can deteriorate more rapidly; they should be kept cool but not refrigerated.

Routes of administration

The first medical use of oxytocin involved soaking a cotton pledget with the drug and placing it in the nostril. It has also been administered in dry form as a snuff powder for the mother to inhale. Buccal wafers impregnated with 200 to 400 μg of oxytocin and placed either inside the cheek or under the tongue were used for decades to induce or stimulate labor; buccal oxytocin was removed from the market in the midsixties because of its unpredictable action. A liquid preparation has been sprayed into the nasal passages to be absorbed by mucous membranes, although absorption is rather sporadic. The nasal spray is still in use to stimulate a letdown reflex during lactation. All methods that involve absorption through mucous membranes are unpredictable in their action on the uterus during labor, and some women have a hypersensitive response that cannot be immediately reversed. Oxytocin is not effective when administered via the digestive tract. Today, oxytocin is administered during labor via the IV route (described below). After birth, it may be given as an intramuscular injection or diluted in an IV and given with or without an infusion pump.

Use during labor

Oxytocin is said to act primarily on the uterine fundus with less effect on the lower uterine segment (although this property is not documented in the pharmacologic literature). Perhaps this statement is related to the understanding that oxytocin produces rhythmic contractions resembling those of normal labor in that they build, peak and subside, although they are typically more abrupt and sharper than natural contractions. It causes the uterine muscle fibers to retract and relax, as occurs in natural labor. When oxytocin is given diluted in an intravenous solution during spontaneous labor, about 90% of women will respond with contractions of increased intensity and about 75% will respond with increased frequency of contractions. This is the drug of choice for stimulating labor at term; however, it is a powerful agent and a tiny amount can have devastating effects in hypersensitive women.

Oxytocin crosses the placenta and enters the fetal blood stream within seconds or minutes. During labor, oxytocin augmentation may produce adverse reactions in the baby such as abnormal fetal heart rate patterns, low 5 minute APGAR scores, neonatal jaundice, retinal hemorrhage, central nervous system damage and death. These problems are related to hyperstimulation of the uterus and the constrictive effects of oxytocin on umbilical vessels. In addition, researchers are now questioning if fetal exposure contributes to the development of autism after birth, although it is hard to separate the effects of the oxytocin from the epidural drugs, such as bupivacaine (brand name, Marcaine [the labeling for which has removed been from the PDR]), that frequently precipitate the need for uterine stimulation (Haire, 2004b).

When used for augmentation, oxytocin is most safely provided in a very dilute dose via an IV infusion pump, a device that carefully regulates the amount of solution the mother is receiving and that can be discontinued immediately if necessary. It is not without consequences, however. The drip is started and the dose is typically doubled every half-hour until the desired contraction pattern is achieved. Kelly and colleagues (1974) (assuming a drug half-life of 3 to 5 min), estimated that a woman receiving 32 mU/min of synthetic oxytocin will have blood levels of 40,000 mU/ml, 130 to 570 times more than during natural labor (70 to 300 mU/ml). This severely disrupts the mother's hormonal milieu. In labor, oxytocin rises during pushing to prepare her to fall in love with her baby; first circulating to areas of her brain and then her body. Synthetic oxytocin given into the blood stream cannot enter her brain. Thus it cannot replace naturally released oxytocin to perform this vital preparation for bonding and grossly disrupts the natural process, whenever it is given (other hormonal drugs are likely to have similar disruptive effects). Synthetic oxytocin does however, provide negative feedback. When the posterior pituitary detects high levels, it slows production, leaving women at risk for postpartum bleeding when the IV is turned off (Buckley, 2004).

In addition, hypersensitive uterine reaction or excessive dosage can both result in hypertonic and often prolonged contractions. This can reduce the amount of oxygen that reaches the baby and risks uterine rupture. Whenever the duration of stimulated contractions exceeds 90 seconds and they are coming more frequently than every two minutes, the oxytocin infusion should be discontinued immediately (Buckley, 2004).

No amount of oxytocin, no matter how small, should ever be injected directly into a laboring woman. Because some women are far more sensitive to its effects than others, even a tiny amount can produce contractions so long and intense as to endanger the baby and risk uterine rupture. In addition, the effect of oxytocin lasts much longer when injected, and there is no way to "turn it off." Thus contractions that are too intense will take some time to calm back down.

Assisting placental delivery and controlling postpartum bleeding

Use of oxytocin with the birth of the first shoulder: In some settings in Europe and England, 5 U of Syntocinon are commonly given prophylactically as an intramuscular injection after the birth of the anterior shoulder to speed placenta delivery and prevent excessive bleeding after the birth. This approach to the delivery of the placenta is highly controversial, and I do not recommend it. The assumption is that women cannot produce sufficient oxytocin to proceed with a physiologic placental delivery. Institutions should be asking themselves why mothers cannot produce sufficient oxytocin on their own, rather than imposing yet another intervention. (Delicate hormonal responses are disrupted by numerous features of routine institutional care.)

Giving IM oxytocin with the anterior shoulder may result in overstimulation of the uterus, leading to premature separation of the placenta, and may cause the uterus to clamp down on the baby. If there is a second twin, that baby would be placed in grave danger for the same reasons. If the cord is still intact, the strong uterine contractions may result in a temporary overtransfusion of placental blood to the baby. The baby may also receive some of the oxytocin as well. Once the baby is born, the effect of receiving a small amount of synthetic oxytocin is probably negligible, since both baby and mother produce copious amounts of oxytocin during labor and since babies who have accidently been given a full dose have had no apparent side-effects (O'Grady, 1998).

Intramuscular route: After the birth, if bleeding is heavy and the placenta is not coming, intramuscular oxytocin can be given. It is widely stated that there is little risk that the cervix will close down and trap the placenta because oxytocin acts primarily on the fundus. The strong rhythmic contractions it produces can often help detach the placenta.

Oxytocin can also be given intramuscularly once the placenta is born, if bleeding remains heavy. Because oxytocin is believed to have its strongest action on the fundus, it is most helpful when the placenta has been implanted in or near the upper portion of the uterus. (See the chapter entitled "Examining the Placenta" for details regarding how to determine where the placenta was implanted.) Ten units is the usual starting dose when given intramuscularly. It should take effect 3 to 7 minutes after administration and last 30 to 60 minutes.

Intravenous route: Oxytocin can be given diluted in solution and given IV to maintain a continuous level in the bloodstream to help deliver the placenta. Oxytocin is diluted by mixing 10 to 40 units into one liter of isotonic crystalloid IV solution such as lactated Ringer's (Hartman's in the UK) or normal saline infusion fluid and given intravenously without an infusion pump (5% dextrose should not be used, see below). Diluted oxytocin given via IV takes effect within one minute but has a shorter duration of effectiveness than when given IM. If you intend to use oxytocin to prevent a postpartum hemorrhage, mix 10 units into 1 liter of fluid after the placenta is born, or give 10 units as an intramuscular injection. To treat an active postpartum hemorrhage via an IV, start with 10 units in 1 liter of fluid and adjust the rate of flow so that about 20 ml/minute is delivered to obtain a 200 mU/min dose of oxytocin (note that 10u/l = 10,000 mU/l = 10 mU/ml). Also see the subchapter entitled "Intravenous Equipment and IV Therapy."

Intraumbilical route: Oxytocin can also be injected into the umbilical vein, where it travels directly up the cord to the site of placental attachment. Wingeier and Griggs (1991) describe their procedure which begins with waiting for 30 minutes for the placenta to deliver spontaneously. Presumably, this wait occurs after the cord has been cut and the placental end clamped, although they make no mention of their protocol in this regard. If the placenta remains undelivered at 30 minutes, they mix 10 units of oxytocin with 20 cc of normal saline and inject it directly into the umbilical vein. They immediately clamp the cord below (distal to) the puncture site and await placental delivery within 5 minutes. Although they do not mention it, reverse milking of the cord would likely speed delivery of the oxytocin to the placental site. If the placenta remains undelivered after 5 minutes, they proceed with a manual removal. Intraumbilical administration requires the cord to be clamped and cut, a practice which, by itself, leaves the placenta engorged with blood and can delay its delivery. In addition, intraumbilical oxytocin is most effective when residual blood is in the umbilical vein, necessitating early clamping, which interferes with the baby's postnatal transition. For these reasons, it is not recommended.

Intramyometrial route: If massive postpartum bleeding occurs after the placenta is born and if circulatory collapse has occurred, the Society of Obstetricians and Gynecologists of Canada (SOGC) guidelines describe giving oxytocin intramyometrially (IMM) as an injection through the abdominal wall directly into the uterine muscle (aspirate before injecting to be sure you are not in a vein) (Schuurmans et al., 2000). This requires at least a 1.5 in needle to achieve sufficient penetration to reach the uterus. This would be done at home only if the hemorrhage was extreme, other methods had failed to control it and you have confirmed that there is not a multiple gestation.

Side-effects of oxytocin use

In general, oxytocin is well tolerated physically; and only a very few minor side-effects are typically noted. These include occasional mild nausea and vomiting, as well as those discussed below.

Antidiuretic effects: The oxytocin molecule is similar to vasopressin (antidiuretic hormone, ADH), the other posterior pituitary neurohormone. Oxytocin also has pronounced antidiuretic effects, promoting water retention in the renal tubule. This is dose dependent and is seen at intravenous infusion rates of 10 mU per minute or more. It is most pronounced when oxytocin is given in large amounts, especially when given continuously by IV over a 24 hr period in a woman who is also taking fluids by mouth. Oxytocin given at rates of 20 mU/min significantly reduces maternal urinary output, and doses of 50 mU/min or more inhibit urinary output by 90%. Neonatal urinary output may also be reduced if an antidiuretic effect manifests during labor. The antidiuretic effect dissipates within 30 minutes of discontinuing the infusion.

The most common cause of a condition known as "water intoxication" in pregnancy is the administration of high concentrations of oxytocin. The risk is greatest when large doses of oxytocin are given mixed with electrolyte-free IV solutions, such as dextrose in water (D_5W), which promotes the progressive resorption of free water. Most cases of water intoxication do not manifest until at least 3.5 liters or more of hypotonic solution have been administered. This results in **hyponatremia**: low concentrations of circulating sodium ions in the bloodstream. This creates a hypoosmolar state, which leads to brain swelling and neurologic symptoms when the serum sodium levels fall below 120 to 125 mEq/L (mmol/L). The fall in sodium concentration exceeds the range predicted by blood volume dilution from the IV fluid alone. Other factors, such as sodium loss via the urine and into the cellular space are likely to play a role as well. This is one more reason never to use dextrose solutions in laboring or postpartum women (see the subchapter entitled "Intravenous Equipment and IV Therapy" for more details).

Water intoxication is easily prevented by close attention to total oral intake when an IV is in place, monitoring urinary output, and using only an isotonically balanced IV solution, such as lactated Ringer's for diluting oxytocin for IV administration. Avoid prolonged infusions of oxytocin concentrations exceeding 20 mU/min. Restriction of oral fluids while the IV is being given will help to avoid this complication as well. Treatment consists of restricting oral fluid intake, discontinuing the IV infusion as soon as water intoxication is suspected and transporting. Less commonly, the use of diuretic drugs or high sodium infusions may be required to correct this problem.

Water intoxication results in acute neurologic dysfunction. Nausea and vomiting followed by confusion and lack of mental clarity with or without seizures are the most frequent presenting symptoms. Other symptoms include headaches, disorientation, lethargy, coma, involuntary rhythmic oscillation of the eyes (either pendular or with a slow-and-fast component), convulsions, pulmonary edema, psychosis and death. Most of these manifestations mimic a toxic central nervous system effect. A history of the use of hypotonic IV solutions to dilute oxytocin for IV administration in a woman who was previously normal and who is now presenting with acute neurologic signs strongly suggests water intoxication, other possible causes being numerous but unlikely in the previously healthy woman. Early symptoms will rapidly progress to seizures, coma and death if prompt treatment is not provided. If you suspect water intoxication, transport should take place immediately.

Hypotension: Constant infusion of oxytocin prepared by dilution in a liter of solution and administering it intravenously within a physiologic dosage range not exceeding 20 mU/minute has little or no effect on the blood pressure. Constant infusion of very large doses diluted in solution results in a slight elevation of the blood pressure, which resolves as soon as the infusion is discontinued. Doses of up to 10 units of oxytocin given either intramuscularly or subcutaneously have no significant effect on the blood pressure.

However, when undiluted oxytocin is injected directly into a vein in a single dose (also called an "IV bolus" or "IV push" dose) it can cause a significant drop in blood pressure, as oxytocin is a potent vasodilator. As little as 2 units given directly into a vein can cause a 30 to 50 mm Hg drop in mean arterial pressure, with accompanying tachycardia, within 2 to 5 minutes of administration. Doses exceeding 2 units are followed by electrocardiographic changes consistent with hypoxia. IV bolus doses of only 5 units consistently produce a precipitous blood pressure drop within 20 seconds, reaching a nadir as quickly as 35 seconds (in one case, BP dropped from 115/60 to 72/38 at is lowest point). A feeling of warmth may also occur. Recovery takes place over the next 3 minutes with a small "overshoot" of blood pressure values above the original pressure; a subsequent return to normal pressure occurs within 10 minutes. The heart rate also increases rapidly as the blood pressure drops but takes more than ten minutes to return to a normal baseline. The pattern of blood pressure decrease and recovery is always the same, but the extent of the decrease is proportional to the amount of oxytocin given. It is obviously inappropriate to further reduce the blood pressure of a woman who is already at risk for shock due to blood loss. IV bolus administration also produces tetanic postpartum contractions. Oxytocin to control or prevent postpartum hemorrhage should only be given either by intramuscular injection or be diluted in solution and administered by controlled intravenous infusion (slow drip). Bolus intravenous doses should never be used (Hendricks & Brenner, 1970; Sultatos, 1997).

Uterine rupture: Uterine rupture is extremely rare when oxytocin is given during labor in appropriate doses via a controlled IV infusion pump to a woman with a normal, unscarred uterus. The risk of rupture rises considerably when oxytocin is given in an uncontrolled fashion or when used in a laboring woman who is hypersensitive to its effects, whose uterus is scarred or who has experienced many pregnancies. Uterine rupture is virtually unheard of when oxytocin is given postpartum to a woman with an empty uterus.

Allergic reactions: Reactions to oxytocin-based drugs are exceedingly rare. Most of the very few on record can be traced to a reaction to chlorbutanol (a derivative of chloroform), which is widely used in injectable drugs as a bacteriostatic preservative. One case of allergy to oxytocin itself has been recorded.

Additional side-effects listed in the FDA approved labeling: Numerous additional maternal side effects are noted on the label, but little information is available about them. These include maternal hypertensive episodes, subarachnoid hemorrhage (bleeding around the spinal cord), cardiac arrhythmias and premature ventricular contraction, fatal afibrinogenemia, pelvic hematoma, increased blood loss, convulsions and coma (Haire 2004a).

Accidental administration to the baby: Accidental administration of oxytocin to the newborn should never happen at home. This has occurred in hospitals when a prefilled syringe of oxytocin has been used instead of a syringe containing a neonatal medication. Giving the newborn baby oxytocin has no apparent short-term effect but, of course, should be avoided. Never draw up a Vitamin K injection prior to its immediate use and always store your neonatal drugs separately from uterotonic drugs.

Ergot Alkaloids

Ergot is produced by a parasitic ascomycetous fungus, *Claviceps purpurea*, which is a pathogen of rye grass and certain other grains. The fungus transforms rye seeds into a compact, spur-like mass containing five or more pairs of alkaloids. These alkaloids enhance the muscle tone of the uterus as well as producing frequent, rhythmic contractions. The myometrial cells are stimulated to contract, which compresses the uterine blood vessels, adding to the efficiency of this drug as a hemorrhage-abating agent. However, this action makes its use during labor dangerous for the fetus because it cuts off blood flow to the uterus over and above the reduction that occurs during normal labor contractions. Traditionally, ergot has also been credited as having more effect on the lower uterine segment than oxytocin, making its use in labor more dangerous for the mother (although this action on the lower segment is not documented in the pharmacologic literature [Pozner, 2004]). It's recognized tendency to more easily produce tetanic contractions may be the origin of this statement. Pronounced contraction of the lower segment or tetanic contraction can both obstruct descent and invite uterine rupture because the lower segment needs to relax and dilate. As is true for oxytocin, the mechanism of its action is still not fully understood.

Ergot is the oldest and most widely used oxytocic substance in the West. Its ability to stimulate the uterus has been recognized by midwives and doctors for at least 2000 years and probably longer. However, by 1822 ergot's actions were better understood and the danger it poses to the fetus was recognized. By the end of the 1800s, it was no longer used during labor. Ergot and its derivatives are now used to control bleeding after birth or abortion and to alleviate certain localized vascular disorders (such as migraine headaches) in nonpregnant persons.

Forms

Ergot comes in several degrees of purification. Ergot-based drugs are well absorbed when given orally and are also used intramuscularly when treating postpartum uterine atony.

Ergotrate maleate (ergonovine maleate): This less-refined pharmaceutical form of ergot was removed from the US market in 2001. It is still available in some countries. The descriptions given for all ergot-based drugs can be applied to Ergotrate maleate as well.

Ergometrine (ergonovine): Ergometrine is similar to Ergotrate. It is available in England and other countries.

Methergine (methylergonovine maleate) by Novartis and Sandoz: This semisynthetic ergot alkaloid is available in the United States and other countries. It is intended to be used for postpartum hemorrhage only. It is sold in sterile 1 ml ampules containing 0.2 mg methylergonovine maleate for use as an intramuscular or an intravenous injection. Methergine is also prepared in a 0.2 mg oral dose as a coated, orchid-colored tablet with "78-54" imprinted on one side and "SANDOZ" on the other. Methergine is more refined than Ergotrate and carries a slightly lower risk of adverse effects.

Methergine is metabolized in the liver and has a half-life of .95 to 2 hours, with peak plasma concentrations occurring within 60 to 90 minutes.

Methergine is approved for use in obstetric care and is indicated for use only after the birth of the anterior shoulder. Its FDA approved labeling has also been removed from the PDR (Haire, 2004a).

Packaging

Ergot-based drugs are supplied in tablets or single-dose ampules. Potency varies according to the country in which it is manufactured.

Actions and effects

Ergot alkaloids are known to act on at least three different types of receptors in the body. Eleven alkaloids and 14 alkaloidal complexes have been isolated from ergot, all of which are built upon a basic nucleus, lysergic acid. Only three of these active alkaloids have made their way into clinical use: ergotoxine, ergotamine and ergometrine. Of these three, ergometrine (Ergotrate, ergonovine) proved the most useful. It has the smallest molecule and acts the most rapidly. Its action persists for up to an hour, after which a second dose will renew its effects.

While oxytocin primarily stimulates uterine contractions, ergots have two primary effects: vasoconstriction and uterine contraction. Its vasoconstrictive action primarily targets dilated arteries. Ergot-alkaloid drugs also act directly on the smooth muscle in the uterus to increase the tone, rate and amplitude of rhythmic contractions until, for all practical purposes, they create a tetanic or sustained contraction. This tetanic effect is dose dependent, with higher doses producing stronger, more sustained contractions. The vasoconstrictive action of ergometrine and methylergometrine, both of which are pharmaceutically similar, is less than that of other ergot alkaloids.

The rapid and sustained tetanic uterotonic effect induced by ergot can shorten the time it takes for the placenta to deliver and can reduce blood loss. As compared to other oxytocic drugs, the lower segment has been said to be more influenced by the action of ergot. Ergot is thought to produce a more total uterine contraction involving the myometrium from the fundus to the cervix. *Because of its possible action on the lower uterine segment, its vasoconstrictive effects, and the more sustained contractions it tends to produce, it should never be used during labor.* Such use could produce an arrest in labor, uterine rupture and fetal demise because there is insufficient relaxation of the uterine muscle between contractions and because its action on the lower uterine segment may interfere with normal dilation.

Metabolism

Ergot-based drugs are metabolized by the liver; the reported half-life ranges from 30 minutes to 2 hours.

Indications

The best use of ergot-based drugs is for postpartum hemorrhage that oxytocin cannot control or in a woman known to have had a low-lying placenta. Its dual action (vasoconstriction and uterine contraction) make it an excellent drug to follow oxytocin. Methergine can be given either as an intramuscular injection or orally after the placenta has delivered. Using ergot before the placenta has been born could result in it becoming trapped because ergot acts so strongly on the lower segment. In addition, the tetanic contraction it tends to produce does not facilitate moving the placenta down and out. Therefore, ergot-based drugs should be given before placental delivery only if oxytocin has been used without effect and the situation is dire, with bleeding so profuse you believe the mother's life to be in danger. In such cases, the primary goals would be to control bleeding as effectively as possible and to get the woman to the hospital for treatment.

Administration

Ergot-based drugs can be given by the intramuscular, intravenous-bolus or oral route. The use of ergot-based drugs in an IV bolus should be reserved for rapid bleeding that oxytocin will not adequately control as this route carries a slightly higher risk of side-effects. When an IV bolus is deemed appropriate, each milliliter of drug should be diluted in 4 ml of normal saline to allow for more controlled administration over the 60 seconds you should take to inject it into a vein. It is best to start an IV first and give the IV bolus into the injection port nearest the puncture site.

Commonly used dosages of ergot-based drugs vary between the United Kingdom and the United States, with the US tending to use lower doses. The Society of Obstetricians and Gynecologists of Canada (SOGC) guidelines describe using Methergine IM in 0.25 mg doses as often as every 5 minutes to a maximum cumulative dose of 1.25 mg if bleeding is severe (Schuurmans et al., 2000). Severe hemorrhage can also be treated with Methergine given as an IV bolus in a 0.125 mg dose or given directly into the uterine muscle through the abdominal wall. This requires at least a 1.5 inch needle to penetrate to the uterus, and you would want to aspirate the syringe prior to injection to make sure you were not in a vein. The intramyometrial route is not to be used at home unless the situation is so severe that there is no other choice; the potential for side-effects is somewhat higher. The guidelines in the following table shows the similarity of use in different locales.

DRUG	ROUTE	DOSAGE	ACTIVE WITHIN	REPEAT
Ergometrine	IM	200 μg (US) 125 to 250 μg (UK)*	2 to 3 minutes	Every 2 to 4 hours, up to 5 doses, as indicated
	IV bolus	200 μg (US) 125 to 250 μg (UK) Diluted in 4 ml saline and given slowly over at least 60 seconds	As soon as 45 seconds	
	Oral	200 to 400 μg (US) 500 μg (UK)	5 to 15 minutes	3 times daily for 3 days (UK) 2 to 4 times daily up to 7 days (US)
Methergine	IM	200 μg	2 to 3 minutes	Every 2 to 4 hours, up to 5 doses, as indicated
	IV bolus	200 μg diluted in 4 ml saline and given slowly over at least 60 seconds	As soon as 45 seconds	
	Oral	200 μg	5 to 15 minutes	3 to 4 times daily up to 7 days

*In some countries such as Ireland, Ergometrine is supplied in ampules containing up to 500 mcg.

Stability and storage

Ergot preparations are unstable and tend to lose potency when stored at room temperature. Some researchers feel that Methergine is slightly more stable than ergometrine. Deterioration is most pronounced at higher temperatures and with exposure to light. Injectable forms may be refrigerated at a temperature of 35.6 to 46.4°F (2 to 8°C) for up to 3 years. Ampules can also be stored at temperatures up to 77°F (25°C) for up to two months when protected from light but then must be discarded.

Regardless of the storage procedure, each ampule should be checked for color by being held over a white background in glare-free natural light. Check ampules when they are first purchased to ensure potency. Check them again during equipment setup at the time of labor. Liquid preparations of ergot drugs are normally clear and colorless, with no particulate matter. The powdered form of Ergometrine is white to very pale yellow. The powdered form of Methergine is white to a pink-tan color. However, to the eye, in solution, these drugs appear colorless. Any suggestion of discoloration usually indicates that the solution contains less than 90% of the stated amount of active ingredient and should not be used (Hogerzeil & Walker, 1996).

Oral tablets show significant loss of potency within weeks, beginning immediately after the tablets are removed from their sealed package or container. Loss of potency is enhanced by increased temperature and humidity. Oral tablets should be stored in their original container, out of the light, at a temperature below 77°F (25°C) and should be discarded if there is any evidence of discoloration or tablet deterioration as well as after the expiration date.

Contraindications

Women who have impaired liver or kidney function, heart or vascular disease, sepsis, severe hypertension, preeclampsia, eclampsia or a history of postpartum depression or psychosis should not be given any ergot-based drugs.

Adverse side-effects

All routes of administration can result in rare but serious side-effects. No more than 1.0 mg (1000 μg) of any ergot-based drug should be given in a single dose. Larger doses and IV administration are more likely to lead to adverse side-effects, including severe uterine cramping, headache, nausea, vomiting, abdominal pain, dizziness, and skin rashes. More rare are hypertension, bradycardia, cardiac arrhythmias and myocardial infarction, transient chest pains, labored breathing, thrombophlebitis, hematuria, water intoxication, asthmatic attack and fetal death (if used during labor). Psychotic effects occur in some women, a by-product of the lysergic acid ergot contains.

Ergotism is an adverse reaction characterized by peripheral vascular constriction. It begins with intense vasoconstriction in the extremities, resulting in tingling, numbness, muscle pain, pale and cool limbs, and weak or absent peripheral pulses. Necrosis and gangrene of the extremities eventually follow. Other rare side-effects include diarrhea, tinnitus (noises in the ears), chest pain, palpitations, brady- or tachycardia, coronary or renal artery spasm, cardiac arrest, respiratory depression, cerebral hemorrhage, convulsions and coma. Long-term use may interfere with lactation by reducing prolactin levels, although this tendency seems more pronounced with the use of ergonovine than with Methergine. Midwives should be prepared to treat allergic and anaphylactic reactions with epinephrine prior to transport whenever any drugs are used. See the chapter entitled "Hypersensitivity Reactions and Anaphylactic Shock" for more details.

Accidental administration to the baby

Mistakenly giving ergot alkaloids to the baby can cause severe complications such as convulsions and oliguria, as well as respiratory depression requiring mechanical ventilation. Convulsions precede apnea and both may present within the first hour after administration. Oliguria may present as late as 19 hours later. The baby would require hospital care and possible treatment with vasodilators. Hemoperfusion or dialysis may help to rid the baby's body of 20 to 50% of the drug within 6 hours, although these are drastic measures. Again, storing neonatal drugs separately from uterotonic drugs, making it a policy never to draw up Vitamin K for the baby ahead of time, and always verifying the labeling of any drug before it is opened eliminates the possibility of such an accident occurring in the home setting.

Oxytocin/Ergot Combination Drugs

Syntometrine is available in the United Kingdom, Europe, Australia and many other parts of the world but is not available in the United States. It is sold in 1 ml ampules containing 5 units of oxytocin (Syntocinon) and 0.5 mg (500 μg) of ergometrine maleate. The brand name for this product varies according to the manufacturer and the country in which it is distributed. The product may be called simply Syntometrine or Syntometrin E (Novartis). Syntometrin or

Syntometrin M (Novartis) contains 5 units of oxytocin and 500 µg of methylergonovine maleate. All these drugs have the same uses and the same basic actions. Check packaging to determine the exact combination and amounts of the drugs it contains. The ones containing methylergonovine can be expected to carry the least risk of ergot-related side-effects. The oxytocin acts within 2 to 3 minutes, and the ergometrine acts within 6 to 7 minutes when administered via intramuscular injection.

The oxytocin quickly produces a uterine contraction soon enhanced by a stronger, sustained contraction when the ergometrine kicks in and lasts approximately two hours. In hospitals in the UK, which practice "active management of third stage," 1 ml is often given IM at the end of pushing as the baby's first shoulder is born, to ensure that effective uterine contractions continue during the birth of the placenta. During the first few minutes, the oxytocin alone is active, producing a fundal contraction and allowing time for the baby to finish being born and the placenta to separate from the uterine wall. Then the ergometrine takes effect, producing a generalized contraction throughout more of the uterine muscle, theoretically reducing the risk of hemorrhage. In actual practice, use of Syntometrine in this fashion runs the risk of placental entrapment if the lower segment clamps down prior to the birth of the placenta. Prophylactic use of combination drugs containing oxytocin and ergot alkaloids during late pushing also increases the risk of separation of the placenta prior to completion of the birth, which poses a small but significant risk for the baby, especially in the event of subsequent shoulder dystocia. This is because, as the uterus becomes empty as the baby emerges, the placental site, which may shrink slightly, can become overstimulated with the drugs, and the placenta may hasten to detach, thus denying the baby optimal oxygen transport during the important period of fetal-to-neonatal transition. Giving drugs to a mother who intends to leave the cord intact until pulsing disappears at the baby's umbilical base may result in the baby receiving a tiny but significant amount. Syntometrine should never be given prior to the birth if the baby is breech or before all babies are out in a multiple birth because of these risks.

In a postpartum emergency, Syntometrine has also been given in a 0.5 to 1 ml dose via slow IV bolus injection over the course of at least 60 seconds (mixing the dose with 4 ml of normal saline prior to administration will make slow administration easier). The intravenous route is *not* recommended as it carries the same risk of inducing hypotension that oxytocin carries when given by itself via the IV-bolus route, plus all the other possible side-effects of IV ergometrine. The theory is that the oxytocin-induced hypotension will not have a chance to develop before the ergometrine affects the blood pressure by producing a rise. In practice, this is a tricky combination of side-effects to be dealing with outside of a hospital.

Prostaglandins

Prostaglandins are one branch of a large family of biologically active hormonal compounds derived from 20-carbon polyunsaturated fatty acids. Arachidonic acid, the most common precursor, undergoes a number of changes to yield compounds with alphanumeric designations according to chemical structure. Those of greatest interest in childbearing are the natural prostaglandins E_2 and $E_{2\alpha}$. Prostaglandins increase the levels of free intracellular calcium which contributes to the production of uterine contractions once labor is underway. However, their primary use in pregnancy is to ripen the cervix prior to labor induction or to empty the uterus during elective abortion or after fetal demise.

Most of the oxytocic prostaglandins have also been used successfully to treat uterine atony and stop severe postpartum hemorrhage after the placenta has been born. The success rate for cases which don't respond to oxytocin and ergot alkaloids is about 80 to 90% for all prostaglandins used. Prostaglandin analogues (carboprost, gemeprost, sulprostone and misoprostol) appear to cause fewer side-effects than natural prostaglandins. A variety of administration routes have been described depending upon the form of the drug used, including intrauterine douche, intramyometrial injection, transabdominal and intracervical injection, transyoni insertion, dilution in intravenous solution, intramuscular injection, and insertion of tablets in the yoni or rectum (Schellenberg, 1999).

A full understanding of the biologic function and action of these drugs has yet to be elucidated. No research has been done to ascertain how these drugs effect the tissue structure of the cervix or uterus, although it is known that profound tissue changes are induced by placing prostaglandin preparations against these tissues. Due to such uncertainties, they should be used with caution for postpartum hemorrhage only after all other means of stopping the bleeding have failed.

Misoprostol (Cytotec [Searle])

Misoprostol is a prostaglandin analogue. An **analogue** is a substance that differs in structure but is similar in function to other members of the same family of agents. Misoprostol has received quite a bit of press in these first years of the new century. It is dispensed in tablets containing either 100 μg or 200 μg of synthetic prostaglandin E_1 analogue. The drug has been FDA approved for oral use as a preventive treatment for gastric ulcers in certain populations, such as those who must take nonsteroidal anti-inflammatory drugs (NSAIDs), the elderly, those with accompanying debilitating conditions and others at high risk for developing gastric ulcers. It is designed to inhibit the secretion of gastric acid and therefore to protect mucosal tissues. It is also highly effective for stimulating the uterus.

In the United States, once a drug is approved for one use, physicians are free to prescribe that drug for any use they see fit, even if the drug has not been tested, found safe and effective, or approved for that use by the FDA. In the PHYSICIAN'S DESK REFERENCE (2000), misoprostol was initially specifically and prominently contraindicated for any use in pregnant women in multiple statements throughout the product description. However, misoprostol is highly effective at stimulating the uterus, especially when the woman is overdue and the cervix unripe. It has a profound action, producing dramatic cervical ripening as well as strong and sometimes intense uterine contractions. Because of its action on the uterus, in the 1990s misoprostol began to be widely used "off label" to induce or augment labor at term. While other prostaglandin products containing the E_2 form have been approved for use to induce labor by the FDA, they are expensive and require refrigeration. In contrast, misoprostol is cheap (about 50 cents a tablet), very stable, storable at room temperature and easy to use. Therefore, misoprostol is a very attractive alternative to managed health care plans trying to keep costs down. In some cases, before publicity about its dangers was widespread, it was given to women to self-administer for induction without medical or midwifery supervision. Some midwives have used it to induce or augment labor both at home and in the hospital.

Dangers and risks of use in labor: While misoprostol has not been through the FDA procedure required for approval for use as a labor stimulant, some obstetrician-led studies have been done. Most of these studies are small and do not address the topic systematically. They often do not look at uterine rupture, maternal death or perinatal morbidity or mortality but focus instead on dosage and the relative effectiveness of the route of administration (oral versus intrayoni) so we cannot be sure that all adverse events were reported. They compare the effectiveness of misoprostol with other prostaglandin compounds as well as with oxytocin rather than with a control group of an unstimulated population of laboring women. Because of all this, the possible adverse effects of misoprostol use have not been fully researched (meaning it is no different, in this respect, than any other drug used on pregnant women) (Gaskin, 2000).

You will recognize the oh-so-familiar tendency to rush headlong into using a drug that has not been proven safe and effective on laboring women and their babies. The behind-the-scenes experience of individual practitioners combined with the little bit of formal research that has been done shows that the use of misoprostol puts women and their babies in grave danger of serious complications.

Misoprostol use has been associated with uterine rupture. One study, by Plaut and colleagues (1999), found uterine rupture occurring in 5 of 89 women who had previous Cesarean scars and were induced with misoprostol. Of the induced women attempting a YBAC, 5.8% had a uterine rupture, compared with 0.2% of those who were not induced. In addition, a review of medical records uncovered several more ruptures associated with misoprostol that did not make it into the final analysis. In some cases, these have been ruptures of the posterior uterine wall, usually a rare event and possibly a result of placing the tablet in the posterior fornix. Ruptures have occurred with dosages ranging from 25 μg to 100 μg, in women receiving both singular and repeated doses. Most cases involved a tablet, or portion of a tablet, being placed in the yoni fornix. In some cases of catastrophic uterine rupture, misoprostol has been described as turning the lower segment to "jelly" (Gaskin, 2000). At a workshop on labor induction at the American College of Nurse Midwives' conference in Anchorage, Alaska, in May 2000, midwives came to the microphone to explain that they had felt changes in cervixes exposed to misoprostol that they had never felt before. "The cervix turned to mush" was how one midwife described it. How does this drug affect the ground substance of the cervix, and does it do permanent damage? No one knows.

The use of misoprostol in labor has also been consistently associated with an increase in meconium-stained amniotic fluid. Tetanic contractions are well known to jeopardize the baby as well as the mother. It is tempting to think such a simple pill might do no harm, especially since many of us know of cases in which misoprostol has been used successfully to avoid a hospital birth for postdate pregnancies. However, these sobering cases cannot be ignored.

In August 2000, Searle, the manufacturer of Cytotec, issued a warning letter regarding the risks to pregnant women and sent it to all medical maternity care providers. Coincidentally, this was shortly after Ina May Gaskin had begun a high-profile campaign on the Web and elsewhere to publicize the dangers of using misoprostol for induction. With an increasing public awareness of the potential harm of the use of Cytotec in labor and its use with mifepristone in an FDA-approved protocol to induce abortion at 49 days or less, the product information was changed to state that it is contraindicated to prevent the development of ulcers in pregnant women who are using NSAID drugs. It also now acknowledges the recognized obstetric uses, in compliance with the FDA ruling that states that any recognized use during labor or delivery must be discussed, even if the drug is not officially indicated for such use. The entire product description under the entry entitled "Labor and Delivery" now reads:

> Cytotec can induce or augment uterine contractions. Vaginal administration of Cytotec, outside of its approved indication, has been used as a cervical ripening agent, for the induction of labor and for treatment of serious postpartum hemorrhage in the presence of uterine atony. A major adverse effect of the obstetrical use of Cytotec is hyperstimulation of the uterus which may progress to uterine tetany with marked impairment of uteroplacental blood flow, uterine rupture (requiring surgical repair, hysterectomy, and/or salpingo-oophorectomy), or amniotic fluid embolism. Pelvic pain, retained placenta, severe genital bleeding, shock, fetal bradycardia, and fetal and maternal death have been reported.
>
> There may be an increased risk of uterine tachysystole, uterine rupture, meconium passage, meconium staining of amniotic fluid, and Cesarean delivery due to uterine hyperstimulation with the use of higher doses of Cytotec; including the manufactured 100 μg tablet. The risk of uterine rupture increases with advancing gestational ages and with prior uterine surgery, including Cesarean delivery. Grand multiparity also appears to be a risk factor for uterine rupture.
>
> The effect of Cytotec on the later growth, development and functional maturation of the child when Cytotec is used for cervical ripening or induction of labor have not been established. Information on Cytotec's effect on the need for forceps delivery or other intervention is unknown. (GD Searle & Co, product insert, revised May 2002)

Midwives have many ways to induce labor (see the chapter entitled "Natural Induction and Augmentation of Labor.") that are far safer and just as effective as using an obviously dangerous drug. Midwives also place themselves at significant liability when using a drug that is not even approved for induction. You can be sure that this fact will not go unnoticed in court cases brought against direct-entry midwives with a bad maternal outcome.

Like buccal Pitocin before it, misoprostol is proving extremely unpredictable and seems to have a cumulative effect. After administration, some women have contractions right away, with or without adverse reactions. Some have no uterine activity for hours, only to have strong labor start much later. The potential for such delayed reactions and complications, even with a single 25 μg dose, significantly increases the potential risk for women encouraged to take multiple doses because "nothing is happening." There no recourse should tetanic contractions begin; once the drug is administered, the effect cannot be reversed. The dose must wear off, which occurs gradually. This makes the effects impossible to control.

Some midwives will agree that the use of any drug in labor is ill advised. Certainly most homebirth midwives feel that drugs should be used judiciously and only when absolutely necessary. As a group, we have been highly critical and vocal in our dismay over the use of unproven drugs on women and babies in hospital settings. Most know that the uncontrolled use of oxytocin in labor is very dangerous. We must not allow the allure of a cheap, easy-to-use fix for induction sway us from our commonsense understanding that, in general, drugs used on laboring women are more often a problem than not. Using misoprostol prior to or during labor is needlessly playing Russian roulette with a mother and baby.

Postpartum bleeding: The one possible use for misoprostol in the home setting is in the rare case of postpartum bleeding that is not fully controlled by either oxytocin or Methergine. Multiple tablets of misoprostol can be given orally or inserted rectally to stop bleeding. Recommended dosages range from 400 to 1000 μg (5, 200 μg tablets = 1000 μg), depending on the practitioner. Sometimes smaller doses are effective.

Bioavailability: Misoprostol must be converted to misoprostol free acid in the liver before it can work. Therefore, the theory that rectal insertion places the drug closer to the site of bleeding where it can act more quickly does not take into account the need for it to circulate through the liver before it becomes biologically available. Thus the rectal route is used when the oral route is contraindicated due to oral intake being ill advised in a woman in shock.

Absorption: Andolina and colleagues (2003) found that misoprostol becomes bioavailable rapidly in postpartum women at term, with plasma concentrations of misoprostol free acid reaching, on average, 89 pg/ml by 5 min, 256 pg/ml by 15 min, and 381 pg/ml by 30 min after oral administration in tablet form. Blood levels were slower to rise when the tablets were crushed and encapsuled (reaching only 20 pg/ml at 5 min), but no significant difference was noted by 15 min. (This is probably because the capsule takes time to break down. Faster absorption may occur if the tablets are crushed, diluted in a little water and drunk.)

Effectiveness: Unfortunately, most of the studies to date focus on the use of misoprostol for prophylaxis rather than for treating hemorrhage. An extensive Cochrane database review (Gulmezoglu et al., 2004) of its prophylactic use to prevent postpartum bleeding found that neither intramuscular prostaglandins nor misoprostol are preferable to conventional injectable uterotonics such as oxytocin and Methergine. Another Cochrane study (Mousa & Alfirevic, 2003) found that 800 µg of misoprostol given rectally seemed useful for treating primary postpartum bleeding with a significant reduction in the number who continued to bleed after administration and those who needed additional interventions (6% versus 34% of those receiving syntometrine IM and oxytocin in an IV). However, there was no difference in the number who required uterine packing or surgical interventions to control otherwise intractable hemorrhage. Joy and associates (2003) found increased rates of shivering and fever in postpartum women receiving misoprostol; they found it generally inferior to oxytocin and other uterotonics given prophylactically, but somewhat effective when compared to placebo. They concluded it would be better than nothing for prophylactic use in less-developed countries. Other studies found conflicting results, with Caliskan and colleagues (2003) concluding that oral misoprostol alone is as effective as oxytocin for the prevention of postpartum hemorrhage but less so that oxytocin plus Methergine. Therefore, you must decide for yourself regarding its use for postpartum bleeding. It seems that the data do not support its prophylactic use at this time.

Administration: Misoprostol is used only after the baby is born. Oral administration should be used only if the woman is fully conscious, when the dose is the same as when given rectally. To administer tablets rectally, the tablets can be crushed, mixed with water and injected into the rectum with a syringe with the needle removed to speed absorption. Alternatively, you can don a glove, apply a water-based lubricant (no oil) to the index finger and touch the tablet to pick it up. It should stick to your finger. Insert each tablet separately by placing the tip of your finger, tablet-first, against the anal opening. Angle your finger toward the mother's navel and push past the sphincter. Insert your finger as high as it will go and press the tablet into her anterior rectal wall, especially if there are feces in the rectum. Continue until all the tablets have been inserted. The exact dosage and best route of delivery is unknown, as the drug has not been officially researched for this purpose, although it is being used this way in US obstetrics. Remember that its use postpartum does not eliminate the unknown risks regarding how or even if misoprostol can adversely affect the tissue quality or integrity of the lower uterine segment, whether it will weaken any scar tissue present and what this might mean for future childbearing. While we do know that extreme tissue softening can occur during labor, we do not know the long-term consequences regarding whether misoprostol, or any prostaglandin for that matter, permanently impacts tissue integrity.

The remaining prostaglandins are noted in the following discussion for your information. They are quite expensive and perishable at room temperature and therefore must be refrigerated until just prior to use, making them are poor choices to be carting around to homebirths. Nevertheless, you may encounter the use of one or more of these agents if you transport a woman to the hospital, so a general idea of their action and use is appropriate.

Carboprost tromethamine (Hemabate [Pharmacia & Upjohn], Prostin 15 in some European and Scandinavian countries)

Carboprost is a prostaglandin used to induce abortion and to control postpartum hemorrhage. It is supplied as an injectable solution in 1 ml ampules containing 250 µg of carboprost. Carboprost given intramuscularly stimulates the full-term pregnant uterus to produce intermittent contractions similar in character to natural labor. Whether this is a direct effect of the drug is unknown.

Indications: Carboprost is recommended as second-line therapy in cases of postpartum bleeding that have not responded to oxytocin or ergot-based drugs and manual means such as massage and bimanual compression. It is currently the only prostaglandin-based drug intended for this purpose. Carboprost should not be used simultaneously with other oxytocics but can be given after other oxytocics have failed to work adequately. An initial dose of 250 µg is given as a deep intramuscular injection. In 73% of cases, the woman's uterus will respond with a single injection. However, more resistant cases have responded to multiple doses given at intervals of 15 to 90 minutes, depending upon the circumstances. The total amount given should not exceed 2 mg (8 ampules). Carboprost levels peak between 15 and 60 minutes after intramuscular injection. IV use is effective after 12.5 minutes and produces less severe side-effects.

Carboprost has been injected through the abdominal wall directly into the uterine muscle. While this may act more rapidly than the intramuscular route, it also carries the risk of intravenous injection, which may lead to cardiovascular effects, including cardiac arrest. It is not a route recommended by the manufacturer.

Adverse side-effects: The use of carboprost has fallen out of favor in some parts of the United States because of its severe side-effects in many women. It stimulates the smooth muscle of the gastrointestinal tract, leading to vomiting, uncontrollable diarrhea or both as major side-effects in two-thirds of those treated. It may also elevate the body temperature within 1 to 16 hours after administration. The temperature returns to normal when treatment is discontinued. Flushing and restlessness may also occur. Large doses can raise blood pressure, although this is not usually a problem when therapeutic doses are used. At this time, the manufacturer does not distribute carboprost to practitioners who work outside hospital settings as they feel the risk of complications is too high.

Precautions: Carboprost administration may be associated with a moderate rise in blood pressure, although it is unclear if this rise is due to the drug or a response to hypovolemic shock. In any event, blood pressure should normalize without treatment. Women with chorioamnionitis may not respond to carboprost. Women with asthma may experience intense bronchospasm, and it is contraindicated for those with major cardiac, pulmonary, renal or liver dysfunction. Women known to be hypersensitive to prostaglandin drugs, those that have acute pelvic inflammatory disease or those with active cardiac, pulmonary, renal or liver disease should not be given prostaglandin-based drugs.

Stability and storage: Carboprost must be stored refrigerated at 36 to 46°F (2 to 8°C) until it is to be used. The solution should be clear and colorless, with no particulate matter. It has a shelf life of 48 months.

Accidental administration to newborns: The literature describes one infant who accidentally received a full dose (250 µg) of carboprost. He was tachypneic and hypertensive within 15 minutes, followed by bronchospasm, and displayed both dystonic movements as well as seizure activity of his upper extremities. He also developed a fever and had diarrhea stools. He recovered within 18 hours with no apparent long-term harm. Other infants who have received lesser doses by accident have remained asymptomatic (Mrvos et al., 1999).

Dinoprostone-based drugs (Prostin E2, Prepidil Gel [both by Pharmacia & Upjohn], Cervidil [Forest])

These drugs all contain prostaglandin E_2, which has proven to be a powerful cervical ripener and uterine contractant. Exogenous prostaglandins have been used orally, intrayoni, intracervically and extra-amniotically to ripen the cervix and induce labor. Each route has its drawbacks. The local application of prostaglandins in the upper yoni or cervical canal is more effective with less than the total dose needed when given systemically, thereby reducing the total dose used and lessening the incidence of systemic side-effects and uterine hyperstimulation. Systemic effects include vomiting, fever and diarrhea, which occur in less than 1% of those receiving topical treatment and, in most cases, can be reversed by removal of the preparation. Caution must be exercised when the woman has asthma, glaucoma or severe liver or kidney impairment. However, bronchial constriction or significant blood pressure changes have not been noted with low doses, and asthma is not an absolute contraindication to the use of PGE_2. Women receiving prostaglandin should be afebrile and have no unexplained yoni bleeding and have no history of allergy to the drug. While each drug contains the same active ingredient, they are formulated differently. The following descriptions are intended to educate you regarding the use of these drugs in labor. Most should never be used in a home setting. The FDA labeling for both Prepidil and Cervidil is still included in the PDR.

Cervidil: This cervical-ripening preparation is FDA approved as a cervical ripener in women at or near term when there is a medical indication (i.e., not for elective induction). It consists of a thin, flat, rectangular disk of the drug, encased in a polyester pouch with a string attached to facilitate removal. A single dose contains a total of 10 mg. The entire pouch is inserted into the posterior fornix of the yoni, where it releases a measured amount of dinoprostone at a rate of about 0.3 mg per hour over a 12 hr period. Cervical ripening and uterine contractions occur gradually and usually develop into active labor several hours after the pouch is first inserted. The risk of hyperstimulation is about 5 to 10%. It must frozen prior to use. Because of its time-release nature, it should never be relied upon to control a postpartum hemorrhage.

Prepidil: Prepidil has the same approved indications as for Cervidil. It is dispensed in 2.5 ml gel doses that contain 0.2 mg of PGE_2. The gel is introduced into the cervical canal using a specialized syringe. First, a speculum is inserted to visualize the cervix, which is swabbed gently to remove any secretions. Then the tip of the syringe is inserted into the os or the posterior fornix, and the gel is ejected. The gel should not be injected above the internal os, as this raises the risk of hyperstimulation of the uterus. The woman is then instructed to remain supine for at least 30 minutes to minimize leakage, during which time careful fetal monitoring is recommended. At least 6 hours should pass before the dose is repeated or IV oxytocin is begun. More than one dose is often required, and the manufacturer warns against using more than 3 doses in a 24 hr period. The gel stimulates contractions similar in character to natural labor contractions, which are often mild and unsustained. The risk of hyperstimulation is less than 1%. Its primary use is as a cervical ripener to be followed by oxytocin administration. It cannot be used for postpartum hemorrhage.

Prostin E_2: This preparation is a suppository containing 20 mg of prostaglandin E_2. Its stated indication is to empty the uterus after 12 weeks gestation for missed abortions, hydatidiform mole and stillbirths up to 28 weeks. The suppository is placed in the upper yoni every 3 to 5 hours until the uterine contents are expelled. The time this takes averages 16 hours, with 85% of labors being complete within 24 hours. It takes slightly longer when the fetus is defective but alive. The time interval is less for multiparous women in the second half of pregnancy. However, it is more dangerous when used to induce women at term. It has also been used for postpartum hemorrhage. It must be stored frozen at a temperature of no warmer than −4°F (−20°C) in its original foil wrapper. It is brought to room temperature, removed from its wrapper and inserted high in the yoni or into the rectum against the anterior rectal wall. Once inserted, other oxytocic drugs should not be given.

Gemeprost (Cervagen [Rhône-Poulenc Rorer]): This analogue of prostaglandin E_1 is supplied in a suppository containing 1 mg of gemeprost. It is indicated for cervical ripening and abortion in the second trimester and has been used for postpartum hemorrhage. It is not available in the United States.

Sulprostone (Nalador): This synthetic prostaglandin E_2 is primarily used for inducing abortion and arresting postpartum hemorrhage. It is supplied in 500 g doses and can be diluted in 500 ml of normal saline and then given in an IV run in at a rate of 60 drops per minute (4 g/min) to stop postpartum bleeding. It is not available in the United States.

Quinine

Quinine comes from the dried bark of the root and stem of various species of *Cinchona*, a genus of evergreen trees (family *Rubiaceae*). They are native to South America but cultivated in many tropical regions. The cultivated bark contains 7 to 10% total alkaloid; about 70% of which is quinine. Quinine first came into use as an antimalarial drug in the 1640s when it was also discovered to be a uterine stimulant. Williams (1930) reports that oral or injected administration during labor promptly produces stronger, more efficient contractions. Today, quinine supplied in tablets or capsules remains a mainstay of malarial treatment, but it is no longer used as an oxytocic. It is mentioned here because I know of at least one midwife in the United States who has used it in the past, and where there is one, there are likely others. While its oxytocic effects are recognized, there is virtually no specific data on its effect on the uterus or the baby. It may, however, produce an artifact fever in the mother, confusing the picture regarding whether she has an infection or not. Other side-effects include nausea, vomiting and diarrhea, headache, ringing in the ears, arrhythmic heart rate and hypotension, to name a few. These side-effects could mask serious maternal conditions that require your attention. In the mid-twentieth century literature, doctors speculated that quinine may injure the ears or eyes of the fetus and may cause fetal death (Titus, 1950). Norris (1895) says that its use will, on occasion, lead to a violent postpartum hemorrhage. With so little to go on regarding the use of quinine in labor, it is ill advised to use it for induction or stimulation. The effects of other herbs are gentler, safer and better understood.

Currently, a concoction made by boiling and pureeing an entire organic grapefruit is being used by some midwives as part of an induction protocol. There is a substance in grapefruit that is a quinine precursor. I have no information on the relative safety or effectiveness of its use, but with the problems with quinine in general, I recommend other remedies for inducing labor (see the chapter entitled "Natural Induction and Augmentation of Labor" for details).

A Word About Drug Expiration Dates

Expiration dates are based upon a 5% maximum allowable loss of effectiveness in the drug. The effectiveness of certain drugs falls off far more rapidly than this. Some drugs also become toxic if kept beyond their expiration date. Therefore, it is always safest to replace drugs in a timely fashion.

Multi-use Skills, Treatments and Related Equipment

Urinary Catheterization

Urinary catheterization involves inserting a tube into the urethra to allow urine to empty from the bladder. Knowing how to catheterize the mother can be very helpful if the urethra becomes occluded and the bladder is full due to pressure from the presenting part or swelling in the area. Note that, even if a woman has voided a large amount of urine, a half-pint or more can still be retained which she may not be able to detect given the myriad sensations of labor. Therefore, if the circumstances of labor increase the likelihood that manipulations may be needed during the birth, and palpation about the pubic bone leads you to believe the bladder still contains some urine, catheterization may be wise. After birth, swelling of the surrounding tissues may occasionally prevent urination as well. Whenever time allows, catheterization is also appropriate when an unexpected emergency arises which requires an empty bladder before further assistance can be given.

Catheterization is an invasive procedure that should be used judiciously, only after all other attempts to empty the bladder have failed or when time is of the essence and flow is occluded. Normally, the interior of the bladder is sterile; inserting a tube has the potential to introduce an infection. Catheterization at home reduces the risk of infection (because the germs at home are familiar whereas those in the hospital tend to be highly infectious and may be resistant to treatment); however, it always requires the use of sterile technique.

Before you proceed, explain to the mother what you propose to do and why. The procedure should not be acutely painful, but she can expect to feel some discomfort and pressure when the catheter is inserted, with perhaps more than usual if the presenting part is pressing on the urethra. Be sure to note latex and iodine allergies before you proceed.

Next, assemble your equipment. Use a straight catheter, which consists of a long, size 10 to 12F tube, flared on one end and with a closed, rounded tip on the other, having two holes on either side of the closed tip. The blunt, rounded tip is designed to be inserted with minimal trauma to the tissues. If the mother has a disability that requires catheterization, she will be quite familiar with the procedure and her needs in this regard and will have appropriate equipment on hand.

You can purchase a tray containing all the disposable items below or they can be purchased separately.

- Sterile gloves
- Sterile lubricant
- Ring forceps
- Flashlight or lamp
- Measuring cup
- Antiseptic solution
- Sterile gauze squares or cotton balls or wool
- Basin to catch the urine
- Sterile field
- Urine analysis dipstick strips

1. If circumstances permit, have the mother wash her vulva and perineal area with soap and water. She should rinse herself thoroughly and pat herself dry with a clean towel. If this is not convenient and the area needs washing, do it yourself. How will you know if she needs washing? Use common sense. If she has just gotten out of a birth pool, she doesn't. If she has been hard at labor for several hours, she may. To do so, use a container of warm water and mild soap. Place towels and then a pan underneath her to catch the water. Wash and rinse from above the vulva downward, gently opening the folds of her labia as you do so. Pat her dry. If time is of the essence, do not waste time with this, as the antiseptic cleanse you do next will suffice in an emergency.
2. Have the mother arrange herself so that she is lying down with her knees flexed and her feet about 2 feet apart. She can position her bottom on the edge of a bed with her feet on chairs. Alternatively, she can position herself on her side with an assistant supporting her upper leg.
3. Arrange your light source so that you can clearly visualize the periurethral area.
4. Wash your hands thoroughly.
5. Arrange a sterile field between the mother's legs.
6. Don sterile gloves.
7. Have your assistant peel back the outer wrapper on several packages of sterile gauze (or cotton, which is less abrasive) and drop the gauze onto the sterile field. Have your assistant peel back the outer wrapper on a catheter so you can pull it out. Have your assistant squirt a dollop of sterile lubricant onto the sterile field. Roll the closed end of the catheter in the lubricant so that 1 to 2 inches of the blunt end are lubricated. Place the blunt end of the catheter on the sterile field.
8. Next, pick up a square of gauze or a cotton ball and have your assistant moisten it well with antiseptic solution. Pick

up the moistened cotton or gauze with the ring forceps. Wipe the labia minora on one side from the upper area toward the lower. Be careful not to scrub, as gauze can abrade delicate tissue. Discard the wipe. Repeat on the opposite side with fresh, saturated gauze or cotton.

9. Spread the labia minora with the thumb and one finger of your nondominant hand, and identify the urinary meatus, which will be near the inner junction of the labia minora below the clitoris. (Maintain separation of the labia with that hand until urine is flowing freely.) Using 3 separate sterile gauze pads or cotton balls held with forceps, cleanse the inner labial fold on one side, then the other and then wipe directly over the meatus. Use one stroke for each wipe, starting at the top and moving downward toward the rectum. Apply enough pressure to clean the area, but not so much that you abrade the tissue.
10. With your dominant hand, pick up the catheter about 3 inches below the tip and place the flared drainage end of the catheter into the basin.
11. Ask the mother to breathe deeply and press downward or cough several times, either of which will cause the meatus to pout slightly. Once you have located the opening, insert the catheter tip 2 to 3 in (5 to 7.5 cm). Guide, rather than shove, the catheter along its path. If the presenting part is blocking the way, you will have to use some pressure. Try rotating the catheter as you slide, rather than force, it in. You may encounter slight resistance as the catheter tip passes the through the urethral sphincter at the level of the urogenital diaphragm. If insertion is difficult, insert the first two fingers of your nondominant hand into the yoni and try displacing the presenting part slightly, or insert two fingers of that hand along the anterior yoni wall. With the pads of your fingers directed upward, splint the urethra on either side as you guide the tube into the opening with your other hand. Watch the other end, and as soon as urine is flowing freely, stop advancing the catheter.
12. Hold the catheter in place while the bladder drains passively. The woman may find she can bear down to help expel urine. However, often the laboring or postpartum woman cannot tell if her bladder is empty, so even if some drainage occurs spontaneously, it is a good idea to palpate above her pubic bone to facilitate the complete emptying of her bladder. To do so, use the flat of your hand and apply pressure starting in the area just inside the pelvic crests and moving toward the area just above the symphysis pubis, first on one side, then the other.
13. Once the bladder appears to have entirely drained, gently and slowly withdraw the catheter.
14. Examine the urine, noting its color and odor. Test the urine with a dipstick. Estimate the amount of urine passed. If there is a question regarding quantity or if the woman has hemorrhaged, pour the urine into a measuring cup and record the amount. (See DIAGNOSTIC TESTS for further information on testing the urine.)
15. Discard your disposable supplies. You can wash rubber catheters in antiseptic soap solution, boil them in water for 20 minutes, then dry and store them in a sterile container such as a sterile specimen cup with a lid for later use on the same woman.

ARTIFICIAL RUPTURE OF MEMBRANES

When you see multiparous women spontaneously rupture their membranes and, in many cases, proceed rapidly to birth, it is tempting to believe that artificial rupture of membranes will speed up a sluggish labor. However, this is by no means a guarantee. There are very few situations in which such an intrusive intervention as artificial rupture of the membranes is warranted. These situations include controlled rupture to prevent cord prolapse; removal of very strong forewaters that are impeding descent; preventing the baby from being born in the caul (with the intact bag over his head), especially if there is meconium in the water; during late pushing in a breech birth to prevent the bag from becoming filled with meconium and thus exposing the aftercoming head to meconium-stained fluid and; on rare occasions, to stimulate advanced but stalled labor. In addition, if induction is medically necessary and absolutely nothing else has worked, you might try breaking the water before you transport for induction. Each of these reasons will be discussed below.

Prevention of cord prolapse is probably one of the only clear midwifery-model indications for performing amniotomy. This procedure is described in the chapter entitled "Cord Problems and Emergencies during Labor."

If the bag is so strong that it is actually impedes descent, or if contractions are strong and there is a lot of pressure down during a contraction, rupturing the membranes may be your only option to keep labor going. Whether strong membranes are truly the reason for a delay must be assessed over a period of hours. A poorly positioned head will not descend upon amniotomy, but rupturing the membranes will eliminate the support of the forewaters and may get the head stuck in a bad position, impair rotation, or both.

Whether to allow the baby to be born in the caul or not is controversial. If the head is on the perineum, it has always been my policy to rupture the membranes to prevent the baby from being born in the caul. This way, if meconium is present, you will know before the head is born. However, many cultures throughout history have singled out those born in the caul as having special gifts, such as psychic abilities. Many midwives therefore allow the membranes to stay intact until after the head is fully born. You can use a flashlight to inspect the membranes for any sign of meconium; clear fluid will reflect back a pearly yellow color while meconium-stained fluid will appear dark.

Inducing or stimulating labor by rupturing the membranes is risky. The chapter entitled "The Placental Membranes and Amniotic Fluid during Labor" discusses the benefits of leaving the membranes intact in most circumstances, and the chapter entitled "Natural Induction and Augmentation of Labor" has a discussion regarding how to assess if amniotomy should be used.

How to rupture the membranes (amniotomy)

See the chapter entitled "Cord Problems and Emergencies during Labor" for specific instructions to minimize the chance of prolapse if you decide to artificially rupture the membranes and the head is not engaged. Do not rupture the membranes in a breech presentation, if you choose to do so at all, until the baby descends to almost a full rump. In a cephalic presentation in which the head is well applied to the cervix and low in the pelvis, and you have determined that artificial rupture is necessary, proceed as follows:

1. Have the mother empty her bladder and lie down flat on a firm surface.
2. Check the fetal heart rate.
3. Be sure you have something white, such as a clean towel, facial tissue, toilet tissue or gauze, to catch some amniotic fluid for examination. Have a receptacle handy, such as a sterile urine specimen container, to collect fluid in order to perform an APT test or other diagnostic procedure, if needed. (For details on this test, see DIAGNOSTIC TESTS.)
4. Don a sterile glove on your dominant hand.
5. Between contractions, insert your gloved hand and assess the tension on the bag, the depth of the fluid between the forebag and the presenting part, and where you will tear the bag. Gently press up into the forewaters and palpate across the surface to rule out a cord presentation, vasa previa or the presentation of a fetal omphalocele mimicking an intact forebag. If the cervix is at least 5 cm dilated and not too posterior, and you are uncertain about the contents or the normalcy of the surface of the forewaters, remove your hand, carefully insert a speculum, and look for signs of a problem with a flashlight. If you suspect a cord presentation or vasa previa, take every precaution not to rupture the membranes. If either is found, place the mother in a position so as to relieve downward pressure. If a cord presentation is discovered, see the chapter entitled "Cord Problems and Emergencies during Labor." If a vasa previa is found, place the mother in a position to reduce downward pressure and transport.

   If you are using an amnicot: Remove your gloved hand, place the rolled amnicot over the tip of the index finger of your dominant hand with the tip of the hook pointing toward your palm. Unroll the amnicot down to the base of your gloved index finger. Make sure the hook is still properly positioned. Insert your hand again carefully so as not to snag the wall of the yoni as you reach for the cervix.

If you are using an amnihook or another instrument: Guide the instrument into the yoni by maneuvering it with your nondominant hand. Withdraw your dominant hand as necessary. Place your index finger parallel with the tip to cup and protect the end of the instrument to avoid snagging the mother during insertion. Reinsert your gloved hand alongside the instrument as you advance it toward the cervix.

6. Press the tip of the amnicot or instrument against the forebag and make a scratching motion to tear a hole in it before the next contraction (the bag will loosen up slightly between contractions). You may find it helpful to use your fingertip to guide the instrument. Or, press the tip of the instrument against the forebag to create a hole (this is easier to do when the bag is tense). Do not stab it into the bag because you have less control this way and risk hitting the baby. If you cannot get hold of the bag or the bag is too tight against the head and you risk poking the baby, wait for a contraction to start before you make your attempt.
7. When the contraction builds, the waters will almost always tense up if the woman is in labor. If not or if water still does not fill the forewaters, apply just enough equalized upward pressure to the presenting part to allow a little water to trickle down into the forebag from above the head. Let the head reseat itself and then poke a hole in the bag with the tip of the instrument. Use your finger to guide the instrument as you enlarge the hole. This may require more pressure than you think. Check the fetal heart rate to be sure you have not caused an occult cord prolapse.
8. Once there is a hole in the bag, remove the instrument by guiding it out with your nondominant hand. Protect the mother's birth canal by cupping your gloved fingers around the tip of the instrument until it is completely withdrawn. If you used an amnicot, guard the tip of your finger as you remove your gloved hand and discard both the glove and the finger cot. Don a new sterile glove and reinsert your hand immediately.
9. Check the fetal heart rate.
10. Use your gloved hand to check the cervix to make sure that the presenting part has replaced the forewaters and to feel how the cervix responds to the ruptured membranes. Rule out cord prolapse. If you are uncertain, keep your hand in place for several contractions and continue to have an assistant listen to the baby until you are reasonably sure that cord prolapse has not occurred.
11. Recheck the fetal heart rate now and again after the mother changes position to rule out occult cord compression.

Cleansing and Retention Enemas

Administering an enema consists of introducing a solution into the large intestine via the anus. Enemas can be used during labor for a variety of reasons. A cleansing enema is used to remove fecal matter from the lower bowel. It may be desirable if a laboring woman is extremely uncomfortable due to constipation in labor, although this is very rare, as the uterus usually stimulates the bowels to evacuate as labor begins. Also, a woman may be concerned about cleanliness of the water if feces are expelled during underwater birth, although solid wastes that are promptly removed from the water have not proven to increase the risk of maternal or newborn infection, and expulsion of liquid from the rectum will make more of a mess.

Any fecal matter in the lower bowel will be expelled as the presenting part descends during pushing, so an enema is not technically necessary. Some women may anticipate embarrassment if they expel feces during pushing. If the fear of elimination significantly impairs a woman's ability to let go, an enema can be helpful. Keep in mind, however, that an enema may not be fully eliminated after it is given and watery discharge may occur, both defeating the purpose and spreading feces during the birth.

Various types of retention enemas come in handy on occasion. An enema may be used to hydrate the mother as an alternative to an IV solution or as a source of nutrition. The intestinal walls are capable of directly absorbing both fluids and nutrient solutions quickly. Enemas of lactated Ringer's (Hartman's) or saline IV solutions are effective in rehydrating a woman following postpartum hemorrhage. To provide a boost of energy, use a warm solution consisting of 10 drops of ginger root tincture and 1 to 2 tablespoons of molasses dissolved in a quart of water (Weed, 1985).

More rarely, an enema may be called for to stimulate labor. In this case, uterine-stimulant herbs can be brewed into a tea for use as the enema solution. Enemas can also create buoyancy in the bowel, which lifts the baby up and facilitates rotation to a more favorable position.

Enemas are generally considered uncomfortable. Some women have been severely traumatized by enemas received in childhood. It is therefore important to explain both your reasons for offering an enema as an option during labor and how it will be done. Go over other options and get the woman's full cooperation and agreement before proceeding with an enema.

Special considerations regarding the use of cleansing enemas

Forgo a cleansing enema if labor is very active and dilation is advanced, especially in women who have had a baby or two. If the presenting part is not engaged or if the baby is breech or premature, use of an enema increases the risk of cord prolapse, whether the membranes are ruptured or not. The water entering the bowel may buoy the baby up even further and may disrupt intact membranes so that the water breaks. Using an enema in the presence of ruptured membranes increases the risk of intrauterine infection via contamination; be extra careful about not contaminating the perineum and introitus. Never administer an enema if the woman is bleeding and you suspect either placenta previa or abruption, as it could make these conditions worse. Transport is then in order.

The method for administering an enema is basically the same regardless of the reasons it is being done.

Enema equipment

Have on hand an enema bag, hose, hose-bag connector, hose clamp, bag hook and rectal tip. You can obtain all the necessary parts with a full-sized hot water bottle/enema/douche bag set at a pharmacy. If a cleansing enema is being given, a disposable enema containing a standard cleansing solution, such as a Fleet's enema, can also be used.

If you use a client's own enema set up, the hose and rectal tip can be washed with antibacterial soap and thoroughly rinsed between uses. Since the rectum is not a sterile area, sterilization is not necessary unless you own a set that is to be used among all your clients. If you carry an enema setup from birth to birth, the tip needs to be sterilized by boiling for 20 minutes, and the hose should be washed in antiseptic solution inside and out. All parts should be thoroughly air-dried before storage. A hair dryer can be used to hasten this process.

You will also need enema solution, the amount and temperature of which will vary depending upon the reason for the enema. For an average cleansing enema, 750 to 1000 ml of fluid at 105 to 109°F (40.5 to 43°C) is commonly used in adults. For a retention enema, where the object is to retain the fluid in the rectum as long as possible, much less solution should be used, with repeated doses of 1 to 2 ounces each. A retention enema should be at room temperature or slightly warmer to minimize stimulation of peristalsis. Other supplies you may need include the following:

- •Bath thermometer
- •Waterproof pad
- •Blanket
- •Large bath towels
- •Water-based lubricant
- •Coat hanger
- •Nonsterile exam gloves
- •Washcloths
- •Pillows covered in plastic and a cloth case
- •Infant enema syringe (can be used to give retention enemas)

Performing the procedure

Setting up: It is best to administer an enema in the largest available bathroom. Arrange a padded surface on the floor near the toilet using blankets, clean bath mats or large bath towels. Cover the end of the padded area, where the mother's bottom will be, with the waterproof pad, arranged so that you can lift up the edge to protect yourself in the event that the solution is forcefully expelled from the rectum while the woman is lying down. Have another sheet or blanket on hand to cover the mother, if she prefers. Use a folded towel or two underneath her belly for support and a pillow under her head. Always have some towels and extra underpads handy in case the woman begins to expel fluid before she gets to the toilet. Make sure the room is a comfortable temperature before you begin, taking into account the temperature of the floor.

Prepare the solution: If you are using a commercially prepared disposable enema for cleansing purposes only, follow the package directions. Since these small, hand-held devices offer the woman the option of administering it herself, make sure to communicate that you would be happy to help and that it may be easier for her to deal with contractions if you assist. If she doesn't want you to assist her, help her get comfortable lying on her left side on the bathroom floor and remain close by in case she does need assistance. A disposable Fleet's-type enema comes with a prelubricated tip, which simply requires positioning the woman, inserting the tip at an angle toward her navel and controlling the flow of fluid by the amount of pressure applied to the container.

If the enema solution to be used is an herbal preparation, steep and thoroughly strain the tea before placing it in the enema bag. Check the temperature with a bath thermometer or on your inner wrist. Ensure that liquid nutrient solutions are mixed thoroughly in a blender or food processor and are thin enough to flow through the rectal tip without difficulty.

Administering a cleansing enema to the mother:

1. Attach the hose to the tip of the threaded connector. Attach the rectal tip (the long, thin tip with one hole in the end) to the other end of the hose. Practice clamping and releasing the hose clamp until you are proficient at doing this quickly and smoothly. To proceed, make sure the clamp is closed.
2. Pour the solution into the bag and screw in the connector.
3. Using a coat hanger, insert the hooked end into the eyelet on the top of the bag, opposite the connector, or put the hook it came with in the eye. For a cleansing enema, find a suitable location from which to hang the bag, such as a towel bar or door knob that is about 12 to 18 inches (30 to 45 cm) above the level of the woman's anus. (For a retention enema, see below.) The higher the bag, the faster the solution will flow. To start with, hang the bag level with the woman's hip.
4. Release the hose clamp and flush fluid through the tube until it comes out of the rectal tip. Reclamp the hose. This removes air from the tube that would otherwise go into the rectum.
5. Have the mother lie on her left side, with her knees slightly bent. Alternatively, have her assume a knee-chest position.
6. Don gloves and lubricate the rectal tip.
7. Wait until there is a space between contractions. Lift or part the woman's buttocks to expose her anus. Ask her to begin deep breathing. Slowly and gently talk her through your actions. Ask her to cough as you insert the rectal tip at an angle pointing toward her umbilicus. If you meet resistance, withdraw the tube slightly and release a small amount of solution. This will help push aside any feces blocking the way. Then continue to insert it. Do not force entry of the tip. Hemorrhoids may obstruct your view. If so, probe gently with your finger to find the anal opening.
8. Introduce the solution slowly as you or an assistant raises the bag to the predetermined level. Infusion time will vary, but expect it to take 7 to 10 minutes to give 1 quart (about 1 liter) of solution for a cleansing enema. Hold the rectal tip in place throughout the procedure. Since the purpose is to cleanse the lower bowel, have her retain a quantity of fluid for several minutes before evacuating. Have the mother give you feedback about how the fluid feels as it goes in. Stop the flow when she begins to feel pressure, and allow her to take a few deep breaths as either you or she massages her belly. The massage should go all around her uterus starting at the lower left-hand corner of her belly, up her left abdomen, under her rib cage and down the right side. This motion will encourage the solution to penetrate

higher into the bowel. Then slowly begin the flow again. This will allow her to retain the maximal amount of fluid. After you are through letting all the fluid in, have her lie still so that she can allow it to make its way up inside her large intestine. Once she feels she is ready to expel the fluid, assist her up and onto the toilet.

9. Once finished, have the mother take a shower so she can wash herself thoroughly, minimizing contamination of the perineum and introitus.

Administering a retention enema to the mother: Fluid is reabsorbed from the stool in the last 6 in of the colon, making an enema an excellent way to hydrate a woman. It generally takes 30 minutes to administer a retention enema of about 600 cc (ml) (about 20 oz) of fluid, depending upon the degree of dehydration (or blood loss) and the woman's tolerance for the enema. If the woman needs the fluid badly, she may completely absorb all the fluid through the walls of the large intestine more rapidly and expel very little. The rate of absorption can be your guide as to how rapidly to give the fluid. If using an enema bag, hang it very low, elevated just enough to keep the fluid flowing.

Encourage the woman to retain the fluid by breathing deeply as previously described. Massage will probably not be required, as she needs the fluid and should absorb it easily. If she feels she cannot do so, assist her to the toilet. Chances are that she will retain and absorb the fluid fairly quickly, thus minimizing the amount that much will be expelled. Try to keep track of how much fluid the woman retains and repeat the dose, as necessary, until the desired effect is achieved.

Hypodermic Injections

Medication can be administered via two basic routes.

Enteral administration refers to absorption by the gastrointestinal (GI) tract. This term generally applies to oral intake but also includes sublingual and rectal routes.

Parenteral (pah-REN-ter-all) administration, which includes the intradermal, subcutaneous (SQ), intramuscular (IM) and intravenous (IV) routes, is used to give drugs that are poorly absorbed from the GI tract and when medications need to be absorbed more quickly than can be accomplished with oral intake. (The exception here is a solution absorbed through mucous membranes, as an herbal tincture or homeopathic remedy.)

Hypodermic syringes are used to give injections when using either the IM or SQ route as well as an adjunct in IV use. Drugs that midwives might inject include local anesthetic, antihemorrhagic agents, Vitamin K for newborns, $Rh_0(D)$ immunoglobulin and sterile water papules for relief of excessive pain in labor. The use of sterile water papules is covered in a separate chapter. This chapter covers how to give an injection. Indications for injectable medications will be discussed throughout the text. Also see the subchapter entitled "Allopathic Pharmacologic Agents for Treating Uterine Atony."

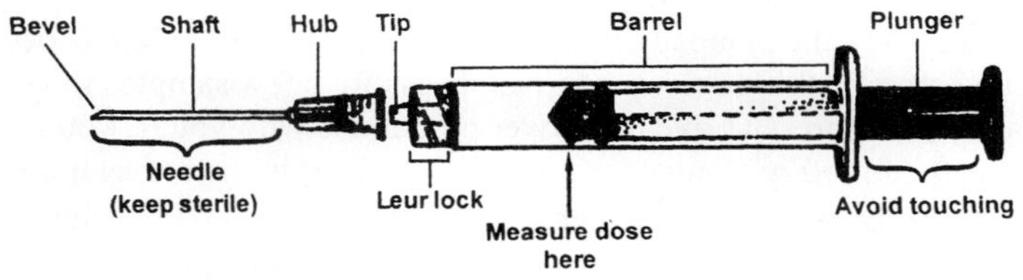

Anatomy of a hypodermic needle and syringe

Equipment for Injections

The equipment used to transfer liquid medication into the person's body is simple and consists basically of a syringe and a needle.

Syringes

A syringe consists of a hollow cylindrical barrel with a narrow, hollow tip on one end. The other end has an opening the same diameter as the barrel and two wings that allow counterpressure to be applied to the plunger, which is inserted into this large opening. The plunger has on one end a silicone rubber tip, which fits into the lumen of the barrel. On the other end, the plunger has a wide flat piece to which finger pressure is applied.

Syringes are available in varying sizes, from 0.3 to 60 ml. A cubic centimeter (cc) equals 1 milliliter (1/1000 of a liter). Use the smallest possible syringe that accommodates the amount of solution to be injected. The outside of the syringe barrel is marked in two scales along the side; one side is divided into tenths of a ml and the other into minims. Tuberculin (TB) and insulin syringes are marked in hundredths of a milliliter (0.01) and minims, and are used to administer doses of less than 1 ml. Insulin syringes hold 0.3 to 1 ml (cc) of fluid. Both types are calibrated in units, a special measurement scale which makes them suitable for delivering very small doses accurately. Each milliliter or cubic centimeter of solution equals 100 units. Frequently, more than one measurement scale is included.

Syringes are classified as being either luer-lock or nonluer-lock (also called "slip-lock"). The lock style refers to how the needle attaches to the syringe. It is best to get luer-lock syringes, which use a specialized needle hub that locks in place over the tip of the syringe and minimizes dislodgement. When you buy extra needles, be sure they are luer-lock needles as well. Nonluer-lock needles simply slip over the tip of the syringe and require replacement needles with a slip-on hub as well. Most insulin syringes have permanently attached needles.

Hypodermic needles

Disposable syringes can be purchased with or without needles attached. Needles purchased separately come packaged in individual wrappers. The advantage to buying syringes and needles separately is that you can easily choose the correct size for the individual client. The advantage to buying them as a single unit is ease of use in an emergency; there is only one package to open and no assembly is required.

Each needle has three parts: the hub, the shaft and the bevel. The needle hub attaches to the narrow tip on the barrel. The shaft refers to the needle length. The bevel is the steeply slanted tip of the shaft that produces a narrow slit when inserted into tissue; it is designed so that the hole it makes in the skin quickly closes when the needle is removed to prevent leakage of medication, blood or serum. Needles vary in length from ¼ to 3 in. The hub and cap will be color coded for ease of selection. Longer needles (1 to 1.5 in or 2.5 to 3.25 cm) are used for intramuscular (IM) injections and shorter needles (⅜ to ⅝ in or 9 to 14 mm) for subcutaneous injections. Select needle length according to the size and weight of the person as well as the type of tissue into which the solution is being introduced.

The gauge is a measure of the needle's diameter. The smaller the numerical value of the gauge, the larger the needle's diameter. For example, an 18 gauge needle used for IVs is many times larger than a 25 gauge needle used to give a newborn Vitamin K.

Selecting safe needle devices: Some syringes are designed with a safety device that covers the needle immediately after it is withdrawn from the skin. The needle cover prevents a needlestick injury. As a midwife working independently, you will not necessarily be exposed to new devices for either hypodermic or IV use as quickly as might a midwife working in an institutional setting. Therefore, it behooves you or your local midwifery organization to cultivate a relationship with a local medical supply distributor. Ask the company to let you know when new products become available that might be useful in your type of practice. If something sounds interesting, ask for a few samples so you can see the new features for yourself. Get the manufacturer's representative to go over proper use with you; if you are duly impressed, arrange for a demonstration for your local midwifery community. Practice on fruit with your samples to see if they better meet your needs than what you are currently using. Arrange for several midwives to go in on a box together to see if you like them. To find out more about currently available devices for sharps injury protection, check "California List of Needleless Systems and Needles with Engineered Sharps Injury Protection" by entering that phrase, in quotes, into the web search engine Google. To reach Google, enter www.google.com.

Filter needles: Filter needles are recommended for drawing medications from ampules. These specialized needles feature a 5 micron filter built into an elongated hub. The filter prevents glass particles from being drawn up with the medication. Once the solution is in the syringe, you must replace the filter needle with a needle designed for use in tissue before the injection is given.

Glass syringes and resusable needles

If you are practicing in an area of the developing world where disposable supplies are not readily available, try to get some glass syringes and reusable needles, as they can be more easily sterilized. Tiny brushes are available for cleaning, and a fine sharpening stone can be used to sharpen the needles. If nothing else, the equipment should be as thoroughly cleaned as possible in whatever antiseptic solution there is on hand (to clean the inside of the needle, draw up the cleaning solution and eject it from the syringe); the needles should then be sharpened, recleaned to remove metal filings and everything boiled for at least 20 minutes between uses or autoclaved if an autoclave is available.

Disposable needles and syringes

Disposable syringes come packaged in a wrapper of paper and plastic. The parts of the syringe that must remain sterile until you administer the injection are the needle itself, the inside of the barrel, and the rubber end and shaft of the plunger. If the syringe comes with a needle, it will be capped. The outside of the cap and of the barrel and the end of the plunger can be touched as necessary to prepare and administer the injection.

If you are "sterile," have an assistant peel back the outer wrapper of the syringe while you remove the sterile syringe from the wrapper. You may, however, handle the outside of the syringe parts, as previously described, without sterile technique.

Medications

Injectable solutions are packaged in three types of containers: ampules, vials and, least commonly, in single-dose, prefilled syringes. A vial is made of glass or plastic, contains single or multiple doses and is topped with a rubber seal. Over this rubber seal is a metal or plastic cap held in place by a tiny plastic or metal band. Vials may contain powdered or liquid preparations. Drugs that are unstable in liquid form are packaged in powder form in single-dose vials. The label should specify the liquid to be used to reconstitute the powder (often sterile water). The appropriate quantity of liquid for a single dose is often included in a separate vial or ampule.

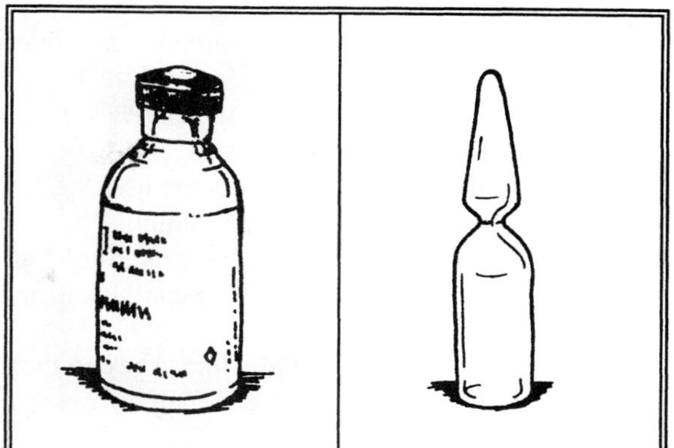

Vial | Ampule

Ampules are single-dose, airtight glass containers. Glass ampules tend to preserve the properties of medications better than vials because they are completely airtight. Some medications come as a single dose in a prefilled syringe.

Giving the wrong medication is a serious, but human mistake that you should take every precaution to avoid. Always double-check the medication, the client's name on the package, the expiration date and the dosage before use to be sure that the medication is correct. The best way to insure that a mistake is not made is to be scrupulous about checking your labels whenever you handle a container of medication of any kind. Be conscious of the color of the container and the specific design and colors on the labels of all your drugs as you receive them from your supplier: double-check that you have received the correct drug in the dosage you expect. The supplier could have made a mistake in your order, especially if individual containers are taken from a larger stock to ship to you. Read labels again as you place drugs in your bags. Read the label once more when you remove a drug from your bag for use. Just because it is where it should be, does not mean it is what it should be. Before drawing up a drug for injection, or preparing to give the baby a drug orally or in his eyes, read the label again, carefully, checking both the type and dose of the drug. As you clean up the packaging, look over the labeling one more time to confirm the dosage and medication was correct.

Should you realize you have given the baby the wrong drug orally (most likely if you had intended to give injectable Vitamin K orally), De Lee the stomach as soon as you recognize the error. If you give the baby an injection of something besides Vitamin K, there is nothing you can do at home. In either case, consult a neonatologist (Anton, 2003). There is also not much you can do about giving the mother the wrong drug by injection except to allow the effects of the drug to wear off. More about the appropriate uses of drugs and how they may affect the mother or baby is covered in the subchapter entitled "Allopathic Pharmacologic Agents for Treating Uterine Atony." That chapter will help you determine what, if any, action should be taken and what effects you can expect in the event that you unintentionally give the mother or baby the wrong medication. Fortunately, homebirth midwives do not carry a wide variety of medications. Confirming that the medication is correct when you receive it, store it, use it and discard it is the best insurance that you won't have to worry about the adverse effects of incorrect administration.

The Use of Injections in Midwifery Practice

The following chart describes the most commonly used medications and syringes in a direct-entry midwifery practice based in the United States.

Solution to be Administered	Recipient	Preferred Needle & Syringe
Sterile water papules (intradermal)	Mother	Tuberculin or insulin syringe, w/27 gauge needle
Anti-hemorrhagic drugs (IM)	Mother	3 cc syringe w/22 gauge, 1.5 in needle
Local anesthetic (intradermal, SQ)	Mother	3 or 6 cc syringe w/22 gauge, 1.5 in needle
Epinephrine (subcutaneous)	Mother	Tuberculin or insulin syringe w/25 gauge needle
Rh_o(D) immunoglobulin (IV bolus or IM, depending on brand)	Mother	3 cc syringe/22 gauge, 1.5 in needle or the prefilled syringe supplied by the lab
Vitamin K (IM)	Newborn	Tuberculin or insulin syringe w/25 or 27 gauge needle

Preparing an injection

To extract medication from a container and give an injection, gather the following supplies:

•Appropriately sized syringe and needles
•Medication in an ampule or a vial
•Filter needles (if an ampule is being used)
•Extra needles in case of contamination
•Antiseptic tincture and gauze pads or cotton balls
•Facial tissue or a gauze pad (if you are using an ampule)

Rubbing alcohol is thought by some to be carcinogenic. Plain 100 proof grain alcohol or an herbal tincture made with grain alcohol and an antiseptic herb such as rosemary, echinacea or other suitable plant can be used to clean surface contaminants from the skin.

Wash your hands before handling equipment.

Withdrawing medication from a vial:

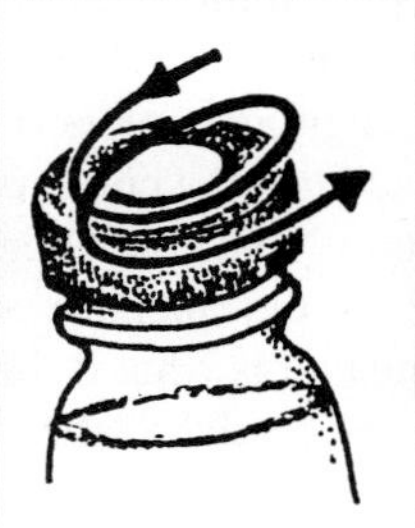
3. Cleaning the top.

1. Determine if you have the correct medication by checking the vial for the name, dosage and expiration date.
2. Examine the medication. Under glare-free light, hold the container over a plain white surface and examine the medication for discoloration, then over a plain colored surface to look for cloudiness and particulate matter. If you find any of these, it should be discarded. If the medication is in a brown container, you will need to carefully examine the medication after it is drawn up.
3. Remove the metal or plastic cap if the vial has not been previously opened. Cleanse the top of the vial with a spiraling motion from the center outward, using a gauze soaked in tincture. This will remove gross contaminants but will not sterilize it.
4. Allow the tincture to dry. This will prevent introducing it into the medication when you insert the needle.
5. Remove the syringe from its package. If you have purchased needles and syringes separately, unwrap the appropriately sized needle and luer-lock it to the barrel by screwing it firmly onto the tip of the syringe.
6. Since the vial is airtight, it will be necessary to inject air into the vial to remove the fluid. The amount of air you inject should be equal to the amount of liquid to be withdrawn. To inject air, remove the needle sheath and hold the syringe at eye level. Draw back on the plunger to the amount of drug to be administered, i.e., if you are to give 1 cc of drug, pull the plunger back so that the edge of the rubber stopper lines up with the 1 cc mark or a bit beyond (if the vial is full, it is best to inject slightly more air). Be careful to touch only the end of the plunger, not its shaft.

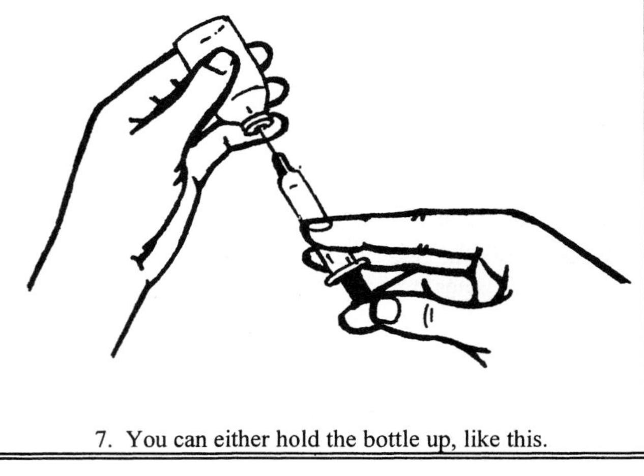
7. You can either hold the bottle up, like this.

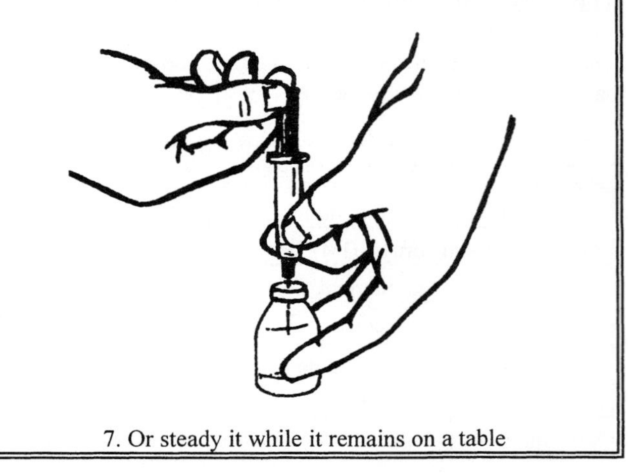
7. Or steady it while it remains on a table

7. Turn the needle so that the bevel is uppermost. Hold the syringe so that the needle is at a 45° angle against the stopper. Apply pressure to slice into the rubber. Then reposition the needle so that it is perpendicular to the rubber stopper and insert it further, but not all the way to the hub (Poznar, 2002). This helps prevent coring the rubber, especially if you are not using a filter needle. ("Coring" refers to slicing a tiny bit of rubber out of the top. A core can become dislodged in the medication, may plug the needle and can be injected into the tissue during administration.) You may hold the vial either up or down as illustrated on the preceding page when you insert the needle (drawings done after the needle has been inserted at an angle and straightened in relation to the vial).
8. Keeping the vial in your chosen position, inject the measured air into the vial.
9. The needle point should remain below the fluid level in the vial to ensure that no air is drawn into the syringe. Air in the syringe will cause your dosage to be inaccurate. While holding the equipment as illustrated above, move the needle tip to below the fluid level and withdraw the exact amount of medication you need from the vial. Be sure to support the plunger if you are using a glass syringe, as the plunger might slip out if you don't. The air you injected into the vial may produce sufficient pressure to allow the syringe to fill passively. If you do get air into the syringe, push up on the plunger and the air will be reintroduced into the vial. Flick the side of the syringe with your fingers to encourage air bubbles to rise to the needle end if necessary.

   Adjust the amount of medication in the syringe until it is just right.
10. Remove the needle from the vial.
11. To prevent leakage from the filled syringe, hold the needle point up and draw about 5 mm of air into the syringe. (The air bubble should be about the size of a small pea.) If you are not ready to use it immediately, replace the sheath over the needle and lay the syringe down.
12. Double-check the medication and expiration date on the vial.

NOTE: If you have not drawn an air bubble into the syringe, you must still hold the filled syringe horizontally or with the needle pointed up to prevent loss of medication prior to injection. The syringe can be replaced in its paper wrapper and propped with the needle slightly elevated until you are ready to use it. It must not be propped so as to put pressure on the plunger.

Once a multi-use vial has been opened, its contents are guaranteed to be sterile for 30 days provided sterile technique is employed each time the vial is entered; that is, a needle or syringe that has been used should not be used to re-enter a vial. Mark the vial with the date on which you opened it. This keeps multi-use vials uncontaminated for future use with other clients.

Withdrawing medication from an ampule: Sometimes a dose will consist of only a portion of the ampule contents; in midwifery, this is primarily relevant to epinephrine administration. If only some of the medication is withdrawn, the rest is considered contaminated and must be thrown away. If you withdraw the entire contents of the ampule into one syringe, it can be used to administer multiple doses to the same woman if aseptic technique is observed during administration. Once you are finished treating that individual, the syringe and any remaining contents must be discarded.

1. Check the ampule to be sure you have the correct medication in the correct dosage and that it has not expired.
2. Look for discoloration, cloudiness and particulate matter just as for a vial. If the ampule is colored or labeled so that you cannot see the fluid clearly, you will need to do this after the medication has been drawn up.
3. Remove your syringe from its packaging. If a needle is attached, secure its cap and remove it. Place the cap on the inside of the syringe wrapper to maintain sterility. Attach a filter needle securely onto the syringe tip.
4. Look to see if there is any medication in the narrow top part of the ampule. If so, hold the ampule by the narrow end. With your arm straight, rotate your arm from your shoulder once or twice in a 360° arc. This will cause all the fluid to go into the base of the ampule. You can also grasp the narrow end and shake the ampule sharply two or three times or flick the narrow tip with your fingers to bounce the fluid down into the base. If these methods fail, however, the rotation method works great.
5. Wipe the ampule, especially the neck, with a tincture-soaked gauze pad and allow it to dry.
6. To open the ampule, locate the break line on its neck. Snap off the portion above the neck by wrapping the entire ampule in a dry sterile gauze pad; grasp the ampule just above the narrowest part of the neck with one hand, grasp it just below the neck with the other hand, point the break away from your body, and snap it in two with one quick, sure motion to minimize shattering the glass.

Some ampules do not have a prescored break line. These may come with a small file to use for filing around the neck before you snap it off. After filing around the neck, wipe off the ampule with tincture to remove shaved glass, allow it to dry and then snap it open. You are most likely to encounter unscored ampules in the developing world.

7. Make sure the plunger of the syringe is pushed all the way down.
8. Withdraw fluid from the ampule using one of the techniques illustrated below. Try not to touch the needle shaft to the ampule lip as you withdraw medication, keep the tip of the needle below the fluid level and keep the bevel flat against the lowermost wall of the ampule throughout withdrawal. If it is an emergency and you do not have access to a filter needle, leave the last drop of fluid in the bottom of the ampule to minimize the chances of drawing up any tiny shards of glass or other invisible particulate matter.

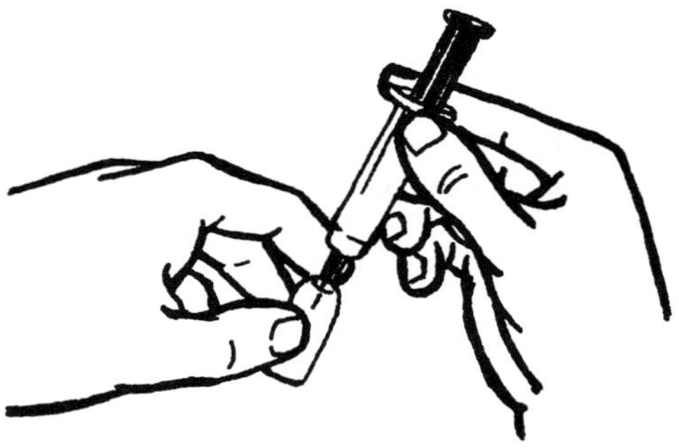

8. You can hold the ampule open-end up.

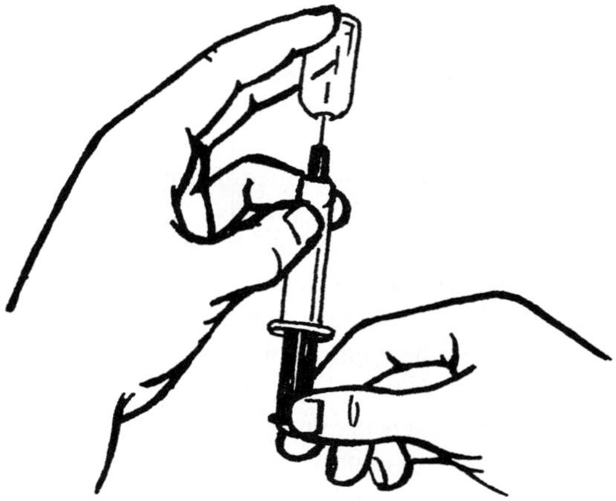

8. You can also hold it open-end down. Surface tension in the medication prevents it from running out.

9. Hold the filled syringe in an upright position to prevent medication from dripping out.
10. Draw about 5 mm of air to equal the size of a small pea into the syringe, to prevent leakage of the medication and to ensure that no medication inadvertently remains in the filter needle or its hub.
11. Cap and remove the filter needle and replace it with the appropriately sized needle for the injection.
12. If you are not using the injection immediately, replace the sheath and lay the syringe aside, needle-end propped up, until you are ready to use it. To prevent leakage from the filled syringe during handling, hold the needle point up.
13. Double-check the medication, dosage and expiration date.
14. If you have not already done so, use good light to examine the medication through the wall of the syringe for discoloration, cloudiness or particulate matter.

Needle recapping technique: You will need to recap a needle when switching from a filter needle to a regular needle, when medication has been drawn up for later use or when no sharps container is available. Note that Official OSHA regulations prohibit recapping needles, so you cannot ask an employee to do so and should instruct them not to.

To safely recap a needle, lay the cap on a table. Hold the syringe by the barrel with the needle pointed away from you. If the needle has not been used, guide the needle into the cap until it is over the hub to maintain maximum sterility. If the needle has been used, scoop up the cap. Now hold the syringe horizontally and press the capped end against a firm vertical surface (the wall, for example) to seat the cap more securely on the hub. Alternatively, hold the syringe upright so the cap falls to the base of the needle hub. Then you may safely secure the cap completely with your other hand.

Reconstituting powdered medications: Occasionally an injectable medication will be packaged as a dry powder that needs to be mixed with an accompanying single-use vial or ampule of fluid immediately prior to administration. In this case, draw up the fluid from the ampule or vial into a sterile syringe. If a glass ampule is provided, use a filter needle to do so.

Uncap the vial of powder, clean the top and insert the needle. Position the tip of the needle against the side of the vial and inject the fluid slowly so that it runs down the inside wall of the vial. (Forcefully squirting the fluid directly into the powder usually produces bubbles.) Remove the needle and gently roll the vial between your hands or tip it end to end until the solution is well mixed. Use only enough motion to mix the solution. Avoid vigorous shaking, which can create many air bubbles that interfere with solution withdrawal. Once mixed, the medication can be drawn up into a syringe as you would from any vial.

Eliminating air bubbles from drawn medications: Sometimes tiny, stubborn air bubbles cling to the inner walls of the syringe after the medication has been drawn up. Flicking the syringe may help, but the quickest way to remedy this problem is to draw the plunger out beyond the level of the air bubbles and then reposition it correctly. This usually eliminates them completely. Tiny air bubbles are sometimes impossible to clear but pose no danger to the person receiving the injection.

Where and how to give an injection

Wherever the proposed injection site, avoid inserting the needle into moles, bruises, thin tissue over bone or inflamed, swollen or discolored areas.

Depths of injection: There are several different depths at which injections are given.

Intradermal (subcuticular) administration: This involves injecting a drug directly beneath the skin surface. This technique is usually limited to the administration of local anesthetic and to perform skin testing, such as TB testing. It is also used to produce sterile water papules to relieve excessive pain during labor. Volumes injected intradermally are usually limited to 1 ml and are given with a 25 to 27 gauge, ⅜ to 1 in long needle. Drugs administered via this route are absorbed slowly and tend to have only a local effect. (See the subchapter entitled "Sterile Water Injections for the Relief of Excessive Localized Pain" for full details.)

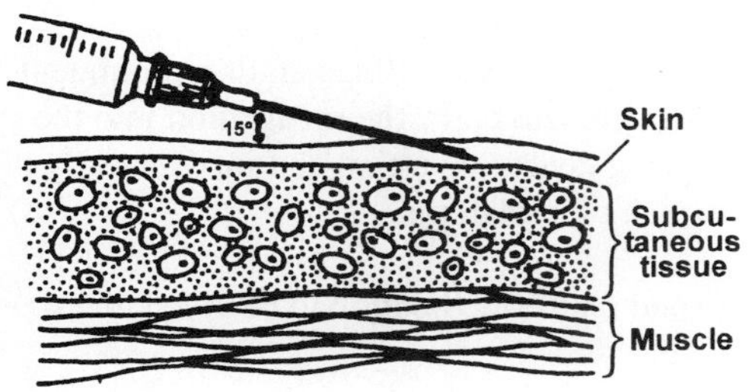

Intradermal injection

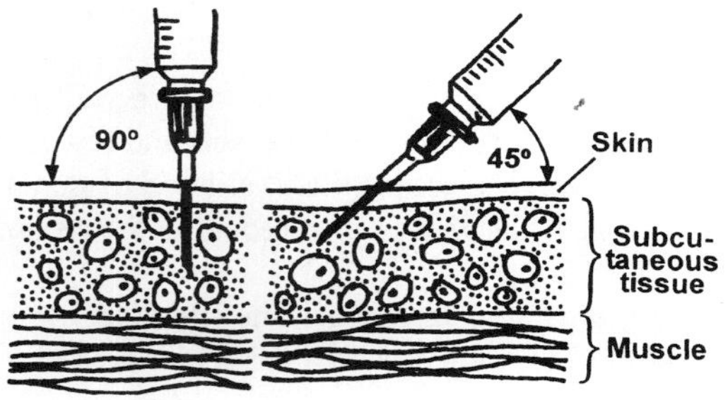

Subcutaneous injection: angles of insertion (see instructions)

Subcutaneous (SQ or SC) administration: This involves injecting medication into the loose connective tissue underlying the dermis. Volumes injected subcutaneously are usually limited to 1 ml or less and are given with a 24 to 26 gauge, ½ to ⅞ inch needle, depending upon the size of the person. Subcutaneous absorption is slower and more sustained than intramuscular administration because this tissue is less vascular than muscle tissue. It is the preferred route for insulin and for 1:1000 epinephrine when used for asthma or allergic reactions. Treatment of anaphylactic allergic reactions with epinephrine is the primary midwifery application for SQ injection.

The best sites for SQ injections are vascular areas, around the outer surface of the upper arms, the abdomen outside a 2 in (5 cm) radius of the navel and the anterior aspect of the thigh. The location and angle of needle insertion depends upon the size and weight of the person. Injections in the abdominal area are given at a 90° angle. To administer a subcutaneous injection, proceed as follows:

1. First, grasp a skin fold between your thumb and index finger at the proposed site of injection. Measure the skin fold across the space between your fingers. The needle length should be one-half the width of the top of the skin fold.
   -If width of the fold is between 2.5 cm (1 in) and 5 cm (2 in), the needle is inserted at a 90° angle.
   -If the width of the fold is 2.5 cm (1 in) or less, the needle is inserted at a 45° angle.

-Do not squeeze the fold, as this will make needle penetration more painful and more difficult.

- **For average-sized persons:** Use a 25 gauge, ⅝ in needle. Gently grasp a roll of tissue to measure. Then either hold the tissue *or* release and spread it tautly and insert the needle quickly and firmly at a 90° angle into the center of the skinfold.
- **For thin persons:** Gently grasp a roll of tissue and insert the needle quickly and firmly at a 45° angle into the center of the skin fold.
- **For women-of-size:** A thick skin fold requires the use of a 25 gauge, ⅞ in needle. Grasp the tissue at the proposed site of puncture. While still holding the skin fold, insert the needle at a 45° angle at the *base* of the fold.

2. After the needle is in the tissue, release the skin fold.
3. Inject the solution slowly. Press the plunger all the way in. Wait a few seconds after injecting the medication before withdrawing the needle. Rapid injections create pressure, resulting in discomfort. Slow injection allows the solution to disperse into surrounding tissues.
4. Withdraw the needle quickly, smoothly and steadily to reduce discomfort and the risk that medication will leak into shallower tissues.
5. Apply pressure with a gauze pad and massage the injection site for as long as two minutes if rapid absorption is desired. This spreads the medication into the tissue and hastens absorption by increasing blood supply to the area.

Intramuscular (IM) injections: These injections involve the administration of small quantities of a drug directly into a muscle. The volume injected into muscle is usually limited to 4 ml or less, as larger volumes may cause irritation. The upper limit of this amount (4 ml) can be injected into well-developed muscles of adults because fluid spreads rapidly through the muscle's elastic fibers. A volume of 1 to 2 ml should be used if the muscle tissue is less than well developed. Only 1 ml or less should be given to an infant intramuscularly. The needle should be 1 to 1.5 in (2.5 to 3.75 cm) in length and 21 to 23 gauge, depending upon the size of the adult; the larger the person, the longer the needle must be, especially if there is a thick layer of fat where you must inject. The needle should be inserted at a 90° angle to the skin surface. Absorption time is determined by the type of drug injected as well as the circulation the muscle receives. For example, water-based (aqueous) solutions are absorbed in 10 to 30 minutes, while oil-based medications (such as some antibiotics) are absorbed more slowly.

Sites recommended for IM injections are well padded with fat, have few nerve endings and no prominent bones. They also have lots of small blood vessels and few large ones. Small vessels will carry the medication into the system. Avoiding large vessels lessens the likelihood of puncturing a vessel during needle insertion and inadvertently giving a drug intravenously, as well as also reducing the risk of producing a bruise or hematoma.

***Sites for intramuscular injection*:** The site of an IM injection will depend on the medication to be given, the size of the woman and the ease of access to a particular area of her body.

Thigh (vastus lateralis) site: One injection site is in the lateral muscle of the quadriceps group, along the length of the muscle body of the thigh, starting a hand's breadth below the greater trochanter and running to a hand's breadth above the knee. You may also locate the region by dividing the length of the outer thigh into thirds and injecting into the center of the middle third. There are some small nerve endings in this area, so some people complain of pain with injections given here, but there are no large nerves or blood vessels and it does not overlie a joint, so the chances of serious injury are slight. It is the safest site to use in a newborn. Have the woman lie on her back with her toes pointed inward or the knee slightly flexed on the side to be injected. Insert the needle on an angle pointing slightly toward the knee (if she is thin) or at a right angle to the muscle. Inject into the outer side of the muscle, not the anterior thigh.

Hip (ventrogluteal) site: The side of the hip lacks major nerve endings and blood vessels yet has dense muscle and a consistent layer of fat. It is therefore considered safer than the dorsogluteal site for adults and anyone over 7 months of age. Have the woman lie on her side to help you locate landmarks. To relax the muscle, the woman should flex her upper leg on the side to be injected and place it somewhat in front of the lower leg. If the woman is lying on her left side, use your left hand; if she is lying on her right, use your right hand. With this hand, find both the greater trochanter at the head of the femur and the superior iliac spine. Place the palm of your hand over the greater trochanter and the index finger on the anterior superior iliac spine (the lateral, anterior corner of the hip bone where the crest curves toward the front). Point your thumb toward her groin and your fingers toward her head. Spread the middle finger back along the iliac crest as far as possible, creating a "V" between your index and middle fingers. Change hands as necessary to spread the tissue to keep it taut, and to give the injection with your dominant hand. Inject into the center of the "V." Angle the needle slightly upward toward the woman's head as you insert it.

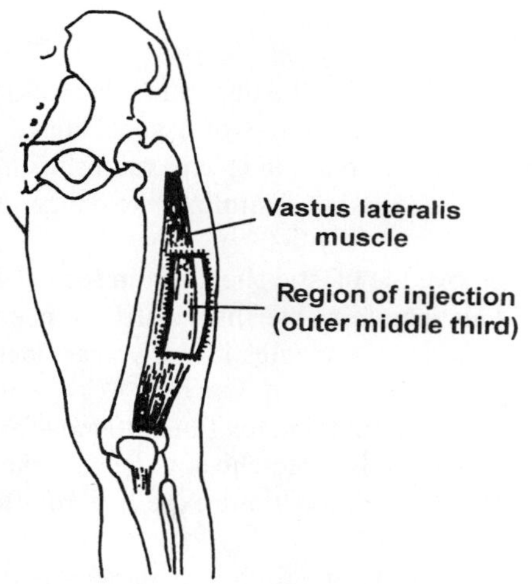

Thigh (vastus lateralis site)

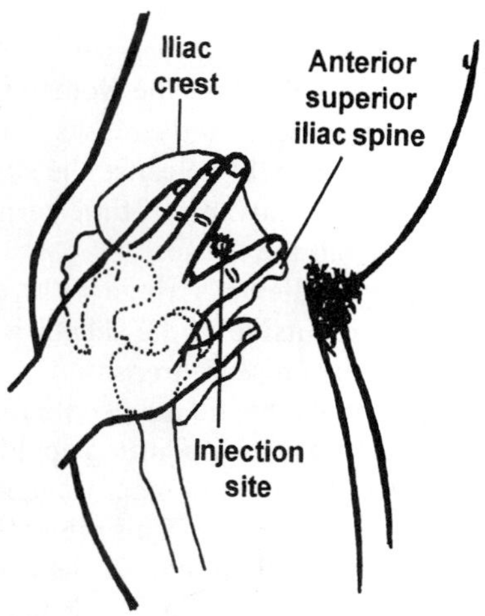

Hip (ventrogluteal site)

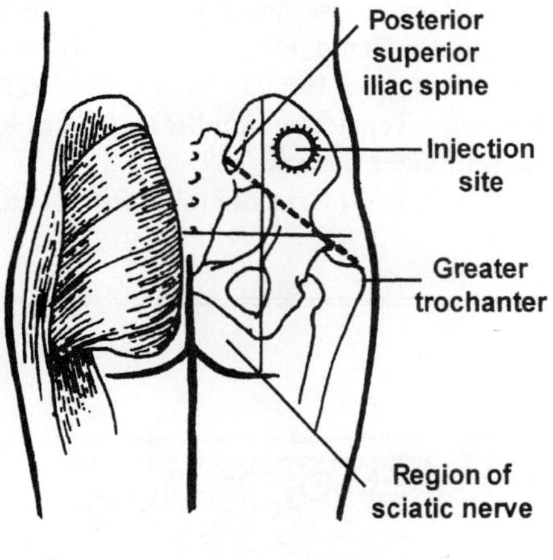

Upper buttock (dorsogluteal site)

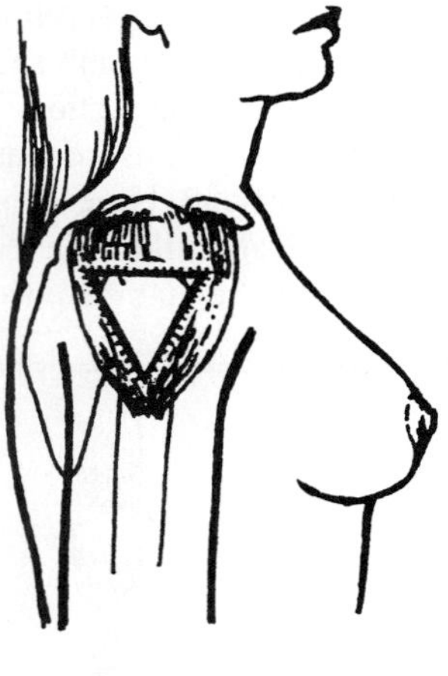

Upper arm (deltoid site)

Upper buttock (dorsogluteal) site: This traditional site for IM injections is in the center of the region of the gluteus maximus muscle, above and outside the diagonal line drawn from the posterior superior iliac spine to the greater trochanter of the femur (the center of the upper outer quadrant of the buttocks).

To use this location, ask the woman to lie on her belly with toes pointed inward or on her side with her upper knee and hip flexed and her upper knee placed in front of her lower leg. Expose the buttocks. Imagine a cross over the center of one buttock, then find the center of the upper outer quadrant and inject there. Insert the needle at a 90° angle to the muscle all the way to the hilt.

This area is particularly difficult to use in large women or those of size, as landmarks are hard to identify and a thick fat layer will prevent the needle from penetrating deeply enough to administer the medication into the muscle with a 1.5 in needle. It works best in thin to average-weight women with small to medium build.

However, use of this site has fallen out of favor. The layer of subcutaneous fat overlying the muscle is inconsistent, which frequently results in the drug not being deposited into the muscle. Even worse, inserting the needle too low or too close to the crease of the buttocks may permanently damage the sciatic nerve or puncture the superior gluteal artery. The newborn is especially at risk for such injuries.

Upper arm (deltoid): The upper arm can only tolerate a maximum of 1 ml of injected solution; making it an unsuitable location for the types of injections midwives typically administer.

Administering an intramuscular injection:

1. Select the site for injection. Have the woman position herself on her side (to inject the uppermost buttock) or on her back (to inject the thigh). This decreases the woman's discomfort and reduces the risk of tissue damage.
2. Using firm friction, thoroughly cleanse the skin at the proposed entry site out to a 2 in (5 cm) radius, using a spiral motion from the center outward. If time permits, allow the area to dry. Cleansing minimizes the danger of forcing organisms and dirt into the tissue.
3. It is probably best to handle the syringe with your dominant hand. Remove the plastic sheath from the needle, being sure not to touch the outside of the sheath with the needle shaft. This maintains sterility. Until the needle enters tissue, there is no risk of disease transmission to either you or your client from a needlestick. If you accidently prick yourself at this point, exchange the needle for a sterile one before proceeding.
4. Hold the syringe with the needle pointing up. Flick the barrel with your nondominant index finger to move air bubbles to the needle end and use the plunger to gently expel all air from the barrel. Double-check to be sure the accurate amount of drug is in the syringe. This minimizes the chances of ejecting medication while expelling air. Be sure the needle is well seated and then remove the cap.
5. If you have drawn up a pea-sized air bubble to prevent leakage, eject it now, watching for the appearance of a tiny drop of medication at the tip of the needle. Modern syringes are designed to deliver accurate dosages without the use of an air bubble to force the last of the medication out of the needle.
6. Some practitioners firmly slap the area to be injected with the flat of their palm before inserting the needle. This serves as a distraction, lessening the perceived pain from the injection itself. Warn the woman if you are going to do this.
7. Z-Track technique: Using the thumb and first two fingers of your nondominant hand, press down firmly on the tissue around the proposed site of injection. Apply skin traction downward or laterally. Be careful not to touch the site of entry itself. Pressure helps ensure that the needle enters the muscle tissue. Tension and pulling reduces leakage of medication into superficial tissues when the needle is removed and minimizes pain.
8. Hold the syringe vertically, like a dart with the needle down, and quickly thrust the needle to its full length into the tissue. This helps ensure that the needle will enter muscle tissue.

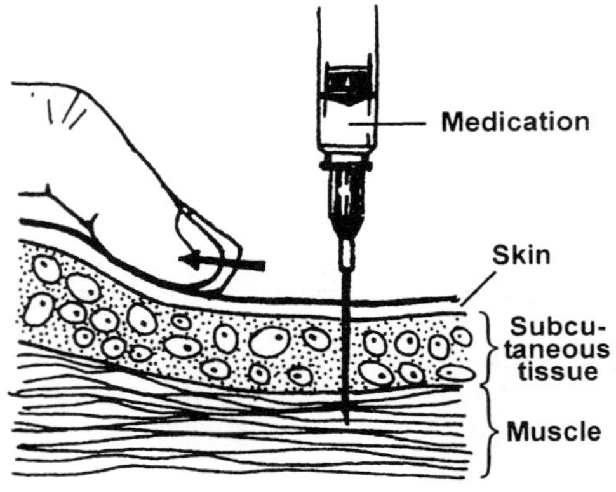

Z-track technique: beginning injection

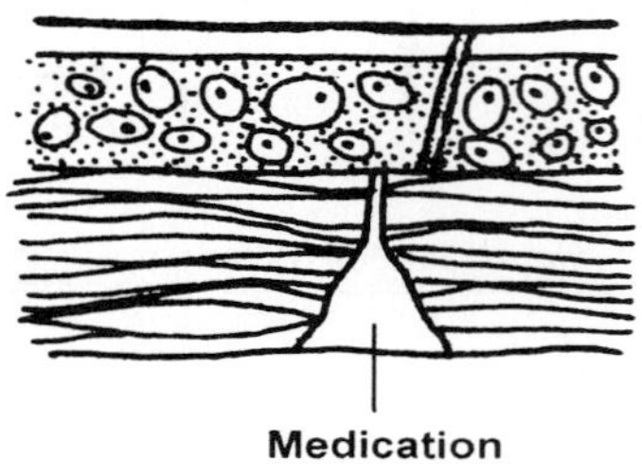

After the skin is released

9. With the needle in place, use your nondominant fingers to steady the lower part of the syringe. Use your dominant hand to pull back on the plunger for 5 to 10 seconds. If you are not in a vessel, the plunger will resist being pulled back (it will feel as though you are pulling against a suction). If the needle is in a blood vessel, blood will appear in the syringe and the plunger will pull back easily. If flashback occurs, remove the needle from the tissue, replace the needle with a new one and select a new site. Drugs injected into a blood vessel are absorbed immediately. IM injections are intended for slower absorption and may be dangerous if injected directly into the bloodstream.

10. If no flashback occurs, inject the solution slowly at a rate of 1 ml every 10 seconds. Press the plunger all the way in, then wait 10 seconds before withdrawing the needle. Rapid injection creates pressure, resulting in discomfort. Slow injection allows the solution to disperse into surrounding tissues.
11. Withdraw the needle quickly, smoothly and steadily to reduce discomfort and the risk that medication will leak into shallower tissues.
12. Z-Track technique: Release the tension on the skin after the needle has been withdrawn. Releasing the tissue allows the layers to realign, which lessens leakage.
13. Apply pressure with a gauze pad and gently massage the injection site for as long as two minutes if rapid absorption is desired. This helps spread the medication into the muscle and hastens absorption by stimulating circulation.

Disposing of Sharps

You must be careful not to puncture yourself with the used needle after giving the injection. Do not recap the needle if you can avoid doing so. Place the needle in a sharps receptacle designed to either cut the needle off or grab the needle, allowing you to twist off the hub before pushing the rest of the syringe into the container. Alternatively, use a sharps container big enough to allow disposal of the entire syringe with the needle attached. Open the receptacle with one hand, move that hand well away from the receptacle, and drop the entire syringe into the opening. Do not attempt to cram a used syringe into a full or nearly full receptacle, as this invites puncture with a contaminated needle. Dispose of empty vials and pieces of ampules in a sharps container as well.

If you have no immediate access to a sharps container, you will need to recap the needle as already explained. Once the cap is firmly seated, twist the hub to remove the needle. Remove the syringe plunger, insert the capped needle into the empty barrel of the syringe, and reinsert the plunger as far as it will go. Save the used syringe in a labeled resealable plastic bag in a safe location, such as a box in your birth bag, where it is not likely to become dislodged or be accidently tossed in the trash. Dispose of it later in a sharps container.

If you have used a small syringe with a nonremovable needle that cannot be properly disposed of right away, scoop up the cap, place a piece of tape over the cap and secure the tape to the barrel of the syringe. Then place it in a resealable plastic bag for proper disposal later.

STERILE WATER INJECTIONS FOR THE RELIEF OF EXCESSIVE LOCALIZED PAIN

Sterile water injections, used properly, can relieve excessive pain during labor. Sometimes called the "midwife's epidural," these injections may relieve pain to the point that the woman can relax sufficiently to allow labor to progress and a transport can be avoided. This procedure will not work to relieve the normal sensations of labor and is most useful when the baby is posterior or when other factors cause the pain of labor to be pronounced in a particular region of the body, especially the back. This technique will work for most, but not all, women with this type of labor. This chapter will cover the use of this technique from two medical perspectives: Western and Chinese.

Will this work?

To determine if a woman is a candidate for this procedure, ask her to rate her level of discomfort on a scale ranging from 0 (no pain) to 10 (the most intense pain she can imagine). A rating of at least 7 is warranted before you can expect this technique to provide any relief.

Injection Therapy, Western Style

Mainstream Western medicine attributes the success of this technique to the gate control theory, first proposed in 1965. Briefly, this theory states that the brain is not a passive receiver of pain messages, but can actually influence the passage as well as the reception of stimuli. Application of this theory entails the injection of sterile water intradermally over regions which are painful. Introduction of the water causes brief but intense pain. This message is relayed to the brain and the brain then "ignores" the pain messages that were coming from the region in the first place.

Equipment

You will need ampules or vials of sterile water with no preservatives. Do not use sterile saline, as it will be much less effective. Remember that a multiple-use 10 cc vial remains sterile for 30 days after the first use when good sterile technique is employed during each reuse. A 1 cc (100 unit) insulin syringe is ideal to use because it can hold enough solution for all four injections. It should be fitted with a 28 or 29 gauge needle. A tuberculin syringe is not appropriate because its capacity markings are unsuited to the tiny quantities you need to inject and the needles tend to be less sharp.

Dosage

Draw up a sufficient quantity of sterile water to allow you to make either four 0.1 cc or four 0.15 cc injections. The lower dosage creates an anesthetic effect that lasts about 45 minutes; the higher dosage lasts up to 2 to 3 hours. It is best to fill the syringe so you will have enough for all the injections should some fluid dribble out while you transfer from one injection site to the next.

Locating the sites for injection

Stand behind the woman and look at her back to locate the diamond-shaped depression in the midline immediately above the buttocks. Place your fingertips on each of her iliac crests (the top of her hip bones) with your thumbs pointing toward her sacrum. Now, keeping your thumbs straight, slide your fingers along the iliac crests toward her spine, feeling along the posterior crests of the bone adjacent to the upper sacroiliac joints with the tips of your thumbs. There are often

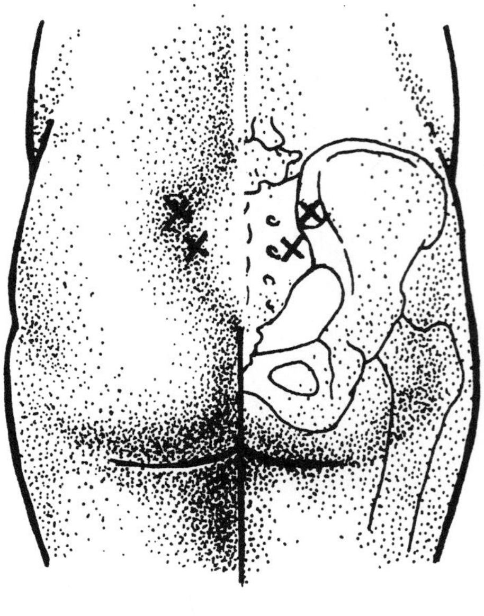

Locating the sites for injection

bilateral dimples overlying the prominences of the posterior superior iliac spines (indicated by two × marks in the drawing). One bleb is injected on each side, over these dimples.

Below each of these points, about one thumb space toward the midline (1 cm down and in from the first points) are two less obvious dimples overlying two much smaller bilateral projections adjacent to each of the 2nd sacral foramina (indicated by the two lower × marks in the drawing). Inject two more blebs over these small dimples; a total of four in all. Inject at least two bilateral sites (either the top two or the bottom two). These dimples are in the region of large acupuncture points, so getting the injections in the vicinity of these points will suffice to achieve the desired effect. Get the mother's agreement that all four points can be injected before you start and always begin with the top two points first. Tell her in advance that at least two blebs that are parallel each other on opposite sides of the back may provide some relief, but in most cases only a single site will not.

You can also place the injections wherever the woman experiences the most pain. This need not be in the back, and midwives have achieved significant pain relief by using this technique in other areas of the body as well. Each injection will cause an intense, localized stinging sensation that lasts 30 to 90 seconds. It is therefore very important to get the mother's fully informed cooperation before proceeding.

Injecting Blebs from a 1 cc (100 unit) Insulin Syringe		
Bleb	**For 0.1 cc blebs, fill syringe to the 50 unit mark and press plunger to the mark for each bleb as indicated below**	**For .15 cc blebs, fill syringe to the 70 unit mark and press plunger to the mark for each bleb as indicated below**
No. 1	40	55
No. 2	30	40
No. 3	20	25
No. 4	10	10

(Filling the syringe as recommended leaves 10 units of water in the syringe after you have given all the injections.)

Once the points are located, proceed as follows:

1. Close the door and warn family members that this will be a brief but painful procedure and there may be some hollering as a result.
2. Cleanse the area with antiseptic herbal tincture on a swab.
3. Have someone focus on the mother. Hold her hands and support her while she breathes deeply. Prepare to administer the injections quickly during the space between contractions.
4. Double-check the barrel of the syringe to note the amount you intend to inject on the gauge. Unsheathe the needle and hold it parallel to the skin surface. Rotate the barrel of the syringe until you can see how much you are injecting. Prepare the woman by telling her you are about to begin and have her start blowing hard into her cupped hands as she focuses on her breathing.
5. Introduce the tip of the needle just barely under the skin at a 5 to 15° angle, until you feel resistance. Advance the needle through the epidermis just below the skin surface and no deeper than 3 mm (1/16 of an inch). If this is done correctly you will be able to see the tip of the needle beneath the skin without poking it through. It is not necessary to aspirate to check if you are in a blood vessel because the dermis is relatively avascular.
6. Inject 0.1 to 0.15 cc of water. Your goal is to raise a bleb (papule) ¼ inch in diameter just beneath the skin. This will appear as an elevated, flattish blister very similar in appearance to a pale mosquito bite or a TB test site. Minimal bruising may result.
7. Remove the needle. Do not rub these blebs in an attempt to aid absorption since you want them to remain swollen.
8. Raise another bleb at the point parallel to and opposite the first, then drop down and repeat the procedure at the other two points. You need not use a fresh needle for each bleb with this type of injection or cleanse the skin again between injections.

Effectiveness and follow-up treatment

The woman should experience a notable decrease in her level of pain with the next contraction. The injections will reach their maximum level of effectiveness by the second contraction. Take this opportunity to encourage the mother to rest a bit, then get her up and do whatever is necessary to facilitate birth. The injections can be repeated without any problem if more pain relief is necessary.

Injection Therapy, Chinese Style

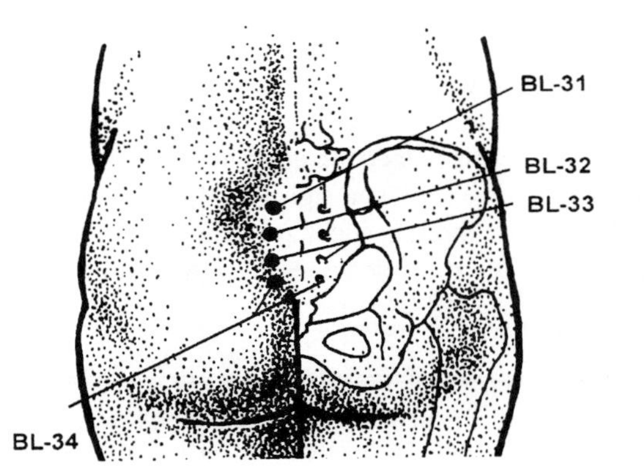

The Baliao points

In general Chinese medical practice, a variety of techniques are used to stimulate acupuncture points. These include pressure, the insertion of a needle, application of heat, and electrical current. The injection of an inert liquid to a depth of 1 to 2 inches can also be used to provide the strongest and longest-lasting stimulation of an acupuncture point.

The Chinese refer to the points used for sterile water injections during labor as the "baliao points." These bladder points are located in the 1st, 2nd, 3rd and 4th sacral foramina (BL-31, BL-32, BL-33 and BL-34), on each side of the sacrum (8 points in all) one of the woman's finger-breadths lateral to the midline, overlying the center of each sacral foramen. The 1st and 2nd foramina (BL-31 and BL-32) are the largest and the easiest to locate. Note that the uppermost dimples of the rhomboid of Venus do not overlie a foramen and are formed where the lowermost tips of the iliac crests meet the sacrum on either side. Bladder 32, however, lies midway between the uppermost dimple and the spine, overlying the 2nd sacral foramina. The baliao points are relatively large regions. Therefore, stimulation at the dimple in the Western technique usually manages to stimulate BL-32 as well.

The sacral foramina are often difficult to find, particularly in a woman at term who has gained weight; neither are they always in a straight line. First locate the lumbosacral junction and the sacrococcygeal junction. Draw a vertical line down the center of the bones, ending at the upper end of the gluteal crease. Divide this line into five equal segments using the four fingertips of one hand, spreading your fingers as necessary to divide the line equally. Each finger should now rest on one of the four sacral spinous processes, which can sometimes be palpated as slight depressions. The foramina lie lateral to the processes, about 1 of the woman's finger-breadths off the midline (or above half the distance between the midline and the border of the sacrum) on either side. Note that the foramina form a gently converging "V" shape from the top of the sacrum downward, as the sacrum narrows toward the coccyx.

Stimulation of the baliao points, especially the ones over the 2nd sacral foramina (BL-32) is known to function wonderfully for the reduction of the excessive pain often produced by back labor. Valerie Hobbs, a midwife and practitioner of Chinese medicine, has noted that marked pain relief can be achieved with little or no painful stimulus at the site of injection if the exact locations of the acupuncture points are used (Hobbs, 2002). If you are not skilled in safe sacral injections to the appropriate depth, you should fall back on the subdermal method. This section is included for those Chinese medical practitioners and others who are skilled enough to use it safely.

Equipment

As with the Western method, needles used for injection therapy should be quite thin, with bores ranging from 25 to 28 gauge. The larger the bore of the needle, the more painful it will be for the mother, with no advantage in effectiveness. The barrel of the syringe will need to be large enough to accommodate 1 cc of sterile saline for each point to be injected. Note that this is a much larger amount of fluid than is required by the Western method. In Chinese medicine, unpreserved 0.9% sterile saline is used instead of sterile water since there is no attempt to increase the painful sensations of the injections.

Injection methods

Chinese medicine uses two injection methods:

1. Inject at the location of the point, just under the surface of the skin (subcutaneously) with a 1 in needle.
2. Inject deeply into the point using a 1.5 in needle.

You may, quite appropriately, be hesitant to use such a long needle in an area that contains as many nerves as does the sacrum. I therefore recommend that you obtain instruction and supervision by a practitioner skilled in this procedure to be sure you are identifying the anatomy and performing the injections correctly. Indeed, in some states, licensed practitioners of Chinese medicine are forbidden to use injections of any kind. You can also restrict yourself to the use of a shorter, 1 in needle or resort to the subdermal method mentioned above, to avoid hitting any large nerves. However, by the end of pregnancy many women have a thick layer of tissue in the sacral region and a 1 in needle may not even penetrate deeply enough to reach the acupuncture point.

Meridians are located at various depths, depending upon the anatomy under consideration. According to Chinese medical theory, the Qi of the point is accessed at the level of the meridian upon which it is located. These sacral points are located rather deep to the surface of the skin. In Japanese acupuncture theory, the Ki (their transliteration for Qi) is believed to rise to the surface and flow back to the depth of the point. The reason that treating at the surface over the point is often effective is that a change in energetic polarity is thought to occur as the Ki rises from and flows back down to the point. Hobbs (2002) has seen value in both theories. In some cases, a shallowly inserted needle may be ineffective, but a more deeply inserted needle at the same point has been quite effective. She has also noted the reverse to be the case. Therefore, the depth of insertion with which you feel comfortable may or may not work for an individual woman. If not, you can use the Western subdermal method.

1. If you are nervous about giving a deep injection, administer subcuticular injections over the baliao points using a 1 in, 25 to 27 gauge needle. Drawing up 3 to 4 cc of sterile water with a small gauge needle takes time; a larger bore needle can be used to load the syringe, you can then switch to the smaller gauge needle for the injection.

   Palpate to locate the sacral foramina. Insert the needle at a 45° angle just under the skin to a depth of 1 in. The skin over the sacrum is thicker than over most of the body, so be sure you are below the skin layer. One cc of saline is injected into the point, and then the syringe is withdrawn. Additional injections are given on the other side of the sacrum, and can be done over all 8 points (in the 4 foramina on each side).

   If you do hit a nerve, the woman will feel a flash of nerve pain. Immediately withdraw the needle, remove it from the syringe and attach a new, sterile needle. Now insert the needle at a more shallow depth before you inject the saline.
2. With practice, a midwife can use Method 2, administering deeper injections directly into the sacral foramina using a 27 gauge, 1.5 in needle. The tip of the needle is inserted to a depth of about 1 in, at a slight angle toward the spine and at an angle between 60 and 90° to the skin surface, into the center of each sacral foramen. One cc of saline is injected. When using this deeper injection method, just one set of bilateral points, at BL-32 at the level of the 2nd sacral foramina, are used rather than all eight injection sites.

Effectiveness and follow-up treatment

Pain relief, when obtained, should be nearly immediate and should last at least 45 minutes or longer. The injections can be repeated every hour if necessary, but it is probably best not to repeat them more than three times.

Acupressure

If you are concerned about using such deep injections, if lay use of acupuncture is illegal in your jurisdiction or if you have no access to supervised training, acupressure can be used to great advantage over the same area. Simply apply pressure to the BL-32 points with your fingertips or knuckles. When the point is located correctly, the woman will report a sensation that lets you and her know you are on target (the area is likely to feel particularly sensitive), confirming that you are not merely pressing on bone. The best location for pressure may move downward along parallel, converging points as the baby moves down during labor.

Practicing the Techniques

To practice the subdermal technique on students or midwives, use sterile 0.9% saline solution (normal saline) for the Western method, which is less painful upon injection than sterile water. Do not practice the Chinese method without experienced supervision.

The TENS Unit

TENS (transcutaneous electrical nerve stimulation) is the transmission of electricity across the skin surface to the nervous system via electrodes attached to the skin. It is used during birth extensively in England and Europe, but less so in the United States. These devices work on the principle of the gate control theory (see details in the chapter entitled "Sterile Water Injections for the Relief of Excessive Localized Pain") to reduce or relieve pain, in part by stimulating the production of endorphins. TENS units produce either symmetrical or asymmetrical bip,hasic pulses of electricity which last from 0.02 to 0.4 milliseconds at frequencies varying from 0 to 200 Hz at a voltage not exceeding 100 mA.

TENS is most helpful during early labor, but can be used throughout. Obstetrics units are available consisting of the TENS machine (which is small and portable), lead wires, electrodes and a battery. You will also need a special electrotransmission gel to establish conduction; substitutes should not be used. Karaya gum, a naturally occurring conductive gum, when moistened, becomes adhesive (it must be stored in a cool place). Manufacturers typically include detailed instructions and sometimes instructional videos with their equipment, which should be thoroughly studied prior to use. Look for a unit that provides a way to alter frequency according to individual needs, a way to change from burst to continuous mode with an additional boost of amplitude and a way to independently control the intensity of each pair of electrodes. Press/release buttons only transmit when finger pressure is maintained and are preferable to press/hold buttons, which may be forgotten and left on or off.

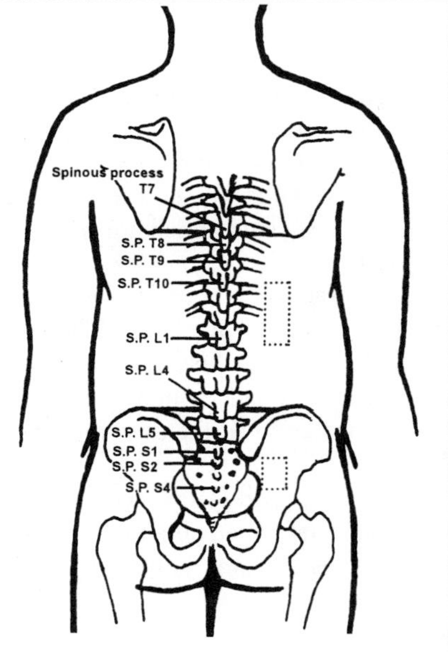

S.P.= spinous process

Use of the TENS Unit during labor

Contraindications and cautions: TENS cannot be used if the person has a cardiac pacemaker or prior to 37 weeks gestation (opinions vary as to the cut-off here; some say the first or second trimester). Epileptics should use TENS only after a full medical consultation. TENS may rarely interfere with readings on a fetal heart monitor. Do not place electrodes over the carotid artery (this can lead to cardiac arrhythmia) over the pharynx (where it may trigger spasm leading to cardiac arrest) or over the eyes, superficial bones (such as the tibia), near the heart (if there are heart problems), over the abdomen or over any skin lesions, open or closed. It should not be used while driving. If skin irritation develops, discontinue use. Its use may result in electrical burns, chemical or mechanical irritation or allergy. TENS cannot be used when the woman is in water. Keep all oils away from the electrodes.

TENS and drugs: Certain drugs are influenced by TENS. Those which enhance its pain relieving effects include tryptophan, tricyclic antidepressants and D-phenylalanine (DPA). Those that may decrease the analgesic affect of TENS include naloxone, benzodiazepines and corticosteroids.

Setting up the unit: Electrodes can be either reusable carbon-silicone (which require tape, gel or Karaya gum for attachment) or self-adhesive and disposable (attached by a conductive gel). Application with tape requires that the tape maintain full contact with the skin. Do not tape over an electrode-lead junction so that a detached lead can be seen; worn leads must not be used. The ideal size for labor is 10 cm × 4 cm. Four electrodes are commonly used over the nerves supplying the uterus and cervix.

Clean and dry the skin. ·Firmly attach the leads to the electrodes. Place the top two on either side of the spine between the spinous processes of T10 and L2 and *no higher*. Ask the woman to fully relax her shoulders with arms to her sides. Find the tips of the scapula. Trace toward the midline, until you hit a bump, which will be the spinous process of T7. Palpate down over three spines to reach T10. For self-adhesive electrodes, peel off the backing, avoid touching the adhesive, and apply to either side of the spine, leaving a space equal to the width of the patch between the two. Press firmly into place. To attach reusable electrodes, apply enough transmission gel to the flat side to cover the entire surface. Press firmly and tape securely into place as above. The lower electrodes are placed adjacent to the spinous processes between S2 and S4 and may require a shorter electrode. Palpate the hips to locate the iliac crests and follow horizontally to the midline to the spinous process of L4. Palpate down over this lump to the spinous processes of L5 and S1 to S2, S3 and S4. The sacral dimples overlie S2 on either side. Attach electrodes as above between the spinous processes of S2 and S4. Remove and reapply gel every 4 hours to prevent drying. (based on Davies, 1997)

OXYGEN DELIVERY DEVICES AND RESUSCITATION EQUIPMENT

Supplemental oxygen is widely used in emergency situations when the partial pressure of oxygen (PaO_2) in the bloodstream drops below 60 mm Hg or when the oxygen saturation of arterial hemoglobin (SAO_2) falls below 90%. At these values, tissue hypoxia is assumed to be present. The primary goal is to correct hypoxemia and thereby increase the oxygen content of arterial blood, which will improve oxygen delivery to the tissues.

Carrying oxygen to a birth allows the midwife to provide oxygen to the mother in the event that she is tired during labor or shocky from blood loss after the birth or if the baby's heart rate is compromised before birth. The midwife may also use it during resuscitation of the baby or mother. How and when to use oxygen during labor will be addressed as appropriate in the rest of this text. Specifically refer to the chapters entitled "Assessing and Supporting the Baby's Well-Being during Labor," "Resuscitating the Mother" and "Evaluating and Assisting the Infant in Need of Resuscitation."

Most midwives carry at least one oxygen tank, masks and tubing for use on the baby and mother and a bag-valve-mask resuscitation device for use on the baby. Midwives should also carry an adult bag-valve-mask for the mother. This chapter will go over the details regarding the basics of oxygen use and the equipment for its delivery, how it is constructed, how to check if it is working properly, how to set it up at the birth, and how to care for it. You owe it to yourself and your clients to be totally familiar with your equipment, how it works and how to use it safely. There is very little information in the medical literature about oxygen equipment. As you go through this chapter, have your equipment handy and practice!

Atmospheric Gases, Oxygen and Altitude

The atmosphere is made up of a combination of gases in the following proportions.

GAS	APPROXIMATE %	PARTIAL PRESSURE AT SEA LEVEL (MM HG)
Nitrogen (N_2)	78.6	597
Oxygen (O_2)	20.9	159
Carbon dioxide (CO_2)	0.04	0.3
Water (H_2O)	0.46	3.7
TOTAL	100	760

Air also contains insignificant amounts of other gases such as argon and helium.

Understanding atmospheric pressure

The total pressure exerted by any given combination of gases is the sum of the individual or partial pressures of each gas in the mix (Dalton's law). The pressure exerted by a single gas is referred to as its partial pressure, which is measured in millimeters of mercury (mm Hg) or torr (1 torr equals 1 mm Hg). Each gas exerts a pressure equal to its own percentage of the total concentration of gases. The combined pressure of the gases in the atmosphere at any given altitude, which is referred to as the total barometric pressure, decreases as altitude rises because the combined weight of the gaseous components decreases. (Just as water becomes heavier the deeper you are submerged). At sea level (0 ft [0 m]), the total barometric pressure is 760 mm Hg and the partial pressure of oxygen (PO_2) is 159.22 mm hg ($PO_2 = 20.93\% \times 760$ mm Hg $= 159.22$ mm Hg). At 10,000 ft (3048 m), the barometric pressure is reduced to 523 mm Hg and the partial pressure of oxygen has correspondingly decreased to 109.57 mm Hg ($PO_2 = 20.93\% \times 523$ mm Hg $= 109.57$ mm Hg).

Understanding how the gas content in the air changes at different altitudes will help in understanding how attending births at a high altitude may affect you and how transport of the mother or baby in an aircraft may impact them. From sea level to 70,000 feet (21,336 m), the percentage of atmospheric gases remains constant. However, as altitude rises, a decrease in barometric pressure results in the gas molecules in a given volume of air moving farther apart or expanding. For example, lets say there are 1000 molecules of gas in a given volume of air at sea level of which 20.9%, or 209, are oxygen. Lets imagine that an identical amount of space contains only 100 molecules of gas at 20,000 feet

(6097 m), of which 20.9% of 20.9 of them are still oxygen. Thus, the percentage of gases remains the same, even though the amount of each gas in a given cubic area decreases the higher up you go.

Facts about Oxygen

Oxygen (O_2) is the most important element to the maintenance of life on earth, comprising about 21% of the volume of atmospheric gas (although concentration varies according to altitude and, to a lesser extent, the amount of surrounding vegetation). It is colorless, transparent, tasteless, odorless and nonflammable. Oxygen makes up almost 50% of the weight of the earth's crust and is present in all living matter, as part of water molecules and in combination with other elements.

The principal source of oxygen for commercial and medical use is distilled, liquified air. Liquid air is a mixture of gases consisting of one-fifth oxygen and four-fifths nitrogen. Once the nitrogen is boiled off, the remaining oxygen can be further purified. The industry standard for medical-grade oxygen exceeds the 99% purity required by the United States Pharmacopeia. (Oxygen of lesser purity is used for some industrial applications.)

While oxygen itself is not flammable, it does support combustion. Materials that will burn in air usually burn more vigorously and sometimes explosively in an oxygen-enriched atmosphere. (See details later in the chapter.)

How the body takes up and carries oxygen

Oxygen enters the body via air inhaled into the lungs, where molecules of oxygen are picked up and carried via the blood to the cells. Some of these oxygen molecules dissolve directly into solution in the plasma. The amount of oxygen in the plasma is the most accurate means of determining whether oxygenation is adequate at the tissue level and in determining the extent to which oxygen combines with hemoglobin. The oxygen saturation level in plasma is designated as the Po_2 value.

Dissolved blood gases are referred to in terms of volume percent (vol %), which indicates milliliters of gas per 100 ml of plasma. In the adult, the average arterial blood level is 0.3 ml of dissolved oxygen for each 100 ml of plasma (or 3 ml O_2 to 1 liter of blood). When the plasma is saturated with this much oxygen, the plasma "compartment" is said to be filled.

Once the plasma is saturated to this degree, oxygen begins to be taken up by hemoglobin molecules, which remove dissolved oxygen from the plasma, allowing diffusion to continue. These oxygen molecules (about 98% or 197 ml) are incorporated into erythrocytes, where they bind to hemoglobin to become oxyhemoglobin. Oxyhemoglobin does not contribute to the Po_2 value of plasma.

Each gram of adult hemoglobin is able to take up and carry a maximum of 1.34 ml (or 4 molecules) of oxygen. A single red blood cell contains about 250 million hemoglobin molecules; each of these tiny cells is capable of carrying about 1 billion molecules of oxygen. However, the quantity of oxygen actually carried, or the content, is dependent upon the oxygen saturation. **Saturation** refers to the amount of oxygen combined with hemoglobin divided by the maximum amount of oxygen the hemoglobin is capable of carrying. (When a single hemoglobin molecule carries four molecules of oxygen, it is said to be fully saturated.) Saturation is expressed as a percentage: the ratio of the actual amount of oxygen the hemoglobin is carrying divided by its full capacity. For example, if the actual amount of oxygen the hemoglobin molecules are carrying is one-half their capacity, the saturation would be reported as 50%. In the normal situation, blood is saturated to an average of 95% of total capacity.

In the adult, oxygen consumption runs about 3.5 ml/kg/min, and in newborns it is about twice this much (7 ml/kg/min). Oxyhemoglobin is an unstable compound that readily releases oxygen to the tissues that need it most. It is released in the presence of elevated carbon dioxide in tissue fluids, at raised temperature and when increased levels of 2,3-diphosphoglycerate (2,3-DPG) are present in red blood cells. Increased levels of 2,3-DPG in the pregnant woman result in reducing the affinity of maternal hemoglobin for oxygen and enhancing the release of oxygen in the intervillous space, thus facilitating transfer to the baby. Fetal hemoglobin has a greater affinity for oxygen, facilitating transport across the placenta but reducing oxygen release to the tissues. (For more details, see the section on fetal hemoglobin in the chapter entitled "The Baby's Journey through Labor to Birth.")

Uptake of oxygen at high altitudes: The ability of the body to transfer oxygen across the alveolar membranes into the blood stream is dependent upon the diffusion gradient. The diffusion gradient is determined by the difference in the partial pressure of oxygen between the blood and the ambient air. The greater the diffusion gradient, the more rapid and pronounced the absorption will be. Thus, absorption is determined by the difference in the partial pressure of oxygen contained in the blood on one side of the alveolar membrane and the air on the other. When air enters the body at a higher pressure than that already in the blood, the oxygen is pushed across the alveolar membrane into the blood.

The partial pressure of the water in the body is 47 mm Hg at normal body temperature. As we inhale, water vapor from the respiratory tract is added to the inspired air. Humidification actually lowers the partial pressure of the inspired air because the addition of the water molecules changes the partial pressure of the inspired air to more closely match that of the blood. Humidification thus reduces the diffusion gradient. At an altitude of 62,976 ft (19,200 m), the barometric pressure is only 47 mm Hg. We cannot absorb oxygen at this altitude because when the inspired gases are combined with water vapor, the resulting barometric pressure of the inspired air falls below 47 mm Hg, thus there is no driving force to diffuse the oxygen across the membrane and into the blood.

Pharmacology

Pure oxygen is classified as a drug because of the profound effects it can have on the body.

Beneficial effects of short-term use: The short-term inhalation of pure oxygen in the form of a few whiffs through a face mask acts as an analgesic, relieving muscle tension as well as pain and nausea. It can calm down a nervous or fearful mother and give her a boost of energy, clear her head if she is tired, and help revive her if she is woozy from blood loss.

Toxicity: Oxygen is nontoxic at normal room-air concentrations. However, breathing a concentration of oxygen that exceeds the amount in room air can eventually lead to undesirable side-effects. Breathing nothing but pure oxygen may produce coughing and chest pains (often the earliest warning sign of toxicity), paresthesias (burning, prickling, tickling or tingling in the extremities), nausea and vomiting, malaise and fatigue within 6 to 24 hours. Concentrations of 60% may produce these symptoms after several days. Lung damage and enzyme disturbances develop as well, and if the concentration is not reduced, the end result is profound central nervous system disturbance, culminating in coma and death.

Infants given oxygen concentrations of 35 to 40% or above for prolonged periods may suffer permanent visual impairment or blindness. Retrolental fibroplasia (RLF) or retinopathy of prematurity (ROP), a condition in which light cannot penetrate to the retina, occurs when the withdrawal of long-term oxygen therapy triggers damage to the immature retinal vessels. When this happens, new vessels form in an attempt to supply the retina. As they grow, these vessels extend into the vitreous body, and retinal bleeding occurs. Together, these complications result in retinal detachment and blindness. While it has long been believed that it was the use of oxygen that caused this, James (1999) has demonstrated that it is abrupt discontinuation of oxygen administration that is the problem, although his findings have been largely ignored and not confirmed with additional studies. He found that when long-term therapy is withdrawn slowly over a period of weeks, retrolental fibroplasia did not occur in his population of babies (Stoller, 2003). Fortunately, midwives do not often need to administer long-term oxygen therapy to preterm newborns and RLF is rare in term infants, in part because they do not often require long-term oxygen therapy. Premature infants undergoing prolonged hyperoxygenation therapy may also develop bronchopulmonary dysplasia, a form of obstruction that may be caused by free-radical damage to lung tissues that is made worse in the presence of hypoperfusion secondary to early cord clamping (Morley, 2002).

However, even the short-term use of high concentrations of oxygen encourages the production of large quantities of free radicals. This occurs when intracellular oxygen concentrations overwhelm the antioxidant defenses of the cells. Free radicals are by-products of oxygen metabolism that can react with and damage important biomolecules, including enzymes, membrane lipids, and nucleic acids, all of which can lead to cell damage and death. Giving the mother Vitamins E and C with bioflavonoids as soon as she is stable can help her body cope with this and may benefit the baby as well. Giving the baby Vitamin E from an opened capsule onto the tongue can help the baby as well.

In healthy nonsmokers, respiration is regulated by the primary respiratory control center in the brain, which reacts to the level of carbon dioxide in the blood. The higher the level of carbon dioxide, the more rapid the respirations. Conversely, high concentrations of oxygen will cause a person to slow down her breathing.

It is important to note that persons who smoke or have chronic medical conditions that affect the lungs have an increased tolerance for elevated carbon dioxide levels. Chronically elevated carbon dioxide levels lead to a phenomenon known as **hypoxic drive**, which causes the body to switch from the respiratory center in the brain to secondary respiratory centers in the carotid arteries to regulate oxygen uptake in the blood. If the person is unconscious and breathing, giving too much oxygen too quickly will cause the carotid centers to shut down, resulting in respiratory arrest; this will not happen if the person is conscious. However, when these individuals experience respiratory difficulty unrelated to their pulmonary condition, such as women who are shocky from birth-related complications, they can be given oxygen at the same levels you would normally use but should be watched closely for signs of respiratory depression.

Do you need a prescription in the United States to carry oxygen?

Interestingly enough, the equipment that is most useful to midwives falls in the category of emergency equipment. Technically, an oxygen dispensing device is considered to be an emergency unit if it is a portable container holding medical-grade oxygen, has a pressure-reducing system for delivery, has a contents gauge, a mask or other means of delivery, and it is able to deliver oxygen at a minimum flow rate of 6 l/min or more for at least 15 minutes. Such units are available over the counter in the United States and refilling them does not require a prescription (FDA policy–Guide 7132a.16). In spite of this, the statutes in local jurisdictions vary and some may be more restrictive than this federal rule.

Medical grade vs. industrial grade oxygen: Both medical and industrial grade oxygen are dispensed from the same source and are identical in processing and purity. However, oxygen known to be for medical use is dispensed only into tanks which are labeled for medical use. Once gas for medical use is in the tank, its purity is tested again to ensure that no contaminants have also entered the tank in the process of filling. An oxygen tank that is not labeled for medical use can be filled at any welders supply house without a prescription in the United States.

Equipment to Store and Dispense Oxygen

Oxygen tanks

A cylinder for storing oxygen must be strong enough to withstand the pressure of the gas it contains. Cylinders can be constructed from seamless, high-quality steel or aluminum, which is 40% lighter than steel and more costly. The material for tank construction must meet chemical and physical requirements of the Department of Transportation in the United States and the Board of Transport Commissioners in Canada. In the United States, steel tanks holding pure oxygen are completely green, and aluminum tanks are often green around the top collar with the lower portion an unpainted gray-silver metal. Internationally, however, the color code for oxygen is white.

The amount of oxygen contained in a cylinder is determined by its pressure and temperature. Generally, the higher the pressure, the more oxygen is contained. Any gas confined in a closed container will increase its pressure as temperature rises. The possibility always exists that a cylinder charged with gas at a safe pressure at normal temperature may reach a dangerously high pressure at warmer temperatures. To prevent this during normal use or storage, federal regulations limit the amount of gas that may be charged into a cylinder.

There are two sizes of cylinders that are practical for portable use, D and E. Larger cylinders can be used in locations such as birthing centers, where the tank can remain stationary. Smaller cylinders are available as well, but their smaller capacity makes them impractical for many midwives to carry, as they must be filled more often and hold less than a half-hour of oxygen at a flow rate of 5 l/min. It is good to have enough oxygen on hand to go to two births in a row without refilling. Busy midwives often have multiple tanks. One regulator can be transferred from tank to tank as oxygen is used.

Cylinder size (diameter X height [including valve])	Gas characteristics of Oxygen Cylinder pressures at 70° F (21.1° C) = 1800 to 2400 psig*			
	Cylinder volume		Running time in minutes	
	Cubic feet	Liters	Approximate at 6 l/min	Best at 6 l/min
D (4.5 X 20), Constant .16	14.0	350-425	66.00	48.0
E (4.25 X 30), Constant .28	23.3	625-679	109.8	84.0

*psig = pounds per square inch, gauge

Approximate running time: Use these formulas to determine the approximate minutes or hours of use a full tank can deliver:

(# liters in cylinder ÷ liter flow per min = number of min of use) ÷ 60 = hours of use

For example, a D cylinder holds about 424 liters ÷ 5 l/min = 84.4 min, 84.4 ÷ 60 = about 1.4 hours of use.

While D and E cylinders are commonly available, note that size does vary among manufacturers. If you obtain an older tank, be sure that it is intended for and has only been used for oxygen storage in the past and that a compatible valve is currently available that will match the threads in its neck. Capacity limitations also differ depending upon whether the tank is constructed of steel or aluminum. Therefore, the values given in the table above are approximate.

Best running time: This is figured by using the size of the cylinder, the flow rate, and the type of pressure regulator. As the pressure in the cylinder falls during use, many regulators will not deliver a constant flow rate. Therefore, it is recommended that the tank be considered empty when the pressure in the tank drops to 200 pounds per square inch (psi) or less. (The remaining gas is referred to as the "safe residual.") Ideally, when the pressure approaches 200 psi, you should switch to a full tank. However, in an emergency situation, continue to use whatever oxygen is on hand until transport is complete, recognizing that the amount delivered to the woman may be dramatically reduced as the tank empties. The formula to calculate best running time is as follows, using an average gauge pressure of 2000 psig:

(Gauge pressure − 200 psi safe residual) X Constant ÷ Liter flow rate = Best running time

The "constant" is a value established for each cylinder size to help calculate best running time. (See the first column in the preceding table.) Thus, the best running time for a filled D tank delivering a flow rate of 6 l/min would be 48 minutes. ([2000 psi−200 psi=1800 psi] X 0.16 ÷ 6 l/min = 48 min.)

Labeling requirements: The tank label should include the name and address of the manufacturer and the distributor/refiller (if different from the original manufacturer), contents in liters or cubic feet, lot number (original source of contents), and method of production (e.g., air liquefaction). The label should also state that the tank has been filled with oxygen, which may be indicated by a yellow diamond on the front, as well as by the words "Accelerates combustion. Keep oil and grease away." The Department of Transportation requires that a cylinder bear a series of identifying marks including the date of its original and subsequent retests.

Valves

The small D and E cylinders that midwives typically use come with a diaphragm-type medical post valve, which is a closure device that screws into the port at the top of the tank. The valve must be professionally installed and is left permanently in place. It acts as a plug so that oxygen won't escape, and it maintains pressure. The valve can be opened or closed to allow gas to flow during use. The valve has exit ports that allow the attachment of a regulator and pressure gauge. The exit port is located above two index holes. The size and position of the index holes identify the valve as being used specifically for oxygen and match the two pins built into the yoke used to attach an oxygen pressure regulator. Valves used for other gases have index holes in other positions to prevent their use with an oxygen regulator.

Valves come in different styles. Western Medica carries a dual-control valve that has a cross-bar knob on the top to open and close the valve. Toggle valves have a lever on top to open and close the tank; a wrench valve requires a separate cylinder wrench (available in nonferrous metal or plastic) to open and close the valve. The advantage of the cross-bar and toggle styles is that there is no need for an additional instrument (and one more thing that can be lost) to open the cylinder valve. The wrench can be attached to the base of the valve with a large rubber band, string or nonferrous metal chain, or it can be carried in your oxygen tank case. Note that metal valve wrenches are constructed of material that will not spark should they strike against a metal object. If you use another type of metal tool in a pinch, it should not be attached to the tank because there is a risk of fire if it hits the tank and sparks.

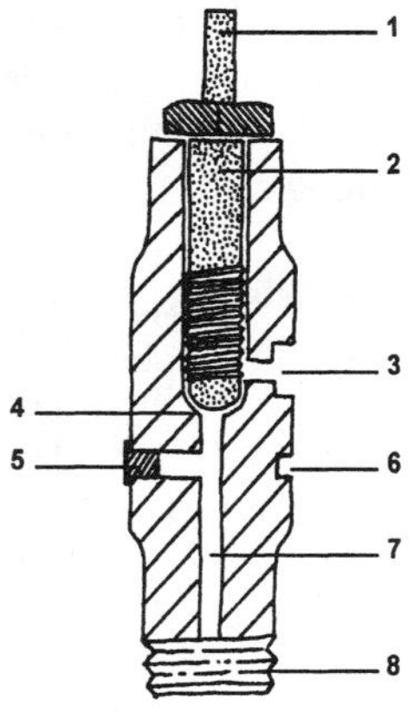

Anatomy of a small cylinder valve
1. Stem to receive a tank wrench
2. Valve plunger
3. Valve outlet (gas exits here)
4. Valve seat (starts and stops gas flow)
5. Meltable plug for emergency gas release
6. Pin-index receptacle
7. Gas flow path from tank to gauge
8. Threads to screw the valve into the tank

Western Medica also carries an all-in-one system that incorporates a valve, flow-control knob and contents gauge in one easy-to-carry unit that includes a built-in handle. A durable cover protects the regulator assembly. This is an ideal regulator to use if you do not wish to purchase a case for your tank, as it is designed to minimize damage to the regulator. This type of regulator can be transferred from an empty tank to a full one. Note that special precautions are necessary to install this type of regulator. Check with your local oxygen supplier to make sure they are familiar with this type of equipment. If not, bring the instruction booklet with you when you go for a refill. Oxygen equipment may be ordered through Cascade HealthCare Products.

Pressure regulators and flowmeters

A pressure regulator is a device that reduces the high pressure of the gas in the cylinder to a safe working pressure for medical use (about 30 to 70 psi). A single-stage regulator has one pressure gauge with a round, "watch-face" type dial that has a ring of marks and a single needle that moves to indicate the amount of pressure in the tank, indicating how much oxygen the tank contains. A two-stage regulator has a tank pressure dial and a flowmeter. The flowmeter measures and indicates the amount (volume) of oxygen delivered to the person over a narrow range of flow rates, usually from 1 to 15 liters per minute (l/min). There are three major types of flowmeters available.

Bourdon gauge: The Bourdon gauge flowmeter has a round "watch-face" type gauge with a ring of pressure marks and a single needle that moves to indicate pressure changes. The pressure gauge is calibrated to indicate flow in liters per minute. This flowmeter is fairly inaccurate at low flow rates and has often been criticized as being unstable. However, it is rugged and will operate at any angle, making it very useful for portable units and is, overall, the best type of gauge for most homebirth midwives to use.

The main problem with this type of gauge is its inability to compensate for back pressure. A partial obstruction (e.g., from kinked tubing) will produce back pressure and result in the flow meter displaying a reading that is higher than the actual flow. (The gauge may read 6 l/min when only1/min is being delivered.) This type of gauge also contains a filter that can become clogged, causing the gauge to read higher than the actual flow. The filter must be inspected and changed as recommended by the manufacturer.

Thorpe gauge: The pressure-compensated flowmeter (Thorpe tube-type) has an upright, calibrated clear glass tube containing a ball float that rises and falls according to the amount of gas passing through the tube. It is more fragile and is gravity dependent; that is, it must be upright to deliver an accurate reading. When it is upright and oxygen is flowing, a change in the position of the float indicates a partial obstruction to gas flow. If the tubing collapses, for example, the ball will drop to show the lower delivery rate. This gauge is not practical for portable units, although it is useful in settings where the tank can remain upright, such as a birthing center.

Constant flow selector valve: The constant flow selector valve has no gauge. It allows for the adjustment of flow in liters per minute in stepped increments (e.g., 2, 4, 6, etc.). When in use, make sure it is properly adjusted to the desired flow rate, and monitor it to make certain that it stays properly adjusted.

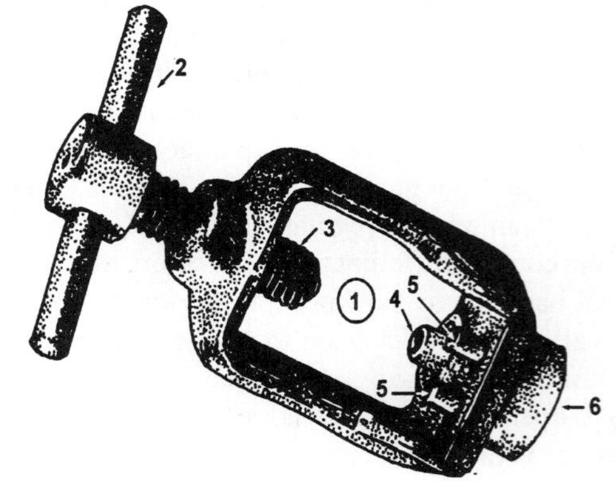

A common style of yoke connector that fits over the valve:
1. Opening that slips over the valve
2. Screw handle for clamping the yoke
3. Screw that holds the yoke firmly in place on the valve
4. Gas receiving nipple that fits into the gas outlet (#3 in the drawing of the valve)
5. Pins that fit into the pin index plugs (#6 in the drawing of valve)
6. An extension for a Bourdon gauge attaches on this end

Basic Use of Oxygen Equipment

Attaching the regulator to the valve

Make sure that the regulator you purchase is compatible with the valves already installed on the tanks that you own. If you change regulators, make sure the appropriate valve is available and have someone install it correctly on your tanks. Do not attempt to change a valve yourself.

The liter flow gauge and regulator must be attached to the tank. The regulator may be attached directly to the valve or to the pin-indexed yoke. The liter gauge is attached to the yoke. The yoke fits over the valve and is clamped into place with a screw fastener. A single gasket or washer called an "O-ring" should be placed between the cylinder valve and the pressure regulator to ensure a tight fit. This gasket is usually supplied with new equipment as well as each time you fill the tank. When the regulator is in place, the pins line up and fit in the holes on the valve on one side and the tip of the screw fastener fits into a shallow, cone-shaped depression on the other side. The washer fits over the nipple on the valve where the gas exits. The yoke held steady while you firmly hand-tighten the screw clamp to secure it in place.

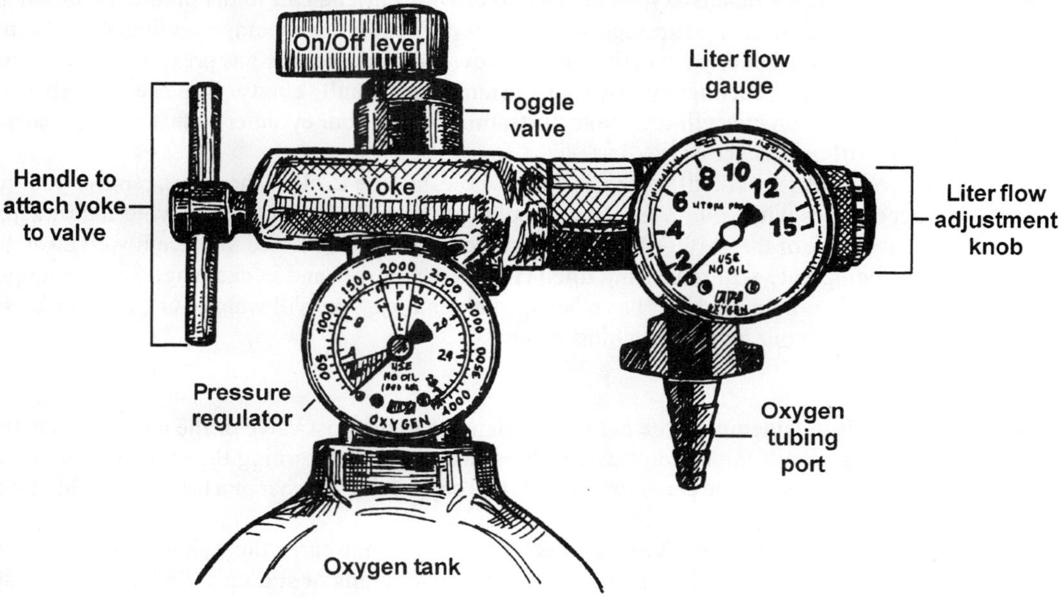

Small oxygen tank with a Bourdon gauge and a toggle valve.
The pressure regulator is attached to the valve and the liter flow gauge is attached to the yoke in this model.

Safety testing and inspection

Cylinders in use exclusively on land may be in service indefinitely without retesting except when refilling is required. You will also want to test the tank if the oxygen level drops without apparent cause. (This is probably, but not always, a problem with the valve. If so, the valve can be replaced.) Cylinders in use on aircraft must be within their last hydrostatic test date to be in use. Hydrostatic tests determine the expansion and leak characteristics of the cylinder to ensure that the cylinder can withstand the pressure of refilling and safely contain the gas. Cylinders must also be inspected visually for damage inside and out. A "+" symbol following the stamped hydrostatic test date indicates that a steel cylinder may be filled 10% in excess of marked service pressure on the cylinder. Aluminum cylinders may not be overfilled in this fashion. When retesting is required, it is performed every five years. (Under certain conditions, retesting is allowed every 10 years, indicated by a "★.")

The midwife should periodically inspect the exterior of the cylinder for rust, corrosion, damage or dents. Rust on a steel tank can flake off inside the tank and deliver particulate matter along with oxygen flow. (Aluminum will not rust.) If any labels are missing or damaged, causing doubt about its contents, replace the cylinder. Periodically review and update your equipment to meet all local, state, and federal regulatory requirements. Fortunately, these requirements are generally stable, and you do not have to replace your equipment every few years.

Regulator calibration should be checked at regular intervals, as recommended by the manufacturer. An independent contents gauge is used to validate the reading on the pressure gauge while it is connected to the cylinder. Periodically inspect the regulator for corrosion, dirt or damage and replace any filters per the manufacturer's recommendations.

Leaks: If you discover a leak in a cylinder that still contains some oxygen, first make sure all valves and gauges are properly shut down. If so and the leak persists, move the tank to an isolated, well-ventilated location, preferably outdoors and away from combustible materials. Open the valve slightly and allow the tank to drain slowly. Do not leave it unattended while it expels gas. Have the valve and system connections checked and, if necessary, replaced before refilling. Leaks are typically a result of valve defects in either the threads, safety devices, stem or outlet.

Refill logistics

Ideally, you should refill your tanks when the contents are estimated to last less than double the anticipated travel time from where the birth is taking place to the hospital at a standard flow rate of at least 6 l/min. Travel time for an ambulance to arrive to transport the mother should also be figured into this equation, since you never know when an ambulance will be necessary. Have sufficient oxygen on hand to provide enriched air to the mother in the event of low fetal heart rate during labor and to cover a postpartum emergency. When returning empty cylinders, close the valve before shipment, leaving about 200/psi of oxygen in the tank to allow for some positive gas pressure. There is more risk of air entering the tank and corrosion occurring if you transport a tank that is totally empty. Replace any valve outlet and protective caps originally shipped with the cylinder. Note the testing date on your cylinder so that you can have the tank retested at the same time as a fill-up, if necessary.

If possible, wait while your tanks are filled. If this is not possible, be sure to close the valve, remove your regulator and take it and all other accessories with you. Use a large label tag to identify your tank with your name, address and phone number and tie it to the neck of the valve. (If you tape a label to the tank, be sure to place it well away from any important markings.) Some companies will return any filled tank they have on hand in exchange for your empty, but if your tank is a more expensive aluminum model or has other special features, you will want your own tank back. Make sure you specify this and point out your label if you must leave it.

Transporting oxygen tanks

Careless handling can result in puncture of the cylinder or damage to the post valve or the connection between the valve and the cylinder. This can cause the rapid release of pressurized oxygen, turning the cylinder into a projectile. Damaged tanks have been known to penetrate concrete walls. If this happens in your car or a house, it could be a disaster.

- If hand-carrying a cylinder, do so carefully, using both hands. Do not carry the cylinder by the valve or regulator, unless your unit is designed for you to do so. Avoid dragging or sliding cylinders, even for short distances. Do not use them as rollers for moving other equipment.
- If possible, move cylinders in a protective case or cart.
- If placing a cylinder next to a mother, secure it to prevent falling, but do not attach it to a bed.
- If transporting a cylinder in a vehicle, keep it in a harness or holder to minimize movement. Never carry unprotected cylinders in a car trunk.

Your other oxygen delivery and resuscitation equipment should be placed in a handy, easy-to-grab bag or box that can be taken with you during a transport. An ideal container allows you to simply open the top and gain easy access to everything you might need without removing it from the container. This simplifies setup and, should you transport in a hurry, you won't be worried about stuffing everything back in your bag before you go.

Storing your oxygen tanks

Oxygen tanks should be stored in a designated area in your home or office away from fire (such as furnaces), heat and the risk of falling or being knocked over. The area should be dry, cool and well ventilated. A large closet or dry basement or garage are good choices. No part of a cylinder should be subjected to a temperature above 130°F (54°C). Do not permit cylinders to come into contact with an electrical apparatus or circuit. Mark and label used cylinders "empty." Do not store full and empty cylinders together. It is best to transport and store larger tanks using a cart with wheels. There are also storage cases designed for D and E cylinders that make them easy to carry to births.

It can be very tempting to leave your equipment in your car, ready to go to a birth. However, if you live in a warm climate or it is a hot summer, the heat will cause the gas in the tank to expand, increasing the likelihood of an explosion. Remember that the temperature in a car can be many degrees higher in full sun, even if the outdoor temperature is quite moderate. It is best to place your tanks in a closet near an exterior door, where they can be grabbed quickly on your way to a birth. If the tanks are in the car and heat is an issue, park in the shade or cover tanks with a white towel. If it is winter, you can leave the tanks secured in your car.

Cleaning your oxygen tanks

Metal components require periodic cleaning. Clean the oxygen exit port on the post valve and the oxygen entrance port on your regulator according to the manufacturer's directions. Avoid commercial cleaning fluids, as they may contain petroleum-based oils. Any part that comes into contact with a person's body fluids, such as the delivery system, must be thrown away after use or cleaned according to the manufacturer's instructions.

Fire-related risks

The regulator releases a surge of oxygen when the cylinder valve is opened quickly and near-adiabatic compression can result. **Adiabatic compression** refers to an immediate, high-pressure flow of gas that can produce sufficient energy to ignite any contaminants or particles in its path. Although this occurs only rarely with portable units, follow the directions outlined in this chapter for setting up the equipment to minimize this possibility. Oxygen should also be kept away from direct contact with petroleum products, such as grease or oil. Never use white, medical adhesive tape or any tape with a thick coating of adhesive on an oxygen tank or valve since the adhesive is petroleum based. The combination can produce a chemical reaction leading to a violent explosion.

If cylinders are located where a fire develops, the heat will expand the gas and the cylinder may rupture, releasing oxygen, which can increase the intensity of the fire. To prevent this, there is a temperature-sensitive fusible plug inside the valve. At the relatively low temperature of 180°F (82°C), the plug melts, venting the oxygen into the air before intense heat ruptures the cylinder.

If a fire should develop, shut off the tank and remove it from the flames, if possible, before fighting the fire; remember that the tank may heat up to an untouchable temperature quickly. Extinguish wood, rubbish and textile fires with water and foam. For oil, solvent, grease or paint fires, use dry chemical powder, such as baking soda, carbon dioxide or foam. For electrical fires, use carbon dioxide or dry chemical powder. If you call the fire department, advise them of the presence and location of your oxygen tanks. Cylinders that have been in a fire must be removed from service permanently.

Oxygen Delivery Devices

Oxygen comprises 21% of ordinary room air. When we exhale room air, our breath contains 16% oxygen, thus we retain only 5%. Oxygen masks and nasal cannulas deliver supplemental oxygen from the cylinder to a breathing person. As a rule, oxygen intake increases by 4% for each single, unobstructed liter of pure oxygen flow per minute (room air 21% + [1 l/min = 4%] = 25%). The regulator's flow setting and the type of delivery device determines the concentration of oxygen. There are five oxygen delivery devices in common use for the care of conscious, breathing persons: the nasal cannula and four types of face masks.

Nasal cannula

A nasal cannula is a vinyl catheter with two short prongs that fit into each nostril. Oxygen enters the nose and passes directly into the back of the throat through each prong. This causes the oxygen to pass into the lungs, even with mouth breathing. Cannulas are suitable for flow rates ranging between 1 and 6 l/min. While comfortable, the small prongs deliver less oxygen than a mask, even if the flow rate is high. Flow rates exceeding 6 l/min cannot be delivered effectively and tend to dry the nasal passages, which can lead to nosebleeds and headaches. If the mother needs more air, she will instinctively gasp through her mouth, which will aggravate mucosal drying. Cannulas are intended for those requiring long-term, low-level oxygen supplementation and are inappropriate for most midwifery applications.

There is, however, one exception. A neonatal sized nasal cannula can be used to provide a small amount of supplemental oxygen to a baby having difficulty with breathing or cyanosis who is born at a high altitude to a mother who is not from an high-altitude acclimated population. In moderately high altitude locations, 25 to 50 ml/min is given via nasal cannula to babies to mimic sea level oxygenation in order to maintain their oxygen saturation levels above 90%. Since this low flow rate requires a special tank gauge, it can be approximated by giving the breathing baby oxygen by nasal cannula at a flow rate of 1 l/min. If no cannula is available, a face mask can be used with an oxygen flow rate of 5 l/min.

Oxygen masks

A mask provides a higher concentration of oxygen than a cannula because masks augment the reservoir capacity of the upper airway. Adult masks come in four basic styles: low, medium, and high concentration and the Venturi. All consist of a soft, molded, transparent, flexible latex or silicone face mask. Adult and pediatric masks come in short and elongated styles, for patient comfort; you need not carry both styles. Masks conform to the contours of the person's face. Maximum performance of any mask requires a tight seal between the mask and the person's face, which is uncomfortable. A snug fit is better tolerated.

Simple face (low concentration [Hudson calls this a medium concentration]) mask: This is the most commonly available type of mask. It has an oxygen inlet port at the base and multiple perforations called "exhalation ports" on both sides to allow room air to enter and the person's exhaled breath to escape. Simple masks deliver moderate concentrations of oxygen (35% at 6 l/min and 55% at 10 l/min).

Partial rebreather (medium concentration [Hudson calls this a high concentration]) mask: This combines a simple mask with a reservoir bag attached to the base. Oxygen flows into and is inhaled from the bag, and room air is pulled in through ports on each side of the mask. This mask is called a "partial rebreather" because a portion of the person's oxygen-enriched exhaled air reenters the reservoir bag to be mixed with fresh oxygen that is taken in by the person on the next inhalation. The rest escapes through the perforations in the mask.

Before placing the mask on the person's face, the reservoir should be filled with enough oxygen so that it loses no more than one-third of its volume when the person inhales. This prevents carbon dioxide build-up in the reservoir. If the bag is not properly filled, the person will not get a full breath on inhalation. This mask provides oxygen concentrations ranging from 35 to 60% when the flow rate is between 7 and 10 l/min.

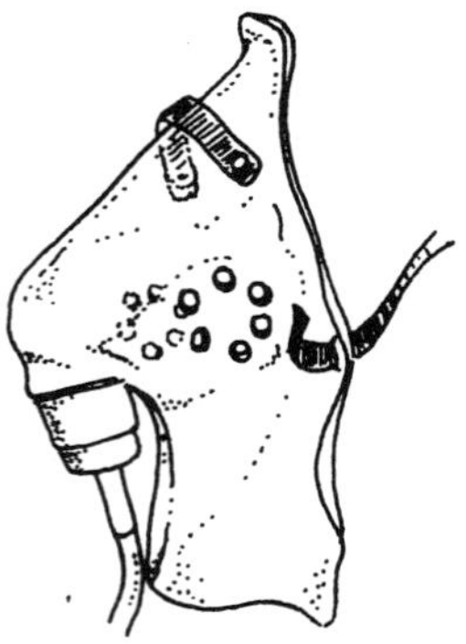

Simple mask (shown larger for detail)

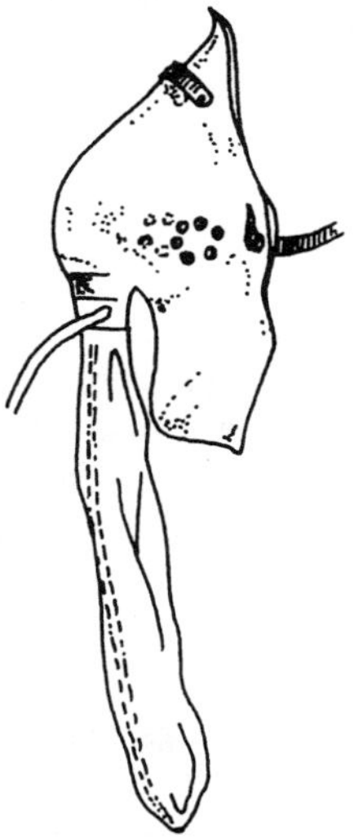

Partial-rebreather mask

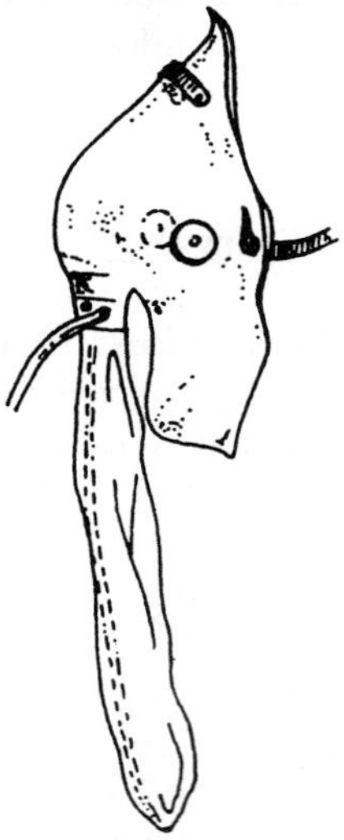

Nonrebreather mask

Nonrebreather (high concentration [Hudson's model is called a Three-in-One]) mask: This consists of a partial rebreather mask equipped with two types of one-way valves. There is a one-way valve between the reservoir bag and mask that allows oxygen to enter the mask from the bag, but prevents exhaled air from flowing back into the bag from the mask. There are two exhalation ports, as in the other masks. One of these functions as the second one-way valve because it is covered with a one-way flap which vents exhaled air so that it does not return to the reservoir. There is also an exhalation port on the opposite side that allows room air to enter the mask should the oxygen supply fail. While this prevents the mask from delivering 100% oxygen, it is a necessary safety precaution in case oxygen ceases to flow. The reservoir bag must be inflated before the mask is placed over the person's face, and it must remain inflated during use, or the person will get little to no air on inhalation. This mask provides concentrations of oxygen ranging from 80 to 95%. The minimum flow rate is 10 l/min. Depending on the manufacturer and the fit of the mask, the maximum flow can range from 12 to 15 l/min. This type of mask is excellent for use on those in shock or for otherwise severely hypoxic persons who do not suffer from chronic obstructive pulmonary disease.

Relationship between Oxygen Flow Rate and Concentration by Type of Delivery Device			
Delivery device	**Flow rate**	**Oxygen delivered**	**Special use**
Nasal cannula	1 to 6 l/min	24 to 44%	For babies born at high altitudes and certain chronic medical conditions
Simple face mask	6 to 15 l/min (8 l/min is the most practical)	35 to 60%	For laboring mothers with no evidence of shock. Assists in correcting depressed FHR and for prophylactic use in breech birth.
Partial rebreather mask	6 to 10 l/min	35 to 60%	For laboring mother with more significant fetal distress, mild hypoxia or shock
Nonrebreathing mask	10-15 l/min	80 to 96%	Useful in treating severe hypoxia and shock

Venturi mask: This mask is designed to deliver precise concentrations of supplemental oxygen from a high-pressure source to those who have a flare-up of a chronic pulmonary condition. It is not suitable for midwifery applications.

Some masks have a special valve that can be adjusted to allow them to function interchangeably in either partial rebreather or nonrebreather mode. The nomenclature for masks varies among catalogues and manufacturers. Be sure to discuss product differences with your sales representative.

Attaching a face mask to the regulator: Connect the oxygen delivery device to a tube that attaches to the oxygen outlet port on the regulator. Some masks already have tubing permanently attached; others have an outlet port for the tube. Most tubing used by midwives is made of clear plastic or pale green latex. These tubes are quite flexible but bend and kink easily. A permanently kinked or bent tube needs replacing as it can alter gauge readings.

Resuscitation Devices

Resuscitation devices deliver or allow the transmission of air or oxygen to a nonbreathing person via positive pressure. When correctly used, these devices are constructed so that no leakage occurs as air or oxygen is forced through the device into the lungs.

Adult, child and infant mouth-to-mask resuscitation devices

Midwives are not usually expected to carry adult resuscitation equipment but are expected to know adult CPR. If you choose not to carry an adult bag-and-mask resuscitator, you will need to carry an adult mouth-to-mask device. These masks are designed to prevent backwashing of air and fluids to the user (which is inevitable when mouth-to-mouth is used) in the event that mouth-to-mouth (or mouth-to-nose-and-mouth) resuscitation is necessary.

Having three sizes will equip you to resuscitate adults and newborns of varying sizes. The long corrugated tube from the mouthpiece to the mask allows you to visually monitor the chest without moving your head. While direct mouth-to-mouth will also work, having a device to protect you from blood-borne pathogens while doing so is desirable. If you have employees that will provide CPR, it is a must in order to comply with OSHA regulations (see the chapter entitled "OSHA Regulations and the Disposal of Biological Waste" for more details).

There are many such masks on the market, and adult and infant models are constructed identically, except adult devices are larger. When selecting a mask, look for one made of a transparent, flexible material that allows a tight seal. The types that have an inflatable or soft-cushioned rim form very good seals. Some inflatable rims can be filled and emptied by attaching the needle port of a luer-lock syringe to the inflation port. The mask should also have a one-way valve to release the exhaled air, a standard 15 mm or 22 mm coupling assembly to receive the one-way valve and an inlet for the delivery of supplemental oxygen.

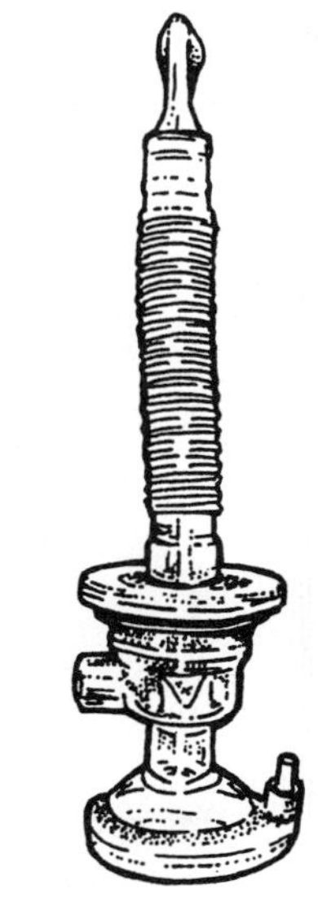

Mouth-to-mask device

It should work well under a variety of environmental conditions, such as extreme heat or cold, and assemble easily for use. These devices deliver 16% oxygen when ventilations are provided with the care provider's breath alone. The oxygen concentration increases to about 50% with supplemental oxygen attached. How to use this device is explained in the subchapter entitled "Evaluating and Assisting the Infant in Need of Resuscitation."

Neonatal resuscitation equipment

Midwives must carry equipment to resuscitate the newborn. It is also ideal to carry a self-inflating bag-valve-mask device, also called a resuscitator, which is a ventilation device to use when two midwives are available to provide ventilations and cardiac massage or when the baby requires only ventilations.

Infant oxygen masks: The three basic types of infant masks you will be using include a simple face mask, the mask on the mouth-to-mask devices for use during CPR and the mask that will come with your self-inflating resuscitator. Newborn masks have cushioned rims. Masks come in a variety of sizes. You should carry at least two sizes of newborn masks to fit term and preterm babies. A suitable mask, which is intended to fit most near-term or term infants, will come with the bag-and-mask unit designed for neonates. If you decide to purchase a child-size bag-and-mask (more on this later), you will need to ensure that you obtain an appropriately sized mask for newborns. The manufacturer often has other sizes for preterm and large term infants available at an additional charge.

Noncushioned-rim masks: If you are working in the developing world, or you acquire older equipment, you may encounter a now-obsolete noncushioned mask. A noncushioned rim requires more pressure to obtain a seal. This increases the likelihood of damaging the baby's eyes or bruising the face if improperly positioned or applied too firmly. They should not be used unless you have no other option.

Cushioned-rim masks: A mask with either an inflatable, a rubber or a soft, rolled rim is by far the best and safest option. Inflated rims are permanently filled and must be replaced when the air, inevitably, seeps out. These types of rims conform most readily to the infant's face, require less pressure to obtain a good seal, and pose less risk of damaging the baby's eyes if the mask is incorrectly positioned.

Round vs. anatomical shapes: Masks come in either round or anatomical shapes. One advantage of round masks is that they do not have to be oriented; however, they may provide an inadequate seal if improperly sized. If too large, round masks may put too much pressure on the eyes.

Anatomical masks are pear-shaped and are fitted with the most pointed end over the bridge of the nose. They pose less risk of eye damage because the rim is contoured to fit between the eyes and nose. Mercury is the only manufacturer that makes an anatomical mask designed specifically to fit the contours of the flat newborn face.

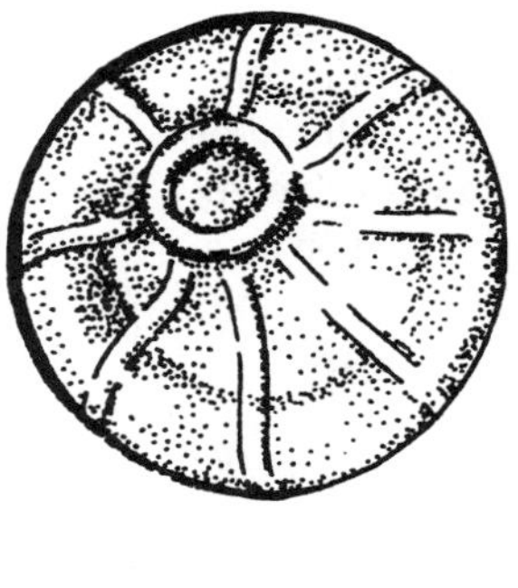

Round mask

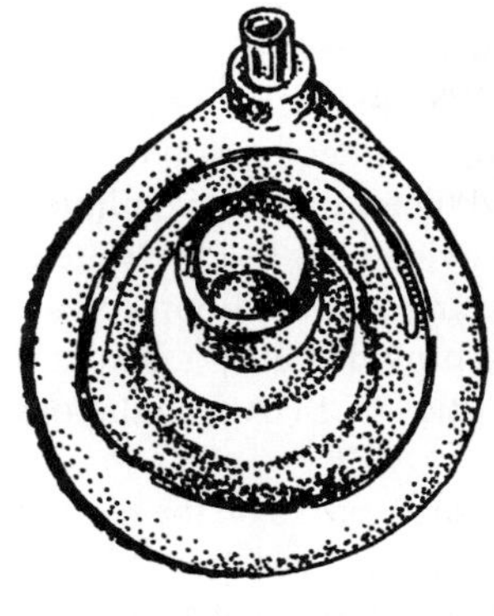

Anatomically shaped mask

Self-inflating resuscitators: Self-inflating bag-valve-mask devices, sometimes referred to as "Ambu bags," are designed to deliver a measured amount of air, air mixed with oxygen, or almost pure oxygen under positive pressure. These units are rarely needed, but when they are, they can deliver a more or less regulated amount of air or air mixed with oxygen. There are four top manufacturers of these devices in the United States: Ambu, Hudson, Laerdal and Mercury. The features of adult and newborn models are identical unless otherwise noted.

Self-inflating bag-valve-mask units are manually operated and come in adult, child, infant (or neonatal) sizes. The device consists of a self-inflating silicone ventilation bag that is squeezed to deliver a set amount or volume of air or oxygen to the baby. Note that in bags that are very soft (as most are), you will probably require a 500 ml ventilation bag to deliver a sustained inflation for a full two to three seconds for the initial breaths if the baby has not yet breathed on his own (inflation breaths are discussed in detail in the subchapter entitled “Evaluating and Assisting the Infant in Need of Resuscitation”). Once the lungs are inflated, term babies require only 20 to 30 ml of air with each ventilation, a tiny fraction of the volume of air in the bag. Therefore, the capacity of a bag for newborn use should never exceed 750 ml. If the bag is larger than this, it is difficult to regulate the small volume of gas needed with each ventilation unless you use a Mercury resuscitator. If you do not get a Mercury unit, with practice you can use a pediatric unit to prolong the important inflation ventilations for the necessary 2 to 3 seconds and give additional shorter duration ventilations by controlling how hard you squeeze the bag. Be sure you order large and small *infant (neonatal)*-size masks if you choose a pediatric unit, as it will be equipped with pediatric masks, which are too large for newborns. Self-inflating units come with at least one “standard” size mask for infant use. Masks of different sizes and shapes that have compatible couplers are also available from Cascade HealthCare Products or the manufacturer.

MAKE AND MODEL	VENTILATION BAG VOLUME	RESERVOIR VOLUME IN ML (TYPE)	POP-OFF VALVE LIMIT
Ambu-neonate	220 ml	100 ml (tube)	40 cm H_2O +/-5
Ambu-SPUR neonate*	220 ml	100 ml (tube)	40 cm H_2O +/-5
Hudson-infant	280 ml	600 ml (bag)	40 cm H_2O +/-5
Laerdal-infant	240 ml	600 ml (bag)	45 cm H_2O +/-5
Mercury-infant*	240 ml	600 ml (bag or tube)	42 cm H_2O +/-5
Ambu-child	700 ml	2600 ml (bag) 400 ml (tube)	40 cm H_2O +/-5
Ambu-SPUR child*	700 ml	+2600 ml (bag) 400 ml (tube)	40 cm H_2O +/-5
Hudson-child	500 ml	2500 ml (bag)	40 cm H_2O +/-5
Laerdal-child	500 ml	2600 ml (bag)	45 cm H_2O +/-5
Mercury-child*	500 ml	2600 ml (bag or tube)	42 cm H_2O +/-5

*single-use, disposable units

An adequate bag-valve unit has the following features:

- •A self-inflating bag that is either disposable or easily cleaned and sterilized
- •A nonrebreathing valve assembly allowing an oxygen inlet flow up to 15 l/min
- •A nonpop-off valve in adult models or a pressure regulating pop-off valve in pediatric and infant models
- •A system for delivering a high-concentration of oxygen through an inlet port at the back of the ventilation bag
- •A nonrebreathing valve
- •An oxygen reservoir
- •Manometer attachment

While Laerdal has long been touted as the best, Hudson’s infant resuscitator is less expensive, with virtually the same design. Ambu and Mercury make single-patient-use resuscitators which are disposable and less expensive than a reusable model. (A disposable adult bag-valve-mask resuscitator comes in handy in the rare event that you care for a mother who ceases to breathe for any reason.) However, Mercury is the only manufacturer in the United States to have produced a bag-and-mask unit with special attention to the requirements of neonates (whereas the other makers tend to simply reduce the size of components). The walls of the Mercury ventilation bag on the infant- and child-size units are designed so that you can actually feel the resistance as the lungs fill with air; a helpful feature when inflating tiny lungs. They are also resistant enough to allow the delivery of sustained inflations, which is not true of any other neonatal bag and mask. All components and accessories of Mercury units are latex-free. *Given the pros and cons of each unit, please note that I overwhelmingly recommend the Mercury neonatal self-inflating bag and their neonatal-size masks. Unfortunately for the planet, these units come only in disposable models, but they are still the best.*

An L-shaped plastic coupler connects the self-inflating bag to the mask at one end of the bag-valve-mask. At the other end, a straight coupler attaches the self-inflating bag to an optional oxygen reservoir bag or tube. In the center of this coupler there is a thin, round "flutter" valve which lets a small amount of room air in when the oxygen reservoir or tube is attached during use.

Manometer: Some self-inflating bags have a port for attaching a manometer or pressure gauge. This is usually a small hole or projection close to the patient outlet. If your bag has such a port, the gauge must be attached or the port plugged, or gas will leak through the opening, preventing adequate pressure during ventilations.

Mercury makes a manometer that attaches directly to the resuscitator unit; this alone is a good reason to go with a Mercury device. It consists of an easy-to-read dial gauge with a pressure range 5 to 60 cm H_2O. A manometer takes the guesswork out of ventilating. It can be used to check the unit and to learn to provide inflation pressures just below the pop-off valve release pressure.

Note that the Mercury resuscitator can be ordered with or without a manometer attached. When ordered with the manometer in place, it comes with a small white silicone sleeve, which is designed to hold the manometer securely during shipping. This sleeve also makes removal and replacement of the manometer much easier and seems to lessen the pressure required to inflate the bag with the manometer in place. Therefore, if you want a manometer, I recommend ordering your resuscitator units so equipped rather than getting it as a separate item.

Note that a pressure gauge with an attached pressure release valve that connects to the resuscitator with small-bore tubing can deliver dangerously high levels of flow that would not be accurately reflected in the manometer reading due to the high resistance of the tubing. These devices are now obsolete as they cannot provide the degree of precision needed to monitor ventilation pressures for infant resuscitation; they should never be used.

Flow-inflating bags (formerly called an "anesthesia bag"): Some hospitals use flow-inflating bags for resuscitation. However, these bags cannot self-inflate and therefore require a compressed gas source. As a homebirth midwife, you want to carry a self-inflating bag.

Can a self-inflating bag provide blow-by or free-flow oxygen? The valve assembly in some self-inflating bags allows gas to flow from the bag through the patient outlet only while the bag is being actively compressed; in others, a certain amount of gas can flow through the mask when the bag is not being compressed. However, the majority of gas entering a self-inflating bag will normally be diverted from the air inlet into the oxygen reservoir and then out of the unit. The amount of oxygen reaching the baby will depend on the relative resistance of the valves in the unit; therefore, even though you may be able to detect gas flowing from the mask, the amount of oxygen reaching the baby will vary widely from unit to unit. Such units should not be depended upon to provide free-flow oxygen.

Familiarizing yourself with the resuscitator: You will seldom need to use your resuscitation equipment. It is therefore important to have the tools best designed for the job because a precision tool helps make up for your lack of experience. Take them out frequently to look at them, use them to practice on manikins (or a newborn-sized doll) and become intimately familiar with how they, and any optional equipment you choose to carry, work. This way, on the rare occasion when you need them, you will know exactly how to use them and be comfortable with setting them up. Once you have your resuscitator (or when checking out which one to buy), you should read the enclosed directions carefully. If you do not understand something in the instructions, call the manufacturer or the person who taught your resuscitation classes to clarify the point. The suggestions below will apply generally to all units, but you should be throughly familiar with the unit you own. First, identify the parts already discussed, then familiarize yourself with the following parts as well:

One-way air intake valve: Air is drawn into the ventilation bag as it expands during compression via an air-inlet port, to which a one-way valve is attached. The air inlet is usually the largest opening located on the far end of the bag. You may need to squeeze and release the bag several times to find it.

Oxygen inlet port: The oxygen inlet is a small nipple or projection, usually located near the air inlet, to which tubing can be attached when oxygen is needed.

One-way valve assembly: The assembly positioned between the bag and the patient outlet opens when the bag is squeezed during ventilation, delivering oxygen or air into the mask. This valve is often positioned above the mask coupler and may be shaped like a pair of lips. Look straight down into the mask coupler; you can see the valve open with each compressed ventilation, then close as you release the bag to allow it to refill via the air inlet port while the breath exits via the exhale port during exhalation. This one-way valve prevents the exhaled air from entering the ventilation bag and mixing with the fresh air or oxygen flowing in to be used during the next ventilation. Squeeze and release the bag several times to see how the one-way valve moves as it opens and closes.

One of two types of valves may be used: a pair of thin flexible plastic or rubber lips, or a tiny, spring-loaded floating-ball valve. The bag should not be used if this valve is missing or malfunctioning.

The thin, circular valve that releases exhaled gas from the resuscitator is also positioned near the mask coupler, usually above it. To see it work, occlude the mask with your mouth and blow into it to mimic exhaling. Watch the valve to see if it lifts slightly as it releases exhaled gas. Movement of this valve is usually harder to detect when you are actually using the device during resuscitation.

Exhale port: The port sticking off the end of the one-way valve through which exhaled air escapes.

Patient outlet (mask port): The coupler that allows gas to exit the bag for inhalation. It is located below the one-way valve assembly.

Manometer (pressure gauge) port: Look for a small hole or projection close to the patient outlet (this port must be plugged if no manometer is attached).

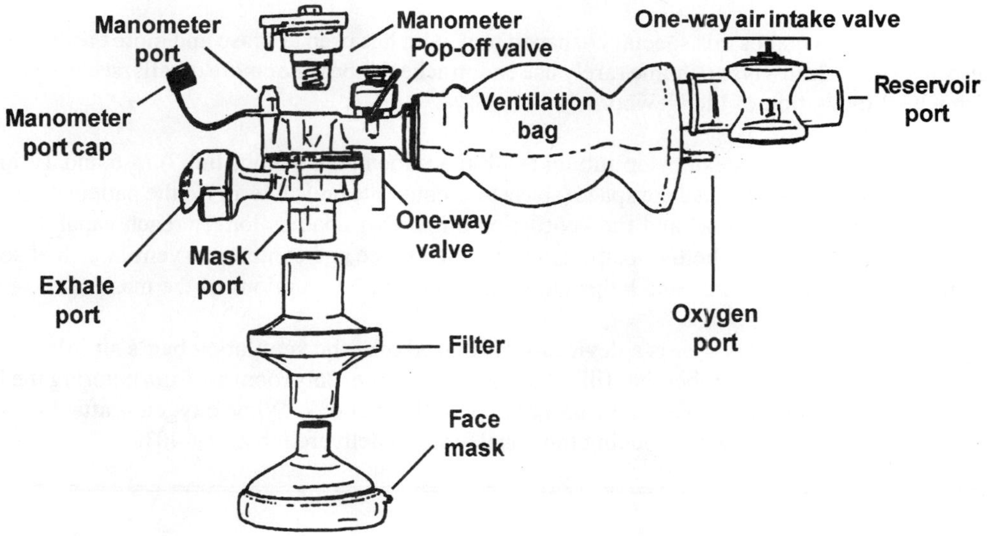

Anatomy of a Mercury neonatal resuscitator

Safety features on newborn units: Infant and pediatric self-inflating bags have either a pressure release valve (also called a "pressure regulator" or "pop-off valve") or a pressure gauge (manometer) or both. Pressure release valves are typically positioned between the ventilation bag coupler and the valve assembly. All newborn units should have at least one of these two safety features. Adult models do not have these features.

Pressure release valves are set to release at 40 to 45 cm H_2O, depending on the manufacturer. The valve opens to expel excess gas if this pressure is exceeded, thus limiting the pressure being delivered to the baby. This prevents overinflation of the lungs, which could result in rupture of the alveoli, and decreases the likelihood of gas entering the stomach and causing distension. There can be a wide variation in the pressure that must be reached before the valve will open. The make and age of the device, as well as the method of cleaning, affect the actual opening pressure. Soapy residue or improper drying can leave the valve sticky and resistant to opening.

In some bags, the pop-off valve can be occluded temporarily or bypassed to allow high pressures to be delivered. This may occasionally come in handy when the baby is born with a limp cord and the lungs have not been aerated at all. Occlusion of the pop-off valve may rarely be necessary to elevate the pressure of the delivered volume of air to mimic the higher pressure of the baby's first few breaths as the baby inflates his lungs for the first time, but there is still the danger of delivering the gas at such a high pressure that it would damage the lungs. Therefore, a manometer should be attached whenever a pop-off valve is bypassed during the first few ventilations.

To locate the pop-off valve, remove the mask and occlude the mask port with your palm or against your bare thigh so that no air can leak out. Now squeeze the bag forcefully. The pressure-release valve will be a small device that releases gas. When the pressure being delivered exceeds 40 cm H_2O or so, you will be able to hear the valve open with a soft "raspberry" sound–you may be able to see the valve open–as the extra pressure escapes through the pop-off valve. Practice occluding the face of the mask as above and compressing the bag using a pressure somewhat less than that needed to activate the pressure release valve. This will give you a feel for pressures of 15 to 25 cm H_2O.

Mercury offers a safety feature in the form of a pathogen barrier called an exhalation filter. This coupler fits between the mask port and the mask and provides filtration of bacterial and viral agents at a 99.5% effectiveness rate. This filter minimizes contamination of your self-inflating unit by separating the baby's exhaled air from the rest of the valve assembly.

***PEEP valve*:** PEEP (positive-end expiratory pressure) valves are optional devices designed to prevent full collapse of the neonatal lung between ventilations. They are most useful in tiny, premature babies whose lungs are immature and in any baby whose cord has been clamped early and is therefore hypovolemic. A PEEP valve should not be used by midwives ventilating babies at home. In the Mercury unit, the PEEP valve fits over the exhale port.

Disconnect wedge: Mercury makes this special U-shaped tool, which is used to grasp and more easily detach a mask port from an endotracheal tube. Midwives at home rarely use endotracheal tubes. For more details, see the subchapter entitled "Digital Endotracheal Intubation of the Newborn."

***Extension tubing*:** Mercury makes extension tubing (with the trade name "Omni-link") in 6 and 12 in lengths. This flexible, corrugated tubing does not add dead space (space to accumulate unusable air) to the patient pathway. It provides a link between the ventilation bag port and the ventilation bag. This enables longer reach capabilities, enabling the midwife to move around or assume a better position in a cramped space and continue to ventilate. It absorbs movement, reduces arm fatigue and airway trauma, and helps eliminate accidental disruptions of the mask seal.

Oxygen reservoirs: An oxygen reservoir is a device that is placed over the ventilation bag's air inlet. When oxygen is attached, the reservoir provides a chamber that fills with oxygen and prevents room air from entering the bag. It recycles the oxygen, keeping the concentration within the unit as high as 90 to 100%. When oxygen is attached and no reservoir is used, air mixes with the pure oxygen, reducing the concentration delivered to about 40%.

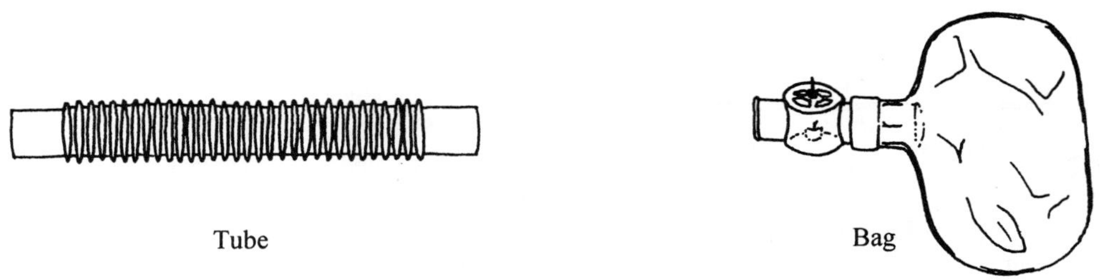

Oxygen reservoirs

There are two different types of oxygen reservoirs. One type is a ribbed, open-ended tube that allows a small amount of room air to enter the ventilation bag during reinflation. It can provide an oxygen concentration of 90% or higher. A closed-end bag supplies almost a 100% concentration. The bag can be observed for fullness, offering a big advantage over a tube. If the reservoir bag is completely flat most of the gas that enters the self-inflating bag will be room air, even if oxygen is attached.

A self-inflating bag can be used to deliver positive-pressure ventilation with or without supplemental oxygen. The reservoir device *must be* removed when room air alone is used because, if left in place, it will adversely affect the refill rate of the ventilation bag, reducing the number of ventilations that can be effectively delivered. When no oxygen is attached, the baby or adult receives 21% oxygenated room air, which is drawn into the bag through the air inlet as the bag reinflates.

Setting up resuscitation equipment:

Checking out a nondisposable resuscitator: You or a trained assistant should assemble the resuscitator and check to be sure it is working properly at each birth. It is a good idea for another midwife to double-check everything once it is set up. This should be done whether you are using a disposable or nondisposable unit. You should also check for damage after each use and with each complete cleaning and sterilization prior to storage. You may want to put a checklist with your resuscitation equipment, with space to write the dates of cleaning and checking and the initials of the person responsible, to ensure that this procedure is not overlooked. The last thing you want is a nonfunctioning unit in the midst of a crisis.

Be sure all parts are present. Attach the mask to the coupler on one end of the ventilation bag and the oxygen reservoir to the coupler on the other end. Throughout your setup procedure, look carefully for any defects, damage or leaks. If the unit is defective, it should not be used. To check your self-inflating ventilation bag, cover the mask with plastic and block it by forming an airtight seal against the palm of your hand or your bare thigh, then squeeze the bag. Answer these questions:

- •Do you feel pressure against your skin?
- •Does the manometer (if attached) register up to 30 to 40 cm H_2O?
- •Can you force the pressure release valve to open by applying excessive pressure to the bag?
- •Is the valve assembly present and moving as it should each time you compress the ventilation bag?
- •Attach oxygen tubing and the reservoir bag. Does the oxygen reservoir bag fill with oxygen? (If the reservoir bag does not fill, check the two valve shutters for problems, look for a tear in the reservoir bag and check the oxygen tubing for kinks.)

Remove the mask. Compress the ventilation bag with one hand, and then place your other palm over the mask-valve coupler. Release the grip on the bag. Does the bag reexpand rapidly, confirming efficient air intake?

Now block the mask valve coupler with one hand and try to compress the bag with the other. If the bag cannot be compressed with reasonable force, or if bag compression forces the air out between your hand and the patient coupler, the valve efficiently prevents backward escape of air. If you have performed all these steps and confirmed that your resuscitator is operating properly, it is ready to use. Attach the appropriately sized mask, and make sure that all connectors are secure. If you plan to use oxygen, attach the tubing and an oxygen reservoir (neither should be attached if you plan to ventilate with only room air).

Setting up a new, disposable resuscitator: A new, unopened resuscitator should be ready to use right out of the package. If it has been opened for any reason but remains unused, the above-mentioned tests can be performed as you set up. Check to make sure that you are not past the expiration date. If so, it should be replaced by a new one; the old one can be used for practice sessions. Expiration dates cover sterility as well as the integrity of components.

Setting up an oxygen cylinder:

NOTE: A loud hissing sound will occur whenever an oxygen tank is opened, especially if the regulator is not attached. This is simply gas releasing under pressure and does not mean the tank is going to blow up. If you have taken precautions to remove combustible materials from the vicinity, as described below, and open the value slowly, there is minimal danger.

1. Be sure your hands are clean and free of petroleum-based oils or grease. This includes mineral oil and mineral-oil-based hand creams and lotions (which most non-health-food-brands contain) and petroleum-based products such as KY. No white medical-grade adhesive tape should be used on or used near the tank. Move the tank away from other combustible materials and open flames. Extinguish all candles, incense, kerosene lanterns, open fires, fuel-powered space heaters, cigarettes, etc. Do not use oxygen in the presence of high levels of static electricity.

2. Examine the cylinder for the oxygen label and lot number as well as the hydrostatic test and visualization expiration dates. In the United States, do not use the tank if it is not green, doesn't have a green (or white) collar around the top, or if the markings indicate that there may be another type of gas inside. (Note that, in the US, the color is green; everywhere else, an oxygen tank is white.)
3. Inspect the regulator and valve post for cleanliness before connecting or using them.
4. If selecting a newly filled cylinder, remove any protective covering on the cylinder valve. As you do so, take care not to discard the O-ring gasket, which is included with each newly refilled tank.
5. Locate and attach the valve wrench to the valve stem or operate the knob, toggle or handle. Turn the valve stem counterclockwise for one second and then turn it off. This brief release of gas clears away any debris that may be lodged in the valve outlet.
6. Ensure that the plastic O-ring gasket is fitted around the oxygen entrance port on the regulator between the regulator and the valve opening. Do not operate the tank without this gasket in place or it will leak.
7. Make sure the regulator knobs are in the off or closed position before attaching the yoke to the valve.
8. Connect and hand-tighten the regulator yoke to the valve on the cylinder. If the two pins on the regulator do not fit the holes on the valve, do not use (or purchase) the equipment.
9. If you are opening a partially used cylinder to which the regulator was previously attached, check that the gauges were fully bled out after the last use (all needles will be on zero). If so, tighten the yoke and proceed with the next step. If not, open the valve on the pressure gauge, bleed it out completely until the needle reads zero, close the valve and proceed with the next step.
10. Connect the oxygen tubing to the regulator's oxygen outlet port (an open-ended, tapered, or stairstep connector). Make sure the tubing attachments on the tank and the mask are seated firmly so oxygen will not leak. Check to be sure the tubing is smooth and free of obstructions such as twists or kinks. Kinked or bent tubing needs to be replaced because it will impair oxygen flow.
11. Position yourself to the side of the regulator, away from the front of the gauges and adjusting knob. Direct the valve away from you and any other persons. Place both hands on the cylinder valve. Turn the handle counterclockwise very slowly until the cylinder pressure builds on the gauge and the needle stabilizes. If there is no handle, use the valve wrench to open the valve to the full limit of its travel. Then turn it back a quarter of a turn, which will back-seat the valve.
12. Check the pressure gauge to determine if the tank has been properly filled or to see how much oxygen you have left in a partially used tank. Now your tank is ready to use. Be sure the liter flow knob is closed; set the tank up where you want it for the birth.
13. When you are ready to use the tank, adjust the liter flow rate to the appropriate volume by turning the liter flow knob counterclockwise. Decrease or stop the flow by turning it clockwise.
14. Check for the unrestricted flow of oxygen through the oxygen delivery device by listening or feeling for escaping gas.

Dispensing oxygen from a cylinder into a face mask for a conscious, breathing mother or baby:

1. First, if using a partial- or nonrebreather mask, fill the reservoir bag. To do so, attach the oxygen tubing to the port on your oxygen gauge. Cover the large port at the base of the face mask with your finger. Start the oxygen flow at 15 l/min and the bag should fill with oxygen.
2. Place the mask over the person's face and the elastic band below her ears and the back of her neck. Pull outward on each of the elastic straps to snug the mask against the face and mould the metal strip down against the nose.
3. The reservoir must always contain enough oxygen so that when the person takes her deepest inspiration, it does not deflate by more than one-third for partial rebreather masks and two-thirds for nonrebreather masks. Gradually reduce the flow of oxygen until the bag is collapsing no more than this with each inspiration and refilling completely between breaths.

Avoiding carbon dioxide build-up in the mask: Always start with at least 6 l/min of flow when using any type of mask. Flow rates of less than 6 l/min can produce an accumulation of carbon dioxide in the mask. Therefore, a mask receiving an oxygen flow rate of 1 l/min gives the person less oxygen than she would get from room air alone.

Using your bag-valve-mask unit to ventilate a nonbreathing mother or baby using oxygen:

1. Attach the oxygen tubing to the oxygen port on the resuscitator.
2. Be sure the mask, connectors and oxygen reservoir are securely attached.

3. Turn the oxygen flow to 6 l/min. Keep turning it up until the reservoir fills with oxygen.
4. Begin to provide ventilations. The reservoir bag should collapse no more than half-way with each ventilation
5. If the bag collapses by more than half its volume, turn up the liter flow until it remains half full during ventilations. If the bag collapses entirely, you are ventilating with room air only.

Turning off and storing your oxygen equipment when the tank is still partially full:

1. Close the cylinder valve by turning it clockwise until the valve is tightly seated (using a valve wrench, if appropriate).
2. Remove the mask from the person's face.
3. Vent (or bleed) pressure from the regulator system completely by fully opening the gauge knobs until all the pressure is released and the needles read zero.
4. Close the gauges and store the equipment.

Removing the regulator: The following steps should be taken if you must remove the regulator for transferring it from an empty to a full tank or for refilling a tank. Whenever possible, leave 200 psi in an "empty" tank to maintain enough positive pressure to prevent it from drawing in moisture and other debris that might cause damage.

1. After following the procedures for shutting down the equipment, disconnect the regulator from the cylinder by loosening the yoke. Replace the cylinder's valve cap and secure in place with regular transparent tape to prevent debris from getting inside the valve. Tape the O-ring in place as well. If no cap is available, tape or rubber band a piece of clean paper around the valve to cover the ports.
2. If you must store the regulator for an extended period of time, protect it from damage or contamination by replacing the plastic covers it came with, or store the regulator in a clean resealable plastic bag inside a clearly marked box.

Cleaning a Self-Inflating Resuscitator: Clean your reusable resuscitator after each use. Unfortunately, you must toss a single-use disposable unit that becomes contaminated as it is not designed to disassemble for adequate cleaning. Cleaning without disassembly risks leaving moisture, which can form a breeding ground for pathogens.

First, disassemble the nondisposable unit according to the manufacturer's instructions. Do not attempt to disassemble parts that are not intended to be taken apart. Units vary as to how much and in what ways they can be disassembled. Usually, infant models have fewer parts to disassemble than do adult models. Laerdal advises leaving the connectors in the couplers of ventilation bags, masks and reusable reservoirs and gaskets in the valve assembly during the entire decontamination procedure. However, you may find it easier to disconnect the mask and reservoir. Wash and rinse the unit thoroughly, using warm water and a detergent that is compatible with the resuscitator materials (see manufacturer's instructions). Rinse all parts thoroughly in clean, running water.

Next, sterilize the parts directly exposed to the expired gases from the resuscitated person: the mask-valve assembly to which the mask attaches and the mask itself. Check your manufacturer's instructions and sterilize these parts using common methods such as boiling in water for 10 minutes, pasteurizing, soaking in a cold sterilization solution or autoclaving up to 277°F (136°C), if appropriate.

Clean the ventilation bag, inlet valve and reservoir bag or tube periodically to remove dust and other surface contaminants. You need not sterilize these parts since they do not come in direct contact with the expired breath. However, if they become grossly contaminated during use, you can cold-sterilize them.

Any parts that have become wet or damp during cleaning should be set out and allowed to dry thoroughly prior to reassembly. Improper rinsing or drying may result in sticky or malfunctioning valves. Once reassembled, check to make sure all valves are working correctly before storing your equipment.

INTRAVENOUS EQUIPMENT AND IV THERAPY

NOTE: This chapter describes the technical details regarding intravenous equipment and its use. For details regarding the theory and treatment of shock, see the part entitled "Understanding and Treating Shock."

Intravenous therapy involves use of specialized equipment to administer fluid or medications directly into a vein. Midwives administer intravenous fluids primarily to prevent or treat maternal hypovolemic shock due to blood loss after birth. Intravenous fluids can also be used to correct dehydration in a mother who has been vomiting or unable to keep down fluids in labor and whose energy is really flagging. A third use is to correct a compromised fetal heart rate when the mother's blood volume is marginally contracted or she has become acutely dehydrated. IVs can be used to administer antibiotics if the development of infection during labor is a concern. If you are practicing in a very rural location far from medical help, there may be rare occasions when you want to place a saline lock just prior to birth if circumstances suggest that the mother is at significant risk for hemorrhage.

The skills you need to insert an IV are, in many respects, very similar to those required to draw blood. However, inserting an IV is trickier than drawing blood, and incorrect technique can result in life-threatening complications. There is less room for error than with many of the other skills you perform as a midwife.

(For a review of the steps entailed in drawing blood, see the chapter entitled "Collecting Blood for Testing" in the Appendix of DIAGNOSTIC TESTS. This chapter assumes that you have already mastered that material.) As with drawing blood, the use of an IV requires adequate hands-on training. The information in this chapter should only be used as an adjunct to such training.

THE BASICS OF IV THERAPY

The Use of IV Fluids for Volume Expansion and Hydration

Hypovolemic shock occurs when blood volume reaches a critical low due to blood or fluid loss. Crystalloid IV solutions (water and minerals) provide fluid volume replacement. However, while crystalloid IV fluids can replace minerals and water, they are not colloids (as are blood and blood products) and will not increase the oxygen-carrying capacity of the blood. They are volume expanders, not blood replacements, and serve as a stop-gap measure that can help to stabilize a woman before she is transported for evaluation. Increasing the body's fluid volume improves and maintains cardiovascular function, which assists in distributing the blood that is still in the woman's system by pushing fluid into constricted peripheral vessels, thus improving blood flow to the cells. However, large amounts of crystalloid infusion may have negative effects on plasma oncotic pressure (pressure exerted by colloids in a solution) and on the blood's coagulation factor and platelet concentration. Because of these risks, IV therapy for volume replacement should be reserved for women showing signs of compromise. If a woman has lost a great deal of blood, she may require a packed red cell or whole blood transfusion in order to ensure adequate oxygenation to her tissues, prevent additional bleeding resulting from reduced coagulation factors, which can lead to DIC (disseminated intravascular coagulation), and otherwise speed her recovery.

Risks

The major systemic risk of giving crystalloid fluids occurs when too much is given too fast. Compared to colloids, crystalloid solutions tend to equilibrate rather quickly between the intravascular and interstitial spaces, which is one type of "third spacing." Fluid overload may occur when large volumes of crystalloids transfer into the interstitial space after having only temporarily restored the circulating volume. This transfer of large amounts of fluid overburdens the tissues, the lungs and heart become edematous, and adult respiratory distress as well as heart failure or bowel edema may result. Excessive swelling in the intestinal tract may lead to bowel obstruction (with accompanying pain and distension), diarrhea or both. If shock has disrupted the protective mechanisms in the brain that prevent fluid imbalances, accumulating fluid may eventually lead to brain injury. These side-effects occur more rapidly when IV fluids are given for reasons other than shock from blood loss or to otherwise unhealthy individuals. However, peripheral edema is a frequent side-effect of fluid replacement, which, when extreme, can affect how oxygen is used by the tissues. This, in turn, can lead to poor wound healing, skin breakdown and infection.

Other risks include systemic infection from the procedure itself. While peripheral IV insertion is generally considered a clean rather than a strictly sterile technique, proper preparation of the puncture site and keeping the parts of the IV setup that will come in direct contact with the blood stream sterile are imperative (Garcia, 2002). In addition, those who have experienced blood loss are less tolerant of small infusions of air into the circulation than those who have not. A sufficiently large infusion of air may precipitate an embolism, which is a serious, life-threatening emergency.

IV Equipment

IV equipment is complicated and quite foreign to those who are not trained in hospitals or emergency rescue work. The following discussion will make the most sense if you obtain a simple IV administration set, a bag of IV fluid and an over-the-stylet catheter unit to examine as you study. Ask a practicing midwife or a nurse who works in the hospital if she can obtain supplies that have passed their expiration date that you can use for practice.

The state-of-the-art in IV equipment has been rapidly evolving since heightened concern regarding blood-borne pathogens was generated in the mid-1980s. Consequently, there are a wide array of products available for IV use. Because there are minor differences in manufacturing techniques among brands, it is best to choose a brand and then have all your tubing, catheters and attachment devices from the same company. If you choose to mix brands, be sure the devices you buy are compatible. The best way to ensure this is to consult a knowledgeable sales representative or to call the manufacturers of the devices in question. Once you and your midwifery community are familiar with basic terminology and equipment, ask a local medical supply sales representative for a group review of current products. Most will be happy to oblige. Once you have selected your equipment, familiarize yourself with its features well before you need to use it by sacrificing one of each item to use for "dry run" practice sessions.

Basic supplies

Safety vs. nonsafety devices: Here, "safety device" refers to built-in mechanisms which prevent or minimize the chances of a needlestick accident during use. Devices designed to reduce the risk of needlestick accidents are primarily relevant when selecting a catheter and when add-on access devices, such as a saline lock, are used.

NOTE: To avoid confusion, note that all IV systems, both safety and nonsafety, whether needle or needleless, utilize a peripheral IV catheter consisting of a rigid steel stylet needle sheathed in a flexible cannula. Catheters are discussed in more detail later in this section.

Needle systems are traditional, nonsafety devices because they require sharp steel syringe needles to puncture through the rubber ends of access ports. The use of needles increases the risk of puncture accidents, damage to surrounding tubing, and a phenomenon called coring, which occurs when a large bore needle tears out a tiny core of rubber on the port, compromising the integrity of the closed system. This may allow air to enter the vein and risks producing an embolus if the core escapes into the circulation. Nonsafety devices are almost all universal, which is to say different parts of an IV setup are interchangeable among brands (for example, threads should match, etc.). However, it is always a good idea to confirm compatibility with a sales representative before ordering unfamiliar equipment. This chapter will focus on the types of devices you are most likely to require in midwifery practice.

Needleless systems are safety devices, the steel stylet in the catheter assembly being the only needle in the system. Other specialized connectors are accessed using blunt-tipped, cannulated spikes to enter the injection ports in IV tubing and locking devices. Having safety ports and needleless adapters is most desirable when using IVs intermittently with a compatible saline-lock device because of the need for entering the IV line more frequently.

Needle-safe systems include additional devices and shields used on catheters to decrease the chance of a needlestick injury. They consist of a traditional IV catheter with a built-in sheathing device to automatically cover the stylet after it is withdrawn. These safety devices may, at first, be a nuisance to use if you are accustomed to nonsafety needles. However, once you get used to them, you may find they promote easier insertion because of their design (Garcia, 2002).

These technologies are changing rapidly, so describing different styles of safety devices in detail in this textbook is not practical. When ordering equipment, ask for information regarding costs and devices available in both nonsafety and safety systems so that you can compare features, prices and the minimum quantity you must purchase at a time. A well-informed sales representative should know their stock well enough to go from there. While there are many different types of IV products available, most medical supply houses do not carry everything, as the cost is too prohibitive. Minimally, you will want to have a few of each of the following items on hand: IV solution, primary administration set and IV catheters. You will need to adjust quantities to suit the size and location of your practice.

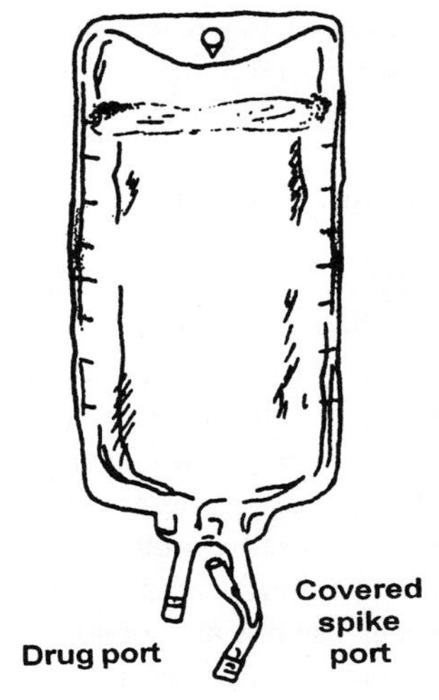

Solution bag

Fluids to infuse: For volume replacement, carry at least two bags (1000 cc each) of lactated Ringer's (in the UK, this solution is called Hartman's) and, ideally at least two bags of normal (0.9%) saline. These bags will be equipped with one or two rubber-topped ports on the bottom: the longer insertion port where the tubing will be attached and usually a shorter port through which medications can be added to the fluid. Some solution bags have an insertion port on the bottom, with a rubber nipple to be used as a drug port, located on the side of the bag.

Regardless of the type of safety system you are using, the drug port on the solution bag is designed to receive a regular syringe needle, even if a needleless safety system is to be used for other parts of the infusion set. Fluids should be packaged in biologically inert, non-PVC and non-DEHP plastic containers. The differences in IV fluids are discussed later in this chapter.

Gravity-flow primary macrodrip IV administration set (IV infusion set or solution set): These are the common names for the main tubing that will carry and regulate the flow of IV solution from the bag to the cannula and its built-in features. You will require macrodrip [macrodrop] IV administration (infusion) sets with standard-bore tubing. (Macrodrip and standard-bore features are explained more fully later in this chapter.) The various parts of the set are described below.

Spike: At the top of the tube is a pointed plastic insertion device, called a spike, that inserts into the tubing insertion port on the bottom of the bag of fluid. The spike should have a finger guard that prevents your hand from slipping during insertion. It both aids insertion and prevents contamination of the tip, which should remain sterile.

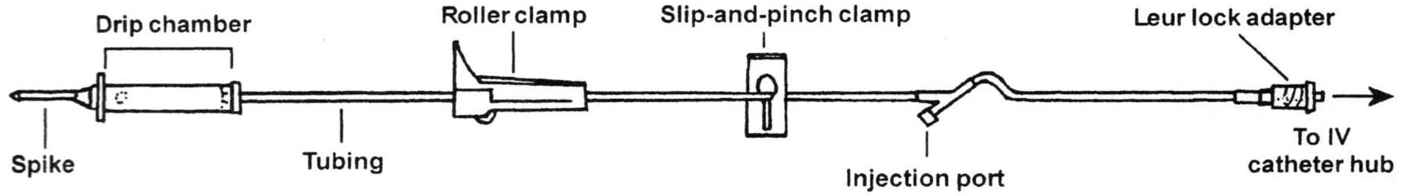

IV administration set

Drip chamber: Under the spike is a drip chamber, which is a large-bore, clear plastic compressible tube. Solution enters the chamber in precisely measured drops. The drip chamber provides a way to see how fast the IV is running and thus gauge the rate of flow. Among the characteristics of the drip chamber, there are two factors to consider:

Vents: Drip chambers come with and without vents. A nonvented set or one with a sealable vent should be chosen when using solutions in flexible plastic to minimize the risk of an air embolism. (Vented sets are designed for use with rigid solution containers.)

Drip factor: The drip chamber allows you to administer fluid in a measurable dose, calibrated in terms of "number of drops = 1 ml." Knowing the number of drops per milliliter allows you to calculate the amount of fluid to be given over a period of time. A common **macrodrip** chamber usually delivers ten drops to one milliliter, but drop size can vary with the manufacturer; be sure to check the labeling. (Note that metered volume drip chambers are designed to limit the amount of fluid infused and are therefore not recommended for emergency midwifery applications.)

Tubing: The tubing or "infusion line" extends from the bottom of the drip chamber to the connector that attaches to the hub of the IV cannula. Tubing length ranges from 60 to 100 in (152 to 254 cm); the shortest tubing that is practical will help speed the replacement of fluid. Microdrop (minidrip) tubing is also available for administering flow rates of less than 100 ml/hour, which is useful when giving antibiotics but should never be used for emergency fluid replacement. Among the characteristics of the tubing, note:

Clamps: Most tubes come equipped with two types of clamps which allow to you regulate or stop the flow of solution through the tubing. There are two types of clamps:

Roller (regulator) clamp: This clamp consists of a roller in a frame fitted around the tubing. It is designed to incrementally occlude the tubing by pinching it as the roller is tightened, which allows you to control the rate of flow in drops per minute. It can be operated with one hand and is accurate to plus or minus 10%.

Slide-and-pinch clamp: This simple push-on, push-off device is placed beneath the drip chamber. It is helpful to shut the IV flow off completely when you need to do so rapidly or when removing the IV from the woman's arm. They can also be used to assist in removing air bubbles from the line (more about this later).

Injection (drug) ports: Most primary administration sets have one or more Y-shaped injection or drug ports along their length. These resealable ports provide a way to administer drugs directly into the IV tubing. A syringe fitted with either a needle or, in a needleless system, a dull plastic cannula is inserted into the port, the drug is injected and the needle or syringe cannula is removed. The port then reseals the hole made during the puncture, maintaining the sterility of the line and preventing the entry of air. Injection ports are designed to tolerate numerous punctures, although excessive use or the insertion of large-gauge needles compromises the seal's integrity sooner, risking the entry of air and bacteria. Needleless ports designed to receive cannulated devices are usually amber colored and have some distinguishing feature such as a color-coded housing or a white circle on the top of the port. Nonsafety ports have an off-white plain rubber covering. Safety features will be clearly marked on the packaging as well.

Back-check valves: Many primary sets have back-check valves, whose sole purpose is to allow fluid to flow in one direction only. They are primarily needed when "piggyback" medication administration devices are being used and are therefore not relevant here, but they pose no problems for midwifery applications.

Adapters (connectors): These devices are permanently fitted to the patient end of the tubing and allow you to attach the end of the tube to the hub of the cannula. They come in two styles:

Male luer-slip adapters: These simply slide into each other and provide a tight connection when twisted, although they can be pulled apart because they do not lock.

Male luer-lock adapters: This type has a straight tip that inserts into the hub as well as a screw connector that then screws down over the hub, making this type of connector much harder to dislodge. They are the connector of choice when a saline lock is in use and are recommended for all applications. Luer-lock adapters are an industry standard and do not increase your cost.

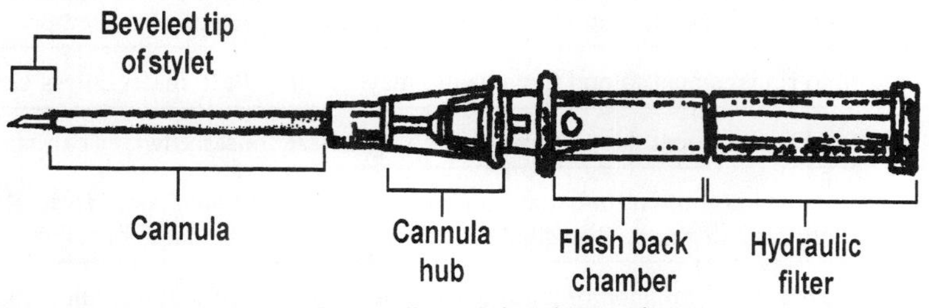

Over-the-needle peripheral IV catheter

Over-the-needle peripheral IV catheters: The next device to consider is the catheter itself, which consists of a soft plastic cannula with a rigid, color-coded plastic or metal hub. A hollow metal stylet (needle) with a beveled tip is preinserted into the cannula, the tip of which extends slightly beyond the end of the cannula. The rigid stylet is used to penetrate the blood vessel and guide the cannula insertion as venipuncture is performed. The terms "catheter" and "cannula" are used interchangeably in the medical literature. To avoid confusion here, "catheter" will refer to the entire unit prior to removal of the stylet and "cannula" will refer to the thin, flexible plastic tube that is left in the vein. Also, the terms "needle" and "stylet" are used interchangeably in the literature to refer to the steel needle in the cannula. Here, the needle in the catheter set will be referred to as a "stylet" to avoid confusing it with a syringe needle.

Flashback chamber: The flashback chamber is a clear, closed chamber attached directly to the end of the stylet. The end of the flashback chamber has a removable plug with a filter in the center through which air enters the chamber to facilitate flashback. When the vein is penetrated, blood appears in the flashback chamber to confirm proper placement. The metal stylet and flashback chamber are then removed, leaving the soft cannula with its color-coded hub in the vein, thereby forming an open channel between the blood vessel and the tube that carries the IV fluid.

Cannula: The cannula is the soft catheter that remains in the vein once the stylet is removed. It fits snugly around the stylet and gently tapers to its tip, which makes it easier for it to be inserted in the vein. Cannula construction varies with manufacturer. The material should be radiopaque to allow visualization of the cannula in place and location of a fragment should a piece get lost in the vascular system. It should be evaluated for its clot-encouraging or thrombogenic properties, as all foreign materials are somewhat thrombogenic. Biocompatibility is also assessed and refers to the body's overall ability to accept the foreign material–the more biocompatible the material, the more bioinert it is. Cannulas are made of various plastics, such as PVC or polyurethane. At present, silicone is the most bioinert material available. Other materials include Teflon (polytetrafluoroethylene), a plastic-coated material that is less reactive than PVC, and vialon, a nonhemolytic, hemocompatible polymer that is very slick when wet and softens after insertion, minimizing vein trauma and clot formation. Use of a catheter suited for peripheral insertion is important; one with too soft a cannula will result in the cannula bunching up on the skin as you try to insert the stylet.

Size: Carry a selection of 1 in to 1.25 in (2.5 to 3.13 cm) standard, peripheral over-the-needle IV catheters in sizes 14, 16, 18 and 20 or 22 gauge. The lower the number, the larger the hollow bore, or lumen, of the cannula, and the quicker the fluid can be delivered. Cannulas that are 18 gauge or larger (that is, with a lower gauge number) are preferred for administering whole blood through the same line. Having a large-bore cannula already in place prior to arrival at the hospital assists in replacing blood as quickly as possible, should it be needed. However, smaller gauge catheters are more comfortable and easier to insert. Therefore, if you believe you will be unable to insert anything larger, a 20 gauge catheter is minimally acceptable for volume expansion, with the understanding that it may have to be replaced with a larger catheter once someone with that skill arrives on the scene. A 20 gauge catheter can also be used when an IV is being given in a nonemergent situation, such as for rehydration or antibiotic administration during labor. Note that 22 gauge and 24 gauge stylets are so fine that they frequently bend during insertion attempts (especially if the skin is thick) and are therefore often impractical (Garcia, 2002).

PERIPHERAL IV CATHETER SELECTION CRITERIA		
COLOR	**GAUGE**	**USAGE**
Orange	14	Rapid fluid replacement, blood transfusion; difficult for even experienced practitioners to insert.
Gray	16	Rapid fluid replacement, blood transfusion; may be difficult to insert unless veins are large.
Green	18	Rapid fluid replacement, blood transfusion; largest size most midwives can insert successfully.
Pink	20	Continuous or intermittent infusion, can be used for blood transfusion. Best, all-purpose size that is relatively easy to insert. The smallest gauge that should be used for volume expansion.
Blue	22	Intermittent general infusion of antibiotics or nonemergent hydrating fluids; may bend during insertion.
Yellow	24	Small or fragile veins or intermittent infusion of antibiotics or nonemergent hydrating fluids; is likely to bend during insertion.

Be well aware of manufacturer's color coding of packaging and cannula hubs for the different gauges of catheters to help avoid accidental misuse. *Color coding allows you to select the proper gauge catheter quickly, but does not indicate length, safety devices or any other features.* While the shades may vary, basic color coding for IV catheters is universal among the following major brands in the United States: Johnson & Johnson (Jelco), B&D (Becton Dickinson),

Abbott and B. Braun (formerly McGaw).

Splints: On rare occasions, if you have placed the cannula in the bend of a joint or if transport will be tricky (going down stairs, for example), you may need to use a splint to stabilize the arm and prevent cannula disruption. Padded disposable arm (3.25 in X 18 in) and wrist (3.25 in X 9 in) splints are available. If you do not have a real splint, one can be fashioned from any long, flat, nonsharp object, such as a folded magazine or section of newspaper, a disposable paint stirrer, or dull-edged ruler. Wrap the item in a small towel and tape in place.

IV pressure infuser: This device fits around the IV bag, providing positive pressure and eliminating the need to hang the bag for gravity feeding. However, pressure infusers are tricky to use and will speed air embolism if air enters the tube while it is in place. Even in hospitals, they are often not used except during administration of blood products (Garcia, 2002). The use of a pressure infuser adds one more risk in an already critical situation and is one more thing that must be carefully monitored when you need to focus on the mother. Therefore, their use is not elaborated here.

Summary of basic IV starter supplies: To summarize, for emergency volume expansion ask for a simple primary macrodrip IV administration set (10 to 15 drops/ml) with a nonvented (or sealable vent) drip chamber, with a roller and a slide-and-pinch clamp, with 70 in (175 cm) or so length of standard-bore tubing and with a male luer-lock adapter. You don't need an injection port, but most supply houses carry administrations sets with at least one. If it comes with one or more, you usually won't use it; their presence poses no problem and they do come in handy for clearing the line of large, stubborn air bubbles. Read the administration set wrapper; it will tell you what, if any, additional devices you need for a basic IV setup using that brand. You will also minimally require several catheters in 18 and 20 gauge sizes.

Needleless systems are really not relevant if you plan to use IVs primarily for emergencies. If you plan to administer drugs intermittently, a needleless safety system may be more desirable. In this case, be sure to obtain all the necessary component parts and be sure they are fully compatible, including the connection devices on the solution bags. A knowledgeable sales representative should be able to confirm compatibility among different brands. While universal adaptability is more common with add-on devices than in primary administration sets, the compatibility of all accessory devices should be verified to ensure the safest connections when in use. More details regarding needleless accessories, including various types of saline-locks, can be found in the section entitled "Devices that can be used for intermittent IV administration" later in this chapter.

In addition to the items listed above, you will need the following items that can be purchased together in a small IV starter kit or that can be assembled separately:

- Gauze pads and grain-alcohol-based herbal antiseptic tincture, prepared rubbing alcohol swabs or iodine swabs. (Be sure to check the prenatal records regarding iodine and latex allergies.)
- Transparent, porus IV tape (2 in × 3 in) such as Tegaderm® (can be used for all taping needs)
- 1 in wide paper or plastic tape suitable for skin application
- Tourniquet
- Labels

Other items that are handy to have on hand include:

- Well-fitting sterile and nonsterile gloves
- Something from which to hang the IV bag so that it is above the level of the mother's heart. This can be a nail in the wall, a coat hanger hooked over a door knob or dresser drawer, or an IV pole. An assistant can also hold the bag, which will probably be necessary during a transport.
- Absorbent underpad or towel to place beneath the puncture site
- Several small hand-sized towels
- Heating pad to warm IV fluids
- Thermometer to tape to side of IV bag
- 3 in gauze bandage for attaching the splint
- 3 cc and 5 cc luer-lock syringes with 18 or 20 gauge, 1 in needles
- Vacutainer tubes for storing blood samples if blood is drawn. (However, most of the time, when using an IV in an emergency, you will probably not want to take the time to collect blood samples.)

Some IV instructions call for iodine swabs to scrub the puncture site before inserting the catheter and antibiotic ointment to apply to the puncture site just before the IV line and cannula hub are taped into place. Antiseptic herbal grain alcohol-based tincture or plain grain alcohol are just as good for cleansing the puncture site. When short-term IV use is anticipated, it is not necessary to use an ointment at the puncture site. It tends to make a mess and prevent adhesion of the tape (Garcia, 2002).

Equipment for intermittent IV use

Another list of supplies falls into this category, including saline locks. These are discussed beginning on page 883.

Carrying and storing IV equipment

Bags that are designed to store and carry IV equipment for homebirth practice are available. Cascade HealthCare Products lists them under IV equipment and supplies in their catalogue. Other options used by many midwives include a tackle or tool box. If you choose to purchase a specialized bag, make sure to store all your emergency IV equipment together in one place and nonemergent supplies in another, even if this means duplicating some items, such as a tourniquet. For example, you might purchase a red tackle box to keep antihemorrhagic drugs, syringes and emergency IV equipment and a blue box to store all nonemergent venipuncture and injection supplies.

Fluid and Electrolyte Balance Within the Body

Fluid compartments

The water in the body is contained is a variety of different types of tissue regions or "compartments" which are referred to by several (sometimes overlapping) terms, as follows:

FLUID	LOCATION OF FLUID	% OF TOTAL BODY FLUID
Intravascular (IVF)	A generic term used for fluids in both vascular systems in the body: blood and lymph. Often refers to the plasma and other blood components within the cardiovascular system.	----
Intracellular (ICF)	Fluids within the cells.	about 63%
Extracellular (ECF)	Usually refers to all plasma and interstitial fluids. This term is also used to mean all fluids outside a cell, excluding transcellular fluid.	32%
Transcellular	Fluids that are not inside cells, but are separated from plasma and interstitial fluid by cellular barriers; e.g., intraocular, cerebrospinal, synovial and pleural fluids.	----
Interstitial	Interstitial refers to fluid in spaces within tissues, or organs, excluding fluid within body cavities (such as ingested water in the stomach). Includes extracellular fluid between cells. Some sources also include transcellular fluids as intersitial fluids.	15 to 16%
Plasma	Fluid component of the blood within the circulatory system (intravascular).	5%

Thus, about two-thirds of the total body fluid is in the intracellular space and one-third is in the extracellular space. Fluid moves back and forth among these compartments as the solute balance in the fluid shifts, always moving from a region with a lower concentration of solutes to one with a higher concentration, until the balance of solutes to fluids in each adjacent compartment is the same (homeostasis). Fluid loss via **dehydration** leads to a greater concentration of solutes in the extracellular spaces. **Blood loss** produces a dramatic reduction of fluid and solutes in the intravascular space. **Fluid retention** in the extracellular area is treated with sodium and fluid restriction. Headache and confusion may indicate intracellular fluid changes. Thirst and nausea may indicate extracellular fluid changes.

Water balance

Water is essential for life. Water content influences blood volume, temperature regulation, the transport of minerals and nutrients to and from cells and plays a role in many biological reactions. Water and mineral solutes (electrolytes) work together to maintain water balance. Water intake is regulated through the sensation of thirst as water and electrolytes are continuously being lost and replaced. The water content of the body depends on a number of factors such as age, sex, body composition and disease processes such as renal or heart failure and gastrointestinal disorders. Adult bodies contain about 60% water, while newborn bodies contain 77%. Women have a lower water content than men because they have proportionately more body fat. Water balance is easily monitored through body weight. Rapid, otherwise unexplained weight changes of a few pounds usually reflect a loss of body water. Normal daily gains and losses of water in an average 150 pd man are as follows:

ROUTE OF ENTRY		ROUTE OF EXIT	
Dietary water	1000 ml	Skin	500 ml
Oxidation	300 ml	Lungs	350 ml
Fluid intake	1200 ml	Feces	150 ml
		Kidneys	1500 ml
TOTAL	**2500 ml**	**TOTAL**	**2500 ml**

Water is lost through the kidneys, lungs, skin and gastrointestinal tract. The kidneys are the organs primarily responsible for regulating the volume and concentration of all body fluids. When fluid intake is normal, the kidneys can maintain water and electrolytes in balance. Water loss increases from the lungs and skin with elevated environmental or body temperature, rapid breathing and loss of skin integrity (from surgery, burns or wounds). Gastrointestinal losses increase in the presence of vomiting and diarrhea. These losses are normally replaced during food and water intake. To assess normal fluid/electrolyte balance, consider the following:

ASSESSING FLUID/ELECTROLYTE BALANCE	FINDING
Compare fluid intake and output	Intake should roughly equal output
Compare daily weight at about the same time on the same scale	A gain or loss of 2.2 lbs (1 kg) corresponds to 1 liter of fluid.
Review serum electrolyte values	Fluid excess: values are diluted Fluid deficit: values are elevated
Observe for clinical status	Evaluate the condition of the mucous membranes and skin, pulse, blood pressure, thirst and mental alertness.

Electrolyte basics

A normal balance of electrolytes is necessary for physiologic functioning, and imbalances can be fatal. The term electrolyte refers to any compound that, when in solution or when liquified by heat, conducts an electric current and is decomposed as the current passes through it. Electrolytes influence four primary physiologic processes: water distribution in the ICF and ECF, neuromuscular irritability, acid-base balance and maintenance of osmotic pressure. The intake of fluids either orally or via IV therapy replaces lost electrolytes and fluid, which restores the body to a normal pH. The three major electrolytes are sodium, potassium and chloride, followed by calcium and magnesium. The following brief discussions introduce the role of these electrolytes in the body. If a midwife suspects an electrolyte imbalance, she should transport immediately. Although conditions known to result in electrolyte loss can be treated at home with balanced mineral solutions, a midwife should never try to treat a severely symptomatic imbalance of an individual electrolyte at home. The treatments given below are not full descriptions of how to correct these imbalances and therefore cannot serve as a guide. They are offered to give a general idea of what would be done in each circumstance. The lab values given below are relative, as actual values will vary depending upon the type of tests used and the woman's condition when tested.

Sodium: Among all the body's electrolytes, sodium has the most influence over the distribution of body fluid because it attracts water. Sodium is the primary determinant of the extracellular fluid volume, and thus sodium imbalances are also extracellular in nature. Normal nonpregnant levels range from 135 to 137 mEq/l or mmol/l (i.e., the numerical values are identical for both unit systems). Sodium values undergo minimal changes within this range during pregnancy.

Elevated concentrations of sodium in the plasma (hypernatremia) result from conditions such as impairment of the sense of thirst, hyperventilation, fever, head injuries, decreased secretion of antidiuretic hormone (ADH), diabetes insipidus and the inability of the kidneys to respond to ADH. Low sodium concentrations in plasma (hyponatremia) involve an increase in the proportion of water to salt in the blood and result from a disturbance of the secretion of ADH. Causes include head injury and severe physiological and psychological stress. Hyponatremia may also occur when hypotonic fluids are given to persons at a time when their ADH secretion is elevated.

SIGNS & SYMPTOMS OF HYPERNATREMIA	SIGNS & SYMPTOMS OF HYPONATREMIA
Serum sodium >145 mEq/l or mmol/l	Serum sodium <135 mEq/l or mmol/l
Hypotension	Hypertension, increased intracranial pressure
Hypervolemia	Hypovolemia
Dry mucous membranes	Increased salivation
Urine output < 30 ml/hr	Low urinary specific gravity
Coma and death	Coma and death
Treatment: normal saline IV infused over 48 hours*	**Treatment:** hypertonic saline (3 to 5%) followed by diuretics

*Hypernatremia can be corrected with a physiologic saline solution because it contains less sodium than the serum of a person with severe hypernatremia.

Potassium: Potassium is the primary electrolyte contained in intracellular fluid. It is required to maintain osmotic balance and the electrical potential of cellular membranes and also assists in moving glucose into the cells. Potassium levels range from 3.5 to 5 mEq/l or 13.7 to 19.5 mg/dl (3.5 to 5 mmol/l) and undergo tiny variations within this range during pregnancy.

Serum potassium (that which is in the ECF and is measured in laboratory tests) levels are influenced by dehydration, blood pH, dietary intake, and diuretic therapy. When the potassium balance between the ICF and the ECF is altered, cellular metabolism is affected along with the cardiovascular, renal, respiratory and neuromuscular systems. Elevated serum potassium (hyperkalemia) occurs when acidosis drives potassium out of the cells. Reduced levels (hypokalemia) occur when alkalosis drives potassium into the cells.

SIGNS & SYMPTOMS OF HYPERKALEMIA	SIGNS & SYMPTOMS OF HYPOKALEMIA
Serum potassium >5 mEq/l or mmol/l	Serum potassium <3.5 mEq/l or mmol/l
Conduction disorders of the heart	Ectopic cardiac activity
Diarrhea, abdominal pain	Decreased bowel sounds, ileus
Neuromuscular irritability	Muscle weakness, burning, prickling, tickling or tingling sensations
Oliguria or anuria	Polyuria
Cardiac failure	Digitalis toxicity
Treatment: potassium chloride IV	**Treatment:** calcium gluconate, sodium bicarbonate, glucose or insulin

Chloride: Chloride is the primary electrolyte in the ECF. Chloride levels in the blood are passively related to those of sodium, so that when serum sodium increases, chloride does as well. During pregnancy, chloride values change little if any from normal, nonpregnant values, which range from 95 to 105 mEq/l (mmol/l).

Factors causing losses or gains of chloride frequently affect sodium levels as well. Chloride levels rise in the presence of dehydration, renal failure or acidosis. Chloride levels fall in the presence of fluid losses from the digestive tract (nausea, vomiting, diarrhea and gastric suction) and excessive sweating. IV chloride solution is always given in combination with sodium and potassium.

Signs & Symptoms of Excessive chloride	Signs & Symptoms of Chloride deficit
Serum chloride > 110 mEq/l or mmol/l	Serum chloride <100 mEq/l or mmol/l
Dehydration	Fever
Hyperventilation	Nausea and vomiting
Urinary output > 30 ml/hr	Tissue wasting (burns)

Calcium: Calcium is the most abundant electrolyte in the body and is primarily stored in the bones. Less than 1% of skeletal calcium is available for daily electrolyte regulation. Calcium is present in the blood in two forms: free, ionized calcium that is circulating and calcium that is bound to protein. The bound form attaches to the plasma protein (albumin) and other complex substances such as phosphates, making it important to correlate the serum calcium concentration with the serum albumin level. Normal calcium levels average 8.8 to 10 mg/dl or 4.4 to 5 mEq/l (2.2 to 2.5 mmol/l) outside of pregnancy and fall gradually to a level at term about 10% below the nonpregnant level, which matches the fall in the serum albumin level which accompanies hemodilution. There is a tiny decrease in ionized calcium within the nonpregnant range as well. Calcium effects neuromuscular and cardiac function and bone formation. Calcium imbalances result from changes in bone metabolism, secretion of parathyroid hormone, renal dysfunction and altered dietary intake.

Signs & Symptoms of Hypercalcemia	Signs & Symptoms of Hypocalcemia
Serum calcium > 10.5 mEq/l (>5.25 mmol/l)	Serum calcium < 8.5 mEq/l (<4.25 mmol/l)
Decreased mental alertness	Neuromuscular irritability, for example, numbness and tingling, hyperactive reflexes, and seizures
Abdominal pain, muscle weakness, nausea and vomiting, and hypertension	Bone pain
Treatment: sodium chloride IV, thiazide diuretics	**Treatment:** calcium gluconate or calcium chloride

Magnesium: Magnesium is normally obtained through the diet and excreted via the kidneys. Some 70% is located in the bones with 30% found in cellular fluids. Magnesium is involved in many essential metabolic processes including the energy production of glucose, vascular tone, muscle impulse transmission, electrical stability of cells, neurotransmission and activity and the absorption and metabolism of other minerals such as calcium, phosphorus, sodium and potassium. It appears to fall gradually by about 10 to 20% below the normal nonpregnant values, which average 1.6 to 2.4 mEq/l or 1.8 to 3.0 mg/dl (0.80 to 1.20 mmol/l).

Signs & Symptoms of Hypermagnesemia	Signs & Symptoms of Hypomagnesemia
Serum magnesium > 3.4 mEq/l (>1.7 mmol/l)	Serum magnesium < 0.3 to 1 mEg/l (<0.15-0.5 mmol/l)
Lethargy	Disorientation, combativeness
Absent deep tendon reflexes	Hyperactive reflexes
Hypotension	Tremors, tetany
Depressed respirations	Altered speech, difficulty swallowing
Treatment: magnesium sulfate	**Treatment:** calcium gluconate

Hypomagnesemia results from prolonged malnutrition or starvation, alcoholism and long-term IV therapy without magnesium supplementation. Symptoms are worsened by hypocalcemia. Elevated levels (hypermagnesemia) occurs most often in those with renal failure, diabetic ketoacidosis and those who take lots of antacids or laxatives.

Characteristics of IV Fluids

There are two main categories of fluids used in replacing volume loss: crystalloids (water and mineral solutions) and colloids (whole blood, blood components such as red cells, and synthetic blood substitutes). Midwives working at homebirths only have access to crystalloid solutions, which are created by dissolving crystals, such as minerals or simple sugars in water. They are readily available, easily stored, nontoxic and reaction-free. Examples of crystalloid solutions include lactated Ringer's (Hartman's), normal saline and dextrose solutions in water.

The movement of bodily fluids among various compartments is accomplished in various ways, including osmosis. **Osmosis** refers to the natural movement of pure water molecules through a selectively permeable membrane from an area of higher solute concentration to an area of lower solute concentration. **Diffusion** refers to the movement of solutes (particles) from an area of higher concentration to one of lower concentration via a semipermeable membrane, which continues until the concentration on both sides of the membrane is in balance. When choosing which crystalloid fluid to use, you must consider the osmolarity of the solution.

Osmolarity is an intrinsic property of bodily fluids, representing all the dissolved particles (or solutes), both colloid and crystalloid, in a solution. The amount and size of dissolved particles will influence how the fluid moves into various parts of the body. **Osmotic pressure** is the pressure required to prevent the movement of pure water into a solution containing other substances when these solutions are separated by a selectively permeable membrane. The more solids a solution contains, the greater the osmotic pressure. Colloid molecules, which are the various protein molecules in plasma, cannot pass through the semipermeable capillary membranes and are responsible for the oncotic pressure of a solution. Oncotic pressure is simply the osmotic pressure exerted by colloids in solution. The review table on page 864 shows the locations of different fluids in the body.

When speaking of crystalloid fluids, the term **tonicity** is used in place of osmotic pressure. Solutions are categorized based on their osmotic properties (the amount of particulate matter they contain) as either hypertonic, hypotonic or isotonic when compared to another fluid, in this case, blood plasma. The type of fluid a woman needs depends on the nature and extent of her condition.

Hypertonic solutions have higher osmotic pressure (i.e., higher solute concentration with an osmolarity greater than 300 mOsm/L [milliosmols per liter]) than does plasma or intersitial fluid. These solutions tend to draw water from inside the cells into the intravascular space, especially when the person is normally hydrated. This means that a relatively small quantity of hypertonic solution is needed to achieve expansion of the blood volume, resulting in the rapid restoration of normal blood flow to the brain and vital organs. Hypertonic saline also leads to selective blood flow restriction to skeletal muscles and causes the capillaries in the digestive, respiratory, urogenital, and endocrine systems as well as the spleen and heart to dilate, resulting in restoration of normal blood flow to vital organs and shunting it from skeletal muscles. Although cardiac output is also restored, how this occurs is not well understood. In the brain, hypertonic solutions not only improve cerebral blood flow but also prevent both cerebral edema and increased intracranial pressure. These solutions include 5% dextrose in 0.9% sodium chloride, 5% dextrose in 0.45% sodium chloride and 3%, 5% and 7.5% sodium chloride solutions.

However, the intravascular benefit hypertonic fluids produce only lasts 15 minutes, after which the fluid becomes redistributed between the intravascular and interstitial space. Hypertonic fluids can damage veins. They can also create imbalances in sodium, potassium, chloride and clotting factor levels. Although these types of problems are most likely to arise with overly aggressive fluid replacement, they require careful monitoring with lab tests to avoid complications. In spite of the theoretical benefits, hypertonic saline is rarely used in obstetrics and is inappropriate for home use due to lack of access to immediate lab testing.

Hypotonic solutions have a lower osmotic pressure, and therefore a lower solute concentration (<280 mOsm/L), than does plasma. When they are given to a normally hydrated person, infused water moves from the solution into the red blood cells, leading to swelling and eventual bursting (hemolysis). These solutions supply calories and replenish salt and water but may lead to widespread hemolysis if too much is given at once. They are used to prevent and treat dehydration, but because of their rapid defusion out of the vascular space, they should never be used for volume replacement. Examples include distilled water, 0.45% sodium chloride, 2.5% dextrose in water and 0.45% normal saline (½ NS). The use of hypotonic solutions for volume replacement carries the highest risk of hyponatremia, or sodium deficiency, which can lead to brain damage and death in its most extreme manifestation. This risk is particularly high in women of childbearing age. In most cases, the infusion must take place over several days to cause this type of imbalance. Prevention of these complications requires electrolyte monitoring using blood tests. Hypotonic solutions should not be used at home.

Isotonic solutions have a solute ratio equal to that of most normal body cells and plasma. The normal physiologic range for isotonicity is about 280 to 300 mOsm/L. When isotonic solutions are infused into a normally hydrated person, they neither draw fluid out of the cells nor do they move fluid into cells. Isotonic solutions are generally used to replace extracellular fluid lost during bleeding, severe vomiting, or any time chloride loss equals or exceeds sodium loss. Examples include 0.9% (normal) saline and lactated Ringer's solution (Hartman's). Five percent dextrose in water (D_5W) is technically isotonic but acts hypotonically in the system (more details below).

Effects of Various IV Solutions on Fluid Volume in Various Locations Compared to Whole Blood				
IV Solution (1 liter/1000 ml)	ICV (ml)	ECV (ml)	ISV (ml)	PV (ml)
Sodium chloride (hypertonic)	-2950	3950	2690	990
0.5% Dextrose/water (hypotonic action)	660	340	255	85
Normal (0.9%) saline (isotonic)	-100	1100	825	275
Lactated Ringer's (isotonic)	-100	1100	825	275
Whole blood (isotonic)	0	1000	0	1000
ICV=Intracellular fluid (volume) ECV=Extracellular fluid (volume) ISV=Interstitial fluid (volume) PV=Plasma (intravascular fluid) volume				

(Carlson et al., 1990)

Crystalloid fluids for use in birth-related situations

Lactated Ringer's or normal (0.9%) saline solution are considered by many to be the fluids of choice for emergency pretransport volume expansion for those in obstetric shock. Because of the increased capillary permeability induced by volume loss, crystalloids are less effective than colloids for expansion of intravascular volume even when given at equivalent volumes. However, many feel crystalloid solutions most effectively replace the interstitial deficits that occur with blood loss (see the chapter entitled "Hypovolemic Shock due to Hemorrhage" for details). They distribute rapidly into intra- and extracellular fluid, decreasing the chance that pulmonary edema will develop. Equilibration within the interstitial space occurs more slowly with isotonic solutions. For example, when an isotonic solution is given to a dehydrated person, equilibration usually occurs within 20 to 30 minutes after infusion. When given to a hypovolemic person, the solution tends to remain in the intravascular space until the body recognizes that it is hemodynamically stable. At this point, the body starts to redistribute fluids to tissues outside the vascular space. Because of this, only 33% of the infused solution remains in the vascular space after an hour or two when the person is otherwise healthy, as is the case with most pregnant women. (When the person is ill, 80% of the infused fluid leaves the circulation quickly; 40 minutes later almost all of the fluid has migrated to the interstitial space.) When a nonpregnant person suffers blood loss (for example, due to trauma), it is expected that 3 to 4 liters of crystalloid solution will need to be given to replace every liter of blood lost. However, when a woman with a well-expanded blood volume hemorrhages after birth, she has a safety margin of extra blood to lose. Therefore, more blood can be lost before shock ensues, and stabilization is more likely to occur without having to replace as much fluid as would otherwise be the case when her bleeding is moderate and can be stopped (Clark et al.,1997). (Normally, women who have not hemorrhaged begin to excrete a large volume of urine soon after birth as their blood volume starts to return to normal, nonpregnant levels.) (Also refer to the chart below comparing different properties and uses of various crystalloid IV fluids.)

There is controversy regarding whether lactated Ringer's or normal saline is best to use. Both solutions infuse easily into the interstitial space, and neither becomes hypotonic in the body. When the kidneys are functioning normally,any excess chloride from either solution is secreted. However, animal studies done by Healey and colleagues (1998) found that the two were equivalently effective for mild to moderate hemorrhage. However, lactated ringers proved superior in those with massive hemorrhage, with significantly more acidosis and a mortality rate of 50% in the saline group.

Normal saline has a pH of 5, making it more acidic than Ringer's. It also does not contain lactate to help neutralize any metabolic acidosis that may already be present from the shock. Saline also has a tendency to produce hyperchloremic acidosis if electrolytes become imbalanced. Hyperchloremic acidosis is characterized by a decreased ability to acidify urine, low plasma bicarbonate and high plasma chloride concentrations, often with hypokalemia.

Lactated Ringer's is a well-balanced solution with a pH of 6.5 that contains many of the minerals found in the interstitial fluid, such as sodium chloride and small amounts of potassium and calcium. It also contains 28 mEq of lactate per liter, which is metabolized by the liver into bicarbonate, thus helping to neutralize the acidosis produced by hypoperfusion. The lactate load from lactated Ringer's solution does not aggravate the lactacidemia (excess lactic acid) associated with shock (Trudnowski et al., 1967), nor has it been shown to affect the reliability of blood lactate measurements (Lowery et al., 1971).

CRYSTALLOID IV FLUIDS APPROPRIATE FOR USE IN LABOR AND POSTPARTUM AND THEIR APPLICATIONS					
IV SOLUTION	**CONSTITUENTS**	**OSMOLARITY**	**ADVANTAGES**	**DISADVANTAGES**	**PRIMARY APPLICATIONS**
0.9% saline	154 mEq Na/L 154 mEq Cl/L	308 mOsm/L isotonic	Fluid & sodium replacement	Pulmonary edema, congestive heart failure; large amounts may cause electrolyte depletion.	Best for hypovolemia, heat-related problems, dehydration, diabetic ketoacidosis, fluid replacement in babies (in hospital only)
lactated Ringer's	130 mEq Na/L 109 mEq Cl/L 4 mEq K/L 3 mEq Ca/L 28 mEq lactate/L	273 mOsm/L isotonic	Approximates electrolyte concentration of blood	Pulmonary edema, renal failure, congestive heart failure	Best for dehydration, fluid replacement in babies (in hospital only), hypovolemia

Solutions containing dextrose: Dextrose, formerly referred to as glucose, is a monosaccharide (simple sugar) that freely dissolves in water. When it enters the system, dextrose is quickly metabolized as glucose and breaks down into carbon dioxide and water. It provides 3.4 calories per gram in solution (170 calories per liter at a 5% concentration). Dextrose solutions are primarily used for rehydration and to provide calories to nonpregnant individuals. Historically, dextrose solutions were given to laboring women to provide energy and to help correct or prevent ketosis. In reality, IV dextrose wreaks havoc with maternal and fetal blood sugar levels.

In particular, infusions of dextrose-containing solutions given to the laboring woman may be harmful to the fetus. The mother is usually rendered hyperglycemic by the infusion, even when efforts are made to monitor glucose levels. This leads to fetal hyperglycemia because glucose from the mother's system easily crosses the placenta, but her insulin does not. The fetal pancreas responds by secreting more insulin, which eventually results in fetal hypoglycemia. This cycle stresses the baby, placing him at risk for being born hypoglycemic and renders him less tolerant of hypoxia.

In most cases, dextrose offers no particular benefit to the mother and baby over solutions that do not contain dextrose. And, while dextrose solutions are still used in hospitals, I recommend that you refrain from giving the mother dextrose-containing IV solutions just before or during labor at home. They are most likely to be problematic for the baby when given an hour before the birth. If the mother is hypoglycemic, it is much safer to give her food, even hard candies or spoonfuls of honey, to raise her sugar level while receiving an IV of lactated Ringer's solution. This is because the sugars you are giving must go through the gastrointestinal tract to be absorbed, a very different process than direct infusion into the bloodstream. Infants whose mothers have received dextrose IV solutions during a hospital labor are usually monitored for hypoglycemia for the first two hours of life (Oxorn, 1986). The best preventive as well as corrective measure for newborn hypoglycemia is nursing soon after birth.

PROBLEMS WITH IV DEXTROSE USE IN LABOR	PROBLEMS WITH IV LACTATED RINGER'S USE IN LABOR
Maternal and fetal hyperglycemia Maternal hyponatremia (sodium loss) Fetal hyperinsulinism, acidosis, reduced tolerance for asphyxia Neonatal hyponatremia likely with rapid breathing Neonatal hypoglycemia Neonatal jaundice associated with maternal hyperglycemia Fluid shift from mother to baby resulting in more weight loss for the baby in the first 48 hours of life	Possible fluid shift from mother to baby when large amounts of IV fluid are given in labor

(Keppler, 1988)

IV fluid storage and preparation

Fluids should be stored at room temperature. Do not leave IV solutions in an excessively hot location for long periods prior to use or anywhere freezing is likely (e.g., you should not leave them in your car between births) because freezing destroys some electrolytes. The packaging should remain clean and undamaged; store the bags in new 1-gallon resealable plastic freezer bags to help protect them.

Tips on sterility: It is imperative that IV fluid be sterile when used. Make sure that expiration dates are monitored closely; expired fluids are not guaranteed sterile.

Warming IV fluids: The viscosity (essentially, the resistance to flow) and temperature of the IV solution affect how quickly it flows. Administering cold fluid takes longer and may worsen the woman's condition, further shocking her system and adversely affecting her core body temperature. Therefore, fluids should be warmed to *no greater than body temperature* prior to use. To raise the temperature of the fluid, lay it on a heating pad with a glass oral or rectal thermometer taped to the outside. Practice heating solutions with layers of toweling between the bag and the heating pad, noting how long it takes for the temperature of the fluid to rise. Make sure to note the appropriate setting on the heating pad. Never microwave IV fluids as it can destroy electrolytes. You can also place the bag port-end up with the thermometer taped in place, into a large new, well-sealed, 1 gallon resealable plastic bag (to protect the ports from becoming wet). Place the bag, sealed-end up, into a sink of clean, warm water no more than 100°F (37.5°C), taking care not to submerge the sealed end. This will work, but it may be more difficult to tell if the fluid has reached the proper temperature in the water.

As a practical matter in an emergency, as long as the solution bag feels lukewarm to the touch, the solution is at a safe temperature to use. If the room is warm, room temperature will also suffice, especially if only one or two liters are to be administered (Garcia, 2002).

When to Administer an IV

The following discussions focus on the use of lactated Ringer's solution during labor. Normal saline can be substituted if that is the only fluid available, but lactated Ringer's, with its balanced mineral content, is a better choice in my opinion for use during labor. Since insertion of an IV is painful, the cannula is uncomfortable and the presence of the IV bag and tubing limit mobility and gives the woman the impression that she is sick, IV use should be avoided whenever possible.

Prophylactic use of IV solutions in labor

The prophylactic administration of IV solutions during normal labor is unnecessary and leads to otherwise avoidable complications, the highest risk being fluid overload. Electrolytes can become imbalanced when they are infused into a woman whose electrolytes are already in balance. Women who have eaten well during pregnancy have plenty of extra blood volume and are well prepared to maintain their fluid balance during labor. The administration of any type of IV fluids should only be considered if vomiting or diarrhea has pushed the woman into a compromised state.

Even if the woman is a candidate for receiving some IV fluid, overinfusion can occur. However, most midwives carry only two or three liters of solution to a birth; this amount of infused solution should not induce a fluid overload in a healthy woman, even if she received it all (Garcia, 2002). In judging when to start an IV, don't deplete your supply of IV fluids when oral or rectal intake could solve the problem, as it may be needed for a true emergency later.

Dehydration and fluid loss

Fluids are normally lost during the day via urination, gastrointestinal activity, breathing and sweating. Whenever a person is urinating frequently, working hard, vomiting, having diarrhea or breathing rapidly, she is losing more fluids than she normally would. Although in a healthy, well-nourished pregnancy, blood volume expands by 50% and additional fluid is held in the interstitial spaces, these extra fluids are protective against dehydration only to a certain extent. Taking in more fluids will help balance out a fluid loss that exceeds the limit of this protection. In addition, a woman who is vomiting or has diarrhea is losing electrolytes as well, imbalances of which will eventually lead to serious compromise if not corrected.

However, nature has built in a margin of safety for the laboring woman. Mild ketosis alone is not a sufficient reason to resort to IV therapy during labor (for details, see DIAGNOSTIC TESTS). If something must be done to address established and symptomatic maternal hypoglycemia involving fluid lost through vomiting or diarrhea, always attempt to have the mother take fluids and nourishment by mouth first. Nourishing retention enemas are another option. When the mother's ketone status is in question, dip her urine every hour or so. If ketone levels rise to +1 or higher, encourage her to increase her intake of water or electrolyte-balancing fluids. If she can successfully keep these fluids down and still has ketone levels in the +2 to +3 range an hour later, an IV may be warranted (Rawlins, as quoted by Newton, et al., 1988). If oral or rectal intake prove impossible, undesirable or unsatisfactory and an IV is opted for, the first choice should be to replace fluids and electrolytes with lactated Ringer's, which will often stabilize the nausea and allow the woman to begin oral intake. As soon as the nausea stabilizes, discontinue administering the IV solution but do not remove the cannula until you are quite sure she is doing better. Instead, attach a saline lock to the cannula hub and resume oral intake of nourishing foods and fluids as soon as possible (Garcia, 2002; Keppler, 1988; Oxorn, 1986).

IV fluids for prolonged labor

The woman who is somewhat dehydrated may have a prolonged labor accompanied by weak contractions. An IV of Ringers (no dextrose) can sometimes cause labor to pick right up and proceed to birth.

IV fluids for hypovolemic shock

Lactated Ringer's (Hartman's) is also the fluid of choice when blood loss is the concern. Hemorrhage causes a depletion of electrolytes, which are carried out of the body with the blood being lost. When a balanced electrolyte solution is given, the electrolytes lost with the hemorrhage are replaced. Normal saline may also be used, as imbalances are unlikely to occur when only 2 or 3 liters of solution are used for emergency volume replacement for acute shock during transport. When the woman arrives a the hospital, the staff will perform electrolyte laboratory studies to determine if any adjustments in the type of solution being used are necessary.

Dextrose solutions and hypovolemic shock: A dextrose and water solution is technically considered to be isotonic and should theoretically produce an immediate volume-expanding effect upon infusion. However, as the solution enters the bloodstream, the dextrose is rapidly metabolized by the adjacent cells, leaving excess free (mineral-free) water behind. This renders the solution hypotonic almost immediately upon entering the body. The free water dilutes the blood and then rapidly diffuses into the surrounding interstitial spaces, producing edema. In an attempt to stabilize the oncotic pressure, more fluid travels from the intravascular to the interstitial space further compromising the circulating volume and resulting in more edema. This is particularly damaging to the brain when ischemia (vascular constriction) is already present from shock because the extravascular swelling puts pressure on the already-constricted vessels, reducing blood flow even more. It is also potentially damaging to the heart, kidneys and other organs for the same reason.

You may wonder if it is safe to use a solution containing dextrose with either lactated Ringer's or normal saline, reasoning that the electrolytes will hold more fluid in the circulation once the dextrose is metabolized for energy. In fact, the presence of the electrolytes does not cancel out the detrimental effects of giving dextrose. First, the dextrose will be metabolized quickly, followed by the escape of free water from the vascular system. Simultaneously, minerals will be drawn into the vascular spaces from the cells. This produces an electrolyte imbalance in the circulating blood volume as well as the tissues and further impairs cellular metabolism. In addition, the presence of additional dextrose in the bloodstream during a hemorrhage could encourage necrosis if even tiny bleeds are taking place into vulnerable tissues, especially the brain. For all these reasons, solutions containing dextrose should *never* be used to treat blood loss.

To Set up an IV

The best way to study the following procedure is the have a full set of all the necessary items and a volunteer on hand so you can practice as you move through the steps. Do not attempt to actually insert the catheter if you have not had any hands-on training by a person with clinical IV experience. You can, however, go through the motions with a partner, which will help clarify the steps involved. If no volunteer is available, use an unpeeled banana as an arm substitute. In an emergency, the person with the most IV experience should insert the IV catheter.

1. **Remain calm:** Take a deep breath and keep breathing. Center yourself. This is probably an emergency. Proceed deliberately and consciously. No matter how desperately a woman needs an IV, do not add an additional

complication to the situation by rushing. Poor technique can be deadly.

2. **Wash your hands.**
3. **Assemble your supplies and equipment:** These items should be checked over and made easily accessible for use during your routine birthing equipment setup. Select the correct administration set and catheter. If you are treating shock, select the largest catheter you think you can successfully insert. If the goal is volume expansion, a 16 or 18 gauge needle would be ideal, but a 20 gauge will do. Set the catheter aside.

Prepare the solution bag and tubing:

1. **Remove the wrapper from the fluid bag:** The inner bag of IV solution may be wet due to condensation, but should not be leaking. Check the type of fluid and the expiration date on the bag, since the fluid *must* be sterile. Do not risk using out-of-date solution.
2. **Inspect the bag:** Apply gentle pressure and look for leaks, punctures or tears. In good, indirect light, rotate the bag from top to bottom and back to dislodge any sediment and hold it against both a white and a dark background to look for discoloration, cloudiness or particulate matter. Both Ringers and saline should be absolutely clear and free of visible particles. If the bag does not check out, use another bag.
3. **Prepare the tubing:**
   A. Open the infusion tubing package.
   B. Be sure the roller clamp is wide open and slide it along the tube until it is few inches below the drip chamber; this prevents accidental knocks from disrupting it during use. If the IV is to be in place longer than 24 hours, move the clamp to a new spot along the tubing each time the rate of flow is adjusted. This avoids tubing "memory," in which either the tube resists compression by the roller, causing the roller to open, or the tubing becomes permanently crimped and thus impairs flow.
   C. Close the roller clamp by rolling the wheel to the bottom of the frame. (It is best to close only one clamp at a time, to avoid inadvertently forgetting to open both of them later.)
   D. Remove the sterile cover from the spike on the end of the drip chamber.
   E. Remove the cover from the tubing insertion port on the bottom of the IV bag. If there is also an injection port, the insertion port will be the longer and larger of the two.
   F. Push the spike into the insertion port to the hilt, taking care to maintain sterility by not touching the spike or the rubber end of the port. This is called "spiking the bag."
4. **Fill the drip chamber:** Use your thumb and index finger to squeeze and release the center of the drip chamber until it is at least one-third to half-full of fluid (or until it is filled to the indicator line on the lower portion of the drip chamber). If you overfill the drip chamber, close the slide clamp below the drip chamber, invert the bag, squeeze the drip chamber to return excess fluid to the bag, turn the bag upright again, and open the clamp. Once it is properly filled, keep the drip chamber vertical at all times to prevent air bubbles from entering the tubing. (If you fill the drip chamber before priming the tubing, you will have far fewer air bubbles to contend with [Garcia, 2002].)
5. **Hang the bag:** Hang the bag or have an assistant hold it by the end opposite the spike at a level above that of the woman's heart. The bag should be a minimum of 36 in (90 cm) above the proposed IV insertion site. (The bag can also be hung prior to filling the drip chamber).
6. **Prime (fill) the tubing:** Place the capped end of the tubing in the outer bag the solution came in to catch any drips. Open the clamps on the tubing to fill the tube with fluid. Usually the entire tube can be fully filled (or primed) without removing the cap on the end. Flick the tube with your finger to encourage air bubbles to move along. Tiny air bubbles are not a problem. If a large amount of air is in the line that cannot be eliminated otherwise, loosen (without removing) the cap on the end of the tubing, which should allow the fluid to flow more easily. Check any injection ports to be sure they contain no air bubbles. If there are, invert the Y injection ports to displace air. Once the tube is full of fluid and free of bubbles, close the clamp and tighten the cap on the end of the tubing.

Locate a puncture site, place and secure the IV cannula

1. **Prepare tape:** You will need four pieces of tape to secure the cannula hub and tubing once everything is in place. Tear off 2.5 in of tape. Split this piece lengthwise and then split one half of it again to create two, ¼ in wide strips. Tear off two more 3 in pieces, leaving each one 1 in wide. Tack them to the edge of a piece of furniture or in another location where they can be reached easily and removed quickly while maintaining their tackiness.
2. **Find a vein:** Examine both of the woman's arms for suitable veins on either the back of the hand, on the side of the wrist above the thumb, or on the forearm. If you are starting an IV because the mother is bleeding, note that venous

valves are not in veins at the level of the antecubital area and above and that these veins are likely to receive a large bore catheter more easily. (You may have a good idea where to look if you have drawn blood during prenatal care.)

Pick the largest, straightest, most visible vein you can find to accommodate the catheter you will be inserting. If an inverted "Y" shaped venous bifurcation can be used, so much the better. Insertion of the catheter at the crotch of the inverted "Y" makes access easier, puncturing through the vein less likely and minimizes rolling (Garcia, 2002). When starting an IV for reasons other than fluid replacement for bleeding, it is best to use a vein that does not cross a joint, as placing a cannula at the bend of a joint can occlude flow. If you are doubtful about being able to start the IV on your first try, the vein should be as far from the heart (i.e., as near to the hand) as possible. That way, if your first attempt to insert the catheter fails, you will be able to choose another site closer to the heart. (If you must make a second attempt along the same vein, do not use a second site of puncture farther from the heart [distal to the first] because this may result in fluid leaking from the hole in the first site.) Many times your best option will be in the antecubital fossa (near the bend of the forearm). The large vein there accepts a large catheter and is capable of handling a substantial volume of fluid, making it the best choice if volume expansion is the goal. However, if you use this site, you need to secure the arm to a splint to minimize joint movement; it is therefore not an ideal site if you anticipate prolonged IV use.

Lastly, you want to avoid inserting the catheter immediately in front of (distal to) or into a venous valve. To determine the location of the valves, place the pad of your finger over the vein a couple inches above the proposed site of puncture. Press your thumbpad over the vein well above the proposed puncture site, flex the woman's wrist to pull the skin taut; then, maintain thumb pressure while slowly moving it in a stripping motion down the vein (away from the body). If there is a valve in the next couple of inches of the vein, the valve will resist the backflow of blood away from the heart, and a single or two parallel lumps will appear where the valve is located. Insert the catheter above the valve. This is, admittedly, a rather subtle exam, and it will take some practice to be able to quickly and accurately locate venous valves. Practice on the hands and arms of everyone who will allow it.

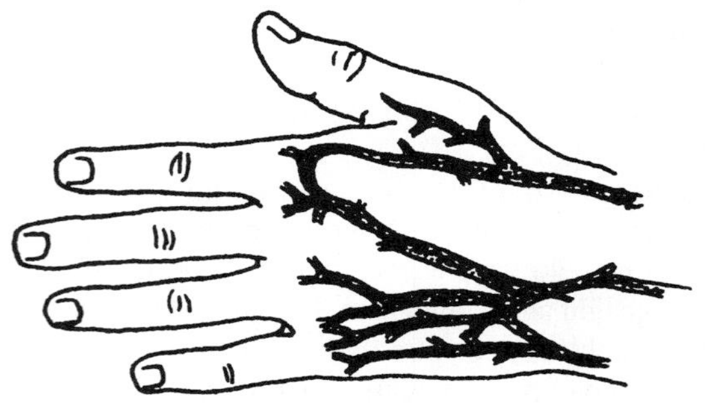

Veins of the back of the hand

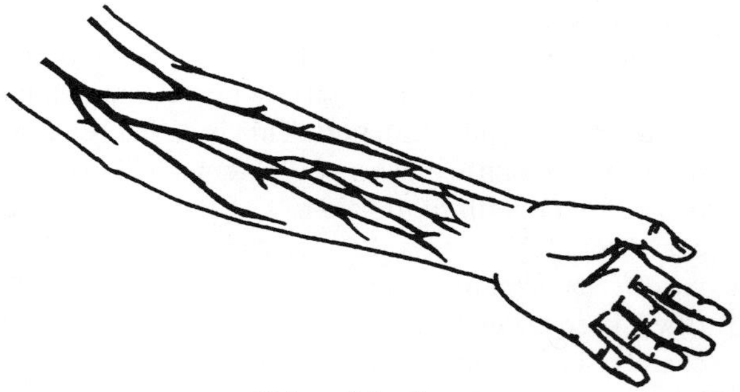

Veins of the forearm

If you are having trouble locating a vein and her condition allows, have the woman get in a warm bath. Her peripheral vessels will dilate and make both locating a vein and inserting the catheter much easier. If this is impractical or it is an emergency, place a towel soaked with very warm water over the lower portion of the arm that appears to have the best veins. Apply the tourniquet, wait about 30 seconds, remove the wet towel and dry the arm. This will distend the veins for a short while, making them more accessible. Note that, generally speaking, hand veins are the easiest to locate and stabilize for access (Garcia, 2002). A 20 gauge butterfly can be used in women-of-size to access a vein on the back of the hand when no other suitable veins can be found (Gilmore, 2003).

3. **Place an absorbent pad or towel beneath the arm under the proposed puncture site to catch any blood drips.**
4. **Clean the puncture site:** Clean the proposed puncture site. Wipe the site with a piece of gauze soaked in herbal antiseptic solution or an alcohol swab. Use a circular motion, starting where you intend to insert the catheter and spiraling outward about 2 in. Repeat this process with a new swab. Allow the area to dry for two minutes, if circumstances allow, although it is not necessary for it to dry completely before proceeding. Do not blow on the site to hasten drying, as this will contaminate the area, although fanning it with your hand is okay. Do not touch the site again prior to puncture or recleaning will be required (Garcia, 2002).
5. **Don non-sterile exam gloves.**

6. Apply the tourniquet: Position the woman's arm so that it is dangling below the level of her heart, which will bring more blood to the extremity. Apply the tourniquet by wrapping and tightening it about 4 to 6 in (10 to 15 cm) above the proposed puncture site. It should be tight enough to restrict venous but not arterial flow. If correctly applied, you should still be able to palpate her radial pulse. A blood-pressure cuff can also function as a tourniquet. Apply the cuff and pump until the needle on the dial is about halfway between her systolic and diastolic pressures. Leave the bulb regulator closed to retain the air.

Allow 30 to 60 seconds for the veins to distend. If they are not sufficiently distended after 60 seconds, release the tourniquet, rest the arm and then retighten the tourniquet. You can also try the other arm to see if a better vein pops up. Remember, however, that if the woman has lost blood, her veins may not distend very much, even with a tourniquet in place. Therefore, you will have to proceed and make your best effort to insert the catheter before she is further compromised. Remember that a vein that is distended may not always be visible, therefore palpate to confirm its location and reclean the site before you proceed. (Note: If you are unfamiliar with venipuncture, it is very unlikely that you will be able to successfully insert an IV catheter into a vein that you can palpate but cannot see. However, if that is the only vein you can find, go ahead and try. This is one reason why it is important to practice venipuncture techniques on a regular basis if you are ever going to use them [Garcia, 2002].)

7. Prepare the catheter: Double-check the size of the catheter. Peel back the outer wrapper and remove the catheter unit. Remove the plastic cap from over the catheter. Inspect the tip of the stylet for barbs and rough edges. Look carefully at the tip of the cannula. It should taper smoothly to its end. (If defective, toss it into the sharps container and use a new one.) Loosen the cannula (the sheath on the stylet) by twisting the hub slightly (do not move the stylet up and down in the cannula). Do not touch the cannula or the stylet tip, as these both must remain sterile.

8. Stabilize the vein. Grasp the woman's arm (or hand) below the proposed puncture site with your nondominant hand. Use your thumb to apply downward traction, being careful to position your traction so that it won't be in the way of your dominant hand when you insert the catheter. To apply traction to the anterior (palm side) of the forearm, apply your thumb and pull down to create tension on the skin of the forearm below the proposed puncture site with your nondominant hand. Too much tension can flatten the vein, especially in the presence of shock; press straight downward into the surface muscles below the puncture site and apply traction toward the hand (or fingers). Veins on the hands tend to move easily when palpated but are also easily stabilized. If you are near a joint, flex the joint away from the vein below the site to help take up any slack in the skin around the vein.

9. Insert the catheter into the vein:

A. Hold the top edge of the cannula hub, or the flashback chamber between the thumb and forefinger of your dominant hand in such a way that the flashback chamber is easily visualized and the bevel of the stylet is facing upward.

B. Place the tip of the stylet, bevel up, near the proposed puncture site (the center of the vein) with the catheter at a 30 to 35° angle to the skin, depending upon the depth of the vein (deeper veins or a thick layer of fat require a greater angle). Warn the woman that she will feel a big poke. Insert the needle. Once you are under the skin, stop and inform the woman that you are in the skin.

C. Advance the stylet forward slowly, maintaining your angle, until you feel a pop.

D. If you are in a vein, you should see an immediate spurt of blood in the flashback chamber above the hub.

Difficult insertion: If you get no flashback and the woman's veins do not appear to be collapsed, you are probably not in a vein yet. When using a large bore catheter, it can easily push the vein down beneath it or to the side. With experience, you will be able to tell where the vein has gone. Using the thumb providing stabilization, change the angle at which pressure is being applied to move and stabilize the vein near the stylet. When "fishing" for the vein, do not fan the needle around, as it is razor sharp and can do considerable tissue damage. Instead, withdraw the needle without taking it out), redirect it, and readvance it until you get flashback.

E. Once flashback is confirmed, do one of the following: reduce your angle and advance the catheter (cannula and stylet) about 1 to 2 more mm to make sure that the cannula sheathing the stylet enters the vein as well. Or, reduce your angle and advance only the cannula about 5 mm to push it into the vein. While doing so, take care not to push the stylet any deeper to prevent it from puncturing through the other side of the vein.

F. Prepare to transfer traction on the vein from your nondominant hand to your dominant hand. To do this, grasp the hub of the cannula with the thumb and forefinger of your dominant hand and use the heel of that hand to apply downward traction below the puncture site as you remove your nondominant hand.

Collapsed vein: Veins collapse when a person loses a great deal of blood. A collapsed vein will be flat like empty, soft tubing. About 5% of the time, a collapsed vein may result in the absence of a flashback when you insert the needle, even if it is correctly positioned in the vein. If you are fairly certain you are in a vein, attach the IV line to the catheter hub and open the roller clamp while watching the puncture site. If the tissue surrounding the catheter swells (referred to as "infiltration"), you are *not* in the vein and will need to start over, selecting a vein on the other arm or a puncture site closer to the woman's torso on the same arm. Reclamp the tubing by moving the roller to the bottom of the frame. Remove the catheter from the woman's arm. Remove the catheter from the IV tubing and recap the end of the tube with the original cap to preserve its sterility. If the cap has been misplaced, a capped sterile syringe needle can be used instead.

Vein collapse is a good reason to insert the IV sooner rather than later if you feel a woman is bleeding too much. This is especially true if you are remote from medical help and cannot rely on an ambulance team to arrive soon with personnel who are more skilled than you are at difficult IV insertions.

NOTE: If you cannot successfully insert the needle, turn the woman on her left side and give 600 cc of solution via a retention enema. Very often, once some of this fluid absorbs and the veins are more filled out, you will be able to start an IV (Marshall & Buffington, 1998).

10. **Advance the cannula into the vein.** With the thumb and forefinger of your nondominant hand, use one of the following techniques:

Method 1: Gently slide the cannula off the stylet into the vein until the cannula hub is almost flush with the puncture site. The stylet should remain stationary and should not advance with the cannula.

Method 2: Withdraw the stylet a short distance and advance the cannula into the vein.

Method 2 or advancing the cannula while holding the catheter at too steep an angle both carry the risk of the cannula hitting the opposite wall of the vein and curling up. Whichever method you choose, once you begin the process, *never pull the cannula back over the stylet or try to reinsert the stylet into the cannula.* You must also *never move the stylet back and forth within the cannula.* Should you lose the vein, do not attempt to reinsert the stylet into the partially advanced cannula. Any of these actions could cause "catheter shear," whereby the sharp bevel on the tip of the stylet either nicks the cannula (creating a rough place and risking venous trauma) or actually cuts off a portion of the cannula, sending a plastic fragment into the woman's circulatory system and creating a potentially deadly foreign-body embolus.

11. **Prepare to remove the stylet:** Before removing the stylet, position the ring finger of your nondominant hand 1.25 in above the puncture site. Grasp the hub of the cannula with the first finger and thumb of your nondominant hand to stabilize it during stylet removal.
12. **Remove the stylet:** Use the tip of your nondominant ring finger to apply firm pressure to the vein and cannula by depressing the skin about 1.25 in (3 cm) above the puncture site after you begin to remove the stylet with your dominant hand. This lessens the likelihood that blood will drain out of the open end of the hub.
13. **Dispose of the stylet:** Place the stylet directly into a sharps container.
14. **Attach the tubing:** Remove the cap from the lower end of the infusion tubing and place it inside its original packaging in case it is needed later (or hand it to an assistant). Use one hand to retract the luer-lock connector (if necessary), revealing the tip of the port. Seat the end of the tube into cannula hub, taking care to maintain sterility and not to move the cannula. If using a luer-lock, move it over the cannula, use your other hand to stabilize the hub while you twist to lock the tubing port in place over the hub.
15. **Release the tourniquet.**
16. **Start the flow:** Open the roller clamp and the slide clamp (if it is closed) and observe the drip chamber. Fluid should flow rapidly without obstruction, and there should be no swelling around the insertion site. Swelling indicates that fluid is leaking from the vein. Slow the rate of flow by adjusting the roller clamp and then retract the cannula slightly to see if the swelling stops; if not, you will have to start over.
17. **Regulate the flow:** Regulate the flow of solution to the desired rate by adjusting the roller clamp as you watch the drip chamber to see how fast the solution is flowing and how it is affected by opening and closing the clamp (more about how to do this follows later).
18. **Secure the cannula hub and tubing:** Stabilize the tubing just below the cannula with your hand until you have it taped in place. This prevents movement in the vein, which may cause irritation and introduce bacteria into the bloodstream from the skin.

This section describes the chevron method of securing the tubing, which is commonly used and is very secure. Start with a ¼ in wide piece of tape. Gently lift the tubing (which will raise the hub) enough so you can slip the tape, sticky-side up, beneath it, just below the puncture site so that the puncture site will remain visible. Center the tape under the hub. Lift one end of the tape, cross it over the hub and tape at an angle toward the woman's body. Lift the other end and secure it in the same manner on the opposite side. This piece of tape should now form a wide "V," the tip of which points toward you. Place a second ¼ in piece of tape straight across the arm so that it covers the infusion line just below the cannula port. It is best not to tape directly over the joint between the line and the cannula port. Taping the hub and the tubing separately lessens the chances that you will dislodge the cannula if you must change the tubing or insert a saline lock later (Garcia, 2002).

For the third tape placement, use a 1 in wide piece, taped over the tubing 6 inches from the puncture site. Finally, form a loop in the tubing just distal to the third piece of tape, and place a fourth piece of 1 in wide tape over the third piece including the loop, securing the loop to the arm. This loop is additional insurance that the tubing will not become dislodged.

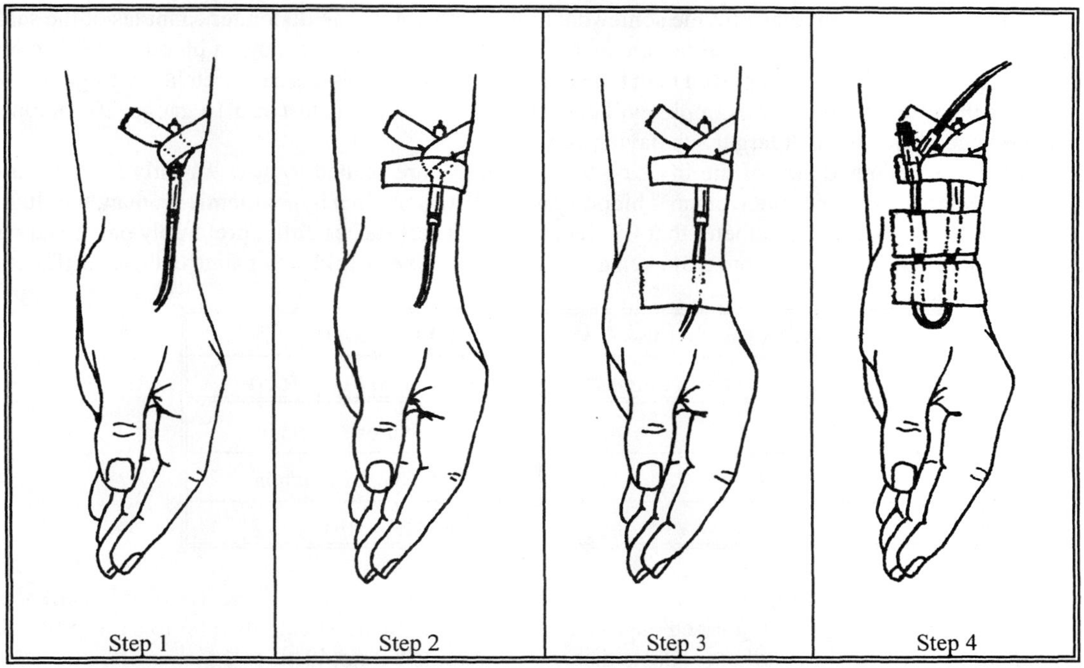

Tape should be changed when it becomes loose, wet or soiled. If the IV site is wet, try to determine where the moisture is coming from before changing the tape as it may be leaking from the IV itself. If the woman is receiving an IV for a nonemergent reason during labor and wishes to enter a bath, some recommend sheathing the arm with the IV in a plastic bag to prevent it from becoming wet. However, if the woman makes an effort not to get the IV site wet, this is usually sufficient. When a bag is used, it usually gets moisture inside of it getting the puncture site wet and loosening the tape rather quickly, all the while giving a false sense of security (Garcia, 2002).

19. **Label the IV.** Record the date, time, cannula gauge, and your initials on both the tape securing the tubing and on a second label secured to the IV bag (this can also be a piece of tape). Be sure to record the type of solution, how many bags have been given (e.g., "lactated Ringers, bag #2, 1000 cc") on each bag of fluid as it is hung. Immediately record the same information plus the location of puncture in your labor or postpartum notes in the woman's chart.
20. **Splint the arm:** A splint is used to ensure that the cannula will not be pulled out or become crimped in the vein. In most cases, a splint is not necessary. However, one may prove useful if the cannula is directly over a joint or if the woman must be removed from a cramped or otherwise hard-to-navigate location. Attach the splint to the arm or hand on the elbow side, using a roll of or cloth to wrap the arm and splint. Do not cover the IV site or the tube with the gauze. Take care not to produce a tourniquet effect when securing the splint; fingers should remain warm and pink.
21. **Stay with the woman the entire time an IV is in place** or until she is in the care of a transport team qualified to monitor her IV. EMT crews will not want the midwife in the ambulance in most cases.

How Much Fluid Should Be Given and How Fast?

As a general rule, a healthy woman can easily receive a liter of IV fluid infused over a 60 minute period without undue risks, although it is inappropriate to give any IV fluid without good reason (Garcia, 2002). If the woman is truly hypovolemic, she would need about 2 liters in a shorter period of time.

Factors that influence IV flow rates

A fluid's rate of flow through a closed channel is directly related the channel's diameter or gauge (to the fourth power) and inversely related to its length.

IV cannula size: A hollow cannula or tube with a large bore allows fluid to flow at a much faster rate than one with a smaller bore. Likewise, short cannulas provide somewhat higher flow rates than do longer cannulas of the same gauge. The size of the vein also affects flow rate, although the rate at which fluids flow through a blood vessel is more related to the size and length of the IV cannula placed than the vessel itself because vessels can stretch. A 14 gauge, 4 cm long cannula placed in the forearm vein, for example, will pass fluids about twice as fast as a 16 gauge, 20 cm long cannula placed in the more central and much larger subclavian vein.

The bore of the cannula and size of the infusion tubing you use are related to how urgently fluid replacement is required and to how large a catheter the woman's blood vessel will accept. In a hypovolemic woman, the fluid needs to be given rapidly. Choose the largest catheter that you feel you can insert successfully, preferably one no larger than 14 gauge and no smaller than 18 gauge. Note that even experienced IV experts find a 14 gauge catheter difficult to insert.

Cannula Gauges and Maximum Fluid Flow Rate	
Cannula Gauge (Internal Diameter)	**Maximum Flow Rate**
18	4.81 l/hr or 88 cc/min
16	7.45 l/h or 124 cc/min
14	9.67 l/hr or 161 cc/min

Internal diameter of infusion tubing: Flow rate is also influenced by the internal diameter (bore or lumen) of the tubing in the administration set. Tubing is categorized based on lumen size. Industry standards refer to a range of inner lumen sizes, and each maker is allowed to market products that are compatible but not identical. Generally, minor differences do not significantly affect performance when the administration of fluids is imprecise, as is the case with volume replacement.

There are three types of tubing: standard, macrobore and microbore. Standard tubing is used most often, and almost all IV therapies can be accomplished with standard-bore administration. This tubing has a common inner lumen diameter that varies very little among manufacturers. Standard-bore tubing can be obtained with either a macrodrip or a microdrip drip chamber attached.

Macrobore tubing (larger than standard) is sometimes used in emergency volume replacement. Microbore tubing (smaller than standard) is designed to deliver precise flow rates, so its use is usually limited to administering IV medications. Both are inappropriate for midwifery applications.

Drop factor: The drop factor is a characteristic of the drip chamber and refers to a specific drop size that is perfected to deliver exact amounts over a long period of time with an accuracy of plus or minus 10%. The speed of flow or "drop factor" is expressed in the number of drops that must be delivered to equal one milliliter. "Drops" is often designated as "gtt," which is the abbreviation of the Latin word *guttae*, meaning "drops." The drop factor in gtt/ml will be printed on the tubing package and is specific according to manufacturer.

Macrodrop infusion set drip factors vary among manufacturers:

Abbott labs:	15 gtt/ml
Baxter labs:	10 gtt/ml
B. Braun labs:	15 gtt/ml

Macrodrop (macrodrip) sets: A "macrodrop" refers to the size of the drops created by the drip chamber; a macrodrop administration set is used when emergency volume expansion is needed. The drip factor ranges from 10 to 20 gtt/ml, depending upon the manufacturer. Macrodrop sets deliver fluids at rates of 100 ml/hr or more. When the tubing is left wide open (i.e., unclamped), a macrodrop set allows you to empty a 1000 cc bag of solution in minutes when used with a 16 to 18 gauge cannula. Macrodrop sets can be used in any application, although their accuracy diminishes as the flow rate per hour decreases and are therefore unsuited to administer precise amounts of drugs.

Microdrop (minidrip) sets: Microdrop administration sets look the same but produce smaller drops in the drip chamber. Infusing fluids much more slowly than do macrodrop sets, they usually deliver 50 to 60 gtt/ml of fluid at rates of less than 100 ml/hr. They are normally used to administer medications at precisely controlled rates. A midwife might use a microdrop set when giving prophylactic antibiotics in labor or with an oxytocin drip after the birth to contract an atonic uterus when bleeding has not been excessive. *Because of their slow infusion rate, a microdrop set should never be used when volume expansion is the goal.* Therefore, microdrop sets and small-gauge catheters should be stored entirely separately from your emergency IV equipment, which is intended for rapid volume expansion.

Figuring the rate of flow

The amount of fluid that will be given over a certain length of time can be determined by the rate of flow of the IV, in drops per minute. Here is the nitty gritty of the math. (Remember that a milliliter [ml] equals one cubic centimeter [cc].) First, determine how much solution is to be given per hour, using the total amount of fluid and the time period over which it will be infused:

Flow rate = Total infusion (volume of IV solution in one bag in ml) ÷ hours of infusion (total time to give all of the solution in ml per hour). For example, to give 1 liter (1000 ml) of fluid over a 10 hr period, you would calculate the flow rate as follows: 1000 ml ÷ 10 hr = 100 ml/hr. To give the same amount in 8 hours: 1000 ml ÷ 8 hr = 125 ml/hr.

The next step is to calculate the drop rate in drops per minute, using the number of ml per hour as the total volume. You must know the drop factor of the administration set you are using to calculate this value (check the packaging). One way to figure these amounts is outlined in the table below.

DROP FACTOR (GTT/ML)	DIVIDE DESIRED RATE PER HOUR BY
10	6
15	4
20	3
60	1

Formula for a macrodrop infusion set: Volume of solution in ml × gtt/ml (often 10 gtt/ml for macrodrop infusion sets) ÷ total time of infusion in minutes = drops/minute. For example:

Total volume to be infused (ml)	100 ml
Drip chamber drop factor (gtt/ml)	10 gtt/ml
Time of infusion (minutes)	60 minutes

(100 ml × 10 gtt/ml = 1000 drops) ÷ 60 min = 17 drops/min (rounded up)

Note that with microdrop infusion sets with a drop factor of 60 drops per minute, the number of drops per minute equals the number of milliliters per hour.

Regulating the flow

To adjust the flow to the desired rate of delivery, first close the regulating clamp until the roller meets the bottom of the frame. Then, slowly open the flow regulator wheel. Watch for the number of drops per minute releasing into the drip chamber. Regulate the flow by adjusting the clamp until you achieve the desired rate of administration. Mark the bag with the time you expect it will take to administer each 100 ml of solution; for example, if you are giving 10 ml of solution per minute, it will take 10 minutes to administer 100 ml.

Volume expansion: If you are expanding the woman's circulating blood volume due to hemorrhage, initially open the roller clamp all the way and allow the first 500 to 1000 cc of fluid to run in as rapidly as possible (how large a bolus you use and how fast you run it in will depend upon the severity of the hemorrhage). This will maintain or restore blood pressure, resulting in more efficient circulation. You can then either slow the flow down, giving the remainder of the bag at a rate of 100 ml every hour, or monitor the woman's blood pressure on the other arm and maintain a rapid flow until the systolic pressure is stable at 100 mm Hg. The option you choose will depend on the overall condition of the mother after she receives the first 500 to 1000 cc of fluid. Once the mother is stable, give the remaining fluid at a rate of 100 ml every hour. Keep in mind that it takes at least three cc of crystalloid IV fluid to replace one cc of blood; therefore, a 1 liter blood loss would require at least three or four liters of IV fluid replacement. However, this calculation does not take into account third-spacing of fluids (seepage into surrounding tissues), which could be problematic later, after transport is complete. Third-spacing can lead to overloading of the interstitial space with accompanying edema while inadequate intravascular volume persists. However, since you probably will not be carrying more than 3 to 4 bags of solution, extreme overloading of the interstitial space is very unlikely to occur, unless no IV fluids were needed (i.e., if shock was misdiagnosed). The overarching goal in an emergency is to stabilize the woman so that transport can be accomplished as safely as possible (Garcia, 2002). How to assess the woman's response to IV therapy is covered in detail in the chapter entitled "Hypovolemic Shock due to Hemorrhage."

Dehydration: For vomiting or fatigue during labor, start with a conservative 500 to 1000 cc of lactated Ringer's at a slower rate than for hemorrhage; then assess the woman for improvement before deciding to give more. How much you start with will again depend on the mother's overall condition.

Prolonged labor and dehydration: Dehydration may result in weak contractions. An IV can sometimes cause labor to pick right up and proceed to birth. The safest solution to use for this purpose is lactated Ringers (no dextrose). Run in 300 ml, then slow the drip down to 125 ml per hour and see what happens to her contractions. To avoid fluid overload, discontinue administration of the IV solution and attach a saline lock to the cannula as soon as labor resumes.

Avoiding fluid overload

When treating noncritical problems such as dehydration, as a general rule give no more than 50 ml of solution per kilogram of body weight (at term) in a 24 hr period. To arrive at this figure in pounds, divide the weight by 2.205. For example, for a weight of 204 lbs use 4650 ml as the maximum total limit ([204 lbs ÷ 2.205 = 93 kg] × 50 = 4650 ml). A weight of 100 lb can take 2250 ml ([100 lbs ÷ 2.205 = 45 kg] × 50 = 2250 ml) (Marshall & Buffington, 1998). Start by giving 300 ml (see "prolonged labor and dehydration") and then reassess the woman's condition before giving more.

To keep the line open: Once the initial fluid load has been delivered, you may wish to keep the line open (that is, prevent a clot from forming in the cannula) so that more fluid can be given later. To do so without using a saline lock, reduce the rate of flow to 10 to 12 gtt/min, which will deliver about 25 ml of fluid an hour.

To Discontinue and Remove an IV

Once the immediate purpose of using an IV has been satisfied, it is always a good idea to attach a saline lock so you can leave the cannula in place in case the IV is needed again later. This way, you need not insert another catheter. Use of a saline lock is covered later in this chapter. The following instructions cover removing the IV completely:

1. Don gloves.
2. Close the flow regulator clamp completely.
3. Gently remove the tape or dressing securing the cannula hub and tubing in the opposite order of placement. Tear the tape down the center, if necessary, to minimize movement of the cannula. Do not use scissors as they may accidently snip the cannula, creating a major complication should the cannula get lost in the vein.
4. Hold a dry, sterile 2 × 2 in gauze pad over the puncture site.
5. Grasp the hub and infusion tubing simultaneously. Smoothly and firmly pull the cannula straight out, keeping the hub as close to the skin as possible.
6. Place the gauze over the puncture site and apply a 3 in (7.5 cm) piece of tape firmly across the center to form a pressure bandage. Have the woman bend her arm and elevate it if she is able.

7. Confirm that the cannula is intact by holding it up against a dark background and examining the tip for splits or missing pieces. The tip may be slightly flared from having been inserted. Note your findings in the chart "cannula intact," "cannula split, but no missing pieces." Examine it with a magnifying glass if you are unsure. If it is not intact, describe and sketch a drawing of the location and extent of the damage or missing piece.
8. Dispose of the cannula in a biohazard or sharps container.
9. Dispose of the tubing and the fluid bag.
10. Record the total amount of fluid administered, the amount and type of any drugs that were added, any problems that were encountered and the time the IV was discontinued in the woman's chart.

Administering Intravenous Medications

Medications, primarily antibiotics or oxytocin, can be added to an IV solution. Antibiotics may be used during labor if the mother has a heart condition for which antibiotics are recommended, such as mitral-valve prolapse or a positive test for group B-strep. Oxytocin can be safely administered in a gravity-flow IV without the use of an electronic infusion pump for postpartum hemorrhage *only*. During labor, oxytocin should always be given with an infusion pump to precisely regulate flow and therefore should never be used to augment labor at home. Read about the use of oxytocin in the subchapter entitled "Allopathic Pharmacologic Agents for Treating Uterine Atony."

Infusing oxytocin directly through the IV fluid (rather than via IM injection) may be very desirable, especially if you plan to transport, as monitoring the mother's uterus in a moving vehicle can be tricky, and dealing with additional bleeding en route is to be avoided whenever possible. Adding oxytocin to the IV will keep a small amount running into the woman's system constantly. The drugs can be added through the drug port on the bottom of the IV bag either prior to set up or after the IV is running.

Equipment needed:

- Medication to be given
- Labeling materials (white adhesive or paper tape will do)
- Gloves
- Two 2 to 5 cc syringes fitted with 1 in, 20 gauge (or smaller) needles filled with normal saline (0.9%).
- Antiseptic swabs (or alcohol-based herbal tincture and cotton or gauze)

Adding medication to the bag prior to starting the IV

The best way to administer oxytocin in an IV is to mix it into the solution prior to starting the IV.

1. Draw up the desired amount of medication into a syringe just as you would to give an injection.
2. Locate the drug port on the bottom or side of the IV bag and clean the rubber cover with an antiseptic swab. Allow it to dry if time allows, but this is not absolutely necessary.
3. Uncap the needle on the syringe and insert it into the drug port.
4. Inject the medication into the IV fluid, taking care not to poke a hole in the IV bag as you do so.
5. Remove the needle; discard it and the syringe in a sharps container.
6. Gently rock the bag from end to end to mix in the drug.
7. Label the bag with the drug, amount, time, date and that it was added to a full bag of solution.
8. Start the IV as you would normally.

Adding medication to an IV that is already running

1. Check the amount of solution left in the bag. If the solution is half used, add half the total dose of the medication. If less than half remains, mix a fresh bag, and replace the bag in use with the new one.
2. Close the tube clamp and lower the bag.
3. Follow steps 1 through 6 above under "Adding medication to the bag prior to starting the IV."
4. Rehang the bag and regulate the drip flow to the desired rate by adjusting the clamp.
5. Label the bag with the drug, amount, time, date, and amount of solution with which it was mixed.

Use of oxytocin for postpartum bleeding

Add 10 to 40 units of oxytocin to a 1000 ml bag of lactated Ringer's or normal (0.9%) saline. How much oxytocin you use will depend upon the gravity of the situation; most hospitals start with 20 units, running at a rate of 10 ml of mixed solution per minute (for a drop factor of 10 gtt/ml, the drop rate would be 100 drops/min [10 gtt/ml × 10 ml/min] = 100 drops/min), which will supply 200 mU of oxytocin per minute. Use a macrodrip infusion set to achieve this rate of delivery. As noted earlier, if the woman is hemorrhaging, open the roller clamp and allow the solution to infuse as rapidly as possible, slowing the rate according to the amount of blood loss and how effectively the bleeding is being controlled. A standard recommendation for continued therapy after a hemorrhage is to mix 20 units of oxytocin into 1000 ml of lactated Ringer's and give it at a flow rate of 40 gtt/min. Always keep in mind how much fluid you have on hand and how quickly help is likely to arrive (Garcia, 2002).

Dosages for antibiotics

Antibiotic dosages must be worked out with your back-up provider, using the current protocols in your community for the condition being treated. Be sure to determine what type of solution would be best to use for dilution; generally speaking, normal saline is preferred. (Consult the chapters on specific conditions in my DIAGNOSTIC TESTS for more details.)

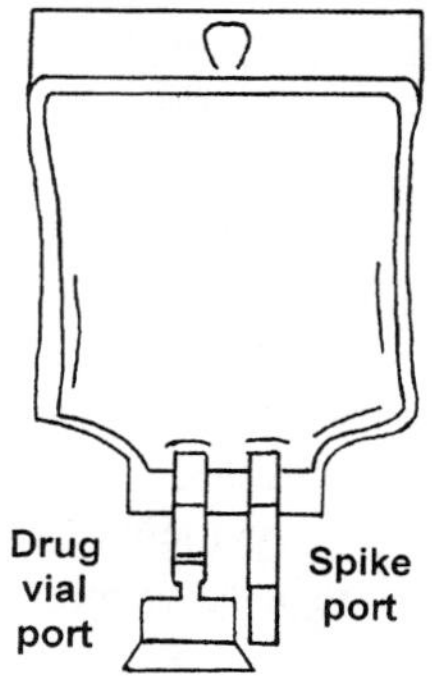

Minibag (Baxter)

Some pharmacies provide small (50 ml) bags of IV fluid with the medication already mixed in. Antibiotics, however, commonly come in powdered form that must be mixed with the IV fluid prior to use. The bag of choice is the Minibag Plus by Baxter Inc. It has a drug port adapted to accept any vial with a standard 20 mm diameter top. The antibiotic will usually come in a separate vial. Proceed as follows:

1. Uncap the vial, cleanse the top and allow it to dry.
2. Open the drug port of the solution bag and spike the rubber top on the vial into this port.
3. Squeeze the bag so that fluid enters the vial. Rotate and shake the bag gently to mix in the powder. With the vial down, squeeze the bag again to wash out all residual powder and rotate the bag until all the powder is mixed in.
4. Leave the vial in place and proceed as you would for setting up any IV.

One bag is used for each IV dose at the recommended intervals for that drug. Since the fluid will drop only to the level of pressure stability between the line and the woman's vein, the last little bit of solution will not infuse. Do not force it. Remove the IV tubing and, if using a saline lock, leave it in place in preparation for the next dose.

Changing IV tubing

Tubing used for intermittent infusion should be changed every 24 hours. Homebirth midwives are unlikely to be called upon to change tubing because we do not typically use continuous IV therapy. Changing tubing is only relevant if a woman requires repeated IV therapy during a long labor, as when prophylactic antibiotics are used for group B-strep colonization. You may wish to use a new tube each time you administer a dose throughout labor. Changing tubing is most easily done when a new bag is being hung. It is also most convenient to mix the antibiotics into the solution if this is necessary before you hang a new bag. These instructions assume that a saline lock is already in place and that a T-connector extension set is also in place and needs replacing as well. Details regarding saline locks and T connectors can be found later in this chapter.

Replacing the T-connector extension set and IV tubing:

1. Connect the new primary tubing set to a fresh bag of solution by spiking the bag, hanging the bag, filling the drip chamber and flushing the line. Attach an extension set to the port on the primary tubing and prime it as well. Close the roller clamp on the new primary tubing and the pinch clamp on the old extension set.
2. Remove tape from the IV site in reverse order of application, leaving the V-shaped piece around the hub in place.
3. Look for evidence of problems at the puncture site. If none are noted, proceed to remove the last piece of tape. Place a strip of tape across the cannula hub to temporarily anchor the hub of the cannula. (If problems are noted, remove the cannula and insert a new one in another location.)
4. Apply gentle pressure using the thumb of your nondominant hand about 1.5 inches (3 cm) above the puncture site and remove the old extension set.

5. Gently attach the hub of the new extension set to the hub of the IV cannula.
6. Release the pressure above the puncture site. Open the clamp on the new primary tubing.
7. Remove the temporary tape and secure the infusion line to the arm, using the chevron method, as usual.

Changing the fluid bag

To minimize the possibility of producing an air embolism, change the solution bag before the one in use is empty. Keeping the drip chamber vertical *at all times* prevents air from entering the tubing during the switch.

1. Be sure the primary tubing is still filled with fluid, then shut of the roller clamp.
2. Unwrap and inspect the new bag. Remove the port cover from the tubing port.
3. Disconnect the tubing from the empty bag (remove the spike).
4. Insert the tubing spike into the tube port on the new bag, taking care to maintain sterile technique.
5. Verify that the drip chamber is appropriately filled. If not, squeeze and release it until it is about half full.
6. Confirm that the tube is full of fluid and free of air bubbles. If you find bubbles, either loosen the cap on the patient end of the tubing or remove stubborn bubbles by using a syringe as described on page 873.
7. Attach the primary tubing port to either the cannula or the saline lock.
8. Reopen the flow regulator wheel and adjust to the desired flow.

INTERMITTENT ADMINISTRATION OF IV FLUIDS OR ANTIBIOTICS DURING LABOR

Use of a Butterfly Needle

Equipment

Primary microdrop administration set: For intermittent use when administering medications, you can use a simple primary *microdrop* administration set (50 to 60 gtt/ml) with a nonvented (or sealable) drip chamber, a roller and a pinch clamp, 70 in (177.8 cm) or so in length with standard-bore tubing, with a male luer-lock adapter or a needleless safety adapter that can be attached to any one of several compatible devices to be used as a saline lock.

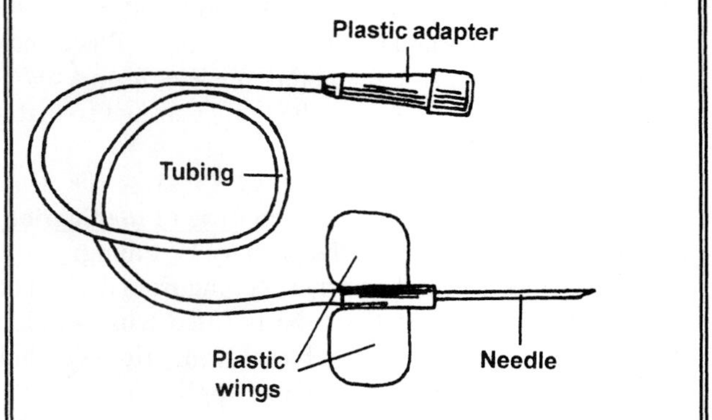

Butterfly infusion set

Butterfly (winged) infusion set: This set consists of a short, small-gauge stylet that extends through the center of two wings. One portion of the stylet is permanently attached to a short length of tubing ending in a cannula hub that luer-locks to the primary tubing port. The butterfly's tubing also serves as a flashback chamber during insertion of the stylet into the vein. The wings are flat, flexible plastic flaps on either side of the hub end of the stylet. There is no flexible cannula and the small stylet itself is inserted and left in the vein. Leaving the stylet in place presents two problems: movement with a stylet in situ is more painful and the needle may puncture through the vein. For this reason, if the device is to be left in place, it is better to attach a saline lock to the hub of a soft cannula than to use a butterfly as a saline lock. However, butterfly stylets are small and less painful to insert than a catheter. Therefore, when giving intermittent doses of antibiotics, many midwives simply insert a new butterfly for each dose and remove it when done, although this does subject the woman to numerous sticks and the midwife to numerous IV insertions. It is best to explain the pros and cons and give the woman the option as to which she would prefer; she will have to remain more still and be more careful if a butterfly is used. If the woman's veins are not well suited for IV insertion, you might encourage her to allow you to place a cannula and leave it in, using a saline lock until the entire course of medication has been completed. Butterfly sets come with tubing in various lengths, 6 inches (15.5 cm) being of sufficient length to bend around easily before securing with tape.

Syringe cannula: Syringe cannulas are universal needleless devices designed to replace regular steel syringe needles for use in any needleless port designed to receive a cannula (it cannot be used in a regular port). A regular syringe needle can be used to withdraw fluid from a vial of saline, as you normally would and is then replaced with the syringe cannula to access the specialized safety port in the IV setup.

Syringes: Small syringes fitted with needles no longer than 1 to 1.25 inches can be used to flush a saline lock. A regular syringe needle can be used with any type of port, however a syringe cannula can *only* be used with safety ports designed for this purpose. The size syringe you need will depend upon the capacity of the saline lock you choose.

Needles: Extra syringe needles (20 to 22 gauge, 7/8 to 1 in in length) can be used to connect the primary tubing to any type of rubber port on a saline lock.

Saline (0.9%) in vials: You will want to carry small, preservative-free vials of saline for use during saline flushes. Small vials can be used for one woman and then thrown away, as sterility expires 30 days after the vial is first opened.

Preparing and inserting a butterfly infusion set: Butterflies are inserted as follows:

1. Prepare the IV bag and affix the primary tubing as you normally would. A microdrop primary administration set can be used if you are administering antibiotics.
2. Locate and prepare a puncture site.
3. Prepare two ¼ in wide and two 1 inch wide pieces of tape, each 3 in long, to secure the IV.
4. Loosen the cap on the hub end of the butterfly tube and sheath on the stylet and set the butterfly aside.
5. Apply the tourniquet.
6. Remove the sheath from the butterfly stylet and insert the stylet as you normally would a catheter. Hold the stylet by the wings, bending them upward with one hand as you anchor the vein with the other hand by placing your other thumb below the proposed puncture site. Gently press down and toward the woman's hand to stretch the skin taut.
7. Introduce the stylet at a slight angle either above or to the side of the vein. Advance the needle carefully into the vein.
8. Release the tourniquet.
9. Look for flashback in the butterfly tube. Allow the blood to completely fill the tube to eliminate air bubbles.
10. Once the tube is full of blood, uncap the cannula port on the primary tubing and screw it over the butterfly hub.
11. Open the tubing clamp and watch the drip chamber. Fluid should flow easily with no swelling at the puncture site.
12. Regulate the rate of flow of solution by adjusting the clamp on the tubing.
13. Secure the wings and the tubing with tape. Place one piece straight across the wings, being sure not to keep the tape only on the wings. Use another piece to form a "V" on the tubing below the wings as illustrated in step 1 and 2 on page 877. Bend the end of the tubing around so that it is not too close to the needle and secure it separately with the third piece of tape.

Removing the butterfly after each dose of medication is completed

1. Close the roller clamp on the primary IV tubing.
2. You may disconnect the primary tubing from the end of the tube on the butterfly, although this is not essential. If you do, be sure the butterfly tube is filled with solution before you do so. Cap the butterfly hub immediately after disconnecting it to prevent blood from dripping from the end. Also recap the cannula port on the primary tubing.
3. Remove taping in reverse order of application.
4. Hold a 2 × 2 in gauze pad over the puncture site.
5. Withdraw the butterfly needle by pulling straight out in line with the insertion angle.
6. Apply pressure with the gauze pad and tape it over the puncture site.

Using an IV (Saline) Lock

An IV lock consists of an adapter that seals off the IV cannula, allowing it to stay in place when the infusion is discontinued or the tubing is removed. During locking, the locking device, hub and cannula are filled with saline which maintains a patent pathway, thus "locking" the vessel, while preventing blood and air from entering the cannula. This avoids the hassle, discomfort and time it takes to reinsert another catheter. Periodic saline flushes are performed to clear away any accumulated blood in the line and prevent clotting. Formerly, locking was performed with a combination of heparin (a blood thinner) and saline; however, pure saline is now preferred for use in peripheral IV devices.

IV locking is invasive, and to a degree, uncomfortable and is therefore seldom used at homebirths. In addition to intermittent IV use, locking the vein can be employed when you are far from medical help and are anticipating a tired mother (and uterus) after birth, which *may* result in a hemorrhage (in which case a macrobore infusion set and an 18 gauge cannula should be used). Although it is best not to start running an IV prophylactically, an IV lock can be inserted so that the IV can be started easily should excess bleeding occur. Once an IV has been used for any reason during labor, a lock allows the cannula to remain in the vein just in case the IV is needed again.

The decision to use a saline lock is best made prior to setting up the IV. When the intention is to insert one device and leave it in place, it is best to place a small-gauge cannula in the vein and attach a device to serve as a saline lock. Do not, however, use anything smaller than a 20 gauge catheter or butterfly.

There are a number of devices that permit intermittent administration of medications or fluids and that attach to the cannula hub. They end in either a rubber port that can be penetrated by a blunt-tipped plastic cannula or a regular syringe needle, depending upon whether it is a safety or nonsafety device.

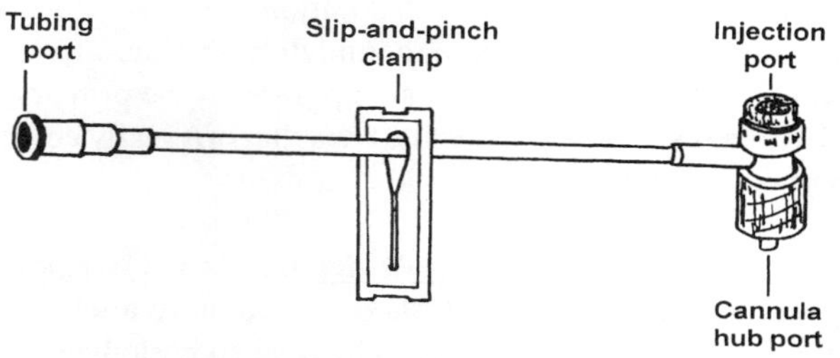

T-connector extension set (Baxter)

Equipment for Saline Locking T-connector extension set (by Baxter) or Clave ™ (by B. Braun): This device consists of standard-bore tubing with two attachment ports; a port at one end of the tube attaches to the luer-lock on the end of the infusion tubing from the primary administration set. At the other end of the main tube is a small, double-ended tube with two ports on either end (the bar of the T). One side is a luer-lock port with a retractable collar to receive the cannula hub; the other port has a rubber port to receive a needle for saline flushes. The tube will have a slip-and-pinch clamp. The size of the tubing for both the primary and the extension set should be standard bore. Extension sets should have luer-lock connectors to minimize the chances of dislodgement when in place. A T-connector extension set attaches the tube to the hub at a right angle and bends around easily for taping on the arm. Extension sets typically come with a slide clamp. Check the packaging for the total volume that the extension set will accept, as this is the minimum amount of saline required for flushing and filling the device. This set does not require any other devices and is considered by many to be the easiest and safest to use, especially for those not using IVs frequently (Garcia, 2002).

Injection ports (caps): These add-on connectors are another type of saline lock, consisting of a short length of tubing (or a hard plastic channel) with a rubber injection port at one end and a luer-lock connector on the other. The rubber port receives a cannula (if a needleless system is used) or a regular syringe needle which is attached to the primary tubing. The luer-lock connector receives the hub of an IV cannula. A short bridge of tubing may span the space between the two ports, which is available in lengths ranging from ½ to 2 in. A shorter port is easier to secure and makes movement easier for the recipient but may allow needles to penetrate the hub of the infusion cannula, potentially compromising the integrity of the cannula or tubing. The use of needleless devices eliminates this concern. Also, when used with regular syringe needles, these devices provide a much less secure connection that do T-connector extension sets. If a port with only a rigid plastic housing is used, it becomes very difficult to manipulate the port without disturbing the cannula. Therefore, T-sets are the device of choice for midwives.

Safe use of regular syringe needles with needleless safety ports

The rubber safety ports on needleless devices can accept either a regular syringe needle or a syringe cannula. When using a needle with a safety port, insert it along the edge of the port to prevent undue damage to the port. If you are using a regular, nonsafety port it should be accessed with a regular metal syringe needle only, and the needle may be inserted anywhere on the port. *Do not* attempt to use a syringe cannula with a nonsafety port. Not only will penetration be difficult but the hole the cannula makes will not reseal properly, risking air embolism and contamination of the IV line.

Using a T-connector extension set when the IV is first set up

These directions assume no IV has yet been inserted.

1. Spike the IV bag as you normally would.
2. Attach the saline lock to the cannula port on the infusion tubing. Uncap the cannula port on the primary tubing.
3. Uncap the hub on the end of the extension tube and luer-lock it to the primary tubing. Loosen the cap on the luer-lock on the cannula port on one end of the T.
4. Carefully set aside the caps by rewrapping them in the original packaging.
5. Prime the IV bag, drip chamber and tubing as usual, flushing the tube and extension set. Check to make sure the extension is filled with fluid.
6. Insert the catheter as usual.
7. Remove the cap and securely screw the luer-lock on the T end of the extension set to the hub of the cannula.
8. Tape the IV site down, taking care not to tape down the attachment joint between the tubing and the end of the saline lock so that the tube can easily be detached.
9. Run the IV as usual.

Removing the primary administration tubing with a T-connector extension set in place

1. Clamp off the infusion tubing.
2. Be sure the tubing is filled with solution.
3. Clamp the extension tubing off completely with the slip-and-pinch clamp. Unscrew the luer-lock on the primary tubing port and disengage the extension port from the primary tubing.
4. To maintain sterility, replace the caps that originally covered the tip on the cannula port of the primary tubing and the port on the end of the extension set.

Performing a saline flush on a device with a rubber port

A saline lock should be flushed immediately after the primary IV line is detached and immediately before it is reattached. In the interim, it should be flushed periodically, according to the size of the cannula being used: for 24 g or smaller, flush every 3 hours, for 20 g, flush every 6 hours; and for 18 g or larger, flush every 8 hours (Gilmore, 2003).

1. Fill a syringe fitted with a 1 in, 23 to 25 g needle with normal saline. Draw up more than enough saline to completely flush the lock and cannula. Replace the needle with a syringe cannula if using a needleless system.
2. Swab the injection port on the saline lock with antiseptic.
3. While waiting for the antiseptic to dry, carefully examine the injection port for evidence of wear, damage or, if using a needle to enter the port, large needle holes. If the port appears damaged in any way, it must be replaced. If using a butterfly, just replace it. If it is attached to a separate length of extension tubing that is part of the cannula, leave the cannula in place. Prepare a new extension set by filling it with saline, apply pressure through the skin to the tip of the cannula, disconnect the damaged device and screw in the new one. You may need help with this.
4. Insert the needle or syringe cannula of the saline-filled syringe into the injection port on the saline lock.
   - If using a needle, take care not to puncture any tubing as you do so. If the port offers little resistance to being punctured, suspect coring or weakening and replace the device immediately.
   - To insert the needle into a nonsafety port: Turn the needle so that the bevel is uppermost. Hold it at a 45° angle and apply pressure to slice into the rubber. Reposition the needle so that it is perpendicular to the port and insert it more deeply (Poznar, 2002). A new puncture site should be used each time the port is penetrated.
   - To insert a needle into a safety port: insert the needle along the edge.
   - To insert a syringe cannula into a safety port, pierce the center of the safety port.
5. Aspirate slightly to confirm that the cannula is still open; you should see a bit of blood in the line when you do this, which indicates that no clot has formed in the cannula. Depress the plunger gently to flush the catheter with 2 to 5 cc of fluid, depending upon the capacity of the locking device. Once you begin the flush, maintain positive pressure on the syringe plunger throughout the procedure in order to prevent blood from entering the cannula.
6. Whether you are using a needle or a syringe cannula, continue to slowly depress the plunger as you withdraw it from the injection port on the saline lock.

If you meet more than slight resistance during a saline flush, do not use forceful positive pressure in an attempt to clear clotted blood from the cannula or stylet. To do so may dislodge the clot and send it into the bloodstream or it may rupture the cannula. The cannula will have to be removed and replaced with a new one.

Reattaching the primary tubing to an T-connector extension set

1. Flush the set with saline, as described above.
2. Make sure the primary tubing is free or air bubbles; if not, flush them out before proceeding.
3. Fill the drip chamber and clamp off the primary tubing.
4. Uncap the cannula hub on the extension set and the port on primary tubing port and connect them.
5. Open the pinch clamp on the extension set.
6. Open the roller clamp on the primary tubing and adjust flow.

Dealing with Complications of IV Use

Air bubbles that develop during administration

You can minimize the chance of an air embolism by ensuring that all tubing connections are secure and that fluid bags are changed before they are completely empty. The drip chamber should remain vertical whenever the IV is in place. If you notice a large quantity of air in the tubing after it is in place, slow the drip down by almost closing the roller clamp. Insert a sterile syringe needle without a syringe attached into the cleansed drug port on the tubing below the air bubble. Reopen the roller clamp slowly. The air will flow down the tubing and naturally seek the path of least resistance, exiting via the syringe needle. Once the air is cleared, remove the needle from the port and discard. Readjust your rate of flow. More about air in the line is discussed on the following page under "embolism."

Overinfusion

There is a danger of overinfusing when using IVs. This is especially true when volume loss has not occurred. Crystalloid fluids will eventually leak into the tissues and can lead to edema, which can ultimately cause heart failure. In addition, fluids can dilute clotting factors, which can contribute to hemorrhaging. Electrolyte imbalances can also occur when large amounts of lactated Ringer's or normal saline alone are used to deal with volume loss. While these types of complications are unlikely to occur in healthy women when only 2 to 3 liters of fluid are infused, you should know the signs that point to problems.

Overhydration: Overhydration is an extreme situation that is less likely to develop in a young, healthy woman, but it should always be kept in mind. When it occurs, there will be subtle warnings well before heart failure ensues. The earliest signs are a bounding pulse and colorless urine. Eventually crackles in the lungs when listening with a stethoscope are noted, reflecting early pulmonary edema, where fluid pools in the lung tissue.

Listen to the heart and lungs every 5 minutes to assess cardiac and pulmonary status. Crackles will first develop in the most dependent region of the lungs which is the lowermost point according to maternal position: near the clavicles if the woman is in a Trendelenburg position (a position not recommended postpartum [see below for reasons why]); at the bottom of the lungs near the costal margin if she is upright and over her back if her torso is supine. Other signs and symptoms include difficulty breathing when lying down, pink frothy sputum, distended neck veins and swelling of the hands and feet. If you think pulmonary edema is developing, transport immediately. Pulmonary edema can be confirmed with a chest X-ray and by the measurement of central venous pressure after transport.

As soon as you suspect overinfusion, slow the drip down and watch the woman very carefully. If crackles have developed which do not resolve with reduced IV flow, discontinue the IV immediately. As the situation becomes more critical, swelling of the face or extremities develops, especially around the eyes. A change in the level of consciousness may indicate cerebral edema but could also be due to worsening shock because of concealed blood loss, so assess the situation carefully. Because the infusion of crystalloid solutions will always result in the transfer of fluid from the intravascular compartment into the interstitial spaces, it is important to remember that a woman can experience significant swelling, indicating too much crystalloid solution has been given, even though plasma volume expansion was only temporarily restored. Such a woman requires immediate transport.

Flow problems

Failure to remove the tourniquet: The number-one reason for lack of flow is that you have forgotten to remove the tourniquet, so be sure and check for that first. If fluid does not flow freely once the tourniquet is removed and the tube clamps are both open, make sure the cannula is not bent by the position of the elbow joint. If straightening the arm does not help, try pulling back slightly on the hub of the cannula while watching for flow through the drip chamber.

If there is little or no flow through an open tube, lower the IV bag below the level of the mother's heart. If blood flows into the tubing, this confirms that the cannula is correctly placed. Raise the bag again, and the blood will flow back into the vein. Fluid will not flow if the cannula is in a muscle or tendon. Placement in either is also quite painful.

If the IV has been placed correctly and it stops running, this is likely to be due to a clot forming in the cannula. Prevent this by always keeping the fluid running, even if only at a very slow rate or by attaching a saline lock. If a clot has formed, *do not* try to blow it out by forcing fluid through the line. You must replace the cannula.

Infiltration: Infiltration may result if the flow of solution through the stylet or cannula becomes displaced. This can occur if the tip of the stylet punctures through the opposite venous wall during insertion or when blood or IV solution leaks from the cannula out of a single venous puncture and into the surrounding tissue (this could happen if the cannula is placed too shallowly in the vein). It can also occur if the cannula is placed in fatty tissue (which will allow some fluid to enter). Infiltration is indicated by coolness and blanching of the skin at the puncture site, swelling–with or without pain–and sluggish or absent flow rate. If allowed to progress uncorrected, more severe symptoms such as numbness, gross edema, discoloration, bruising and circulatory impairment may develop (Garcia, 2002).

Phlebitis: Phlebitis, or inflammation of the vein, is evidenced by pain and tenderness at the IV site with reddening and bruising at the site or over the vein. The insertion site is warm to the touch and the flow of solution may stop. If either infiltration or phlebitis is suspected, clamp the tube immediately, remove the cannula, and bandage the area. Choose another puncture site closer to the torso (that is, proximal to the original site), preferably on the opposite extremity.

Embolism

Embolism is one of the most serious, life-threatening emergencies that can result from poor IV technique. An embolism occurs when a blood vessel becomes blocked by an abnormal mass moving through the circulatory system. It can occur because a thrombus breaks loose into the vascular system, air enters the vein, or a fragment of the cannula escapes into the circulation. The biggest risk is air embolism. Because of this, it is imperative that you stay with a woman at all times when she has an IV or saline lock in place. Air embolism is most likely to occur when the cannula is passed into the central circulation–a technique beyond the midwife's scope of practice–but it is possible for air to enter the circulation during insertion of the peripheral catheter, when the tubing is disconnected to replace solutions, when new extension tubing or a saline lock is added or when an accident such as a needle puncture damages the tubing or bag. Air embolism most commonly occurs, however, when an IV is started through unprimed tubing or when an empty bag is being replaced and air enters tubing that has not been properly handled before starting the new bag (Garcia, 2002).

It normally takes at least 20 cc of air to create a life-threatening emergency, with symptoms more common only after 100 cc have entered the circulation. A 68 in length of macrobore tubing holds 8 cc of fluid, that's 1 cc of fluid per 8.5 in of tubing. Microbore tubing would hold less. This gives you some idea of the small quantity of air contained in the tiny bubbles that frequently cling to the walls of the tubing that you cannot seem to remove. However, a person in shock is more susceptible to an adverse reaction to an air infusion. A sufficient quantity of infused air causes the blood to become foamy as it is agitated within the beating heart. When enough air enters the heart chamber, the heart muscle cannot pump effectively, blood flow is impeded, platelets are damaged, clots may form that eventually enter the lungs and shock results. Symptoms include hypotension, cyanosis, weak but rapid pulse and loss of consciousness.

Pulmonary embolism occurs when a thrombus breaks loose into the circulation and lodges in the lung, cutting off the blood supply to a region of the lung tissue resulting in oxygen deprivation. This produces pin point chest pain, painful breathing and signs of shock including loss of consciousness, coma and death.

A foreign body embolism occurs when a foreign body becomes lodged in a blood vessel or when the body's natural defense reaction results in the foreign material accumulating white blood cells, platelets and blood clots as it travels through the circulation. Eventually, it can form a mass large enough to occlude a blood vessel, leading to signs and symptoms similar to those of pulmonary embolism.

If you are starting an IV for an already shocky woman, be alert for any worsening of her condition that may indicate embolism. If an embolism is suspected, immediately proceed as follows:

1. Clamp off the IV tubing and check it for leaks.
2. Lay the woman supine on her left side. (If air has entered the heart chambers, this position helps keep the air on the right side, away from the cardiac valves. The pulmonary artery may absorb small air bubbles.)
3. Administer oxygen via a nonrebreather mask at a high flow rate.
4. Transport in an ambulance whenever possible.

RESUSCITATING THE MOTHER

You may never be called upon to resuscitate a mother. However, knowing how to do so may be life saving in the rare event that the need arises from such crises as shock secondary to hemorrhage, embolism or brain aneurism. This chapter will focus on the use of resuscitation devices in adults, thus building on the information found in Volume I in the chapter entitled "Cardiopulmonary Resuscitation and Airway Clearance during Pregnancy." This information is not intended to replace adult CPR and bag-valve-mask certification by a reputable credentialing body such as the American Red Cross or the American Heart Association.

Volume I describes delivering emergency CPR to a woman during pregnancy. During labor, your equipment is going to be set up and close at hand. Providing more advanced support until a transport team arrives will thus be possible. Instruct others to make arrangements for ambulance transport while you attend to stabilizing the mother.

Using an adult self-inflating resuscitator

Adult bag-and-mask devices are almost identical in structure and function to their neonatal counterparts. The only real difference is that adult units are larger and have no pressure-release mechanism, since over inflation of the adult lungs with a bag-and-mask unit does not occur. Adult models are equipped with a non-pop-off breathing valve. Adult ventilation bag sizes range from 1600 to 2000 ml; oxygen reservoir bags range from 2500 to 2600 ml. (For a detailed description of bag-and-mask construction, see the subchapter entitled "Oxygen Delivery Devices and Resuscitation Equipment.")

Bag-and-mask technique: Using a bag and mask on an adult is essentially the same as using one on a newborn. Attach oxygen tubing to the oxygen port, apply the mask over the mouth and nose, and ventilate 15 times per minute. Be sure you see the chest rising and falling with each ventilation. If no pulse is detected after the first 5 to 10 seconds of ventilatory support, begin chest compressions at a ratio of 2 compressions to each ventilation. If you have an assistant, the ratio is five ventilations to one compression. (Ventilation and compression-to-ventilation rates change frequently; refer to your certification manual for the latest recommendations.)

Maintaining a tight seal between face and mask while keeping the airway open and ventilating is difficult and requires practice. Two people can provide adult bag-and-mask ventilation most effectively. If you are alone and cannot manage the bag and mask for whatever reason, you should use simple mouth-to-mask CPR as described in Volume I.

Using an adult oral airway

If the mother is completely unconscious or semiconscious with no gag reflex, you can insert an oral airway to maintain an open airway. Oropharyngeal airways are also discussed in the subchapter entitled "Selecting and Using an Infant Oropharyngeal Airway." The technique for fitting adults and infants is essentially the same. Generally speaking, the following sizes work for these body types:

- Large adult: Berman 100 mm or Guedel size 11
- Medium adult: Berman 90 mm or Guedel size 10
- Small adult: Berman 80 mm or Guedel size 8

This list can be used as a guide for which airway to try first when selecting the appropriate size. To size the airway, place it against the side of the face so that the flange is at the level of the woman's central incisors, the bite block segment is parallel to the woman's hard palate and the curve of the hump is directed toward the top of her head. The properly sized airway should extend from the corner of the mouth to the tip of the ear lobe when the shaft is held parallel with the line of the jaw.

Inserting an airway: Note that inserting an airway is an advanced life-support procedure: even when performed properly, the person receiving such support may experience long-term complications such as aspiration, tracheal stenosis, infection, temporary difficulty swallowing and voice changes. Additional problems are described in the chapter covering the use of an oropharyngeal airway in a newborn. Care should be taken not to get bitten during insertion or removal; an airway should only be used if the woman is unconscious or nearly so. Here are the steps to be followed in inserting an adult airway:

1. Place the mother on her back and hyperextend her neck.
2. Use a bulb syringe to clear the mouth and nose of all secretions.
3. Cross your thumb and forefinger of one hand and place them on the woman's upper and lower teeth at the corner of her mouth. Spread your fingers apart to open her jaws and hold her mouth open.
4. Position the airway so that its tip is pointing toward the roof of the mouth. Alternatively, you can insert it at a 90° angle (tip toward the corner of the mouth). Either position avoids catching the tongue on the tip during insertion.
5. Insert the airway and advance it parallel to the roof of the mouth. Once the tip is past the crest of the tongue, gently rotate it 180° (or 90°) into the proper position so that it rests against the posterior wall of the oropharynx. This places the tip past the uvula and soft palate. Now the tip is pointing down into the throat. Be certain not to push the tongue back into the throat during insertion. Occasionally you may need to use a tongue depressor to hold the woman's tongue in place during placement. Watch what you are doing: this procedure should not be performed by feel alone.
6. Place the woman's head in a maximum head-tilt position, as for any type of CPR.
7. Make sure the flange of the airway rests against her lips; this position indicates that it is the correct size. If the airway is too long or too short, remove it and replace it with one of the correct size. Never use an airway if you do not have the proper size.
8. Provide mouth-to-mask ventilation, taking care not to dislodge the airway.
9. Monitor closely. If there is a gag reflex, remove the airway at once. Removal is accomplished by reversing the insertion procedures.

Multi-use Manual Skills

Opening the Pelvis (or the Midwife's Forceps)

The medical profession has devised instruments, such as forceps and the vacuum extractor, to pull the baby's head out during births that are delayed due to a tight fit or when the mother's energy is flagging. Midwives have been busy for centuries developing their own techniques to remedy this difficulty.

There are many problems with using instruments. They are expensive; they require complicated manufacturing before they can reach the hands of the practitioner; and, most important, their use poses significant risks to both mother and baby. Instrumentation is a highly skilled and risky procedure that can result in maternal injury, and fetal injury or death, even in the most experienced hands.

Forceps blades fit around the skull (actually taking up room in the pelvis) and press the bones together as they are locked into place and the head is pulled out. Hematomas, subgaleal or intracranial hemorrhage, palsies from neurological trauma and other types of fetal damage are not infrequent results. A vacuum extractor, on the other hand, takes up no additional room in the pelvis but comes with the risk of mild to severe scalp trauma (including complete detachment of the scalp if improperly used), as well as subdural hematomas and bleeding in the brain. Pulling the head through the mother's pelvis can interfere with proper shoulder rotation; both vacuum extraction and forceps delivery are associated with an increased rate of shoulder dystocia. Both forceps and vacuum cups, if improperly applied, can also do considerable damage to the mother's soft tissues.

This is not to say that the use of instruments is never appropriate. In some situations, the use of vacuum extraction may be important for properly trained midwives working in very rural areas or in the developing world. However, all midwives should have a repertoire of techniques that can be used at home to get babies out without any instrumentation.

When to manually open the pelvis

There are several techniques midwives use to open the pelvis. Foremost and least interventive are position changes and activities that create more space along the pelvic passageway. Given the wide range of options, position changes should always be tried prior to using the manual techniques described here. If you can get the mother into a Birth Sling or have an assistant support her in a dangle position to take all the weight off the pelvis before attempting any of these manipulations, the position alone may remedy the problem. Consider pelvic-opening techniques as a last resort, to be used only after other less invasive and less uncomfortable techniques have been tried to no avail.

Deciding if opening the pelvis will be useful

Most of these pelvic manipulations are only appropriate for use in cephalic presentations when the baby is well into the pelvis and it is felt that there is enough room but a very tight fit or that the pelvic ligaments and joints are not as flexible as they might be. They will not help if the correction needs to occur at the brim. They are therefore usually reserved for when descent is slow and pushing is well underway (exceptions are noted in the discussions below). Some manipulations presented here can help to resolve shoulder dystocia of the midpelvis or outlet (see the chapter entitled "Shoulder Dystocia" for more details). Any of them may be particularly useful for a woman who has a disability and cannot stand for any length of time.

Risks of manual opening of the pelvis

Separation of the symphysis (covered in Volume III of this text) is perhaps the most likely complication that may result from opening the pelvis. Urethral bruising or damage may occur if pressure is applied under the pubic bone. Coccygeal misalignment may also occur with some techniques. However, the strength in a female midwife's hands and upper body is such that significant damage will probably not occur. A postpartum visit to a chiropractor or osteopath should be recommended for any woman who has undergone manual pelvic opening.

If significant cephalopelvic disproportion is suspected, these techniques should not be used because the baby may become quite stuck in the process. Neither should they be used if the mother has been transported and given regional anesthesia such as an epidural. The primary risk of pelvic manipulation is straining and overstretching of the pelvic joints; this risk is particularly high if manual opening is applied abruptly, with brute force or without regard for how much will be enough to accomplish the desired result. The risk is also greatly increased in women who are drugged. Although the pelvis may give dramatically with these techniques, the artificial relaxation of the ligaments produced by the drug makes joint injury likely.

Maneuvers that open the midpelvis and the outlet

Pelvic press: The pelvic press is one of the best of these techniques because it can be done with the mother upright and requires no internal manipulation. It can be used prior to complete dilation to help reposition an asynclitic head or to help an engaged head descend further, or during pushing to facilitate descent with a deflexed head or a compound presentation. The pelvic press is also an excellent way to open the lower pelvis in the event of an outlet shoulder dystocia. A mother who is still in the dilation phase of labor should assume a standing, forward-leaning position. A woman who is pushing and whose baby is deeply engaged may stand, assume a standing squat (feet flat on floor, bottom level with the floor, knees bent), assume a full squat, as illustrated, or get into the Birth Sling. The strongest assistant present should stand behind the woman, place his hands firmly on the iliac crests and press them together firmly until he feels some movement. This position should be maintained during the next contraction.

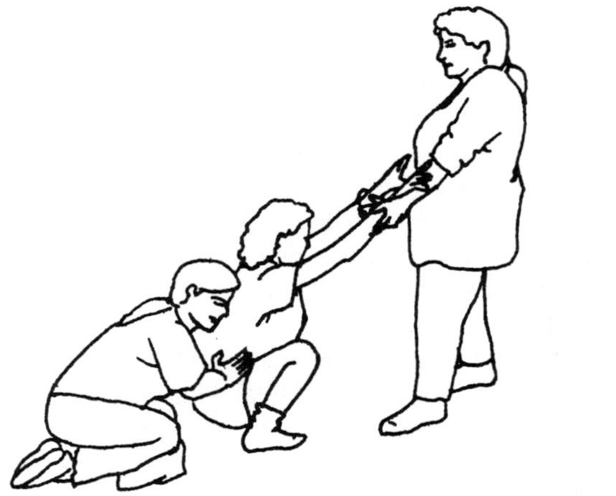

Pelvic press

(Artwork on this page redrawn with permission from illustrations by Stella Cruz, © Ruth Ancheta 2000)

Alternatively, two assistants can position themselves on either side of the mother. Each one should kneel down as close to the level of the mother's hips as possible, and then use the heels of their hands or their fists to simultaneously press inward on the mother's iliac crests while she pushes. The assistants should hold each other's free hands to equalize the pressure and maintain balance.

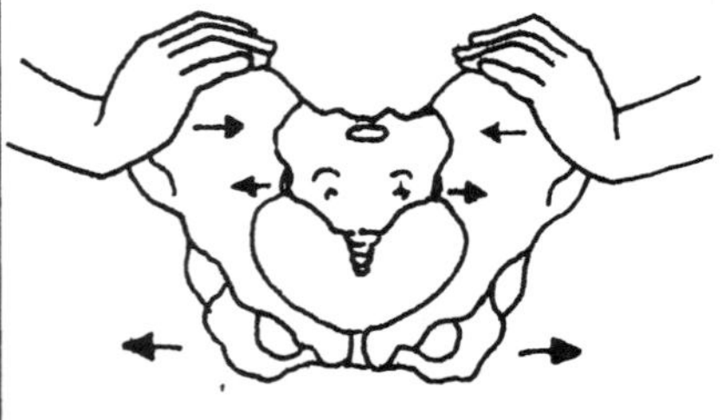

The effect of the pelvic press

Pressure causes the lower borders of the sacroiliac joints as well as the ischial tuberosities to widen, thus opening the midpelvis and the outlet. Applying pressure over the hip joint below the iliac crests may help to open the inlet if the head is very high, but the same thing can be accomplished by having the mother tip her pelvis forward and swaying her back (Koehler, 1985; Davis, 1997). If the pelvic press is going to work, a change in the desired direction should be noted within three or four contractions.

The pelvic press can also be used when the mother is lying on her side, during or even prior to pushing. The mother should assume a side-lying position on a firm surface (a mat or padded floor). If space is needed in the outlet alone, her legs should be flexed up toward her belly; if space is needed throughout the pelvis, her legs should be in a less flexed position, her knees level with or lower than her tuberosities. An assistant should then press the uppermost iliac crest directly down toward the floor. This will significantly lift the uppermost tuberosity; in addition, the sacrum may move backward slightly. However, the pressure can also tend to lock the sacrum in place. The tuberosity pull (see below) may be a better option if more space is needed posteriorly.

Tuberosity pull: This maneuver pulls up on a single tuberosity. The mother lies on her side on a firm, padded surface, deeply flexing her upper leg while an assistant supports it for her. Insert your gloved fingers into the yoni, find the inside surface of the upper tuberosity and pull upward during a contraction. If this is being done to correct a compound presentation, the mother should lie on the side opposite the small part. If used to correct asynclitic descent, have her lie on the side opposite the one to which the head is tilted (i.e., sagittal suture cocked to her left, she lies on her right). The tuberosity is then pulled up to widen the space on that side. Lifting the side of her pelvis where the crown of the head is pointing may create enough room for the head to come down. However, if the head is cocked because there is a hand under the jaw, switch sides and see if you can create enough room for the baby to move his hand.

Hip lift: This is a variation of the tuberosity pull described in the Pink Kit that can be used during dilation or pushing. Have the mother lie on her side, as above, but with her legs together. Use one hand to press straight down on her upper iliac crest. Hook the fingers of your other hand under the tip of her upper tuberosity. Slowly press down on the iliac crest while pulling up on her tuberosity (www.birthingbetter.com).

Sacral press: This maneuver will help to rotate the sacral promontory from above; in some cases, it may actually narrow the inlet but will widen the pelvic passage from below the brim to a certain extent (Gaskin, 1998). The mother should assume any position that does not put direct pressure on the sacrum (squatting, hands and knees or side-lying) on a firm surface. The midwife places two or three fingers inside the mother's yoni and presses against the lower sacrum during pushing. Standing or a hands-and-knees position will allow the entire sacrum to move backward spontaneously, so this technique is most useful when a woman is incapable of standing, thus limiting her sacral mobility to an extent, depending upon the position she chooses.

Techniques that primarily open the pelvic outlet

Scissors-jack maneuver: This technique is performed during pushing and helps to open the outlet. The mother lays supine on a firm surface, legs hyperflexed up on her belly (McRoberts position). Using the index and middle finger of your right hand, position the fingerpads on the inside edge of the mother's *right* tuberosity (which is to *your* left). Position the index and middle fingers of your left hand on the inside edge of her *left* tuberosity (your wrists are now crossed). Now push the pelvic rami apart during contractions (Hobbs, 1982). While this maneuver opens the outlet, it will be impossible to do if the head is already out, so it cannot be used for an outlet shoulder dystocia.

Sheela-na-gig maneuver: This is similar to the scissors-jack maneuver and accomplishes the same thing. Place the pads of your index and middle fingers of your left hand against the mother's right ischial tuberosity (to your left) and the fingers of your right hand on her left tuberosity (to your right; your forearms are not crossed). Now pull the bones apart during contractions. This opens the pelvis to get the head out and can also be used to deal with an outlet shoulder dystocia. (This technique was named by the late Pamela Truzinski, a beloved Oregon midwife who died in 2000.)

Pubic pull-up (pubic expansion): This is a more painful technique which should not be used if the pubic arch is shallow, because inserting your fingers will further decrease space in the anterior pelvis. The mother is positioned as for the scissors-jack maneuver. An assistant stands to the mother's side and above her, reaches down with her strongest hand and inserts two fingers under the pubic arch. These fingers should be spread slightly to avoid applying direct pressure to the urethra. The assistant pulls directly upward during a contraction to widen the pubic arch (Daniels, 1978). By both widening and changing the angle of the symphysis, this technique can help resolve either inlet or outlet shoulder dystocia if the problem is a funnel-shaped outlet. (Scholles, 2000).

Moving the coccyx: If the mother's coccyx is prominent or has previously broken and has healed at an angle that impedes descent, it may need to be pressed backward and out of the way. This should be done with two fingers in the posterior outlet, keeping in mind that this is likely to be very painful. Having the mother lie flat on the floor in a dorsal position (knees up) may also help the baby's head put sufficient pressure down to displace the coccyx backward.

Learning to use these techniques

Good pelvimetry skills will help the midwife decide which, if any, of the various positions or activities, or pelvic opening maneuvers to try first. If the mother has a tight midpelvis, as evidenced by lack of progress around the ischial spines, then techniques that open the midpelvis, such as the pelvic press, may help. Likewise, if the mother has a very tight outlet, spreading the rami along with using the sacral press will get things out of the way from three sides.

Afterbirth care

Any woman who has had her pelvis manipulated in any of these ways should see a chiropractor or an osteopath for evaluation and treatment after the birth. Separation of the pubic bones will be covered in Vol. III of this text.

FUNDAL PRESSURE

Fundal pressure is the application of pressure to the abdominal wall overlying the uterine fundus and is used to augment maternal pushing efforts and thus accomplish the birth more quickly. Whether or not its use is ever appropriate is a matter of controversy for medical practitioners and midwives alike. The need for fundal pressure is rare, especially in light of the increased remembering that midwives have accomplished over the past 35 years regarding maternal position changes and pelvic movements that can facilitate birth. However, midwives practice in all kinds of settings, and in some cases, fundal pressure can quickly and effectively overcome a problem that position changes alone have not resolved. It is thus worth discussing, and important to know how to perform it in a way that minimizes risks.

Obstetrical uses of fundal pressure

Although mention of it in the obstetric literature is nearly nonexistent, fundal pressure was extensively used for decades in hospitals on women who were under full anesthesia and therefore unable to offer spontaneous pushing efforts. Today, fundal pressure to augment pushing is used far less. Women are more often conscious and able to push, even if they must be told when to do so due to the effect of an epidural; in addition, there are more witnesses (such as partners) in the delivery room, who are scrutinizing medical procedures (thus the risk of a law suit is increased). However, fundal pressure is still often used during surgical births to facilitate the birth of the baby through the uterine incision.

Fundal pressure has also been used in institutions and at home by midwives to compensate for situations such as weak contractions during pushing, a mother who is unable or unwilling to push, acute fetal distress that is not responding to corrective measures, shoulder dystocia, a marginally tight fit through the pelvis, or a resistant perineum. Some of these indications may, of course, overlap. It is important to note that fundal pressure should *never* be used by itself to attempt to dislodge a shoulder dystocia. The reasons for this are fully discussed in the chapter entitled "Shoulder Dystocia."

Potential risks

Fundal pressure is not without its considerable dangers and negative consequences. It is most risky when applied forcefully, insensitively and continuously in situations in which it is not effecting an easy resolution of the problem. It is important to recognize the potential risks.

- Uterine rupture: The risk of rupturing the lower uterine segment is great when used in the presence of an incompletely dilated cervix, absolute or even relative cephalopelvic disproportion, pelvic obstruction or an impacted shoulder dystocia. Fundal pressure should never be used on a grand multipara, who is at more intrinsic risk of uterine rupture and who should be able to get her baby out. If she cannot, an unusual obstruction should be suspected; transport.
- Fetal distress: Pressure on the baby and uterus can increase fetal distress, although fetal distress is often the indication for its use. The benefit is getting the baby out faster, crucial if the baby's life is threatened. For example, if the placenta suddenly starts to abrupt or the cord tears, fundal pressure may get the baby out before oxygen deprivation reaches a critical low.
- Crushing the placenta: A placenta that lies directly beneath the area where pressure is being applied can be damaged, resulting in maternal and infant bleeding and impairment of blood flow to the baby. This is especially problematic in the presence of blood incompatibilities, as it raises the risk of maternal-fetal blood mixing. Fundal pressure is therefore only appropriate when the birth is imminent, although the risk of blood mixing remains.
- Fetal damage: Forcing a baby through a pelvis that is too small can cause intracranial hemorrhage, nerve damage in the neck and shoulder area, as well as fracture of the skull or other bones. The application of fundal pressure in an attempt to resolve shoulder dystocia risks brachial plexus injury.
- Strain on uterine support ligaments: Supporting ligaments are taxed whenever the uterus is forced downward. Thus, fundal pressure can be a contributing factor in uterine prolapse; either immediately following birth or later in life.
- Supine positioning: Fundal pressure is most effective when the mother lies supine on a firm surface. This puts pressure on the sacrum, preventing its motion, and manual force from above risks malrotation of the shoulders as the head descends. Getting the mother into an upright position may remedy the problem and eliminate the need for outside force.

Deciding if fundal pressure will help

Fundal pressure is most effective when the problem is that there is not enough force from above. After having tried everything else, fundal pressure might be considered in the following situations:

- The baby is well down in the pelvis, with the biparietal diameter about ready to descend past the pubic bone. You feel the mother could birth the baby easily with a bit more power behind her efforts.
- Birth is imminent, the mother is tired, and the fetal heart rate is not good. The mother has changed positions has taken a break in pushing and may have been offered oxygen by mask through at least one contraction with no recovery of the fetal heart rate.
- You have determined that the perineum is quite rigid and hanging things up and is likely to be overcome with more force from above. However, when the forces are adequate and the perineum is rigid, clitorotomy [i.e., episiotomy] may be a better alternative. Remember neither fundal pressure (nor clitorotomy) will overcome absolute fetopelvic disproportion; it is likely to cause damage in such circumstances.
- You are attending a breech birth, the baby's parts are properly aligned, neither the arms nor the head are extended but the partially-born baby is limp and pale and needs to be born quickly. Frank Louwen, a doctor who has attended quite a number of breeches in Germany, finds it relatively safe and effective to apply fundal pressure to bring the baby down, and feels it is much safer than applying traction (Tully, 2013). This is especially true when only the flexed head needs to be born. *In order for this to be safe, the baby* ***must*** *be properly aligned, with the arms in a good position and not hung-up anywhere.* For this to be safe, you should have considerable experience with breeches. If in doubt, do not attempt to use fundal pressure.

Fundal pressure, applied with sensitivity, might help in any of these situations. It should always be applied as a short-term effort; if significant descent has not occurred within three or four contractions, fundal pressure should be discontinued.

How to do fundal pressure

Fundal pressure should be performed by a woman to prevent the inadvertent application of excessive pressure, which men are more likely to provide because of their greater upper body strength. Fundal pressure is typically performed using the hand or forearm to apply pressure to the fundus in a longitudinal direction with the mother supine. In hospitals, the most popular technique entails the application of a single open hand, palm to fundus and arm held rigid and this is how Frank Louwen has used it for the breech situation described above when you are only facilitating bringing the unobstructed breech down or birth of the aftercoming head. The arm is positioned at a 30 to 40° angle to the mother's spine. Pressure is always applied in the direction of the pelvic cavity.

However, for a vertex birth, using a single forearm across the top of the fundus spreads the pressure out and carries less risk of localized trauma. Another way to apply fundal pressure involves having two assistants stand to either side of the mother, lock their arms by each grasping the other's upper arm just above the elbow and use their forearms to apply pressure to the fundus. This method produces a broader distribution of force across the top of the uterus but also involves the combined strength of two individuals and may reduce sensitivity to how much pressure is being applied. Once the person applying pressure is in place, she applies pressure as the mother pushes. When the mother relaxes or takes a breath, the pressure is reduced or discontinued entirely, so that it is augmenting her efforts without the use of brute force and to give the baby a chance to recover. Fundal pressure should not be done while the receiving midwife is attempting to manipulate the baby in any way, unless the midwife specifically requests some pressure to help rotate the baby or flex the head.

Tully G. "Identifying and resolving obstructed breech birth," MIDWIFERY TODAY, (106);21-23, Summer 2013.

THE USE OF VERSION DURING LABOR

Version, or manually turning the baby, is any procedure in which the practitioner's hands are used to change the position of the long axis of the fetus so that a more favorable part is presenting. Both external and internal version can be used during labor. The performance of internal version during labor is controversial. This procedure varies from that of external version, which is still used during pregnancy and early labor in many areas. Internal version is rarely used in industrialized countries today, and then only sometimes in the case of an easily turned second twin; surgery is considered the much preferred alternative. Therefore, any midwife who performs an internal version is practicing outside of the bounds of standard midwifery and modern medical practice, unless she is working in the developing world, where version during labor is still performed out of necessity. This skill is included here for those midwives who find themselves in circumstances where it is the best or only reasonable option.

That being said, it is really not so farfetched to think that version could be a reasonable option when judiciously used by someone with good manual skills in general and good palpation skills in particular. Today, the majority of obstetric practitioners have very poor hands-on skills, which, no doubt, makes the idea of performing version quite daunting for them. However, this lack of expertise should not be assumed of everyone in the field; indeed, many if not most experienced midwives have excellent manual skills as well as smaller hands than the average male practitioner, not to mention better rapport with the babies with whom they work. All these factors increase the likelihood that a midwife will be able to perform version more safely and more successfully (which is not to deny that this is a very risky procedure).

Indications

Version (especially the external variety) may be indicated whenever the fetus is in an unfavorable position that cannot be corrected by less invasive methods. Version is also useful as a means of facilitating a rapid birth when the need for such is indicated by the condition of the mother or child and timely transport is not possible. Indications include:

- **Transverse or oblique lie:** Yoni birth cannot occur unless the presentation can be converted into a longitudinal lie. If the membranes are intact, external version can be attempted prior to labor or between uterine contractions during early labor. If other methods of fetal rotation fail (such as using a rebozo), internal version can be attempted once the cervix is sufficiently dilated if transport is simply not an option.
- **Version of the second baby after the birth of a first twin:** If the second baby needs to be born rapidly, internal version can be followed with extraction. Indications include nonlongitudinal lie and abruption. Internal version may be life saving, at least for the mother if bleeding is profuse, the baby is not coming down and transport impossible. Internal version followed by extraction is feasible because the birth passages are already dilated. In fact, internal version for a nonvertex second twin may produce less fetal distress than external version in this circumstance (Chauhan et al., 1995).

Note that version is a technique unto itself. Historically, it was usually followed by fetal extraction (the manual facilitation of the birth). However, an urgent indication must be present to warrant proceeding with extraction because it carries its own considerable risks.

Methods of Version

There are two basic types of version; cephalic and podalic. Cephalic version is typically done before the onset of labor or during early labor; its intent is to cause the head to present. In podalic version, the breech (usually as a footling) is made to present; this procedure is typically performed after the onset of labor in situations where the baby needs to be brought out as quickly as possible. There are three methods of performing version:

- **External version:** The turn is accomplished using both hands on the mother's abdomen. This type of version is covered in Volume I of this text in the chapter entitled "Ensuring a Vertex Presentation at Term." Review that chapter before studying this one in depth, as the material presented here builds on that information.
- **Internal version:** One hand is inserted completely inside the uterus while the other manipulates the baby through the abdominal wall.
- **Bipolar version:** Popularized by Dr. Braxton Hicks (1823-1897), this is similar to internal version, but only two

fingers are inserted through the cervix. The opposite hand assists manipulation of the baby through the abdominal wall. All three methods are, in fact, bipolar in that both poles of the baby are manipulated during rotation.

External version in labor (Wigand method)

Only rarely will the presence of a nonlongitudinal lie first be discovered during labor; most will either have been corrected during pregnancy or a surgical birth planned if the baby couldn't be turned. Also on rare occasions a previously longitudinal baby converts to a transverse or oblique lie between the last prenatal visit and the onset of labor. In addition, babies occasionally will turn once labor has begun.

External version can be performed to correct the baby's position, although expect it to go more slowly and be somewhat more difficult than when performed earlier in gestation. It is most likely to be successful during early labor, when the membranes are intact and the spacing of contractions is such that you will have more time to accomplish the version before the cervix is very dilated. The process of turning the baby will produce pressure changes within the bag of waters; thus the support of the closed or nearly closed cervix from below minimizes the chance of inadvertent rupture of membranes. Place the mother in a slight Trendelenburg position by supporting her pelvis with a folded sheet or blanket to lift the baby away from the pelvis and reduce downward pressure, especially if dilation is already underway. Listen to the fetal heart rate before you begin and at least once during the process. Be sure your hands are warm. As you proceed, pause whenever a contraction occurs, but keep your hands in place so as not to lose any progress so far gained. You can resume turning as the contraction subsides. Although having intact membranes is ideal, external version can be performed when a nonlongitudinal lie is discovered upon rupture of membranes, if there is still sufficient fluid and if uterine contractions space out, as they often do when the bag breaks and there is a sudden loss of intrauterine volume. An assistant midwife should insert a hand into the yoni and monitor internally for cord prolapse during the version.

After the version, if the bag is broken press down gently on the fundus to help flex the spine and neck, thus assisting the baby into a vertex presentation (however, if the waters are intact this is unlikely to help). Listen to the fetal heart for a while. Continue to monitor internally to confirm both that the baby is descending in the desired position and that cord prolapse is not occurring. Some authors recommend rupturing the membranes to settle the baby into the new position. This should be avoided when possible (especially if the baby is floating [high risk for cord prolapse]) but you should let the individual situation be your guide; it is usually safest to allow contractions alone to move the baby down. Once the baby is well engaged, gradually remove supports from under the mother's bottom. Either way, the mother can get up and resume normal labor activities once the presenting part is well seated in the pelvis and the fetal heart rate is stable.

Internal version in labor

Risks: Internal version carries two major risks for the mother: uterine rupture and infection. The risks to the baby are numerous. The baby may be injured or killed during attempts to turn him; cord disruption or prolapse may be precipitated when the membranes are ruptured in the presence of a nonlongitudinal lie. Placental abruption can occur if the placental implantation site is disturbed. Entry of air into the uterine cavity during the procedure (an unlikely event) can prompt the baby to gasp.

Contraindications: Internal version is absolutely contraindicated when any of the following are present:

- **Prolonged rupture of membranes:** A relatively dry uterine cavity provides no room to work. If labor is underway, it is likely to be accompanied by a thin lower segment; attempted version can easily result in uterine rupture. The baby's body can become doubled over during version, with the head still in the lower segment when the breech is brought down, placing great strain on the lower uterine segment, especially if the woman has been in active labor for a long period of time.
- **Tight contraction of the uterus around the baby with a well-developed retraction ring:** When the intermittent character of normal uterine activity is lost and the uterus does not relax between contractions, the introduction of the hand (even under full anesthesia) can excite violent expulsive efforts that greatly interfere with manipulations and increase the risk of rupture. Also, a well-developed retraction ring above the head may impair its upward movement; pulling the breech down can result in sudden distension, with possible rupture, of the already thinned lower segment.
- **Obstruction of the birth canal:** This can be caused by maternal tumors or pelvic contraction.
- **Fetal anomaly:** Hydrocephalus, in particular, may result in a persistent nonlongitudinal lie.
- **Fetal demise:** With the baby dead, risks of uterine rupture and maternal infection must be clearly outweighed

by the risk posed to the mother by the indication for version (as might be the case with abruption).

- **Insufficient dilation:** Forceful manual dilation increases the risk of version when it results in cervical lacerations because tears may extend into the lower uterine segment when you insert your hand into the uterus. However, careful manual dilation can be attempted if the situation is dire (for example, if the mother is bleeding from an abruption and transport is impossible). A widely dilated cervix makes version considerably easier. Full dilation is most useful when immediate extraction is anticipated. When the baby is in a nonlongitudinal lie, however, full dilation may never occur, no matter how long you wait, and waiting increases the risk of uterine rupture.
- **Placenta previa:** Historically, podalic version followed by bringing down a leg was used to apply counterpressure to the placenta and slow or stop the bleeding when surgical birth was a much more dangerous option than it is today. This was a desperate attempt to save a mother from bleeding to death by using the fetal body to compress the placenta from above to stop the bleeding. However, internal manipulation of any kind carries considerable risk of cervical tearing, as the tissues will be friable because of their increased vascularity due to the overlying placenta. For this reason, you should *never attempt a version if a woman is bleeding and you suspect previa is the source.* Decades of data have proven that the risk of maternal death is even higher when tissue trauma is added to the situation. See the chapter entitled "Bleeding due to Placental Disruption" for details.

In addition, internal version in a woman who has a history of uterine surgery should be approached with caution. If the uterus is roomy, the membranes are intact or just ruptured and the version anticipated to go easily, it may be perfectly acceptable to proceed. However, always remember that a scarred uterus will be less able to tolerate manipulations of any kind without trauma versus one that is unscarred.

<u>Prerequisite conditions for internal version</u>: Most of the items in the following list were gleaned from various historical sources written by authors skilled at internal version.

- Fully informed consent from the parents regarding all possible options and the risks of internal version. Internal version will be uncomfortable, at best, and the woman should be completely committed and fully prepared. Do not attempt internal version on a mother who has not tolerated other internal exams well.
- Multiparity. Some authors consider first-time mothers unsuited for internal version, as their tissues are tighter and manipulation is thus more difficult.
- Dilation sufficient to admit the hand and allow the necessary internal manipulations without force. If immediate fetal extraction is to follow, full dilation is most desirable.
- Normally sized pelvis.
- Placenta previa has been ruled out.
- Intact or only recently ruptured membranes (that is, plenty of fluid in the uterine cavity)
- An absence of uterine activity or the presence of well-spaced, normal contractions.
- Lax or relaxed abdominal wall (preferably, the mother is a multipara).
- Unengaged and mobile baby who is not in the process of spontaneous evolution (that is, progressively descending through the birth canal as a transverse lie; this would only occur if the baby were very small)
- No suspected fetal abnormalities
- A living baby or a mother in jeopardy
- A mother who is as calm and centered as possible
- An empty maternal bowel and bladder
- Warm examining hands

The safest time to attempt version is as soon as a problematic lie is noted. Early in labor, external version is very likely to accomplish rotation without resorting to this more risky option. Generally speaking, the danger of internal version increases the longer the membranes have been ruptured, although each case must be evaluated individually. Even though hours or days have elapsed, internal version may be accomplished with relative ease if the uterus is lax, with contractions being few or absent. Conversely, the risk is much greater if the uterus is contracting strongly and clamps down around the baby should the waters break during the procedure.

Performing internal version for transverse or oblique lie

The most likely time a midwife will consider performing internal version will be when a second twin is in a nonlongitudinal lie. The cervix is wide open, the birth canal has just been dilated and the uterus is roomy. There is no history of neglected labor, pathologic retraction ring or any similar danger. The chance of success with subsequent rapid delivery of the second baby is excellent. Even so, this is not a procedure to be taken lightly. I expect that only experienced midwives will attempt internal verison and that all others who practice in urban areas will usually forgo it in favor of transport whenever feasible.

If version is being performed merely to correct a nonlongitudinal lie, cephalic version should be attempted first, as a head-down birth is always more desirable and is a simpler procedure. However, sometimes this is difficult to accomplish. If that is unsuccessful or the baby needs to be born very rapidly (such as with an abruption of twin placentas), internal podalic version can be used, which allows more control over bringing the baby out fast with breech extraction.

Podalic version consists of reaching in, grabbing one or both feet and bringing them down; this will cause the rest of the baby's body to follow along, thus converting the lie to a footling breech. It is imperative to make certain that it is a foot, and not a hand, before proceeding. Bringing down an arm will only tend to fix the baby in a transverse position. The opposability of the thumb distinguishes the hand from the foot, but the heel is an even more definitive landmark. Even if you are sure you have found a foot, follow the limb up to where it joins the body for confirmation.

If you intend to follow version with immediate extraction, you should bring down both feet together, gently directing the toes toward the floor (or toward the mother's posterior side) to encourage anterior rotation of the sacrum (Løvset, 1968). However, if you only need to fix the baby in a breech position, you will only bring down one leg. In that case, the next consideration is which leg to bring down; how the baby becomes positioned and subsequently descends will be greatly influenced by which leg is chosen. The proper leg is the one that will result in the baby rotating so her back is anterior. If the baby is transverse and the back is anterior, the lowermost leg should be brought down. If the baby is situated so that the back is anterior but lying across the inlet at an angle, the lowermost leg is moved more posteriorly. When the transverse baby's back is posterior, the uppermost leg should be brought down. If the baby's back is superior (directed toward the fundus) with limbs extended toward the os and the spine transverse, the anterior leg is brought down. If the baby is lying so that the spine overlies the os, the posterior leg is brought down first.

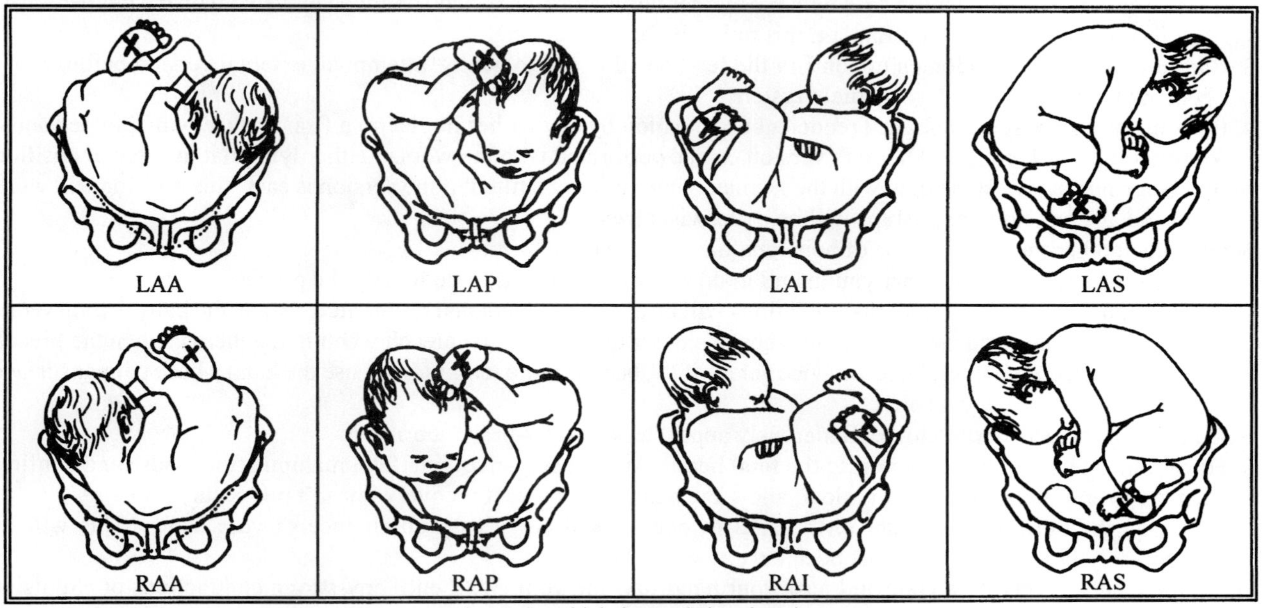

(× marks which foot to bring down)

Note that the direction of trunk rotation is controlled by the choice of leg only when one leg is brought down; bringing both legs down together does not control rotation in the same way. In addition, remember that babies frequently lie with their legs or feet crossed; therefore, the first foot encountered is not necessarily attached to the appropriate limb. The midwife's fingers should be passed up along the leg to the buttocks and the leg followed back down to confirm the desirable foot. To see how bringing the proper foot down works to rotate the back anteriorly, get someone to work with you using a doll with cloth limbs and a model pelvis.

The following drawings show how, when the baby is anterior (in this case LAA), going for the lowermost (in this case the posterior) leg rotates the baby's back to the anterior as the leg is brought down.

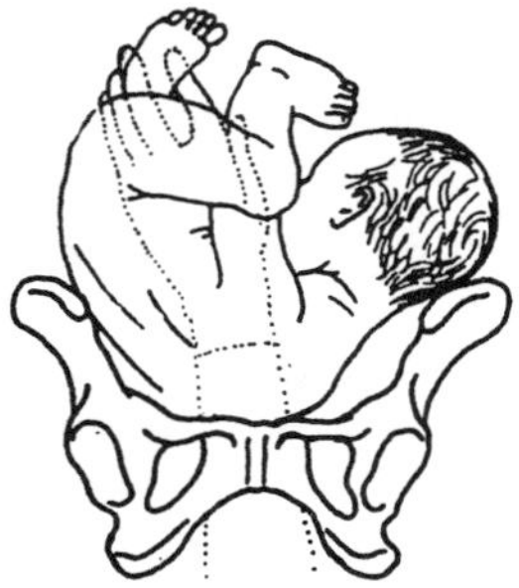

Having gone up over the buttocks, the foot of the lowermost (baby's right) leg is grasped.

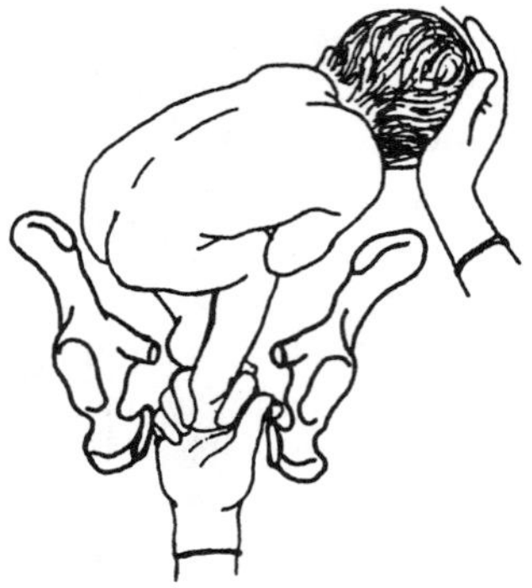

The left foot is gently drawn down; as this happens, the back remains anterior. Note the grip on the foot. Toes should be directed toward the mother's rear.

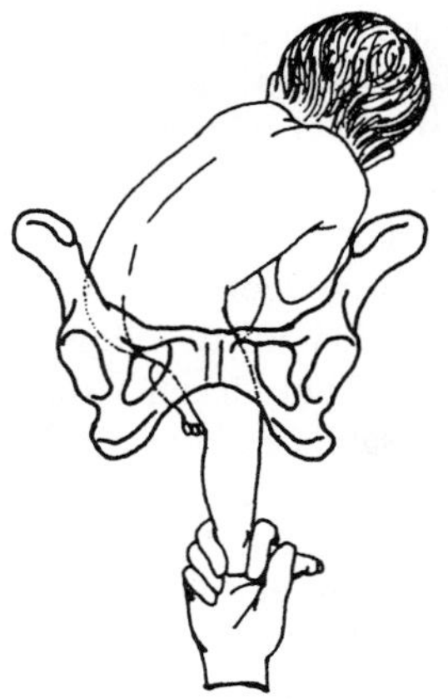

The version is completed as the back assumes a directly anterior orientation.

If internal version remains the best option, even with all the sobering precautions already reviewed in mind, proceed as follows:

1. Obtain the full agreement of the parents. Always discuss the option as well as the feasibility of transport.
2. Have an assistant remain face to face with the mother throughout the version. Sudden movement on the mother's part can result in uterine rupture. Explain this to her before proceeding.
3. Carefully palpate her abdomen to confirm the fetal position and to gently attempt an external version before proceeding with the more risky internal version.
4. Have the mother assume a slight Trendelenburg position by having her lie flat on a firm surface with a folded sheet or blanket under her hips. Although version can be performed with the woman either lying flat in a dorsal position or on her side, it is best to begin with the woman lying supine and tilted; if the version is easy, this position will work well and anatomical relationships will be better visualized.
5. Give the mother the highest dose of homeopathic pulsatilla you have.
6. Talk to the baby. Tell him what you intend to do and what he needs to do to help the process.
7. Which hand you use for internal manipulations will be a matter of personal preference. When the baby is transverse, some texts recommend using the hand whose palm will lie against the breech when in the uterus; when the breech is to *your* left, use your left hand and vice versa. If the baby is more longitudinal, use the hand whose palmar surface will lie against the baby's belly.
8. Don a long-sleeved sterile glove. Generously apply sterile, water-based lubricant.
9. Have someone constantly monitoring the fetal heart. At each step involving fetal manipulation, pause and confirm that the heart rate is good. If it is slow, allow the baby to recover; if recovery doesn't not occur, stop.
10. Massage the introitus and outer birth canal to open it and allow easy admittance of your hand. This will be unnecessary if a first twin has just been born.
11. Shape your fingers into a cone and pass your hand into the yoni. Wait until any strong contractions or expulsive efforts triggered by the introduction of your hand subside before passing your fingertips through the cervix.
12. Rupture the membranes if they are intact and insert your hand inside the bag, rather than against the uterine wall, as this will lessen the chance of infection. Your arm will tend to stop the outward flow of fluid. Have an assistant wrap a towel around your forearm if there is any flow of fluid.
13. Confirm the position of both the baby and the cord. Gently push the cord up above your hand, it will be safer than trapped behind your hand or below it. Take care not to disturb the baby's arms, especially if they are folded over the

chest. Version should be easy; do not proceed if fetal parts are found to be packed together as your hand enters the uterus or if the foot can only be reached with the application of brute force.

14. Slowly and carefully withdraw your hand if you encounter a firm band running around the body of the uterus; such a band is either a well-developed retraction or constriction ring. Further manipulation may injure the uterine wall.
15. Use your external hand to guide and control the motions of your internal hand throughout the version, thus minimizing strain on the uterine wall.
16. Feel which way the baby wants to turn most easily; if one way seems obviously easier, go with that. Depending upon the indication for version, you may attempt to encourage rotation to a cephalic presentation. To do so, go through the same basic movements inside the uterus that you would use abdominally to cup a hand around the head, flex it and bring it toward the pelvis, with guidance from your external hand. If the baby cannot be turned head down, or if you need to get the baby out as rapidly as possible, attempt to bring down a foot. While creating a footling breech is less desirable than a vertex presentation, the baby presumably cannot be born at all in his current position, or you wouldn't be attempting this in the first place. Always go slowly.
17. If you plan to do an immediate extraction, locate both feet and bring them down together, gently directing the baby's toes behind the mother (to the floor if she is supine). If bringing out only one foot, locate the correct limb. Always make sure the limb is not entangled in the cord before you proceed.

    If the baby is transverse with the back anterior: Follow the curve of the lower (or posterior) buttock and thigh until that foot can be grasped. Use your external hand to lift the baby's pelvis to make the leg more accessible.

    If the baby is transverse with the back posterior: Pass your hand over the baby's belly to find the upper hip and leg, aided by your external hand.

    If the baby is transverse with the back superior: Pass your hand up the leg you believe to be the most anterior and confirm that it is attached to the anterior hip.

    If the baby is transverse with the back inferior: Follow the spine down to the sacrum and locate the most posterior buttock and bring that leg down. This is the trickiest of these manipulations because you may have to move the baby to allow room to bring the leg down without injury. Find the posterior thigh, move along to the knee, and press against the back of it to flex the leg, bringing the foot into reach. Now gently nudge the buttocks to the side to make room to bring down the leg, taking care not to move it in an unanatomical direction by working from the hip down as much as possible.

    If the baby is head-down and oblique: Reach for the anterior knee, rather than the foot, because it will usually be lower down and therefore easier to reach. Note that the knee will point downward, while the elbow points up. When the knee is found, press your finger against the back of the knee to flex the leg to the side or hook a finger behind the knee and apply gentle traction to the side. This will flex the knee and bring the foot down across the baby's belly and within reach.
18. If possible, use your external hand to press the foot toward your internal fingers and grasp the foot indicated by the fetal position between the thumb and first two fingers. While grasping the indicated foot is ideal, as a practical matter there may be only one leg you can reach easily. In this case, you should bring down the foot you can grasp and do your best to encourage sacrum anterior rotation as you do so. Do not make a fist to grasp it, as this will unduly strain the lower segment during withdrawal and your sharp knuckles may cause a uterine tear. Bring the foot down very gently. Once the foot is grasped, use your outside hand to push the head up toward the fundus as you bring the foot down. Move slowly and gradually.
19. Should a contraction occur as you are working, flatten your internal hand against the baby's body, making it as small as possible. Make no attempt to move the baby until the contraction is over. Manipulation during contractions will not only be much more difficult for you and painful for the mother; it will also considerably raise the risk of uterine rupture and fetal injury.
20. If you cannot find fetal landmarks with the woman lying flat, have her turn to her side while your hand remains inside. If the baby is oblique, she should lie on the side to which the baby's small parts are directed (the side opposite the baby's back). If the baby is transverse, she should lie on the side of the breech. This should cause the baby's small parts to fall toward your hand. A lateral position also causes the presenting part to fall away from the cervix, making more room for your hand. Prop up her lower hip slightly with a folded sheet or blanket. If the recommended side doesn't make reaching the baby any easier, try having the mother turn to the opposite side.
21. Should an arm prolapse before or during the version, do not attempt to replace it inside the uterus. The act of turning the baby to a breech will naturally draw the arm up along with the torso. In order to keep the arm from being swept

up and above the head as your proceed, use a strip of gauze to apply a clove hitch around the wrist and have an assistant apply gentle tension on the gauze (see next page).

If the other untethered arm should become extended during the version, it will be a simpler matter to deal with one extended arm rather than two. Note that the gauze is merely to encourage the arm not to become extended; if the arm does slip up, do not attempt to pull on the gauze to bring the arm down. This risks major damage to the arm and shoulder; instead proceed as you normally would.

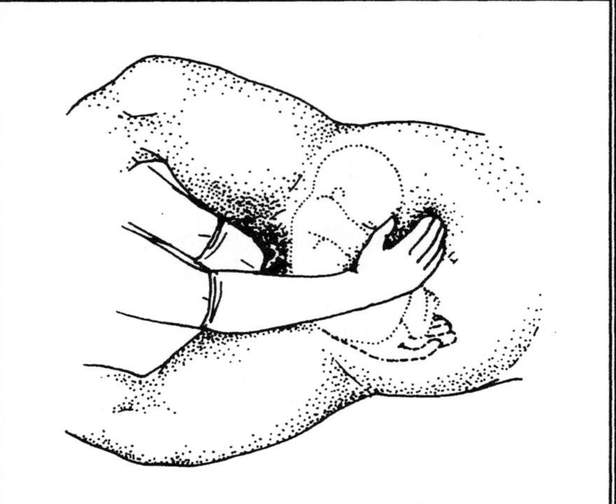

Mother has rolled to her left side to bring the breech into the midwife's hand.

22. Once the leg has successfully been brought through the cervix, confirm that the head has moved into the fundus. It is quite possible to bring a foot to the vulva without dislodging the head from its original position. In this case the baby will be doubled over on himself. Do not pull on the leg any more than is necessary to fix the baby in a breech position. Do not use excessive force; if the baby will not convert to breech, the cause of the delay must be sought. Bringing down one leg leaves the other extended, which allows the breech to form a better dilating wedge as labor proceeds.
23. Check around the lower limbs to see if the cord is there; if so, gently push it upward past the level of the umbilicus before removing your hand.
24. Very slowly withdraw your hand first by flattening it against the baby and then slowly forming your fingers into a cone as you bring them through the cervix. This allows the uterus to gather around the baby as you take your hand out.
25. Once again confirm that the fetal heart rate is normal. It is not uncommon for it to be very slow after the version is completed. Continue to listen; the heart rate will usually return to normal as the baby recovers. Allow the baby to fully stabilize before you proceed with any additional interventions and before the mother arises.

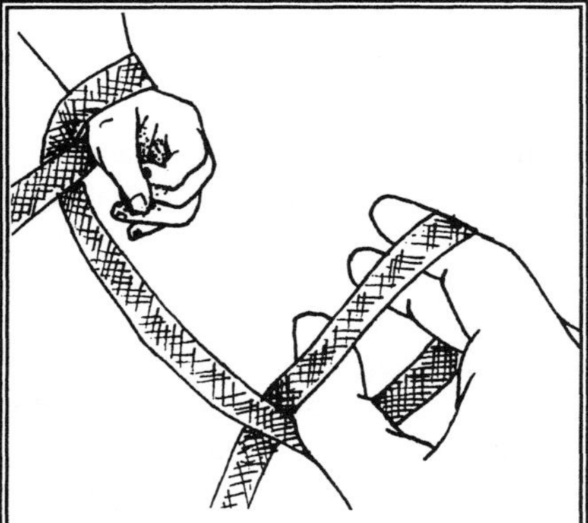

First throw of a clove hitch in place. Midwife preparing to apply second throw.

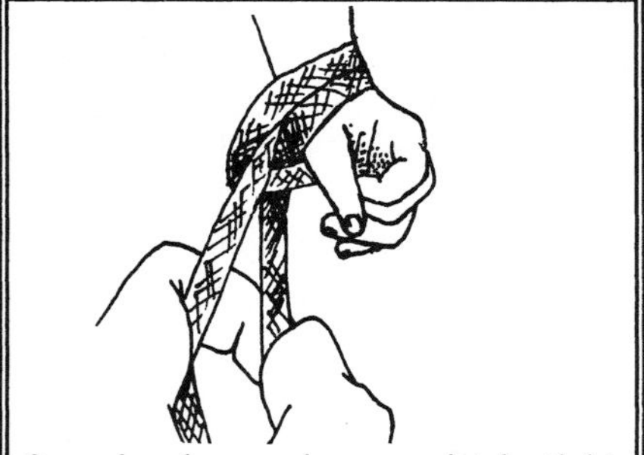

Once in place and appropriately tight, equal traction on both ends will prevent it from pulling taut and constricting the arm.

If version is successful, allow labor to proceed unless you have converted the baby to breech and another indication warrants breech extraction (see the chapter entitled "Assisting at the Birth of a Breech Baby" for instructions regarding breech birth and extraction). Fetal mortality is higher with version and extraction than with version alone.

Bipolar version

Bipolar version is so called because it involves manipulating both ends of the baby at once. It is performed prior to rupture of membranes and before full dilation and requires the cervix only be open enough to admit two fingers. At that point, two fingers are inserted to push the presenting part out of the pelvis, while using your outside hand to help turn the baby around. It was used historically in the management of cord presentation, transverse lie and even marginal placenta previa in those decades when surgical birth was not a very safe option.

Readers experienced in performing internal exams will appreciate that this method is much more difficult to accomplish than external version or internal version; for this reason, it fell out of favor with those who otherwise still practiced other forms of version in the early to mid-1900s. Bipolar version risks rupturing the membranes, and the original indications do not make sense today because of the relative safety of surgical birth. Besides, if the woman is this early in labor, you should have plenty of time to transport, if necessary, unless you are exceedingly remote from medical care.

References and Further Reading on Remedies, Skills and Equipment for Complex Labor Situations

Naturopathic Remedies

Burns E, Blamey C, "4: Soothing scents in childbirth," Internat J Aromatherapy, 6(1);24-28, 1994.

O'Reilly K. Private communication regarding flower essences for birth, Feb, 2002.

Tiran D. Aromatherapy in Midwifery Practice. Baillière Tindall, London UK, 1996.

Weed S. Wise Woman Herbal for the Childbearing Year. Ash Tree Pub, Woodstock NY, 1985.

Traditional Chinese Medicine

Betts D. Acupressure: Promoting A Natural Labour and Partner Involvement. http://home.clear.net.nz/pages/debra_betts/, downloaded Feb 15, 2002.

Deadman P, Al-Khafaji M. A Manual of Acupuncture. Journal of Chinese Medicine Pub, Hove UK, 1998.

Edmonds P. Midwife, Portland, OR, personal conversation, Dec 2003.

Francolini L, LAc. Personal communications, 2002.

Hobbs V. Ancient Medicine–New Tools: Applying Traditional Chinese Medicine to Modern Western Midwifery, unpublished workshop handout, Apprentice Academics Homebirth Conf., Salt Lake City UT, July 1994.

Hobbs V, LAc. Personal communications regarding the use of Chinese medicine during labor, Mar, 2002.

Lowe C, LAc. Personal communications and editing notes, Sept, 2003.

Maciocia G. The Foundations of Chinese Medicine: A Comprehensive Text for Acupuncturists and Herbalists. Churchill Livingstone Inc, Edinburgh UK, 1989.

Maciocia G. Obstetrics and Gynecology in Chinese Medicine. Churchill Livingstone, New York NY, 1998.

Rizack L, Trinidad, U. The "Qi" of the Childbearing Year, unpublished workshop handout, "Moving the Qi/Buying the Herbs," MANA conf., New York NY, Nov 12, 1992.

Skelton IF, Flowerdew MW. "Acupuncture and labour–a summary of results," Midwives Chron, 101(1204);134-137, May, 1988.

West Z. Acupuncture in Pregnancy and Childbirth. Churchill Livingstone, Edinburgh UK, 2001.

Wolfe H. How to Have a Healthy Pregnancy, Healthy Birth with Traditional Chinese Medicine. Blue Poppy Press, Boulder CO, 1993.

Yelland S. Acupuncture in Midwifery. Books for Midwives Press, Hale UK, 1996.

Allopathic Pharmacologic Agents for Treating Uterine Atony

Alliance Pharm. "Syntometrine product characteristics," product information sheet, Wiltshire UK, Jan, 1999.

Altura BM, Altura BT. "Actions of vasopressin, oxytocin, and synthetic analogs on vascular smooth muscle," Fed Proc, 43(1);80-86, Jan, 1984.

Andolina K, et al. "Oral misoprostol is rapidly absorbed in postpartum women at term," J Matern Fetal Neonatal Med, 14(4);229-232, Oct 2003.

Antigen Pharm. "Summary of Product Characteristics: Ergometrine," package insert information, Ireland, 2000.

Bedford Labs. Package insert information and drug characteristics materials supplied on Ergotrate Maleate, rev Mar, 1995.

Buckley S. "Drugs in labor: an overview," Midwifery Today, (71);13-20, 65, 67, Autumn 2004.

Bukowski R, Hankins G."Managing postpartum hemorrhage," Contemp OB/GYN, Sept 1, 2001.

Caliskan E, et al. "Oral misoprostol for the third stage of labor: a randomized controlled trial," Obstet Gynecol, 101(5, Pt 1);921-928, May, 2003.

Day M, Snell B. "Use of prostaglandins for induction of labor," JNM, 38(2S);42S-48S, Mar-Apr, 1993.

Donatini B, et al. "Inadvertent administration of uterotonics to neonates," Lancet, 341(8848);839-840, Mar 27, 1993.

Elbourne D, et al. "Choice of oxytocic preparation for routine use in the management of the third stage of labour: an overview of the evidence from controlled trials," Br J Obstet Gynaecol, 95(1);17-30, Jan, 1988.

Gaskin IM. "The case against Cytotec induction and augmentation," MANA News, XVIII(3);22-24, May, 2000.

Groot A de, et al. "Ergot alkaloids. Current status and review of clinical pharmacology and therapeutic use compared with other oxytocics in obstetrics and gynecology." Drugs, 56(4);522-535, Oct, 1998.

Gulmezoglu A, et al. "Prostaglandins for prevention of postpartum hemorrhage," Cochrane Database Syst Rev, 1;CD000494, 2004.

Haire D, "FDA approved obstetrics drugs: their effects on mother and baby," http://www.AIMSUSA.org, accessed Jan 7, 2004a.

Haire D, "Improving the outcome of pregnancy through science," http://www.AIMSUSA.org, accessed Jan 7, 2004b.

Hardman L, ed. Goodman & Gilman's Pharmacological Basis of Therapeutics, 10th ed, McGraw-Hill, New York, 2001.

Hazardous Substances Databank. Searches for "ergonovine" and "methylergonovine," Jan, 2000.

Hendricks C, Brenner W. "Cardiovascular effects of oxytocic drugs used post partum," Am J Obstet Gynecol, 108(5);751-760, 1970.

Hertog C den, et al. "History and use of oxytocics," Eur J Obset Gynecol Reprod Bio, 94(1);8-12, Jan, 2001.

Hogerzeil H, Walker G. "Instability of (methyl)ergometrine in tropical climates: an overview," Eur J Obstet Gynecol Reprod Biol, 69(1);25-29, Oct, 1996.

Joy S, et al. "Misoprostol use during the third stage of labor," INT J GYNAECOL OBTET, 82(2);143-152, Aug, 2003.
Kelly J, et al., Letter: "Dangers of oxytocin-induced labour to fetuses," BR MED J, 4(5936);101-102, Oct 12, 1974.
Kruse J. "Oxytocin: pharmacology and clinical application," J FAM PRACT, 23(5);473-479, Nov, 1986.
Moir C. "Oxytocic drugs and their use," J OBSTET GYNAECOL BR EMP, 51;247-255, June, 1944.
Morley G. Letter to the editor re Respiratory Distress Syndrome, www.emedicine.com, submitted via e-mail, June, 2002.
Mousa H, Alfirevic Z. "Treatment for primary postpartum hemorrhage," COCHRANE DATABASE SYST REV, 1;CD003249, 2003.
Mrvos R, et al. "Carboprost exposure in a newborn with recovery," J TOXICOL CLIN TOXICOL, 37(7);865-867, 1999.
Munsick R. "The pharmacology and clinical application of various oxytocic drugs," AM J OBSTET GYNECOL, 93;442-463, Oct 1, 1965.
Norris R, et al., eds. AN AMERICAN TEXT-BOOK OF OBSTETRICS FOR PRACTITIONERS AND STUDENTS. WB Saunders, Philadelphia, 1895.
Novartis Pharm. Methergine injection and tablets package insert information, E. Hanover NJ, 2001.
O'Grady J. Section IV: "Neurologic Conditions," Chap. 29: "Water Intoxication," in O'Grady J, Buckman R. OBSTETRIC SYNDROMES AND CONDITIONS. Parthenon Pub Group, New York NY, 1998.
Olin B, III, ed. DRUG FACTS AND COMPARISONS 1991. JB Lippincott, St. Louis MO, 1990.
Parfitt K. MARTINDALE: THE COMPLETE DRUG REFERENCE, 32nd ed. Pharmaceutical Press, London UK, 1999.
Payton R, Brucker M. "Drugs and uterine motility," JOGNN, 28(6);628-638, Nov-Dec, 1999.
Pharmacia & Upjohn. Hemabate package insert information, Kalamazoo MI, rev 1999.
PHYSICIAN'S DESK REFERENCE (PDR), 54th ed. Medical Economics Co, Montvale NJ, 2000.
Plaut M, et al. "Uterine rupture associated with the use of misoprostol in the gravid patient with a previous cesarean section," AM J OBSTET GYNECOL, 180(6 Pt 1);1535-1542, June, 1999.
Pozner J, R. Ph. Personal communications, Apr, 2002-Feb, 2004.
Schellenberg JC. "Primary postpartum hemorrhage," Dept Obstet Gynecol, Geneva U Hospital, web pub, Sept 29, 1999.
Schuurmans N, et al. "Prevention and management of postpartum hemorrhage," SOGC Clinical Practice Guidelines, J SOGC (88), Apr, 2000.
Sultatos L. "Mechanisms of drugs that affect uterine motility," JNM, 42(4);367-370, July-Aug, 1997.
Titus P. THE MANAGEMENT OF OBSTETRIC DIFFICULTIES, 4th ed. CV Mosby Co, St. Louis MO, 1950.
Weis R, et al. "Cardiovascular effects of oxytocin," OBSTET GYNECOL, 46(2);211-214, Aug, 1975.
Williams J. OBSTETRICS: A TEXTBOOK FOR THE USE OF STUDENTS AND PRACTITIONERS, 6th ed. D Appleton & Co, New York, 1930.
Wingeier R, Griggs R. "Management of retained placenta using intraumbilical oxytocin injection," JNM, 36(4);240-244, July-Aug, 1991.

REFERENCES USED FOR THE CHAPTERS ENTITLED URINARY CATHETERIZATION AND CLEANSING AND RETENTION ENEMAS

Elkin M, et al. NURSING INTERVENTIONS AND CLINICAL SKILLS, 2nd ed. Mosby Inc, St. Louis MO, 2000.
Lewis L. FUNDAMENTAL SKILLS IN PATIENT CARE. Lippincott, Philadephia PA, 1976.
Timby B. CLINICAL NURSING PROCEDURES. JB Lippincott, Philadelphia PA, 1989.
Weed S. WISE WOMAN HERBAL FOR THE CHILDBEARING YEAR, Ash Tree Pub, Woodstock NY, 1985.

HYPODERMIC INJECTIONS

Anton S. "Safer handling of medications–a cautionary tale," NARM NEWS, Winder, VI(1);15, 2003.
Elkin M, et al. NURSING INTERVENTIONS AND CLINICAL SKILLS, 2nd ed. Mosby Inc, St. Louis MO, 2000.
Hahn K. "Brush up on your injection technique," NURSING, 20(9);54-58, Sept, 1990: erratum in NURSING 21(1);6, Jan, 1991.
Lewis L. FUNDAMENTAL SKILLS IN PATIENT CARE. Lippincott, Philadelphia PA, 1976.
Poznar J. PHARMACOLOGY FOR MIDWIVES, 2nd ed. Bellpine Pub, Monroe OR, 2002.
Timby B. CLINICAL NURSING PROCEDURES. JB Lippincott, Philadelphia PA, 1989.

STERILE WATER INJECTIONS FOR THE RELIEF OF EXCESSIVE LOCALIZED PAIN

Ader L, et al. "Parturition pain treated by intracutaneous injections of sterile water," PAIN, 41(2);133-138, May, 1990.
Hobbs V. LAc, Personal communications, 2002.
Kurokawa J, Gentry C, Welsh G. "Sterile Water Papules." Proceedings from the Annual Meeting of the ACNM, San Francisco, 1998.
Melzack R. "Prolonged relief of pain by brief, intense transcutaneous somatic stimulation," PAIN, 1(4);357-373, Dec, 1975.
Reynolds J. "Intracutaneous sterile water for back pain in labour," CAN FAM PHYS, 40;1785-1788, 1791-1792, Oct, 1994.
Trolle B, et al. "The effect of sterile water blocks on low back labor pain," AM J OBSTET GYNECOL, 164(5 Pt 1);1277-1281, 1991.
Welsh G, CNM, Portland OR. STERILE WATER PAPULES FOR THE RELIEF OF PAIN IN LABOR. VHS video, 1998.

THE TENS UNIT

Davies R. Chapter 10: "Transcutaneous electrical nerve stimulation." in Moore S, ed. UNDERSTANDING PAIN AND ITS RELIEF IN LABOR, Churchill Livingstone, New York, NY 1997.

Oxygen Delivery Devices and Resuscitation Equipment

American Red Cross. Oxygen Administration. Mosby Lifeline, St. Louis MO, 1993.

Egan D. Fundamentals of Respiratory Therapy, 2nd ed. CV Mosby Co, St. Louis MO, 1973.

James P. Presentation on retinopathy of prematurity and the role of oxygen therapy at the 3rd European Paediatric Neurology Society, Nice, France, Nov 7-10, 1999. Cited in Stoller K. "Oxygen therapy: 50 years of ignorance," http//www.pediatrics.or /cgi/eletters /110/3/615#337, accessed Sept 16, 2003.

Kacmarek R, et al. The Essentials of Respiratory Therapy, 2nd ed. Year Book Medical, Inc, Chicago IL, 1985.

McPherson S. Respiratory Therapy Equipment. CV Mosby Co, St. Louis MO, 1977.

Morley G. Personal e-mail communications, 2002.

Sanders M. Mosby's Paramedic Textbook. Mosby Lifeline, St. Louis MO, 1994.

Sassoon C, McGovern J. Section VII: "Pulmonary," Chapter 120: "Oxygenation strategy," in Grenvik A, sr. ed., Textbook of Critical Care, 4th ed. WB Saunders, Philadelphia PA, 2000.

Schneider K, neonatal respiratory therapist. Personal communications, 1999-2000.

Stoller K. "Oxygen therapy: 50 years of ignorance," http://www.pediatrics.org/cgi/eletters/110/3/615#337, accessed Sept 16, 2003.

Strange K, CPM, instructor neonatal resuscitation for midwives. Personal communications, 2002.

Tiep B. Portable Oxygen Therapy: Including Oxygen Conserving Methodology. Futura Pub Co, Mt. Kisco NY, 1991.

Zaruby J. Colorado Altitude Training. E-mail communications, notes on barometric pressure and altitude physiology, Feb, 2004.

Intravenous Equipment and IV Therapy

Carlson RW, et al. "Fluid resuscitation in conditions of increased permeability," Anesth Rev, 17(S 3);12, 1990.

Clark S, et al., eds. Critical Care Obstetrics, 3rd ed. Blackwell Science, Malden MA, 1997.

Cunningham F, et al. Williams Obstetrics, 20th ed. Appleton & Lange, Stamford CT, 1997.

Elkin M, et al. Nursing Interventions and Clinical Skills, 2nd ed. Mosby Inc, St. Louis MO, 2000.

Garcia L. Editing notes, 2002.

Gilmore E. Personal conversation, MANA conf., Austin TX, Nov 2, 2003.

Hankins J, et al. Infusion Therapy in Clinical Practice, 2nd ed. WB Saunders Co, St. Louis MO, 2001.

Hayes K. "IV fluids in midwifery practice," Birth Gazette, 14(1);43-45, Winter, 1998.

Healey M, et al. "Lactated Ringer's is superior to normal saline in a model of massive hemorrhage resuscitation," J Trauma–Injury Infect Crit Care, 45(5);894-898, 1998.

Keppler A. "The use of intravenous fluids during labor," Birth, 15(2);75-79, June, 1988.

Kwan I, et al, eds. "Timing and volume of fluid administration for patients with bleeding following trauma," Cochrane Database Syst Review, (1);CD002245, 2001.

Lowery B, et al. "Electrolyte solutions in resuscitation in human hemorrhagic shock," Surg Gynecol Obstet, 133(2);273-284, Aug, 1971.

Marshall M, Buffington S. Life-Saving Skills Manual for Midwives: Module 7: Prevention and Management of Sepsis, Module 8: Hydration and Rehydration, 3rd ed. American College of Nurse-Midwives, Washington DC, 1998.

Newton, N et al. "Psychologic, physical, nutritional and technologic aspects of intravenous infusion during labor," BIRTH, 15(2)67-72, 1988.

Oxorn H. Oxorn-Foote Human Labor and Birth, 5th ed. Appleton-Century-Crofts, Norwalk CT, 1986.

Perry A, Potter P. Pocket Guide Basic Skills and Procedures, 3rd ed. Mosby, St. Louis MO, 1994.

Poznar J. Pharmacology for Midwives, 2nd ed. Privately printed, Monroe OR, 2002.

Smith S, Duell D. Clinical Nursing Skills, 4th ed. Appleton & Lange, Stamford CT, 1996.

Trudnowski R, et al. "Effect of Ringer's lactate solution and sodium bicarbonate on surgical acidosis," Surg Gynecol Obstet, 125(4);807-814, Oct, 1967.

Resuscitating The Mother

Jevon P, Raby M. Resuscitation in Pregnancy: A Practical Approach. Books for Midwives, Oxford UK, 2001.

Opening the Pelvis (or the Midwife's Forceps)

Daniels S. Lecture notes, The Maternity Center midwifery training program. Fall, 1978.

Davis E. Heart and Hands: A Midwife's Guide to Pregnancy and Birth, 3rd ed. Celestial Arts, Berkeley CA, 1997.

Hobbs V. Five-day midwifery skills workshop, Informed Homebirth, 1982.

Gaskin IM, Personal conversation, 1998.

Koehler N. Artemis Speaks: VBAC Stories and Natural Childbirth Information, Nan Ullrike Koehler, Sebastopol CA, 1985.

Scholles H. Editing notes, 2000.

Fundal Pressure

Cosner K: "Use of fundal pressure during second-stage labor: a pilot study," JNM, 41(4);334-337, July-Aug, 1996.

Kline-Kaye V, Miller-Slade, D. "The use of fundal pressure during the second stage of labor," JOGNN, 19(6);511-517, Nov-Dec, 1990.
Penney D, Perlis D. "Shoulder dystocia: when to use suprapubic or fundal pressure," MCN, 17(1); 34-36, Jan-Feb, 1992.

THE USE OF VERSION DURING LABOR

Bland P, Montgomery T. PRACTICAL OBSTETRICS, 3rd ed. FA Davis Co., Philadelphia PA, 1939.
Chauhan S, et al., "Delivery of the nonvertex second twin: breech extraction versus external cephalic version." AM J OBTET GYNECOL, 173(4);1015-1020, Oct 1995.
De Lee J. PRINCIPLES AND PRACTICE OF OBSTETRICS, 3rd ed. WB Saunders Co., Philadelphia PA, 1918.
Eden T, Holland E. A MANUAL OF MIDWIFERY, 7th ed. J & A Churchill, London UK, 1931.
Hirst B. A TEXTBOOK OF OBSTETRICS, 8th ed., W B Saunders Co. Philadelphia PA, 1918.
Kerr J. OPERATIVE MIDWIFERY, 3rd ed. William, Wood & Co, New York NY, 1916.
Løvset J. VAGINAL OPERATIVE DELIVERY, Scandinavian University Books, Oslo Norway, 1968.
Mayes B. A TEXTBOOK OF OBSTETRICS. Australasian Pub. Co., Sydney Australia, 1959.
Potter I. THE PLACE OF VERSION IN OBSTETRICS. CV Mosby Co, St Louis MO, 1922.
Shears G, Williams P, eds. OBSTETRICS: NORMAL AND OPERATIVE, JB Lippincott Co, Philadelphia PA, 1920.
Wigand JH. "Uber Wendugn durch äussere Handgriffe," (On an external manipulation whereby, in labor, the malposition of the fetus can be corrected), HAMB MED MAG, 1;52, 1807.

MIDWIFING WOMEN THROUGH UNCOMMON OR CHALLENGING LABOR SITUATIONS

WORKING WITH COMPLEX LABORS

Any type of delay in labor is referred to as dystocia, which literally means "difficult childbirth." You may be called upon to use all your creative resources when a woman has a particularly unusual, long or hard labor, such as one that is made difficult by a problematic fetal position. Difficult labors will challenge you to be there for the *woman*, not for your own agenda or for proving yourself as a midwife. This means that, while all the knowledge and experience you bring to the birth are exceedingly valuable, the mother and her process should be the focal point of your attention. Not every challenging labor presents increased risks for the mother and baby, but some will do so. Therefore, you need to do some soul-searching regarding your beliefs about such situations and your role as a midwife in relationship to them to adequately and safely help women traverse difficult or unusual labor and postpartum situations.

Beliefs about care

Examine your strongest beliefs about your role and obligation as a midwife. Be honest. You might be surprised by what comes up. For example, you may discover that you hold one or more of the following beliefs:

- A competent midwife is able to handle all complications and emergencies.
- A competent midwife should always know what is going on.
- A competent midwife can completely trust her own clinical judgement.
- A compassionate midwife always acquiesces to the parents' wishes.
- A competent midwife never transports.
- A competent midwife never has a mother or baby die under her care.
- A competent midwife transports at the first hint of a problem.
- Birth is normal and natural, therefore problems should be allowed to fully develop before transport is considered.

Most of these beliefs reflect overconfidence, lack of healthy boundaries and magical thinking. If such beliefs are clouding the picture, it can be very difficult to proceed appropriately when a problem arises. You may punish yourself for being unsure in certain circumstances. Your inner critic may work overtime to instill a sense of failure when you finally realize you are in over your head. Your need for self-sufficiency may lead you to keep women at home beyond the point when you should have transported, thereby increasing the risk for all concerned. Furthermore, these kinds of beliefs can make it hard to tell when you are imagining a problem to be worse than it is. A belief that transport should occur at the first sign of a stormy labor is a disservice to the woman who wants to stay at home as long as it is safe and reasonable, to do so and may reflect your own unresolved fears about birth. Such beliefs may be unconsciously influencing your choices and decisions. It is important for you to bring them to consciousness so that the underlying feelings behind them can be dealt with and you can replace them with beliefs about birth that are more realistic. Beliefs that work better for everyone might include the following:

- As a midwife, I support each woman to have the most healthy and healing birth experience possible.
- As a midwife, I remember that what is most heathy and healing is different for every woman and may differ from what might be so for me.
- As a midwife, I need to recognize variations that require care I cannot provide in a home or birth-center setting and to deal with them appropriately by providing physical, emotional and mental support to the best of my ability while transporting to the hospital.
- As a midwife, I must understand that birth, by its very nature, cannot be completely known or predicted.
- As a midwife, I should have appropriate and healthy professional limitations and boundaries regarding the types of situations I am willing and competent to handle.
- As a midwife, I cannot control whether someone lives or dies. I can control only how I prepare myself to take on the responsibility of being a primary attendant and how I respond to the situation in the moment.
- Birth is a powerful event that requires a healthy respect.

Working with the parents

The parents' reaction: Each woman brings to her birthing experience a unique history and perspective that impact her approach and relationship to the birth process. Most likely, you will have developed during prenatal care a relationship with the mother in which you have learned something about her beliefs and desires for this birth, her fears, her hopes, her level of trust in her body and the birth process itself, as well as her previous history. You will have discussed responsibility taking and informed decision making. However, none of these really indicate with certainty how a woman (or her family) will respond to a difficult birth situation or a life-threatening emergency. In addition, you cannot control their response. You can carry with you what you have learned about the woman and her family during prenatals, take appropriate action and support the woman or couple as the birth process unfolds. For those parents who are less trusting of the natural process, it is often wise to have a policy of transporting sooner for variations that pose potential risk but that you might otherwise keep at home.

Keeping the parents informed: When faced with a complex labor situation, it is important to give the parents realistic markers along the way that honestly communicate your sense of how the birth is going, to periodically reassess what is working and what isn't, and to review options, always including hospital transport as a possible course of action. It is very important to communicate honestly and clearly with the parents regarding your experience with their type of labor. Most parents highly respect and trust a practitioner who is scrupulously honest about her experience and her limits. Be sure to let the parents know that a normal outcome is possible if you have seen a labor similar to this one that was completed successfully at home. Conversely, be honest if you have never seen a successful homebirth under similar circumstances.

In the midwifery model of care, parents and midwife work as partners in the decision-making process. It is therefore imperative for the midwife to provide complete information for the parents regarding the situation at hand. This includes a review of the status of both mother and baby, an assessment of labor progress, options available at home, and how the situation might be handled in a medical setting. For example, a midwife assisting a woman whose labor has stalled might say, "I have never seen a woman stay at one dilation for so long before. The medical model expects women to progress at least 1 cm every hour or so, although this is a very artificial standard based only on the most common pattern and does not recognize a broad range of what is normal among individuals. Other experienced homebirth midwives have documented that everything can be okay when women dilate much more slowly than that. You seem fine, you're resting and eating, the baby seems fine, heart tones are good and fetal movement is normal, the amniotic fluid is clear, and we know you are Group-B strep negative. Your labor seems to be slow because of the following factors (tell her whatever you know about that might be causing the delay, for example, that surgery left scars on the right side of her cervix). How are you feeling about being at home? (Give her time to reflect on this and give you an answer.) It is my sense that there is no urgency to transport at this point. We could try these things first (then run down the list of options that have not yet been tried). If we went to the hospital right now, these are the probable things they would do (explain these)." Information presented in such a manner allows the parents to make informed decisions and to examine their own level of commitment to homebirth.

A midwife should not sit and worry in silence and wait until a crisis has developed before informing the parents that their labor appears to be headed for trouble. Parents should be informed as questions arise without the concerns being presented as a full-scale crisis. They need to know what the midwife suspects as the situation unfolds so they can fully participate in any decisions that need to be made. Outline as clearly as possible what you suspect is going on, what further information might be gathered from a more thorough exam and what that exam would entail, including maternal positioning and the degree of discomfort. Findings should be explained, along with the degree of potential risk involved for both the mother and baby, and what, if anything, can be done or needs to happen in the natural course of labor to correct the problem. Hospital transport should be discussed whenever a situation poses a potentially serious risk.

Continued monitoring should then clarify whether the problem will right itself. The mother's intuition about the situation is an important parameter to consider as well. The parents also need continuous communication from you regarding how the situation is changing, for better or worse. It is perfectly acceptable to say that you have no idea what your findings may indicate.

In addition to understanding any potential medical risks to the mother or baby, it is important for parents to be informed when the parameters of labor are getting outside the bounds of the local standard of care or outside the legal regulations for midwives. An example of this is prolonged prelabor rupture of membranes with no history of a negative group B strep culture (that the parents previously refused via informed consent) and no history of antibiotic use during labor (that the parents have also refused). If the transport hospital is unknown to you or if it has an established reputation for hostility toward homebirth transports, they should be prepared for this possibility as well. They also need to understand how their choice may impact your continued ability to practice. In addition, the midwife needs to weigh the risk that parents may later claim they were encouraged to remain at home with a high-risk labor, which may occur if the labor results in significant morbidity or mortality for the baby or mother.

Following the mother's intuition: You may be faced with a circumstance that suggests a problem but in which the clinical picture is uncertain. In these cases, the mother can often, without contemplation, give a direct answer that everything is fine. Using the mother's clear intuitive impression as a guide is the most reliable in cases in which there has been full continuity of care during the prenatal period and the midwife knows the woman well. If the mother is not clear, you must follow your own experiential, intuitive and clinical cues regarding what might be going on and the appropriateness of intervention at home versus transport to the hospital. Do not rely upon the intuitive opinion of a woman who has not been completely honest prenatally.

If the parents request transport: Occasionally, in the throes of a hard but otherwise perfectly normal labor, a woman will request to be taken to the hospital for drugs. (Most often, in women who have chosen homebirth, they just want the baby to hurry up and be born.) Explain to her that hard labor is something from which almost every mother wants to escape at some point, and it is normal to feel that drugs might make things better. She should be reminded that she will have to continue her labor at the hospital, that drugs will reach her baby and affect her labor, and that they may lead to adverse side-effects as well as further interventions. She should be told that if she really wants to go, that is an option. Women will usually change their minds and not wish to go to the hospital.

However, if the labor has stepped outside of average parameters–that is, if it is prolonged, there are signs (such as meconium staining) that point to potential complications, or the mother is unable to cope with the sensations of labor any longer–her requests to be taken to the hospital should be seriously considered. Explain what is likely to happen there and what your experience has been in the past with similar labors, then offer an honest assessment of how the mother is doing. Tell her that transport is perfectly acceptable if that is what she feels is best. It is very important not to make her feel ashamed of her choices or her sense of what is best for her. Not only is this highly inappropriate, but it invites trouble later because women will remember negative comments, especially if the outcome of the birth is somehow disappointing.

When you feel transport is advised and the parents are reluctant: General parameters of care, attitudes about labor complications, and the types of situations that are likely to result in transport should be addressed prenatally. Those discussions help weed out parents who want a more or less conservative approach than your own.

In many ways, parental refusal to transport presents a much bigger problem than a request for transport. You will need to explain in no uncertain terms that the parameters of labor now exceed what you feel comfortable handling at home and that hospital transport is necessary. You need to be clear whether you are suggesting transport for purely political reasons (for example, the case has moved entirely outside the scope of your licensing regulations), for both political and medical reasons (it is a breech presentation during a very slow labor with a big baby when it is outside licensing regulations to do nonemergency breeches at home) or for overwhelmingly medical reasons (the woman is hemorrhaging and nowhere near delivery, putting both herself and the baby in jeopardy).

A midwife must do some soul-searching regarding situations in which parents refuse transport, especially if such cases arise frequently in your practice. Are you transporting because it is truly warranted, because of your own fears regarding birth, because of a lack of faith in birth at home, or because of a lack of experience and training? Have you been unclear in explaining to the parents why they need to transport? Are you feeling conflicted because you don't agree with a midwifery regulation that requires transport? (This will pull in clients that reflect your ambivalence.) Parents may state that they do understand the risks and are willing to take the risks at home. Depending upon your skill level, the legal situation and the relative risks involved, you may be able to allow the parents to sign an informed consent agreement to stay at home. This statement should indicate the complication involved and preferably outline the potential risks as described to the parents (ideally written by one of the them in their own words) prior to signing and dating the document.

For example, perhaps a breech presentation is discovered when you arrive at the home, and everything points to an easy and straightforward birth. However, protocols with the regional government state that you cannot attend non-emergency breeches at home but do offer provision for parents to refuse care; leaving them to fend for themselves would constitute professional abandonment. In such cases, an informed consent document could be employed. It is possible that this birth will proceed without any hitches; however, you must consider your position if everything doesn't turn out well. Having solidly committed parents is a must in these situations.

A midwife must be scrupulously careful not to seem to lead parents toward a particular decision or point of view when on shaky legal ground (i.e., practicing outside state protocols), even if she feels a birth is likely to proceed without any problems. This is especially true if there is any question about her relationship with the parents, and she must later defend the choice to remain at home.

Dealing with partners, relatives and friends during complex labors

Relatives and friends who have been invited to the birth can either be wonderfully helpful or very problematic during difficult labors. Most of the time, these people have little or no reference for the parameters of normal that can occur during any labor, and are even more ill equipped to handle the notion of staying home in the face of a problem. Naturally, they will refer to their own birth experiences, and those of their acquaintances, when trying to decide if the way you are midwifing the situation is appropriate. While your relationship with the parents may be solid, the reactions of the others present must be taken into account when you are proposing to push the limits regarding staying at home in certain situations. This is because well-meaning but poorly informed attendees can decide that what you are doing is inappropriate and report you to regulatory authorities. They may also convince the parents that they should report you as well, especially if the outcome of the birth is undesirable. Therefore, you must be very clear with the parents regarding how things are going as well as with those others present; explain things to them in simple language, ask if they have concerns, tell them explicitly why you believe staying at home at this point is still appropriate. It is prudent to ask others to leave for a period of time to see if this will effect the labor for better or worse.

It is even more serious if the woman's partner has been equivocal about the decision to stay home in the first place. A problem can push these folks right over the edge, and if an undesirable outcome occurs, they are very likely to blame you. Therefore, the relationship dynamics with all present must be constantly considered as you walk the fine line of what to do and when to recommend transport.

Consulting with other practitioners

Practitioners working in a hospital will often call upon others for advice when a situation they haven't seen before arises. It is possible for the homebirth midwife to do the same. It is a good policy to carry an address book with the names and numbers of other experienced midwives who can be called upon for assistance. Prior to calling, let the parents know whom you plan to call, your knowledge of or relationship to her, her background and experience level and if you are aware that she has handled similar labors herself. As much information as possible about the labor and the labor record should be on hand as well as paper and pen to write down suggestions. Remember to respect the confidentiality of your client by leaving out names and other identifying information unless the parents give written permission to divulge it.

You might also consider calling a friendly doctor or nurse-midwife, if there is one available who will not automatically suggest hospital transport. A practitioner who also attends home or birthing-center births is often the most open to exploring ways to continue the labor at home.

It is only common courtesy to call and let her know the outcome of the birth whenever you have consulted with another practitioner. This allows her to mentally complete the process and provides more information about the effectiveness of the suggestions offered, and builds a relationship where she will feel comfortable providing this service in the future.

Coping with Critical Emergencies in Labor: Some Basics

Problems that arise in labor can often be anticipated and either averted or resolved before a crisis ensues. However, this is not always the case. There are times when a critical or life-threatening emergency develops without warning. This chapter covers some primary things to remember whenever a critical emergency requires quick action and clear thinking.

Stay calm

The first step when faced with an unexpected emergency is to take a deep belly breath, center yourself and remain calm. All this takes only a second or two; however, your presence of mind is vital to rational decision making and careful performance of any necessary physical maneuvers. A frantic mental attitude and hasty handling performed without regard for the particular situation is ill advised and most likely to result in damage to the baby or mother.

Know your options

Many techniques that midwives have found successful in dealing with a variety of difficult situations are included in this section. As the severity of a situation increases, so does the amount of intervention and, in some cases, the amount of invasive maneuvering necessary to deal with it. No series of techniques will work in every case; therefore, it is important to be familiar with many different options. In addition, intimate familiarity with the variations in fetal descent and the signs and symptoms of critical maternal emergencies is critical. This combination of knowledge and skill will help you to stay calm, knowing that you have a good understanding of the anatomy involved and a broad repertoire of resources to deal with the situation.

Sometimes a maternal, fetal or neonatal problem may occur that is so rare that you don't know what is going on, only that a critical problem has arisen. In such a case, if the mother is still in labor, transport immediately. If the fetus is in trouble, transport with the mother positioned to maintain as optimal a fetal heart rate as possible. A newborn with unidentifiable distress should be stabilized to the best of your ability and transported without delay.

Being prepared: the reality of your practice location: If you practice in a remote or difficult-to-access location, part of knowing your options is being ready to step in and provide a broader range of and more ongoing emergency care than midwives practicing in urban, industrialized areas. This text aims at helping you do just that. You and all your assistants should take classes in advanced first aid or basic paramedic training to learn how to lift and carry a woman should she require transport and be unable to walk; a folding stretcher and any other helpful devices that you learn of in classes should be part of your basic birth equipment.

Calling time and keeping records

During an emergency having an assistant is much more than just a convenience. Your assistant should call time every 30 seconds to a minute or so during a maternal crisis (such as rapid blood loss) and every 15 to 30 seconds during a birth or neonatal crisis, as well as take notes in the chart. Time has a way of lengthening during a crisis. Calling time will help you know how long you have been dealing with the crisis and how long you have attempted to remedy the problem with a specific technique. In addition, the time table in the chart notes will provide valuable information later as you critique the birth.

The chances of a subsequent lawsuit are increased when a complication develops. Although lawsuits of any kind are rare in midwifery practices, completing a detailed record as soon as possible after the crisis has passed will help tremendously if any questions about the birth are raised in the future.

Be scrupulously careful to record exactly what you did. The midwife who actually handled the emergency should be the one to chart it and should not rely on anyone else to do this for her. If you write "screw maneuver of Wood" to say how you handled a shoulder dystocia, it will be assumed that is what you did, even though you may later try to explain that you actually used the praying hands maneuver. If you used a technique that you have never seen written anywhere, describe exactly what you did instead of imprecisely calling it a maneuver that has an established name. (See the chapter entitled "Record-Keeping during Labor" for more details on charting during unforeseen emergencies.)

When Transport Is Necessary during Labor

The decision to transport is always disappointing to the midwife as well as to the parents. However, the ability to judge when transport is warranted in a timely manner is an essential skill.

Considerations regarding transport

Your experience level: If in doubt about a problem that could have serious consequences, transport. Regardless of the reason, if you feel unsure of the situation, you are almost always better off seeking outside help. If you are inexperienced, what constitutes a necessary transport today may not be the same 200 births down the road. This is nothing to be ashamed of or embarrassed about; you are practicing responsibly to the best of your continuously evolving abilities. Transport will hone your skills by enabling you to compare your own perceptions of what was going on with how things turn out in the hospital. It allows you to observe the interventions used at the hospital to complete the birth as well.

When to transport: Transport should be considered whenever the suggestions you have offered are not working to restore a progressive labor pattern and the mother is headed toward exhaustion due to an inability to rest, eat, drink or eliminate. Early transport is your best and most responsible option when the baby shows signs of compromise. It should also be considered when the progress of labor is not straightforward and the parents are becoming afraid or shaky about their commitment to homebirth, or when you have no more tricks up your sleeve and the midwives you call for suggestions have nothing new to offer. It is always best to transport when the mother and baby are still in good condition. Suspecting trouble but waiting until a concerning situation transforms into an emergency is always a bad idea and will quickly build you a less-than-welcome reputation in your medical community.

Another important aspect of when to transfer has to do with the shift changes at the hospital. If it is a nonemergent transport, you may be able to wait to transfer until a shift change is imminent, thus ensuring the mother of some degree of continuity of care once you arrive. Shifts typically change at 7 am, 3 pm and 11 pm. Arriving for the night shift (11 pm to 7 am) usually means there are fewer staff members on hand. This can be good if the woman is having a prolonged labor and may be bad if it is a dire emergency. Arriving at the end of a shift can mean the woman will fall victim to the tendency of one shift to try and "clean the board" before the next shift comes on. That is, they try to get all the women to deliver before they leave. This can be very bad for a woman who just needs more time and an IV.

Suspected fetal demise: If you believe the fetus has died once labor begins, you must transport to confirm the death. If, once this is accomplished, the parents wish to sign out against medical advice and return home to have the baby, that can be dealt with once transport has occurred, if your jurisdiction looks favorably on such choices. Transport is important to document the demise, to confirm that the baby is, indeed, dead (which it may not be) and to cover yourself in case of future legal action.

Emergent versus nonemergent transport: Fortunately, the need to transport does not always equal a catastrophic emergency. In fact, the overall national average for homebirth transports in the United States is about 11%, with only about 3% of those being considered true emergencies by the attending midwife. Nonemergency transports run the gamut and essentially include any labor that cannot be completed at home for reasons such as maternal exhaustion, a poor contraction pattern, prolonged labor, parental desire to go to the hospital and lack of fetal descent with effective pushing. None of these constitute emergencies unless the situation has been sorely neglected or the baby is compromised.

Only rarely will you be suggesting transport "out of nowhere," with no warning signs suggesting the possible need to go in. In such a case, the need to transport usually arises out of the presentation of an emergency for which you may have no explanation. For example, labor is going along fine, but suddenly fetal heart tones take a nose dive and do not recover; the mother starts losing lots of blood for no apparent reason and birth is not imminent; or the mother's condition suddenly becomes unstable with no obvious cause. These are the types of rare emergencies that prompt you to say, "We're going to the hospital *now*."

Choosing to use a private car, ambulance or specialized transport service: The first order of business is to decide if you need to call an ambulance or if a private car can be used to carry the mother or baby to the hospital. Hopefully, your local ambulance services are midwife friendly. In some cases, it just makes sense to call an ambulance. If you are transporting a severely compromised mother or baby, going in a private car may entail more risk because private vehicles are not recognized by other drivers as emergency vehicles. Driving yourself raises your liability risk considerably should an accident occur and also means you cannot (or can less effectively) monitor the mother en route. Having a frightened or nervous father or a relative drive in a crisis raises the risk of an accident. Therefore, emergencies are ideally handled by a skilled ambulance service. If the baby is in trouble, find out if there is a neonatal transport unit from the nearest Level III or IV hospital. They will be able to most skillfully provide a high level of support in a complex transport situation. Those situations where a professional transport service is best generally include the following complications:

- The mother is seizing or at risk for seizing.
- The mother has bled, is bleeding or is at great risk of bleeding and may go into shock or is already in shock
- Cord prolapse has occurred and the mother needs to be moved in a specific position to keep the cord pulsing. This is especially important if you have no vehicles that would allow the mother to assume the position that best enhances cord blood flow or if she needs to be moved from the house to the vehicle in a certain position. There must also be room in the transport vehicle for the midwife to remain with the mother, monitoring the baby and holding the presenting part off the cord with one hand up the yoni.
- Any other situation that requires maternal care, positioning or both that cannot be accomplished safely and successfully in the vehicles at your disposal.
- The baby is in a respiratory or other physiologic crisis that requires ongoing attention en route.

If the situation is not emergent, transport in a private vehicle if it is feasible and acceptable to all concerned. You can go to the hospital immediately and do not have to wait and (potentially) hassle with ambulance attendants. Record the time of your decision to go in and time of departure. Be aware that there may be times when you believe that transport in a private car is a safe and reasonable choice but the hospital staff disagrees: if you are legal, it is prudent to ask the attending obstetrician for her opinion on whether to transport by ambulance or private car. If a private vehicle is chosen, you might still be liable for suggesting it; car; thus you are better off transporting in the parents' car and having a person of their choice do the driving. If private transport is unacceptable or undesirable, wait for an ambulance to arrive.

These recommendations change if you are working in a state where midwifery is still illegal. Then, you must scope out the attitudes of the local medical community. If it is hostile, transport by private car is usually the best option, unless the mother or baby will be in grave danger unless an ambulance is used. Get advice from other local midwives.

Facility Designation by Level of Obstetric & Neonatal Services in the United States			
Level	**Obstetric services (Providers on staff)**	**Neonatal services**	**Transport scenario**
I	Cares for all laboring women; triages high-risk labors for transfer to higher level facilities. Can perform a surgical delivery within 30 min.* 24 hr laboratory facilities and blood bank. (All those with relevant pediatric skills)	Resuscitation, stabilization and general care of healthy, term and 35-37 week infants who remain stable. Stabilize ill & <35 week infants until transport	Term or near-term laboring woman with failure to progress, cord prolapse, fetal distress
II	Level I services plus care of high-risk mothers & fetuses (babies weighing 3 lb 4.5 oz–5 lb 8.5 oz or 1500-2500 g at 32 to 36 wks gestation). (Pediatric hospitalists; neonatal specialists)	Level I services; moderately ill or immature neonates with problems that are expected to resolve rapidly	Preterm labor or abruption at 32 to 36 weeks
III	Level II services plus comprehensive care for mothers of all risk categories. Evaluation and trials of new high-risk technologies; advanced Dx tests (range of pediatric subspecialists on site or at a closely related institution)	Level II services plus care of extremely small (<1500 g) or critically ill neonates needing sustained support	Preterm labor <32 wks; known fetal anomalies; need prenatal maternal intensive care.
IV	All above care (All types of pediatric subspecialists on site 24/7)	Set up to deal with the most complex and rare problems the quickest	Need for immediate neonatal surgery for severe anomalies

(*Of course this depends upon the number of women needing surgery at the time.)

Working with the hospital

Which hospital should you use? The types of care available in the mother's community should be reviewed during prenatal care. An absolute emergency often requires transport to the nearest available facility. However, not every hospital is equipped to handle all obstetrical and neonatal emergencies. In addition, private hospitals in the United States can refuse care to women who do not have insurance. Federally funded facilities do not have this option and must care for anyone presenting in the emergency room with a crisis, regardless of ability to pay. If you are near the Mexican-United States border and the mother is an illegal alien, she may be refused care unless the situation is dire. If there is time, these women will often be taken back across the border and turned over to a Mexican hospital.

Facilities are ranked according to three levels of care, as described in the preceding table. Be aware that not every hospital that offers a particular level of care offers every possible service within that scope of care. For example, not all Level III hospitals have doctors on call for every variety of neonatal surgery; however, all will be adequately prepared to receive, support and stabilize the most severely compromised infant. Some may transport the baby to another Level III unit that can provide the necessary services or may obtain the services of a suitable practitioner who will travel to their facility. This will usually be relevant only if the baby was born with certain anomalies requiring rarely needed surgery.

Let the hospital and back-up practitioner know you are coming: It is common courtesy, as well as your professional responsibility, to let the back-up practitioner and receiving facility know you are coming before you arrive. If possible, first call the back-up practitioner who has agreed to provide medical coverage for this woman and baby in the event of a problem. The back-up practitioner may offer to notify the hospital himself; you should, however, ask him how to proceed in this regard. If that practitioner is not available and his back-up provider will not talk to you, call the hospital directly. Call the nearest hospital that you feel can handle the situation, given the choices in the mother's area for maternal and neonatal intensive care facilities and the nature of the problem. Ask for the obstetrical department (labor and delivery) and speak to a resident or attending physician on call. If this proves impossible, ask to speak to nursing staff on the labor and delivery floor. As a last resort, speak to a resident or attending physician in the emergency room.

Describe, in the most succinct terms possible, the condition of the mother and baby. Use as much medical language as you can, but do not use terms if you are unsure of their meaning or pronunciation. Knowing the correct definition of terms and how to pronounce them are very important. First of all, you may inadvertently inform them that something is wrong that is not. Secondly, you want to sound like you know what you are talking about. It is better to use terms that you know and otherwise describe to the best of your ability what is going on.

Be sure to explain what may be necessary when you arrive, for example, "I am a licensed midwife attending a planned homebirth. The mother is at term at 8 cm of dilation with a vertex baby. The membranes ruptured spontaneously five minutes ago and a 1 foot loop of cord prolapsed outside the vagina. The mother is stable and the fetal heart rate is good. We have taken precautions to minimize pressure on the cord with maternal positioning and counterpressure on the head from below. An ambulance was called at 8:30 pm, and we will be leaving her home as soon as they arrive. Please have a surgical team ready upon our arrival, which I anticipate will be in approximately 15 minutes. We would like to transfer directly to the labor and delivery unit; can this be arranged?" Request that you be admitted directly to labor and delivery and not have to go through the emergency room, a process that will waste valuable time and require interacting with personnel who are not obstetrical specialists. Get the name of everyone you speak to and her location (or extension number), note the time, and make brief notes about the conversation. Remember to thank her for her help.

Don't leave your back-up hanging: Once you call to announce your intention to transport, things can change fast. The prospect of transport can cause some women who have been absolutely stuck in labor to start progressing rapidly to birth. This doesn't always happen, of course, but if the reason for transport is nonemergent, the situation changes dramatically and the mother wants to stay home, you absolutely *must* call whomever you have spoken with as soon as you can safely leave the mother long enough to do so to let them know that things have changed and you either will not be coming in after all or the mother wishes to wait to see how things develop. If you don't follow-up, the medical community will not think well of you. Call them back once the birth is completed to let them know that everything is fine.

Preparing for transport

Prepare the mother for transport: While one midwife is arranging the transport on the phone, an assistant can be helping the mother get ready to leave. If there is time, assist her with a quick shower. If not, help her clean herself up by wiping away any secretions on her thighs with a warm washcloth, washing her face, brushing her hair, etc. Most of the time the mother will be quite capable of getting up, dressing herself and making her way to the transport vehicle. Avoid transporting a woman in a disheveled state if you can possibly avoid it. A mother who is not able to walk unassisted should be supported to the vehicle. If walking is difficult because birth is imminent, someone who is prepared to receive the baby should he fall out (it can happen!) should accompany the mother in the transport vehicle. If she is unstable on her feet or unable to walk because of blood loss or because of unidentifiable complications, an ambulance should probably be summoned, unless there is an individual strong enough to lift and carry her to the vehicle.

Be sure the mother is dressed appropriately for the weather. It is ideal if she is dressed to allow easy access to her yoni, especially if there is any likelihood that the birth may occur en route. A loose dress or skirt with panties would be appropriate. If she is bleeding, open her supply of sanitary pads for after the birth, place one in her underwear, and bring a spare. If she is hemorrhaging, an ambulance or a vehicle where she can lie down and you can position yourself to monitor blood loss would be ideal.

Carry with you things the mother may need for, hopefully, a short stay. She should have her own nightgown or T-shirts so that she will not have to wear hospital gowns. She should carry warm socks, hair ties, and any other personal items that might make her more comfortable during labor.

<u>Who should go to the hospital</u>? The primary support person should go with the mother. If there are children present, someone should stay at the house with them or take them to their home. At least one and possibly two of the midwives should go as well, depending upon the hospital's policies regarding the number of labor support people allowed to be with the mother. Some hospitals still allow only one additional support person besides the significant other. If the hospital does not allow extra support people to relieve each other, there is really no point in more than one midwife going. In this case, it makes the most sense for the other birth attendants to go home, so at least one person will be rested sufficiently for the full day of prenatals tomorrow or the for next birth. Once the other attendants have had time to get some rest, the midwife who has accompanied the mother should take every opportunity to supply a designated person with progress reports. Phone numbers of all those who need to be kept informed should be gathered by the midwife staying behind so she can keep them apprised of the situation rather than leaving multiple parties to call the hospital for progress reports.

While friends and relatives may wish to come to the hospital and sit in the waiting room, encourage them to rest and wait for word at home. This way, they will be more rested and more able to support the mother after she has had the baby, when she will probably wish to exit the hospital as soon as possible. They can be put to work tidying the home, caring for other siblings and preparing a welcome home meal which can be frozen, if necessary.

<u>Get yourself ready for the transport</u>: The midwives who are accompanying the mother to the hospital should also attend to their appearance. Remember that transports usually occur after long hours of labor support; you will likely be tired and disheveled yourself. Get cleaned up while the other midwives help the mom. If you don't have time to shower (and you probably won't), quickly wash, apply fresh deodorant, brush your teeth, comb your hair, change your underwear and throw on fresh clothes, even if they are just clean sweats. This will increase your presentability as well as gird you for the hours ahead as you support the woman in the hospital and make perhaps a first impression of midwife-attended homebirth on the attending practitioners at the hospital. Your appearance, however, should never take precedence over the well-being of the mother and baby. If a crisis is in process, go as you are and remember that the hospital staff are used to practitioners who look bedraggled after a long shift.

<u>Calling 911</u>: When someone calls 911, an ambulance will be sent. The fire department and the police may also come, even if you say that they are not needed. Response varies among communities, and it is always a good idea to know whom to expect ahead of time. Having all these services show up can be quite disruptive, with the police asking questions and later sending detectives, child-protective services, home nurses and representatives from other agencies who often totally misinterpret homebirth as well as the circumstances of the transport, especially if your region is still in a legally gray status regarding midwifery. It may be best to call an ambulance directly rather than relying on 911.

<u>Ground transport</u>

<u>If an ambulance is coming</u>: Ambulance attendants are frequently very nervous about the prospect of being called to a birthing scene; how you handle things can help relieve some of their anxiety and prevent problems with communication during transport. Assign someone who knows your equipment to tidy up the room. Throw secretion- and blood-soaked disposable articles into a big plastic trash bag and remove any blood-stained linens to a laundry area or another plastic bag. These bags should be placed out of the way. If possible, strip the bed down to the postpartum set of sheets, especially if the top sheets have been soiled with blood. Midwives sometimes have equipment such as needles and medications that are not included within their legal scope of practice; these should be put away in your birth kit or covered with a clean towel or Chux pad so they are not visible. The sight of blood usually causes emergency medical personnel to think in terms of injury, which may prompt them to proceed with that in mind as they enter the home. Having a clean, tidy space that does not look like a war zone will make a better initial impression on the ambulance team. It lets them know that things are under control and also minimizes the shock of complications during a planned homebirth.

Have at least one person right beside the mother. If she has been unstable, a blood pressure cuff should be in place, and the assistant should be prepared to report a recent blood pressure and pulse and the time they were taken.

One of the primary midwives should be selected to be the spokesperson when the ambulance arrives. Take a deep breath or two and remain calm and centered. State clearly that you are the midwife, and that you wish to "give report." This paramedic lingo prompts the ambulance attendants to listen and lets them know you have some idea regarding their protocols. Then state clearly that this is an obstetric situation (woman in labor, etc.), the mother's (or baby's) condition, what you wish to be done and how you want her to be transported. If you are licenced or certified, state that as well. For example: "I am Jane Barnes, licenced midwife. I want to give report. This mother ruptured membranes at 6:05 pm and a loop of umbilical cord prolapsed with the waters. The presenting part is being elevated off the cord by this midwife. The fetal heart tones are stable when the mother remains in this position." Use medical terminology as appropriate. Request that you be allowed to stay with the mother. If she is conscious, have her ask for the same thing. Remain with her until hospital staff takes over. Speak respectfully but with authority; look and talk like you know what you are doing. Don't be timid or arrogant. Explain the arrangements you have made with the hospital and give the name of the back-up practitioner, if there is one, or the person you spoke to at the hospital, if there isn't.

The ambulance staff may not want you to ride with them due to limited space in the back. If you are providing a necessary service to the mother, such as holding the head up off a prolapsed cord or performing bimanual compression to prevent blood loss, you will need to explain to the attendants what you are doing and why. If they still will not allow you to accompany the mother, say aloud that you are now turning responsibility for the well-being of the baby and mother over to them. If the mother requires care that only they can provide, it is best to ride in a car behind them.

En route in a private car: If transport in a private vehicle is your only or your best alternative, be sure the mother is positioned appropriately before taking off. At least one midwife should be by her side if there is a likelihood that the baby will be born in transit. If the baby does start to come, it may be best to pull over at the first safe location, attend to the birth and then proceed based on what happens with the birth. If, however, the baby is in deep distress or the mother is bleeding heavily, continue driving to the hospital. This will get you there faster and may save precious minutes if lives are hanging in the balance.

AMBULANCE	PRIVATE CAR
Advantages	
Speed of transport (recognized emergency vehicles can move through traffic easily and more safely) Medical team on board Easy access for continued care of the baby May provide advanced support beyond your skill Well lit Equipment on board	Good for short trips Immediate transport is possible Good if the baby is stable, requiring minimal support
Disadvantages Both methods are susceptible to delayed arrival due to road conditions, weather or traffic. It may be difficult to distinguish between problems with vital signs and artifacts caused by the vibration of the vehicle.	
Must wait for their arrival Medical personnel may be hostile, especially in places where direct-entry midwifery is not legal More noise than in a private car (sirens, etc.); makes auscultation difficult and may result in hearing impairment	Public does not recognize it as an emergency vehicle Doctor may prefer ambulance transfer Midwife may be liable if her car is used Accessibility is limited Poorly lit No equipment on board; must anticipate all needs in advance

General considerations regarding transport by aircraft

If you live very rurally, such as in a small village in Alaska or in a remote area in the developing world, there may be occasions when air transport is the only or best means available to take the baby to the hospital. If there is a medical flight-transport service with trained technicians on board, you will not be responsible for overseeing and troubleshooting any problems that may arise; the team should know what to do. However, there are midwives who sometimes need to transport an infant in a private aircraft or with personnel who are not medically trained. In this case, the midwife will need some understanding of the types of problems she may face.

Fixed wing aircraft vs. helicopter: Fixed-wing transport (airplanes) and helicopters each offer their own advantages and limitations. These are summarized in the chart below. Both generally lack cabin space, limiting physical accessibility to the baby during flight. Any problems that are ordinarily encountered during ground transport such as temperature control, noise, vibration and motion sickness are often magnified. The weather may also be an interfering factor. Because most people can tolerate an altitude of 8000 ft (2439 m) without difficulty, the cabin pressure of fixed-wing aircraft is adjusted by pumping in air to maintain the cabin altitude just below that level. Modern aircraft flying at higher altitudes are pressurized to 6888 ft (2100 m), which does help to minimize the effects of changing altitude, even though the plane may be flying at 40,000 ft (12,195 m). Helicopters very rarely fly above 1000 ft (304 m) because their cabins are not pressurized, but flying at a higher altitude may be unavoidable in some cases, such as a mountain transport.

FIXED-WING AIRPLANE	HELICOPTERS
Advantages	
Best for distances exceeding 150 to 200 miles Speed Pressurized cabin permits flying above 8000 feet	Good for short trips Minimal requirements for landing Immediate landing is possible Can be used in urban settings Possible to hover
Disadvantages	
Runway required for landing More noise than in ground transport Bad weather may prevent landing or take-off Ground transfers required (must land) Rapid decrease in ambient temperature at higher altitudes; may make thermoregulation tricky	Susceptible to turbulence Marked noise and vibration Limited access to mother or baby in cabin Power conversion problems Limited range of travel Cabin may overheat if it must sit in the sun for a prolonged period before takeoff Unpressurized cabin

(Donn et al., 1985)

Flying at high altitude: In pressurized aircraft, adults experience a 6 to 8% decrease in baseline oxygen saturation levels. This is generally well tolerated because the person is at rest and most flights are of short duration. However, when the crew must be actively caring for a person being transported, hypoxic symptoms may develop. In unpressurized aircraft, all passengers may experience hypoxic effects, which can influence how the crew functions and worsen the condition of those being transported.

Everyone on board may be exposed to significant temperature variations. This can result in an increased metabolic rate and increased demand for oxygen. Prolonged exposure can result in motion sickness, headache, disorientation, fatigue, discomfort, irritability, impaired performance, and reduced ability to cope with other stresses, such as hypoxia.

As the altitude increases, the air cools and the amount of moisture in the air drops. A pressurized aircraft draws in fresh air from the outside dry atmosphere resulting in an extremely low humidity level in the cabin. To avoid dehydration, fluid intake of everyone on board should be monitored carefully, and anyone receiving supplemental oxygen should receive humidified gas. This is especially important during long air transports.

Noise and vibration may be especially problematic, particularly during transport by helicopter. Excessive noise can interfere directly with care-giving. Prolonged exposure to noise may result in discomfort, headaches, fatigue, nausea, visual disturbances, vertigo, temporary or permanent ear damage and poor performance of tasks. Hearing protection can be worn by the crew and supplied to the woman or baby if noise is a problem. Vibration can lead to a slight increase in metabolic rate, fatigue, shortness of breath, motion sickness, chest pain and abdominal pain. It may also interfere with normal body thermoregulation and with the operation of some invasive and noninvasive monitoring equipment.

Gravitational forces: Shifting gravitational forces are pronounced during air transport. One "*g*" represents the pull of gravity on a seated person at sea level at 45° N latitude. Gravitational forces come into play during ascent and descent and during a change in speed or direction. During acceleration (take-off) a person will be pulled to the rear of the craft. During deceleration (landing) of an air or ground vehicle, an improperly restrained person will fall face forward. Securing the person will prevent falling during ascent or descent. For anyone with cardiac disease, myocardial perfusion is enhanced during acceleration by positioning him with his head toward the rear of the aircraft.

As negative *g* forces increase, blood tends to pool in the upper part of the body. In those with head injures or fluid overload, augmentation of positive gravitational forces, which would shift blood to pool in the lower extremities, may be desirable. This is accomplished by positioning the person with his head toward the front of the aircraft, which may also reduce the risk of a transient increase in intracranial pressure during takeoff. It is therefore desirable to do this for a preterm baby as well (Gomez, 1999).

How altitude affects gases in the body: At altitudes a few thousand feet above sea level, the amount of expansion which the gases in the atmosphere undergo is only 10 to 15%. However, at 8000 ft above sea level, gas expansion will be 30%. This change will affect any body cavity that contains gases such as the stomach, intestines, middle ear, sinuses, or a closed pneumothorax. Other potential spaces include the intracranial space and brain (pneumocephaly) and subcutaneous emphysema. The respiratory rate and volume of gas exchange may also be affected. The stomach and small intestines normally contain about 0.95 liters of gas in adults. On ascent, symptoms of bloating from gas expansion may develop, but do not typically become severe if the gastrointestinal tract is normal until an altitude of 25,000 ft (7621 m) is reached, when the volume of gas triples. As gas expansion becomes symptomatic, the person suffers from discomfort, nausea, vomiting, shortness of breath and hyperventilation. Any condition which may increase the amount of gas in the gastrointestinal tract, such as a diaphragmatic hernia, will result in more severe symptoms as the gas expands. A low atmospheric pressure and low oxygen levels also cause anaerobic bacteria to grow rapidly.

Transporting for long distances at a high altitude or very high-altitude medical transport of shorter lengths may also result in third spacing where intravascular fluids seep into other body compartments. A drop in barometric pressure may result in such leakage, which can be further aggravated by temperature changes, vibration and the shifting effects of gravity. Signs and symptoms include edema, dehydration, increased heart rate, and decreased blood pressure. Those with preexisting conditions involving fluid leakage, including heart defects or kidney disease, are at the most risk.

Disturbances of the middle ear (barotitis media) may occur when the barometric pressure changes. During ascent, gas expands in the middle ear behind the tympanic membrane, which usually does not result in pain. As one descends in altitude, the gas in the middle ear contracts, pulling the tympanic membrane inward. Such pressure changes can be compensated for by gas exiting or entering the eustachian tube, unless a person has a cold or sinus problems.

Air transport of the woman in labor: There appears to be no specific risk to the fetus or mother when a pregnant woman rapidly ascends in altitude during air travel. The arterial partial pressure of oxygen in the fetus is already significantly lower than that of the mother. A healthy baby at sea level has an umbilical arterial oxygen level of 32 mm Hg, while the mother's PaO_2 will drop only from 32 to 25.5 mm Hg. In addition to the lower partial pressure of arterial oxygen in the fetus, fetal hemoglobin has a higher affinity for holding onto oxygen than does that of the adult. Thus, fetal hemoglobin is more fully saturated at a lower PaO_2 than is that of the mother (Gomez, 1999). Air transport is further discussed in the subchapter entitled "Transporting the Newborn: An Overview" because babies tend to have more problems that can be adversely affected by high altitude than do adults, but the principles are the same for all age groups.

How altitude affects medical devices: A rise in altitude also impacts the gases contained in medical equipment. The gas in an oxygen tank will expand; thus there are special tests and precautions taken to ensure that tanks do not explode as an aircraft ascends. You will not be allowed to use your tanks during an air transport and should never try to do so unless they have been so tested. Intravenous flow rates, the pressure in medical devices (such as inflatable anti-shock trousers) and endotracheal tube cuff expansion can be altered. The air trapped in containers expands with ascent, thus IV fluids are delivered under a higher pressure. On descent, the flow of IV fluids slows as air volume decreases. The gas in any type of inflatable device will also expand with ascension, risking the production of excessive pressure and possible airway or circulatory compromise. The gas will likewise contract on descent, resulting in a loosening of the device. All this means that medical support interventions, such as IVs, laryngeal mask airways and any other device containing gas will require careful monitoring and will need for monitoring and adjusting throughout the transport.

After You Arrive at the Hospital

Getting there and getting settled

Arriving at the hospital: If there is no emergency, your party may be able to enter the front lobby and go straight up to the labor and delivery floor on foot. However, if the mother needs to be on a gurney, you will probably have to enter through the emergency room, get her situated, and then proceed upstairs. Either way, tell any staff you encounter whom you have spoken to and that you have permission to go straight to labor and delivery. If this was not prearranged, tell the staff exactly what is going on as concisely as possible and request immediate transfer to labor and delivery.

Stay with the parents: Many hospitals allow at least one support person aside from the woman's partner to accompany her throughout labor. One experienced midwife should take this role. If more than one or unlimited additional support people are allowed, two midwives or a midwife and an apprentice can accompany the mother. Do your best to avoid being separated from her. If necessary, the mother should request that you accompany her. It is likely that you and her partner will be asked to leave the room during certain procedures. In some places, this may still be the policy during internal exams, but it usually applies to procedures such as the administration of an epidural. The mother can request that you stay, but if the request is refused, it is best not to insist. Simply rejoin the mother as soon as possible.

Maintain an attitude of gratitude: Regardless of how you feel about hospital birth, you are there because you thought it was the best place to be. Now, act like it. The staff people you interact with may have very distorted views about homebirth or midwifery care or both and may have little firsthand experience. They are often disconcerted by homebirth transports, since they see all the problems, not the hundreds of beautiful homebirths that give you your perspective on the current situation. Be polite, especially to the nurses, as they are low down in the hospital pecking order.

Intake procedures: Prepare the mother for the admission routine, which may include transporting her to the labor ward in a wheelchair. Once she is assigned to a room, she can expect to have blood drawn; to have her vital signs such as blood pressure, pulse and temperature assessed; to have an IV catheter inserted and to be given lactated Ringer's. Hospitals usually require at least 20 to 30 minutes of external fetal heart monitoring as part of their intake procedure to obtain a documented baseline of uterine activity and fetal well-being on admission. An internal exam and numerous history questions can also be expected. If relevant, be sure to mention that the woman has allergies and that she is Rh-negative.

Getting what you came for: Explain to the physician and the nurses assigned to your client (or to her own physician, if her back-up provider is present) the circumstances of labor and why you transported. Be sure to include facts about the baby's and mother's well-being, food and fluid intake, voiding, and general impressions about the mother's ability to cope with labor. The mother will be questioned as well. Let her do the talking as much as possible, filling in the gaps from your point of view. Be sure to emphasize that the mother and baby are fine, if that is the case, especially if labor has been prolonged. Keep in mind that long labors are usually not allowed to proceed without intervention, and hospital staff often believe that a long labor means something is very wrong. Make a definitive request for the intervention you think will help. Be specific. Discuss the matter in "progress-model" terms (see next chapter). Say why you think this is what is needed and then listen to their assessment of the situation. The following is a brief list of interventions that may be warranted in specific situations:

- **Prolonged labor with poor contractions:** Resting the mother with sedatives or oxytocin augmentation, or both.
- **Maternal exhaustion:** Resting the mother with a sedative drug, or augmenting labor and getting it over with quickly (depending upon where she is in labor and the condition of the baby)
- **Uncontrollable vomiting:** IV fluid for electrolyte replacement, antinausea medication
- **Baby low but will not deliver:** Large clitorotomy, forceps or vacuum extraction
- **Questionable fetal heart rate patterns:** Fetal heart monitoring
- **Small suspected abruption:** Fetal heart monitoring, coagulation studies if bleeding has been prolonged
- **Large abruption or cord prolapse:** Immediate assessment, likely surgical delivery
- **Maternal collapse:** Immediate assessment and stabilization or surgical delivery
- **Acute fetal distress:** Immediate surgical delivery
- **Deeply meconium stained amniotic fluid:** Fetal heart monitoring, neonatal care
- **Signs of maternal or fetal infection:** Fetal heart monitoring, IV antibiotics

•**Suspected fetal demise:** confirmation of death. If the baby is dead, consider proceeding with natural labor in the hospital or checking out to return home to labor, depending upon your local legal climate and the wishes of the parents. Either way, do your best to minimize interventions and maximize the uninterrupted time the parents can spend with the baby after the birth. Most hospital staffs realize the importance of spending time after the birth and will be very supportive.

The hospital practitioners may suggest a different course of action than you thought was needed, either based on findings gathered at the hospital or their own perspective. Whenever another intervention is proposed, it is appropriate to ask them to explain the procedure fully or to request additional information. Then, if it is not a dire emergency, say to the provider, "Can the parents have a chance to talk about this for a minute in private?" Do not attempt to refuse an intervention on the woman's behalf. Once the medical personnel are out of the room, explain any potential problems the new intervention could pose and encourage the woman to fully consider all her options. In addition, remind her that she need not accept all interventions offered. For example, very often, the agreement to augment with oxytocin will be followed by an assumption that the woman will not be able to handle the ensuing more intense contractions. An epidural may be ordered without the mother requesting one, which she will then have to refuse (or not). Remind her that she will want to be fully able to participate in pushing.

Once you have an agreed upon plan of action, give the intervention a chance to work. Set a time limit, if necessary, to allow for this and let the doctor know what that limit is. Hospital practitioners usually work well within time limits.

The parents should make their desires known: Other routine procedures can also be negotiated. Requests such as "We wish to avoid any unnecessary interventions" are not as effective as "Do not cut my perineum" or "Do not cut the cord until it has stopped pulsing" (remember that the hospital staff does not view early cord clamping as an intervention).

Postpartum care of the baby: Ask to speak to the nurse who will be overseeing the care of the baby so that the partner can explain preferences and sign release forms regarding such procedures as Vitamin K, eye prophylaxis and metabolic screening. Request that all baby exams take place at the bedside of the mother. If the nurse insists that the baby must go to the nursery, the partner should be prepared to accompany the baby, while the midwife stays with the mother. It is important that the partner be present to advocate for the baby, as the mother can advocate for herself. The midwife cannot make decisions on behalf of either one. Although it is always best to leave the hospital as soon as possible, rooming-in should also be discussed with relevant staff prior to the birth as well.

Depending upon why you transported, there are certain predictable responses you can expect as to the hospital staff's opinion as to how to manage the baby. If there has been meconium staining, expect that the baby may receive laryngoscopy with suctioning at birth. If the mother is suspected of having an infection, or if her group-B strep status is unknown or positive and IV antibiotics have not been started, the baby may be treated as though he is infected after the birth. However, even if the baby is thought to be in severe distress (based on fetal heart rate patterns) during labor, if he is in good shape at birth he will generally be treated as for any other normal, low-risk baby, as long as infection or some other complication is not suspected.

If the baby has died, be sure keepsakes such as a lock of hair, photos, foot and palm prints and the like are obtained. Most hospitals are very sensitive to these types of things and will do them without asking.

Legally refusing consent: Parents may have to be firm in order to have their choices respected. Remarkably, phrases such as 'please don't," "stop," "I don't want that" are not legally binding. The legally binding phrase is "I refuse to give my consent to ____________." They can also add "at this time" to make clear that if circumstances dramatically change, they are willing to reconsider. If they use this phrase, hospital staff is legally bound to respect it or face litigation.

Supporting women in the hospital

Once you are in the confines of a labor room, the woman's ability to change positions and walk may be limited. This may be due, in part, to getting what you came for–IV oxytocin, for example. You can help the mother by talking to the hospital staff about possible position changes and the like. You may have ideas that are totally foreign to the staff; be patient and have the mother ask for these things, then support her choices: "That's a great idea; Nurse, can she move into the shower for a while?" Keeping a woman in the shower or bathroom can provide the small quiet space she needs for privacy and can help cut down on routine procedures and exams. Encouraging the parents to cuddle and kiss can accomplish the same thing! As labor nears pushing, it may become apparent that the mother should give birth in a delivery room or even the operating room if a serious problem is anticipated. Ask if a birthing bed can be wheeled into the room so that the mother can be more comfortable and more easily change positions for birth.

Very often, once hospital staff people are familiar with who you are, they will leave you to your own devices for stretches at a time. What with short staffing in modern hospitals, they are often just as glad to have one less labor to worry about. Staff care providers invite you to catch the baby so they can more fully appreciate what homebirth is all about. This can be flattering, but be very cautious about transports to hospitals that are unknown to you or that have a reputation for being hostile to midwives or when you are transporting in a state or jurisdiction in which midwifery is illegal. In these situations, it is best to err on the side of caution and stick to a strictly labor-supporting role. Even applying a hot compress to the perineum or anything else that smacks of midwifery could land you in big trouble, as you have been witnessed in practice. Don't take the risk.

Drugs that may be offered in labor

You may have come to the hospital so that certain drugs could be used; however, there is great likelihood that the mother will be offered drugs that she had no intention of considering. It is therefore helpful to have a basic understanding of what those drugs may be and how helpful they really are. Any drug you request will also carry risks and benefits as well. The drugs reviewed below are, for the most part, not used by midwives at home in the United States.

The FDA approves only a dozen or so drugs for use during obstetric care, and more than half of these have had their FDA-approved labeling removed from the PHYSICIAN'S DESK REFERENCE (PDR) by their manufacturers. The PDR is the only publication that must publish the text of an FDA-approved drug label exactly as it appears in the package insert. Manufacturers must pay for these listings, so they tend to remove drugs with expired patents so they can replace the descriptions with those of other drugs that are still under patent, and therefore make them the most money. FDA approval status is granted when the FDA determines that a drug's benefits outweigh its risks. The FDA definition of safe is a relative one, based on the known risks, the considered acceptable potential risks and the benefits of a particular drug (rather than the dictionary definition of "free from harm or injury"). No drug approved for use in obstetrics has been proven safe for such use, and no drug approved for an obstetric indication must be tested as to its short- or long-term effect on the baby. Neither are drugs tested for their interaction when used concurrently. While short-term clinically evident side-effects are focused upon below, all these drugs may have a dramatic and lifelong impact on the delicate, rapidly developing fetal and newborn nervous system and brain (Haire, 200a). The following discussion of medications is based on Gaskin (2003), unless otherwise noted.

Labor stimulants: Oxytocic drugs are reviewed in the subchapter entitled "Allopathic Pharmacologic Agents for Treating Uterine Atony."

Tranquilizers, sedatives and sleeping pills: A tranquilizer may assist a woman with contractions through which she cannot sleep, and is therefore helpful in her getting some rest. However, do not expect tranquilizers to make any difference in the pain of active labor. Sedatives, frequently diazepam (Valium), are given to reduce anxiety and tension. In fact, they cross the placenta and affect the baby's ability to establish respirations, her sucking reflex and her muscle tone, so they are best used only during early labor.

Narcotics: Narcotic drugs, if given in sufficient quantity, can reduce the sensations of labor. Meperidine (Demerol) is the most widely prescribed narcotic in the US for use in labor, either intravenously or by injection. However, doses high enough to diminish pain are also detrimental to maternal, fetal and newborn well-being, and it is therefore not given to the point of effectiveness. The amounts that are used tend to produce sleepiness and can make the woman feel as though she is swimming through the sensations of labor, which she can still feel. Narcotics also have unpleasant side-effects such as nausea, vomiting and a reduction in blood pressure. Babies exposed to narcotics in utero tend to be lethargic and irritable and to nurse poorly, side-effects that may persist for some time after birth.

Alphaprodine (Nisentil) is another narcotic agent that has effects similar to those of meperidine. It takes effect faster and wears off more quickly than meperidine, but also frequently causes maternal nausea, vomiting, drowsiness and confusion and newborn depression at birth.

Other narcotic-like drugs approved for labor include nalbuphine (Nubain) and butorphanol (Stadol). Unapproved drugs that are used include hydromorphone (Dilaudid), fentanyl citrate (Sublimaze), and codeine. (Haire, 2004b).

Naloxone (Narcan) is approved for use in infants exposed to narcotic drugs given to their mother, but it is not approved for use during labor. Most sluggish, drugged newborns become alert when given naloxone, but the effect is limited, and if it wears off before the effects of the narcotic do, the baby's condition will be like that of a similarly drugged baby who has not received naloxone (Haire, 2004b).

Antinauseants: Antinausea drugs are used when nausea is overwhelming and otherwise uncontrollable, or to counteract the adverse effects of other drugs, such as narcotics. Perphenazine (Trilafon) and promethazine (Phenergan) are frequently used to treat nausea in labor and are often given as a rectal suppository. They may cause dizziness and sleepiness in women and may impair the clotting ability of the baby. Therefore, the least amount that is effective should be given. Hydroxyzine (Vistaril) is an anti-anxiety, antinauseant that is sometimes used in labor and that may have a potentiating effect when used with other central nervous system depressants (Haire, 2004b).

Nitrous oxide (N_2O) combined with oxygen (Entonox): In the United Kingdom, a 50/50 combination of nitrous oxide and oxygen is used as an inhalant anesthetic to dull labor pain at home or in the hospital. Nitrous oxide is a nonexplosive, weakly analgesic gas that does not cause skeletal muscle relaxation, meaning that the mother can still move around after administration. Its primary adverse effect is to lower blood oxygen levels, which is why it is mixed with oxygen. Hypoxia is exaggerated when Entonox is used with opiates. In high concentrations, pure nitrous oxide can cause cyanosis, vomiting, respiratory depression and death. Higher rates of miscarriage have been noted among care providers repeatedly exposed to it in the work setting. Use for over 4.5 hours in labor has been linked to opiate and amphetamine addiction in the adult offspring (Jacobson, 1990). The gas is administered by mask from a tank (like an oxygen tank). The mother controls the dose by placing the mask over her face and inhaling, usually at the peak of intense contractions. This induces pain relief within a minute, which is short lived. It can also produce dizziness, sedation and drowsiness, especially if used continuously. Overall, nitrous oxide is probably the best allopathic analgesic for use during labor. While it is widely used by dentists in the United States it is, unfortunately, not used in obstetrics. Its widespread use would eliminate a lot of epidurals for women having hospital births (Buckley, 2004).

Anesthetics: Most of the medications listed above may dull or temporarily relieve pain, but do not obliterate pain completely. Anesthesia is intended to do so. There are several forms of regional anesthesia available. These include Bupivacaine hydrochloride (HCl) (Marcaine, Sensorcaine), lidocaine (Xylocaine), mepivacaine (Carbocaine) and chloroprocaine (Nesacaine). These drugs can be used for an epidural, spinal or caudal block (providing anesthesia from the navel to the toes), saddle block (numbing limited to the perineum, inner thighs and buttocks), or pudendal block (numbing primarily genitals) or as a local anesthetic for perineal repair. Each has its own inherent risks. The following is excerpted from the FDA-approved labeling for bupivacaine HCl:

> "**LABOR AND DELIVERY:** Local anesthetics rapidly cross the placenta, and when used for epidural, caudal or pudendal block anesthesia, can cause varying degrees of maternal, fetal and neonatal toxicity. The incidence and degree of toxicity depend upon the procedure performed, the type and amount of drug used, and the technique of drug administration. Adverse reactions in the parturient, fetus and neonate involve alteration of the central nervous system, peripheral vascular tone, and cardiac function . . ."
> **ADVERSE REACTIONS: Neurologic:** Neurologic effects following epidural or caudal anesthesia may include spinal block of varying magnitude (including high or total spinal block); hypotension secondary to spinal block; urinary retention; fecal and urinary incontinence; loss of perineal sensation and sexual function; persistent anesthesia; paresthesia; weakness; paralysis of the lower extremities and loss of sphincter control all of which may have slow, incomplete or no recovery; headache; septic meningitis; meningismus; slowing of labor; increased incidence of forceps delivery; and cranial nerve palsies due to traction on nerves from loss of cerebrospinal fluid . . ." (Haire, 2004a)

These tidbits on the adverse effects of these drugs are just the tip of the iceberg. Since these drugs are not used directly by homebirth midwives, a full discussion of their possible risks and side-effects will not be included here. I refer the student to Doris Haire's web site www.aimsusa.org, where several excellent articles review the dangers of drug use in pregnancy and labor. The following offers an overview of various anesthetic options:

Epidurals: Epidurals are the most commonly used type of pharmacological labor pain relief in North America. The procedure has been touted as the "Cadillac of anesthesia" and has been widely marketed to women as though it has no adverse side-effects. Because an epidural can cause a rapid fall in blood pressure, a bolus of IV fluid is usually given before an epidural is placed. During insertion, the woman lies on her side, hugging her knees to her chest to spread the spaces between her lumbar vertebrae as widely open as possible. A cannula is then placed in the epidural space (the space just outside the dura mater covering the spinal cord). A numbing drug is injected through this cannula. The cannula is then left in place so that the drug can be "topped up" if it wears off. Epidurals do not cause nausea or vomiting. The mother remains conscious, but may find herself feeling detached from the experience of labor. For this reason when a yoni birth is anticipated, many women choose to have the epidural wear off in time for pushing. It provides full anesthetic coverage, and is considered the best choice of medical anesthesia to use during a surgical birth. One of the most commonly used epidural anesthetics is bupivacaine HCl (Marcaine or Sensoracaine).

Epidurals have a number of serious drawbacks. A fall in blood pressure can result in a drop in both maternal and fetal heart rates, although giving continuous IV fluids can help control this effect. An epidural administered in early labor, can significantly slow progress and impair rotation and descent of the baby. The relaxation of the pelvic muscles and ligaments increases the chance of the baby descending in a deflexed or asynclitic position, which the mother cannot change positions in order to correct, thus increasing the likelihood of an instrumental or surgical delivery. Pushing under an epidural is difficult, at best, as the woman cannot feel her body cues and must be told when to push. For this reason, many hospital practitioners add at least an hour to their "normal" time for pushing and wait until the scalp is visible at the introitus before enjoining the mother to begin pushing. This helps relieve unnecessary straining, tension and trauma on the mother's soft tissues during descent. Even so, the lack of ability to push effectively often results in an instrumental delivery. Additional risks of epidurals include injury to the woman's tendons, muscles and ligaments as they are unnaturally relaxed. This means that it is very easy to manipulate her limbs into exaggerated positions that could result in injury. Be aware that hot or cold applications can be especially dangerous to a woman who cannot tell you if the application is too hot or too cold. In addition, the epidural site may become infected, a serious concern since it is a direct path into the epidural space. Twenty percent of women develop total body itching. Many women develop an artifact fever that is indistinguishable from a fever due to infection. This can lead to further intervention both during labor and once the baby is born; the woman may be given IV antibiotics; and the baby may be subjected to tests, including a spinal tap and numerous blood draws, to rule out neonatal infection. This will likely entail mother-infant separation and a course of antibiotics for the baby "just in case." Exposed babies commonly have respiratory or nursing problems.

Just as with any drug, each woman's response to an epidural will be individual. Epidurals fail to work at all 3% of the time. Another 12% of women get some pain relief, while 85% have complete numbing of all sensation. This presents a serious problem when the purpose of the anesthesia is surgical birth. A properly inserted epidural does not result in a spinal headache; however, in up to 2% of all cases, the anesthesiologist punctures through the dural membrane, causing leakage of spinal fluid that can result in a terrible spinal headache, which can persist for hours or even days. When this occurs, an epidural cannot be used to relieve the pain. Finally, on rare occasions (about 1 in 5000 procedures), an epidural can result in permanent paralysis or death.

Spinal anesthesia: Spinal anesthesia is similar to an epidural. First an IV line is established, and then a local anesthetic is given via a needle inserted between the lumbar vertebrae, through the dura mater and into the subarachnoid space overlying the spinal cord. A catheter is not left in place, so the entire procedure must be repeated if the pain relief is to be renewed. Spinal anesthesia provides excellent pain relief, often better than an epidural, while the rates of complication and side-effects are similar. However, spinal anesthesia may result in a sudden and dramatic reduction in blood pressure, and 1% or so of treated women will have a spinal headache after the birth.

General anesthesia: General anesthesia offers the most profound pain relief. It causes loss of consciousness via the injection or inhalation of anesthetic drugs. A general can be administered more rapidly than any type of spinal anesthesia and is therefore still widely used for emergency surgical delivery. It does not cause a drop in the blood pressure, but can result in aspiration pneumonia, nausea and vomiting. The baby frequently suffers from respiratory problems as well.

Antibiotics: Antibiotics are offered to laboring women in a variety of circumstances. Today, a primary reason is a history of a positive intrayoni group B-strep culture. Other reasons include the development of maternal fever in labor, prolonged rupture of membranes or known infection with another agent that poses a risk to the fetus. Antibiotics are usually given via intermittent IV boluses that are piggybacked to the main IV line, each bolus taking about 40 minutes to administer. The type of antibiotic used will vary according to the reason for administration and the mother's allergy history. Specifics regarding the use of drugs to treat infections during pregnancy are discussed in my DIAGNOSTIC TESTS.

Other interventions

Electronic fetal monitoring: In hospitals, fetal monitoring is often performed with a machine either externally or internally. The external monitor uses two transducers, or sensors, both of which are placed on the maternal abdomen. A Doppler transducer is placed over the fetal back or another location where it can clearly register the fetal heart rate by reflecting high-frequency sound waves against the cardiac chambers. The other is a tocotransducer, a pressure-sensitive monitor that is placed on the abdomen where it registers the onset, duration and frequency (but not the strength) of contractions via a pressure-sensitive button that is depressed when the uterus becomes firm during contractions as well as by fetal movement. These sensors are secured with two straps that encircle the abdomen.

External monitoring does not require invasion of the uterus, although irradiation with ultrasound is a form of invasive technology. Ultrasound is easy to set up and provides a continuous recording of the fetal heart rate and uterine activity. It can also distinguish the fetal heart rate from that of the mother. It does, however, limit maternal movement and requires repositioning of the sensors when the mother changes position. It has limited usefulness as a fetal heart monitor as it assesses only relative short-term variability, may double-count a slow heart rate below 60 bpm and may cut the heart rate in half if it exceeds 180 bpm. The maternal heart rate may be detected if the transducer is placed over a maternal artery, and use in obese women is difficult because the thickness of the abdominal wall increases the distance between the fetal heart and the transducer. Readings of uterine activity are not as precise as with an internal tocotransducer either.

The internal monitor uses a 1.5 mm long cork screw-shaped wire electrode that is screwed into the baby's scalp or buttock (but not the face or a limb) to monitor the fetal heart rate by converting electrocardiogram readings into graph tracings. Contractions are monitored via an intrauterine pressure catheter that is inserted through the cervix high into the uterus. The catheter is a soft plastic tube that is filled with saline. Pressure changes register variations in intrauterine pressure to monitor the frequency, duration, strength and resting tone of contractions. This is the gold standard of medical-model monitoring and is often required during a hospital labor in women who have previously had any type of uterine surgery. Use of an internal monitor requires rupture of membranes, an accessible and identifiable presenting part and at least 2 cm of dilation to allow the introduction of the scalp electrode and the uterine catheter. Internal monitoring always requires that the woman be tethered to the machine, severely restricting her movement.

The basics regarding information gleaned during fetal heart monitoring are explained in the chapter entitled "Assessing and Supporting the Baby's Well-Being during Labor." The monitor display will show numerical readings for the fetal heart rate (sometimes two if the unit can accommodate the monitoring of twins) and uterine pressure. Some monitors include maternal noninvasive blood pressure, pulse rate, pulse oximetry and ECG. Fetal movements and oxygen saturation may also be displayed. The fetal heart rate and uterine activity tracings appear as continuous parallel printouts on scaled paper, with the fetal tracing on the upper half and the uterine tracing on the lower. Paper feed rates and other features of the printout differ between North America and other countries described in the table below.

FORMAT OF PAPER GRAPH STRIP	NORTH AMERICA	OTHER COUNTRIES
Longitudinal (vertical) axis: Graph height	Fetal heart rate: 7 cm Uterine activity: 4 cm	Fetal heart rate: 8 cm Uterine activity: 4 cm
Fetal heart rate: Graph height Range Scale	7 cm 30 to 240 bpm 30 bpm per cm of height	8 cm 50 to 210 bpm 20 bpm per cm of height
Uterine activity: Graph height Range Scale	4 cm 0 to 100mm Hg of pressure 5 or 10 mm Hg increments	4 cm 0 to 100 mm Hg pressure or 1 to 13.3 kilopascal units (1 kPa = 7.5 mm Hg) 10 mm Hg increments
Horizontal axis: Recording speed	3 cm of paper feeds per minute, which is divided into six 10 sec subdivisions	1 cm/min, spanning 2 subsections 2 cm/min, spanning 4 subsections

(Adapted from Tucker, 2000)

The time, date and speed at which the paper is feeding is usually marked by the machine at ten-min intervals.

Telemetry provides remote monitoring via radio wave signals that are transmitted to the fetal heart monitor during either external or internal monitoring. The mobile transducer is strapped to the woman with a shoulder harness or something similar, allowing her to be more mobile. Watertight transducers allow continuous fetal monitoring while the woman is submerged.

If you have transported because of concerns regarding the baby, you may want the baby to be monitored full time. If not, unnecessary exposure should always be avoided as an external fetal heart monitor is an ultrasound device. If the parents do opt for monitoring, be sure that an internal monitor (or a human with a fetoscope or Doppler) confirms suspicious fetal heart rate patterns, as external monitor tracings, in particular, can be misleading. Anything that disrupts the transducer can alter the reading; artifacts (tracings created by anything other than the fetal heart rate) frequently occur.

Fetal scalp sampling: A blood sample is obtained by cutting the baby's scalp with a tiny razor. The baby's blood gases and pH are assessed to determine if suspicious fetal heart rate patterns truly reflect fetal compromise. If the monitor tracing is exceptionally alarming, fetal scalp sampling will probably not be performed in favor of immediate surgical birth. (Scalp sampling is further discussed in DIAGNOSTIC TESTS.)

Pulse oximetry: The pulse oximeter measures functional oxygen saturation of arterial hemoglobin via an electronic, light-emitting sensor (using both red and infrared light) that is inserted through the cervix and placed against the baby's cheek. The membranes must be ruptured. It cannot be used during water immersion or with multiple babies. It is used only in the presence of a nonreassuring fetal heart rate (characterized by one or more of the following: persistent late decelerations during more than 50% of contractions; a relative drop of ≥70 bpm for >60 sec; persistent slow return to baseline; long-term variability >5 bpm; tachycardia over 160 bpm; recurrent prolonged decelerations (2 or more of <70 bpm for >90 sec) or either of the following for over an hour: tachycardia >160 bpm with long-term variability of <5 bpm or a persistent decrease in variability of ≤5 bpm. An oxygen saturation of 30% or more between contractions is reassuring, corresponding with a nonacidotic fetus. (Tucker, 2004) It is a good alternative to fetal scalp sampling. See a recent edition of my DIAGNOSTIC TESTS for more details on this test.

Amnioinfusion: Amnioinfusion is performed during labor by infusing warmed saline into the uterine cavity via an open-ended intrauterine pressure catheter. The primary indications are to prevent or correct umbilical cord compression due to a low volume of amniotic fluid, to treat variable or prolonged deceleration patterns in the fetal heart rate, and to dilute or wash out thick meconium from the uterine environment. The membranes must be ruptured in order for it to be used. A soft catheter is inserted through the cervix high into the uterine cavity, and the saline is run into it like an IV. Protocols vary; however, most include beginning with a bolus infusion of 500 to 800 ml of saline followed by a continuous infusion of about 3 ml per hour. Some practitioners administer the saline continuously via an infusion pump.

Amnioinfusion carries all the risks of inserting anything into the uterus, including the introduction of infection and damage to the uterine wall (sometimes with rupture), hypertonic contractions, abnormalities of the fetal heart rate, cord prolapse, maternal cardiac or respiratory compromise, placental abruption, fetal malpresentation and maternal death. In addition, the woman must remain supine, as the water will run out otherwise. Continuous infusion carries the risk of overdistension of the uterus, while intermittent infusion may not fully account for any fluid that is lost per yoni.

Studies on the efficacy of amnioinfusion have produced varying results, with the majority concluding that it doesn't make much difference in the use of other interventions or the well-being of the newborn. Some studies have found amnioinfusion to be helpful in relieving fetal distress, especially when the volume of amniotic fluid is low. However, Owen and colleagues (1990) found no benefit when they performed a randomized control trial. While amnioinfusion for oligohydramnios decreases the frequency and severity of variable fetal heart rate decelerations in labor, there is often no corresponding reduction in the use of surgical birth or the condition of babies born at term (Nageotte et al., 1991). A summary of 13 prospective trials looking at diluting thick meconium found fewer surgical births as well as fewer babies with meconium-related complications in the infused groups (Pierce et al., 2000). In contrast, a study headed by Usta (1995) found no such improvement in infant outcomes. Spong and colleagues (1994) also found that while amnioinfusion does dilute meconium, the perinatal outcomes were unaffected.

Given the significant maternal and fetal risks involved and the lack of consensus as to its value, women may wish to forgo this intervention (Cunningham, et al., 2001).

Clitorotomy (episiotomy): Depending upon who cares for the woman in the hospital, the question of whether to cut the perineum at the time of birth is likely to arise. The woman can express her desire to tear, rather than be cut, but the attending practitioner may be reluctant not to cut because she has little experience with repairing tears and always assumes that tears will always be worse than a cut, which is only rarely the case. In the middle of active pushing may be a time when the woman needs to use the "I refuse to give my consent" phrase.

Instrumental delivery: You may have come to the hospital because you felt this particular woman could proceed with a yoni birth if she had the help of forceps or a vacuum extractor. Even if you did not come to the hospital for an instrumental delivery, the attending practitioner may want to use instruments anyway. Forceps are curved instruments with spoon-shaped cups on the ends that are contoured to fit around the parietal bones of the baby's head in a cephalic birth. Piper's forceps are used to extract the head in a breech delivery. Forceps take up room on the sides of the baby's head, and thus the mother's tissues must stretch to accommodate the blades. The safety of forceps use is very dependent upon the skills of the individual practitioner; misjudgement as to the appropriateness of forceps to a specific case, misapplication of the blades, misjudgement about the depth of descent prior to using forceps and injury of the maternal soft parts can all occur. However, in skilled hands, forceps can, on rare occasions, bring the baby out and avoid a surgical birth, a desirable goal for all concerned.

Vacuum extraction involves the application or a rigid or flexible suction cup to the vertex. The cup is attached to a suction-generating device, which has a gauge to tell how much suction is being created. The vacuum cup fits on the top of the head, and does not require as precise a fit as do forceps, but misapplication can be problematic as with forceps.

Both methods risk serious injury to mother or baby. Forceps use is associated with a higher than average incidence of brain hemorrhaging, skull fractures and facial palsies. Vacuum extraction does not compress the fetal head nor does it take up space along the sides of the birth canal, as do forceps. After a vacuum birth, the baby will have a large iatrogenic caput, which will probably develop into a hematoma; intracranial bleeding can result as well. Both forceps and vacuum cup can also seriously injure the mother if maternal tissues are included under the blades or cup. Instrumental delivery is not wonderful, but it is probably better for the psychological well-being of both mother and baby than a surgical birth (because surgical birth is an even worse interruption of the natural process). It also saves the mother the risk of surgery now as well as the risks posed by uterine scarring should she decide to have more children. Babies and mothers who have had instrumental deliveries should be given homeopathic arnica or bellis perennis after birth.

Surgical birth: With luck, a woman will only wind up with a surgical birth if it is really necessary. In practice, sometimes this is not the case and you know with more support, she could give birth naturally, but the situation is such that you must acquiesce to the status quo. This can be a very difficult pill to swallow.

The partner can usually remain with the mother during surgery unless the circumstances are critical. The parents can request that the midwife also accompany the mother into the surgical suite; however, this is seldom allowed. If it is, eat first, as you may feel queasy if you are not used to seeing surgeries (for example, be prepared for ripping sounds as they open the incision wide enough to bring the baby through). Stay where they put you (usually in a corner). If you feel sick, sit on the floor, put your head between your knees and breathe deeply. Once the baby is out, either take the partner's place beside the mother so the partner can go with the baby or go with the baby yourself. If you were not allowed in surgery and the baby is rushed off, go with him, if at all possible.

Double-layer closure of the uterine scar: Starting in the early 1990s, a single-layer suturing technique has been increasingly used to close the uterine incision after a surgical birth. This may be called either the Misgav-Ladach or the Pelosi method. Single-layer closure has been poorly researched and was initially attractive primarily because it saves time in the operating room. While the research that has been done says that postoperative recovery goes more smoothly with fewer complications, there is anecdotal information suggesting that single-layer closure may increase the risk of two severe complications during any future pregnancies: subsequent uterine rupture (possibly because it produces a weaker scar) and, even more seriously, placenta percreta, an otherwise rare complication that with a 50% mortality rate.

With the jury still out on this issue, the parents may wish to request (i.e., demand) traditional double-layer closure of the uterine scar as well as "delayed" cord clamping. If these requests are trivialized, the parents should be good-humored about it, saying politely, "Well, humor me," and, if necessary, "I will hold you accountable if it isn't done."

Double-layer closure consists of closing the uterine incision with a layer of locked stitches, followed by a second layer of stitches, placed by a process frequently referred to as **imbrication**, which means to overlap the tissues. The second layer is created by forming two rolls of tissue from the unincised surface of the uterus that parallel the incision on either side. The top of each roll is stitched to the other over the closed incision, with a layer of running stitches. This second layer reinforces the region of the incision and relieves tension as it heals. The mother, or, if the situation is dire, possibly the partner, should write the request on the consent form one of them will be asked to sign before the surgery. They should then point out this addition to the person asking them to sign the form before they hand it over. They should also ask to speak directly to the surgeon who will be responsible for closing the incision as well. (Sometimes closing the incision is assigned to a surgeon other than the one who made the incision.) The request for delayed clamping should be discussed with both the surgeon and the neonatal or pediatric staff. The parents can offer to present literature to back up their request at a later time. (Single-layer closure is thoroughly discussed in a recent edition of Volume I of this text.)

Cord to be left intact at the time of surgery: The following protocols for managing a surgical delivery are based on the combined experience of Peter Dunn (1986, 1988), a pediatrician in the UK and George Morley (2003), an obstetrician in the US, both of whom have supervised surgical births during which optimal placental transfusion was allowed.

1. Two members of the pediatric staff attend the birth. One scrubs up and stands by the ob-surgeon with a mucous catheter and warmed towel in hand.
2. The uterus should be contracting as the baby is brought out through the uterine incision. If the woman is in good labor while the surgery is being performed, there may be no need for oxytocin augmentation. If not, an oxytocin IV can be started and maintained at a very slow drip rate when the surgery begins, and then the drip rate can be increased after the head is delivered. (Dunn, assuming the uterus starts out flaccid and the woman is given an injection after the incision is made suggests waiting the 30 sec to 3 minutes it will take for the first uterine contraction to occur before bringing the rest of the baby's body out of the uterus. If oxytocin is started in an IV as described, Morley sees no need to wait.)
3. The obstetrician wraps the baby in a warmed towel and lays him on his side across the mother's legs. The pediatrician clears the airways.
4. The uterus begins to contract rhythmically, causing the placenta to detach and be expelled through the uterine incision. This seldom takes more than 10 minutes with a strongly contracting uterus. The placenta is usually out after two or three contractions. According to Morley, ensuring that there are uterine contractions and waiting for the placenta to detach spontaneously results in far less maternal bleeding than does manual removal from an atonic uterus. It also allows the baby to receive his placental transfusion, which, in turn, allows the placenta to reduce in size, thus minimizing blood mixing at the site of detachment. Dunn comments that the obstetrician should ease the placenta through the incision with minimal handling or traction on the cord, if necessary. If the placenta has been damaged and the cord must be clamped, it should be clamped as near its placental base as possible.

   Morley points out that it will be an educational experience for the doctors to monitor the newborn and the cord during this time. The tension in the umbilical vein rises markedly during a uterine contraction, and if the child has received an adequate placental transfusion, a closed, bloodless portion of the umbilical vein can be seen at the child's umbilicus. The arteries are usually pulseless at this time; in other words, the child's own intraabdominal cord clamp has shut down the cord vessels. The physicians will also see that the placenta functions until the child starts to breathe–the cord usually continues to pulse and remain full of blood as long as the baby is apneic.
5. The placenta and unclamped cord are now placed inside the towel, next to the baby. The baby and placenta are then taken to a prepared warmer for observation and stabilization, where the placenta is placed alongside the baby and the baby is placed on a head-up slope. (Dunn, 1988).
6. If the baby is breathing well, is pink with good peripheral circulation, and shows no signs of inspiratory retraction and has good air entry into the lungs on auscultation; and the umbilical cord is white and has ceased to pulsate at the umbilicus, the cord may be clamped and cut.
7. If those conditions are not satisfied, and especially if the baby is less than 32 weeks gestation, he should be intubated and intermittent positive-pressure ventilation maintained for 10 to 15 minutes, using the minimum positive pressure required to bring about a steady improvement. This is Dunn's recommendation, which is intended to help milk alveolar fluid from the lungs, if the lung fluid is slow to resolve on its own. All the while the placenta is kept alongside the baby in case central venous pressure rises to allow blood to backflow via the intact cord. If the baby is believed to be hypovolemic, the placenta can be held above the baby to the height that the intact cord will allow while the necessary assistance is rendered. Once the baby is stable, the cord may then be clamped and cut.

These requests may be even more difficult to have granted than that of a double layer of closure for the uterine incision, but it is important for the baby. If the surgical team will not agree to this ideal scenario, the parents can request that the mother be given oxytocin and that the baby be allowed to receive at least a minute of placental transfusion while being held below the placenta to speed the transfusion with or without milking of the cord before the cord is cut.

After the birth:

Once the baby is born and both mother and baby are stable, it is usually best for them to leave the hospital at the earliest possible moment. Leaving sooner rather than later will minimize the number of procedures done on the baby and will preserve, as much as possible, maternal-infant contact. Accompany the parents and baby to their home and resume your care where you left off. Plan on coming for all the postpartum visits, as you normally would.

References and Further Reading on Midwifing Women Through Uncommon or Challenging Labor Situations

When Transport is Necessary during Labor

Donn SM, et al. "Neonatal transport," Curr Probl Pediatr, 15(4);1-65, Apr, 1985.

Gomez M, chair. Chapter 7: "Altitude physiology and the stresses of flight," in Guidelines for Air and Ground Transport of Neonatal and Pediatric Patients, 2nd ed. Amer. Acad Pediatr, 1999.

Zaruby J. Colorado Altitude Training. E-mail communications, notes on barometric pressure and altitude physiology, Feb, 2004.

After You Arrive at the Hospital

Bivins H, Gallup D. "C/S closure techniques: which work best?" OBG Management, 98-108, April, 2000.

Buckley S. "Drugs in labor: an overview," Midwifery Today, (71);13-20, 65, 67, Autumn 2004.

Cunningham F, et al., eds. Williams Obstetrics, 21th ed. Appleton & Lange, Stamford CT, 2001.

Dunn P. "Reservation about the methods of assessing at birth the predictive value of intrapartum fetal monitoring including premature interruption of the feto-placental circulation," 130-137, in Rolfe P. Fetal Physiological Measurements, Report of the 2nd International Conference, Oxford, April 2-4 1984, Butterworths Pub, London UK, 1986.

Dunn P. "Perinatal factors influencing adaptation to extrauterine life," Unpublished lecture notes, Plenary session 72: Preterm Birth. XII World Congress of Gynecol Obstet, Rio de Janeiro, Oct 23-28, 1988.

Gaskin IM. Ina May's Guide to Childbirth, Bantam Books, New York NY, 2003.

Haire D. "FDA approved obstetrics drugs: their effects on mother and baby," http://www.aimsusa.org. Accessed Jan 7, 2004a.

Haire D. "How obstetric drugs can affect labor and birth," http://www.aimsusa.org. Accessed Jan 7, 2004b.

Jacobson B, et al. "Opiate addiction in adult offspring through possible imprinting after obstetric treatment," BMJ 301(6760);1067-1070, Nov 10, 1990.

Morley G. Ob-gyn. E-mail communications, 2003.

Nageotte M, et al. Prophylactic amnioinfusion in pregnancies complicated by oligohydramnios: A prospective study," Obstet Gynecol, 77(5);677-680, May, 1991.

Owen J, et al. "A prospective randomized study of saline solution amnioinfusion," Am J Obstet Gynecol, 162(5);1146-1149, May, 1990.

Pierce J, et al. "Intrapartum amnioinfusion for meconium-stained fluid: meta-analysis of prospective clinical trials," Obstet Gynecol, 95(6, Pt 2);1051-1065, June, 2000.

Rinehardt H. "A VBAC primer: technical issues for midwives," Midwifery Today, (57);16-20, Spring, 2001.

Spong C, et al. "Prophylactic amnioinfusion for meconium-stained amniotic fluid," Am J Obstet Gynecol, 171(4);931-935, Oct, 1994.

Tucker S. Pocket Guide to Fetal Monitoring and Assessment, 4th ed. Mosby, St. Louis MO, 2000.

Tucker S. Pocket Guide to Fetal Monitoring and Assessment, 5th ed. Mosby, St. Louis MO, 2004.

Usta I, et al. "The impact of a policy of amnioinfusion for meconium-stained amniotic fluid," Obstet Gynecol, 85(2);237-241, Feb, 1995.

Wenstrom K, et al. "Amnioinfusion survey: prevalence protocols and complications," Obstet Gynecol, 86(4, Pt 1);572-576, Oct, 1995.

ASSISTING LABOR AND BIRTH IN OTHER-THAN-VERTEX PRESENTATIONS, MULTIPLE, PRETERM AND POSTTERM BIRTHS

ASSISTING AT THE BIRTH OF A BABY PRESENTING HER FACE

Babies who present their face with the chin anterior often birth normally. This chapter will go over special considerations to keep in mind when the baby's head is fully extended.

Associated factors

Face presentations are associated with anencephaly and other cranial vault abnormalities (especially when found with polyhydramnios). They are also said to be seen more frequently with high parity. Anything that significantly impairs flexion or encourages extension could be an associated factor. If you suspect that a fetal anomaly may be part of the picture, transport is your best alternative. If none of these factors are present, a wait-and-see attitude is appropriate as long as mother and baby are doing well.

Early labor

The baby's head will be high in the pelvis in early labor, giving the impression that the pelvis is empty on internal exam (rule out oblique or transverse lie). The bag of waters is likely to be large and functioning as the chief dilating wedge; take extra care not to break it if you do internal exams. When fetal features can be felt, the presentation may feel more like a brow than a face because many babies who start out in a brow presentation convert to a fully extended face presentation during descent. Labor is often longer than in vertex presentations as the pliable face does not apply itself firmly to the cervix. The contractions of early labor are often weaker as a result and dilation is thus delayed.

Fetal heart rate monitoring

It is important to listen to the fetal heart rate frequently and carefully throughout labor. There appears to be an increase in the frequency of abnormal heart rate patterns in face presentations compared with vertex presentations. In a study by Benedetti and colleagues (1980), concerning fetal heart rate patterns were noted in 58% of the babies that were monitored with an internal monitor. Some of these babies had improved heart rates with maternal position changes and oxygen administration. Repetitive severe variable decelerations may be due to more severe cord compression if the cord is trapped behind the extended head (where the cord can become pinched under the occiput) or between the face and the bony pelvis or maternal soft tissues. Babies presenting with their chin posterior are most likely to have poor fetal heart rate patterns and low APGAR scores. If the fetal heart rate is consistently concerning, transport is your best alternative.

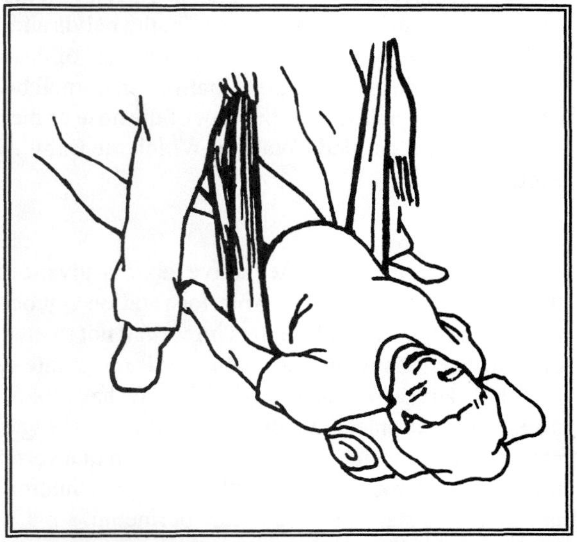

(Adapted with permission from photographs appearing in COMFORT MEASURES FOR CHILDBIRTH: THE REBOZO WAY, © 2001, Guadalupe Trueba.)

Should flexion be encouraged?

When the head is well extended, the presenting facial diameters are almost the same as those for a flexed vertex. Attempting to flex a mentum anterior will result in an occiput posterior vertex presentation, which is actually harder for most mothers to deliver. If labor is progressing, leave well enough alone.

If it is felt that flexion should be encouraged, for example you feel the baby is in a brow-face presentation, Irene Sotelo (2004), a traditional Mexican midwife, recommends the following rebozo technique. It can assist in flexing the head whether the membranes are intact or not. As soon as the presentation is identified, fold your rebozo into a narrow strip 6 to 8 in (15 to 20 cm) wide. Place the center of the shawl on the floor and have the mother lie with her buttocks over the center with her legs straight and slightly open. Then stand over the mother, straddling her hips. Grasp the ends of the shawl and rock back and forth *very gently* beginning at the end of one contraction until the beginning of the next. As you do this, the mother should be panting like a dog. This almost always works to flex the head with only one such session unless the baby is too far down in the pelvis. You will know because progress will be evident.

If the head is only partly extended you can also try some of the techniques in the chapter entitled "Techniques Used to Help the Baby Descend during Labor" to flex the head.

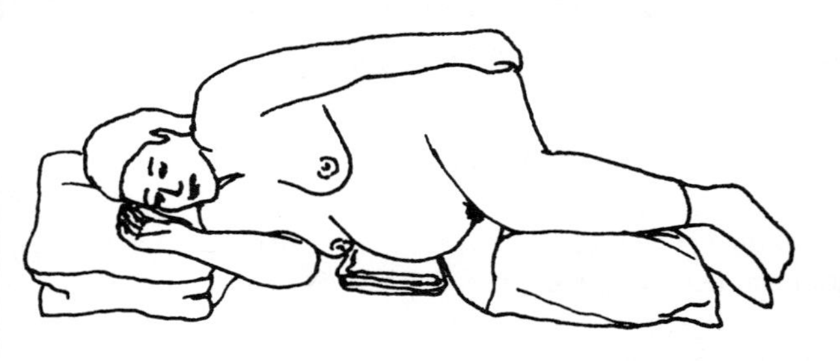

Mother lying on her left side with the baby LMT (brow-face presentation) to encourage the baby to fully extend her spine.

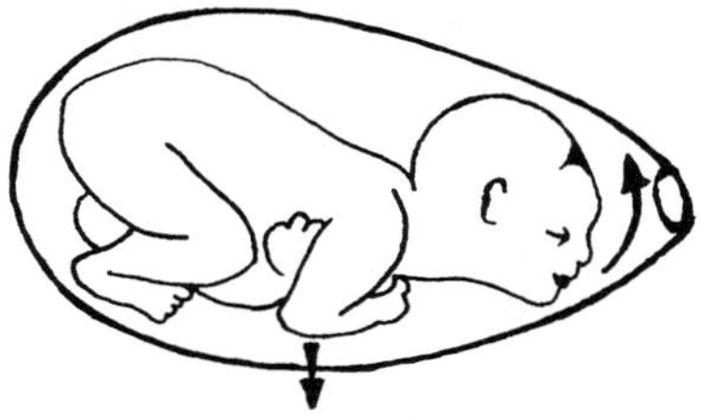

How side-lying with the baby's belly to the bed helps to extend the spine.

(Adapted with permission from illustrations by Stella Cruz, © Ruth Ancheta, 2000)

Encouraging full extension and descent: If the head is already fully extended into a face presentation, have the mother lie on the side with the baby's belly to the bed (e.g., if the baby is LMT, LMA or LMP, have the mother lie on her left side). This will help to encourage or maintain full extension. You might also try elevating her lower hip with a pillow. This should help maintain full extension as well as encourage anterior rotation of the chin.

Avoid rupture of membranes

Early rupture of membranes may occur due to the ill-fitting presenting part. Because of the poor fit, the intact forebag often hangs through the os in a loose pouch. Do what you can to avoid rupture, with careful internal exams kept to a minimum and use of maternal positions that decrease full pressure on the forewaters. However, don't be too rigid about this; allow the mother to go with her instincts and watch to see if the positions she chooses keep labor going. The forewaters will buoy the baby up, which will help with flexion (if it is going to occur) and rotation as well as minimize trauma to the baby's face from direct pressure. Should the membranes rupture spontaneously, check the fetal heart rate and, if indicated, perform an internal exam to rule out cord prolapse.

Engagement of the head

Recall that engagement has taken place when the biparietal diameter has passed through the inlet; face presentations do not engage until the face is deep in the pelvis and continuing to descend. In most occipital presentations, the parietal eminences have just dropped below the level of the inlet when the lowest part of the vertex lies in a line drawn between the ischial spines. In face presentations in normal babies, the parietal bones are still several centimeters above the plane of the inlet when the brow, the root of the nose or the chin (the lowest part) is at the level of the spines (for an illustration, see the chapter entitled "Ways in Which the Baby's Body Adapts during Descent: Anatomical Diameters, Attitude and Moulding").

Signs of progress

Typically, it is only after active labor is advanced that the head descends, extension becomes more pronounced, and the face actually presents. Anterior rotation can occur at any point, but may not begin until the face is well applied to the pelvic floor. Therefore, it is important not to give up hope if labor continues to progress, even if the chin is transverse or posterior. Many of these babies will rotate late in labor.

Gail Hart (2001), an Oregon midwife, has found that almost all posterior faces will rotate to anterior and that rotation takes place extremely late in labor, as the head bulges the perineum, which is much later than rotation with a vertex. This makes sense, considering that late rotation in a vertex presentation typically occurs as the biparietal diameter is passing through the ischial spines. With a face presentation, the parietal diameter doesn't often reach the spines until the chin is visible and starting to bulge the perineum.

Manual rotation of the mentum posterior baby

If the head has descended into the pelvic floor so that it is well within reach, nothing else has worked to rotate the chin, labor seems arrested, and there is still no sign of spontaneous rotation, you can try grasping the baby over the cheekbones or forehead above the temples (above the level of the eyebrows) between contractions and rotating the chin to anterior during a contraction. Have the mother lie supine, with her bottom hanging off the end of a firm surface and her legs supported by chairs or two assistants. Have someone listen to the fetal heart rate as you do this. This maneuver is likely to produce a temporary reduction in the fetal heart rate because pressure on the temples may stimulate a vasovagal response. If this occurs, continue to listen and have the mother breathe oxygen through contractions until the heart rate normalizes.

Daniels (1978) recommends standing between the mother's legs facing to the side to which you want the face to turn (i.e., if the baby is LMP, stand with your left shoulder toward the mother). Extend your arm, insert your hand and grasp the head with the crotch of your thumb and index finger directed to the floor. Now turn away from the mother. Perform the rotation by pronating your arm as you pivot your body to face the mother, using the strength of your entire body to affect the turn. Manual rotation may be surprisingly easy at this point. If rotation proves difficult, discontinue your efforts (Mentzer, 2001).

Birth of the head with the chin anterior

The mother who is completely dilated and ready to push should ideally assume a position that maximizes sacral mobility, so that the occiput can have the most space possible. The birth should proceed without too much problem as long as the chin is anterior (under the pubic arch). Slip one small pellet of homeopathic arnica (30C or 200C) into the baby's mouth, between the cheek and gum as soon as the mouth is visible to minimize further bruising. Keep your hands ready to apply light pressure to the forehead to maintain full extension as the baby's face crowns, then release this pressure after the chin clears the pubic bone.

Birth of the head with the chin posterior

While conventional wisdom states that this is virtually impossible if the baby is at term, on rare occasions the birth of untraumatized babies who are mentum posterior to mothers with very large pelvises do occur. As always, if descent is progressing with relative ease and the baby is stable, allow the birth to proceed, even if the chin is posterior.

Appearance of the baby

Prepare the mother for a baby who has a very swollen, bruised face. A caput-like swelling may form over the anterior cheek and eye. The eyes may bulge and exude a mucoserous discharge; the lips are swollen, the mouth is held open by the swollen lips, and the tongue may protrude. Small hemorrhages often develop in the whites of the eyes and the skin. Cracks in the skin of the neck may also be present. The blood vessels of the neck may be intensely congested. Give additional arnica and bellis perennis 30C or 200C or even 1 M to help with healing this trauma. If the parents had decided prenatally against prophylactic Vitamin K, discuss it again in light of this degree of trauma.

Airway trauma

Trauma to the larynx and trachea may occur during face presentations and can lead to airway obstruction after the birth, although this is a relatively rare occurrence. Fracture of the larynx has been known to occur as a result of excessive pressure as the throat passes beneath the pubic bone. Trauma and pressure can also stimulate a vasovagal response, temporarily depressing respiratory and cardiac functions. Any difficulty the baby may have with breathing could be related to such traumas. Watch the baby closely, and if you suspect damage to the airway has occurred, transport immediately. Passage of an orogastric tube may be difficult due to swelling. Be very gentle if such a baby requires artificial ventilation.

Assisting at the Birth of a Baby Presenting His Brow

Babies descending brow-first present one of the widest possible diameters of their skull. A normally sized, term fetus can rarely birth successfully in this position, unless the mother has a truly huge pelvic capacity.

Take steps to assist with flexion or full extension as soon as a brow presentation is recognized. Abdominal palpation may be the best way to determine deflexion of this degree, as the head will be high in the pelvis, limiting what can be discovered upon internal exam. First, try to flex the head with the rebozo technique in the chapter entitled "Assisting at the Birth of a Baby Presenting Her Face," as this almost always works unless the head is too far down in the pelvis. Brow presentations are, by nature, unstable, and since most will spontaneously convert to a vertex or a face presentation, a little encouragement is often all it takes and conversion to either vertex or face vastly increases the chances of a yoni birth.

If the head is found to be only partly extended in a brow-face attitude, the woman can also lie on the side to which the occiput points (e.g., if the baby is LFP or LMP, have the mother lie on her right side). Make sure the mother's bladder is empty, by catheterizing her if necessary. Side-lying on the side of the occiput encourages the weight of the baby's body to fold back on itself and may result in flexion of the head.

Any of the position changes or movements described in the chapters addressing asynclitic or posterior positioning may also help convert a brow to a vertex or full face presentation. Ideally the mentum or occiput is anterior once the presentation has converted. If not, take steps to remedy this as outlined in the chapters mentioned above.

Labor is typically slow when a brow does not convert because the head remains high during most of labor and there is nothing putting direct pressure on the cervix, making cord prolapse more likely should the membranes rupture. Descent is delayed because of the large presenting diameter and, when it does occur at all, usually begins only after complete dilation and rupture of membranes.

If the position remains stable and the baby descends partway through the brim and stops, consider the possibility that the open fetal mouth could be hung up on the pelvis. (If the head has not entered the brim, the mouth is not yet at a level where it could get hung on the brim.) Try placing the mother in a Trendelenburg position for a few contractions. Have her shake her hips side to side or rock her in a rebozo as described in the previous chapter. If these techniques alone do not result in conversion and the membranes are ruptured, try inserting your hand in the yoni, applying evenly distributed pressure with your entire hand, and pushing the head upward. Be sure not to press directly into the anterior fontanelle or the eyes and check for cord prolapse before you remove your hand.

Borell and Fernström (1960) describe a technique that was first introduced into the literature in 1821 by the French midwife Marie Louise Lachapelle. Have the mother in a Trendelenburg position. Lachapelle recommended inserting a hand far enough to hook a finger under the fetal chin, closing the mouth and removing the hand. This may result in dramatic conversion to a face or vertex presentation. It may also result in dramatic prolapse of the cord, so be careful. Monitor the fetal heart rate closely for several minutes after any of these procedures and before having the mother change positions, to rule out cord prolapse.

If the baby does not convert his position in spite of trying everything and if labor becomes arrested, transport is probably your safest alternative. However, if the head is advancing, labor appears to be moving along and mother and baby are doing well, let nature take its course, being sure to have the mother in a position that puts no pressure on the sacrum during pushing. If the mother has a very large pelvis or the baby is small, a yoni birth is possible. Use of a Birth Sling with the pelvis press would be ideal for this mother. However, if the baby gets stuck during pushing or the fetal heart rate takes a nose dive, have the mother stop pushing, give her oxygen by mask and place her in a position that reduces the amount of downward pressure. Do not force a brow through the pelvis, as the risk of intracranial damage is increased, so do not even consider using fundal pressure. However, opening the pelvis may work in some situations and is worth a try if the head is well descended. If none of the tricks for helping the baby flex his head and otherwise dealing with stuck labor work to remedy this situation in a timely fashion, or the baby appears compromised, your best bet is to transport.

ASSISTING AT THE BIRTH OF A BREECH BABY

NOTE: Preparation for a breech birth, including a discussion of the relevant research, political ramifications and possible complications, is discussed in the chapter entitled "Breech Presentation: General Principles" and in HOLISTIC MIDWIFERY Vol. I, in the chapter entitled "Anticipating a Breech Birth." Review the entire part on breeches entitled "The Birth Process When the Baby is Breech" before studying this chapter.

This chapter will discuss the differences between a breech labor and birth and a cephalic labor and birth. It is included for your review in conjunction with observation and hands-on experience with breech births under the guidance and supervision of a skilled senior midwife. However, whether such instruction is available or not, it is recognized worldwide that midwives must know how to assist at a breech birth because a woman may present with a surprise breech baby during labor. If you do not have access to hands-on training, you should prepare for such an event by getting together with other students or midwives to review the cardinal spiraling movements of breech births. Then watch and wait while keeping your hands off as someone times pushing a doll through the pelvis as in a spontaneous birth. This will give you a feel for how long a normal birth might take as each part of the baby emerges as well as offering valuable experience in observing when and how you want to intervene when nothing is wrong. Finally, practice hands-on techniques with a doll and pelvis until you feel familiar with the maneuvers.

The birth of a breech baby can be a straightforward and simple process, often easier than many a vertex birth. However, when breech birth is difficult, it is every bit as scary and as serious a situation as a severe shoulder dystocia; even more so, in fact, because breech birth is a relatively uncommon event, and we are unused to the head being the last part of the baby to be born. It is therefore important to be knowledgeable about minimizing problems and, at the same time, well prepared to assist if complications occur. How the mother is supported during her breech labor as well as the experience level and common sense of the midwife will affect the ease or difficulty of the birth to a great extent.

Breech births are a political hot potato because of the amount of fear surrounding them in contemporary obstetrics. With the advent of drug use in labor in the early 1900s, large quantities of anesthetics were used during breech births, which also cause muscle relaxation in the baby. This artificial relaxation increases the risk of fetal injury. A knocked-out, supine mother and drugged baby can do nothing to facilitate the birth on their own. These factors, in conjunction with the routine application of massive hands-on interference has fostered the impression that spontaneous breech birth is all but impossible and an increasing trend toward surgical delivery. Thus, there has been a trend toward automatic surgical birth for breeches over the last third of the 1900s. This has left several decades of medical and midwifery graduates with little or no hands-on training in assisting normal breech births (Gaskin, 2004). Fortunately, we have midwives (and some doctors), the world over, who have had the courage to support women in giving birth spontaneously to their breech babies, relearning old skills and experimenting with new ideas to reduce the intrinsic risks to the absolute minimum. Among them, several have published books and videos, notably BREECH BIRTH–WOMAN WISE by Maggie Banks; ASSISTING A VAGINAL BREECH DELIVERY, a video by Ina May Gaskin and The Farm midwives (1992); and NORMALIZING THE BREECH DELIVERY, a video by Valerie el Halta and Rahima Baldwin (1987) (see references for additional sources).

Note: Almost all the existing literature on breeches assumes that the mother is supine. In this chapter, both supine and upright maternal positions will be discussed, with upright positions as the norm. Remember that anatomical references to anterior and posterior refer to the mother's body; her front is always anterior; her back is always posterior. The same goes for the baby. Remember this, use your own body for reference, and have a doll and pelvis on hand when studying to avoid confusion.

Assessing the Prospects for a Breech Birth during Early Labor

Since everyone agrees that the easier the birth is anticipated to be, the better, a variety of scoring systems have been devised in an attempt to provide a cookbook answer regarding whether a particular woman is a good candidate for a breech birth. These scoring systems rely on parity, dilation, station and the size of the baby to make this determination, favoring partially dilated multiparous mothers who have had a breech baby in the past and are now carrying a small, slightly early baby at an advanced station as contractions begin.

However, there are many and varied opinions regarding what constitutes favorable physical signs that a breech labor is likely to go well. A lot also depends upon whether the birth is "managed," or the mother and baby are allowed to follow their own cues about positioning, pushing, etc. Some women carrying breech begin labor at term with a relatively closed cervix, with the baby high until complete dilation, after which the baby moves down and birth proceeds with no problems. While scoring systems suggest a more favorable outcome with a smaller baby, many experienced practitioners do not find this valid either. A large, term, frank breech baby fitting through the pelvis is a good indication that the head can fit through as well. A smaller baby, with a disproportionately large head, may cause more problems because the body can slip through easily without stretching the birth canal sufficiently to allow the head to pass. Also, Mayes (1959) points out that incomplete anterior rotation or posterior rotation of the occiput is more likely to occur when the baby is early. A preterm baby is also more likely to present SP at the onset of labor because she is not yet ready to be born.

As you assess the prospects for a successful labor, palpate the baby's head to determine if it is flexed, using the same techniques described in Volume I for detecting a flexed head. Mayes (1959) notes that the flexed head is usually found to one side of the fundus; in a frank breech, the head is often found in the center of the fundus, indicating that it is less well flexed. A truly hyperextended head at the start of labor is a universally accepted contraindication to proceeding with a yoni birth. As with an extended cephalic presentation, a hyperextended head in a breech is associated with extension of the spine. Likewise, a sacrum posterior presentation is generally considered a contraindication to allowing labor to progress. These babies are unlikely to descend easily, and transport is strongly advised whenever an SP presentation is identified prior to active pushing (Cronk, 2002; Evans, 2002). A military attitude of the head does not necessarily contraindicate yoni birth by itself, but it is something to be aware of during pushing.

When a breech birth is expected, pelvimetry should be performed in late pregnancy and can be reassessed in early labor, when the tissues are at their softest. Gaskin (1992) wants the interspinous diameter to be greater than 9 cm, the pubic arch to be normal, and the anteroposterior diameter of the diagonal conjugate to be ample. If the pubic arch is somewhat narrow, the impact is lessened if the diagonal conjugate of the outlet is large.

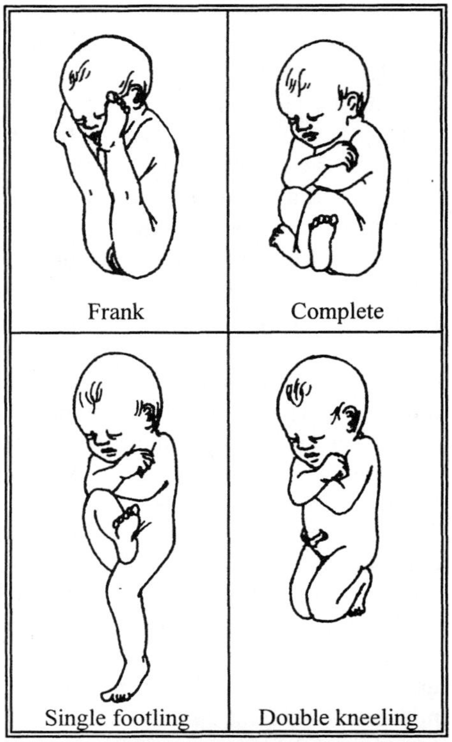

(Babies are shown sacrum posterior to better demonstrate the attitude of the legs.)

Mary Cronk (2002) and Jane Evans (2002) emphasize that their main parameter for a healthy breech birth is good, steady, smooth, unstimulated progress in labor. Progress is measured by regular, increasingly frequent contractions that become longer and more intense, accompanied by steady cervical dilation. If fetopelvic disproportion or other problems are part of the picture, labor will not move along smoothly. If labor slows or stops, the safest and most prudent course of action is to transport as soon as possible. *Breech birth should never be a struggle.*

Surprise breeches

If you arrive at a labor and discover that the baby is breech, what happens at that point will depend upon the phase of labor, your skill with breeches, the desires of the parents, and the proximity of decent hospital backup. The well-being of the baby must be your first concern. Transporting a baby about to be born breech, whether by ambulance or private car, can be risky. Emergency medical personnel often do not let the midwife ride in the ambulance; the baby may be born en route with ambulance attendants whose training in breech birth is cursory at best. Should you choose to transport by private vehicle, there may not be sufficient room for the mother to assume different positions and for you to perform any necessary maneuvers. Either way, having the baby en route will just increase any risks. If it is cold outside, the chances of chilling the baby during birth in a vehicle are great. Birth en route is more likely if the hospital is a long distance away. Keep in mind, as well, that the movement of the vehicle may encourage fetal descent. Consider remaining at home when labor is far advanced and the baby seems fine, with the valid claim that birth was imminent and transport ill advised.

On the other hand, if labor is just getting started and the breech presentation is a surprise, your most prudent move may be to transport. You need to consider the political implications of breech birth, unless your local jurisdiction and regulations allow a mother to choose an attended breech birth at home during labor. Furthermore, it is your duty and obligation to remind the parents of the risks specific to breeches (including the politics of your local hospital regarding breeches, the likelihood of a surgical birth if you transport, with all the risks that entails), your hands-on skill and experience level with breeches (or lack thereof), as well as any didactic education or hands-on training you may have had using models. It is also your responsibility to be totally candid and recommend transport if you feel you cannot attend the birth at home, whether for medical, experiential or political reasons.

Deciding to stay at home with a couple who have not made the choice to have a breech baby at home prior to labor is also risky on many other levels. Assisting a couple who have contracted and expected to give birth at home with a pregnancy considered medically "low risk" is very different from assisting them in an unexpected situation considered more medically risky. They are having to make a difficult decision very quickly; it can be hard to assess full commitment to a new plan in an unexpected circumstance. You must carefully consider the circumstances, remembering that this particular political limb is long and thin. In many jurisdictions, regardless of how conscientious your decision was as a care provider or how clear the commitment of the parents, there will be almost no support for you or the parents if things turn out badly. However, there are many good reasons why you might choose to stay home. For example, maybe you have helped this couple with one or more previous births and have a solid relationship with them; you may know that this woman gives birth easily and staying at home is what she wants to do. It is under such circumstances that staying at home with a big surprise might be the best choice. If so, provide the couple with a written informed consent statement and have them sign and date it.

General Tips on Caring for the Laboring Mother and Breech Baby during Labor

Assuming that the decision is clear to remain at home, review the following tips from a variety of sources. They cover the differences you can expect to see in many breech labors as well as suggestions for attending breech labors.

Arrive early

Women carrying breech should call you as soon as they suspect labor is beginning. Arrive as early in labor as possible and remain at her side until the baby is born. This will give you experience in observing breech labors, and will allow you to immediately attend to any emergency that may arise.

Rupture of membranes as the first sign of labor

Rupture of membranes in the presence of a breech baby increases the possibility of cord prolapse, especially if the station is high. If you are with the mother at the time of rupture, check the fetal heart rate, then check for prolapse of the cord or a foot as soon as possible.

In the event that you are not there, stay on the phone with the parents while someone checks the fetal heart rate and looks at the introitus to see if anything is presenting such as a loop of cord or a foot. If the FHR is within a normal range, ask the mother to lie down on her side or enter a birthing pool on her hands and knees until you arrive. Have the partner recheck the FHR to make sure her new position is not compromising cord circulation; if so, have her slowly change her position (so as not to precipitate a prolapse) until the heart rate is stable. As the risk of prolapse is now increased, get there as quickly as you can to monitor the situation. If you have an assistant who lives closer to the parents and can get there faster than you, notify her at once.

If the parents hear a problematic heart rate that does not resolve with your advice regarding position changes, or if they report that a loop of cord can be seen or felt in the yoni, recommend transport with the mother in a knee-chest position while someone holds the presenting part off the cord, and meet the parents at the hospital. If there are not enough people in the house to perform all these tasks, ask that an ambulance be called. Getting to the hospital as quickly as possible is a top priority.

Assessing the mother's coping skills

The mother's ability to cope with labor, especially during pushing, is of paramount importance to the successful birth of a breech baby. It is imperative that she be able to cooperate fully with any instructions given and with any procedures you need to do to get the baby out safely. If this is a planned breech, the mother should have been well prepared prenatally for the types of position changes she may have to make during pushing, she should understand what you might have to do to facilitate the birth and should be prepared for the possible need for her concentrated effort during pushing.

However, you will not know exactly how a woman will cope until she enters labor, unless you have been her midwife for a previous birth. Even then, you will have no certain knowledge of how she will react now. Therefore, it is a good idea to be present for the entire labor so that you can observe her reactions. If you note that the mother is not coping well, it is most prudent to transport prior to pushing. This is especially important with women who are having their first baby, because you have nothing else to go on regarding how they might respond during pushing.

Even if you do not perform many internal exams during most labors, it is a wise precaution to perform at least one or two during a breech labor. This will give you valuable clinical information and help you assess how the mother will cope with internal manipulations during pushing. Again, if she cannot handle such an exam with ease, transport before pushing begins.

Setting up for a breech birth

Choose a large room with good temperature control for the birth itself. Rearrange or remove unnecessary furniture so that the woman will have quick and easy access to the places you will arrange as options for position changes during late labor and pushing while keeping the path to the door clear.

Very nearby, you will want a very firm, flat surface with a drop of at least 20 inches (51 cm) between the surface and the floor (most beds and couches will meet this criterion). The perfect height allows the mother to get on and off of the surface easily without having to climb or be assisted. It can be a very sturdy, padded low table top or a bed with a large piece of plywood on top and padded with blankets and thin foam. The head of the flat surface should be flat against a wall with plenty of room on both sides or placed kitty-corner in a corner of the room with space on both sides. There should be low chairs or padded milk crates on either side at the end of this flat surface for the mother to prop her feet. The height of the foot supports should allow her thighs to be slightly flexed when she is lying supine. Having the foot props too high will increase tension in the perineum and narrow the inlet. Have her practice getting on and off this surface a couple of times during early labor, so that things can be adjusted as necessary. If climbing is necessary for her to get up on the furniture available, how this will occur should be thought out and provided for in advance. Provisions must take into account her size, ability to balance and ease of movement. It should be noted that supine positions are not used by the majority of midwives with a track record of successful home breeches, even when complications arise (among them Banks, 1998; Cronk, 2002; Evans, 2002). However, experienced midwives know to never say never. The use of supine positions during a breech birth can be viewed as a back-up of last resort. If a birth tub is available, it should be placed in another corner of the room with space all around it to accommodate support people and assistants.

You will want to have space for the mother to move from position to position, to kneel or squat, and a sturdy chair of the right height for her to rest one foot with that thigh parallel to the floor while standing on the other leg. There should be plenty of room for the mother to move from standing to kneeling to hands and knees without moving to another location. Only a step or two should be required to assume another position or to reach the flat surface where she can lie down, and there must be plenty of room for the midwife and at least one assistant to maneuver as well.

Especially if you tend to have cold hands, have a crock pot of plain water available so that your hands can be quickly submerged to warm them before handling the baby. Place a brown paper sack with at least 6 clean receiving blankets and a few soft washcloths or dish towels in a 150°F (65°C) oven. Several warmed blankets or towels should be available so that wet ones, which will get cold quickly, can be replaced. Have your oxygen tank and other resuscitation equipment readily available.

Assessing fetal well-being during dilation

The fetal heart rate should be checked regularly and frequently during breech labors because of the increased risk of cord compression or prolapse. Prolapse can occur more easily because the baby's abdomen is relatively close to the os, especially when the presenting part does not fit well in the pelvis.

Listen with a fetoscope as long as the fetal heart can be heard clearly through the mother's abdomen. The location of the fetal heart sounds are typically higher on the mother's belly than in a cephalic birth. Listen over the back, just past the anterior fetal shoulder. The point of maximum intensity moves down as the upper torso descends and rotates as in a cephalic birth.

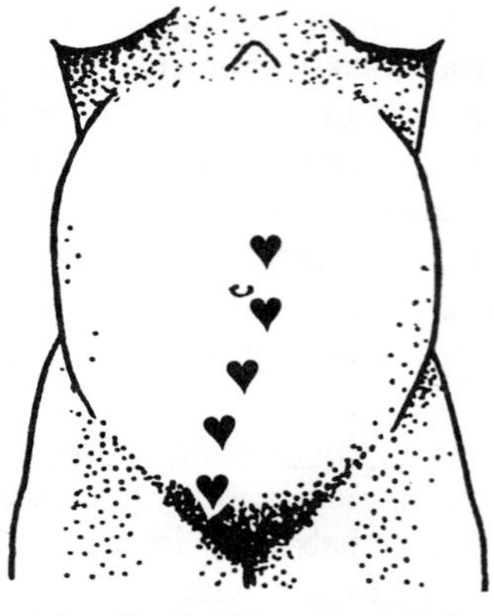

Locating the fetal heart sounds in an LSA baby as descent and rotation proceed.

Prodromal labor

The position of the baby will influence the progress of labor. El Halta

(1989) has found that early labor may be prolonged in breech births if the presenting part is not well applied to the cervix. However, prolonged early labor has not been the rule in births attended by Cronk (2002) and Evans (2002).

In women who have had babies before, early labor may be particularly easy, with minimal discomfort. It is not unusual to discover a multipara to be 4 cm dilated or more before she is aware that her labor has begun (El Halta, 1989).

Rupture of membranes after labor begins

Frequently, the membranes rupture sooner than they would with a vertex presentation, especially in footling or kneeling breeches. This happens because the small, irregular fetal parts near the os cannot plug the pelvis the way a head or a butt can, and the pressure changes on the forewaters from repeated contractions and maternal position changes (and shifts in fetal position) result in rupture. Sometimes the baby will kick a hole in the bag. Note that Cronk (2002) believes that spontaneous rupture of membranes prior to or very early in labor may be a warning sign that things may not go well as labor advances.

Because the presenting part may fit poorly, the mother should immediately lie down upon rupture of membranes and the heart rate should be assessed as soon as possible to determine if the cord has been swept down with the waters. Even if the heart rate is normal, an internal exam should be done to rule out uncompressed cord prolapse before the mother assumes an upright position. Auscultate the fetal heart again once the mother has changed positions to make sure the cord has not become compressed during maternal repositioning.

Do not rupture the membranes. The forewaters help equalize pressure on the cervix and act as a dilator as well as protect the baby from cord prolapse, especially when small parts are presenting. The longer the bag is intact, the better.

Active labor

Breech labors are ideally straightforward. Once underway, active labor should progress normally and even rapidly in many cases. If the first phase progresses normally, pushing can be anticipated to proceed smoothly as well. If active labor is prolonged, many old-time doctors and experienced midwives take this as a warning sign that the birth should not continue at home. A long, drawn-out labor results in a tired mother when it comes time to push, when her full attention and cooperation are essential. It may also indicate that the baby will have trouble coming through the pelvis due to extended arms or a deflexed head.

Maternal positioning during labor: Midwifery opinion varies regarding maternal positioning during breech labors. Cronk, Evans and Banks are all very clear that positioning should be led by the mother, as in any birth. Other midwives try to guide maternal positioning, primarily based upon the attitude of the baby with the intent of minimizing the risk of early rupture of membranes and cord prolapse.

If the baby is term and in a complete or frank attitude with the presenting part filling the pelvis, some midwives encourage upright and walking positions during labor. If the baby is early, footling or kneeling, the chance of cord prolapse upon rupture of membranes is increased. Therefore, the mother may be encouraged to labor in a side-lying or possibly a hands-and-knees position to minimize downward pressure on the membranes. She can also enter a birth pool on her hands and knees or reclining. Laboring in water removes the influence of gravity, lessening both the chance that the baby's torso will descend prior to full dilation and the chance that the membranes will rupture before pushing. Cord prolapse may also occur if the mother moves around a great deal after the membranes rupture because it shifts the baby around. Keeping the mother quiet until active pushing is underway also helps minimize the chance of rupture of membranes or cord prolapse, should the bag break.

Alternatively, Valerie El Halta (1989), who has attended many breech births, has found that the best upright position for the mother is to sit "tailor fashion," with the soles of her feet pressed together and her back straight and well supported. This is an especially good position with footling breeches as it allows gravity to assist the buttocks in becoming better applied to the cervix without the mother having to move around a lot.

Characteristics of active labor contractions: The sensations of the contractions are usually about the same as for vertex labors. Watch for weak, spaced-out contractions. While weak contractions are not desirable during any labor, good, consistent contractions are especially important during pushing with a breech. Weak contractions increase the chance of asphyxia during the birth and the likelihood that you will have to perform manual manipulations to get the baby out.

Encouraging contractions: The labor should take its natural course with no attempt to stimulate contractions prior to a full rump. If active labor slows, wait a reasonable amount of time and then transport if contractions do not resume.

Spontaneous birth can be encouraged once you are beyond the point of safe transport (as the baby is emerging) by doing things that assist the uterus in maintaining effective, closely spaced contractions.

Instruct the mother to focus on having contractions when indicated. A support person can provide nipple stimulation and firm abdominal massage. Slight position changes are also likely to stimulate additional contractions. If contractions slow down after the baby begins to emerge, uterine stimulant herbs can also be given during pushing.

Eating and drinking: The mother may find it particularly uncomfortable to eat and drink during labor because of the pressure from the head pressing into her diaphragm. If this proves a problem, liquid nourishment such as a protein drink or fruit smoothie taken in small sips may be the best solution (El Halta, 1989).

Elimination: There is an increased possibility of the need for manipulation at breech births. Therefore, it is a good idea to have as much space in the pelvis as possible by emptying the lower bowel and bladder. In most cases, the bowels take care of themselves by becoming loose during early labor. If there is any question about the status of the bladder and the mother cannot urinate, catheterization may be wise, as suprapubic pressure may be needed during pushing. Wiping away stool during pushing is contraindicated because it may cause the mother to reflexively clinch her sphincter (Evans, 2012).

Fetal descent during labor: Regardless of parity, the breech baby often remains high in the pelvis until labor is well advanced. Significant descent may not occur until dilation is complete and the membranes have ruptured. Descent is slow because the softer breech cannot wedge itself into the yoni as firmly as does the head (Greenhill, 1951). Mary Cooper, a midwife who practiced in Ohio for several years, observes that a breech baby's station may move up and down more frequently than in cephalic presentations (Cooper, 1992?). Evans (2002) finds that fetal descent varies greatly during otherwise normal breech labors; the baby may remain high until dilation is complete, or progressive descent may occur as the cervix dilates. Therefore, do not focus on station as a criterion of good progress until dilation is complete and pushing has begun.

Situations that may arise during labor:

Localized pains and sensations: El Halta (1989) has found that breech labors often produce more intense back labor than is the case with anterior vertex presentations, although this has not been reported by other experienced midwives (Cronk, 2002; Evans, 2002). Back pain may occur because there is little or no moulding of the head as it descends and passes through the pelvis, or it may occur more frequently among the clients of midwives who encourage reclining positions during labor. However, overall, labor is usually not as painful as with a posterior vertex labor. Schlinger (2002) has noted more flank pain during breech labors. (The flank is defined as the sides of the abdomen between the costal margin and the iliac crest.) As with any birth, pokes from small parts can cause localized pains as well.

Mothers who have labored before may find the sensations associated with breech descent to be quite different from those of their previous vertex births. For example, many women experience a sensation of breathlessness during or after contractions due to the pressure of the baby's head under the diaphragm (El Halta, 1989).

Emergence of a small part prior to pushing: Although this is a rare occurrence, when the baby is a footling or kneeling breech, a foot or knee may emerge well before dilation is complete. Should this happen, first rule out cord prolapse. Some midwives then reposition the extremity back inside the yoni for as long as possible, using their hands to provide counterpressure if necessary. Others gently and loosely wrap any small part that emerges in a warmed cloth to prevent chilling and stimulation of the baby, because they believe undue stimulation may prompt the baby to gasp before birth (El Halta, 1989; Gaskin, 1998). The cloth should to be replaced frequently to avoid chilling the baby. A better option is for the mother to get into a body-temperature birth pool, which will keep the baby warm and eliminate the effect of gravity while she continues to labor. Still others leave the small part exposed and do nothing, having found exposure to air does not prompt the baby to breathe while the rest of the baby's body is still inside (Dzata, 2001).

Cord compression and prolapse: The distance between the umbilicus and the crown of the vertex is 28 cm, while the distance from the umbilicus to the lowest point of the breech is only 9.4 cm. This is why cord prolapse in cephalic presentation is only 0.5%, and why the risk rises with breeches. It occurs in 1% of term, frank breech babies. Frank babies are also more likely to experience increased cord compression from the pressure of the extended legs splinted up on the torso. Complete breeches run a 5% risk of prolapse, and incomplete breeches are the most prone to cord prolapse, with an incidence of about 15% (Collea, 1981).

Cord prolapse in the incomplete breech, while an indication for immediate intervention (which may include surgical delivery), is not usually as immediate an emergency as it is in cephalic presentations. When the cord does prolapse, it typically passes down between the fetal legs. Evans (2002) and Cronk (2002) point out that there is often only minimal compression when the cord is in contact with soft tissues alone in contrast to its being compressed between the hard fetal skull and the maternal pelvis. Thus, cord compression may not occur at all during many labors until the head is deep in the pelvis during pushing. Also be aware that occult cord prolapse or compression occurs more frequently in breech presentations and contributes to asphyxia in the newborn (Cruikshank, 1986). To rule out the possibility of occult cord compression, the fetal heart rate should be followed closely. Cronk (2002) and Evans (2002) point out that, in their experience, cord prolapse is rare during dilation and, when it does occur with pushing, is rarely a problem.

Passage of meconium in labor: Passage of meconium prior to descent (or before 6 cm of dilation), especially prior to 40 weeks gestation, should be taken as a *possible* sign of compromise, as with cephalic births.

Premature urge to push: Women often have a desire to push prior to full dilation. This is especially true for those carrying a footling or kneeling breech because the membranes tend to rupture earlier in labor and small parts often descend and apply pressure in the yoni and rectum long before dilation is complete. If the baby is early, dilation may be incomplete even though the buttocks are visible upon parting the mother's labia. Cronk (2002) and Evans (2002) emphasize they have never seen a full-term, well-grown baby descend like this when dilation was not complete.

<u>Resting phase</u>

As with vertex labors, there is often a natural resting phase between complete dilation and the onset of pushing.

<u>Pushing</u>

<u>Keep the birth room quiet and calm</u>: In hospitals, breech births often take place in an atmosphere of tension and crisis. A quiet and calm environment helps the mother to stay relaxed and allows her to fully open the soft tissues of her pelvis. A tense pelvic floor can restrict the smooth descent of the baby (Cronk, Evans, 2004).

<u>Ensure complete dilation before pushing begins</u>: Many experienced midwives feel that the truly uncontrollable urge to push signals that the cervix is fully dilated and allow the mother's instincts to be the guide as to when pushing begins. However, if there is *any* doubt about the condition of the cervix, the baby is not frank breech or the baby is early, do not encourage a woman to go with the urge without a thorough internal examination to determine if the cervix is fully dilated. If you can still feel any cervix, the mother is not complete. Pushing through a partially dilated cervix, especially if the baby is small or early, increases the risk of the arms becoming caught on the cervical ring and swept upward, and of the head getting hung up on the remaining rim.

The hour of patience: To ensure that the cervix is fully taken up before pushing begins, some midwives impose anywhere from a half-hour to one hour "of patience" after complete dilation. This is done to ensure that the cervix is completely taken up before pushing begins, even if the mother feels like pushing and an examination finds dilation to be complete (Daniels, 1978). This prevents any tiny edges of cervix from becoming hung up on the jaw line or chin of the descending head. In the meantime, the uterus may spontaneously begin expulsive contractions, which the mother should not try to resist nor add to but simply allow to do their work until the bottom is rumping.

<u>Rupture of membranes at the onset of pushing</u>: Banks (1998) recommends rupturing the membranes as the perineum begins to bulge, allowing the release of any meconium that has been passed during descent, thus clearing the birth canal and fluid of meconium before the head enters the pelvis. Cronk (2002) and Evans (2002) caution that you should never rupture the membranes until you are sure which fetal part is behind the forewaters. Use a flashlight to check; wait if you are unsure. This precaution may avoid a cord prolapse. If the baby is small and the cord is floating near the legs, allowing most of the baby to emerge prior to breaking the bag will greatly minimize or eliminate pressure on the cord, especially if she is a second twin, as the birth canal has already been dilated once.

<u>Passage of urine or meconium as descent progresses</u>: As the lower torso enters the deepest curve of the birth canal and the buttocks begin to emerge, it is quite common for the baby to urinate (especially boys) as a result of lower abdominal compression. Abdominal pressure also makes the passage of meconium a normal variation during descent and pushing. This is especially true for a frank breech presentation, where the legs are splinted up against the abdomen, applying additional pressure as the baby moves down.

Pushing contractions: Pushing-phase contractions may not be as strong, long or frequent as they were during active labor. However, descent should occur once the membranes are out of the way. If it does not, reevaluate for disproportion, pelvic obstruction or weak contractions. However, delay once the buttocks have descended to the pelvic floor is not uncommon with a frank breech presentation, as lateral flexion may be hindered. Encouraging the mother to assume an upright position is the best and safest way to overcome this problem as it maximally straightens the birth canal. If there is significant delay, transport if this is reasonable, given the distance you must travel.

Active pushing: Once active bearing down begins, Banks, Cronk and Evans encourage the mother to push as she feels the urge. During descent, pushing proceeds as for a vertex birth, without prolonged holding of her breath.

However, the late Nial Ettinghausen (1981), a Southern California naturopath who attended hundreds of breech births at home, strongly advised that the buttocks be allowed to descend to at least +3 station and ideally to the perineum before active pushing began. He believed that the longer the mother could "pant the baby down" (ideally until the anterior hip is visible), the less likely it would be that complications would develop. The 6th edition of MYLES' TEXTBOOK OF MIDWIFERY (1968) also says to wait until the buttocks are bulging at the perineum before encouraging active pushing.

Continuous pushing? Some women lose the urge to push once the baby is born to the umbilicus, although this is much more likely to occur if the mother is supine or if she is afraid (Cronk, 2002; Evans, 2002). At this point, there will inevitably be some degree of cord compression, as the baby's shoulders and head fill the pelvic cavity. Many practitioners, therefore, have the mother push continuously, even between contractions, until the birth is accomplished, being sure the woman takes time for deep breaths between pushes. The mother is often instructed to suspend pushing once the shoulders and arms are free until the weight of the baby's body pulls the occiput beneath the pubic bone.

Assessing fetal well-being during pushing: Pamela Hunt (2003), Farm midwife from Summertown TN with years of experience attending breech births, has found that, once the presenting part is visible, its color can also be monitored for good oxygenation, just as in a cephalic presentation. It is perfectly normal for the presenting part to be swollen and bruised due to the pressure and impaired circulatory return that occur during breech births (Hunt, 2003), although bruising can confuse your assessment. As more and more of the baby emerges, the boundaries of the most bruised region should end and the color above that level should transition to the more normal lavender pink color that indicates good fetal oxygenation. If unbruised areas are not a normal color, check the fetal heart rate and capillary refill time and responsiveness. In addition, exposed parts often move spontaneously, a good sign, even if the fetal heart rate is slow.

Some midwives switch from auscultation to gently palpating the base of the umbilicus for pulsations after the baby has been born to the midabdomen. Once the torso has started to emerge, it will be far easier, faster and often more reliable to assess the heart rate directly via palpation than to try and listen through the mother's abdomen. However, if you do try to listen, do so directly above or over the pubic bone, over the fetal back, which will be easy to locate based on the positioning of the partially born torso. A prewarmed infant stethoscope, a Doppler transducer or your hand can also be slipped up along the baby's chest or back to feel or listen for the heartbeat as the body is born, but this is a lot more invasive, uncomfortable and awkward than simply palpating the base of the cord.

To palpate the pulse, warm your hand and press the pad of your index and middle fingers into the baby's abdomen to one side of the base of the umbilicus (to feel the pulse just beneath the skin) or straddle the cord base with your fingers (to feel the pulse as the blood enters the cord). The fetal pulse is very strong in this region; you should have no trouble detecting the rate. This is safer than repeatedly palpating the cord itself, which risks causing the vessels to spasm. Palpating the base of the cord gives you valuable information about systemic perfusion; a good pulse at the umbilicus is a reliable indication of adequate circulation, whereas a slow or weak umbilical pulse does not necessarily reflect cardiac activity.

If a foot emerges, it may be tempting to palpate the tibial artery at the ankle to check the pulse. However, newborn peripheral pulses are very subtle, and their palpation is a notoriously difficult skill to master. Furthermore, palpating the ankle stimulates the baby and is therefore not recommended as many midwives feel that any palpation, regardless of how gentle, may startle the baby, causing him to throw his arms upward.

While the heart rate may remain within normal limits throughout the birth, it can drop to as low as 40 bpm after the umbilicus is born. When the pulse is slow, the skin color and responsiveness of the baby and careful monitoring before and during the birth will help you determine how the baby is faring and if intervention to hasten the birth is required. If responsiveness changes or ceases, even if the presenting part is pink, take this as a sign of compromise and proceed as quickly as possible with birth or transport, if it can be done quickly, while the mother receives supplemental oxygen. Birth should be hastened with care. More babies die from intracranial hemorrhage due to ill-advised, hasty maneuvers than from anoxia due to cord compression (Myles, 1968). Mayes (1954, 225) even warns against monitoring the heart rate as the torso emerges. Finding that cord pulsations are invariably slow at this point he states "... if you suddenly realize that it is beating slowly your equanimity may be further disturbed, resulting in hurried vigorous efforts at extraction, thus perhaps defeating your very aim to get a living baby." In short, *be measured and careful in your actions.*

Maternal hyperoxygenation during pushing: There is a diversity of opinion regarding the prophylactic use of maternal hyperoxygenation during the pushing phase of a breech birth. Dr. Leo Sorger and many midwives advocate it because of the associated cord compression; they feel that this will transfer more oxygen to the baby even if the fetal heart rate is slow. The mother may be given oxygen by partial-rebreather or nonrebreather mask at a flow rate of 8 to 15 l/min from the time the rump is being born until the head is out. Cronk (2002), Evans (2002) and Banks (2002) all feel strongly that this is not necessary if all is going well. If the fetal heart rate is normal, supplemental oxygen may do more harm than good (see the chapter entitled "Assessing and Supporting the Baby's Well-Being during Labor" for details). However, if birth is delayed at any point, give the mother oxygen immediately and continue until after the baby's head is born.

Maternal positions for pushing: Midwives who attend breech births at home vary tremendously as to the pushing positions they recommend. Banks (1998) feels strongly that the mother knows which position is best for her and usually does not offer any guidance. Evans and Cronk (2004) concur; from the onset of active pushing until the presenting part is visible, the woman is encouraged to assume the position of her choice. They find that women commonly choose hands and knees or a kneeling leaning forward position, with an occasional woman choosing to squat or sit on a birthing stool.

The rationale for the historical use of supine positions: The medical-model view is that the supine position minimizes the chance of cord prolapse because the full force of gravity is not in effect. Relieving the full force of gravity is also why it may be the best position when extensive internal manipulations, such as bringing down an extended leg, are called for. It also provides adequate access to the abdomen so that an attendant can apply suprapubic pressure to keep the head flexed. It allows the baby's body, once born, to hang so that the weight of the dependent torso will help the head to flex maximally, allowing the occiput to clear the pubic bone first. Finally, it allows access by the midwife to effect a controlled emergence of the head, preventing (to the extent possible) rapid decompression of the cranium, which could result in intracranial hemorrhage. Supine positions are superior to semi-sitting because they do not entail bending the torso, allow more access to the perineum and yoni in case manipulations are required and allow the coccyx to move, as well as allowing for some sacral mobility if the woman's bottom is positioned so that her lower buttocks (and sacrum) are hanging off the edge of the table or bed.

However, there are numerous drawbacks to all types of supine positions. The mother may quickly tire of pushing without the assistance of gravity; she may also develop supine hypotensive syndrome. Increased practitioner access to the mother's belly and perineum invites more hands-on fiddling with the baby than is typically necessary and may wind up creating a problem where there was none to begin with. The supine position does not allow gravity to maximally assist with the birth of the body or shoulders. The baby cannot actively participate in her birth as easily, as her movement is restricted by being acutely bent at the torso and neck as descent proceeds (Banks, 1998). Many midwives with breech experience feel lying flat contributes to many of the complications that necessitate the very interventions that give doctors the impression that breech birth is so dangerous and which makes them so afraid.

Lithotomy position: A full lithotomy position with the woman's thighs raised high in the air and widely spread is *not* recommended. This position maximizes the pelvic curve, pinches off the brim and tightens the perineum (Potter, 1922), although it does open the bony outlet.

Semi-sitting: Semi-sitting is said to eliminate the risk of supine hypotensive syndrome. However, it places maternal weight squarely on the sacrum, severely restricting posterior pelvic mobility, and therefore hinders the birth. This position also elevates the knees well above the tuberosities, pinching off the pelvic inlet; as a result, the torso or head may have difficulty entering the brim. Semi-sitting also maximizes the natural curve of the lower birth canal, requiring the baby to exaggerate lateral flexion, or it may interfere with lateroflexion of the baby's body altogether as well as encourage head deflexion as the head moves under the pubic bone. Although the risk of deflexion is lessened by applying manual suprapubic pressure to keep the head flexed, semi-sitting remains one of the worst positions for any birth.

Modified Walcher position: In the classical Walcher position, the woman lies on a table, buttocks hanging off the edge, with her legs dangling toward the floor, a posture intended to maximally open the brim. However, it is excruciatingly uncomfortable. Therefore, the modified Walcher position has the mother lying supine with her bottom extended beyond the edge and her feet propped on low supports to keep her perineum and pelvic floor relaxed. Her knees can also be raised slightly above the level of her abdomen by assistants supporting and gently spreading her thighs (Potter, 1922). Once the arms are born and the head is below the brim, the legs can be raised a bit more to open the outlet.

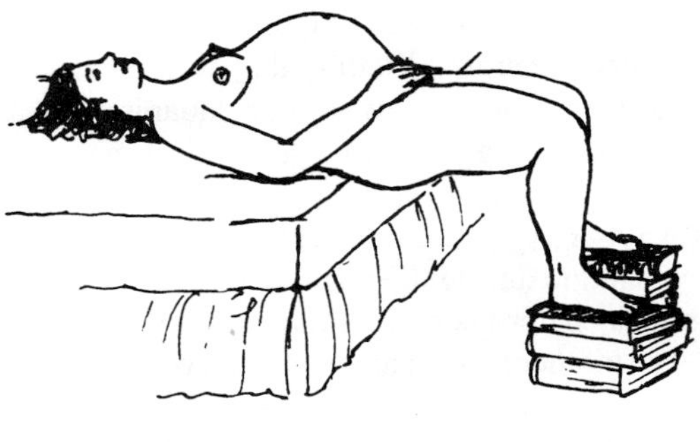

Modified Walcher position as described by Potter (1922)

Standing or standing squat: A standing squat allows gravity to maximally assist the birth. It also tightens the abdominal muscles and therefore may help aid head flexion. The mother's circulation is not compromised, and the pelvis can open in all dimensions to let the baby out. It is an excellent position to use to bring the breech to rumping.

However, there are drawbacks to this position as well. El Halta (1987) believes that descent may occur too rapidly since it is advisable for the head to be born as slowly and in as controlled a manner as possible. However, Banks, who has much experience with standing breeches, observes that upright pushing allows the babies to move and therefore facilitate their own descent (Banks, 1998, 2002).

Cronk (2002) and Evans (2002) have noticed that a fully upright position can lead to immediate placental separation as the baby is born. They feel this occurs because the center of gravity is higher than in a vertex birth and there is no check on the pull of gravity. Early separation increases the risk of anoxia for the baby and of excessive bleeding for the mother. Others have noted that a separation gush often occurs quickly after the birth when the woman is fully upright, regardless of the presentation. If the mother does give birth standing, be sure to ease the baby out and allow plenty of slack on the cord so that the placenta does not become detached prematurely.

Standing with one foot propped, legs well apart: This position affords plenty of room for the baby to come out, with the propped side of the pelvis opened wider. It is a good position to use to bring the breech down to rumping and can be used for the entire birth if descent goes smoothly, although the possibility of early placental separation still exists.

Full squat: Although some practitioners like to do breeches with the mother in a full squat, this position reduces the space at the brim, possibly interfering with engagement of the head. In addition, squatting tightens the perineum. A standing squat, maintained by supporting the woman from behind so that her thighs are held nearly parallel to the floor, the use of the dangle position or the birth sling are all much safer options, allowing gravity full play and keeping the spinopubic angle open. Beware of pulling on the cord at birth as well as the possibility of immediate placental separation.

A deBy birthing stool could also be used with the mother sitting, leaning forward into someone's arms with the open end of the "U" under her bottom, allowing the midwife excellent access to the baby.

Upright, kneeling, (open Christian prayer position): This position, with the mother kneeling with her upper torso inclined forward at about a 45° angle and knees spread, affords advantages similar to those described for standing, without the disadvantage of unchecked gravity encouraging placental separation during pushing.

Hands and knees: The late Dr. Gregory White advocated the hands-and-knees position for breech births. This position allows maximal pelvic mobility, offers an excellent view of the perineum and emerging baby, and facilitates hand maneuvers, should they be called for. Remaining in a hands-and-knees position for the entire pushing phase may, however, encourage some deflexion of the fetal spine as the curled spine falls toward the floor as it emerges. It could also pose deflexion problems if the woman has a pendulous abdomen. Schlinger (2002) has used hands and knees for the entire birth but cautions that it can be difficult for the midwife to shift her thinking 180° when assistance is needed.

Upright kneeling to hand-and-knees: Once the presenting part is visible, Cronk and Evans (2004) encourage the mother to assume an upright kneeling position (as above) for the majority of the pushing phase of labor. They have found that many women assume this position spontaneously without any prompting from the midwife. After the arms are born and further descent of the well-flexed head, the woman will often spontaneously drop forward to a hands and knees position–with her back horizontal. If not, they ask her to do so. This position change moves the mother's pelvis around the baby's head as the baby's mouth and nose clear the perineum (as described later under the Burns-Marshall maneuver with the mother upright). Overall, these are probably the best positions for the majority of breech births.

Proceeding with an Easy, Straightforward Breech Birth

At this point in our discussion, the baby is in the process of emerging, with the presenting part visible at the introitus. An "easy" breech is defined in this text as a baby whose arms are not extended and whose head is flexed, born to a calm and centered mother whose pelvis has plenty of room to let her baby out. The baby requires little or no manipulation.

Please note that the general reference to "upright positions" in this chapter includes all those positions in which the mother is not supine or semi-reclining, including hands and knees, the prayer position, standing squat, etc.

Hands off the breech

Nearly every midwifery and obstetric textbook, both old and new, highly recommends a policy of noninterference with the birth, at least until the baby is born to the buttocks and preferably to the umbilicus. Internationally, there is a strong feeling among most midwives that a hands-off policy is best. In many cases, watching and waiting are all that is needed while the baby is born quickly and easily with no assistance except support of the baby's body to prevent the head from bursting out of the yoni. Ettinghausen (1981) and Oxorn (1986) both state that allowing the baby to birth to the navel without interference allows the fully dilated cervix to become paralyzed, a condition that prevents it from clamping down on the shoulders or the aftercoming head. Other sources recommend keeping hands off the baby until the axilla are born, and Banks (1998) advises no manual intervention until the nape of the neck is seen.

Internal rotation is more variable in breeches, underscoring the importance of keeping your hands off the baby during descent. In addition, pulling or twisting the baby while the head and arms are not yet fixed in the pelvis can dislodge the arms and encourage the head to extend, delaying the birth. It is widely held that hands-on assistance given too early may stimulate the baby to breathe or startle the baby into throwing his arms upward, making for a difficult shoulder delivery.

The above represents the predominate European point of view. On the other hand, Gaskin (trained in breech delivery by a North American physician [Gaskin 2004]) and El Halta (1987) offer two of the best examples of careful use of a much more hands-on approach to the straightforward breech birth in their respective videos on the topic. Women are shown reclining or semi-sitting with more manipulation of the arms and head than is described here for an easy breech with the mother pushing in an upright position. This type of manipulation may include bringing down the arms and assisting with head flexion and birth more routinely than is recommended in this text. It is important to emphasize that neither Gaskin nor El Halta recommend manipulating the baby until she is born to the umbilicus, although Gaskin feels that touching the baby without manipulation lets her know "someone friendly is out there" (Gaskin, 1998) and does not believe this startles the baby.

If you are going to touch the baby, explaining what you are doing and why, as well as what she can do to help with the birth, is always a good idea. Whenever the baby is touched, hands or instruments should be prewarmed. The head of the stethoscope can be prewarmed by placing it under your arm or breast.

Where to position yourself

Cronk, Evans (2004) and Banks (2002) like to place themselves either behind or to one side of the mother. Cronk and Evans note that some women may be threatened or otherwise feel uncomfortable if you are behind them, where they cannot see you.

Should you assist the birth of the scrotum?

If emergence of the buttocks is taking its time, some midwives assist the emergence of the scrotum of a frank breech baby boy to avoid extensive bruising and testicular trauma. Such assistance must be done *very* gently to avoid damaging these delicate parts. Apply a very gentle stroking-pulling motion and very slight pressure on the surface of the scrotum to work it over the perineum. Avoid blindly sticking a finger into the yoni to sweep out the scrotum, as the risk of damage is greatly increased. On the other hand, Cronk (2002), Evans (2002) and Banks (2002) advise leaving the scrotum alone; they find that upright positions usually cause the birth to move along rapidly, so excessive genital trauma is not a concern.

Rumping

The baby's bottom rocks back and forth until the bisiliac has clears the pubic bone, just like the head does in a cephalic birth. When the mother is upright, the anterior buttock typically emerges first from beneath the symphysis. It then advances at a slightly forward angle as the spine bends laterally, and the posterior hip drops down as the perineum retracts. Note that centered buttocks indicate a lack of lateral flexion and that the arms may be extended (Tully, 2013).

Only if descent of the buttocks in a frank breech seems arrested and the hips are not directly anteroposterior, place your index finger against the belly side of the anterior hip and apply pressure to the bone to nudge it toward the mother's midline. This gentle nudge can bring the pelvic axis toward the symphysis and may help the baby rotate fully into the anteroposterior diameter of the pelvis to facilitate lateral spinal flexion. In any event, *do not pull on the baby.*

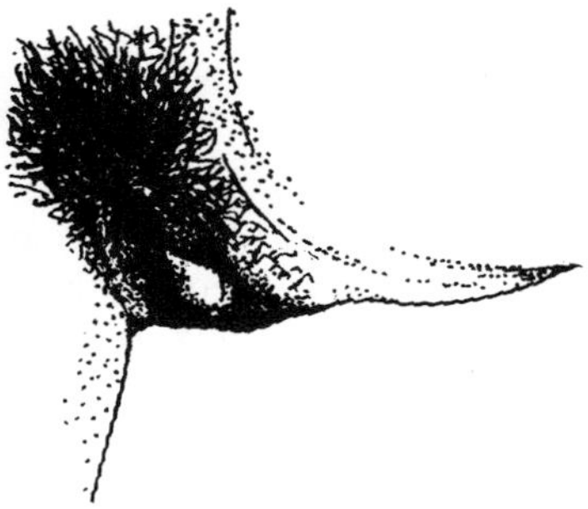	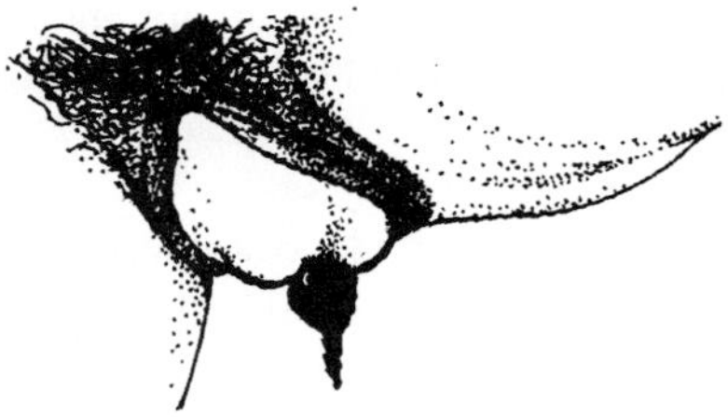	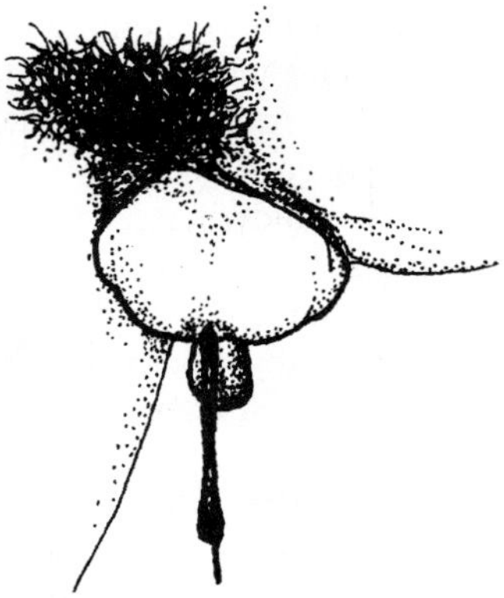
Maggie Banks attended Frank's birth, his mother's third baby. His buttocks are beginning to show.	The anterior buttock is born first, LST. Frank is passing meconium, as is very common.	The buttocks are born and have rotated to SA as more meconium is passed.

Frank's mother was standing on her right leg with her left foot on a chair seat throughout pushing. She pushed 20 minutes from the time she had rectal pressure until a peep of his buttocks was visible. From the time his buttocks were on the perineum (just prior to rumping but well beyond a peep) until he was entirely born took another 18 minutes, total (Banks, 2002).

(Illustrations based on photographs © Maggie Banks 1998, with permission.)

Perineal care during the birth

Some midwives apply hot compresses (take care not to burn the baby) or request that the mother change position to help the tissues stretch. In hospitals large clitorotomies are often performed to remove as much perineal counterpressure as possible which some feel helps lessen the need for lateroflexion in frank breeches; this is not such an issue if the mother is upright. If the perineum is very tight and descent arrested, you could cut a tiny one (you must be very careful not to cut the baby). However, simply having the mother change positions will often get things moving again. El Halta (1989) recommends performing a clitorotomy if the scrotum is very swollen, although Hunt (2003) advises against this, as it is very tricky to do without hurting the baby. Inserting your hand behind the perineum to protect the baby while you perform the incision may compress the genitals, an action that also risks damage.

Birth of the Legs

If you are behind the mother, once the buttocks have emerged, the baby's body will rotate so his belly faces you, then the legs will be born. (If the sacrum remains transverse, the arms may be stuck above the brim [Tully, 2013]). Birth of the legs varies, according to their attitude.

Birth of the extended legs (frank breech): It is tempting to try to assist the birth of extended legs, as they will seem to go on forever after the lower torso emerges. However, in the opinion of many midwives, it is rare that there is any need to free them as long as descent is progressing and the baby is doing well. In many cases, the baby must be born almost to his armpits before fully extended legs will drop out on their own. One leg will finally flop out, then the other. Again, an upright maternal position allows the baby more opportunity to move and work his little legs free.

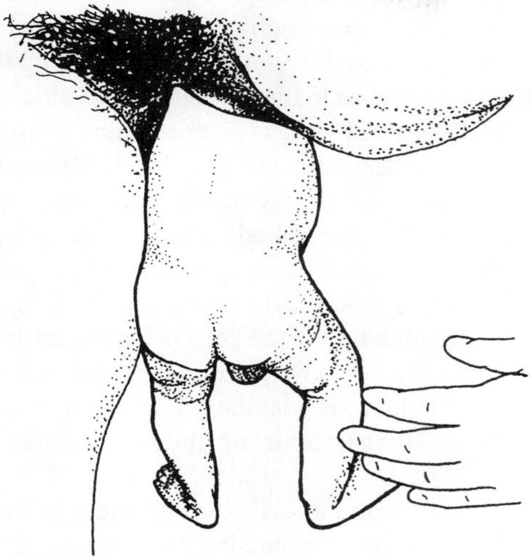

Continuing Frank's birth, his legs emerged suddenly, one after the other. From the time he was born to the umbilicus until the birth of his nose took 3 min.

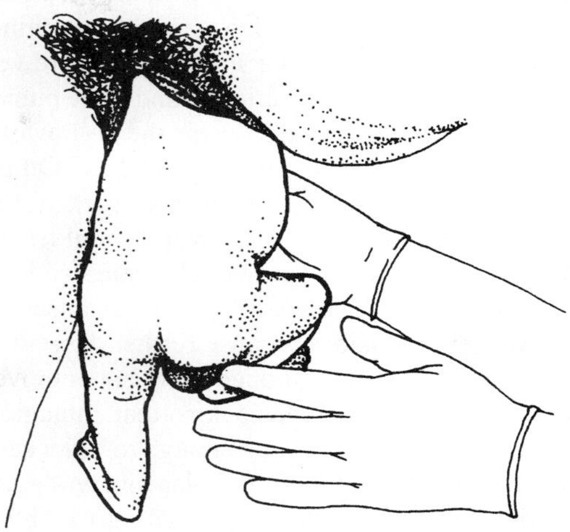

Before the next contraction, he began to bicycle his legs to work his way out. Maggie gently palpates the base of the cord to count pulsations with her left hand.

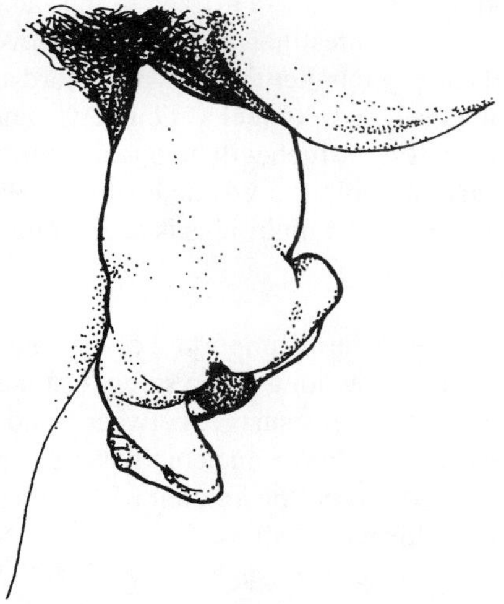

Little Frank continues to work his way down.

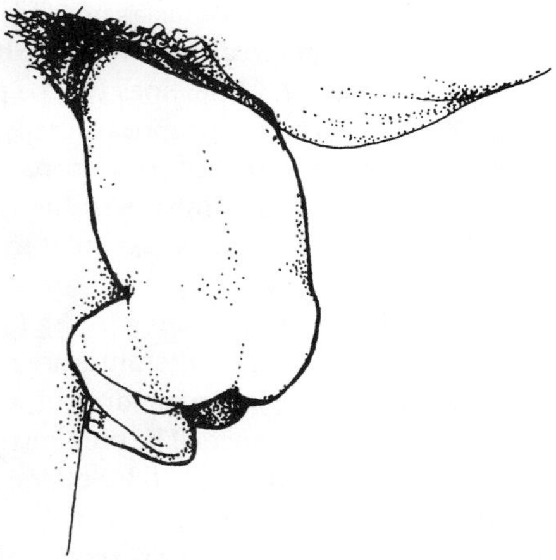

Frank's anterior shoulder is almost born. You can see the edge of his left scapula at only a slight angle, indicating that his left arm is not extended. Color, activity and muscle tone are excellent although cord pulsations are only about 40 bpm.

(Illustrations based on photographs © Maggie Banks 1998, with permission)

Birth of the flexed legs: The legs and feet of the baby in a complete, footling or kneeling position will become disengaged from the introitus as pushing continues. Most of the time this happens easily and spontaneously, with no assistance needed, especially when the woman is upright. Once flexed legs have disengaged, the baby is usually born to the umbilicus during the same contraction. When the mother is upright, once the legs are out, the baby may start wiggling to facilitate descent (Banks, 1998). Evans (2002) notes that the action of flexing the legs curls the spine and tightens the abdominal muscles; both of which help the baby keep his head flexed during descent.

Relieving tension on the cord

When the baby is born to the umbilicus, look to see if the cord is tight against the baby's belly. Only if it is, insert a finger between the baby's belly and the cord and apply gentle outward pressure against the cord (away from the belly) to create some slack to relieve tension on the cord. Do not try to pull down a big loop (although it may happen that a loop comes down, depending on the length and positioning of the cord). Handling the cord roughly or too much, or exposing a lot of it to air, may precipitate spasm in the cord vessels, as might undue stress on the cord from not relieving tension as described. If the cord is positioned under the pubic arch, it should be gently moved to the side and, if possible, around to the perineum, where it will traverse the hollow of the sacrum and therefore undergo less compression. If this is not accomplished easily, discontinue your efforts. Otherwise, keep your hands off the cord (Mayes, 1954; Myles, 1968).

A cord that offers resistance when you attempt to relieve tension or move it aside may be short or simply hung up somehow, either around the neck, over a shoulder or pinched between the baby's upper body and the mother's pelvis. Cord entanglement is often seen with breeches and is one reason why some babies won't assume a cephalic presentation. If descent is proceeding, leave it be. If you can see the cord between the baby's legs, gently loosen it and slip it over to the side whenever possible because further descent is likely to cause it to tighten up. If the cord is entangled around a limb, it should be loosened, slipped down and removed unless the birth is proceeding rapidly, a circumstance that usually indicates that there is enough slack so that entanglement will not pose a problem. Remember, a cord long enough to become entangled is usually long enough to be loosened or removed without having to cut it, and the birth occurs without worry that the cord will tear or the placenta will abrupt.

As with a cephalic birth, it is *exceedingly rare* for a cord to be so tight that cutting it is required, and it is always in the best interests of the baby to leave the cord intact. The cord will almost always start pulsing again once it is free of compression. Cutting the cord necessitates as speedy a birth as possible because there is no possibility of oxygen getting to the baby; it also prevents placental transfusion, thus imposing significant additional risks.

However, if you cannot untangle or loosen the cord and it is becoming increasingly tight, it probably should be clamped and cut. Do so only if you believe that it will either snap or that the placenta will abrupt as the baby continues to descend; in either case, the baby will hemorrhage and so will the mother if the placenta separates. Place cord clamps close together as far from the umbilicus as possible prior to cutting, making sure they are affixed to the same length of cord. Be especially careful not to clamp or cut the baby's finger, toe, genitals or intestines, in the unlikely event that the baby has a gastroschisis defect. (Intestines will be pulseless, darker and usually tougher than a typical cord and will not have a coiled appearance. They may appear lumpy or swollen, and will have a doughy feel.) You may want to place a clean gauze square behind the cord before you proceed with clamping and cutting, which will help you identify what and where to cut. Once the cord is cut, time is absolutely of the essence. If you don't cut the cord and it does break, compress the stump with your fingers and ask an assistant to help you clamp it as soon as the umbilicus is accessible.

Timing from the birth of the umbilicus to the birth of the head

Both the medical and midwifery literature are rather spotty when it comes to the all-important question of timing for the rest of the birth. However, understanding how long birth should take and how long it can safely last are critical to minimizing unnecessary interference. The previously uncompromised baby can usually survive between 5 and 10 minutes of partial cord compression (Myles, 1968; Sellers, 1993; Stevenson, 1993). How long you actually have depends upon the baby's condition when she is born to the umbilicus, the location of her cord (and the amount of compression it has already and must still undergo) and her reserves; all these things vary from birth to birth.

The cord receives a varying amount of compression as the umbilicus begins to emerge. While birth of the umbilicus has traditionally been used as the point to start timing, cord compression actually increases more once the head starts to enter the brim, which roughly corresponds to when the baby is born to the lower angle of the anterior scapula (Künzel & Kirshbaum, 2002, 110-111). The cord receives the most compression as the head engages. This does not happen when the baby is cephalic unless the cord is entangled and compressed or prolapsed or a nuchal cord is pinched behind the neck of a baby presenting his face. The work of Dunn (1967) regarding selective compression of the umbilical vein during the birth of the abdomen in cephalic presentations suggests that impaired venous return may persist for a longer period of time in a breech birth. Stevenson (1993) points out that in a breech, once the baby's body is born, the uterus is relatively more empty for a longer period of time until the head is born than is true in a cephalic birth. He feels this causes the uterine wall to shrink and may interfere somewhat with placental perfusion. This combination of factors may be the main reasons why many breech babies have a lower heart rate from this point on and are prone to low APGAR scores at birth.

As of this printing, it seems that most contemporary obstetrical textbooks in the United States assume that the baby will be born as quickly as possible, since they recommend lots of manual intervention from the birth of the umbilicus on (see WILLIAMS OBSTETRICS [Cunningham et al., 2001]). Apparently, they therefore assume timing is irrelevant and make no mention of it. This rush to birth has to do with the higher risk of brain injury from hypoxia that breech babies face. Oxorn (1986) states that once the baby is born to the umbilicus, you have about 3 to 5 minutes to create an airway before the baby becomes hypoxic; Gaskin (1992) says 4 to 5 minutes. The 14th edition of WILLIAMS OBSTETRICS (Hellman & Pritchard, 1971) cites 8 minutes to get the baby out alive. It is probably ideal for the baby to be born to the point that an airway can be established within 5 minutes after birth to the umbilicus has occurred. Cronk (2002) and Evans (2002) emphasize that their parameters rest *largely* upon the condition of the baby; if the baby seems okay, they allow the birth to proceed, but will intervene after two contractions without progress (Evans, personal communication, 2012).

In spite of recommended time limits, the older literature is also filled with warnings about hastening the birth unnecessarily. As long as the baby seems to be tolerating descent and advancement is steady, it is best to let the birth occur with as little interference as possible. European midwives typically do not intervene unless the baby's progress really seems arrested. Mayes (1954, 224) commented on the dangers of rushing the birth: "Abandoning the old idea 'Deliver the head within ten minutes of the umbilicus or your baby will suffocate,' I adopted *twenty minutes* as the safer time limit. I concentrated rather on breathing space for the doctor–its better for the baby in the end. (If you think of ten minutes as the death-line, you will get your baby out in three minutes, save it from asphyxia and lose it from cerebral hemorrhage.)" In his 1959 text, Mayes adds "You will find that most will still be delivered within 10 minutes (p. 596)." While he knew that twenty minutes is quite a long time, he makes his point. European attendants are urged to "wait and wait again; wait for as long as possible!" until the lower angle of the anterior scapula becomes visible before acting. This allows a little more time for normal shoulder descent and rotation. At this point, allow 3 minutes "at most" for the head to be born (Künzel & Kirshbaum, 2002, 110-111).

A minute can seem like an eternity. For this reason, an assistant should quietly indicate 15 or 30 second intervals as soon as the umbilicus appears. Calling time can be done subtly with a prearranged signal such as a tap on the arm of the midwife who is receiving the baby. It does not have to sound like the ninth inning.

Consider the following parameters, gleaned from a number of medical and midwifery sources, when deciding whether to "do something." They are intended to serve only as a guide. Each is based on the assumption that the preceding events occurred smoothly, with no undue delay. Suggested timing takes into account that a delay will create the need for additional time to resolve the difficulty. What to do (and mostly what not to do) at each step, as well as the recommended maneuvers should labor become arrested, are fully described in the rest of the chapter.

Birth to umbilicus: This proceeds spontaneously with the mother pushing at will. Timing is not critical prior to this point unless descent is completely arrested or fetal distress develops.

From umbilicus to shoulders: Once the umbilicus is born, wait for the next contraction, which will rotate the shoulders. The torso will descend to the level of the lower angle of the scapulae and the arms should start to emerge. If the mother has not had a contraction after two minutes (actual timing depends upon the overall rhythm of her labor), have her shift her position slightly, perform nipple stimulation or do belly massage to get a contraction going. When the mother is upright, the baby is likely to start wiggling, flexing her legs and working to get out on her own. If there is still no progress, proceed to the discussion of how to assist the delivery of the arms.

Once the arms are free: Allow the baby to hang for one to two minutes while waiting for the nape of the neck to appear under the pubic arch anteriorly and the posterior angle of the jaw and the chin to appear at the perineum (Banks, 1998; Sellers, 1993). You should see steady, gradual progress as the weight of the baby pulls the biparietal diameter under the pubic bone to the pelvic floor. If nothing has changed after one minute or if the neck has elongated with no advancement of the head, the head may be deflexed; proceed with maneuvers to encourage flexion and birth of the head.

Once the face is born or you have established an airway: If the baby is in good shape and starting to breathe, bring the vault of the head out over the perineum as slowly as possible, ideally taking 1 to 3 minutes. Have the mother breathe the head out. Practically speaking, such a slow birth of the head is often impossible, as the flexed head usually comes quite easily. Support the baby as you ease the head out as slowly as possible.

Using warmed receiving blankets on the baby's body after he is born to the umbilicus

Many textbooks recommend placing a small warmed cloth around the baby's body as he emerges. This is intended to mitigate the effect of being born into a cold delivery room. Cronk (2002) and Evans (2002) note that if the room is sufficiently warm, a cloth is not usually necessary. The literature also recommends leaving the cloth in place during any manipulations. In theory, this makes the wet, slippery baby easier to grasp. However, some midwives find that a cloth interferes with finding (and seeing) appropriate landmarks on the baby's body and generally makes handling the baby more awkward; this is likely to be more of an issue if you have attended few breech births and are not as familiar with the feel of the baby as he comes out backwards. Thick terry towels contribute to this problem. Hunt (2003) recommends using receiving blankets as they are thinner and softer, making it easier to feel what you are doing. Warm cloth chills quickly once wet. If manipulation is called for, you may wish to dry the baby quickly, remove the cloth and proceed.

The birth of the shoulders and arms

As the shoulders reach the pelvic floor, their long axis will usually rotate to the anteroposterior diameter of the outlet on its own, moving the sacrum to a transverse position. At this point the arms will be born. The weight of the baby's lower body and his movements assist this process. If things are moving along, continue to keep your hands off the baby.

Longitudinal chest crease: A crease between the nipples is a reliable sign that the arms are well positioned for birth (Tully, 2013).

The position of the scapulae: If you are positioned in front of the mother, check the position of the scapulae, which indicate the position of the arms. If the mother is slim, you will probably be able to see the outline of the scapulae as they emerge. If the mother or baby is plump, you will probably have to palpate for them (Løvset, 1968). The scapula is shaped like a "V" with the tip pointing down when the arm is against the side or across the front of the torso. The scapulae remain approximately in this position until the arm is elevated more than 90°. Whether the arm is extended straight out from the body, above the head or across the face, the tip of the "V" will rotate toward the side of the body according to the amount of arm elevation involved. This rotation is obvious from the back or the side of the baby. If the position of the scapulae and other signs indicate normally positioned arms, wait. Chances are no help will be needed. To get an idea of what the scapulae look and feel like with the arms in various positions, practice arranging the arms of a thin child above and behind his head. The following pictures show the rotation of the scapula with the arm in various degrees of extension.

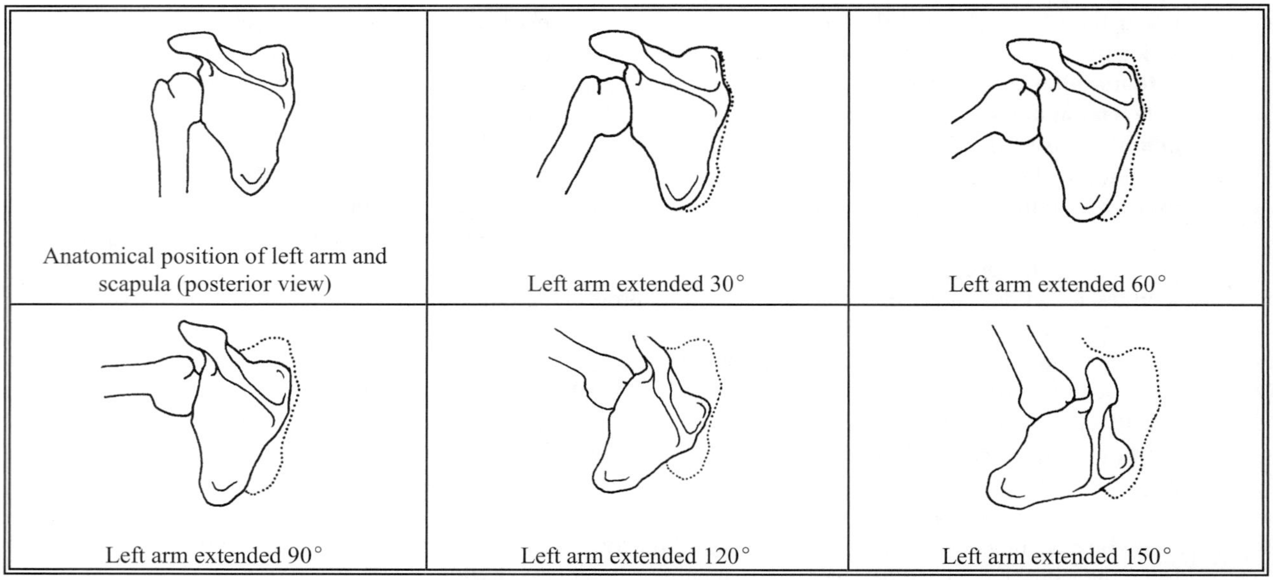

Anatomical position of left arm and scapula (posterior view)

Left arm extended 30°

Left arm extended 60°

Left arm extended 90°

Left arm extended 120°

Left arm extended 150°

The location of the elbows: If you are behind the mother, watch for the elbows to become visible against the chest as it descends. If they cannot be seen and you are beginning to worry about a delay in progress, check the scapula or gently palpate for the elbow on the chest, which indicates that the arm is not extended. If you find both elbows on the chest (or at least no higher than the chin), the arms should come easily with no manipulation. Banks (2002) points out that the baby's arms are frequently lifted so that the upper arm is about parallel with the nipple line. In this case, the arms should still come easily. Wait for their spontaneous birth. If you feel no elbows, be alert for possible problems with the birth of the arms. Keep your hands off as the mother continues to push. The baby may be able to work her own arms out.

Wait for the axillae to appear: Watch for the axillae as well as the elbows. The armpits are also level with the scapulae. If the arms are flexed on the chest, they may fall out before the baby is born to the axillae. If not, wait for the axillae to appear. This may take one or, at the most, two contractions.

Birth of the arms: When the mother is upright, the anterior arm is likely to birth first from behind the pubic bone. The body rotates to a slightly oblique angle and the posterior arm emerges. If descent arrests, one or both arms may be extended, blocking descent. A discussion of maneuvers to assist the birth of the arms begins on page 958.

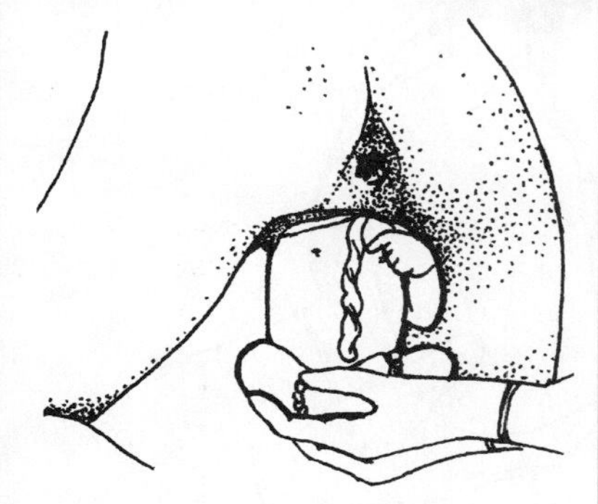

Matt's birth is progressing as easily as Frank's. His left (posterior) arm fell out faster than the camera could catch it. His right forearm is just visible as a horizontal band to your left at the introitus.

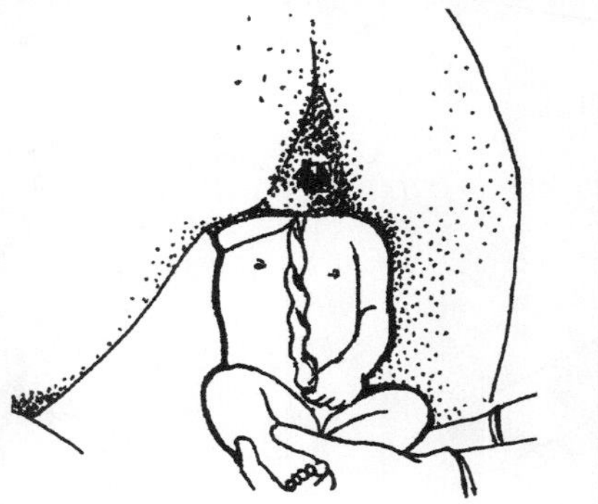

Matt's right forearm is emerging. The midwife gently supports his weight to slow him down just a little.

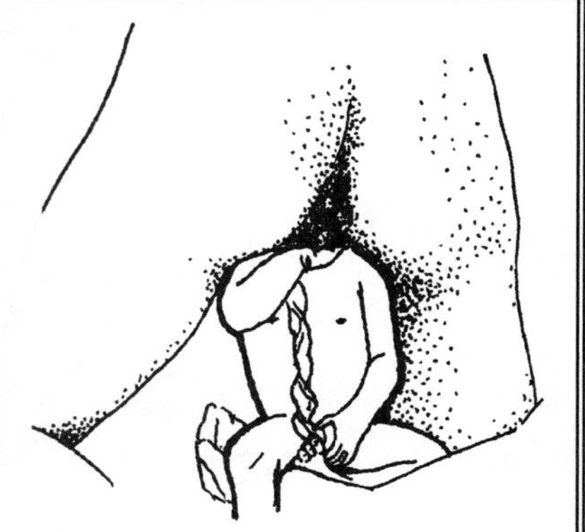

Matt's right arm drops down spontaneously and his hand is almost free. He is now sitting in the midwife's hand, which is resting on the mattress.

This series shows a different birth from behind the mother so you can see the arms coming down. Matt's mother is pushing while leaning forward in an open kneeling position. Matt was of average size, his birth required no manipulation and his APGAR scores were excellent. Maggie did not attend this birth, therefore more specific records are not available. (Banks, 2002; illustrations based on photographs © Maggie Banks 1998, with permission)

Birth of the baby's neck and head

Once the is no longer contained in the fundus, maternal pushing efforts, rather than uterine contractions, provide the primary counterpressure that facilitates the birth of the head from above (Stevenson, 1993). Maternal pushing still helps because the muscles of the pelvis are involved when the mother focuses the pushing energy down and out of her birth canal. The flexed head keeps the perineum full and round, with a pressed-out anus (an extended head leaves the perineum hollow, casting a shadow over the baby's clavicles and the anus appears more closed) (Tully, 2013). In an easy breech birth when the head is flexed and the mother upright, you do not need to do much of anything to assist the birth of the head; simply have your hands ready to support the baby's body if birth starts to progress rapidly.

The head descends comparatively rapidly, and the cranial vault does not have much chance to mould. Once the arms are born, the baby should be born as quickly as is safe, allowing some time for the head to undergo compression and decompression as gently as possible. If the head is not flexed, the Burns-Marshall maneuver will often remedy this.

Basic, minimally interventive maneuvers used during the birth of the head: Many midwives who have an otherwise hands-off policy will provide gentle support or assistance as the head emerges, which can occur quickly, so be ready!

Check for nuchal cord: Look or, if in doubt, feel for a nuchal cord as the neck emerges; a very tight cord could cause the head to extend or lead to arrested descent. In that case, it may need to be cut.

Spontaneous emergence of the head with the mother standing: Position yourself to the mother's front or side, making sure you have plenty of room to move behind her quickly. Allow the baby's body to hang unsupported (for the rationale, read the entry entitled "Burns-Marshall maneuver" below). Be prepared to provide gentle support of the baby's body to prevent the head from bursting out of the yoni. Once the nape of the neck is well exposed and the hairline and suboccipital region can be felt, *and not before*, either move around to the front of the mother or behind her and use both hands to support the baby's chest and bottom, following the baby's own movements downward as she, not you, controls the angle of descent. You are only providing support to prevent a rapid birth and avoid straining the neck (Banks, 2002).

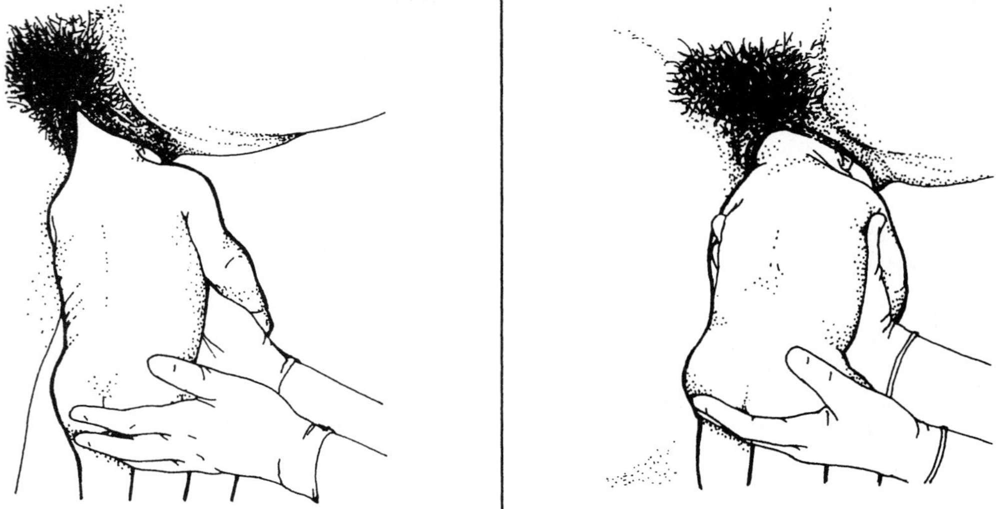

Frank's head is well-flexed. You can see the jaw beginning to emerge at the introitus. The nape of the neck is almost visible. The midwife provides gentle support with her left hand while palpating for cord pulsations with her right.

Maggie continues to provide gentle support as she follows (rather than guides) the movements of Frank's body as his lower jaw and chin emerge. After his nose was born, the rest of Frank's head was born during the following contraction.

At birth, Frank was a little floppy but he was pink, his heart rate was about 100 bpm and he required no resuscitation. He weighed 9 lb 0.5 oz (4110 g) and was his mother's biggest baby (Banks, 1998, 2002).

(Illustrations based on photographs © Maggie Banks 1998, with permission)

Supporting the baby's body as the head is born with the mother on her hands and knees: Once the head is emerging and you are behind the mother, you can support the baby's body by placing one arm under his back as though helping him go to the breast, with the legs straddling your elbow. The baby will be lying belly up on your arm with your palm near the back of his head. Provide gentle support, allowing the baby to take most of his own weight as the head emerges.

Keeping the head flexed (Kristeller maneuver): This maneuver may be used when the mother is in a reclining, belly-up position and the baby is sacrum anterior. An assistant places a hand on the mother's abdomen over the baby's head and applies pressure to encourage head flexion. After both arms are out, the assistant cups her hand over the crown of the head and applies only enough pressure to encourage the head to remain flexed. Positioning the hands will be difficult or impossible during active pushing, so they must be positioned between pushes and left in place during pushing so that the application of pressure can resume after the contraction subsides or when the mother takes a breath between pushes. Irving Potter is probably the most experienced breech specialist in history, since he turned all his client's babies breech unless they fell out first (!). He had performed 920 versions by August of 1920. Potter warned *never* to apply pressure prior to the birth of the arms, as this encourages the arms and head to extend. Pamela Hunt concurs

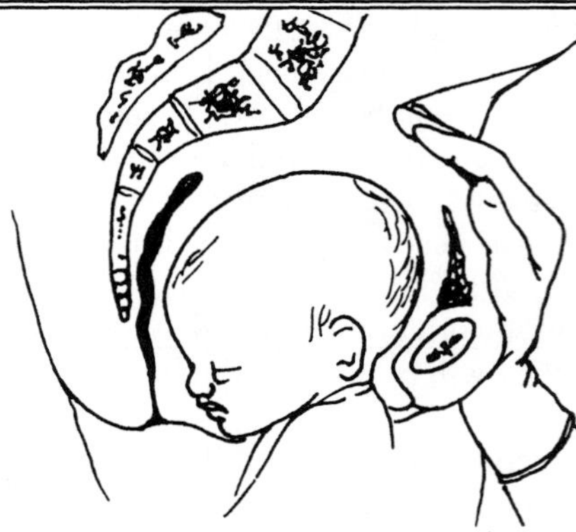

Flexing the head with the mother upright

If the mother is upright, an assistant can try to maintain flexion in the same manner, but this is considerably more awkward. Pressure can be applied to the vertex, pushing it toward the mother's spine (again, after both arms are out). However, with an upright mother, the need for maintaining flexion externally is less of an issue since the mother's abdominal muscles will be more tense and should assist in keeping the head flexed as it descends. When the head rotates to OA in the midpelvis, the occiput is pressed forward by the pubic bone, which also encourages flexion. When hanging free from an upright mother, babies will often assist flexion by lifting their legs after the legs are born.

Fundal pressure: According to Dr. Louwen, direct fundal pressure *is* relatively safe, even if the arms are not yet born, *as long as no part of the baby is hung-up and all parts are lined up correctly*. It should be reserved for a limp baby that needs to descend more quickly. He believes it is much safer than using traction to hasten the birth (Tully, 2013).

Burns-Marshall maneuver: The Burns-Marshall maneuver (1934) is not even discussed in US textbooks but is widely used in Australia, New Zealand and England. It can be used whether the mother is in a supine or an upright position. It avoids traction yet promotes full flexion and gentle delivery of the cranial vault, both of which dramatically reduce the risk of intracranial or spinal injury.

The baby is gently supported while internal rotation of the head occurs. He is then allowed to hang by his own weight. The occiput passes under the pubic arch, which pushes chin to the chest as the face descends to the pelvic floor. The neck elongates as the baby continues to hang. The hairline appears under the pubic arch as the jaw and chin appear at the perineum. The baby may hang for as long as one to two minutes until the suboccipital region is completely below the pubic arch, where it can be palpated, and the head can no longer be felt suprapubically, indicating that the occiput underlies the symphysis or is in contact with the pubic rami. Do not interfere as long as steady progress is noted and the baby is doing well. Specific techniques at this point differ depending upon the mother's position as described in the following entries, but either way, the occiput will pivot against the pubic bone as the face passes over the perineum. The baby may start to breathe. Once the head is born to the biparietal diameter, gently ease it out as the mother breathes (rather than pushes). Ideally, two or three more minutes will pass as the head is allowed to birth slowly. As a practical matter, supporting the body slows the birth of the head somewhat.

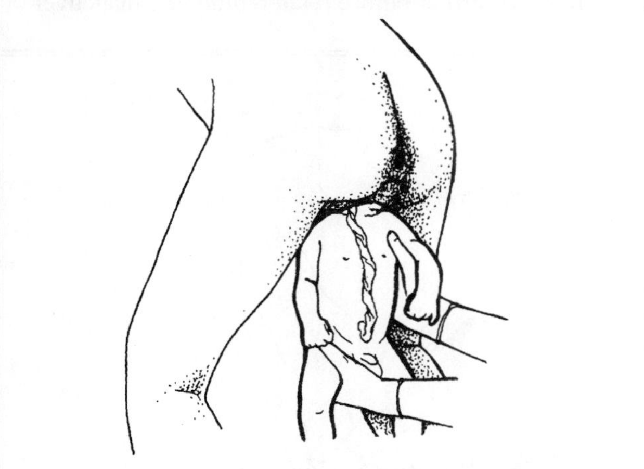

Burns-Marshall (mother upright): Continuing Matt's birth, after his arms were born, the midwife let the baby hang and asked his mother to stand to stimulate a contraction. As the contraction builds, his chin is visible at the perineum.

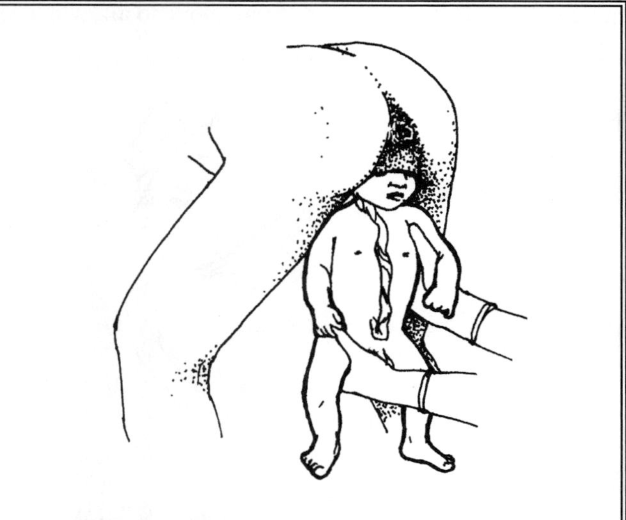

The midwife asks Matt's mother to lean sharply forward, causing his occiput to pivot around her pubic bone.

(Illustrations based on photographs © Maggie Banks, 1998, with permission.)

***Burns-Marshall maneuver with the mother upright*:** If the mother is in an upright kneeling position, when the jawline, the chin or both appear at the perineum, ask her to lean forward into hands-and-knees. If she is standing, ask her to lean forward from the waist. The baby's nose and mouth should naturally clear the perineum as the mother repositions herself. This replaces the maneuver described for a supine mother, below. If maternal repositioning does not bring the mouth and nose out immediately, create an airway while the head continues to descend (see page 965) (Banks, 1998).

Beware of the mother going to hands and knees or leaning too far forward prior to seeing the nape of the neck, chin or lower jaw: If a mother assumes a hands and knees position prior to adequate descent of the head, it is very important to support the baby's back. If the baby's body is allowed to hang dependently, he will be in a "looking at the sky" position, with the pubic bone in the bend of his neck, severely deflexing the head. This can dangerously delay the birth, requiring repositioning of the mother and waiting for the head to flex again. A deflexed aftercoming head may not be easy to flex, as the chin can get caught on the soft tissues. Supporting the baby's body avoids straining the neck and helps prevent deflexion. However, if the chin and jaw are visible before the mother goes to hands and knees, deflexion is virtually impossible (Evans, 2002).

***Burns-Marshall maneuver with the mother supine*:** This is the safest way to assist the birth of the head when the mother is supine because it requires minimal intervention. Some sort of assistance is required because the supine position does not facilitate pivoting of the occiput under the pubic bone by itself. Resort to supine positioning only if you were unable to accomplish the birth of the head with the mother upright and leaning forward.

Have the mother lie flat with her knees somewhat raised and supported, her legs gently spread to open the outlet and her bottom overhanging the edge of the mattress. Position yourself between her legs. Let the baby hang unsupported and wait for the hairline at the nape of the neck to appear, which indicates that the occiput is now beneath the pubic arch, where you will be able to see it bulging the tissues. Suprapubic pressure need not be used routinely. Once you can see the nape of the neck and the jawline, and not before, grasp the baby's feet by wrapping the thumb and index finger of one hand around one ankle and the middle finger around the other ankle, thus bringing the ankles together. Suprapubic pressure can now be applied as you stretch the baby's body straight out, away from the perineum. Provide sufficient traction to keep the occiput well under the pubic arch (otherwise the head recedes and merely rotates within the pelvis, severely straining or breaking the neck or producing suboccipital trauma) as you slowly bring the feet upward in an arc of 180° so that the occipital region above the neck (*not* the neck itself) pivots against the pubic bone as the face passes over the perineum.

If you try to bring the body up before the suboccipital region is past the pubic bone–that is, before the nape of the neck is fully visible–you can easily cause nerve damage, break the baby's neck or produce severe suboccipital trauma. If you begin to bring the body up and find that the neck is bending, gently lower the baby's body and let her hang some more with suprapubic pressure from above to allow the head to descend further before reattempting the maneuver.

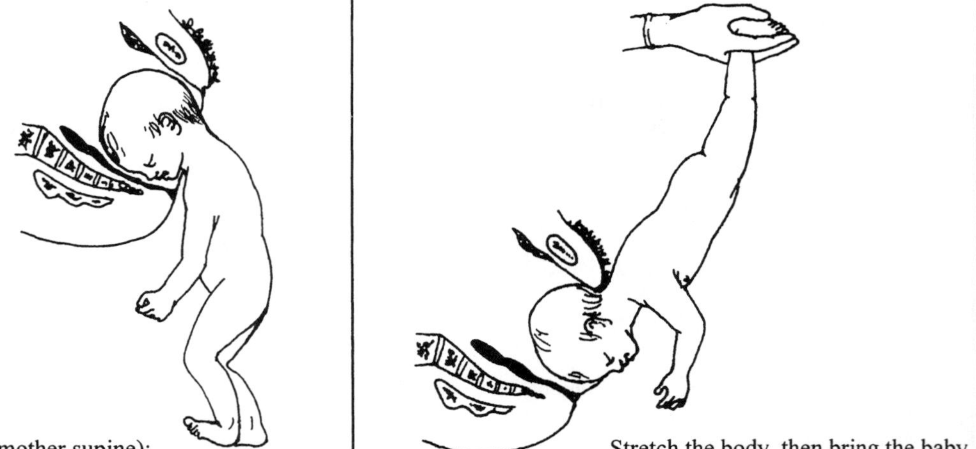

Burns-Marshall maneuver (mother supine): Letting the baby hang until the nape of the neck appears.

Stretch the body, then bring the baby upward in an arc.

Even if the head is deflexed after the shoulders are born, the natural processes respected by the Burns-Marshall maneuver should aid flexion and allow the head to come with relatively little handling if you will just *wait* for it to descend far enough for the natural pivoting action of the pubic bone to do its work. If the head will not flex, proceed to the Mauriceau-Cronk or Mauriceau-Banks maneuvers, depending upon the position of the mother.

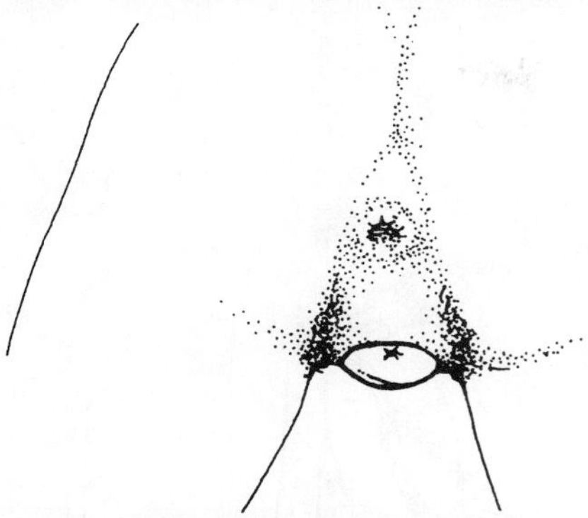

Mary Cronk attended Bill's birth, a first baby. His mother is in a kneeling prayer position, with her elbows supported on a couch. Bill's buttocks are starting to rump with his anus just visible in the midline, next to the perineum. From the onset of pushing until the presenting part was visible took 15 minutes.

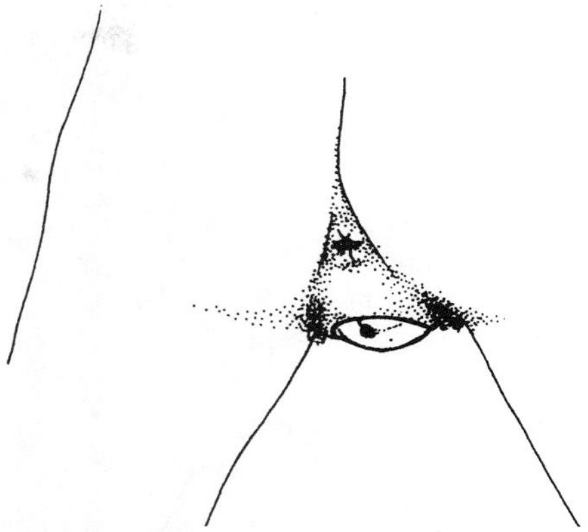

The breech is RST as the anterior buttock emerges first. A spot of meconium can be seen. From the time the butt was visible to full rumping, pushing lasted 6 minutes.

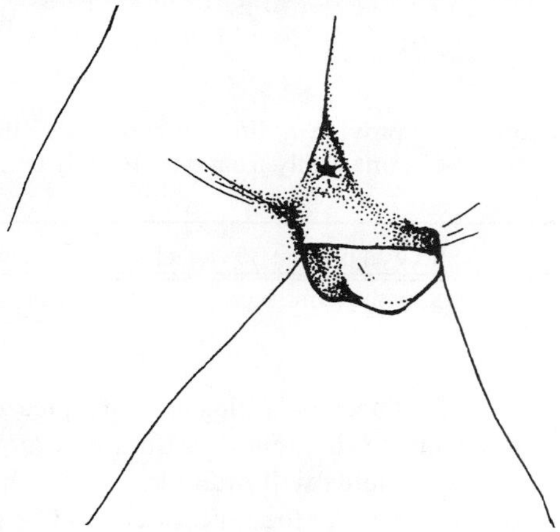

The posterior buttock and scrotum are born. The breech has rotated to SA (camera angle makes it appear RSA).

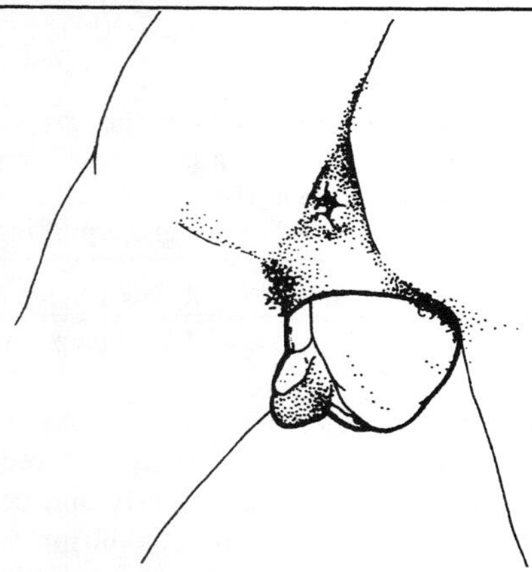

Bill's splinted legs are beginning to emerge. From a full rump to birth took another 9 minutes (from the birth of the umbilicus to the birth of the head took less than 5).

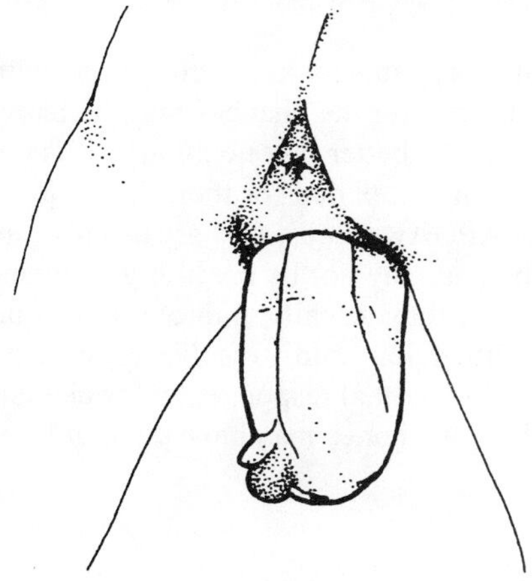

The birth of the legs seems to go on forever; keep your hands off and the legs will birth spontaneously.

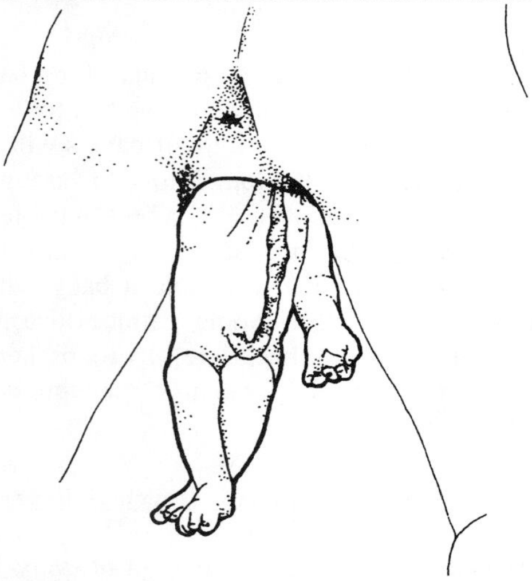

Bill's anterior arm is out and his posterior arm is about to birth.

(Illustrations based on photographs by Mary Cronk ©1998, with permission.)

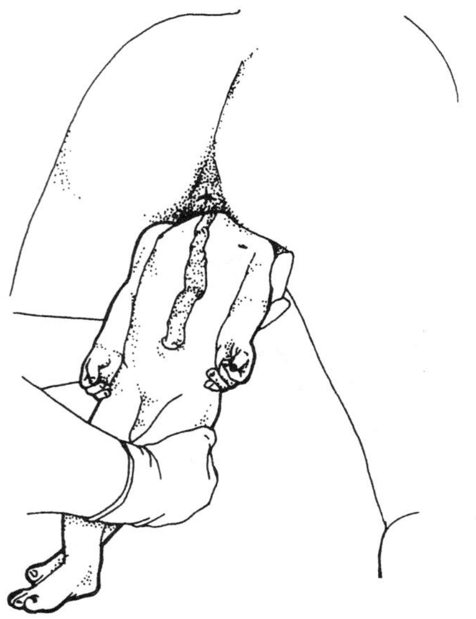

Just after both arms were born, Bill's mother dropped to her hands and knees. Mary provides gentle support, allowing Bill to take most of his own weight as she awaits further descent of his head. His heart rate was 100+ throughout pushing.

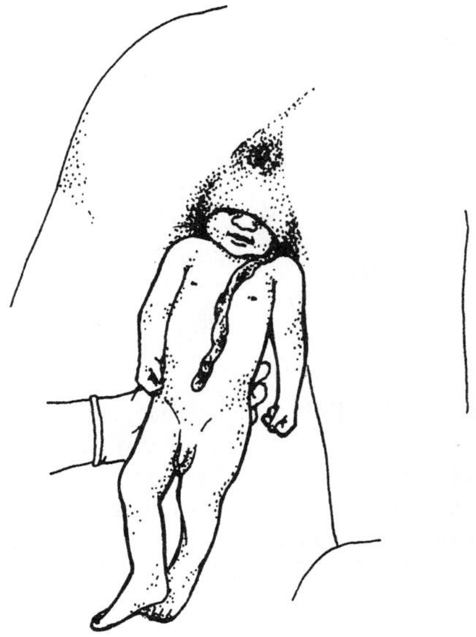

Mary continues to provide a little support, as Bill's chin emerges. His head came easily from nose to fully born in less than 1 min.

Bill's 1 min APGAR was 10. He weighed 7 lb 12 oz (3515 g) and was born at 39+ weeks.

(Illustrations based on photographs by Mary Cronk ©1998, with permission.)

Clearing the airway

Breech babies may need their airways cleared more often than vertex babies because fluids are not squeezed out of the upper airways and nose as efficiently and because their heads are upright in the amniotic fluid and move down nostrils-first, gathering fluid and mucus during descent. Once the face is free, fluids will often drain from the baby's mouth and nose, and the baby can be suctioned, if necessary. Watch for meconium in the hindwaters and be prepared to wipe the face if meconium is noted on the upper body or head. Postural drainage can be used in the term baby immediately after birth.

Immediate newborn care

While you should always be prepared for a baby who is slow to stabilize, you should anticipate one with a breech birth. The more manipulation you have had to do to get the baby out, the greater the chances that the baby will need assistance to stabilize. While a lot of babies will have APGAR scores of 8 or better by one minute, it is common for breech babies to take a little longer to come around than those who are born vertex and for their APGAR scores to be lower at one and five minutes. When breech babies have low one minute APGAR scores, they are usually pink (2) with a good heart rate (2) but may score only 1 on reflexes, 1 on muscle tone and may not be breathing spontaneously (0) (Cronk, 1998). Thus they resemble a baby with serious hypotonia, but they usually improve very quickly with stimulation. Giving the baby homeopathic arnica, 30C or 200C, after the birth helps rapidly resolve any bruising. During the baby exam, be sure to check carefully for broken bones, hip dislocation and normal responses. If the clavicle has been broken accidentally, watch for signs of pneumothorax, as the sharp ends of the bones may have punctured a lung.

Dealing with Complications of Breech Delivery

Stevenson (1993) estimates that out of every 12 breech births, 2 babies will need assistance of some type. Cronk, Evans (2004) and Banks (2002) all find that assistance is needed even more rarely when the mother births in an upright position, as described, and a strict hands-off policy is adhered to.

There are four possible outcomes for breech birth, and three degrees of assistance that apply:

Spontaneous: The baby is born easily and usually very quickly without any assistance.

Assisted: The baby is born spontaneously except for hands-on manipulation during the birth of the head.

Partial extraction: The baby's legs and trunk are born spontaneously, with manual assistance for the birth of the arms, shoulders and head.

Total extraction: The entire baby is manually removed from the mother. This is the most dangerous procedure for the baby because of the increased risk of fetal hypoxia and injury, and it is also the most dangerous for the mother because it raises the risk of uterine rupture and of other soft-tissue injuries as well as infection.

Aside from cord entanglements, the five major complications of breech birth involve rigid extension of the fetal legs, preventing spinal flexion; extension of the fetal arms over or behind the head; posterior rotation of the sacrum (bringing the face under the pubic arch and the occiput posterior); entrapment of the head in the cervix, and extension of the head. These problems become serious very quickly and require a centered and skillful response. When manipulations are required, practiced, competent handling of the baby and the ability to clearly direct the mother are essential to ensure the best possible outcome. You must have a sound understanding of both maternal and fetal anatomy, particularly the range of motion of the baby's arms, legs and neck and take into account what works as well as what doesn't with the mother and baby in a variety of positions.

Read through the following procedures carefully. Several less desirable techniques are described, along with their drawbacks, at the end of the chapter. These are only included so that midwives can understand the hows, whys and why-nots of different options.

Some of the techniques in this section may come in handy when assistance is required during a more or less "easy breech." Learning to use them with the mother in a variety of positions is best accomplished by first reviewing these techniques, as explained, using a pelvic model and a fetal doll with arms and legs that have bendable joints. Practice with a pelvis and doll to simulate the mother in different positions once you have a good understanding of the basic procedures.

All manipulations involve highly interventive obstetrical maneuvers that should be used when and only to the extent they are absolutely necessary. Manipulation of the baby is more likely to result in extension of the arms or head. Pushing in an upright position and never applying traction will usually eliminate the need for such maneuvers. When maneuvers are called for, never resort to brute force to deliver the baby. Try the gentlest approaches first; if one technique is obviously not working, try another, rather than persisting with a technique that is ineffective.

Sterile gloves

The following instructions assume that you will be wearing non-sterile gloves during manipulations performed at or just inside the introitus. Wear long-sleeved sterile gloves during manipulations involving the insertion of a hand higher in the birth canal.

Lubrication

Unless otherwise noted, lubrication of the baby or the yoni is generally not advisable, as it will render the baby even more slippery.

Handling the baby

The breech baby is easily damaged. Injuries include intracranial hemorrhage; stretching or tearing of the spinal cord or brachial plexus nerves; fractures of the spine, femur, humerus, clavicle or skull; damage to internal organs; and joint damage.

Manipulating the torso: Prior to the birth of the first arm, the lower body should be manipulated by grasping the pelvis or inserting a finger in a groin as described later. Grasping the torso over the abdomen can damage soft tissues and organs, such as the liver, spleen or kidneys, that are unprotected by bone. It can also break a lower rib, possibly resulting in lung puncture. Instead, if you are behind the mother, grasp the pelvis by placing your thumbs on the anterior, superior iliac crests and your fingers on the sacrum. If you are in front of the mother, place thumbs on the sacrum and fingers on the iliac crests.

Once the baby is born to the chest, if rotation is required, further pelvic manipulation may result in undue twisting of the spinal column, especially if rotation is difficult. It is then better to manipulate the upper body to facilitate birth of the arms. This, however, is also somewhat risky as the fetal rib cage is very flexible and therefore prone to fracture.

Therefore, grasp the upper body by equally distributing pressure. If you are behind the mother, wrap your fingers around the back and place your thumbs side by side on the sternum; if you are in front of the mother, place your thumbs directly over the scapulae or touching along the spine and your fingers over the upper, anterior rib cage. Keep your fingers over the ribs and do not dig your little fingers into the area just below the costal margin, as the liver or spleen underlie these areas. Once an arm is born, you can hold it alongside the body, which will further protect the ribs from fracture. Never rotate and apply traction simultaneously except when assisting the delivery of the arms with the Løvset maneuver (as described later).

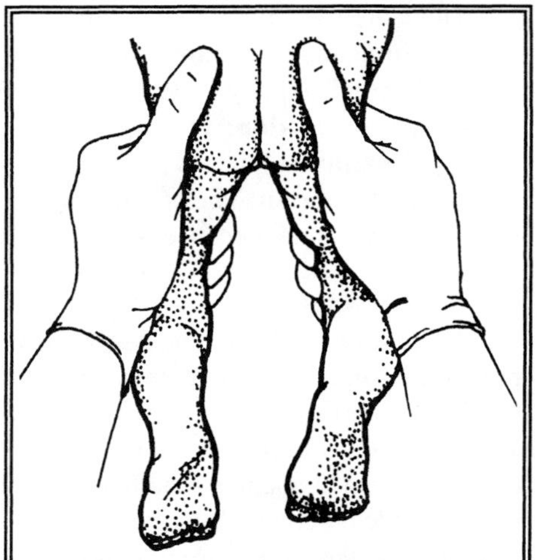

How to safely grasp the pelvis if you are in front of the mother and baby is SA.

Manipulating the limbs: Brachial plexus injury may occur if the birth of the arms is mishandled. Take care not to apply pressure to the anterior neck or in the armpits, not to bring down an arm in an unanatomical direction, and not to put undue traction on a limb or the neck.

Splinting an arm is sometimes required to bring it within reach. This braces the humerus so that it is less likely to be broken. Do this by stretching out your index and ring fingers along either side of the baby's upper arm until you feel the elbow (splinting to the level of the elbow avoids breaking the humerus). If splinting the arm proves impossible, hook two or preferably four fingers around the arm to evenly distribute pressure along the upper arm down to the elbow or reach for the bend of the elbow. Once your fingers are in place, gently nudge the arm downward and splint the humerus as soon as you can. Do not use only one finger to manipulate across the length of a bone at a right angle nor should you hook one finger over the bone to sweep the arm down. Both maneuvers are likely to break a bone. These precautions generally apply to the legs as well, when the knee replaces the elbow as the point of flexion. Refrain from pulling on the limbs (which may dislocate a joint) except as instructed for total extraction later in the chapter (when, of course, you still run the risk of injury).

Maternal position during rotational maneuvers to free the arms or head: Supine positioning is traditionally used when the baby's arms are so impacted that rotational maneuvers are required to free them. While upright positions are very useful in preventing problems and seem safe for use when flexing the head or when gentle rotation is all that is needed, I have questions about their use when rotational maneuvers prove more difficult because of the possible stress on the fetal spine. The spine is very flexible and can easily be twisted and severely damaged without any movement in the parts you are trying to dislodge. If the mother is upright, gravity will be brought to bear on her soft parts, which may exaggerate any resistance to rotation inherently produced by the problem at hand. Therefore, if rotation is difficult, I recommend either a hands and knees position or having the mother lie down to remove the downward pull of gravity on the baby as a precaution against injury to the baby's spine.

Providing traction: Traction should be applied gradually to allow tissues to stretch; never jerk on the baby. Avoid sustained traction for longer than 10 seconds or so at a time. This will help prevent excessive stretching.

Wiggling the baby down: Rather than applying direct, downward traction, you can rock the baby from side to side or up and down slightly, to wiggle him through the pelvis (like working anything out of a tight space). This is much gentler than straight traction and tends to work well. This wiggling technique can be used whenever traction on the torso is required and avoids the use of any direct traction in many cases (Gaskin, 1992). Never wiggle or twist a limb, as this is very likely to damage joints or break bones.

"Stuffing" movement: When rotation of the torso is required to deliver the arms, Künzel and Kirshbaum (2002) suggest it be carried out with what they call a "stuffing" movement. This means that the rotation is not undertaken as one continuous movement (which they say may not be possible anyway) but in a series of short movements, during which the baby's body is pushed up into the birth canal slightly and then pulled back out again as you bring it around. Myerscough (1977) comments that rotation (which he says is often quite easy), may cause the chin to catch if it is too low in the pelvis. If this occurs, the head can become hung up on the retracted uterus and the neck twisted beyond the point of safety. He therefore recommends the same "stuffing" movement. First, push the torso up a little to dislodge the head and arm from the pelvis. Then, alternately rotate and push up on the torso so that the chest is gradually brought around to the hollow of the sacrum. Løvset (1968) also refers to back and forth (rather than in and out) movement to accomplish a difficult rotation. These and other forms of wiggling the baby but must be done gently and not to an extreme degree to minimize stress on the fetal spine.

Manipulating the head and neck: Breech babies are also prone to injury of the sternocleidomastoid muscle; this is the most prominent muscle in the anterolateral region of the neck, extending from the manubrium of the sternum and the medial portion of the clavicle to the mastoid process of the temporal bone. Injudicious or improperly directed traction can cause tearing of this muscle or its fascial sheath, leading to a hematoma and gradual contraction due to scarring.

Do not apply traction and rotation simultaneously when working to deliver an extended head. When the head is engaged, rotation will cause only the neck to turn; simultaneous traction can result in injury to the cervical spine.

Forceful hyperextension of the aftercoming head can produce severe suboccipital pressure, causing the lower edge of the squamous portion of the occipital bone to become displaced and pushed forward over the edge of one or both condyles. This tears the dura and occipital sinuses and may lacerate the cerebellum or spinal cord.

Safely applying pressure to the face: Some techniques require straddling the nose with your fingers and applying pressure to the face in order to deliver the head. Some sources recommend applying the fingers to the cheekbones. In order to apply pressure here, the fingers must be placed on or just above the prominence of the zygomatic arch, very close to the eyes. However, the superior border of the upper maxillary bone (the upper border of the superior jaw bone, on either side of the nostrils) is an equally prominent bony ridge, which is lower on the face and thus further away from the eyes. If the fingers slip or are slightly off target, it is less likely that the eyes will be damaged because the cheekbones provide a speed bump, lessening the chance that the fingertips will slip into the orbits.

To find the maxillary ridge, follow the baby's anterior chest up the midline of the neck, over the chin past the mouth to the nostrils. Spread your fingers at the level of the nostrils and palpate by rocking them up and down until you locate the depressions above the upper border of the maxillary bones on either side. Locate this ridge on your own face.

Hyperoxygenate the mother

Consider providing supplemental oxygen to the mother throughout the period of manipulation. Have someone follow the fetal heart rate closely. Only if the rate is normal, discontinue oxygen when you finish your manipulations. Providing oxygen in the presence of a normal fetal heart rate is generally not recommended. However, because fetal compromise is anticipated in these situations, because birth is delayed and the manipulations themselves may compromise cord flow to a certain extent, supplemental oxygen is expected to lessen the trauma.

Bringing down the other foot in a single footling breech

Mabel Dzata (2001), a CNM who trained in West Africa and has much breech experience, has a unique way of dealing with the emergence of one foot. She brings the other foot down, feeling that the round shape of the baby's torso provides a more uniform dilator than the irregular-bottom-plus-extended-leg combination in a single footling. *It should be emphasized, however, that most midwives leave well enough alone, as this risks cord prolapse, fetal injury, deflexion of the head and extension of the arms.* Løvset (1968) also points out that the leg that remains up inside provides a larger presenting diameter to dilate the birth canal. You may want to consider this more seriously in order to avoid superrotation (see below) if the posterior leg is the one extended downward. Although you will be attempting to bring a leg down during labor, when the baby is higher in the birth canal than is suggested here, the technique is essentially the same.

Bringing down extended legs (Pinard maneuver)

According to Parvin (1895) this technique was originally presented by Madame Lachapelle in 1825 (Vol II, 88, 89) and usurped as his own by Pinard in the late 1800s. It can be used to bring down the legs when descent is completely arrested in a frank breech and for some reason transport is ill advised, or when the baby is halfway born and the birth needs to be hurried because the baby gives indications of compromise. Arrested descent is typically a result of the legs being splinted up against the torso, impairing lateral spinal flexion and causing the baby to have trouble passing under the pubic bone.

Always try flexing the anterior leg first. If descent resumes, stop there. Do not flex the posterior leg by itself, as this increases the chance that the anterior hip will get hung up on the brim, which may result in a full 225° internal rotation of the breech or arrest of descent (see the chapters entitled "Variations in Breech Descent and Rotation" and "The Use of Version during Labor" for more about these recommendations).

To free the baby's leg, use the hand that is on the same side as his belly. It is ideal to wait until the baby is born to the popliteal fossa (the diamond-shaped area behind the knee joint), and then place two fingers along the length of one thigh with your fingertips behind the knee. Confirm that the cord is not entangled around the upper limb. If you do not think you can bring the limb down without pulling down the cord, leave it alone.

If you follow the leg up from the hip, confusing a leg with an arm is unlikely to occur. If in doubt, palpate more thoroughly to confirm the landmarks of the knee, heel and toes (see the chapter entitled "Performing Internal Exams during Labor").

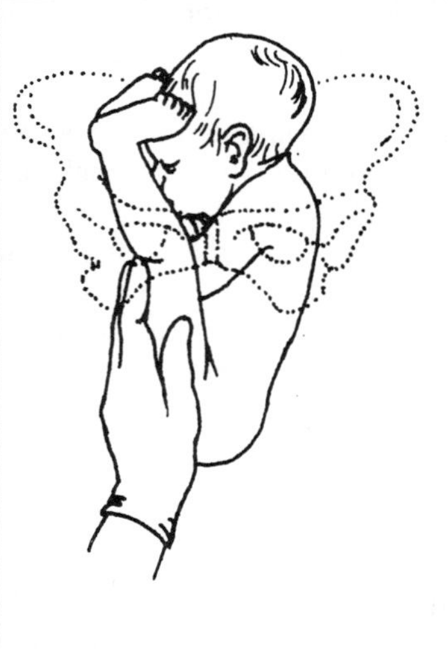

Reaching for the popliteal angle of the left knee.

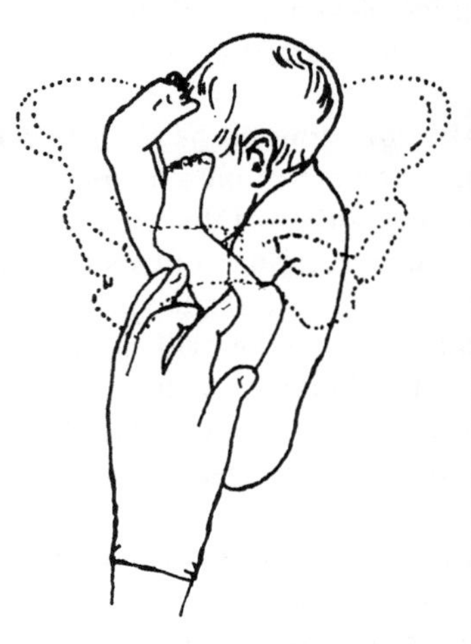

As the leg flexes away from the midline, the foot comes down into reach.

Apply gentle pressure behind the knee or use all four fingers to apply well-distributed pressure along the length of the femur up to the knee to flex the thigh away from the midline. As you do so, the lower leg will sweep down and across the baby's abdomen. This will automatically bring the foot lower; it may be felt touching the back of your hand. The foot may even be born at this point. *Do not pull on the leg* as you may dislocate the hip as well as encourage the head to extend. Flex one leg and then the other.

Once the knees are flexed, the torso should be free to flex and the birth should be able to proceed spontaneously. Unless you are bringing down the second leg to avoid a single footling situation, there may be no need to grasp a foot and bring the leg out further. However, should this be required, slide your fingers up, over the knee and down the shin to the top of the foot. This avoids inadvertently grabbing a hand and reconfirms that the cord is not tangled around the limb. Grasp the ankle between the index and middle fingers and sweep the flexed leg across the abdomen and out, following the natural motion of the leg. Take care to not get it caught on the other leg or the cord. (If the arm on that side is easy to reach, you can extend it down across the chest.) Once the leg is more or less straight, double-check to make sure the cord has not prolapsed, then slowly withdraw your hand.

If simple flexion does not bring down the first leg you reach for, consider the possibility of legs are crossed at the knees or ankles, of feet lodged under the chin, or of undetected cord entanglement. Crossed legs interfere with lateral flexion even more than simply extended ones. Don a long-sleeved sterile glove. Reach up higher to find out if crossing, stuck feet or the cord is a problem. In this case only, disengage the leg that is easiest to maneuver and proceed as above (Mayes, 1954). When you have finished, monitor the fetal heart rate for several minutes to make sure all is well.

Bringing down extended arms

Extended arms are the breech version of shoulder dystocia. They exist when one or both arms are not fully flexed on the chest. There are degrees of extension, from the positioning of one or both forearms over the face to one or both arms being raised completely over the head. Nuchal arms are raised and flexed at the shoulder and elbow so that the forearm is trapped behind the fetal head. Extended arms occur much less frequently than extended legs but are potentially far more dangerous.

A primary cause of extended arms is manipulation. Cronk (2002) comments that she has rarely had to assist the birth of the arms and believes that extended arms are caused by attendants applying traction. Extension can occur during manipulations performed when the head and the shoulders are still freely mobile above the pelvic brim. Once an arm is lifted near the head, further descent tends to sweep it upward even more because the arm or elbow gets caught on the pelvic sidewalls or the brim. This is especially likely when traction is applied while the uterus is relaxed or the mother is not actively pushing. Arms may also extend when the mother pushes through a partially dilated cervix because the elbows catch on the cervical rim and become swept up alongside the head. Descent in a sacrum posterior position brings the elbows through the shallow anterior pelvis right past the pubic bone, where they can easily be caught and nudged upward as the baby moves down, or become lodged and arrest descent.

Extended arms are suspected when you cannot see the elbows on the chest once the baby is born to the lower chest or if there are good contractions with no advancement at this point. Lateral rotation of the scapula confirms extension.

As soon as you suspect extended arms, attempt to bring them down before allowing the birth to proceed. If the arm is over the head or behind the neck, it will be easier to dislodge before it gets jammed in. Besides that, an extended arm will take up additional space in the pelvis and will delay or prevent descent of the shoulders and head.

There are a wide array of techniques offered in the medical literature for resolving extended arms, most of which have some component that is of questionable safety as far as the baby is concerned. I have selected those that seemed the most reasonable, that were recommended in several places and that addressed every possible nuance of serious complications.

Bringing down extended arms from behind the mother: As with shoulder dystocia in cephalic presentations, approaching the mother from behind allows the best access to maneuver the arms. Plus, you don't have the weight of the maternal abdomen bearing down on the fetal parts as you try to dislodge them and you don't have to ask the mother to move to a supine position before you can do anything. Even a pendulous abdomen is not such a problem because most of the baby has already been born, although pillows can always be placed under the mother's belly to provide support.

If the mother is in some sort of upright position but not currently in a Christian prayer position, ask her to assume one. You can let the baby's body hang freely. From behind the mother, place your hands on the baby's pelvis or chest, whichever seems appropriate. Tune into the situation to see if sweeping down the arms or attempting to rotate the baby first seems the best way to proceed. If you feel rotation is in order, test to see which way the baby will rotate most easily by nudging the baby first one way and then the other taking care *not* to pull on the baby. (While it is always theoretically better to rotate the baby back-to-pubes, when working with the mother in this leaning-forward position it may not be as big an issue because gravity will work to help the baby rotate to the anterior.) Gentle rotation alone may be enough to dislodge the arm and resume normal, spontaneous descent. If you sense that you need to evaluate the position of the arms first, or if the baby cannot be rotated easily in either direction, insert your hand over the perineum and press the sacrum back out of your way with the back of your hand. Follow along the torso to the inner angle of the scapula, feel along the humerus to the elbow of the arm you can most easily reach. Hook your finger up and over the elbow joint (not a long bone) and sweep first one arm, then the other, down over the face and chest.

If the arm is still not born and further, more aggressive rotation is required, have the mother drop to her hands and knees. Now, attempt to rotate the baby in the direction he goes most easily; *do not apply traction*. The arm may be born as rotation occurs. If not, go in and sweep the arm down as described above. If you wind up rotating the baby belly-to-pubes, be sure you keep your hands on the baby to feel if spontaneous rotation is resuming to bring the sacrum anterior. SA rotation is the rule, even in this situation. You can, however, help complete the rotation as the arm is born to bring the sacrum transverse as the head enters the brim and then gently assist him to finish rotating to occiput anterior. Have the mother resume a prayer position to allow the head to descend until the chin and jaw appear, or have the mother remain in hands and knees and support the baby's back as the head comes down. Then bring it out with the Mauriceau-Cronk maneuver. *Cronk and Evans emphasize that, with about 100 breeches between them, they have only had to release a single extended arm. The above is based on that situation plus their in depth understanding of breech descent* (Cronk, 2004; Evans, 2004).

Unless otherwise noted, the rest of the techniques in this section assume you are either in front of the mother if she is standing or working between her legs if she is supine. They are based on more aggressive and risky obstetrical approaches. Specific techniques have been reviewed and compared as described in various texts.

Modified classical method to bring down partially extended arms: The original version of this technique was first introduced by Arthur Müller of Munich, Germany, but I could not discover when. It can be used when the arms are raised in front of the face or extended alongside the head. In such cases, the arms can sometimes be brought down without rotation. This technique will not work if maternal muscle tone is rigid or disproportion exists.

Which arm first? Textbooks vary regarding which arm they recommend delivering first. The rationale for delivering the posterior arm first is that it will have the most room for maneuvering, as it is nearest the hollow of the sacrum and, as long as the scapulae are visible, you know it is already below the brim. Dislodging the posterior arm first creates more space for the body to drop down into the pelvic cavity and thus more room to manipulate the anterior arm. The anterior arm has far less room, and it is easy to get it caught at the brim as you try to dislodge it. Trying to work in the shallow anterior pelvis makes reaching in for the anterior arm difficult at best, and increases the chance of breaking the humerus.

On the other hand, bringing out the anterior arm first entails angling the body downward, taking advantage of the room in the sacrum to contain the undelivered posterior shoulder.

Künzel and Kirshbaum (2002) advise using the classical method. This involves delivering the posterior arm first and then rotating the anterior shoulder 180° to posterior before attempting to bring it out to take advantage of the extra room in the sacrum. To do so, you must either rotate the baby's belly under the pubic arch, which helps bring the arm in front of the baby's chest but risks encouraging the aftercoming head to rotate posteriorly, or rotate the baby's back under the pubic arch. They recommend the latter, but this risks further extending the anterior arm, abducting the undelivered shoulder, thus widening the shoulder axis, and perhaps creating a nuchal arm, an even worse complication. For these reasons, the technique described below combines their recommendations for delivery of the posterior arm with those of Myerscough (1977) to bring out the anterior arm with reference to Løvset (1937; 1968).

As a practical matter, it is probably best to attempt to bring out the arm that seems to want to come most easily, noted when an acute angle of traction is not required in order to bring the arm out. This creates more room for the arm likely to cause the most problems. However, quickly shift to working on the opposite arm if you find that the first arm you go for does not come easily. If the following techniques do not bring the arms on the first attempt, abandon them in favor of the Løvset maneuver.

Bringing down extended arms: Position yourself between the legs of the supine mother or in front of her if she is standing. Confirm that the baby's sacrum is in either a transverse or anterior oblique position. Do not encourage rotation during these maneuvers. Make sure the lower border of the anterior scapula is at or just about level with the lower border of the symphysis. If it is not, this maneuver could break the baby's neck (Eden & Holland, 1931). However, if the trunk is too far down, the head and arms will be jammed into the pelvis, making manipulations difficult. Go for the arm you feel will come most easily. If in doubt, go for the posterior arm first.

To deliver the posterior arm:

1. Use the hand on the same side as the baby's abdomen to grasp the feet and the other hand to manipulate the arm.
2. Assuming the baby is LST, flex your left wrist so you can grasp the ankles from behind the feet (palm to your right). Lift the baby's body up, then pull the baby's anterior torso over toward the mother's right (your left). This clears the way for you to insert your right hand along the baby's back. Maintaining the baby's body at this angle also brings the posterior arm and shoulder down closer to the outlet. If you only lift the body without moving it over like this, bringing down the arm is considerably more difficult. Lifting and holding the baby at an angle may bring the posterior axilla into view and allow the posterior scapula, shoulder and arm to pass over the perineum.
3. If the arm is not born, insert two or more fingers of your right hand over the perineum, up the back to the posterior shoulder. Using more fingers makes the maneuver easier and lessens the likelihood of fetal injury.
4. Now push your internal fingers over the baby's posterior shoulder until they are parallel with the upper arm. Splint the humerus and sweep the arm across the chest, down and out. When you reach the elbow, splint or, if impossible, push into the crook of the elbow to sweep the arm down, following its natural range of motion, bending the arm across the chest and down.

To deliver the anterior arm:

1. To release the anterior arm, grasp the baby's pelvis, placing your thumbs over the sacrum, or, if the posterior arm is already born and still assuming the baby is LST, grasp the chest with your left hand and the arm alongside the chest with your right. Direct the baby's torso at a 45° angle or more posterior to the long axis of the mother. If the mother is upright, gently direct the baby's body in the direction of her heels. If the mother is supine, angle the baby's body toward the floor.
2. As the mother pushes, apply only enough downward traction (gentle, slight up and down wiggling can be used) to bring the axilla of the anterior arm into view. The arm may emerge spontaneously with this maneuver.
3. If not, release the pelvis and support the baby's body with the hand nearest his belly, or do so by grasping the baby's ankles. Use your free hand to follow along the upper side of the baby's back, under the pubic bone, over the shoulder and up the arm until you reach the elbow. You can place two fingers along the humerus to prevent the arm from going behind the neck and use the palmar surface of your hand to push the scapula of the anterior shoulder toward the transverse diameter of the pelvis slightly to create more room.
4. Now, splint the humerus if possible. If not, insert more fingers to reach the elbow and push the crook of the elbow to

bend the arm forward toward the midline of the chest. Bringing down the humerus will flex the arm and bring the hand into reach.

5. Splint the arm as soon as you can, sweeping the hand in front of the face and bringing the arm and hand across the chest and out from under the pubic bone, around the side of the torso and out.

If these maneuvers are ineffective because the arm is higher up than you thought, because it is behind the neck, because you can't get your hand under the pubic arch or because retrieving the arm seems to require rotation of the torso, go directly to the Løvset maneuver on the next page (Sellers, 1993).

Bringing down the posterior shoulder (Rosshirt maneuver): If the baby is quite large, his body may prevent you from introducing your hand far enough inside to reach the elbow. If you cannot do so and the shoulders are in the anteroposterior diameter, there should be enough room to the side for you to insert your hand along the baby's back, hook two fingers over the tip of the posterior shoulder and pull it further down toward the introitus (Løvset, 1968). If you meet a lot of resistance stop, as you may damage the brachial plexus. This should be easiest to accomplish with the mother on her hands and knees. Once the posterior shoulder is well below the promontory, you may be able to reach the humerus and sweep the arm down. If not, proceed with the Løvset maneuver or the modified classical maneuver just discussed.

The Løvset maneuver: This technique uses both rotation and horizontal and then downward traction to effect the birth of the arms with the mother supine. While generally not discussed in North American textbooks, it is an anatomically sound and relatively safe maneuver when properly performed. It is widely used in the United Kingdom, New Zealand and Australia. It can be employed whether the arms are extended, bent at the elbow or flexed back behind the nape of the neck. It facilitates the birth of otherwise inaccessible arms and is helpful even when the baby is so large that reaching in to get the arms is impossible. Løvset remarks that it is easiest to perform on a large, firm baby.

How the Løvset maneuver works: The angle of pelvic inclination places the posterior half of the brim and the sacral promontory above the anterior half. In addition, the sacrum is much longer and deeper than the pubic bone. Thus, when the baby's body is born far enough that you can see or feel the lower border of the scapulae at the introitus, his posterior shoulder is below the sacral promontory and his anterior shoulder is above or just behind the symphysis. For these reasons, this multistep rotational maneuver begins with dislodgement of the posterior arm.

The maneuver begins with keeping the baby's body horizontal to the long axis of the mother and rotating her 90 to 100°, moving the long axis of her shoulders from the anteroposterior to the transverse pelvic diameter as her back passes under the pubic arch. Keeping her body horizontal helps to further engage the posterior shoulder and starts the process of dislodging that arm. The hollow of the sacrum allows space for this process to begin. The slight forward and upward angle of the pelvic outlet will force the delivered part of her body into the same angle, causing her posterior shoulder to dip closer to the outlet. As her body is brought around laterally, counterpressure from the sidewalls of the birth canal encourages her arm to sweep across her face and chest. Pressure from the pelvic sidewalls as well as the natural range of motion of the arm prevents it from being swept further upward.

Maintaining the baby's body in a horizontal plane for the first 90° of rotation keeps his posterior elbow below the back and sides of the pelvic inlet, thereby preventing it from gliding above the brim and getting caught. However, if his body were maintained in a horizontal plane during the next 90° of rotation, his elbow could find its way above his mother's pubic bone and become trapped. To avoid this, during the second 90° of rotation, the baby's body is angled 45° or more toward his mother's heels if she is upright or toward the floor if she is supine. Løvset (1968) recommends angling the baby downward as far as possible. Rotation continues for a total of 180 to 200° until the originally posterior elbow is under the symphysis, which allows you to reach in for it with the least risk of breaking his arm.

In his text VAGINAL OPERATIVE DELIVERY (1968), Løvset is clear about applying horizontal traction for the first 90°, then switching to downward traction for the next 90 to 120° of rotation. However, Mayes (1954) and Myles (1968), both enthusiastic advocates of this maneuver, recommend steady traction at a downward angle *throughout* the entire 180 to 200° of rotation. Bower (1967) uses *upward* traction for the first 90° of rotation (with the mother supine) to further ensure that the posterior arm engages well below the brim (however, it seems to me that upwardly directed traction greatly increases the risk of deflexing the head). He then uses downward traction for the second half of rotation. In part, I suspect that these variations reflect what can get lost in translation when practitioners actually start performing maneuvers themselves as well as learning what works for them when using a new technique. Therefore, if the original technique proves inadequate, try using only acute downward traction for the entire rotation. I have added the recommendation to relax tension briefly before redirecting the angle of traction; shifting the angle without doing so may damage the baby's spine if done too aggressively or at too acute an angle. While Løvset makes no remarks on this point, it just seems prudent to me as it allows a split second pause which further ensures gentle handling of the baby.

A hallmark of the safety and success of this technique lies in always keeping the baby's back anterior during rotation and always completing the rotation before making any attempt to deliver the arm. This means that the arm will always have the benefit of the sacral space to begin dislodgement and always have the benefit of passing against the sidewalls of the pelvis and under the pubic arch to aid flexion toward the anterior chest, where the arm is most easily reached. Also, prior to the birth of the first arm, the extended arms are likely to splint the head, helping to keep the spine straight as rotation occurs, thus limiting strain on the neck. The risk of infection is minimized because hands are not inserted to get the arm, and fracture of the humerus is generally avoided, although fracture of the clavicle may still occasionally occur.

This maneuver should not be attempted if the mother has a flat, contracted pelvis, when attempts at rotation will result in the shoulders becoming stuck in the transverse diameter, making further rotation impossible. However, when the pelvis is not contracted in the anteroposterior diameter, or when disproportion between the baby and the pelvis does not make yoni delivery impossible, this is a safe and minimally interventive method of delivering severely extended arms.

Whether one arm is more extended than the other, or the anterior arm is also quite extended or even if you do not think the anterior arm is in a particularly bad position, do not worry about moving it into a more unfavorable position while working to free the posterior arm. Any undesirable repositioning of the anterior arm will be corrected by repeating the maneuver to deliver it.

Performing the maneuver: The Løvset maneuver is performed from between the mother's legs as she lies supine or in front of the mother while she remains upright. Having her lie down will take her out of gravity and may allow you better access to the baby for steps 3 and 6.

We will use a baby who is RST as an example. When the baby is born to the scapulae, the shoulders will still be in the anteroposterior diameter of the pelvis. If descent has stopped, proceed as follows:

1. You may begin rotation as soon as the inferior borders of the scapulae have arrived under the pubic arch (you may have to palpate to be sure they are sufficiently descended as they may be just out of view in some cases).
2. Grasp the pelvis. Keeping the baby's body horizontal to the long axis of the mother, rotate the baby 90° in a clockwise direction (RST to RSA to SA) while applying continuous outward traction. Løvset does not say whether to coordinate traction with pushing or not. My guess is that his clients were under general anesthesia, so they could not participate. Therefore, I recommend that the mother not be pushing, as pressure down may cause the head to become hung up and impair free movement. In any case, traction should **only** be sufficient to maintain the proper angle of the body and achieve rotational movement during each portion of the maneuver. If rotation cannot be accomplished pretty easily with a continuous movement, rearrange your hands to grasp the chest and use the "stuffing" movement described on page 956. Do not wait for contractions because time is of the essence.
3. For the second 90 to 110° of clockwise rotation and traction (SA to LSA to LST), relax your traction and redirect the baby's body so that it is held at a 45° angle or more posterior to the long axis of the mother.
   Mother supine: Lower the baby's body toward the floor 45° or more until the baby's elbow is under the symphysis.
   Mother upright: Direct the baby's body posteriorly in relation to the mother's long axis by angling it 45° in the direction of the mother's heels.
   The sacrum moves from one transverse position to the opposite during rotation. The shoulder axis (which starts out anteroposterior or at an oblique angle) is rotated so that the anterior scapula, the back, and then the posterior scapula pass beneath the pubic arch.
4. During rotation, the arm that was originally posterior should become dislodged and sweep past the face as it flexes at the elbow. It may even emerge spontaneously; if not, it may be within easy reach. You can also pull the baby down toward the floor a little more to see if the arm will come down enough for you to reach it. Even if the posterior arm has not been born during or after the first 180 to 200° rotation is completed, Løvset has you proceed to step 5.
5. As soon as the first shoulder and arm have been delivered, the body is rotated 180 to 200° in the opposite direction. First, move your hands up to the rib cage so that you are holding the delivered arm against that side of the baby's body. Place each thumb on a scapula and be sure no fingers are sticking into an armpit or below the costal margin. When the first rotation has moved the baby from RST to LST, reverse your movements in a counterclockwise direction. Keeping the baby's body horizontal to the long axis of the mother, begin by rotating the baby a quarter-circle from LST to LSA to SA so that the scapula passes under the pubic bone.

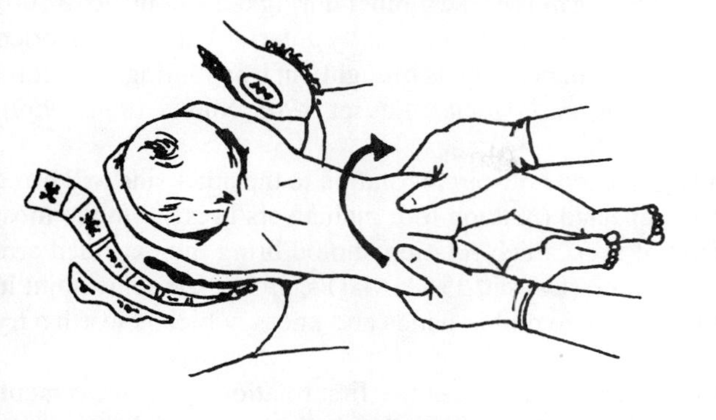

Step 2. The mother is in a modified Walcher position; the baby is RST. The extended posterior arm (baby's left) is already well below the level of the promontory. Grasp the pelvis and hold the body horizontal to the long axis of the mother and begin rotating the back under the pubic arch (in this case, to your right).

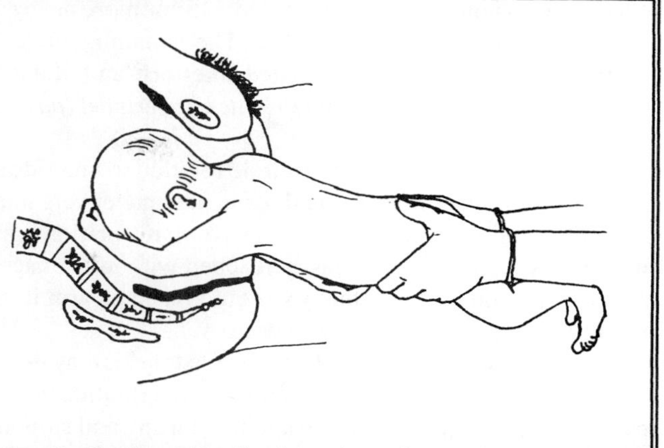

Step 2. The first 90° of horizontal rotation has been completed, bringing the sacrum from RST to RSA to SA and sweeping the posterior arm down toward the baby's face part way.

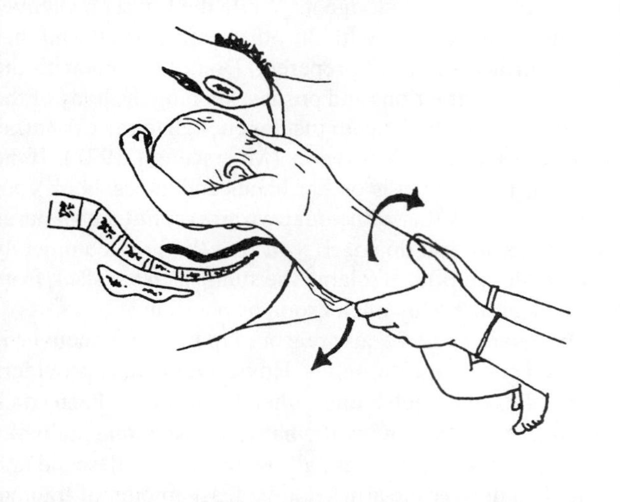

Step 3. The body has now been lowered 45° here but could be lowered more to ensure that the baby's left elbow stays below the level of the symphysis during the next 90° of rotation from SA to LSA to LST.

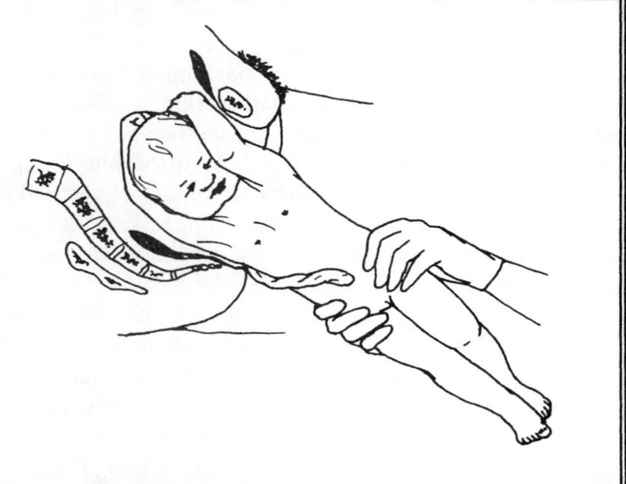

Step 4. After 180° of rotation, the baby's left arm is now within easy reach with the elbow presenting. The next step is to deliver the now anterior arm. The right arm became more extended during rotation, but will be dislodged during the second rotation in the opposite direction.

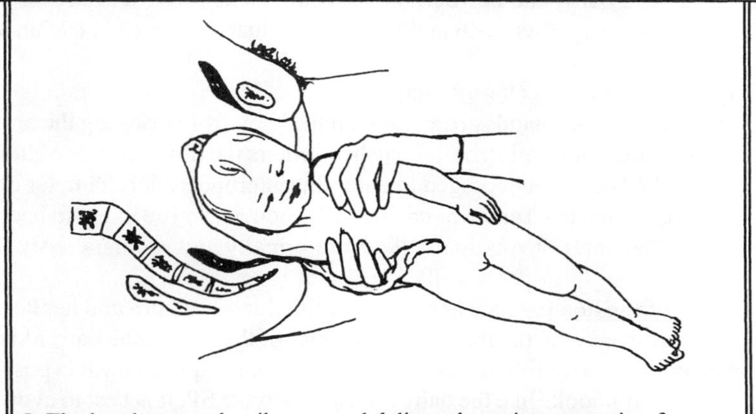

5. The hands grasp the rib cage and delivered arm in preparation for rotating the baby in the opposite direction to bring down the other arm.

6. Release tension and redirect the body 45° or more posterior to the long axis of the mother during the second 90 to 100° of rotation (SA to RSA to RST). The remaining undelivered arm (which was originally anterior but was converted to posterior) is once again rotated anteriorly and, if it isn't born spontaneously, is brought out by splinting, as before. *When rotating, always keep the back uppermost (passing under the pubic bone)* (Løvset, 1968; Mayes 1954, 1959).

In an easy case, the first half-circle rotation to one side and the second half-circle rotation to the other side will bring both arms out. In a more difficult case, the maneuvers must be repeated (making four maneuvers in all). In the most difficult cases, you may need to do two more rotations (a total of six). Each rotation should bring the extended arm further down until it can be easily reached without damage to the limb (Løvset, 1968; Mayes, 1954). At some point in this process, you may feel that you could reach an arm if the mother were on her hands and knees, which is worth a try if multiple rotations have been necessary.

In first-time mothers with firm muscle tone, it may be difficult to complete the entire first rotation in one movement. If you meet significant resistance, reverse the rotation at the point that resistance impedes further rotation, then proceed to rotate in the original direction again. Starting and stopping rotation in this manner can be repeated several times until the first rotation can be completed smoothly (Løvset 1968). The stuffing movement could also be used.

Moving the baby up to facilitate release of a very extended or nuchal arm: An alternative approach to releasing a nuchal arm or reaching the arms of a very large baby, is to move the baby up to dislodge it. While the Løvset maneuver works to dislodge even nuchal arms, it may not if the arm is entangled in the cord or with the other arm. Have the mother quickly assume a hands and knees position or lie down on the flat surface you have prepared. Do not try this with the mother standing because you will be working against gravity. Between contractions and pushes, keeping the body of the baby horizontal to the long axis of the mother, gently push the torso back up into the yoni just far enough to raise the arms above the brim, insert your hand, follow up the anterior torso to the most accessible forearm (Myerscough, 1977). If the arm in nuchally placed , the elbow should be adjacent to the face. If the woman is on her hands and knees, hook your finger over the elbow and pull it at an angle toward the midline of the face (try this with your own arm) splint the humerus and bring it down. Try to feel for a cord or other complicating factor as you do so. If you find the limb completely entangled in the cord and cannot remove it otherwise, cut the cord at the umbilicus (clamp the stump), create slack from below by pulling up on the loose end, pull the cord off the limb and get the baby out as soon as possible.

This is mentioned only because it is something you should be aware of if, for any reason, the Løvset maneuver is unsuccessful. Moving the baby back up like this may deflex the head or damage the spine. However, medical providers in the US have used the Zavanelli maneuver to replace the entire bodies of breech babies when the head has been stuck (Sandberg, 1999). While I do *not* recommend this, it does suggest that gently moving the baby up just enough to make room to move a nuchal arm is not so far fetched. Once the arm is not behind the neck, allow the baby to descend and bring the arm out or perform the Løvset maneuver, which should then deliver the arm with the least amount of trauma.

Break the humerus: If time is running out and you cannot dislodge an arm any other way, hook a finger across the humerus and apply traction to deliberately break the arm. This will collapse it and may facilitate delivery. While this sounds harsh, it is better than a dead baby, and newborn bones heal quickly. It is a last resort measure, but it may save her life. Give the baby arnica right away after birth and have her evaluated by a pediatrician as soon as possible.

Techniques to facilitate the birth of the neck and head

Preventing extension of the head: If their hands are already on the baby from bringing the arms down, some midwives like to keep them there to prevent anterior rotation before the head enters the transverse or oblique diameter of the pelvis, indicated by further descent. If the head is encouraged to enter the anteroposterior diameter of the brim, which is what is likely to happen if the sacrum is turned to an anterior position too soon, it is more likely to become extended. However, if you do let go, it is very likely that anterior rotation will occur normally and spontaneously if the mother is upright.

Preventing posterior rotation of the head: Once her arms and shoulders are born and her head has descended through the brim with the sagittal suture aligned with the transverse diameter of the pelvis, the baby almost always rotates so that her back is anterior. Spontaneous posterior rotation is rare. While a face-to-pubes birth is possible, getting the head out without problems can be difficult. If it looks like the baby is trying to rotate SP, it is best to avoid this challenge by gently nudging the pelvis in the desired direction with a finger or hand.

Women whose babies persist in a sacrum posterior position during labor should be transported before pushing begins.

If a sacrum posterior baby is discovered only after pushing begins, spontaneous rotation to anterior often occurs. If not, Schlinger (2002) recommends grasping the pelvis and rotating the baby to a sacrum anterior position as soon as the umbilicus is born, which can be easy with small second twins if the arms and head were still above the brim. Be careful not to apply any traction as you rotate, as it increases the likelihood of disrupting the position of the arms or deflexing the head. Not every experienced midwife agrees with this intervention, as some babies will spontaneously rotate anteriorly as they move down, but if this does not occur, you may be in for a difficult birth of the head.

Delay at the neck: The baby is in grave danger when the birth of the head is delayed, which may occur at three levels: extended in the anterior-posterior diameter of the inlet (rare); occiput oblique in the midpelvis (even if flexed; also rare) and near the outlet (the most frequently discussed example). If extended at the inlet, reach up and nudge the chin to oblique or transverse; and flex the head by pushing up on the occiput from inside with the other fingers. Let go. If the baby is still not coming, (perineum flat?) the head may be stuck obliquely in the midpelvis, reach in and push the chin toward the mother's anus while pushing up on the occiput (as above) and let go. If the head is extended at the outlet use one of the techniques described in the following pages. (Tully, 2013).

How to create an airway while the head is still inside: If the baby is making gasping movements, first soak up as much birth fluid as possible with gauze, insert your hand, palm toward baby, place spread fingertips on the maxilla and cup your hand pushing the back of your hand into the adjacent yoni wall to create a passageway. The baby may start to breathe on her own at this point. If not, stimulate the baby to get her to breathe. If the baby is unresponsive, you will have to get the head out more quickly. If you cannot get the head out and must transport in this horrible situation, leave your hand in place.

Entrapment of the head in the partially closed os: If the cervix is not completely dilated at the onset of pushing, the baby's lower body can slip through the os, with the head becoming trapped on the cervical rim. This happens most frequently with premature babies, who have little fatty tissue on their bodies and whose heads are disproportionately larger than their bodies, or when the mother has begun spontaneous pushing without attention to signs that full dilation has occurred, or without performing an internal exam when there is doubt, or both. It is a very dangerous situation that calls for a quick and well-calculated response (in other words, don't panic). Have an assistant give the mother the highest potency homeopathic gelsemium you have or 1 drop of the herbal tincture of gelsemium diluted in hot water and have her swish it in her mouth as she drinks all of it. This may relax the cervix. Then, try to reduce the cervix with your fingers. Start by pushing it back over the chin, since it is the sharpest part near the base of the skull and is likely to remain hung up even if you can push the cervix up over the occiput. Reducing the cervix may require a lot of force. If finger manipulation is not working, don't waste time trying as the cervix may be in spasm and resistant to such techniques.

If the cervix doesn't release, you have a major complication. Only in an emergency of this magnitude would you consider making a cervical incision with blunt-blunt surgical scissors, a technique which should allow the head to be born. Make your incision at 2, 6 or 10 o'clock, whichever is easiest to access. These locations avoid the uterine arteries. (Cuts so placed are referred to as "Dührssen's incisions.") You must be very careful not to cut or puncture the baby, the cord or the surrounding maternal soft tissues. Heavy cervical bleeding is likely to ensue. These incisions can be extended if necessary, but one cut is usually all it takes to complete the birth. This type of incision will need stitches and may extend on its own. Clamp a ring forceps over the apex of the incision to stop the bleeding. Transport for repair and be prepared for some serious questions from the hospital staff.

Assisting the birth when the occiput-anterior head is extended at the outlet: If the baby's body has been allowed to hang and the neck has elongated but the nape of the neck, chin or jawline are still not presenting, it is likely that the head is deflexed. This is far less likely to be a problem if the mother is upright because gravity and her abdominal muscles will work to maintain head flexion. The Burns-Marshall technique may help flex the head, even in this circumstance. If not, more complex procedures are given below in order of difficulty.

Mauriceau-Cronk maneuver: When the mother pushes in an upright kneeling position and you are behind her, Cronk recommends a reverse Mauriceau-Smellie-Veit maneuver to encourage the head to flex (reversed because you are behind her). Place the baby belly-up on your nondominant forearm, legs straddling your forearm, buttocks near your elbow, and your palm toward the occiput, as if helping her to go to your breast. Gently slide your index and middle

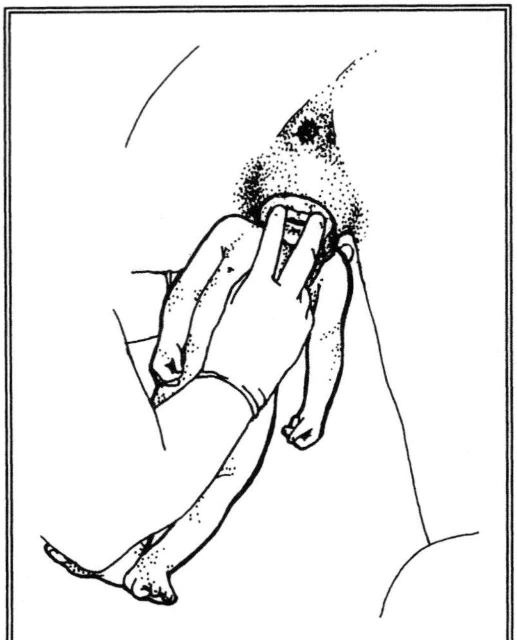

Mauriceau-Cronk maneuver: When the chin is visible, flex the occiput from behind and place fingers on the maxillae to aid flexion of the head.

fingers up behind the pubic arch, inside the birth canal and apply upward pressure on her occiput. At the same time, slide two fingers of your other hand in, past the perineum, onto her maxillary ridge and apply gentle downward pressure, thus flexing her head. Only after flexion has occurred, ask the mother to drop down to a low hands-and-knees or knee-chest position. This opens the pelvic outlet and helps the occiput pivot around the pubic arch as the baby's face and bregma pass over the perineum toward you. Follow the rotational movement of the head as it pivots around the pubic bone.

Mauriceau-Banks maneuver: When the mother is standing and the midwife is positioned in front of her, Banks uses her adaptation of this classical technique (which can also be used if the mother is supine). Place the baby's body astride your nondominant forearm, with your palm supporting his chest and buttocks in the crook of your arm, near the elbow. Brace your index and middle fingers against the upper border of the superior maxillae to flex the head (you can place the ring finger in the baby's mouth to aid stability as well). Insert the index and ring fingers of your other hand into the yoni, under the pubic arch. Spread your fingers, placing one against the posterior side of each of the parietal eminences. To flex the head, apply forward and downward pressure to the parietal eminences while applying downward pressure to the maxillary bones with the internal hand. As the head starts to advance, direct your traction down at a 30° angle. As it descends, redirect your arm in an arc to bring the head around the pubic arch. Once the suboccipital area is under the pubic arch, the mother can lean forward and the face should pass over the perineum. Bring the vault of the head out as slowly as possible to reduce the chances of intracranial injury (Banks, 1998). Suprapubic pressure could be added by an assistant.

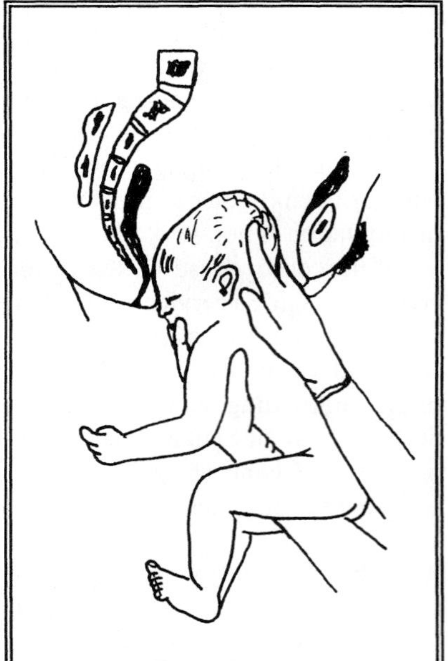

Mauriceau-Banks maneuver

Cronk's and Banks' modifications of the Mauriceau-Smellie-Veit maneuver use pressure on the occiput and parietal eminences respectively and eliminate shoulder traction. This reduces the inherent risks of the classical technique because no traction is applied directly to the neck. (See the entry on the classic version of this maneuver at the end of the chapter.)

ModifiedWigand-Martin maneuver: Assuming that the mother is upright, kneel in front of her or, if she is supine, stand between her legs. Support the baby's body on your nondominant arm so that he is straddling your arm, with your palm on his chest. Place the middle finger of this hand in his mouth and brace your index and ring fingers on the upper border of the superior ridge of his maxillary bones. Use your external hand or that of an assistant to apply suprapubic pressure to his head through the mother's abdomen. Apply traction with the fingers on the maxillary bones, using the finger in his mouth for stabilization (*not* traction). The head is brought out in a natural arc from beneath the pubic bone, downward, around and then upward, following the curve of birth canal. This is considered a relatively safe maneuver.

McRoberts maneuver: In 1992, Shushan and Younis presented a case report involving entrapment of the aftercoming head. The Bracht and Mauriceau-Smellie-Veit maneuvers were used unsuccessfully in an attempt to deliver the head. (They did not attempt to use the Burns-Marshall maneuver.) At that point, McRoberts was employed, which resulted in release of the head. They note that a generous clitorotomy was cut prior to the birth of the head. Since the McRoberts maneuver rotates the perineum up, creating more of an obstacle for the head to have to get past, that the perineum was cut probably facilitated the success of its use in this case. McRoberts does pivot the pubic bone up, where it would press against the occiput, thus aiding flexion. If nothing else has worked, I suppose this is worth a try in conjunction with the Burns-Marshall maneuver. As long as you wait until the head is well down in the pelvis, it is a safe maneuver as it involves no traction on the baby. The mother must be supine, be prepared to guide the head down around and up. (I suppose she could also go into a deep squat if she is upright, but this makes it hard to reach the baby, if necessary. Cronk uses a deep closed knee-chest position to aid head flexion, which gives you excellent access to the baby).

Frank's Nudge: If the head is not coming and the occiput is directly anterior, from behind the mother, grasp the baby's shoulders, place your thumbs in the subclavicular hollow just above the ribs and press toward the mother's pubic bone. This triggers a reflex to flex the head. Someone can apply direct fundal pressure and the head should come. (Tully, 2013)

If the head rotates occiput posterior (face-to-pubes): If sudden occiput posterior rotation should take place once the rest of the baby is born (a very rare occurrence) any attempt at manual rotation to occiput anterior is likely to severely strain or even break the neck once the head is below the brim. If you are going to try to turn the baby at this point, you must use a grip that maintains the head and spine in anatomical alignment (Myerscough, 1977). It would be ideal to have the mother supine with her bottom slightly elevated to take the baby out of gravity and use a modified Mauriceau-Banks maneuver with fingers stabilizing the shoulders, while carefully turning the baby around (however you don't have a lot of time to mess around with this as the baby must be born shortly). Besides, if the occiput and maxillary ridge can be reached to enable such an attempt, the head is poised to deliver relatively easily, making OA rotation unnecessary.

If the head is flexed: If the head is well flexed, the chin and face are permitted to descend past the pubic bone as far as the root of the nose, then the occiput pivots over the perineum. If the mother is standing and you are in front of her, once the occiput has descended so that the nape of the neck is seen at the perineum and the chin appears below the periurethral area, a Mauriceau-Cronk maneuver can be used to lift the body anteriorly and pivot the bridge of the nose around the pubic bone as the occiput passes over the perineum. Alternatively, the mother can assume a hands and knees position at this point, which allows the baby to drop to facilitate this movement spontaneously. Have an assistant get under the mother and apply suprapubic pressure to assist the downward movement of the head. Sotelo (2001) describes rolling one woman over into a crouched hands-and-knees position and pivoting the baby out.

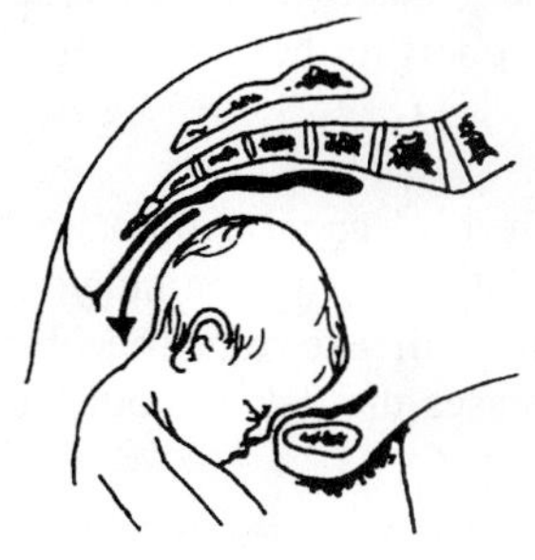

Flexed OP head: mother on her hands and knees

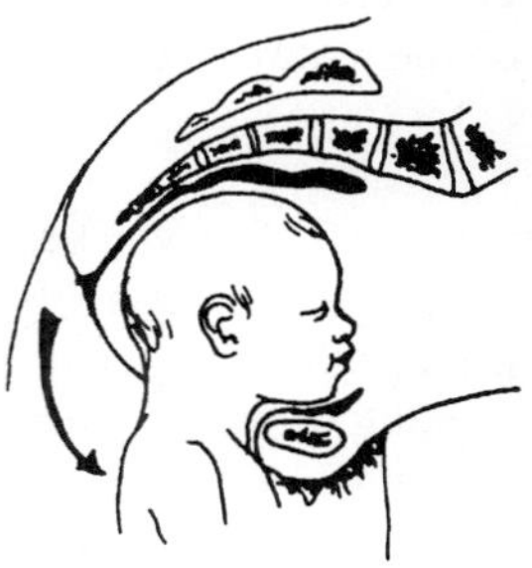

Deflexed head, direction to lift the body to pivot the head: mother on hands and knees.

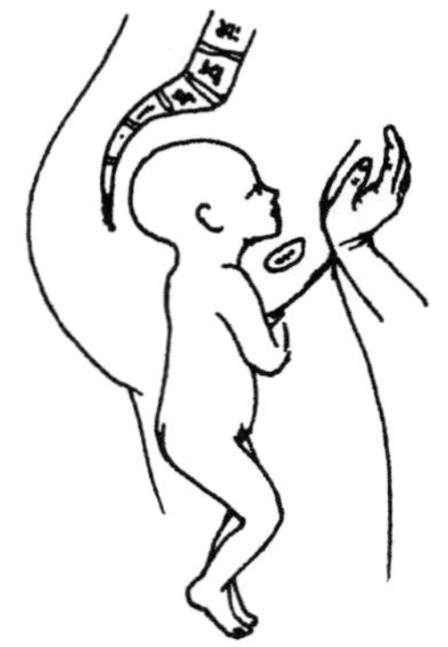

Deflexed head: applying pressure to the chin with the mother standing.

If the head is extended: Unfortunately, the head can easily become deflexed as the chin passes the pubic arch, inviting fetal injury. If the head does extend, the region just below the chin pivots around the pubic bone. The classical method of dealing with this has the mother supine. The midwife lifts the baby's body to allow the occiput to sweep the perineum while the underside of the chin serves as the pivot point against the pubic bone. This greatly stretches the perineum and results in a larger cephalic diameter passing through the midpelvis and outlet. It is a tricky and dangerous maneuver. Having the mother assume a hands and knees position may accomplish this movement spontaneously. In case more help is needed, have an assistant ready to apply suprapubic pressure on your cue. One midwife, who wishes to remain anonymous, describes using suprapubic pressure directed toward the mother's spine to dislodge the chin from the pubic bone, which rapidly delivered the head. In this case, the mother was standing in front of her.

Total Breech Extraction

Total breech extraction is the same as partial breech extraction with the addition of bringing down the feet and legs. Total extraction is potentially dangerous for both mother and baby. Spontaneous descent may occur if you are patient. Conversely, a serious problem, such as complex cord entanglement or a fetal defect may be preventing descent. Extraction should only be resorted to when you are very remote from medical assistance and fetal distress develops rapidly during advanced labor or to bring down a second twin, when it is relatively less risky and more easily accomplished because the passages have been dilated. Only manipulate the baby to the point that spontaneous descent begins, after which the mother should be assisted into an upright position and encouraged to birth spontaneously. Also study the subchapter entitled "The Use of Version during Labor" to gain a better understanding of what to do (and what not to do) and the differences in handling a transverse versus a breech presentation. Obviously the parents must be in total accord with the decision to extract the baby.

How to proceed will depend upon the station and the attitude of the baby. If the baby is out of reach, giving the mother lobelia or other sedative herbs to relax may be helpful. General anesthesia was given when total extractions were done routinely.

Risks of and precautions for extraction

Breech extraction is risky for both the mother and baby. The baby may suffer hypoxia or injury and the mother may suffer uterine rupture. The reason to proceed must be compelling. If the baby is large, extraction is likely to be very difficult. If the baby is dead (especially for more than a day), extraction may pull the body apart.

Positioning the mother

The mother should assume a hands and knees position or a modified Walcher position, which will relax the soft tissues of the pelvic floor. Do not attempt extraction with the mother upright, as you need her out of gravity.

If reaching the fetal parts proves impossible with the mother supine, Shears (1920) recommends rolling the mother onto the side which places the fetal small parts in your palm. This will shift the baby, allow greater access to the uppermost side of the pelvic cavity, and will often overcome the difficulty. If the mother is to assume a side-lying position, she should reposition herself further up on the mattress to provide adequate support for her lower leg.

Preparing the birth canal

The cervix must be fully dilated and the bladder empty before you begin. Even so, the birth canal will not be dilated because the baby is still high. To overcome this barrier, generously apply sterile lubricant to the mother and your hand and insert your fingers and eventually your fist to massage the birth canal open. While this will take some time, bringing the baby through an unprepared birth canal is not going to be quick or easy and increases the risk of both fetal and maternal injury.

Direction of traction and rotation

Regardless of which maneuver you employ, your primary aim is to bring the baby through the curve of the birth canal with minimal trauma. The curve of the canal will be more exaggerated than in a normal situation because the mother is supine and the baby's body has not dilated the passages naturally. As long as the breech remains unborn, the baby's body is aligned with the axis of the pelvic inlet, and this axis should be your main focus during the first part of the extraction. The only part of the baby that is not in the axis is usually the thighs (unless the baby is at a much higher station when you begin). Thus, the angle of traction should be about 30° downward in relationship to the long axis of the mother until the anterior hip is fully born. After that, redirect the angle of

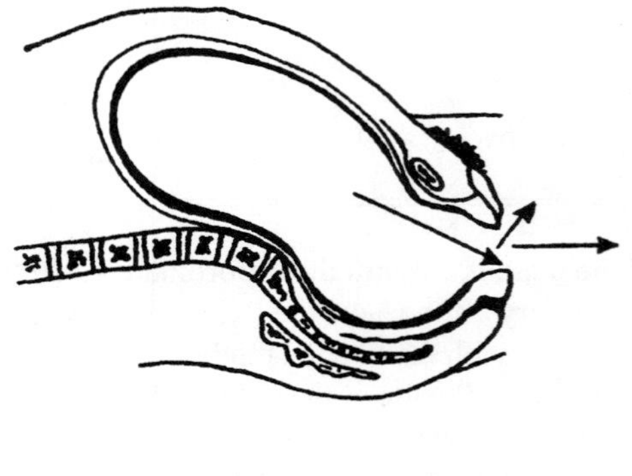

Directions of traction (mother supine)

traction upward briefly to bring out the posterior hip. As soon as the posterior hip is born, the baby's body should be kept horizontal to the long axis of the mother to give equal consideration to the axis of the pelvic inlet and outlet. Remember that the shoulders are entering the pelvis as the umbilicus emerges. Therefore, as the hips are born, the back should be rotated anteriorly, if the baby does not do so spontaneously. The baby's body should be held in the horizontal plane until the scapulae present at the outlet. Then the back is turned to the side it originally occupied for the birth of the shoulders. After the shoulders emerge, the head engages either LOT or ROT and the back is again rotated so the sacrum is anterior for the delivery of the head. If you must maneuver the head out, follow the path around the pubic arch. Never extract the head in the horizontal plane, as that causes a larger cephalic diameter to pass through the outlet and may result in deflection (Løvset, 1968).

How to begin if no leg is presenting

If the baby is a rigidly splinted frank breech, the birth may be delayed due to impaired lateral flexion. In this case, attempt to bring down the legs. If they will not come, bring down the buttocks.

Bringing down a leg: These instructions add to those covered under the Pinard maneuver given earlier in this chapter. Insert your hand high into the uterus between contractions. Avoid the cord. If you feel the cord, maneuver your hand so that the cord is either above or behind your hand to keep it from getting entangled as you bring the leg down. If it is behind your hand, it may get compressed as you proceed; therefore placing it above your hand is much safer. Attempt to bring down the anterior leg whenever possible, as doing so will encourage the baby to rotate with his back toward the pubic bone and will result in the direction of traction corresponding more closely to the axis of the brim.

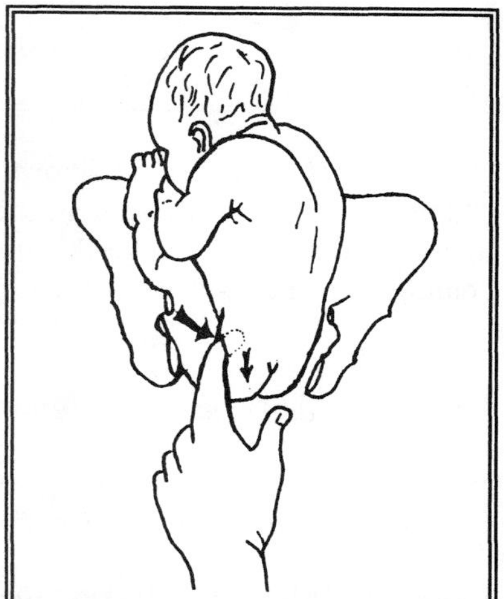

With the mother supine, hook a finger in the anterior groin and apply traction to the anterior hip out in a downward direction.

Bringing down the buttocks: In a frank breech baby, you may be able to bring the anterior hip down without having to reach further up to flex the leg. Wedge one fingertip in the baby's groin (between the upper thigh and the baby's abdomen) and pull, leaning the pressure inward toward the baby's lowermost belly and pelvis rather than out against the anterior thigh. This helps prevent an uncontrolled delivery of the anterior leg. Now apply gentle traction. Never use two fingers on either side of the same hip, as this is likely to damage the hip joint.

Once it is within reach, place your other index finger in the groin crease of the other leg. During contractions as the woman pushes, apply traction with both fingers, leaning the pressure inward toward the baby's pelvic area (as described above). Apply the most downward traction to the groin of the posterior leg, using the finger in the groin of the anterior leg to guide the buttocks. Wiggle the baby down in line with the long axis of mother, then upward in relationship to the introitus as the breech comes under the pubic bone, following the curve of the birth canal. Potter (1922) advises *not* to use fundal pressure even now, as extension of the head is the likely result. If a leg does come down as you apply traction to the groin, grasp the baby's pelvis as soon as possible.

Pulling in the direction of the anterior groin (that is, away from, rather than toward the lower abdomen) is more likely to cause your finger to slip down the length of the femur and result in the leg becoming flexed and popping out, an event likely to produce a tear in the mother and possibly break the femur. It also presses the legs forward against the wall of the birth canal, which will impair lateral spinal flexion. In addition, anteriorly directed traction applied to the posterior groin will encourage the baby's sacrum to rotate posteriorly.

If a leg is presenting: In some cases, a leg will be presenting when you begin a total breech extraction. Always try to bring down the other leg so you are manipulating the baby by grasping the pelvis, as this is, by far, the safest option. When one leg is the *only* part of the baby within reach, you can splint it by grasping it with both hands, placing one thumb above the other on the back of the leg over the center of the femur. Your fingers should be evenly spaced over the limb.

Only enough smooth, steady traction should now be applied to produce descent. Do not attempt to wiggle or rotate the limb as you are very likely to traumatize the hip or knee joint. Traction is coordinated with uterine activity and maternal pushing efforts and directed downward at a 30° angle, following the axis of the inlet until the anterior hip has passed beneath the symphysis. Reposition your hands higher on the leg as the limb appears and redirect traction upward to deliver the posterior hip. Grasp the pelvis as soon as possible. If the other leg has not delivered you may not need to bring it down as it should naturally follow delivery of the trunk.

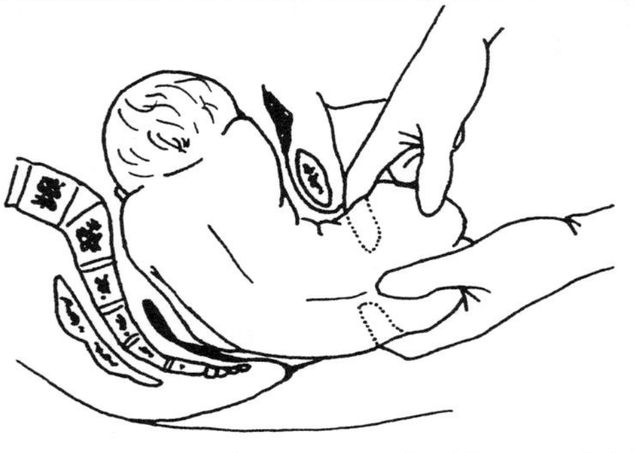

Using two fingers to bring the posterior hip around the pubic arch (mother supine).

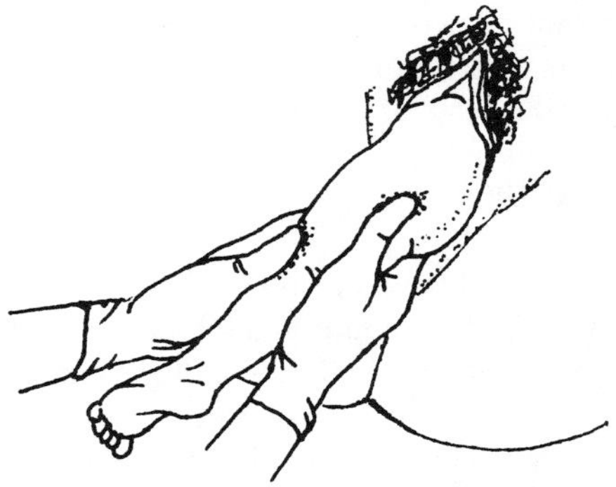

Splinting a leg with both hands (mother supine).

Now check to see if the elbows can be felt on the baby's chest. If so, the mother can be assisted into a standing position, which can help facilitate the rest of the birth. If not, proceed with the techniques described earlier in the chapter to bring out the arms and head. Always be prepared for extended arms and a deflexed head. However, if the baby is coming spontaneously, do not manipulate her any more than is absolutely required.

Techniques that are *not* recommended

The following maneuvers are discussed here only because I know that midwives learn techniques from many different sources and wonder if they are appropriate. They are mentioned only to clarify why they are not recommended.

Classical method of delivering the shoulders

First introduced by Friedrich Scanzoni (1821-1891), the classical method of delivering extended arms begins with the mother supine. The posterior arm is brought out first, then the baby is rotated belly-up to bring the other arm to posterior. In this case, the arms are dislodged by rotating them past the pubic arch, rather than into the roomier sacral area. This risks getting an arm caught up above the anterior brim as well as deflexing the head, or getting the baby stuck in a belly-up position, which creates the additional risk of getting the chin hung up on the pubic bone when the head engages. For all these reasons, it has been abandoned in favor of the modified classical method or the Løvset maneuver, which are both much safer and more effective in all types of extended arm situations. If the posterior arm comes out and the anterior arm is still undelivered, it is safer to use the Løvset maneuver than to rotate the baby belly-up, particularly when the mother is supine and the weight of her abdomen is pressing upon the fetal parts still undelivered.

Bracht maneuver

The German obstetrician Erich Franz Bracht, introduced this maneuver in 1936. It is widely used in Europe. It assumes that the mother is supine. The breech is allowed to emerge spontaneously to the level of the umbilicus. The pelvis and splinted legs are grasped together with both hands, fingers over the sacrum and thumbs over the thighs. Anterior rotation of the fetal sacrum is encouraged. Suprapubic pressure is used to maintain downward movement and head flexion. When anterior rotation is almost complete, the fetal body is slowly lifted up and held, but not pressed, against the maternal pubic symphysis (with a force that is intended to equal gravity) just enough to allow the arms to drop out from behind the perineum. This part of the maneuver is easy and works well if the arms are over the chest and therefore require no manipulation (Hughes, 1972; Künzel & Kirshbaum, 2002).

After the arms are free, the baby is held as described and the torso slowly pivots up and onto the mother's abdomen while uterine contractions and moderate suprapubic pressure effect "spontaneous" birth of the head. As you can tell from this description, this technique risks extension of the head and injury to the spine. It is used to deliver a baby that would be born on his own if his mother were upright and is therefore *not* recommended here.

Breaking the clavicle

If none of the recommended techniques have brought the arms down, traditionally the humerus or clavicle has been fractured. This is done by pressing the thumb into the clavicle until it breaks. This collapses the shoulder girdle on that side, making more room to work the arm down. Breaking the clavicle is impractical for female attendants, many of whom will not have sufficient upper body strength to accomplish it. It is not recommended.

Mauriceau-Smellie-Veit maneuver (Mauriceau-Levret maneuver)

In 1668, François Mauriceau is credited as the first to formally describe the basics of this maneuver. During the 1700s, William Smellie wrote of it in England and Andre Levret revived it's use in France. Gustav von Veit refined the maneuver in Germany in the late 1800s. In looking over a number of texts, there seems to be a lot of confusion about the original maneuver. The following description is the best I could piece together about its origins and is based on original sources whenever possible.

The mother gives birth in a supine position. The 4th edition of Mauriceau's THE DISEASES OF WOMEN WITH CHILD AND IN CHILD-BED (1668) is the most often referenced source of this technique. In it, however, I could only find a description on page 188 of inserting a finger into the mouth and applying the thumb to the chin to extract the head when it has become detached from the body (!). He describes an entirely different technique for getting out the stuck aftercoming head in a living child, which is nowhere discussed in more contemporary literature, but which is very interesting. He states "In this case he must not endeavor only to draw the child by the shoulders, lest he sometimes separates the body from the head, but he must disengage it (the head) little and little, from the bones in the passage, with the fingers of each hand, sliding them on each side opposite the one to the other, sometimes above, and sometimes under, until the work be ended" (1668, 187). (Actually, this sounds like inching the head out with a wiggling motion and appears to be relatively safe [if not particularly easy or always effective] as long as you reach high enough so you are manipulating above the joint of the mandible and don't jam fingers in under the jaw line.) According to Graham (1951), Mauriceau also described (apparently in one of his many untranslated French texts) placing the child astride the forearm and inserting a finger into the mouth to apply traction while an assistant pulls on the baby's feet. The problem with simply applying traction to the jaw, is that the jaw will always drop down while the dome of the skull can remain immobile at the brim; thus traction on the jaw alone does not encourage flexion or descent and may injure the baby.

Smellie describes a similar maneuver, laying the baby over his forearm and placing a finger in the mouth to flex the head into the hollow of the sacrum, allowing the resistance afforded by the pubic bone to assist in flexing the head. However, if more than moderate traction was required, he then placed a finger on each side of the nose and hooked the fingers of the other hand over the baby's shoulders (the index finger goes over one shoulder and the other three go over the other) before applying more traction. This splints the spine and thus reduces direct traction upon it (Smellie, 1752, 312-313). Only sufficient traction to guide the head through the arc of the birth canal is then applied to the shoulders, not the head. The mother pushes as the attendant pulls in a downward posterior direction (about a 30° angle toward the mother's heels). As the occiput passes under the pubic bone and the nape of the neck is seen, the baby is lifted to pivot the occiput beneath the pubic bone. *The classical maneuver places more direct tension on the baby's neck and jaw, posing more risk than either the Mauriceau-Cronk or the Mauriceau-Banks maneuvers previously described.*

Mauriceau-Myers maneuver: In 1986, Myers proposed his own modification of the classic maneuver. The mother is supine. After delivery of both arms, the baby is placed astride the anterior forearm with the index and middle fingers straddling the nose, pressing just above the maxillary ridge. The ring and little fingers of the opposite hand are placed over one shoulder, and the thumb is placed on the other shoulder, while the index and middle fingers are extended as far as possible up the back of the neck for term infants or to the occipital eminence for preterm infants. The fingers of the upper hand push upward while the fingers of the lower hand pull downward, thus flexing the head. The maneuver is then carried out as for all other similar maneuvers, with traction being applied down, around and up to follow the curve of the birth canal. This technique requires a large hand and traction on the shoulders and is therefore not recommended.

Zavanelli maneuver (podalic replacement)

Incredibly, the Zavanelli maneuver, which consists of replacing the partially born baby back up inside his anesthetized mother, has been used on breech babies who could not be delivered normally (usually performed when the head is trapped, but sometimes sooner), after which an emergency surgical delivery has been done (Sandberg, 1999). While this technique is touted by Sandberg as minimally traumatizing, I do not recommend it. Even the newest edition of WILLIAMS OBSTETRICS (Cunningham et al., 2001) generally frowns upon its use.

UNSTABLE LIE, OBLIQUE LIE AND TRANSVERSE LIE IN LABOR

NOTE: Techniques for dealing with these three problems are similar; therefore all presented together in this chapter.

Discovering a Nonlongitudinal Lie in Labor

Unstable lie

A baby who frequently changes her lie is called "unstable." This usually begins prenatally or, much more rarely, it first presents during labor. In fact, the fetus can change position multiple times during the course of labor. While a very unusual occurrence overall, it is more likely to happen when the baby has displayed a tendency toward unstable lie during pregnancy. However, babies do have minds of their own and can decide to change position in labor even when the lie was stable during pregnancy. This should be suspected if large movements of the baby are seen through the mother's abdomen, if the mother reports that the baby is moving a lot, or if she says the baby has turned. Naturally, this occurs most often in women who have had several babies and whose abdominal and uterine tone is somewhat lax, but it is a possibility at every birth and should especially be suspected if two midwives perform abdominal palpation or internal exams and report wildly different findings, in which case multiple pregnancy should also be ruled out.

Oblique lie

Most babies in an oblique lie will have been identified and handled prenatally, but a baby can become oblique in early labor. In most cases, this occurs when the baby's head is near the opening of the brim, but the torso is tilted too far to one side and he is not well flexed.

Another possible cause is an inlet obstruction that pushes the baby to one side. The force of uterine contractions may be required before the baby becomes pressed against the obstruction and diverted to the side, which is why the oblique lie didn't occur during pregnancy. A careful internal exam may or may not reveal the cause. A growth such as an ovarian cyst or a fibroid can prevent the presenting part from entering the pelvis but may not be felt during an exam. Rupture of membranes with an oblique lie, since nothing is filling the pelvis, raises the risk of cord prolapse. The mother may not have any particular sensation when the baby is oblique except a noticeable lack of pressure in her pelvis, especially as labor advances.

Transverse lie

Finding a baby in a transverse lie during labor is typically unexpected and a truly disconcerting experience for all concerned, because no responsible midwife would knowingly allow a woman to enter labor with a stable transverse lie. The baby may have turned between the last prenatal and the onset of labor or may have turned in early labor. You also may be caring for a woman who has not received prenatal care and thus be confronted with a transverse lie for the first time when labor begins.

What to Do

The following steps should be taken whenever a nonlongitudinal lie, whether oblique or transverse, is encountered. Some of these techniques also work to keep the baby in the most desirable position.

Assessment

Palpate the baby: If labor is underway and you or the mother suspect that a large fetal movement has occurred, have the mother lie down and palpate her abdomen immediately to determine the lie of the baby. If the baby has been unstable during pregnancy or has been transverse or oblique at any time, palpate shortly after you arrive at the labor.

Perform an internal exam: If you are unsure of the baby's position or if abdominal palpation confirms that the baby is not vertex, first prop up the mother's bottom with a folded sheet or towel to reduce pressure on the membranes, and then perform an internal exam, taking care not to rupture the membranes. Keep in mind that the presenting part of a baby you can feel may be held in place by a second baby you cannot feel as easily. Take note if you palpated a baby in a distinctly transverse or oblique lie abdominally but now find deeply engaged head on internal exam; this is a good indication that there are at least two babies. Use your other hand to palpate the abdomen while you keep your internal hand in place to see if you can figure out what is going on. In cases in which there is only one baby in a nonlongitudinal lie, you may find no presenting part in the pelvis or you may feel an extremity, a shoulder or some part of the torso presenting. Note dilation and effacement. The further along the dilation, the more risk there is of cord prolapse if the membranes rupture during manipulations (see below).

If you confirm a nonlongitudinal lie

If internal exam confirms a transverse or oblique lie, have the mother remain horizontal and keep her propped up to minimize the risk of uncontrolled rupture of membranes and subsequent cord prolapse while you both discuss how you want to proceed.

Talk to the mother: Explain to the mother what is happening and discuss potential courses of action available both at home and in the hospital. Let her know that if labor is early and the membranes are intact, dealing with the situation at home may be quite successful. However, any such discussion must include both the benefits and risks of such actions.

Tune into the situation: Listen inwardly to see if the baby is trying to tell you something by turning. Maybe there is a reason you should not stay at home. Ask the mother to tune in as well. If either of you feel something is wrong, transport.

Talk to the baby: You, the parents, and preferably both should talk to the baby about what she is doing and ask her to assume a vertex presentation. Babies who are moving around a lot are usually trying to find the best way out. The baby may be afraid of moving through the pelvis or may be picking up on maternal fears. If fears have not come to light and been addressed during prenatal care, they need to be addressed now, making it clear to the baby that creating a drama around the birth will not help the situation.

Rebozo techniques to turn the baby: This technique can be used to turn the baby whether the membranes are intact or not, however, if they are ruptured, the risk of cord prolapse is increased. Fold your rebozo into a narrow strip (about 6 to 8 in wide [15 to 20 cm]) and lay it on the floor. Have the mother lie supine across it with her buttocks over the center and her legs straight and slightly open. Stand over her, straddling her hips and hold the ends of the shawl so they are perpendicular to the floor. As a contraction ends, start rocking gently, periodically jerking the shawl on the side opposite the side to which you want the baby to turn; for example, if the baby is transverse (RAA), the baby's head will be on the mother's right. If you want to try to turn the baby to vertex, jerk on the mother's *left* side. Enriqueta Contreras (2003), traditional Mexican midwife, explains that the rocking motion sets up a current in the amniotic fluid to help bring the baby around as well as opening the first chakra (energy center). Discontinue the rocking during the next contraction. This may need to be continued during the space between two or three contractions to get the baby to rotate completely.

This technique can also be performed with the mother on her hands and knees. The midwife kneels or stands at the mother's head, wrapping the narrowly folded rebozo around the mother's buttocks. The midwife then grasps the ends of the shawl and rocks gently back and forth keeping the rebozo more or less horizontal to the floor. Gentle motions are sufficient in this position because the abdomen is dependent and the baby floats easily.

As you rock her, ask the mother take short breathes with sharp exhales to jerk the abdominal muscles upward and facilitate the turn, regardless of which position is chosen.

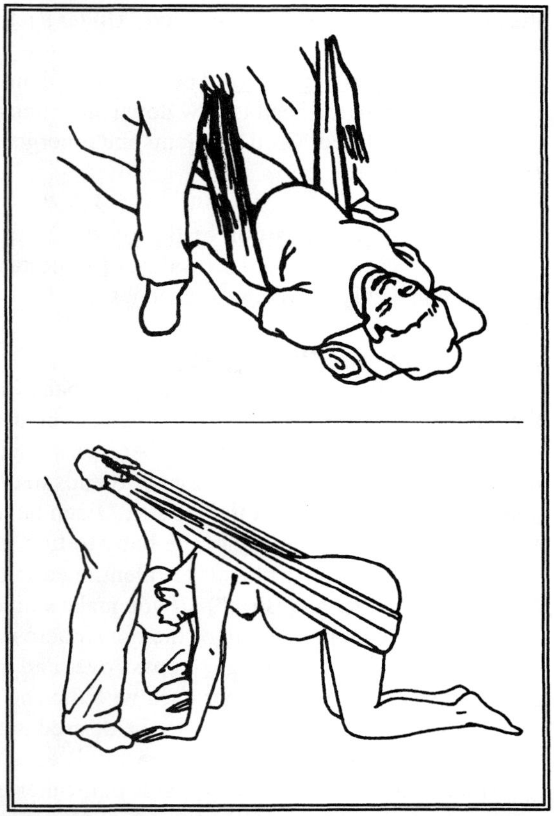

(Adapted with permission from photographs appearing in COMFORT MEASURES FOR CHILDBIRTH: THE REBOZO WAY, © 2001, Guadalupe Trueba.)

Attempt external version: External version can be very successful even in labor, if the membranes are intact. Doing so is described in detail in the chapter entitled "The Use of Version during Labor." Do not persist in your efforts if external version proves difficult or impossible. There may be a cord entanglement or some other reason why the baby won't turn. Keep pressure off the bag by placing the mother in a supine, side-lying or knee-chest position and prepare for transport.

Monitor descent: If you are able to turn the baby externally to a vertex or breech presentation, closely monitor for proper descent into the pelvis by keeping a hand in the yoni. When contractions begin to move the baby down, evaluate descent internally to be sure the lie is remaining longitudinal and the presenting part is contacting the cervix. Encourage stronger contractions to help move the baby down into the pelvis unless labor is very early or contractions are strong already. Once the baby is filling the cervix and moving down, have the mother stand up and lean forward with her pelvis tipped forward to help the baby enter the pelvis. Recheck the lie with palpation and descent with an internal exam until you are satisfied that the baby is well seated in the pelvis.

The status of the membranes

Rupture of membranes: When the membranes rupture, as always, listen to the fetal heart rate to rule out cord prolapse. If version has been successful, recheck to make sure the baby is remaining in a desirable position. If an obstruction is preventing descent into the pelvis, rupture of membranes may cause the presenting part to encounter the obstacle and revert back to an undesirable lie.

The loss of a large quantity of fluid leaves the uterine walls temporarily slack. If this occurs while the baby is still in an undesirable position, and if nothing has prolapsed and the uterine walls are distensible, the midwife may attempt external or internal version at this point. The old textbooks state that version is often easy just after the membranes rupture, with little risk to mother or baby. Be aware that this situation affords *relatively* less risk. External and certainly internal version always carry a certain amount of risk, much more so if the uterus has resumed contracting for awhile and the amount of water is much reduced. Under such circumstances, uterine rupture is a real possibility.

If the membranes are intact: The risk of cord prolapse is high when the membranes are not ruptured when the baby is high, even though the head is now down and contractions are good. You may want to rupture membranes as described in the chapter entitled "Cord Problems and Emergencies during Labor," using the method recommended there to minimize the risk of prolapse.

If the baby changes position or lie again

Repeat all the suggested procedures for reestablishing a vertex presentation. Once accomplished, monitor the fetal position constantly to watch for changes in lie.

Bind the belly with Buist's pads

Using a belly binder can help keep the baby in place, especially if the abdominal tone is loose, and may be tried if the membranes are still intact. Binding may be used to move the baby into position from an oblique lie, to maintain a desirable position when the lie has been unstable, or to keep the baby from reverting to transverse after he has been turned. Roll two towels from their short ends to create two bolsters. Use either large hand towels or small bath towels, depending upon the size of the woman. Each bolster should be small enough to fit snugly against the baby, but large enough to impede the ability of the baby to turn again. Use a rebozo, a strip of bed sheet, any lightweight cloth, or a veterinary elastic support bandage (mentioned in the chapter entitled "Basic and Emergency Equipment and Supplies Using during Labor and Birth"). If you make a binder, it should be about 12 inches (30 cm) wide and 3 to 4 yards long.

- Spread the narrow length of the binder across the bed and roll the rest of it up like a paper towel roll, roll-side down, so it will be easy to pass over and then under the mother's belly.
- Have the woman lie on her back with the end of the binder centered under her upper buttocks and lower back.
- Perform version to the baby to the desired position, if indicated.
- Apply the binder between contractions, as you will then be better able to fit the towels close to the baby.
- Place a towel roll on the right side of the uterus, alongside the baby's body and have the mother hold it in place. Place another towel on the opposite side and have the mother hold it as well.
- Stretch the rolled strip of cloth across the hips and lower end of the towels. Have the mother lift her body and unroll the cloth enough to pass it under her side. Bring the roll around again and do a second pass across her

belly to include the midportion of the towel; pass it beneath her again and come up on the other side for the third pass over the upper end of the towels. You want the binder to be tight at the lower end and looser as it nears the fundus. When it is sufficiently secure, have the mother carefully arise and continue to wrap her in this fashion until you get to the end of the cloth. Attach the ends with safety pins or velcro strips. This should assist the baby in staying in place (Sutton & Scott, 1996); however, be advised that the old doctors who used this technique reported varying success. If the towels don't work, you can try wrapping the belly without the towels.

A good-quality maternity girdle may be used instead of a binder.

If you discover a nonlongitudinal lie upon rupture of membranes

This is a serious situation, especially if the mother is upright at the time the membranes rupture. If the contour of her abdomen suggests a nonlongitudinal lie, have her lie down flat at once on the closest flat surface–on the floor, if necessary. Use folded sheets or a folded blanket to place under her buttocks to elevate her lower body slightly. Immediately check the fetal heart rate. Perform an internal exam to assess what is presenting. If not the head or the breech, check whether there are any limbs or loops of cord in the pelvis and keep your hand inside to monitor the situation. If the baby is high in the uterus and there is nothing pressing on the cord, the cord could still be prolapsed without fetal heart rate problems, so even if the heart rate is normal, it is always a good idea to double check with an internal exam. (See the chapter entitled "Cord Problems and Emergencies during Labor," for more details.)

Turning the baby after the membranes rupture: A baby who is oblique or transverse upon rupture of membranes but who has no cord prolapse can still be turned if the baby is not jammed down into the pelvis. Either way, someone should constantly monitor the fetal heart rate during transport or until version is successful. If you are considering version, do not wait because the more fluid leaks out, the more dangerous version will be for both the mother and baby. Contractions are liable to slack off somewhat as the uterus adjusts to the rapid reduction in size from the escape of fluid; this gives you an opportunity to act. Talk to the baby about moving to a better position; tell the baby he will have to be cut out of the uterus if he does not move. Give the mother the highest potency of homeopathic pulsatilla you have (it is the primary remedy for unstable lie). Continue to monitor what is happening at the os internally with one hand. Either use your other hand to perform external version or have an assistant do so. Consider performing internal version if external version is not successful and the circumstances for transport are not favorable. If turning the baby is successful, continue to monitor descent internally until contractions move the baby down into the pelvis far enough to cause the presenting part to fill the cervix, making cord prolapse less likely. Keep the mother horizontal with her bottom propped up. (More details regarding version during labor can be found in the aubchapter entitled "The Use of Version during Labor.")

If the baby cannot be turned

If the baby cannot be turned, assume that there is some good reason, such as an obstruction or a short cord. The baby may know she needs to be born in the hospital; for example, she may have an anomaly. Do not allow the mother to labor with a nonlongitudinal lie in the hope that spontaneous version will occur. Transport.

ASSISTING AT MULTIPLE BIRTHS

NOTE: This chapter builds on the information in the chapter entitled "Multiple Gestation" found in Volume I.

This chapter is included for your review in conjunction with observation and hands-on experience with multiple births under the supervision of a skilled senior midwife. However, it is recognized worldwide that midwives must have knowledge of birth techniques relevant to multiples even if they have not had access to such training because a woman may present with a surprise multiple birth during labor. It is much more likely that skills for breeches and other unusual presentations will be needed during multiple births. Whether you have access to hands-on training or not, you should get together with other students or primary midwives and practice techniques on a doll and pelvis until you feel familiar with the maneuvers to prepare for such an event.

This chapter will discuss the specific differences between a labor and birth for multiples as opposed to a singleton birth. Much of the discussion will focus on twins; however, most of the information can be applied to higher-order multiple births as well. The planned homebirth of a recognized multiple gestation will most likely have included at least one or two ultrasound examinations during pregnancy. Therefore, certain serious problems will have been ruled out or at least the possibility of such risks will be minimized. (Ultrasound cannot detect every problem, and problems are sometimes missed.) However, a surprise multiple birth may include a number of unidentified complicating factors that would have prompted plans for a hospital birth had they been recognized ahead of time. Therefore, how to deal with problems that can be identified or at least suspected through prenatal testing will be covered in this chapter.

Attending the Labor and Birth

Preliminary Considerations

How many attendants? Ideally, there should be one midwife for the mother and one midwife on hand for each baby. Usually three primary attendants will be sufficient. You should bring at least one skilled assistant and preferably two.

Setting up for a multiple birth: Setting up requires enough receiving blankets, mucus-trap suction devices, oxygen tanks and masks for the mother and all the babies. Ideally, two neonatal bag-and-mask resuscitation units should be on hand as well. Label as many cord clamps as you expect babies with numbers or letters. These should be attached to the cords on the placental side as each one is cut after the birth. You should also be prepared for the possibility of one baby presenting breech or transverse. See the previous chapter for suggestions on setting up for a breech birth.

Notes on fetal positioning and the cardinal movements of birth in twins: Greenhill (1951) explains that the chorio-amniotic sacs of twins usually lie side by side, although one bag may be positioned anterior to the other or even above the other. The babies themselves usually lie parallel to each other with their spines in line with that of their mother, one on either side of her spinal column. However, one baby may lie anteriorly with the other lying behind him, entirely beyond the reach of an internal digital exam. If the amount of amniotic fluid is scant, the babies may overlap each other. If the babies are small and the amount of fluid generous, there is a greater likelihood that the babies will not be vertex and that the second baby will become repositioned once the first is born.

When one placenta is implanted above the other, it is not uncommon to find the lower edge of the fused placentas near or over the internal os. Breech and transverse presentations occur more frequently in the presence of a low implantation of the placentas.

Due to the tendency of the uterus to dextrorotate, which shortens the left side of the uterine cavity, the baby on the mother's left is often closer to the pelvic inlet and presents first. Before contractions that will lead to the next birth resume, the uterine muscle must retract around the next baby after the first is born. The sudden emptying of the uterus by emergence of the first baby's body and amniotic fluid may lead to abruption of the placenta before the next baby is born. The second bag of waters may break as the next baby begins to descend. The second baby is often born more quickly than the first since the pelvic muscles have already been dilated.

The course of labor is more complex when more than two babies are present, but the pattern of one normal birth followed by the next prevails. Typically, the biggest difference is that the babies are small and one or more of them may be in a nonvertex presentation, requiring advanced skills from the midwife. In addition, bleeding and placental separation may jeopardize the babies still in utero.

Caring for Mother and Babies during Labor

Early labor: Have the mother call you as soon as she believes she is in labor and arrive at her home as soon as you can. If you anticipate delay or are facing traffic or other logistical difficulties, call the other birth assistants who are planning to attend and get the closest person there as soon as possible.

Examination of the mother: The exam should include everything you would normally do for a woman carrying one baby. The use of sterile gloves for all exams is advisable, whether the membranes are intact or not, due to the likelihood that additional internal exams will be needed. In addition, you should palpate carefully to try and ascertain the positions of all babies. Ideally, the first baby will be vertex. Determining positions for the babies not in the pelvis will probably not be particularly easy. Pay attention to the mother's reports of large fetal movements in the days before labor or your impressions of a change in positioning when you observe the uterine contour and as you palpate the abdomen. These clues may indicate that the babies have undergone a dramatic change of position, although the crowded uterus of a well-nourished twin gestation at term certainly makes such repositioning less likely.

When you arrive, the position of each baby should be confirmed to the best of your ability. The outlook is most favorable when both babies are vertex. Should you discover that the first twin is not vertex, be aware that medical opinion favors surgical birth in this situation. Therefore, the parents must be well informed about the potential risks of breech birth to make an informed decision. It would be prudent for them to sign an informed consent document outlining what was discussed.

When the first baby is vertex and the second is breech, surgical birth does not change fetal outcomes for the better (Barrett & Ritchie, 2002). If you find the first baby to be oblique or transverse, transport is your safest option. Many would also advise transport if the first baby is breech, because of the exceedingly rare, but potentially disastrous, possibility of locked twins (details below).

Active labor: Active labor should be expected to advance as for a singleton birth. Sometimes a twin labor will have a long prodromal stage; the uterine muscle may not work as efficiently as usual if it is very much distended. If labor is delayed or difficult, take that as an indication that transport is your best option.

Checking the fetal heart rates: Careful assessment of all babies should take place throughout labor. Locate the fetal heart rate for each baby soon after you arrive. It may be helpful for two midwives to listen simultaneously to confirm that different heartbeats are being identified. Differently colored waterproof markers can be used to make small marks on the mother's belly to assist in locating each baby's heart sounds as labor advances, although the location will change as the babies move down, just as they would in a singleton birth.

The resting phase: The uterus may undergo a resting phase after complete dilation, just as for a singleton birth.

Rupture of membranes for the first baby: As always, the membranes of the first baby should remain intact for as long as possible. This is where a daily prenatal dose of Vitamin C with bioflavonoids is so helpful because the membranes will be strong and are not likely to break early.

Pushing for and birth of the first baby

If the baby is vertex, the mother should push as she feels the urge. If the baby is breech, see the chapter entitled "Assisting at the Birth of a Breech Baby" for detailed instructions.

Mother's position during pushing: The mother can assume any more or less vertical position she likes, with one midwife kneeling behind her as the first baby is born. Upright positions tend to keep the second baby in a longitudinal lie and descending with the help of gravity (Evans, 2004). In particular, abdomen-dependent positions such as hands-and-knees and, to a somewhat lesser extent, supine positions, may encourage any babies still in the uterus to become repositioned upon emergence of the first baby. This occurs because both positions take the second baby "out of gravity," leaving him adrift in a large, baggy uterus. This is especially true for multiparous mothers whose abdominal and uterine tone are somewhat lax. This sets the second baby up to move quickly into a different position (I have seen this happen), one that may not be so easy to correct. For this reason, the mother should avoid abdomen-dependent as well as supine positions until the last baby is well down into the pelvis and ready to be born.

Leave a nuchal cord intact: Unless you know that the babies are in separate bags, it is imperative that a nuchal cord be *left alone* until the baby being born has completely emerged. If the babies are in the same amniotic sac, the cord of another baby may become wrapped around the neck or body of the first; if you cut it, the second baby is placed in a life-threatening situation.

Mother's position after the birth of the first baby: Once the first baby emerges, the midwife behind the mother places her hands on the woman's belly and then palpates and guides the next baby into the pelvis as the woman leans back against her. If the mother is upright, wait for the second baby to be well-down in the pelvis before the mother changes positions. If the mother must be supine (for example, if she cannot maintain an upright position for some reason), have her lie on her side until the uterus becomes active once again and moves the second baby down toward the pelvis.

After the first baby is born:

Surprise multiples: In a truly surprise situation, you may not be aware that there is more than one baby until the first one is born. The contours of the maternal abdomen, the roominess of her torso, the positioning of the babies, or the babies being preterm and therefore small may make it hard to tell that another baby is inside. You may be astonished to receive a small first baby, when your prenatal assessment convinced you that the baby was large. In the absence of copious amniotic fluid (polyhydramnios), a small baby from a previously large uterus raises a strong possibility that another baby is still inside. Suspicion should also be raised when the uterine mass is larger than normal after the birth of one baby of average size.

Shortly after every birth, routinely rule out the presence of additional babies by placing a hand on the abdomen. If suspected, palpate and auscultate for the presence of another baby. (Another possible cause of a small baby and a large uterus is the presence of uterine fibroids or a hydatidiform placenta.) Do a quick assessment of the gestational age of the first baby. When multiples are a surprise, dates are often wrong and the babies may be early. If the baby is obviously much earlier than 36 weeks or you are unsure, the best course of action is to transport the newborn plus the still-pregnant mother. Of course if the birth of the next baby is progressing rapidly, it may be safest to remain at home, have all the babies, and then transport. Let the condition of the first baby and the assessment of the next be your guide.

If the first baby is preterm: When the first baby is obviously early (estimated gestation of 36 weeks or less), stabilize him as best you can, discuss with the parents the option of maintaining the pregnancy for the rest of the babies, and transport. The degree to which the first baby is born preterm will dictate whether this strategy will be entertained by physicians in the hospital; however, it has been done with very limited success in a few cases (Cunningham, et al., 1997). If the gestational age of the first baby is such that few problems are anticipated, the other babies should probably be born now. Premature birth in multiples may be prompted by complications such as twin-to-twin transfusion syndrome (discussed below); look the baby over carefully for color and general vitality. If there is any doubt about the condition of the first twin, clamp the cord early and transport the mother and the baby who has been born.

Physiologic closure of the vessels vs. clamping and cutting the cord: It has generally been considered advisable to clamp the first cord as soon as possible after the birth of the first baby due to the risk of acute twin-to-twin transfusion syndrome (TTS). In acute TTS, babies with communicating placental vasculature have more or less equal blood flow between them in utero, which can become disrupted during the birth process. The communicating vasculature allows a rapid blood volume shift to occur between twins after the death or birth of one fetus. Babies with acute TTS may have associated problems such as central nervous system abnormalities, kidney and skin problems and limb defects.

The more such a transfusion is allowed to take place, the more likely the final result will be one reddish, plethoric baby whose blood volume is elevated and one pale, anemic baby who has served as the donor. Clamping the cord quickly has been widely touted as a method of minimizing this rapid fluid shift in these babies, although almost no research has been done to determine what is truly optimal.

In a thought-provoking article, Klebe and Ingomar (1972), differentiate between babies who have suffered chronic TTS from those who experienced acute blood volume shifts at birth. Using a small sampling of twins for data, they postulated that some of the first baby's blood volume is displaced into the placenta and the second twin as the first baby passes through the constriction of the birth canal. If the first baby's cord is clamped early, this volume of blood is lost and she later develops anemia. On the other hand, they felt that late clamping (a maximum of only 3 min) of the first baby results in her receiving a "double" transfusion, leading to polycythemia. Such a double transfusion would occur as the uterine contractions resume to deliver the second twin. Early clamping of the second twin (1.5 min) deprives this twin of blood lost to the first twin as well as the blood squeezed back into the placenta during the second twin's passage through the birth canal, leading to anemia in the second twin. They concluded that timing of cord clamping is obviously significant but made no recommendations.

All of this, plus what is known about placental-to-newborn transfusion in singleton births, suggests that leaving the cords intact until they both stop pulsing in the center and perhaps at the navel base may allow such twins to equilibrate their blood volumes. In fact, Dr. Joe Gilhooley (2003), a neonatologist in Portland, OR, agrees. As long as each baby looks normal as he is born and both babies are about the same size, leave the cord intact and place the babies in a neutral position in relationship to the placenta; that is, level with the placenta or slightly above it. This will minimize dramatic blood volume shifts between babies and give them a chance to balance out their blood supply once both of them are born. However, if you suspect chronic TTS, get the first baby into a placenta-neutral position and clamp the cords immediately as each baby is born.

Also be aware that very rarely a monozygotic twin gestation can result in partial or complete fusion of the cords. If this is the case the fused area and a fork in the cord may be visible once the first baby is born. A fused cord should probably be cut as soon as is feasible after the birth of the first twin, as vessel communications between the babies are more likely. In this case, if the cords are not individually severed and clamped, the unborn twin may exsanguinate into the other once contractions resume. Closely monitor the heart rates of the babies still in utero.

It is extremely important to know which placenta supplied which baby, especially if the placenta is to be taken in for a pathology exam. To make identification easy, attach disposable plastic cord clamps to the cords before each is severed: on the maternal side, place one clamp for baby A, two clamps for baby B and so forth. This way you won't have to worry about running out of hemostats or confusing whose cord is whose while removing hemostats. This eliminates having to use labels, which may fall off. The disposable clamps can remain in place if the placenta must be taken to the lab, making the sequence of births clearly distinguishable.

There is one big advantage of immediate clamping of the placental end of the cord: it keeps the placenta engorged with fetal blood, which means that it will undergo little or no reduction in size. This assists in keeping the placenta attached to the uterine wall until all babies are born. However, this is not reason enough to deny the first baby her placental transfusion or to risk imbalanced blood supplies to either baby.

Talking to the babies: As each baby is born, explain to him that his siblings are still on their way; if they are doing well, say so. Welcome and comfort him. First-born babies are often distressed about leaving their siblings behind. Be sure to tell the babies still inside that those already born are fine, as well.

Issues regarding bleeding and the status of the placentas:

Bleeding between the birth of each baby: The literature is almost silent on the important question of whether any bleeding is normal between babies and, if so, how much. If the placentas are all still attached and there have been no tears, you should see none. If the placenta of the first baby has partially detached along its edge, there may be minimal bleeding, which should stop as the uterus gathers itself around the baby still in utero, pressing her body against the uterine wall. In this case, the fetal heart rate for the babies still inside should remain normal.

It is possible for the edge of a low-lying, fused placenta to slip down over the internal os once the first baby is born, creating what amounts to a secondary placenta previa. This rare event calls for immediate transport unless the birth of the second twin is suddenly in process and birth is unavoidable.

If the mother has torn anywhere in her birth canal, cervix or external genitalia, some bleeding is inevitable. Any type of tear that can happen with one baby can also happen with multiples, including a torn cervix or a blood vessel that won't stop bleeding. In most cases, bleeding from a tear will be minimal and will soon stop. A half a cup or so of blood with a visible tear is not alarming. However, if bleeding continues or has no obvious source, you must ascertain where it is coming from. If it is from a maternal vessel that has torn and cannot be stopped, you may have to transport at this point. If you are in doubt about whether continuous bleeding is coming from the placenta, for the safety of any babies yet unborn you must either transport or quickly facilitate the birth of the second baby (see the section on abruption below). Monitor the fetal heart rate carefully while en route.

If the first baby's cord breaks: The cord stump at the umbilicus must be clamped as soon as possible. The other end of the cord must also be sought (it is likely to be up inside the yoni) and clamped, to prevent the other baby from hemorrhaging. Be very careful not to pull on the end inside the mother to avoid abrupting the placenta.

If the mother has torn with the first baby: Other than trying to determine the orgin of bleeding, it is pointless to try and thoroughly examine or repair a tear before the birth of all the babies is completed. Chances are that any tear that has occurred will not extend; in any case, you have up to six hours to repair a tear before healing is underway to the point that sutures will be less useful. (See my text HEALING PASSAGE for details regarding the delayed repair of perineal tears.)

Birth of the first placenta before the next baby: *The birth of the placenta should not be encouraged until all babies are out.* On very rare occasions, the first placenta separates and delivers spontaneously prior to the birth of the next baby. In these cases, bleeding is usually not severe because the uterus is actively contracting, the site of placental attachment is shrinking and the pressure from the babies still in utero presses against the attachment site of the first placenta. Once delivered, the first placenta should be examined immediately to make sure it is not fused with another. The emergence of an entire placenta and membranes with only one cord is almost always confirmatory of a normal, completely separate placenta.

However, the birth of the first placenta does increase the risk to the next baby somewhat. It further reduces the overall size of the uterine cavity, increasing the risk that another placenta will separate. The uterus cannot close off the open placental site completely while babies are still inside. Bleeding that continues will jeopardize the mother. Finally, it will be impossible to tell if additional bleeding is from the first placental site or another. For all these reasons, if bleeding continues, the birth of the second baby should not be delayed. Once the baby has assumed a longitudinal lie and contractions have resumed (with stimulation if necessary), the second bag should be ruptured and the birth should proceed promptly.

Abruption of the next baby's placenta: If the second baby's placenta has abrupted after the birth of the first baby, the second baby is in grave danger. Check the fetal heart rate. If the baby is already in distress, get her out as fast as possible, as you may have but a few minutes before the baby will be dead. A version and extraction is usually more easily accomplished with a second twin than with a single term baby because the passages are already dilated. This is one case where you may not wish to waste time trying to tell the position of the baby with abdominal palpation. Don a sterile glove, reach inside the uterus, rupture the membranes and determine the lie of the baby. If breech or transverse, perform an internal version and extraction (see the chapter entitled "Assisting at the Birth of a Breech Baby," grab the feet and bring the baby out. If the second baby is vertex, have the mother push and perform fundal pressure, if necessary, to accomplish the birth.

If you are unsure whether there is more than one baby remaining the uterus, this poses an additional problem, as you don't want to do anything to further disrupt any remaining attached placentas, which both internal manipulation or fundal pressure could do. In this case, transport, if possible, might be a better option; if not, you must work to get out the next baby, possibly with version and extraction, then check to see if there is a third baby and proceed from there.

If bleeding is light, the fetal heart rate is good and you are near a hospital, transport may be a reasonable option, especially if immediate delivery does not seem feasible; for example, if the second baby is quite high in the uterus and there are no contractions. Be prepared for a bleeding mother and depressed newborn.

Prolapse of the first baby's placenta: In exceedingly rare cases of fused placentas, the first baby's placenta may become separated from the uterine wall. As the uterus gathers itself together around the second baby, the uterine wall shrinks somewhat. This can move the detached portion of the fused placentas down so that it overlaps the internal os, creating a secondary placenta previa. The second baby may or may not be in great jeopardy as a result, depending upon how much bleeding occurs and whether his placenta is directly affected.

Dealing with this by internal version and extraction will necessitate inserting your hand past the placenta, which risks disruption of the second placenta. Your best bet is transport unless bleeding is so profuse that you feel you must go in after the other baby. In that case, try to insert your hand to the side and around the edge of the placenta, rather than through it, carefully palpating for the edge of the placenta to minimize the chance that you will choose the wrong side and wind up abrupting the placenta of the second twin. (For details regarding internal version, see the subchapter entitled "The Use of Version during Labor;" for details regarding breech extraction, see the end of the chapter entitled "Assisting at the Birth of a Breech Baby.")

Attending to the birth of the second and subsequent babies

Checking the position of the next baby: Once the first baby is born, it is important to check for the position of the next baby as soon as it is practical to do so. However, since the uterus will be quite baggy at this point, checking position may not be so easy until the resting phase is well underway. Even though steps may have been taken to minimize the possibility of repositioning once the first baby is born, up to 20% of second babies do change position, with the greatest likelihood of this occurring in those that are small or preterm. The baby should be in a longitudinal lie. Labor should not be stimulated until the position of the baby is known. If bleeding suggests that the placenta of the next baby is detaching, transport is preferable to forcing labor if the baby should be transverse. External or internal version may also be used to quickly reposition the baby and get him out. External version is performed as it would be prenatally. Internal version is quite a bit more risky for both mother and baby and should only be resorted to if you are far from medical help or it appears that it will be easy to accomplish. It is covered in the chapter entitled "The Use of Version during Labor."

Assess the heart rate of babies still in utero: It is important to check the fetal heart rate as soon as possible after the birth of the first baby. Emergence of the first baby leaves those still in utero at risk for repositioning, rupture of membranes, cord presentation or prolapse, or abruption of the placenta. Normal fetal heart rate findings are very reassuring. If the heart rate is low or questionable and does not quickly recover with the usual corrective measures such as maternal repositioning, transport is your best alternative. Give the mother oxygen by mask on the way.

If the second baby is transverse or oblique: It is best to try and maneuver a transverse baby into a longitudinal lie before contractions resume, while the uterus is still baggy from the birth of the first baby. This should be attempted using external version. Version may be easier said than done, as the uterus is large while the baby is comparatively small and probably still encased in an intact bag. It is more important that the baby be longitudinal than that it be vertex. It is best *not* to rupture the membranes before the baby is longitudinal, since doing so risks cord prolapse as well as stabilizing the baby in a transverse presentation. (See the chapter entitled "Unstable Lie, Oblique Lie and Transverse Lie in Labor" for more details.) If the baby cannot be persuaded to rotate, transport is your safest alternative.

If the second baby is breech: External cephalic version has been used successfully to convert a breech second twin to a vertex presentation. However, studies have shown breech extraction to be safer overall than external version; therefore if the baby is in a longitudinal lie, it is best to leave well enough alone (Barrett & Ritchie, 2002).

Resting phase between babies: The time interval that occurs between the birth of the babies is a matter of much controversy. The medical model tends to rush this along by artificially rupturing the membranes of the next baby to hasten its birth, often giving as little as 15 minutes of lag time between babies. This is predicated on the idea that the second baby is at great risk for placental abruption, hypoxia and death. These risks are primarily associated with early placental separation, cord prolapse, nonvertex presentation and ill-advised maneuvers performed by a nervous practitioner. The medical model is used to seeing preterm and small-for-gestational age babies from multiple gestations. When the mother eats well during pregnancy, the placenta is healthier and implants more securely, thus minimizing the risk of separation once the first baby is born.

Greenhill (1951) states that there can be a space of anywhere from a few minutes to as long as 44 days between babies, with an average of 30 to 40 minutes. Midwives who have attended multiple births have observed spaces averaging an hour to an hour and a half between babies. Time between babies is not critical if there is no bleeding, if fetal heart rate findings remain normal and the mother is doing well. Barring the above-mentioned risks, the most immediate potential risk is the development of intrauterine infection when this interval is much prolonged.

Once each baby is born, the uterus must once again gather itself around the remaining babies so that productive contractions can resume. This is the same process that takes place during the resting phase that occurs at the end of complete dilation in a singleton labor. To force the baby out prior to completion of this process may actually lead to more problems during and after the birth, since the uterus will be larger and more likely to bleed. Allowing the gradual taking up of the uterine cavity also helps minimize an abrupt reduction in size that may occur if oxytocin is started and could prompt placental separation before all the babies are born. Forcing labor may also lead to ineffective postpartum contractions that delay the birth of the partially detached placenta, leading to increased blood loss.

Amniotic membranes of subsequent babies: It is widely recommended to rupture the membranes of subsequent babies to stimulate the uterus to contract and hasten their birth. Whether artifical rupture of membranes is called for as subsequent babies descend must be answered individually. The baby should be well positioned, descending, with her presenting part filling the pelvis before rupture is even considered an option; rupture too soon risks cord prolapse as well as risks fixing the baby in an undesirable position. Keeping the membranes intact reduces the degree of abrupt uterine size reduction after the birth of the first baby. This helps the uterus to more gradually rebalance its capacity, minimizing the chance that the placenta of the first baby will detach.

If there is a delay in the birth of the next baby with signs of fetal distress or unusual maternal bleeding, then rupture of membranes should be considered. If it has been difficult to fix the baby in a desirable position, rupture of membranes may make sense once the presenting part is on its way through the pelvis. The baby must be in a longitudinal lie before the membranes are ruptured. The only exception to this rule is when the decision is made to perform internal version to correct a transverse lie and bring the baby down. (This technique and concurrent risks are discussed in the subchapter entitled "The Use of Version during Labor.")

If the baby is breech, keep the membranes intact for as long as possible, particularly if the baby is footling or kneeling. If the bag is strong and the cord is near the legs, it can float within the bag until the baby is emerging and still receive little, if any, pressure. When it is known that the cord is so positioned, careful fetal heart monitoring should be done every few minutes until the baby is born. If the baby is vertex and the head is well fitted into the pelvis, you may rupture the membranes once contractions resume, but if things are progressing well there is really no need to do so.

Occasionally the bag of the first baby will refill with fluid, giving the impression that the second bag is presenting. That you can see the cord coursing through the fluid in the bag is a tip-off that this is not really the next baby's bag (Edmonds, 2003).

Resumption of labor for the next baby: In most cases, labor gradually reestablishes itself for the birth of the next baby. As contractions pick up, the presenting part descends into position, filling the upper pelvic cavity. How long labor takes, once it recommences, will depend on whether the cervix has closed down at all in the interim. Usually redilation does not take long.

Psychological factors: Resumption of labor for the second baby may be delayed for a variety of psychological reasons. The mother may be in shock that she is having more than one baby, especially if the multiple birth was unexpected. She may be having feelings of being overwhelmed by the responsibility of parenting, the impact on her relationship or financial issues. She may worry that she cannot love both babies equally or that breastfeeding will be difficult. Be sure and let her know that any such apprehension is normal. Encourage her to express her feelings, which will usually unblock the labor energy.

Prompting labor to resume: If the time between babies is extended and no resumption of labor is in sight, consider giving a uterine stimulant, such as cotton root bark, to get contractions going. Nipple stimulation, especially allowing the first baby to nurse, can also be very helpful. If the onset of labor is much delayed, rupture of membranes may stimulate contractions but should only be considered if the presenting part is well placed and fixed and the baby is doing well. The fetal heart rate should be monitored carefully. If the second baby remains high, the lie is transverse, labor cannot be restimulated, bleeding commences or fetal distress develops, transport.

Birth of subsequent babies: Allow the birth to proceed as for any single baby. It is likely that the labor for each subsequent baby will be increasingly more efficient, as the uterus returns to a more normal size. All other babies who may be in utero should be assisted as described above. That the passages are already dilated makes the birth of a second breech baby easier than if it were the first. Assist the birth as you would (or wouldn't) for any baby.

After each baby you must check to rule out whether another baby is still in utero, even, for example, if this is a known and planned twin birth. Ultrasounds do miss triplets and may even miss higher-order multiples if the babies are positioned so that one sibling hides another.

Must subsequent babies cords be clamped? If the second baby is of a different sex than the first and you have ascertained that there are only two babies, you can safely allow the second baby to receive her placental transfusion by leaving the cord intact. Differently sexed babies usually means the twins are dizygotic and twin-to-twin transfusion does not occur in this case. If the babies are of the same sex and the first baby is a normal size and normal color and appears otherwise healthy, it is not necessary to clamp the second baby's cord. If one baby looks ruddy or pale, small and weak, clamping the cord soon, but not immediately, is probably a good idea.

Birth of the placentas: In most cases, the birth of the placentas follows the birth of all the babies, even if the placentas are not fused (Strachan, 1947). The birth of the placentas may take somewhat longer in a multiple birth because the uterus is larger and must again gather itself up to trigger separation and release of the entire placental mass, making for a long resting phase after the birth. If cord traction is to be used to assist in removing the fully detached placentas, it is best to apply most of your traction to the cord of the first baby born, as that placenta is likely to be implanted lowermost on the uterine wall. This will assist the placentas, if fused, to slide out edgewise more easily rather than bringing their collective bulk out at once, which will make passage through the cervix much more difficult (DeWees, 1835).

If birth of the placenta is difficult or delayed and the cords have been cut, remove the clamp on only one of the cords. This will help to drain some of the blood from the placenta without risking confusion regarding which clamp went where. If this doesn't help, you could possibly unclamp more cords, relying on the serrated markings a plastic cord clamp produces on the cord to still be identifiable after the placenta is born (metal cord clamps are less likely to reliably produce a mark in the short time since original clamping). If you unclamp only one cord, you should be able to tell how many clamps to replace once the placenta is born. If the placentas are not fused, birth of the second will generally quickly follow the birth of the first.

Maternal condition and blood loss after multiple birth: The birth of two or more babies is a tremendous psychic and physical shift for the mother. This, coupled with a large and relatively abrupt loss of body mass, makes her more prone to developing symptoms of blood volume compromise, if not true shock. With a larger placental implantation site on the uterine wall and an increased blood volume in the healthy mother, expect more bleeding after birth. Even so, rapid blood loss produces a dramatic shift in the circulatory volume and may send the woman into shock. Therefore, keep a close eye on the mother and be ready with uterine-stimulating herbs and pharmaceuticals should they be needed.

Problems with Multiple Births

In addition to the problems associated with multiple births that have already been addressed, there are other rare but serious problems that can arise.

Obstruction of descent due to fetal positioning: The position, descent or birth of one baby may be obstructed by another. How this manifests depends upon the size and exact positioning of the babies. Predisposing factors may include monoamniotic babies, small fetal size, a very large maternal pelvis, oligohydramnios and uterine hypertonicity.

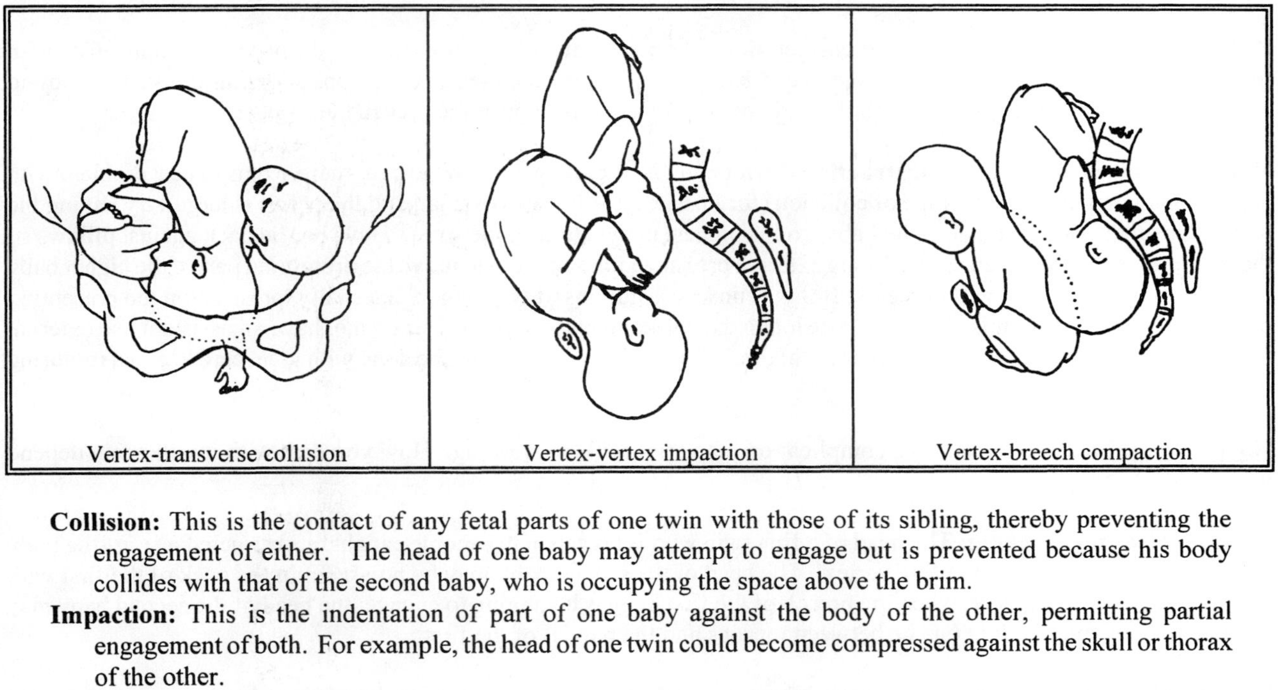

Vertex-transverse collision | Vertex-vertex impaction | Vertex-breech compaction

Collision: This is the contact of any fetal parts of one twin with those of its sibling, thereby preventing the engagement of either. The head of one baby may attempt to engage but is prevented because his body collides with that of the second baby, who is occupying the space above the brim.

Impaction: This is the indentation of part of one baby against the body of the other, permitting partial engagement of both. For example, the head of one twin could become compressed against the skull or thorax of the other.

Compaction: This occurs when the presenting parts of two babies become fully engaged, preventing the further descent of either.

Interlocking: The most dangerous of these complications, this occurs when the further descent of a partially born baby is arrested because a part of his body is caught on that of the second baby. Fortunately, this is a very rare. Interlocking is most common when the first baby is breech and the second vertex and the chins become locked as the first baby's body is born. (Nissen, 1958).

Vertex-vertex collision, impaction or compaction: These types of obstructions are more likely to occur when the babies are small and the pelvis is quite large. They constitute a relatively less dangerous form of obstruction than interlocking because no part of either baby has yet been born. However, sufficient pressure of one baby against another can cause injury; for example, should the head of the second baby become compressed against the neck of the first baby, circulation to the head of the first baby could be severely compromised.

The midwife can try and correct collision or impaction by facilitating the upward displacement of the baby with the higher presenting part, thus allowing the baby closer to the brim to descend. The mother should assume a Trendelenburg position. This will allow thorough palpation to ascertain, as clearly as possible, the positioning of each baby. In addition to Trendelenburg, the mother can also try assuming a hands-and-knees or a knee-chest position; any of these positions will encourage both babies to float away from the brim, increasing the chances that they will reposition themselves, allowing one baby to descend.

If positioning alone doesn't work, have the mother again assume a Trendelenburg position. Displace the fetal pole that is uppermost in the uterus further upward with external manipulation while pressing the upper pole of the lower baby toward the pelvic brim. This will probably take the coordinated efforts of two people and may require more than one attempt. Careful use of a rebozo as described in the chapter entitled "Unstable Lie, Oblique Lie and Transverse Lie in Labor" may help. Internal manipulation may be more effective if the membranes of the lower twin have already ruptured. However, care must be taken not to rupture any unbroken bags of water and not to be too forceful with internal manipulations as the babies may be harmed. Cord prolapse or uterine rupture are also possibilities. When neither baby can be persuaded to descend, transport is advisable.

The babies are probably quite premature if both presenting parts are already engaged. The safest option is transport, since manipulating the small, delicate parts of early babies jammed together in the pelvis is likely to harm them.

Breech-breech collision, impaction or compaction: Both breech babies may try to enter the pelvis at once. Handle this as you would for vertex-vertex collision or impaction.

Breech-vertex collision, impaction or compaction: The breech of one baby tries to enter the pelvis simultaneously with the head of his sibling. In this case, the beech baby should be encouraged to move up, allowing the vertex baby to descend. Whether this is possible will depend upon how easy it is to push the breech back up.

What to do to try and prevent obstruction if transport is not an option: Whenever there seems to be a problem with descent and you suspect some type of collision (for instance, the babies are small and the pelvis is large), try having the mother lie on the side that places the baby who is highest in the uterus uppermost. Have her lie back against pillows so that her back is propped at an angle. Using external pressure alone, attempt to move the presenting part of the higher baby out of the way so the first will descend. If this is unsuccessful, insert two fingers internally, press up on the presenting part of lowermost baby (this will help to dislodge the colliding parts). At the same time, have an assistant use external manipulation to lift the presenting part of the higher baby. This maneuver must be done with great care to avoid rupturing the membranes of either baby.

Interlocking: This life-threatening complication may arise with no warning. How you deal with it will again depend upon fetal positioning.

Breech-vertex interlocking: The head of a first twin who is breech may become caught or obstructed against the body of a second baby who is presenting vertex. The head of the second baby may be pressed into the neck of the first with interlocking of their chins or, when the breech of the first baby is beginning to engage, the head of the second baby may become pressed into the loin (space between the ribs and the pelvis) of the first.

Breech-breech interlocking: This occurs when the head of the first baby cannot descend further because it is caught between the pelvic sidewalls and the lower body of his sibling. For example, his chin could lock on the other baby's pubic bone, with his occiput trapped above the mother's pubic bone.

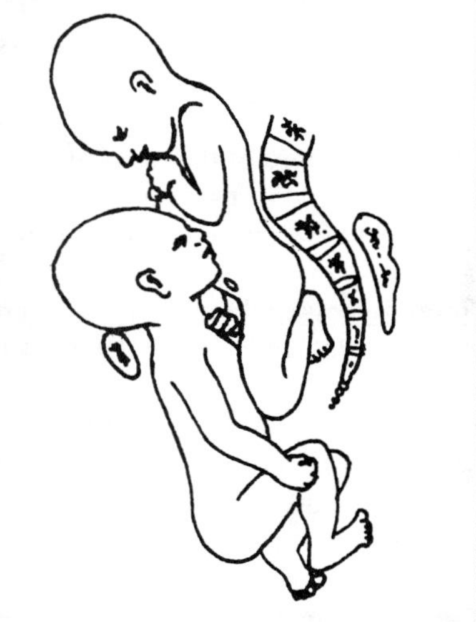

Breech-breech interlocking (rare)

Breech-transverse interlocking: The aftercoming head of the first (breech) baby may become caught on the trunk of a twin who is lying transverse.

Dealing with interlocking: When interlocking occurs, arrest takes place only after the first baby's body has been born to the level of the belly or shoulders. Slow descent of a first baby presenting breech may be your first sign of this problem. Once the body of the first baby be partially born and the problem is identified, you are facing one of the few true obstetrical catastrophes that arise suddenly and almost certainly mean that at least one baby will die. Transporting the mother in a position that minimizes pressure on the babies as much as possible is your best option. Give the mother oxygen by mask and gently wrap the cord of the partially born baby in a warm, wet washcloth to keep it from drying out. Prepare the mother for an emergency surgical birth in an attempt to save both babies once she reaches the hospital.

If you are far from medical help, you will be forced to try and remedy the situation yourself. The object is to disengage the babies so that the first birth can proceed. To do this, quickly get the mother into a Trendelenburg position. Insert your hand internally, pushing the body of the first twin upward. Now attempt to manipulate the heads away from each other. In reality, this is very difficult to do when contractions are strong and always risks trauma to the babies as well as uterine rupture in the mother. In a situation where transport is truly impossible, decapitation of the first baby may be necessary. Whenever possible, even if the first baby has already died, transport is your best alternative.

Monoamniotic gestation: One in every 100 monozygotic twin gestations finds both babies in a single amniotic sac (monoamniotic gestation can occur with higher-order multiples as well). This carries the risk of multiple complications. Both cords may be lethally entangled or, much more rarely, partially or totally unseparated (also less accurately referred to as fused). The cord of one baby may be wrapped around the neck or body of the other, making it impossible to distinguish whose cord is whose when the head of the first twin is born. Anastomoses (vascular communications) can occur between the two fetuses, although the incidence is less than in twins with two chorions. When anastomoses are present, tissue thromboplastins may transfer from a dead twin to the living sibling, placing the survivor at risk for disseminated intravascular coagulation (DIC) and embolism.

During the placental exam, a remnant of membranes can sometimes be found lying between the two cords, suggesting that a separating membrane ruptured during pregnancy. These pseudomonoamniotic twins are at risk for amniotic band syndrome from fragments of the ruptured septum as well as all the other risks listed above.

Monoamniotic twins are at greater risk for interlocking. Failure of one baby to descend or abrupt bradycardia with descent could be due to cord entanglements. If two amniotic cavities were not identified with an ultrasound exam prior to the birth, and you suspect or have identified that only one amnion exists, transport immediately.

Extremely delayed interdelivery periods: There are two reasons for there to be an extremely long delay of days, weeks or even months between the births of the babies. The most likely occurs when the pregnancy is extremely preterm when the first baby is born. In this case, some physicians have allowed the pregnancy for the second baby to continue to term. Superfetation, the extremely rare second reason, occurs when two babies have been conceived at different times; they may even be months apart in gestation. This will probably not have been recognized prenatally and will only be a guess at the time of birth. Ultrasound studies will probably be ordered to further assess the condition and gestational age of the retained baby.

If either of these circumstances presents itself, labor could stop after the first baby is born and not resume on its own. The second baby, unwilling to descend, may remain high in the uterus. Should the first placenta deliver and the second bag remain intact, you may be able to make a case for waiting, *if* you can find a back-up medical care provider who will go along with such a request. However, if the first placenta does not deliver or is fused to the second, the mother and other baby are both at risk for developing an infection; one placenta is no longer functional, one bag is broken and the cervix is wide open. This risk is compounded because the clamped end of the cord from the first baby provides a highway for infection to travel into the uterus. Transport so that the parents can consult with medical personnel and decide on a course that is right for them.

If you are remote from medical assistance, the criteria for waiting include the second baby's membranes remaining intact. The cord of the first baby should be tied off as close to the cervix as possible and reinserted through the os. No attempt should be made to deliver the placenta of the first baby, as this may disrupt the implantation of placentas still in use, or the first placenta may be fused to another.

Fetal defects and anomalies: There are several fetal problems that are more likely to occur with multiple births. Many of these problems will be detected via prenatal ultrasound; you will not be attending these mothers at home.

Stuck-twin syndrome: This term is used when polyhydramnios exists in the amniotic sac of one monozygotic baby and severe oligohydramnios is present in the sac of the other. This causes the baby with oligohydramnios to appear to be stuck to the uterine wall on ultrasound. This situation is associated with twin-to-twin transfusion syndrome and usually gives rise to preterm labor.

Fetal malformation: A higher percentage of babies from multiple gestations have various defects when compared to babies of singleton pregnancies. The possibility for problems still exist even if they were not identified on ultrasound exams during pregnancy.

Twin-to-twin transfusion syndrome (TTS): TTS is a condition unique to monozygotic twins sharing a single placenta with communicating vascular systems. The incidence is about 80% among diamniotic-monochorionic placentas, with the degree of communication varying widely. TTS is very rare when the babies are of different sexes, and impossible when the placentas are entirely separate or when they are joined by membranes alone with no vessels traversing the line of fusion. (Separate placentas in diamniotic-monochorionic gestations are exceedingly rare.) If the anastomoses are balanced, so that the flow of blood through one connection is compensated by an equal amount of flow in the opposite direction, there is no problem. However, babies suffering from imbalanced communicating circulatory systems may not make it to term; if they do, they can be born compromised. While minor, superficial connections usually do not cause problems, when deep shunting takes place, an artery from one twin supplies a cotyledon drained by the venous system of the other baby. Thus the cotyledon is shared by the two fetal circulations and the flow goes directly from one baby (the donor or pump twin) to the recipient. There is usually a net loss of blood in one direction. This loss may be compensated by backflow through superficial anastomoses, but such compensation is limited by the size and number of these small vessels.

Chronic TTS has been defined by a 5 mg/dl (50 g/L) difference in fetal hemoglobins or a 20% difference in fetal weight. The findings in the donor baby include pallor, anemia, hypotension and hypovolemia, resulting in a lowered urinary output and oligohydramnios. This leads to restriction of fetal movement and sometimes facial or limb deformities. The formation of additional blood elements to compensate for this pathology, as well as cardiac failure, may result in changes that resemble nonimmune fetal hydrops (generalized fluid retention). Such developments may cause this severely ill baby to be about the same weight as the recipient twin (the donor twin is usually significantly smaller than the recipient sibling). The placenta of this baby is pale and thin and may, in some cases, show changes compatible with hydrops on microscopic exam. The recipient twin is typically large and ruddy because he is engorged with blood. The internal organs are enlarged, especially the heart and kidneys. The result is often polyhydramnios in the sac of the recipient twin.

In acute TTS, the blood flow to and from both babies is essentially balanced during intrauterine development. A rapid, large twin-to-twin transfusion occurs at birth or after the prenatal death of one twin. The babies are about the same size, but one twin is plethoric and the other pale, even though there is little difference in their original hemoglobin or hematocrit values. As the babies get older, fluid shifts within each baby reveal the donor's anemia and the recipient's polycythemia. The study of other findings such as organ size, fetal weight, amniotic fluid volume and placental appearance may help determine which baby was the original donor and which the original recipient.

TTS can be a killer when associated with prematurity or large anastomotic bridges. When one baby dies, circulatory equilibrium is established and amniotic fluid volume normalizes for the surviving twin. However, the surviving baby is still at risk for central nervous system problems, kidney damage, skin anomalies and limb defects. These risks are related to the size of the dead fetus and the length of gestation at the time of the sibling's death; the later in pregnancy the death occurs, the worse for the surviving baby.

Discordant size of the babies: Babies whose weights differ in excess of a pound should be evaluated for signs and symptoms of TTS, differences in gestational age, and intrauterine growth retardation of one baby. There is more likely to be greater discordancy in birthweights when the placentas of fraternal twins fuse. A disparity of weights is not a concern when each baby is of normal weight for a singleton birth (say, 7 and 8.5 lbs respectively) and appear healthy. Evidence of TTS should be recognizable by the description above.

Conjoined twins: Conjoined twins result when separation of the fertilized ovum is delayed beyond 13.5 days after conception, resulting in a variety of unusual twinning, including incomplete anatomical separation of monozygotic twins. Conjoining occurs in approximately one out of every 500 twin pregnancies (1 in 50,000 to 80,000 deliveries) (Gall, 1996). These babies can be anatomically connected anywhere along the trunk, the head or the extremities. There is a 50% chance of additional malformations as well. Conjoined twins are classified according to the degree and nature of their joining, which can vary widely from those in which two well-developed babies have only a minor, superficial connection, to those in which only a small part of the body is duplicated, to those in which amorphous masses of tissue are attached to an otherwise normal baby (rather than conjoining, this mass is often referred to as a "parasitic twin"). However, the birth of babies with essentially one body and two heads can also occur. The most minor conjoining occurs when the cords are fused just above the level of the chorionic plate. The other major varieties of anatomical conjoining are as follows, listed in decreasing order of frequency (Machin, 1993):

- Thoracopagus–joined at the thorax (33%)
- Thoracoomphalopagus–joined at the anterior abdominal wall from the xiphoid to the umbilicus (15%)
- Dicephalus–joined at the lower body (11%)
- Cephalothoracopagus–joined at the head and chest (6%)
- Craniopagus–joined at the head (5%)
- Pygopagus–joined at the buttocks or rump (4%)
- Ischiopagus–joined at the ischium (3%)
- Other combinations (22%)

Conjoining usually causes the babies to experience significant dystocia during descent. Undetected obstruction can lead to uterine rupture.

Since most twin pregnancies will probably have at least one ultrasound exam, the diagnosis of conjoined twins is likely to be known prior to labor. In the event that conjoined twins have not been identified prior to the onset of labor, several observations during labor suggest this diagnosis. Since conjoined twins always develop within a single amniotic sac, palpation of a second intact bag after the rupture of another rules out conjoining. Conversely, multiple fetal limbs in close proximity, failure of traction on the first twin to effect delivery after complete dilation and inability to move one twin without moving the other, should raise suspicions. Conjoining is confirmed if a bridge of tissue between the two babies can be felt on deep internal exam.

The location of the joining will determine if these babies can be born per yoni. A small, flexible and stretchable region of joining bodes the best for yoni birth, but the attendant potential trauma makes proceeding with a yoni birth unwise. If you suspect that babies are conjoined, transport for the safety of both mother and babies; a surgical birth will be the best alternative for everyone concerned. When the babies are monoamniotic, failure to descend is a problem in any event because it may signify cord entanglement. Your best solution is to transport.

If you are far from medical help in the very unlikely and unfortunate circumstance of needing to assist the birth of conjoined twins outside of a hospital setting, there are a few tips that might help. Lay the mother supine with her bottom at the edge of the bed to minimize the effect of gravity and maximize access to her perineum. Conjoined twins often present breech-breech, which facilitates birth via total breech extraction. When all four lower extremities are within reach and the babies are small, simultaneous traction on all of the limbs at once can accomplish delivery.

The entire bulk of the torsos of breech babies joined at the trunk can often be brought out at once if the babies are small. In larger twins, a clitorotomy may be necessary to provide more maneuvering room (remembering that this will only expand the opening of the soft tissues and have no impact on the bony pelvis). Sufficient mobility at the site of the joining may then allow heads to emerge one at a time. As the trunks are brought out, flex the bodies of the babies over the maternal abdomen. The most posterior head is brought out first, followed by the second head, often without too much difficulty.

If the tops of the heads are joined, one baby will be breech and the other vertex. Birth should not be as problematic as each baby can descend more or less longitudinally, although their bodies will be side by side in utero and some limb entanglement may occur. Cord entanglements are also likely to be present.

The greatest problem occurs when the babies are vertex. The babies may be brought down in a staggered, parallel fashion if the union between them is sufficiently loose by sliding the body of one over the body of the other. Try to position the head of one under the chin of the other so that both heads engage together. This technique works best if the twins are joined at the abdomen or the sternal region. In such cases, if may even be possible for one twin to be born breech and the other vertex.

Destructive procedures are called for when a part of the fused bodies has been born and no further progress can be achieved by ordinary means. Such procedures generally involve evisceration or amputation of body parts. Obviously, a complicated conjoined twin labor and birth would be a nightmare to deal with at home. Whenever possible, conjoined twins should be identified prenatally and surgical birth anticipated. If discovered late in labor, transport prior to pushing (Roddie, 1957; Rudolph et al., 1967). More details on conjoining can be found in a recent edition of the first Volume of this text in the chapter entitled "Multiple Gestation."

<u>Death of one baby</u>: Fetal death happens 3 to 10 times more frequently in multiple gestations. Fetal death may result from uteroplacental dysfunction, cord accidents such as prolapse, damage to a velamentous cord insertion, TTS, or other conditions unique to either fetus.

When one baby has died in the first trimester, the products of conception are usually reabsorbed by the mother's body, placing neither the mother nor surviving baby at any increased risks. Chances are that you will not be aware of the presence of a vanished twin unless evidence of such becomes apparent during the labor or upon examination of the placenta. On the other hand, stillbirth is defined as the death of a baby greater than 20 weeks gestation. It is best to transport if it is known that one baby has died, as the surviving baby is at significant risk for problems after birth. If the baby died late in pregnancy, the birth and appearance of the baby will follow the course of any recent fetal demise.

For general information on handling such a labor at home, see the chapter entitled "Assisting at the Labor and Birth of a Mother Whose Baby is Known to Have Lethal Defects or to Have Died Prior to the Onset of Labor."

Fetus papyraceus: When a baby dies around 16 to 20 weeks gestation, fetus papyraceus (pap-i-RAY-shus) (also known as "fetus compressus" [com-PRESS-sus]) sometimes develops. Optimal conditions must be present, as a fetus papyraceus will not form if the baby is too large. Body fluids are reabsorbed and the fetus is flattened by the continued growth and pressure from the surviving baby. Even so, the mummified fetus can be large enough to delay or block descent of the surviving sibling. This phenomenon can occur in any multiple gestation, but is most commonly seen with monozygotic conceptions. The incidence is said to be 1 in 12,000 live births or 1 in 184 twin pregnancies. The true incidence may be higher due to lack of recognition.

The appearance of these fetuses varies, ranging from a featureless mass to a recognizable, though macerated, baby. The thorax is often flattened on one side, so that most of the anterior surface of the baby's body is concave. The body tends to be a greyish yellow color with a slightly dry, leathery texture. There is usually no bloating or swelling. The skin shrinks to form a thin surface layer. Careful dissection is sometimes necessary to confirm that this is fetal tissue.

Calcification of the entire fetus is referred to as a lithopedion (lith-oh-PEE-de-un) or "stone baby." If the amniotic fluid is absorbed, the fetus can become compressed against the uterine wall as a dry, shrunken mass, which gradually becomes mineralized. Because calcification can take many months to develop, this occurs very rarely.

A sibling surviving in the presence of a fetus papyraceus may present with skin lesions of varying size, as well as bowel atresia and is at increased risk for death. The surviving sibling should be treated emotionally as for any baby whose sibling has died in utero.

The presence of a fetus papyraceus may not be detected until it presents problems with descent during labor or after the birth, when it is discovered during placental exam. Whenever multiple babies are born, be watchful for signs that a fetus papyraceus may be retained in utero. If the placentas are fused, the compressed baby's placenta may appear whitish, hard and fibrous with a marginal cord insertion, in stark contrast to a normal one (although the placenta from a fetus papyraceus may also appear normal). The compressed fetus may be imbedded in the surface of the placenta or retained in utero. A retained fetus will interfere with normal uterine contractions leading to excessive postpartum bleeding. Further decomposition may lead to infection in the mother. If you suspect that a fetus papyraceus has been retained (look for evidence on the placenta, see the chapter entitled "Examining the Placenta" for details), transport for removal.

Twin reversed arterial perfusion (TRAP) (acardius/acardiacus): A baby with this disorder suffers from a severe form of twin-to-twin transfusion syndrome and lacks a normally formed heart. This twin has multisystem malformations and an unusual body shape. The heart is often completely absent or improperly developed. Other anatomical defects range from failure of normal development that proceeds from the upper body downward to a total loss of normal organ development as well as an amorphous body form. Size varies from small placental nodules to that of a term fetus. The lower extremities and abdomen may be minimally deformed, leading to confusion when a fetal part that feels normal is found on palpation. Many of these fetuses are genetically female.

The survival rate for the other twin is about 50%. She is at great risk for heart and liver problems; and may be born with edema. Transport both the acardiac twin as well as the survivor for further evaluation.

Postpartum observation of a single surviving twin: Whenever one baby has died and the surviving sibling is born at home, the surviving baby should be watched closely, even if he is born at term, appears normal, has mature lungs and normal APGAR scores. This baby will be quite emotionally distraught by the loss of the other baby; his distress should be kept in mind by all who work with him. Explain to the baby what has happened and offer unconditional physical and emotional support while he expresses his feelings, which may come out as crying or screaming. Tell the baby that the death of the other twin is not anything he could have controlled. If the reason for the demise of the other baby cannot be determined, the parents may want to consider having the survivor tested to rule out congenital infection and chromosome-related defects. The newborn exam should be done with extra care, with likely anomalies in mind. The baby should be reexamined by a pediatrician as soon as possible. Any variations from normal in the baby's behavior or in physical findings should prompt transport soon after birth for more specialized examination and observation.

WHEN THE BABY IS EARLY OR LATE

NOTE: This chapter builds on the chapter in Volume I entitled "Preterm Labor." Review that chapter before studying this one.

When the Baby is Early

Deciding if immediate transport is indicated

The steps you will take when confronted with a mother in progressive preterm labor will depend, to a certain extent, upon the gestation of the pregnancy, the proximity of the nearest neonatal intensive care unit with Level III facilities, and the parents' preferences.

The viability factor: The official age of viability is still 28 weeks as of this printing. However, the point at which neonatology may attempt to save a baby is constantly being pushed back to an earlier gestational age; a baby as young as 22 weeks is considered sustainable in some locations with advanced neonatal care facilities. However, survival and quality of life may be two different things for these infants. This creates a dilemma for parents who would rather forgo heroic measures that may hold a high risk of permanent disability and that subject their very early baby to painful treatments for many of her first weeks of life. However, having a very early baby at home, regardless of the parents' desires, may be viewed by the authorities as child abuse or neglect, or, at worst, murder. The midwife who supports these parents could be accused of negligent manslaughter. The options you will be able to offer in terms of support at home or in a birthing center for preterm labor will depend upon the support you have from the medical community to allow homebirth parents to make their own choices. The following recommendations are made with these sobering thoughts in mind.

Reassess gestation: The gestational age of the pregnancy should have been determined by history and affirmed by careful prenatal exam. Whenever a woman presents in preterm labor, the factors that went into this determination should be reassessed while doing your best to forestall progressive labor. Be sure to review with the mother and partner all of the following:

- Timing of intercourse near the presumed date of conception
- Menstrual history (review marked calenders or ovulation charts if any are available)
- Familial trends regarding length of gestation on the mother's side
- Any early laboratory or diagnostic tests that may provide information regarding the dating of the pregnancy. Note the date when the fetal heart was first heard. A period of at least 20 weeks since the heart was first heard with a fetoscope or 30 weeks with a Doppler are good indications that the baby is at or near term, as is a positive serum or urinary human chorionic gonadotrophin pregnancy test performed at least 36 weeks ago.
- Mother's past history of gestational ages of previous babies, weights, condition at birth and nutrition during those pregnancies
- Nutrition and stress factors during this pregnancy
- Prenatal records (past and present) regarding pattern of fetal and fundal growth, such as fundal height and the estimated fetal size by palpation. Ultrasound measurement of the crown-rump length that confirmed that the fetus was 6 to 11 weeks gestation at the time of the exam is considered a reliable starting point for assessing the number of weeks gestation the baby is now.
- The familial likelihood of a multiple gestation
- History of maternal infection during pregnancy and group-B strep status. If the mother is likely to have an infection now, the early baby is at higher risk to succumbing to exposure by becoming ill himself.

Regardless of how thorough the initial history taking, often additional facts come to light when a complication such as a too-early baby is looming. Important information is revealed that will significantly contribute to making an informed decision about whether to stay home or transport.

How early is too early to be born at home? First and foremost, consider the possible condition of the baby at birth and the chances that the baby will immediately require high-tech care to stabilize and begin breathing. Even if the baby is able to stabilize, the question remains as to whether the baby can continue to breathe room air on her own. Research appears to confirm that physiologic cord closure goes far to help even tiny babies breathe on their own from birth on; however, the baby must also be able to nurse or at least suck. If the baby can breathe and eat, she can be born at home and stay there. As a general rule, staying at home is safe when the baby reaches 37 completed weeks from the last menstrual period (LMP). At this point, breathing normally is virtually assured. If the dates are off by a week (or two or three) and the baby is actually a 36, 35 or 34 weeker, she is still very likely to stabilize just fine. The dates can be off, so some practitioners feel it best to err on the side of caution with this conservative 37 week cut-off because the earlier the gestational age of the baby, the greater the chances of breathing difficulties. However, with a full placental transfusion on board, you can expect that most of these babies will do fine. In some regional hospitals, 34 weeks is considered close enough to term to say that most of these babies will do well. Just remember that the earlier the baby, the greater the risk of having problems that you cannot handle at home. That being said, talk it over with the parents, look over the gestational ages and condition of the mother's previous children. If they were all born at, say, 35 weeks, and did very well, the chances of another 35 week baby doing well are excellent, especially if the previous babies were born in the hospital and subjected to the additional insult of early cord clamping. However, if respiratory distress does develop, it can become life threatening very quickly.

Another important factor to consider is whether the mother has a sufficient support network to help her care for an early baby. She may need to feed the baby around the clock at 1 to 2 hr intervals for many days or weeks. Not only is an early baby's stomach small, requiring frequent refilling, but continued growth requires lots of fuel, and being "out" when he should still be "in" adds more nutritional stress. This is because the early baby is still supposed to be receiving a constant flow of nourishment from his mother via the cord.

A baby who is at least 36 weeks from the LMP should be able to latch on to the breast, suck and swallow normally but may not be able to sustain nursing for long periods. The size of the mother's breasts or the shape of her nipples may make it difficult for some early babies to latch on with their tiny mouths. In either event, the mother may need to pump her milk for use in a supplemental feeding system or use donated milk for some time.

This means long, exhausting days and nights, which can be almost impossible to get through without a willing and knowledgeable support network to help her. The mother will need to be fed and cared for so that she can feed and care for her baby. Having at least one person on hand around-the-clock for this kind of care means the mother must have a close circle of friends in her community (such as might be available to an Amish, Mennonite, Muslim, Orthodox Jewish or Latter Day Saints woman in some areas), an extended family support system, or the means to hire doulas or other professional support people to fill that role. Unless you attend only a few births a year and she lives close to you, or unless you are running a clinical training program with a ready supply of students who will care for her under supervision, that person cannot be you, as you will need to remain available for the other women in your care. However, even if you don't provide this intensive care directly, you must be prepared to oversee it, to make more home visits and to provide phone consultations throughout the early weeks of the baby's life.

Preterm labor

Care of the mother during preterm labor is the same as during a full-term labor in most respects. Fetal heart rate considerations are reviewed in the chapter entitled "Assessing and Supporting the Baby's Well-Being during Labor." The early fetus is less tolerant of stress during labor and should be auscultated more frequently as a result. Keep in mind that an early baby has more room to assume unusual and, at times, problematic positions, including compound presentations. Even if the presenting part is engaged, cord prolapse is also somewhat more likely when the membranes rupture because the presenting part may not completely fill the cervix, especially in a nonvertex presentation. The baby who is quite early may start to descend and be born prior to full dilation, but such a small baby should be transported before birth whenever possible.

It may be best to have the mother assume a left lateral position at the time of birth to avoid exposing the newborn brain to the sudden influence of gravity in an inverted (head-down) position. Waterbirth is another option that further mitigates the effect of gravity as the baby emerges.

More babies will present breech when labor begins early, and the risks of breech birth to an early baby are greater. The skull being less ossified than a term baby's means the brain is at more risk for damage during rapid compression and decompression, as often occurs during a breech birth. In addition, the baby's lower body is not large enough to serve as an effective dilating wedge, the risk of cord prolapse is increased, and the chance that the baby will start to descend through a partially dilated cervix is higher. Breech birth with early babies must be carefully monitored. The exception to this is the birth of a second early twin because the first twin will have already dilated the birth canal and paved the way for an easy birth of the second baby in most cases.

Newborn and maternal care

The preterm newborn requires gentle handling and the same basic considerations as other babies. Keep the following issues in mind.

Airway considerations: Do not use postural drainage to clear the airways if you suspect that the baby is earlier than 37 weeks post-LMP. Such early babies still have a small region of the germinal matrix active in their brain; inversion could cause bleeding in this area. (For details regarding the formation and regression of this development region of the brain see the chapter entitled "Features of Fetal Anatomy Pertinent to the Birth Process.") Other methods of clearing the airway can be used.

Leave the cord intact: Modern medical insanity has obstetricians cutting the cords of early babies immediately so that they can be transferred to the neonatal staff for stabilization. Leaving the cord intact in a preterm baby is even more important than in a term baby because the placenta contains 50% of the fetal blood volume. The placental transfusion will greatly assist the baby to stabilize and maintain normal respirations. Leaving the cord intact with the placenta placed level with the baby allows the baby to backflow blood to the cord in the event of an increase in central venous pressure as the blood volume equilibrates, thought by Dunn to reduce the chance of intracranial hemorrhage. The baby who appears pale (hypovolemic) should be positioned below the level of the placenta before the placenta is born, with the placenta being raised above the baby after it is born, to encourage more blood to drain into the baby (Dunn, 1986).

Resuscitation considerations: Resuscitation protocols are generally the same as for a term baby. Leaving the cord intact will greatly assist in reducing the effort you or the baby must make to expand her lungs. It is important not to get carried away with the use of high-pressure ventilations because too much pressure can rupture the delicate alveoli. (See the chapter entitled "The Baby's Journey through Labor to Birth" for more details.)

Keep the baby warm: Early babies are much less equipped to deal with temperature fluctuations than their term counterparts. Allowing the baby to receive his placental transfusion will certainly help the baby to optimally maintain his temperature; even so, warmth is an important consideration. Remember that early babies can easily become overheated or chilled because their body core is so close to their body surface. (For more details regarding temperature changes in the preterm newborn, see the chapter entitled "Body Temperature Regulation in the Fetus and Newborn.")

Encourage nursing: While this is important for every baby, early babies are particularly vulnerable to nursing problems during the first weeks of life. This is because they are born when they are not quite "done" and still expect to be on the automatic food pipeline of the cord for a few more weeks. When the cord is no longer functioning, these small babies are particularly prone to hypoglycemia and can easily sleep through feedings. Getting the baby on the breast as soon as possible helps in establishing a good nursing pattern right away and helps prevent hypoglycemia before it begins. The ability to coordinate sucking and swallowing is essential for feeding at the breast or with a bottle; this ability develops at about 33 to 34 weeks gestational age. Without these reflexes, the baby will have to be tube fed until they develop.

Placental delivery: The early placenta may be less ready and willing to detach than at term. First, it is smaller and so is its attachment site on the uterine wall. The baby is also smaller, making for a less dramatic reduction in the size of the uterus after the baby is born. These two factors combine to impair the effectiveness of the reduction in uterine size that shears the placenta off the uterine wall after birth. The placental transfusion reduces the size of the placenta. Allowing the mother and baby as much uninterrupted time as possible to bond ensures optimal oxytocin levels. These measures together can maximize the chances that the placenta will be born without problems.

Postpartum care: An experienced midwife should stay at the mother's home for a prolonged immediate postpartum watch of at least 6 to 12 hours, depending upon the gestational age of the baby and the mother's extended support network. You should ensure that those who are willing to help are adequately instructed on what needs to be done, including monitoring the continued respiratory status of the baby. The delayed onset of respiratory distress syndrome is still a possibility, even if the baby is breathing well immediately after birth. When it does occur, it usually does so within the first 12 hours.

Early babies and infections: An early baby has an even less mature immune system than does one born at term. The baby should be watched very closely for signs of infection, especially if early labor has been a product of early rupture of membranes. The mother should take her own and her baby's temperature 3 times daily for at least 7 days and report any suspicious findings, although she should remember the early baby's susceptibility to becoming overheated or chilled due to environmental factors.

Preterm labor when you are remote from medical assistance

If you are far from medical care, the baby will be born at home and there isn't much you can do about it. Once the baby is out, stabilize her as best you can, leave the cord intact and then wrap the baby up skin-to-skin with the mother for kangaroo care. Even if the baby is quite early, the placental transfusion will give the baby the best chance of being able to sustain respirations. Arrange support for the mother to the extent possible, depending upon your equipment and human resources.

When the Baby is Late

Postterm delivery is defined as that which occurs after 42 completed weeks of gestation (after the 259th day). Refer to the chapter entitled "Postterm Pregnancy and Postmaturity Syndrome" in Volume I for background on this topic. In general, these labors can be attended as you would any labor. In fact, the main thing about late babies is their size, which is often large. Because some postdates babies will have problems, it behooves you to keep a close eye on the fetal heart rate throughout labor. In my practice, if the woman had good dates and was approaching 43 weeks, I discussed natural induction with her. This was because the cultural and medical pressure brought to bear on women who carry three weeks late is intense. Assuming that the woman is well-nourished, if the dates are iffy and the baby is still growing and moving normally, monitor her closely while awaiting natural labor to start and reevaluate the situation every few days.

After the birth do a CANScore to assess fetal nutrition and carefully assess the baby's size in relationship to his gestational age. Large babies and malnourished ones are both prone to hypoglycemia. The best way to prevent or correct this is frequent nursing. If the baby is large, examine her carefully for injuries, especially if the shoulders got stuck.

References and Further Reading on Assisting Labor and Birth in Other-Than-Vertex Presentations, Multiples and Preterm Births

References used in multiple chapters

Cunningham F, et al., eds. WILLIAMS OBSTETRICS, 20th ed. Appleton & Lange, Stamford CT, 1997.

Cunningham F, et al., eds. WILLIAMS OBSTETRICS, 21th ed. Appleton & Lange, Stamford CT, 2001.

Daniels S. Lecture notes, The Maternity Center midwifery training program. Fall, 1978.

Greenhill JP. PRINCIPLES AND PRACTICE OF OBSTETRICS, 10th ed. WB Saunders Co, Philadelphia PA, 1951.

Myerscough P. MUNRO KERR'S OPERATIVE OBSTETRICS, 9th ed. Williams & Wilkins Co, Baltimore MD, 1977.

Sandberg EC. "The Zavanelli maneuver: 12 years of recorded experience," OBSTET GYNECOL, 93(2);312-317, Feb 1999.

Assisting at the Birth of a Baby Presenting Her Face

Benedetti TJ, et al. "Face Presentation at term," OBSTET GYNECOL, 55(2);199-202, Feb, 1980.

Contreras H. Personal conversation, MANA conf., Austin TX, Oct, 2003.

Creasy R. MANAGEMENT OF LABOR AND DELIVERY, Blackwell Scientific Pub, Malden MA,1997.

Cucco U. "Face presentation," AM J OBSTET GYNECOL, 94(8);1085-1091, April 15, 1966.

Hart G, RMA digest #533, web-list serve, June 24, 2001.

Hendrickson F. MIDWIFERY IN 10,000 EASY STEPS, PART 1: A CRITICAL AND CONSTRUCTIVE LOOK AT MIDWIFERY AND OBSTETRICS BY A BIRTH ATTENDANT WITH OVER 20 YEARS UNLICENCED EXPERIENCE. Privately published, Hillman, MN Jan, 1981.

Mentzer J. RMA digest #533, web-list serve, June 24, 2001.

Simkin P, Ancheta R. THE LABOR PROGRESS HANDBOOK. Blackwell Science, Oxford UK, 2000.

Sotelo I. Traditional Mexican midwife, conversation via Anita Rojas, translator, Sept 2004.

Trueba G. COMFORT MEASURES FOR CHILDBIRTH: THE REBOZO WAY, The Rebozo Way, Calle 23, #40, Club de Golf, Mexicao, 14620 Mexico D F, Mexico, 2001.

Assisting at the Birth of a Baby Presenting His Brow

Borell U, Fernström I. "The mechanism of labour in face and brow presentation," ACTA OBSTET GYNECOL SCAND, 39;626-645, 1960.

Jennings PN. "Brow Presentation and Vaginal Delivery," AUST NZ J OBSTET GYNECOL, 8:219-224, 1968.

Lachapelle M. PRATIQUE DES ACCOUCHEMENTS, JB Baillière, Paris France,1821.

Assisting at the Birth of a Breech Baby

Banks M. BREECH BIRTH-WOMAN WISE. Birthspirit Books, Hamilton NZ, 1998.

Banks M. As noted with the drawings, the illustrations of breech birth in the upright and leaning-forward positions are rendered from photos copyrighted by Maggie Banks and used by permission. Permission requests must be directed to her at: Birthspirit Books, 15 Te Ava Road, R.D. 3, Hamilton NZ, (011) 64- (0)7 856-4612.

Banks M. E-mail communication, March 6, 2002.

Burns J, Marshall C. "Breech, its etiology, diagnosis, prognosis and treatment with special reference to the treatment of the after-coming head," (sect Reports of Societies), BMJ, (1);820-821, May 5, 1934.

Bower D. MECHANISM OF LABOR FOR STUDENTS. H K Lewis & Co, Ltd, London UK, 1967.

Collea JV. "The intrapartum management of breech presentation." CLIN PERINATOL., 8(1);173-181, Feb, 1981.

Cooper M. Workshop presentation on breeches and twins, Midwifery Today, Eugene, OR, 1992(?).

Cronk M. "Hands off the breech," PRACT MIDWIFE, 1(6);13-15, June, 1998.

Cronk M. "Midwives and Breech Births," PRACT MIDWIFE, 1(7/8);44-45, July-Aug, 1998.

Cronk M. Illustrations of breech birth in the leaning forward, hands-and-knees position are rendered from photos copyrighted by Mary Cronk and used by permission. Requests must be directed to: Milburn Cottage, Clappers Lane, Earnley, Near Chichester, West, Sussex England, PO20 7JJ. (011) 44-(0)1-243-670-382.

Cronk M. Editorial comments, 2002, 2004.

Cruikshank D. "Breech Presentation," CLINICAL OB GYN, 29(2);255-263, June, 1986.

Dunn P. "Alterations in the distribution of blood between the fetus (and infant) and placenta during and after birth." Unpublished presentation handout. Canadian Pediatric Society, Centennial Commonwealth Meeting, Toronto Canada, Sept 3-9, 1967.

Dzata M, CNM. Personal communication, Aug, 2001.

Eden T, Holland E. A MANUAL OF MIDWIFERY, 7th ed. J & A Churchill, London England, 1931.

El Halta V. ADVANCED MIDWIFERY SEMINAR: MOVING MIDWIFERY FORWARD: ESSAYS AND OUTLINES, workshop manual, Garden of Life, Dearborn MI, 1989.

El Halta V, Baldwin R. "Normalizing the breech delivery," video, Garden of Life, Dearborn MI, 1987.

Ettinghausen N. Unpublished transcript from a workshop on breech birth presented in the early 1980s. No date.

Ettinghausen N. "Delivering a breech," MOTHERING, 21;56-57, Fall, 1981.

Evans J. Editorial comments and personal communications, 2002, 2003, 2004, 2012.
Gaskin IM. "Assisting a vaginal breech delivery," Farm Video Productions, Summertown TN, 1992.
Gaskin IM. Personal conversations, 1998.
Gaskin IM. "The undervalued art of vaginal breech birth: a skill every birth attendant should know," MOTHERING, (125);52-58, July-Aug, 2004.
Graham H. ETERNAL EVE: THE HISTORY OF GYNAECOLOGY AND OBSTETRICS. Doubleday & Co, Garden City NY, 1951.
Hellman L, Pritchard J. WILLIAMS OBSTETRICS, 14th ed. Appleton-Century-Crofts, New York NY, 1971.
Hughes E, ed. OBSTETRIC–GYNECOLOGIC TERMINOLOGY. FA Davis Co, Philadelphia PA, 1972.
Hunt P, CPM. Editing notes, 2003.
Künzel W, Kirshbaum M. "Management of vaginal delivery in breech presentation at term," EURO PRAC GYNECOL OBSTET: BREECH DELIVERY, 2;99-126, 2002.
Lachapelle M. PRATIQUE DES ACCOUCHEMENTS, Vol II. JB Baillière, Paris France, 1825.
Løvset J. "Shoulder Delivery in Breech Presentation," J OBSTET GYNECOL BR EM, 44;696-704, 1937.
Løvset J. VAGINAL OPERATIVE DELIVERY, Scandinavian University Books, Oslo Norway, 1968.
Mauriceau F. THE DISEASES OF WOMEN WITH CHILD AND IN CHILD-BED, 4th ed. 1668. (Translated by Hugh Chamberlen, Andrew Bell, London, England, 1710. (Facsimile ed by Garland Pub, New York NY, 1985.)
Mayes B. PRACTICAL OBSTETRICS, Angus & Robertson, Sydney Australia, 1954.
Mayes B. A TEXTBOOK OF OBSTETRICS, Australian Pub Co, Sydney Australia, 1959.
McNeile L. OBSTETRICAL MANIKIN PRACTICE, Williams & Wilkins Co, Baltimore MD, 1939.
Myers S. "A new technique for flexion of the aftercoming head during breech delivery," AM J OBSTET GYNECOL, 155(1); July 1986.
Myles M. A TEXTBOOK FOR MIDWIVES, 6th ed. E & S Livingstone Ltd, Edinburgh England, 1968.
Oxorn H. "William Smellie and the mechanism of labor," AM J OBSTET GYNECOL, 77(1);41-49, Jan 1959.
Oxorn H. HUMAN LABOR AND BIRTH, 5th ed. Appleton/Century/Crofts, Norwalk CT, 1986.
Parvin T. THE SCIENCE AND ART OF OBSTETRICS, 3rd ed. Lea Brothers & Co, Philadelphia, PA, 1895.
Popper N, Walker P. "Forces at the glenohumeral joint in abduction," CLIN ORTHOP, 58(135);165-170, Sept 1978.
Potter I. THE PLACE OF VERSION IN OBSTETRICS. CV Mosby Co, St Louis MO, 1922.
Schlinger H, CPM, CNM. Editing notes, 2002.
Sellers P. MIDWIFERY, A TEXTBOOK AND REFERENCE BOOK FOR MIDWIVES IN SOUTHERN AFRICA, VOL 2: COMPLICATIONS IN CHILDBIRTH. Juta & Co, Ltd., Kenwyn So Africa, 1993.
Shears G, Williams P, eds. OBSTETRICS NORMAL AND OPERATIVE, 3rd ed. JB Lippincott, Philadelphia PA, 1920.
Shushan A, Younis J. "McRoberts maneuver for the management of the aftercoming head in breech delivery," GYNECOL OBSTET INVEST, 34;188-189, Oct 1992.
Smellie W. A TREATISE ON THE THEORY AND PRACTICE OF MIDWIFERY, VOL. 1. 1st ed. D. Wilson, London England, 1752. (Facsimile ed by Classics of Obstet Gynecol Library, div. Griffon Ed, New York NY,1990.)
Sotelo I. 5-day midwifery intensive, Doña Irene Sotelo, trad Mexican midwife, MIDWIFERY TODAY, Eugene OR, Aug 27-31, 2001.
Stevenson J. "More thoughts on breech," MIDWIFERY TODAY, (26);26, Summer, 1993.
Tully G. "Identifying and resolving obstructed breech birth," MIDWIFERY TODAY, (106);21-23, Summer 2013.
Wagner V, "Birth: a video presentation on childbirth by a Christian lay midwife who has delivered thousands of babies in over twenty years of practice," video, Veronica Wagner, Aptos CA, 1989.

UNSTABLE LIE, OBLIQUE LIE AND TRANSVERSE LIE IN LABOR

Contreras H. Traditional Mexican midwife. Personal conversation, MANA conf., Austin TX, Oct, 2003.
Sotelo I. Traditional Mexican midwife, conversation via Anita Rojas, translator, Sept 2004.
Sutton J, Scott P. UNDERSTANDING AND TEACHING OPTIMAL FOETAL POSITIONING. Bay Print, Ltd., Tauranga, NZ, 1996.

ASSISTING AT MULTIPLE BIRTHS

Barrett J, Ritchie W. "Twin delivery," BEST PRAC RES CLIN OBSTET GYNAECOL, 16(1);43-56, Feb, 2002.
DeWees W. A COMPENDIOUS SYSTEM OF MIDWIFERY, Carey, Lea & Blanchard, Philadelphia PA, 1835.
Edmonds P. Personal conversation, 2003.
Evans J. Personal communication, 2003.
Evans J. "Can a twin birth be a positive experience?", MIDWIFERY MATTERS, (74), Autumn 1997, in web archive: http://www.radmid.demon.co.uk/twins.htm, accessed June 29, 2004.
Gall S. MULTIPLE PREGNANCY AND DELIVERY, Mosby, St. Louis MO, 1996.
Gilhooley J, Neonatologist. Personal communication, 2003.
Houlihan C, Knuppel R. "Intrapartum management of multiple gestations," CLINICAL PERINATOL, 23;91-116, 1996.
Keith L, et al. MULTIPLE PREGNANCY: EPIDEMIOLOGY, GESTATION AND PERINATAL OUTCOME, Parthenon Pub, New York NY, 1995.
Klebe J, Ingomar C. "The fetoplacental circulation during parturition illustrated by the interfetal transfusion syndrome," PEDIATRICS, 49(1);112-116, Jan, 1972.
Machin G "Conjoined twins: implications for blactogenesis," BIRTH DEFECTS, 29(141-179), 1993.

Nissen E. "Twins" Collision, impaction, compaction and interlocking," OBSTET GYNECOL, 11(5)514-526, May, 1958.
Rayburn W, et al. "Multiple gestation time interval between delivery of the first and second twins." OBSTET GYNECOL, 63(4);502-506, Apr, 1984.
Roddie T. "A case of conjoined twins," BMJ, I, 831, 1957.
Rudolph A, et al. "Obstetric management of conjoined twins," pp. 28-37 in Bergsma D, ed. BIRTH DEFECTS ORIGINAL ARTICLE SERIES: CONJOINED TWINS, New York: The National Foundation–March of Dimes, 1967.
Strachan G. TEXTBOOK OF OBSTETRICS, HK Lewis & Co, London UK, 1947.

WHEN THE BABY IS EARLY OR LATE

Dunn P. Chapter 21: "Reservations about the methods of assessing at birth the predictive value of intrapartum fetal monitoring including premature interruption of the feto-placental circulation." pp. 130-137 in P. Rolfe, ed. FETAL PHYSIOLOGICAL MEASUREMENTS. Report of the 2nd International Conf. April 2-4, 1984, Oxford. Butterworths Pub, London UK, 1986.

ISSUES INVOLVING THE FLOW OF LABOR

NATURAL INDUCTION AND AUGMENTATION OF LABOR

To induce labor means to get labor started before it starts on its own. To augment labor means to stimulate the uterus once labor is underway to increase the strength, duration or frequency of contractions so that birth can proceed. Both are discussed in this chapter because most of the techniques used to induce labor can also be used for augmentation.

It may seem inaccurate to claim that any form of induction or augmentation is natural because both are most definitely forms of intervention. Here, "natural" refers to the method used. Instead of dangerous chemopharmacological agents such as oxytocin or misoprostol, natural methods are used such as herbs, acupuncture, nipple stimulation or other nonpharmaceutical remedies that stimulate the uterus safely and can be used at home. "Natural" also refers to the way that most of these methods work with the mother's body to encourage her to open to the energy of birth, gently allowing her body to take over on its own and produce a physiologic contraction pattern appropriate to her phase of dilation, not one artificially intensified. Natural induction is also unlikely to work if the mother or her baby is not really ready to go into labor. While all inductions will have an emotional impact on the baby's relationship to timing and being imposed upon by others, proceeding at home is sometimes your best option to avoid even more disruptive interventions.

In my experience as a midwife, I have had great success with natural induction techniques. I attribute this as much to my personal involvement in supporting the process as I do to the agents used to stimulate the uterus.

Deciding Upon Whether to Proceed with an Induction

There are only a few reasons why a midwife might want to induce labor.

Fetal status

Postterm pregnancy: Chief among these "reasons" is one colored by the politics of doing holistic midwifery in the larger context of a medical-model health care system. The obstetrical community exerts increasing pressure on the woman to have the baby by a certain time in relationship to the calculated due date. This most commonly occurs when the baby is overdue. Careful, individualized assessment of the due date, as described in Volume I of this text, will help to eliminate some of that pressure. Nevertheless, no due date is exact, and it is perfectly normal for women to give birth anywhere between 37 and 42 weeks of pregnancy and sometimes after that, especially if long pregnancies are the rule in the family. Your comfort level with waiting for spontaneous labor to begin when there is no clear indication that induction is necessary must be assessed in light of the circumstances of the individual case, the "medical" indications for induction, the political repercussions in your community of waiting for spontaneous labor to begin and the mother's informed choice. If the mother refuses induction, be sure to get a signed informed-choice waiver from her stating that she was told of the risks of waiting for labor and that she declined interventions. Be sure to update this on at least a biweekly basis as long as the pregnancy continues.

Reduced volume of amniotic fluid: Postterm pregnancy, when accompanied by a reduction in amniotic fluid, also prompts recommendations to induce. Reduced fluid is sometimes associated with impaired blood flow to the fetal kidneys and may result in cord compression. However, it may not reflect compromise in the baby and can often be remedied simply by having the mother drink more fluids. While it alone is not a good reason to intervene prior to term, if the woman is at term or later, and increasing fluids does not make any difference, induction at home is a better solution that transport to the hospital.

Fetal size: When the baby is deemed too small, and therefore possibly suffering from intrauterine growth retardation, or too large, and therefore more likely to develop shoulder dystocia, the medical model often calls for induction. You and the parents must use your own judgment, along with careful palpation for fetal size, to determine what is right for the baby. Shoulder dystocia is notoriously unpredictable; women who eat well are constantly told their babies are too big; conversely babies may seem small who are, in fact, fine. Careful evaluation includes taking into account the stature of the mother; the woman with a long torso might "hide" a much larger baby than expected based on fundal height, while a short-waisted woman can appear to be carrying a larger baby than she actually is. Beware, as well, of "medically" indicated recommendations for induction of a "large" or "small" baby based only on recent ultrasound evaluations of fetal size; after about 20 weeks, ultrasound estimates are increasingly inaccurate as term approaches.

Multiple gestation: Physicians in some medical communities expect multiple births to come early or recommend early induction; however, there is no reason that multiple births can't be carried to term. They certainly do not need to be induced early in the healthy, well-nourished woman whose babies appear healthy.

Direct evidence of fetal compromise: Findings that represent possible fetal compromise, such as a questionable fetal heart rate pattern, a reduction in fetal movement or both, as well as problems such as isoimmunization or severe fetal growth restriction, often lead to a medical recommendation to induce. These babies require diligent monitoring during labor. Oxytocin induction in the hospital will be more traumatic for the baby than a natural induction at home. It may be wisest, depending upon fetal response and your experience level, to transport for in-hospital supervision of the baby's condition during the course of labor once a naturally induced labor is underway. This is especially so if you are a newly fledged midwife; it is always best to err on the side of caution and transport when the potential for problems is increased.

Fetal demise: If the baby has died in utero, some women will want to have the baby out as soon as possible. If the mother is near term, you can try a natural induction. However, if she is not, it may take the extra oomph of oxytocin to push her into labor, which means a hospital birth. Natural induction can be used successfully in the presence of fetal demise, but it usually takes some time to prime the body so that labor can begin.

Maternal condition

The condition of the mother can also play a role in the decision to induce. The primary maternal reason to induce in women who have no preexisting medical conditions is suspicion of toxemia. Be careful to troubleshoot secondary symptoms, such as blood pressure changes and weight gain, so that you are not overreacting to what amounts to a benign symptom picture. If you are convinced a woman is toxemic, vigilant assessment of the status of the baby and mother is important during labor, since the baby has to cope with contractions in the presence of an inadequately expanded blood volume. Medical conditions that may place the baby at more risk if the pregnancy continues include diabetes, renal disease, chronic pulmonary disease or chronic hypertension. The individual woman's total health condition must be taken into account when deciding to induce for these reasons.

If the mother does have a preexisting medical condition that makes carrying her baby to term or beyond more problematic for either herself or her baby, back-up care and options for induction should have been arranged prenatally.

Mother's desire: The woman herself may wish to get on with labor for a variety of reasons. Many first-time mothers feel sure they will start labor early; with this attitude, they can be quite anxious and impatient by their due date, as most well-nourished women will carry past term. If a mother talks of inducing, provided that things are going well, suggest that she wait for spontaneous labor to begin. Pressure from well-meaning but anxious friends and relatives calling to ask whether labor has begun may be a factor in her requesting induction. Suggest that she tell them that the baby will come when he or she is ready and that it is not helpful to get called every day to be asked if she is in labor yet. Be aware, however, that a mother's anxiety may also reflect an intuitive sense that the baby needs to be born now in order for the birth to go well. Sound out the mother to determine if this is a factor prompting her request.

Psychological factors interfering with the onset of labor: Psychological factors or external circumstances may stall the onset of labor, and no induction should proceed without first exploring any and all reasons why the woman might believe she is better off with the baby inside rather than out. The baby, too, may have compelling reasons to remain in utero, such as an awareness of being born into an abusive environment. Both you and the mother can talk to the baby about how delaying the onset of labor will not fix the problem. Also see the chapter entitled "Psychological Impediments to Progress during Labor."

Rupture of membranes: Another reason for induction is prelabor rupture of membranes, which can place both mother and baby at risk for infection. Ideally, labor can be stimulated to avoid additional interventions, especially if there is an increased risk. (The diagnosis and handling of prelabor rupture of membranes is also discussed in Volume I of this text.)

Abruption: When a partial abruption is occurring, induction may help complete the birth before the placenta separates more and therefore avoid a surgical delivery. However, using allopathic methods of induction may lead to hyperstimulation of the uterus and cause the abruption to progress. Getting the baby out sooner rather than later, however, is a good idea. Natural means coupled with vigilant fetal monitoring are probably the best option, but if you believe the abruption is escalating, you will have to transport.

Contraindications to Induction

Do not attempt to induce if the dates are uncertain and the baby is small but growing as evidenced by serial abdominal palpation exams and fundal height measurements. Review the chart and the mother's nutritional status as well as her due date, and continue to monitor over the following week or so to see if the baby and the fundal height continue to grow. If so, the dates are more than likely wrong and need to be readjusted. If the baby does not grow, it may be growth retarded for some reason that is not related to maternal nutrition and may need to be born sooner rather than later.

Other reasons to forgo induction include such obvious things as diagnosed placenta previa or vasa previa, transverse or oblique fetal lie that cannot be corrected, cord presentation or prolapse, major pelvic structural abnormality, active genital herpes, and severe, acute fetal distress. Avoid pharmaceutical induction for mothers with a history of uterine incision or full-thickness myomectomy (fibroid removal that required an incision all the way through the uterine wall) and use gentle techniques in these women to encourage labor at home.

Discussing the Reasons for Induction with the Parents

You and the parents should discuss the reasons why induction is warranted. Make sure that you distinguish between reasons that are truly based on concern for the mother's or baby's well-being and those that have more to do with the political climate in your community. If the political climate is the reason for induction, it is important to tell the woman the truth, so that she will be able to make an informed decision based on your real motives and not assume or be told that the reasons are medical when they are not. Differentiate, as well, between medical-model reasons and midwifery-model reasons (although the two will often overlap).

Preparing to Induce

Modified Bishop's Score to Assess Potential Cervical Responsiveness to Induction of Labor

Parameter	Points assigned			
	0	1	2	3
Dilation (cm)	0	1-2	3-4	5-6
Effacement (%)	0 to 30	40 to 50	60 to 70	80 to 100
Station of presenting part	-3	-2	-1 to 0	+1 to +2
Consistency of cervix	Firm	Medium	Soft	--
Position of cervix	Very posterior	Normally posterior	Slightly off center toward the back	--
+Cervical sensations	None	Slight	Strong and frequent	Coordinated with some or all toning contractions
+Yoni secretions	No increase	Increased mucus	Increase with bloody mucus	--
+Toning contractions	None to slight	Mild	Strong, sporadic, frequent	Almost regular, visible on abdominal observation

+ = items added by the author that have proven helpful from a midwifery-model perspective. All others are original components of the Bishop score.

Total score = sum of all points for each parameter. The meaning of the score:

7 or less: Do not attempt induction without ripening the cervix first.
9 or more: Favorable to attempt induction.
12 or more: She is quite ready for labor or in early labor; a little encouragement should get her going.

(modified from Bishop, 1964)

Assuming there is a good reason for labor to begin sooner rather than later, how do you decide when to induce, what method to use, and whether the mother's body will be receptive to your efforts? A first step would be to assess how ready a woman's body is to go into labor. (This discussion assumes you have already reviewed the advice given in the chapter entitled "Postterm Pregnancy and Dysmaturity Syndrome" in a recent edition of Volume I of this text.) Good indications that a woman's body is preparing for labor include frequent episodes of toning contractions; cervical aches, pains and twinges; and engagement of the presenting part, especially in a first-time mother. If none of these are happening, induction will be that much more difficult and often impossible.

If the membranes are intact, an internal yoni exam can provide useful information regarding the woman's readiness to go into labor. The more changes the cervix has already undergone, the easier it will be to get labor going. As you gain experience, you will develop an intuitive understanding regarding when a woman will be most responsive to induction efforts. In the meantime, the preceding assessment tool is a good place to start. The scoring system on the preceding page was developed by E. H. Bishop to assess a woman's receptiveness to induction. I have added cervical sensations and toning contractions, both of which are very important findings. The higher the score, the more likely it is that the cervix will respond to induction efforts. It is worth noting that this scoring system was originally intended for use with multiparous women; however, it is obvious that a high score in a nullipara is a very favorable sign as well.

Acupuncture induction

Treatments by a practitioner of traditional Chinese medicine, especially one with an obstetrical or midwifery background, can be enormously helpful, especially if the woman is 10 to 14 days overdue. If you have access to one in your community and your client can afford it, send her in for a few labor-encouraging treatments. The practitioner will be able to tailor the treatment to her specific symptom picture, and it is likely to be even more effective than what you can do at home. It is quite normal for several sessions to be necessary before the desired result is achieved, so a woman should be referred sooner rather than later (Hobbs, 1999).

Ripening the cervix

When the goal is induction, the ripeness of the cervix will influence what is suggested first. Ripeness refers first of all to the softening of the cervical tissues followed by the ease of admitting a fingertip if not actual dilation, and ending with effacement. Ripening decreases the cervix's resistance to the forces of labor.

Oils containing prostaglandin precursors: If the cervix is not ripe and the membranes are intact, either the midwife, the mother or her partner can place 4 to 8 whole, unpunctured capsules of evening primrose, borage or black currant oil inside the os or next to the cervix in the fornices, where they will melt on contact. (Borage oil is very concentrated, so you will want to start with fewer capsules.) The mother may use a diaphragm or an Instead menstrual cup to hold them in place if she prefers; however, this is not necessary. The oil will also compromise the integrity of the rubber in the diaphragm. All of these oils provide high percentages of the acidic precursors to the prostaglandins. Theoretically, direct contact with the oil feeds the cells what they need to make more prostaglandin. Since it has now been determined that prostaglandin levels rise after labor begins, it is uncertain how evening primrose oil or any prostaglandin hormone or precursor actually works, but it does produce results. The oil will markedly soften the cervix, making it more receptive to other methods of stimulation. While the capsules are in place, the mother can also take herbal tinctures orally, as suggested below, two or three times during the day. Recheck the cervix in 12 hours and repeat, if needed.

If the mother has ruptured membranes, inserting anything into the yoni increases the risk of infection. One option is to insert the capsules in the upper yoni canal below the cervix using sterile technique, while another is to have the mother take the capsules by mouth. However, neither will result in the same degree of cervical softening that occurs when the oil is in direct contact with the cervix.

Sexual activity: For the woman with intact membranes who feels so inclined, sexual activity such as heterosexual intercourse, female orgasm and breast stimulation can help to both ripen the cervix and initiate labor. Semen contains natural prostaglandins and appears to assist in ripening the cervix. There has even been some research that suggests that the prostaglandins in semen may be absorbed better through the gut than through the walls of the yoni, meaning that swallowing semen may also be of help.

Orgasm can have the effect of opening the woman up psychically, as well as causing uterine contractions. The energy of sex is the energy of birth, and women who are sexually active late in pregnancy have the advantage of opening to the life energy that brings their babies to birth. Kissing softens the cervix (the mouth of the uterus) and the yoni by sympathetic response. If a woman does not wish to engage in sexual activity with her partner or if she has no partner, she can bring herself to orgasm with many of the same benefits.

Watching birth videos: Watching and hearing other women give birth can be a powerful encouragement to get labor going. Make sure any videos you loan or recommend show normal births that include the birth of the placenta.

Prime the uterus

You can begin to prime the uterus several days prior to the actual induction, which will also help ripen the cervix.

Herbal encouragement of uterine activity: Give 10 drops of labor tincture (from Equinox Botanicals or homemade) four times daily or as frequently as every hour, or use a combination of 10 drops of blue cohosh, 10 drops of black cohosh and 10 drops of ginger tincture on the same schedule. Place the tincture in a small amount of water to be taken when the mother is awake (she should not wake herself to take tinctures). Sometimes ingestion of one of these mixtures alone will get the mother into labor, particularly if she has given birth before. Alternatively or in addition, you can recommend red raspberry leaf infusion as a preparatory uterine tonic.

Hydrotherapy: Prior to induction, the woman can take a warm bath every night for one hour, alone. This will help her focus and relax.

Stimulate the nipples: To increase the number of toning contractions, start stimulating the nipples with one- to two-hour sessions several times daily using a manual or electric breast pump (you can even try one on each breast) or the fingers: grasp the nipple with the thumb and forefinger and gently roll it between them. (Note that stimulating the areola will not produce the desired effect.) The woman's partner or a nursing baby can also suckle to accomplish the same thing.

Lift the belly: Once the cervix is ripe, the mother can begin lifting her belly just below the level of her navel with some of her toning contractions. (This technique is described in detail in the chapter entitled "Entering Pains and Back Pain in Labor.") Lifting the belly changes the angle of the uterus and is particularly helpful if the baby is posterior or the mother has a pendulous abdomen because it helps early contractions to be most effective. It may also stimulate stronger contractions (King, 1993).

Acupressure for uterine priming: The following technique is quoted directly from Debra Betts's excellent INFORMATION FOR MIDWIVES on the professional use of acupressure in childbirth:

> To prepare the woman's body, commence contractions and encourage cervical dilation, acupressure on Co-4 [LI-4] and SP-6 every 2 hours (left Co-4, right SP-6, then swapping to the right Co-4, left SP-6 two hours later).
>
> Acupressure, combined with strong massage on GB-21 and BL-32, preferably twice a day, but at least once daily for 10 minutes over each point.
>
> If there is time this regime can be commenced three days prior to a medical induction. While the ideal outcome is for labour to commence spontaneously, I receive positive feedback that on giving Prostaglandins following acupressure, labour proceeds efficiently with no further interventions required.
>
> If an induction is required within a 24 hour period, using Co-4 [LI-4]and SP-6 as above half-hourly is helpful.
>
> If it is felt that the position of the baby is hindering the onset of labor, using ear press needles on BL-67 bilaterally is recommended. (This point is located on the lateral side of the little toe, just posterior to the corner of the nail). A plaster or tape can be placed over the press needle to keep it in place. (Betts, 2002)

These points (other than BL-67) are also helpful in inducing labor when the membranes have ruptured early. See the subchapter entitled "Traditional Chinese Medicine" for details regarding locating these points and for information on how to obtain Debra Betts's acupressure manuals.

Induction Techniques

You are ready to begin induction in earnest once the cervix is ripe. First-time mothers with intact membranes are the most difficult to induce. It is easier to induce a multigravida with or without intact membranes because her body remembers what labor is like and responds more readily to the stimulation.

Setting the intention to get labor going

I get the impression that many practitioners believe nonpharmaceutical induction is not very effective. This may be because the psychological factors that make induction likely to succeed are not taken into account. One of the most important of these is the presence and intention of the midwife.

Go to the mother's home; bring your birth gear and plan to be there until the birth. This way, you give her the clear message that you expect your efforts to work. Make sure she is fed, hydrated and rested so that she is ready physically as well as psychologically. Do not attempt an induction when the mother's energy level is compromised. Since the uterus is most active at night, you can try to have the woman rest during the day by taking a hot bath and sleeping in a darkened room. This would allow you to arrive the next evening for the induction. If she does not feel rested, have her get a good night's sleep, with induction beginning first thing the following morning.

The amount of personal attention from the midwife as well as the ritualized nature of some of the suggested methods are big reasons why such methods work well for the midwives who use them. In conjunction with whatever labor stimulating agents you use, sit with the mother and do belly massage and nipple stimulation to encourage contractions. This provides attention and nurturing as well as physical stimulation and is an integral part of making natural induction efforts a success.

Carbohydrate loading

The effectiveness of any induction method may be enhanced by having the mother eat large amounts of complex carbohydrates for a few days to a week before induction. Even if she has not "loaded up," a meal high in complex carbohydrates about one hour before commencing induction will boost glycogen (stored carbohydrate) reserves. Midwife Valerie El Halta feels this is especially important if the baby is in an ROA position, as having the mother's ascending colon full will help prevent the baby from rotating posteriorly once labor is underway (Wainer-Cohen, 2001).

Sweeping (stripping) the membranes

Sweeping the membranes is an invasive technique that has been used for centuries by physicians to stimulate the onset of labor. Some midwives also find it an invaluable tool that is effective and a far better choice than transport for induction with synthetic prostaglandins or oxytocin. It is done during an internal exam and involves inserting fingers through the os to separate the bag of waters from the lower uterine segment. Obviously the cervix must be very ripe or partially dilated for this to be possible.

This technique works because it tears away fragments of decidua parietalis from the lower uterine segment. These fragments remain attached to the outer surface of the forebag. Exposure of the fragments to yoni secretions prompts the release of inflammatory mediators, including prostaglandin F_{2a}, a promoter of cervical dilation. However, the procedure is painful and carries the risk of inadvertent rupture of membranes and infection, as well as the risk of damaging a marginal placenta previa. Ideally, sweeping the membranes should be attempted only if they are intact, the cervix is ripe, the mother is at least at term and there are no signs of infection and no suspicion of a marginal placenta previa or group B-strep colonization. However, some midwives do sweep the membranes when they have been ruptured for a while with no sign of labor in sight. Sweeping the membranes can be used with or without other inducing techniques.

If you choose to sweep the membranes, inform the mother about what you are proposing to do, including that it is uncomfortable and likely to produce bloody show, especially if done thoroughly enough to be effective. She should feel fully in favor of proceeding so that she does not feel victimized. Sweep the membranes as early in the day as possible. Have her empty her bladder and assume a comfortable position that optimizes your ability to reach the cervix, such as lying on a firm surface with her hips propped up. Have a support person remain eye-to-eye with the mother and help her with deep, relaxed, abdominal breathing. Make sure she is ready before you begin.

Use sterile gloves and sterile technique since you will be coming in direct contact with the lower uterine wall. To begin, gently insert two gloved fingers through the outer os and up, beyond the inner cervical opening. Angle your fingertips to the side so you don't rupture the membranes as you insert your fingertips between the bag of waters and the lowermost region of uterine wall, just beyond the inner os. Slowly sweep your fingers in a full circle to separate the bag from the cervix. The membranes may feel "shiny" or "squeaky."

Proceeding gently and slowly, gradually move your fingers more deeply up along the sides, separating the bag of waters from the lower uterus. Do not press directly against the bag of waters itself. Take your time; five minutes is not too long. If it is too uncomfortable for the mother, stop and wait while she breathes deeply and regains her centered relaxation. You have done a good job if you can get your fingers into the cervical os two knuckles deep. The prostaglandin response is enhanced when the greatest possible membrane surface is dislodged from the inner cervix. Stop if you feel firm adhesions or a grainy surface or if fluid blood appears, any of which could be due to a low-lying placenta or even from an unrecognized previa.

As you go around, gently attempt to stretch the cervix. You may feel it opening and relaxing. Often you can only get one finger in at first; then, after a minute or so, the cervix will open another few centimeters. However, the cervix must be very ripe and somewhat effaced to have this kind of success with stimulating dilation. This will loosen the mucus plug and there may be bloody mucus on your glove as you remove your fingers after the exam. Bloody show is a good sign that you have swept the membranes effectively. Let the mother know she may have more bloody show throughout the day. The plug may reform if labor doesn't begin within 24 hours. When sweeping has been thorough, expect labor to start anytime between 3 hours and 3 days later. On the average labor will begin within 24 hours (Berghella et al., 1996; Midwife list)

Examine the mucus plug carefully for meconium staining, which can be a rare but serious sign of fetal compromise (see the chapter entitled "The Placental Membranes and Amniotic Fluid during Labor for details").

More acupressure priming and induction techniques

Certainly one of the least invasive ways to encourage labor to begin is acupressure. These are good techniques to try before moving on to other, more interventive approaches. There are several different protocols for inducing labor. These techniques can be used alone or in conjunction with other labor-inducing techniques, such as herbs.

- •LI-4 and SP-6 can be stimulated simultaneously on the same side (right or left) or contralaterally (right hand, left foot, then switch) to increase the frequency and strength of contractions. Hold these points for several minutes every half hour or so, or continuously. When using intermittent stimulation, switch sides with each session.
- •Use your thumb to apply direct pressure to SP-6, then use it to massage down the leg from SP-6 to the Achilles tendon. Stimulate both legs 5 or 6 times, counting slowly to 60 each time pressure is applied to SP-6. Labor should begin in 1 to 1.5 hours. (Israeli midwife, Midwifery Today Conf., London England, 1997)
- •Apply pressure to LIV-3, LI- 4 and BL-32. A sharp-tipped object, such as a pen tip or small crochet hook tip can also be used to stimulate Bladder 67 on the little toe, especially if the baby is not in a great position.
- •Stimulate LI-4 by applying firm pressure at an angle toward the uterus, which should help strengthen or regulate contractions. (Bullets 1, 3 and 4 based on Betts, 1997; Lowe, 2003; West, 2001)

To locate these points, see the chapter entitled "Traditional Chinese Medicine."

Hypothalamic point: This point is located by following the coronal sutures down the side of the head to the point where those lines intersect a line drawn around from the brow (in the region of the temple). Feel around for the sensitive point. Massaging here can help bring labor on as well as enhance the effectiveness of other techniques (Enning, 2003).

Nipple stimulation

Nipple stimulation will usually get labor going if kept up long enough, although it may take several hours. Stimulation can be stopped during a contraction but should be continued between contractions until labor is progressing on its own. This technique can be used in combination with herbs taken orally. The time it takes for labor to get rolling varies tremendously among women, with some going into labor quickly and others taking up to several hours to establish an effective labor pattern. Just be sure the mother does not get exhausted with the effort.

Herbal induction

Cotton root bark (*Gossypium herbaceum*) tincture is perhaps the most effective of all labor-inducing herbal remedies. The vast advantage of this herb is that it is very safe and therefore can be used in quantity. It does not produce nausea, nor does it cause the fetal heart rate to fluctuate or maternal blood pressure to drop, all of which are possible when using large amounts of blue or black cohosh. Chinese medicine states that cotton root bark is a good uterine contractant that is likely to work regardless of the overall symptom picture.

First, you can give a dropperful of blue cohosh tincture at 30 minute intervals for one to two doses. Then switch to cotton root bark tincture in dropperful doses spaced as often as every 15 minutes for the next 3 to 6 hours. According to the Chinese medical point of view regarding herbal interactions, using a uterine tonic tincture containing blue cohosh (or both blue and black cohosh) as a prelabor preparation and then using cotton root bark alone for the actual induction is a good combination, especially when the woman is overdue (Hobbs, 1999). Therefore, the prenatal combination tinctures mentioned in this chapter can also be used several days in advance of using cotton root bark to actually induce.

If the membranes are intact or the mother is a primigravida, it may take up to 6 to 8 hours to get active labor going, but you should see some evidence of increased uterine activity after the 3 hr mark. If the bag is broken, labor often gets rolling by three hours, especially in multigravidas. If nothing is happening after three hours, don't exhaust yourself and the mother with an endless effort. Try again another day, or incorporate other labor-inducing techniques.

You can also give the mother either cotton root bark tincture or tinctures of blue and black cohosh and ginger to take home. She should take 1 dropperful of cotton root bark or 10 drops of each of the other three herbs every 2 to 3 hours and increase the dosage to every half hour when contractions start. Although most of the time you will want to be there to nurture the process along, this will be appropriate for some women. This can work rapidly if the woman just needs a little nudge toward labor and can cause a very fast labor in a multipara. Be prepared!

Hydrotherapy

The woman can immerse herself in a birth tub of warm water, which will have two benefits; water supports the interaction of the maternal and fetal hormones and improves blood flow to the uterus and placenta. Both of these effects can increase the success of induction attempts. Herbs, acupuncture, homeopathy or whatever other methods you wish to try can all be used in combination with warm-water immersion (Enning, 2003).

Cold-water induction: Russian homebirth midwives are big advocates of using cold water during pregnancy, birth and postpartum. They feel it balances the system, stimulates the immune system and can be used to stimulate contractions. Most of the women they work with take cold showers twice daily during pregnancy, but a history of cold shower use is not necessary for this to work. A Russian pediatrician and midwife, Zinaida Bakhareva (1999) of Vladivostok, Russia, explained the method used in her community to encourage labor, which she reports is effective for about 80% of the women who are willing to try it.

Turn on a completely cold shower with the water running forcefully. The force of the water hitting pressure points all over the body is a key to the success of this technique. The mother should get in the shower literally a few seconds, just long enough to get fully drenched and have her skin stimulated by the force of the water. Zina emphasized that it works best when the woman is quiet while showering (no hooping and hollering about how cold it is). Some sign of increased uterine activity should be apparent 3 to 5 min after the woman is out of the shower. Zina was quite clear that when this works, you get very fast results. Barbara Harper speculates that the extreme cold may trigger the fetus ejection reflex if used late enough in labor (Harper, 1999). If nothing changes, wait half an hour, giving the mother herbs and doing other things to get labor going in the meantime, then repeat the shower. You can try this 3 to 5 times with a 30 min break between each dousing before deciding it will not work for a particular woman.

When you do get results, wait at least one hour before trying it again, although you may not need to do anything else. This technique can be helpful in women with ruptured membranes who have no contractions as well as those who need stronger contractions in established labor. Note that the use of cold during labor is entirely contrary to the theory of Chinese medicine, which strongly advises against exposing women to cold during pregnancy, birth or thereafter. The Chinese feel that cold can have long-term adverse health consequences by weakening the kidney Qi. However, the mother may prefer to try this instead of going to the hospital. Zina also emphasized that Russian midwives use this only for mothers who truly need to be induced or to have stronger contractions.

Stimulating cervical pressure points

This variation on cervical manipulation can be used to induce labor at term in a normal pregnancy, to augment active labor, and to stimulate the cervix when labor stalls. It can also be used in a woman prior to term if she has experienced a fetal demise.

Barbel Kesting (1999), the German midwife who shared this technique, learned it from a traditional midwife in southern India. Barbel has had a success rate of about 90% using it, although this kind of success is likely to be achieved only after a midwife has become skilled with the procedure. She feels it is so effective that indiscriminate use could start labor early. Barbel does not know why this technique works but speculates that it causes tight cervical and uterine ligaments to release, thus facilitating contractions and the opening of the os. For it to work, you must attend to all the factors described below.

- The cervix must be ripe, although it does not have to ripen on its own. If it is not ripe, use whatever natural means you find useful for producing ripeness, such as evening primrose oil. The degree of effacement is not relevant to success with this technique.

- The cervix must be centered between the yoni walls, although it can be posterior. You can try the technique with the cervix slightly off center; the more central the os, the more successful you will be.
- The bladder and rectum must be empty. The energy flow from the cervix must be unimpeded as it goes up the length of the spine. Therefore, give the mother a warm-water enema to remove any fecal material that may impede this flow. Do not use commercial enema preparations for this purpose.
- The atmosphere must be quiet, cozy and private. Candles, soft music, and one-to-one contact with the midwife greatly increases your chances of success. (It is best to clear out all support people, including the partner, until things really get rolling so that the mother can relax and focus.)
- It is ideal for the mother to be in water that she finds comfortably warm and that is deep enough to submerge her pelvis, at a minimum. If the water is not deep enough to cover the belly, place a towel soaked in warm water on her belly to help keep her warm. The tub in which she rests should be large enough to allow her to stretch out on her back with her spine and neck straight. The straightness of the spine facilitates the flow of energy and is important to the success of this technique. It may work without this, but it works best with the woman in a bath as described. Use folded bath towels to prop her back and neck at a slight angle to keep her face out of the water while keeping the spine as straight as possible.
- The mother's legs should be spread as far apart as is comfortable for her, flopped to the side, supported, and very relaxed.

Sit or kneel beside the tub. First don a sterile glove; then apply a light lubricant and place two fingers inside the yoni. Locate the urogenital diaphragm and check its consistency. If it is quite soft, proceed to the next paragraph. If it is at all tense, very gently move your fingers back and forth all the way around the muscle, applying the gentlest pressure until the muscle starts to soften. Release of this muscle helps to open the energy flow in the spine. (For information about which muscle you are looking for, review the chapters entitled "Pertinent Anatomy" and "Learning to Identify the Perineal Muscles" in HEALING PASSAGE.) Barbel has found that women often start to cry at this point, especially those with a history of abuse. Continue to gently massage this muscle until it is soft.

Next, find the cervix and begin stimulating pressure points in the cervix. To do so, imagine the face of a clock, with the points at 3, 6, 9 and 12. Insert the tip of your index finger into the os up to the level of the first joint. You will be stimulating points located at this depth in the internal cervical canal. Apply firm pressure to each point with the pad of your fingertip. The only way to get good at this is to do it. To get an idea of how much pressure to apply, straighten your index finger and use the pad to apply firm, even, increasing pressure against the solid surface until the tip end of your nail starts to blanche. Once you have achieved that much pressure ease off slowly, then move on to the next point. Note that there is nothing special about the way the points feel to the touch. If the cervix is effaced, you still want to press against the point on the inner surface of the cervix, not merely into the edge of the os. To do so, you may have to bend your finger joint around the edge of the cervix.

In first-time mothers: Apply pressure first to the 12 o'clock point and then the 6 o'clock point. Then press into the point at 3 and then 9 o'clock (up and down, then side to side). Starting with the top and bottom points first and then stimulating each lateral point successively is the most important thing. You could start with 6, then 12, then 9, then 3 as well.

In multiparas: Apply pressure to either the 3 or the 9 o'clock point first, then stimulate the opposite point. Then stimulate the vertical points at 6 and 12 (side to side, then up and down). With a multipara whose cervix is open enough to allow it, you can also spread your fingertips laterally across the cervix and simultaneously stimulate the 3 and 9 o'clock points. Then spread your fingers up and down and simultaneously stimulate the 12 and 6 o'clock points.

Keep this up for at least 20 minutes and no more than an hour, moving consistently from one set of points to the other in the proper sequence. In many cases, if this technique is going to work, it will trigger some uterine activity as quickly as 5 to 10 minutes after you begin. You will know the energy is moving when the baby starts to move and the woman reports an indescribable sensation above her pubic bone.

Start timing contractions when they begin and look for contractions that last one minute. At this point, keep up the stimulation for another 30 to 45 minutes to be sure labor is well established. When using this technique for stalled labor, some change can be expected in about 20 minutes.

Castor oil induction

Castor oil has been used widely for decades to induce labor. Castor oil contains prostaglandin precursors, causes intestinal mucosa to release prostaglandins, and also stimulates the bowels, which begin to contract and cause diarrhea about an hour or two after ingestion. The bowel activity is believed to stimulate the uterus by sympathetic response. The cervix must be ripe for castor oil to be effective, and the mother must be at term or overdue. Be sure to start inducing only after the mother has had a long, restful sleep. Castor oil induction may begin working as soon as an hour or so after administration, but may take 4 to 6 hours. Some midwives report that Metamucil (a fiber-based laxative product that is stirred into water and drunk) is just as effective and more pleasant to take.

Dosage: Various amounts of castor oil are used by different practitioners; ranging from 1 tablespoon to 4 ounces per dose. A good average dose is at least 2 tablespoons and no more than 2 ounces at a time, given one to three times as needed. Wait at least one hour before repeating the dose.

Getting it down: There are many recipes intended to get castor oil into the mother and down into her stomach before she throws it up. While not really bad tasting (it's pretty bland, actually), plain castor oil has a distinctly heavy, oily odor and is thick, viscous and very oily in the mouth, making it unpalatable and hard on a stomach already challenged by pregnancy. Here are a few suggestions for getting it down. Use at least twice as much carrier as castor oil and let the mother pick which of these formulas sounds most appealing. One midwife suggests having a wet washcloth ready to use after ingestion in case the mother wants to wipe her mouth out to eliminate the oily feeling, while another suggests having a mint candy available for the mother to suck on immediately after taking the mixture.

- Scramble three eggs, remove from the heat and add a dose of castor oil. Mix well.
- Add a teaspoon of liquid lecithin (or break open a couple of lecithin capsules) to any solution intended for drinking as this will help to emulsify the oil. Whip with a wire whisk or blend in a blender and drink immediately.
- Have the woman drink the oil straight, followed immediately by hot apple juice.
- Put the castor oil in 3 to 4 ounces of root beer, then place a palm over the glass, and shake it vigorously (or put it in the blender) to suspend the castor oil. Have the mother immediately guzzle all of the foamy root beer.
- Add a couple of scoops of ice cream to castor oil in fruit juice and blend. (Hilary Schlinger notes that women say orange juice "burns on the way out," so she has switched to using nonacidic juices such as grape, apple or cranberry.) The ice cream in this recipe may help to counterbalance the acidity if you use orange juice.
- Add castor oil to fruit juice other than orange and then add ¼ to ½ tsp of baking soda, which will cause the solution to foam, temporarily suspending the oil in the juice. Have the woman drink it immediately.

There is an emulsified, mint-flavored castor oil product on the market, which may or may not be more appealing than any of the above. If the mother really loves mint, she might try it mixed with fruit juice or with cold chocolate or carob milk. Remember that in some people, mint can antidote homeopathic remedies.

Some midwives add a little alcohol both to help with absorption and to relax the mother. The recipe below is a slightly more elaborate method of inducing with castor oil. Since it is more involved, it is probably best reserved for women whose cervices are less ripe than is ideal and for whom the onset of labor is very important (I used it on an overdue multiparous mother who had a very low RH_OD titer). Contractions may start right away or take as long as 6 hours to get going, so start this process first thing in the morning. Labor-stimulating herbs may be given once the initial doses are completed.

Give three 2 oz doses of castor oil in fruit juice spaced out over 3 consecutive hours, 6 in all. Use a pinch of baking soda and a whiz in the blender to help mix in the oil. This can be done with or without a little bourbon or brandy, which helps to loosen the mother up psychologically.

During the hour following the first dose, have her take a walk or a hot shower.

During the hour following the second dose, administer a high, slow, warm enema (you can use blue cohosh infusion).

During the hour following the third dose, repeat the walk or hot shower.

Possible problems: One disadvantage of castor oil induction is the tendency for the mother to become dehydrated, as the oil produces copious loose stools, which may be accompanied by intestinal cramping. Therefore, it is best for the mother to take castor oil under your direct supervision and for you to pay close attention to maternal hydration throughout. Also be warned that the use of castor oil, on rare occasions, has been associated with rupture of membranes without starting labor. It is also most unpleasant for women who already have problems with hemorrhoids, as the diarrhea will only aggravate them. Other methods may be equally effective in many cases.

There is much speculation among midwives regarding whether the use of castor oil can lead to an increased incidence of meconium passage. There is no evidence to support such a relationship. Meconium-stained amniotic fluid is much more common in postterm babies, and for those midwives who limit their use of castor oil to those mothers, what appears to be a correlation may only be circumstantial.

Enema

Simulation of the bowel can also be achieved by using an herbal infusion as an enema solution. (For more details, see the subchapter entitled "Cleansing and Retention Enemas.")

Belly massage

Induction effleurage: Massaging the uterus through the abdomen can be very helpful regardless of the means you are using to start labor. This technique focuses more energy on the uterus, as well as physically stimulating it. You can also consciously channel your energy to the uterus and baby through your touch. Cup your hand slightly and separate your curved fingers. Use your entire hand to firmly (but not roughly) massage the abdomen in a large circle, using your open fingers and the pads of your fingertips to gently grab and knead the uterus as you go. Don't be afraid to use firm pressure, but do not use jerky, abrupt motions or jab the belly with your fingertips, and avoid the navel. Massage oil (see "aromatherapy induction massage" below) can be a nice addition to the massage. The majority of women like this type of stimulation. If the mother does not want you to do it, show her partner or support person how to do it or suggest that she do it herself; otherwise, leave it out.

Aromatherapy induction massage: To induce a full-term mother, use 2 ml of palma rosa essential oil diluted in 100 ml of a carrier oil such as sesame (do not use peanut oil on a pregnant woman). Use this to give the mother a full-body massage, focusing on the back and abdomen 24 hours before you want labor to begin. This is reputed to boost the level of natural oxytocin (Gentlebirth archives, accessed 2000).

You can also add jasmine essential oil diluted in a carrier oil to your acupressure point massage. It should be rubbed into the points noted, as well as on the soles of the feet.

Mechanical dilators

Mechanical dilators of various kinds have been used for centuries in an effort to get the cervix to open. Today, osmotic dilators are available as laminaria tents (made from the seaweed *Laminaria japonicum*) and artificial laminaria (Lamicel and Dilapan [Gynotech, Inc]). These are sold as dried sticks and are inserted into the cervical canal under direct visualization. They absorb secretions and gradually swell up, thereby dilating the cervix. Several can be inserted simultaneously, but often the tents must be removed and the procedure repeated to produce the desired effect. An average of 4.3 Dilapan devices or 9.7 laminaria tents are required. The tents have been known to disintegrate upon attempted removal or become lost inside the uterine cavity.

Also currently used are extra-amniotic Foley-style (balloon) catheters such as a 24 F Foley designed for draining the urinary bladder and a specially designed double-balloon device, the Atad Cervical Ripener. Both have been used successfully to dilate the cervical canal with insufflation of the balloon. With both devices, a speculum is inserted and the uninflated tip of the catheter is placed inside the cervical canal under direct visualization. The balloon is then gradually filled with sterile water and left in place to apply counterpressure to the internal os and produce effacement and dilation. The tube of the Foley-style urinary catheter is then strapped to the woman's thigh so that it applies gentle traction to the filled balloon to effect dilation. The double-balloon device allows placement of one balloon inside the internal os and one outside the external os and is designed so that an optional dose of prostaglandin gel can be delivered via a port in the tubing that connects the two balloons.

While the use of mechanical dilators is probably a more attractive option than transport for induction, they seem invasive for routine midwifery use. Forcing a rigid device through the cervical canal runs the risk of damaging the mother's tissues or rupturing the membranes. Leaving any device in place creates an avenue for the entry of bacteria and it is uncomfortable for the mother. Although sweeping the membranes is also quite invasive, and should not be used casually, leaving a device in place goes one step further. With those precautions in mind, here is a protocol shared by Sister Angela Merdock (2003) for using a large male urinary catheter (24 F or larger) to effect dilation. The cervix must be ripe for this to work; it should not be done if the membranes are ruptured or if the mother is known to be group B-strep positive.

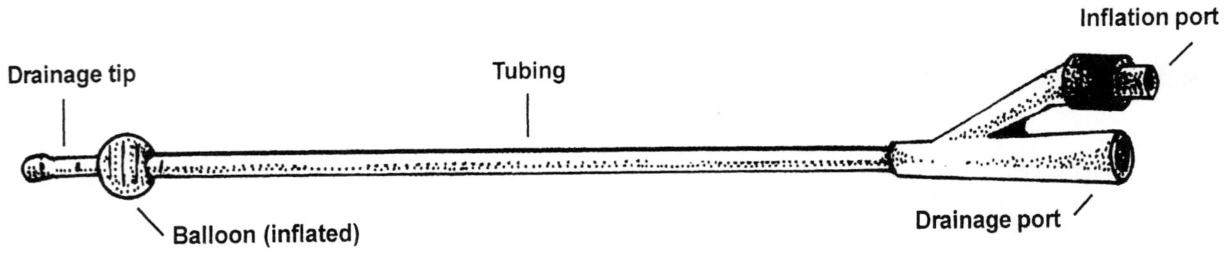

Foley-style catheter (the balloon for induction would be much larger than this)

1. Don sterile gloves and find the inner cervical os.
2. Insert the tip of the Foley through the internal os and advance it until it is between the lowermost uterine segment and the membranes.
3. Use a large luer-lock syringe to fill the balloon with 75 cc of sterile water. To fill the syringe, remove the needle, luer-lock the syringe tip to the syringe port on the Foley and inject the water. Repeat until 75 cc have been injected.
4. Create a deep fold in the flared end of the Foley and tape around it to prevent ascending infection. Form a loose loop with the length of tubing extending from the yoni and tape it to the mother's upper thigh in the same way you would tape the tubing of an IV. The loose loop will assist the mother in normal movement without pulling the balloon.
5. Instruct the mother to rinse her vulva with an antiseptic solution such as rosemary infusion or another type of antiseptic rinse each time she uses the toilet.

The balloon should fall out within 24 hours. Instruct the woman to call immediately when this occurs, as she is often around 5 cm at that time. If the balloon has not fallen out by 24 hours, remove it.

Artificial rupture of membranes (ROM or amniotomy)

I do not recommend rupture of membranes as an induction method; it is too unpredictable. Rupture of membranes starts the clock ticking (because the risk of infection is now increased), and limits the amount of time you have to leisurely work on getting things going. As a rule, artificial rupture of membranes to further progress is contraindicated with first-time mothers because there is no history of it helping in a previous labor. *Always keep in mind that rupturing the membranes is irreversible and one of the most potentially problematic decisions you can make.*

However, when absolutely nothing else is working, there is a good medical reason to induce and you are faced with either rupturing the membranes or going in for a hospital induction, it might be your best option, especially if the mother seems otherwise ready to go into labor and if this is what worked for her in a previous labor. If you transport, you might be faced with more interventive options, and hospital practitioners are very likely to break the membranes as part of their protocol as well. If the mother wants to try induction by rupturing the membranes at home, you should make the decision that if it doesn't work, transport is your next step. Place a time limit on how long you will wait for labor to begin. Sometimes herbs that have not worked before will work after the membranes are ruptured.

Do not rupture membranes if there is evidence of reduced amniotic fluid or if there is knowledge of group B-strep in the yoni. If the amniotic fluid volume is already low, draining more out may result in cord compression. If the woman is colonized with group B-strep, rupture of membranes invites infection to ascend into the uterus. The risks of rupturing the membranes and then having labor stop afterward must be carefully weighed against the hoped-for benefit of getting the baby out. Once dilation is well underway (at least 6 centimeters and preferably 8), rupturing the membranes may be something to consider, especially if this has worked to move labor along for a particular woman in the past. (See the augmentation section below for a discussion of all the things that may indicate whether rupturing the membranes during active labor will help or not.)

Augmenting Labor

Reasons to augment labor

In most cases, labor can take as long as needed, if the mother can eat, drink, rest, cope and maintain her emotional stamina and the baby is doing well. The exceptions to this, of course, are when disproportion is suspected between the mother's pelvis and the baby (when a long labor may eventually compromise both mother and baby) or when you are dealing with a positive group B-strep culture.

A wide variation in normal labor patterns appear when women labor naturally without the constraints of hospital protocols. However, there are times when stimulating labor is called for to minimize problems and allow the mother and baby to stay at home if they so desire. Allowing a slow labor to drag on until the mother is exhausted or otherwise compromised is a setup for transport. When the mother is compromised, the baby is usually not far behind. You must also take into consideration that a tired or compromised mother equals a tired uterus and a much higher risk of problems with getting the placenta out, as well as hemorrhage after the birth.

Other reasons to augment labor include maternal anxiety about how long labor is taking (in some cases, a little external stimulation can help push women past a scary point) and the need to help the woman who is resisting surrendering to the strength of labor. In the presence of a rigid cervix or contractions that are just not strong enough, augmentation can sometimes really turn things around.

For augmentation to work best, it is important to support the mother in clearing up any reasons that make it difficult or problematic to have the baby at this time, such as fears about any aspect of the birth process. Getting clear with the mother that she and her uterus are connected is the first step toward getting labor re-established.

With the exception of castor oil (which produces too much physical discomfort for most women to want to use it during active labor) and the Foley catheter, all of the induction techniques described in this chapter can also be used for stimulating stronger contractions during labor.

Artificial rupture of membranes (ROM)

Whether to rupture the membranes to speed a labor in progress is a tricky question. With intact membranes, if labor stops, everyone can go home and wait for it to resume. If the water is broken, you do not have as much leeway because rupturing the membranes increases the risk of infection for both mother and baby: the longer the bag is broken the more the risk goes up. In almost every case, labor will progress just fine with the membranes intact; ROM is therefore very rarely warranted.

Since there are no guarantees that labor will proceed neatly to birth once the waters are gone, rupture of membranes, in the vast majority of cases, should be considered only after all other options have been tried and proven unsuccessful. In women who have a history of rapid progress after either spontaneous or artificial rupture of membranes, and in whom nothing else has made much difference, breaking the waters may be your best option; however, evaluate for other favorable indications first. In one dramatic case of mine, the woman had felt very interfered with when her water had been broken during her first labor, so we waited patiently at about 7 centimeters for several hours before she decided that rupturing the membranes was something *she* wanted to try. Once the bag was out of the way, the baby came in the next 20 minutes. Women who have a pattern of responding well when something "from outside" is done to them may also do well with artificial rupture of membranes; however, it is important to talk to them first and be clear about the potential risks versus the *potential* benefits.

ROM may cause the cervix to close down: Keep in mind that ROM may cause a temporary regression in dilation by 1 to 2 centimeters and sometimes more. This occurs when the forewaters have been acting as the chief dilating wedge; when they are removed, the presenting part does not always immediately drop down to fill the space. In that case, the cervix frequently recedes to meet the presenting part and in the process closes down a bit. Thus the anticipated immediate benefit to labor does not materialize, and the woman (not to mention, at times, the midwife) gets discouraged. I always wonder if I wouldn't have been better off leaving well enough alone. If all the other factors are favorable, however, ROM may still have beneficial effect with a recovery of previous progress occurring over the next hour or so.

Making the decision: During an internal exam, it is possible to assess whether rupturing the membranes may make a difference. The more you take the entire labor picture into account and the more conservative you are about using this intervention, the less likely you are to have it backfire on you. There are several questions you should ask yourself first.

Is the baby in a cephalic, vertex presentation? Unless you are certain that the baby is in an anterior vertex position, do not rupture the membranes, as you risk cord prolapse, getting the baby stuck in a not-so-great position or both. A breech baby needs the forewaters to equal out the pressure on the cervix, prevent a premature urge to push and protect against cord prolapse as well.

Where are the fetal shoulders and back? If you determine that shoulder dystocia is more likely in this mother, note that some midwives feel that the risk of shoulder dystocia may be further increased when a large baby has undergone internal rotation to OA with his shoulders and body remaining oblique. Intact membranes give the baby more buoyancy, maximizing the possibility that the baby's torso will eventually rotate into the transverse diameter of the brim (Schlinger, 2003). See the chapter entitled "Abdominal Examination Techniques for Use during Labor" for more details.

At what station is the presenting part? Is it filling the pelvis or partially floating, with a big area of space behind or around the circumference? If the presenting part is filling the pelvis, this is a good sign that ROM may help. If not, rupturing the bag may cause a cord prolapse or may fix the baby in an undesirable position. If ROM is necessary, it should be done so that the water drains out slowly. (How to maximize the chances of this is covered in the chapter entitled "Cord Problems and Emergencies during Labor.")

Are you trying to get the presenting part to move into a more favorable position? If you are still trying to get a baby to rotate, breaking the waters will usually not help because the bag helps to buoy the baby up and creates space for her to turn. Once the baby is in a good position, ROM can help her settle in so that she stays there.

What does the bag feel like during a contraction? Does it get tense? Does the presenting part descend with the force of the contraction? If the answers to the later questions are favorable, ROM might help. If not, the contractions are not very strong or labor may not even be underway. If the bag advances downward with contractions but the head does not move down, then the bag is probably acting as the main dilator and rupturing it is not likely to increase the strength of contractions. If the bag hourglasses deeply into the birth canal either during or between contractions, the forebag and the hindwaters are communicating; breaking the bag is not likely to do much of anything in this case.

Is the bag tightly applied to the head? If the bag is tightly applied to the head and the head descends with contractions, the head itself is acting as the dilator and breaking the bag probably won't do much.

Is the bag so strong that it is acting like a trampoline, holding the presenting part back? When this occurs you can feel the baby and forewaters trying to advance with a contraction but unable to do so because of the resiliency of the bag. The bag feels thick and becomes taut during contractions but does not press forward with the force of the contraction. In this case, ROM can *almost always* make a positive difference in the progress of labor.

Are contractions strong and frequent enough for this point in labor? Infrequent, mild contractions may or may not pick up once the bag is broken. If labor is really languishing, it is better to try to get contractions going first or have the woman rest, as appropriate, or you may wind up with no labor and a busted bag. This is especially true in first-time mothers. Try using cotton root bark tincture to stimulate more effective contractions.

Is the mother past 6 centimeters? Breaking the waters early in labor is a real gamble because it is so unpredictable how long early labor will last, especially in first-time mothers. ROM after 6 centimeters is also a gamble, but the further along the mother is at the time of rupture, the better your chances that it will really help, especially in multiparas with a history of it helping before. It is best to wait until at least 8 centimeters or more with good, steady contractions.

If you feel rupture of membranes might help, and the mother is amenable, see the chapter entitled "The Placental Membranes and Amniotic Fluid during Labor" for detailed instructions.

Slow Progress in Labor: An Overview

There are three approaches to the perception of labor; the temporal model, the progress model and the well-being model (Scholles, 2003). The temporal, or time-based, model is popular among doctors and was codified for modern practitioners by Emanuel Friedman in the 1960s to early seventies (Friedman, 1967). Friedman used the rate of dilation and fetal descent to arrive at statistical averages to delineate "normal" progress in labor in terms of the time it takes for these changes to occur. Although Friedman confirmed that there is a huge variation in normal labor, the middle part of the bell-shaped curve he devised has, unfortunately, been focused upon as the range for "normal." It is ironic that his work has been used to force women into a specific timeframe and has perpetuated an artificial standard of normality for women who labor in institutional settings, when, in fact, his work supported the long-held midwifery view that very long or very short labors can also be normal. In midwifery circles, the current manifestation of the temporal model modified by the notion that progress must also be considered promotes use of the "partograph," a complex labor record charted on a graph which plots dilation and descent according to the amount of time labor is taking.

The progress model is popular among childbirth educators, doulas and many nurse-midwives. Born from the constraints placed on laboring women by the protocols and limitations of birthing in hospitals, it puts forth the idea that labor can take more time than average, as long as progress is being made. Although time is still considered, progress moves more to the fore as the focus of when and how to intervene. Thus the time-based focus is modified with the recognition that the progress of labor can be unique for an individual woman and her baby.

The well-being model predominates in the homebirth midwifery model of care. Here, while time and progress are not forgotten, maternal and fetal well-being become the primary concern and labor can take as long as it needs to take if the mother and baby are doing well. Time, in and of itself, is not considered a barrier to allowing labor to take its course. In this model, what constitutes progress is much broader than is possible within most institutional settings, and slow progress in labor is considered in this context. The range of normal among women is understood to be extremely wide. As long as the mother is eating, drinking, eliminating, resting, and coping; the baby is doing well; and there are no signs or symptoms of obstructed labor, no complication, per se, is inferred.

Among homebirth midwives, stories abound of women who, by medical standards, had very unusual labor patterns but still gave birth to perfectly fit and healthy babies and who did well themselves. Labors that have lasted for days have been reported, with women dilating one or two centimeters a day. As a society, we don't hear about such labors because it is only in the environment of homebirth that such variations of normal have been allowed to occur without interference. Women who labor like this often have an ebb and flow of openness to the energy of birth, integrating it in steps that are less overwhelming than a straightforward labor would be.

While holding the space that affirms that most labors are normal, it is equally important to recognize that slow labor can result from numerous underlying problems. The midwife's attunement to the process, as well as her skill and experience, will make the difference in determining which labors fall into the wide range of normal and which are truly headed for trouble unless interventions that she can offer or that are available only in a hospital setting are applied. This discernment helps to avoid allowing a stuck labor to remain that way for fear of intervening thereby winding up with an exhausted mother and distressed baby.

Why labor slows down

The most common problem that midwives and women face once labor begins is a labor that either slows or comes entirely to a standstill. The root of the problem can fall into several broad categories, some of which have been formally recognized in textbooks for decades. These reasons have been categorized according to various players and processes in the event. In medical terms, "the three Ps" have been used to describe these factors: the passenger, the passages and the powers. In midwifery terms, these considerations include BBEEing present as follows:

- B–The mother's whole being; her sexual, emotional, psychological, spiritual and physical milieu, including her soft and bony pelvic tissues
- B–The baby's whole being (she is far from a passive passenger, healthy babies will actively seek the best position for descent whenever they have the opportunity)
- E–The energy of birth
- E–The environment of birth

Hand in hand with problems in labor comes the excessive pain that often accompanies a poorly situated fetal presenting part. Certainly not least are the mother's psychological and emotional responses to labor. Fear, as well as unresolved or completely unconscious issues that can be stimulated by the powerful sensations of labor, can impede if not completely stop progress because the labor brings up feelings that she is reluctant to allow to surface. Anxiety and fear also increase the levels of stress hormones in her body, which contribute significantly to a slow labor as well as make fetal distress more likely.

Another factor is the environment that the mother has chosen for her labor. If her personal needs for safety, privacy, intimacy and trust are not met, labor will invariably be affected for the worse. Sometimes these needs are not met even though her caregivers are aware and sensitive in regard to preserving the environment of birth. This happens when women cannot or will not articulate their thoughts regarding what feels right to them. Some women have grown up and lived in such unsafe environments that they have no reference for how to create a personal "safe space." This is especially true for women whose traumatic body memories are triggered by labor but for whom a conscious recollection of the traumatic and abusive events is missing.

One particularly significant aspect of how the caregivers relate to the woman involves their sensitivity to her background, including cultural and ethnic norms that are familiar and comforting to her. Innocent comments or behaviors from caregivers who are not knowledgeable in this area can bring labor to a standstill. It is the midwife's job to independently educate herself regarding the mother's cultural norms and then ask respectful questions to fill in the gaps. This should have occurred during prenatal care.

Progress may lag at any time during labor. The point in labor when this occurs is an important consideration when evaluating why it has happened and what assistance is needed to get things back on track. It is, of course, possible for several factors to influence the situation at one time; this can sometimes confuse the picture and make it hard to know how to proceed. Fortunately, almost any problem in labor can be overcome (Simkin & Ancheta, 2000).

When to take a second look

Given that the range of variation from woman to woman is so wide, how does a midwife decide when progress in labor is such that some type of specific intervention is necessary? In general, "normal" labor is defined by midwives more by the overall physical, psychological, emotional and spiritual condition of the mother and baby than by the number of centimeters per hour the mother is dilating. The decision regarding when to intervene is also influenced by an individual midwife's experience regarding labor patterns that suggest that something particular is impeding progress, as well as the midwife's prediction of how that might change over the hours to come. Laboring women who resist the energy of birth may strive to remain lucidly in their head, they may be chatty or complaining through most contractions, or they may be psychologically unable let go into that altered state of consciousness that signals that the hormones are in optimal balance to facilitate progress; these women can be expected to have longer than average labors. Clearing the room of all observers, dimming the lights, pulling the blinds and promoting quiet may well help these women "turn off" their neocortex. However, watchful waiting works only to a point.

The midwifery model of care basically moves from a let-nature-take-its course approach for a labor moving along well to carefully selected, minimally interventive techniques intended to gently guide the labor back to a smooth flow toward birth, to midwifery interventions that are more invasive but still avoid the risks of drugs, instruments and surgery. It is not compassionate midwifery to allow a woman to labor long and hard when an internal exam could be done to determine if the cause for the delay is a physical problem. Only when all her midwifery tricks fail, when the mother calls a halt and asks to be transported, or when a complication develops that requires hospital care, does the midwife suggest that medical-model interventions might be appropriate.

(Separate chapters entitled "Don't Just Do Something," "Endless Early Labor" and "When Active Labor Is Slow" also address more specifically how to help women experiencing prolonged labor.)

Endless Early Labor

Latent labor may progress smoothly into early labor which can be quick and easy when the baby is in an ideal position and well settled into the pelvis, but it can easily last 12 to 24 hours and sometimes longer. The impression of how long labor is lasting is often subjective. The mother may have strong toning contractions during the days prior to labor and may become anxious or excited and not sleep. Anxiety will cause the woman to release stress hormones, which may result in an even longer period of early labor contractions as these hormones tend to slow the action of the uterus. The more tired she becomes, the longer the labor seems and the fewer resources she has to cope. The longer early labor lasts, the more an inexperienced midwife begins to think along the same lines, believing something might be really wrong when, in fact, active labor probably hasn't even begun.

Basic considerations

Conditions that may mimic labor: Sometimes what appears to be labor to both the woman and the midwife is, in fact, something else. Chief among these imposters is a urinary tract infection. Symptoms may include pain above the pubic bone, flank (side) and back pain, and frequent urination. Whenever early labor is going nowhere, you should review the woman's prenatal record for signs and symptoms of previous urinary tract infections, then inquire about nausea, vomiting, urgency, pain on urination and blood in the urine. A urinary tract infection may even cause uterine activity due to irritation. Check the mother's temperature and do a dipstick exam of a clean-catch urine specimen for blood, protein and nitrites. (See DIAGNOSTIC TESTS for full details on diagnosing and treating urinary tract infections).

Dehydration will not start preterm labor but can result in an irritable uterus that may have both the mother and the midwife thinking labor has begun. The simple answer is to hydrate the mother and see if the uterus calms down. Lastly, sometimes women near term are so miserable and tired of being pregnant that they convince themselves and their midwives that they are in labor when they are not. In all of these situations, a lack of cervical changes and a uterus that is not changing shape with contractions will help you recognize that this "ain't it." Recall that toning contractions are felt in the fundus as a tightening, while labor contractions are felt low down in front (Sutton, 2001). In any event, the woman needs to relax, get the urinary tract infection or dehydration handled, if either is a problem, and let go of this being labor. Sleep will be a welcome relief. Hot baths, massage with a lavender-scented oil, chamomile infusion (½ oz of chamomile flowers to 1 pint water steeped ½ hour) or a glass of wine may all help her unwind. Hopefully, this will break the cycle and pull her out of "labor" mode if she is not ready (Varney, 1997).

Psychological factors: Women can sometimes experience long early labors due to fear of going into active labor. This stress, once again, causes the release of hormones that further provoke the problem. The solution is to have someone knowledgeable (preferably the midwife herself or an experienced doula) stay with the woman, provide a restful atmosphere and calm the mother down.

It is important to validate the woman's feelings regarding how her labor is going. Previous traumatic birth experiences often leave a woman anxious and afraid to go through labor again. She may have had a set idea about how her labor would progress; there is nothing like a long, apparently unproductive period of tiresome uterine activity to burst that bubble. Encourage her to express whatever she needs to–cry, yell, beat a pillow if necessary–in order to move through and not hold onto stressful emotions. This will help her release tension, move through her feelings, and allow her to be more present with her labor as it is. In fact, being present with the reality of her labor is one of the most important things she can do. Taking each contraction one at a time can really help women not to anticipate and not wear themselves out.

Remember the signs that constitute progress in early labor: Often, within the medical model, dilation and descent are the only recognized signs of progress. Coupled with the rush to get the birth over, it can be forgotten that the contractions of early labor prepare both mother and baby for active labor. Patience during early labor is an essential skill for the midwife. The more posterior, unripe and uneffaced the cervix is, the longer prodromal labor will take; the problem is compounded when the baby is posterior and the fetal spine is deflexed. The midwife must remind herself and the mother that changes are occurring that will soften the cervix and align the os with the force of the contractions, and that progress is indeed being made that will lead to the next phase of labor, dilation and descent. Women and midwives must learn to pace themselves during both early labor and strong prelabor uterine activity.

Determining if there is an underlying physical problem: It is also true, however, that long early labors can signal an underlying problem with the way the baby is trying to descend. Sutton and Scott note that long, painful, erratic bouts of early labor contractions are often associated with posterior babies who are trying to rotate to the front or babies who are having a problem entering the brim. Each contraction may last as long as 15 to 20 minutes. (For more information, see the chapters entitled "Entering Pains and Back Pain in Labor" and "Assisting a Woman Whose Baby Is in a Posterior Position.") Perform a careful abdominal exam to check for engagement and to rule out posterior presentation, remembering that occasionally the baby's back can feel anterior but the head can be twisted around at the neck into a posterior position.

A very posterior cervical os is often associated with a posterior occiput. The force of the uterine contractions comes down on the lower uterine segment in front with the head being driven against the sacrum in back, producing excessive back pain. The baby must turn or the uterus must work for hours bringing the cervix more forward so that dilation can really begin. Likewise, cervical rigidity or scarring can cause slow progress. Mothers can have contractions that are quite strong and long for many hours with a little to no change in such a cervix. These signs should prompt you to investigate with a review of the woman's history and a thorough internal exam. See the chapter entitled "Cervical and Other Soft-Tissue Problems during Labor" for suggestions on how to deal with these problems. Dysfunctional uterine activity can also, in rare cases, be a problem, although this usually doesn't develop until labor is well underway. (See the chapter entitled "Difficulties with Contractions" for more details.)

What to do

When there is nothing specific that needs to be done to assist the situation, the best medicine for a long early labor is time and patience. The mother should be encouraged to relax; to distract herself with reading or light projects, to go to a movie, shop or the like (but not overexert or exhaust herself); and to take naps and go to bed early, even if she feels she cannot sleep. Rest is important. She should avoid semi-reclining positions and sitting with her knees higher than her tuberosities, both of which can prevent normal rotation and engagement (Sutton & Scott, 1996).

Feed the mother: Marginal hypoglycemia can forestall the onset of active labor. Feeding the mother a meal rich in complex carbohydrates may be needed to get labor going. She should eat nonspicy, nourishing foods and drink when thirsty. She can eat any nonsugary food that she wants, keeping in mind that spicy foods may cause heartburn in active labor. If you believe her uterus is tired, also give her electrolyte balancing fluids to help reduce lactic acid levels.

Time contractions: Simkin and Ancheta (2000) recommend timing a few contractions periodically to assess whether labor is picking up. It is best for the partner to do this, preferably discreetly, and only *after* contractions have become strong enough so that distraction techniques no longer work to take the woman's mind off the sensations. The partner can then relay this information to the midwife. By taking a back seat, the midwife will avoid making the woman feel like a "watched pot," and is less likely to feed any anxiety the woman may have about how strong and long her labor may be.

Specific positions and activities for a long early labor: Many positional recommendations in this text are recommended for a variety of labor difficulties. Maternal position changes can work to realign the presenting part in a better position during early labor and may work to transform troublesome, colicky contractions into more effective ones. These positions are described in detail in the chapters entitled "Techniques Used to Help the Baby Descend during Labor" and "Assisting a Woman Whose Baby Is in a Posterior Position." They are reviewed here because those positions that assist later in labor can at times work wonders in early labor.

- Leaning forward may help the head pivot from an asynclitic position and drop down through the brim.
- An open, exaggerated knee-chest held for 30 to 45 minutes may help reposition the head. This can be tried if labor is taking a long time, even if you are not sure what position the baby is in.
- Belly-lifting can be used when the abdomen is pendulous or when the woman prefers to stand; it is performed during a contraction. However, if entering pains are occurring in the suprapubic area, lifting immediately above the pubic bone may interfere with the baby's attempts to engage. To avoid this, lift at the level of the navel. Leaning forward with the back straight, especially in water, is also a good option. (Also see the chapter entitled "Entering Pains and Back Pain in Labor" for more details on this technique.)
- Semi-reclining is suggested by Simkin and Ancheta (2000) as a position for women who have a pendulous abdomen as a way to line up the uterus with the pelvic brim, encouraging better application of the presenting

part to the cervix, and thus more effective contractions. However, unless the baby is in a good position and is already engaged, what is gained in better alignment may be lost by reducing the spinopubic angle. In addition, any reclining position naturally causes the weight of the uterus to shift backward toward the mother's spine. A reclining position may thus lessen the chance that the baby will rotate if the presenting part is poorly aligned with the axis of the birth canal. If you suggest this position, make sure the angle of recline is such that the weight of the uterus is shifted back into the torso but not all the way back toward the spine, and that the woman does not become hypotensive in the process. Belly-lifting or an abdominal binder with the woman standing will accomplish the same thing without reducing the spinopubic angle.

The following additional suggestions can also help labor to progress (Gaskin, 2003).

- •Remember the connection between the mouth and throat and the cervix. Keeping the mouth and throat open and loose, even in early labor, is important to progress.
- •If the woman is tired, resting in a tub of warm water can help her relax. Contractions often quiet down with warm water, and this may allow her to sleep. The hot sitz bath technique described in the chapter entitled "Difficulties with Contractions" may also quiet down early labor and allow sleep.
- •Have the mother watch videos of women in labor, as she may get going by sympathetic response.

Abdominal Pregnancy

It is very unlikely that a mother will make it through an entire course of prenatal care without having an abdominal pregnancy discovered. However, if you are caring for women who have not received prenatal care, as might be the case if you are working in the developing world, you may, on some rare occasion, be faced with detecting an abdominal pregnancy for the first time in a woman believing she is in labor who presents herself to you.

In those few abdominal pregnancies that make it to term, the baby is very easily palpated through the abdominal wall, although this is frequently true in thin women who have normal pregnancies. The women report that fetal movement has been particularly uncomfortable or downright painful throughout the latter part of pregnancy. The uterus may be displaced anteriorly or posteriorly. On internal exam, displacement of the yoni canal may be noted, it may be stretched forward behind the pubic bone or pressed backward or to one side. In any event, the cervix is squashed to the side and difficult to reach. Some minor amount of dilation may occur as a response to the prevailing hormones, but there is only rarely any effacement to speak of. A uterus that is anterior to the fetus may be seen in outline over the lower abdominal wall. Small fetal parts or the head may be palpated through the fornices and are found to be clearly outside the uterine cavity. Abdominal massage over the woman's belly does not cause firming over the baby as it would if the baby were inside the uterus. Toning contractions never progress into active labor.

Uterine Torsion

This is another very rare reason why labor may not progress. Twisting of the uterus, which usually occurs during normal pregnancy to a certain extent (most often to the right) can be extreme, stretching the uterus and supporting ligaments and impairing blood flow, all of which contribute to varying amounts of pain prior to labor and fetal distress. A history of abdominal surgery, pelvic tumors, abnormal fetal presentation and abnormalities of the uterus, spine or pelvis are associated factors, however it can occur without any of these being present. Torsion can mimic a slow, progressive concealed abruption because to the increasing severity of the pain as the uterus enlarges. The onset of labor only worsens the pain. Symptoms will lead to you transport prenatally; therefore you are most likely to encounter this problem in women who have received no prenatal care. It will be impossible to discern if torsion is the cause of the problem, although if the woman is thin and your palpation skills are good you might be able to feel the round ligament abnormally stretched at an oblique angle across the abdomen, although such palpation is likely to be quite painful. Dilation typically does not progress, as the forces cannot pull on the cervix as they should. If neglected, uterine rupture may occur. The only remedy for this manual repositioning of the uterus during surgical delivery.

When Active Labor Is Slow

Active labor is defined in both the medical and midwifery models by contractions that become stronger and longer, that produce progressive cervical changes in the form of effacement and dilation and that result in fetal descent.

The medical temporally based model for normal labor, based on Friedman's work, expects that active labor will take, on the outside limits of normal, no longer than 11.7 hours from the time a woman reaches 4 centimeters to complete dilation. Definitions of normal labor include *minimal* progress at a rate of 1 cm an hour after active labor has become established. At that point, standard North American obstetrics defines protracted, or slow, labor by a rate of dilation of less than 1.2 cm per hour in a primigravida and a rate of less than 1.5 cm per hour in a multigravida. Descent is expected to accelerate when the woman reaches 7 to 8 cm and become more rapid after 8 cm. Protracted descent is defined as a rate of less than 1 cm of descent per hour in nulliparas and less than 2 cm of descent per hour in multiparas. Arrest is defined as a complete lack of dilation or descent. Arrest of dilation is defined as 2 hours with no cervical changes, and arrest of descent as 1 hour with no fetal descent. The World Health Organization defines slow labor as less than 1 cm of dilation an hour but allows a limit of four hours before intervention is recommended to see if the woman's labor gets back on track on its own.

All these medical-model averages are problematic as they do not translate into individual patterns of normal for each woman and as they focus on dilation as the most important criterion of progress, thus presenting an artificial norm. To quote the 21st edition of WILLIAMS OBSTETRICS (Cunningham, et al., 2001), "When time breaches in normal labor boundaries are the only pregnancy complications, interventions other that Cesarean delivery must be considered before resorting to this method of delivery for failure to progress." It is in this arena that midwives excel.

<u>Characteristics of slow active labor</u>

Simkin and Ancheta (2000) have done a fine job of summarizing the features of prolonged active labor. Once labor is underway, it develops the following features:

- •Contractions space out; that is, the time interval between them becomes longer.
- •Contractions become shorter and weaker.
- •Contractions progress to a certain point then plateau out, remaining the same hour after hour, neither building nor diminishing in strength.
- •The mother learns to cope well with the intensity of her labor, dealing with the sensations by using the same approaches over many hours. She may report that her labor is easier to handle.
- •On internal exam, the cervix has undergone little or no change.

<u>Dealing with a slow labor</u>

The factors that can contribute to a slow active labor are similar to those that contribute to slow early labor, such as:

- •Emotional issues about events that occurred in the past or in relationship to others (present or not), including the baby
- •Lack of privacy and quiet, a sense of being observed
- •Poorly positioned fetal head
- •A large baby
- •Weak contractions
- •Maternal dehydration, hypoglycemia or exhaustion
- •Physical variations in the mother

(Simkin & Ancheta, 2000)

Note that a large infant, per se, only rarely prevents spontaneous birth (Cunningham, et al., 2001). Delay with large babies is usually because the baby's head and the mother's pelvis and soft tissues need extra time to mould because there is less wiggle room than with a smaller baby.

<u>How slow is too slow</u>? The medical model of care places a great deal of emphasis on getting the baby out in a given amount of time. Underlying this concern regarding long labor is fear that absolute disproportion may be present, which can lead to uterine rupture and fetal death if labor is left to its own devices. Ultimately, this is a fear that labor usually doesn't work and that it is an accident waiting to happen. In contrast, midwives are much more willing to allow for flexibility and individualization of time parameters during labor. Midwives know from experience that it is safe and even desirable to allow labor to continue as long as mother and baby are doing well. A patient "watch and wait" policy avoids unnecessary interventions and sees many women through to normal births at home. In order for this to happen, the mother must be willing and able to eat, drink, rest and eliminate. A long labor calls upon the midwife to continually reassess what is taking place and how the mother and baby are faring. Allowing labor to take its course is not the same as letting things go to the point that both mother and baby are compromised.

Maintain intact membranes: One of your top priorities should be to preserve the membranes intact for as long as possible to facilitate rotation and descent. This means minimizing exams. Those that are required should be done carefully to avoid accidental rupture. There is a great deal of latitude in how long labor can go on without physical compromise to the mother or baby as long as the membranes are intact.

Environmental impediments to progress: Some women manage to give birth in almost any situation (or else the surgical birth rate in hospitals would be 100%!). However, since midwives have the opportunity to create an optimal environment at home, they should take advantage of it. When labor slows down, try the following:

- Reduce the number of people in the room.
- Eliminate that "watched pot" feeling for the mother by clearing extraneous people out of the house as well. Before you do so, however, get agreements from a few people that they will be available to come back after the birth to help clean the house.
- Eliminate extraneous chitchat conversations audible to the mother.
- Darken the labor room (dim the lights, close the curtains).
- Invite the mother to go into a smaller, more womb-like room, such as the bathroom, if one is available.
- Have only one calm and centered person who understands the mother's need to internalize and won't chat with her stay with her.
- Unless she is very scared and needs to be calmed down or assisted to stay present, avoid eye contact with the mother (thus helping her "go within").
- Ask her to tune into her baby, her pelvis and her soft birth canal and focus on releasing, using any techniques she learned prenatally.
- Offer simple, straightforward and image-based suggestions to her only as necessary to get and keep things back on track.
- Once the situation has been processed verbally, avoid additional, prolonged conversation with the mother. Such conversation will keep her neocortex active.

Slow labor due to physical impediments

Give labor some time to get back on track after emotional issues and the overall environment have been attended to. Then, if indicated, go on to address any specific physical problems that may be complicating the picture.

Characteristics of slow labor due to physical impediments: The following indications should cause you to question if fetal malposition, disproportion or a large baby might be an underlying factor (Simkin & Ancheta, 2000). Non-productive contractions are often associated with a malpositioned head and have the following characteristics:

- Unpredictable variations in intensity and duration occur.
- Contractions bunch up, with two or three very close together, followed by a long pause before the next.
- Contractions get further apart after a period of more typical active labor contractions.
- Back pain that persists between contractions is present.
- Progress slows down or comes to a standstill.
- The woman may have a strong urge to push prior to complete dilation.

Fetal positioning or disporportion: Perform a thorough abdominal and, if indicated, internal exam to determine the fetal position. This may not be easy, especially if the head is high and the forewaters are large and tense. Be careful not to rupture the membranes. Each event which takes place in a well-progressing labor takes time. If the baby must first work with the contractions and his mother to arrive at a better fit between his head and the pelvic cavity before descent and rotation can proceed, then this will take more time. Such situations can be favorably influenced by having the mother remain upright, change positions and move freely during labor.

Changing the baby's position: If you think the baby's position needs changing, see the chapter entitled "Techniques Used to Help the Baby Descend during Labor" or "Assisting a Woman Whose Baby Is in a Posterior Position." If you can't tell for sure if the baby is in a good position, the good news is that suggesting the mother try different position changes will probably not make the situation worse.

If the baby is quite small or quite large: Small babies have plenty of room to get themselves into odd positions. Large babies can also get themselves into odd positions, and correction in these babies is more difficult because there is less room. The things you would do to correct malpositioning in these babies are the same as for more average-sized babies. As well, big babies can just take longer to come down than smaller ones, even if the mother has had babies before. Be patient and be sure the mother pushes in a position that places no pressure on her sacrum.

Physical variations in the mother: Maternal physical factors may be hampering progress. Supporting the pendulous uterus with a binder, lifting the uterus during contractions, and utilizing positions and activities which flair the ilia may help. (See the chapters entitled "Techniques Used to Help the Baby Descend during Labor," "Unstable Lie, Oblique Lie and Transverse Lie in Labor" and "Recognizing and Dealing with Obstructed Labor.")

Weak contractions: Weak contractions can be due to the position of the baby, cephalopelvic disproportion, maternal exhaustion, or a combination of factors. Look for the underlying problem and correct it. If nothing specific can be identified, try either stopping labor entirely or the hot sitz bath treatment described on page 1028.

Maternal exhaustion or dehydration: Rest and rehydration are the obvious solutions to these problems. Do not try to stimulate labor or do gymnastics to reposition the baby if the mother is tired and dehydrated. Rather, give her fluids either by mouth, rectum or via IV, and foods to restore her energy. While waiting for labor to pick up, help her relax and have a nap, if possible. This will renew her, even if she winds up being transported. A warm bath, warm milk, or sedative herbs (such as skullcap, valerian, passionflower, or hops), or both, can be used for relaxation. Encourage her to doze off between any contractions.

Dehydration can also result in weak contractions. An IV can sometimes cause labor to pick right up and proceed to birth. The safest solution to use for this purpose is lactated Ringers (no dextrose). Run in 300 ml, then slow the drip down to 125 ml/hr and see what happens to her contractions. To avoid fluid overload, discontinue administration of the IV solution and attach a saline lock to the cannula as soon as labor appears to be back on track.

If labor does not stop but isn't going anywhere

Very often, when physical factors have been ruled out, there are emotional issues that have not been acknowledged, expressed or dealt with. Emotional issues can lead to physical problems. For example, a woman who is tense and afraid can hold tension in her perineal muscles, causing the fetal head to be pushed over to one side with the force of contractions. This is a classic cause of persistent asynclitism. Having one's life completely in order and being issue-free are certainly not prerequisites for birth, but quite often unresolved emotions can hold up a labor for a very long time.

If labor stops entirely

When a woman dilates to a certain point and labor stops, there is no hurry to have the baby unless the membranes are ruptured or some other situation warrants more haste. In fact, when labor is taking its time, having it simply stop altogether for a while is one of the best possible things that can happen.

Let the woman rest, sleep, eat and go about her daily life. The midwives can go home unless they live very far away. Only leave after thoroughly discussing the mother's feelings about what is going on, including any feelings of abandonment she may harbor regarding your leaving. She may feel "wrong" or that she is disbelieved about being in labor. Point out that some progress has been made, an indication that real labor activity was truly ongoing for a while, but that labor has wide variations from woman to woman and even from pregnancy to pregnancy. Explain that you need to take a break (or take care of your other responsibilities) while there is some time and that you will be fully available to her when she needs you again. Instruct her to call the minute anything changes. When labor starts again, things can move very quickly, especially if the woman has given birth before, so be prepared. If you do live far from the mother, it is best to wait at someone else's home, if possible, so the woman does not feel like she must perform. You might be able to do a few home visits in the area or even see a movie while you wait. Be aware, however, that it could take a day or two or even longer for things to get started again.

UNIQUE LABOR PATTERNS

NOTE: This chapter should be studied together with the one entitled "Difficulties with Contractions."

Midwives have identified some unusual labor patterns which are within the very wide range of normal. These patterns often look like a problem at first, but are not because they lead to birth. Always keep in mind that the nature of the labor may be protective in ways you cannot directly assess until the baby is born. Intervene to "correct" a contraction pattern only when it is clearly impairing progress. Also be aware that dysfunctional contractions are the most common early manifestation of fetopelvic disproportion, both relative and absolute, and that absolute disproportion is very rare in industrialized countries.

Labor when the umbilical cord is short

Midwives have reported that some cases of short, weak or otherwise unusual contraction patterns are associated with such things as velamentous insertion of the cord, short cord or cord entanglement. This phenomenon is discussed in detail in the chapter entitled "Cord Problems and Emergencies during Labor."

Start and stop labor

Women who are allowed to labor on their own will sometimes have contractions that start and stop over a period of days, with the cervix partially dilating with each new series of contractions, finally culminating in birth. This may or may not be related to a cord problem as above, and is not a problem as long as the mother and baby are maintaining themselves with rest, food and fluids, there is no evidence of structural obstruction, the membranes are intact and the fetal heart rate is normal. Such a start-and-stop labor pattern occurs frequently enough to be considered within the range of normal, although it is very culturally unfamiliar, since once dilation is underway, protocols of most hospitals dictate that the baby be born in a timely fashion either with labor-augmenting drugs or via surgery. The pattern is most common in multiparas whose labor appears to have stopped, although they are quite dilated. Be prepared; the baby can come quickly once contractions resume.

Precipitate labor and birth

A precipitate labor lasts less than 3 hours. In some women, very strong contractions result in such rapid labors. However, in most cases, the primary reason why labor is so fast is a lack of resistance of the maternal tissues. Fast labors are also seen among women who had long difficult labors for their first baby, during which they overcame their basic fears of birth. For the next baby, they may have a super fast labor. Conditions that contribute to precipitous labor include multiparity, large pelvis, lax soft tissues, strong contractions, a small baby in a good position and a previous precipitate labor. Of course, some fast labors are due to uterine stimulating drugs.

While precipitous labor has been said to be dangerous for mother and baby with an increased risk of maternal and fetal injury (including brain bleeding, damage and hypoxia from interference with placental circulation from strong frequent contractions), the risk is really no greater than in most labors (Oxorn, 1986).

A precipitous birth occurs when the baby starts to descend rapidly with no detectable labor to warn the mother that the birth is imminent. In such cases, you will probably miss the birth. If women have a history of precipitous birth, their family should be well prepared prenatally to assist in the event that no attendant is present.

DIFFICULTIES WITH CONTRACTIONS

NOTE: Review the information in the chapters entitled "Anatomy and Physiology of Uterine Changes during Late Pregnancy and Labor," "Assessing the Progress and Strength of Labor: An Overview" and "Unique Labor Patterns," before studying this chapter.

Many problems with the quality of uterine contractions can occur. Some of these stem from contractions that have normal characteristics but that are less effective than usual at dilating the cervix and moving the baby down. The primary reasons for poor quality contractions include uterine muscle exhaustion; maternal fear and, with it, pelvic tension; less-than-optimal fetal position and protective labor patterns. When a poor fetal position and poor contraction pattern are combined, a difficult labor is usually the result.

Preliminary Evaluation

Evaluate the woman for the type of contractions she is having; her general condition; the degree, location and timing of pain and the contractions, effect on her labor (Is her cervix changing? Is the baby descending? Is the bag getting tight during contractions?). If the membranes are ruptured and the baby has developed a caput, this indicates forceful uterine action. Weak contractions produce little to no pressure down and have little, if any, effect on the membranes and, if they are broken, no caput forms on the baby's head. Are the contractions normal with the problem centered at the cervix? If so, see the chapter entitled "Cervical and Other Soft-Tissue Problems during Labor." Is there pain in an unusual location? Is it constant? Is it out of proportion to where she appears to be in labor? Is there any bleeding? Assess fetal well-being; is the baby in distress?

Basic approaches to problematic contraction patterns

Look through the rest of the chapter for information about a variety of uterine contraction problems. The following is just an overview of what to do once you have the problem identified. The therapies given here can be used in a variety of situations. Additional considerations for specific findings are given throughout the chapter.

Hypotonic uterine action: If you feel the uterine action is hypotonic, allow the mother to rest if she is tired. Once she is rested, carefully evaluate fetal position, and then stimulate contractions to get some force to assist maternal positions and activities to get the baby to turn.

Acupressure to promote effective contractions and descend the baby: If weak contractions are the only problem and the mother is rested, these techniques can be very effective (Lowe, 2003):

- Stimulating Jianjing (GB-21) strongly descends the Qi, helping bring the baby down during dilation or pushing as well as increasing the strength of contractions during any part of labor. Apply firm pressure to the GB-21 point on one or, preferably, both shoulders.
- LI-4 can be used by itself, or simultaneously with SP-6 to regulate and increase the frequency and strength of contractions. LI-4 also helps bring the baby down during pushing.
- Pressing BL-67 also promotes strong downward movement and is very effective when the fetal position is not ideal.

To locate these points, see the chapter entitled "Traditional Chinese Medicine."

Hypertonic uterine action: If the uterine action is hypertonic, do not try to stimulate it even more. Rule out malpresentation, especially posterior presentation, as the symptoms are similar. Rest the mother with sedative herbs and 2 grams of calcium (El Halta, 1998). Very often, after a period of rest, the uterus responds normally when labor resumes.

Hot sitz bath to relieve painful, ineffective contractions: Stockham (1898) recommends the hot sitz bath, as described in the chapter entitled "Cervical and Other Soft-Tissue Problems during Labor," to relieve nonproductive contractions. She found that the bath caused the uterus to quiet down and later resume normal activity after the mother had rested.

Characteristics, Causes and Specific Treatments for Ineffective Contractions

Attempts to catagorize problems with the strength or duration of contractions have produced the following categories. However, in practice, some of these variations are difficult to define and identify on a clinical level. Therefore, take these descriptions with a grain of salt and always look to the condition of the mother and baby, rather than the definition, when deciding how to proceed.

Contractions that are too weak

Contractions with prelabor characteristics (inverted gradient): Labor contractions that result in progress have three characteristics, called "gradients." An initiating wave comes from a pacemaker region and moves downward; the duration of the contraction is mediated as the wave progressively moves away from the pacemaker; and the intensity of the contraction diminishes starting at the fundus and sweeping to the lower uterine segment. Clinically, this manifests as contractions that are coordinated, with cramping and pulling sensations usually noticed in the suprapubic area.

The uterus cannot do the work of labor when one or more of these characteristics is occurring in an inverted fashion, as they do with prelabor contractions. Inversion of the propagation gradient means that the initiating wave begins in the lower segment and moves upward. Inversion of the duration gradient occurs when contractions last longer in the lower segment than they do in the upper segment. When the intensity gradient is inverted, the contractions are stronger in the lower segment than in the upper.

All three types of activity are known as reversed polarity. When they occur together, the contractions are completely ineffective, producing neither dilation nor descent. When only one or two of the gradients are involved, some dilation occurs but it is very slow. These contractions do not further the progress of labor and produce no effacement or dilation of the cervix. They often occur in bouts during toning activity or just before labor begins. Women with such contractions usually report pain, which may be severe. Backache is often a primary symptom. The baby remains high and the cervix is thick, uneffaced and not well applied to the presenting part.

What to do: Wait for labor to begin. In the meantime, give relaxing herbs to help calm the uterus at night.

Uterine inertia or hypotonic uterine action (weak contractions): These are defined by contractions that are normal in their character yet not strong enough or frequent enough to move labor along. True hypotonic uterine action occurs when active labor has been underway for some time, often with a history of previously strong contractions, but the contractions have subsequently diminished in duration and strength. Otherwise, "weak" contractions are probably just early labor. In such cases uterine inertia may be diagnosed when labor has not really begun.

Hypotonic uterine activity is more common in multiparas, but may occur in first-time mothers who are carrying a posterior or asynclitic baby. These weak contractions usually occur at a rate of less than 2 per 10 minutes once active labor begins. Uterine tonus is normal, muscle activity is coordinated and the lower segment is relaxing between contractions, but the uterus is not active enough and the forces are too weak for progress in either descent or dilation to occur. The normal discomfort that accompanies effective uterine activity is either mild or entirely absent. It may be difficult to tell if the woman is in labor or not. When you perform an internal exam during a contraction, you can feel that the force exerted on the cervix and the presenting part is minimal and, even if the membranes are ruptured and the head is low, no caput has formed. The observable abdominal changes that are usually seen during the effective contractions of active labor may be diminished or absent.

In many cases, however, a uterus that reacts like this is tired, just as any muscle can become tired from exertion. Quenby and colleagues (2004) found that both myometrial capillary pH and oxygen saturation levels were low in uterine blood samples taken from women experiencing hypotonic contractions. Both findings reflect myometrial lactic acidosis.

What to do: The traditional midwifery approach of resting and sleeping the mother whose contractions are flagging has a very sound physiological basis. Recommend food, fluids and rest rather than augmentation if the mother is tired and the contractions peter out after labor has begun. Insistence on moving ahead with poor contractions invites the development of a constriction ring, fetal distress and problems with the birth of the placenta and bleeding afterward. Trying to force a tired uterus to contract is hard on the mother and may be fruitless. Meanwhile, give her electrolyte balancing fluids, such as Recharge, to help to flush out the lactic acid that is built up in the muscle and restore normal activity. A few doses of homeopathic arnica (30C), which is widely used for athletic muscle fatigue, will help as well.

After a rest, if the uterus needs a little boost, some sort of uterine stimulating remedy can be discussed. If the baby is in a good position, other options include cotton root bark tincture which can be used to stimulate stronger contractions. Uterine stimulants such as nipple stimulation, uterine massage and sexual activity may also help get things going. Walking, an enema, or sweeping the membranes to a depth of 5 cm all the way around the internal os may also help (use the last only in women whose last group-B strep culture was negative). In first-time mothers with a deeply engaged head and a thin but posterior cervix, you can try pulling the os forward, sweeping the membranes, and pushing the head up a little to allow some amniotic fluid to run down and create forewaters. This may cause the contraction pattern to improve (Greenhill, 1951). Other techniques, as described in the chapter entitled "Natural Induction and Augmentation of Labor," can also be used in these cases. If the baby is not in a good position and some uterine activity is occurring, you can try position changes and activities to correct this before contractions are restimulated, which may jam the baby into a really bad position. If that doesn't work, contractions should be encouraged as you continue to try and correct the fetal position.

Secondary uterine inertia: Inertia is defined by effective contractions that become weak, infrequent and irregular. Progress ceases and labor may stop entirely. Inertia also occurs with the mother and her myometrium are fatigued and is often associated with prolonged, obstructed labor.

What to do: Treatment involves a thorough investigation regarding whether labor is actually obstructed, hydration and rest. If obstruction is confirmed and is uncorrectable, transport is in order.

Oxytocin dependency: This is a little understood phenomenon seen in women who have had several previous labors artificially stimulated with IV oxytocin. Midwife Shari Daniels (1978), who taught me about this problem refers to it as Pit dependency (Pitocin being the trade name for oxytocin). The woman typically enters active labor and progresses to 5 or 6 cms, at which point her contractions do not increase in strength; they either remain at that level or space out. This is often the point at which the oxytocin was administered in previous labors.

What to do: Should this occur, more oxytocin will get things moving. However, since there is no safe way to administer oxytocin at home during labor, try nipple stimulation, accupressure or other physiological means of stimulating contractions. Cotton root bark tincture is the herb mostly likely to help labor to resume. Use it in combination with the other uterine-stimulating activities mentioned above.

Uterine response to overdistension: Overdistension of the uterus, which can occur in either a multiple pregnancy at or near term with good-sized babies or in polyhydramnios, may be an underlying factor in abnormal uterine action.

Rapid overdistension: Acute polyhydramnios of late pregnancy is the best example of rapid overdistension. The quickly rising volume of amniotic fluid may lead to a rise in tonus and a fall in the intensity of contractions once labor begins.

Slow overdistension: The increase in uterine volume occurs slowly when the mother is carrying more than one baby or has chronic polyhydramnios, where the build-up of fluid has been gradual, allowing time for the uterine muscle to compensate. In this case, the tonus and intensity of the contractions are usually normal.

Contractions that are too strong and very painful or which persist, and which are ineffective

Tetanic contractions (irritated uterus): Constant uterine contraction also causes labor to come to a standstill. This problem arises when the uterus will not relax. Tetanic contractions significantly reduce the amount of oxygen received by the baby as well as the uterine muscle and cause extreme pain to the mother.

Most often, what appear to be tetanic contractions result from pain due to an abrupted placenta. When abruption is the cause, the uterus may not actually be in a tetanic state, but the blood building up behind the separated placenta causes the uterine wall to become constantly rigid as well as so painful and irritated that it is impossible for the mother to distinguish whether her uterus is contracting or not.

When abruption is not the cause, truly tetanic contractions may be caused by overstimulation of the uterus from the use of misoprostol, oxytocin or, more rarely, natural means of augmentation such as herbs (very rare), as well as too-frequent attempts to manually dilate the cervix. The uterine muscle may in a spontaneous spasm, undergoing the equivalent of a charley horse, which could be secondary to lactic acid build-up from overexertion. (See the section entitled "Hypertonic [incoordinate] uterine action" below for suggestions about calming the uterus down.) Act quickly, because if the uterus will not calm down, you will need to transport, as the baby cannot tolerate prolonged lack of blood flow to the placenta. Sustained tetanic contractions can easily lead to catastrophic uterine rupture and fetal demise.

<u>Incoordinate uterine activity</u>: These are varieties of contractions where the uterine muscle activity is not working properly. There are several ways these can manifest. Again, these categories are vague and tend to overlap.

Asymmetrical uterine action: This problem is characterized by localized contraction waves. The pacemakers do not work rhythmically, and each side of the uterus acts independently. Short contractions alternate with long ones, and all are equally ineffective. While the stronger, longer contractions may result in some cervical dilation, they are much less effective than normal uterine activity.

Hypertonic (incoordinate) uterine action: This is usually associated with early labor in first-time mothers and is often related to maternal fear. Symptoms range from mild to severe. Apparently strong, always painful contractions may be frequent but vary as to their strength and length and result in little to no dilation or fetal descent. Pain may occur before the contraction can be palpated and may persist after the uterus softens. Continual pain, especially in the back, is not uncommon. Uterine tone is high; the uterine wall is tender to the touch and cannot be indented by fingertip pressure during a contraction. Tone persists after the contraction subsides. The increased tension and spasm in some parts of the uterine muscle may persist between contractions.

Labor may begin normally, or these ineffective contractions may occur from the beginning. The woman usually complains of intensely painful contractions. As time passes, the colicky nature of the pain increases and the woman may guard her uterus with her hands. The cervix may be thick or thin, applied tightly to the presenting part or hanging loosely in the birth canal. Dilation typically stops around 6 to 7 cm. An early urge to push may develop. Urinary retention and vomiting are also frequently associated factors. While labor is prolonged, full dilation and birth can occur, although frequently something must be done to assist dilation.

<u>What to do</u>: First, assess the mother for placental abruption or obstructed labor. Tumultuous labor with no progress that suddenly changes to weak contractions is a classic pattern in uterine rupture. Once these are ruled out, the best thing to do is to try and relax the mother and her uterus. Calming the woman will allow her to rest in anticipation of normal labor resuming later. Lobelia, motherwort or skullcap tincture and Rescue Remedy may assist with this. Place the mother in a warm bath or shower and turn the lights down low. Give her a massage using an oil scented with lavender. Do whatever she can come up with that normally helps her relax. If nothing else is working, her medical back-up provider may be able to prescribe a mild sedative. Labor will often restart on its own with a more effective contraction pattern after the mother and her uterus have had a period of quiet.

Colicky uterus (fibrillation): This is a type of hypertonic uterine action in which contractions are frequent, ineffective, irregular and erratic. The midportion of the uterus is often contracting more strongly than the fundus, and there may be patches of hypertonic muscle activity scattered throughout the myometrium. Before, during and between contractions the woman feels pain that is out of proportion to their strength. Tonus may be slightly elevated, but the uterine action is not effective and the baby is not pushed down, nor does the cervix dilate well. In some cases, the lower uterine segment is also hypertonic and resists descent of the head, giving rise to persistent lower abdominal pain and severe backache. The os dilates slowly; the cervix may be thick or thin but feels tight and unyielding. This type of pattern is also often related to maternal fear and raises the risk of developing a constriction ring and may also interfere with placental separation.

Constriction ring: A localized spasm of the myometrium may develop secondary to incoordinate uterine action. It is discussed in the chapter entitled "Recognizing and Dealing with Obstructed Labor."

Psychological Impediments to Progress during Labor

Numerous psychological factors can impede progress toward birth. Whenever the energy of labor stops flowing for a while or seems stuck, an emotional or psychological issue may need to be addressed.

Dealing with feeling in the midst of labor: The primary emotion that stalls an otherwise normal, active labor is fear. In early labor, especially in first-time mothers, this is often a simple fear of how strong the labor is likely to become. If a woman has not been through labor before, early labor contractions are already probably the strongest uterine sensations she has ever experienced, and she knows this is only the beginning. How strong will labor get? Can she handle it? She may also have a fear of motherhood, economic concerns, ambivalence regarding the sex of the baby, worry about the ensuing changes in her relationship with her partner, fear of damage or permanent changes in her body (due to stretching or tearing), concerns over her future sexual desirability, fear of uterine rupture (if she had a surgical birth previously), fear that strong labor will damage her baby, fear of losing control or embarrassing herself, a feeling of being overwhelmed, unresolved or unconscious sexual abuse issues, other types of abuse issues or a persistent fear for her own life (as opposed to the intense but fleeting fears that tend to arise in conjunction with the fetal ejection reflex). These are common fears that she may not be able to articulate very well. While a woman does not need a lot of intellectual stimulation in labor, helping her move through her fears will cause her catecholamine levels to drop and allow her to open to the energy of birth, helping to move labor along. In general, fears in labor can be addressed as they arise. It is most helpful to:

- Ask the mother how she is feeling. If she doesn't express fear, ask if she is afraid, letting her know how very normal this is.
- Paraphrase what you have heard her say, to be sure you understood it correctly.
- Assure her that it is perfectly okay for her to feel whatever she is feeling. Invite her to open to the fear, let it become bigger and breathe into it. Ask her to locate the sensation of fear in her body, then breathe into that area, doing so should allow it to diminish. Explain that opening to fear will help to let it expand and move out of her body. Talking though the previous traumatic abortion or birth experiences and helping her see herself dealing with it in a healing way, or helping her understand that this labor offers an opportunity for healing, can help as well. If this does not help, continue to explore with her what her fear may be linked to; sometimes she will not be able to get in touch with the source. In this case, or in women for whom delving into the specifics seems inappropriate, simply helping her stay in the present can get her through.
- Validate her concerns, rather than minimizing them, and let her know she is not the only one who has ever had such a concern. Let her know if you share her concern. Be alert for a mother's gut-level intuitive sense that something may really be wrong, as opposed to a knowledge-based "intellectual" fear.
- Talk to her about where the fear is coming from, especially if she is concerned about damage to the baby. This will help differentiate an intuitive knowing on the mother's part that her baby is not safe from other sources of fear (such as her own unresolved birth trauma). Help her focus on being present with what is happening right here, right now. Have her put her hands (or take her hands and overlie them with your own) on her belly to feel fetal movement or follow a contraction or touch the baby's head, if she is pushing, to ground her in her present reality. Assure her that the baby is well prepared for the stress of labor, and that labor helps make the baby ready to adapt to being outside her body.
- Provide accurate, reassuring feedback, but do not misrepresent the situation.
- Recognize that many fears that arise during labor can be traced back to a woman's early childhood and personal experiences of her own birth. These deep-seated issues will not be fully resolved during labor, but helping her release her fears and focus on the present can help tremendously in getting her through her current labor. (See the chapter entitled "Understanding Physical and Sexual Abuse Issues" in Volume I for more details.)

Prolonged active labor: A woman may have plenty of reasons to keep labor going as long as possible. Other reasons include fears about how strong labor may become, fears for her own safety (tearing, bleeding, etc.), money, changes in her relationship with her partner, fears that the baby will be abused, or concern over having another child or a child of the undesired sex; just about any fear that is of sufficient concern to the mother can delay progress. For example, during one very long labor, the father was being very attentive. I later discovered that he has been having an affair during the pregnancy. The attention the mother was getting was most welcome and she believed it would disappear after the birth.

Prolonged resting phase: If a spontaneous urge to push does not occur after several hours of complete dilation (especially if the mother is unable to eat, drink, rest, and cope) and there appears to be no physical reason for the delay, try to figure out what might be holding things up on other levels. A history of sexual abuse can be a big factor. The pelvic pressure of later labor can bring back body memories of events that are often completely buried subconsciously. Allowing pelvic pressure to build becomes a dilemma as the psyche tries to protect the woman from painful memories that may be restimulated by the sensations of birth. (Just imagine how much pressure a child might experience from the fingers or penis of a grown man. Similar trauma may be associated with childhood enemas or previous genital mutilation.) Therapists report that many women's first memories of abuse surface after they have given birth. Although this is certainly not always the issue, keep this possibility in mind.

Women with such histories may lose it by becoming unable to focus, overwhelmed by the physical sensations of fetal descent or hysterical when they finally start to push or "leave" their bodies (which hold the sensations and the memories) so they can have their baby. Attempt to direct their focus on what is happening *in the present*. Keep them apprised of their progress and give verbal support. Touching the baby's head can help some women relax and stay focused on what they are doing. Wait until after the birth to address the possibility of childhood sexual abuse, if you feel it is appropriate.

One woman I attended stopped her labor for 12 hours at full dilation. As time went on she talked about how, to survive in her dysfunctional family, she ensured success by never trying anything she thought might be too hard. She had previously had a surgical birth for her first baby without ever going into labor. With a clear decision on her part that she wanted to tackle pushing, we used a combination of therapeutic touch, herbs, massage and nipple stimulation to get her labor going again. She expressed a great deal of fear during pushing but pushed anyway and had the baby at home after a 4 hr second phase during which she would push for a while, integrate her experience, and then go back to pushing.

Women may resist the back pressure inherent in the process of the baby descending through the pelvis and opening the bones. Although most of the time this pressure subsides as the biparietal diameter passes below the sacral promontory, sometimes it doesn't. This is especially true if the baby has a hand near the face (the elbow and arm over the chest can increase and prolong back pressure considerably). In any case, back pain represents progress as the baby moves down. Encourage the woman to recognize it as such and welcome it. Fears regarding tearing, parenting, and losing control are also common inhibitors of spontaneous pushing.

Some women resist the feeling of rectal pressure because they are inhibited by the possibility of passing stool. If this is a big issue, the woman can self-administer a small hand-held enema early in active labor (Fleet enemas are available in any drug store). This will cleanse the lower bowel and do away with this concern. If a woman doesn't want to do this, encourage her to realize that passage of stool is a good sign of progress, signifying that the baby is moving down with pushes. Pelvic floor tension resulting from any of these reasons can cause the head to cock into an ill-fitting position and further compound the problem.

At its best, labor induces a primal state that overrides ordinary concerns regarding modesty or inhibitions. Women who are self-conscious about bodily functions have usually not given themselves over to labor in the way that is needed. Encouraging them to get up, out of their chosen position, even to go outside for a walk, can jar their control and help them let go.

Women must make having the baby their top priority, above being comfortable, avoiding pain, or shying away from any underlying fears. If they don't open to the energy of birth and allow it to come through them, their babies simply won't come out!

Cervical and Other Soft Tissue Problems during Labor

There are many births in which the cervix dilates without any problem and the midwife does not find it necessary or desirable to perform even one internal exam. Sometimes, however, the cervix itself resists the force of contractions. Knowing when and how to deal with a cervix that is not dilating can mean the difference between a lovely homebirth and a surgical birth in the hospital. This chapter will cover all types of cervical problems.

Preventing Cervical Problems in Labor

Every midwife will encounter a certain percentage of women who have problems dilating. Techniques that generally assist labor in moving along can prevent the majority of stalled labors due to cervical problems. Encourage the mother to stay as loose and open as possible. The mouth, throat, cervix and yoni are very symbiotically connected. One excellent way to promote cervical softening is to have the mother blow air noisily out of her loose lips. If she feels so inclined, kissing and sexual intimacy with her partner can also loosen things up (Gaskin, 2003). Loving, flowing energy can change the whole quality of labor because it melts away resistance. Another helpful technique is to have the mother tune into her cervix and consciously work on relaxing areas where she senses tension; she will be well prepared to do this if she has had good prenatal education in this regard.

However, there are a few problems, such as scar tissue or a posterior os in a primipara, that cannot always be predicted or eliminated before labor begins and may not respond to the usual labor-enhancing techniques. Typically, problems with cervical dilation fall into predictable patterns according to the advancement of labor, but most of these problems can present at any time during labor. The sections below outline different types of cervical problems, and include suggested methods for resolving them. It assumes that you have exhausted the suggestions found in the chapter entitled "Active Pushing" and now need more specific techniques.

Specific Problems and Solutions

Bleeding as a sign of cervical trauma

Very often, trauma to the cervix results in bleeding, which is usually a deep red and may be slippery with a mucusy feel. However, bright red liquid blood could be from a previa or low-lying placenta, although most of the time, such bleeding is also coming from cervical trauma. In any event, the possibility that it is from the placenta must always be entertained. See the chapter entitled "Bleeding due to Placental Disruption" for more details on differentiating the two.

Notes on recommended treatments

Homeopathic remedies: Homeopathic remedies may be used with great success to treat any type of tissue trauma. The first remedy to give is arnica in 30C or 200C doses orally. In addition, or as an alternative, arnica oil can be applied directly to the traumatized tissues. Arnica relieves symptoms of bruising, swelling and strain. It resolves swelling and helps restore prolapsed tissue to its normal location.

Cervical manipulation: Cervical manipulation is one way to correct a variety of cervical problems. For example, when a stubborn cervical lip is impeding progress, risking trauma and causing undue pain, it can be reduced with the fingers (more on this later in the chapter). Cervical manipulation is controversial because it can lead to tissue damage, but so can many of the problems noted in this chapter if they do not resolve with other techniques.

This chapter assumes that you will resort to manual cervical manipulation of any kind only after having tried other techniques to remedy the situation and have decided, along with the mother, that cervical manipulation is your best option at this point. It is very important that the mother be willing to go ahead with this, because in most cases cervical manipulation is painful for her and it is important that she not feel victimized by it. This is especially true for women who have a history of abuse. Note that midwives who have done their own cervical manipulation during labor with their own children have reported that when they did it themselves it did not hurt. Often a woman can be instructed in how to perform the manipulation herself.

Previous cervical damage

Previous cervical damage may be the underlying cause when severe edema or a stubborn anterior lip develop during labor. Damage is usually secondary to previous surgery (i.e., cerclage, biopsies, cryosurgery, etc.), damage from instrumental delivery (forceps or vacuum extraction), or tearing during a previous labor that resulted in scars that dehisce during labor. Very rarely, previous intrauterine infection or cervical damage leaves such severe scarring that normal dilation is impossible.

Every woman with a history that places her at risk should be encouraged to take prophylactic measures prenatally to maximize the flexibility of scar tissue during labor. If she has not done so, or if those measures did not adequately soften the tissue (as demonstrated by a particularly rigid os on internal exam), use sterile technique and insert several (up to eight) whole capsules of evening primrose oil in the fornices and inside the lip of the os, particularly near the area of greatest rigidity. It is best for the membranes to be intact when the capsules are inserted. The oil will help soften the scar tissue and help labor to progress. This should be done prior to any attempts to manipulate the cervix and may work so well that no further intervention is required.

Posterior os

Whenever a very posterior os is found, the cervix does not dilate as efficiently because the opening force is not centrally located in relationship to the pulling action of the uterus; instead the force of the contraction is directed about 2 to 3 cm in front of the os, into the lower uterine segment. This is like trying to put a T-shirt on a child by pulling straight down on the shirttail with the neck hole over his face; the hole has to be repositioned over the child's head before the shirt will go on. Often an extremely posterior os is associated with a posterior baby. (For details regarding what to do if the baby is posterior, see the chapter entitled "Assisting a Woman Whose Baby Is in a Posterior Position.") A woman who has a long cervix prior to labor may also tend to have a more posterior os during early labor, especially if the head is low, even when the baby is well positioned. Even a cervix that is more than half effaced but quite posterior can take a very long time to be pulled into a less posterior position so that dilation can progress.

If the mother is having good contractions but the os is very posterior, first palpate to determine the position of the baby. If the baby is posterior, use maternal positioning to try to get the baby to turn. If the baby is already anterior and you know the woman has a long cervix, it can be very helpful to pull the cervix into position. Have the mother lie on a firm, flat surface, flattening her lower spine against the surface as necessary so you can reach the os. Insert your gloved hand just as a contraction subsides and reach back or to the side to find the os. Hook two fingers in the anterior rim, pull the cervix forward into position, and maintain it there during the space between contractions. Leave your hand in place as the next contraction builds and pull the cervix toward the center of the pelvis, using all the strength you can muster. Hold it there both during and between contractions. Do this for 2 or 3 contractions, and then stop. It may also help to sweep the membranes as described in the chapter entitled "Natural Induction and Augmentation of Labor."

Have the mother get up, move around, and give her a 30 minute break. During this time, have her stand and lean forward with her back straight. If her abdominal muscles are lax, have her perform the belly-lift technique described in the previous chapter. Then, recheck to see if there has been any change. Depending on your findings, you may elect to manually reposition the cervix as before and repeat this sequence every half-hour or so until the cervix is where you want it to be. If the cervical position has corrected itself, you need not do anymore.

Attempting to reposition the cervix in short but frequent sessions works much better than centering the cervix for many contractions in a row. Prolonged attempts can be much more painful, can cause the mother to become tense and less likely to let it be done again, and can tire both the mother and midwife. The method described allows you to bring the cervix into position, provide time for the uterus to do some work, and then recheck relatively soon. The problem should be corrected in a couple of hours, sparing the mother many hours of prodromal labor. The use of forward-leaning positions between sessions, with or without the belly lift, can make repositioning that much quicker and more effective.

Achalasia (a-kah-LAY-zee-ah) of the cervix

This is an old term for failure of the structurally normal cervix to relax and open. It often reflects maternal psychological resistance to the strength of labor. Maternal fear or control issues may play a part. Physiological factors include a history of hormone-based contraception within six months of conception in first-time mothers or long-term use in the past with no subsequent birth, previous anovulatory menstrual cycles, and a history of extended periods of natural hormonal imbalance. Most of the techniques for dealing with a rigid cervix listed below can also be used when the cervix is structurally normal but refuses to open.

Rigid cervix

A rigid cervix is defined as one with an anatomic abnormality. It can make itself known any time during the dilation phase of labor. Rigidity may be due to scarring from previous infection, lacerations or surgery.

The degree of rigidity can range anywhere from an unyielding region of the edge to a thick "pop-bottle lip," that is, a slightly thickened, quite resistant ring of tissue. You may feel areas of localized rigidity with or without an irregular surface, indicating a scar, but very often the entire opening feels rigid and you cannot localize any particular area of damage. While some rigidity will be broken up by the strength of contractions in active labor, some cervices will hold fast even through contractions that are quite strong. The possibility that the cervix is rigid should be explored whenever a woman remains at the same dilation for several hours when she is past 4 cm. Breaking up the rigidity can cut out hours of very hard labor. Here are some things that might help.

Spasm of the internal or external cervical os

Here the cervix cannot relax and does not dilate and progress ceases. This is a type of incoordinate uterine action which results in contractions that are stronger in the cervix than they are in the lower uterine segment. The only solution for such an event is to rest the mother and do things to relax the uterus in the hope that normal contractions will resume. For suggestions, see the chapter entitled "Difficulties with Contractions."

Acupressure to release cervical resistance: Stimulation of SP-6 is a traditional technique which has a direct action on the cervix, causing the os to yield to contractions; this point also helps establish or enhance active labor. It may be useful if the cervix is rigid. Apply firm pressure to SP-6 with the thumb or index finger (the point may be very sore). Betts suggests "using this point on one leg at a time for approximately one minute (count slowly to 60!) then using it on the opposite leg 20 to 30 minutes later." LI-4 can also be stimulated simultaneously on the same side to increase the frequency and strength of contractions (Betts, 2002; Lowe, 2003; Maciocia, 1998; West, 2001).

Herbal remedies to soften the cervix: In very early labor, 6 to 8 capsules of evening primrose oil placed in the fornices will help soften the cervix considerably over the next 12 hours or so. Another herbal remedy that can be used for a rigid cervix at any point in labor is gelsemium (yellow jasmine root) tincture. This herb can be almost miraculous in its ability to soften a rigid cervix. I have *felt* cervices soften beneath my fingers as a woman took the tincture in her mouth. It must, however, be used *very* carefully (see below) as it is a powerful and potentially dangerous herb. Administer an initial dose of no more than three drops in a small amount of hot water. Have the woman sip this slowly, holding each sip under her tongue before she swallows.

Gelsemium acts on the central nervous system to relieve spasms and in labor seems to direct its energy to the cervix. However, overdoses can depress the central nervous system; in the worst case scenario, it can cause respiratory paralysis. If one tiny dose does not help (you should see some improvement), a repeat dose of 1 to 3 drops may be given again in two hours. If the cervix doesn't show some improvement after the second dose, give up and move on to other remedies. If you do note improvement, a third dose can be given two hours later if you feel it is necessary. *Do not exceed a maximum dose of 10 drops in 24 hours and never give more than 3 drops in a single dose, which is slowly taken as described.* You may also use a homeopathic preparation of gelsemium (30C, 200C or 1M) and then do not need to worry about overdose or adverse side-effects.

Sitz bath therapy: In her book TOKOLOGY (1898), Alice Stockham recommends a hot sitz bath for rigidity of the vulva or cervix. She says this works to relieve neuralgic pains (throbbing or stabbing sensations) and ineffective contractions. It is contraindicated if the woman has a fever. Seat the woman in a sitz bath containing water that seems very hot to her but no hotter than 101°F (38.3°C). You don't want the mother's core temperature to exceed 102°F (38.9°C); however, localized bathing like this should reduce the risk that the core temperature will rise that high (OTIS, 2004). Her feet should be placed in a hot foot bath as well. Remember that laboring women have an increased pain threshold, so monitor the temperature of the water carefully to avoid scalding her. Cover her with blankets and add more water to maintain the temperature as high as she can bear it. Let her remain like this until she is perspiring profusely. Dry her under the blankets and let her lie down while still wrapped up. It is important that she break a sweat, which can take up to an hour but usually happens sooner. The contractions should subside and she may fall asleep. The heat results in local relaxation, the contractions later resume and become more effective, and the labor progresses rapidly from this point on.

Heating the mother in this way may produce transient fetal tachycardia, which should subside once the mother is out of the sitz bath for 20 minutes or so. Check the fetal heart before the bath and after the mother lies down. If the fetal heart rate is elevated, check it periodically to make sure it returns to a normal baseline.

Finger pressure: A localized area of hardening in the cervix usually indicates scarring or an adhesion. Press the adhesion against the presenting part during a contraction. This may cause it to break up under your fingers. Unlike cervical stretching, this is usually painless and may resolve the problem. There may be slight bleeding when you are finished (El Halta, 1998). Sometimes, just opening your fingers inside the os will cause the cervix to "crack" open. Other times, more firm massage can help move the cervix past the stuck point. Massage by inserting two fingers inside the os and using the fingerpads to sweep back and forth across the edge of the anterior os, stretching side to side as you do so. This can loosen up a cervix that has been resisting strong contractions for hours and allow normal dilation to proceed.

Stretching: If pressure alone doesn't work and labor is more active or if the entire cervix feels stiff, break up rigidity with stretching. In order for this to work, the cervix must be well applied to the presenting part, which is ideal, or at least well applied to the bag of waters. (If cervical swelling is part of the problem, it should be addressed first [see later in this chapter]). Avoid stretching a swollen cervix if you can, because swelling increases the likelihood of tearing.) You should have the mother lie on a firm, flat surface. Insert your hand between contractions and place a couple of evening primrose capsules inside the lip of the os. Wait 10 to 15 minutes, reinsert your hand and find the edges of the os. Feel the edges of the cervix to determine where the most rigid area is. Adjust your fingertips accordingly, which may require placing them side by side in the most rigid region of the os. Now adjust your hand so that you can apply maximum pressure during your attempts. For example, if your fingers are near the anterior lip, it may be best to position your hand so that your palm is facing the mother's perineum. If you wish to stretch the cervix laterally, spread your fingers across the center of the opening with your palm facing up at an oblique angle. You are attempting to achieve maximum leverage. Once in position, wait for a contraction to begin. As it builds, press your fingers into the edge of the cervix, against the presenting part, stretching the cervix in the appropriate direction. Hold the stretch after the contraction subsides. Do this for two or three contractions, then stop, unless an emergency demands that you achieve the most rapid dilation possible.

Recheck in half an hour to assess whether more stretching is needed. Depending upon the dilation, you may be able to insert your fingers into the os, hook them under the edge of the cervix, and massage back and forth in a semicircular motion around the anterior edge. It will be less easy to massage the posterior half of the cervix, but it may be equally necessary. Placing the mother in a hands-and-knees position can help, although gravity may cause the presenting part to move away from the cervix, and you need counterpressure from the presenting part to stretch the cervix effectively. If the head recedes as you apply pressure, change the mother's position to supine. Continue to massage as above during and between the next few contractions. Then stop, give the mother a break, and recheck again in 30 to 45 minutes.

You are looking for either a gradual diminishing of rigidity or a sudden "cracking" sensation as the edge of the cervix gives up its rigidity. This cracking feeling is comparable to what you would feel if you folded a length of stretchy cloth, applied a thin film of glue along the edge, allowed it to dry, and then pulled the ends of the cloth in opposite directions. Cervices that respond in this way are typically very effaced, the baby is low, contractions are strong, yet dilation is not advanced. Breaking up rigidity can cause labor to progress very quickly in such cases. The "pop-bottle lip" form of rigidity is not as easy to alleviate but can be done with persistence.

The uterine reflex and cervical rigidity: Block has found that having an assistant massage the uterine reflexology point (found at the top of the center of the heel pad in the foot) while the cervix is being stretched facilitates cervical opening considerably. (For more details on this reflex point, see the chapter entitled "Additional Non-invasive Techniques for Assessing Progress".) This technique is effective once the cervix is more than 3.5 cm dilated (Block, 1984). She also has noted a connection between the cervix and the perineum with regard to this point. This technique is far less effective in women who have had two or more clitorotomies or who have extensive cervical tearing, which, she postulates, is probably due to nerve damage. Massage will offer some benefit to women with cervical scarring if they have a very thin skin layer.

Conglutination of the external os

This is defined as the "sticking together" of the lips of the cervical os, causing the circular fibers around the external os to remain undilated. True conglutination is a rare condition, although cases in which the os remains closed in a similar fashion can occur as well. In both cases, the cervix effaces to nearly paper-thin as labor progresses and the presenting part is usually low in the pelvis and firmly applied to the cervix, with little or no forewaters. Upon examination, you may mistake this situation for full dilation, especially if the cervical os is very posterior, but the surface of the cervix will feel very smooth and no suture lines will be palpable (or will be felt only faintly through the wall of the cervix). Is some cases, the os cannot be identified with the examining finger but may be seen through a speculum as a tiny opening with a red ring around it and perhaps a little mucus in the center. If this condition is not identified, the lower uterine segment can become stretched downward to the point where the external os presents at the vulva.

Upon detection, attempt to insinuate your finger into the os and massage it open. If this proves impossible, insert 6 to 8 capsules of evening primrose oil, wait an hour or so, and recheck to see if there is any softening of the tissues. If the os is truly unresponsive, further attempts are likely to produce cervical tears.

Historically, Dührssen incisions were made in the cervix to allow a yoni birth. Originated by Alfred Dührssen around the turn of the 19th century, these incisions were made at 2, 6 and 10 o'clock after the cervix had dilated to 4 to 6 cm in cases in which rapid cervical dilation was deemed desirable. However, they are usually not done today. The risk of extension into the lower uterine segment is high; such incisions also require extensive repair and may bleed profusely. Do not attempt to perform such incisions at home (the only possible exception to this is when the aftercoming head of a breech baby is trappped in a partially closed cervix and nothing else will cause the cervix to release: this reason is further discussed in the chapter entitled "Assisting at the Birth of a Breech Baby.". It makes more sense to force the cervix open with massage. Even though this may produce a tear, it is less likely to extend than a clean incision.

Closing down of the os

Mainstream obstetrics does not recognize that cervical dilation can reverse; however, midwives know that the cervix can sometimes open to a certain point and then close down. This may be due to fetal positioning but may also result from maternal fear or other psychological factors. It has been known to happen with babies that had congenital defects, seemingly a signal that things weren't quite right. The cervix may close down when a woman who has previously been dilating well is taken to the hospital. Maternal fear of stronger contractions or pushing, a change in fetal position, cervical swelling (which may be caused by fetal malpositioning), or contractions that are not strong enough or that slack off all may result in the cervix closing down. However, in planned homebirths, it most often occurs when the intact bag of waters has been serving as a dilator, the bag breaks, and the cervical os then recedes upward to contact the presenting part. Closure of the os always feels like lost ground to both mother and midwife, and necessitates redilation.

How you assist progress will depend on why you believe the cervix has closed down. If the cervix is not swollen and the reason is simply that the membranes have ruptured, have the mother get into a warm bath, change positions, stand and lean forward or use any of the other means of assisting progress in labor, including the belly lift, and continue laboring in anticipation of redilation. Increasing the strength of contractions may help. (See the chapter entitled "Natural Induction and Augmentation of Labor.") However, if the cervix is swollen, deal with that first. See later in this chapter for details.

Loreen Kingston (1982?), a midwife in the Midwest, recommends the following as a way to get the cervix to reopen: have the mother lie on a slanted board elevated 10 inches off the floor, with her head at the low end. Wait 5 minutes and then let her get off the board from the side that feels most comfortable to her. Recheck the cervix. Try this several times; if there is no progress, try something else.

Arrested dilation

Sometimes women get stuck at a particular dilation. This can happen even if the cervix is not particularly swollen, rigid or scarred, although these are often contributing factors. Those things suggested in the chapter entitled "Techniques Used to Help the Baby Descend during Labor," should be tried first because often this problem is related to either a compound, asynclitic, or posterior presentation. However, arrested dilation can also be related to psychological factors such as maternal fear. Given your knowledge of the woman, you need to talk to her about whatever psychological issues might be contributing to this arrest in progress.

Manual dilation: What if the usual tricks don't work? You might know that if she has the baby in the next few hours she will be fine, but waiting and laboring longer and getting more tired will exhaust her for pushing and put her at more risk for bleeding after the birth. She may be disheartened. If you have tried *everything else* and nothing is working to change the situation, manual dilation may get the woman past her stuck place and help move labor forward. Other situations in which manual dilation can come in handy include emergencies requiring rapid dilation (such as an abruption of the placenta in a setting that prevents rapid transport to the hospital) and when a stubborn anterior cervical lip has developed (see below).

Various methods of manual dilation were widely used in the last century. It has fallen into disfavor in mainstream medical circles and has been called "manual laceration" in modern textbooks because so often the cervix was damaged when manual dilation was performed by doctors. While there is always a degree of risk that the cervix will become lacerated during manual manipulation, the use of instruments or incisions to dilate the cervix, and the large hands and upper body strength of male obstetricians applied to the os, increases the risk considerably.

Manual dilation is accomplished using the fingers of the examining hand and is performed in a similar fashion to breaking up rigidity; in fact, arrested dilation and rigidity often occur together. It works best when the baby is low and the presenting part is well applied to the cervix. Between contractions, insert your index and middle fingers into the os and spread them apart across its widest diameter, as you would to assess dilation. Keep your hand in place to stretch the cervix during the next few contractions to encourage the uterus to work most efficiently to open the os. If the membranes have ruptured, put one fingertip on each side of the cervix and press into the rim, stretching the cervical edges laterally while using the surface of the presenting part for leverage (do not worry about hurting the baby; as long as you are not pressing directly into the membranous region of a fontanelle or a suture line, the term skull can withstand this localized, temporary pressure just fine). If the membranes are intact, press against the cervical rim only and avoid putting pressure against the bag so that you do not break it inadvertently. This is hard to do, and typically you cannot apply as much stretching pressure as you can when the presenting part is well applied. If labor has been stalled quite a while, manually dilate the cervix at least one more centimeter before you give the mother a break. Then, depending upon the overall labor picture, check again in at least 30 to 45 minutes to see if dilation has changed for better or worse.

Manual dilation can be forceful and sustained when being done to deal with an emergency such as massive abruption. In this case, the risk of tearing the cervix is secondary to the risk placental bleeding poses for both mother and baby. Manual dilation should *never* be used in the presence of previa, as the cervix is quite friable and easily torn.

Cervical and other soft-tissue swelling

Cervical swelling may occur during labor because of poor circulatory return, especially before 6 cm dilation. Sometimes other tissues swell as well, with or without cervical swelling, and often respond to the same types of techniques, so they are discussed together here. If the mother has been lying down, having her walk will help to increase circulation and relieve the pressure (Davis, 1997). Fetal positioning may be a factor, and when it is, attending to that is called for prior to any other interventions. (See the chapter entitled "Techniques Used to Help the Baby Descend during Labor.")

If what you have tried so far hasn't worked, get the pressure off the swollen tissue. Have the woman first assume a knee-chest position, then pour arnica oil into her yoni or gently coat outer tissues if they are swollen. If the membranes are broken, you may opt instead to give homeopathic arnica orally in a 30C dose every 15 to 30 minutes. If you get no results after three doses, switch to bellis perennis, another great remedy for deep soft-tissue trauma. Use 30C doses of the most effective remedy every 15 to 30 minutes. Additionally, intact evening primrose oil capsules inserted inside the os and around the cervix often work quickly to relieve swelling. Have the mother remain in the knee-chest position for at least 30 minutes, or until she reports a dramatic shift in the quality of her contractions.

Some women have a hard time assuming a knee-chest position. Other positions they can try include lying on a slant board propped to a height of 10 inches (easily done with folded blankets or couch cushions) with their head at the low end. You can also use the hands-and-knees position. Have the woman maintain the position for 30 to 45 minutes and then recheck to see if this is helping.

Another way to reduce pressure on the cervix is to have the mother labor for two or three contractions in a side-lying position on one side, then switch to hands-and-knees for a few contractions, then switch to side-lying on the other side for a couple of contractions, then switch to a Trendelenburg position for a couple of contractions. Moving around on all sides is intended to equalize and relieve the pressure on the cervix and thus reduce the swelling.

If these things fail to work, massage can help reduce cervical swelling by mobilizing fluids out of the tissue. Grasp the edge between two extended fingers and massage back and forth across the entire anterior lip. As a last resort, place a piece of ice in the finger of an exam glove or a condom and apply it directly to the swollen cervix (admittedly an uncomfortable process) but one that will often reduce the swelling by the time the ice has melted (Davidson, 1997).

Active bearing down before complete dilation

This is a primary cause of cervical trauma and anterior lip formation. While maternal efforts to push before complete dilation may damage the cervix, spontaneous bearing down by the uterus is completely involuntary and impossible for the woman to control. To tell her to stop pushing is counterproductive and will exhaust her as she tries. Instead, encourage her not to add any voluntary efforts, but just "let the uterus do the pushing." The uterus will frequently pull the cervix out of the way rapidly, and she will be fully dilated with the baby low and ready to be born. The body, left to its own devices, will usually not hurt itself. The cervix should be monitored after every few contractions, and cervical swelling, when it does occur, should be dealt with promptly.

If additional bearing down cannot be stopped or the cervix starts to swell, have the woman assume a nonerect position to take pressure off the cervix. This can help relieve the intensity of her pushing urges. Hands and knees and side-lying are two good positions to try first. Once positioned, she should still not try to fight the natural responses of her uterus. If changing positions eases the urge to push, this usually indicates that the woman is not fully dilated; this clue can help you avoid an unnecessary internal exam.

Acupressure for a premature pushing urge: Applying strong pressure to Ciliau (BL-32) can help move the cervix out of the way when the woman develops a strong urge to push prior to complete dilation or when a cervical lip is present. To locate these points, see the subchapter entitled "Traditional Chinese Medicine" (West, 2001).

Anterior cervical lips

Lips often develop when the presenting part is low, contractions are strong and the woman is in a position that puts pressure on her sacrum, compressing the baby forward, against the pubic bone. In addition, women with long cervices whose os was posterior during much of the labor are prone to the development of an anterior lip, as are those carrying a persistently occiput posterior baby.

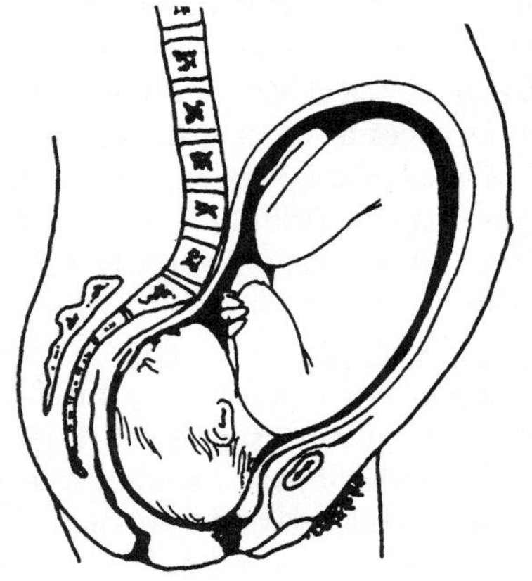

Anterior cervical lip

Lip formation is accentuated if a strong bearing-down urge has established itself before complete dilation, and the presenting part is well applied to the cervix, or the os has been very posterior during labor. The anterior cervical lip can become trapped between the presenting part and the pubic bone. Cervical polyps can also become trapped between the presenting part and the pubic bone and can prevent the lip from moving back. The woman often feels an urge to push accompanied by extreme pain and sensitivity above the pubic bone, indicating that the anterior lip is being dragged down by the baby's head. This causes the woman to behave in a very characteristic manner: she appears to be trying to move away from the her lower abdomen. She will rear up, arching her back; even as her body starts to push, she may throw her arms behind her, lift her head up and away, and appear to be in pain. In addition, there is usually a continuous trickle of red blood that seeps from her yoni during each contraction.

Cervical lips that do not resolve on their own can usually be pushed up and out of the way. To reduce the lip, try any of the suggestions given previously under swelling. Other options include having the mother lie on her back and roll from side to side during or between contractions, exaggerated crawling or a hot bath. Note that edema must often be resolved before any other technique will work. Check the swelling every few contractions, because if one thing isn't helping, another might. On exceedingly rare occasions, a sacculated uterus may mimic an anterior lip. For details regarding this form of obstructed labor, see the chapter entitled "Recognizing and Dealing with Obstructed Labor."

Suprapubic pain may also be caused by an anterior compound presentation. See details in the chapter entitled "Assisting a Woman Whose Baby Is in a Compound Presentation" under "Move the arm."

Position changes to reduce an anterior lip, uneven dilation or to hasten dilation: Uneven dilation and sometimes an anterior cervical lip may indicate that the head is not symmetrically applied (which may be due to unequal pressure from the dilating forces). This is especially true during active labor before full or nearly full dilation. Changing the angle of the fetal head against the cervix before the fundus forces the head through the pelvis at the wrong angle (creating decelerations of the fetal heart rate, possible cervical or yoni tears or both, as well as difficulty with pushing) will benefit labor now and during pushing.

Kathi Wilson (1997?), a Canadian midwife, has the mother lie in a exaggerated semiprone position for a few contractions, then switch to the other side for a few more. Help the mother breathe through any bearing-down sensations as much as possible (let her uterus do what it wants to do, but she should not add any voluntary effort of her own).

Another suggestion comes anonymously from the Gentlebirth archives on the web. Have the mother go through two contractions on her left side, two contractions on her right side, then two contractions on hands and knees, and the last two in an open knee-chest position. If the woman has been transported and has had an epidural, roll her to her right side and adduct the left leg into the frog (McRoberts) position for two contractions, then use the reverse positioning on the left side, instead of hands and knees and knee-chest. Alternatively, her hips can be elevated with pillows so they are higher than her head for the last two sets of two contractions. She should then be checked again. If the baby's head has been asynclitic, at the most two sets of eight contractions as explained above should correct the problem. However, if a hand near the baby's neck is the reason for the lip, other position changes may be necessary.

Attempting to move the lip without attention to the position of the presenting part encourages the baby's head to come down in an unfavorable position. Maternal position changes in general, and the ones noted above specifically, give the baby the highest likelihood of finding the space to move into a better position. Remember that if you can't directly change the angle of the head, then change the angle of the mother. Something will almost always give.

Manually reducing an anterior lip: There will be times when none of your suggestions work to bring about full dilation, but the mother has a strong urge to push and is in a great deal of pain. The best option then is to try pushing the lip back while the mother bears down. This usually works best when the mother is lying flat on a firm surface such as the floor with her legs up and apart (actually this is the first choice of position for any cervical manipulation). This positioning moves the lip as far forward as possible for the purposes of manipulation. Place your fingers on the edge of the lip (palm down) at 11 and 1 o'clock; direct your efforts up and over the head as the mother bears down during a contraction. You may have to push very hard. This works best when the mother has a strong urge (which tends to override the pain of the procedure), the baby is low (at least zero station) and the membranes have ruptured or the forewaters are very minimal. If the lip does not go back easily or reappears between contractions, make a few attempts, switch to other techniques for a few contractions, then continue to alternate between them until the lip is gone.

Manual reduction of a lip is uncomfortable, to be sure. However, it is a better solution than letting the lip swell and be dragged down to the introitus. This is hard on the lower uterine segment, the transverse cervical ligaments, and other connective tissue of the yoni. Dragging on a cervical lip encourages prolapse, hematomas, and lacerations. Since the cervix is weakest along the sides, a laceration is more likely to occur as a result of pushing with a persistent lip than from relieving the tension on the tissue with maternal efforts and manual reduction. The cervix is very elastic and will usually withstand this intervention without tearing, especially when the problem is attended to in a timely fashion.

Detachment of the cervix

Detachment of all or a portion of the cervix may occur when cervical resistance is left unattended for a very long period of time in active labor. A combination of edema, lack of circulation and poor oxygenation may lead to tissue necrosis and cause some or all of the cervix to be sloughed off. The separation of the entire cervical ring is called annular detachment. In other cases, only a portion of the cervix comes away. Detachment usually results from the intense pressure of a persistent anterior lip or an excessively rigid os. This may also occur when a cerclage has been placed and labor begins before it has been removed. However, it happens most commonly in first time mothers who have had prolonged labor with ruptured membranes and a low baby, in combination with a thin, rigid cervix and strong uterine contractions. Detachment is followed by sudden advancement for no apparent reason. A portion of tissue is passed either before or after the birth, that may, at first, be mistaken for placental tissue. If you suspect that detachment has occurred, be sure to check the cervix carefully for bleeding and for tears which extend into the lower uterine segment. Because the tissue has been pinched off due to pressure, bleeding is unlikely, and repair rarely necessary. If bleeding does occur, it needs to be controlled with figure-eight stitches along the edge of the stump, which may require transport; be sure to take the scrap of tissue with you to the hospital. This complication is further discussed in Volume III of this text and in my HEALING PASSAGE. Detachment should not happen during a well-attended labor at home.

Cervical prolapse and labor

When a woman has a uterine prolapse prior to conception, the growth of the uterus during pregnancy always results in it being drawn up into the abdominal cavity into a more or less normal position. On rare occasions, however, a portion of the uterus, most commonly the elongated cervix, protrudes through the introitus. When this has gone on throughout the pregnancy, the cervix is often toughened, swollen and ulcerated. Premature labor is more common, as are urinary retention and infection.

During labor, dilation may begin outside the introitus. This can easily impede dilation, as the cervix cannot stretch to either side as well as it can when it is properly positioned. The cervix is likely to be quite swollen, and scar tissue may lead to problems with dilation. Lacerations of the cervix occur more easily because the tissue is traumatized. If the cervix cannot dilate, obstructed labor may result in uterine rupture; because of this, fetal mortality is increased.

The best remedy is patience and gentle care of the cervix. Most women will still have a normal labor. To maximize the chances, place the mother in a Trendelenburg or knee-chest position in early labor to relieve pressure on the cervix and reduce swelling. This may allow the os to be withdrawn into the yoni so it can dilate more normally. If positioning does not help, you can try using herbs to gradually increase the strength of contractions, which at times will pull the cervix back into the yoni. If none of these techniques are productive, do not let labor go on with no progress; to do so invites uterine rupture. Transport is your best option.

Yoni herniations and the progress of labor

Large herniations into the yoni (cystoceles, rectoceles, etc.) may become trapped in front of the presenting part as it descends. These would appear as outpouching of the wall overlying the hernia. Be sure to check such a prolapse periodically during labor. If it becomes trapped, it should be replaced by pushing it above the presenting part. Do so by inserting your index finger on one side of the tissue and your middle finger on the other. Between contractions, exert pressure upward by supporting the tissue with the flat, palmar surface of your fingers and move it out of the way so the presenting part can descend. This maneuver allows the head to descend unimpeded, as well as avoiding further damage to the wall of the yoni. The presenting part will act as a support once it is displacing the tissue, and your continuous support can usually be discontinued. The mother should push in a gravity-neutral position, such as side-lying or hands and knees, to minimize further trauma to the prolapsed tissue.

Large cystoceles and rectoceles may require reduction before they can be displaced. Getting pressure off the yoni with the types of techniques discussed under "Cervical and other soft-tissue swelling" earlier in this chapter also work well in these cases. This, combined with the application of arnica oil, can produce a gradual reduction in the size of the prolapse. Once it is small enough, it can be pushed up and over the presenting part. This can probably take place only late in labor when the baby is very low.

Maternal tumors in the birth canal

At times, a maternal tumor such as a cervical polyp or a pediculated fibroid will become positioned alongside or in front of the presenting part and prevent further descent. Tumors can also lodge between the presenting part and the pelvis and impede dilation. A tumor that is small and within reach can often be pushed out of the way during an internal exam. To do so, don a sterile glove. Find the point of attachment between the tumor and the maternal soft tissues. If the tumor is attached to a stem and has been pushed out of the uterus, be sure to push it up inside the os, where it may well recede above the presenting part. If this is impossible and the tumor is large and impeding progress, transport is your most reasonable alternative.

If you are attending a birth far from medical help, you can apply primrose oil to the growth to soften it. Check it every 10 to 15 minutes to see how it is softening. Once it has softened, you can attempt to compress the tumor with your hand to see if you can reduce its size (Lim, 2002). A fibroid will respond by emptying of blood. Be aware that this may rupture the tumor, may cause significant pain to the mother, and, if the tumor is cancerous, it could force cancerous cells into her circulation, sending them traveling to distant locations in her body where they may form metastatic tumors. These risks must be weighed against those of obstructed labor, eventual fetal demise and possible uterine rupture. Proceed cautiously and stop if the tumor does not respond to pressure. Have it evaluated as soon as possible after the birth.

Recognizing and Dealing with Obstructed Labor

NOTE: Review the chapter entitled "The Process of Labor for Women with Contracted Pelvises" before studying this chapter.

Obstructed labor can arise whenever there is an anatomical variation that impedes descent. This may be due to a maternal tumor in the pelvic region, an unyielding cervix (as might occur with severe scarring from previous surgery or infection), or a relative problem involving the size of the pelvis in relationship to the size of the baby's head, referred to as cephalopelvic disproportion (CPD). While the vast majority of disproportion occurs between the fetal head and the mother's pelvis, this is not always the case. In this chapter I will refer to fetopelvic disproportion (FPD) to encompass CPD as well as situations where a fetal part other than the head is causing the problem. When CPD is meant specifically, that term will be used. See the chapter entitled "Assisting at Multiple Births" for details on obstructed labor with twins.

The Maternal Pelvis and FPD

There are two perspectives from which to understand obstructed labor caused by FPD. Absolute FPD exists when the pelvis is so small or severely contracted from deformity or disease that the birth of a normally sized baby is impossible. Deformity may be associated with rare congenital abnormalities of the pelvis, dwarfism, nutritional deficiencies during the formative years that resulted in rickets (which can deform an otherwise normal pelvis) or injury resulting in a broken pelvis.

FPD can occur in a very small woman who is proportioned normally but whose pelvis is not large enough to allow for the birth of a normally sized baby. It can also occur in women who have suffered severe, chronic malnutrition resulting in osteomalacia. Most prevalent in the developing world, osteomalacia causes progressive softening and deformity of the adult pelvis with each successive baby until a normal birth is impossible. Sellers (1993) points out that women in the developing world who must carry heavy objects on their heads daily (such as large containers of water, wood or food) tend to develop android pelvises because the weight on the developing bones causes the femurs to press into the sides of the pelvis, narrowing the passageway. Women with severe curvatures of the spine may also have significant distortions in their pelvic anatomy.

Relative FPD occurs when both mother and baby are anatomically normal but the baby, for reasons of size or position, cannot pass through that particular mother's pelvis. She could, however, have another baby who was smaller or even this baby if he were in a more favorable position. When changing the fetal position can be accomplished, relative FPD can usually be overcome and the baby born normally. When the fit is tight but not impossible, maternal position changes, stronger contractions or opening the pelvis manually may allow the birth to proceed without problem. Relative FPD is also operative when the baby has a deformity that prevents passage through a normal maternal pelvis or when the mother has a soft-tissue lesion, such as an ovarian cyst, that blocks the pelvis.

Rickets and other forms of malnutrition leading to bony deformities were the number-one cause of FPD during the 19th and early 20th century. During this era, most FPD was overcome with difficult instrumental delivery that often left both mother and baby damaged and sometimes dead. Thus, the danger of FPD was emphasized. Although rickets is rare in industrialized countries today and most women have normally formed pelvises, the legacy of the early 20th century has persisted and the fear of obstructed labor remains a major concern in many medical-model practices in the West. Many medical-model practitioners have no experience with using maternal position changes and little or no knowledge of pelvic mobility dynamics; hospital providers have been known to diagnose FPD before the head has even attempted to descend into the pelvis. In other cases, problems with fetal position are allowed to progress to the point of the baby's becoming totally stuck, and then his position declared uncorrectable. Time for adequate moulding of a large head may not be allowed. With the option of relatively safe surgical birth, challenging deliveries (which, in the hands of many modern obstetricians, is just about any birth where the baby doesn't fall out), are not allowed to take place. To compound the problem, many women receive drugs that make it hard or impossible for them to change positions or do other things that may help the baby descend.

Older textbooks offer valuable tips for detecting obstructed labor in women with truly contracted pelvises and arrested labor patterns. Although this is important information for all midwives to know, encountering a woman with a defective pelvis in North America or northern Europe is really quite rare. Therefore, FPD should never be diagnosed without careful consideration of the entire labor picture. Relative FPD is much more common and often correctable, given time, patience and the proper midwifery-model interventions. Most experienced midwives have seen many a labor progress to birth that would have been declared CPD and resolved surgically if the woman had been under medical-model care. However, all midwives, especially those working with poor populations in the West or in the developing world, must keep all types of FPD in mind whenever labor is prolonged. Truly obstructed labor that is left to nature or handled incompetently may leave the woman, her baby or both severely injured or dead.

Small women and FPD

It is easy to assume that a small woman is more likely to have trouble getting her baby out. However, while a small woman is likely to have a small (but otherwise normal) pelvis, she is also more likely to have a relatively smaller, but healthy, baby. Thoms (1937) studied 362 small first-time mothers and found their babies weighed, on average, 280 grams less than babies of women with medium- to large-sized pelvises. In addition, pelvic mobility can often overcome marginally disproportionate pelvic capacity when a woman's baby is relatively large.

Technical degrees of disproportion

Different criteria, based on pelvimetry, have been used to define the severity of pelvic contraction. The first classification system does not differentiate between the pelvic planes:

- Mild or minor: One pelvic diameter is 1 cm less than normal
- Moderate: One pelvic diameter is 1 to 2 cm less than normal
- Severe or major: One pelvic diameter is over 2 cm less than normal

Another system gives minimum values for diameters in each pelvic plane:

Inlet (brim): Inlet contraction is present when the shortest AP diameter is less than 10 cm, the greatest transverse diameter is less than 12 cm, or the diagonal conjugate is less than 11.5 cm. Obstruction is more likely when two diameters are contracted than when only one is contracted. Declaration of inlet contraction is based on the average size of the biparietal diameter of 9.5 cm, which can range up to 9.8 cm.

Midpelvis: The definition of midpelvic contraction is less well defined. It is likely to occur when the sum of the midpelvic interischial spinous diameter, which averages 10.5 cm, and the posterior sagittal diameter, which averages 5 cm, falls to 13.5 or below (normally, this value is 10.5 cm + 5 cm = 15.5 cm). Some sources state that an interischial diameter of 8 cm or less denotes contraction.

Outlet: Contraction at this level is usually defined by an interischial tuberous diameter of 8 cm or less. True outlet contraction is usually accompanied by midpelvic contraction.

Of course, all of these estimates are based on the pelvis in stasis, as it were. When the mother's hormones are flowing and she is up and moving around, the pelvic bones can move and open in ways that are impossible to predict or assess during an internal exam performed on a still and supine woman. In addition, the backward motion of the sacrum and the accompanying widening of all pelvic diameters during pushing is not accounted for in this assessment.

Detecting Possible CPD and other types of FPD during Labor due to Pelvic Contraction

Elizabeth Davis, co-founder of the Midwifery Institute of California, offers several valuable tips, incorporated into the following discussion, for detecting CPD in her text HEART AND HANDS: A MIDWIFE'S GUIDE TO PREGNANCY AND BIRTH (1997).

CPD cannot be diagnosed until the head has unsuccessfully attempted to enter or pass through the pelvis. The mere presence of the head above the brim, even in a primigravida, is usually not an indication of CPD unless some obvious spinal or pelvic deformity or a fetal malformation is present. Often this scenario is caused by fetal positioning, particularly posterior positioning, rather than any problem with the pelvis. Very strong or poorly toned abdominal muscles, muscle tension and fear may all hinder descent even when contractions seem strong enough to move the baby down. A history of sexual or other types of abuse, control issues or worries about the baby's well-being may be the real underlying problem.

Descent may become arrested anywhere along the birth canal. The level of the fetus at the time of such arrest will often provide the clue for determining the causative factor. For discussion's sake, we will refer to arrest at the inlet, the midpelvis or the outlet.

Inlet disproportion

This is associated with nonvertex presentations. Shoulder presentation and extreme asynclitism are found three times more frequently and cord prolapse occurs four to six times more often than when there is no disproportion. Breech presentation is not necessarily more common. Oblique lie is common; unable to enter the brim, the head may be pressed aside into one iliac fossa. Prolapse of an arm or foot is also more likely when the presenting part fits poorly, especially in flat (platypelloid) pelvises.

Disproportion at the inlet may also be indicated by a lack of descent past –3 to –2 station, exaggerated asynclitism or a cervix that is not well applied to the fetal head. The cervix may hang like an empty sleeve below the bag of waters. Dilation usually arrests at 6 cm. The cervix may also close down during a contraction because nothing is holding it open. Contractions become weak or incoordinate, and the mother may report asymmetrical, isolated, spastic pain (Davis, 1997).

Such a scenario may not be due to CPD, however. This picture is also typical of a labor in which the membranes are very strong and holding back descent or in which the contractions are not yet strong enough to get the woman past this point. A woman who has taken evening primrose oil prenatally may dilate to around 6 cm with what appear to be early labor contractions that build on their own. A good uterine stimulant, such as cotton root bark tincture, will often remedy this labor pattern. Even if you believe that strong membranes are the problem, hold off on rupturing them until you see if a better contraction pattern can be established.

Early rupture of membranes frequently occurs in true CPD because of the high or poorly fitting presenting part. A head that is arrested above the brim does not block off the forewaters from the hindwaters, as usually occurs. Instead, the entire force of the uterine contraction goes around the head and is brought to bear directly on the forewaters, making early rupture of membranes far more likely to occur, eliminating the only dilating wedge. Afterward, the absence of pressure against the cervix and lower uterine segment leads to less efficient contractions, causing dilation to slow down or plateau entirely.

Of prime significance in whether any type of disproportion can be overcome is the quality of the uterine contractions. Often, the force of the contractions corresponds to the amount of work required. In some women, contractions increase in strength when descent is delayed. Sometimes, this extra uterine effort will overcome minor degrees of disproportion. Likewise, other women start out with weak contractions that never build, no matter what is done. Contractions will also become weak if the mother becomes exhausted. When absolute disproportion is suspected, transport is warranted.

Midpelvic disproportion

Here the head usually enters the brim without difficulty. Dilation proceeds normally, but descent becomes arrested at the level of the ischial spines, either during labor or pushing. There may not be enough room in the midpelvis for the head to rotate to an anteroposterior position; it then becomes stuck either just above or between the ischial spines. Position changes and strong contractions may overcome this problem if the interischial diameter is tight but all other pelvic dimensions seem adequate.

Outlet disproportion

Outlet dystocia usually affects the very last part of descent, after +2 station, and is associated with prolonged pushing. A narrow or low pubic arch will cause the head to dip deeply backward toward the sacrum during late pushing, often resulting in a deep perineal tear. Moulding or caput formation may be extreme if the interischial tuberous diameter is narrowed (Davis, 1997). In these cases, the posterior sacral diameter must be large enough to compensate for a narrow pubic arch. A position that allows maximal sacral mobility is very important before and during pushing. Be prepared for an outlet shoulder dystocia (discussed in detail in the chapter entitled "Shoulder Dystocia"). If descent is arrested during pushing, pronounced labial edema may develop because of obstructed blood flow to the area.

CPD in women who have had other babies

The lower uterine segment forms rapidly and the cervix typically dilates soon after in multigravid women who have had several difficult labors through a marginally contracted pelvis. If the baby cannot descend, uterine rupture is likely because of the thinned lower uterine segment. It is also possible for the cervix to become compressed between the head and the pelvis. The part below the area of compression becomes edematous and may even slough off. The anterior lip is likely to be caught between the head and the pubic bone, particularly in women with flat pelvises and pendulous abdomens; it can become very swollen, bruised and even necrotic if neglected (Greenhill, 1951). These risks indicate the need for more frequent internal exams to make sure therapies are helping and things are progressing normally.

Contraction patterns in obstructed labor and development of a pathologic retraction ring

One of two contraction patterns may develop as obstructed labor continues. Contractions may become weaker, or the uterus may try to overcome the obstruction with stronger and more frequent contractions during which uterine tonus rises. In the latter case, the upper segment continues to retract while the lower segment becomes increasingly thinned and stretched. The physiological retraction ring rises from its usual level. The upper segment thickens and the lower segment becomes dangerously thin. This situation transforms the normal retraction ring into the pathologic retraction ring (Bandl's ring). The upper segment will appear thickened above the naval while the lower segment will be stretched and very thin. The pathologic retraction ring, which is actually the lower border of the thickened upper uterine segment, forms a transverse ridge that can be palpated and is sometimes visible abdominally. It will be found roughly at the level of the umbilicus or higher, running diagonally across the abdomen, and is higher on the side that is most severely stretched. The round ligaments are tense and may be palpable through the abdomen.

If the obstruction is not overcome and these contractions continue for many hours, the upper segment will retract to the point that the baby is contained almost entirely in the lower uterine segment. This area will become very tender; the mother's pulse and temperature will rise. The mother reports severe pain and may be excited or restless. The lower segment eventually becomes thin beyond its tolerance, and there is a high risk of uterine rupture (see the chapter entitled "Uterine Rupture during Labor"). In some cases, the myometrium will become exhausted and uterine inertia sets in before rupture occurs. If not, the strong frequent contractions and high resting tonus may cut off the placental circulation and kill the baby. Transport without delay if you suspect that a pathological retraction ring is developing.

The following table summarizes findings when labor is marginally or profoundly obstructed. Keep in mind that this information is based on labors in which women have not been instructed to change positions in the specific ways described throughout this text. If labor has been going on for hours and the woman appears to be experiencing borderline CPD, position changes, especially those involving asymmetrical movement with frequent shifts in activity, may move labor along to complete dilation. When that occurs, put the woman in a Birth Sling to afford maximal pelvic mobility and be prepared to use pelvic-opening techniques to affect progress during pushing. If CPD appears to be pronounced and the lower uterine segment is very thin, transport. If contractions are still good, try various, frequent position changes and monitor closely for descent. If nothing changes or if the uterine activity seems to be taking a dangerous turn (constant contractions), transport.

The development of severe moulding or formation of a caput with the head still high are hallmarks of true CPD. In most cases, even if the head is markedly asynclitic or otherwise having trouble coming down, moulding will only be moderate and caput formation absent until the membranes rupture and the head is encircled by maternal soft tissues sufficient to impair circulation to the scalp. Severe moulding with or without a caput in a head that is above the brim is an excellent presumptive indication of CPD. Transport.

Assessment	Borderline CPD	Pronounced CPD
Status of membranes	May be intact	Ruptured
Abdominal estimate of descent	2/5 or less of the head can be felt abdominally, with 3/5 or more having descended through the pelvis	4/5 to 5/5 of the head can be felt abdominally
Station by internal exam	Lowermost portion of the skull is near or below zero	Head above the brim
Moulding	Mild to moderate	Severe, often with caput
Dilation	7 cm or more	Usually less than 7 cm
Characteristics of contractions	3 or more every 10 min, lasting 20 to 40 sec or more	Variable, may be very irregular or almost constant

Obstructed Labor from Causes Other Than Pelvic Contraction

Labor can be obstructed for reasons that have nothing to do with pelvic disproportion. For example, a mother has previously had several normal births, but in this labor the baby is not descending at all, even after rupture of membranes. Nothing the midwife does changes the situation. There may be a tumor present blocking descent.

Detecting obstructed labor is a "what's wrong with this picture?" scenario; the best ways to learn are by watchful attention during the course of many labors and experience. Things that can cause obstructed labor include both fetal and maternal conditions. Fetal causes include:

•Dystocia upon attempted engagement of the shoulder girdle
•Abnormal shortening of the umbilical cord due to entanglement or length (see the chapter entitled "Cord Problems and Emergencies during Labor.")
•Fetal abnormalities such as hydrocephaly, enlarged abdomen or body stalk anomaly
•Problems related to multiple births such as fetus papyraceus, locked or conjoined twins (covered in the chapter entitled "Assisting at Multiple Births")
•Shoulder dystocia (could be maternal due to pelvic shape) (see the chapter entitled "Shoulder Dystocia")

Causes which originate with the mother include:
•Maternal tumors
•Obstruction in the yoni
•Rupture of the uterus, with part or all of the baby extruded into the abdominal cavity
•Constriction ring
•Abdominal pregnancy
•Blockage by one half of a double uterus
•Sacculation of the uterus
•Partial dilation of the cervix (birth of a small head through an incompletely dilated cervix followed by arrest as the shoulders become hung up on the os)

Dystocia upon attempted engagement of the shoulder girdle

The fetal shoulders may become hung up on the brim as they try to enter the pelvis. In cephalic presentations, this can delay or arrest descent of the head during late pushing. After making sure the mother's bladder is empty, palpate carefully along the upper edge of the pubic bone to try and identify the shoulder. Move the anterior shoulder by placing the heel of your hand above the pubic bone and pushing straight down or rocking your weight back and forth slightly to help flex the shoulder girdle and encourage transverse rotation. This may be most easily accomplished with the mother lying down, after which she may get back up to resume pushing (Sutton, 2001).

Fetal abnormalities

It is not always possible to know if a baby has an abnormality that may obstruct labor, especially when women do not receive ultrasound scans during pregnancy. Likewise, it is possible for scans to miss an abnormality (or even twins). Newborn defects that cause arrest during labor or birth fall into three categories: enlargement of the head, enlargement of another anatomical region of the fetus, which causes arrest after the birth of part of the fetal body; and absence of the umbilical cord. An early indication that a delay in labor may be due to fetal defects is an abnormal fetal heart rate pattern.

Enlargement of the head (hydrocephalus): Hydrocephalus occurs when there is an imbalance in the circulation or production of cerebrospinal fluid within the ventricles of the brain, resulting in cranial enlargement. Careful abdominal palpation during prenatal care may have detected an enlarged head; if so, further evaluation should have taken place at that time. It is uncommon for babies to reach term with undetected hydrocephalus, as most of these babies will be born prematurely. Affected babies typically have other anomalies, especially along the spinal cord. The normal head circumference at term ranges between 32 and 38 cm; the head circumference of a hydrocephalic baby often exceeds 50 cm and may reach 80 cm, with fluid volumes averaging 500 to 1500 ml but ranging as high as 5 liters in some cases. While babies with minor degrees of hydrocephalus may be born naturally without undue harm, those with more extreme forms can not. Although one-third of these babies present breech, as the smaller pelvis fits more easily into the pelvic brim, these babies may present vertex and be unable to enter the brim or unable to descend. However, regardless of the presentation, gross cephalopelvic disproportion generally results.

Hydrocephalus is somewhat difficult to diagnosis with X-rays as the fetal head tends to appear larger than usual in X-ray exams of normal babies. Sonography eliminates this artifact because the diameter of the lateral ventricles of the brain can be compared to the biparietal diameter. Sonographic exam also allows evaluation of the thickness of the cerebral cortex, as well as comparison of the size of the head to the chest and abdomen.

Detection and transport: When hydrocephaly is suspected before the head is born, transport is your best option.

Cephalic presentation: If labor is delayed because the head will not come through the brim, external suprapubic palpation may reveal a head that is obviously out of proportion to the rest of the baby. Palpate the head and suture lines carefully in an attempt to rule out hydrocephalus; the sutures will be widely separated and the anterior fontanelle will range from larger than normal to huge. Transport is the best option when hydrocephaly is suspected before the head is born. If you can not transport for any reason, continue to have the mother push while monitoring descent closely; with patience, the mildly to moderately enlarged head is likely to be born.

Breech presentation: If the baby is born to the shoulders and the aftercoming head will not come, especially if you can see that the baby has spinal defects, the reason for arrest may be hydrocephalus. You must palpate abdominally, above the pubic bone, to try and detect cephalic enlargement. In an urban setting, where transport is easy and quick, try to insert your hand far into the yoni to the baby's face to create an airway. If you can accomplish this rather difficult task (because the head will be completely above the brim) and the baby begins to breathe, transport with your hand in position. However, forming an effective airway in this situation may be impossible.

If you can not transport: If you can not transport for any reason, and the head seems only mildly to moderately enlarged, continue to have the mother push while monitoring descent closely; with patience, the vertex baby is likely to be born. If the head is stuck, the baby is breech, you feel sure that the head is quite enlarged and you are *remote from medical help*, you can try to do a cephalocentesis to drain off enough fluid to allow birth of the head. The baby is likely to die or suffer intracranial bleeding as a result but will surely die anyway if this situation is not dealt with promptly.

Cephalocentesis: In industrialized settings, cephalocentesis is used only in cases in which fetal demise is anticipated, as there is a 90% mortality rate with the procedure itself. However, in a place remote from medical help, with a woman who has been in arrested labor for some time with a hydrocephalic baby, cephalocentesis is a reasonable option to consider. The lower uterine segment will be thin, and there is a very real risk of uterine rupture if the baby isn't born soon. If the baby is cephalic, palpate abdominally and internally to identify the very widely spaced sutures and huge fontanelle that characterize the grossly enlarged hydrocephalic skull. The ventricles may be tapped with a needle as soon as the cervix is dilated to 3 to 4 cm. While an 8 in, 17 gauge needle is ideal to draw off fluid most rapidly, a pudendal needle and sheath or the largest needle you have can be used. Guarding the needle tip with your index finger, guide it into the yoni and against the fetal skull. Insert the tip into the space between sutures or through a fontanelle (you will have to apply some pressure). Alternatively, protect the mother's soft tissues by sheathing the needle with a 6 inch length of sterile IV tubing.

If the baby is breech, with the head above the brim and the baby facing the sacrum, the needle can be passed up through the yoni and inserted through the widened joint at the base of the occiput. Proceed as above (Cunningham, et al., 2001).

Abdominal defects: The baby's abdomen may be enlarged in the presence of tumors of the liver, abnormal development of the kidneys, urinary retention, ascites, pelvic cysts, or other anomalies. It will be impossible to know if the enlargement is due to a solid or fluid-filled mass. This type of defect may not present itself until the head is born and there is dystocia with the aftercoming body, which, at first, may appear to be a case of shoulder dystocia.

Delay at the shoulders in a small to average-sized baby in a mother who has a normal pelvis that cannot be resolved with ordinary shoulder dystocia maneuvers should lead to a suspicion that a fetal defect might be holding things up (other possibilities include a tight cord around the neck, a limb or the body; a short cord; a hand or foot near the neck impeding further descent or a maternal tumor). You may have to insert your hand into the yoni to investigate the possible cause of dystocia before proceeding. Remember to be gentle, as a baby with a defect can have exposed organs that may be easily damaged.

If the shoulders are positioned correctly for birth and are not impacted, have the mother push. Once the shoulders are born, grasp the baby by them and wiggle gently from side to side, working the body out as you would anything out of a tight space. If the baby still does not come, once the arms are born, use both hands to grasp the baby around the rib cage, have someone apply gentle fundal pressure and have the mother push to see if a little more force will result in advancement (be very sensitive to what you are doing, as you do not want to rupture anything with too much force). Be sure your grasp is evenly distributed and no fingers are pressing into soft parts as you gently move the torso up and down or from side to side just enough to work the baby out of the yoni. The most likely reason for such a delay is a cord entangled around the lower limbs. Remember that you have some time to try and figure out your best option to birth the rest of the baby if the head and chest are born and the baby is breathing. Defects are often soft enough that the baby can be coaxed out with gentle side-to-side outward traction and optimal maternal positioning (upright to maximize the space in the outlet). Be exceptionally gentle. Organs and their vasculature (particularly the liver) are easy to injure when you are grasping the baby like this. If birth proves impossible, you can transport the mother with the baby partially born. If the baby is breathing, she will not die on the way; if she is not, establish an airway and provide respiratory support to the best of your ability.

Paracentesis: If you are *remote from medical help,* the head is out and the baby is dead or the mother's condition indicates that immediate birth is imperative for her well-being and you have detected a massive abdominal defect that does not respond to other attempts at delivery, you can try to drain fluid from the defect. Guide a needle into the yoni (as for cephalocentesis) and insert it into the enlarged area. Be aware that if the mass is solid (more likely if the baby can not be encouraged to advance), this will not help and may create an additional problem for the baby by causing further trauma. The needle is likely to have to pass through solid organs to get to the entrapped fluid when inserted from this direction. This option should be considered only as a last resort when the need is dire.

Absence of the umbilical cord (body stalk anomaly): This is a severe and exceedingly rare form of fatal abdominal defect in which the umbilical cord either does not form at all or is very, very short. These babies typically have a large anterior abdominal defect, with most of the internal organs enclosed in a sac that is directly attached to the placenta. There is a complete lack of fetal descent during labor with no apparent cause. Clues to this problem include minimal fetal movement during pregnancy, a small baby and abnormal fetal heart rate patterns (Benirschke & Kaufmann, 2000; Fox, 1997).

Maternal tumors

Uterine fibroids, cysts of the reproductive organs or adjacent regions or tumors of the yoni may rarely become an obstacle to descent of the fetus during labor. Most of the time, such growths will be pressed out of the way as the uterus enlarges. Internal growths may be pressed to the side or pulled up and out of the way during fetal descent as the upper segment retracts. A cervical fibroid is the most likely tumor to obstruct labor; however, these are very rare. A growth on or in the anterior lip can sometimes be detected before the baby has moved down into the pelvis and can be pushed up and out of the way. Likewise, if identified soon enough, a pediculated polyp or fibroid can be pushed upward. If such an obstruction is large or cannot be displaced upward, a surgical birth may be necessary.

Robin Lim, a midwife who works in Indonesia, reports attending a birth where a pediculated fibroid was blocking the birth canal. Transport was not an option, so the obstetrician who was working with her reached up and squeezed the tumor as hard as she could. This expelled the blood, causing the tumor to collapse, after which the birth proceeded normally. Such a procedure can certainly be tried if you are very remote from medical help, but keep in mind that a solid tumor will not collapse and that collapsing a cancerous one may send malignant cells into the mother's bloodstream (Lim, 2000).

A large growth in the pelvic or lower abdominal region may significantly impair or arrest descent of the baby, although the reason will not be apparent. For example, a large ovarian cyst, displaced bowel tumor or diverticulum, kidney displaced into the pelvis (pelvic kidney), sacrococcygeal tumor or hydatid cyst of the liver may not be detectable prior to surgery, but all can prevent descent into the pelvis. Descent may become arrested for no apparent reason. This may occur in any laboring woman, regardless of the number of babies she has had. If there is prior knowledge of the growth, you can suspect that it is the source of the difficulty, especially if it is known to be quite large (lemon sized or larger). The only recourse then is to transport.

On rare occasions, a cervical hematoma or even a carcinoma may result in obstruction. A constant bloody discharge should prompt an internal exam. A visual inspection may reveal either a swelling like a purple grape or the diseased portion of the cervix. A hematoma will probably allow the birth to proceed. However, if you suspect cancer, transport is in order, as forcing the baby through may cause severe lacerations and infection, as well as encourage the spread of cancerous cells. Hopefully cervical cancer will have been detected prenatally.

It is much less likely for a maternal tumor to delay descent once the head (the hardest part of the baby) is past the level of the growth. However, it can rarely happen that a tumor, moved aside during one part of labor, falls back into the path of descent and prevents further advancement of the baby's body. Unless she was previously aware, for example, that the mother had a growth such as a uterine fibroid, the midwife may not be able to tell if it is a maternal or fetal problem that is causing the dystocia. Changing the mother's position and gently working the baby outward, as above, may remedy this situation. An extensive internal exam may identify the source of the problem. If a maternal growth is found, try to gently push it up and out of the way. If the baby's head and chest have emerged and he can breathe, there is plenty of time. Transport can even occur under such circumstances.

Tumors of the yoni such as cysts or fibroids very rarely cause obstruction. Cysts usually rupture. Glandular abscesses may rupture and spread infection to the baby or the mother's upper genital tract; be sure to treat the baby's eyes after birth and talk to the mother about treatment for herself as well. A calculus is another rare form of tumor, which feels like a stone. However, tumors of any kind rarely obstruct the birth canal enough to prevent descent (Myerscough, 1977).

Obstructions in the yoni

In most cases, you will have identified structural variations which may obstruct labor during prenatal care. Localized stenosis of the birth canal and atresia are rare causes of failure of descent. However, if you do find a band or membrane blocking the yoni canal, it can be snipped transversely. Anterior incision should be avoided to prevent injury of the bladder. More commonly, a longitudinal septum divides the yoni either partly or completely, into parallel canals. Such a septum can stretch during descent but more often tears, so it should be divided with scissors. The head can even pass beyond the septum with the shoulders becoming hung up on the band of tissue, but this is very rare.

Obstruction may occur due to adhesions and scars from previous surgery, fever (especially diphtheria), or injuries from a previous birth. Most such lesions yield during descent. If not, 8 to 10 evening primrose oil caps can be inserted into the yoni to help soften the scars.

Cystocele, rectocele and enterocele may cause minor obstruction during pushing. Simply push up on the prolapsed area, lifting it above the presenting part (Myerscough, 1977). More details about these types of prolapses can be found in my HEALING PASSAGE.

Uterine rupture

If the uterus ruptures during labor, descent of the fetus usually comes to a halt. In exceedingly rare cases, the body of the baby can exit the tear in the uterus prior to the birth of the head. Should the head be born, the result is a very rare type of apparent shoulder dystocia. For more details about uterine rupture in general, see the chapter entitled "Scar Dehiscence and Uterine Rupture in the Third Trimester" in Volume I and the chapter entitled "Uterine Rupture during Labor" in this text.

Uterine constriction ring

A constriction ring exists when a localized band of myometrium goes into tetanic contraction and becomes thickened. It occurs in about 1 out of every 1000 labors. It can develop in either the upper or lower uterine segment, but is usually found near the junction of the two. The chief cause is intrauterine manipulation with procedures such as aggressive massage or pressure on the uterus, internal version, manual removal of the placenta, or manual exploration of the uterus. It can also be caused by failed instrumental delivery or the use of oxytocin or other uterine stimulants when the uterus is already hypertonic. A constriction ring can also develop spontaneously without preceding interventions, although this is rare. Spontaneous constriction rings are usually associated with colicky or hypertonic uterine activity. They may also arise when the membranes rupture early and the uterus becomes irritated by being moulded tightly around the body of the baby. Although constriction rings usually develop during labor, they can also occur before labor begins or immediately after birth.

The constriction ring may form in any area of slight resistance (such as completely below the presenting part) but more often forms around a depression in the body of the baby (such as the neck) or, after the birth, below the placenta. A ring that forms around a fetal part grips that part tightly. Whether around or below the baby or placenta, the grip of the ring prevents descent. A constriction ring that develops after birth can cause the placenta to become trapped partially or completely above the ring (when it is referred to as an "hourglass contraction").

As opposed to a pathologic retraction ring, which arises as the *result* of obstructed labor, the constriction ring is a localized myometrial spasm that obstructs further progress *itself.* The lower segment is neither stretched nor abnormally thin, and the upper segment is not overly thick. There is no risk of uterine rupture if there are no other associated problems, such as disproportion. The woman with a constriction ring has severe uterine pain and tenderness over the upper uterine segment during contractions and has a sense that her contractions have become ineffective. The uterine contractions may be irregular and uncoordinated. In contrast, a pathologic retraction ring causes pain in the lower uterine segment.

The most common site of constriction ring formation is 7 to 8 cm above the external cervical os. While it may form anywhere along the length of the uterine muscle, it tends to form either around the baby's neck at the level of the symphysis (75%), around the body of the child (14%), above the level of the pubic symphysis (14%) or in front of the presenting part behind the pubic bone (9%) according to one old study (Rudolph & Fields, 1947).

Detection: Suspect the formation of a constriction ring whenever there is a delay in labor without apparent cause, especially if the strength and painfulness of uterine contractions are dramatically out of proportion with their effectiveness. The mother is often fatigued. Upon examination, a constriction ring may be palpable abdominally in only about 9% of cases. Although it will produce a depression in the uterine wall and may even be visible in a thin woman, the external uterine surface may feel perfectly normal even when a rigid constriction ring exists (Mayes, 1954). There is no change in station during a contraction. A head that has descended will be loose in the pelvic cavity both during and between contractions. If the head is not engaged, the upper uterus and portion of the baby's body contained therein will move as one mass when palpated. Gentle palpation will trigger the uterus to contract. The cervix is floppy and not well applied to the presenting part; the portion of the uterus between the external os and the constriction ring will remain lax during uterine contractions (this sign is unique to this condition). Because of this, a hand can easily be passed into the uterus and the ring can sometimes be identified (this exam is not recommended as it will increase the chance of infection). A finger can be inserted inside the os between the inner cervical wall and the baby's head; the pressure exerted on the finger by the head during a contraction will be minimal. In fact, the baby may be pulled up, rather than pushed down, during a contraction.

The following chart summarizes the differences between a constriction ring and a pathologic retraction ring.

Constriction Ring	Pathologic Retraction Ring
•Localized ring of spastic uterine muscle	•Result of excessive retraction of upper uterine segment
•May occur in any part of the uterus, although usually occurs at the junction of the upper and lower segments	•Always occurs at the junction of the upper and lower uterine segments
•Myometrium at ring is thicker than that above or below.	•Myometrium is much thicker above than below ring.
•Uterus below ring is neither thin, distended nor tender.	•Uterus below the ring is thin, distended and tender.
•Uterus above ring is relaxed and not tender between contractions but may be tender during contractions.	•Uterus above ring is very firm and may be tender.
•Uterus never ruptures.	•If uncorrected, the uterus may rupture.
•Round ligaments are not tense.	•Round ligaments are tense and prominent.
•May develop before or during any stage of labor	•Usually develops just before or during late pushing
•Position of the ring does not change during labor.	•The ring gradually rises abdominally as labor advances.
•Presenting part does not descend during contractions.	•Presenting part is jammed into pelvis with contractions.
•Fetus may be mainly or entirely above ring.	•Part of the child (usually most of the body) is below ring.
•Woman's general condition is good.	•Woman's general condition is poor.
•Uterine action is inefficient with abnormally polarized contractions.	•Uterine action is efficient or overly so, with contractions of normal polarity for labor.
•Leads to obstructed descent	•Is caused by obstructed descent

Treatment: A constriction ring must relax before labor can proceed. Place the mother in a hot sitz and foot bath, let her rest and give her relaxing herbs such as motherwort or skullcap (for more details, see the chapter entitled "Cervical and Other Soft-Tissue Problems during Labor"). Transport is the best alternative if there is no change; the fetal mortality rate is around 70% when constriction rings are left to nature.

Abdominal pregnancy

Only in the rarest of cases will an abdominal pregnancy progress, undetected, until term (unless, of course, a woman with an abdominal pregnancy first presents herself in labor). Observation of the abdomen may reveal the distinct outline of the contracting uterus, which has been pushed to the side of the fetus. Fetal parts are easy to feel and the baby may not be in a longitudinal lie. A bimanual exam reveals a small uterus with no fetal parts within. Transport immediately.

Blockage by one half of a double uterus

On very rare occasions, the nonpregnant half of a double uterus can become situated below the fetus, thus preventing descent. In some cases, a uterine anomaly of this type may have been identified prior to pregnancy, but this is by no means always true. This situation may be mistaken for obstruction due to a small fibroid, but the presence of two cervical canals (which should have been identified in prenatal exams) points to a double uterus as the real problem. While maternal position changes and digital displacement can be used in an attempt to wiggle the baby past the uterine horn, surgical birth is usually necessary (Gibberd et al., 1965).

Anterior or posterior sacculation of the uterus

Review the chapter in Volume I entitled "Incarceration and Sacculation of the Pregnant Uterus" before studying this section. Sacculation is an exceedingly rare cause of nonprogressive labor. A sacculation is a pouch that forms in the lower uterine segment. This "sac" in the uterine wall most often contains the fetal head but may contain other parts of the fetus, such as a shoulder if the baby is transverse. In anterior sacculation, the sac is in front of the cervix, while in posterior sacculation, the sac is behind the cervix. This condition does not develop during labor; it should have been recognized during prenatal care.

If anterior sacculation has not resolved prenatally, by term the sac and its contents often overhang the symphysis, creating problems with fetal descent. Associated symptoms include pain, with painful or obstructed urination. Contractions produce extreme, increasing pain and sensitivity in the anterior lower segment as the sac is stretched. No uterine action reaches the os, which remains high and often squashed above the symphysis. The sac becomes increasingly thin; necrosis and sloughing of the uterine wall as well as uterine rupture can occur if this condition goes unrecognized.

Descent of the presenting part covered with the portion of the lower uterine segment comprising the sac may occur as the fundus retracts and presses the baby down. A sac that has descended sufficiently may be seen at the introitus; the surface will appear smooth and shiny with a marked vascular pattern. Its presence places the mother at great risk of uterine rupture; the risk is further increased if the sac is inappropriately manipulated as though it were a simple case of a distended anterior lip. With sacculation, the os will be almost impossible to find if posterior. It may be easier to find if it is anterior, but in both cases it will be squashed and closed. Uterine contractions will have no effect on its consistency. Be aware that the appearance of a tissue-covered head at the vulva is *most* likely to be due to a stretched anterior lip, which will appear reddish purple to purple and possibly swollen; the edge will usually be fairly easy to locate by reaching under, around and behind the underlying head. This is a painful, but far less serious situation that can usually be remedied (see the chapter entitled "Cervical and Other Soft-Tissue Problems during Labor" for details).

If you suspect a sacculated uterus, place the mother on a firm surface on her back and elevate her bottom. The following technique can be used if the condition is recognized before the sac has become extremely stretched. The earlier in labor it is employed, the greater the likelihood of success. Insert your sterile-gloved hand into the yoni; open your fingers and gently distribute pressure as evenly as possible to elevate the sac containing the fetal part back up into the pelvis. Be careful; the uterine wall may be exquisitely tender, painful and prone to puncture from the stress it has undergone. As you elevate the sac, search around for the cervix. Insert a finger into the undilated cervix, pull it to the center of the pelvic cavity, and hold it there. Displace the presenting part out of the sac and over the cervix. Hold everything in place during the following contractions until the cervix dilates.

This maneuver is easier to describe than to accomplish. Efforts may be thwarted because the space between the shortened fundus and the lower uterine segment is so reduced that the fetus cannot fit into the uterus in a normal orientation. In addition, the contracting uterus will tend to direct the long axis of the fetus back into the sac, thus bypassing the cervix. The abnormal shape of the uterus may prevent the force of contractions from being properly transmitted to the cervix. Having an assistant hold the baby in position from above, especially if the baby is overhanging the pubic bone, might increase your chances of success. The lower segment will be extremely thin if the condition has gone unrecognized during many hours of labor, and these manipulations will increase the likelihood of uterine rupture. If you suspect that neither the uterine wall nor the woman can tolerate such manipulations, transport for a surgical birth. However, rupture is inevitable if hospital transport is impossible for any reason, so attempting to reposition the cervix offers the best chance of a good outcome. Be careful and sensitive as you proceed.

Incomplete dilation leading to arrest of the shoulders after birth of the head: If the baby's head is unusually small the cervix may give the impression of being fully dilated and allow the head to slip through. However, the incompletely dilated cervix could then become lodged around the aftercoming shoulders. This will mimic a shoulder dystocia. Therefore, if the head is unusually small and the shoulders are delayed, as you check for cord around the neck, slide your fingers around the shoulder girdle to check for a cervical rim as well. If you find one, you will have to work it back over the shoulders, which may take some doing to accomplish; try your best. If that doesn't work snip the cervix it if you have to, preferably at the 12 o'clock point, but be prepared for the possibility that the incision may extend into the lower uterine segment and hemorrhage after the birth. Examine the cervix carefully after the birth and transport if you cannot find the apex of an incision or tear or if bleeding is excessive.

Postbirth Considerations

Inspect the perineum carefully

Whenever the birth is difficult, perineal lacerations are more likely. Perform an especially careful examination of the perineum, anal sphincter and intrayoni. See HEALING PASSAGE for complete details.

Severe maternal injuries

Prolonged obstructed labor may result in injuries to multiple maternal organ systems. This is termed **obstructed labor injury complex**, an incompletely understood range of injuries that can ruin a woman's life. On average, these types of injuries occur after 3.9 days of frankly obstructed labor. Remember, a woman can have a slow and gradual labor without in the absence of obstruction for longer than this. It is the nature of the labor and not simply that it is taking a long time that results in these catastrophic injuries.

The most common injury is an obstetric fistula, which is formed when the maternal soft tissues are trapped between an impacted presenting part and the pelvis for a long period of time. Widespread ischemic vascular damage occurs resulting in tissue necrosis and breakdown, leaving a wide fistula averaging 2.3 cm long (ranging from 0.1 to 8 cm) and 2.5 cm wide (ranging from 0.1 to 10 cm). Postsurgical fistulas are generally small holes surrounded by healthy tissue; in contrast, the damage that leads to large fistula formation means that the hole is surrounded by grossly traumatized tissues that have suffered near-deadly hypoxic ischemia, resulting in wide-spread damage to the pelvic floor and nearby organs. A hole may be created between the yoni and the bladder; there may be to total breakdown of the urethra, stress incontinence, renal failure, a rectovaginal fistula, rectal atresia (where the rectum heals closed), incompetence of the anal sphincter, cervical destruction, pelvic infection, amenorrhea, secondary infertility, yoni stenosis, abnormal hardening in the pubic bone (osteostenosis) and foot drop (inability to dorsiflex the foot due to nerve damage). The level at which the damage occurs varies according to the level at which the presenting part was obstructed. The surgery required to repair such defects is complex and usually not readily available or affordable to the women who are most subject to enduring labor with an obstruction (Arrowsmith et al., 1996).

References and Further Reading on Issues Involving the Flow of Labor

References used in multiple Chapters

Betts D. Acupressure: Promoting A Natural Labour and Partner Involvement. http://home.clear.net.nz/pages/debra_betts/, downloaded Feb 15, 2002.

Cunningham F, et al. Williams Obstetrics, 21st ed., McGraw-Hill, New York, NY, 2001.

Davis E. Heart & Hands, A Midwife's Guide to Pregnancy and Birth, 3rd ed. Celestial Arts, Berkeley CA, 1997.

El Halta V. Preventing Prolonged Labor, Midwifery Today, (46);22, Summer, 1998.

Friedman A. Labor: Clinical Evaluation and Management, Appleton-Century-Crofts, New York NY, 1967.

Gaskin IM. Ina May's Guide to Childbirth. Bantam Books, New York NY, 2003.

Hobbs V, LAc. Personal communications regarding the use of Chinese medicine during labor, 1999 & Mar, 2002.

Lowe C, LAc, CNM. Editing notes, 2003.

Myerscough P. Munro Kerr's Operative Obstetrics, 9th ed. Williams & Wilkins Co, Baltimore MD, 1977.

OTIS, "Hyperthermia and pregnancy," Organization of Teratology Information Services, www.ctispregnancy.org/hyperthermia.pdf, web site accessed Jan 8, 2004.

Oxorn H. Human Labor and Birth, 5th ed, Appleton/Century/Crofts, Norwalk CT, 1986.

Schlinger H, CPM. Editing notes, Nov, 2003.

Scholles H, CPM. Editing notes, 2003.

Simkin P, Ancheta R. The Labor Progress Handbook, Blackwell Sciences, Oxford UK, 2000.

Stockham A. Tokology, rev. ed., Alice B. Stockham & Co., Chicago IL, 1898.

Sutton J. Let Birth Be Born Again: Rediscovering and Reclaiming Our Midwifery Heritage. Birth Concepts UK, Middlesex UK, 2001.

Sutton J; Scott P. Understanding and Teaching Optimal Foetal Positioning, Bay Print, Ltd., Tauranga, NZ, 1996.

Varney H. Midwifery, 3rd ed. Jones & Bartlett Pub, Sudbury MA, 1997.

West Z. Acupuncture in Pregnancy and Childbirth. Churchill Livingstone, Edinburgh UK, 2001.

Natural Induction and Augmentation of Labor

Bakhareva Z. Personal conversation, 1999.

Berghella V, et al. "Stripping of membranes as a safe method to reduce prolonged pregnancies," Obstet Gynecol, 87(6);927-931, June, 1996.

Bishop E. "Pelvic scoring for elective induction," Obstet Gynecol, 24(2):266-268, Aug, 1964.

Davis L. "The use of castor oil to stimulate labor in patients with premature rupture of membranes," JNM, 29(6);366-370, Nov-Dec, 1984.

Driggers R, et al.,"An amniotic fluid index < or =5 cm within 7 days of delivery in the third trimester is not associated with decreasing umbilical arterial pH and base excess," J Perinatol, 24(2):72-76, Feb, 2004.

Enning C. "Birth on Demand," all day workshop on waterbirth, Midwifery Today conf., Springfield OR, Mar, 2003.

Gentlebirth midwifery archives. http://www.gentlebirth.org/archives/. Web site of the Midwife List, international archive of midwifery wisdom, accessed 2000.

Harper B. Personal conversation, 1999.

Hobbs V. Ancient Medicine–New Tools: Applying Traditional Chinese Medicine to Modern Western Midwifery, unpublished workshop handout, Apprentice Academics Homebirth Conf., Salt Lake City UT, July, 1994.

Kesting B. Pegasus, Das Zentrum für ganzheitliche Geburtshilfe Blücherplatz 15-27, 52068 Aachen, Germany. E-mail: pegasuszentrum@t-online.de, Mar, 1999.

King J. Back Labor No More!! What Every Woman Should Know before Labor. Plenary Systems, Inc, Dallas TX, 1993.

Merdock A. Personal conversation, MANA conf., Austin TX, Nov, 2003.

Wainer-Cohen N. Personal conversation, MANA conf., Boston MA, 2001.

Cervical and Other Soft Tissue Problems during Labor

Block P. Polly Block's Birth Book, Hearthspun Pub, American Fork UT, 1984.

Davidson K, CNM. Personal communication, 1997.

Gentlebirth midwifery archives. http://www.gentlebirth.org/archives/. Web site of the Midwife List, international archive of midwifery wisdom, accessed 2001.

Kingston L. Personal conversation, [1982?].

Kolder V. Editing notes, Healing Passage: A Midwife's Guide to the Care and Repair of the Tissues Involved in Birth, Labrys Press, Portland OR, 1990.

Lim R, CPM. Personal communication, July, 2002.

Maciocia G. Obstetrics and Gynecology in Chinese Medicine. Churchill Livingstone, New York NY, 1998.

Wilson K. Personal communication, [1997?].

DIFFICULTIES WITH CONTRACTIONS

Daniels S. Midwifery training program. The Maternity Center, El Paso, TX, 1978.
Friedman E. "The labor curve," CLIN PERINATOL, 8(1);15-25, Feb 1981.
Greenhill J. PRINCIPLES AND PRACTICE OF OBSTETRICS, 10th ed. WB Saunders Co, Philadelphia PA, 1951.
Quenby S, et al. "Dysfunctional labor and myometrial lactic acidosis," OBSTET GYNECOL, 103(4);718-723, Apr 2004. Erratum in: OBSTET GYNECOL, 103(6);1344, Jun 2004.
Rudolph L."Contraction Ring Dystocia," OBSTET GYNECOL BR EMP, 42;992 Dec, 1935.
Rudolph L. "Constriction Ring Dystocia," JAMA, 108;532, Feb 13, 1937.
Stockham A. TOKOLOGY, rev. ed., Alice B. Stockham & Co., Chicago IL, 1898.

RECOGNIZING AND DEALING WITH OBSTRUCTED LABOR

Arrowsmith S, et al. "Obstructed labor injury complex: obstetric fistula formation and the mutlifacited morbidity of maternal birth trauma in the developing world," OBSTET GYNECOL SURVEY, 51(9);568-574, Sept, 1996.
Benirschke K, Kaufmann P. PATHOLOGY OF THE HUMAN PLACENTA, 4th ed. Springer Verlag, New York NY, 2000.
Cehelsky M, Mason V. "Anterior sacculation of the pregnant uterus at term." AM J OBSTET GYNECOL, 99(7);1000-1005, Dec 1, 1967.
Fox H. PATHOLOGY OF THE PLACENTA, 2nd ed. WB Saunders Co, Ltd, London UK, 1997.
Gibberd G, et al., eds. THE QUEEN CHARLOTTE'S TEXT-BOOK OF OBSTETRICS, J & A Churchill Ltd., London UK, 1965.
Lim R, Personal conversation, 2000.
Mayes B. PRACTICAL OBSTETRICS. Angus & Robertson, Sydney Australia, 1954.
Myerscough P. MUNRO KERR'S OPERATIVE OBSTETRICS, 9th ed. Williams & Wilkins Co, Baltimore MD, 1977.
Rudolph L, Fields C. "Constriction ring dystocia," AM J OBSTET GYNECOL, 53;796, May, 1947.
Sellers P. MIDWIFERY, A TEXTBOOK AND REFERENCE BOOK FOR MIDWIVES IN SOUTHERN AFRICA, VOL. 2: COMPLICATIONS IN CHILDBIRTH. Juta & Co, Ltd., Kenwyn So Africa, 1993.
Thoms H. "Obstetrical significance of pelvic variations: a study of 450 primiparous women." BMJ, 2;210, 1937.
Tully G. RESOLVING SHOULDER DYSTOCIA: THE THREE R'S. Spinning Babies Workshops, 10545 Humboldt Ave. So., Minneapolis MN, 2003.

Supporting the Mother Who is Having a Hard Time Coping with Labor

Entering Pains and Back Pain in Labor

Entering pains

This is the term Sutton (2001) has coined to refer to pain in the suprapubic area that occurs for many women as the baby is attempting to rotate to a more favorable position in order to enter the brim. Any mother who enters labor with a posterior baby may have painful early labor as the baby tries to turn. This can be particularly problematic for a woman with a platypelloid pelvis who enters labor with a baby who has not yet assumed an occiput transverse position. As the baby works to find the best position, long, erratic and painful contractions ensue. The use of frequent position changes, leaning forward with the back straight, and asymmetrical pelvic postures will help the baby turn. Use side-lying if the mother must rest. Sutton recommends that the first-time mother lie on her left side. The multipara can choose either side. (See further discussion of how and upon which side to lie in the chapter entitled "Positions and Activities for Labor.") Unless the mother has a pendulous abdomen, it is very important that belly-lifting not be done until the head is through the brim; it will relieve the pain, but it will also lift the baby away from the brim, thus restricting the baby's movements and preventing descent (Sutton, 2001). However, if the abdominal muscles are lax, lifting just below the navel can help better align the baby without restricting movement of the head. Getting in water deep enough to allow the mother to be upright and leaning forward (for example, on her knees) can also be very helpful.

Back pain in labor

Throughout most of labor, as a general rule, the less the back hurts, the more efficient the contractions. However, some back pain occurs during almost every labor. Even a woman carrying her baby in a perfectly flexed, anterior vertex position may experience some back pain related to tension in the lower uterine segment and the cervix. In progressive labors, if back pain occurs, it is often prominent only at the beginning of a contraction during early dilation; between contractions the back does not normally hurt. Late in labor it may occur again as the baby's head descends past the sacral promontory on its way through the pelvis and as the mother's back opens when her sacrum moves back and out of the way during pushing. This is especially true for the mother whose pelvis is being opened for the first time. This results in a modest amount of additional discomfort during contractions but represents good progress. There are, however, five categories of women who experience excessive back pain during labor:

- Women who are carrying an occiput posterior baby. When the head is pressed into the lower spine rather than down into the pelvic cavity (as is usually the case with the baby in an OP position), back pain can be extreme.
- Those who have a pendulous abdomen.
- Those who have a history of back injury or a congenital spinal defect, including women who have a swayback or spinal curvature, typically experience intense back pain. Counterpressure will usually cause more pain.
- Those whose baby has one arm positioned so that her hand is on the opposite shoulder, elbow in front of her chin. Even though the baby's occiput may be anterior, the elbow is pressing into the sacral promontory, causing severe back pain during contractions that may mimic a posterior labor. Back pain is typically more constant in a posterior labor, whereas pain secondary to a compound presentation tends to diminish between contractions. (Sutton & Scott, 1996). (See the chapter entitled "Assisting a Woman Whose Baby Is in a Compound Presentation" for a trick to fix this.)
- Women whose cervix is abnormally resistant to the force of contractions.

See the chapters entitled "Cervical and Other Soft-Tissue Problems during Labor" and "Difficulties with Contractions" for more information.

Severe back pain causes women to move away from their labor rather than sink into it. This is expressed in leaning backward, stretching upright or rising up on the toes while holding tension in the buttocks and thighs, all of which limit sacral mobility. Arching the back is a natural response to this kind of pain, which increases the amount of space in the angle between the spine and the pubic bone, but tightens the abdominal muscles and requires the baby to turn uphill (Sutton & Scott, 1996). Moving away from the energy results in less effective contractions and a labor that is much prolonged. The woman may remark that her back is killing her, that it feels like a knife is in her back, that she wants counterpressure on her back and, not infrequently, will say she cannot stand the pain any longer. Anything that can help better align the baby's presenting part with the pelvic cavity can help move things along and provide blessed relief from often excruciating back pain. Postures that include a straight back while leaning forward will tip the pelvis forward, thus maximizing for most women the space in which the baby can turn.

Special considerations for women with short torsos: Women who have short torsos are almost always short-waisted. That is, they have very little space between the lowermost border of the rib cage and the upper border of the iliac crest. These women carry their babies out in front during pregnancy, as there is less room in the mother's torso to fit the baby as he grows; this problem is compounded if the baby is long (tall). This combination tends to produce pronounced flexion of the fetal spine when the baby's back is anterior because the curve of the abdomen is exaggerated. During labor, a short torso may result in the force of contractions being directed toward the mother's lower spine because, as the uterus leans forward during contractions, the line of force is directed too posteriorly rather than down into the pelvic cavity. Short women may therefore experience more back pain.

Positions that stretch the torso, such as lifting the arms, sagging the lower back forward, tilting the pelvis as far forward as possible, throwing the shoulders back, and maintaining the upper spine in as straight a position as possible, will help create more room in front so the baby can move. The belly lift described below may also be of great benefit to these women (King, 1993). They may also benefit from using the Birth Sling during labor as well as pushing.

Belly lift: This technique was popularized by a mother who was determined to come up with a creative solution to her own difficult back labors. It is based on the understanding that the presenting part must be directed into the pelvic cavity for contractions to work most effectively. When the baby's head is in a cocked position, or when a baby is posterior, the angle of force may push the head against the lower spine or pelvic sidewalls instead. When this occurs, pain is increased and labor is prolonged as the contractions work to reposition the baby and the cervix into a better angle before they can work on bringing the baby down. The belly lift speeds up this process by manually redirecting the angle of descent by moving the baby so that the head is not being pressed into the sacrum but is directed down into the pelvic cavity, sometimes saving the woman hours of work. It may help whenever the head is not ideally placed to move along more quickly, especially if the force of the contraction is centered behind the os (in this case, the cervix would not be unusually posterior).

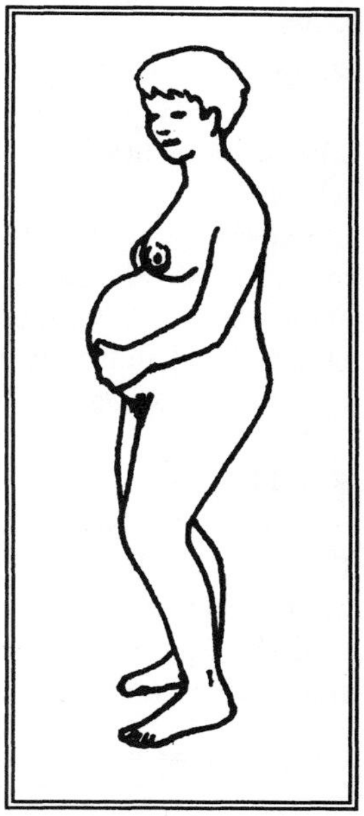

The belly lift can be used after the woman has established effective contractions, which need not be regular but must be affecting the cervix. It is best done standing. The mother places her hands on her lower abdomen between her pubic bone and her navel between contractions. As the contraction begins, she moves her open hands to just above her hips on either side, near where she can feel the contraction starting. As the sensation of the contraction begins to build up the front of her belly, she follows it with her hands. (If she can't feel the contractions in this area, she should just follow the hand movements given in these instructions.) As the contraction becomes more intense, her fingertips should meet at the lower abdomen. She now starts to lift her lower belly, visualizing where the force of the contraction is directed. The lifting is done with the forearms, using the elbow as a hinge, the upper arm and shoulders remain stationary. The higher up the spine the contraction or pain is felt, the higher she should lift her belly, moving the hands up just below the navel. As the uterus is lifted, she will be able to feel the back pain subside, which tells her when to stop lifting and maintain the uterus at that angle. She can also tilt her pelvis forward to help straighten the path of descent or lean forward with her back straight to further facilitate rotation.

Between contractions, the lift should be maintained so that the progress made during the last contraction is not lost. The woman or a support person may find it easier to use the Tummy Lift, which was designed to assist this technique (see the chapter entitled "Positioning-Assist Equipment and Maternal Comfort Items"). Labor may progress rapidly after using this technique, so be prepared. (King, 1993).

The belly lift can be used once the baby's head is repositioned or to try and reposition a head. It can also be used when a woman has a pendulous abdomen. Some women with back labor experience an uncontrollable running or jerking motion of the legs when they lie down. This technique seems to remedy this problem as well.

Acupressure: Stimulating Ciliau (BL-32) can greatly assist in relieving back pain during labor (Hobbs, 2002). For details, see the subchapter entitled "Sterile Water Injections for the Relief of Excessive Localized Pain."

Nausea and Vomiting

NOTE: Read the following chapter entitled "Understanding and Preventing Maternal Exhaustion," along with this one.

Nausea and vomiting can render early labor a miserable experience as well as significantly reduce the chances of staying at home when labor is prolonged. The key to dealing with nausea is to catch it early, before it progresses to vomiting. This will forestall the development of dehydration and electrolyte imbalances, both of which hasten the development of clinical exhaustion.

Nausea and vomiting can manifest in three very different ways during labor. First, there is the woman who enters labor at an intake deficit. She has not eaten well prior to labor and avoided eating in early labor; she then becomes hypoglycemic which leads to nausea. Next, there is the woman who is afraid of the birthing energy. She attempts to stop its flow in the middle of her body, and the energy turns around and comes back up as nausea and vomiting. This usually occurs in early labor in frightened first-time mothers, when labor begins to get stronger than anything they have experienced before. The third woman experiences birthing energy as an "opening up" at both ends. This occurs when the energy is coming through with such force that the woman does not understand at first how to channel all of it down to her cervix. She vomits in transition but usually does not do so persistently, and she quickly progresses into pushing. What follows is a rundown of how to help, in the order of what to do when.

Remind the mother to eat in early labor

It is very typical for first-time mothers to get excited upon the onset of labor and forget to eat. Well-meaning relatives who are present may advise her against eating; she may heed their advice, even if you have told her previously to eat whatever she wants. The excitement of the event, coupled with the fear and the energy, is a setup for the development of nausea. Therefore, emphasize to the first-time mother that she must eat in early labor. If labor is very early, many midwives recommend a high-carbohydrate meal to pack in the calories for the work ahead. The woman should probably avoid highly spicy foods at this time, as she may have reflux as labor becomes more active. Her choices should focus on unrefined, nutritious foods that are easy to digest so they move out of her stomach and into her system more rapidly. Foods such as yogurt, cottage cheese, ice cream (which has sugar but also has protein) or miso soup are good choices.

Fluid intake

The mother should be taking in a minimum of 4 oz of fluid every hour. Health-food brands of electrolyte-balancing fluids, such as ReCharge, are good fluid sources, especially if the mother has been vomiting or has diarrhea. (Mainstream brands contain many additives, food colors and, in some cases, aspartame and should be avoided.). Hot ginger tea can be given for severe nausea (boil 1 Tbsp chopped fresh ginger in 2 cups of water for 10 minutes). Electrolyte-balancing fluids can also be mixed at home. Below are three recipes.

Recipe 1	Recipe 2	Recipe 3
1 tsp miso paste 1 tsp lemon juice 1 tsp salt 1 tsp calcium* 2 cups (480 ml) water	1 tsp salt 1 tsp baking soda 4 tsp honey Lemon or lime juice to taste 1 quart (1 liter) water	⅓ cup (80 ml) lemon juice ¼ tsp salt ⅓ cup (80 ml) honey 1 Tbsp calcium* 1 quart (1 liter) water

*Use powdered calcium lactate or a liquid calcium supplement

It is not necessary to wait for nausea to appear before offering electrolyte-balancing fluids.

If symptoms of nausea have appeared

Stimulate Neiguan (Pc-6), the acupuncture point located on the inner wrists. This point can be used to help relieve all degrees of nausea as well as to curtail vomiting. It is a good first line of therapy and may allay nausea to the point that the woman can eat to help break the nausea cycle. Apply steady pressure to one or both wrists until the woman reports relief, which will often occur within minutes. Seabands™ (or an elastic band with a smooth, rounded button sewn to one side) can be used to provide continuous pressure. Bands are worn like a wristwatch on both arms with the button against the point (Hobbs, 2002; Lowe, 2003). To locate these points, see the subchapter entitled "Traditional Chinese Medicine."

A single drop of peppermint oil can be placed on the woman's forehead. Homeopathic remedies can also be given for nausea. Ipecac works for nausea, especially if it has progressed to vomiting. Give 30C doses every 15 minutes until the nausea has resolved (Schlinger, 2003)

Address emotional issues: Once nausea has set in, treat it as best you can and then discuss fears and concerns. With luck, the treatment will take care of the nausea before it gets worse and any emotional issues can then be addressed.

If the woman can keep nothing down: Discuss the possibility of administering a retention enema (for details, see the subchapter entitled "Cleansing and Retention Enemas"). This can provide vital hydration, stabilize the nausea and allow her to begin to take foods and fluids by mouth once more. It is important to stop persistent vomiting or the woman will have to be transported; it is simply too dangerous to leave her at home. This is not necessary if it is obvious that the vomiting is connected to a rapid transition phase of labor, as the birth will soon be over!

Give a hydrating IV or retention enema: An IV can be used to rehydrate a woman, and will often relieve otherwise intractable nausea allowing labor to continue at home. Do not use glucose infusion; an IV of lactated Ringer's (Hartman's) is preferable. A retention enema accomplishes the same thing, however, and is less risky. (See the subchapter entitled "Intravenous Equipment and IV Therapy" for full details.)

UNDERSTANDING AND PREVENTING MATERNAL EXHAUSTION

Note: Stress in the context of normal labor is discussed in the chapter entitled "Ecstatic Birth: The Maternal Response to the Pain and Stress of Labor."

The greatest threat to continuing with a normal but long labor at home is the development of maternal exhaustion. Once the mother is nearing exhaustion and cannot recover her equilibrium, the only safe course of action may be transport. Understanding adult stress responses outside of pregnancy can help the midwife to be alert for the signs of impending clinical exhaustion and to avert its development.

Adult Stress Responses

The human body has evolved in a generally hostile environment for many hundreds of thousands of years and is thus well designed to deal with the daily stressors of life. In fact, some stress can be productive, as is the stress pregnant women feel as labor begins, an experience that allows them to prepare for birth. During a time of stress, homeostatic processes allow the body to continue to maintain normal parameters of chemistry, temperature and blood pressure while a variety of metabolic activities are modified to prepare the body to meet the crisis.

However, when stress is extreme, unusual or long-lasting, the normal responses to stress may not be enough to prevent metabolic imbalance. In this event, the stress triggers a wide range of changes called the general adaptation syndrome (GAS) or the stress response. This syndrome was first described by Hans Selye, an authority on stress. Once the general adaptation syndrome is triggered, it takes over and changes the normal internal environment so that the body can respond to the higher level of stress. Selye's findings have been expanded on here to include some new information by other researchers regarding the role of hormones such as estrogen, oxytocin and endorphins.

Gender differences in the stress response

The human stress response has been called the "fight or flight" response for many years. This characteristic description was derived from studies primarily performed on male subjects (whether rats, or primates, including humans), who release large quantities of androgens, particularly testosterone, which promote aggressive reactions under stress. It has recently been postulated that oxytocin, produced by the posterior pituitary gland, is particularly high during stress in women. This key hormone is known to be released by both sexes under stress, but does not result in aggressive behavior. For this reason, Taylor and colleagues (2000) have suggested that the female response to stress may be better understood as a "tend-and-befriend" response.

Oxytocin has been found to enhance sedation and relaxation, reduce fearfulness and decrease sympathetic nerve activity, all of which are antithetical to the fight-or-flight response. Expressions of female aggression appear to be less tied to sympathetic arousal than male aggression and are instead more cerebral in nature. Not only is oxytocin released in greater quantity in women, but androgens, which tend to suppress the release of oxytocin, predominate in males, who have less oxytocin to begin with. Oxytocin's actions are also strongly modulated by estrogen, which enhances the antianxiety effects of oxytocin. During labor, when stress may be sustained, additional hormonal influences modulate the progress of labor, as explained in the chapter entitled "Ecstatic Birth: The Maternal Response to the Pain and Stress of Labor." These hormonally mediated differences are important to keep in mind when evaluating research regarding stress, and when attempting to predict the stress response of laboring women. Indeed, the female response to stress requires much more study before it will be fully understood.

General adaptation syndrome (GAS)

The region of the brain known as the hypothalamus monitors daily activities to detect changes in the body's chemistry, temperature and blood pressure. It also "watches" for emotions through connections to the cerebral cortex. When the hypothalamus senses stress, it begins a chain of reactions that eventually produce a stress response. Such stressors include almost any physiological or emotional disturbance, such as a change in the environmental temperature, exposure to toxins, a wound, or a strong emotional reaction such as being startled. The stimuli that produce stress differ among different people and even in the same person at different times.

Stressors stimulate the hypothalamus to trigger the GAS via two pathways. The first is the sympathetic division of the autonomic nervous system and the adrenal medulla, which produce an immediate alarm reaction. The second pathway involves the anterior pituitary gland and adrenal cortex, which produce the resistance reaction.

<u>The alarm reaction</u>: The alarm reaction responds to stress by activating the body's resources for immediate defensive activity. This complex series of alarm responses is immediate and short-acting. They are triggered by the hypothalamus, which sends nerve impulses through the spinal cord and sympathetic nervous system to target the adrenal medulla. The medulla produces catecholamines, which, together with sympathetic nervous system responses, generally increase the circulation and enhance ATP (adenosine triphosphate) synthesis. ATP is the primary chemical involved in the energy transfer system within the body. It can temporarily store and then transfer energy released in exergonic catabolic reactions to cellular activities that require energy; thus it facilitates the changes listed below. The alarm reaction brings tremendous amounts of glucose and oxygen to the organs that are most involved in dealing with the crisis. These are the brain, which must become highly alert; the skeletal muscles, which may have to cope with a physical attack or rapidly escape danger; and the heart, which must pump enough nutrients to the brain and muscles to sustain their increased demands. The alarm reaction triggers the following sympathetic responses:

- The rate and strength of cardiac muscle contractions increase. This speeds the circulation of nutrients and removes waste products from areas where this is needed most.
- Vasoconstriction occurs in nonessential organs and the skin. At the same time, vasodilation occurs in the large skeletal muscles, brain and lungs. Blood is thus rerouted to meet the needs of the most active systems. Circulation to the uterus and other reproductive organs is reduced, as they are not essential for maternal survival; this can severely impact the baby, especially if the stress persists for a long period of time.
- Urinary output falls off as the body conserves fluids.
- The spleen contracts and releases stored blood into the general circulation to increase the blood volume. Red blood cell production is also stepped up, and clotting factors are increased. These reactions prepare the body to deal with a possible injury and help meet the body's increased need for oxygen.
- The liver converts large amounts of stored glycogen to glucose and releases it into the bloodstream. This raises the blood sugar, thus providing an immediate source of energy to the cells.
- The respiratory rate increases and the airways dilate to help inhale more air. This enables the body to take in more oxygen, which is needed by the cells, as well as to discharge more carbon dioxide.
- Production of saliva, stomach fluid and intestinal secretions, all of which contain enzymes, decreases. This reaction slows digestive activity, which is not essential for dealing with the crisis.
- Perspiration increases as a means of thermoregulation.
- Sympathetic nerve impulses cause the adrenal medulla to increase its secretion of epinephrine and norepinephrine. These hormones supplement and prolong the effect of the responses outlined above.

In summary, the alarm reaction rapidly increases circulation, promotes catabolism of energy sources, and decreases nonessential activities. This response may promote survival in the short term but can quickly deplete the body's resources over time. If the stress is extreme and prolonged, the body may not be able to cope and death can result.

<u>Resistance reaction</u>: The other arm of the defense response is the resistance reaction, which begins more slowly than the alarm reaction but lasts longer. It is also initiated by the hypothalamus, which secretes hormones, among them corticotropin-releasing hormone (CRH). CRH stimulates the adenohypophysis (anterior pituitary gland) to increase its secretion of adrenocorticotrophic hormone (ACTH).

ACTH indirectly triggers the adrenal cortex to secrete more of its hormones, including mineralocorticoids. Kidney activity is diminished as blood flow to the kidneys is rerouted. The mineralocorticoids regulate the electrolyte (mineral and salt) balance in extracellular fluids. The most potent of these is aldosterone, which accounts for 95% of the mineralocorticoids produced. Mineralocorticoids help to retain sodium ions and step up the elimination of hydrogen ions, which are produced in high concentrations as a result of increased catabolism and tend to make the blood more acidic. This process prevents the body's pH from becoming dangerously low during stress. Sodium retention also results in water retention, which helps to maintain the high blood pressure that is necessary for an effective alarm reaction. It also helps compensate for fluid lost during severe bleeding, when it occurs.

The adrenal cortex also secretes glucocorticoids, including cortisol, hydrocortisone, cortisone and corticosterone. Of these, only cortisol in secreted is significant amounts in humans. High concentrations bring about these changes:

- Acceleration of protein catabolism and the conversion of amino acids into glucose so that the body has a large supply of energy long after its immediate stores of glucose have been burned.

- Stimulation of the removal of proteins from cells and the liver so that they can be broken down into amino acids. The amino acids are then rebuilt into enzymes needed to catabolize the increased chemical by-products of stress or be converted to glucose.
- Mobilization of fatty acids from adipose tissue, encouraging increased metabolism of fatty acids for the energy needs of most cells, thus sparing glucose for use by the brain. Glucose is the only fuel the brain can use.
- Increased sensitivity of blood vessels to stimuli that cause them to constrict. This compensates for any drop in blood pressure that may result from bleeding.
- Inhibition in the production of fibroblasts, which are immature connective tissue cells. Injured fibroblasts release chemicals that play a role in stimulating the inflammatory response. Thus, stress results in reduced inflammation and prevents it from becoming disruptive rather than protective.
- Slowing in the formation of connective tissues, which retards wound healing during a prolonged period of stress.

The effects of stress, especially when pain is involved, may be modulated by endogenous opiate peptides such as Beta-endorphin, a prohormone derived from the precursor protein preproopiomelanocortin. This protein is found in the anterior pituitary gland and the placenta. The endogenous opioids alter the release of neurotransmitters from afferent nerves and interfere with efferent pathways from the spinal cord to the brain. Thus, when pain is a component of stress, pain signals may be blocked at the level of the dorsal horns and never be transmitted to the brain. In this way, Beta-endorphins increase the pain threshold, provide a degree of analgesia and, in addition, create a sense of heightened well-being and euphoria. Some degree of pain is commonly a part of stressful situations, often due to muscle fatigue from the strain of having to carry out strenuous physical activities in a hurry. Relief of pain is an important component of the resistance reaction because it allows the person to continue to cope with the stress. In addition to playing a role in pain perception, endogenous opioid processes in combination with oxytocin may also be at the core of the tending response in women (Blackburn, 2003; Taylor et al., 2000).

Two other regulating hormones are secreted by the hypothalamus in response to stress: growth-hormone-releasing hormone (GHRH) and thyrotrophin-releasing hormone (TRH). GHRH stimulates the anterior pituitary to secrete human growth hormone (hGH), which increases the catabolism of fats (triglycerides) and the conversion of glycogen to glucose (glycogenolysis). TRH causes the anterior pituitary gland to secrete thyroid-stimulating hormone (TSH). TSH stimulates the catabolism of carbohydrates as it prompts the thyroid to secrete thyroxine (T_3) and triiodothyronine (T_4), which increase the catabolism of glucose to produce ATP. The combined actions of hGH and TSH thus provide more ATP to active cells. These additional thyroid hormones assist the glucocorticoids in supplying and regulating the use of energy to meet the increased physical demand.

In stressed females, the posterior pituitary releases oxytocin, which has been dubbed the "love hormone." Oxytocin is also released in males but to a lesser extent. High levels of oxytocin prompt females to care for immature offspring and other vulnerable females while engaging in community-oriented protective activities to ward off the threat.

The resistance reaction allows the body to continue dealing effectively with a stressor long after the effects of the alarm reaction have subsided. It increases the metabolism, provides functional proteins and enzymes as well as energy in the form of ATP, and triggers the circulatory changes required for dealing with a continuing crisis. Blood chemistry is returned to a nearly normal state during the resistance phase. The cells use glucose at the same rate that it enters the bloodstream, resulting in a normal blood sugar. Blood pH is normalized as the kidneys selectively excrete hydrogen ions, while blood pressure remains elevated because fluid retention increases the blood volume. In most cases, the resistance phase can see a person safely through a crisis until it is over. If not, the person becomes exhausted.

Exhaustion: Exhaustion occurs as the body's ability to meet the stress diminishes and finally gives out. A major cause of clinical exhaustion is the loss of potassium ions. When the mineralocorticoid hormones stimulate the kidneys to retain sodium ions, potassium and hydrogen ions are secreted in the urine in larger than usual amounts. Potassium, the predominant positive ion in the cells, is partly responsible for controlling the water concentration of the cytoplasm. As the cells lose more and more potassium, their functioning is increasingly impaired until finally they start to die. Unless this process is rapidly reversed, vital organs will stop functioning and death will occur. Another component of exhaustion involves the depletion of adrenal glucocorticoids; this results in a sudden fall in blood glucose and a lack of nourishment for the cells. Finally, exhaustion results from weakening organs. A long-term stress reaction places heavy demands on the entire body, particularly on the heart, blood vessels and adrenal cortex. Prolonged exposure to high levels of cortisol and other stress-related hormones results in muscle wasting, suppression of the immune system, ulceration of the gastrointestinal tract and failure of the pancreatic beta cells. These responses are exaggerated if the organs are constitutionally weak or their function impaired from abuse such as the chronic use of drugs or caffeine. This may cause them to gradually or suddenly fail under the strain. Thus, the ability to handle stress and the length of time the reaction can be sustained has a great deal to do with a person's general health. Pathological changes may also persist after the stessors have been removed (Tortora & Anagnostakos, 1990; Tortora & Grabowski, 2000).

Preventing, Detecting and Treating Clinical Exhaustion

The specific recommendations covered elsewhere in this text for conserving the laboring mother's energy, both psychologically and physically, help to stop exhaustion before it gets started. Clinical exhaustion differs from simple tiredness, although tiredness that is not attended to can lead to clinical exhaustion. Doing what you can to reduce the mother's level of fear and anxiety will help. Providing a quiet, respectful and private space helps. Tuning into whether others are hindering the process and, if so, asking them to leave can hasten labor along so that exhaustion does not become an issue. If the proper environment is lacking, some women wind up becoming exhausted and then being transported because that is the only way they can separate themselves from a disruptive labor environment.

Encourage the mother to eat, drink and rest when possible throughout labor. Your alertness for possible signs of exhaustion should be heightened as labor lasts longer and longer. Make sure that the rhythm of the woman's experience is followed: if contractions ease down, encourage her to rest or sleep; if they pick up, encourage her to work with them to get labor moving. Know when to quit; if the woman is not able to keep up with her labor, she needs to be transported.

Signs of impending exhaustion

Performing a simple dipstick check of the urine every time the woman voids is a good way to watch for metabolic evidence of exhaustion. Ketonuria of +2 or more may be the first sign of impending clinical exhaustion and dehydration. Other signs include dry mucous membranes, rising pulse above 100 (note normal range), a rising temperature above 101°F (38.3°C) (which may result in fetal tachycardia) and concentrated urine. Specific gravity denotes the solids-to-liquids concentration in the urine; a high value is an early sign of dehydration (high values may trigger a positive test for proteinuria). Hypoglycemia may be present with or without ketonuria; test with a glycosometer if you are unsure. Contractions also become weaker and spaced more widely apart. Fetal heart rate abnormalities may develop. These signs will appear sooner and become severe more rapidly in women who have a marginally expanded blood volume than they will in those who are well nourished. See my DIAGNOSTIC TESTS for details about how to deal with positive test findings.

Checking for dehydration: The tilt test (postural or orthostatic test) is one way of determining the degree of dehydration. In order to perform this test, measure the pulse and blood pressure with the woman lying flat on her back. Then have her sit upright for one minute with her lower legs dangling off the edge of the bed and reassess her vitals. Then, if you are still unsure, you can have her stand for another minute and reassess vitals a third time.

The pulse and blood pressure should remain approximately the same for each reading, taking the supine readings as the baseline. If the person is dehydrated, exertion from arising results in temporary vasoconstriction which raises the pulse rate. An increase in the pulse of more than 10 bpm with a drop in the systolic blood pressure of more than 10 mm Hg suggests moderate dehydration. This test is strongly positive if the pulse rises as much as 30 bpm or more, a finding consistent with a fluid loss of more than 1 quart (1 liter).

Treating exhaustion

When exhaustion is looming, you must act quickly to turn it around. Use acupressure to stimulate Hegu (LI-4) in women who are tired and are not pushing effectively by applying firm pressure on both hands. Astragalus is another Chinese herb that relieves exhaustion. See the subchapter entitled "Traditional Chinese Medicine" to locate the points and read more about astragalus. You can also give homeopathic arnica, which is good for any kind of exhaustion related to exertion. Encourage the mother to drink a quantity of electrolyte-balancing fluid. If she cannot or will not, either give a nutritive enema or start an IV, giving up to one liter of lactated Ringer's (see the subchapter entitled "Intravenous Equipment and IV Therapy" for details). Once the woman is more stable, eating and drinking are a must. Staying at home with a clinically exhausted mother is foolhardy. With extreme exhaustion, the chances of fetal distress and nonprogressive labor are greatly increased. Even if the mother makes it through the birth, bleeding during or after the placental birth, followed by shock, are much more likely to occur when the woman and her uterus are exhausted.

Blood Pressure Variations in Labor

Acute hypertension or labile blood pressure

Elevations in blood pressure may be noted throughout or at the end of pregnancy. Hypertension that has been determined to be benign prenatally need not be worried about in labor any more than beforehand. Hypertension may be precipitated by anxiety in a particular woman; one way to avoid aggravating her blood pressure is not to check it in labor (especially continuously or excessively), if both the midwife and the parents agree to this plan. However, when there is some reason to be concerned, such as when headaches or other symptoms appear during labor, the blood pressure should always be checked. In addition, any of the remedies already mentioned in Volume I of this text for essential hypertension can be safely used during labor as well.

It can be normal for the blood pressure to be somewhat elevated with the effort of birth, especially if homebirth plans are disrupted with a problem or a hospital transport. Women do not suddenly become toxemic after a perfectly healthy and well-nourished pregnancy, although this myth is commonly supported by medical personnel who may label a hard-working, laboring woman as high risk when she has a rise in blood pressure and a small amount of protein in her urine from the normal stress she is experiencing. However, it *is* possible for unrecognized toxemia to fulminate into a problem during labor. The best way to avoid this problem is to make sure that the woman has been well nourished and that her liver profile tests have been normal.

It is appropriate to transport a laboring woman to the hospital if she is having increasingly severe and unresolvable symptoms associated with high blood pressure or if her blood pressure rises to dangerously high levels (exceeding 150/100), even if no symptoms are present. These symptoms include throbbing headaches, visual disturbances, or other hypertension-related problems that are unrelated to the labor process. Although toxemia doesn't simply appear out of nowhere, it is possible for a woman to have seizure activity or other severe problems precipitated by the stress of labor that are not caused by toxemia but are, nevertheless, very serious.

Some midwives have found that a bath of Epsom salts (pure magnesium sulfate) can help lower the blood pressure in labor and postpartum; use one cup to a tub of water. (There are no published contraindications to this, and the FDA does not have any data on using Epsom salts in a bath.) As a precaution, it is advisable to keep a close eye on the fetal heart rate. Magnesium sulfate is used intravenously in the hospital to control blood pressure because it is a severe nervous system depressant; perhaps as a bath it merely assists with relaxation. Do not attempt to give magnesium sulfate by IV at home. In cases of symptomatic or increasingly extreme hypertension, transport!

Note that magnesium sulfate does not absorb through the intestinal lining (which is why it is given intravenously in the hospital) and therefore should not be used orally for elevated blood pressure; it will only cause loose stools, thus increasing the chance of dehydration.

Hypotension

Whenever the blood pressure drops, first rule out supine hypotensive syndrome. If the mother has been lying on her back, have her change positions. A drop in blood pressure can also be due to overheating, as might occur from a too-hot bath. It may also be associated with bleeding, uterine rupture or amniotic fluid embolism.

Pelvic pain accompanied by a drop in blood pressure and a rising pulse rate, with or without external bleeding, suggests that hemorrhage is occurring and should be thoroughly investigated. Concealed bleeding may occur before birth from an abruption or before and afterward from tears, a hematoma or uterine rupture. If hypotension occurs during labor, check the fetal heart rate immediately, as bradycardia will present if the placenta is detaching. Obvious bleeding usually eliminates the painful pressure build-up that can occur with concealed bleeding and may be due to placenta previa as well as causes directly related to the fetus. Evaluate the situation promptly and transport as necessary.

There are some commonly used herbs, such as blue cohosh and lobelia, that are contraindicated for use in labor when the mother normally has very low blood pressure. Check with some good herbal texts regarding the use of any herbs you are not familiar with if a woman has a blood pressure outside the normal range.

References and Further Reading on Supporting the Mother who is Having a Hard Time Coping with Labor

References used in multiple Chapters in this section

Cunningham F, et al. WILLIAMS OBSTETRICS, 21st ed., McGraw-Hill, New York, NY, 2001.

El Halta V. Preventing Prolonged Labor, MIDWIFERY TODAY, (46);22, Summer, 1998.

Friedman A. LABOR: CLINICAL EVALUATION AND MANAGEMENT, Appleton-Century-Crofts, New York NY, 1967.

Oxorn H. HUMAN LABOR AND BIRTH, 5th ed, Appleton/Century/Crofts, Norwalk CT, 1986.

Schlinger H. Editing notes, Nov, 2003.

Scholles H. Editing notes, 2003.

Simkin P, Ancheta R. THE LABOR PROGRESS HANDBOOK, Blackwell Sciences, Oxford UK, 2000.

Stockham A. TOKOLOGY, rev. ed., Alice B. Stockham & Co., Chicago IL, 1898.

Sutton J. LET BIRTH BE BORN AGAIN: REDISCOVERING AND RECLAIMING OUR MIDWIFERY HERITAGE. Birth Concepts UK, Middlesex UK, 2001.

Sutton J; Scott P. UNDERSTANDING AND TEACHING OPTIMAL FOETAL POSITIONING, Bay Print, Ltd., Tauranga, NZ, 1996.

Varney H. MIDWIFERY, 3rd ed. Jones & Bartlett Pub, Sudbury MA, 1997.

Entering Pains and Back Pain in Labor

King J. BACK LABOR NO MORE!! WHAT EVERY WOMAN SHOULD KNOW BEFORE LABOR, Plenary Systems, Inc, Dallas TX, 1993.

Simkin P. GUIDE TO COMFORT MEASURES FOR CHILDBIRTH, manual for COMFORT MEASURE FOR LABOR WITH PENNY SIMKIN, VHS video, Penny Simkin Inc, Seattle WA, 1995.

Nausea and Vomiting and Understanding and Preventing Maternal Exhaustion

Backburn S. MATERNAL, FETAL AND NEONATAL PHYSIOLOGY: A CLINICAL PERSPECTIVE, 2nd ed. WB Saunders, St Louis MO, 2003.

Hobbs V, LAc. Personal communications regarding the use of Chinese medicine during labor, 1999, Mar, 2002.

Lowe C, LAc. Editing notes, 2003.

Taylor S, et al. "Biobehavioral responses to stress in females: tend-and-befriend, not fight-or-flight," PHYCHOL REV, 107(3);411-429, July, 2000.

Tortora G, Anagnostakos N. PRINCIPLES OF ANATOMY AND PHYSIOLOGY, 6th ed. Harper and Row Pub, New York NY, 1990.

Tortora G, Grabowski S. PRINCIPLES OF ANATOMY AND PHYSIOLOGY, 9th ed., John Wiley and Sons, New York NY, 2000.

Other Special Situations in Labor

Assisting the Relinquishing Mother and Adoptive Family

NOTE: Review the chapter entitled "Adoption Issues" in Volume I of this text, as this chapter will build on that information.

Labor may be difficult for the relinquishing mother. If it is an open adoption and members or the adoptive family plan to attend the birth, they should be well prepared to step out of the room or leave the house, if needed, to give the mother the emotional space she needs to complete the birth. As in the case of a woman whose baby has died, encouraging words should be chosen carefully to respect that the mother is giving up her baby, although the baby's health and safety are obviously of ongoing importance to a woman who has chosen adoption over abortion.

It is possible that the mother will need time during labor to once again process her choice to relinquish her baby, and as much time as necessary should be allowed. This may be the reason for stalls during labor, pushing or placental delivery. Once the baby is born, the baby should remain with the birth mother while she comes to terms with saying goodbye. When she is ready, the baby can be handed over to the adoptive parents. It is important to allow the mother as much time as she requires so that she can have healthy closure around this part of the relinquishing and grieving process. Once the adoptive parents have held the baby, the birth mother may wish to hold the baby again. The adoptive parents need to trust that the birth mother will finally turn over the baby when she is ready. If she should decide to keep the baby, that is her right. Better that she should do so now than later.

As the midwife, you should offer to make yourself available to the adoptive parents to follow the baby as well as to the relinquishing mother for her postpartum care. The postpartum watch is likely to be permeated by complex feelings as the birth mother comes to terms with her decision. In some adoptions, the birth mother has the baby with her for many hours or even days after birth. Sometimes, these mothers nurse or bottle feed the baby during this time. Once the baby has been handed over to the adoptive parents, the birth mother's grieving will extend over the coming weeks, months and even years. How to help the birth mother (and members of the adoptive family, if they are interested) during the postpartum period will be addressed in Volume III.

ASSISTING WOMEN WITH PREEXISTING MEDICAL CONDITIONS OR DISABILITIES

NOTE: Review the chapter entitled "Caring for Women Who Have Disabilities" as well as pertinent chapters on specific medical conditions, in Volume I. This chapter assumes you have reviewed that information.

Prenatal preparation

Serving women who have medical conditions that developed before they got pregnant is a unique and challenging part of midwifery. To practice responsibly, you must establish a thorough history of the mother's condition and the past medical care she has received well before labor begins. The appropriate time to thoroughly research and then discuss the possible risks particular to a woman's health condition is early in the course of prenatal care. Should the woman decide to take any particular risks associated with her condition, you can then evaluate whether you feel competent to take her on. If so, the woman's condition will need to be continually assessed with additional laboratory tests and consultations, as indicated. All necessary medical examinations, laboratory tests and medical back-up arrangements will need to be addressed well before the due date. The number and type of medications required to control the condition should must be investigated as to their possible impact on maternal and fetal condition and response during labor. Whenever possible, medications should be discontinued during the pregnancy and until breastfeeding has been completed. Appropriate specialists can be consulted, and all necessary arrangements made to monitor the woman during labor and transport in a timely manner, should this be necessary. Labor is not the time to try and work all this out. For this reason, an overview of many specific conditions, including suggestions for care during labor, are covered in the last section of Volume I of this text.

Surprise announcements in labor

If a woman in the midst of labor reveals a medical condition of which you were previously unaware, immediate transport should be seriously considered. Even if you are well versed in the condition in question and are certain that there are no ramifications for the mother and baby that place them at particular risk, transport should still be considered. It is one thing to knowingly take on a woman who is honest and well informed regarding her situation and willing to participate in prenatal medical evaluations to determine her current health status and quite another to handle, with the added stressor of labor, such a situation blindly for a woman who has lied to you.

Aside from the physical considerations, questions arise regarding the depth of relationship between yourself and the woman and family. Why did the mother not reveal this condition prenatally? In addition, why would a midwife want to stay home with a woman who has not been completely honest? If the woman or her baby experiences an adverse outcome in the presence of this new knowledge, how will the family react then? What about the local practice regulations? This is a time when you must stand firm and not let the belief that you must be all things to all women overshadow good sense and balanced response.

No prenatal care

Many midwives experience situations where a woman, who was previously unknown to them, walks in to their home or birthing center in active labor. If this happens to you, do the best you can to find out whether any preexisting medical conditions exist and cope accordingly. This is most likely to take place in a permanent birth center, where there should be available reference materials that will, at the very least, provide a succinct description of the condition in question and the mainstream medical approach to it. A book such as the MERCK MANUAL, can offer a basic overview of most conditions as long as the correct medical terminology is known. From there, a triage decision can be made regarding whether you should transport or attend her in labor.

Assisting Laboring Women Who Have Received No Prenatal Care

In industrialized countries midwives with established homebirth practices that offer prenatal care will not usually be confronted with laboring women whom they are meeting for the first time. In fact, in some states there may be political repercussions from assisting women who have had no previous care. In Oregon, for example, providing only birth services is against state regulations for licenced midwives. Even where it is legal, such a situation can potentially be problematic, especially if transport is ultimately required. Therefore, in most urban settings, immediate transport or calling 911 will be the midwife's best option.

However, a midwife working with an immigrant population, such as migrant farm workers, or in a developing country may frequently encounter women in all stages of labor who are absolute strangers to her and the type of care she can provide. These women present during labor, and not before, for a variety of reasons including language barriers, lack of access to transportation, inability to take time off from domestic responsibilities or marginal employment, lack of understanding of what prenatal care can do for them, lack of a cultural context for prenatal care, fear of being deported, distrust of Westerners or Western medicine, cultural or religious preferences, concern regarding strange care providers, disapproval from male relatives, or fears about a provider's reactions to any genital mutilation, to name just a few reasons.

In such circumstances, the midwife must quickly obtain as much history as possible and ascertain the mother's current condition and the position of the baby. If the baby is alive, of normal size, and in a longitudinal lie (preferably head down), and the mother does not have any serious medical conditions and does not appear to be preeclamptic, the midwife is in a fairly good position to provide care on the spur of the moment.

When faced with such a situation, proceed as follows as far as the circumstances allow. Often, such women present themselves in advanced labor and you may have no time to do anything other than protect your hands as best you can, remove any interfering clothing from the mother's lower body and receive the baby.

Whenever possible, first introduce yourself, find out the mother's name, and glean some social history, such as who is with her (or who brought her to you), if she has had any care during the pregnancy, etc. The person who accompanied her may be able to help with questions, history and translating, if necessary. Ask when labor started and the strength, length and timing of contractions. Has the baby been moving? Has there been passage of fluid or blood (color? when? amount?). Assess her level of alertness. Check her reflexes, pupils and vital signs. Ask about any weakness, fainting, severe headaches, blurred vision, vomiting, fever or respiratory distress. Look at her feet and legs for evidence of dried or wet blood or fluids that may have run down her legs and collected on the top or soles of her feet. If she has been bleeding, check her capillary refill time.

The logistics of gathering such information will greatly depend upon the advancement of her labor. Look at the contour of her abdomen to get an idea of the fetal lie. Palpate her abdomen if there is time. If she seems pushy, be as kind and gentle as possible, but explain to her that you need to check her and the baby to see what is going on *now* (the baby could be breech or transverse or anything in between). If there are language barriers, have the person who brought her explain this and assist her in getting in a supine position so you can do a thorough exam. Be as culturally sensitive as possible to issues of modesty and privacy. If a male relative has brought a woman in, for example, try to find out from the woman if she wishes him to stay while you do the exam.

Listen to the baby's heart rate, check the fetal position and perform an internal exam. Even if you normally do not perform internal exams during most labors, doing so in a woman who has received no care is important as it will give you an idea if her pelvis is normal and help confirm the position of the baby and the status of the membranes as well as assess for other abnormalities or a prolapsed cord. Proceed to care for her conservatively, remembering that you will need to explain far more to her along the way because she has not had the benefit of prenatal education.

Keep in mind that this woman may be suffering from any number of conditions including, but not limited to gonorrhea, chlamydia, herpes, hepatitis, intestinal parasites, syphilis, tuberculosis and scabies. Therefore, it is very important to wear gloves, observe universal precautions and to administer eye prophylaxis to the baby. If circumstances allow, arrangements should be made to do a laboratory panel of routine screening tests as soon as possible after the birth. Collect a cord blood sample for syphilis and HIV testing and blood factor testing, in case the mother turns out to be Rh-negative.

ASSISTING THE WOMAN WHO HAS A HISTORY OF UTERINE SURGERY

When assisting women who have had a previous surgical birth or uterine incisions for other reasons, review her records for the reason for the surgery, the type of incision, the type of repair and if any portion of the uterine wall was removed (which may occur if an embedded fibroid has been removed). This situation falls in the same category as for women who have other types of preexisting medical conditions. The specifics regarding what led to the surgery, the type of incision and repair she had at the time and any other pertinent details should have been thoroughly reviewed during prenatal care and are covered in the chapters entitled "Yoni Birth After Cesarean (YBAC)" and "Previous Uterine Surgeries Other Than Cesarean" in Volume I of this text. Again, the revelation in labor that a previous uterine surgery took place suggests that transport is your most prudent course of action. If the surgery was revealed and researched during prenatal care, be prepared to transport if anything does come up in labor.

As far as supporting these women during labor, remember that the point in this labor at which the previous labor was interrupted may be the most difficult time for this woman. Strategies that might help a particular woman are totally dependent upon her history, so this should also have been reviewed prenatally. With luck, a woman's resolve to have a normal birth will carry her through labor rapidly, a happy turn of events which often occurs with these courageous mothers.

See the chapter entitled "Uterine Rupture during Labor" for signs and symptoms of impending traumatic rupture. Remember that many women feel twinges in their scars during pregnancy and sometimes in labor. Be concerned if these sensations appear for the first time in labor or become more pronounced. If the woman tells you something is not right, believe her. Often a sense of maternal foreboding is the only indication that a rupture is going to occur. Be particularly alert for traumatic rupture if the woman has had a single-layer closure of her incision in the past; I recommend no labor augmentation, other than acupressure (not even herbal). Dehiscences or atraumatic separation of the scar may occur, but are not usually a problem in labor unless the opening is so large that fetal parts escape through it.

Working with the Baby Who is Having Problems with Descent

Techniques Used to Help the Baby Descend during Labor

Problems with descent can be caused by a variety of underlying factors. These include a baby in a posterior position as well as other malpositions of the head. Medical-model practitioners often attribute such malpositioning to a problem with pelvic dimensions; however, true cephalopelvic disproportion is rare in the developed world. Deflexion or asynclitism is a more likely culprit. For example, the birth canal may be slightly tight in a one area. Very often, however, such tightness is due to asymmetrical tension in the soft tissue rather than to the shape of the bony pelvis. Maternal fear of pain or of the sensations of fetal descent can cause the mother to unconsciously tighten her pelvic muscles. When the pelvis is tight, so are the sphincters of the rectum, the bladder and the uterus. The baby's head meets a wall of resistance as it tries to descend and is pushed off center. A pelvic floor that is tight from excessive exercise can cause the same problem. These mothers must relax before activities and position changes will assist fetal descent. Small babies, who have more room to move around, can get themselves into some pronounced off-center positions as well.

Signs of Trouble

Labors that involve other-than-straightforward fetal descent sometimes proceed without apparent difficulty. However, they often manifest with the following characteristics:

- Labor is often more painful than usual or painful earlier than is expected, with the mother responding to contractions as though labor is far more advanced. There are often regionalized pains in the pelvic or suprapubic area. Sutton and Scott (1996) comment that women having an asynclitic labor will have pain deep in the side of the pelvis to which the occiput is pointing, just below the iliac crest.
- In spite of good contractions, progress often slows or stops around 6 to 8 cm.
- Impaired flexion and moulding often may be noted once a head in pronounced asynclitism has entered the brim.
- Both increased pain and asynclitism are often associated with compound presentation, especially when a hand is beside the head. The baby may even be sucking his thumb. See the chapter entitled "Assisting a Woman Whose Baby Is in a Compound Presentation" for suggestions for correction.
- Early rupture of membranes may also occur, as unequal pressure on the bag increases its likelihood.
- When a woman resists her contractions, she often tenses the muscles just below her ribs. When she does this, the baby's torso is pressed downward, out of alignment with the head. The baby's body is bent and the force of contractions drives the fetal head toward the mother's spine rather than toward the pelvic cavity. Thus pressure on the cervix is lessened and labor is prolonged (King, 1993). The same thing can occur when a woman assumes any kind of posture that curls her spine forward because curled postures decrease the angle between the spine and the pubic bone (Sutton & Scott, 1996).
- On internal exam, the os may be unevenly dilated, pulled off-center or unevenly swollen.

Things to Attend to in All Cases

Pain in front

By this, I mean pain that occurs above the pubic bone. Early in labor, this may be entering pain from the baby trying to find his way through the brim; late in labor, it may be from a cervical lip, a full bladder, or an anterior shoulder that has not fully rotated to transverse after the head has passed the brim (palpate to see if you can tell if the shoulder is there). Evaluating the source of the pain will help determine what steps to take to remedy the situation.

Back pain

Back pain can impair a woman's ability to relax, and tense muscles will diminish the effect of efforts to correct the baby's position and reduce pelvic flexibility. Therefore, it behooves you to try and mitigate back pain as much as possible before you proceed to any techniques to correct the fetal position. See the chapters entitled "Entering Pains and Back Pain in Labor" and "Sterile Water Injections for the Relief of Excessive Localized Pain."

Positions and Activities to Encourage Positional Correction, Rotation and Descent of the Fetus

One of the most powerful advantages of homebirth over hospital-based birth is that women are not drugged and can change position at will, an ability that is sometimes the only thing that opens the pelvis and repositions the baby, allowing him to descend. The use of several different positions, alternated after every two or three contractions, is often very helpful in working the baby through the pelvis. This is true for labor as well as pushing. While the success of any one technique varies among individual women, the right technique can work miracles on the labor of a particular woman. Therefore, as a general rule, it is best not to recommend techniques that attempt to actively move the baby to a better position until you are present, set up and ready to receive the baby. What you recommend will depend upon the cause of the problem and where the woman is in her labor. Some methods work by positioning the mother so that the angle of fetal descent into the pelvic cavity is redirected, while others succeed by moving the pelvic bones enough to encourage the head to reposition. Of course, many of these postures can be used even when labor is moving along well. Most of these positions are introduced in detail in the chapter entitled "Positions and Activities for Labor" the following discussion focuses on their usefulness for problems with descent.

Basic positions

Leaning forward: Positions that involve leaning forward help align the mother's spine, her pelvis and baby in such a way that rotation and descent are encouraged. The mother's spine must be straight (not arched rigidly forward or slouched backward); in addition, she must be sitting or standing in such a way that the pelvic crests, and therefore the pubic bone, are tilted forward, with her knees below her tuberosities. When these criteria are met, an angle of about 120° which allows maximum room at the brim and just above it for the baby to rotate is created between the mother's spine and the pubic bone.

If the mother is tired, this posture can be easily accomplished even when seated by using a meditation cushion or an ergonomic chair. In UNDERSTANDING AND TEACHING OPTIMAL FETAL POSITIONING (1996), Sutton and Scott suggest using a computer seat with a rocker bottom. If a rocker-bottom seat is not available, a regular ergonomic chair will do. Have the mother gently sway back and forth and side to side as she feels inclined. This will help work the baby's head around and down.

Any other comfortable position that tilts the pelvis forward can be used instead. These include such variations as having the woman sit on the side of a tall bed and lean over a tray table or the back of a chair with her knees low and spread, having her stand and lean forward onto her partner or the bed using her arms for support, or having her kneel with her upper body and arms around a physical therapy ball or bean bag. If the baby's head is already past the pelvic brim, a position in which the woman is off her sacrum is better than a seated position.

Open prayer position: Scholles (2003) recommends kneeling, leaning forward with the knees open as the best of all forward-leaning positions, as it works to open the midpelvis and outlet as well as widen the brim.

Hands and knees: This position is good for relieving back pressure and for helping to turn babies to an anterior position. It works well for some women during pushing and relieves pressure on the pelvic bones, allowing full sacral mobility. The woman can lean forward onto a chair seat, a birth ball or a bean bag to support her upper body. Once in this position, she should sway her back and pelvic brim downward, which will straighten out the birth canal and the direction of force as the contraction applies pressure to the baby.

Open, exaggerated knee-chest: The woman crouches down with her bottom in the air and her shoulders on the floor. A pillow can be placed underneath her to make her more comfortable. This position brings the baby up out of the pelvis and facilitates rotation (El Halta, 1998).

Supine: This position can be helpful to use in combination with others when the engaged baby will not advance during pushing if the head is flexed and the back is anterior. On rare occasions, ironically, it is the only position that works.

Exaggerated semiprone: This position (side-lying, lower arm and leg stretched behind, upper arm and leg bent in front, torso and upper hip rotated forward) opens the oblique pelvic diameters, which encourages the baby to rotate anteriorly. The woman should be lying on the side opposite the baby's back.

Side-lying Trendelenburg: Prop one end of a flat surface onto the seat of the couch or on the foot of a conventional mattress. Have the mother lie on her side on the propped surface, resting her head to the low end and lying on the side to which the baby's occiput is directed. While she is in this position, the midwife can shake her as described below in the section entitled "Chunging." The inverted posture will float the baby's head up out of the pelvis and help it assume a better position.

Exaggerated, asymmetrical movements

When the labor pattern matches that outlined under "Signs of Trouble" earlier in this chapter, the woman often needs to make more space available in the oblique diameter of the entire pelvic cavity. This can be achieved with movement and flexion of her pelvis (Sutton & Scott, 1996). What you recommend will depend upon where she is in her labor:

- Early labor: Have her walk up and down stairs sideways or swing her torso from side to side while lifting the hip in the direction of motion.
- Active labor: Suggest she raise one foot, then flex and bend her torso in the opposite direction during contractions.
- Also try having her lie on her left side, then lift and move her upper leg, if she must be side-lying.

The following movements all open the pelvic dimensions obliquely, while causing the parallel relationship of the bones to change, altering the available space. The inlet, midpelvis and outlet might all be affected, as well as the level of the ischial spines in relation to each other. For example, when one ischial spine is lifted higher than the other, the diameter between them is altered, and this may allow the baby's head to rotate or descend.

Duck walking: Two assistants support the mother on either side as she spreads her legs to broaden her gait, bends her knees and walks forward, swaying her hips from the side to side, rotating each side out and forward with each step. This will often help to correct an asynclitic head (El Halta, 1998).

Stair climbing: This is especially effective to correct asynclitism as well as deflexion of the head. Have the mother climb up and down a flight of stairs, stopping when she has a contraction. Some midwives find it helpful to have the mother exaggerate her gait or to climb every other stair on the way up to move the pelvic bones even more. Sutton and Scott (1996) recommend climbing "sideways." To do this, the woman stands with her feet at a 90° angle to the riser. She lifts the foot nearest the stair up to the next step, and then brings the outside foot up to meet it. The can be repeated up the entire stairway.

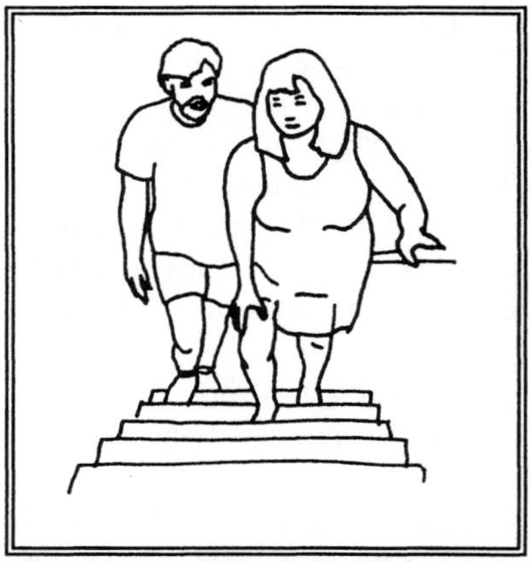

(Redrawn with permission from illustrations by Stella Cruz, © Ruth Ancheta, 2000)

Marching in place: Another way to accomplish the "one foot up" technique is to have the mother march in place, lifting her knees high as she does so. This action is helpful when a woman is discovered to have an asynclitic baby late in labor (Sutton & Scott, 1996).

Moving the pelvis: Any action that moves, bends, rotates, rocks from side to side or otherwise gets the pelvis shifting is ideal for shifting a poorly positioned fetal head, especially one that is asynclitic. It also gives the baby room to get her head past her hand in a compound presentation (Sutton & Scott, 1996). Belly dancing is perfect for this. If the mother is not inclined to belly dance, Sutton and Scott recommend that she swing her hips forward and sideways, first bending her knees, then going up on her toes as she moves and then matching this movement on the other side, making a kind of figure eight with her hips. Doing this in a forward-leaning posture further assists repositioning. Most women will need to plant their hands on a stable object for balance.

The lunge: This technique was perfected by Penny Simkin; it is helpful for turning posterior babies and correcting asynclitism as well as for relieving back pain. It is also useful whenever labor stalls or slows down. Place a chair on a carpeted floor (so it will not slide) at the woman's side, selecting the side on which the baby's back is lying. The side edge of the chair seat should be next to the mother's thigh. Have her stand, facing forward, and place the foot nearest the chair onto the chair seat with her toes pointed to the side. She should then slowly lean sideways in the direction of her raised foot, preferably during contractions; she should remain leaning toward the chair for a few seconds, then return to an upright position. This is repeated through the next several contractions. If she feels a bit unbalanced, her partner can stand behind or in front to assist her. The lunge can also be performed from a kneeling posture, as illustrated below.

A woman who has back labor but is not carrying a posterior baby can try the lunge toward each side and continue with the side that feels most comfortable.

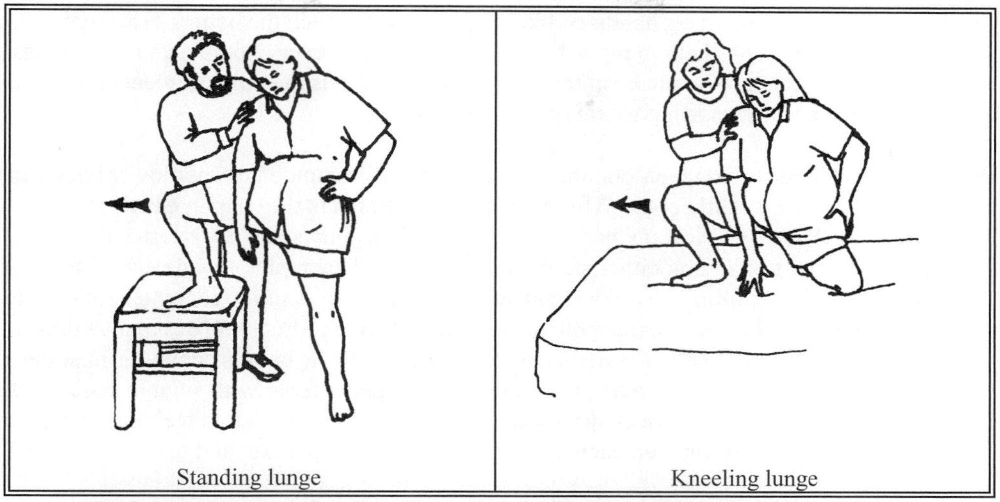

(Redrawn with permission from illustrations by Stella Crus, © Ruth Ancheta, 2000)

Crawling: Crawling here means "walking" on one's hands and knees, and has several benefits. This movement allows the mother's sacrum to move backward. Her belly is dependent beneath her, giving her baby the freedom to move with the maximum assistance of gravity. Her hips move with each advance forward, alternately changing the shape of the pelvis by taking the bones and ischial spines out of their parallel relationship.

The mother should keep her back straight as she crawls and exaggerate her leg motions. Crawling is not as effective if the mother has loose abdominal muscles; using upright postures while moving the hips will work better for these mothers. Alternately, they can crawl while wearing a supportive belly binder.

Asymmetrical positions

Moving one leg out from the center of the body or positioning one knee higher than the other opens the pelvis on the side of the motion, which may allow the baby to reposition his head.

Standing, one foot supported: To correct asynclitism, a posterior presentation, or even a compound presentation, Penny Simkin recommends having the mother stand and place one foot on an elevated surface so that the lifted foot is higher than the opposite knee. The woman should maintain this position for several contractions, then switch her feet and maintain the new position for several more contractions. This simulates stair climbing and raises one ischial spine and tuberosity higher than the other. The dimensions of the pelvic cavity are thus rearranged and the baby is given additional space to rotate or shift position. This maneuver may even provide enough room to allow the baby to reposition a hand that has been up by the baby's head (Sutton & Scott, 1996).

A shoulder can get hung up on the brim and delay descent during pushing if the internal rotation of the shoulders is incomplete. To open the pelvis so that the shoulder can slip under the rami, have the woman raise the leg on the side of the baby's back (if the baby is ROP or ROT, she raises her right leg) while leaning her torso to the opposite side.

Kneeling on one knee: This is an old trick to get the baby to enter the brim (Greenhill, 1951). Keeping her back straight, the mother kneels on one knee and raises the other leg so that the foot is flat on the floor; she then moves that leg away from her body so that her toes are pointed out to her side. She can then lean forward with support in front. Sutton and Scott (1996) have also found this helpful in repositioning the hand in cases of compound presentation. Kneeling on one knee can also be performed with the mother crouched down, bringing her bottom close to the floor. This is recommended by Greenhill (1951) to correct an oblique lie, although the upright kneeling position may be better for this purpose because it keeps the spinopubic angle more open.

Passive movement of the mother

These techniques allow the mother to relax as much as possible while support persons move her in various ways to change the fetal attitude.

Driving over a bumpy road: Put the mother in a car and drive over railroad tracks, an unpaved, unimproved road or similar terrain. If she has space to assume a hands-and-knees position, so much the better. Having the mother in the car and, hopefully, relaxed can sometimes help to reposition the head. Almost every homebirth midwife has seen dramatic changes in fetal position after transport to the hospital. If fetal malposition is the only problem, it is certainly preferable to first try the car ride alone before resorting to transport.

Rebozo technique: Place the rebozo on the floor and have the mother lie supine with her lower back and buttocks over the cloth and her legs straight and slightly open. (This position is illustrated in the chapter entitled "Assisting at the Birth of a Baby Presenting Her Face.") Pick up both ends of the cloth and stand above the mother, straddling her. Alternatively, have two assistants stand on either side of the mother and each pick up one end of the cloth. Now form a hammock with the cloth and, by pulling up on one end and then the other, begin to rock the mother's lower torso and bottom using a rhythmic motion. Encourage the mother to completely relax. Every so often, give the cloth a sharp jerk on the side you want the baby's head to move *away from*. For example, if the baby's occiput is near the mother's right, jerk the side of the sheet on the mother's *right*. Continue to intersperse jerks with regular rocking through several contractions (Vinaver, 1996). Native Americans traditionally used a variation on this technique by laying the woman on a large blanket and having four strong men each pick up a corner of the blanket and toss the mother about.

Chunging: This ancient Chinese technique for correcting malposition involves two or three people placing their hands on the mother and vigorously shaking her all over. The shaking can go on both during and between contractions and can be continued for as long as the support people can keep it up. A good position for the mother to assume is standing leaning over with her arms braced against a fixed object. Chunging can also be done with the mother lying on the side to which the fetal back is directed.

A variation of this technique described by Gaskin (2003) involves placing a hand on each of the mother's thighs or buttocks and rhythmically shaking the soft tissues from side to side during and between contractions. Kneading or massaging the muscles of the feet, calves or thighs is also very effective in helping the mother and her cervix to relax. Softening the voluntary muscles helps to soften the cervix.

Trampoline: The mother can sit in the center of a small, round exercise trampoline and bounce. She can also stand on it and bounce while being supported on both sides by two people holding her hands. This technique will not be suitable for everyone and should not be used by women who are very large or who lose their balance easily. The woman should do this for only two or three contractions and then move on to other techniques, but it can help in the same way as the other passive techniques. Use of a trampoline is another way to provide motion that the mother cannot fully control.

Shake the baby loose with the mother side-lying: A mother who is tired or for other reasons must be in a recumbent position should lie on her side rather than supine. She should always lie on the side nearest the baby's back, *not* on the side to which the baby's belly is pointing. To do so will cause the baby's anterior torso to fall toward the bed and can tilt the head just enough to encourage the head to engage in a deflexed military or brow presentation. This is especially true if the mother is having strong contractions that are likely to cause the head to engage (Hendrickson, 1981). Sutton and Scott (1996) recommend putting a pillow or two under the mother's uterus to bring it in line with her spine.

Shaking can be used in this position to correct an asynclitism. Once the mother is comfortable, the midwife (or partner) stands behind or in front of the mother, grasps her shoulder with one hand and her upper hip with the other and shakes them in opposite directions (shoulder forward, hip back; shoulder back, hip forward) in several strong brisk movements. This will help jostle the baby into a better position while the mother relaxes and remains as limp as possible.

Manual techniques to correct the fetal position

Create a false pelvic floor: The following technique, shared by Sutton (2001), can be used if the cervix is at least 5 cm dilated and the membranes have already ruptured. This is quite painful for the mother, so be sure she knows this and has given full permission before you proceed. The mother can be standing, on hands and knees, or leaning over a bean-bag chair. Because of the awkward positioning of the midwife's hand, the woman could also be supported by the Birth Sling with her knees supported on either side so that you can slip underneath her like a car mechanic. This will allow you to reach up from under her and give you better leverage. Perform an internal exam by introducing your hand, palm anterior, with fingers pointing toward the sacrum. Use two fingers to touch the head. A really stuck baby may require the application of three fingers, which will only be tolerable for the mother if she is in a forward-leaning position. Spread your fingers apart to equalize the pressure, making sure you are not over a fontanelle. As the head is pressed downward during a contraction, apply counterpressure to the head to form a false pelvic floor, otherwise keep your hand perfectly still. The idea is to provide the counterpressure the perineum would provide were the head descended sufficiently to be in contact with it.

Typically, nothing happens during the first contraction. However, on the next contraction, the baby will usually begin to rotate. Keep your hand in place through the next 2 or 3 contractions to see if the counterpressure will provide enough resistance to effect rotation. You should be able to feel the head rotate when it occurs (Sutton & Scott, 1996). Do not attempt this technique before 5 cm because you will not be able to open your fingers sufficiently to form a false pelvic floor. This technique can be used at any time after that to effect rotation or to correct any problematic position. If the head is asynclitic, it may be more effective to apply pressure to either side of the sagittal suture between contractions to start the baby rotating.

Manual correction of asynclitism: Remember that asynclitism, particularly the posterior variety, is the way OT babies usually position their heads to get through the brim and that slight asynclitism frequently persists until internal rotation is complete. Therefore, if engagement or internal rotation has not yet occurred, and you try to correct mild to moderate posterior asynclitism when the occiput is transverse, it is likely to be an unnecessary intervention and may even make engagement harder for the baby.

However, if labor is much delayed or if asynclitism is extreme, correction to a more typical angle often facilitates progress. This technique can be used before or after engagement. Davis (1997) finds it easiest to have the mother assume a knee-chest position. Insert two fingers into the yoni and push upward (i.e., toward the mother's head) on whichever parietal bone is lowermost in the pelvis. Pushing up dislodges the head, rendering it more mobile, thus creating space for the sagittal suture to swing toward midline.

You can also have the mother lie supine. Insert your gloved hand into the yoni. If the posterior parietal bone is lowermost, lift the head up and push it backward by applying pressure to the border of the sagittal suture toward the sacrum. If the anterior parietal bone is lowermost, lift the head, find the sagittal suture and use two fingers to pull the head forward in the direction of the pubic bone (El Halta, 1998).

Promoting flexion: There are many cases of prolonged labor where the head is in a pretty good position, but it needs to be more flexed. Let's assume that the baby is in a median vertex presentation and not descending. Have the mother assume a knee-chest position. Between contractions, insert two fingers and place them on either side of the sagittal suture, pushing upward to lift the head slightly out of the pelvis. Now locate the frontal border of the anterior fontanelle and apply pressure to it in the direction of the pelvic sidewall (so as to bring the baby's chin to his chest) until the head has flexed enough to raise the fontanelle out of reach, or nearly so. (Never apply pressure to the membranous portion of the fontanelle. Palpate until you find a bony edge.) Continue through one contraction. The head should now be flexed, unless something like a hand under the chin is interfering (Davis, 2004).

Acupressure to encourage fetal descent during pushing

Acupressure can be used in conjunction with any of the other suggestions in this chapter. Apply firm pressure to Hegu (LI-4) to bring the baby down during pushing. BL-67 also promotes descent and is especially indicated when the baby's position is not ideal (Lowe, 2003; West, 2001). To locate these points, see the chapter entitled "Traditional Chinese Medicine."

Reversing the Qi

This is another Chinese technique that calls for the mother to concentrate on pulling the baby back up out of her pelvis "up to her throat." She may assume a knee-chest position while she does this. Reversing the Qi can have undesired consequences (like messing up the energy) so choose carefully who you suggest this to and check frequently to see what is occurring. However, when it does work, it can be quite effective (Parry, 2003).

Assisting the Woman Whose Baby Is in a Posterior Position

The incidence of posterior positioning at the onset of labor is 15 to 30%. Most of these babies will rotate spontaneously to an anterior position and be born without any problem. Some will require assistance to facilitate rotation. Approximately 5% of posterior babies will be born "sunny-side up;" in some cases there may be no prior indication of their persistent OP descent. In many cases in which the baby remains posterior, labor can produce excruciating back pain during descent. The head may become arrested in the mid- to lower pelvis and refuse to rotate, often resulting in a surgical birth.

A difficult posterior labor is certainly one of the most trying labor situations for women and midwives alike. Even those women who have given birth before often find it difficult if not impossible to relax during a posterior labor; this adds stress and tension, tightening up the soft tissues of the pelvis and thus further impeding rotation. Although there is no one magic solution that will relax the mother, rotate the baby and get on with the birth, this chapter offers a number of tips to help prevent a long, painful posterior labor and avoid a surgical birth. Many of these suggestions can also be used in any labor where the head is not in an ideal position for birth.

External Signs of Posterior Positioning

The abdomen of a woman carrying a posterior baby looks relatively high and flat. Fetal small parts are in front; the fetal back is usually to the right, in which case the heartbeat is heard on the mother's right side. At the mother's umbilicus, there may be a flat or concave area, which is especially obvious when she lies supine. In addition, the fetal head may be quite high. An unengaged head at term in a nullipara is frequently associated with a posterior position.

Problems That Can Occur during a Difficult Posterior Labor

Sutton (2001) has outlined a series of problems that are often seen in difficult posterior labors. It is interesting to note that posterior positioning is considered highly desirable in at least one indigenous culture, although this is certainly not so in Western cultures.

- Prelabor attempts of the baby to rotate may produce bouts of long, painful toning contractions that bring the mother to the onset of labor already exhausted.
- The mother may complain of back pain in early labor. The onset of labor is likely to be prolonged.
- Failure of engagement in a nullipara may result in the delayed onset of labor and a fetal head that is more ossified, making moulding more difficult.
- Early rupture of membranes may occur more often; the reduced fluid volume restricts the baby's movements. The uterine muscle may take several days to accommodate to the reduced interior volume.
- Contractions are often uncoordinated and irregular, contributing to a long labor.
- Even when the fetal head enters the pelvis, the lordosis of the mother's lower back, combined with the pressure from contractions, still impairs spinal flexion.
- The force of the contraction is usually directed near the baby's anterior fontanelle, encouraging the head to deflex into a military attitude. This tips the occiput back; thus the hardest part of the fetal head is driven directly against the sacrum, rather than down into the pelvic cavity, resulting in a great deal of back pain and hindering descent and rotation.
- Progress is slow because the maximum force of the contraction does not target the os. It is typically misdirected 2 to 3 cm in front of the os. This can displace the os into a very posterior position, resulting in a prolonged effacement and dilation phase. When the force is directed behind the os, as might occur if the abdomen is pendulous or in multiparas, labor is similarly inefficient.
- The misdirected force and traction on the cervix stresses the cervical ligaments, which are attached to the sacrum, contributing to back pain.
- Pulling on the anterior lower uterine segment may result in extreme thinning (to the point where a less than careful internal exam may lead you to believe that the cervix is fully dilated). Alternately, the strength of contractions may be such that the cervix dilates to 5 cm or so before the uterus is exhausted, resulting in what the medical model refers to as "failure to progress."

•The head may remain OP, meaning it cannot take advantage of the best available space to descend. The head cannot make optimal use of the space in the sacral curve due to the shape of the vertex coupled with deflexion. In extreme cases, the head deflexes more into a face or brow presentation.

•Significant moulding must occur for the head to pass through the ischial spines, adding to the length of labor.

•Posterior babies require more space in the birth canal and more dilation in the posterior os to get through the cervix, because the widest part of the head is to the back and the head is deflexed. This takes more time.

•Deflexion of the fetal spine tends to extend the shoulder axis into a more military posture. This encourages the posterior shoulder to become lodged against the sacral promontory and the anterior shoulder to become hung up on the brim, impairing or preventing internal rotation of the shoulder axis to the transverse diameter of the brim. This will interfere with descent as well as prolong labor.

•The release of the sacrum is impaired with posterior descent. (Sutton does not explain why she believes this to be true; however, it may be that the shape of the forehead and face are less effective at triggering the nerve plexus on underside of the pubic bone.)

•Pushing that begins with the posterior shoulder still lodged against the sacral promontory will often result in the anterior shoulder becoming lodged above the symphysis in front. Descent of the shoulder axis is thus delayed and difficult, meaning that the head does not advance.

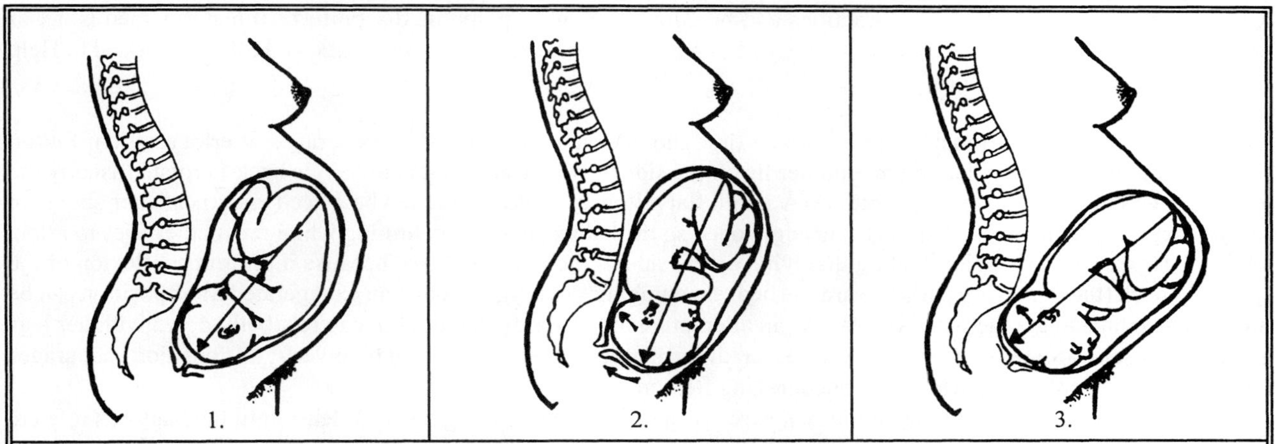

1. When the baby is in an OA position, the force of contractions is usually centered over the os.
2. In an OP baby when the abdominal and uterine muscles are well-toned, the force of contractions may be directed in front of the os by a few centimeters. The baby's spine deflexes and the os may be pulled into an extremely posterior position. The head may be displaced backward where it presses on the sacrum rather than down into the pelvic cavity. Lifting the belly during contractions may pull the cervix forward to center it more directly under the pulling force of the uterus.
3. The direction of uterine force in an OP when the abdominal muscles are quite lax. The baby's spine deflexes and the head is pressed directly against the mother's spine, rather than down into the pelvic cavity. Here the force is centered behind the os and is directed toward the lower sacrum. Lifting the belly may help line up the uterine forces with the os.

•In the mother whose abdominal muscles are more lax, the forward-leaning angle of the uterus is increased (this is most pronounced in women who have had a baby or two or who have a pendulous abdomen). This may cause the baby's spine to be more extended due to the direction of force and the anatomy of the baby's spine. Contractions increase the forward-leaning of the uterus. The angle of the uterus can be so extreme that the fetal head is driven directly into the sacral promontory, resulting in severe back pain.

Coping with Posterior Labor

Regardless of the phase of labor or the technique you use, be sure to explain what you are doing and why to the baby.

Early labor

Signs of posterior positioning in early labor: Sutton and Scott (1996) have observed that women with posterior babies have bouts of strong painful contractions that come and go over a period of hours or days. These may be accompanied by suprapubic pain as the baby attempts to rotate from a posterior to an occiput anterior position. They recommend forward-leaning positions to encourage the baby to turn, explaining to the mother that discomfort near her pubic bone is likely to be the hard occiput moving into an anterior position. Note that forward-leaning positions will only further limit the mobility of the baby in women who are short-waisted; leaning back and opening the spinopubic angle by sagging the lower back while leaning forward will work better for these women (see the chapter entitled "Techniques Used to Help the Baby Descend During Labor.")

All women should avoid semi-reclining and supine positions, seated positions that cause their buttocks to be below their knees (such as bucket seats in cars and soft couches), deep squatting and sitting flat on the floor with their legs crossed. These positions tighten the angle between the maternal spine and the pubic bone.

Preserve the intact bag of waters: Regardless of which techniques you use to try to get the baby to turn, avoid rupturing the membranes whenever possible. The cushioning effect of the forewaters gives space for the baby to rotate most easily. Sudden descent of the head may occur if the waters break prior to rotation to an anterior position, resulting in a deep transverse arrest or the head becoming lodged in another unfavorable position (El Halta, 1998).

What you can do early in labor: If the mother's energy level is good, she should be upright and mobile, leaning forward with her pelvis tilted out during contractions and breathing through suprapubic discomfort. If her abdomen is lax or pendulous, it can be lifted up with the Tummy Lift or a belly binder (see the chapter entitled "Techniques Used to Help the Baby Descend during Labor").

Appropriate resting positions: A mother who is tired should rest in a position that encourages anterior rotation. Sutton (2001) recommends always having the mother lie on the side to which she wants the baby's back to rotate (usually the left side), with her knees below her bottom. A small, flat pillow or folded towel can be placed underneath her abdomen for support. This will keep the spinopubic angle open so the baby can work on turning while the mother tries to relax. Others disagree with this point, feeling that lying on the side of the occiput is best because it prevents deflexion of the spine and neck (the fetal body curls toward the bed, encouraging flexion), although an exaggerated Sims position can be used to advantage to get the baby to turn. As an alternative to side-lying, the mother can rest belly-down with her legs and upper torso supported by pillows to create a cradle so her belly hangs dependent below her; this position encourages the baby to rotate anteriorly while also encouraging flexion.

In any event, standing, leaning and moving are *always* preferable to lying down, at least until the baby has rotated. Work on getting the baby in a better position before she gets pushed down into the pelvis and before the membranes rupture, because the loss of fluid will make rotation more difficult.

Open, exaggerated knee-chest to encourage rotation: Valerie El Halta has made it a goal of her midwifery career to prevent posterior labor whenever possible. She has found a technique that works very successfully to rotate babies early in labor, before they descend into the pelvis and become fixed in a posterior position.

In early labor, the woman is not likely to be experiencing any of the classic signs of posterior back labor. Therefore, at the onset of labor, confirm the fetal position. This is especially important in mothers you have known or suspected to be carrying posterior prenatally as well as those who have been carrying ROT or ROA, because these babies are more likely to rotate posteriorly than those who are LOT or LOA. Remember that the baby's position is determined by the location of the occiput, not by anything else. Rarely, a baby may assume a twisted position in which the back is anterior oblique (suggesting that the occiput is, too) but the occiput is posterior. These labors have classic OP symptoms, even though the baby's back can be felt in the anterior oblique quadrant of the uterus. In this case, the only way to confirm the position of the head is to perform an internal exam.

If the baby's occiput is found to be posterior, have the mother get into a deep, open knee-chest position and remain there for about 45 minutes. The woman should exaggerate the position by placing her shoulders on the floor and elevating her bottom in the air as much as possible. This brings the head further out of the pelvis, relaxes the abdominal muscles, opens the brim and allows the baby plenty of room to rotate. The mother should be supported by pillows and made as comfortable as possible. Although this position is not very comfortable in any event, it is easiest to maintain when labor is not advanced. The contractions may become more regular and effective during this time, which will assist rotation.

If the woman cannot tolerate this position for as long as necessary to turn the baby, alternate it with an exaggerated semiprone (Sims) or "runners" position. Have her lie on the side opposite the fetal back (if the baby is lying LOP, the mother lies on her right if the baby is ROP, the mother lies on her left). Her uppermost arm is crooked in front of her and her lowermost arm is extended backward behind her (not tucked under her head). Her upper leg is bent at the knee in front of her. Her upper leg and arm and her head are all supported by pillows. The object is to lift the baby up and out of the pelvis; rotating the mother's legs encourages a short-arc rotation to an anterior position. A pillow can support her lower hip as well as help get the baby out of the pelvis. Her lower leg should be stretched straight out behind her. Positioning the legs like this helps to shift the pelvic bones around and facilitate rotation. The woman can alternate between this position and the knee-chest position, as she can tolerate them, until you confirm that the baby has rotated (El Halta, 1998). This can correct a posterior positioning as well as asynclitism and transverse arrest.

Early active labor

Signs of posterior positioning in active labor: Once labor is more advanced, the primary indication that a woman has a posterior baby is severe back pain. Women describe extreme, knife-like pains in and near the sacral region as the baby moves down. This is because the hard occiput of the baby is pressing against the mother's lower spine and sacral promontory. Once labor reaches this point, it is impossible for most women to relax. The mother's body language may suggest that she is trying to move away from the pain by rigidly arching her back. The degree of pain she reports will usually not be in sync with her dilation. Her abdominal contour may show the characteristic OP dip in the area of the navel, especially between contractions.

Another sign that points to increased likelihood of a posterior baby is an arrest in dilation. Cervical swelling is an additional marker. An asynclitic presentation can also cause these problems, but a posterior should be ruled out whenever a woman reports severe back pain in conjunction with these symptoms.

Remember that the baby's head can be in a posterior position and the baby's torso can be anterior on palpation. This presents a confusing picture, but the clue that it is an OP is the unusual degree of back pain reported. A deep internal exam will confirm this. This twisted fetal posture is relatively rare, but should be treated like any other OP presentation.

Turning a posterior baby in active labor: There is a variety of techniques used by different midwives to turn the baby in active labor. Whenever the pain of a posterior labor is preventing a woman from relaxing, the sterile water papule injection technique (described in the subchapter entitled "Sterile Water Injections for the Relief of Excessive Localized Pain") may be used prior to any of the techniques below. This will relieve some of the pain, help her relax, increase the flexibility of the pelvis and release tension elsewhere so that the chosen technique will work effectively.

Stroking the baby over: The mother assumes a hands-and-knees position on an elevated surface such as a firm bed. (The floor can be used, but elevating the mother helps the support person to do the stroking most effectively.) You stand beside her on the side opposite the fetal occiput (for example, if the fetus is ROP, stand to the mother's left). Then reach all the way underneath the mother's abdomen to her opposite lateral abdomen above her iliac crest. Firmly and smoothly stroke across the mother's abdomen toward yourself in the direction that the occiput should rotate, using enough pressure to lift the abdomen slightly, stopping when you reach the mother's midline. Repeat the stroking between contractions. While this technique can be used at any point in labor, it works best in early or active labor prior to engagement and before the membranes rupture (Simkin & Ancheta, 2000).

Open knee-chest: The open, exaggerated knee-chest position as described for early labor can still be used when labor has advanced to 4 or 5 cm. The baby may be lower in the pelvis at this point; it can be helpful for the midwife to place her hand on the baby's head and push it up out of the pelvis as much as possible to assist rotation, taking care not to rupture the membranes (El Halta, 1998). This position may be more uncomfortable for the mother to maintain at this point in labor and may need to be alternated with other positions until rotation has occurred.

Hands and knees: The mother assumes a hands-and-knees position. She can creep around, exaggerating her leg and hip movements during and between contractions. This will often encourage anterior rotation.

Exaggerated semiprone position: The woman lies as described at the top of the page almost on her stomach in a runner's position. She should remain in this position for 45 minutes to an hour until rotation is confirmed.

Belly-lifting: See the description of this technique in the chapter entitled "Entering Pains and Back Pain in Labor."

Discovering posterior positioning after 5 cm of dilation

At this point manual rotational techniques become an option. There are many variations of manual techniques that sometimes work to get a stubborn head to turn. They are last resorts since most of the time maternal position changes, the belly-lift or both will work first with less intervention and should always be tried first. In addition, internally rotating the head (usually involving displacing the head upward slightly and moving it) increases the risk of cord prolapse.

Create a false pelvic floor: Try this first. If often works, is a relatively easy and is a minimally risky option as far as cord prolapse is concerned. See the end of the chapter entitled "Techniques Used to Help the Baby Descend during Labor" for a complete description of this technique.

Rotate the head to OA manually: Turning the head by any means can be difficult because it generally results in turning the neck rather than the entire body. If the body doesn't follow as the head is turned, the baby will tend to return to her original position, possibly due to the posterior shoulder being lodged against the sacral promontory. Thus, repeated attempts are sometimes necessary, with a "two steps forward, one step back" type of progress. Therefore, the following techniques include steps to try and ensure full, simultaneous rotation of the head and torso. Regardless of which of these techniques you try, you should always attend to the following:

- **Prepare the mother:** The mother should empty her bladder. Explain your proposed technique and that it may be uncomfortable. Be sure you have her full permission before proceeding.
- **Confirm the fetal position:** Never attempt to manually rotate a baby until you are sure he needs turning! Perform careful abdominal palpation and an internal exam to confirm position, and have your partner check your findings if you are unsure.
- **Assess fetal status:** With any manual maneuvers, listen to the baby before and after the procedure and, when possible, halfway through the procedure as well.

Hamlin rotational maneuver: Hamlin's original maneuver (1959) is presented for an ROP baby:

1. The mother lies on her back with her bottom slightly elevated. The midwife first reconfirms the fetal position.
2. The midwife then stands to the woman's right and an assistant stands to the woman's left.
3. The midwife performs a bimanual maneuver. She first palpates abdominally to find the anterior shoulder and places her left thumb behind it. In an ROP baby, this will be the baby's left shoulder, which lies in the mother's right iliac fossa. She inserts her right hand into the yoni and locates the posterior fontanelle. The following activities then take place simultaneously as soon as one contraction ends:

   Midwife's maneuvers:

   Externally: Forward pressure is exerted with the left thumb to cause the shoulder to roll from the mother's right toward her left (clockwise from below) to rotate of the baby's body to ROA.

   Internally: The fetal head is rotated from ROP to ROA as the midwife's right index finger exerts pressure in an anterolateral direction to guide the head around from the 7 o'clock position to the 12 o'clock (OA) position, similar to dialing an old-style telephone, but using more force (Davis, 1997).

   Assistant's maneuver: As the midwife proceeds, the assistant rolls the woman over onto her left side.

According to Hamlin, the force of gravity the comes into play as the mother rolls on her side assists with the rotation of the fetal torso and shoulders, resulting in the need for the midwife to apply only light pressure during her maneuvers, affecting an easy and gentle rotation. This perception of ease may be due, in part, to the greater upper body strength common to males.

Hamlin-Davis rotational maneuver: Elizabeth Davis (1997; 2004) offers her own modifications on the Hamlin maneuver. She proceeds as follows:

1. Palpate abdominally and perform an internal exam to reconfirm the fetal position.
2. Have the mother lie supine with plenty of space on the side you want the baby to turn toward. For example, if the baby is ROP, the mother will need space to her left; if the baby is LOP, there should be ample space to the mother's right.
3. Have an assistant stand facing the side of the bed that is opposite the one that you want the baby to turn toward (if the baby is ROP, the assistant stands to the mother's right; if LOP, to the mother's left).
4. The assistant palpates abdominally to locate the baby's shoulder and back and leaves her hands resting lightly over these fetal parts.

5. The midwife sits between the mother's legs. Given the desired direction of fetal rotation, the midwife decides which hand to use for this portion of the maneuver. (For example, for an ROP baby, many would find it easiest to use the left hand; for an LOP baby, use of the right hand may afford the best leverage. The hand you choose will depend upon your relative dexterity on either side.)
6. Between contractions, the midwife inserts two fingers and places them on either side of the sagittal suture, pushing upward to lift the head slightly out of the pelvis.
7. Now three simultaneous activities take place as soon as one contraction ends, and on into the next one if necessary:
   A. Midwife's maneuvers: She locates the border of the anterior fontanelle and applies enough pressure to the bony edge to move the head into an OT position. (Never apply pressure to the membranous portion of the fontanelle. Palpate until you find a bony edge.) She then presses against the frontal border of the anterior fontanelle in the direction of the pelvic sidewall (so as to bring the baby's chin to her chest) until the head has flexed enough to raise the fontanelle out of reach, or nearly so. (Often the head turns spontaneously as you do this, but you must still make sure that the body follows.)

   Once the head is OT and the anterior fontanelle is out of reach, the midwife quickly locates the border of the posterior fontanelle, and presses against it to complete rotation to OA. (If, at any point, she meets strong resistance with no movement, she stops attempting to rotate the head.) Throughout these maneuvers, she gives feedback to the assistant regarding when and how to push against the baby's shoulder and back.

   B. Assistant's maneuver: She lifts and pushes the baby's back and shoulder toward the opposite side of the bed, coordinating her actions with feedback from the midwife regarding the current orientation of the head.

   C. Mother's maneuver: As the baby moves from OT to OA, the mother is instructed to lift and swing her uppermost leg up, forward and over in an arc as she slowly rolls away from the assistant, in the desired direction of anterior fetal rotation.
8. Once the mother is fully on her side, the assistant can help her sit up, and then assume a standing, forward-leaning position to help the baby stay in place.

Steps 5 through 7a. can be performed with the mother in an open knee-chest position as well, leaving out the manipulations by the assistant. This is a better option if the placenta is implanted anteriorly, as manipulation of the anterior belly does pose some risk of placental trauma in such cases.

Stevenson lift: Another version of this maneuver is the "Stevenson lift," so named for John Stevenson. An assistant applies upward pressure just above the symphysis pubis to lift the anterior shoulder and the head up while the midwife's internal hand pushes up on the baby's head and a third person manipulates the fetal shoulder abdominally as described above to effect rotation to OA.

Rotational maneuvers using the whole hand: Manual rotation can also be accomplished by grasping the head with the whole hand. This requires considerable physical strength and a large hand with long fingers to grasp and turn the head. It is also a far more invasive maneuver because the whole hand may need to be inserted past the cervix to get a grip on the head, thereby increasing the risk of cord prolapse. Such techniques require patience and a mother willing to put up with a lot of internal manipulation. This maneuver requires an assistant and an exam table or similar furniture (a very sturdy dining room table, a padded pool table, or thick plywood supported by horses could work).
1. The mother must be lying on a table that places her introitus level with the midwife's elbow. She should be on her back, with her bottom slightly off the end of the surface and her legs in a modified Walcher position.
2. The midwife stands between the mother's legs and reconfirms fetal position.
3. If the baby is LOP, the midwife turns to the side so that her left arm is nearest the mother (if the baby is ROP, she turns so that her right arm is nearest the mother).
4. The midwife inserts her nearest hand into the yoni, spreads her fingers and grasps the head over the parietal bones, with the crotch of her thumb and forefinger directed posteriorly (this places the posterior fontanelle between her thumb and forefinger).
5. For an LOP baby, the assistant stands to the mother's left side, reaches over her abdomen, locates the anterior shoulder and cups her fingers behind it so she can pull the baby toward her, or she stands to the mother's right and prepares to push the baby away from her, as the midwife rotates internally. (If the baby is ROP, the assistant reverses her positions, depending on whether she is to pull or push the baby.) (Mayes 1959; Daniels, 1978).
6. Once all hands are in place, the following activities occur simultaneously immediately after a contraction:

A. Midwife's maneuvers: The midwife pushes the head up only enough to get a grip on the baby and allow mobility. Now she rotates the head by pronating her arm as she turns her body to face the mother. This motion turns the head using the strength of the midwife's whole body as the crotch of her thumb and forefinger moves to an anterior oblique position (e.g., LOP to LOT to ROA). She gives feedback to the assistant regarding when and how to manipulate the baby externally.

B. Assistant's maneuver: At the same time, the assistant pulls (or pushes) the fetal shoulder in the desired direction of rotation, guided by the midwife's instructions.

C. Mother's maneuver: If space on the exam surface allows, the mother is instructed to roll over onto her side as all this occurs (to her left if the baby is ROP, to her right if LOP).

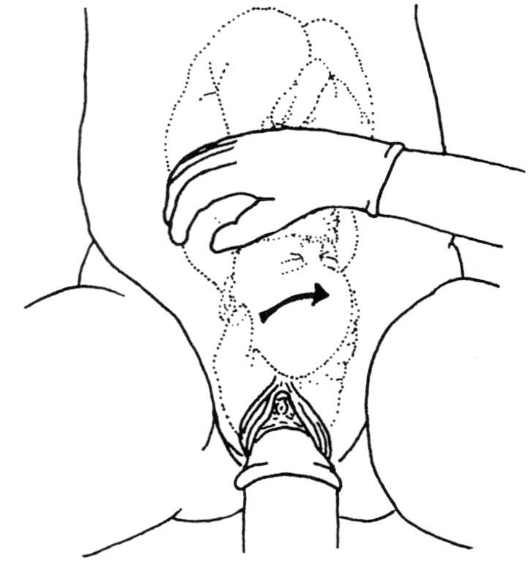

ROP baby with midwife and assistant's hands in place, ready to perform anterior rotation.

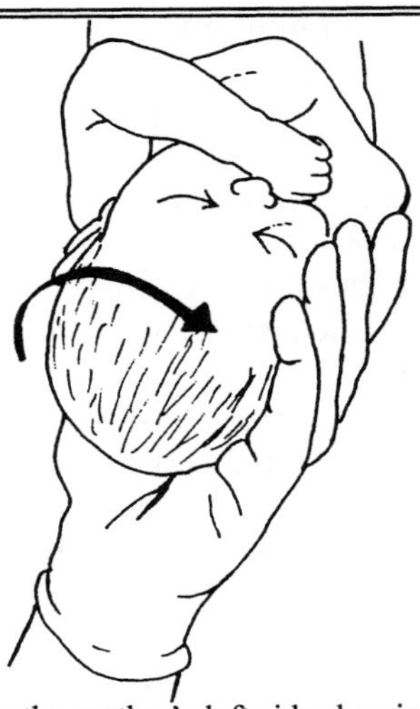

Close-up from the mother's left side showing the midwife's index finger overlapping the posterior shoulder to assist with anterior rotation.

If the head returns to its original position, the midwife can give the mother and baby a break and try again, this time hooking her internal fingers over the anterior shoulder as she rotates the head. This will be *very* difficult unless her fingers are long and very strong. She uses her whole hand to bring the baby around to ROT, then ROA. As she dislodges the shoulder, the head should follow suit.

Getting the baby to remain OA: Sometimes the baby will immediately descend and come quickly after a manual rotation. Other times, the head moves some and then stops or returns to its original position. If the first attempt is not successful (or not completely so), give the mother and baby a break and make another attempt later. Once you have completed the maneuver a second time, have the mother remain lying on her side. Have her lift her lower hip and slide a pillow under her. The mother should then flex her upper leg and bring her knee up level with her lower belly. This moves the pelvic bones into an asymmetrical slant and assists gravity in fixing the position of the baby as well as encouraging full anterior rotation. Hamlin (1959) recommends having the mother maintain an exaggerated left lateral Sims position for 30 minutes or until 6 good contractions have occurred. This will help to remould and fix the head in the new position. If the head still doesn't remain rotated to OA after a few attempts, retry other techniques (Hart, 1995).

Practicing manual rotation: These techniques are somewhat complicated; try working with an assistant, a doll and a pelvis to fully understand the maneuvers.

Discovery of an Occiput Posterior Position After Full Dilation

Knee-chest position and manual rotation of the head: Sometimes a midwife does not discover that the baby is posterior until the mother is completely dilated. It is still possible to turn the baby, although it is more difficult. You can try any of the maneuvers in the previous section. If those fail to help, Valerie El Halta (1998) uses the following maneuver with the mother in an open knee-chest position, with her knees slightly apart. The midwife with the largest hands should be the one to attempt the following maneuver. She inserts her hand into the woman's yoni and attempts to lift the baby up by grasping the head firmly, then waits for a contraction and turns the baby to an anterior position. She should first attempt to turn the baby in a short-arc rotation (for example, ROP to ROT to ROA). If the baby won't go that way, a long-arc rotation can be attempted (ROP to OP to LOP to LOT to LOA). As soon as the head is correctly positioned, it is held in place. During the next contraction the mother should bear down as hard as she can to help the rest of the baby's body follow the head. Membranes that are intact should be ruptured at this point to help ensure that the fetal position remains fixed. When this technique is successful, the baby is often born rapidly.

Promoting anterior rotation during pushing: If labor has progressed to complete dilation, it may be that the mother will give birth with no problems. However, it can happen that pushing is long and essentially nonproductive. The following suggestions are specific to posterior babies who are not descending in spite of effective pushing. It is very important that midwives and parents be patient while the baby finds his way out. Often the use of more than one technique will be required. For example, one midwife tells of a homebirth during which the baby descended to the perineum, almost to crowning, twice over the course of many hours of maternal pushing on and off, interspersed with the mother gently bouncing on a small exercise trampoline. Each time the baby would go back up inside until, finally, the third time the baby came to the perineum, spun around, and came out OA. Remember that time spent at full dilation, in and of itself, does not increase risk for mother or baby; persistent, nonproductive pushing can. For more tips, consult the chapter entitled "Maternal Position during Pushing and at the Time of Birth."

Arch the back: The mother lies flat on the floor and arches her back (pushing her belly up and tipping her pelvic brim forward) during pushing. A padded support can be place, under her sacrum so she can relax more completely. This sometimes helps to turn the baby to an anterior position (Gentlebirth Midwifery list, 1995). This is a version of the classic Walcher position, which was devised by an obstetrician to promote engagement with a tight inlet. It increases the angle between the spine and the pubic arch, thus maximizing space for rotation at the brim. Standing, forward-leaning while tilting the pelvis forward and swaying the back accomplish the same thing far more comfortably.

Side-lying with leg motion: The mother lies on her left side, making sure her knees are at a 90° or greater angle in relationship to her tuberosities. As the baby rotates, the mother lifts her right leg up and out, placing her foot on the bed to help the baby complete rotation and make room for the anterior shoulder to slip under the pubic arch (Sutton, 2001).

Dangle: The use of the dangle position either with partner support or the Birth Sling can help get the baby past the midcavity and outlet by taking all the weight off the pelvis.

Pushing in a full squat: This is a variant of the Bradley technique for turning a posterior baby when all efforts to turn the baby are not working and the baby is already well engaged. The mother goes down into a deep squatting position with feet flat on the floor and knees deeply bent and pushes with everything she's got; this may result in rotation to the anterior within one or two pushes. A squatting bar can be devised using a pull-up bar that fits in a door frame; this will help the mother maintain a full squat while providing her some support. Once the baby has rotated, she may change position.

When the baby is coming out OP

The mother whose the baby is coming down occiput posterior should be in a position that maximally opens her pelvis. Sutton (2001) states that in a persistent posterior, the shoulder axis is often extended. Rotation of the torso to the transverse is hampered when the posterior shoulder and upper torso get jammed against the sacral promontory in back, causing the anterior shoulder to overlap the pubic bone in front. Obviously, this situation will impair or entirely prevent descent. She recommends that the mother lie on her left side and lift her upper leg up and over, planting her foot on the bed to widen the right side of the pelvis and create room for the shoulders and torso to become dislodged. Any variation on this type of oblique movement may do the same; however, side-lying helps the baby rotate in a gravity-neutral position.

Assisting a Woman Whose Baby Is in a Compound Presentation

The baby in a compound presentation still attempts to descend and rotate through the pelvis according to the position of the denominator. However, the accompanying extremity (or extremities) increases the overall presenting diameter, and may delay or prevent progress. Positioning of a limb may seriously impair flexibility and lateral movement of the fetal torso, depending upon which limb or limbs are involved and how the fetal body is otherwise positioned. Thus descent may be delayed for multiple reasons.

Fortunately, babies in simple compound presentations usually descend normally through labor. Spontaneous birth often occurs when the hand lies alongside, rather than over, the head. Spontaneous retraction occurs frequently and obstructive types are rare. If the arm is over the chest, it is likely that the forces of labor and contact with the uterine and pelvic sidewalls will cause the elbow to be pressed down along the baby's chest toward her abdomen, allowing labor to progress. However, when true obstruction of descent is overlooked and if spontaneous resolution does not occur, the dangers are similar to those in transverse lie: membranes tend to rupture early, the lower uterine segment thins, and interventions to replace the extremity invite uterine rupture and cord prolapse. Cord prolapse accompanies the more pronounced varieties of compound presentation as often as 15% to 20% of the time.

Detecting and Dealing with a Compound Presentation

The position of an arm that has prolapsed beside the head may inhibit mobility at the neck and interfere with normal flexion or rotation. Anterior rotation may be impossible if the arm occupies a portion of the pelvis that the occiput needs to traverse. In general, an arm in the anterior portion of the pelvis will obstruct labor more than one prolapsed into the hollow of the sacrum, where there is more room. If the baby is LOA and the baby's posterior (left) arm lies alongside the head, it will take up space in the sacrum and thus assist anterior rotation and, likewise, discourage posterior rotation. If a baby's anterior (right) arm comes down behind the pubis, it will delay or prevent rotation, as it is taking up space that the occiput needs to occupy. The anterior arm seems to prolapse more often when the baby is OP (De Lee, 1940).

Prolapse of a foot beside the head is very rare. When it does occur, the extended leg renders the torso less flexible, and the foot, depending upon its position, may impair head flexion. Slow descent is the rule and arrest in descent is likely to occur. Presentation of a hand and foot together can also significantly impede or arrest progress.

Sutton and Scott (1996) state that a baby descending with his hand beside his head will cause a constant aching feeling on the side where the hand is positioned. The membranes may rupture sooner than usual. As the mother approaches birth, a compound presentation may prevent her from developing an urge to push, and suprapubic pain from the fetal elbow may mimic the pain from a cervical lip. Compound presentation with a hand beside the neck will almost always cause the head to be somewhat asynclitic as it descends and will often pull the cervical os off center as well, usually to the side opposite the small part.

What to Do

The following techniques have been used successfully when compound presentation hampers progress:

Position changes: Changing the mother's position works wonders for all kinds of problems.

Standing, one foot supported: Penny Simkin (2000) recommends having the mother stand and place one foot on an elevated surface so that the lifted foot is higher than the opposite knee (but not higher than her tuberosities). This position can be used to correct asynclitism, a posterior presentation, or a compound presentation . The woman should maintain the position for several contractions, then switch feet and maintain the position for several more contractions. This simulates stair climbing and raises the ischial spine on the side of the lifted leg higher than the other, widening the midpelvis and outlet obliquely on the lifted side, giving the baby additional space to do what she needs to do. Enough room may even be provided to allow the baby to reposition a hand that has been by her head (Sutton & Scott, 1996).

Kneeling on one knee: Sutton and Scott (1996) have found this position helpful to reposition the hand in cases of compound presentation. Keeping her back straight and her bottom elevated, the mother should kneel upright on one knee while placing the other foot flat on the floor; that knee should be held at a right angle to her hip. This position also widens the pelvis obliquely and keeps the brim open.

The mother can also crouch down over one knee, bringing her bottom close to the floor, and lift the other knee so that foot is on the floor, a position that will narrow the inlet but open the midpelvis and outlet more; this may be helpful if the baby is deeply engaged.

Moving the pelvis: Any action that moves, bends, rotates, rocks from side to side or otherwise takes the pelvic bones out of their usual parallel alignment is ideal for changing a poorly positioned head as well as for providing the baby with enough room to move his head past his hand in a compound presentation (Sutton & Scott, 1996). Belly dancing is perfect for this. If the mother is not inclined to belly dance, Sutton and Scott also recommend that she swing her hips forward and sideways as she bends one knee on that side and then goes up on her toes. Then she repeats this on the other side, thus making a kind of figure eight with her hips. The woman should use her hands or the Birth Sling to balance herself so that she can move her hips as much as possible.

Drop one hip: An arm across the chest, with the elbow more or less in the midline, can delay descent. The elbow can get stuck on the sacral promontory if the baby is occiput anterior or on the pubic bone if the baby is occiput posterior. Although this is relatively uncommon, this type of nuchal positioning of the arm is most likely to occur when the mother is multiparous or when the baby is late entering the pelvis, although it is relatively uncommon. If the arm is not caught, pressure against the promontory may cause it to be swept up and out of the way; however, this will require very strong contractions and will be painful for the mother. Impaction at the promontory can be expected if the fetal hand is braced on the opposite fetal shoulder. This positioning produces a characteristic pattern of no pain between contractions, but severe sacral pain during contractions as the arm is pressed against the promontory. To disimpact the arm, ask the mother to drop one hip lower than the other between contractions. She can do so by stepping up on a stair or any sturdy elevated object. Going though the maneuvers to turn around and sit on the toilet may also create space for the baby to move her arm (Sutton & Scott, 1996).

Dangle: The Birth Sling or the dangle position can be used when a small part will not move or when the reason for delay in descent is unknown. The dangling position will often allow the baby to work his way through the pelvis, which is now maximally mobile. This may be helpful during either active labor or pushing. The woman can be supported in the dangle position (by the sling or an assistant) for a few contractions while she moves her hips around and then change position.

Manual techniques: If position changes are not effective, more interventive techniques may help.
Move the arm: An anterior arm may be palpable above the symphysis. If so, you may be able to apply pressure to sweep the arm up and out of the way, especially if the mother is submerged in water. If the hand is palpable on internal exam, the baby may withdraw it if you poke at the fingers and explain what you want him to do. As the mother approaches birth, a compound presentation may prevent her from developing an urge to push. Suprapubic pain from the fetal elbow may mimic a cervical lip. Ask the mother to apply counterpressure over the painful area as she bears down, this will often encourage the baby to move his arm down so he can descend (El Halta, 1998).

Open the pelvis: Some of the techniques described in the subchapter entitled "Opening the Pelvis (or the Midwife's Forceps)," particularly those involving opening one side of the pelvis, can be useful during pushing when a small part won't move.

Replace the small part: If none of the above techniques work, but the cervix is sufficiently dilated, the membranes ruptured, and the small part can be felt, have the woman assume a knee-chest position. Don a sterile glove and insert your hand. Push the small part above the pelvic brim (below the chin) and hold it there until a contraction begins. As the contraction builds flatten your hand against the baby's head and slowly withdraw it, continuing to monitor internally to assess whether the small part stays put. The force of the contraction will (hopefully) push the head down into the pelvis, preventing reprolapse of the small part. Sometimes the baby will spontaneously withdraw the part when it is touched. Explain to the baby what is needed as you do this. To accomplish replacement may require rupturing the membranes, which risks prolapse of the cord (McCormick, 2000).

Irreducible compound presentation

It may be impossible to change the fetal position if the presentation is secondary to cord entanglement or the limbs are too fixed. Transport may be necessary if labor becomes obstructed.

Cord Problems and Emergencies during Labor

Intermittent cord compression, in one form or another, is a frequent accompaniment to labor. It most commonly occurs when a cord is wrapped around the baby's neck or, less commonly, when other body parts are entangled in the cord and is often enhanced if the volume of amniotic fluid is reduced. Usually, these babies have somewhat longer than average cords and thus the entanglement is compensated and the baby does well. The varieties of cord problems will be discussed in this chapter.

Nuchal Cord and Cord Entanglement

A **nuchal cord** is a form of entanglement that occurs when the cord is wrapped around the baby's neck. Other types of **cord entanglement** occur when the cord is wrapped around one or more other parts of the baby. Since nuchal cord is relatively common (occurring in about 20% of all births), what to do when it occurs at birth is addressed in the chapter entitled "Assisting at the Birth of a Vertex Baby."

Signs in labor

Marina Alzugaray (2004) has noticed that, when the cord is entangled or congenitally short, labor may appear to be underway. During and sometimes between contractions, the contour of the abdomen gives the impression that the baby is engaged. However, an internal exam finds that the baby is floating. In a mother who has previously given birth rapidly, contractions that start and stop in the presence of this type of apparent engagement with no other complication may be due to a short cord. She finds this harder to distinguish this pattern in a first-time mother. If the cord is the cause, it is important not to force labor with herbs or drugs, which may result in fetal distress and abruption of the placenta. She has found that the fundus must descend with the baby, and that this takes time.

Once labor is underway, a short (entangled or congenitally short) cord labor pattern may present with contractions that are erratic and of varying intensity or with persistently short, though increasingly intense contractions. Labor is often accompanied by the baby remaining high in the pelvis throughout labor. These short contractions can lead to a long labor, which allows the cord time to stretch and the upper segment time to descend, bringing the placenta along with it.

Impaired cord blood flow is often first heralded by fluctuations in the fetal heart rate as the baby begins to descend, often occurring around 6 to 7 cm of dilation. At this point, ask the mother to assume a hands-and-knees position or lie on her side; the fetal heart rate often responds by normalizing. If not, you can insert a gloved hand and gently lift the head to relieve tension on the cord. If the fetal heart rate returns to normal, you can continue at home, but labor should not be stimulated, to allow the cord time to stretch. If the heart rate does not return to normal, transport. If the cord is very short, transporting the mother in a knee-chest position may help relieve tension most effectively (El Halta, 1998) because it moves the baby back up closer to the placenta.

Upon complete dilation, the baby descends rapidly to birth (O'Conner, 2000). Alternatively, the baby may descend during a push and recede dramatically between contractions, as though she is tethered to a tight elastic rope. Another sign of a baby with a short cord is lots of head movement during pushing (Schlinger, 2003). If fetal distress occurs during late pushing, you should get the baby out as quickly as possible. Always be particularly prepared to resuscitate the baby in these circumstances.

Checking for a nuchal cord: If fetal heart patterns suggest that the cord may be around the baby's neck, you can try to confirm this with the following technique. Have the mother lie supine. Palpate above the pubic bone to locate the fetal neck (assuming the baby is cephalic). You or an apprentice can now apply firm pressure in this area for 30 seconds while listening to the fetal heart. If there is a nuchal cord, the heart rate may drop abruptly but more often will rise 10 or more bpm, which lasts 10 to 15 seconds or longer. Release the pressure. A positive response calls for frequent auscultation until the birth, especially as the baby is descending (Roberts, 1989).

Pushing

If you suspect a tight or short cord, it may be best to have the mother assume a horizontal position (such as side-lying) before pushing resumes. The rationale for this involves slowing the descent of the baby so that any indicated interventions can be carried out before the baby is fully born. Have an assistant check the fetal heart rate constantly, give the mother oxygen by mask if the heart rate is worrisome and have her breathe through a contraction or two. This often restores the fetal heart rate to a normal range. Then, have her resume pushing. Breathing and pushing with alternating contractions may help get the baby out without too much oxygen deprivation. If not, you will have to evaluate how low the fetal heart rate is and if the baby will be born quickly. Keep in mind that a short cord or an extremely tight cord may tear as the baby advances. Be prepared with hemostats, a cord clamp and gauze to apply pressure if the cord should pull away from the umbilical base. If you have any evidence that the cord may have ruptured, be prepared to cut a clitorotomy, if necessary, to speed the birth. Also be prepared to deal with an immediate postpartum hemorrhage, should the placenta be pulled away from the uterine wall during a rapid birth with a short cord. Remember that such complications are very rare.

Be prepared for a hypovolemic baby

Chronic or acute cord compression from any cause can result in impaired return of venous blood flow from the placenta to the baby, while the arteries, which are more active in moving blood, continue to function more or less normally, bringing blood from the baby to the placenta. This results in placental engorgement and fetal hypovolemia. The best way to compensate for this is to leave the cord intact. If the umbilical vein is still patent, the placenta will retransfuse the baby after the birth. If the umbilical vein has completely collapsed, the baby is likely to be quite depressed at birth and require resuscitation. See the subchapter entitled "Evaluating and Assisting the Infant in Need of Resuscitation" for details about how to proceed.

If the Cord Breaks during Birth

On rare occasions, the cord may be quite thin, have a thin or weak area, be congenitally short or be wrapped around the baby in such a way that you are unable to relieve the tension on it, or have a Battledore or velamentous insertion and it tears or breaks as the baby emerges. Alternately, once the baby is born, a sudden move by the mother may snap the cord. When a cord does break, it tends to tear at the weakest point. This takes everyone by surprise and makes a bloody mess that will make it hard to see where the blood is coming from. The baby can lose blood rapidly and doesn't have to lose very much before he is severely compromised. If the break occurs prior to birth, a sudden gush of bright blood will let you know something is bleeding, but it will be hard to know if it is from a tear, the placenta or the cord. Most commonly, the sudden appearance of bright red blood as the head comes out is from a periurethral tear. Look for such damage first, although it will be hard to see. If you can't tell what is bleeding, be prepared for a large gush with the shoulders (if the placenta is abrupting) or for a broken cord. As the belly emerges, check to see if the cord is intact as soon as you can. If it is not or you are unsure, pinch off the stump with your thumb and index finger. If it turns out that the cord is intact, release the cord immediately and continue to search for the cause of bleeding. If the cord is broken, ask an assistant for a hemostat to secure the end as soon as possible once the baby is out. A hemostat will be easy to work with and will be easier than fumbling with a cord clamp at this time.

Once the baby is born and her broken cord is clamped, check for twins. Only in the event of multiple pregnancy is finding the other end of the cord critical (because the placentas may be fused, allowing the second baby to bleed out if there are significant vascular communications between the placentas). If another baby is found, try to find the other end of the cord, which is still inside the mother, and clamp as above. If you have two attendants, one of you can see to the baby while the other looks for the cord inside the mother.

If the translucent portion of the cord stump is too short to clamp properly, someone should apply firm finger pressure to either side of the remaining stump while you get ready to either tie off the end with sterile string or tie off the vessels with suture using absolutely sterile technique. Remember, you should clamp only the translucent portion of the cord. If you have a cord bander, sometimes a cord band will work in these situations as well. If you do not feel confident dealing with this at home, you will need to transport. Apply continuous manual pressure to the cord stump to prevent the baby from hemorrhaging during transport.

Exceedingly Short Cord

Another rare complication involves the baby who is born to the navel with a cord so short that birth is halted. You will have to palpate along the anterior torso for the cord, clamp it with one hemostat (be sure you do not clamp any other part of the baby) and cut beyond the clamp (on the mother's side). This is easier said than done. Be very careful not to cut the mother or the baby in the process. This should allow the baby to be born rapidly. This baby will not have the benefit of the placental pulmonary transfusion, so be ready for a baby who may have a choppy transition to breathing room air.

Cord Prolapse

Cord prolapse is defined as the positioning of the cord beside, beneath or below the presenting part. In most cases, this does not occur because the cord floats in the amniotic fluid and remains high in the uterus, while the lower uterine segment is so evenly applied to the presenting part that there is no room for the cord to slip down. Cord prolapse is divided into three presentations:

Occult cord prolapse: This presentation is present when a portion of the cord becomes trapped between the presenting part and the pelvic walls, where the cord cannot be palpated or visualized upon internal exam. Compression of an occultly prolapsed cord could occur prior to membrane rupture, although membrane rupture will generally result in increased compression because the presenting part is no longer cushioned. This type of prolapse may be more common than is generally recognized. It could cause fetal death without leaving any evidence at the time of birth.

Cord presentation (cord previa): This is present when a portion of the cord is positioned beneath (below or in front of) the presenting part, contained within the intact forewaters. While cord presentation does not technically constitute a prolapse until the waters have broken and the cord drops down into the birth canal, it is included here because the cord will prolapse once the waters breaks. Cord presentation is relatively rare.

Revealed or frank cord prolapse: This occurs during or after membrane rupture. It presents as a loop of cord that can be felt beside or below the presenting part and may extend outside the yoni. Frank prolapse may be preceded by a cord presentation or may occur when the cord is washed down with the escaping forewaters from higher in the uterus.

When prolapse occurs

The highest risk of cord prolapse occurs upon rupture of membranes in the presence of a preexisting cord presentation. The next highest risk (and most common occurrence) happens with forceful spontaneous or induced rupture of membranes in the presence of an average to large amount of fluid and a poorly fitting presenting part, causing the cord to be washed down with the gush of fluid. Cord prolapse can also occur at any point after the membranes have ruptured, particularly if the initial escape of fluid has flushed the cord down closer to the lower part of the uterus and then as the baby shifts, more fluid escapes and washes the cord through the os along with it. Cord presentation, a poorly fitting presenting part or both may also be associated with most of the factors listed below but is present before the membranes have ruptured. Specific predisposing factors in cord prolapse include:

- **A small baby (most commonly due to prematurity):** Preterm babies are also more likely to be in an unusual position when labor begins. Fetal mortality is high, in part because preemies have a low tolerance for anoxia.
- **Fetal positioning:** This can result in a poor fit into the pelvis (as with breech, brow, oblique and shoulder presentations). The highest relative incidence is in the following order: transverse lie, breech and cephalic.
- **Compound presentation or prolapse of an arm:** This causes an imperfect fit of the presenting part in the pelvis.
- **Contracted pelvis:** The poor fit between the baby and the pelvis leads to prolapse.
- **Placental implantation in the lower uterine segment with marginal insertion of the cord near the os:** This causes the cord insertion point and an accompanying length of it to be much closer to the cervical os than would ordinarily be the case.
- **Unusually long cord:** The longer it is, the more easily it can prolapse.
- **Nonengagement of the presenting part:** This creates room for the cord to drop down beside or before the head (most often seen with multiparous mothers).
- **Lax abdominal muscles:** This is a contributing factor because, with or without pendulous abdomen, the uterus tips forward, both hampering normal engagement and leaving a large amount of posterior space where the cord can drop down.
- **Polyhydramnios:** This condition is associated with a high presenting part as well as unusual fetal pre-

sentations. This, in combination with the large amount of amniotic fluid, presents a high risk of cord prolapse upon rupture of membranes.

•**Multiple gestation:** It is associated with unusual presentations, polyhydramnios and rupture of the membranes of the second baby prior to engagement.

•**Spontaneous rupture of membranes:** Prolapse may occur with or, less commonly, without any of the associated factors listed above. After the membranes break, cord prolapse may occur at any time. Most (47% in a study by Murphy, 1995) occur within 5 minutes. Ten percent occurred within one hour and 5% waited more than 24 hours later to occur. Prolapse is least likely to occur when the membranes rupture spontaneously late in labor with the presenting part filling the birth canal.

Cord prolapse may occur as a consequence of manipulations by the practitioner such as:

•Uncontrolled artificial rupture of membranes when the head is high or the fetal position is unusual
•Disengaging the head to facilitate rotation or correction of a compound presentation
•Flexion of an extended head
•External or internal version or fetal extraction

The dangers

While cord prolapse does not jeopardize the mother in any way, the baby is placed in grave danger of hypoxia due to cord compression. The risk of compression is greatest when the cord comes down behind the pubic bone. In a cephalic presentation, if the cord slips down near the sacroiliac joint, the jutting promontory offers some protection, although the pelvic soft tissues and the presenting part can still produce compression sufficient to compromise blood flow. The danger of compression is not as acute in undescended breech and shoulder presentations because small, irregular fetal parts are adjacent to the cord. In addition, the baby is typically very high in the pelvis, and, if the cord prolapses posteriorly, there is ample space in the sacroiliac notches at the rear of the pelvis for the cord to be relatively free of compression. When the cord prolapses alongside an extended arm, the arm may protect the cord from direct pressure to some extent. This is not to say that prolapse is such cases is not of concern. Every case of prolapse is a serious and potentially life-threatening event.

Compression affects the vein first, reducing the amount of blood getting to the fetal heart. If part of the cord falls outside the yoni, temperature change and handling can lead to spasm of the vessels and contribute to impaired blood flow.

The prognosis for the baby: Studies generally conclude that the overall fetal mortality rate for cord prolapse is 35%. However, a large study done by Murphy (1995) in the UK found a rate of 1 prolapse for every 426 total births with a very low fetal/neonatal mortality of 1 in 20,000 births (or an uncorrected mortality rate of 91 per 1000) directly attributable to cord prolapse. There was an apparently low, but still nonspecific, incidence of subsequent handicap among survivors. Out of 132 cases of cord prolapse, 126 babies were born alive. There were 6 fresh stillbirths (4 of whom were alive at the time prolapse was identified and 2 of whom had no heart beat), 6 deaths during the first 28 days of life and one baby who was diagnosed with cerebral palsy at the age of three. Of the 132 babies, 77% were singletons, 9% were first twins and 14% were second twins. Of the survivors, 32 were born per yoni (23 vertex, 9 breech) and 94 were born via surgery. He attributed the low mortality rate to birth within the hospital, where the prolapse was identified and dealt with relatively quickly. The longest diagnosis to delivery interval was 30 minutes.

Overall, any baby's chance for survival depends upon the degree and duration of cord compression and the interval between diagnosis and delivery. If full compression goes unrelieved, the fetus may run out of oxygen in as little as two and a half minutes. The more mature the baby and the better his condition at the time of diagnosis, the more likely it is that he will survive. A strong pulse in the cord is a good sign; a weak or absent pulse obviously bodes ill for the baby. The sooner the baby can be born, the better he will fare. A delay of over 30 minutes increases the mortality rate fourfold, and the longer this interval becomes, the more the mortality rate is likely to rise (Murphy, 1995). Mature babies have a greater tolerance for withstanding traumatic events, especially oxygen deprivation. Even so, every baby whose cord prolapses is at grave risk for brain damage or death.

Preventing cord prolapse

Pendulous abdomen: Place a belly binder to both support the mother's abdomen and assist the baby in entering the pelvis. This alone may help some babies enter the pelvis and eliminate the need to artificially rupture the membranes. Have the woman lie down on the end of the binder and have her or an assistant hold the uterus in place. Wrap a long piece of cloth, starting at her hips and continuing upward. Keep the lower part of the wrap relatively tighter, and gradually make it looser as you move up the abdomen. Once it is wrapped properly, recheck internally to see if the baby is lower. Some time in labor may be needed to bring the baby down. See the chapter entitled "Unstable Lie, Oblique Lie and Transverse Lie in Labor" for detailed instructions about wrapping the belly.

Controlled rupture of membranes: Frank cord prolapse typically occurs suddenly, with no warning, because the bag breaks with the baby high in the pelvis. It is therefore more likely when the baby is early, malpositioned or breech. Prolapse may occur before the midwives have even arrived, especially if the woman has one of the risk factors listed above. Frequently the mother has had several babies and has lax abdominal muscles.

If you are present and have determined that the baby is high with the waters buoying the baby up and preventing engagement, and the woman is at or near full dilation or actively progressing in that direction, you can attempt controlled rupture of membranes. This prophylactic technique can allow the waters to leak out slowly preventing the sudden breakage that produces a large gush of fluid that can wash the cord down with it. It should be done well before forceful pushing begins.

You may be hesitant to break the bag yourself. This is one instance when breaking the bag artificially is likely to considerably lessen the chance of a problem. The bag will break eventually, anyway, and it is better to have the water release gently in these circumstances. You will, of course, want to explain the situation to the parents and be sure they understand that there is a risk of prolapse with either rupturing the membranes or not and that they are in agreement that this is the best course of action.

Have the mother lie in a supine or a modified Trendelenburg position. This can be accomplished by propping her hips up slightly with pillows or folded blankets but keeping her shoulders flat on the bed. This will encourage the cord to stay high without dramatically moving the baby even further from the os, which a knee-chest position would do. Schlinger (2003) makes the point that moving the presenting part further from the pelvis in a reversed gravity position is counterproductive to the aim of facilitating descent. I favor a slight Trendelenburg position because it reduces the pressure down even more and allows the contractions to gently move the baby down after you break the waters. Either position can be used. Have an assistant listen to the fetal heart rate throughout the procedure.

The goal is to allow the water to leak out slowly, avoiding a sudden, large, uncontrolled gush during labor or pushing. Create a small hole in the membranes just after a contraction subsides. To do so, you will need a sharply pointed device. The best tool for this purpose is a long syringe needle. A pudendal needle and sheath is ideal for this purpose, but any long syringe needle will do. If you don't have a sheath, you can cut a length of sterile IV tubing so that the tip of the needle can easily move beyond the edge. Because the tube is plastic and the needle could catch on it as it is inserted, sheath the needle first, then insert both into the yoni, holding the needle in place with the tip recessed below the edge of the tube by pressing the tip of your index finger against the tube to stabilize the needle within. Otherwise proceed as for a pudendal needle and sheath. Either of these tools will allow you to create a tiny puncture. Regular amnicots and amniohooks tend to produce tears rather than punctures and you want to create as small a hole in the bag as possible. Do not rip across it. Creating one small hole allows the liquor to drain slowly with the least amount of forceful pressure, and therefore carries the least risk of the fluid carrying the cord down and out through the cervix. It can be difficult to break the bag between contractions because the bag is typically slack at that point, but don't be tempted to break it at the onset of the next contraction, as this will defeat your purpose. If you have a suitable needle and sheath, proceed as follows:

1. Insert your dominant hand into the yoni first, then guide the sheath in with the other hand.
2. Slide the needle part way through the sheath.
3. Use the fingers still inside to help guide the end of the tube to where you want to place the punctures. Use your other hand to manipulate the needle through the sheath.
4. Poke a hole through the membranes. Poking is less likely to rip and burst the bag than a tear. Schlinger (2003) recommends making only one hole. Several holes may weaken the bag to the point that the holes act as a perforation, ripping between them and creating a long tear. In addition, the flow of fluid from a single hole can be easily controlled with finger pressure if the fluid seems to be escaping too fast. If making a hole proves difficult, have an assistant apply just enough fundal pressure to create only enough tension in the forewaters to allow you to poke through the membranes. Taut membranes give you more control over the size of the hole created. Once you have begun, have her release the pressure.

If you have no IV tubing, a syringe needle can be held between your thumb and two forefingers. Form your fingers and palm into a cone and guard the tip while moving carefully toward the cervix. This will require inserting more of your hand than when using a long needle and will therefore be more uncomfortable for the mother. A small needle will be considerably harder to manipulate for this type of puncture, but it can be done if care is taken. If you don't feel comfortable using a small needle, the next best choice is an amnicot, because it provides more control than an amniohook over how big a hole you make. Scratch the surface gently; an amniocot is designed to create a rip, not a hole, and making a small tear will be tricky.

Once the puncture is made, keep your hand in the yoni until the presenting part moves down and is fully in contact with the os. This may take a few contractions. To be sure there is no occult prolapse, the fetal heart rate should be continuously monitored as descent proceeds. Don't be alarmed by the squishy feel of the posterior cervical canal before the head fills the space. In contrast, the cord would feel firm, smooth and pulsating. You can place your external hand on the fundus to guide the presenting part into the pelvis as the waters leak out. Do not push forcefully; you want to avoid creating a big tear and a big gush.

As contractions continue and the baby begins to descend, slowly remove the elevation below the mother's hips as contractions continue to gently allow gravity to assist in bringing the baby down. The mother may assume any position she desires once the presenting part is filling the pelvis and is applied to the cervix and the fetal heart rate is normal.

Diagnosing cord prolapse

Diagnosis of cord prolapse requires an internal exam. If the membranes are intact, nothing should be felt in the forewaters between the presenting part and your hand. The possibility of a cord presenting in an intact bag of waters should be considered whenever the presenting part is not felt in the forewaters. Differential diagnosis includes an unusual presentation, fibroids, polyps, a compound presentation and a contracted pelvis. Place one hand on the fundus and press the baby down into the pelvis gently to see if any other obstruction becomes obvious. A contracted pelvis is very unlikely if the woman has previously had normal births of normally sized babies. In the event of cord presentation, it may be possible to detect the pulsing of the cord through the bag. Take care not to rupture the membranes if they are still intact.

A structure that is shaped like a cord but is not pulsating may be detected if the baby is dead or if the baby has an abdominal wall defect with exposed intestines and is lying transverse with his belly to the os. In the second case, the loops may have a doughy consistency. An omphalocele may mimic a cord presentation as the intestines are contained within a membrane. Other things that may mimic prolapse are a posterior uterine rupture through which loops of maternal bowel have escaped or a pediculated maternal myoma. Transport is in order whenever any of these is suspected.

Cord presentation is often associated with a marginal insertion point; also feel carefully for a velamentous cord vessel, which will feel like a pulsating worm traversing the membranes. Take care to distinguish vessels encased in the membranes from pulsations that may be detectable in the fornices and from cervical polyps or other unusual growths.

Occult prolapse must be considered whenever the fetal heart rate displays irregularities, particularly variable decelerations, especially if these are first detected when the baby starts to descend. (Note that, especially at first, the heart rate may be normal between contractions and only drop during a contraction.) If the membranes are ruptured, place the mother in a slightly hips-elevated supine position. This may move the presenting part up enough so that is it is now possible to reach inside and palpate the cord beside it. This must be done with great care, as displacing the presenting part may cause the cord to prolapse further. Do not attempt to manually confirm an occult prolapse if the membranes are still intact, as you may inadvertently break the bag and produce more distress. Instead, alter the maternal position and continue to monitor the baby closely.

A frank cord prolapse has occurred whenever the membranes have ruptured and a loop of cord hangs down into or outside the yoni where it is easily recognized by manual and visual inspection. Be sure not to panic. Do a careful exam to make certain that a fetal part is not being mistaken for the cord or vice versa. More suggestions for identifying a cord presentation or prolapse can be found in the chapter entitled "Performing Internal Exams during Labor."

Listen to the baby: It is prudent to listen to the fetal heart rate whenever the bag breaks. If there is a significant change in the heart rate upon rupture of membranes, perform an internal exam to rule out cord prolapse. This is especially important if the baby is high when the bag breaks. If you confirm or continue to suspect a prolapse, the heart rate should be monitored constantly until transport and transfer of care has taken place.

Dealing with cord prolapse

Cord presentation: If you discover that a loop of cord is contained in the forewaters, put the mother in a position that elevates her bottom as high in the air as possible, such as a knee-chest position. It is possible for the cord to float up and out of the way, although waiting for this to occur should not delay transport. Monitoring necessitates careful internal exams coupled with scrupulous fetal heart rate monitoring to make sure that the cord previa has not merely converted to an occult prolapse. Talk to the baby about what needs to happen (ask the baby to grasp the cord and pull it up), and have everyone present visualize the cord being replaced above the baby's neck. If this does not work, transport the mother in the knee-chest position. Consider version to try and replace the cord only if you are remote from any possibility of medical help. (This is discussed in the chapter entitled "The Use of Version during Labor.")

If cord prolapse has occurred: The steps taken when faced with cord prolapse will depend on a number of factors, such as how close you are to medical assistance, the parents' wishes, your skill as a midwife and the individual circumstances of the case. There is usually no attempt to deliver the baby rapidly when the baby is known to be dead, abnormal or so premature that survival is unlikely (less than 22 weeks gestation or 500 g, although the cutoff date or weight in your local community may depend on the proximity and sophistication of your regional neonatal intensive care facilities). You should discuss your findings with the parents. If the baby is alive, the standard treatment is to:

1. Keep pressure off the cord by manually elevating the baby with your hand.
2. Place the mother in the position that best maximizes cord blood flow.
3. Give the mother oxygen by nonrebreather mask at a flow rate of at least 10/lpm.
4. Check the fetal heart rate as often as possible and preferably continuously. This is one time when the emergency use of a Doppler is warranted, especially if the mother's position does not allow auscultation with any other instrument. Cord pulsations, while reassuring, are no guarantee of the fetal condition. Listening to the fetal heart is the best gauge of fetal well-being.
5. If contractions are strong, administer a uterine-relaxing agent such as motherwort or lobelia to the mother.
6. You could place an indwelling catheter to help elevate the presenting part.
7. Transport to proceed with an emergency surgical birth as soon as possible.

More details on these choices are presented below; other, more controversial, options then follow.

Keeping pressure off the cord: Regardless of what actions will be taken, the first order of business is to get pressure off the cord. Quickly position the mother in such a way that pressure on the cord is minimized; choice of position depends upon where and to what extent the cord is prolapsed. Have an assistant continuously monitor the fetal heart rate. Constant monitoring will help determine the maternal position that compromises the baby the least. Monitoring that must stop momentarily due to maternal repositioning should resume as soon as possible.

The best position will vary with the location of the cord. Mechanics dictate that the mother should be in a position that allows the presenting part, aided by gravity, to fall away from the cord. If the cord is positioned between the head and the pubic bone, have the mother assume a deep knee-chest or Trendelenburg position; don a sterile glove (preferably one with a long cuff) and apply counterpressure to the presenting part, if necessary, and gently try to move the cord to the side. This will move the cord away from the pubic bone, where it would have been maximally compressed. Even if the cord is wedged between the pubic bone and the head and cannot be moved, having the mother remain in a deep knee-chest position or a Trendelenburg position may still be the best option. The three most effective positions are side-lying with pillows propping up the mother's hips (especially if the cord is prolapsed along the side of the pelvis; have her lie on the side opposite the cord), lying on her back with her hips propped up, and the knee-chest position (especially if the cord is prolapsed near the sacrum).

Insert a hand into the yoni and apply gentle, steady counterpressure to lift the presenting part off the cord. If the mother is a nullipara and the presenting part is not engaged, apply enough pressure to keep the presenting part out of the pelvis and off the cord; if the baby is engaged, apply only enough counterpressure to relieve compression. If the mother is a multipara, elevate the presenting part out of the pelvis and then keep it off the cord. (Do not attempt to completely disengage the presenting part if the woman is having her first baby; the tissues are too firm to allow this easily, and too much counterpressure can injure the baby.) Whenever possible, lift the presenting part just above the brim and push it over into the iliac fossa opposite the side on which the cord is prolapsed. This helps to minimize the effect of contractions as they try to force the head downward, and it is easier to hold the head off center than if you push straight up. The late Lani Rosenberger (1992?) dubbed this the "Van Deik maneuver" after the Dutch midwife who taught it to her.

If the mother feels like pushing, someone should be in close contact with her helping her breathe or pant through contractions and not bear down. The person elevating the presenting part should be prepared to remain like this until the woman is in the hospital and the baby is removed with surgery or a practitioner there assumes responsibility for the case and specifically for elevating the presenting part.

A cord that has fallen outside the yoni should be carefully and gently placed back inside, unless the length exposed is such that compression would occur if it were replaced inside. In that case, replace as much as possible and then hold a wet warm cloth loosely over the remaining cord. To hold the moisture cover the cloth with a piece of clean plastic wrap and cover that with a piece of space blanket to retain the heat. If you do not have a space blanket, a piece of aluminum foil will suffice.

Using an indwelling (Foley) catheter to displace the presenting part: If the presenting part has been successfully displaced off the cord without undue effort, an assistant can insert a 16F indwelling (Foley) catheter into the urethra to backfill the bladder, which buoys the baby up and takes the place of the supporting hand. (Only attempt this if the presenting part was easily dislodged; if not, manual support of the presenting part should continue until a responsible party at the hospital has taken over.) This technique involves supplies that are not typically used by midwives at home, takes up valuable time, and will be difficult if the woman must be in a position other than supine or Trendelenburg. It is, however, relatively noninvasive and will help buoy the presenting part if transport time is prolonged. I suggest you do a few dry runs with a set of practice supplies before you consider using this technique on a laboring woman.

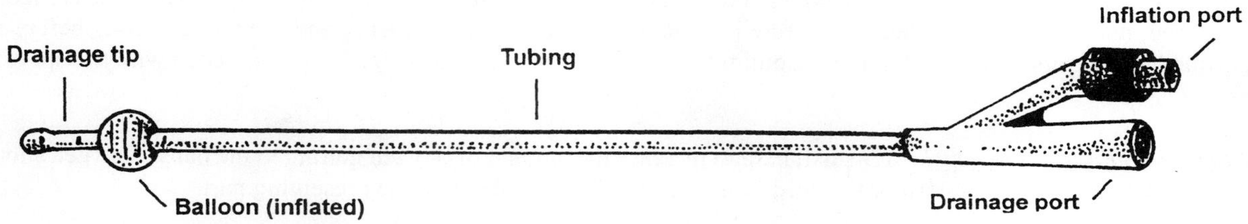

Foley catheter

Equipment: Assemble the following supplies and equipment on a clean Chux pad within easy reach:

- Size16F Foley catheter
- 1 small hemostat
- 3 cc syringe with no needle attached
- Basin to catch urine (a placenta pan will do)
- 60 cc catheter syringe
- Sterile, water-based lubricant
- Prepackaged sterile plastic bowl
- Betadine or Hibiclens (or similar product)
- Catheter plug
- 1 liter bottle of normal (0.9%) sterile saline

Procedure:

1. Open the sterile bowl and pour the sterile water into it. Spread open the bowl wrapper and place it on the pad to serve as a sterile field.
2. Fill the needleless 3 cc syringe with saline and set it on the sterile field.
3. Open the Foley catheter, pulling out its port end while leaving the rest of it in the wrapper to maintain sterility.
4. Firmly attach the syringe tip to the hard plastic balloon port.
5. Push the syringe plunger until the balloon on the other end of the catheter is fully inflated to make sure it does not leak.
6. Deflate the balloon by drawing the solution back into the syringe. Leave the syringe in place.
7. Lay the catheter on your sterile field.

8. Use the Betadine or Hibiclens to cleanse the periurethral area as you would when performing any urinary catheterization.
9. Place a dollop of sterile lubricant on your sterile field.
10. Don sterile gloves. Drape the inside of your glove wrapper over the bowl of sterile saline.
11. Use one hand to hold the labia apart in order to visualize the urethra.
12. Lubricate and insert the tip of the catheter into the urethra, advancing it 10 to 12 cm (you may feel a slight resistance), and then release as the tip passes into the bladder.
13. Release the labia and hold the catheter in place. Inflate the balloon with the preattached syringe. If inflation produces pain, stop, release the air and insert the catheter a little farther up and try again.
14. Gently tug on the catheter to ensure that the balloon is holding it in place.
15. Quickly remove the syringe, keeping the plunger fully depressed. The port should automatically seal in the saline to keep the balloon inflated.
16. Allow urine to drain from the bladder. This prevents you from overfilling the bladder with water and flushes the catheter line, preventing you from injecting air into the bladder.
17. Fill the 60 cc catheter syringe with normal saline. Insert the cannula tip into the drainage tube and inject saline into the tube; this will start to fill the bladder. Use the hemostat to clamp the drainage tube, then remove the catheter syringe to refill it. Repeat until you have filled the bladder with 500 cc of fluid (8 and ⅓ syringes full of fluid).
18. Plug the catheter port with a catheter plug. If no plug is available clamp the tubing above both ports to prevent fluid from escaping from the bladder.

The full bladder will take the place of your hand in elevating the presenting part (Varney, 1997). Once the procedure is completed, make sure that the fetal heart rate is good and that the cord is pulsing and remains that way before the supporting hand is completely withdrawn. Continuously monitor the fetal heart rate as you proceed with transport for a surgical birth.

<u>Give the mother oxygen by mask:</u> This will help to increase the amount of oxygen getting to the baby. Oxygen should be continued until the baby is born or the cord is satisfactorily replaced above the presenting part.

Transport considerations: It is very difficult to move the mother to a transport vehicle while she maintains the optimal position that keeps pressure off the cord and while the midwife maintains counterpressure on the presenting part. An ambulance team experienced at moving accident victims while maintaining their position will provide the best care; if available in your area, call an ambulance with paramedics. Be aware that emergency medical personnel will not transport a woman down stairs in a knee-chest position, as it is impossible in this position to secure the woman sufficiently to prevent her from falling. They will probably want to use a transport chair, which will then be tipped backward and carried by at least two strong men. However, it is difficult to maintain counterpressure on the head when such a device is used. Therefore, if the mother has been in a knee-chest position prior to their arrival, find the next best position that minimizes cord compression. This is usually some sort of reclining position, which will allow better access to the head until the mother can be repositioned in the ambulance. Improvise based on the circumstances at the time and the size of the mother. The fetal heart rate should be monitored as consistently as possible while moving the mother to the transport vehicle. Once there, make sure she is settled in a position that optimizes fetal well-being and is receiving oxygen by mask before departure.

In developed countries, you can expect that a surgical delivery will be performed upon arrival at the hospital. There is virtually no hospital practitioner that will consider attempting to replace the cord (there are always exceptions, but don't expect it).

<u>Controversial methods of handling cord prolapse</u>

A midwife who goes against standard medical procedure in such a serious situation is legally on very shaky ground. However, if the woman has had other children (that is, she has dilated and pushed a baby out before) and is at or near full dilation, if you are remote from help, or if for other reasons (such as a bad storm) timely transport is next to impossible *and* your relationship with the parents is solid, you might want to try one of the following options.

<u>Assess the cervix:</u> The degree of cervical effacement and dilation will clarify your options. When the cervix is not fully dilated (or nearly so), transport to the hospital is you safest option.

Pushing the baby out: This is most likely to be successful when cord prolapse has occurred in a multipara who is fully dilated and has ruptured membranes with the presenting part on the pelvic floor when cord prolapse is identified. The increased surge of stress hormones that is likely to accompany the recognition of cord prolapse may enable the mother to birth her baby rapidly. Give her oxygen by mask until the baby is born. Sutton (2001) advises calling for an ambulance and then demanding that the mother "give me the baby now." This is one time where fundal pressure may help. The mother should arch her back (in whatever position she is in) and push with all she's got. If this doesn't deliver the baby at once, apply counterpressure to the head, elevate the baby off the pelvic floor, alter the woman's position to relieve as much pressure on the cord as possible and prepare for transport.

Cord replacement: Be aware that attempts at cord replacement are not always successful; they may compound the problem by producing additional compression or cord spasm. Do not attempt to replace the cord in a first-time mother, because her passages will be tighter. Midwives who have done this successfully report instinctively pushing the cord above the presenting part upon identifying it during an internal exam. Having small hands helps.

Repositioning the cord: Have the mother breathe oxygen flowing at 8/lpm or more and get into the position that maximizes circulation in the cord, judging by the fetal heart rate. An assistant should be listening to the fetal heart throughout the following procedure.

Don a sterile, elbow-length glove and insert your hand into the yoni. Cup your hand; as gently as possible, collect the cord into the cupped space created by flexing your thumb toward your palm. Insert your hand through the cervix, bringing the cord up as far as you can past the presenting part. If a length of cord remains below the presenting part, walk your fingers along it, drawing it back into the uterus. Leave your hand in place once the cord is repositioned to be sure it is not slipping back down. Confirm that the fetal heart rate is good.

Wait until you are convinced that all is well, then carefully remove your hand. Do so slowly, so that you do not displace the presenting part and have the cord come down again. Once your hand is out of the cervix, keep it in the yoni to continue monitoring for fetal descent. Have the mother begin to push. Confirm that the fetal heart rate is good. If there is still cervix left, push it out of the way. The baby should move down quickly in a multipara. Once the presenting part is filling the pelvis, have the mother move into a more gravity-friendly position. Continue to monitor the fetal heart rate carefully until the baby is born (Felch, 1991).

SHOULDER DYSTOCIA

Dystocia can be defined as a dysfunction in a process. Difficulty with the birth of the shoulders may occur during either cephalic or breech births because of problems in the rotation and birth of the shoulder girdle through the pelvic bones. In a breech birth, the arms and shoulders may fail to deliver after the birth of the lower body. However, the term "shoulder dystocia" usually refers to arrested shoulder delivery in cephalic presentations, when the shoulders fail to emerge spontaneously after the head is born, even with gentle upward or downward traction on the head and strong pushing efforts from the mother.

Shoulder dystocia occurs when there is impaction of one or, more rarely, both shoulders during descent into or through the pelvic brim or midpelvis or when the shoulders do not fit through the bony pelvic outlet. It may also involve malrotation. Shoulder dystocia is most often a bone-on-bone dystocia. It usually represents a relative, rather than an absolute, disproportion between the soft and bony tissues of the baby's shoulder girdle and the mother's pelvic bones. Midwives must know how to recognize and deal with this notoriously unpredictable, life-threatening emergency.

There are many degrees of severity with delay in the birth of the shoulders. What midwives term "sticky," "tight" or "snug" shoulders usually does not involve impaction of the shoulder girdle on the maternal pelvic bones and is therefore *not* true shoulder dystocia. On the other end of the spectrum, shoulder dystocia in its most severe form presents as a complete impaction of both shoulders above the pelvic brim that is complicated by the full abduction of both of the baby's arms. This chapter assumes that shoulder dystocia is the reason the baby fails to descend further after the head is born and not one of the other problems that can also cause a delay (listed later in this chapter).

UNDERSTANDING SHOULDER DYSTOCIA

Normal Birth of the Shoulders (What Shoulder Dystocia Is Not)

It is important to be familiar with the normal process of shoulder birth in order to understand how shoulder dystocia develops (review the chapters entitled "Features of Fetal Anatomy Pertinent to the Birth Process" and "The Process of Birth in Occiput Anterior Vertex Presentations" before studying this chapter). The baby's head and body are sometimes born in one swift spiraling motion when the mother is experiencing a fetus ejection reflex. If not, the head is born and then there is usually a pause, sometimes of several minutes, between the birth of the head and the birth of the shoulders. Usually nothing need be done to try and rush the birth of the body before it is ready to be born. The baby's neck is not unduly compressed and circulation to the head is unimpaired. The next contraction facilitates shoulder rotation and birth; in the upright and mobile mother, the posterior shoulder has descended into the roomy posterior pelvis and is born first; the anterior shoulder quickly follows.

During the normal birth process, many babies wait several minutes before the spontaneous birth of the shoulders and are perfectly fine. Sometimes the baby will even start to breathe during this time. Shoulder dystocia is often diagnosed by midwives only after the contraction that follows the birth of the head has come and gone with no fetal rotation or advancement. Many apparent dystocias will resolve spontaneously simply by awaiting the next contraction.

It is noteworthy that the older medical literature is full of admonitions regarding the wisdom of waiting for the birth of the shoulders. Benson (1974,132-133), who obviously knew that the posterior shoulder normally comes first, states "This portion of the birth process should be slow and deliberate to prevent fetal and maternal complications. . . Once the head has emerged and a clear airway is established, there is no need for haste, the baby will usually breathe, even before it is completely delivered. Deliver the shoulders after proper rotation. . . . Elevate the head toward the mother's symphysis for release of the posterior shoulder. This is often easily done and should be tried." Litzenberg (1947, 126) advises: "Do not yield to the urge to hasten the delivery as soon as the head is born. There is usually a lull in the pains at this time. . . . There is no hurry . . . When sure that the shoulders lie directly anteroposterior and pains have recurred, delivery may be assisted." Myles (1968, 306) says that "In a natural birth the shoulders are born during the contraction following the birth of the head. . . . The tendency to hurry this phase of delivery should be resisted. The baby's face will certainly look reddish blue . . . (but this is okay)." Other older texts express the same understanding (Baer, 1933, 825; De Lee, 1947, 216; Gibberd et al.,1965, 224). All this has been forgotten as fear of birth has risen, as the natural process has been overridden by technology and manual manipulation and as protocols for assembly-line obstetrics have become more entrenched.

A contemporary lack of understanding of this process is reflected in the research by Spong and colleagues (1995) in which they attempted to define shoulder dystocia in terms of the time that passed between the birth of the head and the birth of the body, the need for dystocia-resolving maneuvers or both. They came up with a "normal" head-to-body delivery interval (which included encouraging the birth of the anterior shoulder as soon as the head was born with gentle downward traction on the head) of 60 seconds or less (!). Not surprisingly to midwives, this definition resulted in a shoulder dystocia rate among the births studied of 10.8%. This time limit was apparently based on the assumption that the rest of the baby would always come more or less instantly once the head was out. This notion of instant shoulder delivery has been fostered by the use of clitorotomy with immediate forced delivery of the anterior shoulder via head traction.

Types of Shoulder Dystocia

The medical literature, with rare exceptions, only discusses shoulder dystocia at the inlet. Holly Scholles (2001), founder of Birthingway College of Midwifery in Portland, Oregon, points out that there are, in fact, two varieties. Her views are supported by Pecorari (1999), who discusses these differences in a short article. Knowing how each type presents will help the midwife respond appropriately by selecting the remedial actions most likely to relieve the type of impaction involved.

Inlet shoulder dystocia

Descent is arrested when the shoulder girdle becomes impacted above (behind) the pelvic brim as it attempts to engage. Inlet dystocia is often associated with a platypelloid pelvis because the shortened anteroposterior diameter makes rotation above rather than beneath the pubic bone more likely. However, inlet dystocia can also result from malrotation; late, incomplete rotation of a posterior baby is a common etiology. It can occur in mothers with a large anteroposterior brim diameter and in babies of all sizes, although the risk of dystocia goes up with increased fetal size.

Theory holds that shoulder dystocia occurs when the shoulders attempt to enter the pelvis through the anteroposterior diameter of the pelvic inlet, which measures 10.6 cm, rather than the larger oblique diameter, which measures 12.75 cm. While the shoulders rarely approach the brim in the anteroposterior diameter, when they do, they can become impacted, especially if the pelvis is narrow front to back, if the sacral promontory projects forward into the brim more than usual or if the baby is large. Even if the shoulders approach the inlet in the transverse or oblique diameter they can become impacted if they malrotate behind (or above), rather than underneath, the pubic bone. A wide, shallow pelvis makes this more likely. Either way, further descent is arrested, and the classic signs of shoulder dystocia, as described later in this chapter, occur. Transverse descent of the shoulders through the brim virtually eliminates the possibility of inlet shoulder dystocia in all but the largest babies or the most deformed pelvises. There are two severities of inlet dystocia:

Unilateral (low, anterior) inlet shoulder dystocia: Most commonly, instead of the anterior shoulder rotating beneath the pubic bone, it rotates behind (i.e., above) it. It may be lodged to either side of the symphysis pubis if the shoulders are still oblique, or it may be impacted upon the symphysis if the shoulder axis is in an anteroposterior orientation. The posterior shoulder is below the sacral promontory in the hollow of the sacrum and may be relatively easy to reach.

Bilateral (high) inlet dystocia: Bilateral inlet dystocia occurs when the anterior shoulder is behind (i.e., above) the pubic bone and the posterior shoulder is lodged against or above the sacral promontory. This rare form of inlet dystocia most commonly occurs during aggressive instrumental delivery coupled with a fetus who is drugged and, therefore, extremely relaxed. Because of the relative shortness of the fetal neck and the anatomical improbability of the head fully emerging with both shoulders so far up inside the pelvis, it is hard to conceive of such a situation arising during a spontaneous birth. However, two experienced midwives report that they have seen this type of dystocia after spontaneous birth of the head. Such instances of dystocia are most likely to occur when a large baby passes through a very shallow pelvis, when the shoulders of a large posterior baby incompletely rotate during descent or when a very large baby passes through a large pelvis (Tharpe, 2003). With the sacral promontory in the standing mother about 6.5 cm above the upper border of the pubic bone, bilateral shoulder dystocia stretches the nerves in the baby's neck to their limit, putting the baby at risk for injury both before and during attempts to free the shoulders.

Midpelvic shoulder dystocia

Gail Tully points out that, on rare occasions, shoulder descent can be obstructed by soft or bony tissue anywhere along the mid-pelvic passageway; for example, against a very rigid pelvic ligament. (Tully, 2012)

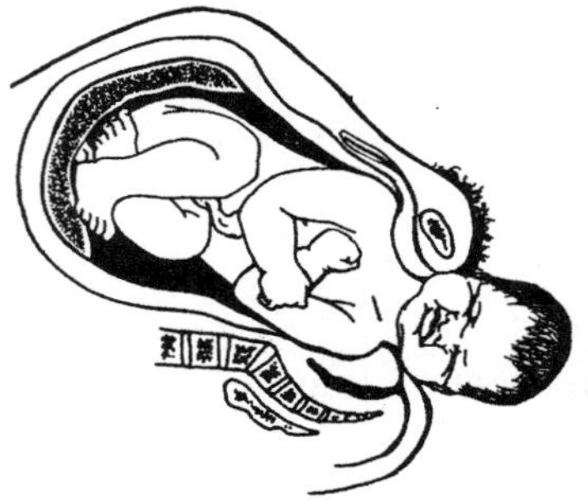

Anterior inlet dystocia in the anteroposterior diameter

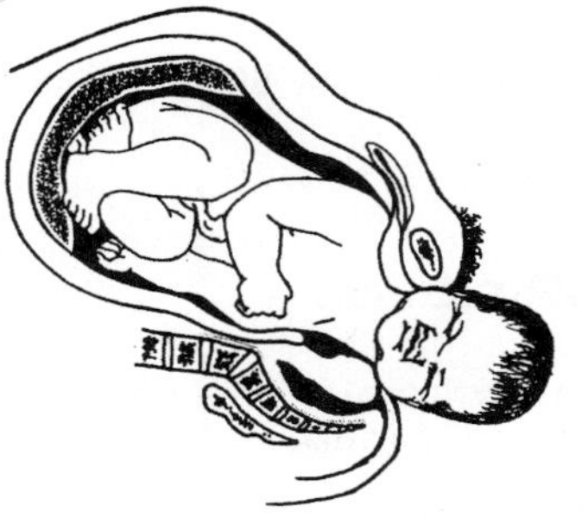

Bilateral inlet dystocia in the anteroposterior diameter

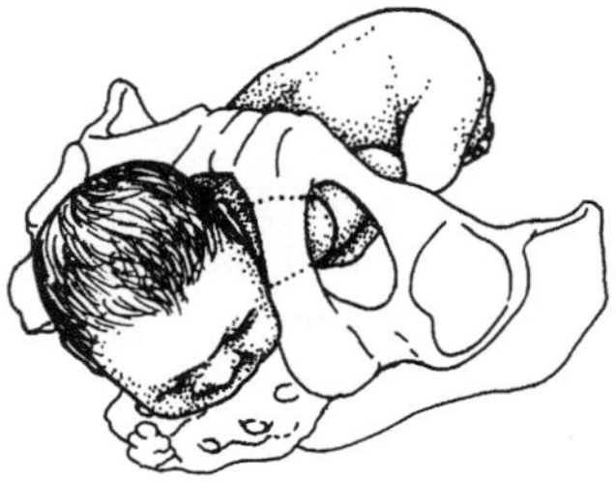

Outlet dystocia: incomplete chest rotation and a narrow pelvic outlet, with anterior shoulder hung up on the left pubic ramus

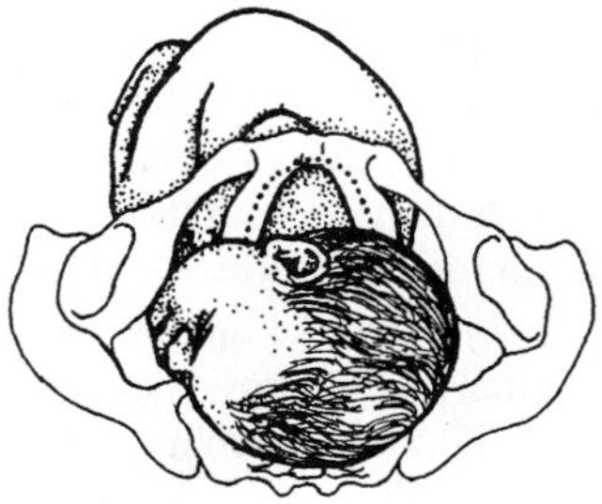

Outlet dystocia with impaction behind a narrow pubic arch

(Since supine positioning tends to encourage shoulder dystocia, these drawings show the woman on her back.)

Outlet shoulder dystocia

Outlet dystocia occurs when the baby's anterior shoulder passes below the brim but becomes arrested at the bony outlet. This is most likely to occur when a woman has a funnel-shaped (android) pelvis accompanied by a shallow sacral curve. The pubic arch is likely to be higher and more acutely angled than usual, allowing the anterior shoulder to pass beneath it with relative ease. However, the steepness of the angle brings the pubic rami and the ischial tuberosities closer together, and the anterior shoulder becomes impacted as it tries to pass through the narrowed passageway. When the outlet is marginally narrow, relative disproportion can occur with a big baby. There are two types of outlet dystocia:

Unilateral outlet dystocia due to incomplete rotation of the chest: The rotation of the baby's upper spine and torso results in the first internal rotation of the shoulders. Any exaggeration of the curve of the birth canal or narrowing of the midpelvis can hamper complete rotation. For example, the shoulder girdle may be able to descend through the transverse or oblique diameter of the brim into the midpelvis, only to have the anterior shoulder become impacted against the pubic rami as it attempts to undergo its second internal rotation to the anteroposterior diameter. The shoulders may pass through the brim in the transverse position, and then the arms could become lodged in the midpelvis between prominent ischial spines, preventing the shoulders from rotating to oblique or descending further, with the shoulders trapped in the transverse diameter behind the pubic rami.

Unilateral outlet dystocia due to the anteroposterior shoulder diameter becoming impacted behind a narrow pubic arch: The shoulders may engage through the transverse diameter of the brim and rotate to the anteroposterior diameter, where the anterior shoulder becomes impacted against the narrow descending angle at the midpoint of the pubic arch.

Bilateral outlet dystocia: This occurs when the shoulders are in the anteroposterior diameter of the pelvis, and anterior shoulder becomes impacted behind the pubic arch and the posterior shoulder gets caught against the coccyx.

Shoulder dystocia further complicated by the position of one or both fetal arms

Both inlet and outlet dystocia are further complicated when one or both of the fetal arms are positioned in such a way that shoulder flexion is impaired. One or both arms may be behind, rather than in front, of the baby's back. The forearms may also be extended across the chest, with each hand braced in the bend of the opposite elbow (Tully, 2003a). Normally, during descent and internal rotation, the shoulder girdle flexes forward or descends at an angle, reducing its diameter by at least one-quarter to one-third. In contrast, the extension associated with full abduction of one or both shoulders increases this diameter. There is a greater likelihood that the shoulders will not rotate correctly or, even if they do, that they will become impacted. This risk is greatest when both arms are so positioned. Getting the baby out may entail repositioning one or both arms in addition to dislodging one or both shoulders.

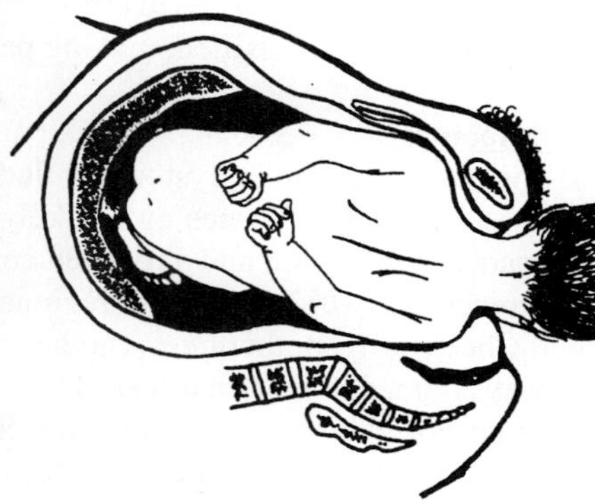

Unilateral inlet dystocia with both arms behind the back

Incidence and Risk Factors in Shoulder Dystocia

Sources vary, sometimes widely, as to the reported incidence of shoulder dystocia. The overall incidence of shoulder dystocia in all yoni births ranges between 0.15 and 0.30%. Within this small population of infants, larger babies are at greatest risk. Among babies weighing over 4000 g (8 lb 13.5 oz), the incidence is about 1.6%. Babies weighing over 4500 g (9 lb 14.5 oz) have about a 1.7% overall risk. However, it is noteworthy that the vast majority of large babies are born with no such difficulties (Golditch & Kirkman, 1978; O'Leary, 1992). Instrumental delivery, either with forceps or vacuum extraction, raises the risk of impaction for large babies because it can interfere with normal shoulder descent and rotation. In addition, babies who suffer shoulder dystocia are more likely to have a greater shoulder-to-head and chest-to-head proportion than either macrosomic babies born surgically due to failure of progress in labor or those born normally without shoulder dystocia.

Risk statistics are derived from institutionally based studies. They include women who may have received a variety of drugs or had instrumental deliveries. In addition, many medical practitioners are taught a limited range of techniques to rectify shoulder dystocia and often do not encourage or allow women to actively alter their position either during pushing or after a delay with the shoulders is recognized. Thus the true risk of shoulder dystocia in women birthing at home may therefore be somewhat lower than these studies indicate.

Fetal risk factors

Macrosomia: There are two main forms of macrosomia. **Symmetric or constitutional macrosomia** occurs when all fetal parameters (weight, length, head circumference and abdominal circumference) are proportionate and exceed the 90th percentile for gestational age. The baby is larger than most and is usually born to a mother who was well nourished or who has a large bone structure. Fetuses who are constitutionally large for gestational age, and therefore symmetrically grown, are not at significantly increased risk of shoulder dystocia. Not all sources agree on this point, however, and Varney states that a fetus whose weight is estimated to be one pound or more larger than a previous baby is at risk (Varney, 1997).

Asymmetric macrosomia occurs in the babies of diabetic mothers. A baby who is asymmetrically macrosomic is large with a disproportional growth ratio. The trunk, especially the chest, is large relative to the head, with chest circumference exceeding head circumference in 80% of cases. The upper arms contribute to a wider upper torso diameter. The head and femur measurements may vary in size and length but generally will fall below the 90th percentile. Abdominal circumference and thigh diameter, however, reflect soft-tissue mass; they will usually be significantly greater than average. Regardless of weight, babies born to diabetic mothers are at increased risk for shoulder dystocia due to this tendency of asymmetrical growth. (Additional information about large-for-dates growth may be found in the chapter entitled "Assessment of the Baby's Size and Its Relationship to Gestational Age.")

Postdates babies: Postdates babies reaching 41 weeks of pregnancy account for 40% of all cases of shoulder dystocia (O'Leary, 1992). The percentage rises to 60% when those born after 41 weeks are included. These babies are often large and their bone structure more ossified, making passage through the pelvis somewhat more difficult.

Maternal risk factors

Maternal risk factors for inlet dystocia include a low pubic arch and a narrowed diagonal conjugate; women with platypellic pelvises are 8 to 10 times more likely to have a shoulder dystocia. The risk of outlet dystocia rises in the presence of a narrow pubic arch and a reduced conjugate of the outlet. Other risk factors include a history of shoulder dystocia (recurrence rate, 10%), the use of regional anesthesia and slow progress during pushing or the birth of the head.

Dr. David Cheek, a hypnotherapist who has worked for many years with pregnant women, believes that shoulder dystocia is always related to maternal fear. He testified in a Canadian fetal death case involving shoulder dystocia that the mother had been told by a doctor that she would bleed to death if she had her baby at home. Once she was in the hospital, her baby, who had been undeliverable at home, fell out (Lemay, 1990?). Indeed, fear can cause the mother to clench her muscles and sphincters and thus interfere with rotation of the shoulders. This means that soft tissues can also delay the birth of the shoulders and hold them back even when there is no bony impaction. Emotional risk factors include maternal fears regarding the baby's condition once she is born and fears for her own safety.

Other associated factors

Additional reasons why shoulder dystocia may occur in a given birth include:

- Other pelvic peculiarity (e.g., prominent sacral promontory, flat sacrum)
- Maternal position during birth (especially if the woman has a pendulous abdomen, if her position does not allow her pelvis to open and her sacrum to move backward or if her posture pinches off the pelvic brim)
- Rapid or forced descent of the shoulders that does not allow for completion of the cardinal movements of the shoulders, resulting in incomplete shoulder rotation. Instrumental delivery with forceps or vacuum extraction may drag the shoulders toward the pelvic brim at an unfavorable angle as well as interfere with or prevent normal, spontaneous rotation.
- Cord entanglement or compound presentation that interferes with normal shoulder rotation
- Drugs given to the mother that interfere with normal uterine action, reduce pelvic muscle tone and thus impair normal rotation.
- Late rotation of a large, posterior baby, especially when a persistent anterior lip has been pushed back and the membranes ruptured, when the woman has been strongly encouraged to push without an urge or both.

Can shoulder dystocia be predicted?

There is a great deal of debate regarding the predictability of shoulder dystocia. Even though it is generally associated with large babies, 50% of all shoulder dystocias occur in babies weighing less than 4000 g (8 lb 13.5 oz); in many cases, it occurs without warning. Although having prior knowledge of the mother's pelvic structure can help midwives recommend advantageous positions for birth, plenty of women with "high-risk" pelvic features do not actually develop shoulder dystocia.

In summary, shoulder dystocia is not predictable. True shoulder dystocia is a rare event, occurring once in every 150 to 300 births. Any midwife who feels she is seeing a lot of shoulder dystocias may not be defining the problem correctly, may be having a run of incredibly bad luck or may be consistently assisting the birth process in such a way that malrotation of the shoulders is encouraged. In any event, all these possibilities need to be explored.

Dangers of Shoulder Dystocia

Risks for the baby: Shoulder dystocia is a highly problematic complication that can lead to fetal injury or death. Several types of injuries can result from efforts to deliver the baby rapidly or with techniques that ignore the anatomy and physiology of the structures involved. These include nerve damage, broken bones, and repercussions from asphyxia.

Excessive or improperly directed traction on the fetal head can cause damage to the brachial plexus of nerves. The brachial plexus originates at the spinal nerve roots of vertebrae C5 to T1. These nerves extend on either side through the

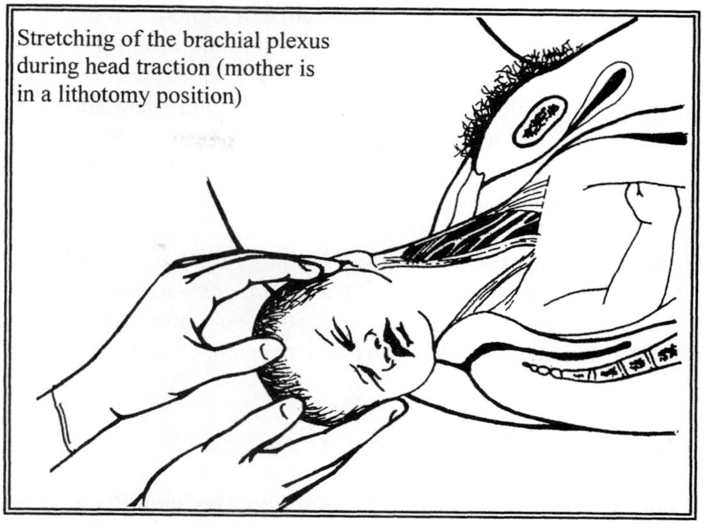

Stretching of the brachial plexus during head traction (mother is in a lithotomy position)

lower neck anterolaterally, through the armpits and down the arms. Injury occurs when strong lateral traction is applied, resulting in stretching, tearing or avulsion of the nerve roots. The brachial plexus injury that accompanies 8 to 23% of all shoulder dystocia cases (Gherman et al., 1999) is typically caused by excessive traction on the head and neck or excessive pressure into the anterior axilla. It does not tend to occur with arm traction because moving an arm up alongside the head relieves tension in the nerves on that side (although arm traction can damage the shoulder joint and is *not* recommended). It has been theorized that severe shoulder dystocia may, in and of itself, produce nerve damage even without any handling by the attendant. During a unilateral inlet dystocia, the neck is stretched from the brim to the introitus, causing extreme lateral traction in this area with excessive stretching of these nerves; this is made much worse during a bilateral inlet dystocia. The posterior arm is most commonly damaged. If, indeed, spontaneous damage actually occurs, its frequency may depend upon the amount of stress the tissues are already under from fetal positioning in the birth canal and the constitutional resiliency of the tissues in individual infants. Additional manual manipulation by the attendant may exaggerate this lateral traction even more, surpassing the limit of nervous tissue elasticity and resulting in damage or increasing the degree of damage already underway.

The injury that results from upper brachial plexus trauma is called **Erb-Duchenne palsy** or simply **Erb palsy**. Wilhelm Erb, a German neurologist, was the first to describe this injury in an adult in 1874. He pointed out that the same injury frequently occurred in newborns due to "moderately energetic manipulation by the obstetrician" at birth. The first to describe this as a birth injury was his contemporary, Guillaume Duchenne (Brody & Wilkins, 1969). While a number of obstetrical maneuvers have been so implicated, 53% of all newborn brachial plexus injuries occur in conjunction with shoulder dystocia (Pollack et al., 2000). About one-third of all cases involve the posterior arm; this may be due to impaction of the posterior shoulder on the sacral promontory or to the frequency of posterior arm extraction as a method of resolving shoulder dystocia.

The level of injury will determine how the palsy manifests. Erb palsy affects the upper plexus nerves at C5, C6 and C7. Erb palsy involving C5-C6 occurs in about 80% of cases. The entire plexus (C5 to C7) is involved in 25% of cases. Injures affecting both sides of the neck are uncommon, occurring in 8 to 22% of cases. Injury to the C5, C6 and C7 nerve roots may result in diaphragmatic paralysis on the affected side, leading to respiratory distress. Erb palsy has a 90% resolution rate by one year of age (Pollack et al., 2000).

More rarely, Klumpke palsy (lower plexus damage) occurs, affecting the nerve roots originating from C8 and T1. It results in weakness of the forearm and hand, especially the wrists and fingers on the affected side. Almost all affected infants will have some improvement of function, although only 40% of those with Klumpke palsy can be expected to resolve by the age of one year. Overall, the baby has a 98.4% chance of complete recovery (Gherman et al., 1999).

Brachial plexus palsies also occur in cases in which there is no history of shoulder dystocia. These are associated with surgical birth, in utero positioning (with accompanying muscular atrophy at times) and situations in which "excessive" traction is believed not to have been used to complete the birth. The posterior shoulder is affected in 67.7% of these cases. Full recovery occurs in only 58.7%, possibly due to the differing etiologies of the injury (Walle & Hartikainen-Sorri, 1993).

The breakage of bones, either inadvertently or intentionally, is another risk of shoulder dystocia. The bones most susceptible to breakage are the clavicle and the humerus. The clavicle may be intentionally broken as a last-resort maneuver to collapse the shoulder girdle and effect delivery, or it may be broken accidentally when the shoulders are manipulated. Breakage may result in puncture of the subclavian vein, leading to internal bleeding, or the underlying lung, leading to a pneumothorax, or both. The humerus may be broken as a by-product of repositioning an arm. In either case, breakage is often signaled by a snapping sound that is usually quite audible. Broken bones heal rapidly in newborns; unless other structures are damaged, they are usually without serious sequelae. Babies with bone fractures should be examined carefully to make sure there are no accompanying brachial plexus nerve injuries or other damage.

Asphyxia is a common consequence of shoulder dystocia. The heart continues to beat and pump blood to the head after it is born. However, if the baby's shoulders are tightly wedged in the pelvis and soft tissue, venous return will be impaired due to pressure on the neck as well as chest compression. As a result, the head will become increasingly congested with blood, reflected by an increasingly darkening skin tone. Such congestion impedes oxygen exchange, can cause blood vessels to rupture, and may even result in brain hemorrhage. The baby cannot tolerate this situation for very long. The result is the birth of a limp baby with a purple head and a white body. Practitioners faced with shoulder dystocia must be ready to deal with a baby who needs resuscitation.

Risks for the mother: Maternal morbidity related to shoulder dystocia can result from soft-tissue injury due to internal manipulations or incision of the perineum, postpartum hemorrhage due to uterine atony (often related to maternal fear), endometriosis and, on rare occasions, uterine rupture. In addition, the mother will experience anxiety, fear and grief over the baby's condition if the baby is compromised, damaged or dies.

Dealing with Shoulder Dystocia

Proposed Methods to Prevent Shoulder Dystocia Prior to the Birth of the Head

Although shoulder dystocia is not predictable and many (if not most) anticipated shoulder dystocias do not occur, there are instances in which midwives take preventive measures for a particular woman they believe to be at higher risk. There is no way to know if a technique actually prevented a dystocia or if it did not occur because it wasn't going to happen at all. However, the midwives who recommend these techniques feel that they help. Most of them have been developed with only inlet dystocia in mind and all of these will not be applied to the same woman; choose those options appropriate to the individual circumstances, the woman's pelvic structure and your personal affinity for various techniques.

Provide prenatal preparation

Review the process of shoulder birth with the mother so she can visualize this as she pushes. Remind her that her cooperation will be essential during the birth; she may be asked to move to another position or push at a certain time. She needs to understand that her immediate response may be essential to her baby's well-being and is not a topic for debate.

Assist anterior rotation of the occiput from the posterior

Addressing rotation of the posterior baby during or before active labor can prevent incomplete rotation of the shoulders during descent. (See the chapter entitled "Assisting a Woman Whose Baby is in a Posterior Position.")

Consider transport

Transport prior to birth is appropriate if you feel a shoulder dystocia is likely to occur and it appears that the mother is too tired or otherwise unlikely to respond appropriately in such an emergency. Although hypnotic suggestion using a quiet voice and simple, positive words can be used during labor when a woman has had a previous shoulder dystocia, the use of language may engage her neocortex and thus interfere with the fetus ejection reflex.

Avoid birthing on soft, indentable surface

Soft beds are never any help at a birth and can compound the problems associated with getting a stuck baby out considerably. Request that a mother who chooses to birth in a side-lying or supine position do so on firm padding such as a futon, a thin camping mattress, or several layers of blankets covered with a sheet.

Avoid birthing in tight space

Many women like to "crawl into a cave" when birth is imminent. However, when shoulder dystocia occurs, a woman may need room to move to another position, and the midwife may need to reposition herself or have an assistant by her side. Always assess the space available around the mother.

Wait for an urge to push

Always allow a spontaneous pushing urge to develop prior to pushing. The resting phase of labor and the development of a spontaneous urge are vital to the normal descent and rotation of both the head and the shoulders. In the absence of other complicating factors that render pushing without an urge the lesser risk, there is no reason to encourage pushing just because a woman has reached full dilation.

Be sure the mother's bladder is empty

A full bladder will reduce the room above the pubic bone and may impede descent of the anterior shoulder, as well as increase the likelihood of bladder damage should the shoulders get stuck. The mother should urinate prior to pushing and whenever pushing has been intermittent or prolonged. She can get up to do so or use a bowl or towel. Catheterization can be performed if the head is too low to allow urine to flow freely.

Postponing pushing when the mother is exhausted

Pushing can be ineffective when the mother is very tired. In addition, her uterus also gets tired, causing her contractions to become weak or spaced out. If a large baby is anticipated, the force of the mother and the uterus together may be needed to get the baby out. Proceeding when contractions are of poor quality only invites trouble with the birth. If there are no signs of obstruction and the baby is tolerating labor well, labor can take as long as necessary. Suggest that the mother eat, drink and rest to rally her forces; when her contractions resume, she will be ready, willing and able to work hard if the need arises.

Apply suprapubic pressure

The technique is used as the head is approaching a full crown and is best performed by an attendant who can position herself so she has access to the mother's lower abdomen. If the mother is supine, and you anticipate the birth of the head with the next contraction, the assistant should stand on a stool to elevate herself above the mother. If the mother is on her hands and knees, the assistant places her hands above the pubic bone and applies suprapubic pressure directly toward the mother's spine during the contraction. Pressure should be maintained until the head is born. This will encourage the shoulders to rotate under the pubic bone rather than behind it. This technique can be used in conjunction with others involving maternal positioning. It may be particularly useful in a woman known to have a shallow anteroposterior pelvic diameter and a history of inlet dystocia with a previous baby.

Birth the head with a contraction

Some midwives encourage mothers to push the head out between contractions as a method of minimizing tears. However, pushing between contractions, even gentle pushing, can interrupt the coordination of the natural forces that bring the shoulders into position for birth. This is not the case when the baby is born spontaneously between contractions without maternal pushing efforts; the birth is then happening without interference, and the necessary rotation is very likely to occur.

Wait for the contraction following the birth of the head before attempting to assist birth of the shoulders

The shoulders *do not* instantly follow the head in many normal births. Slight retraction, or **turtling**, of the lavender pink head back against the perineum after the contraction is also normal. In contrast, impaction is often accompanied by *significant* turtling and darkening of the head. Unless these signs are present, wait for the next contraction before doing anything. The force of the next contraction should rotate the shoulders into position for birth; premature manipulation prior to that contraction can create a problem when none would have otherwise developed. Encourage the mother to relax her pelvic area completely. If there are signs that a shoulder dystocia may be next, you can always firmly massage the mother's abdomen using your open hand and fingers to stimulate another contraction, which should occur pretty quickly. Encouraging a contraction in this way is better than manually interfering or having the mother push without one at this point. However, if there are signs of dystocia, such as a dark head or turtling, and no contraction can be stimulated within a minute or two, proceed to the section entitled "What to Do."

Positions for pushing

Use of the hands-and-knees position prophylactically: This position has become associated with shoulder dystocia because it can be used to remedy impacted shoulders. Some midwives find that hands and knees can be used prophylactically when shoulder dystocia is anticipated. However, its prophylactic use is controversial. Hands and knees exposes the abdomen and the baby to the maximum force of gravity. In a borderline situation, this may encourage the anterior shoulder to rotate behind, rather than under, the pubic bone. Gaskin does not attempt to use the position preventively. She believes once shoulder dystocia has occurred, that moving the mother from another position to hands and knees produces progress in many cases. This is not to say that hands-and-knees births should be avoided entirely; it just may be more appropriate to use prior to pushing to ensure proper fetal rotation but not preventively during pushing in anticipation of shoulder dystocia. If a hands-and-knees position for pushing is chosen, provide support under the woman's abdomen or use a belly binder, especially if her abdomen is pendulous.

Avoid positions that limit sacral mobility: Semi-sitting and lithotomy positions are particularly contraindicated in this regard. The anterior shoulder is much more likely to get stuck when the sacrum cannot move backwards. The descent of the posterior shoulder is more likely to be impeded as well. This is true whether the woman is at risk for inlet or outlet dystocia, as both varieties benefit when there is maximal space in the posterior pelvis. If the mother must birth in a horizontal position, lateral is, by far, the best (Sutton, 2001).

Upright kneeling position, leaning forward: Jean Sutton and Pauline Scott (1996) swear by this as a surefire way to avoid problems with the birth of the shoulders. It allows maximal pelvic flexibility and encourages the posterior shoulder to birth first, creating more room for the anterior shoulder to drop down and pass through the outlet. The shoulder girdle is then born on a slant, naturally encouraging the anterior shoulder to slip past the pubic arch.

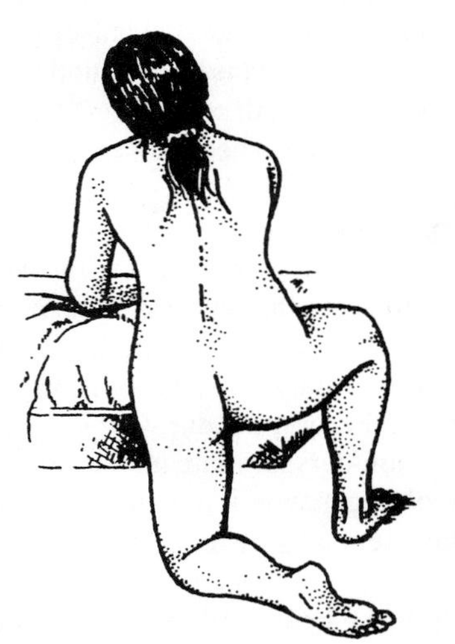

Parker position

Parker position: Karen Parker, CNM, adopted this technique as a preventive measure for shoulder dystocia based on an illustration in the 1951 edition of De Lee's THE PRINCIPLES AND PRACTICE OF OBSTETRICS, edited by Greenhill. The mother first assumes the upright kneeling position, then flexes one leg at the knee and hip so that her foot is on the floor. It is not mandatory to know which side the baby's occiput is on, although elevating the knee opposite the occiput may better facilitate passage of the anterior shoulder under the pubic arch. This position rotates the pelvis, relaxes the pelvic muscles and helps bring about normal shoulder rotation and descent. In addition, it takes the ischial spines and pubic rami out of parallel alignment, a change that can be essential when an outlet dystocia is anticipated. From this position, the woman can lunge toward her elevated knee, further opening that side of the pelvis, if this seems appropriate.

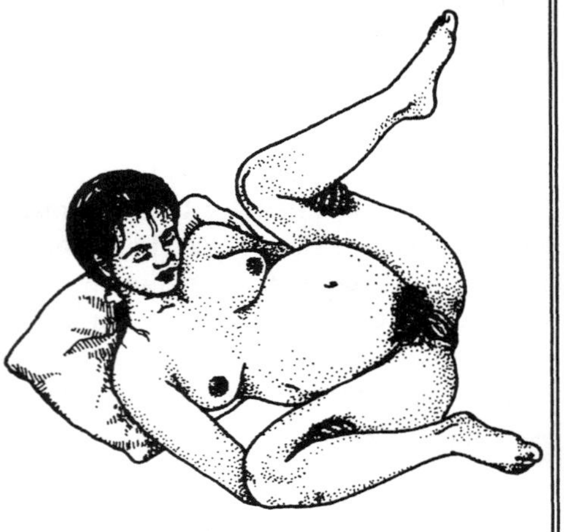

Lateral McRoberts position

Lateral McRoberts position: Although upright postures are most ideal when shoulder dystocia is anticipated, there will be occasions when the mother chooses to lie down. The lateral McRoberts has the woman lying on her side with her lower knee flexed against her abdomen and the upper leg sharply flexed and supported, either by herself or an assistant. This pivots the outlet forward, increasing the curve of the birth canal, but leaves the sacrum more free to move than in a supine McRoberts position (see below). A lateral position also makes getting your hands inside much easier, should manipulation become necessary. The position of the baby is not relevant to which side the mother lies on (Parker, 1996).

Supine McRoberts position: Some practitioners use this position to try and prevent shoulder dystocia. The pros and cons of its use and its appropriate use are discussed in detail later in the chapter.

Recognizing Impacted Shoulders after the Birth of the Head

There are certain classic signs that the birth of the shoulders is impeded. It is vital that the midwife recognize these when they occur, although all of these signs will not always be present even when the shoulders are thoroughly stuck. Simms (1995) notes that, in her experience, moderate to severe shoulder dystocia is always preceded by an extremely painful pushing phase. This may be due to extreme overstretching of the pelvic joints as a large baby moves through.

Inlet dystocia

The signs of inlet and outlet dystocia can overlap; however, generally speaking, signs of inlet dystocia develop almost immediately after the birth of the head. Failure of one or both shoulders to engage can result in the following indications:

- Extremely slow descent of the head
- Either pronounced moulding and a caput or very little moulding (due to the more mature ossification of a postdates baby)
- Very slow crowning
- The appearance of a chubby face (impaction can create the appearance of a chubby face, even if the baby is not overly large).
- The head is only born to the baby's mouth, with the lower jaw becoming hung up on the perineum. (This is more common with bilateral shoulder dystocia.) The midwife must sweep a finger under the chin to bring the lower jaw out.
- Once the head is out, it immediately recoils or retracts snugly against the perineum (the turtle sign).
- Immediate darkening of the head, which becomes increasingly deep purple
- Restitution does not occur or only occurs with manual assistance.
- External rotation does not occur or only occurs slowly and often only partially.
- No further progress toward birth, in spite of maternal pushing efforts, uterine contractions or gently directing the head in the direction it seems to want to go (posteriorly or anteriorly).
- Lack of any subsequent contractions, especially in the case of bilateral inlet dystocia.

The head is born slowly because the neck must stretch to compensate for the anterior shoulder being caught above the brim (which is made worse if the posterior shoulder is impacted above the sacral promontory). In addition, this stretching can cause the head to extend sooner than it otherwise would. Extension presents a larger than usual diameter as the head passes through the outlet. Some tension on the neck is relieved after the head is born. Immediate turtling of the head occurs as the neck recoils; the head snaps back against the soft tissues, which offer less resistance. Excessive turtling causes the baby's jaw to become impinged against the lower lateral pelvic rami and ischial tuberosity as well as the soft tissues on the side to which it is directed, interfering with normal restitution. The head becomes increasingly dark as the heart continues to pump blood to the brain, while venous return, which is passive, is impaired because of the pressure around the neck. Depending upon the degree of impaction, external rotation may not occur at all.

Outlet dystocia

Outlet dystocia can be deceiving at first because it is not usually accompanied by the classic signs of inlet dystocia. It more often presents with the following signs:

- Slow crowning and birth of the head due to the tight squeeze through the outlet
- Baby may have red lines on the side of the head where the head was squeezed through the outlet
- Great distension of the perineum as the head crowns and then emerges may occur, often with a perineal tear
- Normal birth of the head that is frequently followed by normal restitution
- No turtling or only moderate turtling occurs because the shoulders are not held back at the brim but have descended into the midpelvic cavity. Therefore the neck is not stretched as it is with inlet dystocia.
- Darkening of the head may occur, although this usually occurs slowly over the course of a few contractions.
- No further progress toward birth

The head may be born slowly with great distension of the posterior perineum during late pushing. Normal restitution often occurs because the anterior shoulder is not immobilized by impaction at the brim. The head turns dark more slowly than with inlet dystocia because there is less impaction, less tension on the neck and less impairment of venous return.

The anterior shoulder may not rotate to the anteroposterior diameter with the contraction that follows the birth of the head if it is already impacted against the adjacent rami in an oblique or transverse orientation. When this is the case, no external rotation of the head will occur. However, since the shoulders have already descended into the midplane of the pelvis, internal rotation of the shoulders with concurrent external rotation of the head frequently does occur with the next contraction. At this point, further descent can become arrested if the baby's shoulder girdle then becomes impacted in the diagonal conjugate of the outlet, wedged into a narrow pubic arch.

General Considerations Regarding How to Proceed

Rule out causes other than shoulder dystocia

The first step in resolving dystocia after birth of the head is determining whether impacted shoulders are the problem. Most of the time, they will be the issue as those conditions that mimic shoulder dystocia are relatively rare. However, they should be kept in the back of your mind as you proceed. Anything that impedes the spontaneous birth of the shoulders can cause a delay; however, usually these problems will only be searched for when standard remedial maneuvers do not resolve the dystocia or when your index of suspicion for other reasons is heightened because of maternal or fetal history. Other problems or events that can impede advancement and mimic shoulder dystocia include:

- A hand, arm, foot or leg positioned so that further descent is arrested (see the chapter entitled "Assisting at the Birth of a Vertex Baby")
- Tight cord wrapped around the neck or body (see the chapter entitled "Assisting at the Birth of a Vertex Baby")
- A short cord (see the chapter entitled "Assisting at the Birth of a Vertex Baby")
- Spaced-out contractions or a complete lack of further contractions after the birth of the head (This can also happen with a severe shoulder dystocia; see the chapter entitled "Assisting at the Birth of a Vertex Baby.")
- Uterine constriction ring (see the chapter entitled "Recognizing and Dealing with Obstructed Labor")
- A neonatal anomaly such as a tumor or enlargement of the chest or abdomen trapped above the pelvic brim (see the chapter entitled "Recognizing and Dealing with Obstructed Labor")
- A maternal pelvic tumor occupying space in the birth canal (see the chapter entitled "Recognizing and Dealing with Obstructed Labor")
- Situations unique to multiple births (see the chapter entitled "Assisting at Multiple Births")
- Passage of a small head through a partially dilated cervix with subsequent entrapment of the shoulders on the cervical rim (see the chapter entitled "Recognizing and Dealing with Obstructed Labor.")
- A uterine rupture with extrusion of part of the fetal body through the tear (see the chapter entitled "Recognizing and Dealing with Obstructed Labor" for a discussion of this rare complication)

As this discussion proceeds, I assume that none of these things is the cause for the delay.

Stay calm

Once the head is out, a delay in the birth of the shoulders may be the first indication of a problem. If you did not anticipate a dystocia and therefore did not employ any prophylactic measures, you are now suddenly faced with dislodging the impacted shoulders and getting the baby out. Stay calm and take three or four deep breaths to center yourself. Frantic, rough handling done without regard for the particular situation is ill advised and most likely to result in damage to the baby or mother.

Know your options

Each incidence of shoulder dystocia is very individual. This chapter offers a number of techniques midwives have found successful, presented roughly in the order in which they would be used. In general, as the severity of the impaction increases, so does the amount of intervention and invasive maneuvering required to get the baby out. No series of techniques will work in every case. Even large hospital-based obstetrical centers have limited opportunities for studying the effectiveness of various techniques for remedying shoulder dystocia due to its rarity and unpredictability. Therefore, both midwives and doctors are in the same boat when it comes to evaluating which techniques minimize damage to the infant and are truly effective at resolving the problem. A thorough understanding of the physiology of the normal birth of the shoulders, the ways in which the shoulders can become impacted, the ways in which the baby can be injured, and the different techniques available to remedy the situation all go a long way toward helping each midwife devise a safe plan of action. Remember, this is one emergency when hospital-based practitioners have nothing to offer in the way of technological solutions. You have all the things you need to deal with the situation at home, plus the added advantage of an undrugged mother who can change her position at will. Hospital providers are often hampered by the mother's being drugged, by her being on a surface that does not lend itself to movement and by their own lack of understanding regarding normal birth and the help that can be offered by maternal position changes.

Basic considerations regarding procedures and technique

It is important to perform manipulations in such a way that the birth occurs as quickly as possible and damage to the baby is avoided or minimized. Since true shoulder dystocia is rare, practice all hands-on techniques with a doll and pelvis until you are quite familiar with them. It is common for practitioners to rely on one technique that has worked in the past, and often this approach is successful. However, knowing many options will prove invaluable when faced with a situation in which your favored technique proves inadequate.

Your goals: In this order, you need to reposition an arm if it is behind the baby's back and preventing descent; disimpact the shoulder(s) from behind the pubic bone, sacral promontory or both; flex the shoulder girdle and bring the baby out. Repositioning the arm is a separate maneuver since it may be necessary before other maneuvers will be effective.

How much time do you have? About five to seven minutes can elapse before the baby will be in distress (Benedetti, 1995; O'Leary, 1992). This presumes that the baby was in good shape prior to the birth of the head. The pH declines at a rate of 0.04 U per minute once the head is out in a previously undestressed baby. Time is of the essence.

The application of traction or pressure to the head: Since the head is the only fetal part that is readily available for manipulation, many delivery techniques over the years have involved traction on the head. O'Leary (1992) advises never to manipulate the head as pulling it, even gently, risks both brachial plexus and spinal injury. Therefore, if the head *is* manipulated, care must be taken not to use abrupt, jerky movements that are liable to result in brachial plexus injury, fractured cervical vertebrae and no descent. Likewise, no attempt should be made to forcefully turn and twist the head with the thought that the stuck shoulders will follow suit; this is simply not how it works. While it is true that the spine tends to seek anatomical alignment, the neck moves independently of the shoulders; thus manipulating the head in this manner wastes valuable time and risks fetal injury when the shoulders are truly impacted. Avoid placing your hands on the head with your fingers hooked under the jaw or jammed into the side of the neck; this also risks injury to the brachial plexus nerves. Excessive lateral traction, in which the baby's ear is brought near the top of his shoulder (over 40° from the axis of the spine), should be avoided for this reason as well. Finally, the strength behind any manipulation should build slowly and gradually; this has been shown to minimize damage because it allows the tissues to stretch rather than tear (Alan et al., 1994).

The few techniques suggested in this chapter that involve placing hands on the head have been carefully chosen and should be followed precisely as described. While there is always some risk when the head is manipulated, experience has shown that these techniques are reasonably safe when performed as written. It is always best, however, to avoid manipulation of the head whenever possible. Techniques that are excessively dangerous are not even discussed, notably the Hibbard maneuver (Hibbard, 1969, 1982), which involves applying pressure against the anterior jaw and neck, head traction and fundal pressure.

How long should you sustain traction or pressure? Whenever you are unsure about how much is enough, only sustain any manual attempt to relieve the impaction to a count of 15. If there is no progress at that point, release, reassess and begin again, if indicated. However, continue the technique without interruption if it is helping and be sensitive to when and if you meet with definite resistance.

The use of clitorotomy: An extensive clitorotomy is almost universally recommended in the medical literature as a necessary adjunct to freeing impacted shoulders. A mediolateral cut or even proctostomy (deliberately cutting through the anal sphincter and even into the rectal mucosa) is recommended to open up maximum space for internal manipulations. This recommendation is passed down from male obstetricians, who have larger hands than most female midwives. In addition, the traditional supine position of hospital birth leaves the sacrum immobile, hence the need for creating more room. However, shoulder dystocia is primarily a bony, not a soft-tissue, obstruction. While there may be uncommon instances in which a clitorotomy is warranted, cutting the perineum is usually not called for, even when shoulder dystocia is severe.

Even so, one does not stop attempting to get the baby out to spare the perineum. When an incision is deemed necessary, cut from the midline and angle the incision *slightly* off the midline, but otherwise straight down the perineum. Slightly angling the blade encourages any extension to bypass the sphincter. (See my text HEALING PASSAGE for more details.) Mediolateral cuts are not necessary, can also extend, are much more difficult to repair and are painful during healing. While a median cut may lead to extension through the sphincter, the repair is a relatively straightforward process and is likely to heal better than a mediolateral incision.

The use of axillary traction: Contrary to popular opinion, there are safe ways to apply axillary traction. These are discussed in detail later in the chapter.

Working with the mother and baby

Helping the mother know what to do: The explanations below focus on what the midwife should be doing and how the mother needs to be positioned. The midwife needs to clearly explain to the mother what she should do and when. For example, if you are going to insert your hands and grasp the baby, you will want to do so when the mother and uterus are most relaxed. Having her push before your hands are positioned is of no help, and it will only further reduce the room you have to maneuver. When and how the mother pushes will depend upon the situation and what you are trying to do, so some pushing instructions are left to your clinical discretion.

You can explain the situation to the baby, but the baby is in no position to assist with her birth if she is stuck on the pelvic bones. Therefore, the baby is likely to be frightened and may be born with quite a headache if her head became very congested. When explaining the situation to the parents, always remember that the baby is listening too.

Giving the baby oxygen after the head is born: Some midwives report that applying a simple infant mask with an elastic head strap over the baby's nose and mouth with the flow set for at least 8 l/min while working to get the baby out makes a positive difference in the condition of the baby at birth. This finding may be purely coincidental, as most babies are not breathing when so tightly wedged.

Be prepared for a depressed baby: A baby who has experienced a difficult birth is always more likely to need extra support to establish breathing. Be prepared to perform CPR. As soon as the mouth is born, you can give the baby oral homeopathic arnica (30 or 200C, 1 pellet inside the lower lip) and Rescue Remedy (2 or 3 drops) to help minimize bruising and internal bleeding and to calm the baby emotionally. Additional doses can be given after birth. Both during and after the birth, talk to the baby about what happened and tell him it is all right to cry.

Techniques to Prevent or Resolve Shoulder Dystocia Once the Head is Born

Remedies for shoulder dystocia fall into several broad categories:

- Maternal position changes with manual interventions to prevent the anterior shoulder from becoming impacted which are used after the head is born when the midwife suspects inlet dystocia will develop
- Maternal position changes and the movements required to assume the new position
- Combination techniques involving specific maternal movements performed in a specific position
- Maternal position changes plus manual techniques to dislodge an impacted anterior shoulder
- Manual techniques which may be facilitated by maternal position, to deliver the posterior shoulder or arm
- Maneuvers to rotate and dislodge the shoulder girdle (inlet dystocia)
- Surgical or manual intervention applied directly to the baby to collapse the shoulder girdle (inlet or outlet dystocia)
- Maternal surgery to effect the delivery of the anterior shoulder (inlet dystocia)
- Cephalic replacement (inlet or outlet dystocia)

In this chapter, I present the broadest repertoire of techniques to prevent or resolve shoulder dystocia ever published in a textbook in the hope that it will be illuminating for practitioners who are currently aware of only a limited range of options. Techniques are presented roughly in the order in which their proponents recommend they be used. Therefore, the order of presentation does not rigidly follow the list given above, which is intended to clarify the types of maneuvers available. Keeping in mind that an understanding of inlet versus outlet dystocia is all but nonexistent in the literature, I have followed the recommendations of Scholles (2001) in designating which maneuvers are most appropriate for each type of dystocia.

Resolution techniques are presented according to the type of dystocia (effective for either type, inlet or outlet) and their presentation follows the listing in the table on the next page. It was hard to decide how these should be presented because opinions differ widely as to what should be done first. Therefore, I hope that this table assists the reader in understanding the variety of techniques that exist. It is up to you to evaluate all the options and decide which techniques work best for you given the individual situation.

TECHNIQUES TO PREVENT OR RESOLVE SHOULDER DYSTOCIA ONCE THE HEAD IS BORN

PRELIMINARY EXAMINATIONS THAT CAN HELP YOU DECIDE HOW TO PROCEED
- Determining the type of dystocia once the head is born
- Determining the angle of the shoulders
- Determining if one or both arms are behind the baby's back and correcting it

THE USE OF SUPRAPUBIC PRESSURE AS AN AID IN RESOLVING INLET DYSTOCIA

MATERNAL POSITION CHANGES THAT CAN RESOLVE EITHER INLET OR OUTLET DYSTOCIA
- Gaskin maneuver (hands and knees)
- Parker maneuver (one-sided kneeling)
- Standing up
- Duck (wide) walking
- Sutton maneuvers
- Flip-flop maneuvers

TECHNIQUES USED TO PREVENT OR RESOLVE SHOULDER DYSTOCIA AT THE INLET

Techniques intended to prevent inlet dystocia once the head is born
- El Halta maneuver (immediate delivery of shoulders from oblique diameter)
- Malby maneuver (rotate head to OA and apply pressure)

Rotational maneuvers for inlet dystocia (in historical order)
- Screw maneuver of Woods
- Rubin maneuver
- Varney maneuver
- Praying hands maneuver

Methods of delivering the posterior shoulder or arm
- Techniques involving axillary traction
  - Tharpe maneuver
  - Alternative method of axillary traction
- Pull the posterior shoulder down into the hollow of the sacrum
- Deliver the posterior arm

Additional techniques to resolve inlet dystocia
- Scholles maneuvers
- White maneuver (mixing bowl technique)
- Walcher-McRoberts-Pecorari maneuver
- Ramp maneuver

TECHNIQUES USED TO PREVENT OR RESOLVE SHOULDER DYSTOCIA AT THE OUTLET

Maternal positions to resolve outlet dystocia
- Deep squatting
- Upright squatting
- McRoberts maneuver (gravity-neutral, deep squat)

Manual techniques to open the pelvis

To open the midpelvis and outlet:
- Pelvic press
- Tuberosity pull
- Sacral press

To open the outlet:
- Sheela-na-gig maneuver
- Pubic pull-up

MEDICAL MODEL APPROACHES TO SEVERE SHOULDER DYSTOCIA
- Break the fetal clavicle
- Instrumental delivery
- Zavanelli maneuver (cephalic replacement)
- Symphysiotomy
- Abdominal rescue

Preliminary examinations that can help you decide how to proceed:

When and if you use the following techniques will depend on your favored approach to shoulder dystocia. However, it can be very helpful to make the following assessments early on, particularly if your first choice is a change of maternal position that turns out to be unsuccessful. Because these findings are relevant to several of the techniques described below, and individual midwives may wish to use any of these techniques as their first choice of therapy, how to perform these examinations is explained prior to the explanation of any resolution techniques.

Determining the type of dystocia once the head is born: While recalling the features of the mother's pelvis, look for signs that indicate the type of dystocia you are dealing with. Palpate internally for the anterior shoulder, which will either be out of easy reach (above the inlet) or caught in the angle of the pubic arch or on a pubic ramus (behind the outlet). Look for other signs as described above.

Determining the angle of the shoulders: The first thing that many midwives do is have the mother change position without any internal exams, and this often resolves the dystocia. However, if it does not, knowing the angle of the shoulders in relationship to the head is often relevant, regardless of whether you are dealing with an inlet or an outlet dystocia. In addition, if external signs point to a severe dystocia, finding out whether one or both arms are behind the baby's back and resolving this first will increase the success of any resolution techniques you try.

If the head has not restituted, gently manipulate it by placing your hands on either side and turning it slightly from side to side. This may encourage spontaneous restitution or rotation. Pressing in on the perineum around the head may also free up enough space to allow for spontaneous restitution. Either technique merely encourages the head to go where it naturally wants to. Do *not* forcefully twist or pull on the head; just nudge it gently to free it up enough to move. A head that can move will naturally line up with the sagittal suture at a 90° angle to the shoulders; this will let you know where the shoulder diameter is lying. (Sometimes the head will be born, restitute and then turn in the opposite direction, revealing that the shoulders are at an unexpected angle.) If gentle nudging does not produce any movement, the head may already be lined up at right angles to the shoulders or the shoulders may be severely impacted, with the neck twisted.

When restitution or rotation occurs, use the hand on the side you suspect the baby's back to be, hold the fingers together tightly and insert them down the back of the baby's neck Inserting your hand may seem impossible, since everything is jammed in so tight. This is no time to be timid! Remember to insert your hands between contractions or at least between pushes. Check for a cord (which may be the problem). At this point you may be able to tell whether the neck is twisted, meaning that the shoulders and head are not in an anatomical relationship. Feel for the scapulae to determine where the shoulder girdle is (oblique, transverse, or anteroposterior). Feel across the breadth of the shoulders. Assess whether the posterior shoulder is within reach. Rule out an abducted arm by exploring the scapulae (you may be able to detect the angle of the upper arm running from the axilla and across the back). If you find the pelvis entirely empty except for the baby's neck, you probably have a bilateral inlet dystocia (Tharpe, 2003). Feeling for the shoulder girdle gives you an idea of how stuck the baby really is; if the anterior shoulder is very difficult to reach, it is probably caught above the brim. Knowing this now will help you decide what to do next.

The position of the shoulder girdle will influence how you proceed. For example, if the arms are not extended and it is an inlet dystocia, next attempt to push from behind the anterior shoulder forward to flex and disimpact it. If you determine that the shoulders are transverse or stuck on the pubic rami, suprapubic pressure will do nothing since the shoulder is not trapped above the pubic bone (thus confirming an outlet dystocia).

Determining if one or both arms are behind the baby's back and correcting it: While checking for the angle of the shoulders, you may discover that one or both arms are behind the baby's back. This hyperextends the shoulder girdle, further impairing rotation and rendering the torso quite rigid, making any maternal position changes or manipulations less likely to succeed because the shoulders cannot flex. Have the mother assume a hands and knees position, if she has not already done so. This may help the posterior shoulder to drop lower in the pelvis before you attempt to reposition the arm(s). Insert the hand nearest the fetal back and press against the sacrum with the back of your hand to lift it out of the way. If both arms are behind the back, attend to the posterior arm first. Pass the hand nearest the fetal back down the back of the neck, reaching up high enough to find the elbow. (If it is bent across the back, press down on the forearm to straighten the arm.) If you meet resistance, stop and feel along the arm to determine if the cord is wrapped around it. If so, slide the cord along the forearm and over the hand. Now, press against the upper forearm (past the elbow) to assist in maintaining the arm in an extended posture as you nudge it to the baby's side and then toward the front of the torso. If the arm is bent behind the back and you do not straighten it first, efforts to move the arm will be greatly hampered as you will be trying to move it against the range of motion of the joint, and you are more likely to break a bone. If possible, once you have the arm to the side, splint the upper arm with two fingers and sweep it around; this protects the humerus from breakage. Having dealt with the posterior arm, you may now have a little more room to deal with the anterior arm in a similar manner if it is also behind the back, although having both arms behind the back is, fortunately, very rare. If you cannot sweep the anterior arm around to the front of the torso, straighten it as much as you can and nudge it to the baby's side. Then proceed to your chosen option for resolving the dystocia.

The use of suprapubic pressure as an aid in resolving inlet dystocia

Suprapubic pressure is recommended as an adjunct to several of the maneuvers for inlet dystocia, so I will discuss it before I discuss resolution techniques. Suprapubic pressure can be used before the head is born to prevent inlet dystocia by attempting to encourage the anterior shoulder to rotate under the pubic bone. It will do nothing to prevent outlet dystocia. Once the head is out, suprapubic pressure is generally used to assist in dislodging the anterior shoulder by encouraging flexion and rotation to an oblique diameter and hopefully below the brim. This is done in conjunction with maternal pushing efforts and manipulations by the midwife receiving the baby. A major disadvantage of this technique is that its application is almost defeated when used on an undrugged mother. Uterine contractions and pushing combine to make the abdominal surface quite firm, interfering with the ability to apply sufficient pressure.

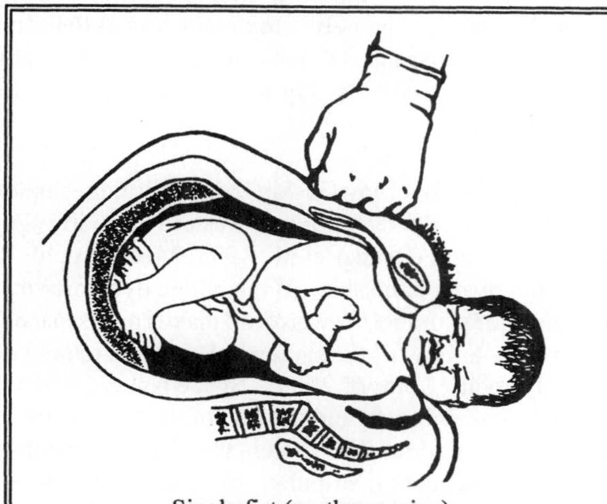

Single fist (mother supine)

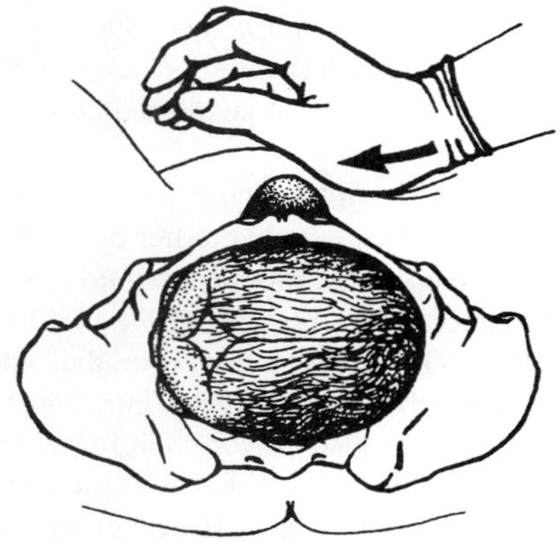

Single hand applying pressure to the anterior scapula at an oblique angle (mother supine)

Suprapubic pressure must be applied just above the top border of pubic bone, not against the bone itself. There it will not do any good and may, in fact, make things worse by preventing separation of the symphysis pubis. Applying pressure slightly above the bone will help ensure that it is directed at the fetal shoulder and upper back, where it will be most effective. The person applying pressure should be positioned to apply pressure directly over the suprapubic area toward the mother's spine (above a mother who is supine; below a mother who is on her hands and knees; in front of a mother who is upright). If the mother is lying supine on a table, the assistant may need to stand on a chair or stool. There should also be room for her to move from one side of the mother to the other if necessary.

Next, the assistant should either make a single fist or make a fist and grasp it with the other hand. The single or double fist is placed above the pubic bone. If the position of the anterior shoulder is not known, pressure is applied directly toward the mother's spine (Mazzanti technique); this is also the safest technique when pressure is applied before the head is out, because the angle of the shoulders will be uncertain, to avoid inadvertently abducting the anterior shoulder. At this point, pressure forces the upper torso toward the hollow of the sacrum, and hopefully assists the anterior shoulder in passing beneath the pubic arch.

Once the head is born, the midwife informs the assistant of the location of the baby's back. The assistant can then apply lateral pressure to the anterior scapula with heel of one hand or with the heel of the other hand on top of it (Rubin technique), although using the heel of the hand may result in a very sore wrist for the assistant. It is important that any lateral pressure be applied to the fetal back, since applying pressure to the ventral aspect of the shoulder may compound the problem by encouraging the shoulder to abduct. Suprapubic pressure is applied at an angle with the intention of pushing the posterior aspect of the anterior shoulder toward the mother's opposite side (for example, if the fetal back to the mother's left, the assistant stands to mother's left and pushes toward the mother's right). Pressure can also be applied using a rocking motion. The rocking should be produced by the weight and movement of the entire upper body so that sufficient force is produced to move the shoulders.

It is important to distinguish between suprapubic and fundal pressure. The application of fundal pressure prior to dislodgement of the shoulders in an inlet dystocia will only further jam the shoulders into the pelvic brim, thus producing more stretching in the brachial plexus area. Likewise, fundal pressure will only further impact the shoulders against the rami in an outlet dystocia. This will reduce the available space and will impede the efforts by the receiving midwife to free the baby. It is also likely to result in fetal injury and invites uterine rupture. If fundal pressure is ever used, it must be used only *after* the anterior shoulder has been freed. In any event, fundal pressure is rarely necessary to accomplish any birth. (A full discussion of fundal pressure may be found in the subchapter entitled "Fundal Pressure.")

Maternal position changes that can resolve either inlet or outlet dystocia

Many midwives do not do any manipulation prior to changing the mother's position, waiting to see if that alone will accomplish the birth. Some first gently direct the head downward laterally to see if they can tell if the anterior shoulder is really hung up (as is standard obstetrical practice). Changing positions is often all that is needed, and is especially useful if you are unsure about the type of dystocia you are dealing with. Whether and how you ask the mother to change position will, to a certain extent, depend upon how willing the woman is to move and how nimble. Position changes all work by jostling the baby around as the mother moves, as well as by opening the pelvic midplane and outlet; thus they may work well on either inlet or outlet dystocia. The huge benefit of this approach is that it often dislodges the baby with no manual assistance, minimizing newborn injury and putting the mother in control. Options for position changes will be limited if the woman has been transported and has received anesthesia.

Gaskin maneuver (hands and knees): This technique was first taught to Ina May Gaskin by a traditional Guatemalan midwife who told her it was revealed to her by God. Gaskin then brought the technique to western midwifery practice in 1976. It involves having the mother assume a hands and knees position (Bruner et al., 1998; Meenan et al., 1991). This alone may disimpact the shoulder girdle in either inlet or outlet dystocia because of the pelvic dynamics involved in changing position. The effect of gravity on the head pulls the anterior shoulder forward and makes more space for the posterior shoulder (which is hopefully not impacted) to glide along the hollow of the sacrum, allowing it to deliver first. The Gaskin maneuver may also be very helpful in bilateral inlet dystocia (Romoff, 2000). Space is increased between the posterior shoulder and yoni wall because the weight of the maternal abdomen and the rest of the baby's body is not resting directly on the posterior arm. However, unless the mother has a pendulous abdomen, the effect of gravity on the rest of the baby's body is relatively small, helping with any needed subsequent manipulations. Hands and knees opens the spinopubic angle (a particularly dramatic benefit when the woman has birthed the head in a supine position), allowing maximal sacral mobility and providing more room to insert your hands, should this become necessary.

The biggest drawback to this position is poor access to provide suprapubic pressure. One option is to straddle the woman's back and use both hands beneath her to provide pressure upward with a double-fisted technique. The size of the woman or the midwife may prohibit this approach. Alternatively, an assistant can lie down under the woman and press upward. Fortunately, hands and knees works well enough that suprapubic pressure is rarely needed. If changing to a hands-and-knees position alone does not resolve the dystocia, see Sutton's recommendations for the use of hands and knees below.

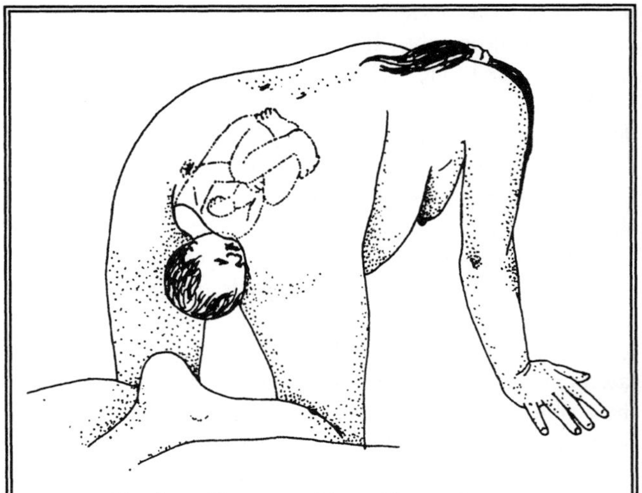

Hands and knees position with spontaneous delivery of posterior shoulder

(Adapted from Davis, 1997)

Hands and knees is not the best position for women who have lax abdominal muscles unless a belly binder is in place. Without one, this position will displace the weight of the mother's belly and the rest of the baby downward. The baby may become dislodged as his body is pulled down into the pendulous abdomen, however, you may have to reach further in for the shoulders or have the mother stand to effect the birth. Theoretically, placing a pillow under the mother to support her belly may help prevent this, but you may not be able to get the pillow under her in time to do so. Applying a belly binder is out of the question as you do not have enough time.

Parker position (one-sided kneeling, one foot up): Either by itself or after hands and knees alone has not resolved the dystocia, the mother can immediately lift the knee closest to the baby's back and plant that foot flat on the floor. This movement twists the bones of the pelvis and pivots the bones of the pubic joint, which can allow the shoulder to "shrug" out from under it. This alone may resolve the dystocia (Tully, 2003a). The mother can also lunge toward the side of the lifted knee, which will exaggerate the rotation of the pelvis. If this does not work, proceed to the "praying hands rotational maneuver" described in that section of the chapter. The one-sided kneeling position can be assumed as the mother moves from a hands-and-knees position to standing.

Standing up: Some midwives recommend having the mother assume a standing position, either instead of or only in the event that hands and knees does not work by itself. They report instances of babies who were otherwise impossible to extract who literally fell out when the mother stood up. A woman must make various asymmetrical movements as she stands up with the baby's head out, and standing twists the bones as well as widening both the brim and the outlet. Again, it is probably as much the movement as anything else that brings the baby. This can work for either inlet or outlet dystocia. Moving the legs asymmetrically takes the rami temporarily out of alignment and may be sufficient to dislodge some outlet dystocias, especially if the shoulders are oblique or transverse.

Duck (wide) walking: Have the woman stand and walk forward, lifting one leg up at a time. She should spread her thighs out to the side with each knee leading the way. This technique works with gravity, widens the pelvis on the lifted side, and reportedly causes the baby to fall out (so be prepared). Although this technique will not necessarily be suitable for all women, Monica Daniel, a CNM in New York State, has found it very effective (Schlinger, 2003).

Sutton maneuvers: Sutton (2001) assumes that shoulder dystocia almost always results from supine positioning during pushing (although this is certainly not the opinion of all midwives). Because her recommendations address both impaction at the inlet and opening of the midpelvis and outlet, this technique may be used in either type of dystocia. Assuming that the woman has birthed the head while on her back, she recommends the following:

1. Ascertain the diameter in which the shoulder axis is located (see above).
2. Extend the mother's legs to straighten her knees, then roll her over on her side; on her right if the baby is LOA or LOT, on her left if the baby is ROA or ROT. Make sure her knees are lower than her tuberosities.
3. Have the mother tip her pelvic brim as far forward as possible by arching her back (sticking her belly out as far as possible). If she cannot do this, have an assistant help her by applying pressure to her posterior upper pelvis, just above level of her buttocks' crease. Alternatively, have an assistant stand in front of her, put her arms around the mother's posterior upper pelvis and pull her lower torso forward. This alone may disimpact the anterior shoulder.
4. If step 3 does not resolve the dystocia, ask the mother to raise her upper thigh as high as possible straight up into the air (knee to ceiling). This increases the available space in the pelvis and often allows the fetal shoulders to rotate.
5. Check to see if the anterior shoulder is visible. If not, press the head downward slightly (toward the mother's buttocks) until the junction of the shoulder and the neck is visible. Confirm rotation to the anteroposterior diameter.
6. Flex the head anterolaterally (moving the baby's anterior ear toward the mother's abdomen). This presses the neck into the pubic arch and the top of the anterior shoulder against the inside of the pubic bone, allowing the posterior shoulder to emerge. The anterior shoulder should then drop down and emerge.

Sutton points out that some midwives prefer to have the woman assume a hands-and-knees position and then rock forward on all fours, bringing her bottom as far forward of her knees as possible and swaying her back toward the floor. This opens the spinopubic angle. The mother simultaneously raises the leg on the side of the baby's back and plants that foot on the bed or floor. If the baby does not come with that leg raised, she should switch to the other.

Sutton's main goal is to confirm disimpaction of the anterior shoulder and then facilitate the birth of the posterior shoulder first, which is usually deeper in the pelvic cavity and therefore easier to get out. This allows for the natural pivoting action of the anterior shoulder against the pubic bone.

Flip-flop maneuvers Gail Tully (2003a) offers a series of steps that may resolve either type of dystocia at any point.

F– **Flip** the mother onto her hands and knees

L–If the baby does not advance, have the mother **lift** the leg nearest the fetal back into a kneeling position. Choose the right leg if you are unsure as to the location of the fetal back (see "Parker position" for more details).

O–If the baby still is not born, insert your hands and rotate the shoulder girdle into the **oblique** diameter of the pelvis using the "praying-hands rotational maneuver," described in detail later in this chapter.

P–If the baby still is not born, deliver the **posterior arm** (how to do so is described later in this chapter).

Techniques used to prevent or resolve shoulder dystocia at the inlet

Techniques intended to prevent inlet dystocia once the head is born: At times, when the head is born, immediate signs suggest that a shoulder dystocia is imminent. Some midwives do not wait for confirmation before manually intervening. Almost all techniques used by medical-model practitioners in such an instance suggest dislodging the anterior shoulder first, rather than delivering the posterior shoulder. This is for two reasons; the medical model believes it is normal for the anterior shoulder to be born first, and direct traction on the posterior shoulder while the anterior shoulder remains impacted may result in nerve damage to the impacted anterior brachial plexus. Both these techniques and the midwifery-model variations used to prevent impaction of the anterior shoulder immediately after the head is born are presented below. Such techniques carry the risk of overuse because they are prophylactic.

El Halta maneuver (immediate delivery of the shoulders from the oblique diameter of the pelvis for inlet dystocia): The El Halta maneuver is intended for use while the shoulders are still in the oblique diameter of the pelvis. The underlying theory is that the anterior shoulder can be directed below the pubic bone before it has a chance to rotate behind it, with the understanding that the oblique pelvic diameter is wider than the anteroposterior, especially in a platypellic pelvis. This technique *must* be employed as soon as the head is born and early signs of dystocia are noted. *Do not* wait for the next contraction to begin. It is simple and does not require manipulating the baby's head, making it a very safe technique. When used in a timely fashion, it may prevent inlet dystocia and eliminate the need for other maneuvers. However, it will not work if the shoulders are already in the anteroposterior diameter.

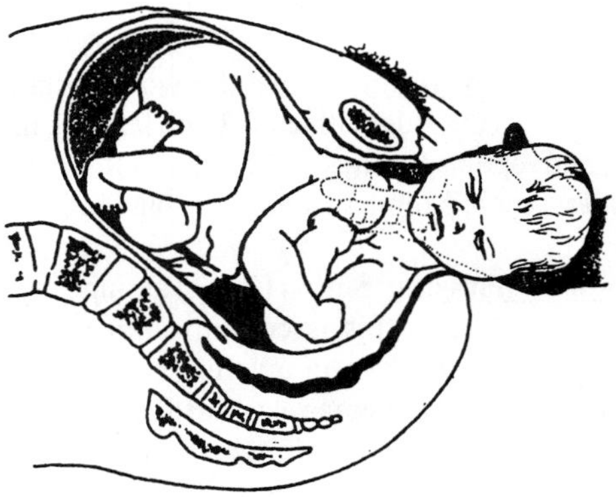

Pushing the anterior shoulder into the oblique diameter before it becomes impacted (mother supine).

Have the mother assume a position that allows easy access to the introitus (hands and knees or McRoberts will work). Use the hand whose palm will be against the baby's back when it is inserted into the yoni. (When the mother is on hands and knees with you kneeling behind her and the baby's back is to your right, use your right hand; if baby's back is to your left, use your left hand.) Insert two fingers into the yoni and place them behind the anterior shoulder, as far up along the baby's back as you can. Now press the shoulder forward with as much strength as you can muster. This flexes the shoulder girdle and prevents rotation to the anteroposterior diameter. Use your other hand to feel for the posterior shoulder at the introitus to see if it is presenting. Encourage the mother to release her pelvic muscles and push. Continue to apply steady pressure on the shoulder; this may cause the torso to rotate as the baby descends. The shoulders should descend in the oblique or transverse diameter. If necessary, once you have your hand positioned against the back of the anterior shoulder or once you have determined that the anterior shoulder has passed under the pubic bone, an assistant can apply fundal pressure if the mother is supine. After the anterior shoulder is born, this maneuver can be repeated for the posterior shoulder, if necessary (technique developed by Valerie El Halta and explained by Susan Claypool, 1998).

Malby maneuver for inlet dystocia (rotate head to OA and apply pressure): Polly Malby, CNM, offers this technique as her first line of defense for inlet shoulder dystocia. She reports success to the point that no other maneuvers are needed as well as minimal fetal injury. This technique assumes that the fetal shoulder girdle is attempting to enter the mother's pelvis in the anteroposterior diameter; however, it can also be used if the shoulders are oblique. When the orientation of the shoulder axis is unknown, the position can be quickly accessed as previously described before proceeding. The steps described below assume that the woman is in (or has repositioned herself to assume) a McRoberts position, that her bottom is hanging slightly over the edge of the birthing surface to allow for space below, and that the baby's head was born occiput anterior. Once the head is out, proceed as follows during the next contraction:

1. Have an assistant place a clean gauze pad or washcloth over the mother's anus.
2. Assuming that the baby's head is now oblique, use both hands to return the baby's occiput to an anterior position, with the chin toward the mother's anus. Do so by placing your palms on either side of the baby's head at about the level of the ears, with your fingers overlapping across the occiput. Reposition the head to OA and then press it directly downward, flexing the chin toward the anus.

3. With your hands still in place, apply steady, even downward pressure to the head while the mother pushes. *Do not pull on the head.* Watch for the nape of the neck (below the posterior hairline) to appear from under the symphysis pubis. If you see advancement, continue to apply pressure. As soon as the nape of the neck has fully cleared the pubic bone, you will know that the anterior shoulder is no longer hung up.
4. Let up pressure slightly, take a breath, and reapply pressure as before. The tip of the anterior shoulder will become visible.
5. At this point, the head may naturally rotate to follow the spine to an LOA or an ROA position. Release the head.
6. Reposition your hands and assist the anterior shoulder to birth. Then lift the body, if necessary, to assist the birth of the posterior shoulder. In some cases, the baby's torso may naturally spiral out so that the anterior shoulder rotates to a posterior position as birth occurs.

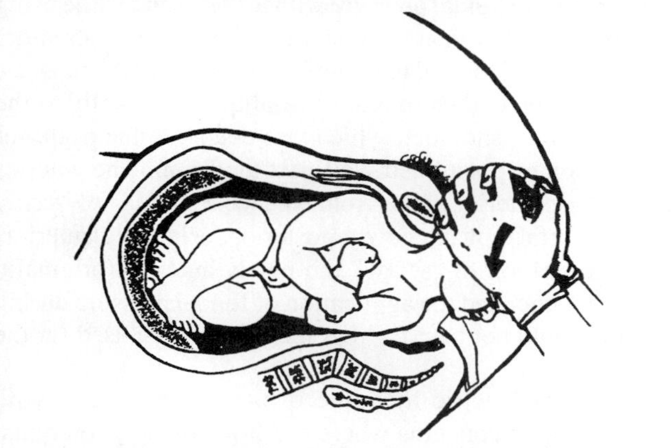

Step 2: After the mother assumes a McRoberts position, interlock your fingers 3 and turn the head to OA(in this case, the head has emerged LOA and restituted to LOT)

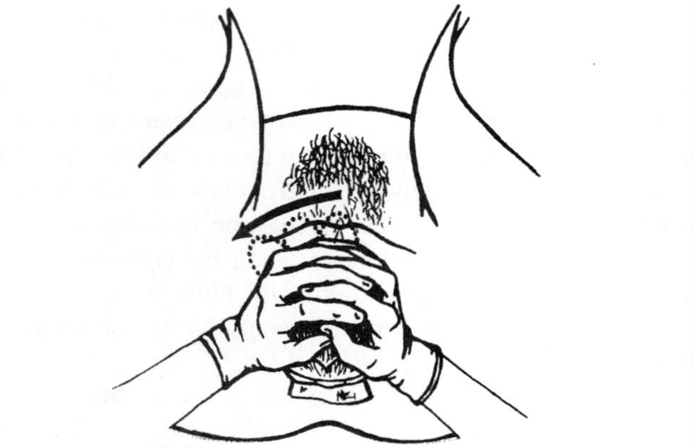

Step 2 & 3: Keeping your fingers in place, press the chin toward the anus.

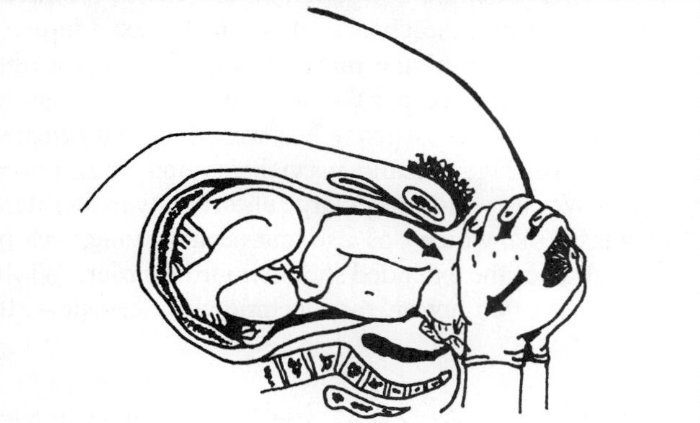

Step 4: The shoulders are now oblique and the nape of the neck is visible. Release and then reapply pressure on the head until the anterior shoulder appears.

Returning the head to an OA position and maintaining steady downward pressure encourages the thoracic spine to realign with the cervical spine. This natural anatomical tendency, in conjunction with the pressure, causes the anterior shoulder to rotate and slide out from behind and under the pubic rami at an oblique angle. By repositioning the head, directing pressure downward (rather than laterally) and by not pulling outward and stretching the neck, the neck is flexed; as a result, minimal tension is placed on the brachial plexus area (Malby, 1996).

Rotational maneuvers to resolve inlet dystocia

The techniques described above should resolve the majority of shoulder dystocias, even those that are very severe. However, sometimes additional internal manipulation is needed to free the baby. When the above techniques have not worked, abandon those that require further manipulation of the baby's head to avoid fetal injury. Manipulation of the baby's posterior arm or upper torso are the procedures of choice when additional maneuvers are necessary. This discussion begins with a review of rotational maneuvers, presented in the order in which they appeared in the medical literature.

Internal manipulations require that the midwife insert her hands into the yoni. When the baby is really impacted, the fit will be tight and thus this is easiest to accomplish between contractions when the mother is not pushing. This is no time to be hesitant. The midwife must get her hands into the mother's yoni for the following maneuvers to be performed.

Screw maneuver of Woods for unilateral inlet dystocia: In 1943, C.E. Woods introduced a technique to resolve shoulder dystocia based on the physics of the screw and thread. It was originally conceived for use in supine women. At the time, direct pulling on the head was the chief means of resolving shoulder dystocia. Woods noted that the fetal shoulders typically descend on a slant. When the anterior shoulder gets hung up, the posterior shoulder has usually descended past the promontory into the curve of the sacrum. He noted that the slanted shoulder axis acts like the threads of a screw, and the staggered projections of the sacral promontory, the symphysis pubis and coccyx act as the pelvis's complimentary threads. The threads of a screw are a continuously spiraled inclined plane; when a screw is in place, it cannot be removed by direct pulling without considerable damage. He reasoned that direct pulling is also not the best way to disimpact the shoulders. He therefore devised a method of turning or rotating the shoulders to effect their delivery. (The image of a nut [the pelvis] and a bolt [the baby] may be easier to visualize and uses the same principle.)

For this technique to work, the posterior shoulder must have descended past the ischial spines so that it is within reach. If the baby is ROA, Woods recommended that the practitioner apply fundal pressure with his left hand while using two to four fingers of his right hand to apply pressure to the anterior (chest or ventral) surface of the *posterior* shoulder to *abduct* it and rotate it 185° (past 12 o'clock) away from the perineum (and toward the symphysis) as the mother pushes. This moves the posterior shoulder to posterior-oblique, then to transverse, then to anterior-oblique and finally to the anterior position as the baby's back passes beneath the pubic bone. This shoulder, which was deeper in the posterior pelvic cavity to begin with, is now rotated anteriorly, where it becomes positioned well past the brim. The anterior shoulder is simultaneously moved from behind the pubic bone into the posterior pelvis from whence it should now easily emerge. Occasionally, a second rotation is called for; the ventral surface of the newly posterior (originally anterior) shoulder is pushed around again using the right hand in the same fashion to "screw" the newly anterior (originally posterior) shoulder out from behind the pubic bone. Woods also recommended the application of fundal pressure during the procedure (probably because the mother was anaesthetized and could not push) which should never be used for the reasons previously stated.

Many descriptions of this maneuver have been presented in the obstetric literature over the years, often with significant departure from the original technique. The primary confusion concerns where and how to apply rotational pressure. Woods's original maneuver involves abduction of the posterior shoulder. This fixes the bisacromial diameter because it hyperextends the shoulder girdle. As the posterior shoulder begins to move, the chest side of the anterior shoulder meets the resistance of the pelvic soft tissues, further extending the bisacromial diameter, thus supplying enough rigidity to effect the rotation and movement of the anterior shoulder from behind the pubic bone. (It also produces maximum pressure against the ventral side of the shoulders, thus increasing the chance of brachial plexus injury.) However, the extended shoulder axis is being rotated against the resistance of the maternal soft tissues, and the simultaneous application of fundal pressure and rotation by the same practitioner, per the original technique, is quite awkward; thus this maneuver requires some serious strength to perform. In 1943, most physicians were male, with greater upper body strength and larger hands than most midwives, making this two-finger technique a viable option. In addition, although he makes no mention of it in his article, we can assume that Woods performed a large clitorotomy to facilitate finding and rotating the posterior shoulder. Finally, use of general anesthesia, which was also routine at the time, greatly relaxes both the pelvic soft tissues and those of the baby, making rotation of the extended shoulder girdle easier. While the principles are sound, for all these reasons, the Woods maneuver is often not an easy technique for female birth attendants practicing at home, nor is it the most desirable.

Rubin maneuver (internal rotation of shoulders to oblique diameter): In 1964, Alan Rubin described a two-step maneuver involving *adduction* to disimpact the shoulders. (To everyone's great confusion, this has been called the "reverse screw maneuver of Woods," leading to misquotes about how it is performed.) First, assuming the mother is supine, he recommended the application of suprapubic pressure to the anterior scapula at an oblique angle using a rocking motion to disimpact the anterior shoulder while the mother pushes. This alone may resolve the dystocia if the shoulder axis is in the anteroposterior diameter or slightly oblique.

If that is unsuccessful, then he recommended inserting the fingers of one hand behind whichever shoulder is more readily accessible (usually the posterior) and pushing the back (dorsal side) of the shoulder toward the fetal chest. This *adducts* the anterior shoulder, flexing and thus reducing the bisacromial diameter. The pressure also causes the shoulders to begin rotation. As the back of the posterior shoulder meets the resistance of the pelvic soft tissues, flexion is enhanced, further reducing the bisacromial diameter. Continued pressure moves the shoulders from the anteroposterior into the oblique or transverse diameter, thus resolving the inlet dystocia. At the same time, the practitioner may be able to hook fingers against the lower border of the scapular wing and nudge it toward the introitus. The midwife's other hand can be used to exert traction in the opposite posterior axillary crease (for the proper way to do this, see "Techniques involving axillary traction" later in this chapter). This technique is facilitated when an assistant applies suprapubic pressure and rocks her body weight through her hands to encourage shoulder rotation. Once the shoulders are free, have mother push.

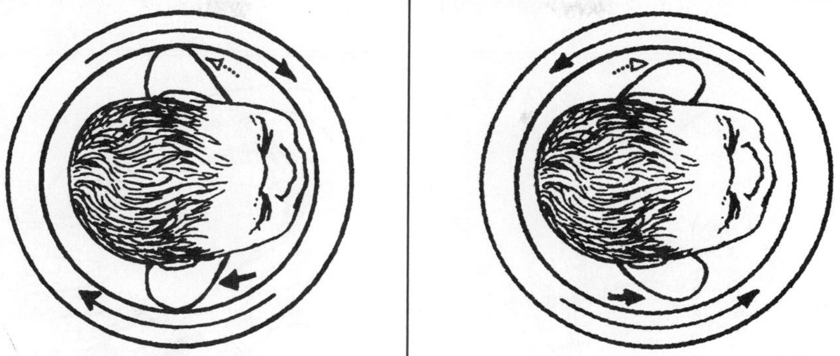

Woods maneuver: abduction forces (ROT) — Rubin maneuver: adduction forces (ROT)

The direction of force applied to the posterior shoulder alters the attitude of the shoulder axis. This tendency is enhanced when the opposite shoulder meets the resistance of the pelvic sides walls. The attitude of the shoulder axis is exaggerated to emphasize these changes.

KEY: Outer double circle = the pelvic cavity, arrows inside the ring represent the direction of rotation.
Small black arrow next to posterior shoulder = the direction of manual pressure.
Small dotted arrow next to opposite shoulder = soft tissue resistance from the wall of the birth canal.

Rubin also studied newborns to determine the diameters of the shoulders in various attitudes (not including hunching, which further reduces the bisacromial diameter slightly). The values for "straight shoulders" and abducted shoulders appear to be reversed at first glance, because straight is said to be larger than abducted (i.e., fully extended). Arching the shoulders posteriorly causes the shoulder axis to bend, resulting in a slight reduction in diameter. Even so, abduction renders the shoulder axis maximally rigid, the other primary problem with this posture.

ATTITUDE OF SHOULDER GIRDLE	AVERAGE BISACROMIAL DIAMETER	AVERAGE CIRCUMFERENCE AT WIDEST POINT
Straight (baby supine)	14.7 cm	36.6 cm
Abducted (Woods maneuver)	14.4 cm	36 cm
Adducted (Rubin maneuver)	12.8 cm	33.6 cm

Varney maneuver: Varney's rotational maneuver (1997) combines the flexion/extension forces of Woods and Rubin and is intended to accommodate the lesser upper body strength of female practitioners. It can be performed with the mother on her back (illustrated) or in a hands-and-knees position. Insert both of your hands, placing four fingers of one hand on the scapula one fetal shoulder to *adduct* it and four fingers of your other hand on the ventral side of the other shoulder to *abduct* it. For example, if the baby is ROT, place the fingers of your left hand on the scapula of the anterior shoulder and the fingers of your right hand on the upper chest in front of the posterior shoulder. (Reverse hand positions and all other directions in the following description if the baby is LOT.) Now apply as much force as necessary (it will likely be a lot) in a clockwise direction to rotate the shoulders 45° into the adjacent oblique diameter of the pelvis by moving the back under the pubic bone. Using four fingers more evenly distributes the pressure over a broad area and gives you more leverage to maneuver. Turning a stuck baby using only your fingers is very hard to do; if no movement occurs, try pushing your entire hands inside and using your palms to facilitate rotation.

Once you have rotated the shoulders into the adjacent oblique diameter, have the mother push. If the shoulders do not advance, complete the rotation of the baby for a full 180°. If necessary, once you have the shoulders in the transverse pelvic diameter, you can remove your hands to reverse their positions, using your left hand to apply pressure anteriorly against the chest on the baby's right anterior chest and your right hand to apply pressure posteriorly to the baby's left scapula. The now posterior shoulder may come out relatively easily once the originally anterior shoulder has been rotated to the posterior position (see the next section for details regarding bringing an arm out). If not, screw the baby out one more 180° turn in a counterclockwise direction by pressing on the scapula of the newly anterior shoulder with your right hand and the chest side of the newly posterior shoulder with your left.

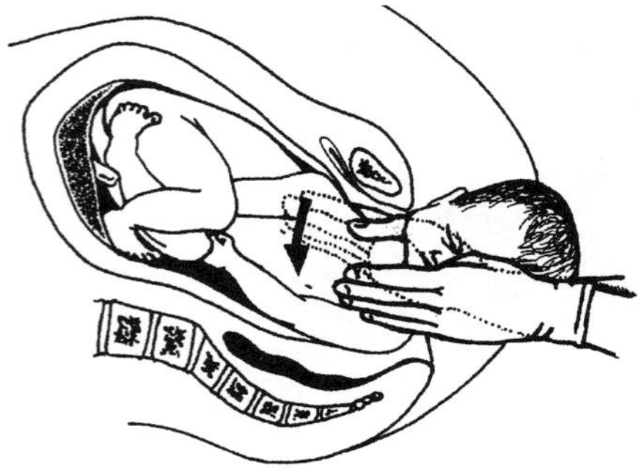

Varney maneuver: With both hands in place, push the anterior shoulder forward into the adjacent oblique diameter and have the mother push.

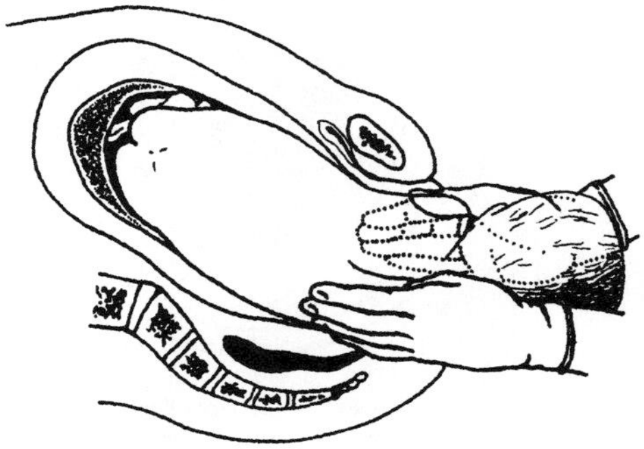

If pushing does not result in descent, continue to rotate the shoulders until the posterior shoulder is under the pubic bone. Reposition your hands when the shoulders are transverse, if necessary, to facilitate rotation, as has been done here.

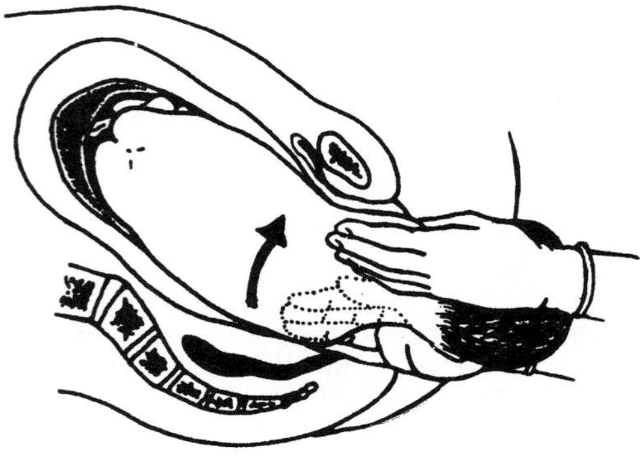

If both shoulders cannot be delivered at this point, reverse your hand positions to prepare for a second 180° rotation in the opposite direction.

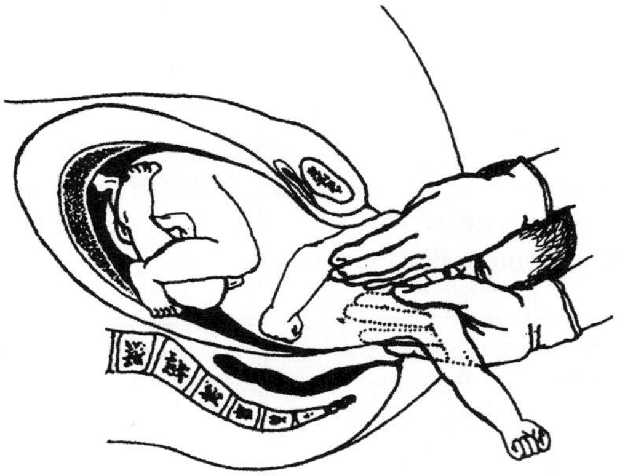

While "screwing" the baby out further, one arm has been born and the currently anterior shoulder has emerged.

This maneuver, which combines adduction forces on one shoulder and abduction forces on the other, probably results in a semiflexed shoulder axis; if so, the resulting shoulder diameter would fall somewhere between those for the Woods and the Rubin maneuvers. It also provides pressure on both sides of the shoulder axis, which makes rotation easier, although some of this benefit is mitigated by forcing one shoulder into abduction, which causes it to create more resistance as it traverses the wall of the birth canal. It is perhaps less stressful on the fetal anatomy than the Woods maneuver but is more stressful and therefore potentially more harmful, than maneuvers that involve only adduction.

Praying hands rotation: This technique is a variation on the Varney maneuver. It works best for an inlet dystocia in which the shoulders are stuck in the anteroposterior diameter and there is room in the transverse diameter to insert your hands. It is most easily accomplished with the mother in a hands-and-knees position, which allows for plenty of sacral mobility. Reach into the mother's yoni with both hands. Grasp the baby around the thorax by placing one hand over the baby's back and one over the chest. Evenly distribute your hands and fingers over the baby's chest to avoid breaking a rib and be careful not to dig your fingers into the soft tissue below the rib cage, where liver, kidney or other organ damage may occur (if your hands are large and your fingers extend beyond the costal border, keep them straight). Rotate the torso an eighth to a quarter turn in the direction the baby is facing while gently applying outward, posteriorly directed (toward mother's sacrum) pressure. This should help move the sacrum out of the way while dislodging the anterior shoulder by rotating it out from behind the pubic bone. Now pull straight outward to advance the torso. If the baby will not advance, rotate the torso an eighth to a quarter turn in the same or even the opposite direction (depending on what appears to be needed) with the same outward, posterior pressure and then pull outward. Be aware that the direction of rotation (with the chest leading) will tend to abduct one shoulder (which one depends upon the direction of rotation). This will broaden the shoulder axis.

Many independent midwives use some form of this technique, grasping the baby's body and then wiggling the torso back and forth to work the baby down and out while the mother pushes. Be sure to grasp the upper torso around the rib cage to avoid putting pressure into the soft abdominal or the lower back area because that can lead to organ damage. Keeping this precaution in mind and taking care not to apply localized pressure or jam a finger into the axilla, you can use this technique very safely.

Methods of manipulating or delivering the posterior shoulder or arm

Do not waste more time trying to dislodge the anterior shoulder when none of the maneuvers above has resolved an inlet dystocia. Delivery of the posterior shoulder is the next step. The posterior shoulder is usually easy to reach, as it is generally found in the hollow of the sacrum. The reason that going for the posterior shoulder is not usually recommended as a first line of therapy is because simply pulling on the posterior arm without disimpacting the anterior shoulder is likely to result in injury to the anterior brachial plexus. However, delivery of the posterior shoulder often works to accomplish the birth when all other attempts at repositioning the baby have failed. Some midwives use delivery of the posterior arm as their first line of therapy when faced with an inlet dystocia.

Techniques involving axillary traction: Techniques to manipulate the baby via the axillary area can be used immediately if an axillary area is within reach. There are numerous warnings in the medical literature regarding the dangers of techniques that involve the region of the axilla because of the very real danger of brachial plexus injury. It is therefore imperative to be absolutely clear as to proper technique. Inserting a finger*tip* into the arm*pit* is dangerous and should never be done. Applying traction to the ventral axillary crease (where the arm joins the shoulder anteriorly) is equally dangerous because the brachial plexus is located in the anterior armpit and axillary fold (where the underarm meets the torso); anterior traction in this area can rip the brachial plexus apart. There are, however, two safe methods to accomplish posterior axillary traction. The first and best of these is offered by Nell Tharpe, CNM, who has observed dissections of the axillary region and understands the anatomy well.

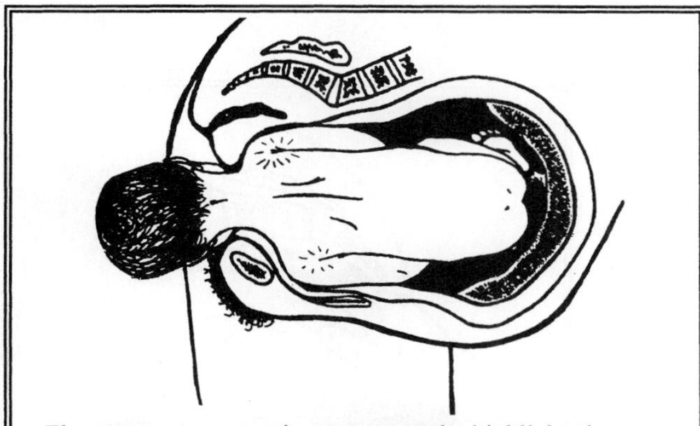

Tharpe maneuver: apply pressure to the highlighted areas.

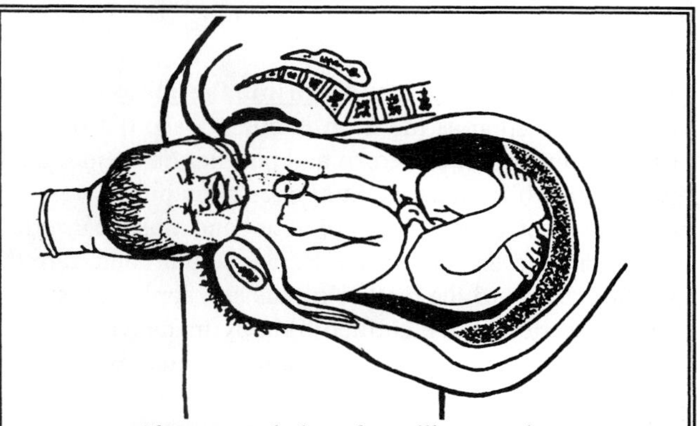

Alternate technique for axillary traction

(Mother is shown on her hands and knees.)

Tharpe maneuver: This maneuver can be performed with the mother on her hands and knees, standing, or in a McRoberts or modified Walcher position. Slide your fingers down the back of the baby's neck, across the upper back, and locate the posterior axillary crease of the most accessible shoulder (which may be influenced by the mother's position). Your fingertips are then pressed against the depression created by the crease to allow you to apply traction and rotation and to reduce the bisacromial diameter of the shoulder. This maneuver avoids applying pressure to the nerves in the anterior axillary area and remains safe as long as none of your fingers slip forward into the armpit. Once your fingers are positioned, gently but firmly rotate the shoulder downward and forward to release it from behind the pubic bone or sacral promontory. If necessary, insert your other hand as soon as possible and locate the posterior axillary crease of the other arm. Using gentle traction, you can now "walk" the baby out by inching one side forward and then the other, wiggling the baby through the birth canal. This technique has been used successfully to dislodge two big babies in bilateral inlet dystocias with no newborn injuries and only a small perineal laceration (Tharpe, 2004).

Alternative method of safe axillary traction: After checking with a chiropractor regarding the safety of this technique, I have used it successfully in my practice on three occasions with no newborn injuries. Infants and small children are often picked up by placing the hands fully under both arms and lifting. Using a similar technique to retrieve a shoulder is very safe. In fact, you can apply a great deal of force while getting a good grasp on the baby and bringing him down without harm to the axillary area, as long as the anterior shoulder is not still impacted. This technique can be used with the mother in just about any accessible position.

Insert your hand down the back of the baby's neck, across the upper back and locate the posterior axillary crease of the posterior arm. Insert a finger completely under the arm so that the tip would be visible on the other side of the baby's body. By inserting a finger fully under the arm to apply traction, rather than applying traction to the head, you are actually bringing the posterior shoulder forward, toward the ear, thereby relieving tension on the brachial plexus of the posterior shoulder.

Once your finger is positioned, keep it as rigid as possible so that you will not accidently hook your fingertip into the axilla if your hand slips. If it does start to slip, straighten your finger (do not curl it, as it may hook into the armpit) and reposition it correctly before proceeding. Now, pull toward the mother's anus and outward. This outward pull at a posterior angle is intended to disimpact the anterior shoulder while advancing the posterior shoulder. Not to disimpact the anterior shoulder risks damage to the brachial plexus of the anterior shoulder, which would be compressed against the pubic arch if you just pulled straight out. Have an assistant provide perineal support below your hand while another applies suprapubic pressure (if the mother's position allows this).

Although you are attempting to get the posterior shoulder to birth first, one disadvantage of this maneuver is that, as the posterior shoulder descends into the hollow of the sacrum, room is created for the upper arm to extend out from the torso, your finger can slip down the upper, inner arm, the elbow bends, the arm extends and comes out. This can jam the elbow down into the perineum, possibly resulting in a bad perineal tear, a broken humerus and possibly brachial plexus injury if your finger slips forward (in other words the technique itself is safe, extension of the arm may not be). If the arm does extend, let it come out. A benefit of having the arm deliver is that the anterior shoulder is likely to become disimpacted in the process. The Tharpe maneuver is unlikely to produce the uncontrolled delivery of an arm; therefore, resort to this technique only when the Tharpe maneuver is unsuccessful. Once the baby has advanced far enough to use the Tharpe maneuver, do so.

Pull the posterior shoulder down into the hollow of sacrum: Insert your hand as soon as the head is out. Grasp the baby around the posterior upper arm and torso and pull her down into the hollow of the sacrum while an assistant applies suprapubic pressure. (This is easier said than done, as most of your hand must be inserted between the sacrum and the shoulder.) Remove your hand, turn the head to OA, flex it toward the mother's anus and apply downward pressure (see the section above entitled "Malby maneuver"). This is most likely to work for an inlet dystocia in a woman who has a gynecoid pelvis.

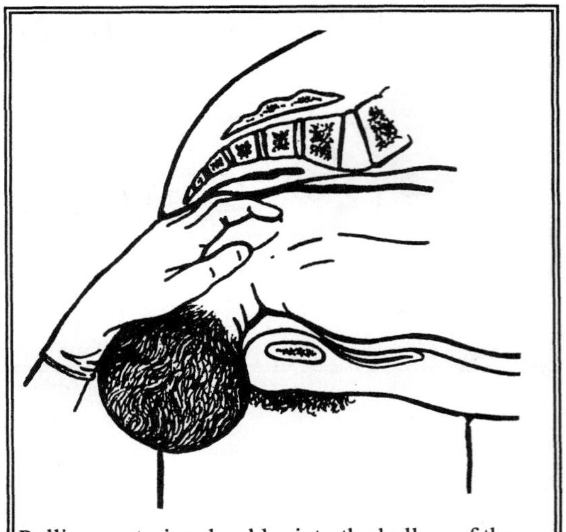

Pulling posterior shoulder into the hollow of the sacrum (mother is on hands and knees).

Deliver the posterior arm: Delivery of the posterior arm reduces the diameter of the shoulder girdle considerably and, in cases of inlet dystocia, will often allow the trapped anterior shoulder to drop down from behind the pubic bone and advance. These changes alone may accomplish the birth. The posterior arm is easiest to do with the mother on her hands and knees. This description assumes that the mother is so positioned.

Insert a hand (left if the baby's back is to *your* left, right if the baby's back is to *your* right) along the back of the baby's neck and to the posterior axillary crease. Inserting your hand into the transverse quadrant of the pelvis makes it more likely that you will be able to advance it far enough to reach the arm. You are trying to reach the posterior arm; however, feel for the shoulder and arm that are easiest to reach. Bilateral dystocia creates the most difficult situation. Once you find the posterior axillary crease, determine if the arm is behind the back, along the baby's side or over the chest by determining the location of the upper arm. Since a posteriorly placed arm will hinder all types of resolution maneuvers, how to deal with that has already been addressed earlier in the chapter.

Assuming the arm is to the baby's side or over the anterior torso (Tully, 2003a):

1. Use three fingers to follow along that upper arm until you find the bend of the elbow (antecubital fossa). As you do so, push backwards against the sacrum with the back of your hand to lift it out of the way.
2. Flex the arm by using the fingertip of your index or middle finger to apply pressure either to the upper arm, pushing it backwards or, if you can reach it, apply pressure to the inner elbow, causing the arm to bend.
3. If necessary, extend your fingers on either side of the upper arm to splint it and sweep it toward the chest. Splinting to the level of the elbow avoids breaking the humerus.
4. Use your index finger to reach for the forearm. As soon as the forearm is within reach, wrap your fingers over it to encourage it to bend. As soon as possible, grasp the wrist or hand (whichever you can grab). If the arm is resistant to bending, check to make sure that the cord is not wrapped around it. If so, nudge it toward the hand with your fingers, sliding it down the arm and off. If this is impossible, proceed to the Tharpe maneuver.
5. Once you have the hand or wrist, sweep the arm across the baby's chest and out of the yoni by applying gentle, steady traction. Pulling on the hand, rather than a long bone, reduces the likelihood of breaking the humerus.

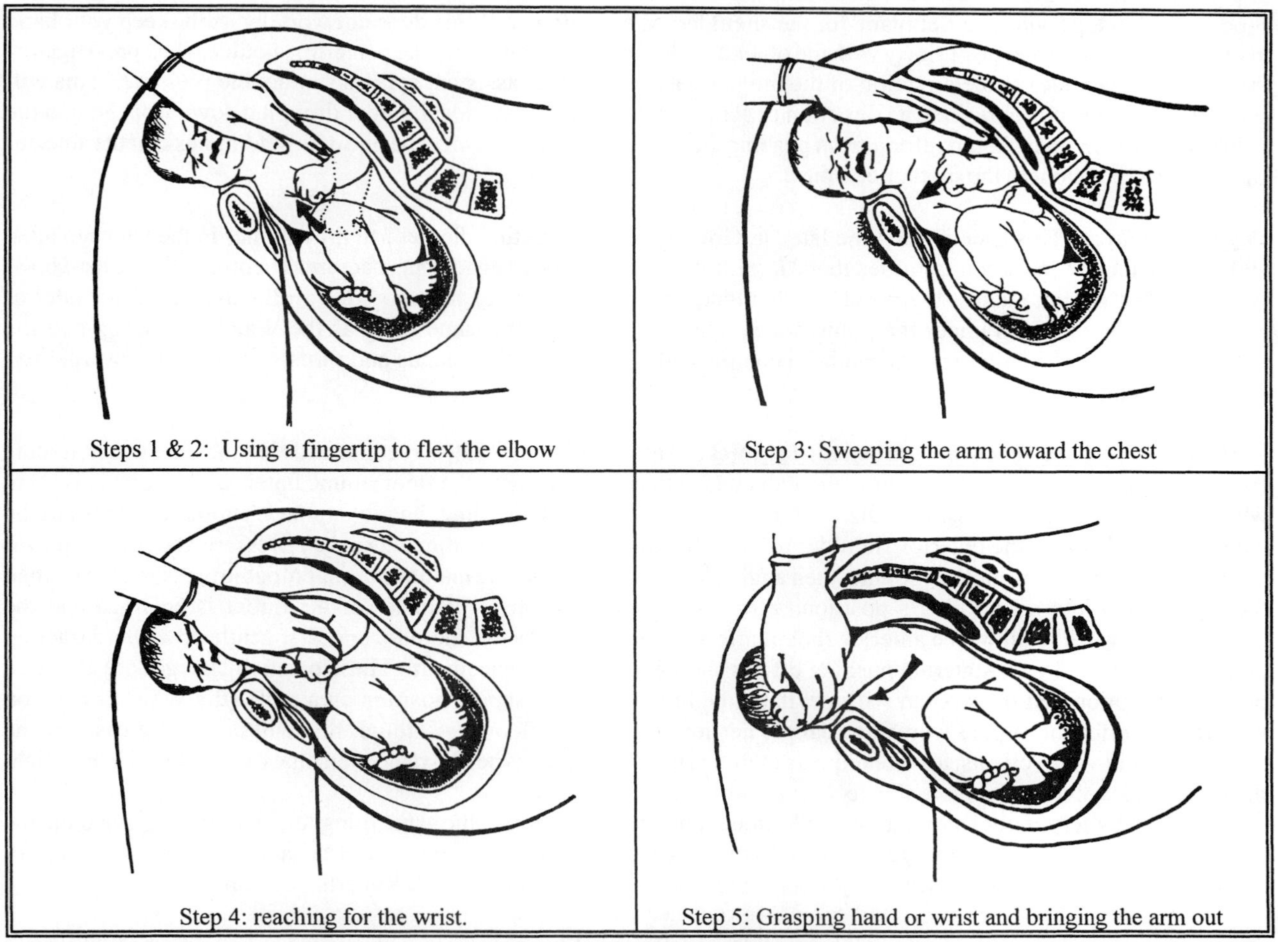

Steps 1 & 2: Using a fingertip to flex the elbow

Step 3: Sweeping the arm toward the chest

Step 4: reaching for the wrist.

Step 5: Grasping hand or wrist and bringing the arm out

(Mother is on her hands and knees)

The act of repositioning an arm carries the risk of breaking a bone in any event. However, broken bones in babies heal within a few days, and a broken bone is more acceptable than a dead baby.

On very rare occasions, the baby will not be born even though one arm is delivered. This is likely to be due to a severe outlet contracture. In this case, the pelvic press (see below) may facilitate the birth. When opening the pelvis is not sufficient by itself, grasp the baby's upper torso by placing one open hand on the chest and one on the back, and wiggle the baby out by using a gentle side-to-side motion, or rotate the baby, literally unscrewing it out of the pelvis, as you apply firm but gentle traction. Be mindful where you grasp; do not press into the baby's lower back or belly, as internal organ injury is possible. Once enough of the body is delivered, wrap a small towel around it to get a better grasp. *Do not pull the baby out by the delivered arm* because you may dislocate it or severely damage the brachial plexus on that side, or both. If you cannot grasp the baby's torso sufficiently to extract the rest of the baby, you may have to rotate the baby 180° to move the anterior shoulder to a posterior position and deliver the newly posterior arm. At this point, enough of the baby should be out that you can insert your hands under each arm and have the mother push.

Additional techniques to resolve inlet dystocia

Scholles maneuvers: The shoulders can become impacted in the anteroposterior diameter of the inlet when they are in the same plane (level with each other); often the head was born relatively easily, but the posterior shoulder is out of easy reach. Holly Scholles, CPM (2003), recommends having the mother in a standing squat, although it can be used with the mother supine. Insert your hand, palm up, placing two fingers up and under the pubic arch. Straddle the urethra with your fingers. Now, pull straight out, away from the mother's body, using as much force as you can muster. This lifts the pubic bone up and back slightly, creating room for the shoulders to dislodge themselves when it is used with the mother in a position so that gravity can assist (Scholles, 2000). The insertion of fingers under the pubic arch also produces a shoe-horn effect, providing a flat plane for the shoulders to slide down. If this does not work by itself, keep your hand in place while reaching in posteriorly with the other hand and pressing inward on the posterior shoulder (i.e., press against the top of the shoulder in the direction of the mother's head) while an assistant applies suprapubic pressure. This will cause the shoulder axis to reverse its direction of slant, resulting in the anterior shoulder dropping down from behind the pubic arch. The mother should refrain from pushing during this maneuver. Once the midwife determines that the anterior shoulder is repositioned, the mother can push.

White maneuver: This trick is from the late Dr. Gregory White, longtime homebirth practitioner in the Chicago area. Have the mother sit on a large, upturned metal mixing bowl with the bowl against her sacrum. Theoretically the hard bowl will press her sacrum against the posterior shoulder, change the angle of the shoulder girdle and cause the anterior shoulder to pop out from under the pubic bone. This accomplishes the same thing as the Walcher position and the Scholles maneuver. Similar results can be accomplished when the mother stands and thrusts her pelvis forward, as in the Sutton maneuver.

Walcher-McRoberts-Pecorari maneuver for inlet dystocia: Pecorari (1999) recommends having the mother assume the Walcher position (buttocks off the edge of the bed with legs dangling to the floor) immediately after the head is born, which increases the anteroposterior diameter of the pelvis. At the same time, he recommends suprapubic pressure be applied to the back of the anterior shoulder to direct it toward the oblique diameter; such pressure should be applied directly down toward the mother's spine, then angled toward her feet. While maintaining suprapubic pressure, the woman then is assisted into a McRoberts position, whereby the anteroposterior diameter of the outlet is enlarged and the symphysis elevated to allow the anterior shoulder to slip beneath it. As the shoulder appears, gentle downward traction on the head coupled with maternal pushing efforts should result in advancement. These position changes are all based on the assumption that the woman will inevitably be birthing from a supine position on a table (the Walcher position requires room for the supine woman to dangle her legs toward the floor). Although this will not be the case for the majority of midwifery clients, his technique is included to illustrate the types of maneuvers that can work and to highlight the anatomy involved. Compare this technique with that of Sutton, above.

In the midwifery-model alternative, the Sutton maneuvers accomplish the same thing, or a woman can stand up and bend backwards as far as possible while someone supports her from behind. An assistant simultaneously applies suprapubic pressure. If the baby is not yet born, the woman then assumes the McRoberts position.

Ramp maneuver: Dr. Donald Coustan uses the complicated maneuver outlined here; it has been dubbed "the ramp maneuver" by the midwives who described it (Afriat, 1994). It is used when shoulder dystocia is anticipated, when the turtle sign appears or when the head fails to restitute after birth. It requires three people to perform, two at the perineum and one to apply suprapubic pressure.

1. The mother assumes the McRoberts position once the chin has delivered.
2. One person inserts a hand, palm up, into the yoni between the fetal neck and the pubic bone to determine the position of the anterior shoulder and announce its location. Finding the anterior shoulder may necessitate inserting the hand palm down to make the shoulder easier to palpate, then taking the hand out and reinserting it palm up.
3. The second person then applies suprapubic pressure directly over the palmar surface of the internal hand, disimpacting the anterior shoulder. The internal hand forms a ramp, preventing reimpaction of the shoulder, which slides out beneath the hand and is born.
4. The third person, who is at the perineum, then applies downward traction on the fetal head.

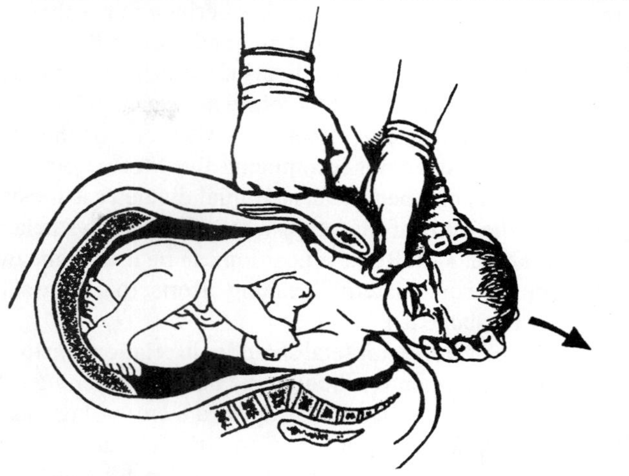
The ramp maneuver (mother in McRoberts position)

The major drawbacks of this technique are that it requires traction on the head, it takes up a lot of room in the pelvis, it requires three people and it requires the woman to birth on a table or an adjustable bed so that the practitioners can access her for the necessary maneuvers. It is therefore most suitable for hospital use in drugged mothers.

Techniques to prevent or resolve shoulder dystocia at the outlet

In outlet dystocia, the shoulder girdle is impacted behind the level of the tuberosities. There are several techniques that widen the outlet and will often move the pelvic bones enough for the baby to descend.

Maternal positions to help resolve outlet dystocia:

Deep squatting: Believing that gravity will greatly assist in bringing the baby down and out, some midwives use the deep squat as a preventive measure when shoulder dystocia is anticipated. A full squat, with feet flat and toes aligned directly under the knees, widens the pubic arch as the tuberosities are pulled up and apart, which may, in fact, prevent an outlet dystocia. However, for modern Western women, sustaining a truly deep, flat-footed squat for a lengthy period of time is tiring if not almost impossible. Squatting is absolutely contraindicated if it is anticipated that the shoulders won't engage, as it narrows the inlet. In addition, with or without gravity, squatting postures can encourage the shoulders to malrotate.

Upright squatting: A standing or hanging squat (dangle position), including using a Birth Sling, opens both the inlet and the outlet and also affords the midwife more room to work when additional manipulations are needed. These positions can be used during pushing or when shoulder dystocia is identified to get pressure off the pelvis and put the woman in an ideal position to maximize the effect of the pelvic-opening techniques described below.

McRoberts maneuver: Dr. William McRoberts (1984) of Houston, Texas, popularized this position for the management of shoulder dystocia. On the positive side, it represents a recognition within the obstetric community that maternal positioning alone can be used to facilitate birth. However, use of this position remains within the limited paradigm of the medical model. The woman remains supine and raises her legs, thus affording excellent physician access to her introitus should additional manipulation be required. It is recommended to correct the factors that tend to produce shoulder dystocia when the mother is in a dorsal lithotomy position; it *was not* the fruit of a search for the ideal position for birth. Note that, like the hands-and-knees position, it was originally intended for use as a response to shoulder dystocia and not as a preventive measure, although many practitioners now use it prophylactically. Although the McRoberts position is recommended for preventing or resolving inlet dystocia, it may, in fact, be more useful for resolving outlet dystocia (further explained in the list below). Because of this, it is included in this section covering position changes to resolve either type of dystocia.

The mother lies on a firm surface such as the padded floor or a very firm mattress (most beds are too soft) and she or her assistants hold her legs sharply flexed against her abdomen, knees to shoulders. Note that her legs should not be spread wide, which would tighten her perineum; her thighs should contact the sides of her belly. This position is said to offer the following advantages and poses the following disadvantages (my remarks are in parentheses):

- (When used prophylactically prior to the birth of the head, it presents the problem of maximally narrowing the spinopubic angle and therefore increasing the likelihood that the shoulder will become stuck above the inlet in the first place. Pecorari (1999), one of the few obstetrical authors who recognizes two varieties of dystocia, does not recommend the McRoberts position as a prophylactic technique for anticipated inlet dystocia or when the bisacromial diameter is impacted above the brim, because it narrows the inlet.)
- (After the birth of the head, when shoulder dystocia is anticipated and the shoulders are still in an oblique position, a McRoberts position can be used right away to widen the outlet, in combination with suprapubic pressure and maternal pushing efforts, to get the shoulder axis down past the brim before it has a chance to rotate above it.)
- It elevates the anterior fetal shoulder in relationship to the mother's pelvis. (This may further impact the anterior shoulder when it is behind the bone by pinching off the brim.)
- The symphysis pubis rotates upward 8 cm, and its angle of inclination is reduced from the angle of 26° (in the supine, lithotomy position) to 10°. Rotating the symphysis up and thus straightening the path beneath the pubic bone reduces the traction on the neck and clavicle produced by lateral flexion, minimizing trauma to the clavicles and the brachial plexus area. (This brings all the pelvic planes into a horizontal, rather than angled, relationship, thus reducing available space.)
- Elevating the pelvic axis flexes the fetal spine up toward the pubic bone and the anterior shoulder. (This interferes with the normal movement that leads to the posterior shoulder being born first.)
- Rotating the symphysis upward after impaction of the anterior shoulder is said to move the pubic bone up and out of the way, allowing the anterior shoulder to emerge. This does seem to work at times, and it may occur without further intervention, although the need for additional maneuvering is not uncommon.
- The lifting and flexion of the pelvis combine to push the posterior shoulder past the sacral promontory and down through the inlet (which could be of great benefit in helping to resolve bilateral inlet dystocia).

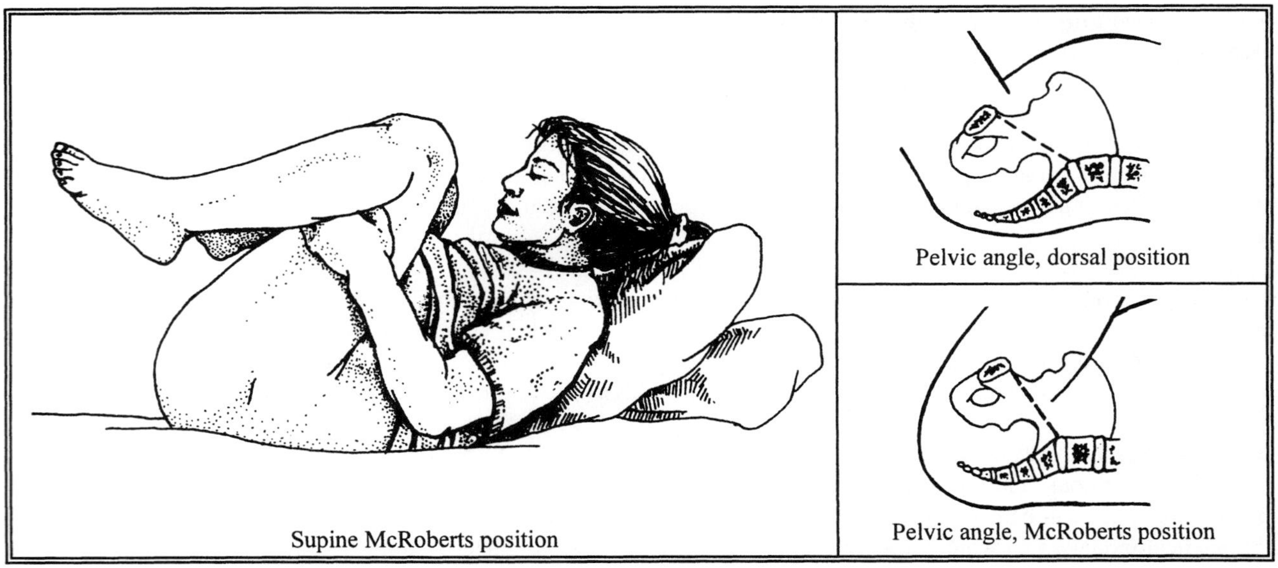

Supine McRoberts position

Pelvic angle, dorsal position

Pelvic angle, McRoberts position

- It straightens the maternal lumbar and lumbosacral curve, thus flattening the spine above the inlet. It is said to cause the sacral promontory to flatten. (Enormously greater sacral movement is possible when the woman is upright.)
- Some weight-bearing force is removed from the sacrum and coccyx by virtue of lifting the legs so high, allowing the sacrum space to rotate backward. (Continued pressure on the upper sacrum and tension in the pelvic soft tissues does not permit the sacrum to move as freely as in an upright position. Pressure from below on the upper sacrum may cause it to impinge on the available space at the inlet.)

- •The outlet is opened to its maximum dimension. (This makes it most useful for the management of outlet dystocia but not necessarily for inlet dystocia. Note that while the outlet may be widened by this position, the inlet is narrowed because it moves the pubic bone closer to the spine.)
- •The inlet is said to be brought into line with the maximum force of the mother's pushing efforts. (This does not line the baby up with the force of contractions, thus interfering with the primary force that moves the baby down.)
- •A full squat is simulated in a gravity-neutral position. (This closes the brim and maximally curves the birth canal, pivoting the sacrum and pelvic floor up into the available space and causing the baby to push through the posterior, rather than the anterior, region of the pelvic floor; a lateral position is preferable when a supine position is required or desired by the mother as it allows much more sacral mobility.)
- •Its use in drugged women may overstretch the relaxed hip and knee joints. This can result in injury and lead to problems after birth. The exaggerated lithotomy position and abduction of the thighs also stretches the articular surfaces of the symphysis pubis and places increased pressure on the femoral nerve overlying the inguinal ligament. Symphyseal separation and transient femoral neuropathy have been noted in one case (Gherman et al., 1998).

Manual techniques to open the pelvis that can resolve outlet dystocia:
Pelvic expansion techniques that open the midpelvis and the outlet: These techniques are useful when the dystocia originates below the brim, somewhere between the midpelvis and the outlet.

Pelvic press: Two assistants stand to either side of the mother and apply pressure toward the midline to the mother's iliac crests with as much force as they can muster. The assistants should join their free hands together in front both to keep balance and to provide feedback to ensure they are placing even pressure on the crests. This technique, because it opens the outlet, can cause the baby to pop out (Rogers, 1996).

Tuberosity pull: The mother lies on her side on a firm surface with her top leg deeply flexed. Insert your gloved fingers into the yoni, find the inside surface of the upper tuberosity and pull upward during a contraction, which widens the pelvis on that side and should work well to relieve an outlet dystocia caused by impaction of the shoulders against the pubic rami.

Sacral press: This maneuver will help displace the sacrum backwards, which could help dislodge a baby whose posterior shoulder is stuck against a flat sacrum or a coccyx that points up into the space at the outlet. The mother should assume any position that does not put direct pressure on the sacrum (such as hands and knees, side-lying or standing). Place two or three fingers inside the mother's yoni and press backward into the sacrum during pushing. Standing or a hands-and-knees position will allow the entire sacrum to move backward spontaneously, so this technique is most useful when a woman is incapable of standing, thus somewhat limiting her sacral mobility, depending upon the position she chooses.

Outlet-expanding techniques: The following three techniques are all useful when the impaction is against the pubic arch or the rami.

Sheela-na-gig maneuver: Face the mother; place two fingers of your left hand inside against her right tuberosity and two fingers of your right hand inside against her left tuberosity. Pull to either side away from her midline. This will separate the bones of the outlet all the way up to the pubic arch, allowing the baby to pass through.

Pubic pull-up (pubic expansion): This is a more painful technique, but it can help resolve an outlet dystocia by widening the symphysis if the problem is a funnel-shaped outlet. It should not be used if the pubic arch is shallow, as it will then decrease space in the anterior pelvis. The mother can be in any accessible, upright position. Insert two fingers, straddle the urethra and pull straight up and out at somewhat of an angle (Scholles, 2000).

Medical Model Approaches to Severe Shoulder Dystocia

Break the fetal clavicle: A shoulder dystocia is sometimes so severe that intentional damage must be done to avert fetal death. While this is certainly a medical-model solution, it is a last resort that midwives are expected to employ should all else fail. Breaking the clavicle is believed to reduce the bisacromial diameter. Whether it actually does or not is debatable because the bone will still be present and could splint itself at an odd angle, injuring the baby and not really causing the shoulder diameter to collapse. The clavicle may break unintentionally as a by-product of other maneuvers; however, intentional breakage can be quite difficult to accomplish, requiring 20 pounds of pressure in the mature fetus. Four techniques are described:

1. Hook a finger around the anterior clavicle and press it outward against the pubic ramus.
2. Use two thumbs to press down into the center of the clavicle. While this technique, recommended by Varney (1997), may be more successful, it also increases the risk of lung puncture or injury to the subclavian vein.
3. Identify the clavicle, hook both thumbs under it to pull up (toward the fetal head) on the middle of the bone. Pulling up is intended to direct the break away from the lungs and the subclavian vein (Marshall & Buffington, 1998).
4. Sever the clavicle by cutting it with surgical scissors. This is also very difficult to accomplish, carries the risk of injuring the mother and producing unintentional injury to the baby. It should be considered only if the fetus is dead, you are very remote from medical assistance and you have run out of all other options.

Instrumental delivery: In 1979, Chavis described an instrument for the relief of shoulder dystocia; the device was similar to a shoehorn with a concave blunt-edged blade attached to a long handle. The lubricated blade is inserted along the anterior fetal neck until it overlies the anterior shoulder. The instrument is then used as a lever, with the pubic bone as a fulcrum, to push the shoulder downward and then, like a shoehorn, the blade provides a continuous passageway along which the shoulder is intended to slide and then emerge. This device is not widely known in North America. It risks injury to both mother and baby, and its use is not recommended.

Cephalic replacement (Zavanelli maneuver): Some medical-model practitioners have resorted to replacing the head back inside the mother once they have run out of other options. This procedure not only sounds impossible but is dangerous. However, it is discussed here because it is accepted medical practice in some settings in desperate cases.

This technique is used by physicians for otherwise irresolvable bilateral inlet dystocia. Anesthesia renders the mother's lower body more relaxed, thus facilitating this maneuver. Needless to say, fetal outcomes are not always good. Severe brain damage and death are likely (Cunningham et al., 2001).

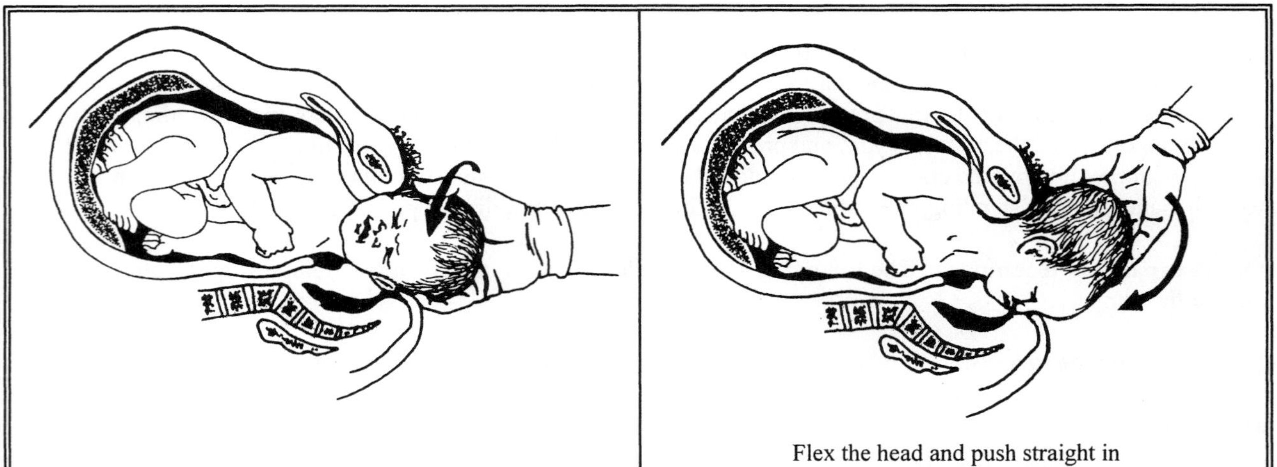

Return the head to OA

Flex the head and push straight in (mother is in McRoberts position)

A deep clitorotomy is cut. A drug that relaxes the uterus is administered. The head is repositioned to OA; the chin is flexed toward the baby's chest. The practitioner's hand is now applied to the occipital region (not over a fontanelle), evenly distributing the pressure as much as possible. The posterior yoni wall is depressed with the other hand. Sufficient pressure is then applied to the head to cause it to retract back inside, replacing it to at least zero station, where it should remain on its own. Some descriptions say this happens easily while others state that replacement is quite difficult, so ease of replacement no doubt varies from case to case. Sources recommend that the mother be supine for this procedure, although it may be easier to perform with the mother on hands and knees to allow maximal sacral mobility. The heart rate is reassessed once the head is back inside and a surgical delivery is then performed (Sandberg, 1985). Homebirth midwives have a wide variety of techniques available to them when faced with shoulder dystocia and should never have to resort to the Zavanelli maneuver at home.

Symphysiotomy: Some physicians resort to transyoni symphysiotomy when everything else has failed, including cephalic replacement. This surgical division of the symphysis pubis to effect a yoni delivery is also used in many developing countries when the pelvis is slightly contracted. The procedure carries a high rate of urinary tract and orthopedic complications and is not recommended (Romoff, 2000).

Abdominal rescue: In this alternative to symphysiotomy, a low transverse incision is made above the symphysis, allowing direct visualization and manipulation of the anterior shoulder. The opening allows the anterior shoulder to pop forward when bilateral inlet dystocia is present. This releases the posterior shoulder and allows it to descend past the sacral promontory where it can be grasped and delivered from below.

Practicing

As with other rare emergencies, hands-on practice using a doll and pelvis can go a long way toward understanding which techniques seem right for you as well as achieving the kind of sure-handed competency you will want to have at births (Deering, et al., 2004). Use of a cloth perineum, available through Childbirth Graphics, will help make practice more realistic. You may also want to line the pelvis with a thin sheet of foam to better simulate the tight fit you will have to deal with in an actual shoulder dystocia.

References and Further Reading on Working with the Baby during Labor

References used in multiple chapters

Cunningham FG, et al. Williams Obstetrics, 21st ed. McGraw-Hill, New York, NY, 2001.

Daniels S. Lecture notes. The Maternity Center midwifery training program. Fall, 1978.

Davis E. Heart and Hands: A Midwife's Guide to Pregnancy and Birth, 3rd ed., rev. Celestial Arts, Berkeley CA, 1997.

Davis E. CPM. Editing notes, Feb, 2004.

El Halta V. "Preventing prolonged labor," Midwifery Today, (46);22-27, Summer, 1998.

Greenhill JP. Principles and Practice of Obstetrics, 10th ed., WB Saunders Co, Philadelphia PA, 1951.

Mayes B. A Textbook of Obstetrics, Australasian Pub, Sydney Australia, 1959.

Schlinger H. Editing notes, 2003.

Scholles H. Editing notes, 2000, 2002, 2003.

Simkin P, Ancheta R. The Labor Progress Handbook. Blackwell Sciences, London UK, 2000.

Sutton J. Let Birth Be Born Again! Rediscovering and Reclaiming Our Midwifery Heritage. Birth Concepts UK, Middlesex UK, 2001.

Sutton J, Scott P. Understanding and Teaching Optimal Foetal Positioning. Bay Print, Ltd, Tauranga NZ, 1996.

Varney H. Varney's Midwifery, 3rd ed. Jones and Bartlett Pub, Sudbury MA, 1997.

Techniques Used to Help the Baby Descend during Labor

Gaskin IM. Ina May's Guide to Childbirth, Bantam Books, New York NY, 2003.

Hendrickson F. Midwifery in 10,000 Easy Steps, Part 1: A Critical and Constructive Look at Midwifery and Obstetrics by a Birth Attendant with over 20 Years Unlicenced Experience. Privately published, Hillman MN, 1981.

King J. Back Labor No More!! What Every Woman Should Know Before Labor. Plenary Systems, Inc, Dallas TX, 1993.

Lowe C. LAc, Editing notes, 2003.

Parry D. "Reversing the Chi," Midwifery Matters, (98), Autumn 2003, accessed at www.radmid.demon.co.uk, Sept, 2004.

Trueba G. Comfort Measures for Childbirth: The Rebozo Way, The Rebozo Way, Calle 23, #40, Club de Golf, Mexicao, 14620 Mexico D F, Mexico, 2001.

Vinaver N. "Traditional Mexican midwifery techniques," Midwifery Today conf., London UK, 1996.

West Z. Acupuncture in Pregnancy and Childbirth. Churchill Livingstone, Edinburgh UK, 2001.

Assisting the Woman Whose Baby is in a Posterior Position

Gentlebirth midwifery archives. http://www.gentlebirth.org/archives/. Web site of the Midwife List, international archive of midwifery wisdom, accessed 2000.

Hamlin H. Stepping Stones to Labor Ward Diagnosis. Rigby Ltd, Adelaide Australia, 1959.

Hart G. Midwifery list, midwife@csv.warwick.ac.uk, Internet list serve communication, 1995.

Assisting a Woman Whose Baby Is in a Compound Presentation

De Lee J. Principles and Practice of Obstetrics, 7th ed. WB Saunders Co, Philadelphia PA, 1940.

McCormick M, ed. Integrated Management of Pregnancy and Childbirth: Managing Complications in Pregnancy and Childbirth: A Guide for Midwives and Doctors. Reproductive Health and Research, World Health Organization, Geneva Switzerland, 2000.

Cord Problems and Emergencies that can Occur during Labor

Alzugaray M. "The cord and the strength of life something extraordinary," Midwifery Today, 70;54-55, 58, Summer 2004.

Felch G. "Prolapsed cord: unusual management," Midwifery Today, (18);27, Summer, 1991.

Murphy D. "The mortality and morbidity associated with umbilical cord prolapse," Brit J Obstet Gynecol, 102;826-830, Oct, 1995.

O'Conner D, CNM, Seattle WA. Personal communication, Sept, 2000.

Roberts J. "Managing fetal bradycardia during second stage of labor," MCN, 14(6);394-398, Nov-Dec, 1989.

Rosenberger L. "Tricks of the trade" questionnaire, Labrys Press, [1992?].

Shoulder Dystocia

Afriat C. "Letter to the editor: the ramp maneuver," JNM, 39(6);337-338, Nov-Dec, 1994.

Alan RH, et al. "Comparing clinician-applied loads for routine, difficult and shoulder dystocia deliveries," Am J Obstet Gynecol,171(6);1621-1627, Dec, 1994.

Baer J. Chapter XXIV: "The conduct of normal labor," in Curtis A, ed. Obstetrics and Gynecology, Vol I. WB Saunders, Philadelphia PA, 1933.

Baskett T, Allen A. "Perinatal Implications of Shoulder Dystocia," Obstet Gynecol, 86(1);14, July, 1995.

Benedetti T. "Shoulder dystocia," Contemp Obstet Gynecol, 40(3);39, 1995.

Benson R. HANDBOOK OF OBSTETRICS AND GYNECOLOGY, 5th ed. Lange Medical, Los Altos CA, 1974.
Brody I, Wilkins R. "Erb's palsy," ARCH NEUROL, 21(4);442-444, Oct, 1969.
Bruner J, et al. "All-fours maneuver for reducing shoulder dystocia during labor," J REPRO MED, 43(5);439-443, 1998.
Chavis W. "A new instrument for the management of shoulder dystocia," INT J GYNECOL OBSTET, 16(4);331-332, 1979.
Claypool S, CPM. Personal conversation, 1998.
Deering S, et al. "Improving resident competency in the management of shoulder dystocia with simulation training," OBSTET GYNECOL, 103(6);1224-1228, June 2004.
De Lee J. DE LEE'S OBSTETRICS FOR NURSES, 14th ed. WB Saunders, Philadelphia PA, 1947.
Gherman R, et al. "Symphyseal separation and transient femoral neuropathy associated with the McRoberts maneuver," AM J OBSTET GYNECOL, 178(3);609-610, 1998.
Gherman R, et al. "Brachial plexus palsy: an in utero injury?" AM J OBSTET GYNECOL, 180(3);1303-1307, May, 1999.
Gibberd G, et al. THE QUEEN CHARLOTTE'S TEXT-BOOK OF OBSTETRICS, 11th ed. J & A Churchill, London UK, 1965.
Golditch IM, Kirkman K. "The large fetus: management and outcome," OBSTET GYNECOL, 52(1);26-30, July, 1978.
Gonik, et al. Objective evaluation of the shoulder dystocia phenomenon: effect of maternal pelvic orientation on force reduction," CONTEMP OBSTET GYNECOL, 27;28, 1986.
Hibbard L. "Shoulder dystocia," OBSTET GYNECOL, 34(3);424-429, Sept, 1969.
Hibbard L. "Coping with Shoulder Dystocia," CONTEMP OBSTET GYNECOL, 20(3);229-233, Sept, 1982.
Lemay G. Personal conversation, [1990?].
Litzenberg J. SYNOPSIS OF OBSTETRICS, 3rd ed. CV Mosby, St Louis MO, 1947.
Malby P, CNM. Faculty member CNM Program, OHSU, Portland, OR, conversations regarding shoulder dystocia, May, 1996.
Marshall M, Buffington S. LIFE-SAVING SKILLS MANUAL FOR MIDWIVES: MODULE 9: VACUUM EXTRACTION; MODULE 10: OTHER EMERGENCIES, 3rd ed. American College of Nurse-Midwives, Washington DC, 1998.
Mashburn J. "Identification and management of shoulder dystocia," JNM, 33(5);225, Sept-Oct, 1988.
McRoberts W. "Maneuvers for shoulder dystocia," CONTEMP OBSTET GYNECOL, 24;17, 1984.
Meenan A, et al. "A new (old) maneuver for the management of shoulder dystocia," J FAM PRAC, 32(6);625-629, June, 1991.
Morrison D."Management of Anticipated and Actual Shoulder Dystocia," MCN, 39(2S);91S-105S, Mar-Apr, 1994.
Myles M. A TEXTBOOK FOR MIDWIVES, 6th ed. E & S Livingstone, Edinburgh UK, 1968.
O'Leary J. SHOULDER DYSTOCIA AND BIRTH INJURY. McGraw-Hill, New York NY, 1992.
Parker K, CNM, Portland OR. Conversations regarding resolution of shoulder dystocia, May, 1996.
Pecorari D. "A guest editorial from abroad: meditation on a nightmare of modern midwifery: shoulder dystocia," OBSTET GYNECOL SURVEY, 54(6);353-354, June, 1999.
Penney D, Perlis D. "Shoulder dystocia: when to use suprapubic or fundal pressure," MCN, 17(1);34-36, Jan-Feb, 1992.
Pollack, RN, et al. "Obstetrical brachial palsy; pathogenesis, risk factors, and prevention," CLIN OBSTET GYNECOL, 43(2);236-246, June 2000.
Ramsey PS, et al. "Shoulder dystocia: rotational maneuvers revisited," J REPROD MED, 45(2);85-88, Feb, 2000.
Rogers S, CNM. E-mail communication, 1996.
Romoff A. "Shoulder dystocia: lessons from the past and emerging concepts," CLIN OBSTET GYNECOL 43(2);226-235, June 2000.
Rosenberger L. "Tricks of the Trade" response form (Dr. Ettinghausen's corkscrew & calling time), Labrys Press, [1992?].
Rubin A. "Management of shoulder dystocia," JAMA, 189(11);835-837, Sept 1, 1964.
Sandberg EC. "The Zavanelli maneuver: a potentially revolutionary method for the resolution of shoulder dystocia," AM J OBSTET GYNECOL, 152(4);479-484, June, 1985.
Sandberg EC. "The Zavanelli maneuver: 12 years of recorded experience," OBSTET GYNECOL, 93(2);312-317, Feb, 1999.
Scholles H, CPM. Personal communications and access to unpublished notes on inlet and outlet dystocia, Nov 8, 2001.
Simms C. E-mail communication, Midwifery list serve, Nov 19, 1995.
Spellacy W. "The Zavanelli maneuver for fetal shoulder dystocia. Three cases with poor outcomes," J REPROD MED, 47(7);543-544, July, 1995.
Spong CY, et al. "An objective definition of shoulder dystocia: prolonged head-to-body delivery intervals and/or the use of ancillary obstetric maneuvers," OBSTET GYNECOL, 86(3);433-436, 1995.
Tharpe N. Personal conversations, Nov 1, 2003; e-mail communications, Feb, 2004.
Tully G. RESOLVING SHOULDER DYSTOCIA: THE THREE R'S. Spinning Babies Workshops, 10545 Humboldt Ave So, Minneapolis MN, Privately published, 2003a.
Tully G. Conversation regarding shoulder dystocia, Oct 13, 2003b.
Walle T, Hartikainen-Sorri AL. "Obstetric shoulder injury; associated risk factors, prediction and prognosis," ACTA OBSTET GYNECOL SCAND, 72(6);450-454, Aug, 1993.
Woods C, Westbury N. "A principle of physics as applicable to shoulder dystocia," AM J OBSTET GYNECOL, 45(5);796-804, May, 1943.

ABNORMAL BLEEDING DURING LABOR

BLEEDING IN LABOR: AN OVERVIEW

Bleeding that occurs during labor is often directly related to an underlying problem that is identified during late pregnancy. Therefore this chapter will build on the information presented in the chapter in Volume I entitled "Bleeding in the Third Trimester." That chapter covers many details regarding the three primary causes of pathological bleeding that occur during late pregnancy and labor: placental abruption, placenta previa and uterine rupture.

Bleeding during labor can be benign, as with normal cervical bleeding from "show" as the cervix first starts to open and again nearing full dilation, or pathological, as described in this part of the text. Details regarding normal show are covered in the chapter entitled "Assessing and Supporting the Mother's Well-Being during Labor."

Pathological bleeding may be either painful or painless. The bleeding can manifest with three basic presentations: concealed (usually painful), in which none of the blood loss is visible; revealed (most often painless), in which all the blood being lost can be seen; and partially revealed (the woman may have some pain), in which only some of the blood loss is visible. Concealed and partially revealed blood loss, if they persist, are most likely to present with fetal compromise, followed by a degree of maternal shock that is inconsistent with the amount of observable blood loss.

Painful bleeding may be related to a partially or fully concealed abruption, uterine rupture, laceration of maternal tissues, or a hematoma. Painless bleeding may be due to normal bloody show, cervical trauma or tearing, placental abruption or placenta previa. If the membranes are ruptured, painless bleeding could originate from a concealed abruption with bleeding into the sac as well as a ruptured vasa previa, torn cord or other sources of fetal bleeding.

Assessing where the blood may be coming from

To determine your course of action, you must try to narrow down where the bleeding is coming from. To do so, review the mother's history and evaluate the situation with the following questions and examinations:

- Ask about pain, its location and character (generalized, localized, of sudden onset, increasing or absent)
- Observe the abdomen during and between contractions. Is anything unusual?
- How far along is labor? (Early, consider abruption, previa, fetal sources; later, think tissue trauma or fetal sources)
- What kind of contractions is the woman experiencing (weak, strong, continuous)? Is the character of labor appropriate for the amount of cervical dilation?
- Perform an abdominal exam.
    - Palpate the position of the baby (note lie, station and whether the baby is unusually close to the abdominal wall).
    - Is the baby moving?
    - Is the abdomen tender to the touch?
    - Is the abdominal wall ballooning anywhere? Is the fundal height rising?
    - Does the abdominal wall feel unusual (rigid, soft, spongy suprapubically)?
    - Listen to the fetal heart rate and for the location of the placenta.
- Note the characteristics of the bleeding (amount, color, clots, consistency). When does bleeding occur (with contractions, between contractions, constantly, when the mother changes position)?
- If the membranes are ruptured, note the color of the amniotic fluid. (Normal, meconium or blood stained?)
- Assess maternal vital signs; are there any abnormal findings?
- Based on your other findings, consider performing an internal exam. Look for:
    - Bleeding: are there clots in the birth canal, does the rate of bleeding change during your exam?
    - Are the membranes intact? If so, check their surface for texture and any unusual features.

The table on the following page will help you determine how to proceed.

Differentiating between blood and meconium in a specimen

To distinguish blood from meconium in stained amniotic fluid, immerse a sample of the fluid from your exam glove into a small clear glass of plain water and swish it around gently. If meconium is present, it will stain the water greenish. If it is only blood, the water will remain pink. Keep in mind that a distressed fetus may pass meconium and thus there may be a mixture of blood and meconium in the fluid. (See the chapter entitled "The Placental Membranes and Amniotic Fluid during Labor" for more information.)

DIFFERENTIAL DIAGNOSIS OF BLEEDING DURING LABOR: FINDINGS ON EXAMINATION	MAJOR CATEGORIES OF LIKELY SOURCES					
	NORMAL SHOW	PLACENTAL ABRUPTION	PLACENTA PREVIA	CERVICAL TRAUMA	UTERINE RUPTURE	PURELY FETAL SOURCES
Characteristics of contractions						
Early labor	✔	✔ (anytime)	✔ (anytime)			✔
Normal	✔		✔	✔		✔
Constant, tetanic		✔			✔ (before)	
Weak, incoordinate			✔		✔ (after)	
Strong, then suddenly cease					✔ (after)	
Observation of abdomen						
Normal during and between contractions	✔		✔	✔		✔
Uterine contour not distinct, fetal parts easily outlined					✔	
Findings on palpation						
Baby is in a nonlongitudinal lie, breech or floating			✔		✔	
Baby is not moving normally		✔	✔		✔	✔
Abdomen is tender to the touch		✔			✔	
Abdominal wall balloons, fundus rises		✔				
Abdominal wall feels rigid		✔			✔	
Suprapubic area feels spongy			✔			
Placental sounds are heard suprapubically			✔			
Fetal heart rate is compromised		✔	✔		✔	✔
Characteristics of blood loss						
Bleeding is accompanied by pain		✔		✔	✔	
Bleeding is painless	✔	✔	✔	✔		✔
Blood mixed with mucus, ropey, thick, gelatinous	✔			✔		
Intermittent	✔	✔	✔	✔		✔
Constant, increasing trickle		✔	✔	✔		
Darker with or without clots		✔		✔		✔
Bright red, with no clot or small clots			✔			
Blood does not clot normally (coagulopathy)		✔				
Bleeding occurs with contractions			✔			
Bleeding occurs between contractions		✔				
Bleeding accompanies maternal position changes	✔	✔	✔	✔		
Amniotic fluid is stained dark red		✔				✔
Maternal vital signs						
Within normal limits: no signs of shock	✔	✔	✔	✔	✔	✔
Signs and symptoms of some degree of shock		✔	✔		✔	
Internal examination						
Clots in birth canal		✔	✔	✔		✔
Fornices feel spongy			✔			
Results in an increase in bleeding			✔	✔		✔
Rough texture discovered inside dilated os			✔			✔

BLEEDING DUE TO PLACENTAL DISRUPTION

Abruption and previa are unique forms of bleeding because each can immediately compromise both mother and baby. This chapter assumes you assessed the situation as outlined in the last chapter before proceeding.

Abruption

An abruption occurs when the placenta separates from the uterine wall prior to birth, resulting in maternal bleeding, fetal hypoxia and fetal bleeding, the amount of which depends upon the damage done to the fetal side. Abruption may occur at any time during pregnancy or labor and can manifest in any of the ways discussed in Volume I. Abruption always causes maternal bleeding which may stop if the site of detachment is small. The blood clots and puts pressure on the attachment site, resulting in the formation of clots in the underlying uterine sinuses.

Varieties of abruption: Pain during contractions that is out of proportion to the degree of dilation and that persists between contractions is a classic indication of a fully concealed abruption, although even these cases may, at times, produce no pain. Concealed abruption can occur when a portion of the middle of the placenta has separated from the uterine wall, leaving only the edges still attached. Blood builds up between the maternal surface and the detached portion of the placenta, but because the edges remain attached, no blood escapes. A concealed abruption may also occur whenever the presenting part blocks the escape of blood. Both presentations result in a build-up of pressure between the uterine wall and the detached portion of placenta. Extravascular bleeding is very irritating to tissues and contributes to the pain that is characteristically present. Accumulating blood causes the uterine wall beneath the bleeding site to become distended, a condition that can cause the overlying fundus or the side of the uterus to expand, depending upon the site of implantation. The onset of pain may occur at any point during labor and may be gradual or sudden, depending upon the amount of bleeding.

The build-up of pressure from concealed bleeding may cause the membranes to rupture near the site of the abruption, especially if it is located near an edge of the placenta. Some or all of the blood will then escape directly into the bag of waters, relieving the pressure and pain and thus confusing the clinical picture. Later, when the membranes break near the os, the blood-stained waters can look like red wine, the "port wine staining" discussed in old textbooks. This is not to be confused with meconium staining, which can sometimes have a brownish appearance. (If you are unsure what is staining the fluid, see the entry entitled "Differentiating blood from meconium in a specimen" in the last chapter.)

Partially revealed abruption occurs when only a portion of the blood loss escapes, working its way down between the uterine wall and the membranes and finally the presenting part, presenting as medium bright red bleeding at the introitus. Because the escape of blood relieves some of the intrauterine pressure, partially revealed abruptions are typically not as painful. A completely revealed abruption occurs when all the blood being lost manages to escape; with no pressure build-up, there is no pain. The minimal to absent pain in these cases presents a more confusing picture, broadening the probable diagnoses to include cervical tearing, previa, a ruptured intrayoni varicosity (rare) and fetal sources such as a ruptured cord or vasa previa (bleeding from a fetal source alone will always be painless).

Prolapse of the placenta: In very rare cases, the placenta separates completely. Blood then seeps between the membranes and the uterine wall, severing the contact points between the membranes and the uterus. Once the placenta is freed of any attachment, it can drift downward, where it may even cover the internal os, producing a placenta previa secondary to premature separation. Such an occurrence is fatal to the baby (unless he is born immediately) and may be life threatening to the mother (Greenhill, 1951).

Presenting signs and symptoms: Abruption can present in all kinds of ways, meaning you must always keep it in mind when evaluating bleeding during labor. Remember that abruption is associated with increased age and multiparity, preeclampsia, chronic hypertension, cigarette smoking, poor diet, cocaine use, prior abruption and uterine leiomyomas, a form of fibroid (especially when the placenta overlies a tumor).

Characteristics of blood loss: Bleeding from an abruption is not usually thick but may be mixed with clots; it may vary in color from bright red to dark cranberry to port-wine red. The darker the blood, the older it is. It is usually not as bright as bleeding from a previa. However, do not take the dark color to mean that the risk has passed. A progressing abruption of any type will eventually cause the fetal heart rate to drop and the mother to become shocky.

Excessive blood loss, especially that which is continuous and prolonged, can cause clotting factors to become depleted due to consumptive coagulopathy, a complication that occurs in 30% women who have an abruption severe enough to kill the fetus and less commonly if the fetus survives. The mother is at serious risk for massive, unstoppable hemorrhage even if the birth can be successfully accomplished at home.

If you are remote from medical care, a significant abruption is suspected and birth is not imminent, a bedside clotting test can be performed to assess the mother's clotting status. At least 2 ml of venous blood should be placed in a small, clean, dry plain glass tube (a plain red-top will do). The tube is then held in a closed fist to warm it. After 4 minutes, the tube is tipped slowly to see if a clot is forming. It is tipped again every minute until the blood clots and the tube can be turned upside down. Failure of a clot to form after 7 minutes or the formation of only a soft clot that breaks down easily strongly suggests coagulopathy. (This summarizes a test that is discussed in more detail in the most recent edition of my DIAGNOSTIC TESTS.) Transport!

Additional evidence of an abruption: The presentation and severity of signs and symptoms other than bleeding depend upon the amount of blood the woman has lost, whether blood is trapped behind the placenta and whether she is going into shock. In a fully concealed abruption, sudden, severe abdominal pain often begins at the site of placental implantation; it starts out as a tearing sensation and then continues as a dull, tense ache. This ache is interrupted by colicky (spasmodic) pains when labor begins because the irritated uterus cannot produce coordinated contractions. If a large concealed abruption occurs suddenly, these contractions are reported by the woman to be intense and of sudden onset; she may feel she is having one constant, excruciating, tetanic contraction. Rarely, pain can be slight or absent, even in severe cases. Nausea and vomiting may accompany the pain and build-up of intrauterine pressure. Dizziness, faintness, shortness of breath, and anxiety that manifests as a feeling of oppression and fear in the upper chest may develop. The woman may yawn and sigh frequently and complain of ringing in her ears, spots before her eyes, darkening of her vision and thirst. She is going into shock. On palpation the uterus feels as hard as wood (ligneous) in 60% of all cases. In others, the uterus is only slightly tense; this is frequently found in cases of partial abruption of a low-lying placenta because blood is escaping. More rarely, the uterus feels flabby and expanded. While you might expect that a tense uterus is a reliable sign of concealed abruption, and a relaxed uterus is found in cases in which the blood can escape, the association is by no means constant. Tenseness of the abdominal wall may occur due to the presence of the underlying distended uterus. Of great diagnostic significance is the tender uterus. The woman can often tolerate only slight pressure. If the fetal heart can still be heard, the separation is only partial.

Differential diagnosis: Also consider uterine rupture, pain from surgical adhesions, embolism, bleeding from a maternal hematoma or other fetal sources as possible sources of a woman's signs and symptoms.

How abruption can effect labor: At times an abruption will irritate the uterus into activity, producing a rapid labor and birth. This is nature's way of fixing the situation.

What to do: If you suspect an abruption, how you handle it will depend on the severity of the blood loss, how far along the mother is in labor and how the baby is faring, as well as your back-up arrangements and how close you are to a hospital. It is always best to transport if there is time.

- If bleeding is heavy and it is late in labor and the mother is a multipara, you may be able to facilitate a rapid birth. This will be more difficult if the mother is a nullipara because her tissues have never stretched before.
- If bleeding is light to moderate, your response depends on the baby's status and the estimated time until birth. Again, transport is best.

If you are supporting a woman with an acute onset of a suspected abruption, follow the guidelines below as you evaluate the situation and prepare for transport:

1. Listen to the fetal heart immediately to determine if there are signs of compromise. Talk to the baby about what is going on, as he is frightened. If the fetal heart rate is concerning, transport. If not, monitor almost constantly until the baby is out or transport is complete.
2. Find the fundus and mark the height with a felt-tipped marker. This will allow you to monitor whether the fundus is rising due to concealed bleeding.
3. Check the mother's blood pressure and pulse frequently. Stay with her. Note her color, respirations and level of awareness. Ask her to report and question her frequently regarding any changes such as visual disturbances, ringing in the ears, loss of hearing, sudden fatigue, dizziness, faintness, numbness, or changes in her awareness, all of which

are signs of shock. (See the chapter entitled "Hypovolemic Shock due to Hemorrhage" for full details.)
4. Start an IV with a large bore catheter and slow the drip to keep the vein open.
5. If the baby is showing signs of compromise, give the mother oxygen by nonrebreathing mask.
6. Evaluate for increasing intrauterine pain or pressure, which indicate that the bleeding is continuing or escalating.
7. Perform an internal exam to assess the progress of labor. Check the lie of the baby. If the baby is longitudinal, rupture the membranes in the hope that contractions will become stronger. If labor is advanced, especially in a multipara, you may be able to manually dilate the cervix and have the mother push the baby out quickly. This is a good choice if both mother and baby are stable and the abruption seems to be mild enough to allow time for this.
8. If the baby is coming, be prepared to resuscitate a hypovolemic baby and to treat hemorrhage in the mother. Remember that this mother will be far less tolerant of blood loss than one who has not been bleeding during labor because her uterus is irritated and her ability to clot may be compromised. Fetomaternal blood mixing may have occurred as well.

If birth is not imminent, transport is your best and safest alternative even if both mother and baby seem to be faring well. If you are remote from medical help, manual dilation of the cervix can be used successfully in any mother, it will just take longer in a first-timer. Once the cervix is out of the way, have the mother push the baby out immediately (this will also take longer in a first-time mother). Fundal pressure may be warranted, especially if the situation is dire and the mother's efforts alone are not sufficient to get the baby out rapidly. However, a woman will get a rush of stress hormones under these circumstances and may be able to push the baby out in short order.

Prior to the birth, you may be tempted to try herbs to stop the bleeding. Because of the type of bleeding, do not expect herbs to do much, although clotting herbs may help the blood behind the placenta to coagulate and tampon off the separated area (note: I do not know this for a fact). They should not be depended upon, however, to remedy the situation. Homeopathic remedies, when properly selected, can work wonders and may temporarily stabilize the woman, buying some time. However, any such remedy should be seen only as a stopgap measure to allow safer transport or to buy a little time to get the baby out.

Transport considerations for abruption: Transport can take place in any vehicle that allows you room to monitor the vital signs of the mother and baby. However, it may be best to call an ambulance as either the maternal or fetal condition can deteriorate rapidly. The mother should be able to lie down to minimize the chance that she will go into shock before transport is complete, especially if bleeding is profuse. Prop her right hip to relieve pressure on her inferior vena cava and maximize blood flow to the placenta. Start an IV if you have one available.

Placenta previa and low-lying placenta

Painless bleeding may have a variety of origins, but placenta previa is the most difficult of all to handle if it is severe. Bleeding from a low-lying placenta, when it occurs, behaves similarly and is treated as for a tiny marginal previa.

Degrees of previa: The degree of previa will guide you as to how to handle the situation. The following drawings show ways in which the placenta may be situated. The drawings look up into the pelvis from below.

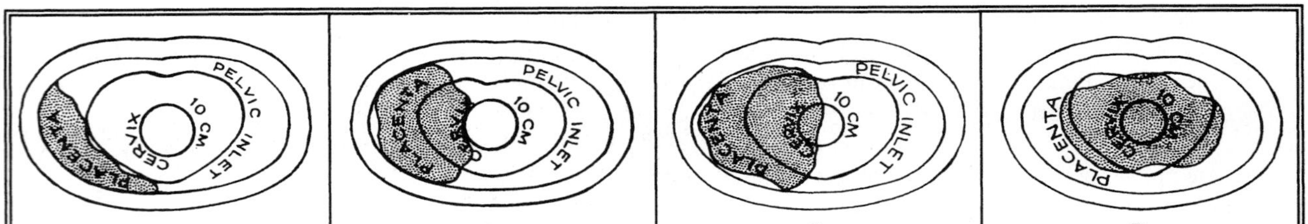

A. B. C. D.

A. The placenta is implanted high on the side of the uterine wall, well away from the pelvis.
B. A low-lying placenta is implanted in the lower uterine segment, but is not exposed even at full cervical dilation.
C. Partial placenta previa: any case where part of the internal os is covered by the placenta at complete dilation. In this case, the placenta covers 50% of the os at full dilation.
D. Total previa exists when, even at full dilation, the placenta completely covers the os.

(After Benson, 1974)

In all cases, bleeding from previa occurs because the placenta overlies the cervix. When total previa is present, placental tissue may grow part way down into the cervical canal. During late pregnancy, cervical changes and the development of the lower uterine segment cause the wall of the uterus to pull away from the placental attachment site and bleeding ensues, making previa an inevitable revealed abruption. For this reason some amount of painless bleeding, which is only rarely fatal, presents during late pregnancy in nearly all cases. Disruption of the placenta results in fetal bleeding as the cotyledons are torn and in maternal bleeding as the open sinuses underlying the placenta continue to function, causing her blood that was supplying the torn area to spill out of the os instead. Prenatal warning hemorrhages usually start and then stop spontaneously.

Once labor is underway, it is possible for the apparent degree of previa to change as labor advances. This depends upon the degree of cervical dilation at the time of examination. For example, the edge of what will later become a partial previa may extend across the entire cervical opening during early labor when the cervix is only 2 or 3 cm dilated, producing classic bright red bleeding and mimicking a complete previa. However, as the cervix opens more, the nature of the partial previa is revealed when the cervix dilates beyond the placenta's edge, uncovering normal membranes. Likewise, a low-lying placenta at 2 cm dilation may become a partial previa by 8 cm of dilation when the cervix dilates beyond its edge. The further along dilation is before the edge is revealed, the more marginal the previa. However, there is no way to tell if what appears to be a total or nearly total previa at an early dilation will turn out to be a marginal previa later on. Therefore, you should transport immediately whenever complete or a substantial marginal previa is suspected.

Total (central or complete) previa: Because of the way bleeding occurs, it is almost impossible for a woman with a total or nearly total previa to go to term and enter labor with no previous warning hemorrhages. You are most likely to encounter an unrecognized total previa during labor in a woman who presents without prenatal care. If questioned, such a woman (or her family) will probably confirm a history of prenatal bleeding episodes characteristic of previa. Since the placenta is occluding engagement, the baby may be vertex but is more likely to be breech, oblique or transverse with the presenting part floating. Bright red, painless bleeding in the presence of these other factors should raise your suspicion of previa. Do not attempt to confirm the diagnosis with invasive exams. Transport immediately.

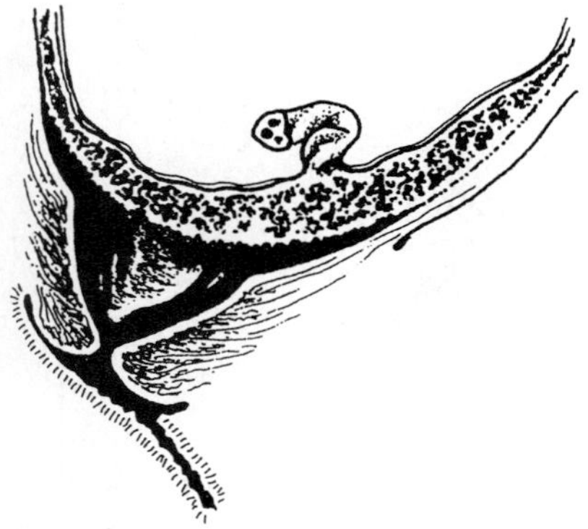

Complete previa: dilation of the internal os has already resulted in bleeding (lateral view, mother standing).

Marginal (lateral) previa: The amount of bleeding produced by a marginal previa depends upon the amount of placenta covering the os. The woman will almost always have experienced third trimester spotting or bleeding because of the changes that occur in the lower segment (Davis, 2004). However, on rare occasions, a marginal previa will not start to bleed until dilation is underway or almost complete, especially if the there is but a small sliver of the placenta involved. The baby may also be in a nonlongitudinal lie or breech presentation.

Low-lying placenta: A low-lying placenta is not technically a previa and may or may not produce bleeding prior to labor.

If you know that a woman has a previa: If a woman calls you in labor who has a confirmed previa, she will probably already be bleeding. Instruct her to go directly to the hospital, where you will meet her.

Bright red bleeding during labor: ruling out undiagnosed previa: When you have provided prenatal care, previa should have already been ruled out in any woman who has experienced painless, bright red bleeding during pregnancy. Although ultrasound is not 100% accurate, when no previa was found, you can be reasonably sure that any bright red bleeding that occurs during labor is not from a previa. It is only when bright red bleeding occurs for the first time during labor that a previa is more likely. However, since warning hemorrhages are rarely absent when previa is severe, the chances of such bleeding being due to a large previa are also quite unlikely; there is an excellent chance that any placental bleeding that occurs during labor will be from a low-lying placenta, an abruption, a ruptured marginal sinus (discussed at the end of this chapter), or a very marginal previa. The following is written with these thoughts in mind. (See recommendations after this section on how to proceed when a woman has had no prenatal care.)

Characteristics of bleeding: The more fully the placenta covers the os, the sooner in labor bleeding will commence and the more dangerous it is to remain at home. Bleeding is bright red because it is fresh. It may be mixed with clots, but these are usually small. If bleeding has been heavy, clots may cling in or near the os. Typically, the blood is more fluid (that is, free of clots) than either bloody show or blood from an abruption. It will present an increasingly heavy flow as dilation gradually tears the placenta. It is always painless because it is coming from the portion of placenta directly overlying or immediately adjacent to the os, and therefore there is no build-up of blood to cause pain. Even if bleeding is heavy, coagulopathy is exceedingly rare; apparently the thromboplastin that causes coagulopathy in abruption escapes through the os rather than being forced into the maternal circulation (Cunningham, et al., 2001).

Characteristics of contractions: Herman (1910) states that contractions are often weak in the presence of previa because direct pressure of the presenting part on the cervix is lacking. He also says that in previa, bleeding tends to occur during contractions (when stress on the placenta is greatest), whereas in an abruption the bleeding, if revealed, tends to occur between contractions (when the uterus relaxes and blood can seep past the forebag). However, because blood can pool in the yoni and come out at any time, these distinctions are not very useful clinically.

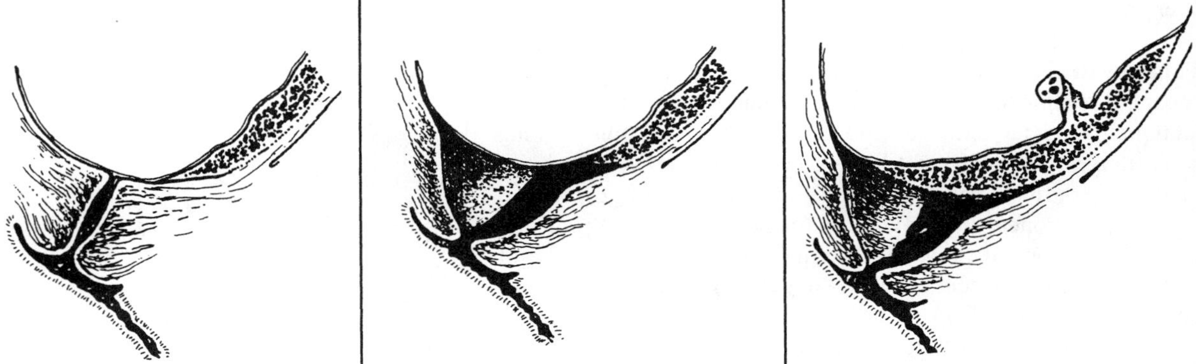

Marginal previa: prior to dilation, bleeding may not occur.

As the cervix starts to efface and the internal os dilates, a trickle begins.

Here, more of the placenta covers the os and bleeding is heavier. With this much coverage of the os, this may present as a complete previa during early dilation.

Abdominal examination: Check the fetal lie and degree of descent. A breech (16%) or nonlongitudinal lie (9%) and a high station are all associated with previa, although 70% of these babies will be vertex (Schmitz, et al., 1954). When the placenta is located anteriorly, Greenhill (1951) points out that experience can teach you to determine when something other than amniotic fluid is between the thin wall of the lower uterine segment and the presenting part without resorting to an internal exam. With practice, the thicker, more substantial but spongy anterior placenta can be differentiated from a fluctuant pocket of amniotic fluid by skilled and careful abdominal palpation, especially if the woman is thin or of average weight. Listen carefully all across the woman's belly above her pubic bone to see if you can hear placental sounds (remember to distinguish placental sounds from those of the cord or uterine artery). (Review the chapter in Volume I entitled "Fetal Heart Rate Assessment and Locating the Placenta" for more details.)

Internal exams with bright red bleeding: are they ever appropriate? Bleeding which accompanies early dilation must be taken much more seriously as cervical trauma is less likely to be the cause at this point unless severe scar tissue is present. The earlier in labor bleeding begins, the more likely a significant degree of previa exists, if previa is indeed the cause. Therefore, if your preliminary external assessments suggest a previa, it is most prudent to forego an internal exam and transport unless previa has been ruled out during pregnancy (in this case, although previa is still a small possibility, the most likely source of serious bleeding in early labor is from an abruption).

In lesser degrees of previa, prior to exposure of the placenta's edge, internal exams will reveal a normal-feeling bag of waters and cervical perimeter. A trickle of bright red blood that is not mixed with mucus is likely to appear when the edge of the placenta is finally exposed. Whenever painless bright red bleeding occurs after active labor has been ongoing for a while, the possibility of a previously unrevealed marginal previa must be kept in mind, although most such bleeding is associated with cervical or other types of tissue trauma.

If all your external assessments appear to rule out previa and you have been seeing the woman throughout her pregnancy and she has no history of painless, bright red third trimester bleeding, a careful, gentle internal exam can be performed, on the assumption that it probably isn't previa for all the reasons previously stated. (Be aware that if previa does exist, even the most gentle internal examination has been known to prompt torrential bleeding, which can be life-threatening).

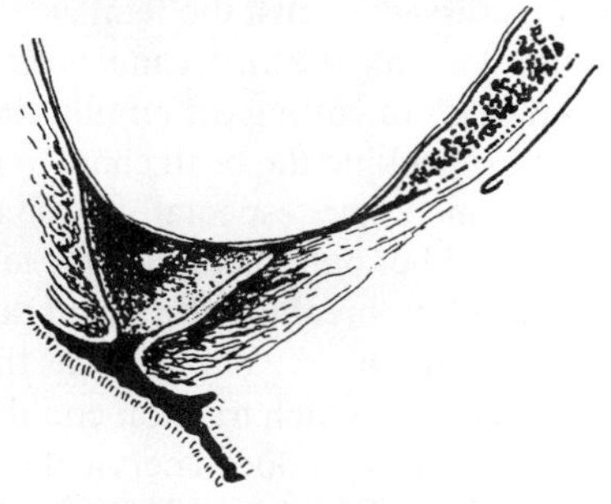

Marginal previa: here the placenta is higher and is not disrupted by early cervical changes.

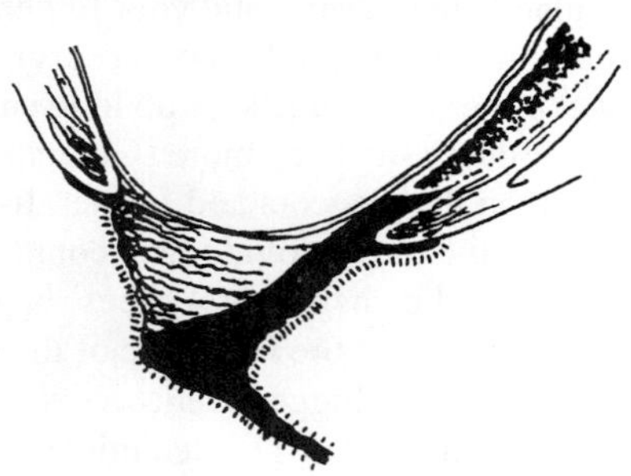

As dilation advances, the placental edge is exposed and bleeding begins.

First perform a gentle speculum exam to try and see if there are other obvious sources of bleeding (a visible cervical tear, a polyp, a ruptured maternal varicosity, etc.). If nothing unusual can be seen or if the cervix is closed and you are still fairly sure that the bleeding is not due to previa, the next step is to perform a digital exam and gently palpate the yoni fornices all the way around the cervix. If the fornices feel spongy, softer and juicier than normal, this tentatively confirms that previa, rather than abruption, may be the source of bleeding. Sponginess must be differentiated from the normal fluctuance present when the forebag is intact. If the firm head is felt through the tissue, this tentatively rules out a complete previa. If you suspect previa, withdraw your hand and transport.

If you found nothing unusual in the fornices, perform a *very gentle* digital exam within the os. Digital examination of a narrow crescent of placenta discovered late in dilation is less likely to provoke massive hemorrhage, but it could. If there is an exposed margin of placenta, you will feel a spongy, fibrous, gritty or meaty texture overlying a portion of the os. The maternal surface may feel similar to several other things such as a firm blood clot (a clot may have formed over the exposed area), thick vernix in matted hair, the exposed brain tissue of anencephaly (which may also be the source of bleeding), hemorrhage into the fetal membranes, and thickened membranes, all of which must be kept in mind. DeWees (1826) points out that the placenta always feels both fibrous and firm. He adds that introducing a finger into the mass (do *not* do so intentionally), reveals a texture that is firmer and more resistant to movement than a clot; pressing your fingertip into the placenta produces a sensation of tearing accompanied by bleeding that feels entirely different than tearing the membranes. A total lack of blood on your glove after an internal exam effectively rules out a revealed previa. In marginal previa, if the membranes are still intact, the margin of their normally smooth surface can be felt adjacent to the distinctly differently textured placental edge. If you think you are palpating placenta, do not continue to touch it.

Once sufficient dilation has occurred to expose the placental edge, the bag may break spontaneously, since there will be a pressure differential at the placental-membranous border. If it does not, before you remove your hand, thoroughly palpate the surface of the intact membranes to rule out vasa previa before deciding your course of action, because there is an increased risk of vasa previa with a low-lying placenta.

Problems of and historical perspectives on handling placenta previa: Before surgical birth was as relatively safe as it is today, placenta previa presented one of the most formidable complications in all of obstetrics. There have been many scary options proposed throughout the centuries to manage previa. In all cases, the goal was to stop or slow the bleeding, usually via compression, while awaiting cervical dilation and spontaneous birth.

Unlike most other complications, just about anything that might help often only makes the situation worse. The cervix and lower uterine segment are highly vascularized and extremely friable when the placenta is implanted over them, rendering the tissue as fragile as wet blotting paper. This means *any* manipulation of maternal tissues, including any attempt to enter the uterus, no matter how careful, is likely to shred the cervix, with tears extending into the lower segment. This rules out internal version and extraction as well as manual separation of the placenta prior to birth, both of which have been tried in the past, often with disastrous consequences. Repeated prenatal warning hemorrhages or continuous bleeding left women ill prepared for the trauma and additional bleeding they would experience during labor, birth and postpartum. In fact, in decades past, maternal death from lacerations and associated blood loss was the primary killer, even more so than bleeding from the placental site (Eastman, 1950).

During labor, digital compression of the edge of the placenta has been used for the temporary control of bleeding, but it requires prodding around to find the edge, breaking the membranes and pinching the edge of the placenta between your thumb, which is placed in a fornix, and your fingers, which are pressed against the fetal side of the placenta. This risks tissue damage, hemorrhage and, if the mother survives, infection. Packing the birth canal with sterile gauze has been used as well. However, either technique kept up long enough runs the risk of cutting off circulation to the cervix, which increases the friability of the tissue even more (Greenhill, 1960). Plus, packing the birth canal to produce compression from below may push up on the placenta and further disrupt the attachment site, especially if the membranes are intact and there is nothing filling the os to provide firm counterpressure. A rubber balloon device the size of the baby's head (called a metreurynter, De Ribes bag or Voorhees' bag) was also used by breaking the membranes and inserting the deflated bag through the os against the fetal side of the placenta, below the head. The bag was then gradually inflated with antiseptic solution so that it plugged the lower segment. It had a tail to which traction could be applied to tampon off the placenta and control bleeding. This technique worked but frequently produced cervical tears, sometimes failed to dilate the cervix completely and often resulted in postpartum infection (Greenhill, 1960).

From the 1800s to 1925, the most consistent recommendation was the Braxton Hicks procedure which involved rupturing the membranes, reaching up through or past the edge of the placenta, performing internal version if necessary, bringing down a foot and attaching a 1 to 2 lb weight to it to compress the fetus against the placenta. In 1925, Willett introduced the use of a de Martell surgical scalp forceps (later, a modified design bore Willett's name, however neither tool is available today), to apply traction to the forecoming head by grasping a fold of the fetal scalp. A cord and a weight were attached to the handle of the instrument. This eliminated the need for internal version when the baby was vertex and, in many cases, was successful at saving the mother and sometimes the baby. This was the best option available up until about 1950 (when surgical birth began to be resorted to more and more) and was used as late as 1975 for marginal cases (Willson et al., 1975). It does involve entering the os, but does not involve manipulating maternal tissues very much, although it may aggravate the bleeding until the forceps is in place. It also risks, at the very least, fetal scalp sloughing, which occurred in at least one-third of babies subjected to this treatment (Eastman, 1950).

In the absence of surgery, attempting to save the mother means letting go of any goal of saving the baby. Therefore, early on, measures were often taken as soon as previa was identified for fear the bleeding would not stop. However, acting prior to term, before the cervix is ready to dilate resulted in terrible maternal damage. Later, viability was awaited if the mother's condition allowed it. However, even if the woman was near term, the baby's condition could not be taken into account *because haste can be deadly with a previa.* If fetal distress developed and delivery was forced with manual dilation, with internal version and extraction, with an attempt to augment labor, or with aggressive fundal pressure, tearing of the cervix and overlying placenta resulted in torrential bleeding, typically killing the baby anyway. Cervical tears, which often extended into the lower uterine segment, bladder or peritoneal cavity, were hard to reach and very difficult to repair because the vascularized tissue is so friable. Meanwhile, the woman was likely to bleed to death.

Once the baby is born, the danger is far from over. The lower segment and the region surrounding the os are not well suited to placental implantation. Therefore, the more central the previa, the thinner and larger the placenta tends to be with a correspondingly larger site of implantation. This results in a large detachment site when the placenta separates after birth. Because of the poor contractility of the lower segment, placental detachment may not occur quickly or easily. Unfortunately, manual removal of the placenta poses the same risks as internal version. In addition, the lower segment is relatively poorly supplied with ligating muscle fibers. This results in inadequate contraction of the open maternal sinuses underlying the implantation site. Both increase the likelihood of severe postpartum hemorrhage that is difficult to control. If the woman did not die during labor, she was very likely to do so after the birth.

<u>If you are in an urban setting: what you can do at home</u>

Talk to the parents and the baby: Thoroughly discuss the risks and options (if previa appears to be very marginal) the parents. Talk to the baby. Placenta previa is a terrifying circumstance for the baby as his source of survival is blocking his way out.

Transport considerations: If vasa previa is discovered or if more than 30% of the cervical opening is covered by placenta (i.e, it is discovered prior to 7 cm dilation), transport immediately. Start an IV. Call an ambulance. Do not perform any (or any more) internal exams. Continuously monitor the fetal heart rate and the mother's vital signs. Get to the hospital as quickly as possible. Even if bleeding is not significant, if you suspect previa, do not delay. Advancing dilation and stronger contractions will inevitably result in more bleeding as long as a portion of the parenchyma is exposed within the opening of the os. The fetus is bleeding too and he has relatively little blood to lose.

Proceeding at home with a small marginal previa: The further along dilation is when the edge of the placenta is exposed, the more likely it is that rupture of membranes will cause the placenta to withdraw from the edge of the os as the placenta follows the retracting uterine wall upward. Rupturing the membranes works particularly well in multiparas. While compression from above may impair some blood flow to the baby with a small marginal previa this is usually not a problem and birth can often proceed without further difficulty since most of the placenta is still functioning normally.

Determine the fetal lie and position and correct the fetal lie with external version if necessary. Go through all the steps previously outlined to assess if previa is present. If you confirm a marginal previa and bleeding is not heavy, once vasa previa is ruled out, the bag should be broken away from the placental edge to avoid damaging it. Take care not to push up on the membranes, as this may result in disrupting adjacent placental tissue, prompting more bleeding. To avoid this, Greenhill (1960) recommends grasping a pinch of membranes with a hemostat and cutting a hole in them. An amnio-cot would probably work as well. In this case, place the amnio-cot on your ring finger and cup it in your palm so you can use your index finger for palpation. Rupturing the membranes will relieve tension on the edge of the placenta. The presenting part drops down, compressing the lower border of the placenta against the uterine wall, the bleeding stops or decreases to the point that it is not alarming and birth can proceed. Fundal pressure can be used momentarily to seat the baby against the placenta, if necessary (do not use it continuously). Greenhill states that this often works well for partial previa.

Do not manipulate the cervix at all and await full dilation. Monitor the baby's heart rate carefully. If fetal distress develops, transport rather than try to resolve the situation. Do not try to augment labor. Start an IV before pushing begins if bleeding was heavy prior to breaking the water. Be prepared for heavy postpartum bleeding and a distressed, hypovolemic baby. Give the mother IM oxytocin after birth and give her 0.2 mg of Methergine IM immediately after the placenta is out if bleeding is not controlled. Women who have a previa are at high risk for all types of placenta accreta, especially if they have had a previous surgical birth. These women and their babies are also at risk for fetomaternal transfusion.

When the placenta is obstructing more than 30% of the os, rupture of membranes may work by itself to slow or stop the bleeding, but it may not, and fetal distress is much more likely to occur.

If you are remote from medical help: A midwife extremely remote from medical help who is confronted with yoni bleeding must ask the mother and family about bleeding episodes during pregnancy. If there is a history of painless, bright-red bleeding, you must assume the woman has a previa. If you are confronted with a woman with profuse bright red bleeding, the recommended course of action is to *forgo an internal exam if maternal history or external evidence leads you to suspect previa.* Initial and even subsequent episodes of bleeding are rarely, if ever, fatal as long as internal manipulation is not performed and transport can occur in a reasonable time frame (Eastman, 1950). Make urgent plans to get to the hospital as soon as possible. Round up healthy friends and relatives to provide blood for transfusion. Start an IV and bring your oxygen equipment with you. Send people out to look for a vehicle to use. Monitor maternal and fetal vital signs en route. These are the steps universally recommended for midwives, regardless of how remote you may be from medical assistance.

Upon researching how to deal with previa, all the books for traditional midwives working in the developing world assume that they are within a reasonable distance from some type of hospital care and that they have access to a vehicle. I know this is not always the case (Davis-Floyd, 2003), but the world-wide standard of care does not acknowledge this and thus there is no provision for this situation. They assume that a "competent" midwife will always transport, ignoring that this may be physically impossible due to impassible roads, lack of a vehicle, inability to get fuel, severe weather, war, natural disasters or other interfering factors. Otherwise, they apparently expect the midwife to stand by and await delivery as the mother pours out blood, based on the assumption that anything you do will likely make the situation worse, at least temporarily. While uterine packing or attaching a forceps to the fetal scalp are both within the capabilities of midwives, they are not recommended. This is probably in part because the tissues of malnourished women will be even more friable than those of a well-nourished western woman, so if the previa alone doesn't kill them, trying to do something may. However, I know midwives, and few will stand by while a woman is bleeding to death. For those horrible circumstances, the following suggestions are offered to help the midwife understand the relative risks of various options and how she might most safely (relatively speaking) proceed if feels she must do *something*.

Possible options if transport is literally impossible: If you do decide to proceed with any of these options, you are on your own. They are included for the purpose of ethical discussion in midwifery schools. As well, there may be local jurisdictions who would support midwives to act in desperate situations if some kind of protocol was outlined in a contemporary text. Most of the techniques described below were standard procedures for many decades prior to 1960, when they were performed in an operating room so that a surgical birth could be done immediately if massive hemorrhage ensued. You will be working without that safety net. One of the guiding principles of care is to save maternal blood, and you will have no access to blood transfusion, making the risks of intervention that much more greater.

If you do decide to proceed, work fast, as bleeding may be profuse and unstoppable until sufficient pressure is applied to the placenta. Be exquisitely gentle, to avoid tearing the mother. *You must ignore the condition of the baby to give the mother the best chance of survival* (see reasons previously stated). Begin by starting an IV, if one is available, and leave it in place until the woman is stable after birth. Talk to the baby, who is terrified at this point. Explain that you are trying to save her mother's life and his as well, but that he may have to leave before birth (there is no point in lying to the baby).

If it is a complete or nearly complete previa: This is what you are likely to be dealing with if massive hemorrhage is occurring during early labor. All options pose high risks for both mother and baby and all have significant drawbacks. See if any of the following make sense under the circumstances:

- If it is a complete previa, or nearly so and the cervix is not very dilated, one of the least invasive ways to compress the placenta is to pack the birth canal firmly with a continuous strip of sterile gauze bandaging (a clean receiving blanket can also work if torn into strips or twisted and inserted). Have an assistant help you feed the strip into the yoni while you make sure that the upper canal is firmly packed. This option may buy some time if transport can be accomplished, but is expected to take a long time. Only do this if bleeding is heavy, as you probably should not remove the packing once it is in place because doing so will disrupt any clots that may form (the historical literature was silent on this point). Be careful not to push the packing through the fragile lower segment. Packing will provide some compression and may slow the bleeding, although not as efficiently as when the membranes are ruptured or when compression is applied from above. The chief dangers are blood building up behind the gauze, masking the amount of bleeding taking place, tissue damage, and infection if the mother survives. Transport must take place right away.
- If the cervix is sufficiently dilated, feel around the rim for a region of normal membranes. If you can find one, rupture the membranes, following the instructions previously given. This is likely to at least slow the bleeding. If the bleeding does not stop, attach a counterweight to the baby if she is vertex (see below).
- If the cervix is fully dilated, traditional Mexican midwives who practice in remote locations used to push the placenta aside to allow the baby to pass before they were as regulated as they are now (Davis-Floyd, 2003). Although this does risk tearing the cervix, the one I spoke with said she never had a problem she could not handle when she did this and never lost a mother or baby. She ruptured the membranes and inserted her fingers past the edge of the placenta. She then applied pressure to the fetal side of the placenta by cupping the palm-side of her hand over it to keep it out of the way as the baby passed. Once the baby was descending, she slowly withdrew her hand. This would only be necessary if the previa was so large as to impede descent.

These techniques disrupt the placenta but will hopefully spare the cervix from trauma and slow the bleeding, conserving the mother's blood. If you manage to find a normal region of membranes and can break the waters but bleeding continues, then consider the following:

If the baby is vertex: If breaking the bag does not stop the bleeding and she is at least a few centimeters dilated, a forceps can be attached to the fetal scalp (this technique was not used by some for first-time mothers, but the literature does not say why, perhaps because tearing was more likely with the previously undilated parts). Willett's forceps (which had grasping bars .5 in [1.25 cm] long with rounded teeth) is no longer manufactured, but Greenhill (1960) says that one heavy or two regular uterine Vulsellum forceps will also work (Teale Vulsellum forceps [Miltex part no. 30-997] may be suitable as they are heavy and have relatively atraumatic teeth). Have someone apply fundal pressure to bring the head in close contact with the os. Insert one hand into the yoni and use it to guide the tip of the instrument as you insert it with your other hand. Have an assistant apply fundal pressure to bring the head down against the cervix as you guide the tip of the instrument to the baby' head. Separate the jaws and, pressing the tips against the scalp, close them, thus grasping a fold of scalp. The grip obtained depends somewhat upon the degree of dilation. It is superficial and never produces a fold that bulges below the jaws. Clamp the rachet completely and tie a cord with the weight attached to the handles.

If you have lighter forceps, first make a whipple-bar by carving three indentations along the edge of an adult tongue depressor; one at each end and one in the middle. Attach the two forceps in the same manner as already described, spacing them evenly in the same area of scalp. Then tie the handles of the instruments to two cords and tie the cords to the around the indented places on either end of the tongue depressor. Tie a third cord over the center indentation and attach a 1 lb weight to it. This equalizes the tension on each forceps. (2 cups of water weighs 1 lb, 1 oz. [495 grams], so a 500 ml bag of IV solution would work.) Once all is in place, the weight hangs over the edge of the bed to apply light traction.

The scalp stretches rapidly at first, and the forceps descend rather quickly, giving the impression of that the head is descending rapidly as well, so take care not to remove the forceps too soon. Do a one-finger digital exam to assess the level of the skull to be sure what is occurring. The use of Willet's technique may result in sloughing or tearing of the scalp or a hematoma, but was successful in achieving a live birth in many cases.

Nothing further is done until the head has descended well into the birth canal, when the forceps are removed and the woman pushes the baby out without further interference.

If the baby is breech: Rupture the membranes. If a leg is presenting or if one can be easily reached at the os (without resorting to sticking your hand inside the cervix), *slowly and gently* bring it down past the placenta until the baby's bottom is well applied to the cervix. This is much more dangerous for the mother because of the stresses brought to bear on her soft parts as you bring the leg down. One little jab from a knee or a foot could rip the fragile cervix. Once the leg is down, tie a rope to the ankle using a clove hitch (for details, see the chapter entitled "The Use of Version during Labor") and attach a 1 lb weight to the rope. If you cannot easily reach a leg, have someone apply only enough fundal pressure to compress the breech against the inner os to help slow the bleeding.

If the baby is transverse: Perform gentle external version to get the baby into a longitudinal lie and rupture the membranes. Do not attempt internal version. Use fundal pressure to seat the presenting part against the cervix.

Regardless of whether you decide to intervene or not, continue to make every effort to get the woman to a medical facility as soon as you can.

The birth and postpartum watch: Even with a total previa, it is possible for a woman to achieve full dilation. Allow the birth to proceed spontaneously, preferably without forceful pushing. Have the mother give birth on her side so she will be lying down as the baby is born, a precaution related to the high risk of shock. The placenta may be born before the baby. Bleeding will be profuse and the baby may be dead. Be prepared for a massive hemorrhage. Give oxytocin as the body is born and allow the placenta to deliver spontaneously whenever possible. If the placenta does not come quickly enough given the amount of bleeding, give another injection of oxytocin. If you must, manually remove it, but take great care so as not to poke a hole through the fragile lower uterine segment. Once the placenta is born, administer a 1 ml ampule (0.2 mg) of Methergine IM and stay with the mother for at least the first 6 hours postpartum if you live close by and at least overnight if you don't. Monitor her constantly for bleeding. Leave her with additional tablets of Methergine to take over the first days postpartum and visit her the next day. This woman is at increased risk for infection and her baby, if he lives, is at great risk of brain damage (Greenhill, 1960). Get them to medical help as soon as possible so the mother can be evaluated for tissue damage and both can receive a transfusion, which they are likely to need if they survive.

Rupture of a marginal placental sinus

Here a small blood vessel along the edge of the placenta breaks prenatally or during labor when the membranes overlying it stretch or break. Painless, bright red bleeding, which is sometimes profuse, may occur, but does not recur as often as it does with a previa. If significant bleeding persists and the mother is not close to birth, transport. Birth may proceed without discovery of the source of the bleeding, except afterward, when the broken vessel containing soft, jelly-like nonadherent thrombi is found. This bleeding would be primarily or exclusively fetal in origin and therefore places the baby at grave risk for hypoxia and hypovolemia.

Bleeding due to Maternal Tissue Damage

Cervical tearing or detachment

The cervix can tear when there is a history of previous cervical scarring, when it is unusually rigid, when a lip is dragged down with the presenting part, when it is diseased, or when it is manipulated. Usually such tearing occurs during active labor, is relatively minor and does not extend. It can, however, produce a rather concerning amount of thick blood that is more than ordinary show. Neither the baby nor the mother will present with any compromised vital signs, and only rarely does such a tear extend into the lower uterine segment. The irregularity in the os where the tear is located may at times be felt on internal exam, thus presumptively confirming the diagnosis. There is nothing to be done during labor except taking care to avoid extension of the tear. To avoid further damage, the tear should be carefully monitored to make sure it isn't extending during any cervical manipulation deemed necessary after the tear is discovered. The cervix should be gently examined after the birth to confirm that a large tear is not present. If it is, transport for repair should occur as soon as possible.

Cervical detachment is a rare complication usually associated with a history of strong contractions in a first-time mother with a very thin, rigid cervix that goes unrecognized or that does not respond to therapy. Suddenly, labor progresses rapidly to birth and a fragment or complete ring of tissue is passed either before or after the baby. Detachment can result in tears that extend into the lower uterine segment. Bleeding from the site of detachment is usually not copious because of the associated necrosis. Examine with this in mind and transport as above if detachment is confirmed. See the chapter entitled "Cervical and Other Soft-Tissue Problems during Labor" for additional information.

Ruptured intrayoni or cervical varicosity

On rare occasions, a maternal varicose vein of the cervix or yoni will rupture during labor, giving rise to dark red bleeding similar to that seen with cervical tearing. Women who have external varicosities of their genitals or legs are the ones most likely to have internal varicosities, although the two can occur independently, and many women who have external varicosities do not have internal ones. Engorged varicose veins feel like fat worms or soft bumps in the tissue. Other sources of bleeding should first be ruled out (the fetal heart rate will remain normal if the blood is not from a fetal source). There is not much that can be done about this complication in labor. The pressure from the descending baby is likely to slow and eventually stop the bleeding, at least temporarily, so giving birth at home is not necessarily contraindicated. Once the pressure is off, however, bleeding may recur. The woman should be carefully monitored for hematoma formation. If bleeding from the vein continues or a hematoma is suspected, transport for repair is indicated.

Hematoma

A hematoma is bleeding under the tissues, often due to a ruptured blood vessel. Hematomas generally develop gradually over the hours postpartum, after all intrapelvic pressure has been relieved with the birth of the baby. However, if a woman, especially one with varicosities, experiences increasing pain and tenderness and a sensation of pressure that begins locally and then spreads, or reports rectal, yoni or perineal pain or pain down her leg a few hours after birth, a hematoma could be the cause. Uterine rupture is another possibility. It is always prudent to transport when the source of unusual pain during labor cannot be confirmed. There will be no way to tell if a hematoma is forming during labor, although changes in fetal and maternal vital signs may suggest that internal bleeding is occurring.

Uterine rupture

Uterine rupture may or may not result in visible yoni bleeding. See the next chapter for more details.

Placenta percreta

Placenta percreta occurs when the placenta grows through the uterine wall and, sometimes, into the bladder wall as well. When percreta occurs in a low-lying placenta, the villia can become ingrown into the bladder wall, in which case it will present with bloody urine. It may thus accompany placenta previa as well. While in most cases bloody urine will become apparent prenatally, it is conceivable for the changing tissue dynamics to result in bleeding from the bladder for the first time during labor, with the sudden appearance of bloody urine heralding this rare form of previa. Predisposing factors include lower segment uterine surgery closed with a single layer of sutures. Blood from the yoni can be differentiated from blood from the bladder by testing a clean-catch urine specimen. If placenta percreta is suspected, transport immediately.

UTERINE RUPTURE DURING LABOR

The chapter builds on information provided in the chapter in Volume I entitled "Scar Dehiscence and Uterine Rupture in the Third Trimester," which includes full details regarding uterine rupture and how it can present during late pregnancy. These details also apply during labor. In-depth information will be covered in the chapter entitled "Hypovolemic Shock due to Hemorrhage" in this text.

Causes of Uterine Rupture

Uterine rupture that occurs during labor is usually associated with:

- Traumatic causes (listed later in this chapter)
- Improper use of uterine stimulant drugs, even in first-time mothers
- Grand multiparity coupled with prolonged labor or inappropriate uterine stimulation
- Neglected obstructed labor due to
  - Absolute cephalopelvic disproportion
  - Nonlongitudinal fetal lie
  - Extended cephalic presentation that is not progressing
  - Fetal deformities such as hydrocephalus
  - Shoulder dystocia
  - Obstruction of the soft parts by maternal tumors, atresia of the cervix or yoni, etc.
- Uterine abnormalities
- Intense, spontaneous uterine contractions
- Extremely pendulous abdomen
- Infusion of fluids intra-amniotically (amnioinfusion)
- Uterine overdistension from hydramnios or multiple pregnancy
- Sacculation of the entrapped, retroverted uterus

While some of these risks are discussed elsewhere in this text, a few bear discussion here.

Grand multiparity (5+ term babies): This is a risk because the uterus becomes more stretched after every pregnancy. Overall, the uterine wall cannot endure as much strain or manual manipulation as the uterus of a woman who has had fewer children. In general, uterine rupture in the grand multipara occurs with artificial stimulation of the uterus with drugs or with internal manipulations.

Uterine abnormalities: Congenital abnormalities of the uterus (a septum, uterine horn or other defects) can leave portions of the uterine wall poorly suited for placental implantation or the stress of labor contractions. Rupture may result from thinning of the muscle layer to the point that the force of labor contractions may exceed its tolerance, or from uneven distribution of the endometrium, leading to excessively deep implantation of the placenta. Both conditions weaken the uterine wall.

Extremely pendulous abdomen: This condition is usually associated with grand multiparity. The uterus hangs far forward during the pregnancy, stretching the posterior yoni wall. Progress is obstructed when labor begins because the head is not centered over the pelvic cavity. Contractions stretch and thin the cervix and lower uterine segment. The resulting tension eventually produces a lesion in the region of the posterior fornix and lowermost uterine segment; this lesion is referred to as a colporrhexis. Unless the force of the contractions can lift the uterus and baby into position over the pelvic brim with only a moderate amount of effort, the weakest point will give way, becoming the site of rupture. Supporting a pendulous abdomen can prevent this type of rupture, as well as lift the baby into a better position, which can greatly facilitate labor.

Spontaneous rupture of the normal, unscarred uterus

Throughout labor, the upper uterine segment retracts and becomes increasingly thicker while the lower uterine segment and cervix are stretched and thinned. The boundary of the upper and lower segments is referred to as the retraction ring. The sacrouterine ligaments stabilize the cervix in the pelvis posteriorly, the bases of the broad ligaments stabilize the cervix on either side and the connective tissue at the base of the bladder anchors it anteriorly. These connective tissues prevent fundal retraction from pulling the lower segment up with it. Instead, during normal labor, contractions take up the slack and then thin in the lower uterine segment and cervix and pull up on upper walls of the yoni, causing these tissues to move over and above the presenting part as it moves down, even while the cervix remains anchored laterally.

If descent is obstructed from below, the upper segment continues to retract in an effort to move the baby down. The fundus may become up to 4 cm thick while the lower segment thins to but a few millimeters. At this point, several types of rupture may occur. If the cervix is rigid and cannot dilate and retract, the lower uterine segment will become stretched dangerously thin. A transverse tear may form across the junction of the cervix and lower segment. If the cervix is dilated, it will continue to retract upward with the lower segment, but it can only be pulled so far because of its anchoring ligaments. When the pulling exceeds the ability of the lower segment to stretch, rupture occurs. Rupture of the lower segment is usually longitudinal or oblique while a fundal rupture is usually transverse. The tear is usually longitudinal if it occurs adjacent to a broad ligament. A tear that begins in the lower segment may extend upward toward the fundus or downward to involve the cervix, upper yoni or even the bladder in some cases.

These same events are most likely to prompt catastrophic rupture of the normal but scarred uterus, which is more vulnerable and may give way with less stress, especially if it is hyperstimulated with drugs. The rupture of a normal, unscarred uterus in a primigravida experiencing spontaneous progressive labor without the use of uterine-stimulating drugs is such an exceedingly rare event that, should it occur, the question of whether the woman underwent a previous, undisclosed pregnancy, uterine surgery or abortion complicated by damage to the uterine wall should be investigated.

Traumatic uterine rupture

Traumatic rupture that occurs during labor is usually a result of:

- Separation of a previous surgical incision involving the myometrium
- Extension of a cervical tear into the lower uterine segment
- Normal labor in the presence of diseased or abnormal uterine tissues or anatomy, including:
  - Pregnancy in an abnormal region of uterine anatomy, such as a uterine horn
  - Gestational trophoblastic neoplasia (cancer)
  - Adenomyosis (a benign invasion of myometrium by endometrial tissue)
  - Placenta increta or percreta
- Ill-advised or poorly performed invasive procedures such as version and extraction
- Difficult instrumental delivery
- Forceful breech extraction
- Destructive operations on the fetus
- Excessive fundal pressure
- Aggressive manual dilation of the cervix
- Difficult manual removal of the placenta

Most commonly, uterine rupture occurs when the uterus is scarred from previous surgery or injury. Dehiscence of a scar is just as likely to occur in later pregnancy as during labor; thus it is covered in Volume I.

Traumatic rupture of the normal uterus is almost always associated with improper invasive manipulations or neglectful midwifery care. Every midwife should be able to distinguish a slow labor from an obstructed one and should be able to judiciously use interventions that she deems are indicated to resolve the problem at hand. She should know when the risks of such interventions are likely to outweigh the benefits and when to transport rather than risk maternal trauma and injury.

The cause and effect of rupture that results from manual manipulations may be apparent, but recognition of the problem is sometimes delayed. Manual dilation of the cervix can produce a tear that extends upward into the lower segment. Internal manipulations can overtax the lower segment when it is already stretched to the limit. Excessive fundal pressure may not be able to overcome an obstruction and may cause the lower segment to give way.

Unrecognized placental problems can produce a traumatic rupture over the site of implantation as the uterus goes about the normal work of labor. Such a rupture is most likely to be mistaken for an abruption and will have similar symptoms, although parts of the baby may be extruded into the abdomen though the tear in the uterus.

Preventing uterine rupture

Understanding the causes, signs and symptoms of obstructed labor and threatened uterine rupture is the most important key to its prevention. Careful monitoring of the fetal heart rate in a woman known to have a uterine scar is important. Transport without delay if you suspect that the uterus is threatening to rupture. Attempting to reposition a baby, even with maternal activities and position changes, is dangerous once an existing scar starts to give way, as well as when obstructed labor has become established, because the uterus may already be dangerously thinned. The uterus may not be able to stand the strain and could rupture at any moment. Transport is essential.

Hopefully, obstructed labor will be detected long before rupture is imminent, and there will be time to address the problem and turn things around. However, a midwife working in the developing world may be faced with a situation in which concerned family members bring her to the bedside of a woman who is in established obstructed labor. The midwife's job is to assess the situation and transport whenever possible to get the help the woman needs.

Transport considerations:

During transport, the jolting over rough roads that can occur in rural locations can actually precipitate a threatened rupture if the thinned and painful lower segment cannot withstand the strain of being tossed about. To prevent this, the mother's abdomen can either be wrapped with a binder padded with a layer or two of towels or the uterus can be held as steady as possible by someone who is assisting during transport. The driver should be advised of the situation and asked to drive as carefully as possible, avoiding potholes whenever he can.

Detecting catastrophic uterine rupture during labor

Typical signs in labor: Spontaneous rupture of the uterus can occur at the beginning of early labor with intact membranes, although this is exceedingly rare. Rupture is typically preceded by a long or very intense labor, accompanied by strong contractions with no fetal descent. Alternately, it occurs when a woman receives injudicious augmentation of her contractions with drugs in the hospital. When labor is obstructed, early rupture of membranes may be accompanied by an enlarging caput on the presenting part.

Threatened catastrophic rupture: Changes in the fetal heart rate are often the earliest sign that the uterus is being stressed to the point of rupture. Abnormal fetal heart rate patterns include isolated, prolonged decelerations and repetitive, deep variable decelerations in active labor, although no one specific pattern is indicative. The woman may experience a sudden drop in blood pressure to one-third its previous level or she may have an unaccountable sudden and marked elevation of her pulse rate.

If rupture is threatening as a result of obstructed labor, abdominal palpation may reveal a hard uterus that is drawn up over the baby. The baby will be contained almost entirely in the lower uterine segment. The upper segment will be thick and hypertonic while the lower segment will be soft. The lower segment tends to balloon outward during contractions, causing the outline of the baby's body to be dramatically distinct and the fetus to appear as if she lies directly under the skin. The entire abdomen and especially the lower segment will be exquisitely tender to the touch. An oblique groove, sometimes visible, can be palpated across the abdomen; this groove can either be the pathologic retraction ring or the upper border of the bladder. The round ligaments are tender, hard and wiry, especially the one that is under the greatest tension. Internal exam will reveal that the cervix is either trapped and swollen under the presenting part or drawn up and out of the pelvis, and the yoni may be stretched taut and feel hot and dry due to impaired pelvic circulation.

Impending rupture: The woman may become restless and anxious or may complain that her suprapubic area is sore as rupture approaches. She may reach to support this area during contractions. Her face may become red, her mouth and tongue dry, and she may have the urge to urinate frequently. She may feel an urge to bear down with contractions. Her temperature may be slightly elevated, her respirations rapid and irregular, and her pulse fast. Brief periods of loss of consciousness probably mean that slight tearing has already begun. The development of constant pain should also prompt the suspicion of abruption, especially in a woman known to have an unscarred uterus and no evidence of obstructed labor, as many of the symptoms are the same.

Detecting actual rupture: Suddenly, at the height of a contraction, the woman may report a sharp tearing or shooting pain has occurred in her lower abdomen, that something has given way or burst inside her or that something is simply not right, although not all women cry out, nor is a sharp pain always felt. At this point, the woman may experience a fleeting sense of relief and the disappearance of any back pain. This will be rapidly followed by a draining of color from her face due to shock and internal bleeding. Her lips will turn white, her features will sink in, a cold sweat will break out on her nose and forehead, her temperature will drop, and her pulse become weak and thready and her respirations sighing. The contractions may stop and the woman become quiet. *When uterine contractions suddenly cease in a woman with a uterine scar, uterine rupture must always be ruled out.* In complete rupture, strong contractions tend to stop suddenly. If the rupture is incomplete, contractions tend to gradually fade away. Any "contractions" she does feel change from those of normal labor to cramps that are more abdominal in character. While abdominal rigidity and tenderness are the rule, on rare occasions the abdomen may become soft. The woman may complain of shortness of breath, labored heart rate, and a feeling of impending doom. Shortly, she may become restless again and may start to vomit, but vomiting usually does not occur until later. If amniotic fluid or blood has spilled into the peritoneal cavity, there may be a dull shifting sensation on palpation or movement as the fluid moves freely in her belly.

Yoni bleeding can appear, although it is often not excessive and may be only slight. The amount of bleeding will depend, in part, on how the baby's body is positioned and whether the baby's weight is applying counterpressure to the site of rupture, or blocking the escape of blood via the yoni, as well as into what region of the body the blood is flowing (uterus, retroperitoneum, etc). More important, the amount of bleeding will depend on the size and location of the tear; lower segment tears that do not involve the base of the broad ligament result in less bleeding than those in the fundus.

Bleeding that distends a broad ligament can cause pain that is felt down one leg. Blood is likely to appear in the urine if the uterine tear extends into the bladder (placenta percreta will also present with blood in the urine); this may or may not appear at the introitus as a scant to moderate flow. Free bleeding into the abdominal cavity may result in discoloration around the navel and a perception of fluid in the abdominal cavity beyond the margins of the uterus. Blood buildup in the abdominal cavity may irritate the diaphragm, with pain referred to the chest. If blood seeps under the liver, the woman may have reflected pain in the shoulder. Slight external bleeding is almost always present, although a slowly enlarging mass alongside the uterus, with increasingly difficult breathing, may indicate an incomplete rupture.

The contour of the uterus may change dramatically upon rupture. Findings will vary depending upon when the rupture occurs during labor and whether the baby is still contained within the uterus. If the baby is completely expelled, the empty uterus may be pushed to one side and may be firmly contracted, or may be pushed posteriorly where it cannot be palpated at all. Once the baby is outside the uterus, it is suddenly distinctly outlined and easily palpated through the abdominal wall, and the presenting part will recede or disappear from the inlet and will be freely mobile on abdominal exam. If the baby was well engaged prior to rupture, only a portion of his body may extrude through the tear rendering the uterus heart-shaped or otherwise distorted, with a loss of fetal station detectable on internal exam. The fetal heart rate almost invariably drops precipitously; sudden death of the fetus may occur as well. Fetal movements may be violent at first and then cease altogether as the baby dies; these movements will be quite obvious on visual inspection if the baby has been extruded from the uterus into the abdominal cavity.

Internal exam may reveal a ragged tear extending upward from the cervix or fornix. You may palpate a doughy-feeling loop of maternal intestines or a pouch of the omentum, which indicates that a complete rupture of all tissue layers has occurred (to be differentiated from a prolapsed cord, which may pulsate). However, lack of ability to identify a tear by no means rules out uterine rupture. If the rupture is incomplete, the tear often stops at the peritoneum; thus the abdominal cavity of the mother is not entered. A hematoma will form at the site of rupture. Additional bleeding can be provoked during an internal exam. This, when added to the already precarious condition of the mother, may cause immediate death.

The signs and symptoms listed above may not appear until several hours after the rupture has occurred. In delayed presentations, the most consistent clinical picture is abdominal pain with tenderness rather than shock. If rupture occurs during labor and goes undetected into the postpartum hours, the first sign may be distension of the lower abdomen from intra-abdominal bleeding.

Weak contractions may continue if the baby has not been expelled from the uterus into the abdominal cavity and, in rare cases, may complete the birth. Symptoms of rupture are often less marked when the baby remains within the uterus. If the baby is born and the rupture goes unrecognized, the woman may die from internal hemorrhage and shock, secondary hemorrhage from a ruptured hematoma, or infection. Shock and anemia in the presence of an obstetrical or labor history suggestive of rupture must always be investigated. Some women may recover spontaneously if the rupture is not extensive.

However, in most cases of catastrophic uterine rupture, the baby dies unless she can be born immediately, as might occur if the rupture occurs at the end of pushing. A baby who is extruded into the abdomen usually dies within a few minutes because placental circulation is impaired as the uterus attempts to contract.

Differential diagnosis

Conditions that may superficially mimic rupture include abruption, placenta previa (frank, revealed bleeding), amniotic fluid embolism (no bleeding), hematoma of the broad ligament (no bleeding) and abdominal pregnancy at term (pain without revealed bleeding). Rule out uterine rupture whenever a laboring woman collapses. It is important to differentiate threatened rupture from tetanic contraction, as the treatment for the latter is rest and relaxing herbs.

Postpartum signs and symptoms of rupture

Uterine rupture usually presents with abdominal pain and tenderness, postpartum hemorrhage or both. Bleeding that persists despite the use of oxytocics should raise the suspicion of uterine rupture or inversion. Blood in the urine suggests that the tear extends into the bladder. Bloody urine with an undelivered placenta should raise the question of whether placenta percreta is involved.

Dystocia during pushing or shoulder dystocia secondary to uterine rupture

This exceedingly rare complication can occur if the head has slipped through the cervix while the body of the baby has become extruded through a tear in the uterus. Pushing may have been unusually painful and the fetal heart rate abnormal, providing a tip-off that something was wrong. With the body outside the uterus, the rest of the baby cannot descend. The uterus becomes contracted and produces soft-tissue shoulder dystocia. If the head is born and the shoulders won't come, you can recognize this problem by the shoulders not being below the cervix. Working the cervix back over the shoulders will be the only way to remedy this problem in the moment, which should be followed by immediate transport (Zisow, 1996). Manipulation of the cervix may further damage the uterus, but if the baby is alive, it is your best option for maximizing the chance that the baby will survive.

Supporting and transporting the woman whose uterus has ruptured

Get the baby out as quickly as possible if he is still in the uterus and can be born. Do so with as little internal manipulation as possible because extraction can cause further damage to the mother. Extension of the tear is likely if a fetal part is caught in the uterine tear. Do not give oxytocics if the baby cannot be born. Transport immediately while stabilizing the uterus as previously described.

If the baby has been born, give the mother oxytocin and Methergine, start an IV, and administer oxygen by mask. The lower uterus and yoni can be packed with sterile gauze. Proceed to the hospital as quickly as possible. It is advisable to use an ambulance due to the accompanying bleeding and shock. If not, lay the mother down in the largest available vehicle and accompany her to the hospital.

SOURCES OF FETAL BLEEDING OTHER THAN THE PLACENTA

Vasa previa

This occurs when a blood vessel from the umbilical cord or the placenta traverses the portion of the membranes that overlies the os. It is most frequently associated with a velamentous insertion of the cord but may also occur when placental lobes are separated by stretches of membranes that contain blood vessels, as in a bipartita placenta or with a succenturiate lobe. The region of the bag containing the vessel is exposed as the cervix dilates. Prior to rupture of membranes, the baby may have bradycardia when the vessel is compressed, which is most likely to happen during contractions. When the bag breaks, the vessel is at great risk of breaking as well. Unless the vessel is a very minor one (as may be found with a succenturiate lobe), this will lead to significant fetal hemorrhage, anemia, hypovolemic shock and possibly death.

A ruptured vasa previa produces painless bright red yoni bleeding that at first may be mixed with lots of clear fluid because the membranes have just ruptured. If the involved vessel is umbilical and it becomes compressed, the fetal heart rate will show compromise prior to rupture. Shortly after the vessel breaks, the fetus will almost certainly show compromise quickly and is likely to bleed to death rapidly, but the mother is not in danger. If it is a placental vessel, the timing and extent of fetal compromise will vary depending upon how large a vessel has ruptured.

A vasa previa may be palpable once the os is partially dilated and may be mistaken for a cord. A careful speculum exam can be performed to visually confirm the diagnosis, although both a cord or a vasa previa will be handled in a similar fashion. If vasa previa is suspected, the best option is to transport the mother in a reversed-gravity position, such as knee-chest or Trendelenburg, before the bag breaks, thus decreasing the risk of fetal distress and death. Inform the hospital of your suspicions.

If the vessel has already ruptured, place the mother on her left side, give her oxygen by mask at a flow rate of 10 l/min to support the baby, and rush to the hospital, unless the baby can be born immediately. Advise the hospital that you think the mother has a ruptured vasa previa and to prepare for surgical delivery.

Torn cord

The cord may tear during the birth as the baby descends. This can be caused by an absolutely short cord that is not long enough to allow the baby to fully emerge without tearing or by a relatively short cord whose length is reduced by being wrapped around the baby. A torn cord is a dire emergency for the baby, who will quickly bleed to death if not born soon enough. A torn cord presents no risk to the mother unless descent also results in a portion of the placenta being pulled away from the uterine wall.

Detection: Tearing of the cord will produce painless bleeding that can only be seen once the membranes have ruptured. Since tearing is most likely to occur as the baby moves down during pushing, blood may not be visible even if the membranes rupture because the presenting part can prevent any fluids from flowing out. In this case, the fetal heart rate may offer the only clue that the baby is compromised. If bleeding has been going on long enough, the presenting part may appear deathly pale from blood loss. These babies will be born hypovolemic, anemic and shocky, if not dead.

What to do: A tear that occurs prior to the onset of pushing (exceedingly rare) or during pushing when birth cannot be facilitated quickly should prompt immediate transport for sudden fetal distress of unknown origin. Oxygen given to the mother en route to the hospital will help to support the baby.

A tear that occurs just prior to or at the time of birth may produce a sudden gush of blood with the birth of the presenting part. Facilitate completion of the birth by instructing the mother to push without waiting for the next contraction, manually rotating the shoulders and providing axillary traction (safe ways to do this are discussed in the chapter entitled "Shoulder Dystocia"), if necessary. Clamp off the torn end of the cord at the baby's umbilicus as quickly as possible prior to resuscitation.

Fetal anomaly

An open fetal anomaly, primarily anencephaly, will produce bleeding with descent and when the brain is palpated. This may be your first knowledge that the baby has a defect. Call your back-up pediatric provider and discuss the situation. Because it is most prudent to seek a definitive diagnosis prior to making the decision to stay home, the mother may need to go in to the hospital to be evaluated. However, since anencephaly is known to be fatal, once it is confirmed she can choose to go home to complete the birth if she so desires.

REFERENCES AND FURTHER READING ON ABNORMAL BLEEDING DURING LABOR

REFERENCES USED IN MULTIPLE CHAPTERS

Greenhill J. PRINCIPLES AND PRACTICE OF OBSTETRICS, 10th ed. WB Saunders Co, Philadelphia PA, 1951.

Greenhill J. PRINCIPLES AND PRACTICE OF OBSTETRICS, 12th ed. WB Saunders Co, Philadelphia PA, 1960.

Marshall M, Buffington S. LIFE-SAVING SKILLS MANUAL FOR MIDWIVES: MODULE 5: HEMORRHAGE, MODULE 6: RESUSCITATION, 3rd ed. American College of Nurse-Midwives, Washington DC, 1998.

BLEEDING DUE TO PLACENTAL DISRUPTION

Benson R. HANDBOOK OF OBSTETRICS AND GYNECOLOGY, 5th ed. Lange, Los Altos, CA 1974.

Cunningham F, et al. WILLIAMS OBSTETRICS, 21st ed. McGraw-Hill, New York, NY, 2001.

Davis E, CPM. Editing notes, 2004.

Davis-Floyd R. "Home-birth emergencies in the US and Mexico: the trouble with transport," SOC SCI MED, 56(9);1911-1931, May 2003.

Dewees W. A COMPENDIOUS SYSTEM OF MIDWIFERY CHIEFLY DESIGNED TO FACILITATE THE INQUIRIES OF THOSE WHO MAY BE PURSUING THIS BRANCH OF STUDY, 2nd ed. HC Carey & L Lea, Philadelphia PA, 1826.

Eastman N. WILLIAM'S OBSTETRICS, 10th ed. Appleton-Century-Crofts, Inc., New York NY, 1950.

Herman G. DIFFICULT LABOR: A GUIDE TO ITS MANAGEMENT FOR STUDENTS AND PRACTITIONERS, 5th ed. Cassell & Co Ltd, New York NY, 1910.

Scholles H, CPM. Editing notes, 2004.

Schmitz H, et al. "Placenta previa: a survey at the Lewis memorial maternity hospital," OBSTET GYNECOL, 3(1);3-10, Jan 1954.

Willett J. "Treatment of placenta previa by continuous weight traction," PROC ROY SOC MED, (sect. Obstet Gynecol), 18(3);90-94, Oct 1925.

Willson J, et al. OBSTETRICS AND GYNECOLOGY, 5th ed. CV Mosby Co, St Louis MO, 1975.

UTERINE RUPTURE DURING LABOR

Torpin R. ed. A TREATISE ON OBSTETRIC LABOR: "Chapter 24: Rupture of the Pregnant Uterus." Augusta Obstetrical and Gynecological Book Co, Augusta GA, 1948.

Turner M. "Uterine rupture," BEST PRAC RES CLIN OBSTET GYNAECOL, 16(1);69-79, Feb, 2002.

Zisow D. "Uterine rupture as a cause of shoulder dystocia," OBSTET GYNECOL, 87(5, Pt 2);881-819, May, 1996.

When Death is a Part of Birth

Assisting at the Labor and Birth of a Mother Whose Baby is Known to Have Lethal Defects or to Have Died Prior to the Onset of Labor

Ettinghausen (1979?) once told an audience of midwives that if they were not prepared to have a baby die, they were not ready to be midwives. Death is part of life and, sadly, sometimes part of birth. Bringing a balanced and compassionate presence to parents facing this tragedy will greatly facilitate their healing process; it is a skill that every midwife should possess.

The parents may wish to proceed with their plans for a homebirth when a lethal fetal deformity or fetal demise is detected at some point prior to the onset of labor. Women who wanted the sanctity of a homebirth in the first place often prefer to go through these difficult labors at home rather than in a hospital. There are a few special considerations to take into account when assisting women through the labor and birth of a baby who will not live or who has already died. The details that follow focus on fetal demise, but most can be applied when the baby has a lethal defect and is expected to die during labor or shortly after birth.

Review clotting panel lab results

Review the prenatal lab reports for the clotting panels that should have been performed periodically since the demise was identified. To safely proceed with a homebirth, the last clotting panel should have been normal; clotting abnormalities usually do not develop within the first four weeks after the demise. (See the chapter entitled "The Clotting Mechanism and Bleeding Disorders" in DIAGNOSTIC TESTS for details.)

Getting labor going

The parents may want to get on with the labor once they have passed the initial shock. The techniques described in the chapter entitled "Natural Induction and Augmentation of Labor" are appropriate to use in these cases, with the exception of rupture of membranes, which you want to avoid. A Chinese medical practitioner can help prime the mother's body to go into labor with herbal treatments and acupuncture.

Birthing energy

First and foremost, the energy of labor and birth will be very different than when the baby is alive. Quite apart from the intense emotions both midwife and parents may be feeling, the baby's physical energy is absent and therefore cannot help move things along. Because of this, the mother's impetus to birth must be strong. Her need to open, release the baby and move through this acute phase of letting go can then be the exclusive focus of your care.

Attend to the mother

Try not to say or do things out of habit that suggest that the baby is alive, such as mention checking the fetal heart rate. While there is no mistake in these cases that the baby is dead, you do not want to inadvertently twist the knife, as it were, as the mother deals with her grief on her own terms. It may be appropriate to talk about the spirit of the baby with certain couples; this needs to be ascertained on an individual basis. Choose your language carefully when referring to the baby who is known to have defects incompatible with life but who has not died, being careful not to disrespect that the baby is still alive.

Grief can manifest in a variety of direct and indirect ways, including maternal complications such as postpartum hemorrhage and infection. It is important to stay focused on the mother throughout the process until she is entirely stable after the birth of the placenta.

Don't rupture the membranes

When the baby has died prior to labor, keep the membranes intact as long as possible to minimize the chance of infection. The forewaters also provide a dilating wedge, which is especially useful if the baby is early, in a breech position, or has been dead for a while, which will cause the brain to liquify and the skull to soften somewhat.

If the baby has a lethal defect and is still alive, the choice to rupture membranes can be made as you would for any other labor. Although the concern regarding cord prolapse is not as critical in these cases, no doubt the parents wish to avoid any undue suffering on the baby's part.

Assisting during labor

Again, focus on the mother. If labor gets stuck, help her to cry or otherwise express herself. After all, the end of labor will mean that she must face the reality of the baby's condition and let her baby go. In addition, if she is not at term, her body is not as ready to enter labor as it would otherwise be, and labor can take more time to become established. If she has been carrying a dead baby for several days or weeks, every day sees a diminishing of her hormone levels back toward her prepregnancy norms. Therefore, her determination and willingness to open to birthing energy are paramount in birthing the baby at home.

The birth

If the baby has lethal defects but is alive, the mother can assume any position for the birth. If the baby is already dead, a side-lying position takes weight off the sacrum while providing a gravity-neutral position to receive a totally limp and possibly fragile baby. Be ready to receive the baby into a towel or blanket as he emerges. The baby should slide right out, but be careful not to pull on the baby if he does not, as the skin may peel away or the body may come apart. Change the mother's position, as necessary, and carefully assess the situation to determine the least traumatic way to get the baby out if labor is truly obstructed. Such obstruction may be due to abnormalities of the lower body, lethal cord entanglements, short cord or other problems. Since you don't have to worry about the well-being of a deceased baby, you have plenty of time.

The appearance of a baby with lethal defects

If the baby with lethal defects is born alive, palliative care includes keeping the baby comfortable, allowing full, uninterrupted bonding time for the parents and the baby and respecting the spiritual being of the baby whose life will be so short. If the baby stabilizes and is doing relatively well, provide care as you would for any mother-baby pair. If the baby is born in distress, an all out resuscitative effort is not called for, but this decision should have been thoroughly discussed in advance with the parents. While the parents may have been prepared prenatally for the type of defect to expect, seeing the baby will bring the problem home on a very real level: your response and lack of hesitation about handling the baby will help the parents do so themselves. Be aware that the parents may change their mind about how the baby should be cared for if the baby is born alive and appears to be doing well. In this delicate situation, you must follow their lead, even to the point of transport for further evaluation if they desire it. If not, the pediatrician should be notified that the baby has been born and informed as to his condition.

The appearance of a deceased baby

Maceration (from the Latin word meaning "to soften") is the process by which tissues waste away or are softened by soaking that causes their parts to separate. **Autolysis** refers to the spontaneous degeneration of tissues or cells by enzymatic action. The body of a dead baby who is retained in utero breaks down by a combined process of maceration and autolysis. These processes occur most efficiently in a moist environment at body temperature or higher, making the intrauterine environment an ideal place for the body to deteriorate via these mechanisms.

A baby who has died during or just before labor will usually look very much like a normal baby. However, as time passes, the tissues will quickly lose all tone. After 4 to 8 hours, vascular permeability increases and the umbilical cord takes on a reddish brown hue. At some point between 6 and 12 hours postmortem, the body of the baby takes on a parboiled appearance. Minimal friction results in the skin slipping off to reveal the shiny, moist, red dermal surface beneath.

Even in the absence of trauma, fluid soon begins to collect under the skin, producing small blisters. This is a normal part of decomposition and should not be mistaken for an infectious process. These may join together to form larger blisters, which can range up to 8 to 10 cm across. Disruption of these blisters releases serous fluid and reveals a raw, weeping surface underneath. Red blood cell breakdown and leakage from the circulatory vessels produces a red brown discoloration of the soft tissues. Seepage of fluid may make the fetus appear more or less edematous. If the fetus suffered from cystic hygroma, fetal hydrops or another condition that produces pronounced edema, the red maroon discoloration may develop more quickly and may persist for several weeks after death.

Joints will be lax. Rigor mortis (hardening of the muscles) does not occur because of the dissolution of both joint and muscle tissues. The muscles of the arms and legs will atrophy, making the extremities thin. The cord will be thin and limp. Weight loss is progressive from the time of death on, due to loss of tissue fluids.

The brain becomes semiliquid and the sutures dissolve. By 4 to 5 days, the dura separates from the skull and the bones easily overlap, causing the skull to become distorted and to finally collapse. The scalp becomes a fluctuant bag containing the skull bones and brain, giving the appearance of hydrocephalus.

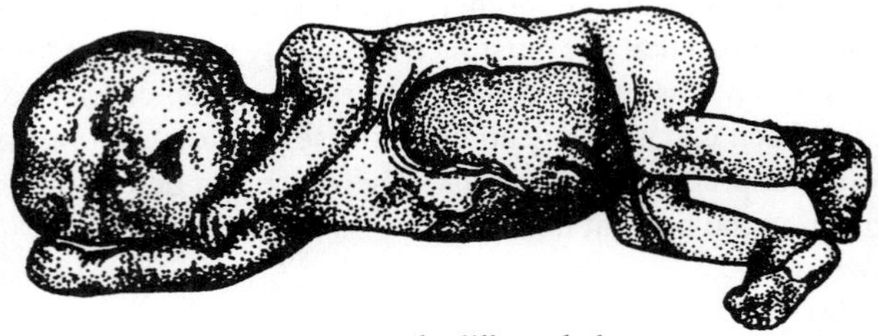

Macerated stillborn baby

Abdominal contents become green as bile pigments seep into surrounding tissues. If the fetus is retained for more than a week or two, the bowel wall may dissolve, releasing meconium into the abdominal cavity. The abdomen may be slightly swollen. When the fetus is retained for over a week or 10 days, the color of the skin gradually fades to a light olive green. Meconium becomes degraded and less sticky the longer the fetus is retained. The younger the fetus, the more rapidly this change occurs. In small fetuses, the abdominal wall may rupture; this should not be confused with intestinal defects.

The baby will be fragile and should be handled with care. If the intrauterine environment has become colonized with bacteria, there may be a strong foul odor upon rupture of membranes. If so, the mother should be watched very closely for infection, as her grief will make her that much more susceptible to problems postpartum. If the cause of death is infection, especially if gas-forming microbes such as *Clostridium perfringens* are involved, the autolysis of fetal tissue may be accelerated, with almost complete dissolution of the soft tissues 12 to 24 hours after death. If you suspect infection, a culture of the fetus and placenta as they emerge is a good idea. (Be extremely careful to protect yourself and the mother from additional contamination. See the chapter entitled "Assisting at the Birth of a Vertex Baby" and my DIAGNOSTIC TESTS for culture instructions at the time of birth.)

As noted in the following table, the appearance of the baby at the time of birth offers only an approximate gauge of the duration of death prior to birth. The rate and nature of the changes that occur will vary depending upon both the gestational age of the baby at the time of death and the underlying reasons for death. The tissues of premature, growth-retarded babies can turn brown and begin to dehydrate after only a few days due to the small amount of soft tissue and blood volume. Decomposition is considerably hastened if the fetus is extremely swollen.

PHYSICAL FINDINGS	DURATION OF DEATH PRIOR TO BIRTH
Normal newborn appearance	0 to 48 hours
Reddened skin	0 to 48 hours
Skin slippage and peeling	0 to 48 hours
Skin peeling of at least 1 cm circumference and brown red discoloration of cord stump	6 or more hours
Peeling of the face, abdomen and back	12 or more hours
Peeling involves >5% of body surface	18 or more hours
Brown skin discoloration	24 or more hours
Extensive peeling, blisters containing red fluid on chest and abdomen	2 to 7 days
Turbid fluids on skin surface, may be mummified	8 days or longer
Mummification	2 or more weeks
Adipocere or calcification formation	several months

(Singer & Macpherson, 1998)

The term **adipocere (ADD-i-poh-sear)** is used to describe a waxy substance that forms during decomposition of bodies interred in moist places away from air. It takes at least 2 to 4 months for fatty acids and salts to form this waxlike coating on the body surface. This condition is found only in some fetuses who die close to term and are then retained in utero for many months prior to birth; it is therefore quite rare.

Mummification of the fetus may also occur. Distinct from rigor mortis, mummification causes the fetus to present with a characteristic mottled brown appearance and a firm to brittle texture. Subcutaneous tissues may have a woody texture. Mummification typically occurs only if the fetus died early in gestation, allowing fluids to be pressed out and reabsorbed over time; however, it can occur at any point in development. **Fetus papyraceus (pap-e-RA-see-us)** and **lithopedion (lith-oh-PEE-dee-on)** are forms of mummification; these occur most often during a multiple gestation when one sibling dies early in pregnancy, typically between 16 to 20 weeks, or much more rarely in a single baby who has died. (See the chapter entitled "Assisting at Multiple Births" for more details.)

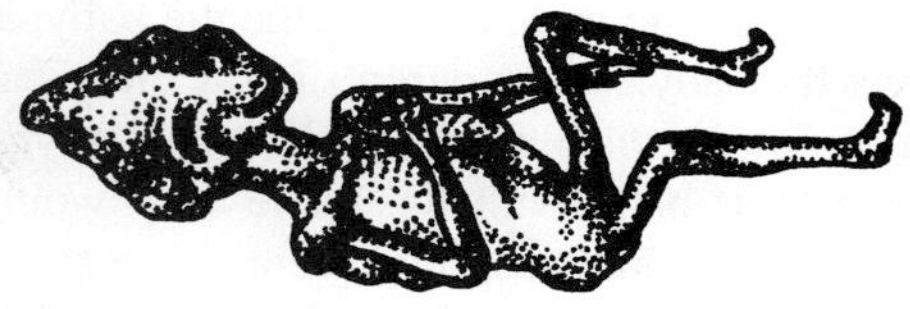

Mummified fetus

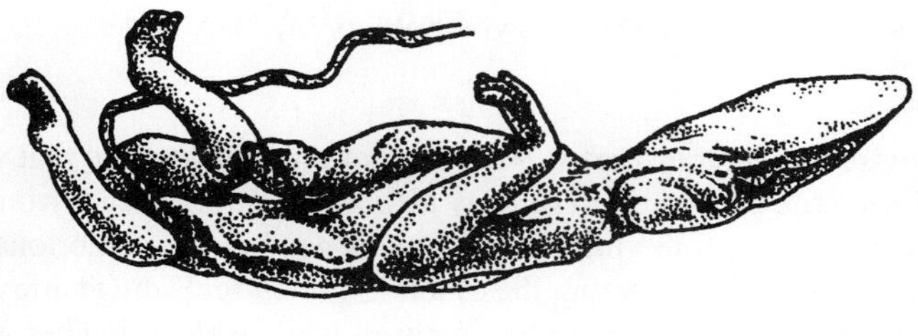

Fetus papyraceus

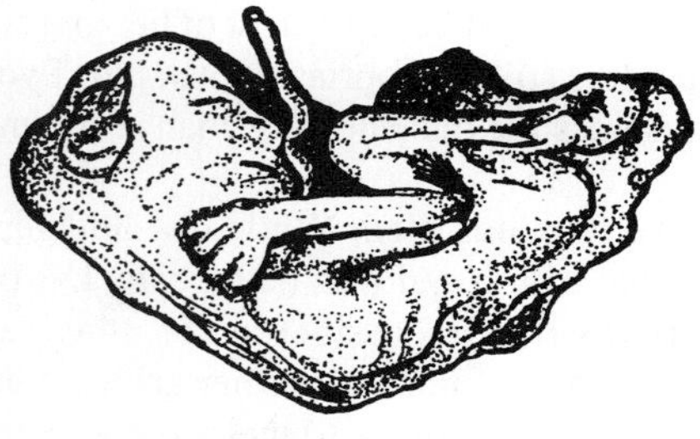

Lithopedion fetus

Birthing the placenta

If the baby is near term and born alive, the birth of the placenta should proceed as it usually does. If the baby is early, the placenta will not have grown to its full size. The area of attachment on the uterine wall will therefore be smaller and the placenta more firmly implanted. It is not programmed to release at this point. The uterus itself will have gradually reduced in size as the baby stopped growing and the amount of amniotic fluid diminished. Therefore, after the birth, the uterus may not have as dramatic a reduction in size as it normally would if the baby were living and full term. For all these reasons, the placenta may not detach as quickly and easily as it ordinarily would. Therefore the midwife must be hypervigilant regarding the safe and timely delivery of the placenta.

Talk to the parents again as the time of birth nears regarding the importance of focusing on the mother's well-being after the baby is out. If the baby is alive, manage the cord as you normally would and hand the baby to the mother, lightly covering any obvious defects with a receiving blanket so that she can examine these areas as she feels ready. If the baby is already dead, cut and clamp the cord on the baby's end and place the baby aside until the placenta is out, the uterus is clamped down and the mother is stable. Only then should the mother be urged to do whatever she needs to in order to deal with the reality of her baby's death.

The placental exam of a deceased fetus: See the chapter entitled "Examining of the Placenta" for details. It is ideal for the placenta to be sent with the baby in the event of an autopsy. A placental pathology exam should be discussed especially if the baby has congenital defects.

Immediate postpartum care

The longer the baby has been dead, the more the mother's blood volume will have had a chance to return to her prepregnancy level. In practical terms, this means that she does not have the large margin of blood loss that she would if the baby were alive. This is even more true if she was not near term at the time of the demise. Be on guard for any degree of blood loss, and be ready with herbs, acupuncture and oxytocics if necessary to stop bleeding promptly.

Saying hello and goodbye: Most mothers will wish to see and hold their baby. Once the placenta is out and the mother is stable, either hand her the baby or help her position herself so that she can begin to relate to her baby at her own pace. Be sure her partner is involved and not left to the side. Many young parents will never have experienced the death (or impending loss) of someone close to them before; even if they have, they may not have had direct contact with the body. Let your intuition be your guide. If the baby is alive, focus on the present circumstances; it is possible for a baby with lethal defects to live for several days or even weeks following birth. If the mother seems reluctant to touch or look at her baby, you can begin by pointing out attractive features of the baby and touching the baby yourself. This is especially helpful in bridging any fear the parents may have, particularly if the baby has physical defects. Have a baby bathtub on hand where the mother can bathe the baby, and baby clothes, preferably an outfit the parents have chosen, in which to dress the baby. Many parents invite close friends or family to see the baby, talk to the baby, hold and rock the baby and have pictures taken while holding the baby, while others simply sit together with the baby and cry. Encourage them to name their baby with the name they would have given were the baby expected to live. This will help them in remembering and keeping special the reality of this baby. For those who are open to the concept, remind them that the baby's spirit is still nearby and receiving all the love they have to give. They may have prepared a basket or other suitable place where they can place the baby when they are ready.

Occasionally, a woman will not want to hold or even look at her deceased or abnormal baby. Gently remind her that this is the only opportunity she will have to say goodbye to this little spirit's body; even though it is hard to do so now, saying goodbye will make the rest of her grieving process easier. If she still refuses, don't push; everyone grieves in their own way. It is still appropriate to ask her if you can hold the baby. Once she sees you holding the baby and expressing grief, it is possible that she may change her mind.

When one twin has died: While it would generally be wise to plan transport in such a situation, it is possible that you could attend a birth and find that a baby has been lost during the pregnancy. You may also be attending such a woman where transport is impossible or for other reasons stayed at home knowing one baby was dead. This emotionally complex situation finds the mother grieving the loss of one baby while greeting the other. She will feel a huge array of emotions, which are likely to include guilt about the death as well as guilt about feeling grief while welcoming her well baby and feeling happy even though she has lost a baby. She may blame herself. You must reassure her that all these feelings are perfectly normal and give her time to relate to both babies. She may wish to hold both babies together, allow the living baby time with his dead sibling and talk to the well baby about the loss. Follow her lead as to how to proceed.

Keepsakes: Regardless of how the parents respond to contact with their baby, keepsakes will provide cherished memories later. Cut off a lock of hair (if possible) and save it. Make ear, foot and palm prints on a keepsake certificate or, if such a certificate is not available, on a 4 × 6 in card. Record the weight, length, head and chest measurements of the baby after the mother and father have had time with the baby. Save the receiving blanket the baby was first wrapped in and any similar items such as the first hat or booties that the baby wore that were replaced later by cleaner items. Do not wash these items, but give them to the mother.

Photographs: Aside from keepsakes, pictures are the most tangible evidence that a baby existed. If the parents have no camera, obtain their permission (preferably ahead of time) to take pictures yourself; the pictures should be included in the chart along with other documents and keepsakes. Take as many pictures as the parents feel comfortable with. If the baby has a known lethal defect and is born alive, try to get pictures of the baby prior to death. Such pictures can include:

- Baby being held by parents, relatives or significant others.
- Head and shoulder photo. Lay the baby on receiving blankets or a pink or blue sheet if the background will be showing and loosely frame the baby by draping the cloth. Avoid using yellow or green, which may accentuate any odd discoloration of the baby's body.
- Baby unclothed, confirming both any obvious defects as well as normal features. Consider the background carefully. Someone can be holding the baby with the blanket unfolded to reveal the body, or the baby can be arranged on a pillow, framed softly by receiving blankets.
- Baby on belly, head turned, hands beside head.
- Close-up of face, hand, ear, nose or a parent's finger in the baby's hand.
- Baby lying on belly resting on a parent's chest.

If the baby has physical defects or the appearance is quite altered from being deceased for some time, make an effort to take the most flattering pictures possible. If the top or back of the head is defective, take a nude photo with the head covered by a cap or by draping. Also take pictures that clearly show the defects. If you are new to photography, practice before the birth with a floppy doll to work on poses, lighting, and background arrangement. Regular lens filters or even a single layer of nylon stocking can be stretched over the lens to soften the effect. A regular 35 mm camera with a 50 mm lens is all that is needed. Lighting should be indirect and natural. A bounce flash, rather than a direct flash should be used if no sunlight is available. A simple light reflector can be made out of white poster board. Arrange the baby near a window, place the white side of the cardboard toward the baby, and bounce the light off of it.

Having these pictures will help parents come to terms with the loss and may help to answer any questions they have later. Get the film developed yourself and put the different types of pictures in different envelopes, so that the parents can look at them as they feel ready. If they do not want the pictures now, save them in their chart in sealed, well-identified envelopes. Most parents will request their photos within the year after birth.

Hand or foot cast: A cast of the baby's hand or foot can also serve as a precious memento (Jung et al., 2003), if the physical integrity of the body will allow this kind of manipulation. You will need dental alginate and dental plaster (die stone peach), both of which can be obtained from a dental supply company. You will also need paper cups, tongue depressors and a small paring or pocket knife. An electric mixer or small whisk are optional.

1. First, use a tongue depressor or the mixer to quickly mix up a batch of alginate (one part alginate to one part water) in a paper cup of adequate size to fully contain the extremity and some of the limb. You want a smooth, soupy, lump-free consistency. The quantity should be sufficient to completely immerse the hand or foot and a short segment of the limb. The colder the water, the longer the setting time. If a base is desired, leave ¼ to ½ in of space in the cup.
2. Place the baby on folded towels so that his arm or leg can hang dependent off the edge into the cup. For a very active baby, swaddling or holding may help keep the baby still enough for the casting. Finger or toe movement does not seem to matter because when the alginate sets, the position is fixed.
3. The baby's extremity is then immersed in the alginate mixture and held there until it congeals, usually 1 to 3 minutes. The alginate will remain flexible enough to carefully remove the extremity from the mold.
4. The next step is to make a positive mold from the alginate impression. Mix the die stone peach dental plaster in another paper cup with water to make a soupy consistency that will pour easily.
5. Fill the alginate impression with the liquid die stone peach plaster. If a base is desired, pour ¼ to ½ in excess into the paper cup containing the alginate. Tap the filled impression firmly and vigorously on the sides to remove bubbles. Or, fill the alginate mold slowly, by adding plaster, tapping the container, then adding more plaster until the air bubbles are gone and the impression is filled. Alternatively, partially fill the mold, rotate it several times and pour it out and repeat this process several times, after which the impression can be completely filled. The drying time for the plaster is 15 minutes to 1 to 2 hours, depending upon the amount of water used.
6. When the die stone plaster is hardened, peel off the paper cup and cut the alginate away with a knife, chiseling off small pieces at a time while being careful not to damage the cast.

Should an autopsy be performed? The parents may have discussed this question prior to the onset of labor. However, the reality of having the baby with them may make them unsure about how to proceed. It is painful to think of the baby's body being examined and cut up to find out what went wrong. It can also be equally painful and frightening to be left in the dark if there is any question about why the baby died, especially if another child is desired later. Encourage the parents to seriously consider the long-term value of the knowledge that the autopsy may provide, but don't try to force them to make any particular decision.

Regardless of whether the parents decide to do an autopsy, state regulations may dictate whether a call needs to be placed to their back-up physician or the state medical examiners office. A plan for collection of the body might already be in place, especially if the fetal demise was detected soon enough prenatally. The agency in charge will send someone to collect the baby's body when the parents are ready to let it go. The parents will have to sign releases to allow an autopsy to proceed. At this time, they may indicate if they want the autopsy to be limited in any way. For example, some parents ask that no incisions be made on the child's head. They should include any such requests on the autopsy permit before they sign it. It is important for the parents to be informed where the baby will be taken, how long the autopsy is anticipated to take and when results will be available. A representative from the funeral home should be informed of these arrangements so she can be called to collect the body once the autopsy is completed.

After-death care and funeral arrangements

To reiterate, the medical examiner's office may still need to be contacted even if the parents want no examinations of the body. Requirements depend on local regulations and the gestational age of the baby. In some jurisdictions, a funeral home with whom the family has prearranged services will need to be contacted to collect the baby. The parents may wish to have a home funeral and follow the traditions of their faith. If they have no ideas about how to proceed, provisions for a gentle death transition are discussed in the book LIVING INTO DYING: A JOURNAL OF SPIRITUAL AND PRACTICAL DEATHCARE FOR FAMILY AND COMMUNITY by Nancy Jewel Poer. This book has many inspiring stories interspersed with the practical information needed to keep the deceased at home for the three days following death. The parents will have to decide if the baby is to be cremated or buried and if they want the baby embalmed. If they have chosen to have an autopsy but want more time with the baby after the autopsy is performed, the body can be returned to them for after-death transition care. The baby can be cremated even if embalming is performed. Parents whose baby has died will need ongoing support. This will be covered in Volume III.

When a Mother Dies during or after Labor

The thought of having a maternal mortality, where a woman in your care dies during labor, frightens even the most experienced midwife. However, maternal deaths do occur. In some cases there is nothing that can be done to prevent them, or only immediate access to advanced care in the hospital would have made a difference. Cerebral aneurism and amniotic fluid embolism are two such killers, both carrying a high rate of mortality–and no prior symptoms for detection.

The list of causes that can take a woman's life but where the woman's life may have been spared had the midwife known more, been more attentive, been quicker to transport or had better access to care is much longer. These include problems associated with medical conditions, such as insulin-dependent diabetes, and the primary killers of pregnant women, full-blown eclampsia and postpartum hemorrhage.

In most cases, a healthy woman is resilient to the risks of childbirth if she is well nourished during pregnancy and well cared for during labor. It is exceedingly rare for a complication to arise out of nowhere and take the life of a woman who, up until then, was apparently doing fine. Most maternal (and fetal) complications provide plenty of warning before fulminating into a life-threatening catastrophe.

The midwife practicing in an industrialized country will have access to a system that can minimize the chances of maternal death. Her actions will depend upon the crisis at hand, the availability of backup and transport options and her knowledge and skill level. Therefore, even if the mother appears near death, transport will usually be underway and the woman's condition addressed by a hospital staff trained and equipped to provide supportive care.

It is the midwife working in remote regions, where timely transport is impossible, who may be faced with the possibility of caring for a dying woman. In this case, the midwife, having done everything she can to preserve the mother's life, including making every effort to obtain medical help, may have to accept that she can do no more. If the baby is not yet born but birth is imminent, manual dilation and fundal pressure may be used in an attempt to rescue the baby. If, however, the birth is not imminent, it is probably best not to attempt to force the birth, as the baby may already be severely compromised. The family wishes as well as those of the mother should be taken into account, but forceful delivery may be futile and render the woman's last moments of life excruciating. As the woman's life ebbs away her pulse will slow, her blood pressure will drop and her skin will become cold and clammy. Her breathing may gradually increase in depth and sometimes in rate to a maximum, followed by a decrease resulting in 5 to 30 seconds of apnea. When this pattern develops, (referred to as Cheyne-Stokes respiration) it occurs in cycles lasting from 30 seconds to 2 minutes in duration until death occurs.

When death is inevitable, the midwife shifts from focusing on the emergency and now-futile physical care to providing emotional and spiritual comfort to the woman and her family. The woman should be talked to, as hearing is the last sense to shut down. She should be shown her baby if he is born, and provided with psychological care as long as she is conscious or even vaguely aware of what is or might be happening to her. She should be treated before (and after) her death with dignity and respect. Assume that she is aware on some level, even if she is apparently in a coma. Her family members should be allowed to be with her for as long as they wish after her passing. The midwife should remain to help with the arrangements for the body and to assist with the baby.

Both you and the family will be devastated by the death. Dealing with death after the birth will be covered in Volume III of this text.

References and Further Reading on When Death is a Part of Birth

Assisting at the Labor and Birth of a Mother Whose Baby is Known to Have Lethal Defects or to Have Died Prior to the Onset of Labor

Eittehausen J. Workshop presentation, [1979?].

Johnson M, et al. A Most Important Picture: A Very Tender Manual for Taking Pictures of Stillborn Babies and Infants Who Die, rev. ed. Centering Corp, Omaha NE, 1995.

Jung A, et al. "Neonatal hand casting method," J Perinatol, 23(6);519-520, Sept, 2003.

Singer D, Macpherson T. "Fetal Death and the Macerated Stillborn Infant" in Wigglesworth J, Singer D. eds. Textbook of Fetal and Neonatal Pathology, 2nd ed. Blackwell Sciences, Malden MA, 1998.

Wigglesworth J. Perinatal Pathology, Vol. 15 in the series Major Problems in Pathology, Bennington J, ed. WB Saunders Co, Philadelphia PA, 1984.

When a Mother Dies during or after Labor

Doyle D, et al., eds. Chapter 18: "The terminal phase," Oxford Textbook of Palliative Medicine, 3rd ed. Oxford U Press, Oxford UK, 2004.

McCormick M, ed. Integrated Management of Pregnancy and Childbirth: Managing Complications in Pregnancy and Childbirth: A Guide for Midwives and Doctors, Reproductive Health and Research, World Health Organization, Geneva Switzerland, 2000.

Maternal Problems That Can Occur during Placental Delivery and the Hours Following Birth

Postpartum Hemorrhage: An Overview

The time between placental detachment and the clamping down of the empty uterus is the most potentially dangerous time for a healthy mother. The well-nourished mother is fully prepared to withstand the normal blood loss that occurs during birth. As a rule, she can lose up to 25% of her *original nonpregnant* blood volume, often with little or no effect on her overall well-being. However, other factors, such as how tired she is and her overall constitutional response to the experience of labor, can reduce her tolerance for blood loss.

The following three chapters will discuss the differential diagnosis and treatment of postpartum hemorrhage. The main bleeding problems that happen during the third and fourth phases of labor can be divided into two clinically relevant categories: those that occur while the placenta is still undelivered and those that occur once the placenta is out.

Some bleeding problems, such as bleeding lacerations, hematomas, ruptured varicosities, cervical tears, coagulation defects and uterine rupture, are unrelated to placental delivery; however, whether the placenta is delivered or not is still a critical factor in being able to identify and address other causes, stop the bleeding and stabilize the mother. The uterus will continue to bleed as long as it is not empty because it cannot clamp down. This part also includes some other problems that are not themselves in any way involved in bleeding but that are intimately related to difficulties with placental delivery.

Regardless of the cause of bleeding or when it occurs, postpartum hemorrhage can be classified as either revealed, partially revealed or concealed.

Types of bleeding

Revealed bleeding: When you can see all the blood that is being lost, the hemorrhage is fully revealed. You have an accurate idea of the extent of the loss, and the mother's responses are in direct proportion to the blood loss. When you find the source and the bleeding can be stopped, the mother can be stabilized.

Partially revealed bleeding: Here you can see only a portion of the blood being lost; the rest is retained within the uterine cavity or is spilling out into the abdomen or pelvis. You could, for example, have bleeding from the yoni due to uterine atony plus an enlarging hematoma. Perhaps clots may be blocking a large quantity of blood that is building up in the uterus, but all you see is a small trickle at the introitus. Such scenarios often entail far more blood loss than is apparent, and the mother's condition may be much worse than her visible blood loss suggests. How much worse depends upon the total amount of bleeding. In such cases, you may find one source of bleeding and get that under control, only to have the mother remain unstable. At this point, there may be no obvious source of the problem. This could mean you have additional concealed bleeding from the same source or from another source. You must continue to search for additional causes of bleeding or transport if the cause of the problem cannot be identified and controlled.

Concealed bleeding: The woman's condition can steadily deteriorate with no external evidence of hemorrhage. The os may be completely obstructed by clots or the placenta; a deep upper vault laceration or uterine rupture may have occurred that is allowing bleeding into the peritoneal cavity; or the only significant source of blood loss may involve an enlarging hematoma bleeding into the pelvic cavity. You must search for the cause of shock, being highly suspicious that the cause is from the type of bleeding likely to be completely concealed. If the source cannot be found, you must stabilize the mother as best you can and transport. Consider that the shock that you suspect is due to concealed bleeding may, in rare cases, be due to another cause. Either way, medical evaluation is in order.

Uterine atony leading to bleeding is the most likely reason for instability or shock. The second most common reason is bleeding related to tissue trauma during birth. Never assume that you can accurately assess the extent of bleeding by visual assessment alone. If the mother is unstable and you can rule out bleeding, you have some other serious problem on your hands and should transport right away. Keep in mind that a deep, enlarging hematoma may not always be detectable and can lead to massive blood loss.

Differential diagnosis

When assessing why a woman is bleeding, you must take into account her medical, prenatal and labor history to arrive at the most likely cause. These diagnostic criteria are mentioned throughout all my textbooks, and the relevant signs and symptoms will be found in those chapters discussing specific prenatal and labor complications in both Volumes I and II of this text. The causes of postpartum hemorrhage can be categorized as follows (the relevant chapters or text in which they are addressed are listed as well):

Uterine sources:

- Atony (See the chapters entitled "The Birth of the Placenta, Cord and Membranes" and "Immediate Postpartum Hemorrhage."). Bleeding in the presence of uterine atony is assumed to be from the placental implantation site until proven otherwise.
- Retained placenta (see the chapters entitled "The Birth of the Placenta, Cord and Membranes" and "Uncommon Problems That Can Interfere with the Birth of the Placenta" and "Immediate Postpartum Hemorrhage")
- Partially detached placenta ("The Birth of the Placenta, Cord and Membranes")
- Abnormal placentation ("Uncommon Problems That Can Interfere with the Birth of the Placenta")
- Lacerations of the uterus or uterine rupture

Nonuterine sources:

- Lacerations of the lower genital tract (see my text HEALING PASSAGE)
- Hematoma (see my text HEALING PASSAGE)
- Coagulopathy (see my text DIAGNOSTIC TESTS)

Uncommon Problems That Can Interfere with the Birth of the Placenta

NOTE: The chapter entitled "The Birth of the Placenta, Cord and Membranes" addresses the most common problems that can occur with the birth of the placenta. This chapter discusses less common problems that can lead to severe hemorrhage before the placenta is delivered. See the chapters entitled "Uterine Inversion" and "Immediate Postpartum Hemorrhage" for a discussion of problems that are unrelated to the placental implantation site, which may occur after the placenta is out.

You must address bleeding and shock, having someone else attend to stabilizing the mother, if necessary, while you attempt to deliver the placenta. If uterine bleeding is part of the problem, the maternal condition will not fully stabilize until the uterus is empty and clamped down; therefore, if the placenta can be delivered, it is extremely important that this be accomplished in a skilled and timely manner. Whenever the placenta does not come out, you must consider uncommon and even rare possibilities, because you want to avoid making the situation worse by ripping off a portion of the placenta in an attempt to extract it. The types of unusual problems that may occur before or during the birth of the placenta include:

- Placenta partially or completely grown within an abnormal region of uterine anatomy and so cannot detach normally
- Placenta of an unusual size or shape that makes detachment or delivery more difficult
- Constriction ring (hourglass contraction)
- Preterm birth with the placenta firmly adhered
- Obstruction from a fetus papyraceus or tumor
- Normally implanted but very adherent portion of placenta
- Partial or total abnormal growth of the placenta into the uterine wall (creta); this can take the form of:
    - Placenta accreta
    - Placenta increta
    - Placenta percreta

<u>Placenta has partially or completely grown within an abnormal region of uterine anatomy</u>

This relatively rare complication occurs when the placenta grows inside a pocket that has formed in the uterine wall, when it attaches to a uterine septum (which is usually thin and provides a poor base for the placental bed, thus encouraging abnormally deep implantation), when it attaches in one horn of a bicornate uterus, or when it is attached to a tumor such as a fibroid. In any of these cases, the placenta is not likely to deliver normally and transport is in order. If bleeding is heavy, give IM oxytocin first. If oxytocin does not slow the bleeding, administer an IM injection of Methergine. While the placenta remains undelivered, Methergine should only be used in the event of profuse bleeding, as it tends to produce a more tetanic contraction of the uterine muscle than does oxytocin.

In many cases, you may already be aware from her medical history or a bimanual exam that a woman has unusual uterine anatomy, but it is quite possible for such a problem to make its presence known only after the birth. If there is no prior history to go on, your suspicion of such a problem will only be a guess unless you discover a uterine anomaly during an attempted manual removal. If the placenta cannot be delivered, these women are likely to require surgery and may need a hysterectomy. Transport!

<u>Placenta is an unusual size, shape or formation</u>

Read the chapter entitled "Examining the Placenta" for a discussion of the different shapes the placenta can assume. Sometimes the placenta has several large lobes that do not detach all at once. It may instead have one small lobe that detaches less readily than the main body because there is little shrinkage of the uterine wall beneath the small accessory portion. Very rarely, the placenta may be shaped like a horseshoe, a ring, or a cap or have some other unusual configuration that makes detachment and expulsion more difficult. However, you will not be able to tell if placental shape is a factor without an intrauterine exploration. If you suspect an oddly shaped placenta, IM oxytocin, an upright position and patience may help the placenta to detach. If not and bleeding is concerning, transport.

<u>Constriction ring (hourglass contraction)</u>

The uterine muscle can form a ring of constriction, either around the body of the placenta or with the entire placenta trapped above it. In either event, the placenta is held back by this band of muscle, which must relax in order for the placenta to be released. This situation may not be discovered until you attempt to perform a manual removal and find your hand cannot advance into the uterine cavity. Try to relax the ring by giving the mother lobelia or skullcap tincture. If bleeding is profuse, transport. If there is no bleeding, keep the mother warm, watch her carefully and wait. The constriction ring often relaxes within two hours. However, if any bleeding should develop or if the mother's condition becomes unstable, transport. If you are far from medical help, do not wait to take her in (Mayes, 1954).

Preterm birth with the placenta adhered

If the baby is born before term, the placenta will be more firmly attached and its size may be smaller. In addition, the baby will be smaller. In this case, as the uterus shrinks beneath the placenta, the amount of shrinkage is proportionately less making it less effective in helping the placenta shear away from its implantation site. The remedy is to stimulate strong contractions, with either an effective herb or oxytocin.

Obstruction blocking descent of the placenta

Any mass in the uterus could be impairing detachment or descent of the placenta. This includes a pediculated fibroid, placental hemangioma, or a small or defective fetus that died earlier in gestation (both of these latter can come out separately). The best way to assess this is to palpate abdominally, then follow the cord up and check to find what is presenting at the os. If the cord is found to go up and around a mass with the placenta beyond, an obstructing mass seems likely. Be cautious about applying cord traction when a mass may be the problem, as the placenta may be attached to it and the uterus may invert. Try pushing it up and to the side; if that doesn't easily resolve the problem and facilitate the delivery of the placenta, transport. A large fibroid can also interfere with uterine contraction once the placenta is out. Transport is probably your best option.

Normally implanted but very adhered portion of placenta

The placenta may be implanted in a normal fashion yet stuck firmly to the uterine wall. This is associated with any infectious process that produced a high temperature during pregnancy, intrauterine infection, disease of the fetal membranes and previous uterine surgery (Varney, 1997). Often the stuck area is very calcified. In these cases, manual removal, described in a separate chapter, is usually effective.

Partial or total abnormal adhesion (ingrowth) of the placenta

The term placenta accreta is used to describe any placental implantation that involves abnormal ingrowth of the villi into the underlying uterine wall. This occurs in regions of the uterine wall where the decidual formation is defective, resulting in a placenta that cannot separate normally, even with manual removal. There is a high correlation with implantation over a previous uterine scar, after uterine curettage, and with parity of six or more; the risk is also increased to 5% with placenta previa, including partial previa or a low-lying placenta.

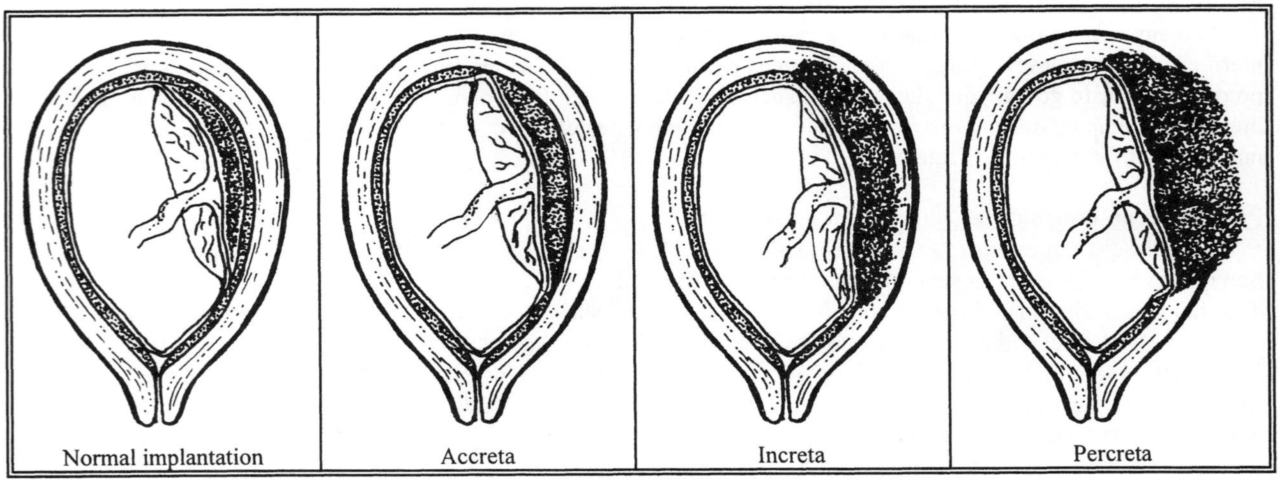

Placenta accreta (ah-CRE-tah): Accreta results in the presence of partial or complete absence of the decidua basalis layer of the uterus, which normally lies between the myometrium and the placenta. In addition, the plane of normal cleavage, the stratum spongiosum (the middle layer of the endometrium), is also absent, resulting in the placenta attaching directly to the surface of the myometrium.

Placenta increta (IN-cre-tah): In this more severe form of adhesion, the chorionic villi have penetrated into but not through the full thickness of the uterine myometrium.

Placenta percreta (PURR-cre-tah): This most serious form occurs when the villi have invaded the full thickness of the myometrium and grown into, and sometimes through, the serosa of the uterus. Occasionally, when the placenta is low enough and implanted anteriorly, it results in growth of the villi through the wall of the bladder, resulting in grossly bloody urine during pregnancy, and sometimes in partial or complete uterine rupture. Intraperitoneal bleeding occurs frequently. There is anecdotal evidence of an increased frequency of this complication with single-layer closure of a uterine incision after surgical birth.

Abnormal adhesion may occur over the entire maternal side, over just a few cotyledons (called "partial placenta accreta") or over a single cotyledon (referred to as "focal placenta accreta").

Clinical presentation: The clinical picture varies, depending upon whether the placenta is partially or completely ingrown. A completely ingrown placenta does not produce any uterine bleeding and will leave the uterus in exactly the same place it was after the baby came out, unless it is being displaced upward by a full bladder. Partially detached placentas bleed beneath the normally detached portion; meanwhile the uterus cannot clamp down properly because the attached portion prevents the placenta from delivering and thus hinders full retraction of the myometrium under the detached portion. In short, there is no definitive clinical evidence that the cause of delay is an accreta. No bleeding whatsoever with prolonged retention of the placenta in the presence of effective uterine contractions should raise your index of suspicion and prompt transport rather than risking manual removal at home.

What to do: The only way to positively identify an abnormally adherent placenta is to perform an internal uterine exploration, to determine if a normal line of cleavage exists between the maternal surface of the placenta and the uterine wall. However, any unsuccessful attempt to manually remove the placenta is very likely to result in a torrential hemorrhage. You may detach part of the placenta, only to find that a portion of it is accreted. This situation is complicated by the placenta still being in the uterus, thus preventing myometrial retraction. Too vigorous attempts to remove the placenta via cord traction can result in uterine inversion; likewise, too vigorous attempts at manual removal can result in uterine rupture (for more details, see the subchapter entitled "Manual Removal of the Placenta"). If you are close to a hospital, transport is your safest alternative.

However, if you are remote from help and the woman is bleeding heavily, an attempt to manually remove the placenta may be your best option. If this cannot be accomplished easily, give oxytocin and Methergine, start an IV and administer oxygen at 10 l/min. Treat the mother as you would for shock and transport as quickly as possible. If the placenta is accreted, surgery will be required with the likely result that the uterus must be removed.

Uterine Inversion

This rare complication (1 in 5000 to 1 in 100,000 births, depending upon the source) occurs when the uterus turns inside out, with or without accompanying hemorrhage. The wide variation of reported incidence may be due to differences in how the problem is recorded as well as varying placental delivery techniques. The placenta may be fully adhered or partially detached when inversion occurs or may have come out at some time prior. Most inversions occur in normal, healthy first-time mothers. Iatrogenic inversion is associated with various interventions designed to deliver the placenta, chief among them being cord traction. Spontaneous inversion, although not completely understood, is believed to be due to a disorder of the myometrium. The two prerequisites for any degree of inversion are cervical dilation sufficient to allow a portion of the uterus to prolapse and uterine relaxation. The demographics include women in their early twenties and term gestation. Women with a history of spontaneous inversion are at greater risk for recurrence at subsequent births. Predisposing factors include abnormalities of the uterus and its contents, such as:

- Adherent placenta (especially accreta)
- Fundal implantation of the placenta
- Short cord
- Congenital anomalies of the uterus
- Weakness of the uterine wall underlying the placental site
- Growths (such as fibroids) within the uterus
- Functional disturbances such as relaxation of the myometrium or problems with normal uterine contractility
- Yoni birth after Cesarean
- Precipitate labor (3 hours or less)
- Large baby (exceeding 8 lb 13.25 oz [4000 grams])

Precipitating events include:

- Ill-advised cord traction to deliver the placenta (too forceful, without regard for signs that the placenta has separated, with the mother in an upright position, or between contractions)
- The application of fundal pressure to deliver the placenta when the uterus is relaxed
- The application of fundal pressure during manual removal of the placenta
- A sudden rise in intra-abdominal pressure when the mother coughs or vomits
- Atonic uterus
- Injudicious use of oxytocin or other uterine stimulants
- Spontaneously, with no apparent precipitating event

Puerperal inversion occurs in the hours after birth and is often associated with traction on the uterine muscle. In a case of spontaneous inversion, traction may be produced simply by the weight of the placenta. Many of the individual factors associated with inversion are common; most often, several must occur at once to produce inversion. The combination of a fundal implantation of the placenta, a flaccid uterine muscle around the implantation site and a dilated cervix predispose a woman to inversion after birth.

Classifying degrees of inversion

Several different formats for categorizing the severity of an inversion are described. First, the inversion is either puerperal or nonpuerperal. Puerperal inversions are associated with abortion, miscarriage, or labor. Inversion can also occur outside of pregnancy. A clinically based, temporally focused classification of inversion follows:

- **Acute:** Occurring immediately after the birth of the baby or placenta, before the cervical os has a chance to close down and extending through the first 24 hours when cervical contraction may or may not be present.
- **Subacute:** Occurs after 24 hours, but less than 4 weeks from birth, with cervical contraction usually present.
- **Chronic:** Occurs after more than four weeks have passed, with cervical contraction always present.

Another classification system is based purely upon timing:

- **Puerperal inversion:**
  - **Acute:** Occurs within the first 24 hours postpartum
  - **Subacute:** Occurs more than 24 hours but prior to 30 days postpartum

•**Acute:** Occurs within 30 days of birth
•**Chronic:** Occurs after 30 days postpartum

Other classification schemes address the severity of the inversion include a system of four degrees, or three descriptive categories shown below in parentheses, which overlap as follows:

1st degree (Incomplete): The body of the uterus or wall descends to the retraction ring.
2nd degree: Protrusion of the corpus or wall through the retraction ring but not to the perineum.
3rd degree: (Complete): The fundus protrudes through the os a variable distance into the yoni.
4th degree (Total or Prolapse): The uterus completely inverts, passing through the cervix and birth canal and presenting outside the introitus.

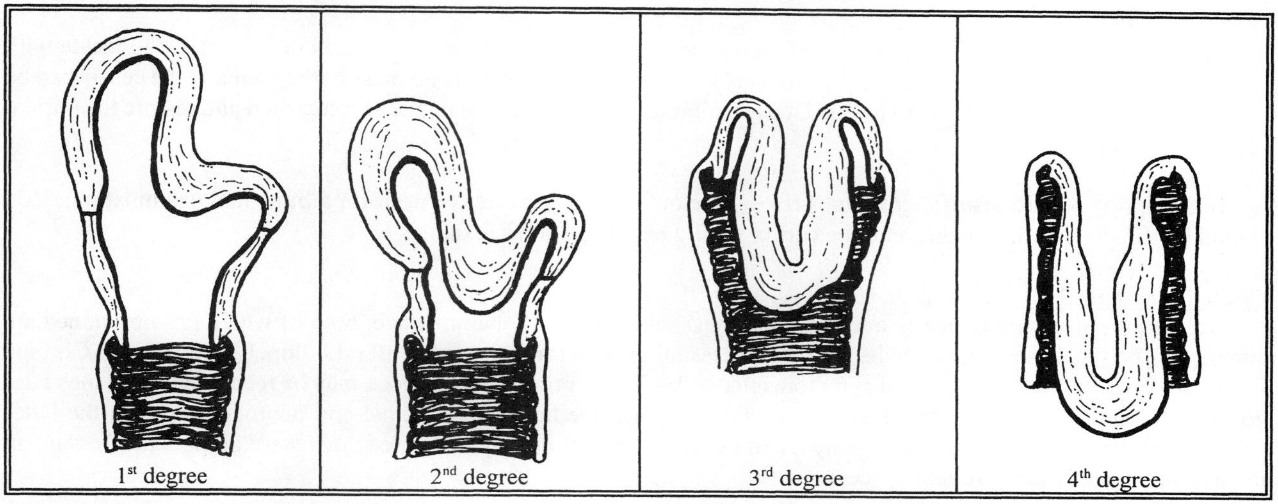

Preventing inversion

Always monitor the fundus for position and for any changes with your abdominal hand when assisting the birth of the placenta. Have the mother lie down, even for spontaneous delivery, if her uterus is boggy. Never apply traction to the cord with the mother upright, as proper monitoring of the fundus is impossible in this position. A dimple, which can often be palpated through the abdominal wall, will develop in the fundus if the uterus starts to invert. The mother is also likely to report pain. As inversion progresses, the dimple will recede more and more under your abdominal hand as the fundus descends through the cervix and yoni and finally makes an appearance at the introitus. *Stop any manipulations at once* if the mother reports pain or even a slight dimple is palpated. Discontinue all efforts to deliver the placenta, place the mother in a Trendelenburg position and transport immediately if you suspect that even a very minor degree of inversion has begun!

Differential diagnosis

Uterine inversion must be distinguished from the following conditions that share some of the same signs and symptoms:

Genital tract laceration: A bad tear revealing a mass of muscle tissue or accompanied by profuse bleeding may confuse the picture.
Prolapse of a uterine fibroid or cervical polyp: A submucous fibroid or other mass can descend through the cervix, partially or completely filling the yoni, thus mimicking a partial uterine inversion.
Ruptured uterus: Profuse bleeding and alteration of the position of the fundus in uterine rupture can confuse the picture.
Yoni, cervical or uterine prolapse: In cervical prolapse, the red, swollen body of the cervix fills the yoni and may be seen at the introitus. Identification of the opening of the os confirms that this is not the inverted fundus. Should the entire body of the uterus descend but not turn inside out, the fundus will move downward, but the cervix will lead the way. If only the yoni walls begin to prolapse, the cervix should still be found in the canal with no mass filling the os.

Gestational trophoblastic disease: A portion of a hydatidiform placenta has a lobulated appearance, like a bunch of translucent bloody grapes of varying size. A cancerous uterine growth (choriocarcinoma) may present as a dark red to purple shaggy mass in the mouth of the cervix and could be mistaken for the fundus. A placental hemangioma may present as a mass that is attached to or separate from the placenta, and its presentation at the os may mimic the descending fundus.

Foreign body: A blood-soaked foreign body, such as a tampon, that was lost up inside the uterus prior to pregnancy, can emerge with the placenta, leading you to believe that the uterus is coming along with the placenta. A wad of gauze pads accidently left in the yoni from suturing may also be discovered as a dark red mass filling the yoni and confuse you as well. In such cases, the fundus will be found where it should be and, with closer inspection, the nature of the foreign object will become clear.

Genital tract laceration: A bad tear revealing a mass of muscle tissue or accompanied by profuse bleeding may confuse the picture.

Uterine atony: In severe uterine atony, the fundus becomes flaccid, rendering it difficult or impossible to locate with abdominal palpation. The body of the uterus is wide and floppy. There is no mass in the yoni and the cervix can be palpated somewhere in the yoni canal. Uterine stimulants should tighten up the myometrium and restore the normal uterine contours.

If the tips above are insufficient to positively rule out a uterine inversion, perform a bimanual examination. You should be able to find the fundus, and the cervix should be felt on pelvic exam.

Clinical presentation

Acute inversions are typically accompanied by shock and usually hemorrhage, both of which prompt immediate attention. The shock is presumed to be neurogenic, resulting from traction on the infundibulopelvic ligaments. Chronic inversion can present with such mild symptoms that it is missed entirely, or the shock may be recognized with the cause going unrecognized, delaying treatment. Inversion may involve both hypovolemic and neurogenic shock, the latter produced by stretching of the broad ligament and peritoneal nerves as they are pulled downward along with pressure on the ovaries created during fundal descent.

Acute inversion: There are generally two ways that acute inversion presents:

Immediate inversion with or without placental detachment: Typically, strong cord traction is used in an attempt to deliver the placenta, during which the mother reports an unusual amount of pain as the placenta emerges. A large mass emerges from the yoni and the fundus cannot be palpated in the abdomen. The uterine fundus appears gray to reddish purple and may be mistaken for a swollen cervical lip. If the placenta is still attached, the mass that presents may, at first, appear to be the placenta that has finally delivered; as the fetal side will be fully visible, the inversion gives the appearance of a Schultz separation. However, the endometrium may be visible above the margins of the placenta, and examination will confirm that the placenta is attached to the mass. The mother will be in an unusual amount of pain. If the inversion is recognized and the fundus replaced promptly, the mother may remain stable and bleeding not be excessive.

Delayed acute inversion after the placenta is out: Another scenario involves difficult but successful delivery of the placenta using fundal pressure and cord traction. A short while later, bleeding is profuse, the fundus cannot be located in the abdomen, and the cervix cannot be located during an internal exam. Instead a dark red to bluish gray mass oozing blood fills the yoni. The exposed endometrium is usually coated with dark blood clots, giving it a ragged or shaggy appearance.

Details regarding presentation: The principle triad of symptoms include hemorrhage (94%), shock (39%) and pain. Complete inversion is generally easy to recognize. It is partial inversion that is likely to go undiagnosed. Partial inversion typically causes profuse bleeding and hypotension of such severity that the mother may have no detectable pulse. However, this extreme picture may not present; a woman may have no bleeding and the onset of shock may be much delayed. Partial inversion may also be more difficult to recognize abdominally, as the egg tubes and ovaries are dragged to the center of the abdomen as the fundus descends, thus filling the region where the dimpling begins and giving the impression that the uterus is still where it should be.

Classically, shock is greater than expected for the apparent amount of blood loss, a circumstance that should prompt the midwife to investigate the cause of bleeding further. Studies have shown, however, that massive hemorrhage often accompanies inversion, and that blood loss is frequently underestimated. Hypotension results from blood loss as well as tension on the nerves of the broad ligaments, egg tubes and ovaries, which are all dragged toward the cervix. Irritation of the peritoneum contributes to shock. Whenever shock is present, uterine inversion should be ruled out by making sure the fundus is at the appropriate height on abdominal palpation. Rapid recognition and deinversion will minimize blood loss, trauma and shock.

Chronic inversion

This term describes uterine inversion that occurs over time, particularly when the inversion goes unrecognized. The fundus begins to collapse in on itself. As the fundus gets lower and passes through the lower uterine segment, the cervical ring contracts and the lower segment of the uterus constricts around the inverted portion of the fundus, typically at the level of the retraction ring. The uterus swells and its blood supply is reduced. If this goes undetected, gangrene and necrosis lead to sloughing of the constricted portion of the uterus.

Key diagnostic tips:

- The fundus is not where it should be; in a thin woman, a cup-like depression may be felt abdominally.
- The cervix cannot be found on internal exam once the fundus has descended through the os. In some cases, a congested, soft, pear-shaped bleeding mass may be felt in the yoni canal.
- The mother may be shocky, with or without blood loss (but not always).

Treatment

What to do in the event of acute inversion: The best way to prevent deepening shock and ongoing hemorrhage is to replace the fundus as soon as possible. While this may exacerbate neurogenic shock by restretching the pelvic organs, it has proven to be the most effective way to avoid the most problems. Shock will usually persist as long as the uterine ligaments are stretched. The longer you wait to resolve the inversion, the more likely it is that a constriction ring will form (or, if one is already present, that it may become more rigid) and that the uterine fundus will become more engorged with blood.

Typically, the placenta will already be delivered. If the placenta has not yet detached, it may be abnormally adhered to the fundus. Although you could try to remove it prior to returning the uterus to its anatomical position, the chances of puncturing a hole in the uterus are much greater with the uterus turned inside-out. In addition, attempts at removal usually prompt profuse bleeding. Since you are very likely never to have seen this complication before, your skill at removing a placenta from an inverted fundus will likely be nonexistent. You are better off repositioning the uterus with the placenta still attached. (Both options are discussed in modern textbooks, although most agree that repositioning the uterus first is the safest option.)

1. Have an assistant start an IV.
2. Lie the woman flat.
3. Give her Rescue Remedy, arnica and bellis perennis in 200C to 1M potencies.
4. Have an assistant remain face to face with her throughout the procedure, keeping her conscious.
5. Don a sterile glove, preferably one with a long cuff. Generously apply sterile lubricant.
6. Insert your hand into the yoni if necessary. Hold the center of the fundus firmly in your palm with your fingertips near the uterocervical junction in the posterior and lateral fornices.
7. Exert even, well-distributed pressure, elevating the entire still-inverted uterus toward the mother's abdominal wall, directing your internal hand toward the mother's navel, while using your outside hand as a guide. Lifting stretches and tautens the uterine ligaments. It also prevents you from driving the fundus into the sacral promontory, which will arrest your progress. As the ligaments are tensed, the cervical ring should widen and the fundus will be pulled up through it. This minimizes the bulk of tissue passing through the cervix at once. Thus the uterus is replaced to its normal position. It may take 3 to 5 minutes for the fundus to gradually recede upward from your fist (or palm).
8. If this seems particularly difficult, a ring forceps can be applied to the cervical lip to provide countertraction.
9. After the fundus is restored to its normal position, clench your internal hand in a fist and begin bimanual compression.
10. Have an assistant administer 10 units of oxytocin IM, which will help contract the fundus.
11. Slowly remove your hand by gradually converting your closed fist into a cone, taking care to let the contracting uterus expel it rather than pulling it out and risking another inversion. It is most prudent to transport once the woman has

somewhat recovered from the experience so that she can be monitored by hospital staff. The woman who has had significant blood loss may require a transfusion. If she cannot be stabilized or if the placenta is still attached, transport immediately.

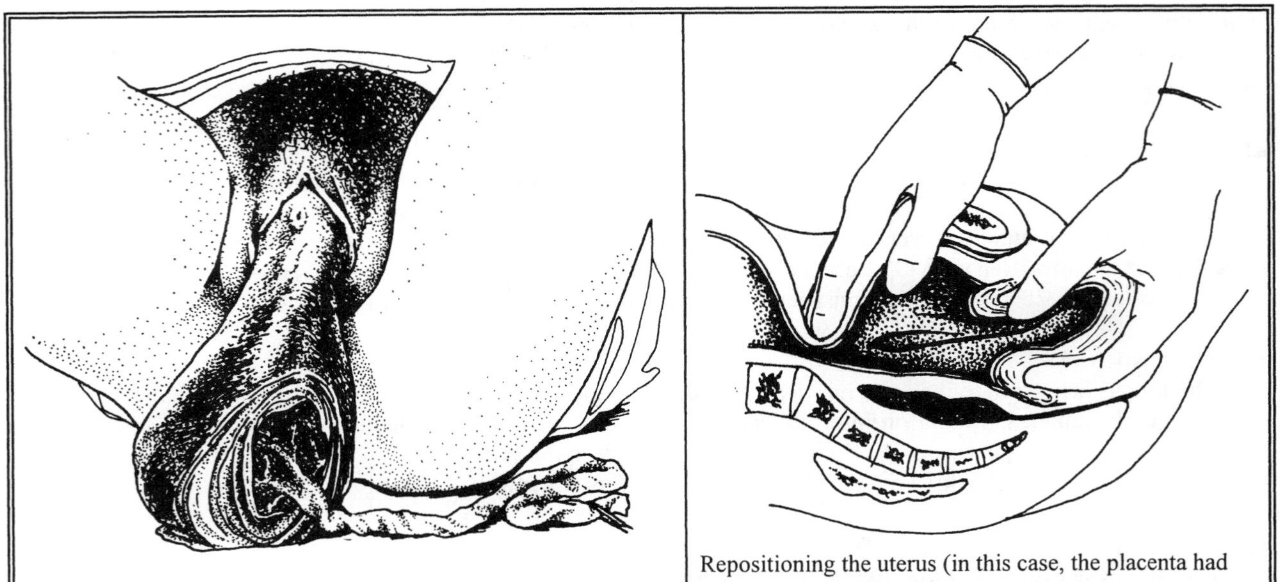

4th degree inversion with placenta attached

Repositioning the uterus (in this case, the placenta had already been born)

If the woman is stable, blood loss has been minimal to average, and the placenta is out, your decision to transport will depend upon the supplies you have on hand, her overall responses and your availability to spend the next 12 to 24 hours monitoring her. If you decide to stay home with her, administer uterine contactants on a regular basis, check the fundus frequently but very gently, place the woman's bottom in a slightly elevated position (propped up on a folded sheet) and accompany her when she gets up the first few times. Do not allow her to get up unless the uterus has been well contracted for at least an hour or so. Meanwhile, she can be catheterized or urinate into a towel or a bed pan. In any event, call the back-up practitioner and let him know an inversion occurred, report the mother's condition and ask what he would like for you to do at this point. A course of antibiotics should be discussed, as the risk of infection is increased.

What to do in the event of subacute inversion

There will be some delay in identifying the situation. Immediate replacement is no longer an option once the cervix has contracted around the inverted fundus or if a constriction ring has formed midway in the inverted uterine muscle. The only time it would be reasonable to consider managing this at home is if the mother is stable, blood loss has been minimal and you are very remote from a hospital. Only in such a situation should you consider giving lobelia to try and get the cervix to relax, but don't prolong attempts to reposition the uterus at home, as necrosis is likely to occur. The longer this situation persists the more danger that the mother will become infected or have circulation cut off to the point that she must have her uterus removed. Transport as quickly as possible while providing stabilizing support; place the mother supine and treat her for shock.

Immediate Postpartum Hemorrhage

This chapter addresses bleeding that occurs immediately after the placenta is delivered. If uterine bleeding is occurring and the placenta is not out yet, first deliver the placenta. (See the chapters entitled "The Birth of the Placenta, Cord and Membranes" and "Uncommon Problems That Can Interfere with the Birth of the Placenta.") If all the suggestions given in those chapters fail and the placenta cannot be delivered, start an IV, give oxytocin (either IM or in the IV solution) and transport. If you are remote from help or the situation is dire, proceed with a manual removal.

Once the placenta is out, bleeding may continue for a variety of reasons. In the majority of cases, something is preventing the uterus from clamping down completely. However, lacerations of the cervix, yoni canal, rectal area or perineum can also cause considerable bleeding and must be ruled out. This is especially true if a larger blood vessel has been torn. Therefore, the causes of postpartum bleeding may be broadly divided into four categories:

- Uterine atony
- Injuries such as lacerations (especially of blood vessels or the cervix), hematomas or uterine rupture
- Uterine inversion (see previous chapter)
- Coagulation failure

In many cases, excessive postpartum bleeding occurs during or immediately after the birth of the placenta. However, delayed bleeding is not uncommon. During the hours following birth, the uterus may contain retained clots, or there may be other reasons why a woman continues to bleed heavily.

Uterine atony

This is, by far, the most common reason for excessive bleeding after birth, accounting for up to 90% of all cases. It may occur before, during or after the birth of the placenta. Even a uterus that has contracted sufficiently to successfully deliver the placenta may not clamp down adequately to control bleeding. Reasons include:

- Disturbance of the mother due to lack of attentiveness or the necessary handling of birth complications that disrupt her delicate hormonal balance
- Long, tiring labor (the uterine muscle is exhausted)
- Polyhydramnios (overdistended uterus)
- Multiple gestation (large placental site; in some cases, the uterus is also overstretched)
- Anemia and malnutrition (lack of oxygen and other essential nutrients)
- Grand multiparity (A stretched uterus is the alleged reason, but this association is debatable. If a grand multipara is healthy, her uterus usually clamps down without a problem.)
- Induction or augmentation of labor for primary hypotonic uterine action
- Antepartum hemorrhage
- Low-lying placental site (The lower segment is not designed to close off bleeding as effectively as the upper segment.)
- Abruption (which causes damage to the uterine muscle by bleeding into the tissue)
- Rapid labor with a large baby
- Uterine rupture
- Adenomyosis (rare cause of postpartum bleeding; this is a form of endometriosis consisting of benign invasion of the myometrium by endometrial tissue which usually develops in multiparous women)

If the uterus is atonic, it will feel large and boggy on palpation. That is, the uterine shape will be ill-defined and, in extreme cases, large and squishy, like a soft, wet natural sponge. The fundus will be high in the abdomen, often at the level of the navel or above, and may be displaced to the right or left. Bleeding will not stop until the uterus clamps down. Therefore, if simple uterine stimulation with light fundal massage does not produce immediate firming, give the mother herbs or drugs to stop the bleeding. Only uterine contractant herbs will be helpful in this situation.

Sometimes uterine contractants do not work or something needs to be done to slow the bleeding while treatment has time to take effect. In this case, there are several things that can be done to help:

Give the mother a remedy to stop bleeding: Your remedy of choice may be an herb or herbal combination, homeopathic remedy or an oxytocic. If bleeding continues, immediately proceed with one of the compression techniques below. Torrential bleeding would be a reason to consider using misoprostol (Cytotec) intrarectally (2 to 6 tablets).

Stimulate SP-1: A most effective remedy for postpartum hemorrhage is to puncture Spleen 1, which is noted for its empirical effect of stopping uterine bleeding. It can be needled with an acupuncture needle, have moxa burned on it, or can be punctured with a lancet, much as you would puncture a finger for a blood draw. (See the chapter entitled "Traditional Chinese Medicine" for how to locate this point.)

There are three basic symptom patterns in Chinese medicine for a postpartum hemorrhage. Stimulating SP-1 works for all of the patterns without having to differentiate them. It is quicker and easier to prick this point with a lancet compared with needling or the time-consuming application of moxa. Keep some lancets with your delivery instruments; very quickly prick both toes at the beginning of a hemorrhage. This takes seconds; and, if it is going to be effective, works in just a few seconds more. The point is pricked only once, so if the hemorrhage is not controlled, move on to other protocols (Hobbs, 1999).

Compression techniques to control bleeding: There are three manual compression techniques that can be used to reduce blood loss: two external or abdominal methods and one internal or bimanual method. The goal of the two methods involving uterine compression is to firmly compress the bleeding placental site against the opposite uterine wall and, at the same time, reduce the blood flow to the uterus by compression of the entire organ and the large arteries that supply it. Either of these techniques can be very useful as a first-line manual therapy for hemorrhage due to uterine atony and can be performed until herbs or an injection of an antihemorrhagic agent takes effect or an IV with oxytocin can be started. The woman should be supine for each of these procedures. You may have to sustain compression for as long as 20 minutes to ensure that clotting has occurred at the placental site and the oxytocic drug or herbs have taken effect.

Abdominal uterine compression: This alone may be enough to stop the bleeding. Make a fist and press it into the abdomen, just above the symphysis. Angle your arm so that you are compressing the midportion of the uterus against the sacral promontory.

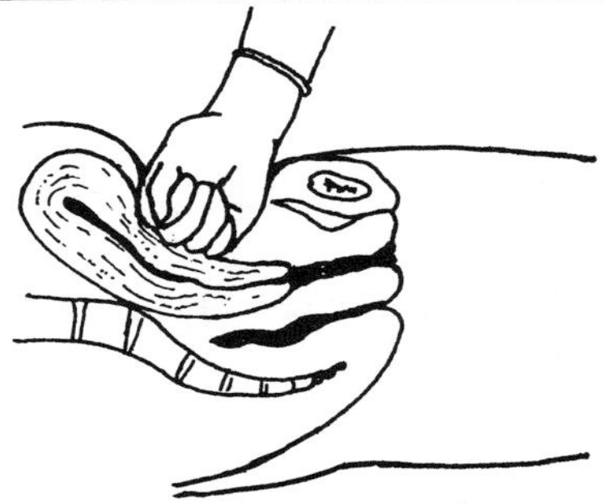

Abdominal uterine compression

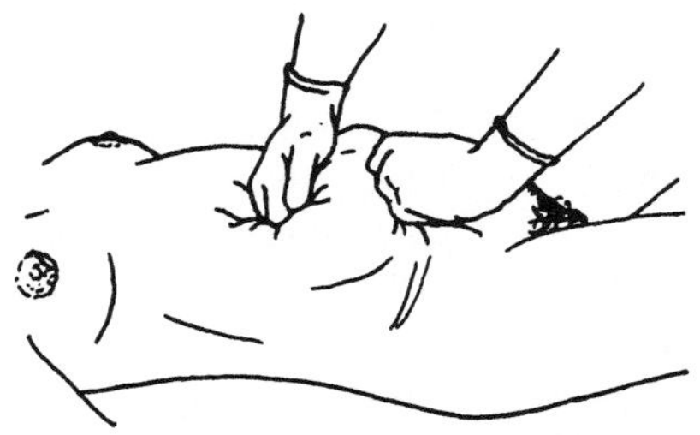

Bimanual abdominal compression

Bimanual abdominal uterine compression: This technique has the advantage of not increasing the risk of infection. To perform abdominal compression:

1. Stand to the woman's side, with your dominant hand at her head. Turn your body toward her head. Press your nondominant fist deeply into the abdominal wall just above the symphysis and press the uterus against the sacral promontory to help cut off blood flow to the uterine arteries. Now, pass your open dominant hand down behind the fundus (fingertips toward mother's spine, heel of palm on fundus) and use this hand to bend the fundus over your lower hand toward the symphysis. Compress the uterus between the palm of the hand on the fundus and the back of the other hand.

   If the above compression is not sufficient, you can use the suprapubic hand to grasp the lower part of the uterus just above the cervix, encircling the lower segment with your fingers. In most women, this should be easy to do as the abdominal wall is quite soft at this point. Squeeze the lower portion of the uterus and lift the organ upward toward the sacral promontory. If you are unable encircle the lower segment, place one hand behind the fundus and use the edge of your lower hand to press firmly downward into the abdomen just above the pubic bone, palm toward the fundus, and compress the uterus tightly between your palms.
2. Maintain compression for at least 5 and as long as 20 minutes before you gradually attempt to release it, all the while monitoring for bleeding (Mayes,1950; Marshall & Buffington, 1998).

Internal bimanual uterine compression: This technique is very effective in the event that abdominal compression fails to control the bleeding.

1. Don a sterile glove on your dominant hand. Rest this elbow on the bed and insert your dominant hand into the yoni.
2. Find the cervical os, which will be large and floppy. In grand multiparas, it may be extremely large and floppy. Pressing on the floppy cervix alone will not stop the bleeding. If the large cervix is hard to move out of the way, open your hand and use your fingers to massage the lower anterior part of the uterus (as high as possible in the anterior fornix) such massage frequently stimulates a contraction.
3. Clench your fist and place it in the anterior fornix (as far above the cervix as possible against the lowermost uterine wall). Gently push upward in the direction of the woman's navel (too much pressure will strain the uterine ligaments).
4. At the same time place your open nondominant palm on the abdomen, over the posterior side of the fundus, and apply pressure toward the yoni, with the heel of the external hand on the fundus.
5. The nondominant elbow points upward toward the ceiling. Compress the uterus between the two hands for at least 5 minutes or until you feel the uterus contract and find that the bleeding is controlled.

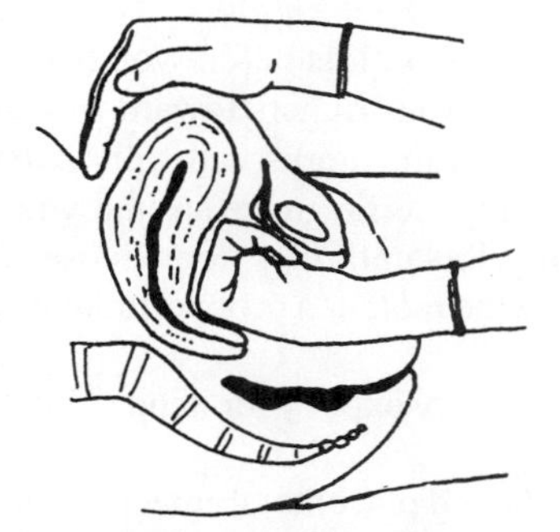

Internal bimanual uterine compression

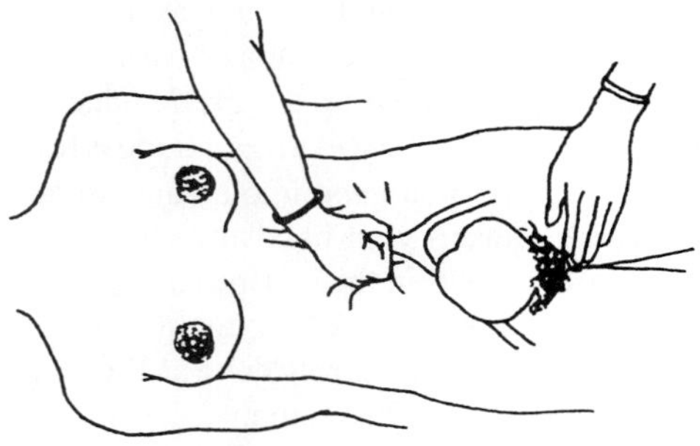

External aortic compression

External aortic compression: This is a last-resort technique that may work particularly well on thin women when nothing else is working to control the bleeding. External compression can be supplied as follows:

1. Stand to the side of the woman with your dominant side to her head.
2. Apply downward pressure with the closed fist of your dominant hand over the abdominal aorta directly through the abdominal wall at the point just above and slightly to the left of the woman's navel. (Aortic pulsations can usually be felt easily through the anterior abdominal wall in the immediate postpartum period.)
3. Use your other hand to palpate for the femoral pulse (upper inner thigh) to assess the adequacy of compression: increase the pressure on the aorta until the femoral pulse disappears.

It may be possible to have an assistant perform external aortic compression while another midwife performs internal bimanual compression if bleeding is torrential and otherwise uncontrollable.

Other causes of uterine bleeding

Bleeding may also be due to a variety of other factors, which may present at the time the placenta emerges or during the first few hours after the birth:

Retained placental fragments: Immediate postpartum hemorrhage due to small retained placental fragments is rare. However, a large piece of retained placental tissue can prevent complete closure of the placental site, making continued bleeding likely. Examine the placenta. If you choose to transport, take the placenta with you to the hospital so that it can be examined there. Generally speaking, retained fragments of membranes do not cause postpartum bleeding, although, on rare occasions, they can. If you suspect retained parenchyma, transport is your best alternative as removing small fragments may necessitate curettage. Give the mother uterine contractant herbs or drugs and use any other means necessary to control bleeding during transport.

Retained intrauterine clots: The midwife should have a high index of suspicion that bleeding is continuing if the mother reports that she feels weak, faint, queasy or vaguely uncomfortable; reports pressure in her abdomen (may have the urge to urinate); becomes unstable when in an upright position; or if she simply keeps slipping in and out of a marginally shocky state. This clinical picture is often associated with retained intrauterine clots. Clots become trapped inside the cervix; this may be seen with or without a trickle of bright red blood or more significant external flow. Flow from behind the clots typically looks somewhat thin and watery, but may appear as a darker red flow interspersed with small clots. The uterus is either somewhat high, globular and firm (suggesting that a full bladder is the only reason for difficulty) or intermittently firm and soft.

If you suspect clots are filling the uterus, first, examine the maternal side of the placenta and the extraplacental membranes to determine if retained placental fragments are the likely cause. If nothing appears to be missing, you can first try to evacuate the clots by pressing firmly downward on the uterine fundus while gently guarding the uterus. If this does not expel the clots and you feel sure clots are the problem or you suspect that pieces of the placenta are retained, perform a digital evacuation as follows:

1. Don a sterile glove on your dominant hand and insert two fingers into the yoni.
2. Place your nondominant hand on the fundus.
3. Locate the cervical os (it will be large, indistinct and flaccid). Insert your fingers into the os, gently pressing the uterus down toward your examining hand as much as necessary to accomplish this. Feel for clots. They will feel firm to semi-firm, slick, and gloppy, like clumps of warm gelatin. You may encounter clots before you reach the os.
4. Straighten your fingers, slide them up the inside edge of the cervix and curl your fingers toward the center to scoop the clots down and out. You may evacuate quite a few. Monitor the size of the uterus with your external hand. If some clots are stuck, form you hand into a cone, remove it gradually, wrap sterile gauze around your index finger (or first two fingers), reinsert your hand and wipe under and around the clots until they come loose.
5. Once no more clots are felt within the uterine cavity, have an assistant give the mother a dropperful of cotton root bark tincture or administer an injection of oxytocin.
6. Form your internal fingers into a narrow cone as the uterine contractions slowly expel your hand. Withdrawing your hand forcefully invites uterine inversion.
7. Carefully examine all the clots by dissolving them in water to see if any retained placental fragments can be identified. If you suspect retained fragments that cannot be identified in the clots, they are probably still attached to the uterine wall. Removing them will require a full-scale intrauterine exploration, which means more pain, and another invasion of the uterus, which raises the risk of infection even more. Therefore, it is best to take the mother and the placenta to the hospital for a curettage (scraping of the uterine wall to remove all placental fragments).

If the placenta was low lying or the oxytocin alone does not slow the bleeding to normal lochia, administer an IM injection of Methergine. Continue to monitor the mother frequently to make sure more clots are not accumulating in the uterus. Once the uterus is empty, most women have a remarkable and rapid recovery of their sense of well-being.

Lacerations

Yoni lacerations: It is good to remember that lacerations are more likely whenever the birth has been assisted with any type of manual intervention. Occasionally lacerations of the yoni will bleed profusely, especially when a blood vessel has been torn. It may be necessary to tie off the bleeding vessel before you can proceed with repair. See my text HEALING PASSAGE for a complete description of how to handle a bleeding laceration.

Cervical lacerations: While small tears of the cervix usually are symptom free, larger tears of the cervix are even more likely to bleed profusely. The flow from a cervical tear seems to be precipitated by maternal movement as well as uterine checks. The blood will be bright red and quite liquid. These types of tears can bleed on and off for weeks after the birth. Large cervical tears should be clamped at the apex with a ring forceps and the woman should be transported for repair. See HEALING PASSAGE for details regarding how to deal with cervical lacerations.

Uterine lacerations: Manual interference can produce cervical tears that extend into the lower uterine segment or tears in other parts of the uterus. Uterine rupture can produce similar injuries. If you suspect or detect such damage, transport immediately.

Hematomas

A hematoma forms when a blood vessel is torn and bleeds out under the skin surface. A blood blister of varying size produces pain, irritation of the surrounding tissue and tenderness. These sensations will usually be worsened by maternal movement, external pressure and palpation. A fluctuant swelling will also be found in the area of the damaged vessel, although enlargement may produce swelling that is distant from the bleeding source. Sometimes the clot of a small hematoma will produce enough counterpressure to stop the bleeding from the torn vessel it contains. In these cases the hematoma is simply left to be reabsorbed. If the hematoma is large, however, internal bleeding can be profuse and may continue, leading to hypovolemic shock. Hematomas are discussed in detail in HEALING PASSAGE.

Coagulopathy

A woman who has experienced a significant amount of ongoing bleeding during labor (for example during an abruption), either as an outright hemorrhage or in a persistent trickle, or who has bled excessively postpartum, may have depleted clotting factors. The blood she passes will not clot normally and will probably be thin and watery. Such women are at grave risk for shock and death. If you suspect that clotting factor deficiencies are interfering with a woman's ability to stop bleeding, given Yunanbiao or shepherd's purse tincture and transport immediately, regardless of the condition of the uterus.

Trickle hemorrhage

Slight but steady bleeding that persists in the immediate postpartum hours may be due to a variety of factors, such as a retained piece of placenta, an unrecognized cervical tear, an unrecognized torn yoni blood vessel (even if the overlying laceration has been repaired), a partially atonic uterus, retained intrauterine clots with blood seeping out around their edges or depleted clotting factors. A trickle hemorrhage that goes on long enough may lead to depleted clotting factors. So note whether the blood lost is clotting normally. Avoid a slow, steady bleed by administering the proper herbs or drugs (Methergine is the best remedy for normotensive women) as necessary. Troubleshoot these other possibilities.

A trickle hemorrhage can be insidious, resulting in severe blood loss that quietly pools under the mother who is not properly monitored postpartum. A woman can slip into a coma and die if the bleeding goes unrecognized long enough. The mother may be losing far more blood than is apparent. Check the uterus and other sources of bleeding. You may have to remove the sutures in order to identify and ligate a seeping blood vessel. (See HEALING PASSAGE for more information.) Trickling will also occur in the presence of a well-contracted uterus if clotting factors are depleted. If you cannot stop a trickle bleed, transport.

SPECIFIC SKILLS

MANUAL REMOVAL OF THE PLACENTA

Manual removal of the placenta is an invasive procedure that can be used as a last resort to remove a placenta that is adhered normally but has not been delivered. It should be performed only after all other attempts to get the placenta out have failed, in situations in which the woman is rapidly losing blood and transport means losing valuable time, or in which you are remote from medical help. If the placenta simply will not come out and there has been little or no bleeding, the safest and most prudent course is to transport rather than attempt to perform a manual removal yourself.

Manual removal carries the risk of introducing infection, rupturing the uterus or causing torrential hemorrhage if the placenta is abnormally implanted. It can be extremely painful and may push a woman over the edge into shock. With all this in mind, many midwives who felt they had no other choice have successfully accomplished manual removal in the home. The following instructions are based on interviews with midwives and the study of various textbooks, particularly Greenhill (1951), Mayes (1954), Varney (1997) and Willson (1961). To perform this procedure:

1. Have the woman's partner or someone else hold the baby and explain to the baby what is happening. The baby may be very frightened. This person should maintain good contact with the baby and allow the baby to cry if necessary. If the baby is very distressed, take the baby from the room but continue to talk to the baby and give him permission to express his feelings.
2. Have the mother lie down flat on a firm surface with her bottom just over the edge. This position will afford you the best access. If possible, flex her knees, with legs apart and her feet supported on either side below the level of her buttocks.
3. Start an IV. Have an assistant draw up an IM injection of 10 units of oxytocin to be given after you have finished the removal. Your assistant should have Rescue Remedy on hand to give the mother throughout the procedure. Before beginning, give the mother a dose of arnica 200C and bellis perennis 200C, both of which are for deep tissue bruising, swelling and general tissue trauma.
4. The assistant should be face to face with the mother at all times, establishing continuous eye contact with the intention of keeping her conscious.
5. Catheterize the bladder, unless you are quite sure it is empty. A full bladder will render the procedure even more uncomfortable and can result in trauma to the bladder.
6. Be sure the anal area is clean. Place an absorbent underpad, plastic side up, across the lower perineum and rectum to avoid contamination of your examining hand.
7. After thoroughly washing your hands and arms, don a sterile, long-sleeved glove on your examining hand. If you do not have a long-sleeved glove, first make a plastic sleeve for your forearm with a long thin plastic bag (such as a bread bag). Then don your sterile glove and tuck the end of the bag into the cuff. It is probably best to use the hand that gives you the most control over fine motor activity. To discover which hand works best, experiment performing manual removals with a knitted uterus and a cloth placenta (see instructions regarding how to make model placentas in the chapter entitled "The Birth of the Placenta, Cord and Membranes.") However, as a practical matter, the location of the placenta may determine which hand will work best. If the placenta is implanted on the mother's left, your right hand will have better access; if it is on her right, your left hand will probably work best. Posterior implantation is most common. Your dominant hand may work best if the placenta is implanted anteriorly or posteriorly.
8. Lubricate your glove with sterile, water-based lubricant. If you are unsure if the lubricant is sterile, don't use it.
9. Form your fingers into a cone, tucking your thumb into your palm, and insert your entire gloved hand into the yoni. Avoid touching the perineum as much as possible and do not touch the anus. Using your external hand to hold the cord taut, use your internal hand to follow the cord inside.
10. Try to get your fingertips under the membranes. Once your examining hand is inside the yoni, spread your fingers enough to allow the cord and membranes to pool in your hand. If you can get the membranes into your hand, your fingertips will move along their maternal side (between the uterine wall and the membranes), which will naturally lead you to the edge of the placenta. Once your fingertips are under the membranes, endeavor to keep the cord and membranes in your palm while bringing your fingertips together into a cone (hold them together in a point) to make your hand as small as possible as you advance it all the way through the cervix. Insinuate your fingertips under the membranes as you follow them to the lowermost edge of the placenta.

If you could not get under the membranes: Hold the cord taut with your external hand so that it is parallel with the mattress. Form your internal fingers into a cone around the cord and advance them along the cord to where it attaches to the placenta. Now, form your fingertips into a straight line. You may need to turn your palm to the fetal surface to use the pads of your fingertips to palpate along it, first to get a sense of the size of the placental disk and then to find the edge of the placenta. The extraplacental membranes form a barrier to direct contact with the uterine wall. Once you find the edge of the placenta, your hand will need to navigate around and under the membranes in order to identify a line of cleavage between the fetal surface of the placenta and the uterine wall.

Practitioners experienced with manual removal can sometimes manage to perform the entire procedure with the membranes remaining between their fingers and the line of cleavage, allowing the membranes to act as a glove. Advocates of this feel that it further protects the mother from infection (Mayes, 1954). However, because you will rarely, if ever, do manual removals, it is most prudent to move around the membranes and have your fingers in direct contact with the line of cleavage.

If the cord was broken at birth: Insert your gloved hand and find the end of the cord. Maneuver your hemostat into the yoni with your external hand and attach it to the end of the cord. It may be helpful to use the longest hemostatic instrument that you have. Ring forceps will help prevent trauma to the mother's soft tissues. Leave the forceps attached as you proceed as above.

11. As your hand advances into the uterine cavity, you may encounter a constriction ring, which may feel similar to a partially dilated cervix. Your cone-shaped fingers should pass through it easily. If the constriction ring is tight, exert gentle but steady pressure with the point of your hand to gain entrance to the upper portion of the uterus. If you cannot gain entry, stop and refer to the comments below.

    When you have located the edge of the placenta, search around to see if you can find a portion that has already started to separate. This will make it easier to start and will help define your line of cleavage.
12. Once you have identified a plane of cleavage, release the cord you have been holding taut with your external hand. To prevent the uterus from receding as you continue the procedure, place your open external hand on the abdomen over the place where your internal hand is. This hand can also be used to grasp and pull up on the uterus to provide countertraction, which will help to prevent uterine inversion. However, as the manual removal is being done, it is more important to provide guidance for the internal hand than countertraction. Providing this guidance is very important because the uterus is very soft at this point. Your external hand will also help the uterus maintain at least some degree of contraction, which will help define the wall and make your job easier as well as lessen the chance that you will poke a hole in the wall.
13. If the mother is bleeding heavily and the uterus is boggy, once you have found the edge of the placenta you can give an IM injection of oxytocin to help bring the uterine muscle together. This should reduce bleeding by tightening up the myometrium somewhat. Better contractions will also thicken the uterine wall, lessening the chance that you will damage it while trying to get the placenta out.
14. Now cup your hand and form your fingertips into a straight line, holding them tightly together. Place the back of your internal hand against the uterine wall, with your fingertips wedged beneath the placenta's edge. Cup your hand slightly so that the back of your hand follows the contour of the uterine wall. Gently attempt to insinuate your fingertips between the edge of the placenta and the uterine wall, making sure to keep your plane of cleavage horizontal to the surface of the uterine wall; doing so makes it less likely that you will pierce the wall. If you find a partially detached edge of the placenta, start there.

    Use the palmar surface of the external hand to press the uterus down and over the fingers inside the uterus. This pressure should be applied as sensitively and as gently as is consistent with accomplishing your purpose. Remember that the postpartum, poorly contracted uterus is very easily punctured. The external hand should provide support and counter pressure as it follows the movements of the internal hand.
15. Keeping your internal fingers together, detach the placenta. You can use a slow and gentle side to side "slicing" (or "beauty-queen waving") motion. Alternatively, you can use a gentle lifting motion by curving the tips of your fingers up slightly to lift the placenta off the uterine wall. Then wedge your fingers beneath the area you just separated until you find the next attached region; lift or slice again, continuing until the entire placenta comes away. *Never claw at the placenta with your fingertips, as this may produce a tear in the placenta or a hole in the uterus.* If the placenta will not detach, you may have to use your external hand for support as you sever tough strands of collagen with your internal fingers. Always keep your plane of cleavage horizontal to the line of separation to avoid boring a hole in the uterus. Remember that the uterine wall will be curved, how curved depends upon how boggy the uterus has become

(a uterus that is contracting will be smaller and have a more curved wall). As you move your hand to remove the placenta from the uterine wall, you are likely to become aware of abdominal organs adjacent to the uterine wall. This can be a frightening sensation. Keep breathing and keep going.

Different midwives have described the feeling of detaching the placenta using the following analogies, all using the same hand motions described above:

•Removing the meat of an orange from the peel
•Removing the skin from a chicken breast (skin is the uterine wall)
•Removing the membrane from a fresh calf liver (membrane is the uterine wall)
•Handling corn meal mush (no line of cleavage in the case of a placenta accreta)

16. The placenta will feel spongy, and there will be a sensation of give as the placenta is removed from the wall. The wall of the uterus in the region beneath the detached placenta may have rounded indentations where the cotyledons were implanted. One midwife has described them as similar to indentations made in soft clay by golf balls. This area of indentations feels smaller than the cotyledons appear on the delivered placenta because the area of implantation will contract. Kerr (1916) says to expect the region of implantation on the uterine wall to feel ragged after the placenta is detached. It cannot not be rendered smooth, even after scraping with the fingers (which he strongly advises against, as it increases the likelihood of weakening the uterine wall).
17. Continue to use a slicing or lifting motion until you have detached the entire placenta. The placenta in utero often feels larger than it looks once it is delivered. Therefore, be aware that there is probably more placenta to detach after you have covered an area that seems to be the size of most placentas (Mayes, 1954).

    Do not remove your hand until you are certain that the entire placenta is detached. Once most of the placenta is detached, do not pull on it with the idea that the rest will also come away; this notion is just plain illogical given the need for a manual removal in the first place. Although the rest of the placenta may detach if pulled, it is unlikely to. Pulling also increases the chance you will need to go back in for fragments, thereby increasing the risk of infection and more bleeding as well as of shock because of the pain. In addition, if you pull it off, you will not be able to tell if you have the entire placenta when you do your exam. The manually removed placenta is ragged; therefore it will be harder to determine if it is intact. If you have not satisfied yourself that it is fully detached while your hand is still in the uterus, you will always question whether you covered the entire implantation site.
18. Once you have detached the entire placenta, grasp it in your hand. Then, use both hands to stimulate a contraction cupping your abdominal hand over your internal hand and gently rocking the uterus. Now use your external hand to provide as much countertraction as you can by pushing upward slightly, toward the mother's head (to prevent inversion). Allow the uterus to expel the hand that is holding the placenta as you gently withdraw it. Insertion of your hand may have created some suction within the uterine cavity and yoni canal. Quick withdrawal may be impossible or unduly painful, as well as invite uterine inversion and additional bleeding. As you bring the placenta out, be aware of the membranes trailing on all sides, do the best you can to deliver all of the membranes as you would during a normal placental delivery.
19. Have your assistant give an IM injection of 10 units of oxytocin once the hand carrying the placenta is completely withdrawn through the os.
20. Examine the placenta as soon as possible. If you suspect that fragments or a portion have been retained, transport immediately. If transport is impossible, perform an intrauterine inspection (see next chapter). Wear a new sterile long-sleeved glove.

After the placenta is removed, treat the mother as you would for shock and watch her closely for the next several hours. Administer another dose of oxytocin or give Methergine IM if the oxytocin is not sufficient to control bleeding. You may want to keep one hand on her uterus for the first hour to detect any uterine relaxation, depending upon how the mother and her uterus responded to the procedure and how much blood was lost (Mayes, 1954).

Give the mother arnica 200C or 1M and bellis perennis 200C or 1M for trauma once the procedure is completed. Notify the back-up provider that a manual removal was performed. Carefully monitor the mother for infection in the two weeks following birth.

Postpartum Intrauterine Exploration

Intrauterine exploration is a painful and risky procedure described in detail by Varney (1997). It should only be done by a midwife who suspects that placental fragments are still attached to the uterine wall or have been retained in the uterus when she is far from medical help and the mother is unstable and is continuing to bleed. There is no point in subjecting a woman to uterine exploration without benefit of anesthesia unless you are truly have no other choice and you believe a significantly large piece of placenta is still inside. It is always be best to transport for intrauterine exploration if the mother is currently stable and transport is feasible.

In order to fully appreciate the steps taken during intrauterine exploration, read about manual removal of the placenta in the preceding subchapter, as the rationale for many of these suggestions is the same.

1. Have someone else hold and comfort the baby.
2. Lay the mother flat on a firm surface.
3. Start an IV if blood loss has been excessive.
4. Give the mother Rescue Remedy, arnica 200C and bellis perennis 200C.
5. Have an assistant maintain face-to-face contact with the mother at all times during the procedure.
6. Catheterize the mother, if necessary.
7. Don a sterile glove with a long cuff.
8. Place your ungloved hand on the fundus in the same manner and for the same reasons as during a manual removal.
9. Wrap sterile 4×4 in gauze around two or three of your fingers, keeping in mind that the back of your fingers will be used to wipe the uterine wall. Hold the edge of the gauze against the side of your index finger; hold the other side of the gauze between your ring and little fingers. Only one piece gauze is used to prevent leaving any gauze in the uterus. Shape your gloved fingers into a cone and insert your entire hand into the yoni, work it through the cervix and into the uterine cavity.
10. Sweep the uterine wall with the back of your hand, cupping it slightly to match the contour of the uterus. After exploring the entire uterine cavity, withdraw your hand slowly, preferably during a uterine contraction.
11. Examine the debris on the gauze and differentiate placental and membranous fragments from blood clots. Repeat the exploration with fresh gloves and gauze only once more should you suspect remaining fragments.
12. When you note this procedure in your record, be sure to mention that one gauze square went in and came out during each procedure and the number of procedures performed.
13. Monitor the mother closely for uterine atony, shock, bleeding and postpartum infection.
14. Administer uterine contractant herbs or drugs.

References and Further Reading on Problems That Can Occur During Placental Delivery and in the Immediate Postpartum Period

References used in multiple chapters

Bennett VR, Brown LK, eds. Myles Textbook for Midwives, 13th ed. Churchill Livingstone, Edinburgh UK, 1999.

Doolittle J, Moritz, R. Obstetrics and Gynecology. 1966.

El Halta V. Moving Midwifery Forward. Garden of Life Pub, Dearborn MI, 1989.

Greenhill J. Principles and Practice of Obstetrics, 10th ed. WB Saunders, Philadelphia PA, 1951.

Hobbs V. Personal communication, 1999.

Kerr JM Munro. Operative Midwifery: A Guide to the Difficulties and Complications of Midwifery Practice, 3rd ed. William, Wood & Co, New York NY, 1916.

Marshall M, Buffington S. Life-Saving Skills Manual for Midwives: Module 5; Prevention and Treatment of Hemorrhage; Module 6; Resuscitation, 3rd ed. American College of Nurse-Midwives, Washington DC, 1998.

Mayes B. A Textbook of Obstetrics. Australasian Pub Co, Sydney Australia, 1950.

Mayes B. Practical Obstetrics, new ed. Angus & Robertson, Sydney Australia, 1954.

Oxorn H. Oxorn-Foote Human Labor and Birth, 5th ed. Appleton-Century-Crofts, Norwalk CT, 1986.

Varney H. Varney's Midwifery, 3rd ed. Jones & Bartlett, Sudbury MA, 1997.

Walsh S. "Maternal effects of early and late clamping of the umbilical cord," Lancet, (7550);996-997, May 11, 1966.

Willson J. An Atlas of Obstetric Technic, deluxe ed. CV Mosby Co, St. Louis MO, 1961.

World Health Org. (WHO), McCormick M, ed. Integrated Management of Pregnancy and Childbirth: Managing Complications in Pregnancy and Childbirth: a Guide for Midwives and Doctors, Reproductive Health and Research, WHO, Geneva Switzerland, 2000.

Uterine Inversion

O'Grady J, Buckman R, eds. Obstetric Syndromes and Conditions. Parthenon Pub Group, New York NY, 1998.

Wendel PJ, Cox SM. "Emergent obstetric management of uterine inversion," Obstet Gynecol Clin N Am, 22(2);261-274, June, 1995.

Immediate Postpartum Hemorrhage

Riley D, Burgess R. "External abdominal aortic compression: a study of a resuscitation maneuver for postpartum hemorrhage," Anaesth Intens Care, 22:571-575, 1994.

Understanding and Treating Shock

An Overview of Shock Syndromes

One of the most serious complications faced by midwives is the development of shock and, while most of the time shock is considered a maternal problem, a baby who is born pale, limp or otherwise compromised from asphyxia or hypovolemia is in shock as well. Shock is a life-threatening emergency that requires immediate attention. This section presents basic information regarding what shock is, the types that can occur, how the body responds to it and how to recognize and treat it. Throughout the book, when shock is mentioned, refer to this section for those basics.

What is shock?

The term "shock" encompasses a wide variety of physiologic derangements that share the common denominator of inadequate tissue perfusion leading to impaired metabolism at the cellular level. Shock is not a systemic phenomenon but a cell-by-cell deprivation of oxygen. When the body is unable to deliver blood to all of the capillaries, the amount of oxygen and nutrients reaching the tissues falls, and cell death eventually occurs. When enough organ systems are so affected, systemic shock develops. Toxins begin to accumulate as oxygen levels fall because the toxins are not being adequately removed. Shock may result from a problem with the heart, the blood vessels or an insufficient circulating blood volume prompted by blood maldistribution or loss. When enough cells in a single organ die, organ death takes place and shock becomes irreversible.

Shock syndromes

There are several types of shock. These can be categorized according to their specific pathology, although overlap does occur among these classifications. All types of shock can be caused by conditions that occur during pregnancy.

Hypovolemic shock: This occurs because of reduced cardiac preload (decreased ventricular filling because not enough blood is flowing into the heart), leading to decreased stroke volume and cardiac output. These trigger compensatory catecholamine release, which leads to an increase in systemic vascular resistance and heart rate. The reduction in preload may be due to internal or external hemorrhage or to extracorporeal loss, which most commonly occurs through the gastrointestinal tract or via urinary fluid loss. Initial treatment is fluid replacement and might include blood replacement in severe hemorrhagic shock.

Hemorrhagic hypovolemic shock: This occurs after an acute loss of blood due to internal or external hemorrhage. A newborn can experience blood loss when blood that he needs remains in the placenta for any reason. It is the most common type of shock among childbearing women and is covered in detail in the next chapter.

Nonhemorrhagic hypovolemic shock: This term encompasses several subcategories of shock including dehydration and conditions that involve capillary leak.

Dehydration can be caused by loss of body fluid due to severe vomiting or diarrhea or both. Excessive urination, such as that occurring in uncontrolled diabetes, can lead to this type of shock as well.

Capillary leak produces another form of nonhemorrhagic hypovolemic shock. Capillary leak is a type of "third spacing" resulting from tissue damage that causes endothelial cell junctions to become loose, allowing fluid to leak from the intravascular space to the extracellular spaces, resulting in a net loss of intravascular volume. This may occur as a result of conditions that involve no actual bleeding, such as sepsis or plasma loss due to burns, pancreatitis or anaphylaxis. It also occurs when intravascular fluid leaks into the interstitial spaces. It may develop as a late secondary response in severe hemorrhagic shock.

Cardiogenic shock: This condition occurs when the heart muscle cannot deliver enough circulating blood to perfuse the tissues because its function fails for some reason. In an adult, this is usually the result of a myocardial infarction (heart attack), which can be due to necrosis in a region of heart tissue. In midwifery, it usually presents in the form of heart failure or congenital cardiac defects in the newborn. The remedy is to normalize the heart function and correct precipitating factors. Decreased contractility may result from inflammation, ischemia, and toxins that can injure the heart muscle. Infection or sepsis may be an associated factor in some cases.

Severe arrhythmias can change the heart rate, either speeding it up or slowing it down, which can decrease cardiac output. They are therefore not a direct cause of cardiogenic shock but can be a contributing factor. Extreme tachycardia does not allow the ventricles to fill adequately; hence they cannot eject enough blood to produce an adequate stroke volume. A heart rate that is persistently too slow results in an insufficient output over time and is an end result of irreversible shock.

Anatomic obstructive shock: This is a type of cardiogenic shock that occurs when the output of the left ventricle is reduced. It is unique to infants during the first weeks of life and is associated with certain congenital heart defects.

Restrictive shock (external obstructive shock): This is caused by obstruction of arterial or venous flow at any point in the circulation. For example, a tourniquet can result in restrictive shock to the distal tissue if left in place too long or applied too tightly. Common causes include massive pulmonary embolism, pericardiac tamponade (increased pressure around the heart from abnormal accumulation of fluid in the pericardium), tension pneumothorax, atrial valve stenosis, cardiac injury, inflammation or disease. Hemodynamic findings vary with the cause.

Distributive shock: This results in a decreased cardiac preload because of redistribution of capillary blood supply. This form of shock is seen with sepsis, anaphylaxis and neurogenic shock. Generally, distributive shock is characterized by an increased heart rate, rapid, weak pulses and, in most cases, cool extremities with signs of peripheral vasoconstriction. This leads to uncompensated shock with reduced systemic vascular resistance characterized by a fall in mean arterial blood pressure. Cardiac output is generally increased at first, but myocardial function might become depressed if shock is advanced. Treatment starts with fluid replacement and may include vasopressor drugs.

Anaphylactic shock: This is the most common type of distributive shock in adults. It is the most extreme form of allergic reaction, which occurs when an antigen interacts with an antibody. In severe cases, the chemicals released (e.g., histamine and bradykinin), produce widespread vasodilation and constriction of the smooth muscle in the bronchial tubes (bronchospasm). This reduces the diameter of the airway and thus the amount of air entering the lungs. Finally, intravascular fluid leaks into the intersitial spaces (capillary leak), producing both edema, which further constricts the airway, and relative hypovolemia. Venous return and cardiac output are dramatically reduced. (More details about this type of shock can be found in the chapter entitled "Hypersensitivity Reactions and Anaphylactic Shock.")

Septic (bacteremic or endotoxic) shock: This condition has many features of distributive shock, with elements of hypovolemic and cardiogenic shock. It is usually caused by a severe systemic bacterial infection during which endotoxins are released into the circulation from dead gram-negative bacteria, or exotoxins are released by the host organism (toxic shock). These toxins stimulate the release of complex vasoactive agents that affect arterioles, capillaries and venules, altering microcirculatory pressure and capillary permeability. Septic shock may develop as a result of staphylococcal and streptococcal infections (including pneumonia), postoperative or intrauterine infection (either after an abortion or birth), and infections resulting from indwelling catheters. The first line of therapy is treating the underlying infection. Because septic shock is most relevant in the postpartum period, it is covered in Volume III of this text.

Neurogenic shock (vasovagal stimulus, spinal shock or fainting): This kind of shock occurs in adults with sudden, acute pain, severe emotional trauma, spinal anesthesia, spinal cord injury, or massive drug overdose, especially with tricyclic antidepressants and barbiturates. Any of these precipitating factors can result in a clinical picture of distributive shock with hypotension and vasodilation. Vasodilation produces a relative hypovolemia which enlarges the cardiovascular "container" and reduces the preload that enters the heart, and therefore the cardiac output. Spinal cord injury can result in vasomotor paralysis below the level of insult. Neurogenic shock may occur with uterine inversion, regional anesthesia, or aspiration of gastric contents. In newborns, the vasovagal response can be triggered by stimulation of the posterior pharynx (which can occur during deep suctioning), leading to bradycardia and respiratory depression.

Whatever the cause, nerve impulses reduce the heart rate and, in turn, cardiac output. Venous return may also be reduced by vasodilation, causing the pooling of blood in dilated veins (resulting in relative hypovolemia). These changes work to reduce the blood supply to the brain, causing fainting. The period of unconsciousness is usually short. If the vasomotor disturbance is fleeting, recovery is complete in a few minutes.

When normal vasomotor tone is lost, however, peripheral vascular resistance decreases. In turn, vasodilation can increase vascular space to the point that even normal blood volume cannot fill it. If the underlying cause is serious enough, neurogenic shock can lead to coma and death.

Causes of maternal shock during pregnancy, labor or birth

Causes directly related to birth include:

•Inadequately expanded blood volume, bringing the woman into labor already in a state of borderline hypovolemia, coupled with blood loss after birth. In some cases, blood loss may appear to be within normal limits or even less than usual. However, if the preexisting hypovolemia is substantial, the mother will be physiologically compromised as a result.

•Bleeding from the placental site due to:
- -Miscarriage
- -Abruption
- -Placental problems such as previa, increta or percreta
- -Retained placenta
- -Postpartum uterine atony

•Trauma due to:
- -Ruptured ectopic pregnancy
- -Lacerations of the yoni, cervix or perineum
- -Uterine rupture
- -Uterine inversion
- -Hematomas, especially extraperitoneal hematomas of the broad ligament or paravertebral region

Causes that are related to the process of pregnancy include:

•Emotional shock (for example, the unexpected birth of a baby who has a defect or requires transport)
•Embolism due to thrombosis, amniotic fluid or air
•Eclampsia
•Sepsis
•Neurogenic insult (such as that occurring with acute pain secondary to abruption, uterine rupture, etc.)
•Severe nausea and vomiting

Iatrogenic causes include:

•Anesthetic complications
- -Aspiration of gastric fluid
- -Extended spinal or regional nerve block

•Drug reactions

Of course, numerous medical conditions may coexist with pregnancy and can lead to shock. These include:

•Cardiac complications leading to myocardial infarction
•Compromise to the respiratory system (e.g., spontaneous pneumothorax)
•Cerebrovascular accidents, such as aneurism
•Abdominal conditions:
- -Rupture of the appendix or spleen
- -Torsion or rupture of an ovarian cyst
- -Perforated peptic ulcer
- -Acute pancreatitis

The chapters in this section cover the various types of shock, complications of labor and birth in which shock is a primary presenting symptom, and the appropriate action to take when shock occurs. Septic shock is covered in Volume III of this text, as it is most likely to occur postpartum.

HYPOVOLEMIC SHOCK DUE TO HEMORRHAGE

While anyone can tolerate a certain amount of blood loss, there is a minimum amount of circulating blood volume that is required to maintain adequate cardiovascular function. The amount of blood the heart moves into the arterial system with each beat (cardiac output) depends upon several factors. These include the strength of cardiac contraction, the rate of contraction and cardiac preload. The heart fills during diastole and requires an adequate incoming supply of blood from the venous circulation, or preload, in order to pump effectively. Cardiac preload describes the force or pressure that propels the blood as it flows to fill the heart in preparation for the next heartbeat and is determined, in part, by the volume of blood entering the ventricle. Preload is technically defined as the degree to which the myocardial fiber is stretched as it fills at the end of diastole. If preload pressure is reduced, the heart cannot function normally and the amount of blood that will reach the tissues is reduced. In hypovolemic shock, preload is reduced as vascular fluid volume diminishes.

Hypovolemic shock is generally defined as a fall of the blood volume by 15%, based on blood loss in an adult male weighing 154 pounds (70 kg). This definition does not take into account individual responses to blood loss or the expanded blood volume of pregnancy. Therefore, the best gauge of shock is the development of signs and symptoms.

General Considerations Regarding Blood Volume and Cardiovascular Function

The adult body is a closed system. Normally, fluid moves throughout the system without the need for constant addition or removal of fluid. About 7% of the total body weight in the average-sized adult male consists of blood. One of the main variables in the actual amount of blood in a given individual is the percentage of body fat. Blood volume per kilogram of body weight varies inversely with the amount of excess body fat. This means that the less fat a person has, the more blood he or she has per kilogram of weight. Women normally have a higher percentage of body fat than men; therefore, they have less blood per kilogram of body weight, and therefore a lower normal blood volume relative to their total weight. Blood volume makes up about 6.5% of total body weight in nonpregnant women of normal weight, with about two-thirds in the venous side of the circulation.

To determine the approximate amount of blood volume for a nonpregnant woman, use the following formula:

Weight in pounds ÷ 2.2 = kilograms of body weight
Kilograms of weight × 65 = milliliters of blood volume
Milliliters of volume ÷ 1000 = liters of blood volume

For example, a nonpregnant woman who weighs 125 pounds would have about 3.7 liters of blood: ([125 ÷ 2.2] = 56.8 × 65 =3693 ml) ÷ 1000 = 3.7 liters. This chart provides general parameters for the total amount of blood volume for women of different weights.

NORMAL AVERAGE BLOOD VOLUMES (INCLUDING PLASMA AND RED BLOOD CELLS)	
WOMEN AT DIFFERENT AGES AND WEIGHTS	TOTAL BLOOD VOLUME (ADULT VALUES ROUNDED OFF TO NEAREST 100 ML)
Nonpregnant adolescent (105 lbs/47.7 kg)	12.4 cups/3.1 liters (3100 ml)
Young nonpregnant adult woman (140 lbs/63.6 kg)	16.8 cups/4.2 liters (4200 ml)
Well-nourished pregnant woman at term (190 lbs/86.4 kg)	23.6 cups/5.9 liters (5900 ml)
Term infant of normal weight range	10+ oz (300+ ml)

One liter equals about 2 pints. One milliliter (ml) is approximately 20 drops from a medicine or eye dropper.
15 ml=1 Tbsp 30 ml = just over 1 oz; 1000 ml = 1

Normal cardiorespiratory function

An understanding of hypovolemic shock is based on knowledge of normal physiology. Normal blood distribution and oxygen delivery involve the following factors, known as the Fick principle:

Binding of oxygen by hemoglobin across the alveolar membranes in the lungs: To ensure hemoglobin saturation, an adequate amount of oxygen must be available in the alveolar sacs. This means that breathing must be adequate, the pressure of inspired air must be normal and there must be minimal obstruction to the diffusion of oxygen across the alveolar capillary membrane.

Delivery of oxygen to the tissues by the red blood cells: This requires adequate circulation, good cardiac function and normal blood volume with proper routing of blood through the vessels. Red blood cells must be able to pick up oxygen in the lungs and unload it into the tissues. This requires normal hemoglobin levels, circulation of oxygenated red blood cells to the tissues in need, close approximation of the tissue cells to the capillaries to allow for diffusion of oxygen, maintenance of normal electrolyte balance (pH), proper temperature and other factors.

Arteriolar constriction: This factor is the main determinant of vascular resistance. Blood pressure is maintained by a combination of cardiac output (the amount of blood pumped by the heart) and systemic vascular resistance. Adequate mean arterial pressure is necessary for the proper function of the microcirculation. The wall tension of the ventricle during its ejection phase is called **afterload** (best reflected by systolic blood pressure).

Condition of venules and venous beds: These structures are largely responsible for the capacitance function of the vascular system. **Capacitance** refers to the electrical charge that maintains vascular tone, which, in turn, assures an adequate return of venous blood to the heart (preload).

Adaptations of pregnant physiology that prepare a woman for blood loss after birth

Blood volume at the end of pregnancy is expanded over nonpregnant levels. The extent of this increase depends upon the quality and adequacy of the mother's diet during pregnancy as well as the number of fetuses she is carrying. In the ideal situation, the average mother who carries one baby to term increases her plasma volume by 50%, from a nonpregnant level of 2600 ml to about 3900 ml by term. Her red cell volume increases from a nonpregnant average of 1400 to 1650 ml by term if she has not had an iron-rich diet or taken iron supplements and may rise as much as 1800 ml if she has. In addition, the levels of certain blood coagulants rise. These changes in blood volume and coagulation factors provide her with a margin of protection against hypovolemia, should she bleed excessively after birth.

Normal blood loss after birth for most women usually exceeds 600 ml. This value was derived from the study of hospital births; expect it to be closer to 500 ml if the woman has not had a perineal incision. Most well-nourished women who bleed at term bleed postpartum and have a margin of volume loss up to 1000 ml before signs of shock (such as tachycardia and, eventually, hypotension) become apparent. This is possible because the physiologic hypervolemia of pregnancy modifies the response to blood loss. The healthy woman will usually remain hemodynamically stable in the face of blood volume reduction as long as she does not lose more than 25% of her prepregnancy blood volume. This is not true for women experiencing blood loss who are not well-nourished in pregnancy or for those who are not at or near term at the time of birth because their blood volume is not fully expanded; nor is it true for those who experienced significant bleeding prenatally and did not have enough time to rebuild reserves before labor began. None of these women can afford to lose as much blood as those who reach term without problems.

An easy way to figure out both the total blood volume and the relative margin of safety for a well-nourished woman at term is to calculate her prepregnancy blood volume based on her weight at that time. Then divide that blood volume in half and add this number to the total nonpregnant blood volume; this gives you her approximate expanded blood volume at term. Divide the nonpregnant value by 4 to get a general idea of what she can afford to lose before shock ensues. Here is an example using the formula on the previous page: a woman who weighed 150 lbs before pregnancy had a total blood volume of 4433 ml when she is not pregnant.

$$4433 \text{ ml} \div 2 = 2216 \text{ ml};\ 4433 + 2216 = 6649 \text{ total ml at term}$$
$$4433 \text{ ml} \div 4 = 1108 \text{ ml of blood loss before signs of shock become apparent}$$

This calculation is a ball-park figure that does not take into account the exact ratio of plasma to red cell expansion. This does not mean that a midwife should sit and watch a woman bleed this much before doing anything, but it does give an idea of the degree of blood loss that is possible in the postpartum period at term. In essence, once the healthy woman has lost about half of the extra blood volume from her pregnancy, her body will respond to the rapid fall. Even though, theoretically, a woman should be able to lose all of her expanded surplus of blood and not experience shock, the rapidity of the loss and the need for the circulatory system to adjust to the sudden decrease in volume will, in itself, be traumatic and result in the manifestation of shock symptoms, even though she technically has that much blood to lose. Women who go into preterm labor or who have a poorly expanded blood volume at term, as well as any woman who is anemic, will respond much sooner and much more severely to any blood loss. The earlier the gestation, the more the woman will respond to blood loss as though she is not pregnant.

Postpartum recovery: If postpartum blood loss is within a normal range, there will be no compensatory increase in blood volume to make up the loss in the days following birth. Instead, plasma volume will gradually decrease after delivery via the physiologic diuresis that occurs via increased urination. The red cell mass will fall to nonpregnant levels more slowly as the red cells produced during pregnancy come to the end of their 120-day life span. Thus, in the immediate postpartum days, the hematocrit gradually rises as plasma volume falls. *If* blood volume expansion has been adequate, a first-day postpartum hematocrit is usually not altered significantly from the prelabor hematocrit, even with a loss of large magnitude (Clark et al., 1997).

Maternal organ perfusion, blood loss and placental function

Maternal cardiac output increases by 10% to 45% in pregnancy, while total peripheral resistance decreases. This occurs because of hormonal changes that reduce the vasomotor tone as well as create a low-resistance arteriovenous shunt for the placenta at the site of implantation in the uterine wall. About 20% to 25% of the maternal cardiac output goes to the placental bed, resulting in a blood flow of 500 ml per minute. Placental blood flow is directly proportional to the uterine perfusion pressure, which, in turn, is proportional to systemic blood pressure in the mother. Any decrease in maternal cardiac output results in a proportionate decrease in placental perfusion.

While all maternal organs receive increased blood flow during pregnancy, three are particularly susceptible to damage when perfusion is decreased. These are the anterior pituitary gland (which enlarges during pregnancy), the kidneys and the lungs. When a pregnant woman bleeds excessively, cardiac output is redistributed via selective arteriolar constriction controlled by the central nervous system to maintain perfusion of the heart, brain, and adrenal glands. This results in diminished perfusion to the kidneys, gut, skin and uterus as well as to the anterior pituitary gland, which can lead to ischemic necrosis.

From the standpoint of maternal survival, perfusion of the uterus becomes relatively unimportant in the presence of bleeding. In the pregnant woman, volume redistribution may result in fetal hypoxia and distress even before the mother becomes overtly shocky. Conversely, significant shock is highly unlikely in the absence of fetal distress, regardless of the absolute maternal blood pressure. However, continued blood loss will eventually place the fetus in grave danger; blood should be replaced promptly to avoid fetal distress and death.

The Pathology of Hemorrhagic Shock

When blood volume drops even slightly below normal, the body initiates a series of responses both to compensate for the loss and to restore adequate blood flow. As discussed above, healthy adults can lose at least 10 to 15% of their total volume without significant effect on arterial pressure or cardiac output; well-nourished pregnant women at term can lose somewhat more.

If that threshold of protection is exceeded, shock will ensue. Shock can be thought of as progressively diminishing tissue perfusion resulting in anaerobic (oxygen-free) metabolism at the cellular level. As blood volume falls, several responses are triggered as the body attempts to restore homeostasis; the individual response depends upon factors such as age, relative health, hydration, level of exhaustion, other conditions that compromise the body's responses (such as reduced clotting factors), the amount and rapidity of blood loss, and the body's ability to physiologically compensate for the problem. Most midwives are blessed by working with women of childbearing age who are robust and healthy and, therefore, likely to respond optimally to treatment even if they start to go into shock. In spite of these reassuring factors, all excessive blood loss must be taken seriously. A woman with an atonic uterus can bleed to death in less than two hours and may die in less than one hour if she is also anemic (Marshall & Buffington, 1998).

Compensated shock

In compensated shock, the body adjusts to blood loss by trying to normalize body functions in the presence of a less-than-adequate blood volume. Early on, the body tries to expand the blood volume by shifting fluid from the interstitial spaces and intestinal tract into the capillary beds, by conserving water and salt via the kidneys (thus concentrating the urine) and by increasing both thirst and the desire for salty foods. These changes may contribute in small ways to the other compensatory processes described below. In addition, an early response is seen in the tissues, which increase the amount of oxygen they extract from the red cells that reach them.

As blood loss proceeds, a drop in arterial pressure stimulates baroreceptors, triggering a sympathetic reflex response. This occurs within 30 seconds after a hemorrhage is detected. Baroreceptors are sensory nerve endings in the walls of the auricles of the heart, vena cava, aortic arch, and carotid sinuses that are sensitive to fluctuations in the pressure exerted on the walls of the vessels as blood flows through them. The activation of this sympathetic reflex increases the body's ability to tolerate blood loss to about twice that which would otherwise be possible, requiring three steps to happen more or less simultaneously. The first is an increase in the strength of cardiac contractions (the heart beats harder). The second is an increase in the rate of cardiac contractions (the heart beats faster).

The last step is an increase in peripheral vascular resistance, which makes best use of the remaining blood volume by narrowing the vessels. The cardiovascular system can be thought of as a container for blood. Normally, at least 70% of the total blood volume is found in the venules or small vessels of the venous circulation, but during a hemorrhage, catecholamine release results in constriction of arterial vessels, pushing the reduced blood volume into the body's core. Arteriovenous shunts divert blood from the kidneys, gastrointestinal tract, skin and uterus, resulting in less flow to their capillaries. This increased vascular resistance effectively reduces the size of the vascular container, reducing the amount of fluid required for adequate perfusion, improving systolic and diastolic blood pressures and increasing cardiac preload. These effects provide a relative autotransfusion to the system. However, they also produce an irregular vasoconstriction, leading to unevenly distributed microcirculatory flow.

It is significant that the sympathetic response does not cause significant constriction of vessels in the brain, heart or adrenal glands. The autoregulatory mechanisms inherent in coronary, adrenal and cerebral vascular beds further prevent moderate decreases in blood flow from significantly affecting the perfusion of these vital organs. Maintenance of normal arterial pressure also works to protect the brain and heart in the presence of decreased cardiac output. These organs are thus the last to be affected by shock, becoming compromised only when the systolic pressure drops below 70 mm Hg.

These compensatory mechanisms help maintain a normal systolic blood pressure. The diastolic pressure, however, may increase, resulting in a narrowing of the pulse pressure; that is, the difference between the systolic and diastolic pressures may become smaller (there is normally a 30 to 40 mm Hg difference between the systolic and diastolic pressures). The woman may exhibit delayed capillary refill and cool skin as the blood is redistributed from the peripheral circulation to her vital organs. In spite of maintaining normal blood pressure, the woman may show signs of decreased central nervous system perfusion (lethargy, confusion or combativeness) even at this stage.

If the bleeding can be stopped, compensation eventually results in a full recovery. However, if there is a very large and rapid blood loss, compensatory changes may not have time to produce a positive effect. If blood loss continues or too much is lost, these compensatory systems collapse.

Uncompensated shock

If the blood loss is rapid enough, uncompensated shock can happen at any time. However, in most situations, uncompensated shock takes anywhere from 10 minutes to 1 hour to become fully established. It represents an exhaustion of the body's ability to compensate for the blood loss when it continues or is very rapid. Circulation to the brain is impaired, and signs of shock become more pronounced because the compensatory mechanisms are no longer able to maintain systolic pressure or do not have time to activate at all. Organs already suffering hypoxia from reduced and uneven blood flow due to vasoconstriction receive even less oxygen as more blood is lost and vasoconstriction intensifies. In the absence of adequate oxygenation, cellular metabolism switches to less efficient anaerobic pathways.

The amount of time the tissues are partially deprived of oxygen is directly related to the accumulation of the by-products of anaerobic metabolism. Damage to the capillary endothelium (walls) may also occur, although this phenomenon is more commonly seen in septic shock. Should such damage occur, it leads to capillary leak as the lining of the capillaries lose their ability to retain large molecular structures within their walls, permitting protein-containing fluid (such as albumin) to leak into the interstitial spaces, thus further reducing the circulating blood volume.

The identifiable turning point in uncompensated shock is a fall in systolic blood pressure, usually to 60 mm Hg or less. The heart rate and breathing increase even more as both systolic and diastolic pressures begin to drop and capillary refill is increasingly delayed. Shunting of blood to vital organs as well as hypoxia may cause the woman to have cold extremities and cyanosis. Effects on the cardiovascular system include a decreased preload and a further increased rate of cardiac contraction secondary to increased catecholamine release.

As shock progresses, the tiny precapillary sphincters that control flow into the capillaries relax, allowing more blood to flow into and enlarge the capillary space. However, postcapillary sphincters remain closed, causing blood to pool or stagnate, resulting in capillary engorgement. Increasing hypoxemia and acidosis lead to the opening of additional venules and capillaries, expanding the vascular space even more. This dilation produces a relative hypovolemia, which, combined with the blood loss, may be enough to reduce the volume of blood available for the large vessels and vena cava, resulting in decreased venous return and a fall in cardiac output. The viscera (lungs, liver, kidneys and gastrointestinal mucosa) may become congested with blood. Sluggish blood flow and reduced delivery of oxygen result in increased anaerobic metabolism and the production of lactic acid. These changes lead to a chemoreceptor response that increases the rate and depth of respirations (an attempt to reduce acidosis by decreasing carbon dioxide levels). Acidosis worsens and pH falls. The red blood cells may cluster together, further compromising perfusion in the organs. Clotting mechanisms are now affected, leading to hypercoagulability.

The strength of cardiac contractions decrease as a result of ischemia from a reduction in circulating red blood cells, poor oxygen saturation of the red cells that remain and decreased coronary perfusion secondary to hypotension (especially on the diastolic side). Hypoxia leads to necrosis of heart tissue, with a reduction in preload leading to decreased contractility. Acidosis can also contribute to decreased contractility as well as cardiac rhythm disturbances.

Disseminated intravascular coagulation occurs as stagnant blood begins to coagulate in the microcirculation. This clogs capillaries, prevents both tissue perfusion and the removal of metabolic wastes, and leads to fluid leaks, rupture and hemorrhage. Hypovolemic shock causes increased platelet aggregation, which results in the release of vasoactive substances. This leads to small vessel occlusion and impaired microcirculatory perfusion. Clumped platelets can embolize to the lungs and contribute to the respiratory failure that often results from prolonged shock.

Tissue cells use anaerobic metabolism; thus, lactic acid production increases. Lactic acid accumulates around the cell membranes, which can no longer maintain homeostasis, allowing water and sodium to leak in and potassium to leak out. The cells swell and die, producing tiny dead areas (microinfarcts) in the visceral organs. Edema develops in the lungs as pulmonary capillaries become permeable, interfering with oxygen uptake and carbon dioxide elimination.

Irreversible shock

At some point in the ischemic process of anaerobic metabolism, the cells in the vital organs become so compromised that they can no longer function in their various specialized capacities. Irreversible shock is an organ-by-organ phenomenon. The amount of cellular necrosis required to produce organ failure varies with each organ as well as with the constitutional sensitivity of an individual's organs to ischemia. If capillary occlusion persists for one to two hours, the cells nourished by the capillaries involved undergo changes that rapidly become irreversible. Metabolic toxins accumulate and damage cells. If the blood volume is not restored in time, hypoxia and low blood pressure cause irreversible brain damage and capillary dilation. When hypoxia persists, there is widespread cell damage and a release of chemical substances that further increase the permeability of the capillaries. More fluid enters the interstitial spaces, leading to further hypovolemia, further reduction in blood pressure and increased hypoxia.

As blood pressure continues to fall, less and less oxygen gets to the brain and heart muscle. A corresponding drop in the arterial pressure causes the coronary blood flow to decrease below that required to sustain adequate nutrition for the heart muscle. This results in a depression of function with a further decrease in cardiac output and falling arterial pressure. In addition, accumulating metabolic toxins, as outlined below, contribute to cardiac depression.

Liver failure is common and often presents early in this stage. The liver is particularly vulnerable because of its high rate of metabolism along with its dense vascular supply being flooded with toxins coming in from cellular degeneration throughout the body. As shock worsens, blood flow to the kidneys is further reduced. Glomerular pressure falls below that required for filtration of fluid, resulting in tubular necrosis. Sloughing and blockage of the renal tubules leads to total loss of function of the damaged nephrons. Acute kidney failure is heralded by a reduction in the secretion of urine. The resulting retention of damaging metabolic waste products leads to life-threatening uremia.

The enzyme that regulates sodium and potassium transport in and out of the cells becomes disrupted; sodium and chloride accumulate in the cells while potassium is lost, causing the cells to swell. Mitochondrial activity is depressed, and lysosomes in the cells release hydrolase enzymes, which cause more cellular degeneration. In the last stages of shock, glucose metabolism at the cellular level becomes disrupted, resulting in a 200-fold reduction in insulin activity. In the lungs, these changes can lead to pulmonary edema and reduced oxygen uptake, further compromising cardiac function. In addition, as anaerobic metabolism proceeds, large amounts of lactic acid are formed, and hydrogen ions accumulate, reaching dangerous levels in just a few minutes. These changes lead to the severe metabolic acidosis that occurs immediately prior to and following cardiac arrest (Hofmeyr & Mohlala, 2001).

Reduced blood flow to the intestines enhances the absorption of endotoxins released by the dead gram-negative bacteria normally found there. This leads to vascular dilation and an increase in cellular metabolism even though nutrition to the cells is inadequate. Gastrointestinal bleeding and sepsis may result from necrosis of the mucosa. Necrosis in the pancreas may lead to further clotting disorders and severe pancreatitis. Clots in the lungs may produce hemorrhage and fluid loss into the alveoli.

A person can live for only a few hours once cardiac output has fallen to 40% of normal (after losing an average of 60% of her circulating blood volume). The actual length of survival depends on a number of factors; for example, a compromised individual will enter irreversible shock much sooner with much less blood loss than an athlete in the peak of health. The clinical symptoms of irreversible shock include bradycardia, serious dysrhythmias, frank hypotension, evidence of multiple organ failure, and pale, cold and clammy skin. Cardiopulmonary collapse is usually imminent in these individuals. If effective treatment is not possible, these irreversible changes become progressively worse and the woman goes into a coma and dies.

This, the third stage of shock, is characterized by the progression of necrosis and subsequent organ death, even if adequate oxygenation and perfusion are restored with transfusions. Those who have suffered from irreversible shock accompanied by massive cellular damage do not survive. Decompensation can occur suddenly, or it may be delayed from one day to three weeks after the onset of irreversible shock. During this time, the person generally feels unwell and typically experiences kidney pain and rapid breathing and may lapse into stupor or coma.

It is impossible to distinguish between uncompensated and irreversible shock by the clinical picture. Assistance should always be directed at resuscitation, especially since irreversible shock is more a function of the duration of hypovolemic compromise rather than the amount of blood loss.

Fetal response to maternal shock

Fetal well-being depends upon the maintenance of adequate oxygenation and uterine blood flow. When either of these is compromised by maternal shock, fetal hypoxia and acidosis ensue. The normal maternal Po_2 (partial pressure of oxygen) is near 100 mm Hg. As long as it exceeds 60 mm Hg, the baby will experience no significant fall in his saturation levels. The fetus can offload acids via the kidneys and initiate other compensatory processes (as outlined in the subchapter entitled “Understanding Fetal and Neonatal Asphyxia”), thus adequately responding to mild hypoxia for a period of time. However, any further drop in maternal oxygen saturation will result in a drastic decrease in the oxygen saturation of the fetus. Administering oxygen to the mother can compensate for marginal fetal hypoxia to a certain extent by producing significant increases in fetal oxygen saturation due to the enhanced ability of the fetus to take up oxygen. Administer oxygen to the mother at a flow of 10 l/min with a nonrebreather mask while transport is underway.

Near term, uterine blood flow approaches 500 ml per minute, accounting for 10% of a woman’s total cardiac output, with circulation to the placenta accounting for 85 to 90% of uterine blood flow at term. The uterine arteries have remarkably little capacity for autoregulation. Thus, as maternal systemic arterial pressure falls, so does uterine perfusion and placental blood flow. Maternal hyperventilation in response to the crisis will reduce uterine blood flow even more. In the hypotensive mother, peripheral vasoconstriction, which maintains blood flow to her vital organs, reduces uterine blood flow even further. Because the mother’s body will tend to maintain systemic arterial pressure and perfusion of her vital organs at the expense of the uterus, abnormal fetal heart rate patterns may develop, even in the absence of maternal hypotension. Therefore, it is often the case that a devastating maternal condition such as internal hemorrhage or uterine rupture or amniotic fluid embolism first manifests with abnormal fetal heart rate patterns.

If the mother collapses during labor and requires cardiopulmonary resuscitation, cardiac compressions produce a cardiac output that is, at best, only 30 to 40% of normal. Under such circumstances, uterine blood flow is severely impaired. The baby will be severely damaged or die unless the mother’s blood pressure and pulse can be restored promptly or a surgical birth can be performed immediately. In short, the mother who presents with evidence of bleeding with a poor fetal heart rate pattern has a baby in serious jeopardy. Transport immediately! Conversely, the mother who is having some bleeding with a normal fetal heart rate is compensating well, for the moment. You may choose to monitor the baby closely and await the birth, if the mother is close to delivery. Transported immediately if a worsening of the fetal heart rate or the mother’s condition becomes apparent before you can get the baby out (Clark, 1990).

Assessing and Treating Hemorrhagic Shock

The initial assessment for signs and symptoms of shock

As a woman is going into hemorrhagic shock, there are numerous signs. The order in which these manifest depends upon whether shock develops during or after labor. These signs and symptoms include:

- Changes in the level of consciousness, such as:
  - Extreme fatigue with muscle weakness
  - Anxiety
  - Diminished responsiveness (confusion, wants to sleep, or unconsciousness)
- Altered pupil reaction (indicates severe shock)
- Cardiovascular changes such as:
  - Poor perfusion (prolonged capillary refill time, ashen skin, blue lips, blanched gums, white nail beds)
  - Cooling skin temperature (may feel cold and clammy)
  - Breaking out in a cold sweat
- Changes in vital signs such as:
  - Rapid breathing (30 rpm or more)
  - Fetal heart rate abnormalities (if blood loss begins prior to birth, this is the most important indicator of both the maternal and the fetal condition)
  - Maternal heart rate (fast, weak or thready pulse which rises to 110 bpm or more)

When shock develops with no revealed bleeding, amniotic fluid embolism must also be considered as a possible etiology.

Recognizing shock: Now we will look at these signs and symptoms in detail.

Changes in the level of consciousness/responsiveness:
Extreme fatigue: It is typical for a shocky woman who has just been through labor to state that she feels suddenly fatigued and just wants to sleep. Muscular weakness due to reduced oxygenation and lactic acid accumulation produces severe fatigue when the woman tries to move. If the woman tries to arise from bed, her legs may give out from under her or she may faint as blood is displaced from her upper body.

Anxiety: A woman may become anxious, a response to the catecholamine surge as her body attempts to compensate for the blood loss. This is often the earliest indication of shock.

Diminished responsiveness: The circumstances surrounding shock during labor or immediately postpartum are unique because the symptoms of shock appear in the context of the work and consequent fatigue of labor. Changes in a woman's level of responsiveness reflect her energy level as well as possible circulatory compromise to her brain. One of the first signs is often a sense of light-headedness. The woman feels woozy, and she must lie down when she attempts to assume an upright position. The color drains from her upper body. This occurs because her system has not had time to equilibrate the blood flow following blood loss from the uterus, even if the blood loss is otherwise within tolerable limits.

The mother may report that she has ringing in her ears or that she cannot hear you. Her vision may also be impaired; she may say she cannot see you. She may experience tingling or numbness in her extremities. These symptoms may come and go or, if you are not vigilant in treating her, progress to unconsciousness. She may have a dreamy response or be unable to understand what you are saying. Her eyes may take on a glazed appearance, progressing to a dull or staring appearance as shock deepens. She may lose track of the present and be unable to state where she is or to relay information she should know readily, such as the day of the week or the name of the president. Keep in mind, however, that labor produces a naturally altered state of consciousness. Ask questions that she is likely to know, such as the names of her relatives, rather than time- and date-specific information, time being altered in labor. Should she lose consciousness, she may be impossible to rouse as she goes into a coma.

Pupil reaction: Check the pupils by holding the upper eyelid open with one hand while passing a penlight across the visual field with the other. The pupils dilate at the onset of shock in response to adrenalin release; they will still constrict in response to light but will remain more dilated than they normally would. The pupils will appear more normal as shock becomes most severe and adrenalin levels fall, with some response to light. At the time of death, the pupils dilate completely, with no response to light.

Cardiovascular signs and symptoms:

Assessing perfusion: Skin color is an important way to assess perfusion since it indicates the blood flow to the capillaries. Pink skin is well perfused and well oxygenated. If the skin is pale, perfusion is lacking and the capillary bed is probably in the ischemic phase. Because the body differentially constricts blood vessels in the extremities, the hands and feet are the most likely areas to show early circulatory changes. The lips tend to lose color next.

The capillary refill test is a good way to judge the rate of blood flow through these peripheral capillary beds. Compress the nail bed of the big toe or thumb or the skin on the palm at the base of the fingers to squeeze blood out of the capillary beds. Release the pressure and count how long it takes for normal color to return. Two seconds or less, about the time it takes to say "capillary refill," is normal; longer than this reflects poorly perfused extremities. The woman has already lost quite a bit of blood if the nails do not blanch with compression. Women-of-color also get pale; however, this may be more difficult to discern. It is helpful to check the conjunctiva of the lower eyelid and gums as well as the nail beds for color.

The skin may at times take on a mottled appearance, which is the result of blood congestion in the peripheral circulation. This correlates with an extreme drop in blood pressure, markedly decreased peripheral perfusion and systemic metabolic acidosis, the manifestations of severe shock. Assessing skin perfusion is a good initial evaluation tool; however, once perfusion becomes abnormal, it will not improve until the person is hemodynamically stable, a condition that can take many hours to restore, depending upon the severity of the blood loss. Therefore, it should not be depended upon as a continuous gauge of recovery.

Skin temperature: The skin should feel warm and dry. It may feel cold and clammy as shock progresses as she breaks out in a cold sweat and becomes more pale. Temperature may fall to a subnormal level in the extremities; however, core temperature will remain within normal limits as long as uncompensated shock does not ensue because blood is being shunted to the body's core.

Vital signs:

Respirations: Breathing may at first become deeper with a sighing quality. An increase in the respiratory rate to more than 30 rpm or shallow breathing is characteristic of a person who is trying to compensate for metabolic acidosis by rapidly discharging carbon dioxide. Note that abdominal pain, which could be present with an abruption or uterine rupture, may also cause the woman to breathe shallowly because excursion of the diaphragm increases pain. Pulmonary edema is unlikely to develop if the woman is receiving IV fluids to compensate for blood loss but should always be kept in mind (for more details see the subchapter entitled "Intravenous Equipment and IV Therapy").

Fetal distress (the fetal pulse): When maternal blood loss occurs prior to birth, the baby has been compared to a miner's canary. Significant maternal shock due to blood loss is highly unlikely if the baby is not in distress, regardless of the apparent amount of maternal blood loss, blood pressure fluctuations or other signs. If the baby is in distress, there is not a moment to lose in transporting immediately while stabilizing the mother en route to the best of your ability. *Do not attempt to keep a shocky woman at home if she is still in labor.* If bleeding is coming from an abruption or placenta previa, you will not be able to stop it prior to birth. If only the baby is losing blood, the mother will not be affected. However, the baby has a comparatively tiny blood volume and is in grave danger; immediate transport is warranted.

Maternal pulse: Feel the woman's pulse; changes in the pulse are a much earlier indicator of compromise than hypotension. To help maintain adequate output, the pulse rate increases fairly early in shock. The strength of cardiac contraction may also increase, although this is often canceled out by the decrease in preload. These types of changes are characteristic early responses to either a hypovolemic (volume loss) or relative volemic shock (which produces distributive shock with vasodilation). A pulse rate over 90 in a nonpregnant person is generally considered abnormal. However, the pulse typically rises near term, and the woman's pulse at term and during normal labor must also be taken into account. As shock deepens, the pulse will continue to rise and grow weaker and thready (that is, a fine, small pulse, feeling like a thread or cord under the finger). In heart failure, the pulse will usually be slower and stronger than in volume deficiency but will still be faster than normal.

Where the pulse can be felt along the extremities is a good indication of the amount of peripheral vascular resistance and how much of the cardiovascular system the heart can still perfuse. Although a mean arterial pressure of 60 mm Hg may be adequate outside of pregnancy, the effect of any given blood pressure on uteroplacental perfusion in individual women is related to gestational age and placental condition. Thus, a blood pressure of 80/50 may be normal for one pregnant woman, while another with uteroplacental insufficiency and hypertension may have inadequate placental perfusion and fetal distress even if her blood pressure exceeds 90 mm Hg systolic. For these reasons, shock in pregnancy is more reliably diagnosed by taking into account the overall clinical picture, including fetal condition, maternal pulse, mental status and urine output than by an absolute blood pressure value. Reference the woman's most recent blood pressure values from her prenatal records when guidance is needed regarding the degree of shock she may be experiencing and her response to recovery. As a ball-park guide, once the systolic pressure drops below 70 mm Hg in a woman whose term systolic pressure equaled or exceeded this value, your primary focus must be to stabilize the mother. When blood flow is redirected away from the uterus, the baby is in grave danger and will probably not survive.

The following table offers average values regarding how to interpret maternal pulse rates during a rapid assessment. This requires skill in finding pulses in all these areas of the adult body. Nevertheless, the fetal heart rate remains your most sensitive indicator of both maternal and fetal well-being.

IF THERE IS NO PULSE FELT HERE	SYSTOLIC PRESSURE IS PROBABLY LESS THAN	REFLECTING COMPROMISED BLOOD FLOW TO THESE ORGANS
Radial pulse (wrist)	80 mm Hg	Gastrointestinal tract, pancreas, muscles
Brachial (midway between elbow and armpit) or femoral artery (in the groin)	70 mm Hg	Kidneys (blood flow decreases to try and conserve fluid), uterus, liver
Carotid artery (anterolateral neck)	60 mm Hg	Heart, brain, lungs

As the primary crisis is dealt with, recheck the pulse. If fluid is not being given, a slowing of the pulse may indicate that shock is becoming irreversible, especially if other signs are not resolving and fetal distress is apparent. If fluid resuscitation has begun (by IV or retention enema), slowing of the pulse is an early indicator that hypovolemia is being corrected, although slowing down below normal indicates severe cardiac ischemia.

Assessing the severity of shock: Two things are evaluated when assessing shock: the amount of blood loss and the woman's response to it. Initially, the well-nourished woman at term can tolerate a larger blood loss than the woman in earlier pregnancy. However, as blood loss progresses, the severity of her reaction to the loss is more closely matched to that of nonpregnant individuals. Even though the woman at term technically has more blood to lose, the body has trouble equilibrating the flow as blood loss becomes more severe. The vasodilation the woman has experienced during pregnancy is a contributing factor; the "container" is bigger. The vascular system must reduce to nonpregnant norms, and may need to further reduce to compensate for the bleeding.

The table below provides a general idea of how severe the response may be to certain amounts of blood loss postpartum. The early pregnancy values have been modified from a trauma chart that accounts for blood loss in a 154 lb (70 kg) male. The near-term values have been estimated using an average based on 25% of the woman's nonpregnant blood volume. Therefore, they should only be taken as approximations; remember that the most important consideration is the woman's overall condition and response to the blood she is actually losing.

TRIMESTER	BLOOD LOSS	DEGREES OF SHOCK			
		COMPENSATED	UNCOMPENSATED		
		(Class I)	Mild (Class II)	Moderate (Class III)	Severe (Class IV)
1st, 2nd or early 3rd	Volume of loss	up to 700 ml	700-1400 ml	1400 to 1800 ml	over 1800 ml
	% total volume	(10 to 15%)	15 to 30%	30 to 40%	more than 40%
Term	Volume of loss	500 to 1000 ml	1000 to 1500 ml	1500 to 2000 ml	2000 to 2500 ml
	% total volume	up to 25% at term	25 % to 35%	35 to 45 %	more than 45%

(Modified from Schuurmans et al., 2000)

After your preliminary assessment, evaluate the severity of shock. Remember that each person's response to blood loss will be very individual. It is important to note that once a woman has reached her shock threshold, even a small amount of additional blood loss may deepen the severity of her condition considerably.

SIGNS & SYMPTOMS	STAGES OF SHOCK		
	COMPENSATED	UNCOMPENSATED	IRREVERSIBLE
Fetal status	Normal	Distress or death based on heart rate	Death
Pulse	Slightly fast, strong	Very fast, weaker	Slow, thready, irregular
Heart rate	Mild tachycardia (>100 bpm)	Moderate tachycardia (>120 bpm)	Bradycardia, severe dysrhythmias, failure
Blood pressure	Normal (esp. if supine) or slight diastolic increase (80-100 mm Hg systolic)	Normal or slight decrease, tilt test positive (70-80 mm Hg systolic)	Frank hypotension (50-70 mm Hg systolic)
Respirations	Slightly fast or deep (≥30 rpm)	Extremely fast and/or shallow breathing, air hunger	Pulmonary edema (lungs sound like Rice Crispies in milk with rhonchi [rattles])
Level of consciousness	Nervous, anxious, may be faint, sleepy, lethargic, confused or combative	Confused, combative, restless, weak; stupor or unconsciousness	Seizures, coma, death
Skin	Early on, skin is still warm, becomes cool & moist with shivers	Cold extremities, cyanotic, deeply chilled	Pale, cold, clammy, may be mottled
GI symptoms	Queasy in an upright position, desire for salty foods, thirst	Nausea and thirst may persist; however, GI & renal systems tend to shut down as blood flow is rerouted to vital organs	
Capillary refill	Normal (< 2 sec)	Positive (> 2 sec)	
Urine output	Normal (>30 ml/hr)	15-30 ml/hr to none, concentrated	0-5 ml/hr; pale as water
Hemoglobin	≥8 g/dl (4.9 mmol/L)	≤8 g/dl (4.9 mmol/L)	Very low
Hematocrit	≥26% (.26)	≤26% (.26)	Very low

<u>Treating shock</u>: The findings gleaned during the primary survey provide the information needed to begin treatment. Early shock is generally reversible and usually responds well to the resuscitative measures outlined here. Late shock is more difficult to treat and usually requires transport for intensive care. Whether the baby has been born or not, treating shock must involve stopping the bleeding (or getting the baby out if that is impossible) and assisting the mother to stabilize. There are a few special considerations if the baby is not yet born; these are outlined below. To treat shock, the primary midwife should:

1. Identify the cause of shock and correct the problem. Most of the time, postpartum shock will be due to visible, excessive bleeding which, in the presence of an atonic uterus, is most likely to be from the placental site. If the uterus is well contracted, visible bleeding is likely to be coming from a laceration. Be aware that a uterus filled with clots can feel firm, confusing the clinical picture. A woman who has experienced vomiting or diarrhea during labor may succumb to blood loss sooner because her blood volume may already be reduced by dehydration. Concealed bleeding could be from a uterine tear or hematoma.
2. Tell the mother why she is bleeding and ask her to focus on what needs to happen (clamping down the uterus, for example) and to remain conscious and here in the room.
3. Tell the mother what is being done for her and why.

The help of an assistant is invaluable with shock present. If there is no trained assistant on hand, the primary midwife should attend to stabilizing the mother as much as possible as outlined below, enlisting the assistance of anyone who may be present. These steps should be taken by the midwife or assigned to an assistant and should take place as simultaneously as possible.

Call for help: Consider calling an ambulance as soon as acute shock is identified so that the mother can be transported for advanced care as soon as possible. This is especially important if the mother is remote from term or if the baby has not yet been born.

Open the airway: Make sure the woman's airway is open. Tilt her head back or pull her chin forward if necessary.

Give supplemental oxygen: Give the mother oxygen by nonrebreather mask, beginning with a flow of 15 l/min (10 liters delivers 100%); step down the flow until the reservoir bag fills between breaths and collapses no less than 50% on inspiration. This will help compensate for the lack of blood flow by saturating all available hemoglobin and plasma so that more is transported to the unborn baby as well as the mother's brain, thus helping to keep her conscious.

Begin volume replacement: Start an IV of lactated Ringers or normal saline (sodium chloride) using the largest-bore needle you can insert successfully (18 to 16 gauge). If the mother is bleeding heavily, you should forgo collection of blood samples in favor of stabilization as soon as possible. Infuse 500 cc of solution as quickly as possible by leaving the tubing clamps wide open. If an IV cannot be started because the mother's veins have collapsed or are hard to find, a retention enema of unflavored Pedialyte, lactated Ringer's or normal saline (¼ tsp salt to 1 cup water) should be given to help restore circulating fluid volume; IV insertion is often possible afterward. You can also place a 20 gauge butterfly in the woman's hand, where veins are shallow and easier to hit, and begin to infuse IV fluids until the veins are filled enough to insert a large bore catheter.

Reassess vital signs after the mother has received 500 cc of fluid. As a rule, when dealing with a woman postpartum, a systolic pressure of 100 mm Hg is the goal. (See discussion below regarding the use of blood pressure as a gauge for shock recovery in pregnancy and immediately postpartum.) If there is no change after infusing 500 cc of fluid or if the cause of bleeding cannot be determined or the bleeding cannot be stopped, and emergency services are not on their way, call for help now.

While it is true that the body generally requires 3 liters of crystalloid solution for every liter of blood lost, as midwives we are providing acute care. This means we provide fluids at a volume and speed which restores the woman's vital signs and state of consciousness to normal, then slow down the flow to maintain the woman in a stable condition. Giving a woman the full 3-to-1 replacement volume too rapidly risks overloading her system, especially if blood flow through the kidneys is impaired and urinary output is thus diminished. Fluid overload occurs when the system is overwhelmed and cannot assimilate the fluid as fast as it is being given. The excess goes first to the lungs, and pulmonary edema is the dangerous result. Generally speaking, full 3-to-1 volume replacement should be titrated over a 24 hour period to allow the tissues to equilibrate the fluid gradually. Of course, this partly depends upon the woman's condition when volume replacement begins and the total amount of blood she has lost as well as her state of dehydration prior to the bleeding episode. If the woman was normally hydrated to begin with, a small blood loss leaves a narrower margin for overload. If the woman was dehydrated and then bled a lot, she can tolerate receiving more fluids at a relatively faster rate of flow. Continuous monitoring of a woman receiving an IV is required so that you can judge how her body is accepting the fluids.

Position the mother: Lay the woman on her left side or prop her right hip with folded blankets or towels. This reduces pressure on the inferior vena cava. It also maximizes blood flow to and from the uterus. This will help the baby if she has not yet been born. If the baby has been born, it helps blood return from the uterus to the rest of the body rather than flowing out. If the mother is to remain more or less supine, turn her head to the side and elevate her legs to a 20 to 30° angle using folded blankets or pillows.

In the event of postpartum bleeding, raising the foot of the bed, her pelvis or entire torso into a full Trendelenburg position encourages blood to pool in the uterus, which is not desirable. Such pooling is especially likely when the uterus is atonic, but can also occur when the bleeding is coming from a laceration, as there is nothing to pump blood that has pooled in the yoni out. When there are no uterine contractions, the inverted position is likely to result in blood collecting in the fundus instead of being pushed out through the cervix. The blood causes the fundus to balloon which interferes with your assessment of how much blood the woman is losing. It also encourages the formation of clots (that then must be removed) and impairs the ability of the uterus to contract, which is the only thing that will stop the bleeding.

Raising her lower extremities while leaving her torso flat encourages blood to flow passively out of the cervix. It also increases venous return to the vital organs in her upper body and to her brain, where the body is trying to move the blood anyway. Laying her on her side reduces the chances of aspiration should she vomit. If lying down causes severe breathing difficulty, heart failure and pulmonary edema may be present. If this occurs, lower her legs and raise her head somewhat to relieve fluid pressure on the lungs.

Keep the mother warm: She is cold because her body is redirecting all available blood to her vital organs, away from her peripheral circulation. Trying to maintain her body temperature will use oxygen and can increase the depth of shock. Cover her with blankets and increase the heat in the room to keep her warm. It is equally important not to overheat her. Warming the skin until it is flushed may deepen the shock by drawing blood flow away from vital organs to the skin surface, thus depriving vital organs of needed blood supply (Sweet, 1997). Do not apply any localized, intense sources of heat such as electric heating pads or hot water bottles. A person in shock may burn easily because peripheral circulation is impaired, which also impairs the dispersal of heat from the skin.

Keep the mother conscious: Maintain close eye-to-eye, face-to-face contact with her at all times. This person's job is to keep her conscious. He should talk to her, ask her questions, talk about the baby, do whatever it takes to keep her awake. Rubbing the sternum, applying finger pressure to the base of the nail beds, and twisting her ear lobes are appropriate noxious stimuli that can be used if the woman is losing consciousness. These types of stimulation produce varying degrees of pain, which helps to bring women back quickly. The purpose is to avoid coma and death; a little discomfort is nothing to be squeamish about in such an emergency.

Give remedies for shock: Acupuncture can easily be used in conjunction with all these other therapies. Apply firm pressure to Du-26, which is very effective for shock. HE-7 can also be pressed on one or both hands (Lowe, 2003; West, 2001). Rescue Remedy (or a similar emergency flower essence combination remedy) can be given immediately and repeated every few minutes.

If the woman is still in labor: If the baby is not yet born, check the fetal heart rate as soon as possible and then continuously. If the baby is compromised, the heart rate may be slow or rapid and sound weak or faint compared to how it has sounded during pregnancy or earlier in labor; large, rapid, jerky fetal movements are an ominous sign of impending demise.

Secondary assessment

Once the cause of shock has been identified and treatment has begun, continuous evaluation of the signs and symptoms discussed under the primary assessment should take place at five-minute intervals. In addition, the following things should be assessed.

Blood pressure: The body can maintain the blood pressure in the face of decreased cardiac output using various reserve responses. Usually the blood pressure is maintained until 30 to 40% of the blood volume has been lost. Recall that blood pressure has two components: systolic pressure reflects the strength of the cardiac contractions, while the diastolic pressure is an indicator of peripheral vascular resistance and coronary artery perfusion.

The normally expanded blood volume of pregnancy coupled with the usual increase in the baseline heart rate of 10 to 15 beats per minute results in a 45 to 50% increase in resting cardiac output at term. These changes are accompanied by a significant decrease in systemic vascular resistance, which results in a decrease in the blood pressure during the second trimester.

In nonpregnant persons, hypotension is often defined as a systolic pressure equal to or less than 90 mm Hg and a mean arterial pressure equal to or less than 60 mm Hg. These levels are usually required to maintain adequate blood flow to the adult heart and brain. During pregnancy, some women can have very low blood pressure, with 80/50 a common finding in healthy women. It is reasonable to assume, however, that a bleeding woman who has very low blood pressure at term will have less tolerance for any further decrease in her pressures than a woman who started out with a blood pressure that is in a more average range.

During shock, the diastolic pressure increases slightly as peripheral vascular resistance reaches its maximum, before systolic and diastolic pressure drop together. Hypotension is usually the most dramatic clinical sign of shock, regardless of the cause. Thus, checking the blood pressure is an important step after initial treatment has begun. Take the blood pressure and count the pulse rate and respirations. Continue to check the blood pressure and pulse every 5 minutes for at least a full hour after her condition has stabilized. This monitors for signs of recovery as well as the development of secondary shock. Remember that the blood pressure may rise temporarily before it falls. A fall of 15 points in either diastolic or systolic pressure or a reading of 80/40 or less is often reflective of shock, unless this was the woman's preshock norm. A pulse that is thready, fast, thin or faint indicates significant blood loss. Aim for a systolic pressure of 100 mm Hg when gauging how much fluid to replace via IV. Once the systolic pressure is holding at 100 or better, slow the rate of flow from the IV solution and continue to monitor. If the cause of shock is volume loss, the blood pressure should rise to the woman's normal baseline after fluid replacement. If the blood pressure does not rise, continue to look for internal sources of bleeding; the most common cause during the postpartum period is a concealed hematoma.

Urinary output: Encourage the mother to urinate into a placenta pan or a towel. If she cannot, catheterize the bladder once the situation allows. Check the labor notes to see when the woman last urinated. If she has not urinated for a while, catheterization will empty the bladder, which will assist the uterus to clamp down after birth.

Urinary output is directly related to renal perfusion and, in turn, perfusion of other vital organs. After fetal distress, it is the second most reliable indication of the degree of shock as well as of recovery in the pregnant woman, especially in one whose blood pressure has been quite low during pregnancy. Urine production is especially sensitive to blood volume changes. Little or no urinary output is a sign of critically low blood volume, such as that seen with severe shock from hemorrhage or dehydration, and reflects impending kidney failure. Urinary output is ideally monitored with a Foley catheter in place. However, an indwelling catheter is usually not inserted at home. Urinary output can also be collected and measured with a pan. If collecting urine is not possible, note the color (concentrated urine is darker; urine looks almost like water as kidney function falls off) and amount. Urine flow of at least 30 ml and ideally 60 ml an hour reflects adequate renal perfusion.

Assessing signs of recovery or deterioration: The woman should stabilize once the source of the shock has been identified and brought under control, the procedures outlined above have been followed and fluid volume has begun to be restored. Even so, in most cases, it is advisable to transport the woman to the hospital as soon as possible, especially if the baby is not yet born. It is still important for the midwife to be able to recognize signs of improvement as well as signs of deterioration. One person should be assigned to assess the mother every five minutes. This allows for quick detection of improvement or deterioration. If the mother is still in labor, have someone monitor the fetal heart rate constantly prior to and during transport. Using the critical care record chart at the end of the chapter, the table below can help you detect trends in the mother's condition and treat her accordingly.

HEART RATE (PULSE)	BLOOD PRESSURE	RESPIRATIONS	SIGNIFICANCE
Drops to normal (below 90 bpm); no fetal distress	Stabilizes to woman's normal or around 100/70	Drops to normal range	Woman is stabilizing; fluid resuscitation is working; bleeding is controlled
Rising or remaining elevated; no fetal distress	Rising or remaining elevated	Rate remains high (over 30 rpm)	Compensated blood loss is continuing; continue to seek sources of bleeding; start an IV, consider transport
Rising; weak & thready; fetal distress develops	Drops and remains the same or drops more	Rate rises to very fast, becomes more shallow	Uncompensated blood loss is continuing; continue to replace fluids & look for source; transport
Falling; severe fetal distress or baby is dead	Falling	Crackles or rhonchi heard on auscultation	Shock may be becoming irreversible; continue to replace fluids and attempting to control bleeding; transport.
Falling	Remains same or rises	Remains same or rises	Reflects central nervous system trauma

Expect to see the following encouraging signs within 20 to 30 min (or sooner) after treatment has begun:

- **Increasing blood pressure:** If shock occurs during labor, aim for a reading corresponding to a woman's prelabor norms. If birth has occurred, aim for a systolic pressure of 100 mm Hg. After birth, do not attempt to raise the blood pressure much higher, as a higher pressure may result in dislodging clots that have formed at the bleeding site. This is most relevant for sources of blood loss other than the placental site (which will also be closed by uterine contraction).
- **Improving mental status:** (lessening confusion or anxiety and increasing alertness)
- **Increasing urinary output:** Aim for a urine output of at least 100 ml (about 3.5 oz) every 4 hours.

If a woman fails to stabilize after 20 to 30 minutes, continue to offer support as follows:

1. Continue giving oxygen and IV (or rectal) fluids.
2. Monitor her condition closely.

3. Perform another complete clinical assessment as the real cause of the shock may not have been identified. The pelvic tissues or the peritoneal cavity (where occult blood loss typically occurs postpartum) can hold several pints of blood. If massive blood loss is occurring in the abdominal cavity, it should feel fluctuant on palpation.
4. Transport if you cannot treat the underlying cause (including a lack of IV fluids for volume replacement).

When an IV is being given, the following signs and symptoms help troubleshoot whether body fluids are in balance once the bleeding has stopped.

ASSESSMENT	FLUID DEFICIT	OVERINFUSION
Blood pressure	Fall in blood pressure, postural hypotension	Increased blood pressure, no postural changes
Pulse	Weak, thready pulse, tachycardia	Bounding, rapid pulse, tachycardia
Jugular vein	Flat neck veins	Venous distension, pulsation visible 2 cm above sternal angle when head of bed is raised 45°
Respirations	Rare crackles and wheezes, dry thick secretions	Crackles and wheezes, moist secretions
Edema	Infrequent	Edema, develops first in most dependent regions (scapula, buttocks if supine)
Skin turgor	Loose, toneless skin, tenting	Good, immediate recoil
Intake and output	Output greater than intake, slow urine output, high specific gravity	Intake greater than output, rapid urine output, low specific gravity

When to begin oral fluids: Use good judgement when deciding if and when a woman is a candidate for oral fluids or foods. *If the woman is in shock (any degree of impaired consciousness), do not give oral fluids or foods as she may vomit and aspirate the vomit.* In addition, if shock is severe, the ability of her kidneys to filter the blood will also be impaired; oral fluids will unnecessarily burden them and, if the tissues cannot handle the volume being given, fluid will be diverted to the lungs, especially if she is already receiving fluids IV. If in doubt, withhold oral fluids until she is more stable. If oral intake makes her nauseous or is otherwise contraindicated and starting an IV is impossible, you can give her a retention enema using saline solution or IV fluid to help rehydrate her and restore her circulating fluid volume.

However, if the blood loss is now under control, the woman is fully conscious and can swallow, and you believe that she is stable or not yet in shock, she may then be given oral fluids or food as she desires them. Her body will quickly absorb the fluids, and eating will result in increased blood flow to the gastrointestinal tract, thus drawing blood away from the uterus. A solution of 1 quart of electrolyte-balancing fluid (see the chapter entitled "Nausea and Vomiting" for recipes) can be given in doses of 4 oz every 15 minutes.

Deciding whether to transport: Transport is your best and safest option whenever a shocky woman is hard to stabilize or when significant bleeding is occurring prior to birth. Internal bleeding that has not or perhaps cannot be identified may be complicating the picture. Transport is also warranted when bleeding has been controlled, but hypotension still persists. *Remember that a woman can survive severe shock initially, only to succumb in the days following birth due to irreversible organ damage.*

Once a woman has displayed signs of shock, it is important to stay with her to make sure that she is truly stable and that the problem does not recur, even if the reason has been resolved. In most cases, however, signs of shock, even if resolved, indicate that the mother should be taken to the hospital as soon as possible. She may need additional fluids or a blood transfusion. If the baby has not yet been born, it is even more important to transport as stability in the mother does not necessarily reflect fetal status; depending upon the reason for the bleeding, the baby may be in grave danger and require immediate intensive care at the time of birth. Transport in an ambulance whenever possible to afford the woman the best possible support until she reaches the hospital, should she become unstable en route.

Post-transport laboratory tests

Generally speaking, the homebirth midwife will not be ordering lab work to determine the woman's status.

Circumstances that warrant lab work to monitor the situation also warrant transport, after which hospital personnel will attend to lab work. However, if you have hospital privileges, you may find yourself in a position to order labs, and if not, it is always good to know what might be ordered and why. Lab work can give you an indirect measurement of the degree of blood loss and determine whether clotting has been compromised. Most of these tests are explained in detail in my DIAGNOSTIC TESTS. Basic tests would include:

- •Complete blood count
- •Hemoglobin and hematocrit
- •Blood type and cross-match (if transfusion is needed)
- •Platelet count
- •Electrolytes
- •Blood urea nitrogen (BUN)
- •Glucose
- •Creatinine
- •Arterial blood gases
- •Serum lactate
- •Prothrombin time
- •Chest X-ray (for heart failure or pulmonary edema)

A clotting panel should also be ordered if there is seeping from wounds or bleeding that will not stop. No attempt is made to correct acidosis unless it is very severe (pH <7.0), because aggressive bicarbonate therapy may worsen tissue oxygenation and cause other metabolic and electrolyte problems.

Follow-up care

Any woman who has lost a great deal of blood or who has gone into shock should eat well and should take iron supplements and antioxidant vitamins (especially E and C) for at least a month after the birth. The impact of excessive bleeding on milk production and the postpartum period in general will be addressed in Volume III of this text.

Maternal critical care record for ______________ Date ______ Time recording began ______ Page __

Time	Pulse	Blood pressure	Respiratory rate/quality	Pupil reaction	Oral Temp.	Responsiveness	Blood loss	Urine output	Fluid replacement Other comments	Midwife's initials

Amniotic Fluid Embolism (Anaphylactoid Syndrome of Pregnancy)

An embolism is defined as the entry of foreign material into the bloodstream. If this material becomes lodged in the pulmonary circulation, it can cause obstruction or constriction. Amniotic fluid embolism (AFE) occurs when fetal cells and amniotic fluid, together with attached platelet-fibrin thrombi, enter the maternal circulation and wind up in the pulmonary vasculature. There they obstruct circulation, resulting in acute cardiorespiratory failure and profound shock. Thus the label "obstetric shock" was first used to describe this condition.

AFE is a catastrophic and deadly occurrence with a mortality rate of at least 60 to 80%. It is relatively rare, with an incidence ranging from 1 in 8000 to 1 in 30,000 pregnancies. Only 15% of those women who survive AFE are neurologically intact. The fetal survival rate is about 80% for hospitalized laboring women when the baby is not born prior to the onset of the embolism. However, only half of these babies survive neurologically intact (Clark, 1990).

Pathology

AFE was first described in 1941 by Steiner and Luschbaugh, who studied a group of women who died during labor. They found debris of fetal origin in the pulmonary circulation of these mothers and concluded that the entry of amniotic fluid and associated debris (such as fetal hair, vernix, skin cells and meconium) from the uterine environment into the maternal circulation resulted in massive physiologic disruption and death.

AFE is still not fully understood. New theories regarding AFE were proposed during the 1990s. Studies using animal models, although not perfect, have shown that, in many cases, the entry of amniotic fluid into the circulation, even in large amounts, is not necessarily harmful. Further studies have theorized that AFE presents a clinical picture that is similar to that seen in human anaphylactic and septic shock and is therefore unlike other embolic accidents. Because of this, it has been suggested that AFE would be more appropriately referred to as "anaphylactoid syndrome of pregnancy."

Anaphylaxis typically involves the introduction of a foreign substance into the system (such as bacterial endotoxin in the case of sepsis or a specific antigen in the case of allergy-provoked anaphylaxis) to which the body responds. The foreign substance prompts the release of mediating substances within the body (endogenous agents), which cause the physiologic derangements that ensue.

Normally, amniotic fluid does not enter the maternal circulation except in very small amounts. When a breach in the physiological barrier that normally prevents mixing does occur, the effect is usually benign. Such small breaches appear to occur frequently, if not universally, and both fetal cells and trophoblasts (early placental cells) are commonly found in the maternal circulation.

Such fetal debris, or some as-yet unidentified substance, may also have an opportunity to enter the mother's bloodstream during a variety of events, including normal labor and birth. Other risk factors include maternal age of 35 years or older, instrumental vaginal or surgical delivery, intrauterine manipulations, polyhydramnios, cervical laceration or uterine rupture, placenta previa or abruption, eclampsia, and fetal distress (Kramer, 2006). Meconium staining and rapid labor are also associated factors.

In most cases, the entry of amniotic fluid and associated fetal debris into the maternal system poses no problem. Some women, however, respond with a series of catastrophic physical reactions similar to those seen in anaphylaxis and sepsis. No evidence exists to suggest that anything can be done to avoid AFE when it occurs.

Uterine stimulation and AFE: It was held for many years that hypertonic uterine action posed an increased risk for AFE, thought to be prompted by the use of oxytocin or other labor-stimulating drugs such as misoprostol. It is now postulated that AFE leads to a release of catecholamines into the maternal circulation, which, in turn, produces intense uterine contractions. Prior to the occurrence of AFE, strong contractions reduce or temporarily cut off blood flow within the uterine muscle, making this is the least likely time for amniotic fluid to be forced into the maternal circulation. For these reasons, definitive statements appear in modern textbooks that there is no causal association between the use of oxytocin and AFE. ACOG has latched on to the notion that uterine stimulants have nothing to do with AFE, and a lack of such an association certainly lets doctors who want to induce and augment at will off the hook for liability.

Marsden Wagner (2005) calls this hypothesis into question, pointing out numerous flaws in the methodology of the studies upon which this assertion is based. In fact, Kramer and associates (2006) did a carefully constructed population-based cohort study of 3 million Canadian births and found that medical induction does indeed pose an increased danger of AFE; nearly doubling the risk of overall cases, with an even stronger association with fatal cases. US authorities, as far as I can tell, have completely ignored this research.

Clinical presentation

AFE is a complex condition. How it actually manifests varies greatly among individual women. Variations in presentation are apparently related to differences in both exposure to amniotic fluid (and its contents) and individual maternal response.

Progression usually occurs in 2 phases. In phase I, pulmonary artery vasospasm with pulmonary hypertension and elevated right ventricular pressure result in hypoxia, which can lead to permanent neurological damage if the woman survives. Hypoxia causes myocardial and pulmonary capillary damage, left heart failure, and acute respiratory distress. Often this initial respiratory distress passes, leaving survivors with damaged lungs and problems with oxygenation. Women who survive these initial insults may go on to enter phase II which is characterized by massive hemorrhage with uterine atony and DIC.

In the most dramatic cases, a woman who is in labor or has just given birth suddenly starts gasping for air, rapidly develops seizures, cardiorespiratory arrest and massive bleeding secondary to consumptive coagulopathy. There may be extremely severe pinpoint, knife-like chest pain that she can point to with a finger, indicating where the embolus is stopping the blood flow. Presentation varies, however, and sometimes respiratory distress is absent. Severe consumptive coagulopathy with a decrease in compliment levels is the most consistent feature and is frequently fatal.

In vitro studies have shown that amniotic fluid can shorten whole-blood clotting time, can have a thromboplastin-like effect, can induce platelet aggregation and release of platelet factor III, and can activate the complement cascade. Amniotic fluid also contains a factor-X-activating factor, although studies conflict as to whether it is present in sufficient quantities to induce the kind of massive intravascular coagulation seen with AFE.

Differential diagnosis

Other serious conditions that may mimic AFE include heart attack, other types of embolism, septic shock, uterine rupture, placental abruption (especially when coagulopathy is the primary symptom), aspiration pneumonia, anaphylactoid reaction and a ruptured cerebral aneurism.

What to do

There is no evidence that any type of intervention improves the maternal prognosis with AFE. This means you will do the best you can to stabilize the woman while praying hard and arranging for immediate transport. Recommended supportive care is as follows:

1. Transport as quickly as possible. The mother will be unable to cooperate in her care or in moving to a vehicle. Therefore, have someone else call an ambulance service if one is readily accessible, while you provide supportive care. If you are far from help, transport in a private vehicle in which the mother can remain supine.
2. Give cardiopulmonary resuscitation using high concentrations of oxygen, as indicated (O_2 saturation below 94%).
3. Left ventricular heart failure is likely to occur even in those in whom respirations and heart function are restored. Provide volume expansion via an IV to optimize ventricular preload.
4. Consider both the mother's and baby's well-being if AFE occurs during labor and the woman is unstable but has not experienced cardiorespiratory arrest. However, when a choice must be made, the mother's survival takes precedence over the baby's. Listen to the fetal heart as often as possible while transporting the mother.
5. If the baby is not yet born and the mother has experienced cardiorespiratory arrest, consider the baby anoxic at all times following this emergency, regardless of efforts to resuscitate the mother. Even in the best of circumstances, complete resuscitation of the pregnant woman is difficult, and CPR only provides 30% of the normal cardiac output. This means that the amount of blood reaching the uterus and placenta approaches zero. A postmortem surgical delivery may save the baby, but the baby is likely to be dead or severely neurologically impaired unless it is done immediately following cardiac arrest. The sooner the baby can be born, the better, with 67% of babies surviving intact if surgery is performed within 15 minutes and less than half surviving intact when it takes longer to get them out.
6. If the mother has given birth, transport her in a supine position that allows bimanual uterine compression during transport. Even if maternal resuscitation efforts are successful, a massive, uncontrollable hemorrhage should be anticipated due to coagulation derangement.

Definitive diagnosis

Once the crisis has passed and the mother has either succumbed or survived, the question will arise as to what actually caused her collapse. In the past, microscopic examination has sought out fetal debris in the distal port of a pulmonary artery during catheterization or at autopsy. Several studies show that such findings are common, however, even in women who have experienced normal labor and birth. Thus, histologic specimens revealing the presence of fetal debris are neither sensitive to nor specific for AFE. The diagnosis, therefore, remains clinical and is based on secondary signs and symptoms. When women survive, a number of tests are generally done in the hospital to try and determine the woman's clotting status and to look for features of disseminated intravascular coagulation; arterial blood gases are drawn to determine if PaO_2 and $PaCO_2$ are reduced and to check for metabolic acidosis.

An echocardiogram (ECG) will be performed to evaluate cardiac function, checking for a right ventricular strain pattern and tachycardia. A chest X-ray can look for pulmonary edema and perihilar infiltrates. These findings are suggestive, but not conclusive, of AFE.

HYPERSENSITIVITY REACTIONS AND ANAPHYLACTIC SHOCK

Hypersensitivity is another term for allergy or allergic reaction. A normal, adaptive immune response occurs in an exaggerated or inappropriate form following ingestion, injection or other exposure to a sensitizing substance, resulting in cellular destruction and tissue damage. Reactions can range from annoying symptoms such as watery eyes and sneezing to extreme life-threatening reactions involving sudden difficulty breathing, heart malfunction and very low blood pressure, leading to shock. In most cases, the person must have had previous exposure to the substance for an abnormal immune response to be triggered by a current exposure. It is common for serial exposures to produce increasingly severe allergic reactions. Four types of hypersensitivity reactions, which may overlap, are described:

Type I (immediate hypersensitivity): This nomenclature is somewhat misleading because a previous primary exposure must have occurred before a Type I hypersensitive reaction will occur with a subsequent exposure. Common causes include exposure to antibiotics, insulin, anesthetics, certain foods, seminal plasma, latex proteins and bee, wasp or ant venom. The original allergic reaction, induced by a specific antigen, results in the production of IgE antibodies. The antigen binds and cross-links to immunoglobulin E (IgE)-sensitized mast cells and basophils upon reexposure to the same antigen (by contact, inhalation, ingestion, or injection) leading to the release of mediators such as histamine, serine proteases and cytokines. This results in an anaphylactic reaction within seconds to minutes of exposure. Type I atopy (another word for "allergy") may be genetically determined, especially when it involves environmental allergies such as hay fever, asthma or atopic dermatitis.

Type II (antibody-dependent cytotoxic hypersensitivity): In Type II reactions, antibodies are formed that can recognize and bind to antigens that are part of the person's own cells. This may result in acute inflammation of the affected tissues, leading to cell damage or death. Type II reactions occur with any kind of blood incompatibility.

Type III (immune-complex-mediated hypersensitivity): Type III occurs in immune complex diseases. Immune complexes are antigens combined with a specific antibody. When they are deposited in tissues, an intense inflammatory reaction occurs, promoting complement activation and resulting in tissue damage. These conditions include pulmonary disorders as well as glomerulonephritis, systemic lupus erythematosus (SLE) and rheumatoid arthritis.

Type IV (delayed hypersensitivity reactions): This variety of reaction is slow to develop, appearing one to ten days after an exposure. Antigen-sensitized T-cells release lymphokines following contact with an antigen to which the person has been previously exposed, producing an exaggerated immune response. Familiar examples include allergic contact dermatitis following skin contact with plants such as poison ivy, sumac, or oak, some heavy metals or certain chemicals. This response is also protective against viruses, bacteria, fungi, cancer and protozoa.

Anaphylaxis is an acute, generalized, potentially deadly allergic reaction. The term "anaphylaxis" usually refers to IgE-mediated, Type I hypersensitivity. More rarely, an **anaphylactoid reaction** (anaphylactoid crisis, pseudo-anaphylactic shock), which does not require the presence of IgE antibodies or previous exposure to the inciting substance and is unrelated to antigen-antibody interactions, may occur. Both forms manifest and are treated in much the same way.

Pathology

Anaphylactic reactions may be local or systemic. Mast cells (a type of white blood cell) are found in large numbers in connective tissues of the skin and beneath the mucosa of both the respiratory passages and the gastrointestinal tract. These areas are common sites of local allergic reactions. Histamine causes blood vessels to dilate and fluid to leak from their walls during localized reactions such as contact dermatitis or hay fever. This results in runny nose, watery eyes, itching and redness. Asthma symptoms may also appear when the allergen is inhaled because smooth muscle in the bronchioles contracts, restricting air flow. Smooth-muscle contraction in the gastrointestinal system causes symptoms such as cramping, vomiting or diarrhea when the allergen is ingested (in foods or drugs).

Researchers have had the opportunity to study this syndrome closely because many severe anaphylactic reactions occur secondary to the administration of drugs in medical settings. Systemic responses are usually precipitated by the introduction of an allergen directly into the bloodstream either via an insect bite or an IV. Two phases of reaction have been described; the first is a hyperkinetic phase, which lasts 2 to 3 minutes and involves a fall in systemic vascular resistance and blood pressure, a rise in the heart rate and an increase in the volume of blood ejected from the heart during systole, resulting in rapid cardiac output. Central venous pressure and pulmonary capillary pressure initially remain stable. This is followed by a hypokinetic phase, involving continued vasodilation, low blood pressure and tachycardia. Central venous pressure and the pressure in the left atrium of the heart both decline. Stasis of blood in the capillaries leads to interstitial fluid accumulation. Loss of intravascular fluid accompanies the relative hypovolemia resulting from vasodilation, and cardiac output eventually falls. The picture may be further complicated by the development of myocardial depression and disseminated intravascular coagulation.

Grade	Signs and Symptoms of Hypersensitivity Reactions
I	Skin symptoms, mild fever, or both
II	Measurable but not life-threatening cardiovascular reaction (tachycardia, hypotension), gastrointestinal or respiratory disturbance (or both); early or mild anaphylaxis
III	Shock; life-threatening spasm of smooth muscle, such as bronchi or uterus
IV	Cardiac or respiratory arrest

Common Causes of Anaphylaxis during Pregnancy

Exposures that commonly occur during pregnancy that may precipitate anaphylaxis include the following:

Foods: Any food preserved with sulfites (typically salad greens, fruits, wine, beer, dehydrated soups and fish) may cause allergic reactions in some individuals. Similar reactions can occur in those sensitive to a variety of other foods, especially nuts, eggs and shellfish. Peanuts are one of the worst offenders.

Salicylic acid (aspirin family drugs): These drugs can prompt anaphylactoid reactions, especially in persons who have chronic sinusitis, nasal polyps and asthma. About 5% to 10% of these people will react with vasomotor collapse when given nonsteroidal anti-inflammatory drugs.

Antibiotics: Penicillin and its derivatives are the most common causes of allergic drug reactions, with 0.6 to 10% of all persons having some form of hypersensitive reaction to penicillin. Most of these are mild reactions, with anaphylaxis reported in only 0.04 to 0.2% of this population. Of these, approximately 0.001% die of anaphylaxis, 15% of whom have a history of other types of allergies. Seventy percent of those with fatal reactions have had penicillin before, with two-thirds of them having had no previous reaction while one-third did.

Although some 20% of those with known penicillin allergy show cross-reactivity to cephalosporins, only about 1% show actual clinical reaction to this class of drugs. Sensitivity to penicillin cannot be determined on the basis of skin tests. Therefore, those with a history of minor reactions to penicillin may be given cephalosporins when clinically indicated. If there is a history of anaphylaxis, cephalosporin should be withheld unless no acceptable alternative antibiotic is available (Clark et al., 1997).

Latex: Latex allergy resulting in anaphylaxis has been noted with increasing frequency. Both delayed (Type IV) and immediate (Type I) hypersensitivity reactions have been attributed to latex exposure. Items such as latex gloves, Foley catheters, and endotracheal tubes can cause such reactions. Infants with spina bifida are at increased risk for severe, systemic reactions to latex and should be treated using nonlatex gloves and supplies whenever possible.

Exertion: Exercise-induced anaphylaxis has been observed, apparently related to elevated temperature and water loss leading to typical hypersensitive responses. On very rare occasions, labor may trigger such a reaction.

Methotrexate: This agent is used to treat ectopic pregnancy in women who want to preserve fertility. It is also used for persistent gestational trophoblastic disease and as an IV infusion to treat breast cancer. Systemic anaphylaxis from low doses of this drug have occurred. Symptoms come on quickly, with burning in the mouth followed by diffuse redness, shortness of breath, cyanosis, low blood pressure, rheumatoid arthritis and respiratory arrest.

Colloid IV solutions: This terms refers to any blood or blood-like product, such as human serum albumin, dextran, gelatin and hydroxyethyl starch, used during volume replacement. These may provoke anaphylactoid reactions. Fetal death has been documented after a mother has had an apparently mild reaction to dextran. Dextran is used for its antithrombotic effect; however, the risk of its use in pregnant women exceeds the benefits.

Nonimmunologic mast-cell activators: These substances lead directly to anaphylactoid reactions. These include radiocontrast media, narcotics, depolarizing agents, dextrans and amniotic fluid emboli.

Oxytocic drugs: These can cause reactions as well, although fortunately this is a rare event. The main problem seems to be the additive chlorbutanol, a bacteriostatic preservative that causes sensitivity on very rare occasions. However, there is a case on record (Kawarabayashi et al., 1988) of a woman who apparently reacted to oxytocin itself. Her condition was successfully reversed with 0.05 mg of epinephrine.

Fortunately, most women will be aware of their sensitivity to a substance due to a previous exposure. For example, a woman may have received a caine-based anesthetic at the dentist and experienced swelling, edema or a skin reaction. This tells you that a more severe reaction is likely should she be exposed to any drug with a similar composition again. It is very rare for an anaphylactoid reaction to occur when no previous exposure has taken place. Therefore, you will be able to anticipate and avoid nearly all anaphylactic surprises during labor or thereafter.

Assessing and Treating Anaphylaxis

Signs and symptoms

Anaphylaxis during labor is an emergency requiring prompt recognition and treatment if the mother and baby are to survive. Although sensitivity to several substances does raise the risk, there are no specific risk factors that can assist in the early identification of women who may have a severe reaction other than a history of a reaction to a particular substance. Symptoms manifest in a variety of organ systems including the cutaneous, gastrointestinal, respiratory and cardiovascular. The hallmark of true anaphylaxis is the onset of symptoms within seconds or minutes after exposure to the offending agent. The woman may report a sense of impending doom with the simultaneous onset of flushing, tachycardia and, often, itching. These symptoms may progress to an outbreak of spots on the skin, swelling, nasal and bronchial discharge, abdominal bloating, nausea, vomiting, cramps, arrhythmias, faintness, cardiovascular collapse, and finally death. Most important, laryngeal edema and asthma may develop; these constitute the life-threatening component of an extreme hypersensitivity reaction.

Anaphylactic and Anaphylactoid Reactions		
Organ System	**Symptoms**	**Signs**
Not life threatening (may occur with or without more serious symptoms)		
Skin	Itching, burning, tingling, numbness, flushing, chills	Rash, swelling, hives
Gastrointestinal	Abdominal bloating, cramps, nausea, vomiting, diarrhea, incontinence	Abdominal pain, metallic taste in mouth
Life threatening		
Cardiovascular	Faintness, malaise, weakness, palpitations, chest discomfort, collapse	Tachycardia, low blood pressure, arrhythmia, *cardiac arrest*
Respiratory	Congestion, painful breathing, choking, gasping, coughing, hoarseness, lump in throat, difficulty swallowing or talking	Tachypnea, rhonchi, laryngeal swelling, pulmonary edema, *respiratory arrest*
Fetal	Decreased fetal movement	Late decelerations, tachycardia, reduced variability, bradycardia

The manifestations of an anaphylactoid reaction are similar to anaphylaxis and include increased secretion from the mucous membranes as an initial warning sign. Itching, burning, tingling, and numbness commonly follow. A raised, red rash on the face and upper trunk develops and may progress rapidly to a generalized rash. Swelling around the eyes and mouth commonly occur. Associated symptoms include runny eyes and nose, as well as engorgement of the conjunctiva. Gastrointestinal symptoms such as nausea, vomiting, diarrhea and abdominal pains develop. Hypothermia (between 95 to 96.8°F [35° and 36°C]) is seen, and rarely, fever (100.4 to 102.2°F [38° to 39°C]). Respiratory signs often present in the form of a dry cough, rapid breathing, and wheezing secondary to bronchospasm. Laryngeal edema may make breathing, positive-pressure ventilation and intubation difficult. Pulmonary edema causing severe respiratory distress can also interfere with ventilation efforts. Cardiovascular collapse is common despite aggressive treatment. Hypotension and tachycardia are the rule. Disturbances of the cardiac rhythm and of conduction within the heart muscle frequently occur early on. Cardiac arrest is usually due to lack of oxygen from bronchospasm and prolonged shock.

Assessment

Physical examination: Assessment depends upon the affected organ systems and the severity of the reaction. Anxiety, tremor, and feeling chilled or warm are common unless hypotension or hypoxia results in loss of consciousness. The person may be agitated or combative; therefore reassurance is key to getting the person to cooperate. General appearance varies with the severity of the reaction; the classic skin reaction is hives, consisting of red, raised, intensely itchy lesions.

First, evaluate the woman's respiratory status by listening to the lungs. Anaphylactic shock is distinguished by cardiovascular and respiratory crises. Vital signs may be normal or significantly abnormal, with tachypnea, tachycardia and hypotension. Upper airway obstruction may occur when the lips, tongue or oropharynx become swollen. Nonpitting, swollen mucosal lesions (angioedema) involving the surface and deeper tissues of the lips, palms, soles and genitals may develop. Difficulty with breathing, coughing, hoarseness, stridor or a quiet voice may be noted, indicating upper airway compromise. Wheezing occurs when the lower airway is constricted due to bronchospasm or mucosal edema. Coughing up of blood-tinged mucus, the use of accessory muscles to breathe and tracheal tugging during inspiration indicate more severe compromise of the lower respiratory tract. Speaking ability may be lost altogether as the swelling becomes severe. Complete airway obstruction is the most common cause of death.

Assess the cardiovascular system next via pulse, blood pressure and capillary refill time. Check the pulse for rate, regularity and quality (bounding, thready, etc.); the pulse quickens to compensate as the vascular system dilates and becomes more permeable; then blood pressure eventually drops. Once the blood pressure has fallen, latter stages of shock are underway. Assess capillary refill time, which should not exceed 3 seconds. The heart rate is normal in mild cases, but severe reactions result in tachycardia due to loss of vascular tone, although bradycardia sometimes occurs. Intravascular volume depletion may occur due to capillary leakage. Shock can occur without either dramatic skin reactions or a history of exposure, therefore an anaphylactoid reaction must always be considered in the differential diagnosis of shock that has no obvious cause.

A person may react within seconds of exposure to an allergen, but the response can be delayed as much as several hours. The severity of the initial reaction does not correlate well with the eventual severity of the reaction; however, the earlier the onset of symptoms, the more severe they are likely to become. Injected allergens typically produce symptoms after 5 to 30 minutes, although a reaction can occur immediately. Ingested allergens usually cause a reaction within 2 hours. Because of this, any evidence of a reaction requires continuous reassessment of pulse, respiration and other vital signs, including level of consciousness and the progression of other signs and symptoms.

Differential diagnosis: Usually a potentially offending substance will have been introduced to the woman preceding the reaction. However, whenever a woman is experiencing what appears to be an anaphylactic response, you must also consider amniotic fluid embolism, heart attack, congestive heart failure and pulmonary embolism as possible causes.

What to do

If you suspect an anaphylactic reaction, the best course of action is to stabilize the mother as well as possible and transport immediately, by ambulance whenever feasible. In addition:

1. Discontinue exposure to the suspected offending substance. When the offending substance has contacted the woman distally (on her forearm, for example), apply a tourniquet to obstruct the blood flow from the source of the antigen or inciting medication. Release the tourniquet every 15 minutes or so.
2. Place the woman in a supine position and keep her warm. If she is still pregnant, place a folded towel under her right hip to shift the weight of the uterus off the inferior vena cava.
3. If the woman is conscious, tell her you are going to help her breathe until the emergency service arrives and ask her to try to cooperate. She is likely to be combative or highly agitated.

4. Measure and record vital signs (pulse, blood pressure, capillary refill) every 5 minutes.
5. Administer aqueous epinephrine (0.3 to 0.5 ml of 1:1000 concentration) subcutaneously or use an auto-injector per package instructions (see discussion of epinephrine below). Repeat every 20 minutes for a total of three doses.
6. If the woman is unconscious, maintain an open airway with jaw thrust and head tilt. If the mother is breathing, give 100% oxygen at flow rate of 15 l/min with your adult resuscitator. The woman should receive artificial ventilation until she is breathing comfortably, even if she is trying to breathe. During an anaphylactic reaction, her airways will be constricted; positive-pressure ventilation can help overcome this resistance.
7. Start an IV and give 2 to 4 liters of a crystalloid solution such as sterile saline.
8. If the baby is not yet born, monitor the fetal heart rate closely. Fetal hypoxia can be expected as blood flow to the uterus is reduced (see the chapter entitled "Hypovolemic Shock due to Hemorrhage" for details). Fetal heart rate abnormalities reflect insufficient maternal oxygenation or relative hypovolemia. They can generally be corrected with maternal position changes and oxygen administration in the hypoxic mother.
9. Call the hospital and let them know the situation, the suspected antigen, and your expected time of arrival.
10. If the baby has been born, be alert for uterine bleeding. *Do not* administer oxytocin (as epinephrine and oxytocin are antagonists); instead use manual methods of controlling hemorrhage until transport is complete.

Post-Transport Laboratory Tests

Once you get to the hospital, it can be helpful to know what tests may be ordered. Standard laboratory tests include arterial blood gases, complete blood count, platelet count, fibrinogen, fibrin-split products, prothrombin time and partial thromboplastin time.

If the cause of shock is in doubt, tests for urinary methylhistamine and plasma tryptase release in serum are warranted. These tests help determine if an anaphylactic reaction has occurred. Methylhistamine is a histamine metabolite which is discharged in the urine and is more stable than histamine collected in blood specimens. Tryptase release in serum or plasma samples can be measured sequentially over the first 24 hr period. This substance is only produced by mast cells. Its presence in the blood parallels histamine. Assessment of these markers helps to confirm an anaphylactic reaction. Skin tests to track down the specific offending agent can also be performed: keep in mind that an inactive component of a solution, such as a preservative, may be the problem. This is vital information for the woman to have for her future medical care providers.

The remainder of the chapter summarizes the important details regarding the use of epinephrine in midwifery.

Epinephrine (Adrenalin [Parke-Davis])

The hormone epinephrine, or adrenalin, is a major hormone involved in stress response. It is also the drug of choice for counteracting an acute anaphylactic reaction; this is its primary indication for use in midwifery practice. It is a sympathomimetic catecholamine with a chemical formula of β-(3,4-dihydroxyphenyl)-α-methylaminoethanol. It can be given to counteract severe allergic reactions to foods, insect bites or stings, drugs and other allergens. In midwifery, it is primarily used to treat a woman who is having a severe allergic reaction to an anesthetic used during perineal repair but may be given in the event of other, more rare reactions, such as latex allergy, as well. Epinephrine has a wide range of other uses. It is sometimes added to local anesthetics to promote local vasoconstriction to localize the anesthetic during suturing, a use that is not recommended in perineal repair. This discussion will focus on its use to treat anaphylactic shock. Midwives will only be using epinephrine in an acute, life-threatening emergency as it is a potentially dangerous drug that can have severe cardiac effects.

Packaging
Ampule doses: Inexpensive amber glass ampules that contain 1 ml of 1:1000 epinephrine (that is, two to three doses) are available. The amount given must be titrated to a precise dose of 0.3 to 0.5 ml (a little under one-third to one-half of the ampule). This can be measured by using a tuberculin or an insulin syringe to draw up the exact amount in cubic centimeters (cc, which is the same as milliliters). Both of these types of syringes have 100 unit markings per milliliter

on their measurement scale (30 marks for 0.3 and 50 marks for 0.5 ml). Dosage is gauged by the severity and acuteness of the reaction, coupled with body size. If you are unsure regarding how much to give, administer 0.4 ml (40 units). It is best to draw up the entire contents of the ampule and then inject the required dose. If only a portion of the ampule is withdrawn, the rest is now considered contaminated and must be thrown away. Repeated doses can be given to one person using the same syringe if aseptic technique is observed during administration.

Premeasured doses: The easiest way for individuals susceptible to severe allergic reactions to carry and use epinephrine is in a prepackaged auto-injector intended for use by anyone faced with assisting a person in anaphylactic shock. The EpiPen is widely available in the United States but is distributed only to patients known to have severe allergies. Therefore, if your client has a severe allergy, she may have an auto-injection dose on hand. These devices consist of a preloaded auto-injection syringe that contains 2 ml of epinephrine for use in emergency situations to be given as an intramuscular injection. It contains no latex. Each adult EpiPen delivers a single dose of 0.3 mg in a 1:1000 (0.3 ml) dosage, suitable for use in persons weighing at least 66 lb (30 kg). EpiPenJr is available for use in persons weighing less than 33 lb (15 kg). The remaining 1.7 ml remains in the unit after use. Each 0.3 ml EpiPen contains 0.3 mg epinephrine, 1.8 mg sodium chloride, 0.5 mg sodium metabisulfate, hydrochloric acid to adjust the pH and water for injection. The pH range is 1.2 to 5.0. The Anapen is a similar product available in Canada and the United Kingdom. As of this printing, auto-injection devices cost around $25.00 in the United States. A number of similar products are available in the United States and other countries.

PRODUCT NAME	MANUFACTURER	COUNTRY OF DISTRIBUTION	DOSE	COMMENTS
Ana-Guard	Hollister Stier Labs	US, some others	Two 0.3 mg doses; other doses possible	Standard prefilled syringe that comes in a sturdy, compact protective tube
Ana-Kit	Bayer	US (?)	Two 0.3 mg doses; other doses possible	Established history; includes a standard prefilled syringe; also comes with antihistamine tablets (chlorpheniramine maleate), alcohol prep pads & tourniquet (for use with stings)
Anapen*	Lincoln Medical Ltd (UK); Quorum Allergy (Canada)	Canada, UK	Adult: One 0.3 mg dose	Easiest device to use and least likely to malfunction if not used quite correctly
EpiPen*	Dey Labs (US); ALK (Europe)	US, Europe	Adult: One 0.3 mg dose	Established history
EpiE-ZPen*	Meridian	US, Canada	Adult: One 0.3 mg dose	Smaller, easier to carry than EpiPen and activated manually, which reduces chances of accidental injection
Min-I-Jet	IMS (UK)	UK	One 1 mg dose; other doses possible	Designed for medical professionals, this high dose is not usually needed and may cause significant side-effects.

*Auto-injector devices that have a dummy "trainer" available from the manufacturer for practice.

EpiPen: The EpiPen has a unique design, so it is important to familiarize yourself with it before you need to use it. A spring-activated prefilled syringe 14.5 cm long by 1.8 cm in diameter comes housed in a outer casing that hides the needle and is sold in a protective tubular case. (The tube is yellow for the adult dose and white for the EpiPenJr.) Upon removal from the case, the pen itself is a narrow cylinder with a black tip on one end and a gray activation cap on the other; between these ends is the auto-injector, which has a clear window through which you can check the color and clarity of the drug. The black tip is where the needle comes out; to avoid inadvertent injection, take care not to put your thumb, fingers or hand over that end. Accidental injection into your hands or feet may result in loss of blood flow to those areas. If this occurs, you are now in a critical emergency situation as well and require immediate care. Epinephrine can shut off the entire blood supply to a digit and can result in gangrene. Be careful!

The pen is designed for intramuscular use only. Do not attempt to use an EpiPen to give the drug intravenously and never inject epinephrine into the buttocks. Because the dose is preset for specific weights, there may be a stronger or weaker reaction in a person whose weight differs greatly from the target weight of the premeasured dose.

When you are ready to use the EpiPen, grasp the unit in the middle with one hand, with the black tip directed downward. Pull off the gray activation cap with your other hand. Place the black tip at a 90° angle against the woman's outer thigh. Push firmly and hold to a count of 10, then remove. Alternately, grasp the pen in such a way as to swing and jab the black tip firmly (3 lb of force) into the outer thigh at a 90° angle and count to 10. The 22 gauge needle is propelled by a spring that generates 16 lb of force, which could injure bone if the wrong site for injection is chosen. Withdraw the unit and massage the site of injection for several seconds. Check the black tip; if the needle is exposed, the person received the dose. If not, simply repeat the steps outlined above; you need not open another pen. Note that most of the drug will still be in the pen even if the intended dose was properly delivered. Dispose of the unit in a sharps container or bend the needle back against a hard surface and replace the unit back into the carrying tube (do not replace the gray cap). Recap the carrying tube. Proceed with transport.

Anapen: The unit is 16.5 cm long and 1.8 cm in diameter with a shelf life of 18 months. The adult unit is bright green and the pediatric unit is bright yellow. When ready to use, pull off the needle cap on one end and then pull off the safety cap on the other, exposing a red button. Position the needle end at a 90° angle to the chosen injection site on the outer thigh. Depress the red button to trigger the automatic injection. The spring action of the Anapen is much less forceful than that of the EpiPen. Unlike the EpiPen, the Anapen can be stored under refrigeration, which is very useful in hot climates.

Inhalant: An inhaler device that may have been effective against allergic reactions (Medihaler Epi by 3M sold in the United Kingdom and other countries) was on the market for a short time, but it has been withdrawn because of stability problems. The currently available inhaler devices available in the United State are not effective for allergic reactions and should not be used.

Stability and storage

Store at room temperature between 59 and 86°F (15 to 30°C). Epinephrine deteriorates rapidly upon exposure to light or air, turning pink from oxidation and brown from the formation of melanin. Protect the solution from light, extreme heat and freezing. Do not remove ampules or prefilled syringes from packaging until you are ready to use them. Examine each dose over a white and a plain-colored background in good light prior to use to confirm that the fluid is not discolored or cloudy and that it contains no particulate matter. Discard any unused portion after the container is opened.

Preservatives

Some epinephrine preparations are preserved with sodium bisulfate, which may cause allergic reactions, including anaphylaxis, in some individuals. However, the general medical opinion is that this should not deter the use of epinephrine containing this preservative in a life-threatening emergency, as the epinephrine itself will counteract any allergic reaction to the sodium bisulfate.

Actions

Epinephrine, whether given subcutaneously or intramuscularly, works rapidly and has a short duration of action. Epinephrine's reaction is highly complex; for midwifery purposes, it can be understood by its two most basic effects. It acts on *beta* receptor sites of sympathetic effector nerve cells to a variable degree, producing a relaxing effect that is most pronounced in the smooth muscles of the heart, blood vessels, irises, bronchial tubes and urinary bladder wall, as well as other smooth muscle, including the pregnant or postpartum uterus. This relaxes the bronchospasm that interferes with breathing.

During labor, epinephrine may also interfere with contractions due to its relaxing effect on the uterine muscle. After the birth, its uterine relaxing effects can increase postpartum bleeding. Administering oxytocin to counteract this effect can result in a drug interaction that produces severe and prolonged hypertension; therefore, nonpharmaceutical means of controlling the bleeding, such as bimanual compression and nipple stimulation, should be the first line of therapy. If an antihemorrhagic is absolutely required, oxytocin, rather than Methergine, which also increases blood pressure, is the drug of choice.

Epinephrine's other primary action involves a pronounced vasoconstrictor effect, acting as a physiological antagonist to histamine through its effect on *alpha* adrenergic receptors. This action halts the generalized vasodilation produced by histamine, reversing the increased permeability of dilated capillaries to plasma and quickly restoring circulating blood volume by constricting the capillary bed and correcting hypotension. As a by-product, vasoconstriction also decreases blood flow to the uterus, which can quickly lead to fetal hypoxia.

Administration of epinephrine alleviates burning, swelling and itching secondary to allergic reactions and may help relieve gastrointestinal and genitourinary symptoms associated with anaphylaxis. It causes the blood glucose levels to rise by prompting glycogen conversion in the liver. The drug becomes fixed to the tissues and is inactivated by enzymatic breakdown into metanephrine or normetanephrine, both of which are then conjugated by the liver and excreted in the urine in the form of sulfates and glucuronides. This results in the formation of vanillylmandelic acid (VMA), which is detectable in the urine.

Side-effects

Trembling, palpitations and a sensation of tension or extreme anxiety and fear commonly occur after the recommended dose is administered; these symptoms will soon wear off. Reassure the woman that this is the fight-or-flight hormone and that these responses are a normal reaction. Expect a transient but extreme elevation in blood pressure to as high as 200/130 mm Hg. The higher the dose of epinephrine, the more exaggerated these effects, which in sufficiently high doses may be dangerous to the heart. Epinephrine may result in hypertension when given following administration of oxytocic drugs. If used during labor, it can produce sloughing of any yoni or cervical tissues that are under direct pressure because of vasoconstriction, in conjunction with a delay in pushing (this is most likely to happen when epinephrine is given in conjunction with spinal anesthesia).

Contraindications

Epinephrine should not be used if there is known hypersensitivity to the drug or *in the event of hypovolemic shock* or coronary insufficiency. Even though amniotic fluid embolism is now referred to as "anaphylactoid syndrome of pregnancy" in some sources, the mechanism of this type of reaction is different than with conventional allergic reactions, and epinephrine should not be used in an attempt to treat it.

Epinephrine should be used with caution in those with cardiovascular diseases, cardiac arrhythmias, hypertension, diabetes, hyperthyroidism, psychoneurosis, bronchial asthma and emphysema with degenerative heart disease and thyrotoxicosis. Remember that there is an increased possibility of precipitating a cardiac event during administration after the age of 40, so it should not be used on older mothers unless the indication is clear.

Inadvertently induced high arterial pressure secondary to epinephrine administration may result in angina pectoris (heart pain), aortic rupture or cerebral hemorrhage. It may also cause potentially serious cardiac arrhythmias in persons who do not have heart disease and in those with organic heart disease or receiving drugs that sensitize the myocardium (such as digitalis, mercurial diuretics or quinidine). The effects of epinephrine may be exaggerated by tricyclic antidepressants and monoamine oxidase inhibitors. The peripheral vasoconstriction and cardiac stimulation produced by epinephrine may lead to pulmonary edema in some individuals.

The use of epinephrine together with *beta*-blocking drugs (used to treat high blood pressure in both pregnant and nonpregnant persons, some heart arrhythmias, glaucoma [in eye drops], migraine headaches and other conditions) can worsen asthma and may make otherwise tolerable skin reactions to an allergen escalate into anaphylactic shock. *Beta*-blocking drugs may also make treatment with adrenaline-based drugs less effective. Those on *beta*-blocking medications should consult the prescribing physician regarding what to do in the event of a severe allergic reaction during pregnancy. *Beta*-agonist drugs, used to treat asthma, have an effect similar to epinephrine. If the woman has a rescue inhaler and her reaction is mild, use of her inhaler may calm the reaction. If the attack is more severe, epinephrine should be given immediately.

Administration of epinephrine by injection or IV during labor and birth can cause the fetal heart rate to rise and should not be used when the mother's blood pressure exceeds 130/80 mm Hg. It is not known if the drug is excreted in breast milk.

Pregnancy category C: Epinephrine is teratogenic in small animals at doses approximately 25 times the human dose. There are no adequate and well-controlled studies of its effect during human pregnancy. It should only be used if the potential benefit justifies the possible risk to the fetus.

Dosage and routes of administration

Treatment of anaphylaxis consists of both short-term therapy to stabilize the woman prior to transport and long-term therapy, which will be administered by medical staff once transport is complete. As the midwife, you will be endeavoring to stabilize the woman and maintain an adequate airway and blood pressure while preparing to transport.

Epinephrine should be given as soon as an allergic reaction is deemed the probable cause of symptoms. The standard dose is 0.01 ml/kg of a 1:1000 solution up to a maximum of 0.3 to 0.5 ml, given subcutaneously every 10 to 20 minutes until the woman's condition stabilizes. Epinephrine can be given high in the deltoid muscle, in the anterior thigh or in any location close to the torso where a layer of fat allows some skin mobility. It should *never* be given distally in an extremity or in the buttocks. Administration into a distal extremity can result in severe vasoconstriction and tissue necrosis and may result in hitting a bone with the needle. Administration into the buttocks can be complicated by the development of gas gangrene infection with *Clostridium welchii*, an organism commonly found on the skin surface in the area (tissue changes secondary to vasoconstriction promote the growth of this anaerobic bacteria). The subcutaneous route is preferred for out-of-hospital, emergency use as absorption is somewhat more reliable from fat layers, skeletal muscle absorption being highly variable. Subcutaneous administration is said to produce bronchodilation within a few seconds but may take up to 5 to 10 minutes, with a peak effect after 20 minutes. However, the literature suggests that subcutaneous administration may result in a more prolonged effect of up to 150 minutes. *Subcutaneous administration is always the route of choice when an auto-injection unit is not being used.*

Intravenous administration is sometimes used in reactions involving full-blown shock with cardiac arrest; however, this route is more dangerous as it poses a greater risk of ventricular arrhythmias and myocardial ischemia. Advanced cardiac life-support guidelines recommend concurrent monitoring with electrocardiography during an IV infusion; it is therefore inappropriate to give epinephrine by any type of IV route in midwifery practice.

Auto-injection devices are designed to deliver an intramuscular injection that is said to wear off in 15 to 20 minutes, although this effect may last longer if given into the outer thigh.

Transport after administration

Any woman who has required epinephrine should be transported for continued cardiac monitoring.

Accidental newborn administration

This should not happen if different classes of medications are stored separately from each other. The baby would develop extreme tachycardia, irregular heartbeat and fainting, become pale and sweat, giving the appearance of a heart attack that may lead to death. The baby will likely recover because the young heart is so strong, but she should be transported right away.

References and Further Reading on Understanding and Treating Shock

References used in multiple chapters

Asensio J, et al. Chapter 4: "Exsanguination," in Grenvik A, et al., eds. Textbook of Critical Care, 4th ed. WB Saunders, Philadelphia PA, 2000.

Bonner J. "Massive obstetric hemorrhage," Baillière's Clin Obstet Gynaecol, 14(1);1-18, Feb, 2000.

Clark S. "Shock in the pregnant patient," Semin Perinatol, 14(1);52-58, Feb, 1990.

Clark S, et al. Critical Care Obstetrics, 3rd ed., Blackwell Science, Malden MA, 1997.

Cunningham F, et al. Williams Obstetrics, 21st ed. McGraw-Hill Pub., New York NY, 2001.

Grant H, et al. Brady Emergency Care, 5th ed. Prentice Hall, Inc, Englewood Cliffs NJ, 1990.

Hofmeyr G, Mohlala B. "Hypovolemic shock," Best Prac Res Clin Obstet Gynaecol, 15(4);645-662, Aug, 2001.

Marshall M, Buffington S. Life-Saving Skills Manual for Midwives: Module 5: Hemorrhage; Module 6: Resuscitation, 3rd ed. American College of Nurse-Midwives, Washington DC, 1998.

Moss M. Chapter 11: "Shock," in Handbook of Pediatric and Neonatal Transport Medicine, 2nd ed. Hanley & Belfus Inc, Philadelphia PA, 2002.

Pearlman M, Tintinalli J eds. Emergency Care of the Woman. McGraw-Hill, New York NY, 1998.

Schuurmans N, et al. "Prevention and Management of Postpartum Hemorrhage," SOGC Clinical Practice Guidelines, J SOGC (88), Apr, 2000.

Shoemaker W. Chapter 8: "Diagnosis and treatment of shock and circulatory dysfunction," in Grenvik A, et al., eds. Textbook of Critical Care, 4th ed. WB Saunders, Philadelphia PA, 2000.

Hypovolemic Shock Due to Hemorrhage

Lowe C, LAc. Personal communications and editing notes, Sept, 2003.

Sweet B. ed. Maye's Midwifery: A Textbook for Midwives, 12th ed. Baillière Tindall, London UK, 1997.

West Z. Acupuncture in Pregnancy and Childbirth. Churchill Livingstone, Edinburgh UK, 2001.

Amniotic Fluid Embolism (Anaphylactoid Syndrome of Pregnancy)

Clark SL. "New concepts of amniotic fluid embolism: a review," Obstet Gynecol Survey, 158;1158-1169, 1995.

Cunningham F, et al. Williams Obstetrics, 23st ed. McGraw-Hill Pub., New York NY, 2010.

Cunningham F, et al. Williams Obstetrics, 22st ed. McGraw-Hill Pub., New York NY, 2005.

Kawarabayashi T, et al. "Anaphylactoid reaction to oxytocin during cesarean section," Obstet Gynecol Invest, 25(4);277-279, 1988.

Kramer M, et al. "Amniotic-fluid embolism and medical induction of labour: a retrospective, population-based cohort study," Lancet, 368(9545):1444-1448, Oct 21, 2006.

Steiner P, Luschbaurgh C, "Maternal pulmonary embolism by amniotic fluid," JAMA, 117;1245-1253, 1941.

Thomson A, Greer I. "Non-hemorrhagic obstetric shock," Baillière's Clin Obstet Gynaecol, 14(1);19-41, 2000.

Wagner M. "From caution to certainty: hazards in the formation of evidence-based practice–a case study on evidence for an association between the use of uterine stimulant drugs and amniotic fluid embolism," Paediatr Perinat Epidemiol, 19(2): 173-176, Mar, 2005.

Hypersensitivity Reactions and Anaphylactic Shock

"Ana-Kit," www.RxMed.com, accessed May 15, 2003.

"Anapen," information from UK manufacturer, posted on www.cargaryallergy.ca, accessed May 15, 2003.

Dey Inc. Patient insert: EpiPen and EpiPen Jr, Columbia, MD, Dec, 2000.

"EpiPen: consumer medicine information," E Merck, CSL Ltd, Aberdeen, Australia, Sept, 2002.

Facts comparisons staff, ed. "Epinephrine," in Drug Facts and Comparisons. Walters Klumner Co, St Louis MO, Oct, 2002.

Kawarabayashi T, et al. "Anaphylactoid reaction to oxytocin during cesarean section," Gynecol Obstet Invest, 25(4);277-279, 1988.

Poznar J. Registered pharmacist. Editing notes on epinephrine section, 2003.

Stern M."Anaphylaxis: life-threatening allergy," www.users.globalnet.co.uk/~aair/anaphylaxis.htm, accessed May 15, 2003.

Walsh P, et al. "Epinephrine," in Physician's Desk Reference, 55th ed. Medical Economics, Montvale NJ, 2001.

Wyatt R. "Anaphylaxis: how to recognize, treat, and prevent potentially fatal attacks," Postgraduate Medicine Online, 100(2), Aug, 1996 accessed on www.postgradmed.com, May 15, 2003.

When the Newborn Develops Respiratory Distress

Anatomical and Physiological Considerations Regarding Respiratory Distress

Understanding Fetal and Neonatal Asphyxia

NOTE: Review the chapter entitled "The Baby's Journey through Labor to Birth," which explains initiation of breathing in healthy newborns, before studying this chapter.

What is Asphyxia?

STEDMAN'S ELECTRONIC MEDICAL DICTIONARY (Rybacki, 2004) defines asphyxia as impaired or absent exchange of oxygen and carbon dioxide on a ventilatory basis, leading to elevated levels of carbon dioxide in the blood. This eventually produces **anoxia**, which is the absence or almost complete absence of oxygen from inspired gases, arterial blood, or tissues. Anaerobic respiration (that occurring in the absence of oxygen) and accumulating carbon dioxide both lead to a rise in lactic acid production and thus contribute to acidosis.

Although the term "birth asphyxia" is widely used, it has no universally accepted definition. The standard definition of asphyxia reveals the imprecision with which this term is applied to fetal and newborn distress that is really caused by varying degrees of hypoxia. "Perinatal asphyxia" has been proposed as a more precise term, as most oxygen deprivation with serious consequences begins in utero. The World Health Organization has rather vaguely defined perinatal asphyxia as a "failure to initiate and sustain breathing at birth." A more biophysical definition includes impaired or absent exchange of carbon dioxide and oxygen, progressive tissue hypoxia (oxygen deprivation), accumulation of carbon dioxide, fetal bradycardia and acidosis. Thus, established asphyxia is associated with a degree of shock, which is technically impaired oxygen delivery at the cellular level. (For more details see the chapter entitled "Hypovolemic Shock due to Hemorrhage.") If allowed to progress uncorrected, oxygen deprivation leads to permanent brain damage, impaired functioning of other vital organs and, eventually, death.

Causes of adult and fetal or neonatal respiratory impairment

The only essential difference between adult and neonatal asphyxia is in how oxygen delivery is typically interrupted. In adults, respiratory distress causes an increase in respiratory rate (gasping) as the victim searches for air in an effort to bring more oxygen to the tissues. Adult respiratory arrest almost always results from a failure of heart function due to myocardial infarction (death of heart muscle cells), severe arrhythmia or both. Breathing ceases because oxygen is no longer being delivered to the medullary brain stem, where the nerve centers controlling respiration are located, therefore no gasping will ensue (although adults may gasp during hypovolemic shock). Since heart malfunction is almost always the cause, successful resuscitation is achieved by using cardiac massage interspersed with ventilation. The problem with the heart can be diagnosed once circulation and respirations are reestablished.

Newborn asphyxial events occur differently. As a rule, the baby's system is perfectly normal and healthy; in most cases, the heart is still beating efficiently. The problem is almost always one of impaired gas exchange, at least at first. In utero, the fetus is held at a constant temperature and puts few demands on the environment of the womb; as a result, the normal state of the fetal circulatory system is one of vasodilation. When a normal fetus is confronted with an abnormal level of stress, however, her demand for oxygen increase, but the fetus has only a limited capacity to influence the amount of oxygen available. The supply cannot be increased by enhancing placental blood flow via vasodilation of the placental bed nor by increasing her right ventricular output. Instead, the baby must rely on her ability to alter the amount of oxygen reaching certain regions of the body by increasing oxygen extraction from the hemoglobin, by decreasing oxygen utilization and by redistributing blood flow (Teitel, 1998). Thus, fetuses and newborns have unique responses that allow them to deal with periods of oxygen deprivation.

- After the initial period of hypoxia, newborns will begin spontaneous, spinally generated, reflexive gasping. If air is available, the infant will begin breathing.
- The newborn heart has a high concentration of glycogen. Oxygen deprivation triggers anaerobic glycolysis,

which allows the heart to continue to beat for up to 20 minutes or more in the presence of hypoxia. The heart can continue to provide adequate circulation even when there is significant biochemical disruption resulting in such low oxygen levels that the breathing mechanism fails and the reserve system for gasping stops functioning. Only when severe acidosis develops will cardiac output fall off.

- The fetal and newborn brain and heart can withstand a low level of oxygen much longer than the four minutes an adult can tolerate, due, in part, to the protective effects of noradrenaline. During periods of hypoxia, vasoconstriction in nonessential organs leaves them minimally perfused, selectively rerouting circulation to the most vital organs: the heart, lungs, adrenals and brain, with the brain and heart receiving the most highly oxygenated blood. These important mechanisms conserve energy when oxygen is at a premium.
- The fetal and neonatal brain has several protective features that make it exceptionally resistant to the effects of hypoxia. It has rich glycogen stores and is capable of anaerobic glycolysis. EEG studies indicate that energy dependent processes are shut down during hypoxia. Preferential blood flow to the brain stem helps maintain the most basic vital functions.
- The fetus responds to hypoxia by slowing his heart rate, especially in the last trimester. This, coupled with the selective organ perfusion described above, helps conserve energy and oxygen.
- It is also worth remembering that the normal intrauterine environment is "hypoxic" by adult standards. Thus, the fetus normally thrives at a lower oxygen saturation level than does an adult.

The above physiological adaptations mean that the newborn who does not breathe right away rarely needs more than brief assistance with ventilation in order to establish and maintain normal cardiopulmonary function. In very unusual cases, cardiac compressions may be called for, but the development of significant arrhythmias in newborns is virtually unheard of, making the types of drugs commonly used in adult resuscitations unnecessary (Morley, 2004; Northern Neonatal Network, 1993; Richmond, 1996; Richmond et al., 2001)

Causes of perinatal respiratory impairment

The baby who has been compromised during labor may be depressed at birth and may have difficulty beginning to breathe on his own. Leaving the cord intact provides him with the optimal opportunity to begin breathing and to restore any insult to systemic perfusion from impaired blood flow that may have occurred prior to birth. However, establishing adequate respirations as placental respiration tapers off and the placenta detaches is vital to preventing further hypoxia from lack of oxygen. The underlying cause of nearly all perinatal hypoxia is either loss of circulation to the baby from the placenta or loss of pulmonary oxygenation after birth. There are six basic ways this may occur:

1. Impairment or complete interruption of umbilical blood flow (cord prolapse, compression)
2. Impairment or failure of gas exchange across the placenta (e.g., abruption, previa)
3. Impaired maternal blood flow to the placenta (e.g., severe maternal hypotension or disease-related hypertension, abnormally intense uterine contractions)
4. Alteration in maternal arterial oxygen levels (maternal hypoventilation, hypoxemia or cardiopulmonary disease)
5. If the baby is otherwise compromised and cannot tolerate the intermittent hypoxia of normal labor (e.g., an anemic or growth-restricted baby)
6. Impaired fetal-to-newborn transition (frequently a result of cord clamping) with failure to begin breathing

The following causes of impaired oxygen exchange in the fetus or newborn may, unless otherwise indicated, be either acute or chronic; any insult that persists long enough will result in chronic oxygen deprivation.

- Cord compression or prolapse
- Placental insufficiency (chronic)
- Prematurity with accompanying central nervous system immaturity, inadequate surfactant and accompanying lung immaturity (acute)
- Drugs administered to or taken by the mother
- Sepsis
- Congenital neuromuscular diseases
- Certain congenital malformations, especially any involving the heart, lungs, airways or the nerve supply to

those organs
•Intrapartum hypoxemia (poor oxygenation of arterial blood) (chronic)
•Placenta previa or abruption
•Fetal isoimmunization (chronic)
•Maternal vascular disease (chronic)
•Maternal hypotension (acute)
•Hyperstimulation of the uterus (acute)

The progressive fetal response to oxygen deprivation leading to perinatal asphyxia

The fetal and newborn response to impaired oxygen delivery is an ongoing and reversible process, the speed, progression and extent of which can be highly variable. Sudden, complete absence of oxygen can be fatal in less than 10 minutes. Mild oxygen deprivation may progressively worsen over 30 minutes or more. Repeated episodes of brief, mild, acutely impaired delivery of oxygen may reverse spontaneously but can produce the cumulative effect of progressive impairment. A chronic lack of sufficient oxygen can persist for many days or weeks, providing enough oxygen for survival to continue while depriving the tissues of optimal levels and sometimes producing permanent damage. A chronic lack of sufficient oxygen also leads to a variety of compensating responses in the fetus.

There is a fairly predictable progression of responses in the fetus or newborn experiencing an acute lack of oxygen, regardless of the cause or severity. Asphyxia triggers the most extreme manifestation of the mammalian diving reflex (the normal, nonasphyxial mammalian diving reflex is discussed in the chapter entitled "Hydrotherapy and Waterbirth"). The progressive response of the fetus and newborn to impaired oxygen delivery was first elaborated in the decade that spanned 1957 through 1967. It is divided into two phases, primary apnea and terminal (secondary) apnea, and is based on research done on a primate model in which total acute asphyxia was induced in fetal rhesus monkeys near term. This was accomplished by allowing the normal birth of rhesus monkey infants to undrugged mothers. The cord was tied immediately and their head was covered with a bag of warm saline (Dawes, 1968). The progression of their distress was then monitored until they either died or were revived. Thus, the classic understanding of asphyxia is based on the progression of sudden and total oxygen deprivation and severe hypovolemic shock in a previously uncompromised newborn who is prevented from taking a breath. The following description interweaves the original findings with additional understandings that have come to light since 1968.

Insulting event: For whatever reason, the baby undergoes a significant reduction in oxygen delivery. The fetus or newborn deprived of oxygen experiences fear and panic, triggering a rise in stress hormones.

Blood-volume redistribution: As oxygen tension falls, the fetal or newborn peripheral blood vessels dilate even more than usual, and blood is mobilized from the liver and spleen in an effort to get more oxygen to the tissues. These changes result in less blood returning to the placenta.

Asphyxial gasping: Within 30 seconds, the baby will attempt to get oxygen by pulling blood into the lungs and heart with a few gasping breaths, resulting in a slight increase in heart rate (Dawes, 1968; Morley, 2004). If the baby has already begun breathing before the insult, he will begin gasping more deeply and rapidly prior to losing consciousness. If the airway is clear and oxygen is available, the baby will revive himself. Intrauterine oxygen deprivation triggers the fetus to begin spontaneous gasping efforts as well, which will not help if no air is available and may complicate matters further if the baby inspires meconium-stained fluid into the lungs.

Primary (first-degree) apnea: Primary apnea, or cessation of breathing efforts, develops within two to three minutes of the onset of oxygen deprivation and lasts for 30 to 60 seconds (Dawes, 1968). The respiratory region in the medulla at the base of the brain shuts down as gasping efforts are suppressed by the higher centers of the brain responsible for normal breathing. Up to this point, the heart rate remains in a normal range. Soon, however, it begins to fall to about half its normal rate, although blood pressure is only minimally affected. This initial fall in heart rate is probably due to a vagal reflex. During primary apnea, oxygen deficiency prompts an activation of the sympathetic-adrenergic system and triggers the onset of anaerobic metabolism, which begins to take over to maintain the heart rate. Anaerobic metabolism is less fuel efficient than aerobic metabolism.

Vasoconstriction: Generalized vasodilation is no longer an effective means of oxygenating the tissues. Catecholamines, which help maintain the blood pressure despite a lower heart rate, rise and peripheral vasoconstriction takes over as circulation is dramatically reduced to all but the most vital organs. The skin color transitions over these few minutes from bluish pink, to blotchy and finally to white.

Lowered oxygen and elevated carbon dioxide levels lead to selective vasodilation of the cerebral vascular bed, resulting in hyperperfusion to the brain stem in particular, while the blood flow to the rest of the brain remains about the same. Cerebral hyperperfusion can reach 2 to 3 times the original rate of blood flow, depending upon the degree of oxygen deprivation and the maturity of the baby. Immature fetuses seem to be particularly endangered by their limited ability to increase cerebral circulation through vasodilation.

The reduction in heart rate conserves energy, allows more time for the ventricles to refill during diastole and increases stroke volume somewhat. (Stroke volume is the amount of blood pumped out of one ventricle per heartbeat. It is relatively fixed in the newborn; thus, cardiac output is determined almost entirely by heart rate.) As a result, cardiac output decreases, although not as much as one would expect from the fall in heart rate. Slowing the heart rate maintains circulation to the vital organs at the expense of the biochemical milieu, which becomes increasingly poor because of the rise in lactic acid levels that occurs as a by-product of anaerobic metabolism. This prompts the release of more catecholamines, causing the blood pressure to rise in an effort to equalize blood flow as neuromuscular tone gradually diminishes.

It is almost unheard of for the newborn's circulation to shut down completely before all respiratory effort ceases. This resilience is a feature of all newborn mammals, largely due to the glycogen reserves stored in the heart. Resuscitation that begins before the baby is so anoxic that all respiratory effort stops is usually easy and straightforward. In most cases, stimulating the baby and exposing her to room air are all that are required to bring her around and start her breathing on her own.

If the oxygen supply is not restored, primary apnea persists for a variable number of minutes. This time span can be influenced by a variety of factors–among them, certain obstetric drugs. For example, certain anesthetics administered to the mother can increase the duration of primary apnea but reduce the amount of gasping that follows. In some cases, primary apnea may persist for as long as 10 minutes. It is impossible to know when this 10 minute window starts, and it often begins while the baby is still in utero. In most cases, last-gasp efforts commence after one to two minutes.

Last-gasp efforts: If oxygen deprivation continues, the higher breathing centers in the brain cease to suppress the spinal nerve pathways governing autonomous gasping. These primitive spinal centers are still able to respond in spite of the increasingly poor biochemical state. After 30 to 60 seconds of primary apnea, gasping starts again. Four to 5 minutes after the onset of oxygen deprivation, the rate of gasping increases somewhat, with deep, body-shuttering gasps that occur 6 to 12 times a minute (every 10 to 20 seconds) and involve all the accessory muscles of respiration in a maximal inspiratory effort (Dawes, 1968). A baby born just prior to or during this gasping phase should still be able to resuscitate himself if his airway is clear. His gasping efforts must be sufficient to pull blood into his pulmonary circulation and inflate his lungs.

Cardiac output is maintained during gasping, but if oxygen deprivation persists, the blood pressure will remain stable only temporarily. Increasing acidosis and hypoxia interfere with synaptic communication between nerve cells. As gasping commences, the heart rate may increase slightly, but as gasping tapers off, the heart rate declines with it and continues to fall. As the minutes pass, the heart rate continues to drop, the blood pressure continues to fall, and the baby becomes nearly flaccid. (The muscle relaxation that accompanies hypoxia also increases the vulnerability of the infant to traction-related injuries during birth.) Vigorous gasping becomes weaker and less frequent as the baby becomes increasingly acidotic. Gasping ceases altogether when anoxia interferes with the ability of one nerve to pass synaptic messages to another. At this point, the baby will take his last gasp and enter terminal or secondary apnea. The baby has now exhausted all of his reserves and is unable to resume respiratory efforts on his own.

Terminal (secondary or second-degree) apnea: The heart may beat slowly for up to 10 minutes after the final gasp. Gradually, however, the blood pressure and oxygen level continue to fall and finally fade away. Prolonged asphyxia results in increased lactic acid production, which accumulates rapidly in the heart muscle. This leads to myocardial malfunction as cardiac output drops and all circulation ceases, even though regular but ineffective ventricular activity is still detectable on an ECG (electrocardiogram). Ineffective cardiac activity reduces and finally eliminates blood flow to vital organs and leads to progressive organ damage. Myocardial failure usually does not occur until pH drops to about 6.9 and P_{O2} drops to 20 mm Hg. There is an increasing impairment of cerebral circulatory autoregulation when the arterial pressure falls below 25 to 30 mm Hg, leading to a reduction in cerebral blood flow. This affects the parasagittal region of the cerebrum and the white matter most of all. The drop in blood pressure closely parallels the fall in heart rate.

All that may be required to revive the failing heart muscle even at this stage is a little artifical ventilation and a short period of cardiac compressions to move blood through the pulmonary circulation, into the left side of the heart and into the coronary arteries to supply the heart muscle with oxygen. An intact umbilical cord supplies the needed blood volume. Occasionally, however, the delivery of oxygenated blood to the heart muscle is not, by itself, enough to revive cardiac contractility because accumulated lactic acid progressively inhibits cardiac function.

If perfusion is inadequate and no oxygen reaches the heart, the baby will be unresponsive to stimulation of any kind. Death will occur unless artificial ventilation and cardiac compressions are initiated promptly. Once the baby is thus compromised, even a short delay in providing ventilation and compressions can result in a long delay in establishing spontaneous and regular respirations. The progression from initial asphyxia to death takes about 20 minutes in the normal term baby (Berger & Garnier, 2000; Kattwinkel et al., 2000; Northern Neonatal Network, 1993; Richmond, 1996; Richmond et al., 2001).

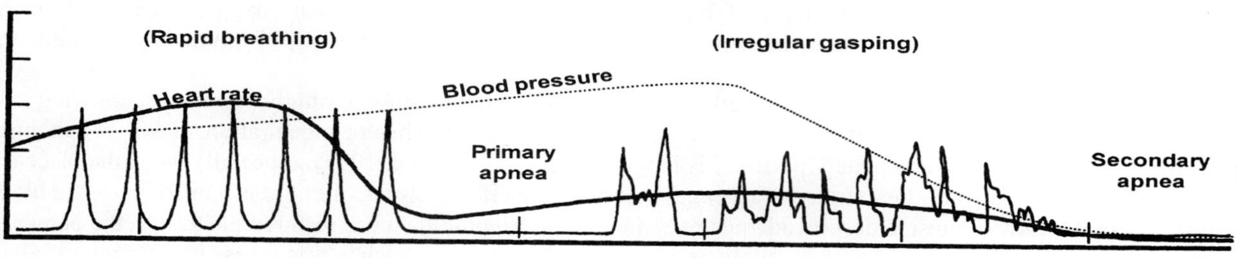

Summary of progressive responses to complete asphyxia

The influence of acidosis: A degree of hypoxia is normal at birth; typical umbilical artery blood gas values when the head is on the perineum appear below (see my DIAGNOSTIC TESTS for details regarding blood gas values in the chapter entitled "Fetal Scalp Sampling").

- •pH 7.175 to 7.295
- •Base excess –12.6 to –5.6 mmol/l
- •$PaCO_2$ 6.9 kPa
- •$PaCO_2$ 2.4 kPa

From the onset of total oxygen deprivation, pH falls constantly. This occurs due to the accumulation of lactic and other acids produced as a by-product of anaerobic glycolysis in hypoxic tissues. There is, however, a poor correlation between umbilical artery pH, the condition of the baby at birth, and long-term prognosis. Often, cord pH suggests significant hypoxia and yet the baby is vigorous and breathes spontaneously at birth.

Hypoxia during Labor and at the Time of Birth

Hypoxia is a decrease below normal levels of oxygen in inspired gases, arterial blood, or tissue, short of anoxia. Hypoxia experienced during labor can cause a fetus to go into primary apnea. The fetus may enter secondary apnea before birth as well, depending upon the degree and duration of oxygen deprivation. A compromised baby can be born anywhere along the continuum between early hypoxia and death.

Is the newborn in primary or terminal apnea?

A baby who has not begun regular breathing within a minute or two of birth and whose heart rate is around 100 bpm, may be in either primary or early secondary apnea. If the baby has progressed to primary apnea at the time of birth, she is about to begin gasping. Manual stimulation should assist her to do so, and she should be capable of resuscitating herself if her airway is clear. Her initial breathing efforts must be sufficient to overcome the fluid in her lungs, fill them with air, dilate the pulmonary capillaries and expand the alveoli to establish functional residual capacity before her circulation fails. When the pulsating cord is left intact and the heart is still beating, the incoming placental transfusion flows in under pressure from rhythmic uterine contractions. This brings blood flooding into the pulmonary vessels as the baby begins to breathe and thus greatly facilitates initial lung inflation while allowing cerebral perfusion to proceed unimpaired. For all this to occur, the first breaths must be of sufficient pressure to compliment the effect of the influx of blood to the lungs: the baby must supply most of this pressure if her cord is not pulsing at the time she takes her first breath. Since the heart is still beating effectively, oxygenated blood reaches the heart quickly and the heart rate rises. Normal regular breathing will replace apneic gasping as oxygenated blood reaches the brain. If the baby is born in the midst of last-gasp efforts, a similar sequence of events will occur, although recovery will be slower.

However, if the baby has progressed into terminal apnea, he has already undergone the last-gasp stage prior to birth. This baby does not have the reserve capacity to initiate the first breaths that will establish pulmonary respiration on his own. An intact cord carries blood from the placenta to provide some of this "opening" pressure for the lungs. But if the cord is cut, the baby must supply all of this pressure. Once the baby enters terminal apnea, he will die unless artificial (positive-pressure) ventilation begins promptly and may die in spite of it. However, effective ventilatory assistance often produces a rapid recovery *if* the circulation is still functioning well enough to transport some oxygenated blood from the lungs to the heart and to mobilize blood to the lungs from the placenta; here the uterus helps by pumping blood into the baby under high pressure.

Severe, persistent hypoxia results in the walls of the capillaries becoming increasingly permeable, allowing salt, water and albumin to leak from the intravascular circulation. This can result in hemoconcentration, making it that much more difficult for the baby to adequately perfuse his lungs (Wardrop & Holland, 1995), especially when the placental transfusion is terminated. If the heart is no longer capable of pumping effectively and the cord is limp, oxygenated blood will not reach the cardiac muscle despite adequate ventilations. Stripping the cord to force blood into the baby and external cardiac massage combined with ventilations may, in some cases, be enough to bring these babies around. Once the heart is pumping adequately, a period of intermittent ventilations may be necessary before these babies fully recover.

Clinical assessment of compromise: Over the years, numerous attempts have been made to develop criteria for distinguishing between primary and terminal apnea at birth. Unfortunately, there is no totally reliable way to determine how far advanced the hypoxia is by looking at the baby. The baby is not breathing and the heart rate may be near 100 bpm in both primary and early terminal apnea. An infant in primary apnea will be deeply cyanotic but is generally well perfused. (This means the baby will be a shade of bluish pink to bluish purple, which indicates that neither circulation nor blood pressure have completely failed, although oxygen saturation is less than optimal). An early gasp or cough in response to stimulation in a baby who can still move usually indicates that the baby is in primary or early secondary apnea. Nearly all babies who are compromised to the point of terminal apnea will have at least a mild degree of metabolic acidosis. They are typically completely limp and pale blue or ashen, indicating neurological compromise and poor peripheral perfusion with a low blood pressure and a heart rate below 80 beats per minute (Stevenson, 1987). Most of these babies are also already hypovolemic due to vasoconstriction that is often secondary to impaired blood flow in the cord, which may have persisted for minutes or even hours before birth.

The APGAR score and distinguishing primary from secondary apnea: An APGAR score cannot be used to describe the degree of hypoxic insult. The APGAR assesses the degree of responsiveness but does not indicate why. A low score does not differentiate compromise due to shock from hypovolemia, the secondary effects of drugs taken by the mother, or such factors as neonatal infection, hypoglycemia or immaturity rather than shock from asphyxia.

Recovery: The most reliable and relevant index of how prolonged or serious the period of shock and asphyxia really was is revealed retrospectively in the way the nervous system (i.e., the brain) responds during the period of recovery. The length of time it takes from the return of a normal heart rate to the onset of regular respiration gives some indication as to the magnitude of the hypoxic insult, with longer periods indicating greater compromise. Signs of recovery occur in reverse order in relationship to the sequence of their failure during asphyxia. Once the heart is beating, vasoconstriction in nonvital organs is still operative and the baby may remain pale; the vessels relax with continued oxygenation and correction of acidosis. A baby who was in terminal apnea does not cough or gasp until circulation is restored, and always has a period of gasping before normal breathing movements controlled by the medulla begin. Respiratory acidosis will be rapidly corrected by the baby's lungs and kidneys once circulation is restored and respiration (or at least adequate ventilation) is established in all but the most compromised babies.

Acute vs. chronic oxygen deprivation

Acutely severe and sometimes complete oxygen deprivation usually occurs during sudden cord compression or shoulder dystocia. If treated promptly, the baby usually recovers completely. Most babies who require continuous artificial ventilations begin to breathe on their own within 20 minutes after the heart rate has been restored to 100 bpm via either spontaneous recovery or chest compressions. It is, however, very rare for a baby who is still only gasping after 30 minutes of resuscitative efforts to survive intact. The majority of these babies die within days and almost all the survivors suffer severe neurological damage (Steiner & Neligan, 1975).

In reality, many more babies suffer from prolonged periods of chronically impaired oxygen delivery in utero. However, the consequences of prolonged stress are potentially more damaging than those of short-term, acute oxygen deprivation. Severe hypoxia of any duration can be damaging. Intrauterine hypoxia that persists for 3 to 7 days is sufficient to induce hypertrophy of the musculature in the pulmonary vessels. This prevents normal rerouting of blood to the lungs after birth and results in persistent pulmonary hypertension. (For more details see the chapter entitled "The Placental Membranes and Amniotic Fluid during Labor.") Chronic oxygen deprivation is also more likely to lead to asphyxial gasping, causing the baby to aspirate vernix or meconium deep into the lungs as well as potentially fatally damaging all the major body systems. Term infants who have suffered from chronic asphyxia may have renal, central nervous system, heart and pulmonary dysfunction, the extent of which largely determines the outcome. The original insult is multiplied many fold if the baby is then subjected to immediate clamping and is born in a state of iatrogenic hypovolemia which may be superimposed on a state of intermittent intrauterine hypovolemia, the usual cause of which is cord compression. Complications can manifest as follows (based on Hatch et al., 1995 unless otherwise noted):

Renal effects: The kidneys are one of the first organs to be permanently affected by hypoxia, which may result in kidney failure with acute tubular, medullary, cortical or papillary necrosis. There may also be a delay in spontaneous urination after birth. Detecting renal damage is often difficult, but particular attention to urinary output is essential. Hypovolemia is a primary cause of kidney compromise and failure when low central venous pressure triggers the release of large quantities of antiduretic hormone and the kidneys shut down in order to conserve body fluid. Prolonged hypotension and hypoperfusion may result in lower nephron nephrosis and, in some cases, cortical necrosis (Morley, 2004).

Cardiovascular effects: Hypoxia can bring about hypovolemia produced by vasoconstriction, low mean arterial blood pressure and metabolic acidosis. Reduced venous return lowers cardiac output and causes the blood pressure to fall (Morley, 2004). Heart problems may include tricuspid insufficiency due to muscle necrosis (suggested by a systolic murmur and enlargement of the liver and spleen), heart failure and dysrhythmias.

Hematopoietic effects: Babies who experience chronic intrauterine hypoxia attempt to compensate by producing additional red blood cells to trap and carry more oxygen, resulting in polycythemia. Severe asphyxia may also lead to disseminated intravascular coagulation (DIC), with bleeding from multiple sites.

Endocrine effects: These include adrenal hemorrhage, transient hypoparathyroidism and inappropriate antidiuretic hormone production.

Respiratory effects: Hypovolemia results in the diaphragm and other respiratory muscles lacking sufficient perfusion to function well causing them to become exhausted. The respiratory center in the brain may be underperfused, leading to apnea. Retraction respirations may develop as the baby tries to reflexively fill the heart with blood by creating negative intrathoracic pressure to pull blood from the systemic circulation (Morley, 2004). Additional complications include respiratory distress from ischemic damage to the alveolar lining and surfactant production, bleeding in the lungs, meconium aspiration and persistent pulmonary hypertension.

Gastrointestinal tract disorders: Digestive function may be impaired, and ischemic mucosal damage makes GI infections more likely. Giving the baby vasoconstrictor drugs to maintain the blood pressure in the presence of hypovolemic shock does not increase tissue perfusion and may also encourage tissue infarction, leading to necrotizing enterocolitis. Diminished perfusion of the hepatic portal vein and liver impairs the liver's ability to convert glycogen into glucose. This results in hypoglycemia and produces other biochemical signs of liver failure (Morley, 2004).

Metabolic disorders: Hypoglycemia and general electrolyte derangement make the baby less able to deal with temperature fluctuations. The establishment of breathing and nursing is usually the best means of correcting these imbalances unless the case is severe.

Central nervous system damage: Neurological evidence of hypoxia includes a decreased level of consciousness, muscle tone, spontaneous activity, as well as alterations in deep tendon reflexes, and in complex primitive reflexes such as the Moro, suck and oculovestibular responses; the respiratory pattern such as apnea that may range from periodic breathing to respiratory arrest. Other signs include alterations in brain stem functions including pupillary response, extraocular movement, and impaired suck-and-swallow response, the presence of seizures and, over time, signs of raised intracranial pressure.

Hypoxic ischemic encephalopathy (HIE) refers to the central nervous system damage associated with perinatal asphyxia. **Ischemia** is defined as localized anemia or reduced flow of red blood cells due to the loss of blood supply to a region of the body. HIE can potentially cause serious long-term neuromotor dysfunction among survivors. Hypoxic ischemic brain damage evolves gradually, beginning during the hypoxic insult and extending beyond the immediate period of recovery (Aggarwal et al., 2001).

Over the past two decades, the data collected regarding hypoxic ischemic injury has increased dramatically. Unfortunately, most of it is fragmented and uninformed because of the lack of appreciation for the role of the placental transfusion at birth. Thus, any research into the pathology of these events is skewed. While poring over the minutia of the biochemistry with a focus on oxygen deprivation as the primary insulting event, the role of the placental transfusion is being ignored in the same way that the importance and physiology of blood volume expansion in pregnancy has so often been ignored.

Some mainstream thoughts on HIE related brain damage: It is now assumed that, initially, brain injury results from diminishing oxygen delivery to the tissues. If the supply of oxygen to the tissues can be improved, cerebral hyperperfusion is brought about by the corresponding sudden increase in cardiac output. Cerebral vasodilation induced by acidosis and a reduction in blood viscosity at higher rates of blood flow may contribute to hyperperfusion. This initial hyperperfusion is followed by a phase of hypoperfusion, which may be caused by tissue-damaging atomic particles produced in high numbers as by-products of the metabolic process during the reperfusion phase after ischemia.

A no-reflow phenomenon can be observed after severe cerebral ischemia. This failure of reperfusion in various regions of the brain occurs due to the greater viscosity of stagnant blood, compression of the smallest blood vessels resulting from swelling of the perivascular glial cells, formation of endothelial microvilli, increased intracerebral pressure, postischemic arterial hypotension and increased intravascular coagulation. The extent of the no-reflow phenomenon depends upon the duration and type of cerebral ischemia; it is most pronounced when the vessels are engorged with blood due to venous congestion. The cerebral blood flow either recovers immediately after postischemic hypoperfusion or overshoots into a second phase of hyperperfusion, which is often accompanied by a lack of brain wave activity, an extremely ominous finding (Berger & Garnier, 2000). These perfusion dynamics have not been examined in babies whose cords were left intact.

The importance of adequate perfusion: The fetus thrives at a low oxygen saturation relative to an adult and compensates for hypoxia by ensuring adequate perfusion to the most vital organs, in particular, the brain. Just as the newborn is uniquely adapted in other ways, perfusion may be more important than oxygenation per se in maintaining physiologic and neural integrity. The work of Cowan and associates (2003) found that events in the immediate perinatal period are apparently most important in the majority of cases of neonatal brain injury. In reviewing their work, Morley (2003) states these events are related to some degree of perineal hypoxia in conjunction with hypovolemia, which can begin prior to birth due to acute or chronic cord compression as well as after birth when further insult occurs if the cord is clamped immediately. Cord compression in utero results in blood becoming sequestered in the placenta as blood flow through the umbilical vein is impaired. When the baby is born, oxygenated blood is likely to flood the baby's system once cord compression is relieved, correcting the hypovolemia before breathing commences. If the cord vessels have already shut down completely, the baby needs immediate volume expansion via a transfusion.

It would seem that the baby can compensate well for variable levels of oxygen saturation; there is little evidence that hypoxia, unless extreme, results in brain damage (Morley, 2003). However, the baby is far less resilient to the effects of hypovolemia with accompanying hypoperfusion. Morley (2003) points out that, when the newborn begins to breath in a hypovolemic state, he must recruit blood from other compartments to perfuse the lungs; this throws his system into hypovolemic shock, resulting in a dramatic drop in both systemic blood pressure and cerebral perfusion. Either acutely or over the days following birth, as the baby struggles to cope with hypovolemia, inadequate flow to the brain can lead to necrosis in its most metabolically active areas as well as multi-organ failure, oliguria or total anuria and progressive kidney damage. These sequelae worsen if blood volume is not restored. Therapeutic hypothermia may help slow this process (see the chapter entitled "Body Temperature Regulation in the Fetus and Newborn") but may be unnecessary or, in some cases, rendered far more effective if the additional insult of cord clamping is eliminated. Normal blood flow allows the brain to dissipate its own heat. Good perfusion also minimizes inflammatory processes as metabolic wastes are removed most efficiently.

Furthermore, the use of supplemental oxygen during ventilation, especially in the presence of hypoperfusion, is apparently detrimental. Cellular injury is aggravated during reperfusion when cells are bathed with blood containing excessive levels of oxygen free radicals (superoxide and hydrogen peroxide) produced by the xanthine oxidase system. These reactive oxygen molecules damage cells in a process known as **oxidative stress**. Damage may be exaggerated in newborns, whose oxygen saturation is low compared to an adult. The switch to adult oxygen saturation levels is not instantaneous and certainly is not completed during the first minutes of life when the cord is supposed to be intact; thus, resuscitating newborns with supplemental oxygen may add to this type of stress and misses the point of the importance of perfusion over high oxygen levels to their recovery immediately following birth.

Oxidative stress contributes to ongoing brain injury over the following hours and days. The initial insult results in an area of infarction. The region around the infarction is called the "**penumbra**," which continues to show adverse changes in the form of neuronal necrosis or apoptosis (programmed cell death) even after oxygen delivery is restored (Aggarwal et al., 2001). Prolonged hypoxia can also result in serious cerebral hemorrhage, especially in preterm babies. In term babies, cerebral ischemia can lead to secondary cerebral edema after a brief latent period. All these complications are minimized when normovolemia is restored via an intact umbilical cord. Intrinsic damage resulting from asphyxia is also minimized by inhibiting the production of oxygen free radicals after ischemia, which can be accomplished by not using oxygen at all during ventilation or by using concentrations below 100% when the baby does not otherwise respond. While all hypoxia always leads to the production of free radicals, levels are lower in babies resuscitated with room air (Vento et al., 2003). (The controversy regarding the use of 100% oxygen during neonatal resuscitation is further discussed in the subchapter entitled "Evaluating and Assisting the Infant in Need of Resuscitation.")

Intermittent oxygen deprivation: Most neonatal resuscitation protocols are based on physiological evidence derived from research on adults or on fetal and newborn animals experiencing sudden, total anoxia without ischemia. However, intermittent partial asphyxia that varies as to degree, frequency and duration, with or without accompanying ischemia, is more typical of fetal distress that occurs during labor. Repeated periods of asphyxia may also result in a degree of muscular hypertrophy of the pulmonary vessels, as described above.

The response of a healthy, well-nourished term baby encountering such stress for the first time in labor, as might occur with partial cord compression during contractions, is different from that of a preterm baby or a baby who has coped with chronic hypoxia in utero, either of whom will have fewer reserves. (See the explanation of the fetal response to stress in the chapter entitled "The Baby's Journey through Labor to Birth.") Although you would expect the healthy baby to respond more quickly and require less vigorous resuscitative efforts, the best approach is to treat all asphyxia seriously, make sure the cord stays intact until well after the baby is stable and to observe or assist babies as necessary until regular respirations, a good heart rate and normal color are well established.

Weak respiratory effort: Human babies are especially prone to the rapid development of hypoxemia. Unlike many newborn animals, the human baby has poor skeletal muscle control and a highly flexible rib cage. This results in an exceptionally compliant chest wall, with an outward recoil near zero. Nearly all the air will be expelled from the baby's lungs as she passively exhales unless she uses her chest muscles and vocal cords to actively compensate in order to retain a small amount of air. The healthy term baby must maintain the ability to retain air in the lungs by taking rapid, shallow breaths and tightening her vocal cords slightly to avoid full expiration until the fluid clears from her lungs.

Well-perfused alveolar vasculature assists in holding the alveoli open in an expanded state. With the development of functional residual capacity and with the rapid removal of lung fluid, the baby is relieved of doing all this work with respiratory efforts alone. Apparently shallow respirations during the first 3 to 5 minutes of life are not so concerning in a baby whose cord was allowed to remain intact until pulsing ceased and who is pink.

For babies who suffered cord compression sufficient to cause hypovolemia in utero and whose cord is cut too soon, initial inflation of the lungs is difficult. The baby may begin breathing with intermittent, weak, ineffective respirations. These gasping, irregular, low-pressure respirations are not sufficient to maintain alveolar expansion or to pull blood into the pulmonary vessels. This limits blood flow to the lungs, hinders absorption of lung fluid and restricts the amount of oxygenation that occurs. (Note we are talking gasping here, not quiet regular, breathing.) Even after the first normal breath, if the baby is unable to actively maintain FRC because of perfusion, drugs received via the mother or loss of consciousness, when the baby exhales, loss of all lung volume is immediate. The lungs collapse, especially if the pulmonary capillary beds are poorly perfused. Loss of FRC causes a drop in pulmonary oxygen stores and oxygen saturation drops rapidly, even with brief periods of apnea.

Acidosis and hypoxemia also contribute to the constriction of the pulmonary arterioles, leading to ischemia in the lung tissue. This results in the ductus arteriosus remaining open. The fetal circulatory pathways remain operative and reduced blood flow to the lungs persists. Proper oxygenation is impossible as long as decreased pulmonary perfusion exists. This condition, formerly known as "persistent fetal circulation," is now termed "persistent pulmonary hypertension in the neonate" (PPHN). Neonatal infection and preterm birth can also lead to PPHN.

Long-term consequences of oxygen deprivation

The baby and subsequent young adult whose birth was exceptionally difficult is left with an overwhelming belief that life is difficult, especially when the emotions surrounding these events are not resolved in a healthy way. Teenage suicide is more common among those who experienced birth asphyxia requiring resuscitation than among those who did not. These teens frequently employ a form of asphyxiation to commit suicide. Violent suicides have also been linked to mechanical birth trauma, especially among young men. Some of these outcomes probably have to do with the separation of mother and baby following resuscitation efforts and subsequent trauma during procedures performed in the hospital.

Preserving as much uninterrupted time for interaction between the mother and her newborn as well as helping the parents understand that talking to the baby about his birth, telling the story of his birth in a straightforward way as he grows older, and allowing the newborn to express pent up emotions such as anger and fear by crying and moving while being lovingly comforted will help to mitigate the effects of such trauma. The parent can validate how difficult and scary it was not to be able to breathe while the baby is expressing himself. If the baby was born in hospital and the cord was cut to soon, the emotional and physical ramifications of this should also be acknowledged (Jacobson & Bygdeman, 1998; Jacobson et al., 1987; Salk et al., 1985).

THE ANATOMY OF THE NEONATAL AIRWAY AND UPPER RESPIRATORY TRACT

NOTE: Review the basic adult anatomy in HOLISTIC MIDWIFERY, Vol. I, before studying this chapter.

The respiratory tree can be divided into three regions:

1. **The supraglottic airway:** nose, nasopharynx, hypopharynx, and epiglottis
2. **The glottis:** vocal cords, region immediately below the cords and the cervical trachea
3. **The intrathoracic airway:** thoracic trachea, larger bronchi and bronchioles

The first two items above comprise the upper airway. The structure and function of the newborn airway differs considerably from that of the adult (maturational differences between term and preterm infants are important as well). Appreciation of these differences will help in understanding the "whys" behind certain neonatal resuscitation protocols and suctioning techniques. This chapter describes these differences, the most important of which are summarized below.

ANATOMICAL PART	NEWBORN	ADULT
Nose and nares	Small, soft and pointed slightly upward	More cartilaginous, nares pointed downward
Tongue	Large, almost fills oral cavity, contained within oral cavity (does not extend down the throat)	Smaller, leaves space in oral cavity, one-third of the tongue extends down the throat
Inlet of the larynx	Opposite 2nd and 3rd cervical vertebrae	Opposite 4th, 5th and 6th cervical vertebrae
Epiglottis	U-shaped, short, stiff, inclined 45° toward the posterior pharyngeal wall	Flat, flexible, erect
Hyoid/thyroid separation	Very close together	Further apart
Glottis	50% cartilage, softer and more pliable	25% cartilage, more rigid
Arytenoid cartilage	Inclined downward	Horizontal
Vocal cords	Concave and slanted forward and downward at a 45° angle	Straight and horizontal
Thyroid & cricoid cartilages	Sidewalls form a funnel	Sidewalls are vertical
Average airway diameter	3 mm at term	7/16 to 1 inch (8 mm to 2.5 cm)
Nasopharynx/oropharynx angle	122 to 129°	Nearly 90°
Size of oropharynx	Very tiny; soft palate and epiglottis may touch at rest	Extends from body of 2nd to upper 3rd cervical vertebrae.
Smallest diameter	Lowermost border of cricoid ring (below the vocal cords)	Space between vocal cords
Consistency of cartilage	Soft and flexible	Firm
Shape of posterior skull	Pronounced occiput	Flatter occiput

(Adapted from Whitten, 1989)

This chapter references Scammon (1923) and the landmark anatomy work of Crelin (1973), unless otherwise noted.

<u>**Structural features of the airway**</u>

The skeletal axis of the airway is formed by the base of the skull below and the hard palate from above. The mandible (jaw bone) serves as the anterior boundary to the floor of the oral cavity. In addition, a series of cartilaginous rings connected by muscle and fascia form the airway tube, or trachea, which extends from the base of the skull to the extrathoracic trachea. The epiglottis and the hyoid, thyroid and cricoid cartilages are quite flexible in the fetus and newborn. In the term baby, these structures are stabilized by fat-laden fascia located between the skin and underlying musculature of the face and neck; in preterm infants, these structures are far less stable. Connective tissue support is provided by the auditory tubes, the larynx, the lower pharynx, the soft palate and the tongue. Opposing muscles maintain the position of the individual cartilages and promote an open airway. The following descriptions assume the child is in the anatomical position: standing, face forward. The drawing is from the side. Remember that the trachea and upper airway form a relatively rigid cartilaginous "hose" anterior to the esophagus, which is a soft, muscular tube.

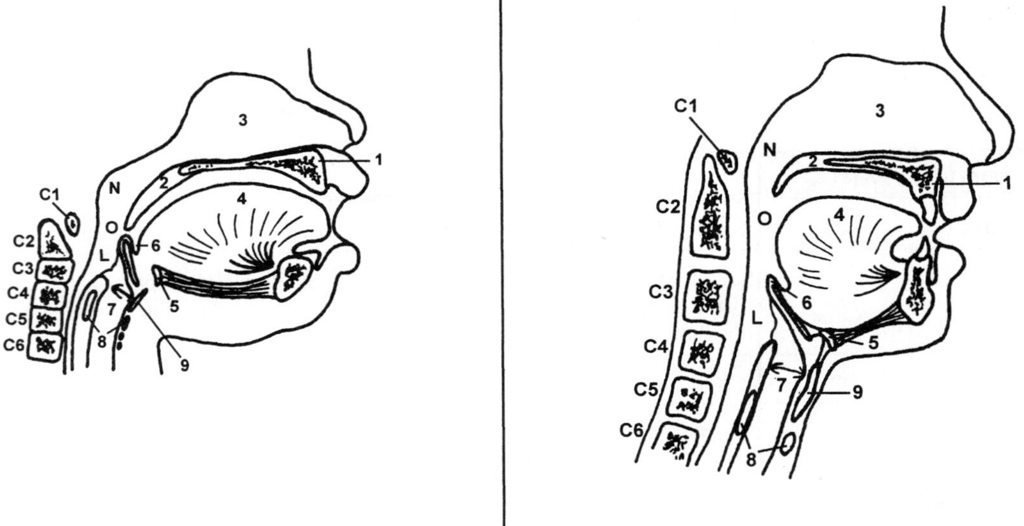

Neonatal airway | Adult airway

Key: 1–Hard palate; 2–Soft palate; 3–Nasal passage; 4–Tongue; 5–Hyoid bone; 6–Epiglottis; 7–Vocal cords above (number in subglottic region); 8–Cricoid cartilage; 9–Thyroid cartilage; **N**– Nasopharynx; **O**–Oropharynx; **L**–Laryngopharynx

(Kent & Vorperian, 1995; Omari & Rudolph, 1998)

<u>**Nose:**</u> The nose of an infant consists of a large bony region and a small cartilaginous region, although the nasal septum is almost entirely cartilaginous at birth, save for the vomer bone. The nares are more vertical than in an adult and the bony nasal cavity is short. Each nasal cavity is wide, short (18 to 19 mm) and long, relative to the adult. The inferior wall of each averages 7 mm in length, and the nasopharyngeal openings of the nasal canals average 5 to 7 mm in diameter.

The external, lateral wall of each nasal cavity is formed by the conchae or turbinates. These are 3 or 4 thin, spongy membrane-covered bony plates with curved margins that project from the lateral walls of the nasal cavity; the channels formed by the underside of these folds are called the **nasal meatuses**. The inferior concha separates the middle from the inferior meatus and articulates with the ethmoid, lacrimal, maxilla, and palate bones; its lower border often touches the inferior wall of the nasal passage in babies. The middle concha forms a portion of the ethmoidal labyrinth, separating the superior meatus from the middle meatus. The superior concha is also part of the ethmoidal labyrinth, separating the superior meatus from the sphenoethmoidal recess. One or more small supreme concha may be located posterosuperiorly above the others, overlying the supreme nasal meatus (its location is not exposed in the illustration on the following page). The turbinates increase the mucosal surface of the passage and enhance air turbulence; as gases pass through these folds, particulate matter gets trapped, preventing particles larger than 4 μg from entering. The resistance to air passage of the newborn nasal cavities accounts for one-third to one-half of the total pulmonary resistance. (Resistance here refers to the passage of air through the various small structures that inhibit its free flow.) Nasal flaring causes pulmonary resistance to fall. For many years, it was thought that neonates were obligate nose breathers. However, they will often resort to mouth breathing if the nasal passage is congenitally obstructed, as in choanal atresia. Studies have shown that full-term infants are able to establish oral breathing in an average of 7.8 seconds in the presence of nasal occlusion, although they may display considerable distress prior to doing so (Rodenstein, 1985).

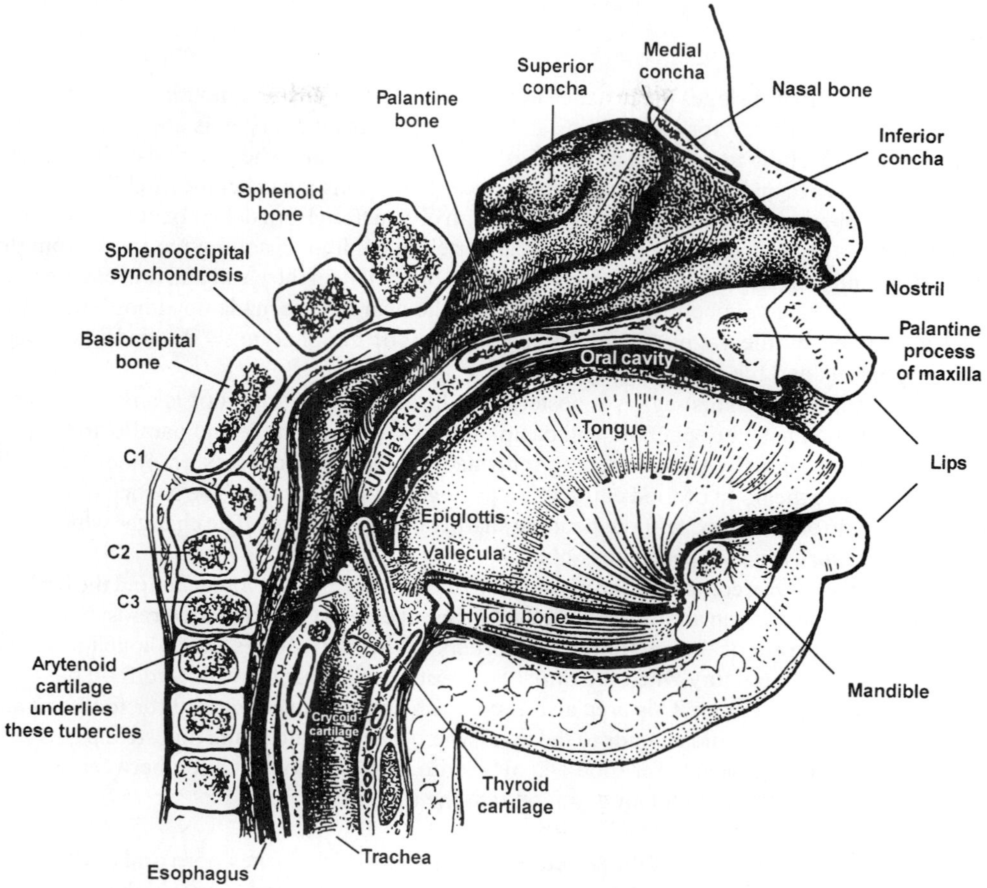

The airway of a newborn breathing quietly: closely paramedian section from the right with nasal septum removed to reveal the three conchae (turbinates) in the left nasal passage.

(Adapted from Bosma, 1986)

Oral cavity: The tongue is short and broad, being 1.5 in long, 2 in wide and 3/8 in thick (4 cm long, 2.5 cm wide and 1 cm thick). The tongue contacts the gums on either side and the palate above, thus nearly filling the infant's oral cavity when the mouth is closed. The newborn tongue is contained entirely within the mouth; it does not extend down into the pharynx because the infant's larynx is placed high in the neck compared with an adult. As the baby matures, the neck and posterior third of the tongue both become longer, resulting in the tongue forming a portion of the anterior pharyngeal wall. However, the newborn's tongue is attached directly to the epiglottis; thus the opening of the larynx is directly below the oral cavity. This causes the epiglottis to be elevated in the throat, relative to the adult, allowing it to touch the soft palate, separating the lowermost portion of the tongue from the oropharynx. The elevation of the larynx at rest and its further elevation during suckling repositions it in line with the nasopharynx, enabling babies to breath while fluid fills the pharynx. Respiration must cease briefly for the infant to swallow. The side walls of the mouth, the cheeks, are supported by a mass of subcutaneous fat that lies between the buccinator and masseter muscles (Crelin, 1973).

Palate: The hard palate forms a gentle arch at birth and usually features five or six irregular transverse raphe which help the baby maintain latch on to the nipple during nursing. A cone-shaped elevation in the midline of the palate behind the superior gumline is present in infants. The soft palate consists of a sheet of mobile, pliable tissue that extends from the posterior edge of the hard palate into the oropharyngeal cavity. Contact between the soft palate and the base of the tongue closes the opening posterior to the soft palate, permitting nasal breathing. This region posterior to the soft palate where the nasopharynx and oropharynx communicate is called the **isthmus of the pharynx** or **oropharyngeal isthmus**. Little is known about the activity of individual muscles of the palate in newborns, despite the important role they play in partitioning the oral and nasal airflow. The specific factors influencing a baby's ability to open the oropharyngeal isthmus remain a mystery.

Pharynx: The pharynx (or throat) bridges the distance between the nasal cavity and mouth to the larynx and esophagus below, serving as a common pathway for food, fluids and air. The neonatal pharynx is about 1.5 in (4 cm) long, only one-third that of an adult's, reaching to the level of the 5th or 6th cervical vertebra when in repose. The pharyngeal airway is short and wide in the newborn and gently tapers from top to bottom. This area becomes stabilized early in gestation, although the more pliable pharynx of preterm infants is subject to obstruction from debris or compression. The posterior wall of the pharynx is the portion that parallels the cervical vertebral column, spanning the space from the level of the uvular attachment to the entry to the larynx. The anterior wall is split between the nasal and oral cavities above and joins both at the level of the tip of the uvula below. The sidewalls of the pharynx are made up almost entirely of pharyngeal constrictor muscles supplied by the vagus nerve. The passageway of the pharynx is divided into three regions: the nasopharynx, the oropharynx and the laryngopharynx.

Nasopharynx (velopharynx): This region is posterior to the nasal cavity. Its roof is a narrow tube about ¾ in (2 cm) long that contacts the sphenoid and occipital bones and lies above and parallel to the soft palate. Anteriorly, it is continuous with the opening (choanae) of the nasal cavities on either side. Since the nasopharynx is above the point of food entry, it is a passageway only for air. The nasopharynx curves very gently as it meets the oropharynx, without bending sharply until adulthood. The changes which the pharynx undergoes with maturity make speech possible.

Oropharynx: The oropharynx comprises the midportion of the pharynx. It is found behind the oral cavity and is continuous with it through an archway called the **fauces**. It extends from the lowermost border of the soft palate to the uppermost tip of the epiglottis; the borders of these structures nearly touch in the newborn, making the oropharynx very tiny when the throat is at rest. Both air and swallowed food pass through it.

Laryngopharynx (hypopharynx): This area also serves as a common passageway for food and air. It lies directly behind the epiglottis and extends to the level where the respiratory and digestive passages diverge. The close proximity of the portals for food and air requires precise coordination between the larynx and upper esophageal sphincter to direct air and food into the right tube.

Tonsils: There are several specialized lymphatic structures called "tonsils" in the newborn oral cavity, as there are in the adult. At birth, the posterior roof of the nasopharynx has a small central depression from which a series of ridges fan out to the front and laterally. The adenoids, or pharyngeal tonsils, develop as these ridges become permeated with indistinct collections of lymphoid cells near term. The newborn palatine tonsils are also small at birth, being well tucked into depressions in the lateral walls of the oropharynx. They measure 5 mm across and 3.5 mm long. The lingual tonsils are a collection of lymphoid follicles on the posterior or pharyngeal portion of the surface of the tongue. The tubal tonsils are a collection of lymphoid nodules around the pharyngeal opening of the eustachian tube.

Larynx: The inlet of the larynx is located at the level of the C2 and C3 at the entrance to the extrathoracic trachea. The larynx is divided by the vocal cords into supraglottic and infraglottic (or subglottic) regions. At term, the newborn larynx is ¾ in (2 cm) in length, about one-third the size of an adult's. Its maximum width, at the level of the upper margin of the thyroid cartilage, is almost equal to its length. Although the larynx is proportionately larger in the neonate than in the adult, its cavity is short and funnel-shaped. Its primary function is that of a protective sphincter for the lower airways, with phonation a secondary function.

Cartilaginous structure: The neonatal larynx is a box-like structure made up of an intricate arrangement of ten cartilages connected by membranes and ligaments. Starting from the top, these cartilages include the epiglottis, hyoid (ossifies into bone) and thyroid, which are bridged by the lateral thyrohyoid membrane, the corniculates (2), arytenoids (2), glottis, cricoid and trachea. The major cartilages are the hyoid, epiglottis thyroid and cricoid. The thyroid cartilage of the neonate is shorter and broader than that of the adult and lies closer to the hyoid bone. Neither its superior notch nor the laryngeal prominence is as marked. The lowermost laryngeal cartilage proper is the cricoid, which forms the only complete ring in the laryngo-tracheobronchial tree. It is the same shape as in the adult, but its lowermost internal diameter is the narrowest portion of the infant airway. It is located anterior to the fourth cervical vertebra (as opposed to the 7th in adults). In addition to these large cartilaginous structures, three pairs of smaller cartilages (the arytenoids, cuneiforms and corniculates) form part of the lateral and posterior walls of the larynx. In terms of airway management, the most important of these are the arytenoid cartilages.

Arytenoids (2): The arytenoids are a pair of irregularly shaped pyramids mounted on top of the upper posterior aspect of the cricoid cartilage. The little projection, called the **signet flange**, on the cricoid separates them from each other. The arytenoids are relatively large in the newborn. Together, they help to form the scalloped posterior entry to the larynx. They pivot in all planes from their attachment point, where they tense, relax and swing the vocal cords from side to side, allowing vocalization, coughing and swallowing. The cone shaped corniculates attach to the apex of the arytenoids, and the elongated cuneiforms attach to the posterior arytenoids. These cartilages add bulk and shape to the arytenoid outline.

Epiglottis: The epiglottis is a leaf-shaped projection of elastic cartilage covered with mucous membrane. It is located at the root of the tongue, where it projects at an upward angle over the entrance to the larynx. It serves as a diverter valve over the superior opening of the larynx during the act of swallowing (the details of infant swallowing are covered in Vol. III of this text). The newborn epiglottis is 7/16 in (1.2 cm) long and inclines to the posterior pharyngeal wall at an angle of 45°. The upper border of the epiglottis is level with the second or third cervical vertebra when the larynx is at rest; it rises to the level of the first cervical vertebra when the larynx is elevated, as it is when the baby sucks. The tip of the newborn epiglottis often extends into the nasopharynx, separating the respiratory and digestive passageways. The larynx is placed higher in the neck of the neonate than in the adult, reducing the size of the pharyngeal chamber and allowing the top of the epiglottis to overlap the soft palate. This positioning of the epiglottis provides airway protection by diverting liquid laterally around the laryngeal opening.

Hyoid bone: The hyoid is a U-shaped bone that provides support for the base of the tongue and the upper larynx. It lies between the mandible and the larynx, suspended from the more horizontal styloid processes by slender stylohyoid ligaments, which are attached to the lesser cornu on either side. The hyoid is closely attached below by the thyrohyoid membranes to the thyroid cartilage. It is relatively higher and more anterior in the neonate than in the adult. It has a small ossification center in the body of the bone, which is mainly cartilaginous at birth. Its two constituent parts can be identified by the horizontal groove along the body. The distance around the body from one upswept tip to the other (greater cornu to greater cornu) is 1 3/16 in (3 cm). It is 5.0 mm in height and 2.0 mm thick.

Cricoid cartilage (cricoid ring): The cricoid ring is the lowermost of the laryngeal cartilages and is located below the vocal cords. It is shaped like a signet ring, being expanded into a nearly quadrilateral plate (lamina) posteriorly; the anterior portion is called the "arch." Although the trachea is roughly the same diameter as the ring, the trachea can stretch, whereas the cricoid forms a complete ring of cartilage, rendering it inflexible. The cricoid forms the narrowest part of the newborn airway; at term the diameter is about 3 mm, which is about the diameter of a large cocktail straw. If you palpate your trachea by moving your fingers up from your sternal notch, the first distinct elevation you come to is your cricoid ring.

Glottis: The glottis is the vocal apparatus of the larynx. It includes the vocal cords of mucous membrane covering the vocal ligament and the vocal muscle on each side, the free edges of which are the vocal cords. The space between the cords is called the **rima glottidis**. The vocal cords or folds are 1/8 to 3/16 in (4 to 4.5 mm) in length; they are short relative to surrounding structures. The infant glottis, more anterior and higher in the neck than in the adult, is behind a soft and often "folded" epiglottis.

Vocal cords (folds): The cricoid membranes run between the arytenoids and the thyroid cartilage. The upper, free edges of these membrane form the vocal cords, which are partially separated when at rest, although loss of muscle tone causes them to partially close (Whitten, 1989). The vocal cords in the infant and child have an upwardly curved shape. The arytenoids incline backward, causing the cords to be slanted more forward and downward, with the anterior attachment lower than the posterior attachment. (The cords are horizontal in adults.) This can pose difficulty during artificial ventilation; see the chapter entitled "Evaluating and Assisting the Infant in Need of Resuscitation" for details. The newborn can partially close her vocal cords to maintain lung volume on expiration. This activity has been identified in compromised preterm babies as well as healthy term infants.

The ventricle or cavity of the larynx is small; however, the saccule of the larynx is often considerably larger. The saccule is a small pouch provided with mucous glands that extends upward from the upper boundary of the laryngeal cavity between the vestibular fold and the lamina of the thyroid cartilage; it is a vestigial structure. The subglottic cavity below the level of the vocal cords extends backward as well as downward in the newborn, whereas it is almost vertical in older children and adults; this is an important fact to be considered when passing an endotracheal tube. The subglottic larynx is bounded by the complete circular ring of the cricoid cartilage and extends from the free edge of the underside of the vocal cord (where the conus elasticus muscle inserts) to the lower border of the cricoid cartilage below. The mucosa of the larynx readily becomes swollen when irritated, which can lead to obstruction of the already small airway.

Esophagus: The esophagus is a muscular tube that is 3 1/8 to 3 15/16 in (8 to 10 cm) long at birth, extending from the cricoid cartilage to the gastric cardiac orifice. It begins and ends 1 to 2 vertebrae higher than in the adult, extending from between C4 and C6 to the level of the ninth thoracic vertebra. Its average diameter is 3/16 in (5 mm), and it has the same constrictions seen in adults. The narrowest area is found at the junction of the pharynx, where the inferior pharyngeal constrictor muscle functions to narrow the lumen; it may be easily traumatized with instruments or catheters.

Trachea: The trachea, or windpipe, is an open cartilaginous tube extending from the lowermost border of the cricoid ring into the thorax, where it divides into the right and left main bronchi at the level of T3 or T4. In the newborn, compared to an adult, the tracheal walls are thick, flexible and pliable. The average length is about 4 cm, three times shorter than in the adult. Its upper border is at the level of C6 when the head is erect and the larynx at rest. Both adult and newborn tracheas are broader at the top. The width of the newborn trachea from side to side is greater (5.0 mm) than from front to back (3.6 mm), and small in relation to the larynx at birth. It is composed of 16 to 20 closely spaced rings of hyaline cartilage connected by a membrane (annular ligament); posteriorly, the rings are deficient for one-fifth to one-third of their circumference, the interval is closed by a membrane containing smooth muscular fibers. The growth of the tissues interspersed between the rings will result in the lengthening of the trachea to adult proportions. Internally, the mucosa is composed of a pseudostratified, ciliated columnar epithelium with mucous goblet cells; numerous small mixed mucous and serous glands occur, the ducts of which open to the surface of the epithelium.

Lungs: The newborn lungs are shorter and broader than those of the adult. This difference is related to the differences in the shape and capacity of the thorax. The height of the medial surface of the lung at rest is about 2.5 cm. The anteroposterior length of the base is about 4 cm, and the greatest transverse width of the base is 2.2 cm. There is little change in the relationship of the skeletal landmarks to the lungs from birth to adulthood, with the fissures and lobes in the same relative position. When the baby begins to breathe, the uppermost apex of each lung lies 5 to 8 mm above the level of the superior border of the sternum; the inferior margins lie at the level of the eleventh rib posteriorly.

The lungs do not fill the entire potential pleural cavity, especially the costodiaphragmatic pleural recesses, in the full-term infant. The point where the two pleurae bend back to form the costomediastinal recesses anteriorly are quite variable. They may not touch at any point along the midline. When they do not, a portion of the anterior surface of the thymus gland, along with the pericardium, is in direct contact with the endothoracic fascia lining the sternum.

Bronchi and alveoli: The lowermost border of the trachea forms a ridge known as the **carina**. Here the airway divides into the two main bronchi, which lead into the lungs. As in adults, the right main bronchus is wider, shorter and more vertical than the left main bronchus. The right bronchus is 4.6 × 5 mm in diameter and 9 mm long; the left is 3.9 × 4.1 mm in diameter and 21 mm long and crosses the midline at a sharper angle than the right. The basic branching of the bronchi into bronchopulmonary segments is present at birth. The number of bronchioles and alveoli within these segments increase until just before puberty. At birth, there are about 25 million alveoli in each lung; there are about 300 million in the mature lung.

Vagus nerve: The vagus or "wanderer" is the 10th cranial nerve. It is the only cranial nerve to extend beyond the head and neck to the thorax and abdomen. The vagus nerve emerges from the medulla oblongata in 8 to 10 rootlets, descending vertically through the neck along the carotid arteries to the upper border of the thyroid cartilage, and then continues on down to the base of the neck.

Here the nerves divide into right and left branches, one supplying the heart and lungs and the other supplying the liver, spleen, stomach, kidneys and gut. Parasympathetic branches extend to the heart, lungs, and abdominal organs, where they regulate heart rate, breathing and digestion. They transmit sensory impulses from thoracic and abdominal organs, from the carotid sinus (which helps regulate blood pressure), from the carotid and aortic bodies (regulating respiration) and from the taste buds of the posterior tongue and pharynx.

Vagus motor fibers also supply the smooth muscles and secretory glands of the pharynx, larynx, trachea, heart, esophagus, stomach, intestines, pancreas, gallbladder, bile ducts, spleen, kidneys, ureter and blood vessels in the thoracic and abdominal cavities. Afferent vagal nerves are found all along the respiratory and gastrointestinal tracts. The cardiac and respiratory systems, therefore, react to a broad range of laryngeal, esophageal, and pulmonary stimuli.

Nearly all vagus motor fibers are parasympathetic efferent nerves except those supplying the skeletal muscles of the pharynx and larynx that are involved in swallowing. Almost all the muscles of the larynx are innervated by branches of the vagus nerve. The oropharynx is a particularly sensitive area; during the first five minutes or so of life, a neurological reaction called the vasovagal response may be stimulated if an object is introduced into the posterior pharynx. This response produces respiratory depression, laryngospasm and bradycardia, temporarily suppressing spontaneous respirations for a variable but relatively brief period of time.

Clinical significance

All structures in the infant airway are much smaller than those of the adult, making them more prone to damage and providing far less leeway for error when introducing tubes or instruments into the airway. The typical adult airway is no less than 5/8 in (8 mm) in diameter at its narrowest point. One millimeter of circumferential edema from trauma leaves an airway of at least 6 mm in diameter, a 25% reduction. The level of the cricoid cartilage is narrowest point in the neonatal airway and is only 3/32 in (2.38 mm) in diameter (the size will vary slightly with the size and maturity of the baby). One millimeter of circumferential edema leaves an airway of 1 mm in diameter, a 68% reduction. Even minimal trauma can create life-threatening airway obstruction.

An infant's tracheal cartilage is very soft and pliable. Unintentional pressure on the cricoid cartilage during resuscitation or tipping the head too far back can pinch off the airway, resulting in obstruction and rendering ventilation impossible. The large newborn tongue fills the oral cavity, makes visualization of the back of the throat more difficult and may interfere with insertion of an oral airway or visual examination of the palate.

The small size of the oral cavity also makes stimulating a vagus nerve more likely. Vigorous or deep stimulation of the posterior walls of the lower nasopharynx, oropharynx and laryngopharynx can trigger a vasovagal response, leading to a temporary depression of respiratory and cardiac activity. When this occurs, a baby in need of assistance to initiate respirations can be thrown into an even greater degree of distress. For all these reasons, it is unwise for midwives to attempt intubation, especially using a laryngoscope.

(Refer to the DVD that comes with the 6th edition of the TEXTBOOK OF NEONATAL RESUSCITATION [Kattwinkel et al., 2011] by the American Heart Association for a visual exploration of the neonatal airway presented in the section on laryngoscopy.)

Autonomic Neuromuscular Reflexes and the Baby's Response to Resuscitation

The baby's response to resuscitation efforts, in particular artificial ventilation, is a product of complex autonomic neuromuscular reflexes that are present throughout life, which have been reviewed by Halbower and Jones (1999). In infants, however, these responses are more complex because the newborn and infant is undergoing rapid growth and development. A stimulus that results in a mild cardiorespiratory response in an adult can have a profound effect in a newborn. By the same token, immature pulmonary physiology increases the likelihood of respiratory compromise.

Changes in pressure, airflow and osmolarity in the airways trigger autonomic reflexes that play a central role in apnea and bradycardia in response to hypoxemia. These complex responses target the source of stimulation as well as the heart, lungs and carotid bodies, reflected in changes in blood pressure, heart rate and respiratory effort.

Neonatal reflexes pertinent to resuscitation

Laryngeal chemoreflexes: There is an age-related reflex response to sensory stimulation of the larynx. The laryngeal chemoreflex induces vagally mediated hypertension and bradycardia via stimulation of afferent sensory neurons in the superior laryngeal nerve. This reflex is triggered chemically by introducing water, saline solution or milk into the larynx (irrespective of the pH of the solution) or mechanically with tactile stimulation. A laryngeal protective reflex is also present in humans, manifesting with profound bradycardia and laryngospasm during deep pharyngeal suctioning. Associated responses include repeated swallowing, central apnea, airway obstruction, cough, and, occasionally, prolonged apnea. Reflex bradycardia stimulated by hypoxemia (low levels of arterial oxygen) is enhanced if the oxygen deprivation is due to apnea caused by the laryngeal chemoreflex and can occasionally result in death.

Carotid body reflex: When the newborn lungs fill with air, arterial oxygen tension slowly rises. If the lungs do not inflate, hypoxemia persists and newborns, especially those who are preterm, respond with an initial increase in ventilatory effort followed by a decrease. As hypoxemia worsens, apnea develops. Systemic hypoxemia stimulates the carotid bodies, which are peripheral chemoreceptors located at the bifurcation of the common carotid arteries on either side of the neck. These bodies are inactive during normal respiration but are stimulated by hypoxemia to increase the respiratory rate. As carbon dioxide levels rise, so does the respiratory effort. The carotid reflex also induces vagal bradycardia and peripheral vasoconstriction. Hyperventilation, in turn, inhibits the carotid body reflex; thus if hyperventilation does not occur, stimulation of the carotid reflex can lead to profound bradycardia.

Distal esophageal reflex: Distinct from the laryngeal chemoreflex, the stimulation of distal esophageal vagal sensory nerves produces marked laryngospasm and stridor, raises the blood pressure, and induces tachycardia.

The role of lung inflation: Hypoxemia does not usually progress to bradycardia in the newborn because it ordinarily results in increased ventilation which stimulates pulmonary stretch receptors in the airways. This, in turn, decreases vagal tone and causes the heart rate to rise. Even marked bradycardia and hypotension induced by stimulation of both the laryngeal reflex and carotid bodies is promptly corrected by lung inflation alone. Central vagal neurons have been found to resist stimulation by carotid chemoreceptors during the inspiratory phase of respiration. Thus, even severe apnea and bradycardia, which may result from a complex interaction of reflexes, may be reversed by the simple act of lung inflation.

How these reflexes impact resuscitation

Though seldom mentioned in resuscitation literature, mechanical inflation of the airways and lungs emerges as the single most important treatment for apnea and persistent bradycardia. The apneic baby quickly develops hypoxemia and chemoreceptor-mediated bradycardia. Laryngeal stimulation from suctioning or attempts at intubation, should these occur, worsen the apnea and further depress the heart rate. The lungs may contain fluid, especially if the cord is cut, which makes inflation more difficult. Artificial ventilation mechanically stimulates stretch receptors in the airways and lungs and reverses vagally mediated bradycardia, *independent of a rise in arterial oxygen levels* or chest compressions. Inadequate ventilation is the most likely cause of continued bradycardia.

In 1868 Hering and Breuer discovered that inflation of the lungs results in a decrease in frequency and probably the force of inspiratory efforts, leading eventually to apnea (the inflation reflex) and that deflation of the lungs causes stronger and more frequent inspirations (the deflation reflex). These reflexes together play a role in modifying the breathing pattern in the neonatal period (Hassan, et al., 2001) and are also stimulated during artificial ventilation.

SPECIFIC SKILLS

CLEARING THE BABY'S AIRWAY

Since the early 1950s, when neonatal resuscitation protocols received a major overhaul, it has become routine to suction the newborn airway at birth. In reality, the healthy term baby, born through clear or nearly clear amniotic fluid, only very occasionally requires any assistance to clear his mouth and nose of fluids and mucus. Barring neonatal anomalies that prevent normal newborn efforts to clear the airway, the only reason to clear it is if it is obstructed or if it contains copious amounts of a material that may cause obstruction should it be inhaled. Even when there is meconium in the amniotic fluid, one should suction only when necessary. (See the chapter entitled "The Placental Membranes and Amniotic Fluid during Labor" for more details.)

The pros and cons of suctioning

One of the main dangers of suctioning a newborn is causing or aggravating apnea. This can occur when the vagus nerve in the posterior pharynx (back of the throat) is inappropriately stimulated by suctioning or intubation. Deep, prolonged catheter suctioning has been found to reduce oxygen saturation levels in the first minutes of life, while removing very little fluid in the process (Carrasco, et al., 1997). Vigorous or deep suctioning may also abrade the delicate mucous membranes of the mouth or nose and can remove the protective, antibacterial secretions, such as lysozyme, that line the upper airway.

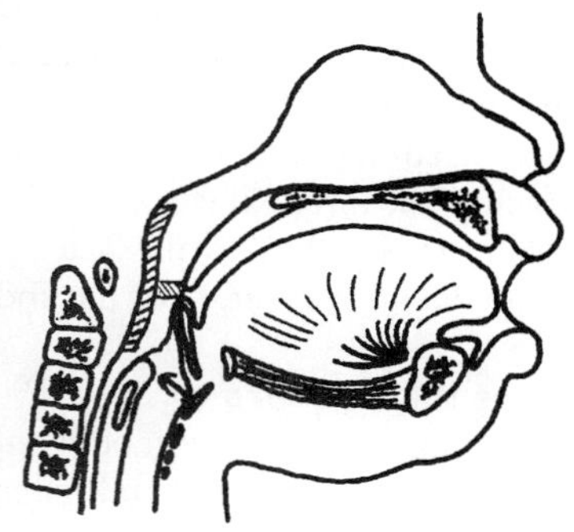

Posterior pharynx (longitudinal shaded region)
Oropharynx (tiny horizontal shaded region)

In addition, the stimulus of suctioning can result in future problems with nursing. If muscles receive a "superstimulus," neural patterning can occur, which is permanent, producing "muscle memory." The tongue muscles can be affected by early superstimuli from deep or repeated suctioning, leading to anteroposterior peristalsis, resulting in tongue thrusting. Irritation of the posterior palate (supplied by the glosso-pharyngeal nerve) can result in the baby using her tongue to reflexively guard her airway, reversing the anterior-to-posterior peristalsis required to draw the nipple deeply into the mouth during suckling (Boshart, 2001; Woolridge, 1986).

In the term newborn, the aforementioned problems can be avoided by using inversion drainage as a first-line therapy to clear the airways. However, inversion drainage is contraindicated if the baby is very preterm; in addition, tactile stimulation of any kind should be performed with the greatest gentleness and care. The germinal matrix is a developmental feature of the brain which undergoes rapid changes from the 24th week until the 37th week of gestation. The matrix's network of tiny, fragilely supported capillaries is prone to rupture if the early baby is handled too vigorously. The head should not be placed in a very dependent or inverted position because this increases intracranial blood pressure. Rupture of vessels within the germinal matrix results in intracranial hemorrhage, which may lead to lifelong disability or death. The earlier the baby, the more potentially dangerous inappropriate handling could be, with the risk being much less as the fetus matures and very minimal past 37 weeks; therefore, to be on the safe side, consider this a risk for any baby born before 38 weeks. This recommendation is given, in part, because US neonatal resuscitation recommendations (Kattwinkel, 2001) advise against the use of inversion drainage, regardless of gestation. They do not, however, say why. Therefore, I have researched in an attempt to come up with a rationale for the safe use of inversion drainage in the term infant. Most very early labors will have been identified prior to birth, allowing timely transport to take place.

Postural Drainage

John Stevenson, a homebirth physician from Australia, prefers postural drainage to suctioning when clearing the airway is necessary. *Remember, inversion should not be used if the baby is earlier than 38 weeks.* In early babies, postural drainage can be performed by briefly placing the baby flat and on her side to facilitate pooling of secretions in the cheek where they can run out or be suctioned.

Inversion drainage can be used when the term baby's airway is partially or completely blocked with secretions. If ventilations are required, the baby should be drained as soon as possible after birth before he is placed supine to provide ventilatory assistance. Stevenson (1987) recommends drying your hands and the baby, or placing a receiving blanket over your hand so you can support the baby without slipping. Place the baby astride your arm, with your palm on his chest and your thumb under his arm (but not jammed into his axilla). Your other fingers can grip the other side of the chest. Spread your fingers beneath his chest to distribute the weight. Allow the baby's face and head to hang dependently. (Do not support the baby under the throat, as this might constrict the airway or stimulate a vasovagal response.) Support the head with your other hand by lifting the upper forehead into the sniffing position, so that the mouth is hanging open toward the floor. Lower the baby's head gently until the body is sloping fairly steeply at a 45 to 60° angle (face lower than waist). Any secretions in the airway should drain out rapidly.

Stevenson feels that a sufficiently acute angle of incline is the key to effective inversion drainage. A conscious baby will work with you to bring up mucus while being held in this posture. If done correctly, inversion drainage will not stimulate a vasovagal response, which should help the baby to recover more quickly if respiratory assistance is needed. Sutton (2001) likes to keep the baby in this position until he sneezes.

Inversion drainage should only be employed briefly as described. Resuscitative efforts should never be attempted with the baby placed in a supine position with the head lower than the body. Also note that a prolonged head-dependent, supine posture may cause secretions to pool in the back of the throat, raise cerebral as well as central venous pressure, diminish venous return to the heart and can impair excursion of the diaphragm due to the weight of the abdominal contents.

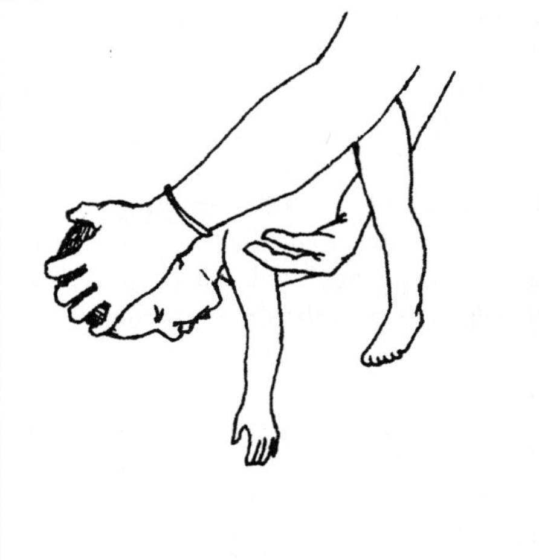

Inversion drainage at a 50° angle

Suctioning the Newborn

Suctioning with a device should only be used if postural drainage has proven insufficient or is deemed inappropriate for a particular baby or circumstance.

Types of suction devices:

Bulb syringes: There are two different types of bulb syringes. An **ear syringe** consists of a large rubber bulb with a long tapered tip. It is designed to lavage the ear canal. It can also be used to suction the baby's mouth and nose after birth to remove mucus or meconium. Syringes come in 1, 2 and 3 oz sizes. The 1 oz size is usually sufficient for clearing small amounts of mucus, although the larger syringes generate more suction. The narrow end of an ear syringe is easily placed in the infant's nose and mouth but can also be easily misplaced too far back in the throat if one is not careful. This can cause emotional distress for the baby as well as tissue trauma and may stimulate a vasovagal response.

An infant **nasal syringe** has a clear plastic, flexible, tapered bulb on the end attached to a larger rubber bulb that is compressed to create suction. The plastic tip is more difficult to empty of mucus between suctions than an ear syringe and is awkward and not very effective when used in the mouth. It does, however, create an excellent seal around the nostril and, when nasal suctioning is all that is required, it may be quite useful. You may want to have one on hand as a second option for suctioning the nose. (A "Little Noses" brand by Little Remedies Products, Velco, Inc., is illustrated on the next page and can be obtained at regular retail stores in the US)

Mucus-trap (De Lee style) suction device: These devices consist of a lidded container with two tubes exiting the lid. The suction tube is inserted down the baby's throat and negative pressure is applied to the other tube to create suction through the container and in the suction tube. The suction tube, like feeding tubes, is sized according to the French scale; an 8F or 10F is usually used to suction term infants. Mucus-trap suction devices can be used for shallow suctioning as well as when the baby has excessive amounts of mucus that cannot be sufficiently cleared with either postural drainage or an ear syringe, or when profuse meconium is in the oral cavity and esophageal suctioning is necessary. Approved devices have a mechanism of some kind that prevents the user from coming into contact with the contents of the mucus trap. For example, the Argyle De Lee style has a trap with a filter to prevent backwashing, although many midwives find these inefficient. The Res-Q-Vac is a DeLee style device that prevents cross-contamination by removing mucus via a hand-pumped mechanism. Dry your hands thoroughly before attempting to pump the Res-Q-Vac. To test a new style of mucus-trap, try to suck up raw egg, thin gravy or pudding with one to see how it performs with thick fluids.

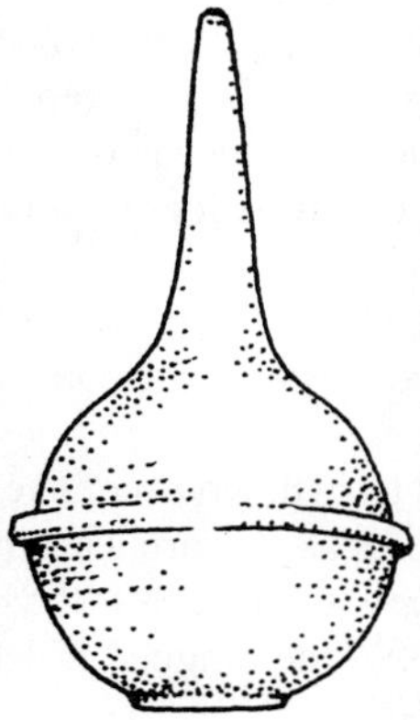

Ear syringe

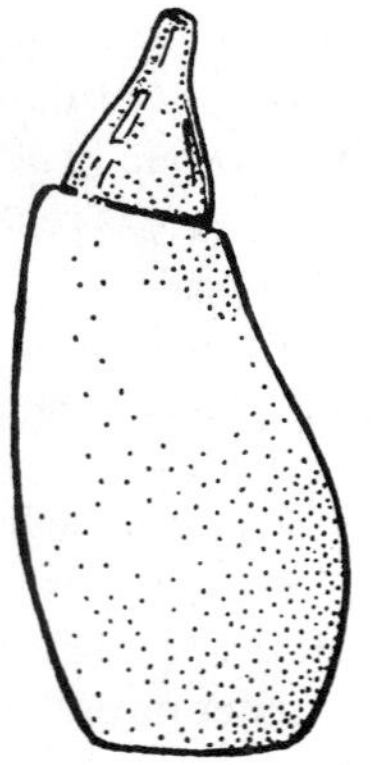

"Little Noses" syringe

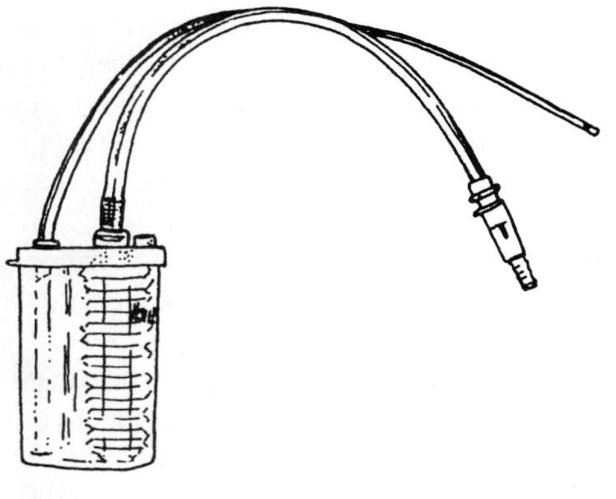

DeLee type mucus trap (the narrow tip goes down the baby's throat, the midwife sucks on the mouthpiece on the other tube).

Schuco aspirators are costly, electronic devices for portable use. They run on batteries and have an adapter that can be plugged into a car cigarette lighter (handy during newborn transports). Electronic suction devices produce a loud noise and a stronger suction than a De Lee and may be more effective at bringing out thick meconium. These types of devices have a variable setting to control the strength of suction. For newborns, it should be set no higher than 100 mm Hg (13.3 kPa or 136 cm H_2O) or as the manufacturer recommends for neonates. Regardless of which suction device you choose, with each use you will need to replace or sterilize the parts that come in contact with the infant or her body fluids.

General considerations:

Is suctioning necessary? You should only attempt suctioning when the baby's airway is blocked and postural drainage has not cleared the airway sufficiently or when prematurity or some other factor causes you to choose suctioning as the safest option for clearing the airway. Suctioning may remove thick meconium, a blood clot or a lump of vernix, as well as thick mucus. Use suction as a last resort. However, it is less likely to trigger a vasovagal response if done properly.

Always suction the mouth first: Currently, it is recommended to suction the mouth first and then the nose. While babies are preferential nose breathers (seemingly an argument in favor of suctioning it first), the first inspiration is frequently in the form of a gasp (especially when the cord is clamped immediately), during which any debris in the oral cavity can be aspirated. In addition, suctioning the nose first is believed by some to be likely to precipitate a sneezing reflex which may also result in aspiration of any debris in the mouth (Sheehy, 1990; Somerson, 1990). To remember the currently recommended sequence (mouth, then nose), note that they are in alphabetical order. Another way to remember is one hole (mouth), two holes (nose).

How much suction should be used? The midwife can judge how much suction to use based on the results of her efforts when suction is supplied with her mouth via a De Lee-type device. Generally speaking, students are surprised by the amount of suction required, which is usually much more than they believe should be adequate. As long as the tip of the tube is not blocked by contact with the baby's tissues or a huge clump of meconium, blood, vernix or mucus, the midwife should be able to adjust the amount of suction she applies so that the maximum amount of secretions are extracted. If a blockage cannot be extracted, the diameter of a firm lump may exceed the capacity of the tube. A larger tube may be needed. If a mechanical suction device is used, the suction should not exceed 100 mm Hg (13.3 kPa or 136 cm H_2O).

Shallow suctioning:

Most of the time, a shallow suctioning will be all that you need to use on the few infants who require mechanical assistance to clear their airways. While the vast majority of babies needing airway clearance will be those who passed meconium into the amniotic fluid, a rare baby has thick mucus that must be removed.

Using a tube for shallow suctioning: A 8F or 10F flexible suction catheter, such as the one on a mucus-trap suction device, is less traumatic and more effective for pharyngeal suction than a bulb syringe (Gage et al., 1981). A tube is also easier to use and control than a bulb syringe, especially when suctioning prior to the birth of the shoulders. Even in the presence of meconium-stained fluid, insert the tube into the oral cavity only, not into the posterior pharynx. Once the tube is in position, apply suction on the mouthpiece to draw mucus into the trap. Reinsert the tube and repeat as necessary. Have another mucus trap on hand in case you fill the first one before you are done. An electric or manual suction device can be used in the same manner. (See text below for details regarding the use of a tube for suctioning.)

Using a bulb syringe: If using a bulb syringe, suction the newborn in a gentle fashion, taking care not to cram the tip of the bulb in as far back into the throat or nose as it will go (which you can easily do out of anxiety if you are concerned about the condition of the baby).

The depth of oral insertion should be a maximum of 1.5 in (3 cm) from the lips in a normal term newborn of average size, and the duration of each suctioning attempt should not exceed 5 seconds. It may be helpful as you are learning to make a permanent mark on the syringe indicating how far to insert the tip. The depth of insertion will be less if the baby is small or early. A bulb syringe can be used to clear the cheeks, anterior oral cavity and back of the tongue. If deeper suctioning seems required, it is least traumatic to use a tube.

1. Begin by turning the baby on his side, or at least turning his head to the side, so that secretions can pool in the lowermost cheek; from here they will be easier to remove without stimulating the vagal nerve. Turning the entire baby has the advantage of maintaining a straighter airway and helping to drain fluids from the posterior airway.
2. To suction the mouth, hold the bulb in the palm of your hand with the tip pointed toward the ends of your fingers. Expel air from the bulb. Then insert the tip along the inside of lower cheek and release the bulb. If you use an ear syringe, do not insert the tip to the hilt, but only about three-quarters (for a 1 oz syringe) to two-thirds (for a 3 oz syringe) of its length, depending upon the size of the syringe and the size of the baby.
3. Withdraw the tip and expel the contents of the bulb into a towel or the underpad beneath the mother.

Continue to suction in this fashion (compress bulb, introduce into orifice, release bulb, remove from orifice, compress to release contents) until you are suctioning little or nothing from the mouth or until the baby is breathing and clearing his own airways with sneezing and spitting up. Stand by in case the baby needs more help. If necessary, repeat this procedure, this time inserting the tip no more than .5 in (1 cm) into first one nostril, then the other.

Deep suctioning:

Deep suctioning of the newborn consists of inserting a tube through the baby's mouth or nose into the esophagus, stomach or trachea. For many years, deep suctioning has been thought to be more effective at preventing meconium aspiration than shallow suctioning. However, it is no longer recommended to suction before the birth of the shoulders when the amniotic fluid was stained with meconium. Choose to deep suction based on the circumstances of the birth or the condition or gestational age of a particular baby, rather than on the belief that is a superior method of clearing the airway.

To deep suction, use a tube attached to a mucus-trap suction device. You should have at least two or three suction trap sets on hand at every birth in the event that one gets filled before all the mucus is out. If you do run out, you can have an assistant uncap and dispose of the contents of a filled trap so that you can use it a second time on the same baby. Discard all disposable items after you are finished.

Gauging the length of tube to insert: To determine how much of the tube to insert, place the tip of the tube on the bridge of the baby's nose and stretch the tube to the tip of her ear lobe and down between the xiphoid process and the umbilicus. Mark the length of the tube with your finger, a piece of tape or a marker. This distance approximates the length of tubing needed to reach the stomach. (See the next page for an illustration.) It is not critical that the measurement be exact for term babies. Small or early babies need a shorter length and require more careful measurement.

Inserting the tube: Insert your finger in the baby's mouth along the inner cheek and use it to hold down the tongue. Use your other hand to gently guide the tube into the back of the throat and down until you have inserted it to the mark or until

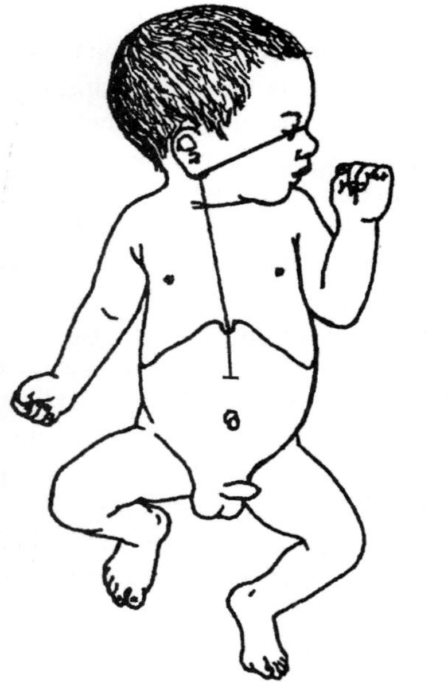
Measuring the length of tubing to insert.

it naturally stops. Do not force the tube. Using your finger to guide the tube will minimize the chances the tube hitting the side of the throat and coiling. If coiling occurs, partially withdraw the tube and try again. When inserting a tube or bulb syringe on a baby whose head is still on the perineum, you will often need to pry open the baby's mouth with a finger. Use that finger to guide the tube. While many midwives are daunted by the idea of sticking a tube down a baby, it is really very simple. Furthermore, the chances of the tube accidently entering the trachea are remote, as the epiglottis will tend to guide the tube into the esophagus. Tips for confirming tube placement can be found in the next chapter.

Applying suction: Place the mouthpiece on the other tube into your mouth or grip the hand pump and apply suction while slowly withdrawing the tube. It is important to keep the tube moving, by rolling the tube from side to side between your fingers as you withdraw it or by simply pulling the tube straight out slowly. This prevents tissue damage if the end of the tube contacts the sides of the passageway. Reinsert the tube and suction repeatedly until the fluids are clear or nearly so or until that trap is full and you must use another.

Endotracheal intubation: Inserting a tube directly into the trachea which is to be left in place for a period of time is termed "intubation." Newborn intubation is used to remove meconium from the around and below the vocal cords. It is also used if ventilatory efforts are ineffective because of a birth defect or lack of ability to maintain an open airway with manual positioning alone. This procedure was formerly performed using a blind, digital technique with a finger inserted down the baby's throat to locate the trachea and guide the tube. This is a relatively safe procedure when performed on a completely unconscious baby. With the advent of the laryngoscope, digital intubation has gradually been replaced in favor of more technology. For details see the subchapter entitled "Digital Endotracheal Intubation of the Newborn."

If the airway is totally clogged:

It is extremely rare to find the baby's airway so clogged with thick meconium, mucus, blood clots or vernix that the usual methods of clearing the upper airway will not work. In such cases, someone else can begin chest compressions if the heart rate is below 60 bpm. Chest compressions will help circulate oxygenated blood from the still-attached placenta, which will be better than nothing until the airway can be cleared.

Meanwhile, explain what is happening to the baby and how you propose to help. If neither postural drainage nor suction have been effective, you should first try to use a larger suction tube inserted deeply into the throat, such as a 10 or 12F tube (most suction devices, like the De Lee, have an 8F tube), which in many cases will dislodge large chunks of debris. If thick, dry mucus, meconium, vernix or even blood is impacted in the throat cavity, all you can do is mechanically remove the blockage with whatever tools you may have on hand. A tiny blunt-edged scoop would be ideal; a long-handled, plastic-coated infant feeding spoon might work, as might any small-diameter, blunt-tipped instrument. One doctor who attended a birth where the baby had a thick, tenacious blockage of meconium curetted it out of the mouth, although a curette has a sharp edge and I do not recommend its use. If you can see the debris that is producing the blockage in the oral cavity, attempt to remove it. If you are using an instrument, it may be helpful to cover the tip with a sheet of gauze to provide more traction, but do so only if attempts to use the instrument alone are unsuccessful. If you do use gauze, arrange it so it does not obstruct your view by covering the end with one thin layer of gauze and dipping it in water so the gauze clings to the device being inserted. Be sure you are not pushing the obstruction further back into the airway with whatever you use. To avoid this, insert the tip of the spoon or hemostat along the inner cheek wall with the convex side of the spoon against the cheek. Advance the tip of the instrument to the edge of the obstruction. Wedge the tip under the edge of the obstruction and, with a scooping motion toward the midline of the oval cavity, lift the blockage up toward the lips to dislodge it. Continue scooping it toward the lips until it comes out. Dislodge the blockage in layers. As soon as it seems feasible, suction the remaining material and begin resuscitation, if necessary.

OROGASTRIC INTUBATION OF THE NEWBORN

Knowing how to insert an orogastric tube can be useful in some situations. It is primarily used to allow for gastric decompression following the birth of a baby who requires artificial ventilation for longer than a few minutes. Insertion of a tube is also employed when meconium or mucus needs to be removed from the posterior airway, when certain defects are present, and when a baby requires tube feeding in the first weeks of life.

In this chapter we will focus on the benefits of inserting a tube during resuscitation, since this is the primary reason you will use this technique in the immediate postpartum period; however, the technique of tube insertion is the same, regardless of the reason it is being inserted.

Air entry into the stomach during ventilatory assistance

Artificial ventilation forces air into the oropharynx, where it is free to enter both the trachea and the esophagus. Proper positioning of the head and neck results in most of the air entering the trachea; however, it has been thought that some air is likely to enter the esophagus and stomach no matter how skillfully the resuscitation is handled. Air in the stomach interferes with ventilation by putting pressure on the diaphragm, preventing full lung expansion. Such air can travel through the gastrointestinal tract to the bowel, producing abdominal distension for several hours, adding more pressure on the diaphragm and making breathing difficult. Air in the stomach can also cause regurgitation of stomach contents, which may be aspirated. Thus it has been recommended to place a tube, which allows suctioning of gastric contents and provides a way to passively vent air from the stomach during resuscitation.

Gas usually reaches the stomach when the conscious baby swallows in response to pressure within the pharynx. For example, preterm infants who receive continuous positive pressure swallow continuously, allowing large amounts of air to enter the stomach. There being very little research addressing this issue, Vyas and colleagues (1983) did a study to clarify the extent to which gastric distension occurs in newborns who receive ventilations just after birth. They aspirated the gastric contents immediately after face-mask resuscitation to determine if air had entered the stomach in a group of babies who were born flaccid and unresponsive. The normal esophagus has a high opening pressure, resisting the passive entry of gas. The pressure required to force the esophagus open during resuscitation at birth was found to average 54 cm H_2O initially (a pressure rarely reached in the typical resuscitation scenario). However, once this had occurred, lower ventilatory pressures averaging 21 cm H_2O resulted in more air entering the stomach intermittently as resuscitation continued. The total number of ventilations these babies received ranged from 21 to 67. The maximum amount of air recovered was 5 ml (which is very little). Therefore, plan to insert an orogastric tube if the baby is not completely flaccid but does require ventilations at birth, if the baby requires resuscitation for more than a few minutes (which would result in more ventilations than were given in this study), if high ventilatory pressures are used, or if gastric distension is noted (the area just below the sternum, slightly to the left of the midline, will start to swell). Insert a tube immediately in babies known or suspected to have a disorder, such as diaphragmatic hernia, in which even a small amount of gastric distension can prove life threatening because the infant's lung capacity is already compromised. If you need to provide ongoing ventilatory assistance to a previously stable newborn, it would be appropriate to insert a tube then as well.

Orogastric (OG) vs. nasogastric (NG) catheterization

Orogastric catheterization is preferred for use by midwives in an emergency situation because it is easier and less traumatic for the baby to have a tube put down his throat than down his nose. Further, orogastric catheterization can be used in a wider variety of neonatal defects. The baby's cheek is soft and provides a good place to tape the end of the catheter. Placement of a nasogastric tube is much more likely to interfere with the seal that must be created around the perimeter of the mask to achieve adequate ventilation. The exception to this general rule is babies who have Pierre Robin syndrome or others involving a small mandible; these babies usually benefit from nasopharyngeal (NG) catheterization. Providing initial support for these babies is described in the subchapter entitled "Complicated Respiratory Distress."

Complications: The first problem arises from stimulating the vagus nerve during insertion. This is almost impossible to avoid and will prompt apnea, with a concurrent reduction in heart rate, and may worsen hypoxia. After placement, the primary complication results from having accidently inserted the tube into the bronchial tube rather than the esophagus. This can result in aspiration, although that is most likely to occur when the tube is inserted for feeding. Careless technique can also result in perforation of the esophagus, posterior pharynx, stomach or duodenum.

Equipment: You will need a 5F and an 8F feeding tube and a 20 cc (or larger) syringe with the needle removed. An

8F tube is small enough not to interfere with the mask-to-face seal if it is placed to the side over the soft part of the baby's cheek, and is still large enough not to clog with secretions. You would only use a 5F tube on a very small baby. The catheter will have a closed, rounded blunt end with small holes on both sides; this is the end that goes into the baby. The other end has a plastic coupler, usually with a plug attached. The tip of a needleless syringe fits perfectly into the coupler.

If you do not have a feeding tube, the tube can be removed from a De Lee and used in the same way. De Lees have permanently attached tubing, which will need to be cut off at the base. The disadvantage is that the tip of the syringe may not fit snugly into the cut end, making suctioning more difficult.

A 20 cc syringe or larger is ideal for suctioning because it is large enough to minimize the need for multiple aspirations. However, any smaller syringe can be used as described below.

Inserting a gastric tube: In case a nasogastric tube is deemed more desirable in an individual baby, the following directions include both orogastric and nasogastric insertion.

1. Check the tube for defects such as cracks or blockages. If all you have is an endotracheal tube, remove the stylet, if there is one, before you proceed.
2. Monitor the baby's heart rate and respirations throughout insertion.
3. Place the infant on her back on a firm surface.
4. Measure the length of the catheter. It must be long enough to reach the stomach, but not so long as to perforate it. Place the tip of the catheter that will go into the baby's stomach on the bridge of the nose. Stretch the tube down to the earlobe and then on down to the xiphoid process. Hold a finger on the tube at the proper distance, then mark it with a permanent marker or a small piece of tape. To minimize interruption of ventilation, the length of the tube can be approximated with the mask in place. (See the previous chapter for an illustration showing how to measure.)
5. **Orogastric placement:** Insert your finger in the baby's mouth along the inner cheek and use it to hold the tongue down as you use your other hand to gently guide the tube into the back of the throat until you have inserted it to the mark or until it naturally stops. Do not force the tube. Using your finger to guide the tube will minimize the chance of the tube hitting the side of the throat and coiling. Make sure the tube does not coil in the back of the throat. If it does, withdraw it and try again. It is usually very easy to insert an orogastric tube. Resume resuscitation as soon as the tube is in place.

   Nasogastric placement: Flex the baby's neck slightly. Elevate the tip of the baby's nose with your finger to widen the nostril and straighten the nasal turbinates (otherwise the tube may run into the turbinates, preventing advancement). Hold the tube in your fingers as you would a pencil and direct the tip of the tube toward the occipital eminence as you pass it along the floor of the nasal passage and into the nostril to the determined length.
6. Leave the end of the catheter open to provide a vent for air entering the stomach.
7. Tape the catheter to ensure that the tip remains in place. Paper skin tape from your IV equipment will minimize trauma to the baby's delicate skin.

   Taping an orogastric tube: Tape the tube to the baby's cheek.

   Taping a nasogastric tube: Wrap a long, thin piece of tape around the tube near the nostril and tape this to the skin between the nostril and the lip. Then tape the tube to the side of the cheek.
8. Confirm the placement of the tube by doing one or both of the following:
   - Inject 5 ml of air into the tube while listening with a stethoscope over the stomach for a rush of air.
   - Aspirate stomach contents and test with pH (Nitrazine) paper; gastric contents should be acid (1.5 to 3.5)
9. Suction the tube, as described below.
10. To remove the tube, remove the tape from the baby's cheek and hold the end of the tube directly above the mouth or nose as you gently withdraw the tube.

To aspirate the tube

Once the tube is in place, it should be aspirated every 5 to 10 minutes during ventilations. First, make sure the syringe plunger is pressed all the way down and that the needle, if any, is removed. Attach the syringe to the coupler on the end of the tube and gently pull the plunger outward. Gastric contents should enter the syringe. If you are uncertain whether you are in the stomach, use a stethoscope to listen over the stomach. You should hear gurgling sounds as you aspirate. If there is resistance to withdrawing the plunger, twist the tube and try again, as the tube may be lodged against soft tissue. Do not continue to try to aspirate if the plunger is very resistant, as you may do tissue damage. Once the syringe is full or no more secretions come out, detach the syringe, note the amount of fluid withdrawn (in cc) and push the plunger to empty the syringe. Repeat as necessary to clear excessive mucus, meconium or trapped air.

Selecting and Using an Infant Oropharyngeal Airway

The use of an oropharyngeal airway to maintain an open airway is only appropriate in a baby who is unconscious and for whom positive-pressure ventilation is proving difficult. Oral airways are rarely needed in neonates and are most often used when the baby has a structural defect, such as bilateral choanal atresia (both nostrils blocked by bone), or a severe deformational defect, such as prolonged in utero nasal compression, that effectively blocks the airways at birth. In this case, the mouth must remain open in order to provide effective ventilation.

The airway is a curved plastic device that is inserted through the mouth and extends to the back of the throat. One end has a flange that rests against the lips. The other end is curved to hold down the tongue as it extends into the back of the throat. Properly used, it holds the tongue in a forward and down position, away from the posterior pharynx, which greatly reducing the chance that the tongue will obstruct the airway. An airway also provides easy access for suctioning and maintains the infant's airway in the event of convulsions.

Two types of airways are most frequently used in the United States. The Guedel (Cath Guide) is distinguished by its flexible, oval, tubular design. It has a rigid bite block (that fits between the teeth) with a color coded insert in the mouth piece that indicates size. The Berman has two open channels along each side to serve as guides for tube placement and is made entirely of rigid plastic. You will want to carry two infant sizes: one for a preterm or small baby and one for an average-sized newborn. A complete set has a range of sizes from adult to newborn.

Patient	Guedel airway sizes	Berman airway sizes
Small neonate	000 Violet (40 mm)	0 (40 mm)
Average neonate	00 Blue (51 mm)	1 (50 mm)
Child	0 Black (63 mm)	2 (60 mm)
Youth	1 White (77mm)	No equivalent
Small adult	2 Green (85 mm)	3 (80 mm)
Medium adult	3 Orange (95mm)	4 (90 mm)
Large adult	4 Red (100 mm)	5 (100 mm)
Extra-large adult	5 Yellow (110 mm)	6 (110 mm)

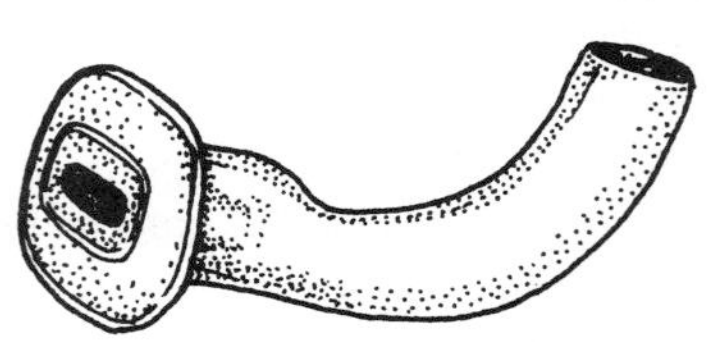

Guedel airway

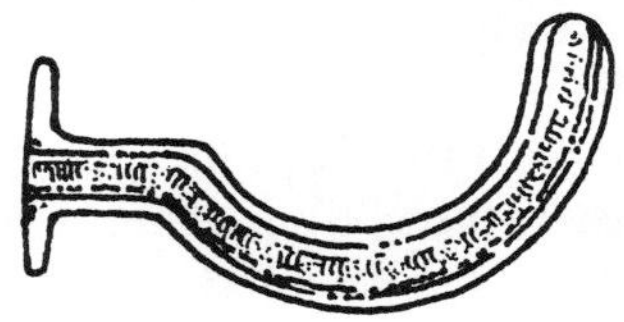

Berman airway

Limitations in the use of an oral airway

This device cannot be used effectively unless you select the correct size and *should not be used* if the proper size is not available. One of the major disadvantages of this device is that there is a not a perfect size for everyone. A device that is too small may fall back into the oral cavity or force the tongue backward into the airway, thus occluding it; it may also be swallowed. If the oral airway is too long, it can press the epiglottis against the entrance to the trachea, which also blocks the throat. One that is too large in diameter can injure the oropharynx. Placement of an oral airway also runs the risk of stimulating the vagus nerve, which exacerbates breathing difficulties, or in a conscious person, of stimulating the gag reflex. An airway should never be used unless deemed absolutely necessary.

If no airway is available or the proper size cannot be identified, an oral airway can be maintained by securing a baby bottle nipple with a large hole cut in the tip in the mouth until the baby can be prepared for surgery at a tertiary care center. This eliminates concerns about damage being done by a rigid plastic airway, but you must keep a close eye on the nipple to ensure that it is remaining patent.

Selecting a properly sized airway

Hold either type of airway parallel with the jaw, direct the hump of the airway down (toward the baby's feet). Place the airway against the side of the cheek with the flange flush with the corner of the mouth. The properly sized airway should extend from the corner of the mouth to the tip of the ear lobe. This method can be used for any age individual. Remember, never use an airway if you do not have the proper size.

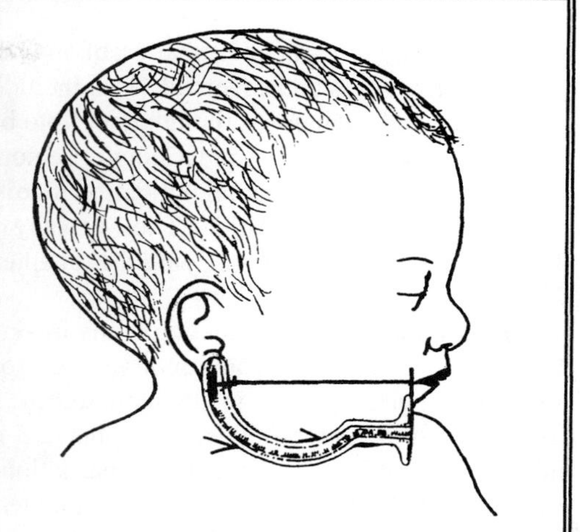

Fitting an airway in a newborn

Inserting the airway

1. Fold a small towel or receiving blanket to create a full-length support for the baby's torso and legs. Lie the baby supine on the towel with the base of his occiput at the edge, so his head falls back naturally into a sniffing position. The use of a full-length towel minimizes the chance that the baby will shift positions. (Be careful if you use a rolled towel to position the head; if it should shift, the angle of the head may change for the worse.)
2. Place the forefinger of one hand between the gums at the corner of the mouth to hold the jaws open.
3. Position the airway in the baby's mouth with the hump toward the baby's hard palate, and carefully direct the tip of the airway back over the tongue. Be certain you are not forcing the tongue back as you do so. (In newborns, it is not necessary to reverse the position of the airway when it is first introduced into the mouth, as is appropriate for an older child or an adult.) If you cannot get the tongue to lie flat against the floor of the mouth with the airway alone, use your finger or a tongue depressor to hold the tongue down while you place the airway.
4. If the airway is the correct size, the flange will rest against the lips. If the airway is too long, the flange will protrude past the lips; if it is too short, the flange will compress the lips. If the airway is not the correct size, carefully remove it and replace it with the correct size or forgo use of an airway.
5. Provide mouth-to-mask ventilation, taking care not to dislodge the airway.
6. Monitor closely. If there is a gag reflex, remove the airway at once.

Removing the airway

Removal is accomplished by reversing the insertion procedures.

DIGITAL ENDOTRACHEAL INTUBATION OF THE NEWBORN

NOTE: Endotracheal intubation of any kind is a risky procedure and whether it should ever be performed by midwives is controversial. It is included here because information on digital ET intubation is scarce but deemed by many (although not all) to be safer than use of a laryngoscope. This technique may therefore be useful to midwives practicing in remote regions, far from medical help. You should not attempt it before practicing on neonatal intubation manikins under the supervision of a qualified instructor. Carefully study the subchapter entitled "The Anatomy of the Neonatal Airway and Upper Respiratory Tract," including the drawings, prior to studying this chapter.

Endotracheal (ET) intubation is the insertion of a tube directly into the trachea. It is used to facilitate removal of debris (mucus, blood, meconium or vernix) from the glottis, to maintain an open airway during artificial ventilation, or both. Although often used in US neonatology, it is very rarely needed. In a Swedish study of 100,000 births, only about 10 babies out of every 1000 who weighed 2.5 kg or more received mask inflation or intubation. ET tubes were placed only in those babies for whom initial ventilations were unsuccessful. Only 2 out of every 1000 babies weighing over 2500 grams required ET intubation (Palme-Kilander, 1992).

With an ET tube maintaining an open airway, the practitioner doesn't have to worry about the exact placement of the head during resuscitation. Intubation can make ventilating hard-to-inflate lungs easier. Preterm babies often have such lungs, as does any baby whose lungs have not yet been filled with air, especially those whose cords have been cut too soon. ET intubation is also used when the insertion of an oral airway has not been sufficient to maintain patency in cases of certain fetal anomalies.

Indications for intubation

In many regions of the United States, hospital staffs no longer routinely perform endotracheal intubation on normal babies born through meconium-stained fluid unless they are born with absolutely no respiratory effort, in which case laryngoscopy and intubation are performed to visualize and remove any meconium near the vocal cords prior to the initiation of artificial resuscitation. However, many now believe that checking the vocal cords is useless if the baby has made any respiratory effort whatsoever, since aspiration, if it is going to occur, has already taken place. At that point, laryngoscopy only runs the risk of stimulating a vasovagal response (Schneider, 1999-2001).

There are only four situations that warrant the insertion of an endotracheal tube by a homebirth midwife. These are described below, in order of importance:

When diaphragmatic hernia is suspected: Direct ventilation into an endotracheal tube will prevent air from entering the stomach and further compromising lung capacity. Since air in the gastrointestinal tract can critically compromise these precarious infants further, it is one of the best reasons to intubate a newborn.

When the airway is thickly clogged or structurally obstructed: Tracheal suctioning is indicated when it is suspected that a blockage is preventing adequate ventilations and nothing else has cleared the debris.

When bag-and-mask ventilation with an airway inserted is still ineffective: Intubation may overcome the difficulty if ventilations are ineffective despite other attempts to establish an open airway.

When prolonged ventilations are necessary: Prolonged ventilations are easier to provide if the baby is intubated. However, when a baby's response to initial resuscitation attempts are such that it appears he will require prolonged ventilation, transport should occur as soon as possible and intubation becomes irrelevant. A midwife who is far from medical assistance might need to intubate for this reason.

In spite of such indications, it is always best to support the baby as best you can and transport as quickly as possible rather than attempting to insert an endotracheal tube at home.

Disadvantages of any method of intubation

- Use of an ET tube requires a bag-valve-mask resuscitation device.
- Inserting anything into the posterior pharynx is likely to trigger a vasovagal response, thus temporarily suppressing respiratory activity. Since ET intubation is done to facilitate positive-pressure ventilations and the vasovagal response is temporary, you should not hesitate to do it if it is otherwise indicated.
- Any type of intubation is relatively safer and best performed *only on a completely unconscious baby.* A conscious baby will tend to fight the introduction of the finger (or laryngoscope) and then the tube, making

insertion much more difficult or impossible as well as more dangerous.

- Blindly inserting your finger or unskillful use of a laryngoscope may more firmly lodge a blockage in the back of the throat. The airway should be cleared as much as possible prior to intubation. Deep suctioning can always be done once the ET tube is in place.
- Laryngeal edema, damage to the larynx or vocal cords, or both may occur from poor placement or forcing of the tube. This risk is minimized if you wait until the baby is apneic before attempting to insert the tube. Apnea depresses the reflexes and causes the larynx to relax. Do not confuse gasping with rhythmic respiratory efforts. If the baby is weakly gasping but is primarily unconscious, go ahead and attempt to place the tube between gasping efforts.
- Bronchial puncture can occur if the tube is inserted too far. One centimeter beyond the glottis is all that is required in most babies.
- Once the tube is in place, it is easy to provide ventilations through the tube at too high a pressure. Be careful.
- Once the endotracheal tube is in place, positive-pressure ventilations must be resumed. The tube creates an artificially narrowed airway that increases expiratory resistance; therefore spontaneous breathing is made more difficult. Offering positive-pressure ventilation compensates for this resistance.
- Sore throat or other localized irritation is likely to occur in some infants as a by-product of intubation, regardless of technique.

As you can see, intubation by any method should never be undertaken lightly, and it is only appropriate as a technique of last resort when the situation is dire and there is no other choice.

Laryngoscopy (lar-in-GAS-co-pee)

Endotracheal intubation is carried out under direct visualization using a laryngoscope in hospitals in Western industrialized countries. A laryngoscope is an L-shaped device consisting of a handle with a light source directed down a long blunt-edged medal blade which extends from the handle at a perpendicular angle. The baby's head is held in the sniffing position to maximally straighten the angle between the posterior pharynx, the larynx and the trachea. The blade is then carefully inserted into the baby's throat, the trachea is identified and an endotracheal tube is inserted between the vocal cords and into the trachea under direct visualization. All this must ideally be done in 20 seconds with a maximum of 30 seconds before the baby must be ventilated between attempts.

The popularity of laryngoscopy as the intubation method of choice is partly a result of the prevailing medical opinion that whenever the amniotic fluid is meconium stained, visualization of the vocal cords must be carried out to determine if meconium is present on the cords, meconium staining being overwhelmingly the most common reason to employ endotracheal intubation in the newborn. Meconium on the vocal cords has been taken as evidence that the baby may already have or be at risk to inhale meconium in the bronchial tubes, requiring direct tracheal suctioning prior to the first breath. The intention has been to prevent aspiration of meconium into the lungs and thus minimize the incidence of meconium aspiration syndrome. The wisdom of inflicting laryngoscopic examination on every baby born through meconium-stained fluid is now widely questioned. In many hospitals today, babies who make any respiratory effort at all are not being intubated before spontaneous breathing is allowed or before artificial ventilations are initiated. If any breathing efforts have begun, it is now thought fruitless to try and remove meconium because if aspiration is going to happen, it probably already has.

Risks of laryngoscopy: Laryngoscopy is a dangerous, delicate and highly skilled procedure that must be practiced on a daily basis to maintain proficiency. Indeed, those professional respiratory therapists who perform intubations for a living still feel the need to practice on stillborn babies or anesthetized cats on a regular basis to maintain their competency. This is because inserting a metal blade down a newborn's throat carries a significant risk of injury. Contusions or lacerations of the tongue, gums, pharynx, epiglottis, trachea, vocal cords or esophagus may occur. Improper pivoting of the blade presses it up against the hard palate, damaging nerves and sometimes impairing later tooth formation. These types of injuries may result from improper technique or the use of the wrong size of laryngoscope blade. The trachea or esophagus may be perforated if the tube is inserted too vigorously, or if a rigid stylet (which can be used to hold the shape of the tube during insertion) protrudes beyond the end. The potential for such complications is increased by the urgency surrounding the need for intubation and the speed with which it must be accomplished, especially if the practitioner uses this technique only rarely. As with any invasive procedure, there is also a risk of introducing infection.

Because of the highly skilled nature of this procedure and the few times, if ever, a midwife would need to intubate a baby, the use of a laryngoscope is considered by many to be outside the scope of home-based midwifery care.

Digital intubation

Intubation can be performed using a blind technique with a finger inserted down the baby's throat to locate the epiglottis and guide the tube past it into the trachea for intubation by touch alone. Although not widely discussed in the United States, where laryngoscopy is favored, digital intubation is recognized in the United Kingdom as a valid procedure that reduces (but doesn't eliminate) the risk to the baby because an instrument is not used. Even though midwives will rarely, if ever, be called upon to intubate a baby and the procedure carries significant risk in any event, the finger technique is probably a safer alternative when opportunities for practice are rare and intubation is absolutely necessary.

Advantages and disadvantages of digital intubation: There are numerous advantages of using one's finger rather than an instrument:

- The digital method is typically faster than laryngoscopy.
- It can be performed with the practitioner standing to the side of the baby or at the baby's feet in cramped quarters. (Although it can theoretically be done from either side of the baby, it works best to have your nondominant side to the baby's feet.)
- It is a blind technique. This has several benefits:
  - Good lighting is unimportant
  - It is easier to perform in the presence of copious secretions.
  - The use of a lighted instrument to open the airway is not required
  - Digital intubation does not require the midwife to maneuver herself or the baby to obtain a decent view of the airway.
- There is better control of the tongue and less risk of injury to delicate tissues.
- Use of your finger is safer than the use of an instrument if you are not an expert. Since midwives are used to touch examinations, use of your finger and a thorough understanding of the anatomy should increase your chances of success, especially since you will be feeling your way directly rather than struggling to use a rarely used instrument as an extension of your hand.
- Finger intubation is sometimes resorted to in hospitals when laryngoscopy fails, meaning it is often more useful in difficult situations. Therefore, you need not be concerned that you are sacrificing quality of care by resorting to an inferior technique.
- It reduces reliance on equipment that is expensive and subject to failure or to being misplaced.

The specific disadvantages and risks of digital intubation include:

- Large hands are a disadvantage and long fingernails are an absolute contraindication. If you have large hands, you may find digital intubation impossible on very small preterm babies, although it has been successfully used on babies as small as 500 grams.
- Some airway deformities make visualization of the trachea desirable.
- Digital intubation offers no assistance in visualizing the vocal cords to check for the presence of debris.

Digital intubation procedure: Digital endotracheal intubation should only be resorted to when the baby is limp, unresponsive to ventilation and unconscious, and you feel you have no other choice. However, if the baby is reflexively gasping (that is, last gasp efforts), he is not rhythmically breathing. Endotracheal intubation may be attempted between gasping efforts if deemed absolutely essential.

Not only is this technique safer than laryngoscopy, a skilled practitioner can accomplish it in 3 to 5 seconds in term babies with normal anatomy. However, as a midwife who may use it rarely, if ever, do not expect to be able to do it this rapidly. The good news is that you are not likely to sacrifice much time with this method, even if you are not an expert with the technique.

Equipment: You will need an unshouldered, precurved endotracheal tube, some sort of medical skin tape to secure, the tube once it is in place and well-fitting, sterile exam gloves.

Endotracheal tubes: Endotracheal tubes consist of a flexible, slightly curved blunt, angled, tube with a rigid, removable plastic coupler attached to the other end. The coupler fits directly into the mask port of a standard neonatal resuscitator. The tube is marked in centimeter increments along its length. There will also be marks indicating size as well as depth of insertion for nasal or oral use. It has a line of color (often blue) that can be seen on an X-ray to check proper placement. There is also a thick black line about a centimeter from the tip which is level with the vocal cords when the tube is inserted to the appropriate depth. This marking is not useful during digital intubation, because it is a blind technique.

The pros and cons of shouldered (tapered or cuffed) tubes: A shouldered tube has a short, narrow length of tubing at the tip, which broadens to a wider diameter above a certain level. A shouldered tube theoretically provides a good seal at the larynx as well as a tactile landmark for how far down past the vocal cords to place the tube. However, there are several problems with using shouldered tubes in newborns. The shoulder increases the external diameter of the upper portion of the tube; this may necessitate the use of a smaller tube, thus increasing airway resistance and the work of breathing. The narrowest portion of the adult airway, the area between the vocal cords, is shaped like a slot; a round tube will therefore not seal the adult trachea, while a shouldered tube will provide a better seal. In contrast, the smallest diameter of the newborn airway is below the vocal cords at the level of the rounded cricoid ring; a tube with an outer diameter that approximates that of the cricoid ring will seal the trachea without applying excessive pressure to the tracheal wall (in other words, the newborn airway is naturally tapered). Furthermore, if a tapered tube becomes obstructed with debris, the chance of tracheal damage is increased. For all these reasons, cuffed or tapered tubes are not recommended for use in newborns.

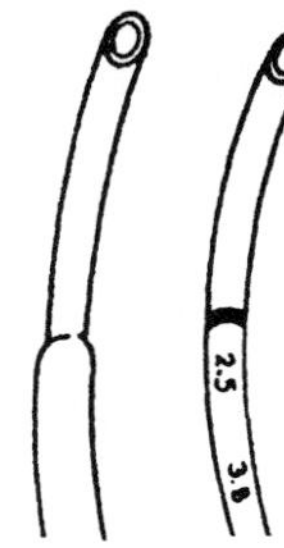

Shouldered tube (left)
Straight tube (right)

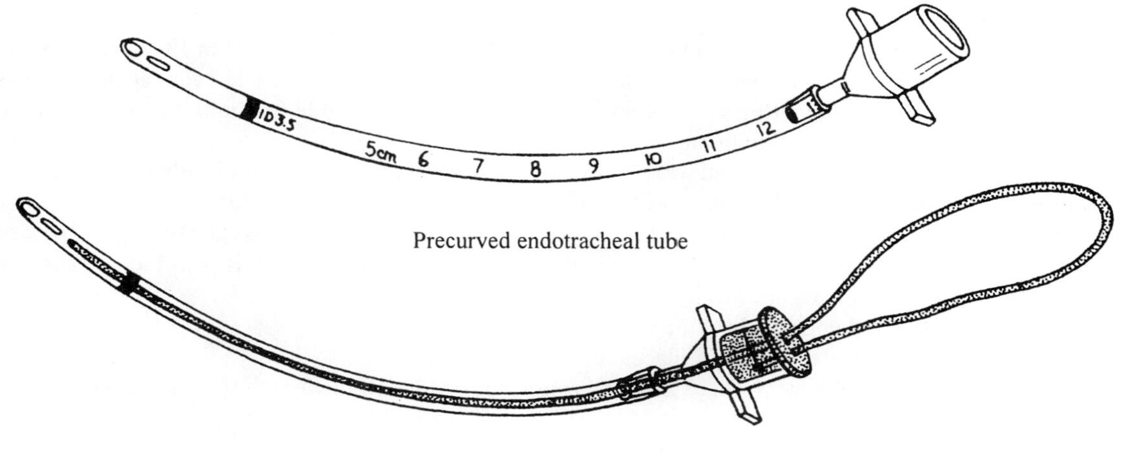

Precurved endotracheal tube

Endotracheal tube with stylet: the tip of the wire is properly in place; a plug keeps the wire from moving during insertion.

Stylets: Sometimes a flexible metal stylet (wire) is inserted into the endotracheal tube. The stylet is formed into a curve; this holds the tube in shape for easier insertion. It is removed once the tube is in place. Although designed to bend, stylet wire is stiff; once shaped, it is hard to reshape. It is best to use an endotracheal tube that has a preformed curve (such as those by Portex, available through Cascade HealthCare Products). If these are not available, keep in mind that your finger itself functions as a guide for the tube. Therefore, you do not have to run the additional risk of injuring the baby by using a stylet if you do not want to. To gain the benefit of the stylet without additional risk, form the tube into a curve through the unopened package with the stylet in place, then place the tube on ice, which will allow it retain the curve when the stylet is removed. When you are ready to use it, open the package, remove the stylet, and otherwise proceed as outlined below. This means chilling an endotracheal tube at every birth because there will not be time to do this in a real emergency. It also requires access to ice, which may be unavailable in some remote settings. If you must use a tube with a stylet in place, make sure the metal tip is well within the open end of the tube, then gently form the tube into a curve.

Bend the end of the stylet that is sticking out of the ventilation coupler to the side to insure that the end does not advance toward the tip of the tube during use. The stylet, if used properly, can facilitate insertion when the technique is unfamiliar. The description below assumes you have a precurved tube.

Selecting the correct sized tube: Take into account the baby's approximate weight and gestational age (assessed by visual inspection, not only by the due date). The ideal size allows a tiny air leak around its circumference during positive-pressure ventilation; this is an additional safety measure to ensure that excess pressure can escape from the airway during artifical ventilations. It also assures that undue pressure is not being exerted at the level of the cricoid ring. A tube that fits too tightly is likely to damage the mucosa, resulting in edema and stridor. Ulceration of the mucosa may progress to subglottic stenosis. However, the use of too small a tube (one that is much smaller than the infant's airway) can actually restrict the amount of air the baby receives; it also causes too much air to escape through the gap between the tube and tracheal wall, worsening respiratory distress (Sniderman et al., 2001).

WEIGHT OF INFANT	GESTATIONAL AGE RANGE	ENDOTRACHEAL TUBE SIZE	EQUIVALENT FRENCH CATHETER SIZES	DEPTH OF INSERTION FROM UPPER LIP
Less than 2 lb 12 oz (<1250 g)	Less than 28 weeks	2.5 mm	5F to 6F	6.5 to 7.5 cm
2 lb 12 oz to 4 lb 6.5 oz (1250-2000 g)	28 to 34 weeks	3.0 mm	6F to 8F	7 to 8 cm
4 lb. 6.5 oz to 6 lb 9.75 oz (2000–3000 g)	34 to 38 weeks	3.5 mm	8F	8 to 9 cm
Over 6 lb 9.75 oz (> 3000 g)	over 38 weeks	3.5 to 4 mm	8F to 10F	9+ cm

(Fletcher & MacDonald, 1993; Kattwinkel et al., 2000)

Tube insertion: Proceed as follows:

1. Prepare the tube for insertion. If the only tube you have is quite long, you may cut it off to 13 cm prior to use. Using sterile surgical scissors, cut the tube at a slant. Remove the plastic connector on the end and replace it securely over the new end. Cutting on a slant makes this much easier. Look at the table and note the appropriate depth of insertion for the baby you are working on.
2. Unless you suspect the airway to be clogged with thick debris, ventilate before attempting intubation. Then temporarily discontinue resuscitative efforts because they will interfere with placement of the tube.
3. In case the baby tries to breathe, have an assistant hold a tube to deliver free-flow oxygen during the procedure.
4. Don well-fitting sterile gloves. If the baby has a spinal defect, use latex-free gloves, if possible, as these babies are particularly susceptible to latex sensitivity.
5. Select an appropriately sized endotracheal tube, as already described.
6. Prepare tape to secure the tube once it is in place. You will need:
   - -Two pieces ½ cm wide, 8 to 10 cm (3.25 to 4 in) in length with half the length split down the midline to form two tails
   - -One piece, 10 to 15 cm (4 to 6 in) in length, unsplit.

   Tack these pieces of tape to a nearby object that will allow for easy removal.
7. Measure the amount of tube to insert. There are two methods that can be used:
   - **-Nasotragus length (NTL):** Place the tip of the tube level with the tip of the tragus of one ear and stretch it to the center of the base of the nasal septum.
   - **-Sternal length (STL):** Measure from the suprasternal notch (dip between the clavicles) to the tip of the xiphoid process (Shukla et al., 1997).

   Nasotragus length is usually the preferred method because obtaining sternal length interferes with chest compressions. In addition, severe chest retractions make it difficult to measure sternal length accurately. However, in babies with facial deformities (such as a cleft lip or palate) or ear deformities, sternal length will yield the most accurate measurement.

   Whichever method you use, add 1 to 2 cm to this measurement and mark the coupler end of the tube with a piece of tape or a fine-tipped permanent marker. Trim the tube to the desired length by removing the ventilation coupler and cutting the tube at an angle at the mark. The angled cut facilitates secure replacement of the coupler before you proceed. Do not cut the baby's end of the tube because it has a rounded edge, designed to minimize trauma.

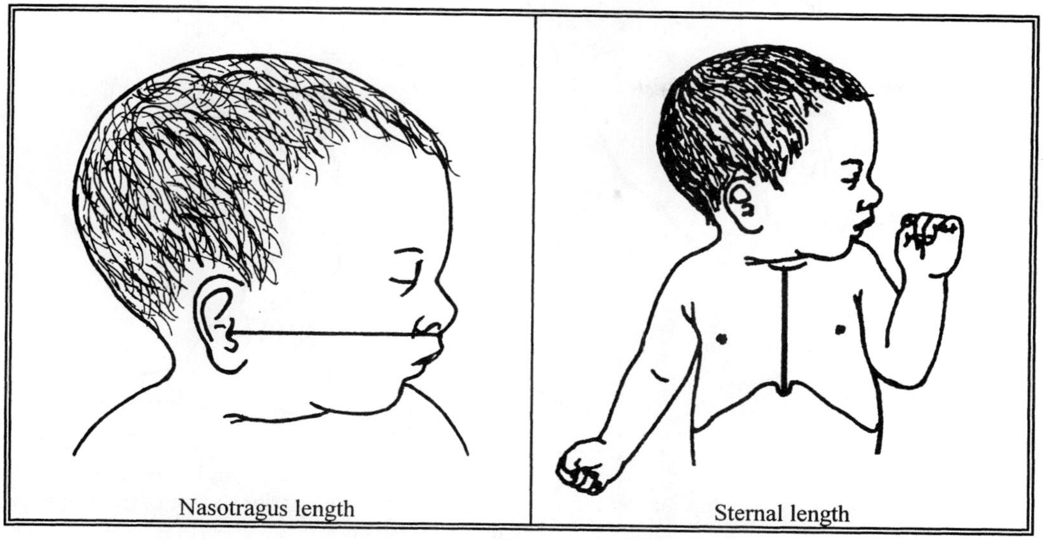

8. Although head extension is not critical with digital intubation, if you prefer, place the baby on a firm, flat surface on a 2 cm (0.75 in) thick folded towel placed under the length of the body with the edge level with the top of the shoulders. Secure the baby's head in a sniffing position in line with his spine.
9. Stand to either side of the baby, preferably on the side that will place your nondominant side to the foot of the baby. You may also stand at the foot of the baby.
10. If an oropharyngeal tube has been placed previously, remove it now. Having it in place may confuse your findings and may make placement of an endotracheal tube more difficult. Insertion of an ET tube will eliminate the need to vent air from the stomach unless the baby has a diaphragmatic hernia; in this instance, the other tube should be reinserted once the ET tube is in place.
11. Suction the baby as best you can before you begin, especially if you feel the primary problem is an airway obstruction.
12. Lubricate the index finger of your nondominant hand and the tube with sterile water (alternatively, an assistant can spray both your hand and the tube with sterile contact-lens saline solution without preservatives).
13. Turn your nondominant hand palm down and insert that index finger into the baby's mouth. Use your little finger if the baby is quite small.
14. Slide your finger along the midline of the tongue until you are touching the epiglottis. This will feel like a small horizontal band running across the root of the tongue. It will be *under* the tip of your finger. If you run into a dead end at the base of the tongue, your fingertip is in the vallecula. Keeping your hand in place, lift your fingerpad up until you feel the band (see the illustrations on the following page).
15. Lift your fingertip just enough to raise it above the edge of the epiglottis. Now slide your finger a little further back, until the fingerpad is above the opening of the larynx. The fingertip should now be beyond the larynx and above the esophagus, with the nail touching the posterior wall of the pharynx (the back of the throat) and the fingerpad above and behind the opening of the trachea. Be sure the baby's head is maintained in the midline position throughout this procedure. You may be able to move the epiglottic flap by using your fingertip to pull it forward before advancing further. However, it is less traumatic if you can lift your fingertip over the epiglottis.
16. Use your dominant hand to slide the tube into the baby's mouth between the underside of your finger and the baby's tongue. Advance the tube until its tip is level with the underside of your fingerpad.
17. Without removing your internal finger, place your nondominant thumb on the baby's neck in the suprasternal notch, just below the cricoid cartilage. Apply gentle pressure to the baby's neck in order to grasp the larynx between your thumb on the outside and your fingertip on the inside. If this seems awkward from this position, move your body around toward the foot of the baby until your thumb is well placed. Use thumbs and fingertip to stabilize the larynx in the midline and prevent movement while the tube is being inserted. This maneuver presses the trachea backward, placing it more centrally in the throat and pinching off the esophagus, both of which help to insert the tube into the trachea, rather than the esophagus.

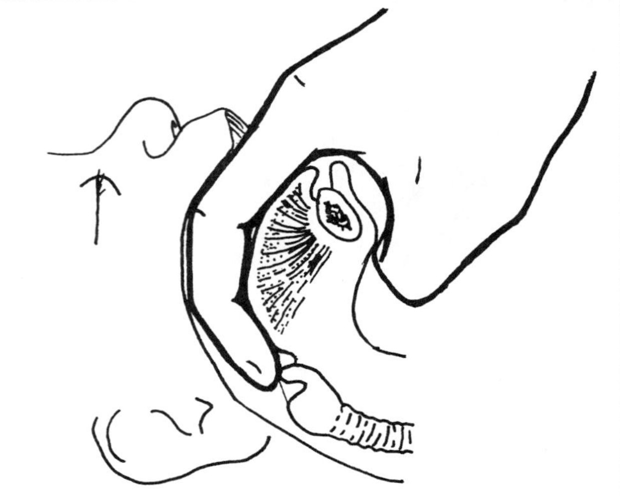

Step 14: The fingertip is touching the top border of the epiglottis.

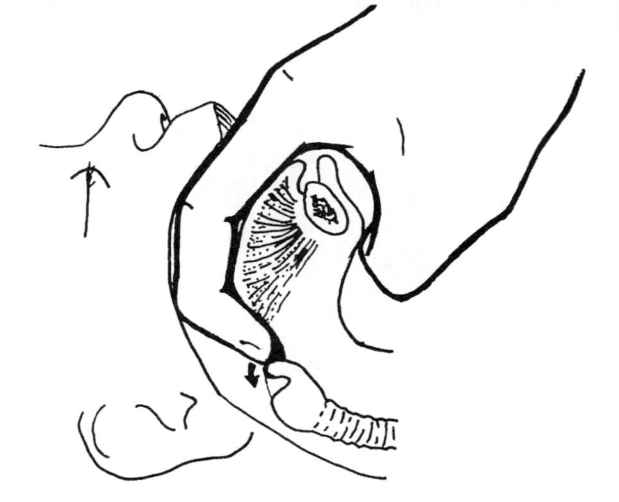

Step 14: Here,the fingertip has landed in the vallecula. Lift the tip up and over the anterior surface of the epiglottis and feel for its upper border.

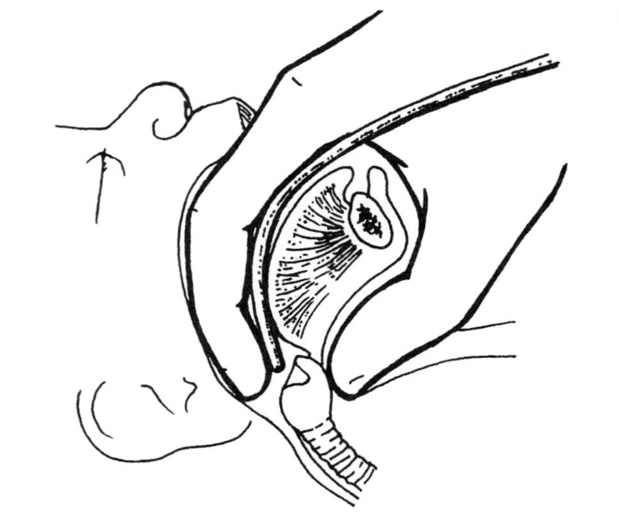

Steps 15, 16, 17: The fingertip is now over the opening of the larynx. The tube is in place to be inserted. The thumb is pressing against the larynx.

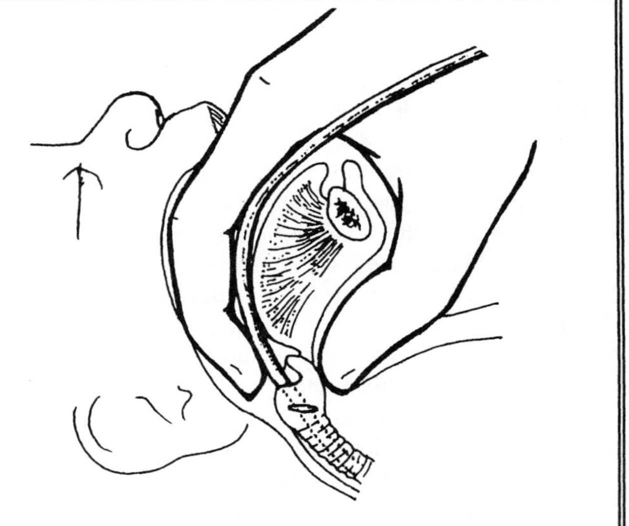

Step 18: The tube has been guided between the vocal cords and down past the larynx.

18. Use your dominant hand to grasp the tube between your thumb and forefinger as you would a pencil and begin to feed it along the underside of your index finger. You may bend your internal fingertip slightly as the tube passes under it to direct it into the larynx. Gently advance the tube a distance of 1 to 2 cm. A slight give will sometimes be felt as the tube passes between the vocal cords into the larynx, *but no force is necessary for proper insertion.* Continue to advance the tube to the previously determined depth.
19. The laryngeal cartilages can be felt to encircle and tighten around the tube when it is in the trachea. You should also be able to feel the tube passing down past the entrance to the trachea with your fingertip. A tube that has mistakenly entered the esophagus can be felt behind the posterior wall of the larynx, under your finger.
    (**If using a stylet:** Once the tube is in place, carefully withdraw the stylet so as not to move the tube.)
20. Check tube placement (as described below) while an assistant holds the tube in place. Note the centimeter marking on the tube at the level of the midline of the baby's gum. Shorten the tube if more than 4 cm extends from the

gumline by cutting it off the coupler end at an angle and then securely reattaching the connector.
21. When the tube is properly placed, tape it securely to the baby's face so that it cannot move, or hold it in place while someone else ventilates.
22. Remove the mask from your bag-and-mask set and attach the mask port on your bag-valve-mask resuscitation device to the tube connector.
23. Ventilate as you would with a mask in place.

Confirming the correct placement of the tube

Ideally, the tip of the tube is now located midway between the vocal cords and the tracheal carina. It is important to verify correct placement because a misplaced tube is worse than no tube at all. In the hospital, ET location is confirmed by X-ray examination; an option unavailable at home. The tube's position can also be confirmed by watching for the following signs:

•A bilateral rise of the chest wall with good breath sounds on both sides
•An absence of gastric distension (no swelling in the area just below the sternum and rib cage).
•Mist formation in the tube
•Improvement in the baby's color and heart rate

An assistant can listen for breath sounds by placing the diaphragm of the stethoscope high on the lateral chest wall in the axillary area (air entering the esophagus stomach or abdomen may be confused with lung sounds if she listens closer to the midline or lower down). She should hear air entering both sides of the lungs with equal intensity; no air should be heard over the stomach. While mist in the ET tube during exhalation usually indicates that the tube is in the trachea, this does not necessarily indicate that the tube is correctly located in the midtracheal area.

If the tube is in a bronchus: The tube may be incorrectly placed if it is in either the right or left main bronchus or in the esophagus. When the tube is in a main bronchus, the following problems may be noted:

•Breath sounds are unilateral or unequal, with most lung sounds coming from the side into which the tube extends. Typically, the tube will be diverted into the right side due to the angle of the main bronchial tubes.
•No air is heard entering the stomach.
•No gastric distension is observed.
•There is a poor response to ventilation with the tube in place.

If you suspect the tube is in the main bronchus, withdraw it little by little while an assistant ventilates. Listen for equal breath sounds; when you hear them, stop withdrawing the tube and secure it with tape.

When the tube is in the esophagus:

•No breath sounds are heard over the lateral chest walls, and there is little or no chest movement on ventilation.
•No mist is seen in the tube.
•Air can be heard entering the stomach with a stethoscope.
•Gastric distension may be observed as the stomach swells just below the sternum and rib cage.
•There is a poor response to ventilation with the tube in place.

If the tube is in the esophagus, remove the tube completely, ventilate the baby with bag and mask, and reinsert a new, sterile tube. Take a deep breath and try a third time. If you still can't get it in, don't waste any more time. Ventilate the best you can and transport. Repeated attempts result in bruising and edema, further narrowing the already tiny airway.

To remove the tube

Once spontaneous respirations are established, remove the tube by gently withdrawing it. Most of the time, you will have placed the tube and then transported the baby, so you will probably not be the one removing the tube.

THE LARYNGEAL MASK AIRWAY

The laryngeal mask airway (LMA) is a device that was originally developed as an aid to maintaining an open airway during anesthesia. It can also be used to maintain an airway during artificial ventilation. It consists of a tear drop-shaped mask with an inflatable cuff. (The same type of device is called a laryngeal airway device [LAD] by Marshall in the UK. Unless otherwise noted, this chapter discusses the LMA, although these devices are essentially identical.) The mask looks and works very much like a miniaturized conventional inflatable-cuff resuscitation mask for the face, except that the LMA is much smaller as it is designed to fit into the back of the throat over the larynx. A 15 mm diameter tube attached to the dome of the mask extends backward at a gentle curve and ends in a hard plastic mask-port coupler, which fits into the mask port on a resuscitator. A smaller tube, which ends in an inflation port, is used to add air to the mask cuff. The deflated mask is inserted, tip-end first, into the mouth and is positioned to overlie the lower oropharyngeal airway; the broad anterior edge of the cuff rests on the base of the tongue in front of the epiglottis. The dome of the mask overlies the opening to the larynx. When inflated, the sides of the cuff press against the lateral walls of the oropharynx and the mask tip projects behind the posterior larynx, where it rests against the upper esophageal sphincter plugging the esophageal orifice. The mask thus seals off the perimeters of the posterior pharynx, and the attached tube provides an open channel to allow for ventilation.

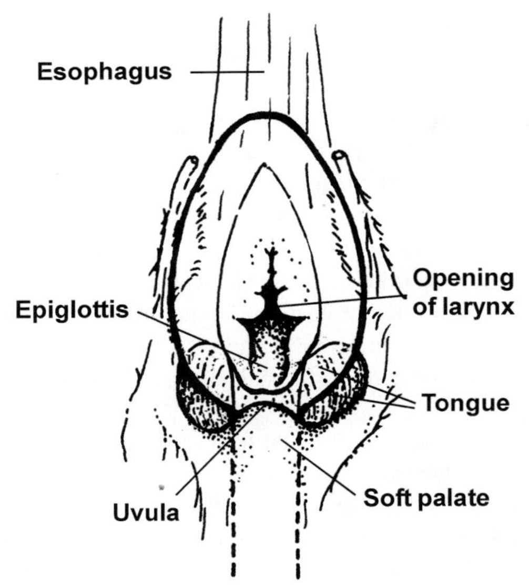

Standing at the foot of the baby, looking down into her throat, showing the outline of a correctly placed LMA (anatomy actual size at term).

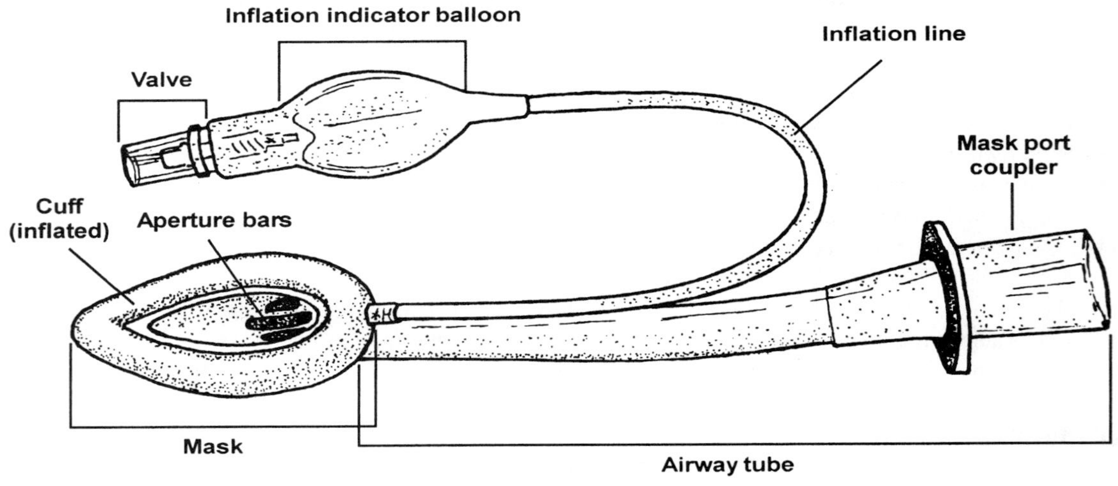

Anatomy of an LMA-Unique (Neonatal size 1, shown actual size, mask facing up)

The LMA comes in a variety of styles and a wide range of sizes, all of which are made of medical-grade PVC and are latex free. The LMA-Classic™ (reusable up to 40 times) and the LMA-Unique™ (single-use, disposable model) are both available in sizes small enough for use in term infants. Size 1 is intended for babies weighing up to 11 lb (5 kg) and size 1.5 is for those weighing between 11 to 22 lb (5 to 10 kg) (sizing is the same for the LAD). The lower limit of birthweight for the size 1 has not been determined, but it has been used in some preterm infants with success by adjusting or eliminating the inflation of the cuff. The LMA-Unique™ comes packaged either with or without a syringe (to inflate the cuff) and lubricant. A regular syringe with the needle removed can also be used to inflate or deflate the cuff.

The procedure for using the LMA is not as exacting as using a laryngoscope, but it does involve several steps and specific skill. It also requires some getting used to because the device looks big, even when deflated, and sticking it down the baby's throat may take a leap of faith.

Advantages and disadvantages

The LMA, as with any device, has advantages and disadvantages. The advantages are as follows:

- It is indicated as an alternative for endotracheal intubation, although it does not replace it. An ET tube may be more appropriate for some applications.
- It can be used for otherwise difficult airway insertion.
- Insertion is an almost blind technique and doesn't need bright light, although some visualization is necessary.
- The LMA is relatively easy to insert for trained but inexperienced residents. In one study, a clear airway was achieved in an average of 9 sec, followed by easy bag-and-mask ventilation (Paterson et al., 1994).
- Oxygen saturation increases rapidly, often more quickly than with face mask ventilation (Margaria, et al., 1995).
- The device is soft and therefore poses less likelihood of injury or stimulation of the vagal nerve than the use of a laryngoscope, which is metal.
- The LMA avoids exerting pressure in the eye region, thereby lessening the chance of injury.
- The device is not inserted directly into the larynx, reducing the risk of swelling or injury to these tiny parts.
- It can be used during resuscitation when inserting an ET tube is not possible. As with an ET tube, the LMA will be easiest to insert if the baby is profoundly unconscious so that protective airway reflexes are absent. Otherwise, the baby may fight the insertion of the device, just as she will an ET tube.

Disadvantages include:

- Insertion may result in gagging, regurgitation and aspiration. This would only be relevant for babies who have swallowed a lot of fluid and thus have a full stomach.
- The device forms a low-pressure seal, and ventilatory pressures must not exceed 20 cm H_2O or air will escape around the cuff. This low pressure may be inadequate for some babies and is usually inadequate for initial inflation breaths. Babies who have never taken a breath and those with meconium aspiration may be inadequately ventilated.
- The LMA is unsuitable for use during the removal of meconium from the throat.
- It should not be used in morbidly obese adults. Therefore, don't use it in asymmetrically grown LGA infants.
- Short-lived, mild sore throat has been reported in 10 to 70% of cases among adults.
- Rarely, neurovascular events such as hypoglossal nerve injury, tongue numbness or paralysis due to lingual nerve injury, cyanosis or swelling of the tongue and vocal cord paralysis have been observed in adults.
- Other adverse events noted in adults include hiccupping; transient glottic closure; airway obstruction; laryngeal spasm; coughing; retching; breathholding; arytenoid dislocation; trauma to the epiglottis, larynx (including hematoma formation), posterior pharyngeal wall, uvula and tonsils; parotid gland swelling; dry mouth; difficulty with swallowing; mouth ulcer; hoarseness; stridor; edema of the head or neck; myocardial ischemia and dysrhythmic heart rate.
- Experience using the device with newborns is limited.
- The manufacturer does not provide specific instructional materials for use with neonates.
- The LMA sizes for infants are miniaturized versions of the adult model. No attempt has been made to adjust the design to match the unique anatomy of the neonatal airway.

Preparing to use the LMA

The rest of the chapter gives you an idea of what using an LMA entails. The distributor only provides detailed written and video instructions for use in adults (not infants). Review their materials thoroughly and practice use on a newborn resuscitation manikin designed for practice of endotracheal intubation before you attempt to use this device on a baby. Obtain hands-on supervised training whenever possible as well.

Testing the device: The LMA-Classic™ should be examined prior to each cleaning. Look for damage, including cuts or tears in the cuff. Look down the airway tube to make sure it is not blocked by debris; shake out any found. The mask connector should be tightly inserted into the flexible tube; if it is not, it should be discarded. Do not twist the coupler, as this can break the seal. Completely deflate the cuff by inserting the tip of a 20 cc syringe into the end of the bladder on the small tube and withdrawing the air. Examine the cuff for excessive wrinkling, suggesting that part of the wall is weakened. Overinflate the cuff, using 6 ml of air for size 1 and 10 ml for size 1.5. Examine the contour of the cuff for bulges. Leaks should be apparent within 2 min. The inflation indicator should be smoothly shaped and elliptical, not round. If it does not check out, it should not be used. Once it is examined, it can be sterilized according to manufacturer's recommendations. It can be washed in a 10% solution of baking soda, although the inflator valve should not be allowed to get wet. A soft bristle bottle brush can be used to scrub the inside of the tube through the mask end, taking care not to damage the little bars of plastic over the opening. The cuff is then fully deflated and the unit is autoclaved and kept sterile until it is needed. A record should be kept of each use so the unit can be discarded after its 40th use. If you are using the LMA-Flexible™, it can be used right out of the package and then discarded.

Deflating the mask rim or cuff: Completely deflate the cuff. To do so:

1. Don sterile gloves to maintain sterility.
2. Attach a syringe with the plunger fully depressed, to the port on the inflation indicator.
3. Hold the mask as illustrated and gently stretch the inflation tubing as you withdraw the air with the syringe. You can also place the inner, sterile glove wrapper on a smooth, flat surface. Press the rim of the mask firmly against the wrapper and stabilize it with your fingertips by pressing them into the margin between the cuff and the ventilation tube on top. Use your other hand to slowly withdraw the air from the syringe until the cuff is completely empty.
4. Check to see that no wrinkles are forming in the cuff as it deflates. If you see a crease, stop deflation and smooth the crease out, either toward the tip or the back end of the cuff. Then hold the mask face up and place your index and thumb tips on either side of the mask where the wrinkle had formed and smooth the rim as you continue to deflation.

When deflated, the cuff walls should be tightly collapsed, forming a smooth wedge shape. The sides should be smooth and evenly curved with only a small longitudinal crease at the tip and perhaps a small longitudinal crease at the other end where the inflation tube is attached. If there is a wrinkle in the side of the cuff, inflate it slightly and use your fingers to smooth the surface as you deflate it again. A smoothly deflated cuff facilitates insertion and avoids the tip catching on the epiglottis. Discard the LMA if the mask reinflates immediately or spontaneously, even if only slightly.

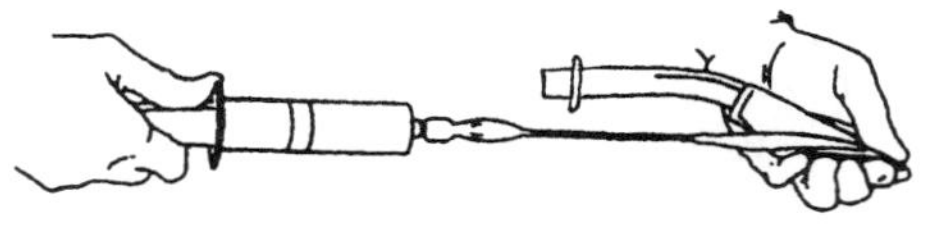

Deflating the LMA mask

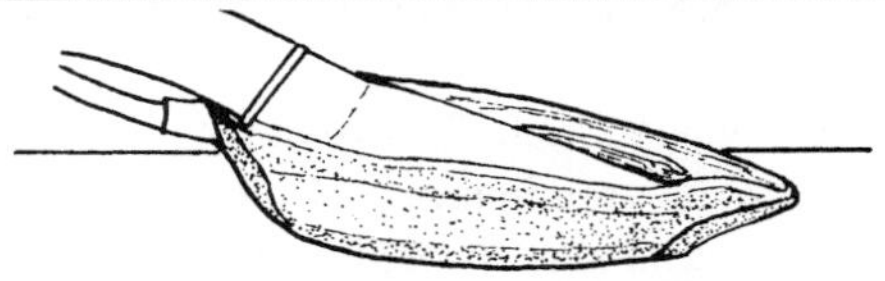

The appearance of a properly deflated mask.

The use of an orogastric tube with the LMA

When this is necessary, it is recommended that the tube be passed prior to insertion of the LMA. The tube remains outside the LMA mask and should not interfere with the mask seal. Placement of a tube does, however, increase the likelihood of regurgitation; this risk is lessened if the stomach is suctioned prior to insertion of the LMA (Gilmore, 2004).

Inserting the LMA

To position the LMA correctly, one must avoid dislocating the tip into the vallecula, the opening to the larynx, or any defects in the baby's palate or getting it caught against the epiglottis or the arytenoids. Also ensure that the tip does not curl backward during insertion and that it properly covers the laryngeal opening. The index finger technique is the recommended method of insertion and should be used whenever the baby can be approached from above the head. The manual also describes a thumb technique, which can be used when it is difficult to access the baby from above his head. It is less desirable because it encourages extension of the head. Therefore, the index finger technique is the only one described here.

Lubrication considerations: Although lubricating the sides of the cuff is recommended for use in adults, the newborn mouth is typically wet enough so that lubrication is unnecessary (Gandini & Brimacombe, 1999). If you feel it is needed, plain, sterile water (such as sterile contact lens solution) can be used. A water-soluble lubricant that is not silicone or petroleum-based could also be used. Never use lubricants containing lidocaine because this may delay the return of normal oral reflexes, and do not lubricate the face of the mask, as this may result in aspiration of lubricant or airway blockage.

1. Prepare your tape: divide a strip of paper IV tape down the middle (see page ?). Do not use medical adhesive tape.
2. Place the baby on folded towels sufficient to form a platform so the occiput tips back off the edge, in the sniffing position. Stand facing the top of the baby's head.
3. Suction the stomach and insert an OG tube.
4. Hold the LMA in your dominant hand by the tubing like you would a pencil. Place with the tip of your index finger to the side of the junction of the tube and the mask. The mask should be facing upward.

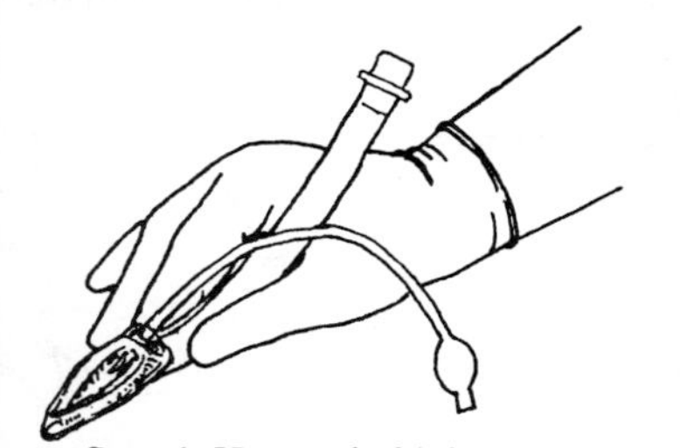
Step 4: How to hold the LMA

5. Look directly down into the mouth. Flex your wrist so that the mask opening is over the mouth with the tube facing the hard palate and the tip pointing toward the posterior fontanelle (a 45° angle). Cradle the occiput in your other hand. Align the black line on the airway tube with the baby's nose. Insert the pointed tip of the cuff into the mouth by pressing it against the hard palate just past the gum line. Keeping the tip-end of the cuff pressed against the palate prevents it from catching on the tongue.
   Most problems with insertion stem from performing step 5 incorrectly, often resulting in the tip of the mask curling in the throat.

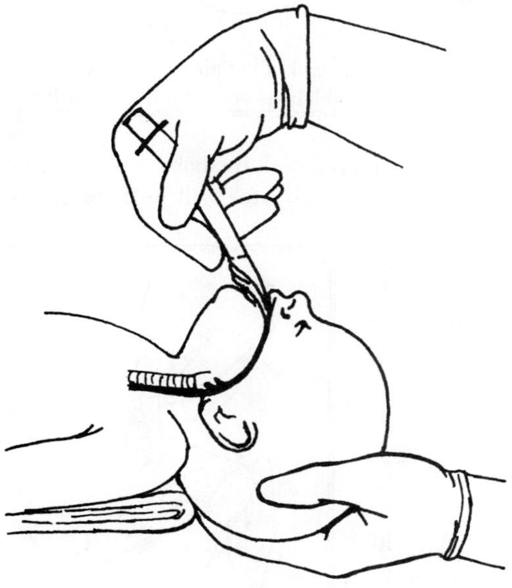
Step 5: Maintain the head in the sniffing position. Introduce the mask into the mouth by pressing it against the hard palette (note the wrist posture).

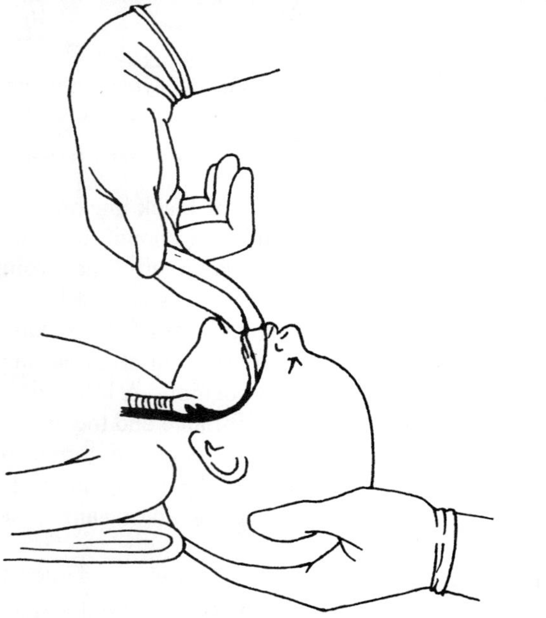
Step 6 & 7: As you slide the mask inward, extend your index finger, using its entire length to press the mask against the hard palette. As you reach the back of the throat, supply counter-pressure with your other hand to aid advancement.

6. Use your finger to press the cuff and then the tube against the palate throughout the procedure. Palpate as you advance the cuff to make sure it is not catching and curling backward toward the lips. If the cuff will not flatten against the palate or it begins to curl, withdraw the LMA and start over. If the baby has a high, arched palate, direct the tip at a more horizontal angle while looking carefully to ensure that the tip is not curling. You may open the mouth by pushing the jaw downward with your middle finger (or have an assistant do so) while you confirm correct

positioning of the mask.

7. As the tip of the mask reaches the back of the throat, use your index finger to press against the front of the mask to prevent it from curling, directing pressure toward the occiput. Supply counterpressure with your other hand against the occiput. *Never use force.* Continue to advance the LMA until you feel resistance. Do not hold the jaw open as you do so as this may cause the tongue and epiglottis to drop downward, blocking the passage of the mask.
8. Once you think you have the mask in position, hold it steady. Use your other hand to press the airway tube against the palette just enough to allow you to withdraw your index finger without disturbing the position of the mask.

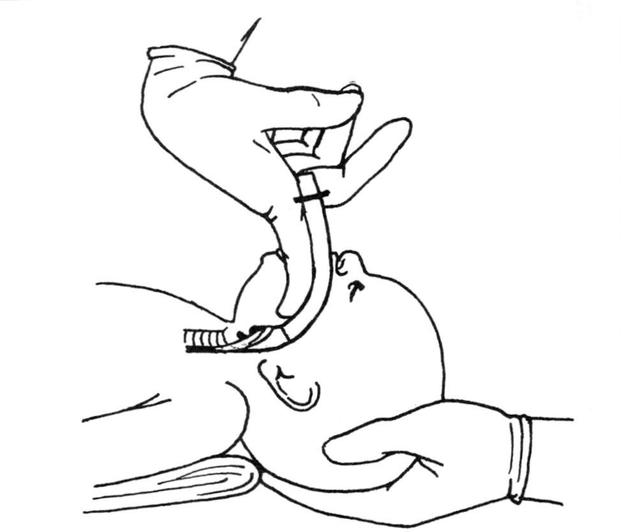

Step 7: Advance the LMA tip into the hypopharynx until you feel resistance. Apply counterpressure to the occiput with outside hand to help guide it in.

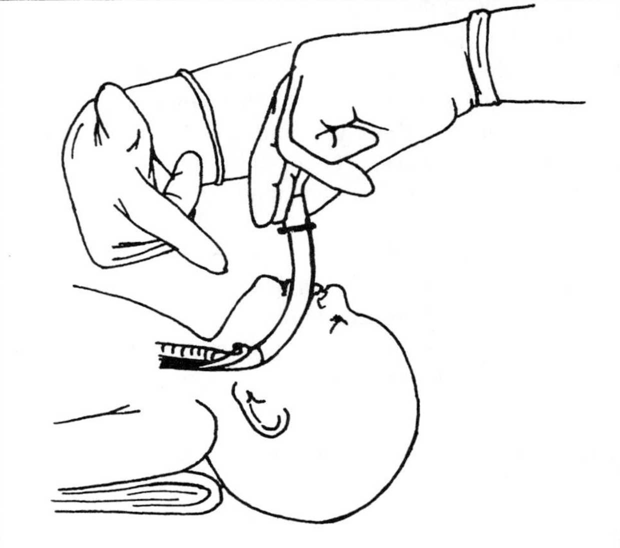

Step 8: Hold the outer end of the airway tube to keep the mask firmly applied to the palate as you withdraw your index finger.

9. Once the LMA is in place, the black line on the airway tube should be centered with the baby's nose. Let go of the tube and inflate the cuff just enough to form a good seal. The inflation indicator will puff up as you do so. Frequently, only half the maximum clinical volume is necessary to achieve a good seal. If you are using a size 1 LMA, the inflation volume should not exceed 4 ml. (If using a size 1.5, the volume should not exceed 7 ml.) Do not hold the tube during inflation as this prevents the mask from settling into the correct position. A little outward movement of the tube may occur as the cuff is inflated and the device becomes seated.
10. Confirm correct placement. Signs of correct placement include a slight outward movement of the tube during inflation, a visible oval swelling in the neck at the level of the cricoid ring and no cuff being visible in the oral cavity.
11. Create a bite block by rolling a gauze pad into a tube, taping around it with IV tape and inserting the roll between the jaws. Do not use a plastic airway for this purpose.
12. Gently press the LMA's tube against the posterior palate and tape the external portion into place by wrapping the tape around the base of the tube where it enters the mouth, forming a crossed-V by bringing the ends of the tape up by the cheek bones on either side of the face (the first step of the chevron taping pattern used to secure an IV cannula).

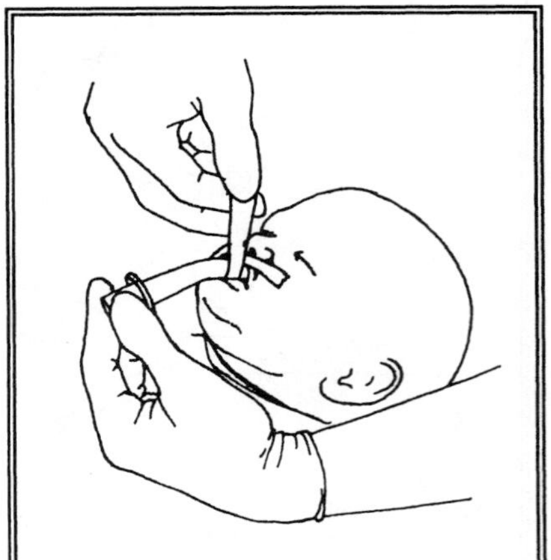

Step 12: Taping the LMA in place

13. Attach the coupler to the mask port on your bag-and-mask device, hold the LMA steady and begin ventilations.

To remove the LMA

Deflate the cuff by fully depressing the plunger on a syringe, attaching it to the inflation port and aspirating the air. Then withdraw the device slowly in the reverse order of insertion. After the baby has stabilized, he may spit it out.

Problems and Solutions

The LMA must be correctly seated over the larynx to work properly. The following chart shows correct placement and the three categories of incorrect placement.

ENSURING CORRECT PLACEMENT	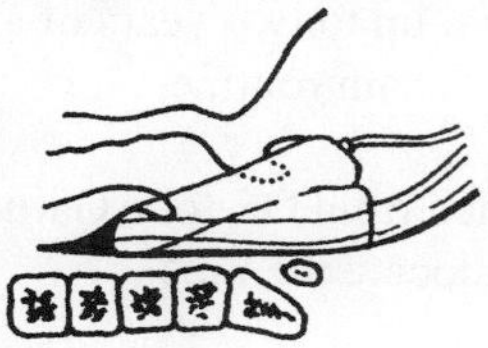	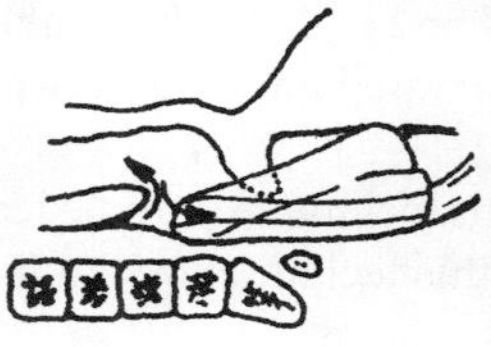	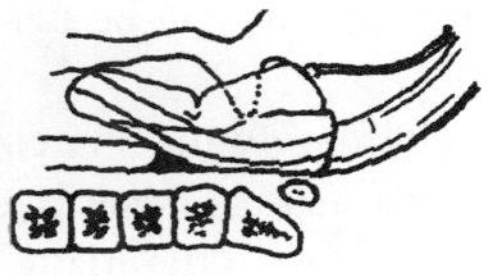	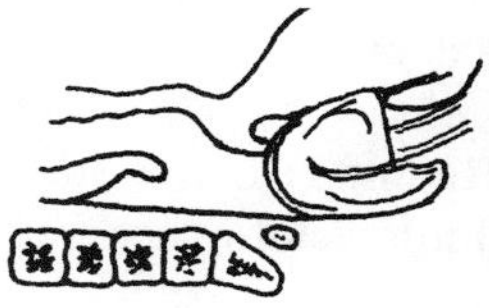
MASK POSITION	Correct: tip behind arytenoid & cricoid cartilages	Tip too high in pharynx	Tip in laryngeal vestibule	Tip folded backwards
BITE BLOCK POSITION	Midway between gums	Too high	Midway between gums	Too high
OTHER SIGNS	Effective ventilation	Pressing the device in further eliminates leaks	Pressing in further increases obstruction	Difficulty passing OG tube

Troubleshooting tips: The following table describes numerous problems that can arise with the use of the LMA. Most of these are not serious and can be corrected. Unfortunately, there are no specific tips from the company regarding problems that can occur in infants.

PROBLEM	POSSIBLE CAUSE	POSSIBLE SOLUTION
Poor airway seal or leakage during ventilation	Mask seated too high in pharynx	Advance mask further and re-secure tube with tape
	Poor fixation	Ensure palatal pressure and secure taping
	Overinflation of cuff	Deflate slightly to see if that helps
	Herniation of cuff	Device may be defective, try inserting a new one
Airway obstruction (difficult ventilation)	Tip of mask is jammed in laryngeal vestibule	Remove and reinsert
	Tip of mask pressing on glottic inlet, forcing the vocal cords closed	Adjust cuff inflation, be sure the head is in a sniffing position and reattempt ventilation
	Wrinkling of cuff walls in the midline	Size too large; ensure correct cuff inflation pressure
Air enters stomach during ventilation	Tip of mask folded backward	Remove and reinsert
	Mask seated too high in pharynx	Advance mask further and re-secure tube with tape
Device moves, rotates or pops out of the mouth	Overinflation of cuff	Deflate slightly
	Herniation of cuff	Disposable device may be defective, try inserting a new one
	Accidental displacement	Ensure secure taping of tube
	Tip of mask folded backward	Remove and reinsert
	Poor fixation	Ensure palatal pressure and secure taping

Spinal Alignment Techniques for Newborns

Two spinal alignment techniques have been brought to my attention by midwives. These can be used on term babies who are having respiratory difficulties and who have not sustained any birth injuries. Both techniques help align the vertebrae, relieve subluxations, optimize the circulation of cerebral spinal fluid and relieve pressure on the medulla, which helps facilitate easy breathing. The inverted position also allows spinal fluid to fully expand the cerebral ventricles, helping the skull to "reinflate" and the skull bones to realign themselves, which may be particularly useful in babies who have experienced pronounced moulding during descent. Either technique can be used on any term baby who is having trouble breathing as part of a resuscitation protocol and both can be beneficial up to two years of age. When the baby is doing well, one of these techniques can be incorporated into your newborn exam routine.

Method 1: Lonna Smoot, a Utah midwife, shares this technique that she learned from Dr. John Garuder, an experienced chiropractor in her area. Performed as described, this technique will not dislocate the hips.

1. Start with the baby lying face-up on the mattress.
2. Lift the baby's lower legs and grasp the back of the ankles with your thumb and index fingers so that your thumbnails "face" each other on the inside of each ankle.
3. Slowly lift the baby so he is hanging by the ankles with his head suspended slightly above the mattress.
4. Check for tension in each leg by gently stretching upward on one leg, then the other. You can also rotate the ankles to bring the soles of the feet together and then pull up on each leg. Bringing the soles together will accentuate any tension in the legs, making it easier to detect.
5. Alternate gently pulling on one leg, then the other until the tension in the legs is balanced. This should take no longer than 10 to 20 seconds.
6. Gently lay the baby back down on the mattress, facing up.
7. Next, have someone hold the baby upright, facing you.
8. Cup your hands around the base of the skull on either side and gently stretch upward for 10 to 15 seconds. This helps to strengthen and realign the cervical vertebrae.

Method 2: Carol Gautschi, of Sequim, Washington, has used a similar technique for years whenever a baby experiences respiratory difficulties or has an otherwise rocky transition after birth. She emphasizes that she explains what she is going to do and why to the baby before she proceeds and talks to the baby throughout the procedure. This technique can be used briefly, prior to or after beginning resuscitative efforts. She has mothers follow-up with this at least once a week whenever babies have difficult births.

1. Lay the baby on the mattress, facing up, with her head toward you.
2. Reach over her and lift her up by the ankles so she is facing you, with her head suspended slightly over the mattress.
3. Once the baby is lifted, sway her very gently forward and backward in an 8 to 12 inch arc by rotating your wrists to swing the baby gently in a pivoting motion (like a swing at the playground) to a count of 12 to 15 seconds.
4. The baby should be awake and content after you lay her back down, facing up.

With either technique, a baby who is benefitting from it will act like it. Put the baby down right away if he complains by fussing or trying to pull his legs away or by fighting and not relaxing. These signs indicate that he needs a more specific adjustment than the technique can provide. Refer him to a chiropractor or osteopath who is experienced with newborns.

EVALUATING AND ASSISTING THE INFANT IN NEED OF RESUSCITATION

NOTE: Review the subchapters entitled "Understanding Fetal and Neonatal Asphyxia" and "The Anatomy of the Neonatal Airway and Upper Respiratory Tract" before studying this chapter.

This chapter discusses neonatal resuscitation from an international perspective. It should therefore be enlightening for midwives everywhere. While neonatal resuscitation is presented as a fairly rote process with minimal discussion of the pros and cons of techniques used in the United States (NEONATAL RESUSCITATION TEXTBOOK, [Kattwinkel et al., 2000]), the RESUSCITATION AT BIRTH: NEWBORN LIFE SUPPORT MANUAL (Richmond et al., 2001), used for the neonatal resuscitation workshops in the United Kingdom, emphasizes different aspects of the process and offers more detail regarding rationale.

Today's resuscitation protocols are predicated on a pathological model of neonatal transition due to the routine practice of immediate or early cord clamping in institutional settings. Therefore, this chapter is an attempt to sort through standard protocols as they apply to the baby who is having difficulty establishing respirations incorporating what is known and theorized about physiologic transition with the cord intact.

Learning Resuscitation

Taking classes

The basic steps in resuscitation are covered in this chapter, with special emphasis on a midwifery-model approach. However, this information does not eliminate the need to attend current classes with a qualified instructor who teaches mouth-to-mouth-and-nose and mouth-to-mask techniques as well as ventilation using a bag-and-mask resuscitator. Such training should cover both adult and newborn protocols, in order to prepare the midwife to assist either the mother or the baby. Training and sufficient practice on models helps to avoid an overly aggressive response when called upon to actually use these skills at a birth. Protocols for resuscitation are constantly being refined, and new recommendations can be expected almost every year. *Never* attempt to practice resuscitation techniques on a normal, living infant. Practice manikins should be provided with formal instruction. (See the resources list at the end of the text for details about courses designed for midwives.)

CPR and bag-and-mask resuscitation

CPR stands for "cardiopulmonary resuscitation." It is emergency first aid used in the field to revive an individual on the spot. It can be performed using a one or two person technique on an infant, child or an adult with or without equipment. Cardiopulmonary resuscitation that includes the use of a bag-and-mask resuscitator (and, when indicated, the provision of cardiac compressions) is generally considered preferable to mouth-to-mouth CPR. However, full CPR cannot be provided by one person alone when a resuscitator is used because one hand must be available to secure the mask to form a good seal around the baby's face and the other must pump the ventilation bag. This leaves no hand free to provide cardiac compressions. Thus, you must be competent in both manual CPR and bag-and-mask use because you have no control over whether there will always be two trained people available, especially as a homebirth midwife. This situation may present itself regardless of how carefully you try to avoid it. For example, you may be the first to arrive at a precipitous birth, or your midwifery partner may have to deal with a maternal complication while you resuscitate the baby by yourself. For reasons such as these, it is a good precaution to have any apprentices you work with attend classes that cover both CPR and bag-and-mask techniques. They can then help if full resuscitation is called for; but this is no guarantee of always having assistance, either. While the chances of a baby needing full resuscitation are remote, you must be prepared to offer it, regardless of the circumstances.

Resuscitation Equipment

Your equipment should be checked, set up and ready for use well before the birth. Details regarding the selection and use of resuscitation and oxygen equipment are given in the subchapter entitled "Oxygen Delivery Devices and Resuscitation Equipment." Setting up your equipment is discussed in the chapter entitled "Setting Up Equipment and Preparing the House for Birth."

Spiritual and Emotional Considerations

When a baby has difficulty establishing respirations, it is a frightening time for everyone, *including the baby*. Once placental respiration falls off for any reason, the baby's response is the same as that of anyone who cannot get air.

The birth may have been hard for the baby, even if it was perceived by the midwives and others present as having been relatively easy for the mother. The baby may not be fully in his body due to trauma and, for that reason, may not actually be asphyxiated. For example, if all the people in the room are holding their breath or very afraid, the baby may become confused about what to do next. The baby may be apneic (not breathing) after birth if the parents have ambivalent emotions and the baby feels unwanted or unwelcomed. Of course, if the mother has been transported to the hospital, any drugs she may have received for pain or sedation could be contributing to the baby's condition as well.

Calling the baby in

The baby is a conscious being; it is important to let her know she is welcomed, wanted and cared for. The parents should call the baby, by name if they have chosen one, just as they would do if an older child fell unconscious, and ask her to come into her body and begin to breathe. This has a powerful effect on many babies and may be all that is needed to bring the baby around. The midwife can very quickly prompt the others in the room to do this–"Everyone, breathe; focus on the baby. Mom and Dad, tell your baby how glad you are to see her; call her name"– as she also attends to the physical well-being of the baby. At the same time, focus your mental and emotional intention on reviving the baby and helping her come into her body.

Validate the baby's condition

Many times, in their concern, midwives will tell a baby who is obviously distressed that everything is okay. This is not true, and the baby knows it. Instead, acknowledge the baby's condition: "I can see you are having trouble breathing and I am going to help you get started." Encourage the baby as he makes his own efforts to stabilize. Explain each intervention in simple, straightforward language as you proceed, addressing both the baby and the parents.

Keep the baby and mother together

Removing the distressed baby from her mother is contrary to everything we know about the spiritual needs of the situation and the psychological and physical needs of bonding. Leaving the cord intact eliminates the option of removing the baby to another location. The baby should be separated from her mother only if transport is required.

Center yourself

Breathe deeply and take this process one step at a time. You want to proceed consciously, intentionally and carefully whenever a baby is in trouble. You could injure the baby or provide ineffective care if you panic, hurry or use equipment carelessly.

Physical Care and Assessment

Adjust room temperature

The room should already be appropriately warmed to at least 80°F (26.6°C) but no warmer than 89.6°F (32°C), except as discussed in the chapter entitled "Hydrotherapy and Waterbirth." Have an assistant attend to making sure the room remains warm by minimizing persons coming and going from the room to prevent excessive air movement, closing doors and windows to eliminate drafts, etc., as appropriate.

Set a time clock

Have available a timer or stopwatch that an assistant can start at the time of birth and watch to see how long your efforts are taking during the resuscitation process. Use a kitchen timer if nothing else is available. The assistant can quietly indicate the time in 30 sec intervals.

Leave the cord intact

Whenever possible, leave the cord intact to maximize perfusion of vital organs as well as the amount of oxygen the baby will receive, allowing for a more gradual transition to breathing. When the cord is cut immediately, adequate oxygenation depends entirely upon the establishment of respirations.

Leaving the cord intact is even more important when the baby is asphyxiated to begin with. Remember that all "standard" (read "hospital") protocols call for cutting the cord quickly (removing the only possible source of oxygen to a nonbreathing baby) so the baby can be removed to another location for resuscitation. Because of this underlying assumption, previous resuscitation protocols have recommended that respiratory effort be evaluated before heart rate.

When the cord is actively pumping at birth, the baby is receiving oxygen via the cord for at least the first 2 to 3 minutes of life and probably until the placenta separates. Blood moving into the pulmonary circulation under positive pressure may expand the alveolar capillary beds before breathing begins; the baby may be rosy pink and not in respiratory distress unless compromise becomes evident with a drop in heart rate or diminishing muscle tone. The medical profession does not recognize this variation on normal transition because they never allow it to happen.

Cutting the cord quickly eliminates placental blood flow to the fluid filled lungs. The hypoxic baby must then redistribute his existing blood volume to accommodate lung perfusion, thus contributing additional systemic insult as blood is syphoned off from the brain and other vital organs. Cutting the cord right away virtually guarantees that the baby will panic and gasp deeply if she is capable of doing so in an effort to inflate the fluid-filled lungs.

Blood volume alterations in hypoxia: When fetal hypoxia first develops, a generalized vasodilation occurs; the baby also mobilizes sequestered blood from his liver and spleen into the circulation. The net result is more blood pooling in her system, stepping up perfusion and providing more red blood cells to deliver oxygen to the tissues. This decreases blood return to the placenta. Soon, however, the hypoxic baby begins to vasoconstrict peripherally to redirect blood to vital organs. This results in the body allowing less inflow of blood from the umbilical artery and a disproportionate amount of blood being retained in the placenta. Vasoconstriction coupled with little or no lung inflation allows fetal circulatory pathways to remain open. Placing a vasoconstricted baby lower than the placenta ensures that blood preferentially flows to the baby and does not remain pooled in the placenta between contractions (Morley, 1998). Once respirations begin, if the cord is intact, the uterus is contracting and the baby's heart is beating. The blood will naturally flood the circulatory pathways in the lungs, expanding the capillary framework around each alveolus.

Chronic hypoxia leads to prolonged vasoconstriction. Chronic cord compression results in the birth of a baby who is in a state of hypovolemia. If newborn distress is due to a tightly wrapped or knotted cord, relieving tension on the cord or loosening the knot is likely to result in renewed cord circulation. Venous return may also be impaired because of other problems, such as severe maternal hypotension interfering with the mother's contribution to the placental pumping action. These situations can cause blood to remain sequestered in the placenta limiting blood return to the baby. At first, the placenta vasculature becomes engorged. Maximum vascular engorgement leads to the transfer of fluids into the maternal tissues because the placenta has no tissues into which the fluid can be absorbed. This process leaves the placenta engorged with red blood cells but with little or no plasma to transport the cord transfusion to the baby. This condition would be heralded by poor fetal heart rate patterns (likely starting out with variable decelerations and leading to late decelerations as the fetal condition deteriorates) and would probably prompt transport prior to birth. If such a baby is born at home, how to help is described below.

Provide postural drainage or suctioning

A plug of thick mucus, meconium, vernix or even a blood clot from the birth may be blocking the airway and preventing inspiration. In rare cases, a structural defect may be the problem. If the baby is at least 38 weeks gestation, first use inversion drainage to clear the fluids. If the baby is earlier, place her on her side and suction the mouth and then the nose with a tube or bulb syringe (see the subchapter entitled "Clearing the Baby's Airway" for details). Excessive or deep suctioning should be avoided whenever possible because either may induce a vagal response, which will lead to further apnea and bradycardia. Suctioning should only be used to clear the airway of obstructions. Extensive suctioning of normal amounts of clear fluids may lead to pulmonary collapse, cause trauma or impair the establishment of normal respirations. If, however, the baby has copious material that is too thick to drain, it should be removed even if clear. Continuous production of copious fluids should alert you to the possibility of a congenital airway or esophageal obstruction (see the subchapter entitled "Complicated Respiratory Distress" for details).

Dry the baby and maintain normothermia

Dry the baby with warmed towels or blankets. Replace wet blankets with dry ones. Remember that the intact cord is carrying warm blood to the baby, that he will stabilize more quickly than one who has had the cord cut quickly, and that a baby who is in primary apnea will often begin breathing while being dried off. Continue to monitor for chilling once the baby is dried. During a prolonged assessment, resuscitation or transport, cover the baby's body with food-grade plastic wrap will help to retain heat and still allow you to see the baby to assess color, tone and chest wall movement.

Research regarding the protective effects of hypothermia in hypoxic babies brings up the question of how to manage the baby's temperature during the initial period of resuscitation. To date, experimental data suggest that small changes in temperature during the active period of initial resuscitation are not particularly important. The newborn is remarkably thermally inert. For example, during therapeutic hypothermia active head cooling requires half an hour or more before the core temperature drops to the desired zone and an hour before temperatures stabilize after additional thermal adjustments. Thus, the primary determinant of the newborn's temperature is her mother's during labor. Neonatal hyperthermia, however, can be very damaging and should be avoided. In light of this research, it probably makes sense to keep the room warm and free of drafts while leaving the baby's head uncovered if she requires resuscitation, to allow the brain to eliminate heat (Gunn & Bennet, 2001).

Positioning the baby

Where you place the baby will depend on the length of the cord and degree of distress. In any event, the baby should be as close to the mother and as far below the level of the placenta as is practical considering the assistance needed.

Lateral positioning: If the baby is starting to breathe, place her on her side. As normal breathing is becoming established, the baby's head may be slightly lower than the body and tipped slightly back in a sniffing position for the first several minutes to help drain fluids from her airways. The baby should not be placed in full Trendelenburg nor should she be left in the recommended position because the weight of the abdominal organs can press against the diaphragm, making breathing more difficult. If the baby is not severely distressed, putting her on her mother's chest or on a warmed baby tray at her side will help maintain her temperature. However, if resuscitation is required, a firm, flat surface is needed, so the mother's body will not do.

Supine positioning: If she is showing no respiratory effort, place the baby on her back on a warmed baby tray. First, support the head in the sniffing position by placing a receiving blanket or a small bath towel folded to 2 cm (¾ in) thickness on the tray to match the full length and width of the baby's body with the occiput positioned off the edge. Placing the padding under the full length of the baby's body minimizes the possibility of displacing the infant if ventilations or cardiac massage are required. Hold the tray at a level below the placenta. The tray can be moved while you are working, even for transport if necessary. (Placing the baby on the mother's lower abdomen immediately after birth tends to push the large uterine mass against the inferior vena cava, impeding blood return to the upper body and thus encouraging uterine bleeding.)

Open the airway

Unlike adults, babies have large, bumpy occiputs. When a flaccid baby is placed on her back, the occiput tends to cause the chin to tip toward the chest, collapsing the airway. If the baby has some muscle tone, the head will tend to assume the correct tipped-back position on its own. If the head does tip forward, tip the forehead back *slightly*, into the sniffing position. The ideal angle is called the "sniffing position" because it is the posture one assumes when catching a scent on the air. It is a much less extended position than is required to open the adult airway. In England, this is called the neutral position. It is achieved when the tip of the nose is pointing straight up in the air.

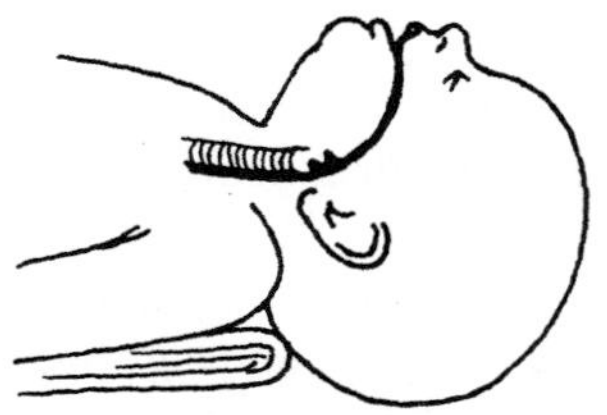
The sniffing position

If the baby is very limp and unconscious, the pharynx tends to collapse and the tongue fall into the back of the throat, even if the head is properly positioned. This can be remedied by moving the jaw forward, which elevates the base of the tongue and maximizes the diameter of the airway. To elevate the jaw, position yourself facing the top of the baby's head; use either your index or ring fingers on either side of the baby's jaw to press forward on the corner of the mandible beneath the ears on both sides. Alternatively, the chin can be brought forward by placing a finger on the bony underside of the tip of the chin and pulling up. Take care not to apply pressure to the soft tissue under the chin or jaw when using either of these maneuvers, as this can put pressure on the base of the tongue (which can close the airway).

Note that both overextension as well as inadequate extension can constrict the extremely flexible newborn airway. Proper positioning elevates the tongue out of the posterior airway as well as maximizes airway diameter and may, by itself, prompt the baby to begin breathing. If the heart is still beating, which it probably will be, the circulatory system will promptly distribute any inspired oxygen to the heart muscle and the brain. The heart rate should rapidly respond. Once the airway is opened, you should maintain the baby in this position until spontaneous respirations begin and he is otherwise stable.

It is possible for the baby to have a birth defect that occludes the airway. The trachea may also be swollen or damaged if the baby was born by a difficult face or breech presentation or the cord was very tight around the neck (this is rare but possible). If you suspect this, see the subchapter entitled "Complicated Respiratory Distress" in the part entitled "Assessing, Supporting and Transporting the Baby in Need of Specialized Care."

Check vital signs

Evaluating whether a baby requires resuscitation takes place immediately after birth and is based upon the status of the baby's airway, color, muscle tone, respiratory effort (including cord pulsations) and heart rate. Although most of these are the same parameters of assessment as those included in the APGAR score, providing physical assistance for a baby clearly in respiratory distress should not be postponed until after the 1 minute APGAR scoring. (Therefore, APGAR scores mentioned in this chapter are intended to be on-the-spot assessments, not the traditional 1 and 5 minute scores, unless otherwise indicated.) The experienced practitioner makes these assessments intuitively and simultaneously in the moments following birth.

Respiratory effort: Approximately 75% of normal babies establish regular respirations by 60 seconds of life. Twenty percent of normal babies take from 60 to 180 seconds to begin breathing well on their own. To evaluate breathing, you must look for and listen to breath sounds. Midwives do not always listen to the lungs with a stethoscope; however, if the baby is breathing shallowly or very quietly, it can be difficult to assess the adequacy of respiratory effort based on visual clues alone. Very often, a baby who appears to not be breathing effectively will have good breath sounds upon auscultation. Breath sounds are judged by listening on both sides of the chest in both the upper and lower lobes of the lungs. Breathing may be irregular for the first minute or so; however, if breath sounds are good, there is no need to begin artificial ventilation. If is important to remember that the first 5 or so inhalations must be of sufficient pressure to expand the lungs; only after this has been accomplished can adequate pulmonary oxygen exchange begin.

Gasping respirations (labored, sighing inhalations with long pauses in between) indicate that the onset of primary apnea or the progression toward secondary apnea started prior to birth. A brief period of tactile stimulation may be all that is needed to bring the baby fully into her body and begin breathing. This can be accomplished by drying the baby and either flicking the soles of her feet or rubbing her back. Improvement should be noted within a few seconds. Continue to provide tactile stimulation while listening to the lungs and heart with a stethoscope, talking to the baby and having the parents talk to her. Depending upon other findings, you may also wish to provide blow-by oxygen to enrich the air she is breathing. However, if there is no response or if the responses of the baby seem to be less and less vigorous, begin positive-pressure ventilation using either mouth-to-mask resuscitation or a bag-and-mask.

Placental respiration in the first 3 minutes of life continues as long as the cord is pulsating. This can be taken as a good sign as long as the other vitals are good or improving. It is important to recognize that simply administering free-flowing oxygen or continuing to provide only tactile stimulation to a baby who is not breathing, who is merely gasping, or whose heart rate is below 100 bpm–especially if accompanied by a nonpulsating cord–will significantly delay the full recovery of the baby and can lead to a worsening state of acidosis.

Heart rate: With the stethoscope in place, evaluate the baby's heart rate, even if the respiratory efforts appear effective and you observe overall improvement. The presence of respiratory effort does not, by itself, guarantee that enough oxygen is circulating to sustain heart activity at a rate of 100 bpm or more. Evaluating the heart rate is especially crucial during positive-pressure ventilation as this will indicate if your efforts are proving effective.

Place the diaphragm of an infant stethoscope over the midsternum, slightly to the left of center. The newborn heart is large compared to the rest of the chest; this makes it easy to hear the heart just about anywhere in this general area, so positioning is not critical. Palpating the base of the cord or the brachial artery to monitor heart rate is not as reliable as listening through the chest wall; there may be no palpable pulsations at the base of the cord if the heartbeat is weak, and the brachial artery can be hard to find even in a stable baby. However, if you *can* feel pulsations at 100 bpm or more at the base of the cord, all is well. If the heart rate is slow and the baby is not breathing, you may be able to see the chest pulsate with each heartbeat. You can often feel the heart rate with your fingers through the chest wall, as well; this method can be used to continuously evaluate the heart rate. *If you are unsure, always listen through the chest.* The heart rate should be at least 100 bpm.

Muscle tone: A baby who has some muscle tone or grimace response will usually, but not always, have the reserves to begin breathing on his own once the airway is clear. However, the baby who is limp is likely not to respond to stimulation. Muscle tone can be evaluated by checking the resistance to limb extension, release and the degree of recoil while other resuscitative actions are being taken.

Color: The baby's skin color indicates whether the heart is delivering adequate blood flow to the tissues. Regardless of race, babies are typically lavender pink at birth and quickly change to a rosy pink as arterial oxygen levels rise with the transition to pulmonary respirations and the heart rate stabilizes. This typically occurs during the first 60 to 90 seconds of life. Vasoconstriction may be present if either the respirations or the heart function is compromised, causing the baby to appear pale, to be unable to maintain good color or to display varying degrees of cyanosis. Some babies may still need extra oxygen to maintain good color even though they are breathing on their own and have a heart rate above 100 bpm. Whenever there is doubt, the best places to assess color are the lips and mucous membranes of the mouth. If the baby's torso is bluish, stimulation and perhaps oxygen are called for. If only her extremities are bluish, make sure the baby is warm and dry and continue to observe to make sure cyanosis does not spread to the torso and progress to central cyanosis. Peripheral cyanosis is caused by a combination of a temperature change at the time of birth plus sluggish circulation, but it does not indicate true hypoxemia (poorly saturated arterial blood).

Various Presentations of Neonatal Depression and How to Respond

From here, you must decide how much more, if any, assistance the baby requires.

First, lower the baby below the placenta

If the baby's color is poor at the time of birth, you can assume that vasoconstriction is occurring, although in many cases this may be difficult to access. Therefore, make sure the baby is kept below the level of the placenta the distance which the length of the cord allows, or at least at the same level as the placenta, during resuscitative efforts to help drain blood to the baby if vasoconstriction is active. Leaving the cord intact affords the baby the opportunity to equilibrate his blood volume as he stabilizes; in most cases, you do not have to worry about momentary over- or undertransfusion.

If the baby's heart rate is approximately 100 bpm, there is good muscle tone, the baby is pink and the cord is intact with a good pulse, but there is little perceptible respiratory effort

Provide gentle stimulation, monitor the heart rate and observe. Intervene further only if the baby's heart rate, muscle tone or color do not continue to improve. Spontaneous breathing is likely to start within 60 sec (Richmond, 1996).

If the baby's heart rate is slow and not rising (<100 bpm), the baby is blue pink, the cord is intact and pulsing mildly and there is reasonable muscle tone but little or no perceptible respiratory effort

Provide tactile stimulation, which will often cause a prompt improvement. Lower the baby to the full length of the cord. Begin positive-pressure ventilation immediately to help expand the lungs, even if the infant is making spontaneous breathing attempts. The midwife who is providing ventilations or an assistant should listen to the chest with a stethoscope to ensure that air sounds are heard on both sides of the chest. (See the discussion under the topic "Initial inflation breaths and the newborn lungs," later in this chapter, for details.)

If the baby's APGAR score at birth is 0 to 4, or cord pulsations are sluggish or absent, and the baby is blue

In this case, immediate transferral to pulmonary respiration *is* imperative, although the cord should still remain intact. Even the umbilical vein of a nonpulsating cord may contain a fair amount of blood that can be a valuable source of oxygen and other nutrients and which will gravity-feed to the baby if she is lowered the full length of the cord. Begin ventilations and check the heart rate through the chest wall. Begin full CPR, if indicated. Even a cord that is limp at birth will usually begin to pulse again once the baby comes around.

If the baby is white, limp and cord pulsations are absent

Lower the baby to the full length of the cord. This baby is likely to be severely vasoconstricted or hypovolemic or both. If the cord is white and limp with thin, collapsed vessels (appearing as thin red threads in the cord), it is not likely to start pulsing again, although I recommend you leave it intact until the baby is stable, just in case some blood flow is still possible. Provide CPR, as indicated. Full stabilization will require some sort of volume expansion; if the baby is transported, this will be provided with a transfusion. If the baby is at home, volume expansion with a retention enema is not recommended as absorption and electrolyte effects are too unpredictable in babies, whose total blood volume is so small (Gilhooly, 2003; Morley, 2003).

Stripping the pulseless cord

If the cord is limp, blood can be actively transferred to the baby via cord stripping. Do this by placing your thumb and forefinger on either side of the mother's end of the cord and sliding them down toward the baby while pinching the cord. This provides a bolus of blood to the heart. If there is sufficient blood in the cord, this may, by itself, cause the heart to restart (Morley, 1998). Be aware that babies who are depressed often have limp cords at birth. Gently, slowly and firmly strip the cord five times, releasing it between passes to allow it to fill, or have an assistant do the stripping, and then proceed with ventilation. Do not waste a lot of time trying to milk blood that isn't there. Again, *do not* cut the cord, even though it may be limp, and *do not* delay resuscitative efforts just because the cord is intact. A limp, empty cord delivers no oxygen but can serve as a conduit for blood that will be pumped out of the placenta by the postnatal uterine contractions as long as the placenta remains undelivered and the vessels have not already collapsed. Once delivered, the placenta can be held above the baby, like an IV, until the baby has fully stabilized.

Providing stimulation

The process of labor, being born, being handled, being dried and being talked to all provide a significant amount of stimulation to the newborn. Additional stimulation can be provided choosing one of the methods described here. If the baby does not respond quickly, assume he is in secondary apnea and begin positive-pressure ventilations. While all of these methods have worked, the spinal massage is by far the gentlest and is the method I would recommend.

Stimulate the baby's back by placing your open hand along the spine; use two fingers on either side of the spine and move them up and down, gently but firmly. Another option is to gently insert the very tip of a feeding tube or a bulb syringe in the baby's nostril to stimulate the mucosa. Or, hold one of the baby's feet at the ankle with one hand and briskly slap it with the palm of the other hand or flick it with your fingers on the sole of the foot in the region between the mounds of the big toe and the second toe.

The exception to the general rule of keeping the baby warm is a brief period during which the cold-crying reflex can be stimulated. Briefly place a 4 × 4 in gauze that has been soaked in ice water and then wrung out on the baby's chest for a few seconds. This may get the baby going (Morley, 2002). Remove the gauze once the baby is breathing, or if this has not been enough to bring the baby around, and proceed with warming.

Acupressure or acupuncture techniques: In Chinese medicine, Kidney 1 (K-1) is a primary point used for restoring consciousness, especially concerning the intake of a first breath. According to Chinese medical theory, the kidneys have a special relationship with the lungs, functioning to assist the lungs in drawing in a breath. K-1 is grouped in a special classification of acupuncture points that are the most distal on the extremity, known as "jing well" points. As the jing well of the kidney meridian, Kidney 1 is most suited for resuscitation due to apnea. Applying pressure to this point or inserting an acupuncture needle during resuscitation is a safe and effective means of providing stimulation to breathe. A 25 mm long acupuncture needle is inserted perpendicular to the skin surface to a depth of about ¼ to ½ inch. Alternatively, apply firm finger pressure to the Du-26 (GV-26) point. (For point location, see the subchapter entitled "Traditional Chinese Medicine.") Stimulating this point provides a much stronger stimulation than rubbing the foot or spine. If there is no immediate response, assume secondary apnea, and proceed with appropriate resuscitation protocols.

Homeopathic stimulation: There are several homeopathic remedies that address respiratory distress. The highest available potency should be used. A single pellet can be placed inside the cheek; however, when ventilations may be necessary, crushing a pellet between two clean spoons or dissolving a pellet in a small amount of water will help prevent choking. The crushed pellet can be placed directly in the mouth; it will dissolve almost instantly. A few drops of the liquid can be placed on the tongue with a clean spoon. The dose can be repeated after 10 to 30 seconds; if there is no improvement after three doses, try another remedy. Babies respond extremely well to homeopathy because their constitutions have usually not been influenced by numerous exposures to environmental, dietary or medical contaminants.

Aconitum napellus–fear (did the baby have a scary birth? Shoulder dystocia or the like?)
Antimonium tartaricum–lungs sound full of fluid, difficult resuscitation
Arnica montana–shock from a rapid or difficult birth
Carbo vegetablis–called the "corpse reviver"; for pale, flaccid, death-like appearance
Laurocerasus–face blue or dark, body pale (shoulder dystocia), difficulty with breathing, pulse failing

Rescue Remedy or another emergency flower essence combination can always be given to a baby in distress.

Providing Ventilatory Assistance

Subsequent actions will depend on the baby's response to stimulation; these include handing the baby to her mother, continuing to stimulate and observe, providing blow-by oxygen and beginning artificial ventilations. A midwife who is alone can provide ventilations using a bag-and-mask device but will need to switch to mouth-to-mask ventilations in order to perform chest compressions if these are required. A midwife with an assistant can have her provide compressions while continuing to provide ventilations with a bag-and-mask.

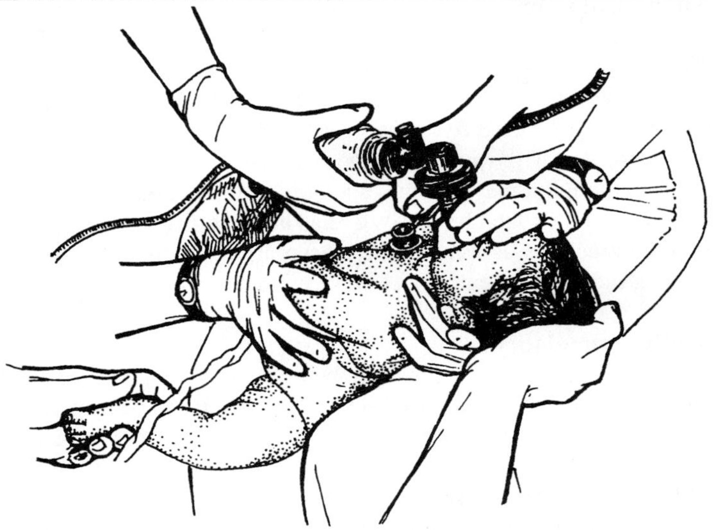

A hands-on resuscitation at home: this 11 lb 8 oz waterbirth baby experienced a 9 min shoulder dystocia and had a 1 min APGAR of 2, 6 and 7 (10 min). The primary midwife has climbed into the tub and holds the baby on her lap and steadies the mask. An apprentice, reaching down from the left, holds the neck in a sniffing position and provides ventilations as the father cradles the head in his hand. The mother is stimulating the baby's foot. Another apprentice auscultates the heart. The cord is intact. This photo was taken near the end of the resuscitation. Color is excellent but the baby is still floppy. The baby is now doing well.

Types of assistance

There are three types of respiratory assistance that you may provide. Please note that the use of oxygen for neonatal resuscitation is increasingly controversial. The following discussion explains various techniques; later in the chapter, the issues regarding whether to use supplemental oxygen at all will be addressed.

Free-flow oxygen (blow-by or wafting oxygen; oxygen-enriched air): This refers to allowing oxygen to escape over the infant's nose from the end of the delivery device so that he breathes oxygen-enriched air. This can be done for a short time by using an oxygen mask or simply oxygen tubing. The oxygen source sends through the tubing 100% oxygen, which then mixes with room air. The concentration of oxygen reaching the baby depends upon the device used, the liter flow of oxygen and the amount of room air it must pass through to reach the baby. Room air contains 21% oxygen. Thus, when 100% oxygen is mixed with room air, the concentration is greater than 21%. An oxygen mask held over the baby's mouth and nose delivers more oxygen because the flow from the tube is closely contained by the mask. Do not use the mask that comes with your resuscitator for this purpose. Never attempt to attach oxygen to a self-inflating resuscitator and hold the mask over the face to deliver free-flow oxygen to the baby. The valve assembly will not allow enough oxygen to flow to the mask, even if a closed-end reservoir is attached.

A simple infant oxygen mask can be slipped onto the end of the oxygen tubing. Alternatively, the oxygen can be concentrated near the baby's nose by holding the tube, pointing down, between your thumb and index finger and cupping your hand around the baby's face. The oxygen flow should be set to 6 l/min; a higher flow rate is not useful and will only serve to chill the baby if the oxygen is not heated. Hold the mask firmly over the baby's face. Close to 100% oxygen can also be delivered when the end of the tubing is connected to an oxygen source and held in this manner. The objective is to provide enough oxygen for the baby to become pink. A baby who requires continued oxygen supplementation will have to be transported to a setting where there is a sufficient supply; the desired oxygen concentration can be determined more accurately and the oxygen can be heated and humidified prior to delivery.

Mouth-to-mask positive-pressure ventilation with your own breath: Mouth-to-mask ventilation replaced mouth-to-mouth-and-nose ventilation with the advent of the AIDS crisis. The mask is placed firmly over the baby's face, covering her nose and mouth; the midwife then forces two cheekfuls of air into the mouthpiece at the other end of the assembly for each ventilation. Two cheekfuls of air per breath approximates the capacity of the newborn lungs. The American Heart Association recommends a rate of 40 to 60 puffs per minute as of this printing in the US (20 to 30 in the UK).

Mouth-to-mouth-and/or-nose ventilation can be used if no equipment is available or if the midwife must perform a full resuscitation by herself on a baby who requires a jaw thrust to maintain an open airway. Wipe or suction fluids from the baby's mouth and nose; cover the baby's mouth and nose (or nose alone while holding the mouth closed) with an open mouth and ventilate using two cheekfuls of air, as above. Gas-permeable barriers are available that can be laid over the baby's face to avoid contamination.

Selecting and positioning a mask on the baby's face: In most circumstances, a mask will be placed over the baby's face to perform ventilations. A properly fitted mask covers the nose and mouth well without putting pressure on the eyes. The pointed end of an anatomically shaped mask is placed over the bridge of the baby's nose, while the wide end cups around the edge of, but not under, the chin. Round masks are applied by centering the mask over the nose and mouth, with the top edge of the rim no higher than the bridge of the nose. The mask is first held at a 45° angle to the face with the edge (the wider edge of an anatomical mask) level with the cleft of the chin, and then laid over the face to cover the nose. Apply just enough pressure to form a good seal around the rim so that air will not escape. Be sure you are not applying excessive pressure or pressing into the throat. Do not let your fingers, parts of your hand or the inflation stem of a cushioned rim rest on the baby's eyes. Use at least one finger to hold the mask against the chin. The seal can be tested by ventilating two or three times and feeling for air leaks around the rim of the mask. Observe for a rise of the chest as the lungs are inflated, which indicates that air is entering the lungs and not escaping around the rim of the mask.

Oxygen concentration of delivered gas

Resuscitation can always begin by ventilating with room air regardless of any later needs of the baby. Whether oxygen is used will depend upon the condition of the baby and her responsiveness. The amount of oxygen delivered using various methods follows. (Actual percentages depend on your equipment, technique and the flow rate of the oxygen):

Mouth-to-mask: 16% to 50% oxygen: Mouth-to-mask resuscitation with expired breath delivers 16% oxygen. Attaching oxygen to the oxygen port on the mask raises the concentration to about 50%.

To deliver room air (21%): A bag and mask can be safely used to ventilate with room air if the reservoir bag is removed first. *Never ventilate with room air alone when the reservoir bag or tube in place, as this will recycle exhaled air and actually decrease the amount of oxygen delivered to below 21%.*

Approximating sea level concentrations of oxygen at moderately high altitudes: In moderately high altitude locations, oxygen is given at a flow rate of 25 to 50 ml/min by nasal cannula to babies to mimic sea level oxygenation in order to maintain their saturation levels above 90%. This can be approximated by giving the breathing baby oxygen by nasal cannula at a flow rate of 1 l/min (Duster, 2004). If no cannula is available, give oxygen by face mask at a flow rate of 5 l/min.

To deliver between 21 to 40% oxygen: Blow-by delivers more than 21% and usually less than 40% but may be much higher, depending upon how closely and effectively the oxygen source is held over the baby's nose.

To deliver 60 to 70% oxygen: A Mercury neonatal resuscitator delivers 60 to 70% concentration when oxygen tubing is attached (flowing at 11 l/min) and the reservoir is removed. The faster and deeper you compress the bag the more room air you will draw in, diluting the oxygen concentration.

To deliver 100% oxygen: A resuscitator delivers nearly 100% oxygen when the oxygen tubing and the oxygen reservoir bag or tube are attached.

Altitude considerations: Boosting the oxygen content of room air is particularly helpful when you are attending births at altitudes where the oxygen content of the air is less than that found at sea level.

Positioning of the person providing ventilations

The person performing either mouth-to-mouth/mask or bag-and-mask ventilation needs to be positioned properly both to hold the mask over the baby's face comfortably and to visualize the baby's chest. There must also be room for a second person to provide chest compressions, if required. Standing to the side of the baby, near to or above the head, will make it easy to watch the chest and will also allow a second person access for providing either two-thumb or two-finger cardiac compressions. Hold the ventilation bag with your dominant hand and the mask with the other. During direct mouth-to-mouth/mask ventilation the baby will have to be supported with one arm under his back or on a baby tray, with the person providing ventilations positioned at the baby's side that she can easily observe the chest and hold the mask over the baby's face comfortably.

Initial inflation breaths and the newborn lungs

Inflation breaths are a concept from the protocols of the United Kingdom and other European countries; they are not discussed in standard US protocols. Uninflated fetal lungs contain about 30 ml/kg of fluid. Labor prompts a variety of physiological changes that halt the production of fluid and begin the process of reabsorption. Although some fluid is squeezed out of the baby's mouth and nose during the birth process, normally more than 100 ml (over 3 oz) is reabsorbed through the alveoli walls into the lymphatic and capillary systems within minutes of birth when the baby begins to breathe. This process occurs most effectively when the baby is allowed to receive his full placental transfusion. The combination of the expansion of the capillary framework around each alveolus and the air provided by the first few breaths expands the alveoli further and helps lung fluid to be absorbed. When a baby has made no effort to breathe on her own or has made only weak efforts, the first several artificial ventilations must overcome pulmonary vascular resistance and assist in the absorption of lung fluid by stimulating blood flow to the alveoli. For this reason, they are often more difficult to perform effectively. Unchallenged pulmonary resistance may result in diverting the flow of gas into the esophagus. In addition, the placental transfusion from an intact cord may be significantly slower in the compromised infant than in the baby who is breathing spontaneously, thus engorgement of the pulmonary capillary beds is often delayed or impaired.

Current recommendations suggest sustained inflation pressures averaging 20 to 30 cm H_2O. Physiological measurements have shown that these pressures, maintained for up to one second, result in mean inflation volumes of approximately 5 ml/kg, which is less than half of that achieved by infants starting to breathe on their own and often insufficient to produce adequate alveolar inflation. In addition, such pressures rarely lead to the development of functional residual capacity. This main reason for these problems is that the inflation volume doesn't reach a plateau. This problem can be overcome by prolonging the first inflation for at least 2 to 3 seconds without increasing the pressure. This more closely approximates the volumes achieved via spontaneously breathing efforts and results in the formation of functional residual capacity. *During the first few ventilations, the most important factor in reviving the baby is delivering sustained inflation at sufficient pressure, not oxygen per se.*

Some authorities recommend ventilating the baby at pressures over 30 cm H_2O during these initial inflations in order to deliver the air at a higher flow rate. However, lung inflation depends more on the volume of air delivered, which is a result of flow and time, than on pressure. Air delivered at a lower pressure for a sustained rate of flow will be just as effective as that delivered in shorter bursts under higher pressure as long as the pressure delivered exceeds the opening pressure of the lung. In fact, preterm infants are at risk for damage to the lining of the alveoli if too great a volume or too great a pressure of gas is used (Milner, 2001). The first two or three inflation ventilations will only help press fluid down through the respiratory tract where it can be absorbed but will not significantly alter the volume of the lungs. The chest will usually not start to rise until the fourth or fifth initial ventilation.

Direct mouth-to-mask ventilation: Ventilations are provided in the same manner as when using a resuscitator. Sustain the ventilations during the first 5 to 6 breaths by giving the baby slightly more air, more slowly than you normally would, stretching it over a 2 sec interval. Then allow the air to escape. After the chest is rising, continue with ventilations as described below.

Using a bag-and-mask resuscitator

To stabilize the mask: Use your nondominant hand to secure the mask over the baby's face. Spread your thumb and index finger and place the stem of the mask in the crook of these fingers. Distribute the pressure from your hand around the part of the mask that flares just below the stem; this will most effectively assist in sealing the rim against the baby's face. Avoid applying direct pressure to the rim with your fingers. Rest stray fingers on bony regions of the baby's face (such as the upper mandible), avoiding the eyes. Use your ring and little finger to assist in keeping the mouth open or in bringing the chin forward, if necessary, to maintain a sniffing position. Do not rest any part of your hand on the baby's neck, and take care not to depress the jaw backward with the weight of your hand. Do not jam the mask down over the baby's face as this can cause bruising. Be sure the baby's neck is slightly extended as described above in "Open the airway." If an assistant is available, she can listen for lung inflation and heart rate with a stethoscope and check for oxygen saturation with an oximeter while you provide ventilations. This can be most informative as you proceed.

To compress the ventilation bag: Use your dominant hand to manipulate the ventilation bag. Place your thumb on one side of the bag and your index and middle fingers on the other. Using two fingers opposite the thumb provides effective stabilization of the bag, preventing dropping or slippage. Compress the bag with the fingertips. Do not grab the bag and squeeze it with your whole hand, as this is likely to deliver gas at too high a pressure, and you will not be as sensitive to resistance in the bag as you will be using your fingertips.

The pressure required to inflate the newborn lungs varies depending upon the baby's size, the condition of his lungs, and whether he has already taken a breath. The volume of a resuscitation bag far exceeds the volume of the newborn lungs, which averages about 20 to 30 ml. For the baby who has made no attempt to breathe on his own, sustained inflations are given during the first 5 or 6 initial ventilations.

Providing inflation breaths: Sustaining an inflation can be tricky when using a self-inflating bag and is something you should practice with your own equipment. Slowly compress the bag by placing your thumb on one side and two fingers on the other to lightly bring your fingers together halfway toward the center. The edges of the valve assembly (over the mask coupler) should part for a full two to three seconds. The pop-off valve need not release, as these ventilations are usually adequate when delivered at about 30 cm H_2O after 30 weeks gestation. Ventilations that are too short will be ineffective while those delivered at too high a pressure can injure the baby's lungs. Squeeze the bag slowly and firmly while slowly counting "One-one-thousand, two-one-thousand, three-release," to sustain the pressure for 2 to 3 seconds. The limited volume of the bag will make overinflation unlikely. These sustained ventilations should be sufficient to overcome the resistance of the uninflated, fluid filled lungs.

After a few of these long ventilations, the lungs should be cleared of fluid and the chest should rise. As soon as you see the chest rise, continue to ventilate, using ventilations of shorter duration. Watch for an easy rise and fall of the chest, although adequate ventilation is also indicated by a rising heart rate, lung sounds and rising oxygen saturation.

Infant response to face-mask ventilation: Studies have shown that self-inflating bags vary widely in their ability to deliver effective ventilations, primarily a result of insufficiently sustained pressures, which do not achieve adequate tidal exchange. In spite of this, most infants respond favorably to ventilation efforts due to the inflation reflex described in the subchapter entitled "Autonomic Neuromuscular Reflexes and the Baby's Response to Resuscitation."

Ventilatory rate: Opinions vary as to the ideal ventilatory rate. That recommended in the United Kingdom is 20 to 30 ventilations/min, while the American Heart Association recommends a rate of 40 to 60 ventilations/min. UK sources emphasize that both inflation and time to allow the lungs to deflate are equally important. A study done in 1999 by Whyte and associates (1999) found that competent, experienced providers have difficulty maintaining a rate of 40 vpm, even over a 5 min period. Out of 33 rescuers, none could deliver 40 ventilations per minute for 5 full minutes. Only 4 out of 18 two-person teams could give 40 ventilations/min during the first minute. All ventilations were counted, even those that were not totally effective.

The phrase "breathe-two-three-breathe-two-three" (waltz time) can be used to maintain the proper rhythm of ventilations. A compression is provided with the word "breathe," the bag released for the count of two-three, then compressed again on "breathe."

VENTILATIONS	COMMENTS & PROTOCOLS
First 5 to 6 breaths	Initial lung inflation may require pressures of about 30 cm H_2O after 30 weeks gestation sustained for 2 to 3 seconds with each ventilation.
Succeeding breaths	Pressures of 15 to 20 cm H_2O are often adequate after the lungs have been inflated the first few times. These are delivered at a rate of 20-30 ventilations/min (UK) or 40 to 60 ventilations/min (US).
Pulmonary disease	Babies with respiratory conditions that interfere with normal lung function may require pressures of 20 to 40 cm H_2O for each ventilation. These babies may also require a slower rate as well.

Dangers of high-pressure ventilation: To avoid damage to the lungs, it is imperative to use the minimum positive pressure sufficient to bring about a steady improvement (Dunn, 1988). Excessively high ventilatory pressures are generally only required when the alveolar capillary beds are totally collapsed from established hypovolemia, cord clamping or both. Air delivered at too high a pressure or at too great a volume can injure the baby's lungs. It is therefore imperative to remain calm and go through the steps of resuscitation in an orderly fashion. By moving smoothly from one step to the next, you are unlikely to hurt the baby. Be sure to focus on the baby, rather than the equipment (e.g., do not watch the manometer and lose track of what is happening with the baby's chest).

Ventilate for 30 seconds: The vast majority of babies will come around during the first few seconds. Even in babies whose heart rate was below 100 bpm, the rate will almost always begin to rise as soon as adequate lung inflation is established, thus ventilation is recommended for a full 30 sec before cardiac compression is even considered.

Check the heart rate: After the first 30 seconds of ventilation, recheck the heart rate by listening with a stethoscope or by feeling for the pulse either at the umbilical base or over the chest wall. To minimize the time required, you can listen to the heart for 5 seconds and multiply by 12, as you do when listening to the baby during labor.

It is rare that a baby will require chest compressions. A slow heart rate usually reflects severe myocardial compromise due to prolonged lack of oxygen, so the heart rate of most babies will immediately improve once ventilations have begun. It is exceeding rare for the heart rate to remain low if adequate ventilations are provided. In most cases, a lack of cardiac response indicates that the lungs have not been adequately inflated. If the heart rate remains low, reassess whether you are adequately ventilating the baby by observing whether the chest is rising.

It is impossible to use a self-inflating device for ventilation and provide chest compressions simultaneously. If chest compressions are needed, you must either set aside your resuscitation device and use direct mouth-to-mouth/mask ventilation or enlist the assistance of a second person.

Assessing the effectiveness of ventilation

Watch to be sure the baby's chest is rising and falling with each ventilation. Once the lungs are have been inflated initially, chest rise is the best gauge of adequate ventilation. If the chest is not expanding or if it expands too much, you need to make some adjustments. If the contour of the chest is uneven or enlarged with a sunken belly, see the subchapter entitled "Complicated Respiratory Distress." If the chest does not expand, it may be due to the following reasons:

- The seal around the rim of the mask is inadequate.
- The airway is blocked.
- You not have adequately inflated the lungs during the initial ventilations.
- You are giving inadequate puffs or not using enough pressure.

Is there a good seal? A poor seal around the mask is the primary cause of inadequate ventilations. If this is the problem, you will feel air escaping around your lips or the rim of the mask. Reposition the mask and try to form a better seal by increasing your pressure on the mask slightly. The most common point of leakage is between the cheek and the bridge of the nose. Squeezing the ventilation bag harder and harder will not compensate for a poor seal. You must reposition the mask until an adequate seal is established. Switch to a differently-shaped mask if you cannot achieve an adequate seal with the one you are using. Overall, round masks tend to produce a better seal on newborns.

Is the airway blocked? The neonatal trachea is relatively compressible, and simply having the neck flexed too far forward will result in obstruction. If you suspect a blocked airway, check the position of the baby's head and reposition as necessary. Try extending it slightly more. Check the nose, mouth and oropharynx for secretions. Meconium may be so thick as to completely block the airway. Suction if indicated. Once blockage is ruled out, you can try ventilating with the baby's mouth slightly open. Placement of an oral airway will facilitate this.

If there is no evidence of debris blockage, consider hypoplastic lungs, a diaphragmatic hernia, pneumothorax or some other defect that prevents normal respirations. Suspect a structurally blocked airway if the baby is gasping with sternal retractions but cannot establish respirations. See the subchapter entitled "Complicated Respiratory Distress" for details.

Laryngospasm: Laryngospasm is a part of the distal esophageal reflexive response to stimulation; such spasm can prevent lung inflation. Positive pressure can be used to treat partial airway obstruction or laryngospasm. This works because the positive pressure pushes the vocal cords downward and slightly apart. Once the cords separate even slightly, the positive pressure expands the space below them, which forces the arytenoids apart, opening the airway. However, the concavity of an infant's cords can cause them to overlap under positive pressure, whereas adult cords, being more horizontal, usually separate more easily. Therefore, to break laryngospasm in a baby, combine positive pressure with chin thrust. Thrusting the chin forward puts tension on the arytenoids and pulls them apart, producing a gap between the vocal cords. This allows air to enter the laryngeal cavity and usually breaks up the spasm. While you will not be able to tell if laryngospasm is the problem, this technique is not harmful and should be tried if the airway seems to be otherwise clear.

Inadequate inflation: You may not be able to provide enough opening pressure for the initial few ventilations if the volume of your bag is less than 500 ml (although the neonatal bag and mask by Mercury should allow you to do so). Do not use an adult bag; you may need to resort to mouth-to-mask ventilation for a few breaths to ensure that adequate ventilatory pressures are sustained sufficiently to open the lungs. Then go back to using a bag-and-mask.

Persistently inadequate ventilation: If the mask seal is adequate, you have carefully delivered several inflation breaths and there is still no chest rise, try increasing the pressure of each compression until the pop-off valve activates. If you still do not have adequate inflation, recheck the airway and consider congenital defects of the airway as a possible cause. Try inserting an oropharyngeal airway and try to ventilate again.

Does the baby require continued positive-pressure ventilation?

The following recommendations assume that the cord is intact and the baby is positioned at or below the level of the placenta.

If the heart rate is 100 bpm or more and the baby is breathing well: Discontinue ventilations and observe the baby closely. Continue to provide tactile stimulation and possibly blow-by oxygen, depending on the baby's condition. If the baby's breathing once again becomes irregular or shallow or tapers off, immediately resume ventilations.

If the heart rate is rising or is steady at 100 bpm or more, the baby's color is good or improving, and some spontaneous breathing efforts have begun: Move the mask aside for a second or two. This will allow you to see if the baby is making respiratory efforts on her own. If so, stand by, ready to provide ventilatory assistance again if needed. Based on the baby's heart rate, color, oxygen saturation and muscle tone, you may choose to give the baby blow-by oxygen; observe for continued improvement. If none is seen, quickly resume ventilations.

If the heart rate is between 60 and 100 bpm: Continue to listen to the heart for more than 6 seconds. If the rate is rising, continue to ventilate, watching closely for signs that the baby is trying to establish spontaneous respirations.

If the heart rate is 60 to 100 bpm and not increasing or is dropping: Continue ventilating while checking for adequate inflation. Have an assistant listen to the chest with a stethoscope to make sure breath sounds are adequate. If the heart rate is below 60 after an initial period of ventilation with room air, the baby is in serious trouble.

If the heart rate is less than 60 bpm: Begin chest compressions (see details below). There is no longer adequate tissue perfusion when the newborn heart rate drops below 50 bpm. Therefore, the American Heart Association and the American Academy of Pediatrics have chosen 60 bpm as the cut-off for the initiation of chest compressions (Kattwinkel et al., 2011). Compression of the heart between the chest wall and the spine moves blood in and out of the ventricles.

Orogastric intubation

If ventilations are required for longer than several minutes, insertion of an orogastric tube is recommended. However, if the baby's condition is improving and you anticipate being able to discontinue ventilations shortly, do not place an orogastric tube, as this may trigger a vasovagal response. Placing a tube is most useful in babies that have deformities of the mouth, throat or gastrointestinal tract but helps to prevent gastric distension in all babies. If you notice that the stomach is becoming distended, placement of a tube will increase the effectiveness of ventilations. See the subchapter entitled "Orogastric Intubation of the Newborn" for details about how to do so.

Providing chest compressions (external cardiac massage)

Assess the heart rate after 30 seconds of effective ventilations. Begin chest compressions if the baby's heart rate is below 60 bpm. Minutes after all spontaneous gasping has ceased, systemic blood pressure falls to the point that all circulation stops. Even though regular but ineffective ventricular activity may still be occurring and, at times, may be detectable with a stethoscope, pulmonary circulation stops if the heart rate fails to accelerate once ventilations have begun. This leads to reduced perfusion as well as a fall in the amount of oxygen that reaches vital tissues; there is no pulsation at the umbilicus and the skin is pale. Even at this point, all that is usually required to revive the heart muscle is sufficient oxygen; a short period of cardiac compressions may be enough to restore cardiac perfusion and pump a little oxygenated blood into the coronary arteries where it will supply the heart muscle (Richmond et al., 2011).

Chest compressions manually pump the blood. This pumping action is not as efficient as spontaneous cardiac activity but is often enough to sustain life until the heart begins to beat again on its own. Appropriate movement of the blood occurs because compression increases the intrathoracic pressure as the heart's ventricles are squeezed between the sternum and spine. The pulmonary and aortic valves direct the blood forward into the arterial circulation rather than into the veins because of the venous valves at the thoracic inlet and because the muscular arterial walls keep the lumen of the arteries open while the thin-walled veins collapse. Blood is also squeezed from the chest by the increased intrathoracic pressure. Releasing pressure for a sufficient amount of time allows the elastic recoil of the chest to pull blood from the aorta into the ventricles. Chest compressions should begin *only* after effective ventilations have been established. Positive pressure ventilation should always be interspersed with chest compressions so that the blood being artificially circulated contains oxygen. Do not attempt to provide a ventilation and to compress the chest simultaneously. To do so compromises tidal volume in the lungs and increases the risk of injuring the lungs and producing a pneumothorax as well as diminishing blood flow to the heart muscle, thus rendering both activities ineffective (Richmond et al., 2011).

Dangers of chest compressions: Enough pressure must be provided to pump the heart while avoiding damage to surrounding organs, particularly the liver, which partly underlies the lower border of the rib cage on the baby's right. Misplaced pressure over the xiphoid can result in laceration of the liver. The newborn ribs are easily broken, especially if the baby is preterm, although breakage in a term baby is most likely when disease is present. Misplaced pressure over the ribs can crack a rib and produce a pneumothorax.

The goal of chest compressions: The American Heart Association (Kattwinkel, 2011), recommends that compressions be performed at a rate of 3 per second, with a pause after every third compression to allow time for one ventilation (overall, 3 compressions and one ventilation in a 2 sec period). This provides 90 compressions and 30 ventilations per minute for a total of 120 resuscitative events. Fewer ventilations are thus performed with compressions than when given alone to prevent breaths and compressions from being delivered at the same time. If a ventilation appears to have been inadequate, take time to deliver a second ventilation before resuming compressions (Aloan, 1987).

The UK Resuscitation Counsel's guidelines (Richmond et al., 2011) point out that both compressions and chest recoil are equally important. Attempts to reproduce a normal neonatal heart action are useless because compressions are not as efficient as normal cardiac function. Therefore, while also recommending the 3:1 ratio, they acknowledge that slowing the rate of compression is often necessary to allow the heart to fully refill. They also acknowledge that the goal of resuscitation in newborns is different than in adults. In adults, a primary cardiac arrest requires that oxygenated blood be circulated to the brain and heart because there is a problem in the heart muscle that must be corrected. In babies, physiological limits have been exceeded in a body that is otherwise in perfect shape (in most cases); thus it is oxygenation and perfusion and not the heart muscle itself that has failed. The goal is therefore to provide enough oxygen to the heart muscle to "jump start" the system, after which it should work normally. Therefore, the purpose of compression is to move a few teaspoonfuls of oxygenated blood from the pulmonary veins to the coronary arteries, a distance of about 5 cm, providing enough oxygen to the heart muscle so that it can then resume functioning on its own.

The American Heart Association states that properly performed cardiac massage *will* move blood to vital organs. An EMT with 15 years of experience reports that newborns with no spontaneous cardiac function can become pink to the toes with compressions and ventilations alone (Schleiff, 2002). This suggests that heart massage effectively circulates blood throughout the body, although the points regarding the importance of compression plus recoil are well taken.

Positioning your hands for chest compressions: There are two ways to provide chest compressions; with two thumbs or with two fingers. With either method, the baby's back must be firmly supported and the neck slightly extended. Each compression should be delivered in the same location and to the same depth. The torso should be bare to facilitate visual monitoring to confirm that the hand position does not migrate as compressions are given and to prevent slippage on cloth.

Two-thumb technique: The thumb technique appears to be the best, safest and least tiring if compressions are required for a prolonged period. It has been shown to result in a higher mean arterial pressure (Peliowski & Finner, 1992), higher coronary perfusion pressure and may provide better cerebral perfusion pressure. The two thumbs are used to compress the sternum, with the hands encircling the torso. The thumb *tips* can be placed side by side or, on a small baby, one pad overlies the other. The rest of the hand and fingers encircle the upper torso to offer back support. To minimize the chance of injury, pressure should be applied with the thumb tips *only*. The fingers should simply provide support, with the pressure exerted directly down toward the spine with the thumb tips from the chest side. This technique can be performed from the head or the foot of the baby, although working from the head end may interfere with ventilations.

This method has some drawbacks. It cannot be used effectively if the baby is large and your hands are quite small. Care must be taken to avoid squeezing the thorax, which may result in changes in intrathoracic pressure, compromising circulation or ventilation or both. Because it requires two hands, this technique cannot be used for one-person CPR.

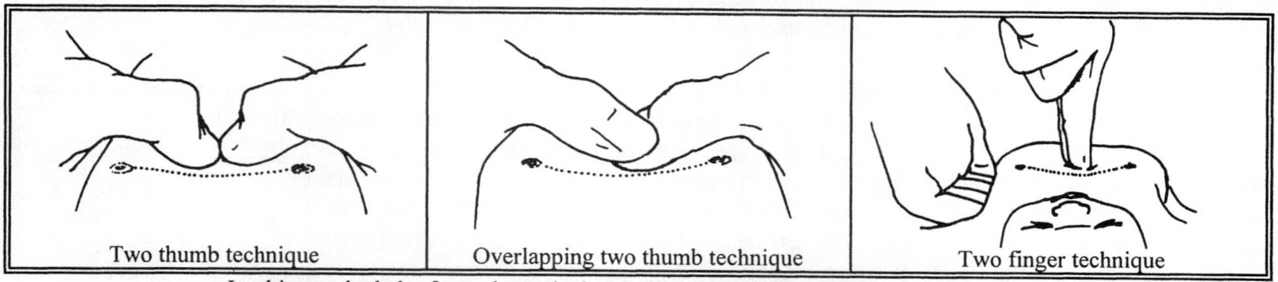

Looking at the baby from above the head. (illustrations after Richmond, et al., 2000)

Two-finger technique: The tips of the middle finger and either the index or ring finger of one hand are used to compress the sternum. You will probably find it easiest to use your dominant hand for compressions. Position the two fingers at a right-angle (perpendicular) to the chest wall and press with your fingertips. Long nails will interfere with proper compressions and can injure the baby. If your nails are long, use the two-thumb technique. The other hand is used to support the infant's back, unless the infant is on a very firm surface. The supporting hand can also monitor the pressure and depth of compressions. This method is preferred if the baby is large or your hands are small. This is the only method you can use if you must provide full CPR by yourself.

Chest compressions are easy in newborns, as the rib cage is very flexible. Pressure is applied to the lower third of sternum, taking care not to press on the xiphoid process. To locate the proper site, draw an imaginary line between the baby's nipples; the proper region of the sternum lies between this line and the upper border of the xiphoid process. It is safest to press the area just below the nipple line, which is still recommended in the UK. The US protocols now suggest that the region just above the xiphoid is preferable; this requires vigilance to make sure your hands to not drift downward over the xiphoid itself. Compressions should be performed to a depth approximately one-third the depth of the torso (or one-third of the distance between the sternum and the spine). The compression should be a firm, rapid stroke downward. Release should be slower. The fingertips or thumbs should remain in continuous contact with the sternum during release so that they do not become misplaced.

Realistic ventilation/compression ratios: The recommended rate for full CPR is three compressions for every breath, with 90 compressions and 30 rpm, thus 3 compressions and one ventilation are to be delivered every 2 seconds. The suggested rhythm for delivery is "one-and-two-and-three-and-breathe." However, there is nothing magical about the chosen ratio of 3 compressions to 1 ventilation for neonates. The current recommendation for adults is 15 compressions to 2 ventilations, while for children of all other ages it is 5:1. In the United States, a 5:1 ratio is recommended when performing chest compressions combined with mask-to-mouth-and-nose ventilations on a newborn. The 3:1 ratio is *only* recommended for newborns receiving chest compressions and ventilations with a bag-and-mask device. However, the results of the 1999 study of ventilatory rates by Whyte and colleagues indicate that this rate is virtually impossible to sustain for the majority of skilled providers. In their paper they state that, based on analysis of the number of truly effective ventilations they observed, "... only 75% of paired rescuers and only 25% of single rescuers would be able to achieve the lower rates advocated by the American Heart Association."

There is apparently no scientific justification for these varying neonatal protocols. Therefore, let practicality and effective care be your guide. If you feel you can deliver more effective resuscitative events, whether they be ventilations or chest compressions, using a slightly slower rate, then do so. Focus on quality rather than quantity. Hastily performed, sloppy procedures will not provide better support even if they accomplish the 120 events-per-minute goal and are more likely to damage or further compromise the baby.

Assessing circulation: After 45 to 60 seconds of effective compressions plus ventilations, stop all activities and check the heart rate for 6 seconds and add a zero to the result. Resume ventilations only if the baby is not breathing on his own. Resume compressions only if the heart rate is still below 60 bpm. In almost every case, the heart rate will rise dramatically once the delivery of adequate ventilations and the stimulation of chest compressions have begun.

Peripheral circulation can be assessed by using your fingerpad to blanche the skin on the sternum and the arm. Check to see how long it takes for the original color to be restored. The skin should pink up within 3 seconds if perfusion is adequate. Ideally, a pulse can be detected with each and every cardiac compression.

Using oxygen during neonatal resuscitation

Minutes of Age	O_2 Saturation
1 min	60 to 65%
2 min	65 to 70 %
3 min	70 to 75%
4 min	75 to 80%
5 min	80 to 85%
10 min	85 to 95%
1st 24 hrs	95 to 99%

Oxygen is not necessary for basic resuscitation and most newborns can be successfully resuscitated using room air alone (Saugstad, 1996). Fetuses thrive in a relatively low oxygen environment. During the first minutes of transition to pulmonary respiration, the baby's brain can still be supported at a relatively lower oxygen concentration than that of an adult but seems to fare very poorly in the presence of poor perfusion; keeping the cord intact helps to maintain perfusion. It is now recommended to use a pulse oximeter to assess oxygen saturation, the goal being to use only enough oxygen to match the normal saturation in an uncompromised term baby. It takes time for oxygen levels to rise from fetal to newborn levels. (The values in this table are from hospital-born babies whose cord was cut. We do not yet have normal values on babies with intact cords and no hospital interventions.) A probe attached to the right hand, which receives blood from the aorta before it reaches the ductus arteriosus, measures the oxygen levels delivered to vital organs. (See your oximeter manual for exactly how to use it). Oximeters must be used carefully, are tricky to master and notorious for false readings. Always look at the baby first.

High oxygen concentration can be damaging (Thornberg et al., 1995). Overuse encourages the increased production of free radicals. These highly reactive oxygen metabolites are produced as a by-product of normal cell respiration and are converted to water by cellular antioxidants, through pathways involving the mitochondrial respiratory chain enzymes (Clark, 1999). However, following prolonged periods of hypoxia, tissue levels of hypoxanthine (a by-product of protein breakdown) increase markedly in any event. When animals or humans are exposed to high levels of oxygen, excessively high levels of reactive oxidants (e.g., superoxide, hydrogen peroxide, and perhydrol radicals) are formed. This tendency is enhanced in the presence of high hypoxanthine levels. Very high levels of oxidants overwhelm the antioxidant system and can oxidize enzymes, inhibit protein and DNA synthesis, decrease surfactant synthesis and cause lipid peroxidation. The preterm infant is particularly vulnerable to free-radical-induced lung and brain injury because the antioxidant system develops during the last trimester. Thus, overproduction of oxygen free radicals can quickly exceed the antioxidant capacity of the preterm neonate and initiate a lung-injury sequence that, if uninterrupted, leads to the development of diffuse alveolar damage and progressive pulmonary dysfunction and may result in death (Clark, 1999). Nitrogen, the most abundant room air gas, is responsible for surfactant secretion, the chemical that prevents collapse of the alveoli at end expiration. Too much oxygen displaces nitrogen and can result in decreased surfactant production, leading to alveoli collapse, especially in preterm infants.

However, if the newborn's oxygen saturations remain below normal despite effective ventilation, ventilation should be augmented with oxygen to bring the saturation up to age-appropriate levels. Oxygen concentration sufficient to raise the saturation levels into the 90s may also warranted in the presence of severe lung complications, such as pulmonary defects or immature lungs that are not responding to ventilations with room air alone. Supplemental oxygen should be discontinued as soon as possible and the baby monitored to see if his oxygen saturation is maintaining itself in a normal range (Saugstad, 2001).

Monitoring the Baby Who Has Required Resuscitation

Monitoring recovery

In general, the baby recovers function in reverse order from the sequence of loss. For example, for the baby who has been in terminal apnea, once the heart is pumping at a rate of 100 bpm or more, the next sign of recovery will be anoxic gasping once every 10 to 20 seconds. Normal, regular breathing will then be established. Color will improve within 3 to 5 minutes and tone return to the limbs in 15 to 20 minutes, depending, of course, on the degree of compromise to begin with. Once the heart rate normalizes, the length of time before normal respiration begins (with or without intermittent gasping) is important because this is a very direct measure of the insult to the central nervous system. Once the baby is quite stable and in no further need of assistance, break open a vitamin E capsule and give the baby a few drops on her tongue. You may also apply it to the mother's nipples. This potent antioxidant will help the baby's body detoxify antioxidants formed during resuscitation (Ettinghausen, [1981?]).

Signs of stabilization: Immediate improvement is indicated by an increasing heart rate and oxygen levels, improving color and spontaneous respirations. The next steps depend on the baby's response to ventilatory efforts. Ventilations should be continued as the heart rate rises toward normal, with ongoing monitoring of the chest to avoid over- or underinflation of the lungs. The rate and pressure of assisted ventilations should gradually be reduced when the heart rate stabilizes above 100 bpm, especially if there are signs that the baby is trying to breathe on his own. When the baby begins breathing spontaneously, blow-by oxygen can be given if indicated, especially if the heart rate has been low.

Ventilations can be discontinued when the baby is breathing on her own and her heart rate is above 100 bpm. Continue to provide gentle tactile stimulation until the rate and depth of respirations is adequate. The baby should be carefully observed to be sure that she is able to maintain a normal breathing pattern on her own and that the heart rate remains stable. With improvement, the baby should have normal oxygen levels and become completely pink.

If there is no improvement or the baby's condition worsens: Have someone else call for transport to the nearest neonatal intensive care facility with a Level III nursery, if one is within a reasonable distance. Do not attempt to provide prolonged resuscitation at home. It is better to transport sooner rather than later, when you may be too tired to continue to offer adequate support. Resuscitation is tiring. Provide continuous support until you can transfer care to skilled personnel or until the hospital staff can take over. Transport by ambulance is preferable to a private vehicle because there must be sufficient room for both people who are providing support to the baby to position themselves for continued effective care while en route. You must anticipate that the baby may require cardiac compression even if that hasn't been the case prior to leaving the house. You will need help in getting the baby out the door and into the transport vehicle, possibly with oxygen tank in tow, while continuously performing resuscitative efforts.

If the baby is not responding, when should resuscitation efforts cease?

This is a difficult call to make in any event and is not one that the midwife should decide unless she has no other choice. A baby who has not stabilized very shortly after resuscitative efforts begin is in grave danger either from pronounced asphyxia, from an injury such as a pneumothorax or from an anomaly. Transport the baby to the nearest neonatal intensive care unit, even if you are fairly certain that the baby will not survive. Refer to the transport protocols in the chapter entitled "Transporting the Newborn: An Overview."

Those midwives who are far from medical help or working where no such help is available may have to decide for themselves when to stop. The 2011 American Heart Association recommendations state that discontinuation of resuscitation efforts may be appropriate after 10 minutes of absent heart rate in spite of complete, timely and adequate resuscitation (Kattwinkel et al., 2011) . Current data shows that resuscitation of newborns after 10 minutes of absent heart rate is very unlikely to result in survival without severe disability and that many of these babies will die soon after birth. Discontinuing your efforts may be warranted if you have exceeded these time limits and the baby is still totally unresponsive. However, the parents should be the ones to make the final decision. If they request that you continue in your efforts, you are obligated to continue for as long as you are physically able to do so. Be sure to scrupulously document your procedures, parental discussions and the baby's condition as soon as you can.

Unusual circumstances that hinder effective resuscitative efforts

There are a number of uncommon and rare disorders that may impair your ability to effectively resuscitate some infants. These are covered in the subchapter entitled "Complicated Respiratory Distress."

Evaluating the Apparently Normal Baby Who Develops Respiratory Distress

This chapter gives you an overview of what might be causing acute respiratory distress that develops in an infant who appears normal at birth and has previously been stable. Normal parameters and assessment for newborn breathing are covered in the chapters entitled "The Healthy Full-Term Newborn in the First Hours of Life" and from a slightly different perspective in the subchapter entitled "Examining the Chest, Lungs and Heart." As many as 10% of all babies have some form of respiratory distress in the first hours of life, but most recover quickly. Many of these babies are born prior to term. In addition, this statistic is derived from populations of hospital-born babies subjected to traumatic hospital routines and is thus higher than it will be at home.

When faced with respiratory distress, you must consider the entire situation when making your assessment. Most term infants who display what is considered minor respiratory variations are experiencing normal transitional respiratory adaptations secondary to physiological cord closure. Adaptive signs and symptoms may become more pronounced when the baby experiences stressful emotions from the birth process. Gentle supportive measures that help the baby clear the airway, integrate the feelings and transition into normal diaphragmatic breathing are appropriate as long as the heart is around 100 bpm, the baby is breathing well, the airway is open, skin color is good and the baby is making continual improvement. These measures include remaining with his mother, nursing and being cuddled, talked to and kept warm. Sometimes a warm bath is very helpful to calm these infants as well.

However, there are other reasons why a baby might experience respiratory distress. Excessive fluid in the lungs is the most common, followed by infection (especially pneumonia), immature lungs coupled with poor perfusion, meconium aspiration or, much more rarely, an abnormality of the pulmonary system that can lead to respiratory distress after birth. Narrowing down what the problem might be can help you decide how to proceed and if transport is warranted. This chapter introduces some problems covered in more detail in the subchapter entitled "Complicated Respiratory Distress."

Distinguishing Normal Transitional Respiratory Signs, Symptoms and Behaviors from Pathology

Normal transitional respiration is covered in the chapter entitled "The Healthy Full-Term Newborn in the First Hours of Life." Since babies who receive a full placental transfusion often experience breathing patterns that mimic respiratory distress after birth, difficulty arises in trying to differentiate a sign or symptom that reflects a healthy variation from those that reflect a serious problem. Our understanding of the normal transitional respiratory symptoms has been altered because in the medical model, cords are clamped immediately, thus physiological respiratory transition is not fully appreciated by mainstream neonatology. You must be alert for signs of normal respiratory transition while keeping an eye out for those babies whose symptoms reflect pathology. Normal respiratory transition has these characteristics:

- Auscultation reveals normal, well distributed breath sounds through clear or minimally junky lungs.
- Symptoms are generally mild and transient.
- The baby's skin color and appearance are consistently normal.
- Heart rate is normal and varies normally with activity.
- The baby's temperature is stable (assuming the baby is suitably clothed or skin to skin with the mother in a reasonably warm environment).
- The baby's behavior, facial expressions and general demeanor are those of a normal term infant and do not suggest that the baby is stressed or struggling to breathe.
- The baby makes normal transitions from one state of consciousness to another.
- Respiratory symptoms do not become worse with activity or handling.
- If the distress is due to chilling, anger or fear, the symptoms dissipate with warmth, maternal contact and comforting.
- Symptoms gradually resolve over time.
- The baby can nurse easily with no aggravation of her respiratory symptoms.
- Breath sounds, vocalizations and crying all sound normal with a normal pitch.
- The baby sneezes intermittently (rather than coughs) to help clear her airways.
- As signs and symptoms resolve they do not return.
- The only symptom that lingers past the initial transition period is shallow, rapid breathing.
- Rapid breathing slows somewhat when the baby is asleep.

These things plus your overall impression of the baby's well-being should be continuously assessed until you are satisfied that the baby is well and healthy.

Assessing respiratory distress

Consider the following when evaluating the possible reasons for respiratory distress in the otherwise normal baby:

History: Review maternal and fetal history to rule out certain serious causes of respiratory distress.

Estimated gestational age: Review the probable gestational age of the baby, based on maternal menstrual and intercourse history, presumed date of conception, fetal growth during pregnancy and the appearance and behavior of the baby. Preterm babies are prone to breathing difficulties, and dysmature and postterm babies are more likely to pass meconium, making aspiration a possibility.

Quantity of amniotic fluid: A history of chronic leaking of fluid or frank oligohydramnios can be associated with pulmonary hypoplasia and other fetal anomalies such as tracheoesophageal fistula, nonimmune hydrops, pleural effusions and myotonic dystrophy.

Labor and birth: A febrile mother, prolonged rupture of membranes, foul-smelling amniotic fluid or the use of excessive manipulation during the birth are all associated with neonatal pneumonia. Placenta previa or abruption, as well as cord rupture or hematoma, increase the likelihood of hypovolemia. Meconium passage is a prerequisite for aspiration and is also seen with asphyxia causing transient cardiac ischemia. Traumatic birth from shoulder dystocia, severe extension of the head, or breech delivery may result in intracranial hemorrhage or phrenic nerve palsy, which can produce RDS.

Time of onset of signs and symptoms: Babies who develop acute respiratory distress and transient tachypnea usually present in the first few hours of life. Sepsis, heart defects and intracranial hemorrhage must all be considered as possibilities if respiratory distress develops after several hours of normal breathing. Choking and coughing with the first attempt to nurse may be due to a cleft palate or tracheoesophageal fistula.

Respiratory scoring systems

Like the APGAR score, the Downes system (1970) below and the Silverman-Andersen scoring system (1956) that follows both offer a means of quantifying respiratory symptoms that takes into account many visible signs of distress. These scores are best used at the onset of distress so that a baseline can be established, with repeated assessments to be performed at regular, frequent intervals until the distress resolves or until the decision to transport has been made.

DOWNES RESPIRATORY DISTRESS ASSESSMENT	0	1	2
Respiratory rate per minute	60	60-80	>80 or apneic episode
Cyanosis	None	In room air	Breathing 40% oxygen
Retractions	None	Mild	Moderate to severe
Grunting	None	Audible with stethoscope	Audible with naked ear
Air entry (inspiratory sounds heard in midaxillary line)	Clear	Delayed or decreased	Barely audible

The Downes scoring system can be used when the distress is mild. The Silverman-Andersen score was developed through researching preterm infants who were ill. I have modified it slightly to more accurately reflect the types of findings that are within a normal range for term babies who have received a full placental transfusion. A total of zero means no evidence of respiratory distress is present, while a score of 7 or more indicates impending respiratory failure. These are not the only criteria to observe, however, and an oversimplification of the baby's condition can lead to misinterpretation. For example, prolonged respiratory distress tires the baby, who then makes less vigorous respiratory efforts. The score in such cases may go down, even though the baby's condition is actually worsening. Such a baby would show no improvement, and other signs and symptoms such as the level of alertness, muscle tone, temperature stability and your general impression of a stressed infant will still be present.

CRITERION	MODIFIED SILVERMAN-ANDERSON SCORE		
	0	1	2
Chest movement	Upper chest and abdomen rise in unison	Lag or minimal sinking of upper chest as abdomen rises	See-saw breathing: pronounced sinking of upper chest as abdomen rises
Intercostal retractions	No intercostal sinking on inspiration	Barely visible sinking of intercostal spaces on inspiration	Marked sinking of intercostal spaces on inspiration
Subxiphoid retractions	No subxiphoid sinking on inspiration	Barely visible subxiphoid sinking on inspiration	Marked subxiphoid sinking on inspiration
Expiratory grunting	None	Grunting heard only with stethoscope	Grunting heard with naked ear
Nasal flaring	None to minimal but intermittent	Minimal and continuous	Marked

Score is calculated by adding values (0, 1, 2) assigned to each category. A score of 0 shows no respiratory distress. A score of 7 or higher indicates impending respiratory failure. A score of 10 indicates severe respiratory disease.

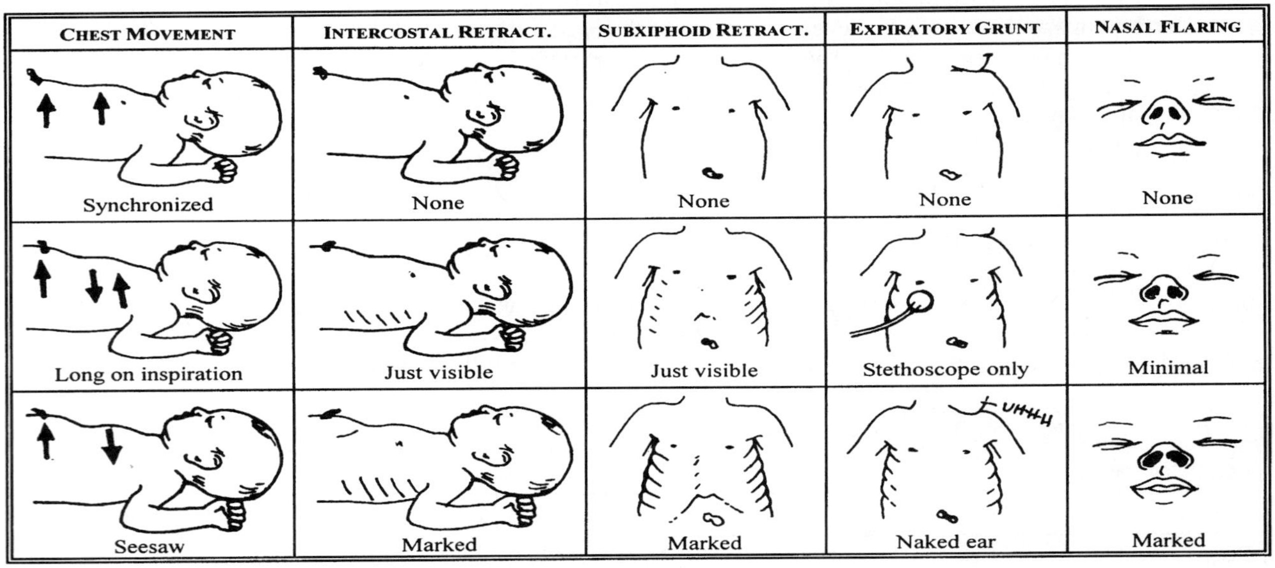

Specific signs and symptoms

Rapid breathing (tachypnea): This can occur for a wide variety of reasons, but by far the most common is residual lung fluid that the baby cannot clear on her own. An increase in the rate of respirations may also be a sign of respiratory distress or even failure. Rates over 80 rpm at birth or over 60 rpm after six hours of life are cause for close observation. However, any baby who is able to nurse without undue distress is unlikely to be seriously compromised, although an airway obstruction may still be present. Be sure the nostrils are clear by lifting the tip of the nose and doing a visual inspection with a penlight. (In one case, a homeborn baby was hospitalized for three days with tachypnea and finally sent home with no cause having been found. The mother looked up the baby's nose, found and removed a big ol' dried booger, and the baby's respiratory rate immediately fell to normal!) Sticky mucus can be removed by placing one or two drops of warm saline into the nostril to encourage sneezing, which may dislodge mucus or at least make it soft enough to be removed with a cotton swab. If no blockage can be found, you can also try giving the baby five inflation breaths with your bag and mask, which will often clear up any respiratory distress due to residual lung fluid. If nothing helps consider that something more serious is the cause and consult or transport for further evaluation.

Chest movement: A baby who is having trouble breathing will often have to work harder to inflate her lungs. Changes in chest movement, most severely seen in the form of seesaw breathing, demonstrate an effort to reinflate the lungs with each breath when the lungs or airways are not working properly. This type of breathing can be caused by poor perfusion of the pulmonary vasculature.

Retractions: Retractions occur when the softest parts of the thorax are pulled inward during inspiration. Mild degrees of subcostal retraction are considered normal variations in newborns, the depth of retraction indicating the amount of diaphragm activity. However, even these variations are minimal unless the baby has a less than optimal blood volume. Subcostal retractions may become more pronounced in any normal baby who is upset or excited but should resolve as the baby relaxes. Homeopathic remedies that may help include aconite (for terror), antimonium tart (for general respiratory distress) and Rescue Remedy (for fear and shock).

Morley (2004) explains that pathological retraction respirations consist of short, strong inspiratory efforts using accessory muscles, such as the sternomastoid, to elevate and expand the rib cage. This produces rhythmic caving-in of the subcostal abdominal wall and intercostal skin as the baby breathes. The ribs and xiphoid process also become more visible during severe retractions, with caving-in of the suprasternal and intrasternal spaces, as well as the sternum itself.

Clinically, such retractions are a form of gasping respiration, and the two terms are essentially interchangeable. It results from the increased respiratory effort required to raise negative intrathoracic pressure when the lungs are poorly perfused, in combination with a relatively flexible chest wall. Retractions are a reflex reaction to hypovolemia, hypotension and low venous return to the heart. This type of breathing generates pulses of negative intrathoracic pressure that pull blood into the heart and increase venous return. Morley (2002) states that retraction respiration, which is seen in the initial stages of RDS at any age, is a reflexive effort to draw more blood into the thorax. It presents as gasping secondary to "air hunger" in adults with terminal hypovolemic shock. There are several varieties of retraction patterns (see table). The degree of retraction correlates with the amount of negative pressure generated in the thorax and corresponds with the severity of the respiratory distress. Normal newborns with optimal blood volumes from placental transfusion do not usually exhibit this type of retraction respiration unless their airways are blocked (Kinmond et al., 1993).

TYPE OF RETRACTION	ANATOMY AFFECTED	IMPLICATIONS
Intercostal	Lung tissue, upper airway	Lung tissue disorders*
Subcostal	Insertion of diaphragm	Lung tissue disorders; indicates lower airway blockage if pronounced and seen without intercostal retractions.
Subcostal on one side only	Reduced movement of opposite side of diaphragm	Pneumothorax, fluid in the chest cavity, nerve disorder, diaphragmatic hernia, muscular disorder
Suprasternal	Upper airway	Obstruction due to structural abnormalities, secretions and edema; paralysis of vocal cords
Sternal	Sternum	Lower airway obstruction, prematurity with very pliable cartilage in the rib cage

*Lung tissue disorders" are usually the direct result of hypovolemia. This is usually ruled out if the baby received a full placental transfusion. However, partial airway obstruction or structural defects may also be causative.

Morley (2004) goes on to explain that, when the cord is clamped immediately at birth, the blood pressure, central venous pressure and cardiac output all fall. How much depends on the degree of hypovolemia. The net effect of retraction respiration is that it pulls blood into the thoracic organs, establishing adequate pulmonary circulation at the expense of systemic circulation. In extreme cases, blood in the carotid and vertebral arteries may be well oxygenated, but when gasping is combined with severe hypotension, flow in these vessels may be tidal, with very little blood flowing though brain capillaries at the height of left ventricular systole. In this scenario, brain damage can ensue in a matter of 5 minutes. Thus, pathological retractions are an absolute indication of some degree of hypovolemia, for which a transfusion is urgently required. They indicate pronounced respiratory distress and require transport.

Expiratory grunting or whining: Mild, intermittent grunting may be transiently present in the baby whose cord has been allowed to close physiologically. This expiratory sound is often heard in all babies during the first minutes of life. It is considered to be within normal limits when it is intermittent and not accompanied by other signs of distress. Mild intermittent grunting can also occur in a cold, frightened or otherwise upset baby; such grunting will resolve when the baby is calmed and warmed up.

However, grunting can also be an alarming sign, as it is also seen when respiratory distress is most severe. Grunting that is loud or persistent should be carefully evaluated, as it usually indicates moderate to severe lung disease. Grunting can occur when the first portion of exhaled air is forced through a partially closed glottis and functions to increase the pressure in the airways in an effort to increase alveolar volume. The baby tightens his glottis in an effort to retain some residual air in the lungs. In pathological situations, this is usually done to prevent complete collapse on exhalation, as is typical of babies with poor pulmonary perfusion, hyaline membrane disease or pulmonary edema. Grunting may also occur in the presence of hypothermia, sepsis, acidosis, polycythemia and other lung disorders as well as with abdominal disorders. Grunting prolongs expiration, so the respiratory rate is usually slowed. Periods of grunting with respiratory rates ranging from 40 to 60 breaths/min may alternate with periods of rapid breathing with rates between 80 and 100 breaths/min. If due to sepsis or other underlying pathology, grunting will not resolve (Fletcher, 1998). Note that grunting in the term infant is an important sign of pneumothorax.

Whining is similar to grunting but entails less complete closure of the glottis during exhalation. Whining may be a normal variation, a sign of pain, or a mild form of grunting.

Nasal flaring: Visible but very slight flaring of the nostrils is normal in babies, especially when asleep and dreaming, when up to half of all breaths may involve flaring. Increased flaring is often indicative of a problem and represents an attempt to increase the airway diameter. This decreases upper airway resistance and thus increases airflow. A significant degree of nasal flaring is usually accompanied by significant chest retraction.

Snoring or snorting: Partial nasal or nasopharyngeal obstruction may produce snoring or snorting sounds during inspiration with no changes in the cry or in the ability to swallow. Total nasal obstruction causes severe distress with cyanosis and retractions; narrowing or partial collapse of the larynx and upper trachea result in prolongation of the inspiratory phase of breathing and a distinctive stridor.

Stridor with breathing: Stridor is a high-pitched, noisy respiratory sound similar to the blowing of wind. It is a cardinal sign of partial airway obstruction and may be associated with a variety of conditions. Obstruction of the upper airway may lead to acute respiratory distress with or without stridor. An expiratory component to the stridor may be noted (grunting or wheezing with stridor) as the level of the obstruction moves down toward the level of the cricoid ring. When severe, this can cause the surrounding tissues of the chest and neck to vibrate or rattle. Try to determine if there is any relationship between the type and duration of stridor and nursing, as supraglottic obstructions may adversely affect the baby's ability to swallow. Immobile disorders of the airway such as tracheal stenosis, the diameter of which is essentially unaffected by respiration, may produce a combination of inspiratory and expiratory stridor.

LOCATION OF OBSTRUCTION	TIMING OF STRIDOR	QUALITY OF CRY	SWALLOWING
Supraglottic	On inspiration	Muffled	Difficult
Glottic	On inspiration and sometimes expiration	Abnormal	Unaffected
Subglottic	On inspiration and expiration	Unaffected	Unaffected
Tracheal	On expiration	Unaffected	Unaffected

Severe obstruction of the upper airway quickly produces hypoxia, which can lead to brain damage. Immediate assessment is called for; the degree of stridor is not, by itself, the most significant feature because stridor will diminish as the baby gets tired, and babies near death may be almost silent. Stridor is further discussed in the subchapter entitled "Complicated Respiratory Distress."

Pitch of breath sounds and crying: Normal vocalization depends on subglottic air pressure, the length, tension and size of the vibrating vocal cords, and the ability of the inner edge of each cord to vibrate freely. Any change in these variables results in an abnormal sound. High-pitched sound is usually associated with a disorder of the larynx while a lower pitch tends to be produced in the trachea or pharynx. A normal cry generally rules out lesions affecting the vocal cords while a weak, aphonic, or hoarse cry suggests vocal cord paralysis or, more rarely, an anomaly such as a laryngeal cyst or cleft.

Central cyanosis: Cyanosis of the mucous membranes is a common and significant indication of respiratory distress that is severe enough to effect oxygen saturation. It can be difficult to identify. The buccal membranes of the mouth should be examined in natural light. Blue discoloration indicates central cyanosis, which is evidence of severe distress.

Supplemental oxygen should be given, either using blow-by or a mask, until the baby's lips and tongue are pink. Do not exceed the concentration necessary to achieve this result. If you suspect heart disease, do not exceed a concentration of 85% in any event. Any baby who requires oxygen to remain pink or who receives oxygen for more than 1 to 2 hours or at a concentration exceeding 40% for longer than a brief period of stabilization should be further evaluated and have blood gas studies done (Ziai, et al., 1984).

Air entry: Listen to the lungs with a stethoscope to evaluate alveolar ventilation. Inadequate air entry is a useful means of determining the severity of respiratory distress. A decrease in breath sounds that occurs on only one side suggests a pneumothorax, diaphragmatic hernia or other obstructive thoracic lesion. Palpate the position of the trachea at the suprasternal notch and listen for the location of maximal intensity of the heart sounds. Deviation of these findings from their normal locations indicates a shift due to one of the above disorders.

Head bobbing: Labored breathing sufficient to involve the accessory muscles of the upper thorax may cause the head to bob with each breathing cycle. This signifies significant distress when seen with other respiratory symptoms.

Coughing: Coughing is a primitive reflex that protects the lower respiratory tract and is part of the body's defense mechanism. Coughing occurs as a response to a variety of respiratory stimuli but is not usually present in disorders of the respiratory tract in babies, as infants typically clear their airways by sneezing. When it does occur, however, it is an important diagnostic sign. The onset, frequency, and force of the cough and the presence of secretions should be noted. For example, coughing associated with feeding or with drinking may be caused by aspiration or a sucking disorder (which may be associated with severe head moulding involving pinching of nerves or with extensive suctioning, which can disorganize the normal sucking reflex). A persistent barking cough with or without stridor is a prominent characteristic of tracheal narrowing and is suggestive of tracheomalacia or tracheal compression. In tracheal compression or collapse, the head and neck may be held in hyperextension, and attacks that are cyanotic, apneic or both may occur. Unless the baby has aspirated a little milk, spontaneous coughing is usually abnormal. The mnemonic CRADLE is used to remind oneself of the primary serious causes of neonatal coughing:

Cystic fibrosis (1 in 1600 live Caucasian births)
Respiratory infection (especially with respiratory syncytial virus or chlamydia)
Aspiration (also reflux, swallowing disorder, and tracheoesophageal fistula)
Dyskinesia of cilia (the cilia in the respiratory tract are not moving properly)
Lung, airway or vascular malformation
Edema from heart failure or bronchopulmonary dysplasia

Of these options, the most likely reasons are respiratory infections and aspiration.

Hiccuping: Occasional episodes of hiccuping are normal in infants and last an average of 8 to 9 minutes per session. Frequent bouts of hiccuping may be a normal variation but can also be associated with low carbon dioxide, irritable diaphragm, seizures, drug withdrawal and encephalopathy.

Differential diagnosis

The midwife must not only assess the degree of distress, but must also determine why the baby is in distress. Most of the time, the baby will be experiencing transient, mild and benign respiratory distress that will resolve with supportive measures at home. However, it will be important to identify or at least suspect if the cause of the problem is serious so that proper care can be sought without delay. You want to eliminate as many confounding factors as possible so that the baby's true condition can be evaluated. The following table describes the constellation of signs and symptoms typically seen in a variety of common neonatal respiratory problems.

Patterns of Respiratory Effort	
Pattern Observed	**Associated Condition**
Intercostal and sternal retractions, flaring, tachypnea, grunting, increased work during breathing	Lower airway obstruction or disorder of the lung tissue
Suprasternal and subcostal retractions	Upper airway obstruction
Tachypnea without effort, quiet but not sleepy, may be cyanotic	Cardiac disorders
Poor respiratory effort compared with physiologic need, apnea	Neurological depression
Tachypnea, apnea, lethargy, whining, minimal retractions	Metabolic acidosis secondary to sepsis

The questions below will help in separating the benign causes from more severe respiratory problems.

What is the baby's temperature? Is the baby chilled or too hot? Either of these situations will result in rapid breathing and grunting as the baby attempts to either warm up or cool off. Adjust the baby's clothing and the ambient temperature accordingly and see if the respiratory symptoms change. If they improve, temperature was at least a component of the problem. If you note no improvement, you must assess the baby's overall condition to decide if transport is warranted.

Is the baby septic? When the baby is septic, respiratory distress often manifests very subtly. Be alert for rapid breathing and slight, persistent grunting. A septic baby may never develop a truly pink color. Grunting that persists despite warming, calming and nursing should not be ignored. Be even more suspicious if the baby refuses to nurse, as this often indicates that breathing is requiring so much energy that she cannot breathe and nurse at the same time. If the circumstances of labor point to the likelihood of sepsis and the baby's respiratory signs or color do not improve and resolve, transport may seem like an overreaction but is often prudent. (See the subchapter entitled "Detecting and Differentiating Newborn Hypoglycemia, Sepsis and Heart Defects.")

Is the baby hypoglycemic? The first respiratory symptom of a baby with low blood sugar will be rapid respirations, which can evolve to more serious distress if the hypoglycemia is not resolved. Other factors such as a long labor, a traumatic birth (e.g., shoulder dystocia or difficult breech) or cold stress may also come into play. Fortunately, nursing can eliminate this problem. If the baby cannot or will not nurse, give soy-based formula, sterile molasses water (1 tsp to 1 cup water) or glucose water with an eyedropper or teaspoon. Do *not* give honey to a baby less than 1 year old, as it can carry botulism. If still in doubt, a simple blood test using Dextrostix or a glucose monitor can determine if hypoglycemia is a factor. (See the subchapter entitled "Detecting and Differentiating Newborn Hypoglycemia, Sepsis and Heart Defects" for more details.)

Will the baby nurse? The baby's ability to nurse and maintain adequate respirations at the same time is a good indication, although not a guarantee, of a benign process. Nursing helps bring up mucus and secretions, lowers the heart rate and improves oxygenation, thus signs of benign respiratory distress may be lessened during nursing. The baby who cannot breathe and nurse at the same time is in significant distress. Adjust the baby's position and try nursing again. If the baby refuses to nurse, further evaluation is a prudent move. (See the subchapter entitled "Complicated Respiratory Distress" for more details.)

Is the baby early? An early baby can become chilled quickly, even in a room that is warm by most standards. Thermal environment is the first parameter to assess and correct whenever an early baby develops respiratory distress. Next, the baby should be assessed for hypoglycemia. If the baby is not too hot or too cold and is not hypoglycemic, immature lungs *must be assumed to be the reason for respiratory distress* until it is ruled out. Early babies who received a full placental transfusion are protected to a great degree from pulmonary dysfunction, but even in these babies, the possibility must always be kept in mind (see the chapter entitled "The Baby's Journey through Labor to Birth" for more information). Babies weighing less than 3 lb 5 oz (1500 g) and those born at less than 36 weeks gestation are most prone to being born with immature lungs. The baby may appear to be breathing normally at birth, only to succumb later to a lack of surfactant, usually before 6 hours of age. The baby will present with increasing tachypnea, nasal flaring, grunting, seesaw respirations and cyanosis, and will become progressively more lifeless and flaccid. Auscultation of the lungs will reveal diminished breath sounds. Characteristic "sandpaper" breath sounds can be heard on inspiration and expiration as the problem becomes more severe. Don't wait. Respiratory distress can quickly become life threatening. The baby should be offered blow-by oxygen as indicated and transported without delay, taking care to maintain a normal body temperature in the process.

Did the baby require any artificial ventilations? While any baby can develop a spontaneous pneumothorax, or hole in the lung, this is most likely to occur in those babies who have received artificial ventilations. Unequal breath sounds, expansion of one side of the chest, distant heart sounds, very rapid breathing, the sudden development of grunting and worsening distress are suspicious signs. See the subchapter entitled "Complicated Respiratory Distress" for details.

Does the baby have a congenital defect or obstruction affecting the respiratory or cardiovascular systems? Consider an abnormality as the underlying cause of respiratory distress if all of the above have been eliminated as possible factors. (See the subchapter entitled "Complicated Respiratory Distress" for more details.)

Possible Underlying Causes of Respiratory Distress

The most common problems underlying respiratory distress in the normal term newborn are as follows:

Transient tachypnea of the newborn (TTN)

The most likely reason for rapid breathing in the otherwise healthy, term newborn is transient tachypnea of the newborn (TTN). This presents as rapid respirations. It occurs in 1 to 2% of all newborns, especially in those who are full term. TTN can also occur in preterm babies, in whom it is hard to distinguish from respiratory distress syndrome resulting from immature (often, poorly perfused) lungs.

Those babies who are preterm and those who have experienced asphyxia or cord prolapse are more susceptible to TTN, as are those whose mothers have experienced sedation, overhydration with IV fluids, asthma, exposure to beta-mimetic drugs, bleeding, diabetes, or surgical birth. Any of these factors can be associated with an infant who is somewhat depressed at birth, resulting in an accumulation of mucus and secretions. Cord compression and vaso-constriction secondary to hypoxia or cord clamping can both cause the baby to be born hypovolemic, making the placental transfusion vital to the establishment of normal respirations, an achievement especially difficult for these infants. Swallowing and coughing reflexes may be diminished. Lack of adequate inspiratory effort may lead to delayed circulatory changeover and closure of the foramen ovale, as well as to decreased absorption of fetal pulmonary fluid. Irregular alveolar inflation and poor pulmonary capillary circulation with interstitial and pulmonary edema occur.

Whereas rapid breathing related to normal transition generally is fastest following birth and drops after the first six hours or so of life, TTN has a slightly delayed onset. Otherwise untraumatized babies who were born to undrugged mothers and who develop TTN usually have good APGAR scores at birth. However, two to six hours later, nasal flaring, slight grunting and minimal retractions develop. Cyanosis may also be present, although the baby pinks up with blow-by oxygen. Rapid breathing, with respiratory rates rising as high as 100 to 150 rpm, are typical. Auscultation of breath sounds reveals adequate air entry, and the lungs sound clear unless significant pulmonary edema, which produces scattered crackles, is present. The tachypnea peaks by 6 to 12 hours and resolves over the next 24 to 48 hours. More severe forms may result in persistent pulmonary hypertension of the newborn (PPHN). TTN is diagnosed by excluding other possible causes and by its natural course. Consider other causes such as a heart defect or unilateral choanal atresia as possible sources of either persistent tachypnea or breathing problems for which no other explanation can be found.

Meconium aspiration

Any baby born through meconium-stained fluid who develops respiratory distress may have aspirated meconium. See the following chapter for details.

Sepsis with or without pneumonia

Sepsis must be considered in any infant with respiratory distress who is born to a febrile mother, who is preterm, or whose mother labored with prolonged rupture of membranes. Fetal tachycardia, other fetal distress, low APGAR scores and perinatal asphyxia are frequently associated findings. Respiratory distress develops at or soon after birth, with tachypnea, tachycardia and generalized signs of infection including temperature instability, lethargy, poor peripheral perfusion, apnea, metabolic acidosis and early-onset jaundice. Symptoms may rapidly worsen as the baby goes from mild respiratory distress to septic shock with persistent pulmonary hypertension of the newborn and, in some cases, pulmonary hemorrhaging and disseminated intravascular coagulation.

Pneumothorax

An air leak injury is the most common, serious reason why an otherwise normal infant is suddenly thrown into acute respiratory distress. All types of thoracic air leak injuries and their management are covered in the subchapter entitled "Complicated Respiratory Distress."

Other causes

A wide variety of serious conditions can impact the respiratory system of the newborn. These are discussed in the chapter "Complicated Respiratory Distress."

If in doubt, transport.

MECONIUM ASPIRATION

Meconium aspiration refers to the inspiration of meconium below the vocal cords. About one-third of all babies born through meconium-stained fluid will aspirate meconium below their vocal cords and possibly into the bronchi and lungs. Some of these babies become seriously ill.

Most of the time, fetal breathing motions are shallow and regular, producing a flow of lung fluid out of the respiratory tract. Ten percent of the time, fetal breathing motions are deeper, resulting in a slight inward movement of fluid. Although the frequency with which these deeper breathing motions occur increases with gestational age, fetal breathing is normally not sufficient to draw in amniotic fluid.

The stress of hypoxia can change this picture. Meconium aspiration, long assumed to occur primarily at the time of birth in conjunction with the onset of respiration, is now felt to happen most often in conjunction with intrauterine passage of meconium associated with periods of fetal asphyxia sufficient to prompt gasping. At the onset, poor oxygenation tends to quiet fetal breathing activity. Then, as carbon dioxide levels rise, the baby passes out of primary apnea, and last-gasp efforts are triggered. The same stress and asphyxia that ultimately result in gasping can also lead to the passage of meconium, as well as the inhibition of swallowing, thus impairing normal clearance of the amniotic fluid. Fetuses also experience episodes of gasping 24 to 72 hours prior to intrauterine death. Meconium in the fluid can be aspirated into the trachea.

Thirty-five percent of those babies born through meconium-stained fluid have meconium in their lungs and 55% have abnormal findings upon chest X-ray, yet not every baby becomes sick. Respiratory disease develops in only 5% to 10% of all babies who have meconium below the vocal cords. In other words, out of the 7 to 22% of babies born through meconium-stained fluid, only 2 to 8% (or 0.2% of all babies born alive) develop respiratory disease associated with meconium aspiration (known as "MAS," meconium aspiration syndrome). It is also noteworthy that some babies diagnosed with MAS have *no evidence* of meconium aspiration and no pulmonary inflammation.

Meconium Aspiration Syndrome (MAS)

The theoretical understanding of the pathophysiology of MAS has changed in recent years. Aspirated meconium, though capable of causing chemical inflammation, rarely causes problems in the lungs of healthy babies. The development of MAS is strongly associated with hypoxia and is characterized by mild to severe respiratory distress at birth. It is most commonly associated with abnormal fetal heart rate patterns before or during labor. Hypoxia and apnea result in relaxation of the vocal cords, increasing the likelihood that meconium will enter the trachea. In its mildest form, MAS presents with rapid breathing, normal blood pH and low P_{CO2} (partial carbon dioxide pressure) and resolves in two to three days. When present, meconium-stained amniotic fluid is usually characterized as thin in those babies who experience mild MAS.

More pronounced illness that has historically been designated as MAS apparently stems from prenatal episodes of hypoxia, with additional hypoxia after birth. Prenatal hypoxia of sufficient duration (3 to 7 days) causes the musculature of the pulmonary arteries to hypertrophy, leading to pulmonary vasospasm. Vasospasm prevents normal dilation and rerouting of the blood from the umbilical to the pulmonary circulation when breathing is initiated after birth, leading to increased pulmonary vascular resistance and decreased pulmonary artery blood flow and oxygenation. Pulmonary vascular obstruction in the newborn mimics the fetal condition of the lungs, resulting in right-to-left shunting of blood through the still patent foramen ovale and ductus arteriosus. This diverts blood away from the lungs, which results in further hypoxia. In severe cases, hypoxemia (poorly oxygenated arterial blood), acidosis, convulsions, disseminated intravascular coagulation, and heart, renal and respiratory failure may occur within minutes or hours after birth. This is the result of the pathological changes brought about by prolonged hypoxia; whether there is meconium in the lungs or not has no bearing on the development of these changes.

When these hypoxic changes are accompanied by meconium aspiration, the vasospasm of asphyxia impairs the normal ability of the lungs to clear meconium, and chemical inflammation ensues. Meconium also provides a breeding ground for bacteria. This, in combination with poorly oxygenated tissues, makes the baby prone to infection. Respiratory distress may be worsened by the displacement of pulmonary surfactant by free fatty acids from the meconium (Clark et al., 1987) or by the direct inhibition of surfactant's surface-tension-reducing properties by meconium (Moses et al., 1991). The more severely the tissue reacts to the presence of meconium, especially in the presence of pulmonary vasospasm, the longer it will take for the baby's body to clear meconium from the lungs.

A larger quantity of aspirated meconium will obviously slow down clearance even more. Thick meconium-stained amniotic fluid was recorded at birth in 95% of babies who developed MAS. This does not mean that a baby who has thick meconium will necessarily get sick, but that if the lungs have undergone pathological changes from hypoxia, the aspiration of thick meconium will only make matters worse. Impaired clearance prolongs pulmonary inflammation, impairs alveolar healing and progressively disrupts respiratory function. The combination of meconium aspiration, infection and asphyxia is a life-threatening situation. Depending upon the severity of the MAS, the baby will either need to be ventilated or put on ECMO (extracorporeal membrane oxygenation) a device which reroutes the blood through a machine for oxygenation in order to bypass the lungs, thus allowing them to heal. Drugs may be used to assist the healing process.

The additional blood volume an intact cord provides greatly enhances the baby's ability to overcome the increased vascular resistance of MAS by holding the capillary framework around each alveolus in an expanded state (thus compensating for the disrupted surfactant), as well as assisting him in recovering from the hypoxia and clearing meconium debris from the alveoli.

Signs and symptoms of meconium aspiration

Respiratory distress appears at birth and often presents after perinatal asphyxia with metabolic acidosis and hypoglycemia. The respiratory distress may increase over the next few hours, with markedly rapid breathing, cyanosis and variations in oxygenation with the stress of handling. The chest may be hyperinflated (barrel chest) with diffuse crackles and rhonchi on auscultation. Pneumothorax occurs in some 20% of these babies as well. The symptoms resolve after 2 or 3 days in mildly affected babies. More severely affected infants present with tachypnea and increased oxygen requirements that persist for days or even weeks.

Meconium-stained amniotic fluid that enters the trachea and airways can produce mechanical obstruction. Meconium may travel to affect smaller, distal airways with plugging, air trapping and alveolar collapse. The resulting problems include some areas becoming hyperinflated while others collapse and chemical irritation from the meconium itself, which may be superimposed on the effects of any asphyxia that has precipitated fetal gasping and entry of fluid into the airways. Lack of adequate lung inflation can result in an inadequate fall in pulmonary vascular resistance leading to persistent pulmonary hypertension of the newborn. Meconium may also inhibit surfactant function by interfering with its surface-tension-lowering properties, thus further complicating alveolar collapse. If you detect signs and symptoms you believe to be secondary to meconium aspiration, transport.

References and Further Reading on When the Newborn Develops Respiratory Distress

References used in multiple chapters throughout This Section

Aloan C. Respiratory Care of the Newborn: A Clinical Manual. JB Lippincott Co, Philadelphia PA, 1987.

Bloom R, et al. Textbook of Neonatal Resuscitation. American Heart Assoc. Elk Grove IL, 1996a.

Bloom R, et al. Textbook of Neonatal Resuscitation, errata. American Heart Assoc, Elk Grove IL, 1996b.

Crelin E. Functional Anatomy of the Newborn. Yale U, New Haven CT, 1973.

Dunn T, et al. "DeLee suction. Does it have clinical significance?" J Reprod Med, 46(10);905-908, Oct, 2001.

Halbower A, Jones M. "Physiologic reflexes and their impact on resuscitation of the newborn," Clin Perinatol, 26(3);621-627, Sept, 1999.

Hatch D, et al. The Surgical Neonate: Anaesthesia and Intensive Care, 3rd ed. Edward Arnold, London UK, 1995.

Kattwinkel J, et al., ed. Textbook of Neonatal Resuscitation, 6th ed. American Heart Assoc, Dallas TX, 2011.

Marieb E. Human Anatomy and Physiology, 4th ed. Benjamin/Cummings, Menlo Park CA, 1998.

Morley G. "Cord closure: can hasty clamping injure the newborn?" OBG Management, 7:29-36, July, 1998.

Morley G. "Retraction respiration: the multiorgan dysfunction that causes hypoxic ischemic encephalopathy," (electronic letter to the editor re: Shah P, et al., "Multiorgan dysfunction in infants with post-asphyxial hypoxic-ischemic encephalopathy," Arch Dis Child Fetal Neonatal Ed, 89(2):F-152-155, Mar, 2004), http//fn.bmjjournals.com/cgi/eletter/89/2/5152, accessed 5/27/2004.

Richmond S, ed. Principles of Resuscitation at Birth, 5th ed. Northern Neonatal Network, Newcastle upon Tyne UK, 1996.

Richmond S, et al. Resuscitation at Birth: The Newborn Life Support Provider Course Manual, 3rd ed. Resuscitation Council, Rochester, Kent UK, 2011.

Schneider K, Neonatal respiratory therapist. Personal communications,1999-2001.

Stevenson J. "Resuscitation of the shocked baby," Birth Gazette, 3(4);26-28, Summer, 1987.

Whitten C. Anyone Can Intubate: A Practical Step-by-Step Guide for Health Professionals. Medical Arts Press, San Diego CA, 1989.

Ziai M, et al., Assessment of the Newborn: A Guide for the Practitioner, 1st ed. Little, Brown and Co, Boston MA, 1984.

Understanding Fetal and Neonatal Asphyxia

Aggarwal R, et al. "Post-resuscitation management of asphyxiated neonates," Indian J Pediat, 68(12);1149-1153, Dec, 2001.

Berger R, Garnier Y. "Perinatal brain injury," J Perinat Med, 28(4);261-285, 2000.

Cowan F, et al. "Origin and timing of brain lesions in term infants with neonatal encephalopathy," Lancet, 361(9359);736-742, Mar 1, 2003.

Dawes G. Chapter 12: "Birth asphyxia, resuscitation and brain damage," Foetal and Neonatal Physiology. Yearbook Medical Pub, Chicago IL, 1968.

Jacobson B, Bygdeman M. "Obstetric care and proneness of offspring to suicide as adults: case-control study," BMJ, 317(7169);1346-1349, Nov 14, 1998.

Jacobson B, et al. "Prenatal origin of adult self-destructive behavior," Acta Psychiatr Scand, 76(4):364-371, Oct, 1987.

Morley G. "Neonatal encephalopathy, hypoxic ischemic encephalopathy, and subsequent cerebral palsy: etiology, pathology and prevention," www.cordclamping.com, Aug 5, 2003, accessed Nov 23, 2003.

Morley G. Ob/Gyn, E-mail communication, recd. Jan, 2004.

Northern Neonatal Network. Principles of Neonatal Resuscitation, 4th ed. Northern Regional Health Authority, Newcastle upon Tyne UK, 1993.

Phibbs R. Chapter 18: "Delivery room management," in Avery G, et al., eds. Neonatology: Pathophysiology and Management of the Newborn, 5th ed. Lippincott, Williams & Wilkins, Philadelphia PA, 1999.

Rybacki H, ed. Stedman's Electronic Medical Dictionary, Version 6.0, based on Stedman's Medical Dictionary, 27th ed. Lippincott Williams & Wilkins, Baltimore, MD, 2004.

Salk L, et al. "Relationship of maternal and perinatal conditions to eventual adolescent suicide," Lancet, 1(8429);624-627, Mar 16, 1985.

Steiner H, Neligan, G. "Perinatal cardiac arrest. Quality of the survivors," Arch Dis Child, 50(9)696-702, Sept, 1975.

Teitel D. Chapter 81: "Physiologic development of the cardiovascular system in the fetus," in Polin R, Fox W. Fetal and Neonatal Physiology, 2nd ed., Vol 1. WB Saunders Co, Philadelphia PA, 1998.

Vento M, et al., "Oxidative stress in asphyxiated term infants resuscitated with 100% oxygen," J Pediatr, 142(3);240-246, Mar, 2003. Erratum in J Pediatr, 142(6);616, June, 2003.

Wardrop C, Holland B. "The roles and vital importance of placental blood to the newborn infant," J Perinat Med, 23(1-2);139-143, 1995.

The Anatomy of the Neonatal Airway and Upper Respiratory Tract

Bosma J. Anatomy of the Infant Head. Johns Hopkins U P, Baltimore MD, 1986.

Crelin E. ANATOMY OF THE NEWBORN: AN ATLAS. Lea & Febiger, Philadelphia PA, 1969.
Crelin E. FUNCTIONAL ANATOMY OF THE NEWBORN. Yale U Press, New Haven CT, 1973.
Crelin E. "Development of the upper respiratory system," CLINICAL SYMPOSIA, 28(3);1-30, 1976.
Kent R, Vorperian H. DEVELOPMENT OF THE CRANIO-FACIAL-ORAL-LARYNGEAL ANATOMY: A REVIEW. Singular Pub. Group, San Diego CA, 1995.
Omari T, Rudolph C. Chapter 125: "Gastrointestinal motility," pp. 1373-1383, in Polin R, Fox W, eds. FETAL AND NEONATAL PHYSIOLOGY, 2nd ed., VOL. 2. WB Saunders Co, Philadelphia PA, 1998.
O'Rahilly R, Müller F. HUMAN EMBRYOLOGY AND TERATOLOGY, 3rd ed. Wiley-Liss, New York NY, 2001.
Rodenstein D. "Infants are not obligatory nose breathers," AM REV RESPIR DIS, 131(3);343-347, Mar, 1985.
Scammon R. Chapter 3: "A summary of the anatomy of the infant and child," pp. 257-444, in Abt I, ed. PEDIATRICS, VOL 1. WB Saunders, Philadelphia PA, 1923.
Snell R, Smith M. CLINICAL ANATOMY FOR EMERGENCY MEDICINE. Mosby, St. Louis MO, 1993.

AUTONOMIC NEUROMUSCULAR REFLEXES AND THE BABY'S RESPONSE TO RESUSCITATION

Cross K, et al. "The response of the new-born baby to inflation of the lungs," J PHYSIOL, 151:551-565, June, 1960.
Halbower A, Jones D. "Physiologic Reflexes and their impact on resuscitation of the newborn," CLIN PERINATOL, 26(3);621-627, Sept, 1999.
Hassan A, et al. "Volume of activation of the Hering-Breuer inflation reflex in the newborn period," J APPL PHYSIOL, 90;763-769, 2001.
Olinsky A, et al. "Influence of lung inflation on respiratory control in neonates," J APPL PHYSIOL, 36(4);436-439, April, 1974.
Widdicome J. "Respiratory reflexes in man and other mammalian species," CLIN SCI, 21;163-170, 1961.

CLEARING THE BABY'S AIRWAY

Boshart D. THE PACIFIER: MAKING THE DECISION. Speech Dynamics, Inc, Temecula CA, 2001.
Carrasco M, et al., "Oronasopharyngeal suction at birth: effects on arterial oxygen saturation," J PEDIATR, 130(5);832-834, May 1997.
Dunn T, et al. "DeLee suction. Does it have clinical significance?" J REPROD MED, 46(10);905-908, Oct, 2001.
Gage J, et al. "Suctioning of upper airway meconium in newborn infants," JAMA, 246(22);2590-2592, Dec 4, 1981.
Kroeger M. IMPACT OF BIRTHING PRACTICES ON BREASTFEEDING: PROTECTING THE MOTHER AND BABY CONTINUUM. Jones & Bartlett, Boston MA, 2004.
Sheehy S, ""Suctioning a neonate: Nose or mouth first?," (section ed response), J EMERG NURS, 16(6);379, Nov-Dec, 1990.
Somerson S, "Suctioning a neonate: Nose or mouth first?," (letter), J EMERG NURS, 16(6);379, Nov-Dec, 1990.
Sutton J. LET BIRTH BE BORN AGAIN! REDISCOVERING AND RECLAIMING OUR MIDWIFERY HERITAGE. Birth Concepts UK, Bedfont UK, 2001.
Waltman P, et al., "Building evidence for practice: a pilot study of newborn bulb suctioning at birth," JMWH, 49(1);32-38, Jan-Feb 2004.
Woolridge M. "Anatomy of infant sucking," MIDWIFERY, 2(4);164-171, Dec, 1986.

OROGASTRIC INTUBATION OF THE NEWBORN

Vyas H, et al. "Efficacy of face mask resuscitation: does it lead to gastric distension?" ARCH DIS CHILD, 58(5); 373-375, May, 1983.

DIGITAL ENDOTRACHEAL INTUBATION OF THE NEWBORN

Fletcher MA, MacDonald MG, eds. ATLAS OF PROCEDURES IN NEONATOLOGY, 2nd ed. JB Lippincott Co, Philadelphia PA, 1993.
Hancock P, Peterson G. "Finger intubation of the trachea in newborns," PEDIATR, 89(2);325-327, Feb, 1992.
Palme-Kilander C. "Methods of resuscitation in low 'Apgar' score newborn infants–a national survey," ACTA PAEDIATR, 81(10);739-744, Oct, 1992.
Shukla HK, et al. "Rapid estimation of insertional length of endotracheal intubation in newborn infants," J PEDIATR, 131(4);561-564, Oct, 1997.
Sniderman S, et al. Chapter 38: "Resuscitation of the newborn," in Hughes S, et al., eds. SHNIDER AND LEVINSON'S ANESTHESIA FOR OBSTETRICS, 4th ed. Lippincott, Williams & Wilkins, Philadelphia PA, 2001.
Woody N, Woody H. "Direct digital intratracheal intubation for neonatal resuscitation," J PEDIATR, 73(6);903-905, Dec, 1968.

THE LARYNGEAL MASK AIRWAY (LMA)

Brimacombe J. "Airway rescue and drug delivery in an 800 g neonate with laryngeal mask airway," PEDIATR ANESTH, 9;177-179, 1999.
Brimacombe J, Brain A. THE LARYNGEAL MASK AIRWAY: A REVIEW AND PRACTICAL GUIDE. Saunders Ltd, Philadelphia PA, 1997.
Ferson D, et al. "The laryngeal mask airway," INTERNAT ANESTH CLIN, 36(2);101-102, Spring, 1998.
Gandini D, Brimacombe J. "Neonatal resuscitation with laryngeal mask airway in normal and low birth weight infants," ANESTH ANALG, 89;642-643, 1999.

Gilmore E, CPM. Editing comment, July 2004.
LMA AIRWAY INSTRUCTION MANUAL, Laryngeal Mask Airway Co, Ltd, San Diego CA, Aug, 2003.
LARYNGEAL MASK AIRWAY INSERTION VIDEO, Laryngeal Mask Airway Co., Ltd., San Diego CA, Nov, 2001.
Margaria E, et al., "La maschera laringea nella rianimazione primaria del neonato,"MINERVA ANESTESIOL, 61;453-454, 1995.
Park C, et al. "The laryngeal mask airway in infants and children," CAN J ANESTH, 48(4);413-417, Apr, 2001.
Paterson S, et al. "Neonatal resuscitation using the laryngeal mask airway," ANESTH, 80;1248-1353, 1994.

EVALUATING AND ASSISTING THE INFANT IN NEED OF RESUSCITATION

American Red Cross. CPR FOR THE PROFESSIONAL RESCUER. Mosby Lifeline, St. Louis MO, 1993.
Angell-James J, Daly M. "The effects of artificial lung inflation on reflexly induced bradycardia associated with apnea in the dog," J PHYSIOL, 274:349-366, Jan, 1978.
Avery G, et al., eds. NEONATOLOGY, PATHOPHYSIOLOGY AND MANAGEMENT OF THE NEWBORN, 4th ed. JB Lippincott, Williams & Wilkins, Philadelphia PA, 1987.
Bloom R. "Delivery room resuscitation of the newborn," in Fanaroff A, Martin R, eds. NEONATAL-PERINATAL MEDICINE: DISEASES OF THE FETUS AND INFANT, 5th ed. Mosby Year Book, St. Louis MO, 1992.
Bloom R, et al. TEXTBOOK OF NEONATAL RESUSCITATION. American Heart Assoc, 1995.
Chamberlain R, et al. Chapter 4: "The first breath," in BRITISH BIRTHS, VOL. 1: THE FIRST WEEK OF LIFE. Heinemann Medical, London UK, 1975.
Clark R. "Support of gas exchange in the delivery room and beyond: how do we avoid hurting the baby we seek to save?" CLIN PERINATOL, 26(3);669-681, Sept, 1999.
Dunn P. "Perinatal factors influencing adaptation to extrauterine life," Plenary session 72: Preterm birth. XII World Congress of Gynecology and Obstetrics, Rio de Janeiro, Oct 23-28, 1988 in Belfort P, et al., eds. ADVANCES IN GYNECOLOGY AND OBSTETRICS, VOL. 5, PREGNANCY AND LABOR. Proc. 12th World Cong Obstet Gynecol, Parthenon Pub, Carnforth Lancs UK, 1989.
Duster M. "Pulmonary hypertension, high altitude," http://www.emedicine.com/ped/topic2783.htm, updated Sept 25, 2002. Accessed Apr 4, 2004.
Ettinghausen N. Cited by Khalsa DK, personal communication regarding working with him, [1981?].
Fletcher MA. PHYSICAL DIAGNOSIS IN NEONATOLOGY. Lippincott-Raven, Philadelphia PA, 1998.
Gilhooly J. Neonatologist. E-mail communication, recd. 2003.
Gunn A, Bennet L. "Is temperature important in delivery room resuscitation?" SEMIN NEONATOL, 6(3);241-249, June 2001.
Head H. "On the regulation of respiration," J PHYSIOL, 10;1-70, 1889.
Marieb E. HUMAN ANATOMY AND PHYSIOLOGY, 4th ed. Benjamin/Cummings, Menlo Park CA, 1998.
Medbo S, et al. "Pulmonary hemodynamics and plasma endothelin-1 during hypoxemia and reoxygenation with room air or 100% oxygen in a piglet model," PEDIATR RES, 44(6):843-849, Dec, 1998.
Milner A. "The importance of ventilation to effective resuscitation in the term and preterm infant," SEMIN NEONATOL, 6(3);219-224, June, 2001.
Morley G. Ob/Gyn, E-mail communications, 2002.
Morley G. Ob/Gyn, E-mail communications, Nov-Dec 2003.
Peliowski A, Finner N. "Birth asphyxia in the term infant," pp. 249-273, in Sinclair J, Bracken M, eds. EFFECTIVE CARE OF THE NEWBORN INFANT. Oxford U, Oxford UK, 1992.
Polin R, Fox W, eds. FETAL AND NEONATAL PHYSIOLOGY, 2nd ed., VOL. 2. WB Saunders, Philadelphia PA,1998.
Ramji S, et al. "Resuscitation of asphyxic newborn infants with room air or 100% oxygen," PEDIATR RES, 34(6);809-812, Dec, 1993.
Roberton N, Rosen M. "Safer resuscitation of the newborn," CLIN OBSET GYNECOL, 9(2);415-435, Aug, 1982.
Sanders M. MOSBY'S PARAMEDIC TEXTBOOK. Mosby Lifeline, St. Louis MO, 1994.
Saugstad OD. "Resuscitation of newborn infants: do we need new guidelines?" PRENAT NEONAT MED, 1;26-28, 1996.
Saugstad OD. "Resuscitation of newborn infants with room air or oxygen," SEMIN NEONATOL, 6(3);233-239, June, 2001.
Saugstad OD, et al. "Resuscitation of asphyxiated newborn infants with room air or oxygen: an international controlled trial: the Resair 2 study," PEDIATR, 102(1);e1, July, 1998.
Schleiff J, EMT. Personal communication, 2002.
Steiner H, Neligan G. "Perinatal cardiac arrest. Quality of the survivors," ARCH DIS CHILD, 50(9);696-702, Sept, 1975.
Tappero E, Honeyfield, M. PHYSICAL ASSESSMENT OF THE NEWBORN: A COMPREHENSIVE APPROACH TO THE ART OF PHYSICAL EXAMINATION. NICU Ink, Petaluma CA, 1993.
Thornberg E, et al. "Birth asphyxia: incidence, clinical course and outcome in a Swedish population," ACTA PAEDIATR, 84(8);927-932, Aug, 1995.
Vento M, et al. "Oxidative stress in asphyxiated term infants resuscitated with 100% oxygen," J PEDIATR, 142(3);240-246, Mar, 2003. Erratum in J PEDIATR, 142(6);616, June 2003.
Whyte SD, et al. "Neonatal resuscitation–a practical assessment," RESUSCITATION, 40(1);21-25, Jan, 1999.
Williams, P, ed. GRAY'S ANATOMY, 38th ed. Churchill Livingstone, New York NY, 1995.

World Health Org. Basic Newborn Resuscitation: A Practical Guide, Safe Motherhood Unit, Div. of Reproductive Health, Geneva Switzerland, 1997.

Evaluating the Apparently Normal Baby Who Develops Respiratory Distress

Downes J, et al. "Respiratory distress syndrome in newborn infants. I. New clinical scoring system (RDS score) with acid-base and blood-gas correlates," Clin Pediatr (Phila), 9(6);325-331, June, 1970.
Kinmond S, et al. "Umbilical cord clamping and preterm infants: a randomized trial," BMJ 306(6871);172-175, Jan 16, 1993.
Mahaffey LW, Rossdale PD. "A convulsive syndrome in newborn foals resembling pulmonary syndrome in the newborn infant," Lancet, 1(7085);1223-1225, June 13, 1959.
Mercer J. "Current best evidence: A review of the literature on umbilical cord clamping," J Midwif Women's Health, 46(6);402-414, Nov-Dec, 2001.
Morley G. "How the cord clamp injures your baby's brain," www.cordclamping.com, Feb 26, 2002.
Oh W, et al. "The effects of placental transfusion on respiratory mechanics of normal term newborn infants," Pediatr, 40(1);6-12, July, 1967.
Silverman WA, Andersen DH. "A controlled clinical trial of effects of water mist on obstructive respiratory signs, death rate and necropsy findings among premature infants," Pediatr, 17(1);1-10, Jan, 1956.
Yao AC, et al. "Expiratory grunting in the late clamped normal neonate," Pediatr, 48(6);865-870, Dec, 1971.

Meconium Aspiration

Ciftci AO, et al. "In-utero defecation: fact or fiction?" Eur J Pediatr Surg, 9(6);376-380, Dec, 1999.
Clark DA, et al. "Surfactant displacement by meconium free fatty acids: an alternative explanation for atelectasis in meconium aspiration syndrome," Pediatr, 110(5):765-770, May, 1987.
Clark P, Duff P. "Inhibition of neutrophil oxidative burst and phagocytosis by meconium," Am J Obstet Gynecol, 173:1301-1305, Oct, 1995.
Cunningham A. "Let's rethink meconium suctioning," Contemporary OB/GYN, 38(7);23-26, 30, July 1993.
Galan H. "Meconum-stained amniotic fluid: meaning and management," OMG Management: CME article, http://www.obgmanagement.com/799/cme/799.html, July 1999, accessed Aug 3, 2001.
Moses D, et al. "Inhibition of pulmonary surfactant function by meconium," Am J Obstet Gynecol, 164(2);477-481, Feb, 1991.
Ramón y Cajal C, Martinez O. "Defecation in utero: A physiologic fetal function," Am J Obstet Gynecol, 188(1);153-156, Jan, 2003.

ASSESSING, SUPPORTING AND TRANSPORTING THE BABY IN NEED OF SPECIALIZED CARE

WHEN A BABY IS BORN WITH SERIOUS PROBLEMS

Note: You will need immediate care protocols for babies in obvious trouble, often prior to when you would ordinarily perform the newborn exam. Therefore, most relevant techniques and exam procedures are explained here, with an emphasis on immediate recognition and support. These same procedures may or may not have been explained elsewhere in the text, depending upon their relevance to care of the normal newborn. This section covers problems due to trauma as well as to anomalies and genetic disorders.

Today, 1 in every 28 babies born in the United States has a birth defect of some type. Many of these are minor, and all of them are relatively rare when considered individually. Some produce gross physical anomalies or other evidence of serious acute or chronic conditions while others result in subtle signs or symptoms that manifest during the first hours of life and that you will notice only if you know what to look for. Because, as midwives, we seldom see babies with serious problems and because many women we work with may choose not to have routine ultrasound exams, the defects and serious problems we do encounter will often be on the order of surprises. This is traumatic for all concerned. Having a well-rehearsed thought process in mind as you attempt to determine how best to deal with the situation will help immensely.

The conditions discussed in this section are the most serious newborn problems, although their occurrence varies from uncommon to very rare. While many of these are reviewed, the range of problems that can occur is huge, and every nuance is not included in this section. However, the discussion is thorough enough to give the midwife a broad repertoire of knowledge and skills to draw on whatever the newborn's condition may be. Although a variety of possible causes are discussed, it is beyond the scope of midwifery to ascertain an exact diagnosis of every newborn difficulty, and care should be taken not to appear as though you know more than you do. In spite of this, a range of specific causes are introduced so that the well-schooled midwife has a good idea of what might be causing the problem as well as offering sufficient background information to prepare her to talk to neonatal care providers and the parents during and after transport.

Communicating with the parents

You will need to quickly evaluate what the problem appears to be and whether and how quickly the baby must be transported to the hospital. In that process, how you respond and communicate with the parents and others attending the birth regarding the baby's condition, as well as how you relate to the baby, will have a huge impact on how the parents integrate the experience. Remember that you can either significantly assist or detract from their ability to bond with and accept their baby. Every parent has a vision of a perfect infant prior to birth. Even the most perfect infant will not always meet the expectations generated by the fantasy baby of pregnancy, but a baby born with problems, especially visible physical defects, can be devastating to the parents' ability to embrace their baby. Labels, such as "Down syndrome," where the specter of "retardation" and all that it implies looms large, can be equally frightening. When one major defect is present, it is more likely that others will be found. Such additional problems may not be immediately obvious, although some (such as metabolic derangement) may become obvious over a relatively short period of time. This should be explained to parents when they are weighing the pros and cons of immediate transport versus waiting a while. The desires and intuitions of the parents, the midwife's intuition about the baby, the proximity of the nearest neonatal intensive care unit, and the availability of the consulting pediatrician should all be taken into account when deciding upon the appropriate means and timing of transport or when establishing outpatient services. However, transport and evaluation should not be delayed because the parents are in denial about the possible condition of the baby.

Transport or consult?

Whenever a newborn does not look or act normally, or there are obvious physical problems that do not appear to be life threatening, advise the parents to seek a medical consultation soon after birth. Such evaluation can usually wait until an hour or two after birth if there is no danger of infection from fully exposed organs and the baby's vital signs are stable, and this wait may safely extend into the first few days of life, depending upon what the problem seems to be. If you decide to allow time for bonding, you can be contacting a back-up provider and explaining the situation during this time. If the baby's condition is unstable, is suggestive of major defects or includes the possibility of major systemic disruption, evaluation must take place as soon as possible.

You should transport to the nearest Level III neonatal intensive care unit, or to one that is relatively close, where you know the providers and the type of the care the baby will receive. If you are very rural, you may need to go to the nearest hospital that handles obstetrics, where they will be responsible for stabilizing and then transporting the baby on, as appropriate. An important consideration is the proximity of the Level III unit to the parents' home, as they are likely to be making many trips to the hospital over the next days and possibly weeks. The exception is when the condition is known to be fatal, and the parents desire for the baby to be allowed to die at home. If the condition was diagnosed with ultrasound or genetic testing during pregnancy, the back-up physician should be aware of the parents' plans. If not and the condition can be easily diagnosed, you can contact a pediatrician who is willing to make a house call to confirm the diagnosis. Once the fatality of the condition is confirmed, you will also need to contact your local medical examiner to avoid an investigation.

The need for a neonatal specialist: It is important to seek services from a practitioner who knows more than you do. You will usually contact a neonatologist whenever a baby has problems that you cannot handle or that you cannot identify. Even if the parents have lined up a family physician or pediatrician, such practitioners usually have only limited experience with newborns prior to six weeks of age and may often not be knowledgeable or up to date regarding serious neonatal concerns. Older doctors may possibly be the exception because they may have been in practice before neonatology was a specialty and may therefore have more firsthand experience with seriously ill newborns. However, neonatologists are specialists in caring for babies in trouble during the first 28 days of life. They work in hospitals because that is where seriously ill babies receive care.

Using this part of the text

This portion of the book assumes that you have a working knowledge of normal anatomy and terminology; it may be helpful to have Volume I (normal adult anatomy) and Volume III (neonatal anatomy), another source of anatomical information, and a medical dictionary on hand as you study. It assumes complete familiarity with the subchapters concerning the complete physical examination of the newborn.

There are three ways every type of neonatal emergency can be approached: by the location of the defect, by symptom picture, and by precise diagnosis. As a midwife, you will not be able to make a precise diagnosis unless the defect is visible and identifiable, thus these chapters outline your course of action based on primary signs and symptoms. In addition, associated defects are given for many of the major conditions, giving you an idea of what else to look for or be aware of when examining the baby and to aid in deciding upon the advisability and timing of transport. Other serious problems (such as sepsis and hypoglycemia) that may show up in an otherwise normal newborn can mimic heart defects, so these are presented together to aid in differentiating the problem at hand. Study this section of the book much as you would study cardiopulmonary resuscitation, thus preparing yourself for rare newborn emergencies.

The incidence of problems: The conditions mentioned are listed roughly from the most common to the least common. Where possible, the incidence of each condition is given. This is to give the student an idea of the relative likelihood of occurrence. For example, you might suspect a simple cleft palate to be causing a feeding problem and rule that out before suspecting another, more rare condition.

It must be kept in mind that data are influenced by the number of affected babies who are discovered in utero and subsequently aborted, who die on their own or who are born preterm, as well as geographical, environmental, nutritional, racial and ethnic variations. All these factors together mean that there can be no absolute statement regarding how many affected babies can be expected per given number of pregnancies or the number of affected babies born in a group who are all born alive. In addition, the total number of affected babies would be higher in pregnancies among women who decide against or have no access to prenatal ultrasound or who choose not to abort an affected baby. The incidence of certain conditions, such as spina bifida, can be influenced by maternal nutrition or supplementation, which will alter the number of babies affected according to the nutritional status of the mothers surveyed. In most cases, the absolute difference in affected babies would be small. Some conditions are so rare that the only incidences to be found mention the total number of reports of the condition that could be counted from a review of the literature spanning a certain number of years. These data are also given whenever possible.

The material covered here should be considered advanced midwifery knowledge. These descriptions assume you are already quite familiar with normal newborn appearance and behavior, can perform a complete newborn exam, understand the diagnostic techniques described in the chapters covering newborn examination and are familiar with transport procedures for normal babies (protocols for which are included in the following chapter). Ideally, this familiarity will include observation and assistance at a number of births and direct observation or experience in assisting a number of normal baby exams. Only with such a background can you retain a balanced view regarding the wide variations in normal infants, appreciate the rarity of these conditions and recognize the nuances of signs and symptoms as they evolve.

Note that this section of the book is intended more for intensive study than for quick reference. My "Quick Reference Cards for Newborns with Problems" are helpful to have as a ready reference for proper care that can be reviewed at a glance, since some of these problems require deviations from standard care that would be offered the otherwise normal but compromised newborn. These cards are intended to complement and serve as reminder notes for the material presented in this chapter.

There are hundreds of congenital anomalies, genetic disorders and other conditions from which the baby may suffer, and conditions can present atypically. The symptoms given are the most common ones associated with the conditions discussed. It is important to keep perspective and realize that most midwives go through an entire career having only seen a handful of the more common of these conditions.

Transport considerations

The following chapters will address specific signs, symptoms and special considerations, if any, in supporting and transporting babies with the condition in question. If no special transport suggestions are made, follow the recommendations addressed in the chapter entitled "Transporting the Newborn: An Overview."

TRANSPORTING THE NEWBORN: AN OVERVIEW

These protocols give a comprehensive overview regarding appropriate newborn transport procedures for all babies, including special considerations for a wide variety of neonatal complications that you may encounter. Most of these recommendations apply whenever newborn transport is necessary, whether the baby is suspected of having anomalies or not. Protocols for specific anomalies are also included where appropriate. The later chapters in this section also review, in much more detail, transport protocols for many of these conditions. This chapter can be used by itself to prepare most babies who are in trouble for transport without further investigation into what the problem may be.

Parental involvement

The parents will, of course, be intensely concerned about the welfare of their baby. Depending upon the circumstances, the mother may or may not be able to accompany the baby to the hospital immediately. Keep in mind that, because adrenaline is an antagonist to oxytocin, women typically become woozy and unfocused and often start bleeding once the baby leaves the house. At a minimum, the placenta should be delivered and the mother should be stable before attempting to travel. It may be advisable to give her an antihemorrhagic agent before she gets up to go, as her preoccupation with the baby makes continued bleeding more likely. The partner can accompany the baby immediately, either in the ambulance or by private car. If the decision is made to transport the baby via car, it is probably best for the partner to let someone who is not so immediately involved do the driving.

Alerting the hospital

Someone with a basic knowledge of the situation and a good medical vocabulary should call the hospital to alert them of the impending transport. First, contact the back-up pediatrician, if the parents have chosen one. She may be able to make all the hospital arrangements and meet you there. If not, call the hospital and ask to speak to staff in the neonatal intensive care unit. Briefly describe the nature of the problem, using appropriate medical terms *only to the extent you are sure you are using them correctly*. Describe what you see or have experienced in trying to get the baby stabilized, rather than names of conditions, unless the condition is obvious and unequivocal (such as open neural tube defect, omphalocele or anencephaly). Tell him how you intend to arrive (by ambulance or private car) and how long you expect it will take you to arrive. Obtain the name of the person you talked to, thank him and get underway as soon as possible. Once the hospital is alerted, it is best to carry through with transport, so do not call until you are certain that transport is appropriate. If you are unduly delayed or for some reason decide against transport (for example, an extremely malformed baby dies), call them back and explain the situation. Then, call the back-up pediatrician and ask her how she would like you to proceed at that point.

Use nonlatex gloves and other supplies

Eighteen to 73% of babies with spinal defects are prone to latex allergy, although latex allergies can develop in any baby. Therefore, to be on the safe side and eliminate one problem the baby does not have to deal with, use nonlatex gloves and other supplies whenever possible.

Explain to the baby what you are doing and why

Ambulance attendants and hospital personnel are likely to talk about the baby in his presence as if what they are saying will have no impact. It is therefore up to you and the parents to relate to the baby as a conscious, sensitive being by being respectful and telling the baby what is being done. Avoid making statements in the baby's presence that you would not make if the baby were old enough to respond verbally. This will assist you in not imprinting the baby with attitudes that could impact his self-esteem and beliefs about who he is and of what he may be capable as he matures.

Keep the baby warm

A space blanket can be cut to size for covering a baby who has been placed on the "newborn transport surface" (cookie sheet) or, if the baby's condition allows it, a baby bunting space blanket which fits over the body like a sleeping bag (foil can be used in a pinch but is not as effective). If resuscitation is required, use clear plastic food wrap so you can monitor chest movement and color and then wrap the cookie sheet lightly in a space blanket. Even if the baby has received a full placental transfusion (which certainly helps him maintain his temperature), the presence of prolonged stress and the excessive heat loss that may occur during transport or via any exposed organs or tissues makes warmth a top priority during transport. No attempt should be made to overwarm the baby. Maintaining a neutral thermal environment is the desired goal.

Clamp and cut the cord long

Depending upon what the problem seems to be, you may or may not have time to allow the cord to finish pulsing at the umbilicus. Unless you have a multiple birth in which you suspect twin-to-twin transfusion, you should always leave the cord intact as long as possible. Ambulance attendants are not informed regarding the benefits of placental transfusion and may think you are crazy if you try to leave the placenta attached during transport; if they walk in and it is still attached they may cut the cord shorter than you would. Therefore, cut the cord just before you expect them to arrive, leaving at least 5 centimeters of translucent cord between the clamp and the baby to allow the hospital plenty of room to cut the cord vessels down to insert an umbilical intravenous line if necessary. If a gastrointestinal defect is suspected, cut the cord off at the placental base and clamp the very end. When intestines are contained within the baby's end of the cord, they may, in exceedingly rare cases, extend up the length of the cord for quite a distance, even if the cord appears normal.

Clear the airway

You may need to clear the airway periodically throughout stabilization and transport if the baby is unconscious, having difficulty breathing, or has a defect that causes secretions to collect in the throat. If the baby is near term, postural drainage can be used initially; if the baby is preterm or appears to have an intracranial injury or cranial defects, suctioning should be performed, as postural drainage may result in the rupture of intracranial blood vessels. If the airway will not remain open, insert an oropharyngeal airway.

Positioning the baby

The baby without obvious defects: Place this baby flat on her back or on her right side. Side-positioning minimizes choking if baby is vomiting or likely to do so. Lying the baby on her right relieves pressure on the heart.

The baby with defects: Place this baby in a position that minimizes trauma to the defective areas and maximizes pulmonary air exchange:

- Minimize pressure on defective areas that do not interfere with breathing by positioning the baby to reduce pressure on the anomalous region.
- **For internal upper body defects (such as masses or a diaphragmatic hernia):** Prop the upper body with a small folded towel to relieve pressure on the lungs and assist air exchange.
- **For small to medium-sized defects of the chest or abdomen:** Place the baby supine.
- **For large anterior or posterior defects (those large enough to slide off to the side if the baby is supine or prone):** Lie the baby on the side (left or right) that most effectively minimizes strain on the lesion.
- **For spinal defects:** Position the baby prone and turn his head to the side or place him on his side, depending upon the size and location of the defect and any other defects present.
- **If the baby has a small jaw:** Place the baby prone and elevate the forehead with a folded washcloth under the forehead or with your hand. This may allow the tongue to fall forward and open the airway.

If internal structures are exposed or are only membrane-covered:

1. Lay a piece of plastic wrap flat across the transport surface. It should be sufficiently long to wrap around the baby and defect once the baby is positioned on the transport surface. You will place the baby over the center of the plastic wrap in a supine, side-lying or prone position, whichever puts the least pressure on the defect.

2-A. *If the defect is very large and extends away from the body, or if the defect may fall to one side and be strained: place the baby on her side.* Before doing so, prepare the underlying surface as follows:

A. Place enough sterile gauze on the plastic to cover the underside of the defect. Place on top of the gauze sufficient moistened nonadherent, nonwicking pads to fully cover the underside of the defect.

B. Place the tip of a sterile feeding tube on top of the pads, with the tube's end extending off to the side, where it will be easily accessible.

C. Soak the center of the gauze and pads thoroughly with warmed saline. If you must make your own saline solution, add ¼ tsp of salt to each cup of water. It should taste no more salty than tears.

D. Position the baby on her side on the tray with the defect overlying the prepared surface.

E. Place more moistened, nonadherent nonwicking pads over the top and sides of the defect so that it is

completely and loosely covered. Place the tip of another sterile feeding tube on top of the pads.
F. Lift the ends of the plastic wrap around the baby and overlap them; avoid compacting the defect.

2-B. *If the defect is such that the baby can safely be placed lying supine or prone with the defect uppermost, position him in the center of the plastic wrap.* Proceed as follows:

A. Place wet nonadherent, nonwicking pads directly over the entire exposed surface of the defect, followed by dry sterile gauze. Thoroughly soak the gauze and pads with warmed saline.
B. Place the tip of a sterile feeding tube over the defective area, outside the gauze.
C. Loosely bring the sides of the plastic wrap up and around the baby and defect and overlap the ends to retain heat and moisture, with the end of the feeding tube hanging out.

3. In either case, attach a warm saline-filled syringe to the tube port in order to remoisten the dressings as necessary.

More specific protocols for managing exposed organs can be found in the subchapter entitled "Externalized Organs and Neural Tube Defects."

Skin-covered lesions and intact omphaloceles: These defects do not require constant moisture. To keep them wet only risks chilling the infant.

Prevent shifting: Place small (preferably warmed) rolled towels or blankets around the baby as necessary to prevent shifting, which would put pressure on any defective areas. If the baby is supine or prone, spread the legs and place a small rolled towel between them to help prevent rolling.

If gastrointestinal blockage or metabolic disorders are suspected or if the baby is convulsing or vomiting, stop all oral intake until after evaluation.

If the baby requires artificial ventilation

Use mouth-to-mask breathing or a bag-and-mask to ventilate the baby. If there is no improvement or if the heart rate is less than 60 bpm, perform CPR, using a bag-and-mask if you have an assistant or mouth-to-mask CPR if not.

When to place a nasogastric or orogastric tube: Place a gastric tube to passively vent air from the stomach during ventilation in a normal baby who is not completely flaccid but does require resuscitation and in a baby whose lung capacity is known or suspected to be compromised for any reason.

Short-term positive-pressure ventilation normally results in a very minimal amount of air entering the stomach (Vyas et al., 1983). However, if the baby's lungs are hypoplastic or are compressed due to misplaced organs, any air filling the stomach during positive-pressure ventilation can further compress the lungs. In this case, it is important to actively remove air by aspirating the tube with a syringe every few minutes and to record the number of ccs withdrawn. If you suspect a heart defect, do not place a tube and otherwise avoid stimulation of the vagal nerve whenever possible by minimizing poking around in the back of the baby's throat. This could interfere with the heart rate or rhythm.

Place an oral airway if indicated: If the baby is unconscious or having a hard time breathing, place an oral airway to prevent the tongue from obstructing the airway.

Supplemental oxygen concentration for babies with suspected heart defects: Supplemental oxygen is a potent vasodilator of the newly expanded pulmonary capillaries and may therefore adversely effect babies who have abnormally high pulmonary blood flow due to certain types of heart defects. A face mask can be used to titrate any oxygen offered the baby to make sure it does not exceed a concentration of 80 to 85% (Marino & Wernovsky, 1999). Providing ventilation with a Mercury bag and mask with oxygen attached (11 l/min) but no reservoir provides an oxygen concentration of 60 to 70%. Use a pulse oximeter to monitor oxygen saturation, aim for a reading in the low 90s.

Method of transport

This section builds on the material covered in the subchapter entitled "Oxygen Delivery Devices and Resuscitation Equipment" and the chapter entitled "When Transport is Necessary during Labor." Study those before going over the remainder of this chapter.

Ground transport: Once she is positioned and all necessary support procedures are established, the baby should be carefully moved to the transport vehicle, be it private car, ambulance or aircraft. If the baby does not require extensive life support, transporting by private car will usually be quicker than calling an ambulance and will involve less interaction with personnel who may not be helpful. However, if you are practicing legally, the back-up physician should always be consulted as to what mode of transport he prefers that you use. Use of a private vehicle, unless it is a large van, makes it harder to maneuver to provide neonatal support. It also leaves you liable if the vehicle should be involved in an accident. The use of an ambulance with a team trained to transport newborns is obviously the best solution when the baby needs continuous ventilatory support or full CPR. In this case, the midwife will turn over care to the transport team. Many large cities have neonatal transport ambulances.

Air transport: Babies born to mothers who live at a low altitude are more likely than adults to develop hypoxia as the partial pressure of alveolar oxygen falls during ascent. Although the usual alveolar-arterial difference in the partial pressure of oxygen in adults is about 10 mm Hg, the difference in newborns is much greater (about 25 mm Hg), thus even a modest drop in PaO_2 will result in newborn hypoxia. In addition, the relaxation of pulmonary constriction as well as closure of the ductus arteriosus may be delayed. The solution is to provide supplemental blow-by oxygen during transport. To approximate sea level oxygenation, it is recommended to offer the baby 25 to 50 ml/min by nasal cannula, but such a low flow rate will require a special gauge that you will not have, although an air-transport service may. If one is not available, offer the baby a very small amount of oxygen by setting the gauge to 1 l/min given by nasal cannula (this delivers somewhat more than the recommended range, but that should not be a problem) or 5 l/min if a face mask is all you have with you.

Respiratory insufficiency may be aggravated at high altitudes. During the ascent from sea level, there is a continuous fall in barometric pressure and the partial pressure of oxygen, with an associated expansion of gases. If this is not compensated for, it can lead to hypoxemia and the worsening of any existing respiratory difficulty. This occurs in a linear fashion as ascent progresses, and may occur regardless of the concentration of inspired oxygen. For example, at 14,000 ft (4268 m) the partial pressure of oxygen is half that at sea level. Babies who are breathing on their own and augmented with blow-by oxygen running at a low-flow rate at sea level may still require artificial ventilation or continuous positive airway pressure (which you will not be able to provide with the midwifery equipment you carry) to avoid hypoxia at higher altitudes.

As in adults, the reduction in barometric pressure that occurs with ascent results in the expansion of any gases contained within body cavities. Adverse effects may develop if there is a collection of gas in the body, such as may result from artificial ventilation or air-leak injuries (pneumothorax, etc.). This is especially dangerous if a pneumothorax or a congenital defect prone to trap air, such as a diaphragmatic hernia, already exists. A 30% expansion of intrathoracic trapped gas within the gastrointestinal tract can force the gas past the pyloric sphincter (at the outlet of the stomach). Such an expansion takes place in an aircraft cabin pressurized to an atmospheric pressure of 8000 feet. Placement of a nasogastric tube with active suctioning every few minutes and flying at the lowest possible altitude will help minimize these adverse effects. The same type of expansion occurs in the air space above intravenous fluids in glass containers during air transport (Donn et al., 1985).

Infants have small, straight eustachian tubes which can collapse with the pressure changes during descent. This can interfere with the release of pressure on the tympanic membrane, resulting in an acute, stabbing pain until the pressure equalizes. Giving a conscious newborn a pacifier or a finger to suck as descent begins until landing can help keep the tubes open.

NEONATAL TRANSPORT: AFTER YOU ARRIVE AT THE HOSPITAL

Carry the baby in yourself or accompany the transporting attendants (if an ambulance was called) to the receiving area. If arrangements were made in advance to meet a neonatal specialist, inform the hospital staff and ask for the person by name whenever possible. Be prepared with your chart, the parents' names and the status of the baby. Give a presumed diagnosis only if the problem is obvious and unmistakable (such as gastroschisis). If not, describe in as much detail as possible what you have observed and the reason you felt transport was warranted. You may or may not be asked your opinion, depending upon the care providers and general opinion of the local medical community regarding midwifery and homebirth. Most of the time, the midwife is pretty much out of the picture once the baby's care is assumed by the hospital staff.

Both parents should be introduced to the specialist, and they should ask for one or both of them to be allowed to accompany the baby. The degree of emergency will dictate if and to what extent the parents are allowed to be with the baby. For example, if the baby requires immediate surgery, preparations will occur fast and furiously, precluding much familial involvement until the baby has stabilized after the surgery is completed. In many cases, however, the situation will not be this dire, and the parents may be able to stay with the baby most of the time. The parents should ask questions and request that any procedures be explained, with the understanding that many babies transported for the types of problems outlined in this section will require extensive diagnostic workups to determine the exact diagnosis, range of problems that may be present and the options for treatment. It is important that the most complete understanding of the baby's condition possible be obtained before options are discussed, as the presence of multiple problems can dramatically affect the best options for a particular baby. Also, any conditions that do not require immediate treatment for clearly medical reasons should be postponed until the parents have had an opportunity to research the pros and cons of all treatments proposed as well as no treatment. This is especially important for babies born with atypical genitalia.

Diagnosis

In most cases, the same types of diagnostic tests that are used in adults are also used for newborns. Some babies will require multiple tests to look for problems in different organ systems. Here is an overview of such tests:

- Blood tests (red and white blood cell counts; liver and kidney function; blood cultures for infection, hormone, glucose, electrolytes, and endocrine tests)
- Genetic tests
- Urine tests of various types to look for infection, blood, specific gravity minerals, metabolites and quantity
- X-ray studies of various types to detect respiratory, renal, cardiac and gastrointestinal disorders (including CT scan, which shows slices of the anatomy)
- Electrocardiography (ECG) studies, often augmented by the use of Doppler ultrasound and color blood flow mapping, to analyze the heart rate, rhythm and general function; cardiac catheterization may be necessary to detect coronary arterial defects.
- Ultrasound (renal, urinary, cardiac and other suspected vascular disorders)
- Dye studies (dye is fed or injected and its pathway tracked via X-ray)
- Electroencephalogram (EEG) (brain or neurological disorders)

SPECIFIC NEONATAL DEFECTS AND DISORDERS

EVALUATING THE NEWBORN WITH SUSPECTED NEUROLOGICAL COMPROMISE

You will be constantly assessing the baby for normal responses and behavior during the first hours after birth. These responses reflect the health of her nervous system and brain. Some of the ways in which the nervous system is evaluated are included in the chapters covering the complete examination of the newborn. In general, a midwife needs to look deeper, using more specific neurologically oriented assessments only if she suspects a problem. However, as a student, you should familiarize yourself with the range of evaluative tools available. Knowing what to look for allows you to observe the baby more astutely and may allow you to satisfactorily answer the question of whether further evaluation is needed.

The baby's central nervous system is one of the least developed at birth; nevertheless, it is far more sophisticated than many people realize. Although the baby's range of vocal communication is limited, as is his control over muscular activity, the baby is learning rapidly to interpret input from the extrauterine world (a continuation of the learning process already begun in utero). The nervous system warrants careful evaluation as it offers evidence of abnormalities of the brain as well as injuries that may have occurred during pregnancy or birth.

The examination of the nervous system may be divided into two general parts. The first involves assessment of structures outside the brain, which can help determine if the baby has a neurological disorder. The second involves systematic testing of various functions of the central nervous system. This chapter is based on Illingworth (1970, 1975, 1987) unless otherwise noted.

If you have questions about the baby's neurological well-being in the immediate postpartum period, you should proceed with a complete newborn exam (covered in the subchapters included in "The Complete Physical Examination of the Newborn") before leaving the house.

Historical Review

Review the following details from your prenatal history and newborn examination prior to beginning a neurological evaluation:

Prenatal findings of significance include:

Quality and quantity of fetal movement: Diminished fetal movement may be the first evidence of muscle weakness due to infantile spinal muscular atrophy, congenital myotonic dystrophy, or congenital myopathy.

Abnormal positioning: Breech positioning may be due to lack of fetal muscle tone or movement seen in the disorders listed above as well as others.

Polyhydramnios: This may be due to decreased swallowing from bulbar (hindbrain) weakness.

Abnormal heart rate patterns: These may reflect abnormal neural mechanisms controlling the heart rate.

Maternal history of certain medical conditions: Myasthenia, thyrotoxicosis, and myotonic dystrophy are among the maternal conditions that have a direct effect on the central nervous system of the newborn.

Family history of siblings affected with neurological disorders: Several disorders involving weakness and hypotonia due to peripheral nervous system problems are genetic in origin.

Ask yourself the following questions while reviewing the newborn examination:

- Do the gestational-age assessments by dates and by examination match?
- Does the labor history suggest that the baby suffered hypoxia or asphyxia?
- Were there signs of trauma or undue moulding of the head or spine?
- Is the baby's cry unusual in any way?
- Are head circumference, fontanelles and suture lines normal?
- Do the suture lines and the anterior and posterior fontanelles appear of to be of normal size without evidence of fusion or of acute intracranial volume expansion or reduction?
- Is the baby asymmetrically large or is she small for dates?
- Does it appear that the baby was malnourished in utero?

- Are there skin lesions associated with neurological conditions (more than 6 café-au-lait spots, port-wine stain over the area of the face supplied by the trigeminal nerve [eyelids, nose, jaw], areas of depigmentation or other dermatological signs suggesting associated syndromes)?
- Is there evidence of spinal defects?
- Are there any bruits audible over the skull? (These suggest arteriovascular malformation.)
- Is the baby at increased risk for infection or other illness? Sick babies are relatively inactive, sleepy, lack interest in nursing, cry less and present with generalized depression of the nervous system.

Have you noticed any of the following abnormalities that are often associated with significant brain injury?
- Persistent failure to latch onto the breast or suck. This may occur in normal babies immediately postpartum.
- Irritability, staring or persistently holding the hands in a clenched fist
- Persistent head retraction with abnormal muscle tone in the extremities. This must be distinguished from posture due to intrauterine positioning, which would be accompanied by normal muscle tone.
- Hypo- or hypertonia
- Lack of spontaneous or symmetrical movement
- Seizure activity

Testing Neurological Function

These assessments are covered in more detail in the subchapter entitled "Observing the Infant and Evaluating Posture, Muscle Tone." Because of this, only certain central points and abnormal findings are highlighted in the following review.

State of consciousness

You will be constantly evaluating the baby's state of consciousness throughout your interaction with and observation of the baby. Alertness includes variables such as turning the head toward a variety of stimuli from the environment, widening of the eyes, brightness (an expression of attentive interest on the baby's face), and the ability to shut out interfering or extraneous stimuli. Such responses range from very dull and slow to fairly long, attentive periods.

The state of alertness determines the way the baby will respond to various assessments. The more alert the infant, the better he will respond to any stimulus offered and the better will be the score. His state should be noted as each assessment is made. While assessing the infant, look for smooth transitions from state to state with appropriate stimuli; persistent lethargy or irritability is not normal. The baby should be able to calm himself, and any crying should be well modulated and expressive. Abnormal findings include a strong preference for a single state with transition to another state difficult or impossible, hyperalertness or persistent crying without reason (keeping in mind that babies do cry if they are frightened or angry), failure to achieve a fully awake state or a weak or monotonous cry. Keep in mind that environmental factors such as ambient temperature, light and noise will impact the baby's state of consciousness.

Depressed response: A decreased level of responsiveness must be assessed in relationship to gestational age and the behavioral state of the baby. When charting, the type of stimuli used to try and change the state should be described, such as "physical handling," "loud noise" or "exposure to cold or heat."

A decreased level of consciousness may result from the following conditions:

Hypoxic ischemic encephalopathy (HIE): This is the most common cause of an altered level of consciousness in the immediate newborn period. (The states associated with various levels of severity are outlined in the chapter entitled "The Healthy Full-Term Newborn in the First Hours of Life.")

Intracranial hemorrhage: Bleeding may be associated with a difficult birth or unusual fetal position. Trauma may result in localized or general signs of central nervous system compromise, including a decreased level of consciousness, which may fluctuate over the first few hours or days of life. Trauma and hypoxic ischemic encephalopathy may occur together in term babies; therefore, babies with any degree of nervous system depression that cannot be explained by an asphyxial event alone should be evaluated for intracranial bleeding. (Intracranial hemorrhage is discussed in the subchapter entitled "Cranial Injuries.")

Infection: Babies born with an active infection may be less responsive, especially when the central nervous system is involved. Any baby with an abrupt change in neurological status should always be evaluated for sepsis or meningitis.

Drug intoxication: Babies exposed to maternal drug use may display a decreased level of consciousness, lethargy, hypotonia, decreased respiratory response and sluggish reflexes. Drugs such as narcotics, alcohol, magnesium sulfate or anticonvulsants may be causative. See the subchapter entitled "Drug Withdrawal."

Metabolic disorders: Metabolic problems of all types commonly produce alterations in the level of consciousness. Hypoglycemic infants may be stuporous, hypotonic or irritable and may have seizures and jitteriness. Hypocalcemia may result in decreased responsiveness plus hypotonia and seizures. It is very rare for an inborn error of metabolism to manifest itself in the first few hours postpartum, but it can happen if the disorder is sufficiently severe. Sufficient intake of the problematic substance results in lethargy, stupor or coma and may result in seizures. Other signs include vomiting, an unusual odor to the skin or urine, and family history.

Electrolyte disorders: A type of metabolic derangement, both sodium and sometimes potassium imbalances may cause alterations in the baby's consciousness. This is particularly relevant to babies who are born jaundiced and those with intersex conditions, who may have a sodium-losing adrenal imbalance. Hyperbilirubinemia, when severe, may also result in lethargy and hypotonia.

Clinical classification of a persistently diminished level of consciousness may fall in the following categories:

LEVEL OF ALERTNESS	BEHAVIORAL STATE OF BABY	AROUSAL RESPONSE	MOTOR RESPONSES	
			QUANTITY	QUALITY
Normal	Awake; normal variations in states	Rouses with gentle manual stimulation, may rouse spontaneously with environmental stimulation	Normal	Normal, high level
Lethargy or slight stupor	Persistently drowsy	Moderately difficult to rouse to more alertness, soon returns to lethargic state without stimulation	Slightly diminished	Normal, high level
Moderate stupor	Persistently sleeping	Difficult to arouse, vigorous or repeated stimulation is required to rouse	Moderately diminished	Normal, high level
Deep stupor	Persistently sleeping	Can be aroused only if continual stimulation is used, with immediate resumption of sleep when the stimulus is removed	Markedly diminished	Normal, high level
Coma	Persistently sleeping	Unable to rouse, only responds to motor stimulation	Markedly diminished	Normal, high level
	Unconscious	Impossible to rouse	Absent	Abnormal, low level

Behavioral evaluation

Babies can respond to a variety of sensory stimuli and integrate input in a relatively sophisticated manner. Behavioral activity can be used as a clinical tool to assess overall neurological health. Responses are dependent upon the baby's state of consciousness. One of the primary transient negative influences on newborn behavior and on her state of consciousness is maternal drug intake during labor. Since babies born at home are not exposed to maternal drug intake (unless the mother is taking recreational drugs without your knowledge), any variations from normal newborn behavior are highly suspicious of an underlying problem. The discussion that follows is intended to help the midwife hone her observational skills so that spontaneous newborn behavior can be interpreted intelligently and thus reduce the need for formal assessments.

Behavioral assessment encompasses most of the other aspects of the exam. These include muscle tone, level of alertness, level of receptivity to stimuli, the baby's ability to alter his state of arousal, the ability to suppress repetitive or intrusive stimuli, other social interactions, and physiological responses such as changes in skin color, tremors, respirations and heart rate.

Most of the following behavioral assessments are discussed elsewhere in this text. Those that are not are discussed in more detail here. Most responses have two components. First is local flexion, or withdrawal of the stimulated limb. The other is generalized and may include trunk or limb motion, color change, increased alertness or crying. Scoring of the response is graded from 0 to 3 and is based on withdrawal of the stimulus. The ranges are none (0), weak and delayed (1), fair but slow (2), and brisk, easily elicited response or withdrawal (3).

Habituation (decrement): The normal baby has the ability to filter meaningless stimuli, especially when the same stimulus is presented repeatedly. Response decrement or habitation is such a response. For example, when a new, simple sensory stimulus is presented to the baby over and over, the initial response evoked diminishes over time and finally extinguishes or disappears. The original response will reappear when a another stimulus is presented, even if it is only slightly different. The types of observable responses that habituate include changes in muscle tone, head and trunk turning, and autonomic nervous system alterations such as decreased heart rate and changes in breathing pattern. Responses to painful stimuli do not habituate in the normal infant and should never be used.

The number of stimulus responses required to observably alter the general response is noted as the habituation score. Always allow the response to subside before offering the stimulus again. Do not give more than 12 to 14 repeated stimuli before deciding that habituation has not occurred. This eliminates the possibility of fatigue becoming a confounding factor in your assessment. The ability to habituate to stimuli is an important criterion for a normal response. An obligatory response to an original stimulus and unvarying repetition without any change or shutoff of response is not usually seen and may indicate an abnormality.

Pinprick response: Because the intention is to stimulate without causing pain (in part because the baby will not habituate to pain in the same way as she will to a benign stimulus), most midwives and parents will not like the idea of using a pin for this test. Instead, touch the foot with the tip of a blunt-pointed object or one that is cold; this may suffice to elicit the same response. Apply gentle pressure to the sole of the foot while the baby is lying in a supine position. The baby should withdraw her foot right away.

Resistance to passive motion: This can be assessed with four examinations. While these are also tests of muscle tone, here the focus is on the baby's behavioral response.

Pull-to-sit: Head flexion is scored in a range from complete floppiness to weak resistance to extreme resistance with a stiff neck. Normal head control at term consists of a forward tilt with little lag when the infant is supported by the hands into an upright sitting position.

Forearm recoil: The infant's passively extended forearm is suddenly released. Here the score is based on absent recoil, weak recoil or recoil to 45°. Normal recoil at term is marked and symmetrical. An asymmetrical or very strong response or rapid, bilateral recoil may not be completely normal and may be evidence of hyperreflexia or hypertonicity.

Scarf sign: Hold the head and torso in a semireclining position by supporting the neck and head with one hand. Bring one of the baby's arms across the chest as if to place the hand on the opposite shoulder. See how far over the elbow reaches in relationship to the midline and evaluate resistance. It may be more informative to apply pressure just above the elbow to push the arm over. A normal response is symmetrical from side to side and appropriate for gestational age (there is increasing resistance to this maneuver as the baby approaches term). If the baby is obese, hydropic or has a shortened humerus or fractured clavicle, the movement of the arm will be inhibited and not truly reflective of muscle tone or responsiveness. An abnormal scarf sign manifests as failure to reach the position expected for gestational age or an exaggerated response. Asymmetry suggests weakness on the side which the elbow reaches the farthest. Unusual resistance on one side is likely to be due to something other than neuromuscular tone, such as a fractured clavicle. Bilaterally exaggerated responses are noted with increased tone in the shoulder girdle. Also see the chapter entitled "Assessment of Gestational Age."

Truncal tone: The baby is suspended horizontally with a hand under the abdomen. Scoring ranges from extreme floppiness or hypotonia, to progressively increasing attempts to extend the head or neck, to vigorous straightening of the trunk. The most extreme response is complete rigidity, which may be abnormal. The normal newborn can maintain his head and sacrum in the same plane for at least 3 to 5 seconds.

General body tone: This is a subjective assessment of the baby's muscle tone during the truncal tone exam. Scoring ranges from complete hypotonia to weak tone to normal strong tone and finally to hypertonicity.

Primitive reflexes: Polysynaptic reflexes such as the Moro, grasp, palmomental and symmetric tonic neck are normally present. Overreactive reflexes produce abnormal postures which may be sustained (dystonic) and can be confused with seizures. Hypotonia, hypertonia or abnormal primitive reflexes delay or interfere with the development of more mature reflexes.

Rooting reflex: Start with the baby supine and the head in the midline. As a finger touches the corner of the baby's mouth, the baby is scored on head turning and lip movement. Scoring ranges from no response to increasingly vigorous head turning and sucking movements with the mouth.

Sucking reflex: With the infant lying down or in your arms, insert your index finger, pad up, into the baby's mouth. Rub the hard palate to stimulate latch on if the baby does not latch on immediately. Scoring ranges from no response to a weak response to 1 to 3 sucks per group. Long periods of vigorous sucking are normal.

Difficulties include persistently slow or poor sucking, prolonged feeding, or regurgitation and choking with feeding. This requires an evaluation of the suck-swallow reflexes (described fully in the subchapter entitled "Developmental Reflexes and Other Neuromotor Evaluations"). Unresolved fetal head moulding, central nervous system damage from hypoxia or trauma and anatomical or functional disorders of the gastrointestinal tract are the primary causes of difficulty with nursing.

Moro response: Hold the baby in your hands so she is supine and let her head fall back rapidly about 10 cm. The baby should reflexively extend her arms, then flex them more slowly, bringing them in front of her body to create a complete embracing motion. Normal infants respond in this manner on the first or second try. Scoring ranges from no response to the response described. The Moro reflex can be used to assess habituation to determine when the maximum response becomes altered; however, since it is one of the most distressing newborn evaluations, most midwives will not want to repeat this test 12 times.

Response to light: Shine a dim penlight in the baby's field of vision or briefly into his eyes until you have his attention. The baby should close his eyes in response. After this has occurred, repeat the test until the baby obviously changes his response. This test is also rather intrusive but becomes important if there is any question about the baby's ability to see.

Response to sound: Quiet the room before you begin. With the baby lying on her back, hold a bell or toy frog clicker in the midline but out of sight behind the baby's head, then make a continuous sound a few inches from the baby's ear. Be careful not to disturb the examining surface, which will provide additional stimulation. Observe the baby's attentiveness to the sound. The scale ranges from no reaction to a slight change in attention level with some head turning to search or other alerting behavior to the fully normal response of definite searching with almost immediate response to the sound. This stimulus can be repeated as each response subsides up to 12 times to see when the baby's response changes. At that point, the habituation to sound number is recorded.

In addition, the assessments described in the subchapter entitled "Developmental Reflexes and Other Neuromotor Evaluations," can be performed, as indicated, to further evaluate the baby. The baby's response to those evaluations can be scored as discussed in this chapter.

Neuromuscular evaluation

Both the central and peripheral nervous systems contribute to the control of muscular movement and tone. All of these nerves originate in the cerebral cortex and terminate in individual muscles, and together comprise what is known as the motor system. Usually there is no evidence of brain damage as the cause of neuromuscular disorders. Assessment takes into account muscle size, tone, deep tendon reflexes, localized contraction (if any) and how easily the baby becomes fatigued. Arthrogryposis, which presents with fixation of position and limitation of movement in the limbs, is often a primary finding when neuromuscular disease is present. Atrophic or hypoplastic muscles and decreased deep tendon reflexes are also frequently seen.

Posture: Normal posture for various gestational ages is discussed in the chapters entitled "Assessment of Gestational Age" and "Observing the Infant and Evaluating Posture and Muscle Tone." Abnormal postures include persistent extension of the neck, obligate flexion of the thumb, and splaying of the legs with the outer thighs resting on the mattress and knees flexed, called "frog-leg positioning," which is abnormal after 32 to 36 weeks gestation. Other abnormal postures include:

Opisthotonic posture: The head is tilted back or cocked at an extended angle, the back is arched, and the upper limbs, the lower limbs or both are extended. This suggests abnormal hypertonicity of the extensor muscles of the neck and may be seen with bacterial meningitis, severe hypoxic ischemic brain damage, massive intraventricular hemorrhage and tetanus (although probably not at birth). Note that a baby born by face presentation may mimic the head position of this abnormal posture, but in this case, the head can be gently guided into a normal position and the other muscles have normal tone.

Decorticate posture: The legs and arms are extended with the wrists flexed and hands clenched.

Decerebrate posture: The arms are flexed and the legs are extended.

Other abnormal postures to which formal terms are not assigned include:

- Lying with the limbs flat on the mattress
- Elbows flexed with the backs of the hands on the mattress
- Exaggerated flexion of the extremities
- Shoulder abducted and arms flexed with the hands constantly in front of the mouth
- Marked or persistent asymmetry in limb posture (for example, the asymmetrical tonic neck reflex held for 30 seconds or more). Turning the head consistently to one side with an asymmetrical overall posture suggests nerve damage such as a brachial palsy.
- Hands always held in a tight fist

<u>**Muscle tone**</u>: This evaluation includes observation of the resting tone, passive tone and active tone of the major muscle groups. Both passive and active tone should be assessed separately and may vary independently. The tests for muscle tension are directly related to the baby's state of alertness and are also influenced by gestational age. They should be assessed when the baby is awake and alert.

Phasic or **passive tone** is a brief, forceful muscle contraction in response to a large (high-amplitude) stretch of short duration when moving a joint at rest. It is tested by evaluating the resistance of the upper and lower limbs to movement and by the activity of the deep tendon reflexes. Resistance to passive movement can be assessed with the scarf sign and with arm and leg recoil maneuvers. Minimal resistance is normal at 28 weeks and progressively increases with maturity. Deep tendon reflexes are discussed in the subchapter entitled "Deep Tendon Reflexes." Passive tone can be evaluated with the ventral suspension, scarf sign, heel-to-ear, popliteal angle, recoil of the forearm and square window maneuvers.

Active or **postural tone** is a long-duration, small (low-amplitude) stretch in response to gravity. Normal postural tone requires the integrated functioning of the entire central nervous system. Thus, hypotonia usually reflects disorders involving the central or peripheral nervous systems or skeletal muscles. Active tone can be evaluated with the palmar grasp, pull-to-sit maneuver and ventral suspension.

These assessments may reveal that the baby is normotonic, hypotonic or hypertonic:

Pull-to-sit maneuver: Postural tone is best evaluated using the pull-to-sit maneuver, which assesses the baby's ability to resist gravity. Grasp the baby's hands and slowly pull him from a supine to a sitting position. At term, the baby assists by contracting his shoulder and arm muscles and flexing his elbows, knees, ankles and neck in an attempt to keep his head in line with his spine. His head should leave the mattress almost simultaneously as the head is pulled up, lagging only slightly behind his body. The head should remain erect for a moment when the baby achieves a sitting posture. When the trunk is tilted forward, the head falls forward as well. At term, more than minimal head lag is abnormal and usually reflects postural hypotonia. Note that neck flexion is absent prior to 33 weeks gestation. Abnormal responses include asymmetry in pulling back, with flaccidity on one side, in one limb, in the arms but a strong response in the lower limbs, or the reverse; complete lack of resistance; full head lag; pull to stand rather than sit; or failure of the head to fall forward once a seated posture has been achieved. An unusually strong response in the neck and trunk extension, especially if seen with failure of the head to drop forward in the sitting position, suggests abnormally increased extensor tone.

Ventral suspension maneuver: Hold the baby by placing your palm under the chest and suspending the baby in a prone position with the head slightly higher than the pelvis. Note the posture of the head, neck and limbs. A healthy term baby can hold her head in line with her body for at least 3 seconds (or should at a minimum attempt to lift her head), with the back straight, hips slightly extended, and arms and legs flexed. Abnormal tone may manifest as less flexor tone in the arms than the legs, generalized floppiness with the legs splayed frog fashion, or extensor hypertonus.

Hypotonia: Central or nonparalytic hypotonia is the most common abnormality seen in infants during the neurological exam. It describes a baby who is flaccid and offers abnormally weak or no resistance to passive movements. It often predominates in the axial muscles of the neck and trunk and proximal muscles of the limbs, possibly because their muscle tone and function develop last and are therefore vulnerable to perinatal insults. The evaluation is subjective; based on the examiner's perception of weak resistance to movement, which widens the normal range of motion. Hypotonia is found with a wide range of problems, most commonly acute encephalopathy resulting from a major insult to the central nervous system such as hypoxic ischemia, birth trauma, intracranial hemorrhage, infection or hypoglycemia. It may progress into normal tone or even hypertonia over the following days or weeks, depending upon the cause. Persistent hypotonia is also seen in lesions of the midline cerebral structures and basal ganglia. Associated signs include convulsions, a decreased level of consciousness and depressed primitive reflexes, although varying levels of deep tendon reflex response are usually present.

Chronic causes of central or generalized hypotonia include many chromosomal and genetic disorders, such as Down and Prader-Willi syndromes. Consciousness is usually *not* affected in such disorders. Central hypotonia may also be a prominent feature in babies with metabolic, nutritional, endocrine, connective tissue disorders or other conditions, such as familial dysautonomia. In problems involving the metabolism or endocrine system, consciousness may be profoundly affected once the disorder has progressed to the symptomatic stage.

Paralytic hypotonia is usually found in babies that are hypotonic with weakness, have an absence of reflexes and have an alert state of consciousness. This generally results from trauma to the upper levels of the spinal cord, disease of the spinal anterior horn cells, or abnormalities of the neuromuscular junction or of the muscle itself. The categories of causes include:

Spinal cord or nerve trauma: Spinal cord trauma presents with respiratory depression, generalized hypotonia and flaccid weakness of the limbs. The baby cannot feel anything below the level of injury and no deep tendon reflexes can be elicited, as the baby is in spinal shock. A baby with normal facial and cranial nerve function in the presence of either quadriplegia or paraplegia must be evaluated for spinal cord injury. Damage to spinal nerve roots results in localized weakness; the area affected will be determined according to the nerves involved.

A localized injury to one side of the cerebellum on can result in weakness of the muscles of the face, arm and, to a lesser extent, the leg on the opposite side. Injury in the parasagittal cerebral region, often caused by perfusion disorders in the brain, results in weakness of the arms more than the legs.

Infantile spinal muscular atrophy (ISMA): In the acute, fulminating form of this disorder, the baby presents with generalized, profound weakness, absent deep tendon reflexes and an alert, expressive face. The tongue is atrophied and involuntarily twitches or contracts. Weakness results in respiratory difficulty and makes the baby prone to aspiration pneumonia. There is no loss of sensation or of sphincter control.

Transient myasthenia gravis: This is seen only in babies born to myasthenic mothers. It causes early feeding problems, generalized weakness, respiratory difficulties and hypotonia, although deep tendon reflexes are normal. Weakness of the muscles around the eyes and droopy eyelids are usually not noted in the transient form but are common in congenital myasthenia, which may occasionally cause neonatal hypotonia. The diagnosis is confirmed if the symptoms reverse after injecting anticholinesterase drugs.

Congenital myopathies: Quite a few congenital muscle disorders present with hypotonia in the newborn. These disorders cannot be distinguished from each other by symptoms alone; brain function and responses to sensation are usually normal.

Congenital myotonic dystrophy: Babies with this disorder have respiratory and nursing problems, paralysis on both sides of the face, severe contracture in the joints of the limbs, and hypotonia. A history of polyhydramnios and a mother with facial features associated with myotonic dystrophy and in whom myotonia can be elicited helps confirm the diagnosis.

Werdnig-Hoffmann disease: This disorder of the lower motor neurons causes flaccidity and weakness of the limbs, with normal tone in the face and normal cranial nerve function early on. Spontaneous contraction of a group of muscles, which presents with continuous rapid twitching movements known as **fasciculation**, may be noted in the tongue.

In a hypotonic baby, inspect and palpate the muscle groups for loss of mass and the associated joints for range of motion.

Flapping of the extremities: This test can be helpful in assessing the relative tone from side to side but should not be performed if spinal injury is suspected. With the baby lying on his back, grasp both of the arms or both of the legs simultaneously above either the wrists or ankles and gently shake them while comparing the movements of the free portion of the limbs on either side. An increase in floppiness indicates a decrease in muscle tone. While amplitude may vary by gestational age (with earlier babies having a wider range), the degree of floppiness should be the same on both sides. If it isn't, this suggests paralysis of the limb with the greater degree of floppiness (Fletcher, 1998).

Hypertonia: Hypertonia is less often a feature of disorders in the neonatal period. When present, the baby is extremely stiff and has marked resistance to passive movements of the limbs, which, when performed, may increase the tone even more, with limited range of motion. It may predominate in the flexor or extensor muscles. It is commonly generalized but may be unilateral or effect only the legs. Flexion hypertonia is more common than extension, especially in the upper limbs. Extension hypertonia is always abnormal. The limbs may be held in rigid postures, and the head may be maintained in an extended or even a backward position (neck extensor hypertonia) during ventral suspension, as described in the section covering posture, above. Typically, the baby appears stiff, tight and "too strong." The arms are flexed, the shoulders thrown back and the thumbs are tightly clenched in the palms. The legs may be tightly flexed or extended. While giving an appearance of strength due to the force required to move the limbs, the baby shows little spontaneous movement, which is slow and poorly controlled. Generalized hypertonia is usually asymmetric with one side more affected than the other; unilateral hypertonia is far less common. Hypertonia of only the legs may be due to lesions of the lower cervical or upper thoracic spine (Ziai et al., 1984). Hypertonia may represent severe neurologic compromise and requires prompt referral and evaluation.

Muscle strength: While there are several scales for recording muscle strength, that in the following table seems the most useful for midwives because it is highly descriptive.

GRADE	DESCRIPTION OF MUSCULAR RESPONSE
Zero	No detectable contraction of the muscle
Trace	Palpable contraction without motion of the part the muscle should move; no joint motion occurs when gravity is eliminated.
Poor minus	Muscle able to move part;, but not through a complete range of motion and not against gravity
Poor	Muscle able to move part through a complete range of motion when gravity is eliminated, but not against gravity
Fair minus	Muscle able to move part against gravity, but not through a complete range of motion
Fair	Muscle able to carry part through a complete range of motion against gravity, but not against added resistance
Good minus	Muscle able to carry part through a complete range of motion against gravity with minimal added resistance
Good	Muscle able to carry part through its complete range of motion against gravity with moderate resistance
Good plus	Muscle able to carry part through its complete range of motion with almost full resistance
Normal	Normal strength; able to carry part through its complete range of motion with full resistance and without evidence of fatigue

Strength is usually correlated with muscle tone, although in some infants muscle weakness may be present with extensor hypertonus. Strength is difficult to evaluate in babies because it is hard to distinguish weakness (a reduction in strength or power) from abnormal tone (diminished or increased tone with tone defined as the tension present when the muscle is at rest). Hypotonia produces a soft, flaccid muscle. Hypertonia produces an extremely rigid muscle. In babies, muscle strength and tone are evaluated together with the palmar grasp reflex, the pull-to-sit maneuver and the stepping response.

Spontaneous movement: All movements are assessed, especially those of the limbs, for quality and symmetry. The term baby is normally active, moving her limbs smoothly in an alternating fashion while awake. The baby who is 28 weeks or less will have only short periods of activity, with three types of movement usually seen: an entire limb is moved rapidly through a large arc; the baby may make slow, twisting movements of limbs, neck and spine, with grimacing; and there may be occasional jerking motions of an entire limb. By 32 weeks, symmetrical flexor movements of the knees and hips are replacing more primitive movements, and the baby begins to turn his head. By 36 weeks, flexor motions of the legs are more prominent and are no longer asymmetrical.

Jitteriness: Tremors of the arms and legs are seen in some normal full-term babies when crying. Normal, mild jitters present as rhythmic, symmetrical shaking of the limbs. Abnormal responses include bicycling of the legs; swatting of the arm without any stimulus; asymmetric, weak and jittery movements while sucking; and a flat facial expression. Moderate jitters may be seen in a variety of conditions including birth asphyxia or hemorrhage, small-for-gestational-age infants, metabolic disorders, hypoglycemia, hypocalcemia, hypomagnesemia, hyperviscosity syndrome, drug withdrawal and congenital central nervous system defects. Extreme or persistent jitters in a baby with normal blood sugar and electrolyte balance may indicate irritation of the central nervous system; the baby should be evaluated as for seizure activity. (Jitteriness is further discussed in the subchapter entitled "Observing the Infant and Evaluating Posture, Muscle Tone.")

Seizures: Seizures are often the first indication of a central nervous system problem and are the most distinctive sign of neurological disease in newborns. They are clinically defined as spasmodic alterations of neurologic function that may affect behavior, motor or autonomic activity.

There is wide variation in the presentation of newborn seizure activity. It can be subtle, differing considerably from those in older children. In addition, a variety of neurologic presentations may mimic seizure activity in newborns because the newborn brain is less capable of propagating generalized or organized electrical discharges. These include jitteriness (described above), clonus, rhythmic alternating movement of the limbs of equal velocity, tonic posturing movements and apnea. There are four types of seizure activity described by Volpe (2001):

Subtle seizures: These motor automatisms are common and repetitive. They include movements of the mouth, face, tongue or eyes, such as lip smacking, facial muscle movement, tongue thrusting, or eye deviation, and autonomic nervous system signs, such as changes in vital signs. Subtle seizures often occur in conjunction with other types. In term babies, they are frequently related to asphyxia. However, they are more commonly seen in preterm than term infants. Subtle seizures are often not epileptic, rarely interfering with heart or respiratory function and not appearing to cause brain injury.

Clonic seizures: This type may be focal or multifocal. Focal clonic seizures are rhythmic, repetitive jerking movements of the face, or one or both limbs on one side of the body. They may be associated with localized cortical disorders or generalized disorders such as metabolic encephalopathies. Multifocal clonic seizures are movements in several different parts of the body, often with the seizure activity moving from one part of the body to another. They are usually associated with asphyxia in term babies.

Tonic seizures: Focal tonic seizures involve only one limb. Generalized tonic seizures involve the entire body, presenting with a sudden increase in muscle tone, usually manifesting as extension. The are often seen as posturing of a limb or symmetric positioning of the trunk, neck or both. They are found with intraventricular hemorrhage in preterm babies and may occur as an adverse reaction to anticonvulsant therapy.

Myoclonic seizures: These seizures differ from clonic movements in that they present with a more rapid jerking and are more likely to occur in flexor muscle groups. They may be focal, multifocal or generalized and are characterized by single flexion of an arm, or asynchronous twitching of several parts of the body or bilateral jerks of flexion in the arms or the legs.

The timing of onset as well as any associated physical abnormalities and the overall neurological status of the baby can help in determining the possible cause of the seizures, which may include:

Perinatal asphyxia: This accounts for most seizures in term newborns, with 50 to 70% of all acutely asphyxiated babies having seizures. They are often subtle, tonic or multifocal clonic seizures and usually occur within the first 6 to 24 hours. They often disappear on their own, even though they may resist therapies. In perinatal asphyxia, the baby's responses between convulsions are usually abnormal.

Intracranial hemorrhage: Bleeding may occur due to birth trauma, hypoxic ischemic injury, low platelets (thrombocytopenia), coagulation disorders, vascular defects or tumors, or injury from invasive procedures after transport. The baby will start to seize 24 to 48 hours after birth with focal, clonic or subtle events. The baby may appear normal between seizures, or may display systemic collapse with anemia, shock, hyper- or hypotonia, lethargy, vomiting, apnea, bradycardia, localized neurological signs and a bulging fontanelle. External evidence of birth trauma may be present. Intraventricular bleeding in preterm babies occurs within 17 to 72 hours of life, with sudden deterioration and tonic or multifocal clonic seizures. See the subchapter entitled "Cranial Injury."

Cerebral infarction or stroke: Localized necrosis in well-defined arterial locations has a high correlation with seizures, especially in full-term babies. Strokes involve the acute impairment of cerebral circulation that lasts more than 24 hours. They occur in a variety of cerebrovascular disorders such as asphyxia, polycythemia, acute severe hypertension and embolization. The majority of these accidents occur after apparently normal births. The infarct may go undiagnosed unless cranial imaging studies are done.

Infection: Seizure activity is often found in conjunction with sepsis, particularly acquired bacterial meningitis. This may occur at any time after birth through several weeks of age.

Metabolic derangement: Hypoglycemia may result in seizures during the first hours or days of life. Hypocalcemia (low serum calcium) may present in the first 3 days.

Cerebral dysgenetic disorders: Malformations of the brain are suggested by more obvious dysmorphic findings in the infant such as abnormal head circumference, size or shape. Seizures may present any time during the neonatal period and tend to be of mixed types. Dysgenetic disorders are those which have a detrimental effect upon hereditary qualities.

Eye movement: Abnormal eye movements are usually involuntary and include the following variations (Fletcher, 1998):

Seizure activity: Tonic deviation of gaze to one side or downward, often seen with fine jerking eye movements.

Ocular bobbing: Intermittent upward and downward eye motion

Opsoclonus: Obvious rapid, irregular, multidirectional jerking of both eyes in unison

Ocular flutter: Rapid, irregular, conjugate jerking in the horizontal plane

Nystagmus: Rhythmic, conjugate (simultaneous), pendulum-like motion of the eyes in a horizontal plane. This may occur as a single finding due to structural defects of the eye; it is also seen in albinism and optic nerve hypoplasia.

Abnormal head circumference

A head that is larger than normal is described as **macrocephalic**. It may be secondary to a collection of fluid in the subdural space, **hydrocephalus** that results in dilation of the ventricles of the brain or, more rarely, **megaloencephalus**, in which the brain is abnormally large.

Congenital hydrocephalus is often associated with spinal defects, especially myelomeningocele at the level of the thoracolumbar, lumbar or lumbosacral levels. In such cases, there is about a 95% chance of significant ventricular dilation if the head circumference falls above the 90th percentile. There is about a 65% chance of hydrocephalus if it is less than the 90th percentile. Defects of the ventricular drainage system, such as aqueduct stenosis, may also result in congenital hydrocephalus. Clinical signs of increased intracranial pressure include a bulging anterior fontanelle and separation of the cranial sutures. However, signs of increased pressure may not be apparent if the spinal lesion is leaking spinal fluid. Other causes of congenital hydrocephalus include TORCH infections (toxoplasmosis, other, rubella, cytomegalovirus, and herpes), vascular defects and other developmental defects of the central nervous system as well as, on rare occasions, cerebral tumors.

Acquired hydrocephalus is usually a product of intracranial hemorrhage, especially if it occurs in the ventricles in small preterm babies or in those with bacterial meningitis.

Megaloencephalus may be familial or associated with disorders such as cerebral gigantism, Beckwith-Wiedemann syndrome, achondroplasia and the neurocutaneous syndromes that may cause brain enlargement (these include phakomatoses such as Sturge-Weber and tuberous sclerosis). Megaloencephalus is also caused by a build-up of metabolic products such as the lipidoses, which may occur in Tay-Sachs disease, and in the mucopolysaccharidosis disorders, such as Hurler syndrome.

Microcephalus describes a baby with a head circumference below the third percentile but whose crown-heel length is normal. It may occur due to craniosynostosis (premature fusion of one or more suture lines). Generally the head is small or normal at birth, but fused sutures can often be detected during palpation. The other cause, microencephaly, may reflect either a primary defect in brain development or may occur due to serious injury either during pregnancy or after birth as a result of infection, teratogenic exposure (maternal alcohol intake), meningitis, trauma or hypoxic ischemia.

Microencephalus usually results in poor psychomotor development.

Autonomic nervous system

Information about the function of the autonomic nervous system is gathered during the complete newborn exam. This includes assessments of the heart rate, temperature, respiratory pattern, sweating, skin perfusion and capillary refill time, positive peristaltic sounds and pupillary response to light. Blood pressure would also be included in this assessment but is usually not checked by the midwife at home. All of these parameters speak to the health of the autonomic nervous system, which must adapt each of these functions to achieve a balance among the organ systems. Neurological health is reflected in multiple assessments that show that the system is able to adapt to changes in the environment over time.

Problems with the autonomic nervous system, such as a contracted pupil in connection with a local injury such as brachial palsy, must be differentiated from generalized abnormal responses, which are indicated when there are overall signs and symptoms of a sick baby. The baby's autonomic responses are usually fine when all the parameters of the vital signs mentioned above are normal.

Evaluating impairment in babies with spinal cord involvement: The types of impairment seen with spinal cord injuries or defects are listed below. All of the following parameters are evaluated to determine the extent of damage.

LEVEL OF LESION	NERVE SUPPLY	SKIN SENSATION	MOTOR FUNCTION	MUSCLE FUNCTION	SPHINCTER FUNCTION	REFLEXES
Cervical-thoracic	Varies	Variable	None, complete paralysis of lower limbs	None	None	Absent
Thoracic-lumbar	T12	Low abdomen				
	L1	Groin	Weak or moderate hip flexion only	Iliopsoas		
	L2	Anterior upper thigh	Strong hip reflexion and moderate hip adduction	Iliopsoas & sartorius		
Lumbar	L3	Anterior outer thigh & knee	Normal hip adduction and moderate knee extension	Quadriceps		Knee jerk
	L4	Medial leg	Normal hip adduction, weak abduction, normal knee extension, absent flexion, moderate foot dorsi-flexion, absent plantarflexion			
Lumbo-sacral	L5	Lateral leg & inner knee	Normal hip adduction, flexion/lateral rotation, absent extension, normal knee extension/moderate flexion; normal foot dorsiflexion, absent plantar flexion; flexed thigh and a dorsiflexed foot	Medial hamstrings		Ankle jerk
	S1	Sole of foot	Normal hip movement except only moderate flexion; strong knee flexion and extension; normal foot dorsiflexion, moderate plantar flexion; weak toe flexion, presents with clawing of toes, flat sole	Anterior tibial (paralysis of most intrinsic muscles of foot)		
Sacral	S2	Posterior leg & thigh	Weak foot intrinsics, otherwise normal lower limb function; difficult to defect abnormality clinically	Gastrocnemius soleus, posterior tibial	Bladder & rectum	Anal wink
	S3	Midbuttock	None			
	S4	Inner buttock		Flexor hallucis		

(adapted from Volpe, 2001)

Deep tendon reflexes

Certain of these may be relevant, depending upon other signs observed in the baby. They are discussed in the subchapter entitled "Deep Tendon Reflexes."

Cranial nerve function

For full details about these assessments, see the subchapter entitled "Assessment of Cranial Nerve Function."

Skin (skin-muscle) reflexes

There are 28 skin reflexes that produce stereotypical motor responses in the limbs with specific stimulation of various regions of the skin (Fletcher, 1998). These may include reflexes that also fall in other categories, such as developmental reflexes, which include skin stimulation during elicitation, such as the palmar grasp. Skin reflex responses are most pronounced in preterm babies and least reactive in adults. The muscles involved may be located either beneath or at a distance from the site of stimulation. The stimulation of specific skin reflexes induces complex motor responses that, to a certain extent, substitute for voluntary activity. Many skin reflexes are described in the subchapter entitled "Developmental Reflexes and Other Neuromotor Evaluations."

Developmental (primitive) reflexes

Many of the most commonly assessed of these reflexes are described in the subchapter entitled "Developmental Reflexes and Other Neuromotor Evaluations." The most important of these are the Moro, the asymmetrical tonic neck response, and palmar and plantar grasp reflexes.

Interpreting the Neurological Assessment

The baby who will have long-lasting brain damage can be identified over the weeks and months following birth through a combination of reviewing predisposing factors and observation of an altered pattern of behavior. Significant risk factors include low birthweight, difficult labor and birth, asphyxia, and congenital abnormalities, especially those involving the skull, face and brain. Observe the baby closely for normal adaptation and behavior as she progresses through the first days of life. More about this ongoing evaluation will appear in Volume III of this text.

Diagnostic Tests

One or more of the following tests may be performed to more accurately determine the cause of neurological disorders:

Examination of the cerebrospinal fluid: This is particularly important if meningitis is suspected.

Cranial ultrasonography: This can diagnose many brain disorders and may eliminate the need for more tests.

Computed tomography scanning (CT): This specialized X-ray technique produces images of thin planes of the region of the body being studied. It is useful in assessing brain disorders and neurologic disease.

Magnetic resonance and ionic (MRI) imaging: A non-X-ray technique using magnetic fields and radio frequency waves to visualize anatomic structures. It gives information on brain structure and function. It produces detailed images of slices of the brain and is useful in diagnosing babies suspected to have congenital brain disorders and other brain problems. Among other things, it can provide the exact location of lesions.

Electroencephalography (EEG): Brain wave studies can help confirm the reasons for seizure activity and the presence of structural abnormalities.

Evoked potentials: These evaluate critical responses to external stimuli by assessing the brain wave patterns when the stimulus is presented. Visual, brain stem (such as auditory) and somatosensory (percutaneous stimulation of peripheral nerve endings) stimuli may be used for this assessment.

Disorders That Affect the Respiratory Tract: An Overview

Respiratory distress is the primary presenting symptom in a wide variety of serious defects. Overall, birth defects that directly involve the respiratory tract occur in one out of every 900 births. The respiratory system can be affected by conditions that arise from any point along the airway as well as defects that have nothing to do directly with the airway. The following list is offered for the student as a reference for where a defect may be located. It will be helpful in understanding the anatomy of the various disorders but not when looking at primary presenting symptoms because sometimes these factors overlap or do not present in "anatomical order." Both direct and indirect causes of the abnormality are listed according to their approximate order of frequency in each anatomical category.

1. Nasal passages and nasopharynx

- Nasal congestion: excessive nasal mucus, swollen nasal passages, infection with mucopurulent discharge (snuffles of syphilis)
- Nasal compression: from birth trauma (deviated septum, etc.), craniofacial anomalies of the nose and nasal passages
- Choanal blockage (choanal atresia): may be an isolated defect; may be associated with a constellation of disorders in CHARGE association (coloboma, heart disease, atresia (choanae), restricted growth, genitourinary anomalies, ear anomalies)
- Intranasal masses: dermoid, encephalocele, glioma (tumor consisting of central nervous system tissue)

2. Oropharynx and hypopharynx

- Abnormalities of the tongue: macroglossia (large tongue), congenital hypothyroidism
- Glossoptosis (displacement of the tongue backward): Pierre Robin syndrome
- Lingual thyroid
- Thyroglossal duct cyst
- Masses within the oropharynx and hypopharynx: hemangioma (does not manifest at birth); lymphangioma

3. Laryngeal: supraglottic, glottic, subglottic

- Congenital: laryngomalacia (75% of all laryngeal anomalies), vocal cord paralysis (unilateral or bilateral), subglottic stenosis, congenital laryngeal webs, laryngeal cleft, laryngeal atresia
- Masses of the larynx: hemangioma, laryngeal cyst, laryngocele, papilloma, lymphangioma, fibroma
- Traumatic: hematoma, fracture

4. Tracheal

- Congenital: tracheomalacia; tracheal stenosis, fistula or atresia; tracheoesophageal duplication (of the trachea or esophagus)
- Tracheal masses: angioma, chondroma, mediastinal tumor
- Extrinsic causes of compression: cervical teratoma, goiter (hypothyroidism), lobar overinflation, vascular ring or sling

5. Bronchial

- Intrinsic bronchial obstruction (35%): bronchomalacia; inspissated mucous plugs, bronchial torsion, bronchial atresia
- Extrinsic bronchial compression: aneurysmal or aberrant blood vessels, enlarged heart chambers due to congenital heart disease, bronchogenic cysts, mediastinal lymphadenopathy

6. Thoracic (chest) cavity

- Congenital pulmonary anomalies: pulmonary hypoplasia; renal agenesis; diaphragmatic hernia; pulmonary sequestration
- Pulmonary masses: cystic adenomatoid malformation; pulmonary cysts
- Air-leak injury: upper airway injury, interstitial emphysema, pneumomediastinum, pneumothorax, pneumopericardium, pneumoperitoneum, air embolism
- Infection with pneumonia

- Extrinsic compression: diaphragmatic hernia; large liver tumor; liver enlargement due to heart disease; hydrops, etc.; eventration of the diaphragm; pleural effusions; pulmonary lymphangiectasia; chylothorax
- Extrinsic organ malfunction: brain injury, bilateral paralysis of the diaphragm, neuromuscular disorder, spinal cord injury or defect
- Other extrinsic causes: maternal drug intake

Aids to the differential diagnosis of complicated newborn respiratory disorders

Given the complexity of the topic of complicated respiratory distress, here are tables that approach the problem from different points of view. Clues to the cause of the problem in the newborn may be derived from the mother's health or labor history.

MATERNAL HISTORY	LIKELY ETIOLOGY OF RESPIRATORY SIGNS IN THE BABY	REFER TO THIS CHAPTER FOR MORE INFORMATION ON POSSIBLE ETIOLOGY
Preterm delivery	Respiratory distress syndrome	Complicated Resp. Distress, #8
Diabetes	Respiratory distress syndrome	Complicated Resp. Distress, #8
Diagnosed intrauterine infection	Sepsis	Complicated Resp. Distress, #5, 8, 9
Premature rupture of membranes	Pneumonia	Complicated Resp. Distress, #5
Prolonged labor	Hypoglycemia	Detecting and Differentiating Newborn Hypoglycemia, Sepsis and Heart Defects
Meconium-stained fluid, dysmaturity	Meconium aspiration syndrome	Meconium Aspiration
Polyhydramnios	Esophageal atresia Tracheoesophageal fistula	Complicated Resp. Distress, #14
Oligohydramnios	Pulmonary hypoplasia	Complicated Resp. Distress, #1, 5
Traumatic birth	Central nervous system damage	Complicated Resp. Distress, #9
	Phrenic nerve damage (paralysis of the diaphragm)	Complicated Resp. Distress, #7
	Intracranial hemorrhage	Cranial Injuries
Fetal heart rate abnormalities Prolapsed umbilical cord Abruption of the placenta	Asphyxia	Complicated Resp. Distress, #9, 10

("#" refers to topic number found in the subchapter entitled "Complicated Respiratory Distress")

Studying complicated respiratory distress: Respiratory distress is a primary presenting symptom in a wide variety of neonatal emergencies, making the subject matter of the following chapter the most complex in this section of the text. I suggest you set aside time and perhaps form a study group just to review these two chapters by themselves. Most of these conditions overlap in their presentations and many are anatomically related or have to do with anomalies of other major organ systems; therefore, the topic of complicated respiratory distress is presented next.

Additional presenting signs in the newborn with respiratory distress that point to these likely diagnoses are included in the following table.

SIGNS IN THE BABY	LIKELY UNDERLYING CONDITION	REFER TO THIS CHAPTER FOR MORE INFORMATION ON POSSIBLE ETIOLOGY
Scaphoid abdomen/barrel chest	Diaphragmatic hernia	Complicated Resp. Distress, #6
Unilateral upper limb paralysis	Brachial plexus damage involving the phrenic nerve	Complicated Resp. Distress, #7
Unable to breathe with mouth closed, pink when crying	Nasal blockage (swelling, lesions), choanal atresia	Complicated Resp. Distress, #3
Stuffy nose ("snuffles")	Congenital syphilis	Complicated Resp. Distress, #3
Gasping with little air exchange	Obstruction of upper airway	Complicated Resp. Distress, #2
Overdistension of chest	Aspiration, lobar emphysema, pneumothorax	Meconium Aspiration Complicated Resp. Distress, #5
Shift of apical pulse	Pneumothorax or thoracic mass lesion	Complicated Resp. Distress, #5
Fever or unstable temperature in a thermally stable environment	Sepsis	Complicated Resp. Distress, #5, 8, 9
	Pneumonia	Complicated Resp. Distress, #5, 8, 9
Shrill cry, hypertonia or flaccidity	Central nervous system disorder	Complicated Resp. Distress, #8, 9, 10, 15
Atonia	Trauma, weakness or absence of muscle tone (myasthenia or amyotonia)	Complicated Resp. Distress, #7, 9
Extension of head in absence of neurological findings	Laryngeal obstruction	Complicated Resp. Distress, #2, 11
	Vascular ring	Complicated Resp. Distress, #2, 14
Choking and vomiting during or after feeding	Gastroesophageal reflux	Complicated Resp. Distress, #13
	Tracheoesophageal fistula	Complicated Resp. Distress, #14
Quiet, cyanotic baby with rapid breathing	Congenital heart defect	Complicated Resp. Distress, #12 Cyanosis, Rapid Breathing Congestive Heart Failure, Shock or Arrhythmia: Detecting Heart Defects at Birth

"#" refers to a specific symptom picture found in the chapter entitled "Complicated Respiratory Distress"

COMPLICATED RESPIRATORY DISTRESS

NOTE: Study the subchapters entitled "The Anatomy of the Neonatal Airway and Upper Respiratory Tract" and "Evaluating the Apparently Normal Baby Who Develops Respiratory Distress" before studying this chapter.

A congenital defect may be a contributing factor when you cannot stabilize a baby born with respiratory distress with standard respiratory support techniques, when a baby's condition continues to deteriorate in spite of effective resuscitative efforts, when respiratory distress develops and persists in a newborn during certain activities, or when it presents atypically.

The preceding chapter gives a list of where each type of problem may be located anatomically. This chapter focuses instead on major categories of presenting symptoms, although the actual symptoms of many conditions overlap. The following primary presenting symptom pictures are offered in no particular order of likelihood. The presentations are numbered to help you locate them in the chapter more easily.

1. Complete inability of the baby to breathe through the mouth or nose with an inability to inflate the lungs during artificial ventilations
2. Some or all of the air will not pass through the upper airways, producing moderate to severe respiratory distress or failure; baby gasps with little air exchange.
3. Respiratory distress that is only relieved during crying or mouth breathing; baby cannot nurse and breathe at the same time.
4. Mild to severe respiratory distress or failure in a baby with a large tongue and a recessed jaw
5. Air passes through the airway, but the lungs do not inflate or there is poor, irregular, or overinflation (air enters but does not exit the lungs).
6. Severe respiratory distress in a baby with a caved-in abdomen and enlarged chest; ventilation is difficult and ineffective or impossible.
7. The baby cannot maintain spontaneous respirations, but responds well to being ventilated.
8. The baby has persistent or increasing difficulty with breathing, sometimes leading to respiratory failure.
9. Baby with respiratory distress is weak, pale and shocky.
10. The baby with a history of chronic intrauterine asphyxia is weak, ruddy or cyanotic with varying degrees of lethargy, respiratory distress and neurological signs.
11. Respiratory stridor, sometimes with an abnormal cry and difficulty swallowing
12. Baby looks otherwise normal with persistent central cyanosis and may have a slow heart rate in spite of effective spontaneous but rapid respirations.
13. There is intermittent respiratory distress, with coughing and choking or vomiting prompted by nursing.
14. Persistent, profuse saliva and/or difficulty with swallowing; coughing and choking aggravated by nursing
15. Apnea (cessation of breathing)

The primary causes of these symptoms can be divided into those caused by respiratory tract obstruction and those caused by abnormalities of the lung tissue itself.

Diagnostic Aids for Assessing Complicated Respiratory Distress

Take a breath, center yourself and observe the baby. Look for obvious defects such as clefts of the oral cavity, or swellings in the mouth, or of the anterior neck or near the midline of the upper chest. Listen to the lungs and heart with a neonatal stethoscope to isolate lung sounds. The two other primary tools you will use are percussion and transillumination. By performing these exams, you can often narrow down what the problem may be. Even though many specific types of problems are described in this chapter, do not expect to make a definitive diagnosis. The purpose of these descriptions is to help you better understand the different types of conditions that may come into play in various symptom presentations. Your goal is to troubleshoot the condition of the baby as quickly as possible so that you can provide appropriate support while transport is underway.

1. **COMPLETE INABILITY OF THE BABY TO BREATHE THROUGH THE MOUTH OR NOSE WITH AN INABILITY TO INFLATE THE LUNGS DURING ARTIFICIAL VENTILATIONS:** There are a few disorders that involve complete anatomical obstruction of the airway, rendering any type of ventilation impossible.

General presentation

In these cases, you will have done everything possible to correct for an obstructed airway. No tumors or other obvious defects can be detected; nevertheless, air cannot pass through the airway. Passage of a tube may also be impossible. Use of a oropharyngeal airway offers no improvement. Some of these babies may attempt to take a breath on their own, with no success. These disorders are likely to be fatal at home.

General transport considerations

Leave the cord intact to buy as much time as possible and call 911. In case something else is the problem, or there is a tiny space that admits air or there is a small region of functional lung tissue, attempt to ventilate and continue to do everything you would normally do to correct ineffective ventilations.

Specific conditions

Tracheal atresia: Tracheal agenesis occurs when a segment of the trachea does not form or contains no lumen, producing complete respiratory failure at birth. Tracheal defects occur in 1 out of every 3000 births and are often associated with multiple cardiovascular anomalies.

Assessment: Intubation into the trachea is unsuccessful with coiling of the tube in the back of the throat.

Transport considerations: Ventilation may allow survival for a few hours if there is a fistula (hole) between the esophagus and a lower, patent portion of the trachea; this is present in 80% of these babies.

Complete blockage of the larynx: Laryngeal webbing, consisting of a web of mucous-membrane-covered connective tissue that extends for varying distances between the vocal cords from front to back is rare. A complete web, located above, in or below the larynx, covers the entire glottis and results in severe respiratory distress or failure at birth and is rapidly fatal. Laryngeal atresia is another rare disorder in which the larynx is not patent, resulting in complete respiratory failure at birth. It presents with dilated airways below the blockage, enlarged lungs and ascites or hydrops fetalis.

Pulmonary agenesis or complete hypoplasia: The lungs may be absent or so underdeveloped that ventilation is impossible. Either condition is fatal. Both are associated with oligohydramnios and renal agenesis.

2. **SOME OR ALL OF THE AIR WILL NOT PASS THROUGH THE UPPER AIRWAYS, PRODUCING MODERATE TO SEVERE RESPIRATORY DISTRESS OR FAILURE; BABY GASPS WITH LITTLE AIR EXCHANGE:** Suspect partial or nearly complete obstruction, compression, or dysfunction of the upper airway. See also item 8.

General presentation

Airway obstruction may present with immediate and absolute respiratory failure or it may develop gradually or sporadically over the first minutes, hours or days of life.

Signs and symptoms of respiratory obstruction include:

Rapid breathing (over 60 breaths/min): This is especially true after neonatal transition has stabilized.
Vigorous attempts at inspiration: These are accompanied by marked chest retraction.
Abnormal breath sounds: These include stridor during inspiration, expiration or both and asthma-like wheezing (usually heard only during auscultation).
Severe intercostal and subcostal recession
Paradoxical movement of the chest and abdomen: The abdomen protrudes and the chest sinks on inspiration and the abdomen sinks and the chest rises on expiration (seesaw breathing).
Tracheal tug: The midline of the neck presents an observable inward tug during inspiration.
Central cyanosis: Pulmonary causes are accompanied by other signs of respiratory distress and include venous

desaturation due to ventilation or perfusion imbalances in the lungs, or airway obstruction preventing normal gas exchange. Persistent central cyanosis without dramatic respiratory distress may be related to a heart defect. It may also be related to hematological disorders (e.g., anemia) as well as metabolic or central nervous system disorders, neuromuscular problems or mechanical respiratory disturbances.

Slow capillary refill time (indicates poor peripheral perfusion)

Head retraction or hyperextension

General restlessness

Cardiac signs: Cardiovascular distress develops early as obstruction continues with tachycardia and pallor or cyanosis progressing to bradycardia and cardiac arrest. Cardiac compromise is especially likely to result in brain damage if it is preceded by a period of hypoxemia (which is usually the case).

General assessment

Listen over the airway at all levels with the diaphragm of a stethoscope. Listening over the nose, the midline of the throat and the upper chest may help you determine where the air is stopping. If there is an obvious problem, such as a swelling of the neck, listen immediately above, over and below the lesion. You will also need to open the mouth and examine the oral cavity and back of the throat and tongue for the presence of tumors that may be blocking the airway. Also check the size of the tongue and jaw. Examination may reveal an obvious cause of the difficulty, such as malformation of the nares; small lower jaw; cleft palate; swelling of the neck, face or tongue; or a tumor in the oral cavity.

General transport considerations

Most of these conditions will require immediate transport or transport within a few hours of birth. Basic support measures will suffice for most conditions, and specific considerations for the transport of babies with various anomalies are mentioned under each condition below. If no transport protocols are discussed below, refer to the chapter entitled "Transporting the Newborn: An Overview."

Special precautions for babies with oral tumors or airway compression: If the tumor is compressing the airway, prior to transport, gently pass an orogastric tube to bypass the blockage.

Whenever suctioning or intubation is attempted, take extreme care to avoid puncturing an intranasal mass or one that protrudes from the midline of the upper oral cavity. Such a mass could be an encephalocele, which would be fluctuant and could be easily damaged. Rupture could be life threatening to the baby. These lesions are discussed in the subchapter entitled "Externalized Organs and Neural Tube Defects."

Specific conditions

The main causes of airway obstruction fall into two categories: basically mechanical problems with no preexisting anomaly and congenital anomalies. It is estimated that less than 5% of all cases of persistent newborn respiratory distress are caused by congenital anomalies of the upper respiratory tract. The following conditions may be involved:

- •Meconium or other substance blocking the airway (relatively common–see the chapters entitled "Assisting at the Birth of a Vertex Baby" and the subchapter entitled "Meconium Aspiration.")
- •Cleft lip or palate (1 in every 750 births)
- •Partial or complete airway compression or blockage from various causes, including positioning, trauma, tumor, oropharyngeal bleeding and vascular compression (incidence varies widely according to cause)
- •Tracheal stenosis (1 in every 4000 live births)
- •Subglottic laryngeal stenosis (see also item 11)
- •Partial laryngeal web (rare) (see also item 11)

Cleft lip or palate: This is, by far, the most common structural anomaly to affect the upper airway, with cleft lip and palate occurring once in every 750 live births and a cleft palate by itself occurring once in every 2500 Caucasian births. A cleft palate may produce respiratory distress at birth from accumulated oral secretions and from the tongue occupying the cleft space. When this occurs, it is treated as for Pierre Robin syndrome (see item 4).

Partial or complete airway compression: Airway compression may result from many different conditions, some of which are much more common than others. Most of the time, compression occurs when something outside the airway is pressing against a portion of the airway. This complication may be associated with:

Positioning: Pharyngeal obstruction may be caused simply by having the neck flexed forward, which increases the opening pressure the baby must exert to move air through the pharynx. The obvious solution is to reposition the head and see if that helps.

Trauma: Airway compression may also result from severe bruising and swelling secondary to birth trauma, which may require the placement of an endotracheal tube or an oral airway along with immediate transport.

Facial flattening: Severe flattening of the facial features occurs in a number of disorders and, when extreme, produces obstruction in the nasal passages. Placement of an oral airway may help such a baby maintain normal respirations while transport is underway.

Tumor: A nasopharyngeal tumor may, on very rare occasions, completely occlude the airway. More commonly, however, these babies present with signs of partial upper airway obstruction such as snorting or snoring sounds.

Nuchal cyst: Cystic hygroma is a cystic swelling with multiple cavities that arises from lymph vessels. It is found in the neck or, more rarely, the axilla. It is a smooth, soft, fluctuant, diffuse, compressible, nontender mass that frequently invades nearby tissues and may span the neck from ear to ear. It may extend around the trachea or brachial plexus. Involvement of the base of the tongue or oropharynx is a frequent complication resulting in respiratory distress. Babies with cystic lesions or other growths in the neck may present with acute or progressive respiratory distress, including coughing, wheezing or stridor, resulting from pressure on the tracheobronchial tree. Esophageal compression occasionally occurs as well, resulting in difficulty swallowing (which may be associated with polyhydramnios).

Hemangioma: Subglottic or laryngeal hemangiomas are rare but, when present at birth, may present a visible lesion on the anterior neck. These can cause difficulty with breathing and stridor, with crying, increasing vascular engorgement and exacerbating symptoms.

Esophageal duplication: Esophageal duplication takes the form of a cyst that can cause airway or, less commonly, esophageal obstruction.

Bronchogenic cyst: These are usually single-lobed cysts that develop next to the major bronchi. If they compress the trachea or a major bronchus, they occasionally cause respiratory distress at birth, resulting in noisy breathing, overinflation of alveoli because air cannot escape (emphysema), or collapse of alveoli because air cannot enter (atelectasis). For these last two conditions, see item 5.

Sublingual ranula: A large sublingual ranula presents as a blue-grey swelling that can fill the mouth and force the tongue against the hard palate, causing respiratory difficulty from birth.

Encephalocele: Any intranasal or upper-midline oral mass should be assumed to be an encephalocele until this is ruled out. These masses are fluctuant and may pulsate. Suspect this especially in a baby whose face looks unusual in any way. Encephaloceles are discussed more completely in the subchapter entitled "Externalized Organs and Neural Tube Defects."

Nuchal teratomas: Teratomas of the neck, hard palate (epignathus) or nasopharyngeal area can cause significant obstruction of the pharynx via either extreme deflexion of the head or direct pharyngeal obstruction. A teratoma of the neck is rounder and less diffuse than a cervical hygroma. An epignathus is a highly organized teratoid tumor that arises from the palate or the pharynx and protrudes from the mouth. It may contain well-formed organs and limbs. These tumors are typically associated with massive polyhydramnios and a deflexed head, which may obstruct descent and necessitate transport in labor. Teratomas are further discussed in the subchapter entitled "Visibile Defects and Anomalies (Other Than Externalized Organs)."

Both ventilation and intubation can be extremely difficult in these babies. If one or both are impossible, an immediate tracheotomy is the baby's only hope for survival. Leaving the cord intact to sustain oxygenation buys you a little time to evaluate the situation. Transillumination of the neck may help locate the tumor. *Do not attempt to perform a tracheotomy at home.* Transport immediately.

Thyroid or thymus growths: Thyroglossal duct cysts or an ectopic thyroid gland or tissue can occur at the base of the tongue near the level of the hyoid bone and may cause airway obstruction by crowding the esophagus backward, producing severe supraglottic laryngeal obstruction. A congenital goiter may rarely cause airway obstruction via compression as well. Cysts may also develop on the thymus gland and result in respiratory distress. All are exceedingly rare.

Epulis: Congenital epulis (granular cell myoblastoma) is a benign tumor usually arising from the upper midline of the gum, presenting as a lobulated pink, pediculated mass that protrudes from the mouth. It may be small, but when sufficiently large, it can produce respiratory obstruction from birth on.

Oropharyngeal bleeding: Thymus hemorrhage may occur because of coagulation defects, producing acute respiratory distress. Transport the baby on his side and aspirate frequently to minimize choking.

Vascular compression: While you will not be able to determine this cause at home, be aware that a variety of vascular malformations can compress the airway. About 3% of the general population have some sort of variation in their mediastinal vascular anatomy, but only 1 in 2500 have a vascular ring, which is the type of vascular anomaly that most commonly causes airway compression. A vascular sling can also produce compression. Either produces nonspecific signs of respiratory distress similar to those occurring with other forms of compression.

Tracheal stenosis: Tracheal stenosis involves a narrowing of a segment of the respiratory passageway. It can present with either mild distress or progressive, severe respiratory insufficiency. Establishing an airway will be difficult in these babies, who should be transported as soon as possible. Provide the best ventilation you can manage; the good news is that many of these babies respond well to ventilation even though passage of an endotracheal tube may be difficult or impossible.

Subglottic laryngeal stenosis: Although congenital subglottic stenosis is the third most common congenital laryngeal anomaly (after laryngomalacia and vocal cord paralysis), it is the most common laryngeal abnormality causing serious respiratory obstruction requiring a tracheotomy in infants. Subglottic stenosis exists when the anatomic caliber at this level is less than 4.0 mm in a full-term newborn infant. Conditions such as neoplasms, inflammatory conditions, and acquired strictures following endotracheal intubation are excluded from this definition.

Partial laryngeal web or cleft: Laryngeal clefting is an exceedingly rare cause of partial airway obstruction. A partial laryngeal web produces hoarse, weak or absent cry and breathing problems that worsen with exertion. Congenital webs or partial laryngeal atresia are relatively rare, accounting for only 2 to 4% of all laryngeal anomalies.

3. RESPIRATORY DISTRESS THAT IS ONLY RELIEVED DURING CRYING OR MOUTH BREATHING; BABY CANNOT NURSE AND BREATHE AT THE SAME TIME.

This is due to a blockage in the nasal passages.

General presentation of complete upper airway obstruction

Regardless of the cause, complete obstruction of both nasal passages can lead to death from asphyxia. The tongue becomes applied to the palate as the baby attempts to take a breath, thus obstructing the oral airway. Vigorous respiratory effort produces marked chest retraction, increasing cyanosis and, eventually, death. The airway obstruction may be momentarily relieved if the baby cries or if she opens her mouth and takes a breath. When crying stops and her mouth closes, the cycle resumes.

Assessment for nasal obstruction

Press up on the chin to close the baby's mouth and see whether the baby can continue to breathe normally. Block one nostril at a time with finger pressure against the alia; assess breathing by holding a thread in front of the unblocked nostril and looking for air movement against the thread. Use a penlight and visually inspect the nasal passages for obstructions, such as tumors (see item 2) while pressing against the tip of the nose to lift it up to straighten the nasal turbinates. If none of these tests are definitive but a problem is obvious, attempt to pass a small-caliber (5F to 8F) suction catheter into the posterior pharynx through first one, then the other, nostril. Note that the insertion of a nasal catheter is difficult even in normal babies. Be gentle, as the mucosa is easily damaged and you do not want to inadvertently rupture an encephalocele. If the baby can breathe at all, do not insert a tube and transport. To insert a tube:

1. Place the baby supine.

2. Lift the tip of the baby's nose by pressing the tip of your finger against the end of the nose and pushing it up. Pushing up on the nose lifts the nasal turbinates out of the way, thus allowing the tube to pass unobstructed. If this is not done, the tube can caught on the turbinates of the nostril walls, giving the impression of an obstruction.
3. Insert the end of the catheter toward the occipital eminence, so that it passes along the floor of the nasal passage. If the catheter cannot be advanced into the pharynx, some sort of obstruction is present. Reasons for this include:
   Swelling: The catheter will usually pass through each nasal cavity into the oropharynx even if a total or near-total functional blockage is present.
   Deviated septum: The obstruction occurs on one or both sides 1 to 2 cm from the anterior nares.
   Choanal atresia: The tube is stopped by a typical "solid" feeling as it abuts the bony obstruction, usually 1 to 2 cm anterior to the posterior end of the septum (deeper than for a deviated septum).
4. If you cannot pass the tube or you detect an obstruction, insert an oral airway to maintain patency and transport.

Specific conditions

Blocked nasal passages: Nasal or postnasal obstruction in a newborn results in respiratory distress and cyanosis that may be relieved temporarily during episodes of crying. It may be due to:

•Meconium or other birth debris (a possibility that is covered elsewhere in this text)
•Generalized swelling of the nasal mucosa
•Excessive mucus (stuffiness), which may be seen when the baby has an infection, especially congenital syphilis (producing a copious, purulent, highly infectious discharge), or choanal atresia
•A severely deviated nasal septum. The overall incidence of deviation is less than 1%, with most of these not resulting in blockage. See the subchapter entitled "Examining the Head and Neck."
•Intranasal tumors (including dermoid, encephalocele, hamartoma, chordoma, developmental cyst, teratoma, rhabdomyosarcoma, glioma and others (also see item 2).

Choanal atresia: Nasal obstruction may be caused by choanal atresia, a congenital blockage of the nasal passages with bone (90%) or a membrane (10%). This relatively rare condition occurs in about 1 out of every 6000 to 8000 live births, with 2 girls affected for every boy. The right side is affected twice as often as the left. Babies normally do not attempt to breathe through their mouths; however, a baby with bilateral choanal atresia may. These babies pink up with crying but often become cyanotic when quiet and when their mouths are closed. Respiratory distress typically becomes much worse when these babies attempt to nurse because they cannot breathe and nurse at the same time. In unilateral cases, symptoms may also worsen when the baby tries to sleep. Unilateral choanal atresia may be the cause of persistent tachypnea or a mucoid discharge and may be discovered in babies who have breathing problems for which no other explanation can be found.

***Associated defects*:** About 50% of babies with choanal atresia have other craniofacial anomalies. It may also be part of CHARGE association (colobomata, heart defect, choanal atresia, restricted growth, genital anomalies in boys and ear defects).

Congenital nasal pyriform aperture stenosis: Narrowing of the nasal passages results in symptoms similar to, but less severe than, choanal atresia. This is a rare condition.

4. MILD TO SEVERE RESPIRATORY DISTRESS OR FAILURE IN A BABY WITH A LARGE TONGUE AND A RECESSED JAW

Possible causes

Small, recessed lower jaw (Pierre Robin, Treacher-Collins and other syndromes): Pierre Robin syndrome occurs once in every 2000 to 50,000 live births, depending on the study. It consists of small jaw (micrognathia), downward displacement of the tongue (glossoptosis) and incomplete cleft palate, although sometimes one of these defects is absent. Any baby with an abnormally small lower jaw has a chin that is even more receded than that of a normal baby. The small mandible critically narrows the pharyngeal airway, creating the illusion that the tongue is enlarged and causing it to be pressed backward, where it blocks the pharynx just above the larynx.

Presentation: Symptoms worsen with inspiration, supine positioning (when gravity pulls the tongue backward), sleeping (when the baby works less to maintain his airway) and nursing (when swallowing increases the negative pharyngeal pressure pulling back the tongue). Wedging of the tongue into the cleft palate may occur, further complicating the situation.

Assessment: Regardless of the cause, when a baby appears to have an abnormally recessed jaw, open the mouth for a quick inspection of the relative size of the tongue, check the palate, and evaluate the size of the lower jaw.

Specific transport considerations

1. Place the baby on her stomach on the padded transport surface.
2. Place a hand on her upper forehead and lift her head into a reverse sniffing position or a bit higher. This should cause the tongue to come forward and free the airway. If the baby can breathe, transport in this position. If immediate transport is impossible, support the head in this position by using paper IV tape to secure an infant stocking cap to the scalp and suspend the tip above the baby to maintain this posture until transport can be arranged.

If prone positioning and lifting the head does not work to open the airway, turn the baby over on his back and create an airway by inserting a nasopharyngeal tube. Use a large feeding tube (12F) or endotracheal tube with the stylet removed. Placement of a nasopharyngeal tube deep into the posterior pharynx, past the tongue, may relieve the suction that the tongue tends to produce as it rests against the posterior airway. With or without a laryngoscope, the placement of an endotracheal tube is usually difficult in these babies and attempting to do so is not recommended. Once the airway is inserted, the baby should remain supine.

Abnormalities of the tongue: Babies with neurological defects that affect tongue coordination may suffer from intermittent obstruction. A mass such as thyroglossal duct cyst or lingual thyroid may be located at the base of the tongue. Very rarely, the tongue is "welded" to the edges of a palatal defect by bands of tissue, resulting in severe respiratory distress and feeding problems.

Assessment: Visually inspect the oral cavity with a penlight. Palpate the base of the tongue to detect a mass. Blockage may occur if such a lesion is sufficiently large.

Specific transport considerations: An enlarged or "welded" tongue can block the airway and may be treated with prone positioning as for a small, recessed jaw (above). You can also try other positions to see if any facilitate spontaneous breathing; if not, try to insert an oropharyngeal airway. Be sure to hold the tongue flat with a tongue depressor so that the airway does not push the large tongue to the back of the throat as you insert it. Transport right away. If the tongue is welded to the palate, an orogastric tube or a nasogastric tube can be placed to bypass the obstruction in some cases, but this will not aid artificial ventilation. Transport as soon as possible.

5. AIR PASSES THROUGH THE AIRWAY BUT THE LUNGS DO NOT INFLATE OR THERE IS POOR, IRREGULAR OR OVERINFLATION (AIR ENTERS BUT DOES NOT EXIT THE LUNGS)

General presentation

The baby's lungs should fill with air if the airway is clear, the head is correctly positioned, the mask is well seated on the face and sufficient ventilatory pressure is used. If not, a disorder of lung function or capacity may be complicating the situation. The most common cause of such emergencies in neonates is a problem with the lung tissue. These types of disorders fall into three categories:

Good air entry with unequal inflation: This implies that air is leaking somewhere rather than entering both lungs and therefore indicates an air-leak injury.

Poor inflation: This can result from defects of lung tissue or impairment of lung volume due to pressure from enlarged or misplaced structures.

Complete lack of inflation: Inadequately developed lung tissue prevents expansion.

General assessment

Whenever air passage in the lungs is not clearly heard, try transilluminating the chest and percussing the chest wall.

You are trying to determine if the lungs are normally developed and inflated.

Possible causes

Any of the following complicating factors may be present:

- Thoracic air leak due to injury of the lung tissue (occurs spontaneously in 1 to 2 of every 100 live births of normal babies, with incidence rising with associated respiratory distress or malformations)
- Air-leak injury to the upper airway
- Diaphragmatic hernia (covered under item 6)
- Congenital pneumonia
- Congenital pleural effusions (1/15,000 births)
  - Congenital chylothorax
- Congenital lobar overinflation ("emphysema")
- Pulmonary atresia or hypoplasia (partial or complete)
- Congenital pulmonary cysts
  - Congenital cystic adenomatoid malformation (accounts for 25% of all congenital lung tumors)
- Pulmonary sequestration
- Pulmonary lymphangiectasia (less than 100 cases reported as of 1993)
- Large liver tumors
- Eventration of the diaphragm
- Mediastinal or thoracic cystic tumors

Thoracic air leak: The most common organic reason for impaired lung inflation is an air-leak injury with subsequent escape of air into regions where air is normally not present. Alveolar rupture is induced when high intra-alveolar pressure is produced during spontaneous breathing or artificial ventilation. Spontaneous air leaks occur in 1 to 2% of all newborns but are thought to cause symptoms in only 0.05 to 0.07% of those affected. Spontaneous leaks are more likely to occur in babies whose lungs are somehow compromised to begin with–for example, from infection or hypoplasia–but can occur in otherwise completely normal babies. Migration of escaped air occurs through layers of tissue that offer the least resistance. There are a variety of air-leak injuries, almost all of which have been found in spontaneously breathing babies, but symptoms occur most commonly and are usually most pronounced when the baby has received positive-pressure ventilation. Clinical evidence varies according to the volume of the air leak, the site of air accumulation, and the overall status of the baby prior to the onset of leaking.

Different types of air leaks: Air travels in a more or less predictable fashion from one thoracic compartment to the next and is sometimes diverted into other body compartments along the way.

Interstitial emphysema: All types of thoracic air leaks begin when alveoli rupture, allowing air to enter the sheaths surrounding the adjacent disrupted capillaries. Rupture of alveoli is most likely to occur when neighboring airways are blocked, resulting in the uneven distribution of high intrapulmonary pressures, as might be the case in a ventilated, asphyxiated infant who did not receive a full placental transfusion. The perivascular sheaths stretch as air accumulates; this stretching results in blood vessel compression, leading to decreased lung compliance, pulmonary congestion and ischemia (tissue damage). Continued ventilation can make the problem worse. Air may accumulate at the hilum (a wedge-shaped depression on the mediastinal surface of each lung, where the bronchus, blood vessels, nerves and lymphatics enter and exit the lung), to form large blebs in folds of the pleural lining of the lung, or it may migrate to other compartments.

***Presentation*:** Interstitial edema results in decreased chest wall movement, especially when it occurs bilaterally. There is a dry, crunching sound on auscultation (as though walking in dry snow or cutting Styrofoam) which may be especially apparent if the condition is present bilaterally.

Subcutaneous (nuchal) emphysema: Air may travel through mediastinal structures and pool under the skin of the neck.

***Presentation*:** This may present as a bumpy appearance of the anterior neck, with crepitance on palpation of the skin and underlying soft tissues of the neck. Crepitation, a feeling of "bubbling" under the skin, may also sound like bubbling or crunching on auscultation. The overlying skin may be pink in an otherwise cyanotic baby if the air leak is high in oxygen. There may be a crunching sound as the stethoscope head is moved over the area of involvement. Subcutaneous emphysema is rarely the only manifestation of thoracic air leak, and symptoms are much more likely to result from the associated air leak and its cause (Fletcher, 1998).

Pneumomediastinum: Once air enters the interstitial spaces, it dissects the tissue layers as it moves through the perivascular and peribronchial sheaths into the hilum. Here, the air enters the mediastinum directly or accumulates in a bleb and then ruptures, resulting in the abnormal presence of air in the tissues underlying the sternum. Pneumomediastinum can also be caused by perforation of the cervical or thoracic esophagus or airways, cervicomediastinal infection, or a perforated abdominal organ.

***Presentation*:** Pneumomediastinum is usually asymptomatic. If the amount of accumulated air is significant, the baby may present with tachypnea or other signs of mild respiratory distress. Occasionally an increased anteroposterior chest diameter at the sternum is found; this presents with a loss of the normal inward sternal curvature. Heart sounds may be faint due to the air trapped in the anterior mediastinum, but there will be no shift in their location. Severe respiratory distress and shock do not usually develop because the pleura of the mediastinum is easily ruptured, making it rare for enough tension to develop to impair venous return to the heart and result in cyanosis or hypoperfusion.

Transillumination reveals clearly evident cardiac activity within the halo of light. Large collections of air in the mediastinal area become visible when the light is placed next to the lower lateral costal margin.

Pneumopericardium: Air from the mediastinum migrates through the tissue lining the thoracic cavity into the sac that encloses the heart (the pericardium), where it becomes trapped. The pericardium generally does not rupture under these conditions. Pneumopericardium is fortunately rare and usually does not occur in the absence of mechanical ventilation.

***Presentation*:** A spontaneous air leak is likely to be small and may not result in clinically evident changes. However, maximum distension of the pericardial sac puts pressure on the compressible right heart chambers, resulting in poor filling and low cardiac output. The only evidence of pneumopericardium would be diminished heart sounds and a dampening of peripheral pulses. Heart function will be significantly impaired if the air accumulation is sufficient to produce cardiac compression, presenting with sudden, deepening cyanosis, muffled or inaudible heart sounds, a fall in blood pressure, diminished or absent peripheral pulses, and bradycardia, all of which lead to metabolic acidosis.

Transillumination can be used to confirm a pneumopericardium. Place the light in the third or fourth intercostal space, in the left midclavicular line, and angle it toward the xiphoid process. When the angle of the light is changed so that the light passes over the thorax, the corona will be brightest over the area of pericardial air and the silhouette of the heartbeat can be seen. In some cases, a pneumomediastinum cannot be distinguished from a pneumopericardium. Remember that an accumulation of blood will not transmit light.

Pneumoperitoneum: Pneumoperitoneum is the least common air-leak injury. It occurs when air passes from the mediastinum along the sheaths of the aorta and vena cava and finally ruptures into the peritoneal cavity. In rare instances, air may travel as far as the scrotum (pneumoscrotum). Free air in the peritoneum suggests that an abdominal organ has ruptured, requiring immediate surgery. However, no such emergency exists when the cause is a simple air leak from the lungs. A ruptured abdominal organ is usually preceded by persistent intra-organ distension, lack of bowel sounds, visible bowel loops, or bloody stools. The absence of these signs prior to air entering the abdomen and the simultaneous presence of air in the chest is a good indication that a pneumoperitoneum is the cause. In addition, bowel perforation is not always associated with free air; if there is no air in the area of perforation, none will escape.

Presentation: The primary symptom of pneumoperitoneum is abdominal distension. This may occur asymptomatically at the onset. As air accumulates, the upward pressure can immobilize the diaphragm, resulting in lung compression and decreased venous return to the heart by putting pressure on the inferior vena cava, requiring a peritoneal catheter to drain off air to allow effective ventilation (you will not be able to offer this remedy at home).

There are no unusual findings on auscultation, and bowel sounds may still be audible even if the air leak is due to bowel perforation from infection, although in this case peripheral pulses will be harder to find. Transillumination of the most elevated portion of the abdominal wall may distinguish free air, but it can also detect air risen from a distended organ if the abdominal wall is translucent enough and the air pocket sufficiently large. Air that has escaped into the peritoneal cavity will move to the highest point when the baby's position is changed. This is not true of air contained in an organ, even though the bowel is relatively mobile.

Air embolism: This very rare life-threatening emergency occurs when air enters the blood vessels, where it can travel to the heart and disrupt circulation. It typically only occurs when extremely high pressures (up to 55 cm H_2O) are used to ventilate very stiff lungs.

***Presentation*:** Air embolus presents catastrophically with sudden cyanosis and slowing of the heart rate. The air-blood mixture of each beat can be heard to crackle and pop, followed shortly by circulatory collapse. Support the baby as best you can, providing full CPR, and transport right away.

Pneumothorax: This is the most common air leak injury. When a bleb of air that has accumulated in the pleural fold grows large enough to exceed the pressure tolerated by the pleura, the pleural membrane ruptures, releasing air into the pleural space, where it is trapped between the lung and the chest wall, producing a pneumothorax. This may also occur when an alveolus ruptures directly into the pleural space. Pneumothorax may occur for a variety of reasons, most of which also apply to other types of thoracic air leaks as well.

Spontaneous pneumothorax in the well baby: Spontaneous pneumothorax is most common at term and usually occurs with the first few breaths, with the majority of these infants being asymptomatic (nontension pneumothorax), although a few will have a serious underlying pulmonary disorder. Rapid cord clamping with resultant sudden, panicky, high-pressure breathing efforts may be a contributing factor when pneumothorax occurs in otherwise healthy infants. Pneumothorax should be suspected when the apparently normal baby who has been doing well after birth or has been stable after being resuscitated at the time of birth suddenly starts to destabilize.

Spontaneous pneumothorax in the sick baby: Hypoplasia of the lungs may result in pneumothorax. Air-leak injuries due to other types of lung disorders usually appear in the days following birth; however, if an established infection is present, the lung tissue may not be able at the time of birth to tolerate air inflation without rupturing. Other possible causes of these signs and symptoms include lobar overinflation (or emphysema, discussed later in this chapter) and congenital cystic adenomatoid malformation, both of which are very rare.

Tension (or symptomatic) pneumothorax: When air leaks into the pleural space, the injured lung becomes increasingly compressed as the baby breathes or (if the pneumothorax goes unrecognized) as artificial ventilation continues. If the accumulation of air becomes large enough, trapped air will prevent the lung from expanding and will interfere with pulmonary blood flow, leading to worsening respiratory distress, bradycardia, reduced cardiac output and a fall in blood pressure, all resulting in cyanosis.

Pneumothorax that occurs during artificial ventilation usually results in a tension pneumothorax, with preterm birth, respiratory distress and high ventilatory pressures as the main predisposing factors. Other causes include breakage of a clavicle or rib, leading to puncture of the lung, as well as significant pulmonary infection or other disease. Partially hypoplastic lungs cannot expand even with normal ventilatory pressures and will frequently develop a pneumothorax during resuscitation efforts.

***Presentation*:** Tension pneumothorax presents with the following signs and symptoms, in increasing order of severity:

- Tachypnea (>130 rpm). While not every sign will present in every baby, tachypnea presents very consistently.
- Chest bulge and decreased movement on the affected side
- Asymmetric breath sounds, with decreased or absent sounds over the side of the leak
- Grunting and retractions as the baby works harder to breathe
- Cyanosis, duskiness (abrupt onset with tension pneumothorax)
- Displaced heart sounds to the side opposite the leak
- Decreased breath sounds over the affected lung
- Acute distension of the abdomen due to depression of the diaphragm
- Bubbling sound as air enters the pleural space
- Mottling, poor capillary refill time, or other evidence of poor perfusion
- Restlessness and irritability
- Declining heart and respiratory rates with a drop in blood pressure

•Loss of breath sounds and chest excursion on the affected side during inspiration

Pneumothorax varies in its presentation and may be subtle. The chest wall on the affected side may appear enlarged on examination, depending upon the location of the injury; there may be less movement on that side during ventilation or breathing. In a supine baby, air usually becomes trapped in the anterior chest wall, although air can also collect along the lower border of the lung and in the interlobar fissures. The trapping of air during a tension pneumothorax results in high intrapleural pressures that may be sufficient to compress or even collapse the opposite lung, impairing venous return and producing acute pressure on the heart.

Assessment: Look at the chest in profile from the foot and then the head of the baby to see if the transverse contour is asymmetrical. You may observe flaring of the anterior, interior edge of the rib cage and bulging or separation between the intercostal spaces as air accumulates and pressure builds. Abdominal distension may occur, because air is being diverted into the esophagus and stomach. The chest wall will be hyperresonant on percussion. Listen over the entire chest to ascertain if breath sounds are unequal. Auscultation reveals unequal breath sounds, with decreased or distant breath sounds on the side of the injury, and in some cases, bubbling sounds. The heart sounds may be shifted slightly from their normal position away from the side of the injury. This common injury mimics the much more rare condition of congenital lobar overinflation (emphysema). Compare the description and assessment of these conditions when evaluating the baby (see next page 1313).

An air leak sufficient to cause a tension pneumothorax should be large enough to identify with transillumination, presenting a wide corona (over 3 cm) of very bright light that penetrates into the chest cavity, shining through the trapped air. This is referred to as the "Chinese lantern sign." Gross edema of the chest wall or an excessively thick fat layer may interfere with your assessment because both transmit light well, expanding the normal corona over the chest wall and interfering with intrathoracic transillumination. Otherwise, this has proven a very reliable diagnostic aid. Note that edema produces an increased corona over dependent anatomy, which in a supine baby includes the occiput, back, and posterior surfaces of the arms and legs, whereas air tends to move to the most anterior location. Be sure the room is completely dark to make the most accurate assessment possible. See the "Presentation" entries above under each description of various air leaks for more information about transilluminating less common injuries.

Support and transport of a baby with a thoracic air leak: Tension pneumothorax, pneumopericardium and, more rarely, severe tension pneumomediastinum, require quick recognition and action to prevent brain damage or death. A baby who can breathe and who does not develop significant respiratory distress may have a nontension air leak or some other condition. If it is an air leak and the baby appears otherwise normal, supporting him is relatively easy. The air contained in a pneumothorax will have the same nitrogen concentration as room air. By allowing the baby to breathe pure oxygen, a gradient for nitrogen is created from the extrapulmonary to the intrapulmonary space. The nitrogen will diffuse across this gradient back into the lung, allowing the trapped air to reabsorb more rapidly. Be aware that the risk of oxidant injury exists whenever high concentrations of oxygen are used. Giving the baby vitamin E from a capsule (a few drops on the tongue) can help minimize the adverse effects of the oxygen. Positive pressure will increase the amount of air that leaks into the chest cavity; therefore, artificial ventilation should only be used if absolutely necessary. Even normal breathing will increase, to a certain extent, the amount of air which leaks. Transport for evaluation and treatment.

If a tension condition develops, support should focus on not making it worse. If the baby requires continued ventilation, decrease the pressure at which air is being delivered and increase the rate. If the problem appears worse on one side than the other, position the baby with the more affected side lowermost, which is intended to relieve pressure on the affected lung and promote resolution of any overinflation (Donn & Faix, 1991).

Paracentesis: If significant respiratory distress develops and you are not close to your transport hospital, and the baby's condition is obviously worsening, you can insert a needle into the affected chest wall and aspirate the trapped air, a technique generally referred to as "paracentesis." *Needle aspiration is a potentially dangerous and invasive procedure. It should only be performed in the home if the need is urgent, transport is impossible or a prolonged wait for hospitalization is anticipated, and you believe that the baby may die without it.* It is not considered within a midwife's scope of practice. Prior to venting air from a tension pneumothorax, consult with your anticipated back-up provider and get verbal agreement that aspiration is warranted. *This procedure should not be used merely to try and confirm an air leak.* It is ideal to have four people to perform the aspiration. One to comfort the baby and hold her still, one to manipulate and stabilize the butterfly needle, one to handle the syringe and be in charge of aspiration and a fourth to hold the flashlight for transillumination.

Aspirating air from a pneumothorax (thoracentesis): In spite of the warnings above, venting a pneumothorax, the type of paracentesis you are most likely to need, is relatively easy and the least likely of all types to produce serious injury. You will need a good flashlight, a 21 to 25 gauge butterfly needle with a 12 in extension tube; a standard bore, three-way stopcock with a rotating luer-lock adapter (Baxter part no. 2C6240); and a 50 or 60 ml luer-lock syringe (no needle attached). Transillumination can be used to identify the location of the trapped air, guide the needle and monitor the aspiration procedure.

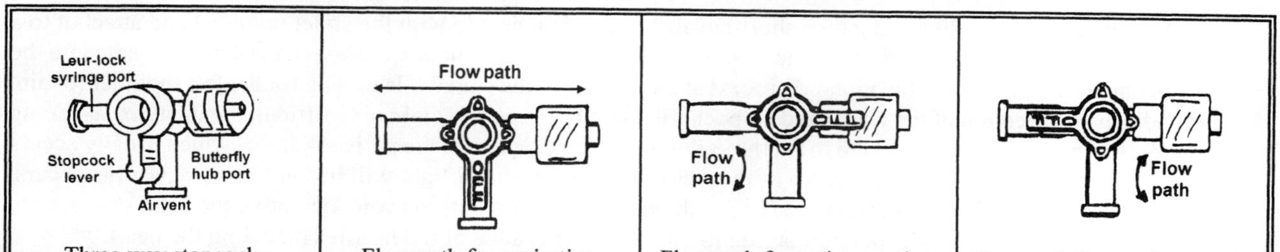

Three-way stopcock | Flow path for aspiration | Flow path for active venting | Flow path for passive venting

(Note that the position of the stopcock lever controls the flow path)

1. Have someone hold the supine infant still on a firm surface and talk to him about what is being done and why.
2. Locate the third or fourth intercostal space on the chest wall on the affected side (the fourth should be in the same horizontal plane as the nipple, if the nipple is normally placed). Longitudinally, the site should be in the midclavicular area. Carefully avoid the nipple and breast bud to prevent scarring. Confirm the site of air entrapment with transillumination; if it is not under the anterior chest wall, the needle can be inserted over the center of the air pocket fairly safely, as long as the needle does not pass through blood vessels or organs. The anterior chest wall is the recommended site because it minimizes the chances that blood vessels or other organs will be punctured. You can try repositioning the baby to see if you can get the air to rise to this optimal location before you insert the needle. *If you cannot identify the site of the air leak visually, do not proceed.*
3. Swab the puncture site with antiseptic tincture or grain alcohol and let it dry.
4. The nerves and blood vessels of the rib cage run along the *lower* border of each rib. Therefore, you will insert the needle perpendicular to the chest wall just over the *top* border of the third or fourth rib. To do so:
   A. Connect the hub on the extension tube of the butterfly needle to the luer-lock port on the three-way stopcock. Connect the syringe's luer-lock end to the opposite port on the stop-cock. Be sure the lever is set to allow aspiration between the two ports.
   B. Slowly insert the needle at a 90° angle to the skin surface over the *top* border of the chosen rib. As the needle enters the skin, have your assistant begin to aspirate by pulling outward very slightly on the syringe plunger to create negative pressure. Stop advancing the needle as soon as air enters the syringe. Continue aspirating until the syringe is full or until air no longer aspirates easily.
   C. When the syringe is full, close the valve on the side to which the butterfly tubing is connected and depress the plunger to empty the syringe.
   D. Redirect the flow path and withdraw more air until ventilations or spontaneous breathing is easier. The needle can be held in place in case air reaccumulates. If it does not, remove it.

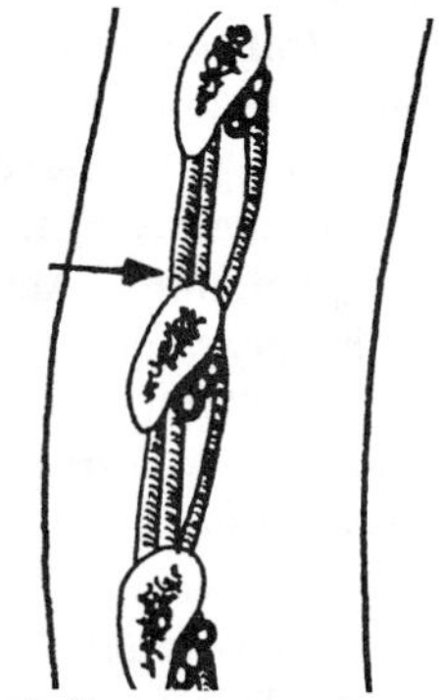

Arrow indicates how going over a rib avoids vessels and nerves on the opposite side.

Note: Aspiration of a nonclotting, clear, light yellow to milky fluid suggests chylothorax (lymph fluid does not become milky until the baby has ingested sufficient milk containing long-chain triglycerides). Other possible sources of fluid include infection or a malignant tumor. Save a sample of the fluid in a red-topped tube for later analysis. If the baby's condition worsens with aspiration, the underlying problem may be lobar overinflation (see page 1313), rather than pneumothorax.

Aspirating air from a pneumomediastinum (thoracentesis): In the extremely rare event that a severe tension pneumomediastinum develops, a subxiphoid location is the preferred site of puncture. Otherwise proceed as for a pneumothorax.

Aspirating air from a pneumopericardium (pericardiocentesis) : *As this risks puncturing or tearing the heart muscle or vessels, it should only be attempted as a last resort when transport is impossible.* When the situation is dire, needle aspiration can result in dramatic and complete relief of symptoms. First, identify the air pocket with transillumination. Use a 20 to 22 gauge short-bevel, 1.5 in spinal needle with the stylet removed and attach it to a 30 to 50 cc syringe. Proceed with the basic steps outlined for venting a pneumothorax, but insert the needle into the anterior chest wall just below the xiphoid process at a 45° angle to the skin while aiming for the left shoulder (or aim the needle in the direction of the visualized air pocket). The fibrous pericardial sac is difficult to puncture, and doing so requires some force. Air will begin to fill the syringe as the needle enters the pericardial sac, which usually occurs as it advances just beyond the left border of the sternum. The corona of light will become smaller; as this occurs, promptly withdraw the needle straight out (i.e., without lateral movement) to avoid lacerating the heart or coronary vessels. Leave a little air in the pericardial sac to minimize the chance of the needle contacting the heart.

Large amounts of blood upon aspiration may be because there is blood (rather than air) in the pericardial sac or because the needle has been advanced too far and pierced the heart. Withdraw the needle slowly while maintaining a slight negative pressure on the syringe. A sudden rush of air into the syringe as the needle is withdrawn confirms the presence and location of a pneumopericardium.

Aspirating air from a pneumoperitoneum (peritoneocentesis): When symptoms are severe, transilluminate the abdomen to locate the trapped air and guide needle aspiration. Use a butterfly as described for pneumothorax. The insertion point should avoid surface blood vessels, underlying organs and bowel; choose a location that goes directly through the skin and underlying tissues into the air pocket. You want to *avoid puncturing the bowel at all costs*, as this could result in peritonitis. Advance the needle only until air enters the syringe, then promptly withdraw it to avoid puncturing any organs as they move forward to fill the space.

***Complications of paracentesis*:** The following complications may ensue when thoracic air leaks are aspirated:

- Misplacement of the needle outside the pleural cavity or across the mediastinum (more likely to occur when a tube is placed)
- Subcutaneous emphysema resulting from a leak at the pleural puncture site
- Trauma to the lung or heart (laceration or perforation) or bleeding
- Infection, either at the puncture site or systemically

***Support for a baby with suspected interstitial emphysema*:** This type of air leak cannot be vented. There is no specific support for intersitial emphysema. The best thing to do is administer 100% oxygen to help diffuse trapped nitrogen and to transport as soon as possible.

Air leak injury to the upper airway: Injury to the upper airway may occur during descent in a face presentation, during labor with a very tight cord around the neck or possibly during rough manipulations in a breech birth. You will have some warning of this due to your knowledge of the baby's presentation at birth and any manual help that was needed to get the baby out. The throat may be visibly bruised. Injury or iatrogenic esophageal perforation may also occur during the difficult placement of an orogastric tube. Esophageal perforation can also occur spontaneously, with no obvious precipitating factors. Symptoms may appear within minutes of birth, or the baby may appear to be well initially, with symptoms developing over the next 30 hours or so. The first signs are increasing respiratory distress followed by cyanosis, a result of pneumothorax or hydropneumothorax, which develops as air and fluids leak from the esophagus into the chest cavity.

Presentation: These babies have difficulty swallowing, with drooling, increased oral secretions and difficulty with nursing, mimicking esophageal atresia, stenosis or duplication. Clear or blood-stained mucus or altered blood (odd in color or consistency) may be suctioned from the mouth. Needle aspiration of the chest, as described in the previous section on thoracic air leaks, yields a serosanguinous fluid and may provide only temporary relief. These babies may require placement of an endotracheal tube or, in rare cases, a tracheotomy. *Emergency tracheotomy is particularly difficult and dangerous to perform on a neonate because of the tiny anatomy. Do not attempt it.* Support the baby with passage of an endotracheal or nasotracheal tube, ventilate as best you can, and transport without delay.

Specific transport considerations: Position the baby on her side to help drain accumulating fluids. Monitor respiratory efforts and ventilate only as necessary, being aware that ventilation may aggravate the problem and force fluid into the airways, causing choking. Transport as rapidly as possible.

Congenital pneumonia: Although most pulmonary infections show up in the days following birth, on rare occasions established infection leads to respiratory failure at birth. Pneumonia is characterized by inflammation leading to the solidification of lung tissue into a condensed mass because the alveoli are filled with exudate, inflammatory cells, and fibrin. Percussion is dull over the airless regions of the lungs and auscultation reveals loud inspiratory crackles over the same area with amplified vocalizations. Pulmonary infection makes the baby more prone to an air-leak injury. These babies may present with fever in a stable temperature environment. Pneumonia may be seen with group B-strep infection. Be particularly suspicious if the baby continues to grunt audibly, even if no other symptoms are present. (See the subchapter entitled "Detecting and Differentiating Newborn Hypoglycemia, Sepsis and Heart Defects" for more details.) Support the baby and transport immediately.

Pleural effusion (hydrothorax): Primary pleural effusion, seen in one baby out of every 15,000 pregnancies, occurs when fluid accumulates in the pleural space, with an increase in either systemic or pulmonary venous pressure and associated hypoproteinemia. It presents with respiratory distress and signs of congestive heart failure. Small pleural effusions may accompany pneumonia or transient tachypnea of the newborn. Babies with hydrops have large effusions that impair respiration and require drainage. A unilateral lesion is suspected when there is a decrease in breath sounds on one side only and a shift of the mediastinum away from the side with the fluid accumulation. Hydrothorax mimics pneumothorax in many respects and will transilluminate brightly.

Congenital chylothorax: Congenital chylothorax is a very rare condition in which a defect in the lymphatic system causes the lymph fluid from the lower body to drip into the chest cavity rather than into the bloodstream. Primary chylothorax is thought to result from absence of the thoracic duct. Secondary chylothorax can occur if the duct is compressed by a tumor. Misdirected lymph fluid builds up in the pleural space, forming a pleural effusion, where it compresses the lungs and impairs inflation. It presents with typical signs of respiratory distress.

Assessment of pleural effusion: If the baby's breathing sounds as though you are listening through water, especially if this finding is more marked at the top of the chest, the baby is likely to have a hydrothorax or, much more rarely, congenital chylothorax. When this is suspected, percuss and transilluminate the chest. If there is dullness on percussion, light transilluminates brightly and there is no evidence of an airway injury, hydro- or chylothorax is a possible diagnosis.

Support and transport: To transport a baby with suspected pleural effusions from any cause:
1. Place the baby on a flat surface and keep him warm.
2. Elevate the baby's upper body to relieve fluid pressure on the lungs.
3. Use blow-by oxygen or positive-pressure ventilations as necessary.
4. Place an orogastric or nasogastric tube and suction every 5 to 10 minutes.

Congenital lobar overinflation (emphysema): This accounts for about 50% of all congenital lung malformations. There are five major causes of overexpansion of the lungs' lobes:

Intrinsic bronchial obstruction: This can be caused by bronchomalacia (collapse of the softened bronchi on expiration), inspissated (hardened) mucus plugs, bronchial torsion and bronchial atresia.

Extrinsic bronchial compression: Causes include defects in major blood vessels, heart enlargement due to heart defects, bronchogenic cysts or enlarged lymph nodes in the mediastinum. Any of these may lead to softening of the bronchial tube and its subsequent collapse on expiration.

Alveolar fibrosis: This may be congenital or secondary to infection.

Pulmonary hypoplasia from too few bronchial branches: Here the total number of bronchioles are reduced, amounting to localized pulmonary hypoplasia. Air becomes trapped in the underdeveloped region without crowding of the adjacent lung and with no mediastinal shift because the total number of alveoli are so reduced.

Pulmonary alveolar hyperplasia (polyalveolar lobe): These may be caused when too many alveoli develop in a region of the lungs which then become overdistended with air and compress adjacent parts of the lung.

Congenital overinflation allows air to enter but not exit lungs, producing massive overdistension of at least one pulmonary lobe. There may be compression of adjacent lung tissue, shifting of the mediastinum and compression of the opposite lung. No cause can be found in 50% of cases. The upper left lobe is most frequently involved, followed by the right middle lobe, with lower lobes rarely affected. The term "overinflation" differentiates air entrapment due to a congenital condition from true emphysema, which is caused by tissue destruction and is largely acquired.

Associated defects: It is associated with heart defects such as patent ductus arteriosus and ventricular septal defect.

Presentation: Lobar overinflation presents similarly to pneumothorax in the first five days of life. Interstitial involvement produces characteristic crepitation (like crushing Styrofoam or walking on dry snow). There may also be an increase in thoracic volume, but unlike pneumothorax, the enlargement is limited to the affected area because the trapped air is within the lung, rather than overlying it. This is accompanied by rib flaring, an increase in chest diameter over the area and decreased breath sounds. This condition usually becomes apparent within the first hours or weeks of life, although it is possible for a severe case to present during the postpartum watch. Respiratory symptoms range from slight tachypnea and restlessness in mild cases to cyanosis and episodes of bradycardia in severe cases.

Assessment: Careful inspection of the chest reveals unilateral hyperexpansion with decreased but clear breath sounds on the affected side and heart sounds displaced to the other side. The trachea may be displaced to the opposite side as well. Differentiating this disorder from the much more common pneumothorax is probably impossible at home. In pneumothorax, both the upper and lower lobes collapse to the midline and lie against the mediastinum; in lobar emphysema, only the unaffected (usually lower) lobe of the lung collapses. This may be detectible during skilled transillumination, although I could find no mention of it in the literature.

Differential diagnosis includes congenital lung cysts, pneumothorax, diaphragmatic hernia and bronchial obstruction (which may occur if the baby inhales exceptionally thick mucus, a blood clot or meconium) with compensatory emphysema. Placement of a needle within an emphysematous lobe may result in acute decompensation, whereas with pneumothorax, it provides relief.

Specific support and transport protocols:

- Place the baby on a flat surface and keep her warm.
- Elevate the baby's upper body to relieve fluid pressure on the lungs.
- Use blow-by oxygen as necessary.
- Use positive-pressure ventilation only when clearly needed. Artificial ventilation may produce sudden expansion and entrapment of air in the affected portion of lung, leading to abrupt cardiorespiratory failure. Use low-pressure, rapid ventilations (20 to 25 cm H_2O) with a high oxygen concentration.
- Place an orogastric or nasogastric tube and suction every 5 to 10 minutes.

This protocol is designed to relieve pressure on the lungs by maintaining an open airway all the way past the constricted area. Positive pressure or even normal breathing may increase the amount of air that is trapped in the chest cavity. Artificial ventilation should only be used if absolutely necessary.

Pulmonary atresia or hypoplasia: Primary pulmonary hypoplasia is found in 0.6% of all babies admitted to neonatal nurseries, and in 15 to 20% of all babies who die in the early neonatal period. Severely hypoplastic lungs can manifest in a variety of ways, depending upon the degree to which the lungs are underdeveloped. Primary hypoplasia, which is not associated with other defects, is rare. Secondary hypoplasia results when another anomaly produces compression due to encroachment of other organs into the lung field. There is often a history of severe oligohydramnios associated with renal agenesis or dysplasia (Potter syndrome), obstructive uropathy (preventing urination) and prolonged leakage of amniotic fluid, as well as other conditions associated with oligohydramnios, such as prune-belly syndrome. Lung compression and impaired growth may also be found with diaphragmatic hernia (see item 6); eventration of the diaphragm; pressure into the thoracic cavity from abdominal organs, ascites or pleural effusion; and skeletal disorders that involve abnormalities of the rib cage and neuromuscular disorders (see item 7). Bilateral agenesis often accompanies anencephaly. Also see the entry for persistent pulmonary hypertension of the newborn in item 12.

Presentation: Complete bilateral absence of lung tissue or severe underdevelopment results in increasingly severe, irresolvable respiratory distress with persistent pulmonary hypertension. This condition is usually fatal. Attempts to inflate the lungs quickly result in pneumothorax.

Potter syndrome is characterized by bilateral renal agenesis. It presents with a senile appearance, with a prominent fold of skin over each eye that may extend to the cheek. The nose is blunted and deviated, and the baby has flattened facial features. There is a prominent depression between the lower lip and the chin; marked creases under the eyes; apparently low-set, crumpled ears; a small chin; positional deformities of the arms and legs with bowing and clubbing of the feet and occasional limb fusion; and a small, shortened bell- or dog-shaped chest, reflecting the lack of normal lung development. The skin is very dry and loose. Some of these babies may void once after birth, but the bladder remains empty with no voiding thereafter. Some may live hours or days, with the rate of renal failure dictating survival.

In Jeune syndrome, the rib cage is short and narrow, displacing the liver into the abdominal cavity, resulting in a large, round belly, as if the baby swallowed a small basketball. Kidney defects are also associated with this disorder. If the baby also has a diaphragmatic hernia, a barrel (large and rounded) chest and scaphoid abdomen are usually present.

Unilateral pulmonary agenesis, as an isolated finding, is compatible with survival. It is more often seen in boys and occurs on the left side in about 70% of cases.

Specific support and transport considerations: These babies should be transported immediately:
1. Place the baby on flat surface and keep him warm.
2. Use, as indicated, blow-by oxygen or positive-pressure ventilation at a low pressure (20 to 25 cm H_2O). These babies are prone to pneumothorax because their lungs do not inflate normally.
3. Insert an orogastric or nasogastric tube and aspirate every 5 to 10 minutes.

Congenital pulmonary cysts: These rare cysts may be single or multiple, but they are confined to one lobe of the lung. They communicate with peripheral airways; thus when a cyst enlarges rapidly, it may produce progressive respiratory distress due to trapping of air. Alternately, it can rupture, resulting in a pneumothorax. Large air-filled cysts may be mistaken for tension pneumothorax on exam. Symptomatic babies require immediate surgery to remove the affected lobe.

Congenital cystic adenomatoid malformation: First described in 1949, this is an exceedingly rare developmental abnormality of the lung bud, with 200 cases reported in the English literature as of 1993. In spite of its rarity, it accounts for 25% of all congenital lung tumors. It combines features of abnormal tissue development and tumor-like growth, resulting in nonfunctional lung tissue and sometimes lung hypoplasia due to compression of the opposite lung. The cyst is usually located in one or both lobes of one lung. It results in preterm birth, stillbirth, acute progressive respiratory distress in newborns, or protracted childhood pneumonias.

Associated defects: Additional defects are found in 42% of babies with congenital pulmonary cysts. Associated cardiac defects occur 21% of the time and funnel chest (depression over the lower chest causing backward displacement of the xiphoid) occurs 16% of the time. Twenty-five percent will have polyhydramnios during pregnancy.

Presentation: Three presentations may occur at birth:

Stillbirth: About 25% of these babies will be stillborn.

Preterm birth: About 50% are born too early. Early neonatal death often occurs in affected preterm babies with pregnancies complicated by polyhydramnios and fetal hydrops. (Also see the subchapter entitled "Pallor with Generalized Edema; Swollen, Fluid-Filled Abdomen and Respiratory Distress: Hydrops Fetalis."

Respiratory distress: In term infants at birth, respiratory distress ranges from mild to severe, as air becomes trapped in the cyst, causing it to enlarge. Severe distress may present at birth with tachypnea, grunting, cyanosis and bradycardia. In some of these babies, feeding may prompt the first difficulties with breathing. This condition may mimic a diaphragmatic hernia and lobar emphysema.

Assessment: Physical exam reveals enlargement of the thorax on the affected side, hyperresonance on percussion, decreased breath sounds, distant or shifted heart sounds, all of which mimic pneumothorax, although these symptoms occur with spontaneous breathing. In some cases, the liver appears enlarged (which is not typical of pneumothorax); this is caused by hyperexpansion of the thorax, displacing the liver downward.

Support and transport: Attempt to distinguish this condition from the much more manageable and more common pneumothorax, although this will probably be impossible at home. Ventilatory support may be warranted in cases of severe respiratory distress, but positive pressure tends to fill the cysts with air and further compromise breathing. Use rapid, low-pressure ventilations (20 to 25 cm H_2O) with a high oxygen concentration.

Pulmonary sequestration: This disorder accounts for 6% of all congenital pulmonary malformations but presents only very rarely in newborns. It is found in 1.1 to 1.8% of all resected lung-tissue specimens. In this disorder, a mass of nonfunctioning lung tissue, most commonly associated with the lower left lobe, is separated from the tracheobronchial tree; its circulatory supply comes from anomalous systemic vessels. The sequestered region of tissue may be within or outside the lobes of the lung, each variety being associated with other characteristic malformations. If the areas are sufficiently large, signs of severe respiratory distress, which include tachypnea, grunting, cyanosis or, rarely, congestive heart failure, appear in the newborn. Less severely affected babies first present with breathing difficulties during feeding.

Associated defects: These babies are relatively free of associated anomalies, although a few will have heart defects. Infants with extralobular sequestration (where the defect develops outside of otherwise normal lungs) have a higher incidence of associated anomalies (15 to 40%), most commonly diaphragmatic hernia. Other related anomalies include cardiac defects, funnel chest, pulmonary hypoplasia on the side of the lesion and (intestinal) duplication.

Assessment: A bruit may be heard over the mass. (A bruit is an intermittent, harsh or musical auscultatory sound, especially an abnormal one.) The precordium may be hyperactive (visibly pulsating) if the baby is in cardiac failure.

Pulmonary lymphangiectasia: This is caused by cystic dilation of the pulmonary lymphatics and results in a wide array of respiratory symptoms.

Associated defects: It may be associated with congenital heart disease (especially total anomalous pulmonary venous return [TAPVD]), hypoplastic left heart syndrome and pulmonary stenosis.

Presentation: When not associated with heart defects, it produces severe respiratory failure in the first hours of life, although this may manifest later in infancy. The lymphangiectasia is usually found on both sides. It is generally not compatible with life.

Large liver tumor: Metastatic neuroblastoma is the most common liver tumor in newborns. These babies may be born with an enlarged liver and abdominal distension that may impair ventilation of the lungs due to upward pressure into the chest cavity.

Transport considerations: Position the baby so the head is higher than the torso (on an upward slant) to take as much pressure off the lungs as possible, ventilate and transport.

Eventration (elevation) of the diaphragm: The exact incidence of this defect is not known. Beck and Morsay (1952) reported a 4% incidence of diaphragmatic elevation in 2500 newborn chest X-rays, a rate that seems high, but all but three of these cases were asymptomatic. Symptomatic eventration results in extreme elevation of all or part of the diaphragm, which impairs lung function on the affected side. The diaphragm is usually poorly developed and abnormally thin and has little or no ability to contract. Complete absence of the diaphragmatic musculature is the most severe form of this disorder and is incompatible with life. Symptoms vary greatly; some babies have severe respiratory compromise, while others are asymptomatic. You will not be able to tell precisely what is going on with such a baby; listen to the chest to try and rule out diaphragmatic hernia and ventilate during transport as necessary.

Mediastinal or thoracic cysts and tumors: A variety of different types of rare cysts and tumors may arise in the mediastinal region. Many of these will be asymptomatic at birth, but if sufficiently large can cause lung compression with signs of respiratory distress.

Masses within the thorax may be completely asymptomatic. If not, symptoms range from quite subtle, with no more than restlessness at first, to progressive tachypnea and finally respiratory failure during the first hours, days or weeks of life. (For a more detailed discussion of obstruction and compression, see items 1 and 2 in this chapter.)

6. SEVERE RESPIRATORY DISTRESS IN A BABY WITH A CAVED-IN ABDOMEN AND ENLARGED CHEST; VENTILATION IS DIFFICULT AND INEFFECTIVE OR IMPOSSIBLE.

Diaphragmatic hernia

Congenital diaphragmatic hernia, appearing in 1 out of 2200 to 5000 live births, occurs when the diaphragm does not form properly, leaving an opening that is most commonly located posteriorly and to the side of the sternum on the left. This allows abdominal contents to migrate into the chest cavity, compressing one or both of the developing lungs and thus impairing proper respiration at birth. There are two main types of diaphragmatic hernia, with the posterolateral (Bochdalek) variety described here being the most likely to present at birth as well as the most severe. The hernia usually involves migration of the entire midgut, a portion of the descending colon, the left kidney, stomach, spleen and, less commonly, the left lobe of the liver. This results in displacement of the heart over to the right in 90% of these babies and some degree of cardiac hypoplasia. The degree of distress will depend upon the degree of migration of abdominal contents to the lung field and the degree to which the lungs and heart have been compressed and their development thus impaired. Thirty percent of affected babies are stillborn.

Associated anomalies: Associated nonpulmonary malformations are found in 95% of affected stillborn babies and up to 60% of those who die within 24 hours of birth. Additional anomalies will be found in about 40% of other surviving babies. Major associated problems include pulmonary hypoplasia, chromosomal defects, congenital heart defects (10 to 25%), neural tube defects, skeletal and urinary tract anomalies, sequestered pulmonary lobes and intestinal defects, principally malrotation of the gut (nearly always).

Presentation: These babies usually present with persistent respiratory distress in the first 24 hours of life, with many experiencing persistent pulmonary hypertension, resulting in persistent cyanosis. Lung sounds are hard to hear on the affected side and, on rare occasions, bowel sounds may be heard in the chest cavity once some breathing or ventilation has been established. Heart sounds are deviated away from the defect, most often to the right side of the chest. The midgut fills with air when the baby first attempts to nurse, resulting in further displacement of the mediastinum to the right and compression of the right lung. Efforts at diaphragmatic breathing also tend to draw the abdominal organs higher into the chest cavity. The degree of respiratory distress depends upon the degree of lung compression and impairment, which usually occurs in both lungs because the more normal lung receives pressure from the displaced organs on the other side. The belly will appear caved in or flat (scaphoid) while the chest will be large and round. These findings strongly suggest that the baby has a diaphragmatic hernia. Transillumination may reveal displaced abdominal organs in the chest cavity, helping to confirm the diagnosis. Mortality is 50% among those babies who develop respiratory distress in the first 4 hours of life. These babies are at risk for sudden changes in pulmonary vascular resistance as well as pulmonary hypertension. Even though many of these babies will die because of poor lung development, they should be taken to the hospital immediately for evaluation, possible surgical correction and advanced supportive care.

Support and transport protocols:

1. Transport immediately on a flat surface and keep the baby warm.
2. Elevate the head by positioning the baby at a 45° angle, supporting the back with a rolled towel, or put her on her side with the affected side lowermost.
3. Prevent gastrointestinal distension by inserting a large-bore (8 or 10F) orogastric tube and aspirating it every 5 to 10 minutes.
4. If you have been trained to insert an endotracheal tube, do so, and use it for ventilation.
5. Place an oral airway or use blow-by oxygen as necessary.
6. Do not use positive-pressure ventilation unless clearly indicated. When it is necessary, use low-pressure ventilations with 100% oxygen at a rapid rate of delivery.

These protocols are designed to position the baby so that gravity aids in pulling the misplaced organs in the chest cavity downward, allowing maximum inflation of any normal lung tissue that may be present. An oral airway is placed to make sure the baby's trachea remains open.

Because the lungs are defective, positive-pressure ventilations are more likely to route air into the stomach or intestines, causing them to enlarge and further compress any functional lung tissue that is present, compounding the problem and further compromising the baby's ability to breathe. High-pressure ventilations must also be avoided. Incapable of full expansion, hypoplastic lungs are susceptible to trauma and rupture; a tension pneumothorax on the side opposite the defect may be fatal because the lung capacity is already so compromised. A combination of low-pressure, rapid respirations and a high oxygen concentration will help minimize overdistension of the lungs. Ventilatory pressure should not exceed 20 to 25 cm H_2O, and the baby should be allowed to breathe spontaneously as much as he is able.

An orogastric tube should be placed as soon as a diaphragmatic hernia is suspected. Aspirate every 5 to 10 minutes to remove both secretions and any air that has entered the stomach before it travels to the intestines where it can become trapped and compress the lungs. Passage of an endotracheal tube is also indicated if transport cannot take place immediately. Blow-by oxygen is given by mask to maximize oxygenation for any baby who is able to breathe on her own, because reduced lung capacity will minimize the oxygen that is reaching the tissues.

7. THE BABY CANNOT MAINTAIN SPONTANEOUS RESPIRATIONS BUT RESPONDS WELL TO BEING VENTILATED

The baby does well while receiving artificial ventilations and can maintain a normal heart rate. However, the baby collapses into complete respiratory arrest when respiratory assistance is withdrawn and cannot recover on his own.

Possible causes

Bilateral paralysis of the diaphragm: Since breathing is so dependent upon the excursion of the diaphragm, bilateral paralysis will not allow the baby's distress to resolve. It may be seen with injury to or congenital absence of the phrenic nerves at the 3rd, 4th, and 5th cervical nerve roots (injury may occur during a difficult breech birth). Brachial plexus damage may manifest with paralysis of the arm on the affected side. It is also found in 5 to 10% of all babies with brachial plexus injuries, although in that case, the paralysis is usually unilateral; 80 to 90% of all cases of diaphragmatic paralysis are associated with such injuries. There may be respiratory distress, lack of lung inflation and mediastinal shift.

Neuromuscular disorders affecting the respiratory system, rib cage or diaphragm: The baby may be unable to assume spontaneous respirations because she does not have adequate musculature to move her chest wall without being ventilated. Another form of neuromuscular dysfunction, Plott's syndrome, is a hereditary disorder with congenital laryngeal adductor paralysis as a feature. The disorder is X-linked and is associated with mental retardation. There is nothing you can do to further troubleshoot a neuromuscular disorder. Babies so affected will not stabilize. The prognosis for life is poor.

Support and transport

Continue to provide artificial ventilation or full CPR and transport immediately.

8. THE PREVIOUSLY UNCOMPROMISED BABY HAS PERSISTENT OR INCREASING DIFFICULTY WITH BREATHING, SOMETIMES LEADING TO RESPIRATORY FAILURE.

Specific causes

The baby who has no evidence of asphyxia prior to birth, was relatively stable to begin with and who is now struggling to continue respirations may have one of the following problems:

- Lesser degree of diaphragmatic hernia (see item 6)
- Infection (sepsis or congenital pneumonia)
- Respiratory distress syndrome (preterm baby?)
- Partial or progressive airway compression or obstruction (see items 1 and 2)
- Maternal drug intake
- Brain injury

•Tracheal stenosis
•Pulmonary lymphangiectasia (less than 100 cases reported as of 1993)

Infection: Respiratory distress with labored breathing is one of many nonspecific signs of infection. See the subchapter entitled "Detecting and Differentiating Newborn Hypoglycemia, Sepsis and Heart Defects" for more information.

Respiratory distress syndrome Type I (formerly hyaline membrane disease [HMD]): Respiratory distress syndrome (RDS) occurs whenever the lungs cannot fully meet the oxygen requirements of the body. In preterm babies, this is often due to an immature level of surfactant coupled with an inadequate blood volume. The symptoms are those of classic respiratory distress: rapid breathing, retractions, grunting and nostril flaring. In the term newborn, the usual cause is hypovolemic shock due to circulatory compromise prior to birth followed by immediate cord clamping.

Babies most prone to suffer from RDS are those with immature lungs. This includes a small minority of babies in the 36 to 37 week range; the earlier the baby, the greater the chances of immature lungs. Babies with immature lungs have more difficulty keeping their lungs adequately inflated between breaths. Mainstream neonatology regards surfactant as the most important factor in mature lung function. In contrast to this widely held view, both Dunn and Morley have observed that an adequate blood volume is much more critical to normally functioning lungs (Dunn, 1989; Morley, 2002b). This is explained in more detail in the chapter entitled "The Baby's Journey through Labor to Birth."

Even though you have ensured that the baby receive an optimal placental transfusion, you must still be alert for signs that normal respirations are continuing. A slightly preterm baby who has received his full placental transfusion, who can breathe on his own and can suck at the breast might be able to remain at home. When weighing whether transport is warranted, keep in mind that babies weighing less than 3 lb 5 oz (1500 grams) are the most prone to the development of respiratory distress. If the baby is this small and unstable, she needs to be kept warm, given full cardiopulmonary resuscitation or blow-by oxygen as required, and transported. Remember that these babies may have "stiff" lungs, and a higher opening pressure may be required for initial inflations during artificial ventilation. As always, watching for chest movement and listening for breath sounds over the lower rib cage are the best measures of adequate ventilatory pressure.

The onset of respiratory distress may be delayed in a baby who appears stable at birth. This is especially true of preterm babies. Preterm babies should be calmed down and watched carefully for the first 8 to 12 hours of life, transported as appropriate, or evaluated by a pediatrician. Assess the baby by listening to the degree of lung inflation with a stethoscope and observe him for continuing or worsening respiratory distress, apnea and poor thermal regulation. Duskiness can also be the first sign of persistent pulmonary hypertension of the newborn, which can easily become serious if not recognized and dealt with right away. Should you choose not to transport, it is best to spend the night and monitor the baby at regular intervals to make sure everything is okay. Prior to leaving, the signs and symptoms of respiratory distress should be explained to the parents.

Partial or progressive airway compression or obstruction: See item 2 in this chapter.

Maternal drug intake: Drugs, especially sedative medications, such as magnesium sulfate, nonnarcotic analgesics and general anesthetics, that are given within four hours of birth may result in significant respiratory distress and lethargy (This is only relevant for hospital births in which maternal drugs are given during labor, for a mother who has taken some form of neuromuscular depressant drug without your knowledge.) See the subchapter entitled "Drug Withdrawal" for details.

Brain injury: Intracranial trauma may result in respiratory distress. Injury may be suspected after a birth in which the mother's pelvis is contracted, after a breech birth, or after instrumental delivery. The only evidence that points to possible intracranial injury as the cause of respiratory distress may be birth history and newborn behavior. Look for a shrill cry, hypertonia or flaccidity. Spinal cord injury can also present this way in some babies (see details in item 9, and in the subchapter entitled "Cranial Injuries.")

Tracheal stenosis: See item 2.

9. Baby with respiratory distress is weak, pale and shocky.

Presentation

This baby is likely to be suffering from hypovolemic shock, which can spring from many causes such as a ruptured placental or cord vessel, which may be missed at first glance because the blood may be assumed to be from the mother. Partial occlusion of the umbilical vein but not the arteries (where the blood flows at a higher pressure) can also result in blood reaching the placenta but not returning to the baby. Hypovolemia from chronically impaired placental blood return will present with a white, limp baby and a pulseless cord with thin, tightly-constricted vessels. Intra-abdominal bleeding from trauma to the spleen or liver may not be immediately obvious. In small babies, large, benign liver tumors can shunt a significant quantity of blood, resulting in congestive heart failure. Fluid and electrolyte loss may occur in conjunction with complications associated with atypical genitalia and a number of other disorders; it is most likely to develop some hours following birth. Septic shock also results from a number of infectious diseases. A 20% or greater loss of total blood volume results in the following signs:

- Pallor persisting in spite of oxygen supplementation
- Persistently weak pulses in spite of a good heart rate
- Poor response to resuscitative efforts
- Decreased blood pressure (although you will not usually take blood pressure at home)

General support and transport recommendations

These babies require continued respiratory support, immediate transport, neonatal evaluation and probably a transfusion with blood or a volume expander once they are in the hospital. Do not attempt to give a newborn an IV or a retention enema.

Specific causes

A baby who is not stabilizing or is stabilizing poorly may be suffering from acute blood loss or disruption. Neonatal hypovolemic shock may be seen with:

- Interruption of the placental blood flow from cord rupture, hematoma or early clamping
- Chronic cord compression or hypoxia from other causes leading to peripheral vasoconstriction and hypovolemia
- Acute fetomaternal hemorrhage such as placental abruption or previa
- Twin-to-twin transfusion
- Blood incompatibilities with maternal sensitization (resulting in a lack of functioning red blood cells)
- Internal hemorrhage due to birth trauma
- Coagulation disorders
- Sepsis
- Disseminated intravascular coagulation (which may develop due to severe, established infection)
- Large benign tumors of the liver (primarily hemangioma and hemangioendothelioma, which can trap platelets, resulting in massive internal bleeding)

Spinal cord defect or injury: Any manipulations required to complete the birth have the potential to overstretch the baby's spine or overrotate the body in relation to the head and cause spinal cord injury. Chief among births that require such manipulations are breech births and those involving shoulder dystocia. If something was broken, a loud pop or crack may have been heard at birth. Clinical signs and symptoms depend upon the level and severity of the injury. A state of shock and difficulty establishing respirations is a common finding. Damage above C3 or C4 paralyzes the diaphragm. Damage further down the spine in the lower cervical or upper thoracic segments cause flaccidity of the legs and portions of the arms. Lack of response to a pinprick will be noted below the level of injury.

Support and transport: An ambulance should be called whenever possible. If you must transport the baby yourself, the baby must be moved carefully to a transport surface, without moving the spine. The spine should be stabilized by strapping down the head, chest, arms and legs with the baby supine to prevent spinal movement and the possibility of causing further damage. See the subchapter entitled "Birth Injuries (Other Than Cranial Injuries)," for more details.

10. A BABY WITH A HISTORY OF CHRONIC INTRAUTERINE HYPOXIA IS WEAK AND RUDDY OR CYANOTIC WITH VARYING DEGREES OF LETHARGY, RESPIRATORY DISTRESS AND NEUROLOGICAL SIGNS

Polycythemia (hematocrit over 65 to 70%) presents in babies who have experienced chronic fetal hypoxia, prompting the overproduction of red blood cells in an effort to increase the oxygen carrying capacity of the blood. However, excessive red cells by themselves may not cause symptoms; Drew and colleagues (1997) found that excessive hyperviscosity (which is often the direct result of hypovolemia) is more problematic than polycythemia per se. Symptoms in macrosomic babies born to diabetic mothers may be due to hypoglycemia rather than polycythemia. When symptoms do develop, the central nervous system is the one most often affected. These babies may display plethora (an excess of any body fluid; in this case, blood), rubeosis (tomato-red to red-purple coloring, sometimes accompanied by cyanosis), weak sucking reflex, lethargy and difficulty rousing with irritability upon arousal, poor response to light, respiratory distress with tachypnea, excessive jitteriness, hypotonia, vomiting, easy startle, heart murmur due to cardiac enlargement, and liver enlargement. A few infants may display persistent bradycardia, persistent erection of the penis and seizures.

11. RESPIRATORY STRIDOR, SOMETIMES WITH AN ABNORMAL CRY AND DIFFICULTY SWALLOWING.

There are numerous reasons the baby may present with stridor, which is characterized by the rapid, turbulent flow of air through a narrowed segment of the respiratory tract. The sound may be high- or low-pitched, noisy or soft, whistling, musical or harsh, depending on the type and degree of obstruction. Generally, stridor on inspiration is produced by an obstruction above the thoracic inlet or in the larynx itself. This results in inward collapse of these structures from the negative pressure created during inspiration. Expiratory as well as biphasic stridor (occurring during both inhalation and exhalation) usually indicates that the obstruction is below the larynx. Defects that narrow the trachea may prompt the baby to hold her head in a hyperextended attitude and may produce a barking cough, cyanotic episodes, apneic spells and aspiration. They often have repeated, prolonged atypical croup as they get older. The characteristics of the breath sounds give clues regarding where they may originate.

BREATH SOUNDS	INSPIRATORY OR EXPIRATORY?	LIKELY LOCATION OF PROBLEM
Harsh, high pitched, crowing	Inspiratory only	Usually supraglottic laryngeal; may be subglottic laryngeal
Low pitched, snoring, excessive secretions	Inspiratory only	Pharyngeal or nasopharyngeal
Prolonged, low-pitched expiration	Both	Tracheal compression or collapse

General transport considerations for babies with stridor

Since the primary presentation is abnormal breath sounds, these babies usually do not require extensive support. Feeding should be withheld until the baby can be evaluated. A consultation should be sought. Position the baby on his right side and transport for evaluation soon after birth to determine the exact diagnosis and whether it is safe for the baby to return home.

Possible causes

- Simple hoarseness is usually due to irritation from suctioning or excessive crying
- Laryngeal disorders, which occur in approximately 1 out of every 1000 births. These conditions include:
  - Laryngomalacia (60 to 75% of all laryngeal disorders), usually asymptomatic at birth and may occur with or without congenital subglottic stenosis
  - Paralysis of the vocal cords (15 to 20% of all laryngeal disorders)
  - Congenital subglottic stenosis (15% of laryngeal disorders; usually asymptomatic at birth), often associated with webbing or laryngocele
  - Laryngeal webbing or atresia (2 to 4% of all laryngeal disorders)
  - Partially obstructive laryngeal tumors, such as saccular cysts (25%) and hemangiomas (1.5%)
  - Laryngeal cleft (less than 0.01% of all laryngeal disorders)

-Hyperexcitability of the laryngeal abductors
•Tracheal stenosis or tracheomalacia (both very rare)

Laryngomalacia: This is the most common cause of congenital laryngeal stridor at birth, accounting for up to 75% of all laryngeal anomalies, with two-thirds of those affected being male. It is probably due to immaturity of the laryngeal muscles and cartilages, causing the airway to be abnormally soft and pliable. This results in intermittent inspiratory collapse of the arytenoids, arytenoid folds and epiglottis, which occlude the glottic opening during inspiration. This produces a high-pitched, harsh, crowing stridor that is at times low-pitched and fluttering.

Presentation: The signs and symptoms of laryngomalacia tend to be variable and occur in phases; the baby may sometimes be able to sleep quietly while at other times he sounds "mucusy," but suctioning does not resolve the symptoms. The stridor tends to worsen with straining, feeding, crying or other agitation, or when he is placed supine with the head and neck flexed. It improves when he is placed on his belly with the head and neck extended, allowing the tongue to pull the supraglottic structures forward. It also improves when the baby is relaxed or when the jaw thrust maneuver is employed. The voice and cry are otherwise normal, and there is usually no cyanosis or difficulty with swallowing due to aspiration; in fact, both are so uncommon that other conditions should be considered if either does occur. The increased tidal volume that occurs during vigorous crying may cause the stridor to temporarily resolve. Feeding difficulties and frank respiratory distress occur occasionally, with suprasternal and lower sternal retractions occasionally severe enough to cause in-pulling over the xiphoid process. Uncomplicated laryngomalacia usually resolves around 18 to 24 months of age as the cartilage becomes stiffer. Laryngomalacia may occur in association with congenital subglottic stenosis.

Paralysis of the vocal cords: Paralysis of the vocal cords is the second most common laryngeal anomaly, accounting for 6 to 15% of all such disorders. It may be unilateral (20%) or bilateral (80%). Causes include dysfunction of the brain stem nuclei, of a vagus nerve, or of the recurrent laryngeal nerve supplying the affected side. The left side is more commonly affected, as the left recurrent laryngeal nerve follows a longer, more circuitous route than the right and is thus more susceptible to trauma. The cause of most vocal cord paralysis is unknown.

Associated defects: Congenital paralysis is associated with Arnold-Chiari malformation and cardiovascular malformations. Acquired paralysis is usually secondary to birth trauma, more rarely resulting from tumors of the neck or thorax. Bilateral involvement suggests central neurological lesions and may be seen with hydrocephaly, lesions of the fourth ventricle, bulbar paresis, Arnold-Chiari malformation and other problems affecting the central nervous system. Unilateral involvement is more likely due to peripheral lesions.

Presentation: Unilateral paralysis often produces a weak cry and mild to severe stridor, which is most prominent during inspiration. The one functioning vocal cord will provide adequate laryngeal function; a weak cry and occasional stridor are often the only clues to the problem. Bilateral paralysis causes a high-pitched, crowing, inspiratory stridor. Because the vocal cords rest in adduction, the cry may be weak and breathy but otherwise normal. Intermittent aspiration and cyanosis during feeding occur with both types. Loss of sensation on the affected side probably contributes to aspiration. Symptoms are generally worse with bilateral paralysis; acute respiratory distress may be present since paralysis leaves both vocal cords in the paramedian position, unable to abduct to allow adequate inspiration. The narrowed airway results in persistent stridor and cyanotic attacks from the moment of birth. When paralysis is associated with birth trauma, the trauma is usually severe enough to affect other cervical nerves or to produce a hematoma.

Congenital subglottic stenosis (subglottic laryngeal stenosis): Congenital subglottic stenosis is a rare cause of airway obstruction at birth, found most often in association with tracheoesophageal fistula or Down syndrome. The most common site of stenosis is the area 2 to 3 mm below the true vocal cords, where the cricoid ring may be small or in an unusual position, resulting in compression of the subglottic lumen. While the stenosis itself may not result in obstruction, slight inflammation can lead to acute and critical obstruction because the cricoid cartilage is rigid and restricts edema within the airway.

Presentation: Stridor may also result from swelling at the level of the cricoid ring after poorly performed ET intubation or when the wrong intubation equipment is used. The relaxed supraglottic larynx is drawn into the glottis during inspiration, causing the characteristic inspiratory stridor. This condition is not life threatening, although it often causes problems with nursing.

Congenital laryngeal webs or atresia: Congenital webs or partial laryngeal atresia are relatively rare, accounting for only 2 to 4% of laryngeal anomalies. Webbing may be located above, in or below the larynx. Size varies, with large webs covering the entire glottis and producing marked obstruction resulting in severe respiratory distress or failure at birth (see item 1).

Presentation: A small web may only cover the anterior corner of the vocal cords producing a hoarse, weak or absent cry. Other symptoms include persistent inspiratory stridor, cyanotic attacks and respiratory distress which worsens with exertion.

Partially obstructive laryngeal tumors: There are several varieties of such tumors.
Papilloma: Papillomas of the larynx are the most common cause of acquired airway obstruction, although these are rarely present at birth. If sufficiently large, they produce a weak or feeble cry or stridor. The mother would have a positive history of papilloma infection.

Laryngeal saccular cysts: These lesions arise when drainage of the mucous glands of the mucous membranes lining the air-containing saccules are obstructed. The saccule does not drain into the laryngeal lumen and becomes filled with mucus (and very rarely, air [laryngocele]), usually forming to the side and extending supraglottically into the aryepiglottic fold. Anterior saccular cysts are smaller and extend into the midline laryngeal lumen between the true and false cords.

Presentation: A large cyst or laryngocele may cause airway obstruction with severe respiratory distress, stridor, cyanotic episodes and a muffled cry. They produce more pronounced obstruction if irritated due to edema, bleeding or both.

Ductal cysts: Mucous retention cysts develop when the duct of a mucous gland becomes obstructed. They may occur in the vallecula, the larynx, the vocal fold or the subglottic region.

Presentation: If large enough, these cysts cause airway obstruction. Those in the vocal folds result in a seriously altered cry or voice.

Subglottic hemangioma: Subglottic hemangioma is rarely present at birth; it occurs more often in girls. Symptoms include stridor that is intermittent at first. Other laryngeal hemangiomas should be suspected whenever the baby has a prominent surface hemangioma over the neck or anterior chest wall; these rarely cause breathing problems at birth. Crying, struggling or partial airway obstruction will increase the size of the tumor due to venous engorgement.

Hyperexcitability of the laryngeal abductors: This is aggravated by hyperthermia and may cause stridor in preterm babies.

Tracheal disorders: Intrinsic narrowing of the trachea (stenosis) is another rare cause of predominately expiratory stridor. Tracheomalacia is an uncommon lesion that results from immaturity and abnormal flexibility of the tracheal cartilage, allowing collapse of the trachea during expiration. This produces asthma-like expiratory wheezes, biphasic stridor and a barking cough, with cyanosis and apnea. It only rarely occurs as an isolated disorder. Symptoms depend upon the length of trachea affected and the degree of weakness.

Transport considerations for babies with stridor

Since the primary presentation is abnormal breath sounds, these babies usually do not require extensive support. Feeding should be withheld until the baby can be evaluated. A consultation should be sought. Position the baby on his right side and transport for evaluation soon after birth to determine the exact diagnosis and whether it is safe for the baby to return home.

12. Baby looks otherwise normal with persistent central cyanosis and may have a slow heart rate in spite of effective spontaneous but rapid respirations

If you have ensured that the baby's chest is moving well and that breath sounds are audible and equal in both lungs and you have augmented with oxygen but when it is taken away the baby once again becomes blue with a slow heart rate, a congenital heart defect must be considered. Cyanosis that improves when the baby exerts himself by crying effectively rules out a cardiac cause; upper airway obstruction is the likely reason. For more information about the presentation of heart defects at birth, see the subchapter entitled "Cyanosis, Rapid Breathing, Congestive Heart Failure, Shock or Arrhythmia: Detecting Heart Defects at Birth."

General presentation

It is rare for congenital heart disease to be obvious this early, although some cyanosis may be present in many of these babies from birth on. Affected babies may not be able to maintain good color and may be quite pale even though they are apparently breathing normally, although often rapidly. Congenital heart disease may also be present when a baby becomes bluish while exerting herself (crying or nursing), although she may have no other symptoms. (See the subchapters entitled "Detecting and Differentiating Newborn Hypoglycemia, Heart Defects and Sepsis" and "Cyanosis, Rapid Breathing, Congestive Heart Failure, Shock or Arrhythmia: Detecting Heart Defects at Birth" for more information.) **Cardiac disease produces central cyanosis with rapid breathing in the absence of other signs of respiratory distress.** The rapid breathing is an attempt to compensate for hypoxia. Cyanosis that is associated with lung disorders usually presents with retractions, grunting and nasal flaring and may not improve with oxygen augmentation. Those with heart defects may pink up with oxygen, only to become cyanotic once the oxygen is taken away.

Specific transport considerations

These babies should be taken to the hospital as soon as possible. Keep supplemental oxygen concentrations below 85%.

Possible causes

- •Malfunction of the cardiac muscle from asphyxia, arrhythmias or myocardiopathies
- •Mechanical restriction of heart function or venous return due to tension pneumothorax, diaphragmatic hernia, pressure, etc.
- •Disturbance of the transitional circulation resulting in persistent pulmonary hypertension of the newborn
- •Certain congenital heart defects

Persistent pulmonary hypertension of the newborn (PPHN): Persistent pulmonary hypertension occurs when the pulmonary arterioles remain constricted or return to a constricted state after birth. It presents with hypoxemia that is disproportionately severe compared to the extent of any associated pulmonary disorder. These babies are usually AGA and born near term. The possibility of PPHN is increased when the fetus has suffered chronic hypoxia; it is a feature of many neonatal disorders. The problem is compounded when the blood volume is compromised from early cord clamping or for other reasons. When sepsis, perinatal asphyxia and meconium aspiration are associated with cyanosis, PPHN may be the underlying cause. PPHN should be assumed when pulmonary hypoplasia is suspected. Categories include:

1. Cardiac: congenital heart disease; depressed myocardial function; shock
2. Pulmonary: meconium aspiration syndrome; retained fetal lung fluid; respiratory distress syndrome; sepsis with pneumonia (especially group B-strep); diaphragmatic hernia; oligohydramnios and associated defects; primary pulmonary hypoplasia
3. Prenatal conditions: intrauterine growth restriction; maternal aspirin or indomethacin use; acute or chronic asphyxia, dysmaturity
4. Miscellaneous: asphyxia, hypocalcemia, polycythemia or hyperviscosity, unidentifiable causes, idiopathic.

Presentation: Signs of respiratory distress are usually present from birth, although it often starts out with mild symptoms that progressively worsen over the next 6 to 12 hours, with cyanosis and tachycardia. Any term or postterm baby with cyanosis that shows little or no improvement during oxygen supplementation should raise the suspicion of PPHN, whether respiratory symptoms are present or not. Lability of the systemic arterial saturation, which, when severe enough, may be reflected in color changes when the infant is handled, is a key clinical feature. Hypoxemia results in further vasoconstriction in the lungs and a vicious cycle of hypoxia and acidosis ensues, leading to impaired cardiac function, low cardiac output and further tissue hypoxia.

Pulmonary arteriovenous malformation: This defect consists of one or more vascular communications that bypass the pulmonary capillary bed, thus creating a right-to-left shunt. Symptoms vary according to the size of the fistula and the amount of shunting. Large, multiple lesions produce frank cyanosis. These babies have a normal pulse, blood pressure and venous pressure with no cardiac murmurs. The heart size is normal.

13. THERE IS INTERMITTENT RESPIRATORY DISTRESS, WITH COUGHING AND CHOKING OR VOMITING PROMPTED BY NURSING.

A number of conditions can intermittently interfere with otherwise normal respirations in a baby who has normal lungs. The baby may be doing well otherwise, but when he attempts to nurse, he develops one or more signs of significant respiratory distress, with coughing and choking or vomiting.

Specific transport protocols

Babies with any of the following problems should have feeding withheld until they can be evaluated. Transport should take place soon after birth, as follows:

1. Place the baby on his right side on a flat surface and keep him warm.
2. Use blow-by oxygen or CPR, if indicated.
3. Insert an orogastric tube and aspirate every 5 to 10 min.

Possible causes

- Gastroesophageal reflux
- Upper airway clefts: cleft lip, palate or both; laryngotracheoesophageal cleft
- Choanal atresia (see item 3)
- Achalasia

Gastroesophageal reflux (GER): Reflux is the most common esophageal disorder of neonates. Reflux is a physiological process that often occurs after nursing, when the baby has swallowed some air and then burps. This does not usually produce any irritation of the esophagus because acid secretion in the stomach does not reach adult levels until 3 months of age. However, for some babies, the process of backward passage of stomach contents into the esophagus can become pathologic; the reason for this is hard to define, especially when the esophagus is not inflamed from contact with stomach acids.

Gastroesophageal reflux is caused by either a loose lower esophageal sphincter or a rise in intragastric pressure that overcomes the resistance of the sphincter. It is accompanied by respiratory distress symptoms and esophagitis in 60% of those affected. Vomiting is the major symptom; this ranges from spitting up to forceful, frank vomiting that may manifest at birth or later. Respiratory symptoms occur acutely, due to aspirated vomitus, and secondarily, due to stimulation of the vagus nerves during aspiration, resulting in apnea, bradycardia and arrest, which may lead to death. GER may be secondary to pyloric stenosis or other obstructive conditions of the gastrointestinal tract. Many of these disorders are discussed in the subchapter entitled "Abdominal Distension and Vomiting at Birth: Detecting Gastrointestinal Disorders."

It has been suggested that this problem is a product of modern Western infant-feeding practices, which give large volumes of artificial milk every 2 to 4 hours, thus increasing intragastric pressure. Women in preindustrial cultures tend to nurse for two minutes every 13 minutes or so and keep the baby upright between feedings (Konner & Worthman, 1980). Keeping the baby is a semi-seated or upright position does seem to help prevent this problem. Any baby presenting with frank vomiting associated with respiratory distress could have a wide variety of serious defects; the baby should be evaluated by a neonatologist without delay.

Upper airway clefts

Cleft palate: A baby who has a cleft palate will often breathe normally until she attempts to nurse; this may produce choking and coughing. She may also experience a degree of airway obstruction from retained oropharyngeal secretions or from her tongue becoming lodged in the cleft space. The obstruction can be relieved by inserting an oral airway, hooking the tongue forward with a finger, or suspending the baby in a ventral or inverted position, as described for Pierre Robin syndrome (see item 4).

Laryngotracheoesophageal cleft: Another cause of intermittent distress precipitated by nursing is laryngotracheo-esophageal cleft, a rare anomaly in which the posterior wall of the larynx and a variable length of trachea fail to separate from the esophagus, resulting in a communication where the two meet. Coughing and choking ensues when milk spills over from the esophagus into the trachea; there may also be a weak or absent cry.

Assessment of upper airway clefts: First, visualize the baby's palate. Look and feel for defects throughout the length of the roof of the mouth using a penlight to aid visualization. These defects range from a pinhole-sized opening in the palate to an external defect involving the upper lip and nostrils. Most babies with a cleft lip alone can nurse normally, but most who have a cleft palate will not be able to create sufficient suction to nurse. If a cleft palate is the problem, the baby will need to be bottle-fed breast milk with a special nipple or prosthetic device designed to be used with presurgical clefts; these allow normal swallowing while preventing milk from getting into the nasal passages. Some severely affected babies may require tube feeding.

Achalasia: This is a motor disorder of the esophagus in which there is absent or diminished peristalsis and failure of the lower esophageal sphincter to relax. It is exceedingly rare, affecting 1 in 100,000 to 200,000 persons in the general population, with only 3 to 5% of them being children. Difficulty with swallowing, choking and coughing while nursing, and aspiration prompting respiratory distress make it indistinguishable from other, more common, causes.

14. PERSISTENT PROFUSE SALIVA AND/OR DIFFICULTY WITH SWALLOWING; COUGHING AND CHOKING AGGRAVATED BY NURSING, USUALLY WITH A HISTORY OF POLYHYDRAMNIOS DURING THE PREGNANCY.

Oral secretions should never be significant beyond the first few minutes of life. When they are, a defect involving normal swallowing should be suspected. Defects that prevent normal swallowing are associated with preterm birth as well as polyhydramnios; the amniotic fluid balance is usually altered when the baby cannot swallow normally in utero.

General assessment for suspected tracheoesophageal (TE) and swallowing defects

Persistent drooling occurs due to TE obstruction. As liquid pools in a blind pouch, coughing and chocking ensue. A fistula produces signs of aspiration with pooling of saliva or of breast milk upon nursing. To confirm a TE defect, insert a soft 10 or 12 F catheter down the throat. If it coils in the back of the throat after several tries, if it consistently becomes obstructed approximately 9 cm from the mouth (10 or 11 cm from the nostril) or if it does not reach the stomach, a gastro-obstruction is very likely. To assess if the tube has reached the stomach, listen over the stomach with a stethoscope while air is forced into the tube with a syringe; you should hear gurgling sounds. If the tube does reach the stomach and cranial nerve exam is abnormal, suspect a neuromuscular disorder.

Support and transport considerations for TE defects

These babies are at high risk for aspiration. Withhold oral fluids and transport soon after birth. To transport:

1. Insert a large bore catheter into the upper esophageal pouch. Check to make sure the tube is not in the trachea (listen for air flow over the chest).
2. Position the baby prone and place a hand across the upper forehead and elevate the head; this facilitates drainage of the upper pouch. *Do not position the baby prone if she is intubated.* If prone positioning is ineffective, try a supine position with the resting surface tilted to a 30 to 45° angle.
3. Avoid artificial ventilation whenever possible as it may cause enlargement of the fistula and passage of air through the fistula into the GI tract, possibly without inflating the lungs.
4. Avoid palpation of the abdomen as this can result in the reflux of stomach contents into the lungs via the fistula.

Possible causes

- Tracheoesophageal fistula (1 in 3000 to 4500 live births)
- Esophageal atresia

- •Other rare esophageal defects
- •Extrinsic esophageal compression, including vascular defects of the aorta (may not be associated with polyhydramnios)
- •Neuromuscular swallowing disorder

Tracheoesophageal fistula (TEF): A tracheoesophageal fistula is a hole between the trachea and the esophagus, with most affected babies being male. It is the most common anomaly of the lower respiratory tract. Most of these defects (85%) involve an esophageal atresia above the connection between the lower trachea and the esophagus (distal TEF). The remaining varieties of this class of defects occur in less than 10% of cases. A TEF joining the trachea and esophagus at the level of the lower neck (H-type) occurs in 4 to 5% of cases. A TEF may join the lower part of a proximal esophageal atresia in 0.5% of cases, and a distal atresia is present in 0.5% of cases.

Presentation: The fistula results in the accumulation of milk and oral secretions in the mouth. Leakage of these fluids through the hole in the esophagus into the trachea causes choking and respiratory distress, possibly leading to aspiration. The risks of all of these problems increase with nursing, which is often accompanied by vomiting. Delayed diagnosis leads to recurrent pneumonitis. Therefore, assume there is a fistula and withhold oral feedings until it is ruled out.

Esophageal atresia: This occurs when the esophagus terminates in a blind pouch. Esophageal atresia alone, with a gap between the two closed ends, is the second most common variety of this defect, occurring in 10% of all cases of tracheoesophageal fistula.

Associated defects: Thirty to fifty percent of babies who have an esophageal atresia have associated congential anomalies such as heart disease, especially tetralogy of Fallot; pulmonary atresia; atrial or ventricular septal defects; patent ductus arteriosus; coarctation of the aorta; vascular anomalies or some combination of these disorders. Upper airway problems such as laryngo- or tracheomalacia (softened cartilages) are fairly common. Cleft lip and palate as well as vertebral, renal and anorectal defects are also frequently found in these babies. At least one-third are born preterm and are of low birthweight.

Presentation: Esophageal atresia results in the production of excessive amounts of white, foamy mucus that does not diminish over time, producing constant drooling.

Other rare esophageal defects: Esophageal stenosis or a web may also result in the same type of symptoms and occurs once in every 25,000 to 50,000 live births. A membranous stenosis of the esophagus is found between the middle and distal thirds of the esophagus. Even more rarely, a laryngotracheoesophageal cleft, resulting in a linear communication between the airway and the esophagus, begins at the larynx and extends distally for a variable length. These more rare forms present in basically the same way as those that are more common.

Esophageal duplication takes the form of a cyst that can cause airway or, less commonly, esophageal obstruction. An esophageal diverticulum occurs with an outpouching of the esophageal wall and presents as for esophageal atresia.

Associated defects: About 50% of these babies have an associated anomaly. Cardiac defects (30%); trisomies 13, 21 and especially 18 (7%); VATER complex (vertebral, anorectal, tracheoesophageal, radial limb, and renal) or VACTERL syndrome (as above but including cardiac defects, variable limb anomalies, and in some cases, hydrocephalus [VACTERL-H]); CHARGE complex (colobomata, heart defect, choanal atresia, growth or mental retardation, genital hypoplasia, ear defects); and hydronephrosis and other urinary tract anomalies may also be present.

Extrinsic esophageal compression: Esophageal compression may occur from pressure applied by a large tumor, mediastinal vascular anomaly, cyst of the neck or a thoracic mass. (See item 2.)

Vascular defects: Vascular anomalies of the aorta are an extrinsic source of compression of the trachea, esophagus or bronchial tube. They are relatively rare, accounting for less than 1% of all cardiac malformations. Many variations of this defect exist, ranging from incomplete to complete vascular ring. Some are asymptomatic while others can cause anything from biphasic stridor to dramatic respiratory distress from birth that is aggravated during nursing.

The most problematic and common type is a true vascular ring around the trachea and esophagus, which may make swallowing difficult. Flexing the head forward may totally occlude the airway. The baby may lie in a hyperextended position, which stretches the trachea taut, reducing the constricting effect. Infants with laryngomalacia or other causes of stridor will not be affected by position in the same way.

Neuromuscular swallowing disorder: Normal infants may have temporary problem with drooling, uncoordinated swallowing and spitting up of feedings. However, swallowing should improve in a day or two. Excessive oral secretions may also be due to an isolated neuromuscular swallowing disorder related to cranial nerve problems, although this is rare.

15. Apnea (Cessation of Breathing)

It is normal for newborns, especially those born preterm, to breathe irregularly with brief pauses lasting 3 to 10 seconds followed by effective respirations for at least three cycles of inspiration and expiration. There is no associated bradycardia. This is referred to as **periodic breathing**.

Apnea is defined as a cessation of breathing for a period of time sufficient to interfere with gas exchange. Such a cessation in neonates is usually termed apnea when it lasts for more than 20 seconds or for a briefer period and is associated with either bradycardia of less than 100 bpm and cyanosis or pallor. Apnea is considered primary when due to preterm birth by itself and secondary when another cause can be identified. Apnea may be of the following varieties:

Central (40% of cases): This is characterized by no respiratory movement for more than 20 seconds.

Obstructive (10% of cases): Breathing efforts continue, but airflow ceases because the upper airway is blocked.

Mixed central and obstructive (50% of cases): In these cases, obstruction is followed by brief periods in which the infant tries to breathe, followed by a cessation of breathing efforts.

Primary apnea in preterm babies does not present in the first 24 hours and usually does not present at all after 34 to 36 weeks of gestational age. Therefore, you are unlikely to encounter a baby with primary apnea in a homebirth practice. Apnea in term or near-term babies may be an early sign of a serious problem and requires prompt investigation.

Specific causes

- Environmental temperature that is either too hot or, more likely, too cold
- Stimulation of the vagal nerve due to nursing, pressure, passage of a tube, suctioning, gastric distension or newborn anomaly (such as a growth pressing on the vagal nerve)
- Discomfort or pain
- Metabolic disorders such as severe hypoglycemia (most likely at home), hypocalcemia, and sodium imbalances (not likely at home where nursing can be established soon after birth)
- Obstruction of the upper airway from excess secretions, laryngeal or pharyngeal stimulation or anomalies. Apneic attacks occurring with innominate artery compression of the trachea or with tracheomalacia associated with tracheoesophageal fistula have been called "reflex apnea" attacks or "dying spells." These prolonged apneic attacks can lead to cyanosis, bradycardia, or even cardiac arrest.
- Decreased oxygen delivery to the tissues because of hypoxemia, anemia or congestive heart failure, with patent ductus arteriosus being a very common cause
- Pharyngeal or laryngeal dysfunction
- Pulmonary disease, such as respiratory distress syndrome or pneumonia
- Sepsis, either bacterial or viral; including meningitis
- Central nervous system compromise (i.e., brain injury, asphyxia, drugs or cerebral malformation)

Support and transport

All apnea in term babies should be taken seriously. Correct the ambient temperature, wait for any vagal nerve stimulation to subside, eliminate discomfort, and evaluate for simple hypoglycemia. If the apnea seems to be obstructive or the baby seems otherwise normal, attempt to clear the airway by De Leeing the baby. If all of this does not immediately resolve the problem, offer resuscitation assistance as indicated and transport.

CYANOSIS, RAPID BREATHING, CONGESTIVE HEART FAILURE, SHOCK OR ARRHYTHMIA: DETECTING HEART DEFECTS AT BIRTH

NOTE: Heart defects, hypoglycemia and sepsis can mimic each other, and all may include respiratory distress. Therefore the chapters covering these problems should be studied together.

One in every 115 to 150 babies has some form of heart or circulatory defect, making heart defects one of the two most common types of birth anomalies (the other being genitourinary tract anomalies). The worldwide incidence of major congenital heart disease is 8 per 1000 live births. There are at least 35 distinct congenital heart defects currently recognized, ranging from simple anomalies to complex malformations. Keeping in mind that even the most severe heart defects are rarely symptomatic at birth, the midwife should focus on deciding if a heart defect is the likely cause of distress. They may manifest anytime in the first years of life. Heart defects fall into three typical symptom pictures: cyanotic, acyanotic and heart failure. *Babies whose heart defects are symptomatic at birth typically look and act normally except that they breathe rapidly and cannot maintain good color. They may even be blue all over.*

An Overview of Congenital Heart Defects

Contributing factors

The following maternal disorders are associated with congenital heart defects:

- Lupus (congenital heart block)
- Diabetes (a wide array of heart malformations and a specific form of hypertrophic cardiomyopathy)
- Phenylketonuria (congenital heart disease of various kinds)
- Rubella in the first trimester (congenital heart disease, especially patent ductus arteriosus and peripheral pulmonary artery stenosis)
- Viral infection in the third trimester, especially Coxsackie virus (myocarditis)

In addition, the following factors increase the likelihood of a cardiac anomaly:

- Maternal drug use, including alcohol, various anticonvulsants, or retinoic acid
- Family history of cardiac malformation, especially in siblings or the mother
- Polyhydramnios, because nonimmune hydrops caused by supraventricular tachycardia can, in some cases, lead to a sudden rise in amniotic fluid over one to two weeks

General signs, symptoms and associated findings that may be present after birth

Perinatal distress or low APGAR score: These may be associated with poor myocardial function in the first hours or days of life, manifesting as congestive heart failure or cardiogenic shock with or without cyanosis.

Persistent cyanosis of the lips and oral mucosa, with or without rapid breathing

The appearance or exacerbation of cyanosis upon exertion: Crying or nursing leads to blue extremities or a blue ring around the lips. Conversely, pinking up with exertion may occur in the presence of pulmonary problems.

Skin mottling: The skin has diffuse white and pink variegation, indicating perfusion problems. This may occur in normal but chilled babies and is also seen with Down syndrome.

100% oxygen improves the baby's color only temporarily: Give 100% oxygen for 10 minutes and see what happens to the baby's color. If the color improves, only to return to cyanotic once the oxygen is discontinued, suspect a heart defect. If the color improves only partially or not at all, suspect a serious pulmonary problem. This is a crude form of the hyperoxia test, which requires arterial blood gas tests to be done precisely.

Evidence of a dysmorphic syndrome or chromosomal disorder: Heart defects are often a component of such syndromes, especially trisomies 12, 18 and 21, Turner syndrome; DiGeorge and related syndromes; cat-eye syndrome; VACTERL and CHARGE associations (complexes).

An audible heart murmur

Abnormalities of the femoral or brachial pulses: These include bounding; decreased, weak or undetectable pulses; and rhythms that are out of sync with each other only in the legs or in all the limbs.

Respiratory distress: Rapid breathing and increased depth of inspiration are often the only symptoms. If the breathing rate increases with activity such as nursing and the baby has difficulty with feeding or exhaustion after nursing only a short time, especially with sweating and a rapid heart rate, suspect congestive heart failure. A full stomach may precipitate or aggravate respiratory distress because it puts pressure against the diaphragm which then presses against the heart.

There may be a delayed onset of signs and symptoms of some heart defects in waterbirth babies (Enning, 2003).

Anomalies associated with heart defects

Malformations in other organ systems occur in some 25% of babies with structural heart defects. The most common of these are listed below (the incidence of associated heart defects is given in parentheses).

- •Tracheoesophageal fistula and esophageal fistula (15 to 40%)
- •Duodenal atresia (30%)
- •Biliary atresia (20% have associated anomalies; 60% of those are cardiovascular and tend to be associated with polysplenia, in which the spleen is equally divided or totally absent)
- •Small bowel atresia (5%)
- •Imperforate anus (60% have an associated anomaly [most commonly genitourinary], with cardiovascular lesions occurring in 8 to 22%)
- •Hirschsprung disease (8%)
- •Congenital diaphragmatic hernia (10 to 25%)
- •Oropharyngeal clefts (incidence varies with the location of the cleft)
- •Omphalocele (19 to 32%)
- •Skeletal anomalies
  - -Upper limb: Highly associated with congenital heart defects
  - -Lower limb: Less frequent association
  - -Vertebral anomalies: High incidence
- •Genitourinary anomalies (8%)

About 8 to 13% of babies with heart defects have inherited syndromes with associated cardiovascular anomalies while 13% have chromosomal syndromes associated with cardiovascular malformation.

Assessment

Assess the baby by looking for central cyanosis (both at rest and with activity), breathing difficulties (assess respiratory work and rate, especially looking for tachypnea) and slow capillary refill time. Palpate the chest for precordial activity. Auscultate the heart for murmurs (intensity, quality, timing and pitch), and the cranium and liver for bruits. Do not depend on the absence of suspicious heart sounds to rule out a defect. Palpate the liver for distension or downward displacement. Check the femoral and brachial pulses. Observe the baby for color changes and breathing problems.

Tachypnea: Persistently rapid breathing (rates of 60 rpm or greater after the first 2 hours) is often the first and may be the only sign of congenital heart disease. Anomalies that involve excessive pulmonary arterial flow or pulmonary venous hypertension cause pulmonary vascular engorgement, edema and decreased lung compliance that often result in an increased rate and effort in breathing. Defects involving decreased blood flow often present with intense central cyanosis associated with rapid breathing that is often minimally labored but persistently fast with an increased depth of inspiration but no other signs of respiratory distress. Cyanosis due to respiratory distress from pulmonary disorders usually manifests with retractions, grunting and nasal flaring.

Systemic perfusion: Decreased systemic cardiac output is an ominous sign that requires rapid assessment. There are many possible causes other than a heart defect, the primary one being sepsis. Signs of decreased perfusion include:

- •Cyanotic, pale, cool or mottled skin, indicating poor perfusion
- •Listlessness
- •Diminished intensity in the peripheral pulses
- •Lowered systolic blood pressure
- •Decreased or absent urinary output

•Metabolic acidosis

Examine the skin color and mucous membrane color under natural or incandescent lighting against a white background. Peripheral perfusion can be assessed using capillary refill time. Apply finger pressure over the sternum, then on a leg and an arm; if it takes 3 seconds or longer for the blanching to disappear, diminished perfusion is confirmed.

Blood pressure can be roughly assessed in all limbs using the flush or palpation method described in the subchapter entitled "Examining the Chest, Lungs and Heart." A low systolic blood pressure indicates shock. The blood pressure in the legs should be equal to or slightly higher than that measured in the arms. A systolic pressure in the upper body that is more than 10 mm Hg above that in the lower body is abnormal, suggesting coarctation of the aorta, aortic arch hypoplasia, or an interrupted aortic arch. However, while the finding of such a discrepancy is diagnostic of an arch abnormality, the absence of such a discrepancy does not rule it out because an accompanying patent and unrestricted ductus arteriosus will render the pressures more equal, as can shock with hypotension secondary to a low cardiac output.

Peripheral pulses should also be assessed. Cardiac output is most likely to be poor if all pulses are low in amplitude. Aortic obstruction results in femoral pulses that are diminished when compared to brachial arterial pulses. Bounding arterial pulses are found with severe anemia, arteriovenous fistula, or a completely patent ductus arteriosus. A cardiac anomaly is strongly suggested if, in addition, a murmur, galloping heartbeat, heart enlargement or cyanosis are present.

Cyanosis:

Acrocyanosis: Peripheral cyanosis of the hands and feet is frequently noted in normal babies during the first 24 to 48 hours of life. It is a persistent finding in many conditions that involve a prolonged circulation time and an increased rate of oxygen extraction in the tissues in the presence of normal arterial saturation. These conditions include poor cardiac output, sepsis, polycythemia and metabolic acidosis.

Central cyanosis: Central cyanosis is defined as blue discoloration of the mucous membranes due to a reduction in circulating hemoglobin and therefore a lowered oxygen concentration in the blood. (However, cyanosis is clinically diagnosed with arterial oxygen saturation tests, meaning that it can be technically present even if the baby does not appear blue.) Cyanosis that presents or worsens during crying in the first 24 hours of life may not indicate heart disease, but it must be watched to see if it persists or is associated with any other cardiac signs or with respiratory distress. Crying will increase the depth of cyanosis in some forms of right-to-left shunting because of increased intrathoracic pressure. Concerning cyanosis is particularly apparent in the lips. Cyanosis around the mouth or of the nailbeds but not in the lips or mucosa is usually not associated with cyanotic heart disease. However, some types of right-to-left shunts are associated with increased blood flow through the lungs, causing these babies to have nearly normal oxygen saturation (and therefore normal color), rendering the identification of cyanosis very difficult.

The clinical recognition of cyanosis depends upon the degree of oxygen desaturation of arterial hemoglobin and is influenced by the total hemoglobin concentration. The visual perception of cyanosis is usually possible only when there is a 5 gram reduction in capillary hemoglobin. In babies with normal hemoglobin levels, cyanosis becomes visibly apparent at an oxygen saturation of 70%; however, an experienced observer can sometimes detect cyanosis with the saturation between 80 and 85%. If the baby is anemic, there may be severe arterial desaturation with no cyanosis. Polycythemia causes the baby to appear cyanotic at normal arterial oxygen levels. Persistent cyanosis is rare in hypoglycemia and methemoglobinemia, but it may occur.

Central cyanosis reflects critically severe compromise. It may be the only indication of congenital heart disease, especially during the first week of life. It is invariably a sign of serious heart abnormality when it occurs without pulmonary disease. Cyanosis is a more threatening symptom than a heart murmur. One-third of infants with potentially lethal congenital heart defects have cyanosis as their primary presenting symptom; another third have cyanosis associated with respiratory distress. Central cyanosis is either due to heart problems, such as venous blood bypassing the lungs, or desaturation of venous blood in the lungs caused by either ventilation or perfusion problems. Finally, airway obstruction may be a factor.

Differential cyanosis: Differential cyanosis occurs when there is either a visible color difference or varying oxygen saturation levels between the upper and lower portions of the body. Deoxygenated blood is perfusing one region of the body while saturated blood is perfusing the other.

When the baby has persistent pulmonary hypertension or left heart outflow tract obstruction with right-to-left shunting through the ductus arteriosus, differential cyanosis may be noted with the upper body pink and the lower body blue below the umbilicus. The reverse picture, with a pink lower body and cyanotic upper body, is seen with transposition of the great arteries and a large, patent ductus arteriosus.

Other possible causes of cyanosis: While early-onset central cyanosis is most often associated with heart disease, the following causes, which are unrelated to heart defects, must also be considered:

- **Birth at a high altitude:** Some babies who are born to mothers who are not from a population with a long history of living at a high altitude may display slight cyanosis at birth. Giving these babies a small amount of supplemental oxygen should result in immediate improvement.
- **Shock, sepsis, hypothermia, hypoglycemia and acidosis:** Any of these conditions may alter peripheral circulation and produce cyanosis.
- **Persistent pulmonary hypertension of the newborn**
- **Diaphragmatic hernia:** Herniated abdominal contents encroach on the space usually occupied by the lungs, resulting in varying degrees of respiratory distress, cardiac compression and cyanosis.
- **Hyperviscosity or polycythemia:** These blood abnormalities, meaning increased resistance to flow and too many red blood cells respectively, develop as a response to chronic hypoxia in utero. Peripheral vasoconstriction, which develops during hypovolemic shock, aggravates the effect of hyperviscosity because it narrows the vessels. When either occurs, it may mimic heart disease by causing cyanosis because the sluggish blood flow results in capillary stasis, reducing delivery of oxygen to the tissues.
- **Central nervous system depression or neuromuscular disease:** These conditions may result in inadequate lung ventilation and cyanosis. Other indications of nervous system involvement will be present.
- **Abnormal hemoglobin:** This may be a factor in a cyanotic baby who shows no other signs of heart or lung problems. Associated findings are little or no improvement in color with oxygen administration and the blood remaining dark when exposed to air.
- **Defects of the lung tissue:** When cyanosis is due to defects of the pulmonary system, other signs of respiratory distress, including rapid breathing, tachycardia, nasal flaring, retractions and grunting, are also present.

Cyanosis that improves with exertion effectively rules out a heart disorder. These babies are likely to have a respiratory-related cause.

Heart sounds and murmurs: The nuances of differentiating heart sounds and murmurs take time and experience to master. In addition to listening to all your babies, teaching tapes on auscultating heart sounds are also available. When you transport the baby, describe what you think you heard. After transport, once the baby is relatively stable, ask the neonatal cardiologist, if she seems willing, to assist you in hearing the sounds under her guidance. This will help you hone this complex skill. Note that birth at a high altitude may alter blood flow pressures within the heart and minimize or eliminate certain murmurs until the baby is brought to a lower altitude.

Prognosis

Babies who have a heart defect that becomes symptomatic in the first hours or days of life may decompensate quickly. Although many of these babies may not appear to be in great distress early on, they may be near death in a matter of hours. The earlier symptoms appear, the more likely the baby's condition will decline rapidly. Among those that survive, organ damage from lack of oxygen is the principal problem that occurs when treatment is delayed.

General transport procedures for suspected heart defects

If you suspect a heart defect, it is important to transport the baby right away. Cardiac compromise can quickly lead to metabolic derangement, which must be stabilized promptly. Keep the baby warm. Administer blow-by oxygen or full resuscitation, as indicated (see below). If the heart rate is over 180 bpm, attempt to bring the rate down into a more normal range by applying a cold, wet cloth to the baby's face for 15 seconds or so, an action that will stimulate the trigeminal nerve and activate the mammalian diving reflex. The baby's condition may worsen if he must be transported from a moderately high altitude to one closer to sea level (more details about this phenomenon are discussed below under "ventricular septal defects").

Special considerations regarding airway support and oxygen use in babies suspected of having a congenital heart defect: The baby should be stabilized quickly with as little additional stress as possible. Intubation in the out-of-hospital setting (without the use of sedatives) should be avoided. These babies are particularly vulnerable to the adverse effects of increased levels of catecholamines (stress hormones), which usually rise during intubation attempts. High levels of stress hormones raise the risk that the baby will respond with significant dysrhythmias in the at-risk heart muscle. Secondly, stimulation of the vagus nerve with resultant bradycardia, hypoxemia, hypercapnia or laryngeal stimulation, may lead to asystole in these babies. Finally, the use of sedation and neuromuscular blocking medications prior to intubation dramatically reduces the rate of oxygen consumption, thus raising the mixed venous oxygen saturation and improving oxygen delivery, a benefit you will not be able to provide prior to hospitalization.

Note that supplemental oxygen is a potent vasodilator and therefore may adversely affect babies who have abnormally elevated pulmonary blood flow. Any baby suspected of having a congenital heart defect should be given oxygen by face mask to titrate the delivered dose to that which resolves the cyanosis. Do not allow it to exceed 80 to 85%.

More Details Regarding Signs, Symptoms and Types of Heart Defects

Heart defects of different types typically present during certain age windows after birth. Cardiac emergencies that present in the newborn are invariably life threatening because they mean that the heart is so abnormal that it cannot sustain normal functioning outside the womb. The table below contains the top five heart defect diagnoses that usually present during the first six days of life as well as miscellaneous additional disorders all of which are most likely to be symptomatic at birth. Most of these present with cyanosis as a major symptom.

HEART DEFECT	CASES PRESENTING IN FIRST SIX DAYS OF LIFE (%)	INCIDENCE (PER 1000 LIVE BIRTHS)
D-transposition of great vessels (arteries)*	19	0.3
Hypoplastic left ventricle*	14	0.16-0.36***
Tetralogy of Fallot*	8	0.3
Coarctation of the aorta*	7	0.3
Ventricular septal defect**	3	2
Miscellaneous, individually less common defects	49	Varies according to anomaly

*Cyanotic **Acyanotic ***Includes all types of hypoplastic left heart syndrome (Flanagan et al., 1999)

Definitions and presentations

Cyanotic congenital heart disease: Cyanotic congenital heart disease can be divided into two categories: those involving normal or increased pulmonary blood flow and those associated with decreased pulmonary blood flow.

Normal or increased pulmonary blood flow: The first category includes conditions in which there is normal or increased pulmonary blood flow with poor mixing of separate parallel circulations. These defects include:

Transposition of the great vessels (arteries): This malformation occurs when the aorta arises from the right ventricle and the pulmonary artery arises from the left ventricle, resulting in two separate and parallel circulations. The condition is lethal unless some communication exists between the systemic and pulmonic circulation after birth; otherwise, unoxygenated venous blood inappropriately enters the systemic circulation while oxygenated pulmonary venous blood is inappropriately directed to the pulmonary circulation. The life-sustaining communication may be an intraatrial passage or a patent ductus arteriosus.

This is the most common type of cyanotic heart disease presenting in the immediate newborn period and it is more common in boys. TGA usually presents in the first two days of life, although this depends upon the degree of mixing between the pulmonary and systemic circulations. Those babies with an intact ventricular septum present with early, extreme hypoxemia when the ductus arteriosus closes. The presence of a ventricular septal defect will lessen the hypoxemia to a certain extent. A large ventricular septal defect results in congestive heart failure, no significant murmurs, cyanosis and minimal respiratory distress between birth and 6 weeks of age. The same is true for other cyanotic heart defects that are sufficiently severe.

Hypoplastic left ventricle: In this form of hypoplastic left heart syndrome, there is underdevelopment of the left ventricle with severe mitral valve stenosis and aortic stenosis. Two to five percent of these babies present at birth with respiratory distress and profound central cyanosis. This defect is lethal unless corrected and sometimes cannot be corrected due to poor development of the affected structures.

Total anomalous pulmonary venous drainage (TAPVD): In obstructive cases, this produces cyanosis and extremely rapid breathing, often leading to a misdiagnosis of pulmonary disease on initial evaluation.

Truncus arteriosis: This uncommon defect involves absence of the tricuspid valve causing the entire cardiac output to enter the right atrium and exit through the foramen ovale into the left side of the heart, where systemic and pulmonary streams mix. Other defects alter the amount of blood flow to the lungs, which determines the depth of cyanosis. This condition is marked by bounding peripheral pulses and a loud, single second heart sound with an ejection click.

Presentation: Defects involving increased blood flow to the lungs tend to cause cyanosis, heart failure with accompanying distress, a pulsating precordium, and systolic murmurs.

Decreased pulmonary blood flow: The second category of cyanotic heart disease includes conditions with significantly decreased pulmonary blood flow, with right-to-left shunting of some unoxygenated systemic venous blood to the systemic arterial circulation. These babies may fare poorly if they must be exposed to altitude-induced hypoxia (Duster, 2004).

Tetralogy of Fallot: Four congenital cardiac defects occur together, including ventricular septal defect, pulmonic valve stenosis or infundibular stenosis, right ventricular hypertrophy and dextroposition of the aorta so that it overrides the ventricular septum and receives venous as well as arterial blood. Tetralogy of Fallot is associated with severe stenosis or atresia in the lungs.

Hypoplastic right heart syndromes (tricuspid and pulmonary atresia or stenosis)

Epstein disease of tricuspid valve: This is associated with tricuspid regurgitation, a hugely enlarged heart and cardiac congestion.

Presentation: In all the conditions listed above, the baby presents with cyanosis but not heart failure. The precordial area is quiet; the baby displays no other signs of distress; and pulmonary outflow obstruction leads to undetectable pulmonary valve closure and a single second heart sound.

Acyanotic defects: These conditions generally present with signs of shock.

Coarctation of the aorta: The simple form of this anomaly is characterized by constriction at the aortic isthmus; sometimes a patent ductus arteriosus is inserted just at or below the constriction. The complex type involves tubular hypoplasia of the aortic arch, with or without regional narrowing, and one or more of the following defects: patent ductus arteriosus, ventricular septal defect, endocardia cushion defect, aortic stenosis, subaortic stenosis, mitral stenosis or regurgitation, hypoplasia of the left ventricle and ascending aorta, other cyanotic anomalies, and endocardial fibroelastosis.

Some babies are asymptomatic but later develop congestive heart failure. The femoral and pedal pulses are weak or absent compared with the brachial or carotid pulses. One of the brachial pulses may be decreased. Systolic blood pressure is high in the arms compared to the legs. A systolic ejection murmur may be heard over the back at the left interscapular area or at the left upper sternal border. Feeding intolerance and mild tachypnea are other early signs. Presentation varies from slowly progressive congestive heart failure to profound shock, metabolic acidosis and ischemia in vital organs, especially of the brain (intracranial hemorrhage), kidneys (acute renal failure) and gastrointestinal system (necrotizing endocolitis). Note that coarctation of the aorta may or may not present with cyanosis.

Ventricular septal defect: This is a defect in the septum (membranous or muscular) located between the cardiac ventricles, usually resulting from failure of the spiral septum to close the interventricular foramen. An audible harsh systolic murmur develops at the lower left sternal border, followed by tachypnea, fatigue with nursing, decreased oral intake and sweating leading up to heart failure. The murmur is caused by flow disturbance as blood moves from the high-pressure left ventricle through the defect into the lower-pressure right ventricle.

Altitude-related details: At higher altitudes, the delayed fall in fetal pulmonary vascular resistance and a genetic predisposition to hyperreactivity may maintain an elevated pulmonary vascular resistance and result in right-sided pressure within the heart that approaches normal, systemic levels. Thus, even with a large ventricular septal defect or an atrial septal defect, or a patent ductus arteriosus, little or no shunting may occur from left to right, thus reducing or eliminating the typical cardiac murmur that is usually present. In addition, babies with a large ventricular septal defect who have significantly increased pulmonary vascular resistance secondary to the hypoxic environment at moderately high altitudes (defined as 5000 to 10,000 ft [1524 to 3048 m] above sea level) may be at risk for increased symptoms when traveling to lower altitudes. Improved oxygenation may result in a decrease in pulmonary vascular resistance which results in abnormal pulmonary blood flow and the presentation of related symptoms (Duster, 2004).

Aside from a lack of a murmur, these babies may not have the usual symptoms associated with an abnormally increased pulmonary blood flow, such as sweating, tachypnea, and (as they mature) delayed growth. Thus, missing a very large defect is possible in these infants. One must maintain a high index of suspicion and exclude an increased right ventricular impulse when a single loud second heart sound is detected during clinical examination. (For more information on oxygen and altitude, see the subchapter entitled "Oxygen Delivery Devices and Resuscitation Equipment" and the chapter covering high altitude problems in a recent edition of Volume I of this text.)

Atrioventricular septal defect: The atrioventricular septum is the small part of the membranous septum of the heart just above the septal cusp of the tricuspid valve. It separates the right atrium from the left ventricle. This condition results in an extremely enlarged heart. The incidence of atrial septal defect has been reported to be higher in populations living at moderately high altitudes (Duster, 2004).

Congestive heart failure (CHF): Congestive heart failure reflects an inability of the heart and circulatory system to meet the metabolic demands of the body without compensatory changes. Clinical symptoms result from the compensatory responses. The heart muscle is inadequate as a pump and fails to maintain the circulation of blood; as a result, congestion and edema develop in the tissues. The presentation in newborns can vary from mild symptoms to shock, depending upon the severity of the underlying defects. The signs of congestive heart failure in the neonate include:

- Central cyanosis, progressing to ashen gray
- Tachypnea, shortness of breath, painful or labored breathing or abnormal breath sounds (wheezing or crackles). It occurs as pulmonary function is impaired secondary to interstitial congestion or pulmonary edema.
- Tachycardia (a galloping heart rhythm in response to a fall in cardiac output)
- Poor feeding
- Sweating
- Poor peripheral perfusion with abnormal peripheral pulses (weak or intermittent)
- Enlargement of the heart (due to increased diastolic volume, which leads to cardiac dilation)
- A liver that is enlarged with a rounded, full or firm edge that extends more than 3 cm below the right costal margin, that is soft with a poorly defined border (which occurs with low cardiac output resulting in edema of the liver, rendering the capsule soft and distensible) or that has a palpable pulse. All suggest congestion and are all early signs of congestive heart failure.
- Difficulty with nursing because the baby becomes tired
- Little difference between the systolic and diastolic blood pressures (referred to as narrow pulse pressure)
- Lethargy or irritability
- Edema that may not pit with pressure around the eyes (and, in some cases, in the limbs), although this is rare.
- Shock with pallor, mottling, cool extremities, hypotension and oliguria

Noncardiac conditions that can cause congestive heart failure: CHF can occur in a variety of conditions unrelated to heart defects, such as anemia, polycythemia, hydrops, hypoglycemia, arteriovenous fistula, intracardiac and intrapericardial teratoma and fluid overload from too much IV fluid. Signs present at birth suggest an intrauterine arrhythmia, anemia or overtransfusion of the plethoric (tomato red) twin from twin-to-twin transfusion syndrome.

Arteriovenous fistulas: These usually result from an aneurysm of the great vein of Galen in the brain or, in some cases, the rupture of a vein in the liver. These babies present with congestive heart failure, bounding pulses and cerebral or hepatic bruits on auscultation.

Macrosomic infants of diabetic mothers: These babies may present with an enlarged heart and mild congestive heart failure secondary to hypoglycemia with associated respiratory distress. They may also have a structurally abnormal heart, most commonly transposition of the great vessels, septal defect, coarctation or hypertrophic cardiomyopathy.

Nonstructural heart disorders that cause congestive heart failure:

Transient myocardial ischemia (TMI): Evidence of TMI may be present following intrauterine hypoxia during labor. These babies are often born at term after a complicated labor; they have low APGAR scores, early-onset respiratory distress and congestive heart failure with or without cyanosis. A variety of associated cardiac signs may develop, including congestive heart failure with a galloping rhythm and systolic murmurs, persistent pulmonary hypertension with right-to-left arterial shunting, cyanosis and marked hypoxemia, and lowered cardiac output with cardiovascular collapse and shock.

Arrhythmias: Serious arrhythmias either during labor or after birth may result in varying degrees of heart failure or death. Prolonged supraventricular tachycardia commonly results in congestive heart failure. In about 50% of these cases, congenital heart block results in enlargement of the heart.

Myocardial dysfunction: This occurs when the heart is infected, particularly with Coxsackie or rubella viruses, as well as in glycogen storage disease type II, a metabolic disorder; endocardial fibroelastosis, a congenital condition characterized by thickening of the left ventricular wall endocardium (chiefly due to fibrous and elastic tissue); thickening and malformation of the cardiac valves; subendocardial changes in the myocardium; and hypertrophy of the heart. The chief symptoms are cyanosis, dyspnea, anorexia, and irritability. Clinically, arrhythmia is a primary presenting sign.

Cardiogenic shock (heart failure): Cardiogenic shock results from a decline in cardiac output secondary to serious heart disease and may be the end result of congestive heart failure, although cardiogenic shock may occur independently. The first presentation of severe congenital heart disease may be cardiovascular collapse and cardiogenic shock, both of which present similarly to septic shock. Heart failure develops rapidly in newborns due to the limited intrinsic reserve capacity of the heart muscle. The newborn heart has a limited ability to compensate by enlarging. Fetal hemoglobin also limits the ability of the red cells to unload oxygen at the tissue level. Nonstructural heart disease may present as acute shock, with the development of tachypnea and poor feeding that fulminates into acute cardiovascular collapse, with gasping, poor pulses, a gray or mottled skin tone, indistinct heart sounds, enlarged liver and heart, and acute metabolic acidosis. Reasons for neonatal heart failure include:

- Congenital heart disease
  - Severe mitral or tricuspid valve insufficiency
- Myocarditis (inflamation of the heart muscle)
- Arrhythmia
  - Supraventricular tachycardia (rate is too fast, usually over 220 bpm)
  - Complete heart block (rate is too slow, usually less than 60 bpm)
- Arteriovenous fistula
- Asphyxia
- Hypoglycemia or hypocalcemia
- Anemia (blood incompatibilities, acute blood loss at birth)
- Sepsis (especially group B-strep)

Abnormalities of the heart rate

Murmurs: A variety of normal heart murmurs are often found in the first few days of life as the baby's cardiovascular system makes the fetal-to-newborn transition. The nature of the defect determines when and how a murmur will present. Obstructive lesions, such as stenosis of the pulmonary valve, pulmonary artery or aorta, are more likely to present with a murmur soon after birth. A loud systolic murmur that radiates widely and persists regardless of activity or position change is suspicious. A loud systolic ejection murmur over the left upper sternal border suggests pulmonary stenosis. This often occurs in babies with certain heart defects, some of whom will also exhibit true central cyanosis. A soft systolic flow murmur may be present without structural heart disease.

Persistently low heart rate: There are several forms this problem can take.

Sinus bradycardia: Sinus bradycardia is a heart rate of less than 100 bpm. Transient bradycardia may occur with nursing, sleeping, yawning, passing stool, hiccuping or suctioning, all caused by stimulation of the vagal nerve.

Persistent or prolonged sinus bradycardia is seen with generalized abnormalities including increased intracranial pressure, hyperkalemia, acidosis, hypothermia, hypoxia, obstructive jaundice (as might occur with bile duct obstruction) or hypothyroidism.

Heart block: A dysfunction of the nerve impulses within the heart muscle that impairs the contraction of the heart muscle is referred to as a "heart block." Second-degree heart block is found with anoxia, metabolic disorders, hyperkalemia, hypocalcemia, sepsis, supraventricular tachyarrhythmias and digitalis toxicity. It may lead to symptomatic bradycardia.

Third-degree or complete heart block is rare (1 in 20,000 live births). The ventricular heart rate is slow and regular, in a range of less than 60 bpm (usually 45 to 60 bpm). About 25 to 35% of these babies will have concurrent congenital heart disease. The mother may show evidence of a connective tissue disorder, especially lupus, at the time of birth or develop such a disorder later.

Presentation: At birth, these babies appear normal with a heart rate around 60 bpm but with no evidence of structural heart disease. If the baby is otherwise well, symptoms do not develop until the heart rate falls below 50 to 55 bpm; however, rates of 60 to 80 bpm may be inadequate for babies with associated systemic illness, such as respiratory distress or sepsis, because they require a greater cardiac output. In those babies with heart rates of less than 50 bpm or with associated structure cardiac defects, the prognosis is not very favorable.

The exact heart rate should be assessed, as should blood pressure, since hypotension reflects the physiological impact of the low heart rate and the need for immediate transport. Rapid breathing and an enlarged liver support a diagnosis of congestive heart failure.

Persistently high heart rate: Tachycardia over 160 bpm may be seen in normal babies; many stimuli can temporarily increase the heart rate into the 200 bpm range.

Sinus arrhythmia: In sinus arrhythmia, there is a variation of the heart rate with respiration. This is commonly seen in association with irritability, infectious illness, dehydration, anemia, congestive heart failure, fever and shock. It may also be a side-effect of a number of neonatal medications. The rate seldom rises above 220 bpm.

Supraventricular tachycardia: Supraventricular tachycardia occurs as either a primary arrhythmia or in association with structural heart defects, and occasionally is present in babies with viral myocarditis. It may be life threatening if not recognized in time. The heart rate ranges between 240 and 360 bpm and often occurs in spasms; that is, with episodes of tachycardia that begin and end abruptly. Note that heart rates this high cannot usually be counted accurately without an electrocardiogram. The baby will often develop clinical signs of congestive heart failure, including rapid breathing, shortness of breath, sweating, pallor, irritability, poor nursing, respiratory distress and enlargement of the liver. Most of these infants have no structural heart defects.

Support and transport for babies with an elevated heart rate: Persistently high heart rates greater than 200 bpm result in decreased cardiac output and constitute a progressive problem that can fulminate into a medical emergency if not dealt with in time. Spurts into these high ranges may precipitate congestive heart failure if they continue for more than 12 to 48 hours, or when associated with structural heart defects. Application of a cold washcloth or ice to the face, left in place for 15 seconds or so, will stimulate a vagal response and may cause the heart rate to drop during transport. Continue to listen to the heart; if it slows to a normal range, use of the cold cloth can be stopped while you continue to monitor to determine if the heart rate is once again rising; if so, reapply the cloth.

It will be impossible to tell what type of heart defect the baby may have without sophisticated evaluation tools. Tell the parents that you suspect a heart defect and that the baby should be evaluated right away.

PALLOR WITH GENERALIZED EDEMA; SWOLLEN, FLUID-FILLED ABDOMEN AND RESPIRATORY DISTRESS: HYDROPS FETALIS

"Hydrops fetalis" literally means "water of the fetus" and occurs when there is an abnormal accumulation of serous fluid in the fetal tissues. In the developed world, hydrops fetalis has an overall incidence of 3 to 10 per 10,000 births. If you are working in a developing region where prenatal care is scarce, the incidence is likely to be higher because women will not have access to comprehensive prenatal screening for blood incompatibilities or infections. You may encounter babies who are born suffering from severe blood incompatibilities, certain hereditary anemias, syphilis or other problems that can lead to hydrops fetalis. Fluid may be found in both the extravascular spaces and the body cavities, around the heart and lungs, in the abdominal cavity (ascites [ah SITE-eez]) and in the subcutaneous connective tissue.

Forms of hydrops

Isoimmune hydrops: Isoimmune hydrops is the end result of a hemolytic process usually brought about by a blood incompatibility secondary to maternal sensitization during a previous pregnancy. Red blood cells are destroyed at a rate that exceeds the liver's ability to process them, and they accumulate in the baby's system. The resulting anemia and hypoxia cause the fetal system to try and compensate by accelerating the production of more blood cells. The liver, spleen and lymph nodes are converted to sites of production. This causes changes in the liver, as the cells that can produce blood cells enlarge, resulting in compression of the intrahepatic blood vessels and bile ducts. This leads to compromised liver function and impaired synthesis of protein and albumin, as well as portal and umbilical vein hypertension. Liver malfunction is now thought to be the primary cause of the development of isoimmune hydrops. As the hemoglobin falls below 6 to 7 g/dl (3.7 to 4.34 mmol/l), signs of hydrops begin to develop. Increased venous and capillary hydrostatic pressures may contribute to edema, and the hypoproteinemia may result in decreased oncotic pressure, allowing fluids to seep from the intravascular to the extravascular spaces. As the anemia becomes more severe, congestive heart failure develops. Umbilical vein flow is markedly elevated as a result of the fetus trying to transport more oxygen to compensate for the decrease in oxygen delivery to the tissues. Hypoxic tissue damage allows fluid to cross damaged blood vessels, contributing to the development of hydrops and edema.

Nonimmune hydrops: Nonimmune hydrops occurs with a wide variety of maternal, placental and fetal disorders. Among Caucasian populations, 20% of cases are due to congenital heart disease or arrhythmias and 15% to chromosomal defects. Among Asians, homozygous alpha thalassemia is the most common cause. In these infants, heart defects, arrhythmias, hereditary anemias or blood loss with subsequent anemia can all lead to chronic heart failure. Infections may lead to increased capillary permeability from chronic tissue hypoxia. However, in some cases of nonimmune hydrops, the exact cause is difficult to determine. Renal disorders may produce hydrops, although they more commonly result in isolated ascites and not full-blown hydrops. There is a high rate of associated fetal anomalies. Anemia commonly occurs in all types of nonimmune hydrops, although the reasons for this are not fully understood.

Presentation

Babies with hydrops fetalis have a constellation of signs and symptoms that typically include preterm birth, pallor, gross edema and severe anemia. Polyhydramnios and decreased fetal movement may have been noted during pregnancy. Pressure from an enlarged liver reduces the space in the chest cavity, as does accumulated fluid in the abdominal cavity and occasionally pleural effusions (fluid in the lining of the chest cavity). This pressure compresses the lungs and other organs in the chest cavity. Unequal breath sounds may be noted if the baby has a pneumothorax. Distant heart sounds are indicative of fluid build-up around the heart. The abdomen may need to be drained and ventilatory pressures of 35 cm H_2O may be required to inflate the lungs. *Do not try to tap the fluid off the abdomen at home!*

Support and transport

Obtain a cord blood sample in both a red-topped and a lavender-topped tube. Peripheral perfusion is often impaired because the intravascular blood volume is decreased; therefore leave the cord intact for as long as you can to give the baby an optimal placental transfusion prior to transport. Full-scale stabilization of these babies may not be possible without intervention to release fluid trapped in the abdominal space. Therefore, ventilate to the best of your ability using oxygen and high pressures, pass an orogastric tube or place an endotracheal tube if you feel you can, assess and treat for pneumothorax if indicated, and transport.

METABOLIC EMERGENCIES AND SEIZURES

Metabolic derangement commonly precedes seizures in the uninjured newborn; therefore these are considered together. Catastrophic metabolic disease may be caused by defects in the metabolism of a variety of chemicals and compounds including amino acids, organic acids, fatty acids, carbohydrates and substances produced during the urea cycle. Mitochondrial and lysosomal disorders may also present with acute illness. Early treatment minimizes brain damage from all metabolic disorders.

Simple hypoglycemia is the most common metabolic problem encountered in neonates. It is easily correctable and harmless when recognized and addressed early. It is rare for uncomplicated hypoglycemia to be profound at the time of birth and exceedingly rare for other metabolic disorders to present with catastrophic symptoms in the first 24 hours of life. In most cases, the blood levels of a substance that the body cannot properly utilize must rise to levels that exceed the baby's tolerance before symptoms present. In utero, the fetus is spared because the placenta clears the offending substance, which is then metabolized by the mother. However, metabolic disorders, if severe enough, can manifest within the first 24 hours of life. This is possible because the catabolism of body tissues that takes place to a minor extent during the first days while the mother's milk supply is being established can release enough of the offending substance into the blood to throw the baby with a very low threshold of tolerance into a metabolic crisis. Disorders of energy metabolism, such as pyruvate dehydrogenase complex, pyruvate carboxylase, electron transport chain deficiencies and respiratory chain enzyme defects are examples of rare disorders that may present in the first few hours after birth.

Differentiating metabolic disorders from more common problems

It is difficult to recognize metabolic disorders because the clinical signs and symptoms are nonspecific and mimic other more common illnesses. Severe hypoglycemia, sepsis, cardiopulmonary defects or central nervous system disorders, which commonly occur in the aftermath of severe asphyxia, are the most likely causes if a baby displays lethargy, vomiting, seizures, hypothermia and respiratory distress within the first 24 hours. Such severe hypoglycemia could be secondary to asphyxia or sepsis, as it is unlikely to occur as an isolated finding in a homeborn baby who receives a full placental transfusion and who begins to nurse in the first hour or two of life. Symptoms could also be due to neurological damage (such as intracranial hemorrhage) or anomalies.

Typical presentation of progressive metabolic derangement: Common signs and symptoms include:

Central nervous system signs: poor suck, lethargy, abnormal tone, loss of reflexes, seizures, coma

Gastrointestinal and hepatic signs: poor feeding, diarrhea (unlikely in first 24 hours), vomiting, enlarged liver, jaundice (unlikely in first 24 hours)

Respiratory signs: tachypnea, apnea, respiratory distress or failure

Other signs: dysmorphic features (many disorders include metabolic derangement); abnormal odor to urine, breath or body; metabolic acidosis or ketosis (determined with blood tests after transport)

Intracranial hemorrhage: These babies may be born depressed but appear to improve until about 12 hours of age. They then may become drowsy and increasingly pale and listless with a weak, feeble or unsustained cry or a high-pitched, irritating cry. Failure to nurse, respiratory distress, cyanosis, vomiting and convulsions may soon follow. These findings may mimic a metabolic disorder. A baby who has severe brain damage may alternately sleep and cry as his only activities. Any infant should be transported as soon as progressive deterioration is noted, regardless of the presumed reason.

Atypical genitalia: Babies with atypical genitalia may appear otherwise well at birth. However, they should be transported without delay as those with salt-losing adrenal disorders can become metabolically deranged relatively quickly.

Recognizing neonatal seizures

Neonatal seizure activity differs in many respects from that noted in older children and adults. Clinical manifestations of central nervous system hyperirritability are variable in newborns due to the structural and functional immaturity of the cerebral cortex. Seizures may accompany many types of neonatal problems such as asphyxia, birth trauma, defects (especially to the brain or spine), metabolic derangement such as acidosis and defects of metabolism, sepsis and drug withdrawal in babies of addicted mothers.

Jitteriness, which is a normal finding in newborns, must be distinguished from seizure activity. Jitteriness is a form of tetany most commonly seen when the baby is sleepy, active or crying. It is least common in babies who are quietly alert and is absent during deep sleep. It is characterized by high-frequency, low-amplitude movements that occur as activity tremors primarily within the range of their normal Moro response. This affects one or more limbs in a baby who is awake and looking around.

In contrast, seizure activity usually presents with low-frequency, high-amplitude tremors that constitute clonic movements. Clonus is a form of movement marked by contractions and relaxations of a muscle that occur in rapid succession. At times, it will be hard to tell these two apart. Jitteriness will stop when the baby sucks, when the limb is grasped firmly and placed at rest or when the noncrying baby is otherwise soothed; seizure activity cannot be stopped in this manner. Excessive jitteriness may stop when the baby sucks but can resume if the sucking stimulus is removed; this baby is more likely to be hypoglycemic or hypocalcemic (low calcium level, a less likely finding in a homeborn newborn). Tremors that persist may also reflect peripheral nerve dysfunction. Jitteriness is also discussed in the subchapter entitled "Evaluating the Newborn with Suspected Neurological Compromise."

Subtle seizures are more difficult to recognize as they present with deviation of the eyes, repetitive movements of the eyes or face, such as blinking or lip smacking; drooling or excess secretions; respiratory pauses (apnea); sudden changes in muscle tone or bicycling movements of the legs. Seizures are also discussed in the subchapter entitled "Evaluating the Newborn with Suspected Neurological Compromise."

Causes of seizures: Babies may have seizures for a variety of reasons, including perinatal hypoxia, birth injury to the brain, intracranial hemorrhage, infection, metabolic abnormalities, congenital cerebral malformations, drug withdrawal, local anesthetic intoxication (during inadvertent scalp administration when the mother is given a local block in labor), familial factors and unexplained reasons.

Support and transport procedures

The most common metabolic problem in the newborn is hypoglycemia, which is correctable with rapid resolution of symptoms when the baby is fed; this should be attempted. Feeding will only result in a worsening of symptoms in many other metabolic disorders. Any newborn who presents with this dramatic array of symptoms shortly after birth and who does not respond to feeding is seriously ill and should be transported without delay, regardless of the presumed reason for the deterioration.

To transport:

- Discontinue feeding until the baby is evaluated.
- Keep the baby warm.
- If the baby is vomiting, place her on her side and clear her airway as indicated.
- Provide an orogastric or nasogastric tube and aspirate it every 5 to 10 minutes.
- Insert an oral airway if indicated and administer full CPR as necessary.

DETECTING AND DIFFERENTIATING NEWBORN HYPOGLYCEMIA, SEPSIS AND HEART DEFECTS

Hypoglycemia, sepsis and heart defects can mimic each other. All may be life threatening. It is therefore very important for the midwife to be able to recognize the subtle differences between them as well as to be alert for those babies for whom sepsis is a greater possibility. The primary value in being able to tell these conditions apart is that hypoglycemia, which will be, by far, the most common problem, can often be corrected at home while the other conditions will require immediate transport. Each of these conditions have a few common predisposing factors associated with them.

PREDISPOSING FACTOR	HYPOGLYCEMIA	SEPSIS	HEART DEFECTS
History of prolonged rupture of membranes (>24 hours)		✔	
Maternal infection during pregnancy		✔	✔
Signs of maternal infection in labor (tender uterus, fever, rapid pulse)		✔	
Persistently elevated fetal heart rate with lack of variability during labor		✔	✔
Persistent bradycardia in labor			✔
Meconium aspiration		✔	
Long, exhausting labor with membranes intact until late labor or pushing	✔		
Poorly controlled maternal diabetes	✔		✔
Preterm birth	✔	✔	✔
Poor maternal health or inadequate nutrition prenatally or during labor	✔	✔	

Sepsis (generalized infection)

Overall, the incidence of sepsis in babies born at term is 0.8 per 1000 live births and 4.3 per 1000 for preterm births. Sepsis is defined as infection in the blood or tissues. Infection, which is usually isolated to one area of the body, easily leads to sepsis in babies because their immune system is immature. Most of these infections are bacterial, but some are viral or, very rarely, fungal. Newborns with sepsis usually present many subtle and nonspecific signs and symptoms. There is often a known history of maternal exposure to an infectious organism to which the fetus is particularly vulnerable during pregnancy or labor. The specifics regarding various types of maternal exposures and the risks to the fetus and newborn are detailed in my text DIAGNOSTIC TESTS. An infection that is established and severe may manifest with any of the following signs. The first four are the most common.

- Temperature instability: Although fever is unusual in the neonate, core temperatures above 100°F (37.8°C) (98°F/36.7°C axillary) are significant; those above 102.2°F (39°C) (100°F/37.8°C axillary) are especially concerning. Be sure, however, that the baby is not too hot because of environmental factors.
- Lethargy
- Poor feeding
- Respiratory distress (may be due to pneumonia)
- Enlargement of the liver (hepatomegaly), spleen (splenomegaly) or both
- Skin lesions (especially rashes, sores or blisters)
- Swollen joints
- Pallor
- External or internal abnormalities of the eyes
- Hypotonia or hypertonia
- Poor perfusion (See the subchapter entitled "Cyanosis, Rapid Breathing, Congestive Heart Failure, Shock or Arrhythmia: Detecting Heart Defects at Birth")
- Foul odor of the amniotic fluid, placenta or baby

<u>Signs and symptoms</u>: Hypoglycemia, sepsis or a heart defect may be present at birth or during the first days of life with one or more of the symptoms in the table below.

SIGN OR SYMPTOM	HYPOGLYCEMIA	SEPSIS	HEART DEFECTS
General			
Inability to regulate body temperature	✔	✔	
Hypothermia (<96.8°F/36.0° C core or <94.8°F/34.9°C axillary)		✔	✔
Hyperthermia (>100°F/37.8°C core or <98°F/36.7°C axillary)		✔	
Jaundice		✔	
Petechiae or mucosal bleeding at sites of minor trauma		✔	
Low blood glucose (<40 mg/dl or 2.22 mmol/l)	✔	✔	
Lesions or generalized body rash		✔	
Foul odor of amniotic fluid, placenta or baby		✔	
Cardiovascular and respiratory signs			
Poor APGAR scores		✔	✔
Respiratory distress	✔	✔	✔ (tachypnea only)
Cyanotic, pale or mottled appearance	✔ (rare)	✔ (if severe)	✔
Tachycardia (>160 bpm)	✔	✔	✔
Capillary refill time more than 3 seconds		✔	✔
Neuromuscular signs			
Stiffness in the neck or lower limbs		✔ (meningitis)	
Swollen anterior fontanelle when baby is supine		✔ (meningitis)	
Sleepy, lethargic baby or hyperactive and irritable one	✔	✔	
Poor muscle tone, limpness, eye rolling	✔	✔	
High-pitched, weak cry	✔	✔	
Seizures	✔	✔	
Sweating	✔	✔	✔
Gastrointestinal			
Vomiting		✔	
Poor nursing or loss of interest in nursing	✔	✔	✔
Abdominal distension		✔	
Enlarged liver, spleen or both		✔	✔

If signs and symptoms or history strongly point to sepsis as the likely problem, transport immediately. A septic newborn who is symptomatic at birth is usually in grave danger. Other signs that point to sepsis include:

Poor APGAR scores: Babies who are born with established infections often have APGAR scores less than 7. Any baby with a 1 min score of less than 7 that does not improve to normal with routine support should be transported and evaluated carefully for the possibility of sepsis.

Low blood glucose: A low blood glucose cannot reliably differentiate septic babies from those with simple hypoglycemia since the stress of sepsis can produce hypoglycemia. The value that defines neonatal hypoglycemia is a matter of much debate. Minimum values ranging from 40 to 47 mg/100 ml (2.22 to 2.6 mmol/l) on heel stick with test strips are used to define hypoglycemia, depending on the source. The good news is that, with adequate nourishment, the symptoms of a baby who has uncomplicated hypoglycemia should improve within an hour or so after feeding, and all symptoms should resolve by the time the baby is feeding normally. While the blood sugar may rise, other symptoms will not resolve completely if another metabolic disorder is causative or if the baby is septic.

Lesions or a generalized body rash: Certain infections produce skin lesions that are obvious at birth. A generalized body rash should prompt you to suspect syphilis. Strictly observe universal precautions as the baby could be highly contagious. Some congenital genetic syndromes also involve noninfectious skin lesions.

Signs of neurological compromise: Signs such as sleepiness; lethargy; hyperactivity or irritability; a weak, high-pitched cry and seizures are associated with neurological involvement and may indicate brain damage. The baby should be transported without delay.

Signs of meningitis: Stiffness in the neck or lower limbs is highly associated with meningitis. A baby with a stiff neck will hold her head rigidly and may cry when moved. A swollen or tense anterior fontanelle with the baby lying down is another highly suspicious sign of meningitis. It is normal for the anterior fontanelle to have a gentle pulse that is detectable on palpation and for it to bulge very slightly when the baby is in a seated or upright position, but it should not be tense.

Dealing with glucose imbalances

Hypoglycemia: Check capillary glucose, feed the baby and recheck glucose in 1 hour. Feeding the baby may require giving the baby a supplemental formula because many women cannot pump colostrum. You can use either prepared 5% glucose water, soy-based formula (follow package directions for powder) or molasses mixed with sterile water (1 tsp to 1 cup). Molasses is preferable to maple syrup as it contains more minerals. Honey should never be used in infants less than 1 year of age as it can carry botulism, which the infant gut is less prepared to deal with. Feeding soy-based formula or pasturized goat's milk will result in a more stable glucose level for a longer period of time because these fluids contain protein. Feed the baby with a teaspoon or an eyedropper. Just a few spoonfuls or droppers-full should prompt improvement if the baby has uncomplicated hypoglycemia. Once the baby rouses, strongly encourage him to nurse. You will see a rebound hypoglycemia (glucose rises and then falls rapidly) if the baby does not begin nursing, especially if a sugar-based fluid is used.

Persistent hypoglycemia is rare in babies. Babies with complicated hypoglycemia may have a rare pancreatic disorder causing their insulin levels to be abnormally elevated. They are usually large for gestational age and present with jitters, myoclonic jerks, cyanotic episodes, apnea and seizures from birth, with persistent hypoglycemia that does not improve with feeding.

Hyperglycemia at birth: It is very rare for babies to manifest overt diabetes in the first week of life, even among those who develop juvenile diabetes. Most elevated glucose levels in the newborn period are due to interventions such as the use of glucose IVs and certain drugs. The overall risk of hyperglycemia is less than 2% among all infants, regardless of gestational age, 5% among those receiving glucose IV and 20 to 40% among very low birthweight infants receiving glucose infusion; since you won't be giving babies glucose IVs at home, the chance that you will test a baby who turns out to be hyperglycemic is very unlikely. Should you discover hyperglycemia in a homeborn baby (whole blood sugar over 125 mg/dl in term babies and over 150 mg/dl in preterm), the most likely reasons include sepsis (especially from *E coli* and group B-strep) or a history of asphyxia or respiratory distress syndrome. Sepsis prompts a release of catecholamines, corticosteroids and cytokines, which leads to an inadequate insulin supply. High glucose levels increase the osmolarity of the blood, resulting in electrolyte disturbances, osmotic diuresis and, in extreme cases, intraventricular hemorrhage at levels exceeding 300 mg/dl. Because of these risks, if you do discover that the baby is hyperglycemic, transport for evaluation right away (Pati et al., 2001).

Transport procedures

If hypoglycemia does not resolve with feeding or is severe enough to cause extreme symptoms that do not respond, if the baby begins to have seizures or if sepsis is suspected, transport immediately. Any of these conditions, if not treated, could lead to brain damage or death. During transport, keep the baby warm, provide an oral airway, insert an orogastric or nasogastric tube and aspirate every 5 to 10 minutes, and administer full CPR as necessary. Carefully observe universal precautions in the event that the baby has a communicable disease.

ABDOMINAL DISTENSION AND VOMITING AT BIRTH: DETECTING GASTROINTESTINAL ANOMALIES

Abdominal and urogenital defects cause a variety of similar signs and symptoms. Intestinal obstruction is a very common emergency of the neonate, accounting for 25% of all emergency neonatal surgery. The exact condition may not be clear, but the likelihood of a gastrointestinal problem can be recognized based on certain abnormal findings. Evaluate by observing the infant, examining the abdomen and genitalia, listening to the abdomen with an infant stethoscope and using transillumination when indicated. The onset of symptoms may be delayed two to three days or as late as one month, depending upon the specific gastrointestinal or urogenital problem.

General Signs and Symptoms Pointing to Serious Gastrointestinal (GI) Problems

The baby may display a variety of signs and symptoms that are associated with gastrointestinal defects:

Polyhydramnios: This occurs in about 50% of babies with esophageal, duodenal and proximal jejunal atresia, as well as in some with ileal or colonic obstruction. Any baby whose birth is accompanied by over 2000 ml of amniotic fluid should be examined by passing an orogastric tube to confirm patency of the esophagus.

Vomiting: This is one of the most important signs (see detailed description below).

Abnormalities of the abdomen

- •Abdominal distension may be present with no passage of meconium but no evidence of distress.
- •Visible loops of bowel may appear distended and lumpy as a result of an intestinal obstruction.
- •Abdominal distension (especially of the upper abdomen) with tenderness may be present.
- •The swollen abdomen may be tense and shiny if the GI tract is obstructed. Obstruction can be due to a congenital defect or an internal injury.
- •The abdomen may be flaccid and wrinkled due to defective abdominal muscles.
- •The abdomen may also be swollen and tense because of an obstructed urinary tract (see next chapter).
- •If the birth required lots of manipulation, the abdomen is darkened and swollen and the baby is lethargic and shocky, internal bleeding may be causative. See the chapter entitled "Birth Injuries (Other Than Cranial Injuries)."

Abnormal gastric secretions

- •Persistently copious quantities of clear gastric secretions may be noted (associated with upper GI atresias or other types of blockage).
- •Green gastric juices at birth in a baby that had clear amniotic fluid is a strong indication of a GI defect. (Swallowing of amniotic fluid stained with meconium that was normally passed per rectum may result is a false positive finding for this sign; however, vomiting of bile-stained mucus in utero can mimic meconium-stained fluid. If abdominal distension is also present, be suspicious.

Cyanosis and choking: When these occur during a feeding, suspect a gastrointestinal blockage.

Abnormal meconium: Meconium may be unusual in color or consistency. Stool may or may not be passed normally in a baby with a gastrointestinal defect.

- •Bloody stools may be due to volvulus (twisting) or any obstruction that involves either the venous or arterial blood supply of the GI tract. Associated abdominal tenderness is seen with peritonitis or intestinal infarction, which may rarely be present at birth; other causes include bleeding disorders such as hemorrhagic disease or DIC. The baby who is otherwise well may also swallow maternal blood during birth; this possibility can be confirmed with an APT test (see my text DIAGNOSTIC TESTS for details).
- •Complete failure to pass stool (normally, stooling occurs within 48 hours of birth) suggests either functional or structural bowel obstruction.
  - -Functional bowel obstruction or ileus, is associated with sick, preterm, LBW infants.
  - -Structural bowel obstruction is usually accompanied by abdominal distension and vomiting.

Shock

Small for gestational age growth

Anal opening may be absent or misplaced

Failure to urinate by 24 hours

Assessment

The two primary signs of gastrointestinal disorders are abdominal distension and vomiting.

Abdominal distension

Distension is the single most important sign of GI tract dysfunction. The normal newborn abdomen is mildly concave at birth but becomes soft, symmetric and slightly rounded quickly as the baby begins to breath and swallow some air. Mild gastric distension is common and, when not found with other suspicious signs and symptoms, is most often benign.

Moderate to severe distension that persists is a reliable, although nonspecific, indication that something is wrong. It may be caused by an increase in intraperitoneal volume or by an increase in the size of thoracic or pelvic contents.

Distension caused by air: Swallowed air is the most common cause of abdominal distension without tenderness. Many normal babies swallow air during feeding, crying or vigorous sucking on their fist; this may cause mild gastric distension. In babies with GI defects, air accumulates as the result of either paralysis or functional bowel obstruction.

Mechanical obstruction with signs of bile-stained vomitus, abdominal wall resonance on percussion, visible peristalsis or delayed passage of meconium will result in distension, the amount of which depends on the site of the obstruction. Air may also be released into the peritoneal cavity if an abdominal organ ruptures. This will produce signs of peritonitis, such as distension, tenderness and absence of normal bowel sounds, as well as redness and swelling of the abdominal wall. Pneumoperitoneum is one cause of air in the abdominal cavity (see the subchapter entitled "Complicated Respiratory Distress," item 5).

Distension caused by fluid: Abdominal distension may be caused by the accumulation of several different types of body fluids, including blood, chyle (lymph fluid), urine or free fluid in the abdominal cavity. Following a difficult birth during which an abdominal organ was injured, blood is usually present as the result of intra-abdominal hemorrhage from the liver, spleen or an adrenal gland. Although a coagulation defect may also result in intra-abdominal bleeding, in these cases there should be abnormal bleeding from other sites as well. Chylous ascites occurs when the thoracic lymphatic duct is obstructed, causing chyle to accumulate in the abdomen. Ascites (the accumulation of serous fluid in the peritoneal cavity) due to the passage of fluid through membranes or oozing of fluid in the peritoneal cavity is found in several conditions such as Rh hemolytic disease, nonimmune causes of hydrops fetalis, congestive heart failure, hypoproteinemia and peritonitis. If ascites is found with severe jaundice, the biliary system is likely to be involved and may require surgery. Urinary ascites occurs when the urinary tract is obstructed or has been injured. It most commonly occurs when posterior urethral valves are present. (See the subchapter entitled "Abdominal Mass, Single Umbilical Artery, Edema, Atypical Genitalia: Detecting Kidney and Genitourinary Tract Disorders.")

Free fluid flows down, causing it to pool in the flanks in a supine infant. Prominent flank distension also occurs when the abdominal muscles are flaccid. The sides of the abdomen widen without an equal increase in the anteroposterior diameter. Free fluid in the abdomen will also move to the lowest point, so that if the baby lies on his side, the abdominal contour will shift a bag downward unless there is so much fluid that the abdominal wall is too tense to allow this.

Distension caused by masses: Enlargement of any of the abdominal organs may result in a palpable, and, at times, visible, mass. The distension caused is usually more localized than that caused by either accumulated fluid or gas. A mass presents as a discrete, regional object within an otherwise normal abdomen, although generalized distension and a mass can occur together. The two most common causes of abdominal masses in the neonate are kidney defects that do not involve vomiting. These are both covered in the subchapter entitled "Abdominal Mass, Single Umbilical Artery, Edema, Atypical Genitalia: Detecting Kidney and Genitourinary Tract Disorders."

GI masses may be asymptomatic at birth but can quickly lead to partial or complete intestinal obstruction. An enlarged pyloric muscle (the cause of infantile pyloric stenosis), which feels like an olive located where the stomach empties into the small intestines, is one such lesion that can sometimes be palpated at birth. Midgut volvulus (twisting of a portion of the intestines), malrotation of the colon or, more rarely, intussusception (telescoping), may present with an abdominal mass. However, the presence of the mass is usually a less important sign than the more obvious ones indicating obstruction.

Rarely, parts of the gastrointestinal tract (often called a duplication cyst) may be duplicated during development, resulting in a copy of the part lying adjacent to the normal one. Duplications may occur anywhere from the tongue to the anus. When in the chest cavity, they may cause respiratory distress and mediastinal shift as they fill with secretions.

However, they typically do not perforate or ulcerate in the neonatal period. Duplicated portions of intestines are usually mobile on palpation and may lead to intestinal obstruction. Abdominal duplications may mimic the olive-shaped mass associated with pyloric stenosis because they are located in the same general area. They may become the starting point for an intussusception or cause intestinal obstruction by ribboning or twisting, leading to perforation and bleeding.

Masses of inspissated (thickened or condensed) meconium may occasionally be felt on palpation in babies with imperforate anus, meconium ileus or Hirschsprung's disease. Injury may involve any of the abdominal organs and usually presents with abdominal distension, lethargy and pallor, as well as with a mass or with an increase in the size of the liver or spleen due to a subcapsular hematoma. A midline mass in a baby girl may be due to fluid distension of the uterus and yoni secondary to an imperforate hymen, especially if the mass remains once the bladder is empty. Metastatic neuroblastoma is the most common liver tumor in newborns; a baby with this form of cancer may be born with an enlarged liver and abdominal distension that may impair ventilation of the lungs due to pressure. A liver tumor is often found in association with petechiae secondary to thrombocytopenia.

Distension with tenderness: A distended and tender abdomen is a potentially emergent problem. These babies will cry when palpated and may cry or fuss when any pressure is applied to the abdomen, as might occur during positioning.

Location of distension: Where the distension occurs and how extensive it is gives clues to its possible cause, as follows:

CHARACTERISTICS OF ABDOMINAL DISTENSION	POSSIBLE CAUSES
Widening of both flanks with little or no increase in the anteroposterior abdominal diameter; fluctuance detected on palpation, organs may be seen floating on transillumination	Intraperitoneal fluid; flaccid abdominal muscles (prune belly syndrome)*
Widening of one or both flanks	Kidney enlargement, injury to bladder or adrenal gland
Localized mass, surrounding abdomen is normal	Organ enlargement, tumor
Suprapubic region, anteroposterior diameter enlarged	Boys: Distended bladder due to posterior urethral valves* Girls: hydrometrocolpos due to a transverse yoni septum*
Lower abdomen, anteroposterior diameter enlarged	GI obstruction, ovarian mass*, interior sacrococcygeal teratoma, anterior meningocele
Lower abdomen, anteroposterior and transverse enlargement producing a single- or double-sided, localized flank bulge.	Kidney enlargement on one or both sides, renal vein thrombosis, kidney tumors, ovarian mass*
Upper left abdominal quadrant extending from beneath rib cage	Stomach enlargement (due to gas or recent feeding?), duodenal obstruction, jejunal atresia; spleen, adrenal or kidney enlargement
Left upper quadrant of abdomen, extending from beneath the rib cage and across the upper right abdomen	Spleen enlargement (often accompanies liver enlargement)
Upper right abdominal quadrant extending from beneath the rib cage and across to the left upper abdomen	Liver, kidney or adrenal enlargement
"Double bubble" with one swelling overlying the stomach in the upper left quadrant and one overlying the upper duodenum in the upper right quadrant; abdomen otherwise normal	Duodenal obstruction (may increase due to trapped gas) due to atresia or stenosis; malrotation with Ladd bands, or an annular pancreas
Visible bowel loops that look like ripples or ladder rungs across the upper abdomen, visible peristalsis	Air distension of organs from breathing, ventilation or normal digestion; seen in thin or preterm infants (benign); if persistent, could also indicate bowel obstruction
A few dilated loops of small bowel	Jejunal atresia
Generalized enlargement	Imperforate anus;* massive amounts of intraperitoneal air or fluid outside of the GI tract (GI perforation? large pneumothorax with escape of gas into abdomen?)
Generalized enlargement with darkening	Meconium peritonitis with rupture of the bowel, internal bleeding into the peritoneal cavity

CHARACTERISTICS OF ABDOMINAL DISTENSION	POSSIBLE CAUSES
Abdominal wall is stretched (may be taut and shiny) over the organs, revealing irregular shapes; distension is not relocated at all or only minimally when the infant changes position	Gas or fluid inside of organs
Abdominal wall is lifted up off underlying organs, resulting in more generalized, rounded swelling; with position changes air rises to highest point, fluid pools to lowest level.	Gas or fluid in the intraperitoneal space. If distension is caused by air, it is leaking from the lungs or the GI tract. If caused by fluid, the baby could be bleeding or intraperitoneal fluid could have accumulated over time in utero with no organ rupture.

*See subchapter entitled "Abdominal Mass, Single Umbilical Artery, Edema, Atypical Genitalia: Detecting Kidney and Genitourinary Tract Disorders"

Vomiting

Nearly all newborns regurgitate some milk during or after nursing (that is, they spit up, often accompanied by a burp), but when it presents with other signs or symptoms pointing to problems, it should not be overlooked. Persistent, true vomiting of copious amounts of stomach contents is rare and usually not normal, especially in fully breastfed babies. Spitting up or frank vomiting in the first hours of life may occur with a severe gastrointestinal disorder or may be secondary to a wide array of other causes. If seen with an enlarged liver, hepatitis, galactosemia or congestive heart failure may be an underlying cause. If found with a distended abdomen, intestinal obstruction, peritonitis or hypokalemia may be the problem. Other causes include drug withdrawal (in babies of addicted mothers), sepsis, meningitis, perinatal asphyxia and sometimes other inborn errors of metabolism, although it is exceedingly rare for these to manifest immediately after birth.

Upper GI obstruction usually produces bile-stained vomitus with less abdominal distension. (Defects near the hepatopancreatic ampulla [also called the ampulla of Vater, where the common bile duct of the gallbladder and the major pancreatic duct empty into the duodenum] usually produce bile-stained vomit.) Lower GI obstruction (that is, distant from the hepatopancreatic ampulla) typically presents with unstained vomitus and more abdominal distension. Vomiting secondary to a structural defect of the GI tract is more likely to result in bile-stained or bloody vomitus as well as to be excessive or persistent, usually totaling more than 15 to 20 ml of fluid obtained by gastric aspiration at the time of birth. The more fluid that is aspirated, the higher the likelihood that an upper GI obstruction exists. Nursing may lead to further abdominal distension and vomiting because normal digestion is obstructed. Vomiting is a major symptom in the disorders shown in the table below.

INTESTINAL DEFECTS THAT FREQUENTLY PRESENT WITH BILIOUS VOMIT	
WITHOUT ABDOMINAL DISTENSION	WITH ABDOMINAL DISTENSION
Duodenal stenosis Duodenal atresia Obstructions due to an annular (ring-shaped) pancreas Proximal jejunal atresia	Ileal atresia Meconium ileus Meconium plug syndrome Hirschsprung's disease

Bilious vomiting in a newborn who was born through clear amniotic fluid or who shows other signs of GI defects should be assumed to have a serious GI obstruction until proven otherwise; this baby requires immediate transport.

In addition, several mechanical gastrointestinal obstructions may result in nonbilious vomit:

Gastroesophageal reflux: esophageal chalasia (incompetence of the lower esophagus) often produces unstained vomit with significant respiratory distress after nursing from birth on. As an isolated condition, it is not associated with abdominal distension, but it may accompany GI disorders, especially pyloric stenosis (which usually does not present at birth). See the subchapter entitled "Complicated Respiratory Distress," item 13.

Esophageal atresia with tracheoesophageal fistula: This condition presents with feeding problems and excess oral secretions. Feeding prompts aspiration, coughing, choking and, at times, cyanosis and respiratory distress.

Swallowing disorders: Failure of the upper esophageal sphincter to relax (cricopharyngeal achalasia) may result in feeding problems with coughing, gagging, regurgitation and aspiration. A lack of coordination between the pharyngeal and esophageal phases of swallowing occurs in pharyngeal-cricopharyngeal incoordination.

Vomiting always makes the infant more prone to choking and aspiration, leading to dehydration and hypoglycemia. Any infant with vomiting and two of these five signs–pain, excessive crying, bloody stool, oliguria, and abdominal distension should be transported for evaluation. Conditions requiring surgery usually cause severe vomiting and include other distinct presenting signs.

Gastrointestinal bleeding

Vomiting of blood and rectal bleeding are both alarming symptoms that may be associated with a variety of acute problems such as perforation of the GI tract. Most benignly, vomiting of blood may occur either because the baby swallowed maternal blood during the birth or from trauma during resuscitation. If the baby spits up blood, the amount and color should be assessed for the possibility that it was swallowed during the birth process, when it will appear bright as opposed to darker red. Any blood that is copious, dark, or passed via rectum should be assumed pathological until proven otherwise. Any stained fluids or stool should be saved in a clean glass container, covered and taken with the baby to the hospital. There, the sample can be tested to determine whether the blood is from the mother or baby, and the baby can be further evaluated. Spontaneous perforation of the GI tract or gastrointestinal injury, although rare, are other causes of GI bleeding. These are discussed at the end of this chapter.

Atypical genitalia

While the presence of atypical genitalia is not, in itself, diagnostic of a GI defect, babies with atypical genitalia often have associated urinary and lower gastrointestinal defects. Even if there are no other obvious defects, the baby should be evaluated as soon as possible to rule out adrenal hyperplasia, which can cause the baby to lose sodium rapidly and thus seriously disrupt the metabolism. (Details regarding the detection of atypical genitalia can be found the subchapter entitled "Examining the Genitalia, Perineum and Anus.")

Transport procedures for All Types of Suspected Intestinal Obstruction

The baby may appear relatively stable at birth, when the electrolyte balance is likely to be normal. However, fluid can pool in the intestinal space and be absorbed, leading to rapid dehydration and electrolyte disturbances. Increasing abdominal distension may put upward pressure on the thoracic cavity, leading to respiratory distress with the risk of aspiration. In fact, aspiration pneumonitis is a common cause of early death that may develop before other problems have had time to present themselves. Delaying evaluation in a baby suspected to have a gastrointestinal obstruction is dangerous and may mean the difference between saving a normal gastrointestinal tract and losing a large portion of bowel due to damage and infection. Whenever a gastrointestinal or genitourinary defect is suspected, all oral intake must be stopped until the baby can be evaluated. Transport soon after birth as follows:

1. Leave the cord intact or cut it off at the placental base (see below).
2. Position the baby with her head low on her right side or on the side opposite the mass or swelling and keep her warm. (This positioning will help relieve pressure on the lungs and help drain the mouth if vomiting should occur during transport.)
3. Insert an orogastric tube to vent air and aspirate it every few minutes; record volume.
4. Complete CPR, including positive pressure, may be administered as necessary. Watch for further distension, which may indicate that the obstructed structures are filling with air. If this occurs, stop momentarily and aspirate the tube before continuing. Try using rapid, low-pressure ventilations of 100% oxygen to maximize tissue perfusion with minimal force.

Leaving the cord intact after the placental transfusion is complete

Transporting a baby to the hospital is complicated enough without trailing the placenta along with you; however, there are good reasons to leave the cord as long as possible in these babies. There may be loops of bowel herniated into the base of the cord. A patent allantoic duct may still communicate with the bladder, causing urine to dribble out of the umbilicus. Very rarely but perhaps most important, a portion of bowel may extend into the umbilical cord for a variable distance, even though the cord may appear normal. The safest thing to do whenever you suspect a gastrointestinal disorder or a urinary tract anomaly is to cut the cord where it connects to the placenta and clamp the very end.

Possible Causes and Differential Diagnosis

The following descriptions can help differentiate between a number of specific gastrointestinal defects. **Atresia** refers to the absence or closure of a passage, while **stenosis** denotes the narrowing or stricture of a duct or canal. Gastrointestinal obstructions can be divided into high and low categories.

Upper (high) gastrointestinal disorders

The upper GI tract consists of the oral cavity, pharynx, esophagus, stomach, liver, pancreas, gallbladder and duodenum.

General signs and symptoms of high gastrointestinal obstruction: Copious vomiting or regurgitation of milk occurs early when there is an obstruction in the upper portion of the small intestines, but it may be delayed if there is only a stenosis. About 40% of obstructions occur above the hepatopancreatic ampulla ("preampullary," that is, above the level where the duct empties into the duodenum); in this case, the vomit will not be bile stained. Postampullary obstruction occurs about 60% of the time and usually produces classic bile-stained vomit. Some blood may be present. Jaundice may also develop due to biliary atresia. A large gastric tube should be passed immediately to empty the stomach and duodenum and to prevent aspiration of vomit. Dehydration is a major risk with active vomiting, so do not delay in transporting. Infants with Down syndrome are at increased risk.

Specific causes

- Congenital gastric outlet obstructions and disorders, including hypertrophic pyloric stenosis (may present at birth; occurs in 1 out of every 300 to 1000 live births)
- Intussusception
- Stenosis (75% of all stenoses) or atresia of the duodenum (40% of all atresias; 1 in 10,000 live births)
- Midgut malrotation with Ladd's bands (abnormal mesenteric ligaments that cross over from the cecum to the duodenum and that may cause obstruction of the duodenum or volvulus)
- Duplications of the upper GI tract
- Pancreatic anomalies and disorders
- Atresias, stenosis or microgastria of the stomach (all very rare; 125 cases reported as of 1989)
- Gastric volvulus (exceedingly rare; 16 acute neonatal cases reported as of 1987)

Congenital gastric outlet obstructions and disorders: Although the gastric outlet can be obstructed, most forms are very rare. The major types of gastric disorders are discussed below.

Pyloric disorders: Infantile pyloric stenosis is one of the most common conditions requiring neonatal surgery in the Western world, with 3 out of every 1000 liveborn infants affected. Although it most commonly presents during the 3rd to 4th week of life, it may present at birth in 3.7 to 6.5% of affected babies with nonprojectile vomiting of nonbilious matter that progresses into projectile vomiting over the first days or weeks or life. The baby nurses vigorously and may have a "worried" look prior to vomiting. Since it is so common and tends to present in the weeks following birth, it is covered in more detail in Volume III of this text.

Congenital aplasia, atresia, membranes and webs of the pylorus or antrum are all exceedingly rare. Polyhydramnios may develop prenatally and low birthweight may be present in any of these conditions. Complete obstruction results in unstained vomitus, stomach distension, failure to pass meconium, and eventual metabolic alkalosis, with partial obstruction often going undiagnosed into adulthood.

Gastric duplications: Discussed later in this chapter.

Gastric teratoma: A gastric teratoma, which is very rare (61 cases reported by 1986), arises from the posterior stomach wall. It may grow into the stomach cavity but more commonly grows toward the outside. It usually presents with an abdominal mass (75%), abdominal distension (56%), vomiting (18%) and respiratory distress (15%). It may also cause premature labor and even dystocia if quite large. Growth into the stomach wall may result in ulceration leading to the vomiting of blood, arm or leg pain and anemia.

Gastric ulcers: Multiple, shallow gastric (peptic) ulcers may present in healthy full-term babies with gastrointestinal bleeding, and sometimes vomiting alone, in the first two days of life. These are rare, with one Japanese study finding 225 cases over a period of 17 years (Kamagata et al., 1990). Stress ulcers may also occur secondary to sepsis or anoxia.

Other gastric defects: These rare defects present with acute epigastric distension, vomiting or unproductive attempts at vomiting. Gastric volvulus is also associated with unproductive attempts at vomiting as well as inability or difficulty in passing an orogastric tube.

Intussusception: Intussusception occurs 1.6 to 4 times in every 1000 live births in Great Britain. It is characterized by a length of the intestines becoming folded back inside another, creating a double-sleeve effect, like a deep cuff on a sock. This is rare in neonates except in the presence of duplication cysts. Intrauterine intussusception has been found to be a cause of intestinal atresia. When intussusception does occur, it is an emergency, resulting in vascular compression and rapidly leading to necrosis if not recognized. It presents with signs of shock.

Duodenal obstruction: Obstruction of the duodenum is the most common type of intestinal blockage. It occurs in about 1 out of every 6000 to 20,000 births (1 in 10,000 to 40,000 live births), with two girls affected for every boy. Polyhydramnios is present in half the cases. The first sign is vomiting of fluid, usually bile-stained, with no abdominal distension, although the dilated stomach will sometimes create a fullness under the ribs, while the rest of the abdomen is scaphoid. Visible gastric peristalsis is common. No passage of meconium is a sign of complete obstruction, although 1 to 2 small stools may pass at the beginning of symptoms.

Associated defects: Associated anomalies include malrotation of the gut, which is quite common (found in 1 out of every 500 adult autopsies; only 50% of all children who are eventually identified present in the neonatal period), Down syndrome (30%), esophageal fistula, anal atresia, heart or urinary tract defects, and limb, vertebral and spinal malformations. As many as 60% of these babies are born preterm.

Types of duodenal obstruction: Obstruction of the duodenum may be due to complete atresia, stenosis, the presence of a diaphragm in the lumen of the canal or a ring-shaped pancreas. The stomach and duodenum above the defect dilate rapidly, resulting in the classic "double-bubble sign," where two lumps appear in the upper abdomen. Vomiting usually begins early on and becomes copious and forceful. The vomit will become bile stained if the obstruction is below the hepatopancreatic ampulla; however, in many cases it is located above this level. Duodenal obstruction may also result from volvulus or Ladd's bands. Most cases of obstruction without stenosis become symptomatic early in infancy with bilious vomitus and abdominal pain. The abdomen is generally caved in (scaphoid) and not distended. The baby may pass meconium.

Duplications of the upper gastrointestinal tract: Duplications are rare lesions that can occur anywhere along the GI tract from the tongue to the anus. They have three common features: they are hollow, they are lined with gastrointestinal tissue, and this tissue includes a layer of smooth muscle wall. This wall is often shared with adjacent gastrointestinal tract structures. It can take the form of a length of a duplicated part that runs alongside the normal length of the primary part, or it can form a cyst. Symptoms vary depending upon the location and size of the duplication and are produced by pressure.

A cyst may cause obstruction of the GI tract or the airway. Hemorrhage or perforation of a cyst may also occur because of acid secretions from gastric mucosa inside the cyst. Anomalies of the spine and of the external genitalia can be associated with duplication. Duplications most commonly occur in the ileum and next most commonly in the esophagus. Large lesions may rupture after distension with mucosal secretions or may cause intestinal obstruction.

Esophageal duplication: This causes respiratory distress and difficulty in swallowing, especially if located in the cervical esophagus or between the trachea and esophagus in the upper mediastinum. Many, however, are asymptomatic, being found only during chest X-ray.

Thoracoabdominal duplication: Large lesions in the thorax may communicate distally with the duodenum or intestine. Respiratory distress, sepsis from intestinal colonization and bleeding from peptic erosion may occur. Large lesions extending up through the diaphragm into the thorax are often attached to the spine and are associated with spinal anomalies.

Gastric duplication: Gastric duplications are also rare, with fewer than 100 cases reported in the world literature as of 1994. They produce a palpable abdominal mass seen with abdominal distension, vomiting (the vomitus being sometimes blood stained), as well as weight loss, abdominal pain, anemia, arm and leg pain, and fever. Duplication of the pylorus may be mistaken for the "olive" of pyloric stenosis and may present in a similar fashion.

Pyloric duplication: These rare lesions present with gastric outlet obstruction (see above).

Duodenal duplication: This is also rare, occurring primarily in the first and second portions of the duodenum on the pancreatic margin.

Peripancreatic duplication: This presents with nausea, vomiting, weight loss and abdominal pain. Most contain gastric mucosa, which bathe the pacreatic duct in acid secretions and produce pancreatitis. This should be ruled out in all children presenting with idiopathic pancreatitis.

Pancreatic anomalies and disorders: Pancreatic disorders are rare in neonates. Complete absence of the pancreas is usually only found in nonviable fetuses. Most often a ring-shaped pancreas is found; less commonly, there are anomalies of the duct system, duplication of the pancreas or fusion with nearby organs. Symptoms of duplication may mimic pyloric stenosis. A ring-shaped pancreas presents with duodenal obstruction. Ductal anomalies present with abdominal pain. The baby with a pancreatic cyst may present with an abdominal mass; signs of gastroduodenal or gastrointestinal compression and biliary obstruction may also be present, with jaundice, respiratory distress, bowel obstruction, dark urine and pale stools. Pancreatic anomalies often accompany trisomy 9, 12 and 18; cystic fibrosis; and Cornelia de Lange, Ivemark, and Meckel syndromes, as well as a few other rare disorders.

Lower gastrointestinal disorders

The lower GI tract includes the small intestines (jejunum and ileum), the large intestines (transverse, ascending and descending colon), cecum, appendix, sigmoid colon, rectum, and anal canal.

Possible causes:

- •Meconium impaction (1%)
- •Meconium ileus (1 in 1000 to 1600 live births; 10 to 15% of these babies have cystic fibrosis)
- •Anorectal anomalies (1 in 2500 to 20,000 live births)
- •Hirschsprung's disease (1 in 5000 to 8000 live births)
- •Prune-belly syndrome
- •Jejunal, ileal or colonic atresia or stenosis (overall incidence of 2 to 4 per 10,000 births)
- •Small bowel atresias and stenoses (1 in 5000 live births)
  - -Ileum: stenosis (20%); atresia (35%)
  - -Jejunum: stenosis (5%); atresia (25%)
- •Malrotation of the intestines
- •Meconium peritonitis (1 in every 20,000 to 40,000 live births)
- •Duplications of the lower GI tract and other cystic swellings of the mesentery
- •Omphalomesenteric remnants at the umbilicus
- •Functional immaturity of the large intestines in preterm babies and infants of diabetic mothers (may have meconium plug syndrome or small left colon syndrome)
- •Intestinal injury with bleeding (due to birth trauma–very rare)

Meconium plug impaction: Meconium plugs occur in about 1% of all babies, although only 1 in 500 show symptoms. These babies are frequently small for gestational age. The lower third of the plug consists of clear mucus while the upper two-thirds is green meconium. This baby usually presents with a distended abdomen and vomiting that may be secondary to immature gastrointestinal motility. Gently inserting a lubricated thermometer into the rectum will frequently result in the passage of normal meconium. The passage of normal meconium with relief of other symptoms does not require immediate transport, but cystic fibrosis and Hirschsprung's disease should be ruled out with evaluations soon after birth.

Meconium ileus: Meconium ileus is the most common cause of bowel obstruction in newborns and is the primary cause of intrauterine intestinal perforation. It causes between one-tenth and one-third of all congenital small bowel obstructions and occurs in 15% of babies with cystic fibrosis; the majority of babies with meconium ileus also have cystic fibrosis. Polyhydramnios is present in about 15% of cases. Approximately 25% of babies with meconium ileus are born early. The overall incidence of meconium ileus is 1 in 20,000 live births.

Cystic fibrosis is the most common autosomal recessive disorder among individuals of Northern European descent, occurring in 1 out of every 2500 live births in these ethnic groups and in 1 out of every 3300 Caucasian births. It causes pancreatic secretions (as well as other body secretions) to be abnormally thick and sticky, resulting in pancreatic obstruction and leading to autodigestion of acinar cells. This results in abnormalities in the composition of meconium. It becomes inspissated (thickened, similar to dehydrated) in the lower ileum due to the absence of proteolytic enzymes, excess albumin and thick ileal mucus. The obstructed ileum fills with lumps of meconium that have a consistency similar to thick, sticky chewing gum, causing the ileum to become dilated and enlarged. The meconium beyond this point tends to form small hard pellets, which fill the rest of the bowel as far as the colon, which has a microlumen and is essentially empty.

Presentation: The baby with meconium ileus is born with a distended abdomen. In one-third of cases, there may be visible, palpable, doughy, indentable loops of intestines upon abdominal exam, usually with little pain or tenderness. In over 75% of cases, there is marked vomiting of bile-stained matter in the first two days of life. Meconium is not passed, although vomiting of bile-stained fluid in utero can mimic meconium passage. Lack of meconium passage by 24 hours and abdominal distension suggest meconium ileus or another lower bowel obstruction. Some babies may have respiratory distress due to counterpressure from the distended bowel.

Associated defects: Meconium ileus may be simple and isolated or complicated and associated with other problems such as volvulus, peritonitis, necrosis or bowel perforation, all of which are the product of progressive impaction of meconium. Volvulus or necrosis that occurs during early gestation leads to resorption of the involved segment of bowel, resulting in atresia and loss of bowel integrity, allowing meconium to spill into the abdominal cavity, leading to peritonitis.

Transport: Stabilize the baby with ventilatory support, if indicated, and pass an orogastric tube to vent air from the stomach and to prevent regurgitation and aspiration.

Once transport has been accomplished, a Gastrografin enema, which contains a wetting agent to soften the meconium, may be used to try and clear the bowel. An enema should not be attempted at home as bowel perforation may occur. Surgery, however, is often preferred, as complications can be hard to detect. Surgery is done to clear the bowel, resect nonviable segments of bowel and create an ileostomy.

Anorectal anomalies: An anorectal anomaly occurs in about 1 in every 2500 to 20,000 live births, depending on the study. It is rarely an isolated defect. The anal opening may be completely absent or may be adjacent to its normal site either internally or externally. There is no universally accepted classification system for these anomalies, however, once such a problem is defined, the parents should seek out the most experienced surgeon available to perform any corrective surgery. The first surgery is tricky and can result in permanent, uncorrectable damage if done poorly.

High anomalies are more common and result from rectal agenesis, with the rectum ending above the levator ani. A fistula usually connects the blind pouch to the skin, and the anal sphincter is usually intact in its normal location. High anomalies that end in a rectourethral fistula communicating with the prostatic urethra or bladder are more common in males by a ratio 3 to 1. In females, a high defect manifests with a fistula high in the yoni or as a blind end with a rectal atresia.

Low anomalies result in an imperforate anus (membranous atresia). The rectum passes through the levator ani sling, but ends close to the perineum, where a thin membrane blocks the anal opening. This results from a failure of the lowermost gastrointestinal tract to reach the perineum and form a true anal canal with adequate size and voluntary sphincter control. Low anomalies may also terminate on the perineum in an external fistula or present as anal stenosis; the incidence is more evenly balanced between the sexes than that for high anomalies. Intermediate anomalies, which are between high and low anomalies, end in a fistula to the bulbar urethra in males or to the lower yoni in females or as an anal atresia without a fistula.

Associated anomalies: Over 60% of babies with anorectal anomalies, especially those that are high ones, have one or more associated anomalies. Genitourinary defects are common accompaniments because the two systems are so closely associated during development. Genitourinary anomalies occur more often with high defects (66 to 71%) than with low defects (25%). In boys with a high imperforate anus, the most common associated anomalies are ureteral reflux (14 to 20%), renal agenesis (17%) and other urethral anomalies such as duplex urethra, megaureter, ureterocele (8%) or undescended testes (27%). In girls, urethral reflux (21%) and renal agenesis (19%) are also common; the yoni and uterus may be septate (28%). With a low, imperforate anus, urethral reflux is the most common associated anomaly (5 to 12%) in both sexes. Anorectal anomaly is also part of the extrophy of the cloaca anomaly.

Imperforate anus and a urogenital sinus with urinary obstruction may present in an otherwise normal baby girl. This represents an arrest in the embryonic development of the cloaca into the mature genitals and is not an intersex state. It is often associated with esophageal atresia; to check for this possibility, observe the baby for excessive oral secretions, which are highly indicative of an esophageal obstruction. In addition, vertebral and skeletal defects (30%), congenital heart defects, and Hirschsprung's disease may be found in these babies. Any baby found to have an anorectal defect should be examined for esophageal atresia with the passage of an orogastric tube.

Anorectal anomalies are one of the VACTERL association anomalies. Cardiac defects are also found in 50 to 80% of these children. Esophageal atresia is found in 10%. Imperforate anus accompanies a number of other conditions, syndromes and associations as well. Low defects are common in Down syndrome. Other associations are cat-eye syndrome, trisomy 18, monosomy 13q, several Mendelian syndromes, teratogen exposure such as thalidomide or progestational drugs, and maternal diabetes.

Assessment: Inspect the baby's perineum for anorectal defects by first placing the baby on his back and flexing his knees so as to bring the soles of the feet together. This relaxes the perineum.

High (rectal) imperforate anus: Gently spread the buttocks and look for an anal opening. If a high anorectal defect is present, no orifice will be visible. Attachments of the external sphincter to the perineal skin result in a localized pucker or dimple that may appear to be a normal anal opening, but no actual opening will be found. If meconium is found on the perineum, the location of a perineal fistula should be identifiable. A perineal fistula rules out a high defect.

The lack of a normal nerve supply to the sacrum may create a smooth "rocker-bottom" perineum that is slightly convex and rounded, and the gluteal cleft is less pronounced or absent. Meconium may enter the urinary tract through a urorectal fistula; this may result in visibly stained urine or may be seen as meconium oozing from the urethra. In girls, meconium may ooze from a fistula in the hymen causing a misplaced anus to be mistaken for a normal yoni orifice.

Low (anal) imperforate anus: The anal canal stops just before it reaches the perineum, with meconium oozing onto the skin surface though a fistula in either sex. Spread the buttocks to either side around the normal location of the anus and carefully inspect the midline of the perineum anterior to the normal anal location, looking for a spot of meconium that locates the fistula. The fistula may also exit in the center of the anal pucker, giving the appearance of a normally patent anal canal. However, careful inspection finds an inadequately small opening. A normal anus should be able to admit the closed end of a hemostat and dilate to the diameter of an 18 to 24 F catheter at term. (Do not, however, insert a hemostat or a little finger into the anus at home as you may tear the delicate anal mucosa. You may use the tip of a lubricated cotton swab to gently probe the external anus to test the sphincter, which still risks tissue trauma but to a lesser degree. If you suspect stenosis, transport.) A true fistula will not dilate normally. A vertical bridge of skin, which always indicates a low anomaly, often spans the opening of the fistula (this is called "bucket-handle deformity"). The opening of the fistula is often found just above the anal "wink" (the pucker of the sphincter muscle). The perineal body may appear smaller or flat and less substantial than in normal cases, with bulging or crying; it may look more normal, with a deep gluteal cleft and anal dimple. The shape noted can give a clue to the development of the underlying muscle complex.

Typical presentation in boys: A fistula usually produces a dot of meconium just above the anal wink. The fistula may also form a path extending up the perineum for a distance through the midline raphe that sometimes reaches the raphe of the scrotum. The fistula becomes filled with either a white material, meconium, or both in the first day or two of life, creating a white or black tract in the midline of the perineum. The opening of the fistula or the tract usually becomes visible after a few hours of life.

A remnant of the anal canal may present as a small dimple on the skin surface where the anal opening should be in either sex. In boys, this results in the fistula joining with the bladder (resulting in green urine) or urethra (causing undiluted meconium to trickle from the tip of the penis).

Typical presentation in girls: The outlet is more often located at the fourchette, in the posterior aspect of the vulva, than on the perineum. If it joins the yoni, meconium may freely ooze from the introitus. The size of the fistula is usually adequate for defecation, but its proximity to the urethra and yoni make infections more likely and warrant surgical correction soon after birth.

Anterior displacement of the anus: Anterior displacement can be subtle; when undetected, it can later give rise to chronic constipation. The perineal body is short and the anus lies anterior to its normal location in the center of the anal wink. There may be associated anal stenosis. The closed tip of a hemostat placed into the anus finds a prominent lower shelf just inside the anal opening (do not try this at home).

Intermediate ectopic anomalies: The rectum ends at a level closer to the perineum than it does in high anomalies, but it does not come down to where low anomalies end. A fistula that opens just behind the hymenal ring indicates an intermediate anomaly. In boys, the rectum ends in a urethral fistula at the level of the bulbar urethra. In general, the fistula does not reach the perineum, but intermediate lesions with a rectoperineal fistula have been seen.

Hirschsprung disease (congenital aganglionic megacolon): This is the most common structural cause of intestinal obstruction in the neonate, occurring in 1 in 5000 to 1 in 8000 live births. It occurs when there is a lack of nerve fibers in a segment of the colon or rectum, resulting in an inability to relax the muscles in that area. Symptoms appear only after feeding begins, and therefore usually do not manifest in the first few hours postpartum. Symptoms include failure to pass meconium within 24 hours, distension of the abdomen, bile-stained vomitus, tumultuous peristaltic sounds on auscultation, and a smooth abdominal wall on palpation. Associated disorders (present in 5 to 21% of these babies) include Down syndrome (5%) and genitourinary anomalies (<5%), including imperforate anus.

Prune-belly syndrome: This condition is marked by the absence of abdominal muscles giving the abdomen a wrinkled, baggy appearance. It is explained in more detail in the subchapter entitled "Abdominal Mass, Single Umbilical Artery, Edema, Atypical Genitalia: Detecting Kidney and Genitourinary Tract Disorders."

Jejunal, ileal and colonic atresia or stenosis: Together, bowel atresia or stenosis occur in 2 to 4 per 10,000 births. A web, scar or fibrous cord of tissue obstructs the small intestines, or the intestines terminate in a blind pouch at the jejunum, ilium or, occasionally, the colon. Jejunoileal atresia (95%) and stenosis (5%) of the small intestines occur in about 1 out of every 270 to 400 live births and account for a third of all cases of neonatal intestinal obstruction. Multiple atresias are present in 10% of these cases. In some cases, the intestines form a spiral around the central mesenteric vessels; these defects, known as an "apple peel" or "maypole" atresia, tend to be familial.

Regardless of the specific type of atresia, all forms cause gross dilation of the intestines above the defect, which may impair venous return from the bowel, causing congestion and necrosis. These babies often present with polyhydramnios in pregnancy (jejunal obstruction, 38%, and ileal, 15%) followed by rapid, severe abdominal distension (78% of jejunal atresias and 98% in ileal atresias) accompanied by bile-stained vomitus. The degree of distension depends on the level of obstruction; the lower it is, the more pronounced and generalized the distension, which can become severe enough to cause respiratory distress. These symptoms tend to develop earlier when the obstruction is higher. The length of bowel above the defect is always dilated and enlarged, with atresia producing more dilation than does stenosis. The bowel below the defect is collapsed because there has been no normal filling with meconium or swallowed air to distend it. The colon above the atresia becomes massively dilated with abdominal distension. Immediate transport is required.

If a stenosis is present, the bowel may contain some meconium and air, which may be passed as gas (this occurs about one-third of the time in jejunal or ileal stenosis). However, 60 to 71% of these babies fail to pass meconium within 24 hours. Although meconium can appear normal when it is passed, it is more common for the baby to pass grey plugs of mucus instead. Meconium peritonitis is present in about 30% of these babies, secondary to bowel infarction. The presentation of stenosis is usually delayed by days or even years. Associated anomalies include other intestinal defects such as volvulus.

Associated defects: Jejunoileal atresia is usually not associated with other complicating conditions, although one in four of these babies may have another condition that is the probable cause of the atresia: malrotation (9%), volvulus (4%), gastroschisis (3%) or intussusception (2%), as well as meconium ileus (8%) or meconium peritonitis (5%), both of which are associated with cystic fibrosis.

Transport considerations: Jejunoileal atresia is not a surgical emergency, although dehydration may develop if it goes unrecognized; the baby should be transported soon after birth. An orogastric tube can be placed to vent air from the stomach and to prevent regurgitation and aspiration. Abdominal distension may result in mild respiratory symptoms that improve with blow-by oxygen. The recognition of a jejunoileal stenosis may be delayed because small amounts of meconium can squeeze past the obstruction, giving the early impression that everything is normal. Colonic atresia is a rare cause of lower intestinal obstruction (Nakayama et al., 1997).

Malrotation of the intestines: This occurs during early gestation when the developing intestines fail to rotate and become fixed in their normal position or do so incompletely. Clinical problems are associated with nonrotation, where the intestines return to the abdominal cavity but do not properly rotate or become fixed, as well as incomplete rotation or incomplete fixation. Malrotation is found in 1 out of every 500 autopsies. In symptomatic cases, small bowel obstruction is the problem. Malrotation tends to have two major clinical problems: volvulus and duodenal obstruction, the manifestations of which most often occur in the first year of life. Ninety percent of volvulus cases occur in the first year of life, with half of these presenting in the first 7 days.

Malrotation is associated with other anomalies such as diaphragmatic hernia, abdominal wall defects, duodenal or jejunoileal atresia, imperforate anus, pyloric stenosis, Hirschsprung disease, anomalies of body symmetry, complex heart defects that involve rotation, reversal of the position of other organs, biliary atresia or misplacement, preduodenal portal vein and abnormalities of the spleen.

Malrotation with midgut volvulus: This combination is the most common to present during the early neonatal period, occurring once in every 500 live births, although many cases remain asymptomatic. It usually results in the duodenum lying behind or to the right of the superior mesenteric artery, with the cecum in front of it and with abnormal folds of peritoneum attaching the cecum to the posterior abdominal wall; these tend to obstruct the second part of the duodenum. The resulting midgut mesentery is abnormally narrow, allowing volvulus to occur. As a result, either improper attachment within the abdominal cavity or twisting can interfere with the blood supply. There are two primary presentations. In acute volvulus, the baby has sudden onset, intermittent vomiting; the vomitus may be unstained at first but then progresses to bile stained. The abdomen may be soft and undistended at first; however, volvulus is a closed obstruction, causing the intestines to fill with fluid and distend the abdomen. These babies usually pass normal meconium in a timely fashion, which can become blood-stained once symptoms appear. Abdominal pain is often absent in newborns. Digestion will produce more trauma, as filling the bowel will cause the tissue to be stretched and eventually lead to acute distress with abdominal pain, tenderness and grunting respiration. Eventually, the twisted bowel produces systemic collapse with profound shock as fluid is sequestered in the obstructed loops, resulting in hypovolemia. This leads to severe acidosis and low sodium levels (hyponatremia) with an ischemic, infected and prenecrotic midgut. In the second presentation, intestinal strangulation presents with bloody stools and abdominal distension. In either case, palpation of the abdomen is uninformative.

Associated defects: Omphalocele, diaphragmatic hernia and duodenal atresia are sometimes found with malrotation.

Meconium peritonitis: This occurs in about one out of every 20,000 to 40,000 live births. It results from prenatal perforation of the colon from any cause, most commonly meconium ileus, that releases meconium into the peritoneal cavity. Infection does not usually develop immediately since meconium is normally sterile; however, it produces an intense chemical inflammation that may result in calcifications, dense adhesions resulting in bowel obstruction or, rarely, the formation of a pseudocyst that effectively seals the meconium off from the rest of the abdominal cavity. Bacterial peritonitis will develop after birth if the perforation remains open.

Signs and symptoms: Meconium in the peritoneal cavity produces an inflammatory reaction involving the parietal peritoneum and the thin abdominal wall, causing the abdomen to be distended at birth. The overlying skin becomes bright red, swollen, taut and shiny, with pain and tenderness on palpation. Petechiae may be present. These babies may have severe dehydration and hypovolemic shock. Intestinal obstruction is also present 90% of the time. Continued leakage of intestinal contents results in free air and bacterial sepsis of the peritoneal cavity.

Duplications of the lower GI tract

Intestinal duplications: These are found within the leaves of the mesentery, with the blood supply draped over their surface. They present as either long, tubular duplications extending along a significant length of small intestine or as small, spherical cysts. Obstruction results from round cysts and sometimes from intussusception. Less commonly, when extopic gastric mucosa is present, bleeding, perforation or abdominal pain develop.

Colonic duplication: This takes two forms: limited round cysts at the cecum or long tubular duplications extending from the ileum to the anus. They are often found with other anomalies (80%), including spina bifida and duplications of the bladder, urethra or external genitalia. The proximal end of the colonic duplication always empties into the lumen of the bowel, with half having a fistula at the distal end, connecting to the urinary tract, yoni, vulva or perineum. Duplications of the anus are rare. Tubular duplications without a distal fistula become massively distended.

Rectal duplication: These round cysts occur between the rectum and the sacrum. They may appear to be either a myelomeningocele or a sacrococcygeal teratoma.

Mesenteric duplication: These duplications arise from the mesentery of the intestines. They cause pain as a result of traction on the mesentery but are soft and only rarely palpable. They may also produce partial intestinal obstruction, vomiting, and failure to thrive; obstruction develops due to recurrent segmental volvulus or chronic partial obstruction.

Presentations in various types of abdominal masses: In newborn boys, an abdominal mass arising from structures located within the peritoneal cavity is most often due to a duplication cyst of the intestines, a lymphangiomatous dysplasia of the mesentery or swollen bile ducts (from a simple liver cyst or a choledochal cyst). In girls, a mass is most often related to an ovarian cyst or duplication defects.

Mesenteric lymphangioma often (60% of the time) presents as a discrete abdominal mass that is mobile and obviously intraperitoneal. The attachment points are hard to identify, even for one skilled at palpation. It may produce simple abdominal distension or a diffuse "filling in" of the abdominal cavity with no obvious swelling that can be felt. The abdomen, in these cases, is dull on percussion, although resonant areas, from displaced intestines, can sometimes be identified. Pressure or torsion caused by the cyst may manifest with an acute abdomen.

Omphalomesenteric remnants at the umbilicus: A patent omphalomesenteric duct results in meconium and gas leaking from the umbilicus. See the subchapter entitled "Visible Defects and Abnormalities (Other Than Externalized Organs)" for a full discussion.

Intestinal injury with bleeding: An intestinal hematoma forms only rarely but may result from a traumatic birth injury. This presents with anemia, difficult feeding or intestinal obstruction, but it usually does not progress to shock.

Spontaneous perforation of the GI tract in the newborn

Although not caused by an obstructive GI defect, perforation mimics obstruction and therefore is included here.

Gastric perforation: The quoted incidence is 1 in 2900 live births, but it is probably less since hospital reports of the condition are rare. A spontaneous rip occurs in the stomach wall, presumably because of a gap in the musculature. This, combined with increased tension from distension, results in the stomach wall splitting open with the release of large amounts of free air into the abdomen, usually within the first 5 days of life. It occurs slightly more often in boys. The size of the opening ranges from 0.5 to 7 cm in length with little inflammation and no necrosis, as distinct from necrotizing enterocolitis. The abdominal wall becomes suddenly distended but may remain soft with tympanic sounds on percussion, especially over the liver. The baby may also refuse to nurse, have bile- or blood-stained vomitus, pass stools containing fresh or recently passed blood, develop respiratory distress or have hypothermia or lethargy (Holgersen, 1981).

Perforation of other regions of the GI tract: A perforation may also occur anywhere else along the gastrointestinal tract, either spontaneously or as the result of obstruction, infection (especially from necrotizing endocolitis), ulceration or intrinsic weakness of the organ wall. It may or may not be symptomatic at first, although some infants will develop respiratory distress. Some types of perforation produce abdominal distension, pneumoperitoneum and sepsis. Appendicitis manifests with refusal to nurse, associated with mild to severe abdominal distension; a mass may be found in the lower right quadrant and blood may appear in the stool.

Abdominal Mass, Single Umbilical Artery, Edema or Atypical Genitalia: Detecting Kidney and Genitourinary Tract Disorders

Fetal genitourinary tract anomalies make up 30% of all defects found during several large studies, making them the most common of all identified fetal anomalies. One out of every 135 births involves a baby with a clinically evident genital or urinary tract disorder, and some 15% of neonatal deaths can be attributed to gross congenital malformations in this region. An abnormality of the kidneys or genitourinary system should be suspected in the presence of the following:

Oligohydramnios: Too little or absent amniotic fluid is found when the kidneys do not develop at all, are hypoplastic or the urinary tract is obstructed.

Maternal drug use: Antihypertensive drugs, indomethacin before birth or prenatal cocaine use may damage the baby's kidneys.

Family history: Familial disorders such as polycystic kidneys, the Finnish form of congenital nephrotic syndrome, and nephrogenic diabetes insipidus may present at birth. The baby may be more likely to have a renal disorder herself if a sibling has a history of a chromosomal or genetic disorder.

Signs and symptoms

Severe respiratory distress after birth with multiple organ compromise and little to no urine output: The baby may void once and then have no further urine output or may have none at all. This combination strongly suggests severe renal dysfunction or agenesis. The other organ systems most often affected are the cardiovascular, respiratory and nervous systems.

Abnormal urine stream: The urine stream should be continuous. A weak, intermittent or dribbling stream suggests the presence of valves in the urethra, congenital stricture of the urethra, a ureterocele or a neurogenic bladder. Minor disorders in these categories may result in normal voiding.

Abnormal urine output: Babies who receive their placental transfusion usually void frequently after birth. In the event of a problem, urine output may be normal or greatly increased but is more commonly reduced or absent in renal failure. Continuous dribbling, urination that occurs only during crying or straining, or urination during the application of suprapubic pressure usually indicates a problem with the innervation of the urethral sphincter. (Suprapubic pressure may provoke a hyperreflexive response that mimics a problem.)

Little to no flow may be related to illness or unusual stress (perinatal asphyxia, hypotension or hemorrhage), resulting in reduced perfusion of the kidneys secondary to redistribution of the cardiac output to the most vital organs. Oliguria is therefore a sensitive marker of the severity of neurological involvement in perinatal asphyxia and correlates with outcome.

Wet cord or leakage of urine: These rare complications can occur in either sex as a result of a patent urachus. It may cause slow ballooning of the base of the clamped cord or constant oozing of urine from the cord stump. In girls, an ectopic ureter can be located just outside the urethra, resulting in incontinence.

Edema: The accumulation of significant extracellular fluid in the subcutaneous tissues is abnormal in a term baby but is often seen in preterm babies without serious disease. Mild to moderate edema may be due to illness in babies whose kidneys or heart have been damaged by asphyxia, hypotension, respiratory distress or congenital heart disease.

Abnormal abdominal wall musculature: Prune-belly syndrome results in absence of the abdominal muscles, causing the abdominal wall to be baggy and wrinkled. It is associated with an enlarged ureter and cystic renal formations, which may present as palpable soft masses to one side of the abdomen, especially in boys.

Single umbilical artery: A single umbilical artery is associated with congenital malformation of the genitourinary, musculoskeletal and cardiovascular systems.

Abdominal abnormalities: Palpate for abdominal masses, ascitic fluid (fluid in the abdominal cavity) and the presence and normal size of the kidneys. Enlarged kidneys are associated with a number of disorders such as renal vein thrombosis, acute cortical or medullary necrosis and cystic abnormalities. The difference between a large, normal kidney and an abnormally enlarged one may be difficult to distinguish on exam. In such cases, an ultrasound exam is called for.

In contrast to abdominal distension, which is usually of GI origin, most abdominal masses are due to genitourinary disorders. Dilation of the pelvis and calices of one or both kidneys, or hydronephrosis, is the most common type of abdominal mass in the newborn. It may result from obstruction of the flow of urine, vesicoureteral reflux (1/100 births), or it may be a primary congenital deformity without an apparent cause. It usually presents as a unilateral, soft and often cystic round mass. Bilateral masses in a male infant in the presence of a distended bladder suggest posterior urethral valves; in girls, ureteroceles are more likely. Multicystic, hypoplastic, lobulated kidney is usually only found on one side. Large bilateral, symmetric, firm masses without a distended bladder are found with infantile polycystic kidney disease. Renal venous thrombosis has a poorly defined incidence of about 2 in 100,000 live births and is associated with an enlarged, firm, smooth kidney in association with birth asphyxia, bloody urine and kidney failure. Adrenal hemorrhage usually occurs only on one side and presents as a lateral mass with impaired kidney function. Other masses include mesoblastic nephroma, teratoma, neuroblastoma or Wilms tumor. Obstructive urinary tract disorders occasionally cause urinary ascites, possibly due to rupture of the kidney, presenting with generalized abdominal swelling.

Other causes of abdominal masses include a retroperitoneal or ovarian teratoma. A neuroblastoma may present as either the primary tumor or an enlarged liver (sometimes with polyhydramnios and nonimmune hydrops). Pelvic neuroblastomas may compress other pelvic organs and cause hydronephrosis or intestinal obstruction. Neuroblastomas are rare, occurring once in every 36.5 to 57.8 million live births.

If the birth required lots of manipulation, the baby has a flank mass and the baby is lethargic and shocky, internal bleeding may be causative. See the chapter entitled "Birth Injuries (Other Than Cranial Injuries)."

Other congenital anomalies: Renal dysfunction is frequently associated with a wide variety of anomalies other than those of the abdomen. A high index of suspicion should be prompted when you find low-set or abnormally formed ears or supernumerary nipples.

Atypical genitalia: Atypical genitalia are highly associated with disorders of the lower urinary tract (bladder and urethra). The upper urinary tract and kidneys, which develop earlier in gestation, are much less commonly involved when the genitals are atypical. A midline mass in a baby girl may be due to distension of the uterus and yoni with fluid, especially if the mass remains once the bladder is empty. Epispadias and hypospadias are types of genital defects most commonly found in boys. Any or all of the following features may be noted: the glans is partially or completely exposed, there may be no foreskin or the urethra may be misplaced (either on top of or underneath the penis).

The parents should understand that an infant with such a defect should not be circumcised! A pediatrician should be consulted soon after the birth whenever atypical genitalia are found. There is no need to transport if no other defects are found and two testes are identified in the scrotum.

Abnormal placental findings: The presence of amnion nodosum (small whitish specks, ranging from 1 to 5 mm in diameter), on the fetal surface is thought to be a result of the abrasion of keratinized fetal skin against the amnion, where it will adhere in the absence of fetal urine. They may be associated with renal agenesis.

General transport considerations

Babies suspected of having any genitourinary disorders should be transported right away. They are at high risk for fluid and electrolyte imbalances. Withhold fluids until evaluation can be obtained.

The most common disorders of the genitourinary tract

Neuropathic (neurogenic) bladder: Neuropathic bladder is characterized by difficulty with the passage of urine due to impaired innervation. It occurs in conjunction with a variety of newborn defects including (in decreasing order of likelihood) myelomeningocele, sacral agenesis, lumbosacral lipoma, other spinal lesions and unknown causes. It may be acquired secondary to severe vascular damage affecting the blood supply to the spinal cord, a tumor or dermal sinus formation with an intradural abscess.

Hydronephrosis: Hydronephrosis is the most common cause of an abdominal mass in the newborn; it can vary in severity from insignificant to life threatening. Hydronephrosis occurs when the ureter is obstructed as it exits the kidney (at the pelvic-ureteric junction), causing urine to back up into the kidney. Extreme damage to the kidney tissue may result; the extent of the damage is, to a degree, proportional to the duration of the obstruction. It has been found via prenatal ultrasound in 0.5% of all fetuses, 60% of which will resolve on their own prior to birth. However, it has also been seen in 3.8% of all autopsies with a renal pelvic dilation over 10 mm. Most cases of hydronephrosis are not serious and can be handled without surgery, but all babies who present with a palpable flank mass should be further evaluated. Not all babies with this condition have an obstructed ureter, and some will have good renal function. The most common presenting symptom is a palpable abdominal mass, but this defect may not be apparent at birth. Associated disorders include vertebral, anorectal, cardiac, tracheoesophageal, renal and limb (the VACTERL association anomalies) malformations, several chromosomal anomalies and fetal environmental syndromes and associations.

Abdominal masses of genitourinary origin: A retroperitoneal teratoma may present as an asymptomatic abdominal mass, more often on the left than the right, with one-third extending across the midline. A renal tumor may result in a palpably enlarged kidney.

In girls, an ovarian cyst, when large enough, presents a fairly large, usually smooth, mobile and nontender mass that can be displaced into the upper abdomen. Systemic symptoms are rare but can include respiratory distress and ascites. The vascular pedicle attaching these cysts is usually quite thin, and twisting may result in symptoms of an acute abdomen. A cystic ovarian teratoma may also present a palpable mass.

Obstruction of the yoni by a transverse septum can produce massive abdominal enlargement causing displacement and obstruction of the urethra, intestines and bladder. Unlike an imperforate hymen, the external genitalia appear normal and there is a perineal bulge due to a build-up of fluids in the peritoneal cavity.

Renal vein thrombosis occurs most often in children of diabetic mothers. The affected kidney is enlarged and hemorrhagic. The thrombosis originates peripherally and spreads to the center of the kidney. It may occur suddenly in a previously well baby but is more often caused by traumatic birth, hypoxia, sepsis and dehydration. It presents a palpable smooth, firm mass along the side of the abdomen (flank) with blood-stained urine in an otherwise unwell newborn. Massive adrenal hemorrhage also produces a firm mass in the flank with signs of hypovolemic shock.

Renal agenesis: Absence of a kidney on one side occurs once in every 500 to 1500 live births and once in every 150 stilllborns. There is a slightly higher incidence among males, and it is more common on the left. There are no specific symptoms, although clinical findings that prompt urological examination are often due to the absence of one kidney.

Bilateral renal agenesis is more rare, occurring once in every 4000 to 5000 births, with a ratio of 3 boys affected for every girl. Since these babies have hypoplastic lungs, they present with acute respiratory distress; they are further discussed in the subchapter entitled "Complicated Respiratory Distress," item 2.

Lower urinary tract obstruction:

In boys: Posterior urethral valves are the most common cause of lower urinary tract obstruction. They are thought to occur in 1 out of every 5000 to 8000 boys, although the true incidence is obscured by the wide variety in presentation and age of diagnosis. They have not been identified in girls. These valves are thick and rigid; they tend to be directed downward and to the side around the lumen of the urethra and fused at a lower level. The valve cusps obstruct the flow of urine, leading to kidney damage. The most likely symptom at birth is an abnormal urinary stream, although there may be a midline abdominal mass due to bladder distension, a flank mass due to an enlarged kidney, or ascites. Note that an intrapelvic sacrococcygeal teratoma may also produce obstructive uropathy. Anterior urethral valves and anterior urethral diverticulum in boys are far less common but present a similar clinical picture.

In girls: Obstruction may be caused by a variety of anomalies in girls as well. Urethral duplication is rare and is usually found with bladder duplication. When occurring with a single bladder, the primary urethra can exit on the perineum or in the yoni while the other urethra is phallic or both urethras may be placed perineally or in the yoni, and there may be a double clitoris. Although most cases are asymptomatic, a double urine stream or urinary obstruction may be present.

Congenital obstruction of the yoni may occur due to an imperforate hymen, transverse yoni septum, yoni atresia, and rarely, yoni agenesis. Complete obstruction of the yoni (1/16,000 female births) causes secretions to build up and is an important consideration when an abdominal mass is found. Yoni obstruction can also result in urethral obstruction, presenting as a symmetrical abdominal mass and leading to hydronephrosis, compression of adjacent organs with venous stasis in the lower extremities, and respiratory distress. Yoni atresia can be associated with multiple anomalies.

A urogenital sinus exists when the urethra and yoni have a common channel with a single shared opening at the vulva. It is found in virilized female babies and also as an isolated defect. Anomalies of the vestibule, urethra and bladder are often found as well. Yoni obstruction may occur due to the angular junction of the urethra and yoni or from stenosis, causing secretions and urine to accumulate.

Cloacal defects occur when a single perineal opening leads to an anterior urogenital sinus into which the rectum opens. The labial folds may be malformed and the clitoris enlarged. About 30% of these babies also have retention of genital secretions and urine, resulting in an irregular abdominal mass composed of both bowel and bladder contents.

Two cases of urethral diverticulum in the neonate had been reported in the literature as of 1994. A diverticulum is a saccular outpouching from the wall of any tubular organ. It may present either as a cystic mass at the introitus or with urethral symptoms, although upper urinary tract obstruction does not occur.

Urethral atresia: Absence of the urethra prevents urination. It presents with a grossly enlarged bladder and very little amniotic fluid. Most of these babies are stillborn. Those that are born alive usually succumb to pulmonary hypoplasia.

Multicystic dysplastic kidney (MCDK): This disorder occurs in about 1 out of every 3000 to 4300 births, making it the second most common cause of an abdominal mass in the newborn. This mass is the primary presenting symptom, although the presentation of this disorder may be delayed into the first two years of life. Those babies with bilateral anomalous kidneys often present with Potter's syndrome.

Prune-belly syndrome (Eagle-Barrett syndrome or triad syndrome): This disorder involves defective muscle development of the anterior abdominal wall and the urinary tract, often accompanied by several other errors of development. Its overall incidence is 1 out of every 29,000 to 40,000 live births, with 95% of these being male. It is presumably caused by obstruction of the lower urinary tract. The severity varies and may involve only one or both sides of the abdomen. The mild form occurs with definite but mild or incomplete features of the syndrome; urinary tract dilation is less pronounced and drainage is good. Most affected babies fall in the moderate group, which results in moderate urinary tract dilation with or without renal dysplasia. The severe form results in stillbirth or neonatal death from severe pulmonary hypoplasia and renal dysplasia. Oligohydramnios is frequently an associated finding.

Presentation in boys: The deficiency of abdominal musculature varies considerably and may be patchy or asymmetrical. The lower recti muscles are most often affected; the lower center of the belly may consist only of skin, fat and fibrous tissue, with the umbilicus placed above its normal location. The skin over the affected parts is often wrinkled, like a prune, with abnormal transverse creases but may be soft, lumpy and distended. The lower border of the ribs is flared, and the sternum is typically prominent. The upper portions of the recti and oblique muscles are usually present. Associated gastrointestinal defects include volvulus and intestinal obstruction. Changes in the genitourinary system are frequently seen; their severity is proportional to the deficiency of the abdominal wall musculature. The bladder is enlarged and the urachus patent to the umbilicus. The ureters and pelvises of the kidneys are often dilated; the degree of dilation depends upon the amount of back pressure from obstruction of the lower urinary tract. One or both testes are undescended. These babies have renal failure, acidosis and dehydration, and may be septic. They may also have respiratory impairment due to the absent abdominal muscles, with an inability to cough and clear the chest of secretions. The full presentation of this disorder occurs only in boys.

***Associated defects in boys*:** Associated defects include pulmonary stenosis or hypoplasia, deformities of the feet (such as club feet), hip dislocation, cleft lip, spina bifida, compression marks on the lower abdomen, dimples on the knees and elbows, impairment of the lower limbs, cardiac anomalies (10%), deafness and mental retardation.

Presentation in girls: Fewer than 50 cases of prune-belly syndrome were reported in girls by 1990. The affected females have the same type of abdominal wall defects found in boys, but most have a normal urinary tract. Only rarely have genitourinary and anorectal anomalies, including yoni atresia and various urinary tract defects, been found.

Exstrophy of the bladder: This rare defect involves an externalized bladder that is split down the anterior midline. It is discussed in the subchapter entitled "Externalized Organs and Neural Tube Defects."

Renal failure: Acute kidney failure is a clinical syndrome that follows a decrease in renal function of sufficient magnitude to result in retention of nitrogenous waste products. It occurs in about 8% of all babies sick enough to require neonatal intensive care. Anuria (no urine output) is the primary clinical sign. When it goes unrecognized, a clinical picture of increasing metabolic derangement develops with general nonspecific signs of a sick baby, such as lethargy. There are three different types:

Prerenal failure: The most common neonatal cause of failure in normal kidneys is inadequate renal blood flow or blood oxygenation, usually resulting from some type of shock or heart failure. The major causes are shown in the table below and are not rare. Inadequate perfusion of normal kidneys occurs when blood flow to the kidneys is reduced due to hypotension or hypovolemia, either alone or together. Allowing the baby to receive a full placental transfusion will help obviate some of the effects of acute hypoperfusion that may have occurred in utero. If poor perfusion is the problem, IV therapy begun after transport should produce urine flow; *do not attempt to give the baby an IV at home.*

Intrinsic failure: The kidneys themselves are structurally abnormal from congenital or acquired defects. Many of these babies have already experienced significant perinatal asphyxia; they often present with compromise of other organ systems (especially central nervous, pulmonary and cardiovascular systems). Dehydration and shock, which may occur in a number of neonatal disorders, often lead to intrinsic failure, especially in very low birthweight babies.

Postrenal failure: In postrenal failure the kidneys are functioning normally, but there is an obstruction of the flow of urine after it is filtered that can usually be corrected. Long-standing obstruction may lead to kidney damage, especially when due to the presence of posterior urethral valves and ureteropelvic junction obstruction. Renal failure may present in these cases despite normal or even increased urinary output.

Primary Causes of Renal Failure in the Newborn

Prerenal failure	Intrinsic failure	Postrenal failure
Asphyxia Dehydration Hypotension due to Maternal hemorrhage Fetal or newborn hemorrhage Early cord clamping Twin-to-twin transfusion Congestive heart failure	Congenital anomalies Cystic dysplasia Renal hypoplasia, dysplasia or agenesis Polycystic kidneys Inflammatory: Congenital syphilis or toxoplasmosis Pyelonephritis Vascular disorders: Venous or arterial thrombosis Disseminated intravascular coagulation Acute tubular necrosis: Perinatal asphyxia Dehydration Shock Nephrotoxins Renal ischemia: Hypotension Congestive heart failure Sepsis Hypoxia Nephrotoxins	Urethral obstruction Posterior urethral valves Imperforate foreskin Urethral stricture Urethral diverticulum Megaurethra Ureterocele Ureteropelvic or ureterovesical obstruction Extrinsic tumors compressing bladder outlet Neuropathic bladder

The most common cause of both prerenal and intrinsic failure is decreased renal perfusion. This usually occurs when a prerenal condition has caused kidney damage, resulting in an intrinsic defect.

General presentation: Although renal failure can be associated with a normal or increased urinary output, acute renal failure in newborns usually presents with minimal to absent urination. The typical case involves a severely asphyxiated baby who has compromise in multiple organ systems. The baby may void once and then subsequently fail to produce any urine; alternatively, there may be no urination at all from birth onward. When this combination is present, renal failure should be assumed, fluids withheld and transport undertaken immediately.

Patent urachus: If urine is leaking from the umbilicus, the baby has a patent urachus. This defect is discussed in the subchapter entitled "Visible Defects and Abnormalities (Other Than Externalized Organs)."

Transport considerations

Babies suspected of having any genitourinary disorders should be transported right away. They are at high risk for fluid and electrolyte imbalances. Withhold fluids until evaluation can be obtained.

NEONATAL HYPERTENSION

The incidence of hypertension in the total newborn population (both term and preterm, sick and healthy babies) is 0.2 to 3%. In term babies, the incidence of hypertension is extremely low, with the vast majority of affected babies having other identified problems. For this reason, standard newborn exam protocols do not call for routine assessment of the neonatal blood pressure; even if symptoms are acute and life threatening, the midwife will focus on stabilization and transport. However, it is helpful to understand the reasons why hypertension may develop in newborns, the conditions in which it is likely to arise, and the ways in which it will present. As with adults, hypertension is not a diagnosis in itself, but indicative of an underlying condition. Such conditions include:

Vascular problems: Vascular disorders causing hypertension include renal artery thrombosis, aortic thrombosis, congenital renovascular anomalies, coarctation of the aorta, and hypoplasia of the aorta. Suspect hypertension due to aortic thrombosis in asphyxiated infants with hypertension, especially if there are additional risk factors such as polycythemia, maternal diabetes, severe dehydration, congenital heart disease or sepsis. Hypertension may be caused by a lesion of the renal artery or its branches that impairs blood flow to all or part of the kidney. Renal vein thrombosis alone does not usually result in hypertension; it more typically presents with sudden enlargement of the involved kidney, shock, hematuria, and uremia.

Renal anomalies: Disorders of the kidneys often lead to hypertension, including infantile polycystic kidney, hypoplastic kidneys, obstructions of the urinary tract, acute and chronic renal insufficiency, renal tumors, medullary cystic diseases and multicystic kidney. Congenital renal artery stenosis accounts for 20% of cases of newborn hypertension. Congenital anomalies of the urinary tract may occasionally cause hypertension. Bilaterally enlarged kidneys may be due to polycystic kidneys (usually associated with hypoplastic lungs), which often cause hypertension.

Medications: Steroids, vitamin D, ocular phenylephrine and pancuronium can cause hypertension.

Endocrinological disorders: Endocrinological causes of neonatal hypertension are generally rare. Pheochromocytoma causes sustained hypertension. Cushing disease commonly presents with hypertension from abnormally high blood levels of cortisol produced by a hyperfunctioning adrenal cortex. Primary hyperaldosteronism is exceedingly rare in infancy and is usually associated with an increase in both diastolic and systolic blood pressure due to an increase in blood volume from excessive secretion of aldosterone from the adrenal gland.

Other causes: These include increased intracranial pressure, neural crest tumors and maternal cocaine intoxication.

Presentation

Cardiorespiratory and neurological signs are common in babies presenting with hypertension. However, most symptoms are nonspecific and may result from other medical conditions.

Congestive heart failure is a frequent reason for hypertension. Neurological signs include lethargy, coma, tremors, apnea, opisthotonos posture (extended head, arched back), seizures and one-sided paralysis, symptoms that may also be caused by intracranial hemorrhage in some babies.

Coarctation of the aorta is frequently associated with hypertension. It is characterized by elevated blood pressure in the arteries closest to the coarctation and decreased blood pressure in vessels more distant from the defect. As a rule, the baby has hypertension in the arms and hypotension in the legs (normally the blood pressure is slightly higher in the legs). Occasionally, the left subclavian artery will be involved and the blood pressure will also be low in the left arm. Palpating the femoral arteries can rule out coarctation. On rare occasions, these babies also suffer intracranial bleeding, thought to be from systemic hypertension, which may be only moderate. Coarctation of the aorta is often associated with multiple cerebral arteriovenous malformations (although without bleeding), which may be a contributing factor (Volpe, 2001).

Complete thrombotic blockage of the aorta, an extremely rare event, is heralded by the sudden onset of ischemia of the lower extremities and loss of femoral pulses. Characteristic changes in the appearance of the retina may also occur with an increased ratio of venous to arterial caliper, vascular twisting and superficial and deep hemorrhages. These findings may normalize once the blood pressure is under control.

NEONATAL SHOCK AND HYPOTENSION

Note: The chapter entitled "An Overview of Shock Syndromes" and the subchapter entitled "Understanding Fetal and Neonatal Asphyxia" should be studied prior to studying this chapter. This chapter builds on that information.

Shock from blood loss is the primary reason an otherwise healthy baby may become hypotensive. Babies may also become hypotensive with conditions such as respiratory distress, asphyxia, sepsis or congenital heart disease. Here is a list of conditions what result in neonatal shock, hypotension or both:

Umbilical cord accidents Cord compression leading to fetal hypovolemia Iatrogenic: clamping before the placental transfusion is complete, especially in preterm or asphyxiated babies Tearing or breaking of the cord Prolapse Entanglement Anomalous vessels Vasa previa Velamentous cord insertion **Abnormalities of the placenta** Previa Abruption Multilobar **Fetal or neonatal hemolysis** Maternal blood group incompatibility Erythrocyte membrane abnormality (such as hereditary spherocytosis) Erythrocyte enzyme abnormality (such as glucose-6-phosphate dehydrogenase deficiency)	**Fetal or neonatal hemorrhage** Fetomaternal hemorrhage Twin-to-twin transfusion Intracranial hemorrhage Subgaleal hemorrhage Intraabdominal hemorrhage **Maternal factors** Infection Hypotension General anesthesia Spinal anesthesia Vasoactive drugs **Other contributing factors** Intrauterine asphyxia Infection Intrathoracic air leak Positive-pressure ventilation with high airway pressures Structural heart disease Patent ductus arteriosus Arrhythmia

<u>Organ perfusion in the newborn</u>

Systemic hypotension allows increased right to left blood flow through the ductus arteriosus, especially when the pulmonary artery pressure is quite high. As a result, hypotensive infants are often poorly oxygenated. Cardiac output is the product of heart rate and stroke volume. In adults, the output of the left ventricle is emphasized; however, in newborns the output of the right ventricle is important because of the frequent concurrence of abnormally elevated pulmonary vascular resistance. The newborn heart rate is high, ranging from 120 to 160 bpm. Elevations above this range may result in minimal increases or even decreases in cardiac output in infants because higher rates shorten ventricular filling time and thus result in a lower diastolic volume. In addition, myocardial oxygen consumption rises with the extra work. Since myocardial perfusion occurs during diastole, any further rise in the heart rate reduces the amount of myocardial perfusion and may lead to undesirable ischemia and ventricular dysfunction. A low heart rate can also compromise output, although some normal infants have mild bradycardia with no impairment.

Finally, the blood reaching the tissues must carry the necessary oxygen and nutrients. The oxygen content of the blood is directly determined by lung function. The delivery of glucose and other energy sources are determined by dietary intake and mobilization of stored fat and glycogen by the liver and other organs. No matter how much blood goes to the tissues, the cells will not be nourished if the blood is deficient in nutrients. Improving blood perfusion and function of the lungs as well as the baby's energy status are necessary to restore tissue perfusion. The ability of the blood to carry oxygen is greatly influenced by the hemoglobin concentration. A hemoglobin of less than 13 g/dl may result in a low oxygen-carrying capacity in the acutely ill infant. Hemoglobin concentrations exceeding 22 g/dl may sometimes reduce oxygen delivery because of hyperviscosity with blood flow. Fetal hemoglobin has a much higher affinity for binding oxygen than does that of the adult, which results in a decreased ability to unload oxygen into the tissues. Other factors that affect unloading include acidosis, hypothermia and hypocapnia (decreased arterial carbon dioxide tension).

Neonatal shock

Shock due to inadequate tissue perfusion is a common problem of seriously compromised neonates. In some of these babies, the process will have begun in utero. Babies who have already suffered an injury to the heart or vascular system, or whose intravascular blood volume is severely compromised to the point that the heart muscle and vascular system cannot fulfill their function in delivering blood to the tissues, may respond poorly or not at all to attempts at resuscitation. Additional problems such as systemic infection, persistently patent ductus arteriosus or thoracic air leaks may result from attempts to ventilate the unresponsive baby.

Presentation: The progression of newborn shock roughly parallels that of the adult. In the early stages, the newborn exhibits prolonged capillary refill time (over 3 seconds), excessive temperature gradient between the surface and the core (core 7.2°F [2°C] or more above the surface temperature), a respiratory rate well over 70 rpm and a heart rate above 160 bpm. Pallor may be present with acute blood loss. Urine output is often minimal (less than 0.5 ml/kg/hr) or absent. As shock progresses, blood pressure falls (hypotension is a late sign of shock in neonates), and tachypnea, persistent oliguria, tachycardia and progressive enlargement of the liver result in a baby who is increasingly listless, dull to sensation and unresponsive. Extremely narrow pulse pressure (the difference between the systolic and diastolic blood pressure readings) and decreased core and surface temperatures develop with continued deterioration.

Evaluation: Assess capillary refill time, color of the skin and mucous membranes, pulse quality and heart rate. In the hospital, blood pressure would be determined; you will generally not take the time to check it at home. In the newborn, supportive measures may normalize perfusion. Dry and warm the baby, give supplemental oxygen or full CPR as indicated, and transport.

Type of shock: Hypovolemic shock is typically associated with events such as abruption or previa, umbilical cord compression from intrauterine pressure or prolapse, or significant maternal hemorrhage. Internal or external fetal or newborn bleeding from accidents such as cord breakage, hematoma or ruptured vasa previa may produce massive blood loss yet not be apparent. Findings include pallor, narrow pulse pressure (presenting as a fast, thready pulse on palpation) and tachycardia. Unresolved hypovolemic shock may evolve into a form of cardiogenic shock as the heart muscle becomes damaged; eventually, cardiac activity fails. If the cord is still intact, hold the placenta up to the length of the cord to allow as much blood as possible to drain back into the baby, and transport.

Newborn cardiogenic shock is usually associated with severe perinatal asphyxia, structural heart defects or arrhythmias. Myocardial ischemia reduces contractility and causes muscle dysfunction, resulting in tricuspid valve insufficiency. The body's attempts to compensate may result in further depression of cardiac function. Increased systemic vascular resistance via vasoconstriction maintains blood pressure and vital organ perfusion but increases left ventricular afterload, resulting in increased myocardial oxygen consumption. Sodium and water retention occur because of a perceived decrease in circulating volume. Decreased left ventricular output in combination with the increased flow of blood to the heart may lead to pulmonary edema. Right ventricular dysfunction may lead to peripheral edema, venous stasis, enlargement of the liver and decreased blood flow through the lungs. This results in worsening hypoxemia and acidosis, which perpetuate this vicious cycle. Clinical findings include peripheral edema, narrow pulse pressure, liver and heart enlargement, and heart murmur, which suggests tricuspid insufficiency.

Distributive shock is most frequently caused by sepsis in the newborn. Clinical findings often include maternal fever or other signs of maternal infection. Toxins and mediators released by the invading microorganisms cause multiple hemodynamic disruptions. Complement, coagulation, and other chemical pathways are activated in early septic shock, resulting in increased permeability of the microvasculature and extensive capillary leakage. The baby initially presents with tachycardia, tachypnea, wide pulse pressures and peripheral edema in the absence of an enlarged liver. Myocardial function deceases as the infection progresses; findings similar to those seen in cardiogenic shock ensue.

The differentiation of the type of shock is not always possible. Support should focus on allowing the maximum amount of placental transfusion possible, maintaining warmth, providing resuscitative assistance as warranted, and transporting without delay.

VISIBLE DEFECTS AND ABNORMALITIES (OTHER THAN EXTERNALIZED ORGANS)

Some of the conditions described in other chapters also have visible signs and symptoms; however, visibility is the predominant symptom for the defects presented here. Babies with gross anatomical defects should not be left in the unsupervised care of their parents right after birth, as the parents are in total shock regarding this finding in their newborn.

Anatomical deformities

Bizarre, malformed facial features

The most severe types of malformation syndromes and disruptions are associated with disfiguring craniofacial defects. The incidence is 1.43 to 4.85 per 100,000 live births (excluding cleft lip, cleft palate or both, which occur in 1 out of every 750 live births). Extensive facial clefting that runs at an oblique angle across the head is likely to be due to a disruption from an amniotic band. The nose and eyes may be severely malformed to the point that a single nostril or single eye opening may be present, or none at all. Facial clefts that run in a longitudinal or transverse direction are more often due to malformations associated with syndromes. The baby may have such severely altered facies that normal methods of resuscitation are rendered impossible. Do the best you can to stabilize the baby and transport. Severely deformed facial features are one of the most difficult fetal defects for parents to grapple with; be as reassuring as possible and stabilize the mother so that she can join her baby at the hospital as soon as possible.

Abnormally protruding eye: Certain congenital syndromes and metabolic disorders can cause the eye to protrude from its socket. An orbital teratoma, while rare, presents an alarming clinical picture, with marked protrusion of the affected eye and enlargement of the bony orbit. The eyeball may be distorted or even completely prolapsed by the tumor, and the optic nerve can be damaged due to stretching. Apply normal saline to the eyeball, cover it with a saturated sterile nonadherent dressing (do not use gauze, as it is very abrasive) and transport immediately.

Missing feet, hands, limbs, or digits

The two primary causes of missing parts of an extremity are amniotic bands and congenital exposure to a teratogenic substance that interfered with limb formation.

Amniotic band syndrome (ADAM [amniotic deformities; adhesions; mutilation], sequence or complex): This problem occurs in approximately 7.7 out of every 10,000 live births. Typically the amnion ruptures at some point during pregnancy and rolls up into a string or band. This band becomes wrapped around a fetal part, which may be eventually amputated. In addition to outright amputation, amniotic bands may result in constrictions presenting as grooves of varying depth, with underlying necrosis or linear erosions of tissue. Unilateral, nonuniform amputation suggests this as the cause. The areas affected, from most to least frequent, include the fingers, toes, limbs, cranium, and abdominal wall. Strangulation of the umbilical cord can kill the fetus. Severe cases result in combinations of craniofacial malformations such as clefting of the face, palate, eyelids, and other eye deformities, as well as absence of portions of the skull and brain. Such disruptions are thought to be caused when a strip of amnion is caught in the mouth during fetal swallowing, the strip damages the delicate fetal structures that it contacts. Amniotic disruption (tearing) may result in a hole that exposes the embryo to direct contact with the much rougher inner surface of the chorion, to which the body may adhere.

Other causes: Vascular accident or intrinsic defects of the skeleton, usually resulting in missing extremities, commonly show bilateral involvement as well as damage from a teratogen, and an inheritance pattern. The most notorious example of a teratogen is thalidomide, a sedative that causes severe limb deformities in babies whose mothers take it during early pregnancy.

Fused legs

Sirenomelia, or mermaid fetus, is a lethal defect always found with oligohydramnios due to renal agenesis. These babies have a single lower limb (fused legs) and may have one foot, two feet or no feet; they lack an anus, have abnormal genitalia and commonly have postural deformities. The incidence is 1.5 to 4.2 per 100,000 live births.

V-shaped hands or feet; missing or fused digits

Clefting of the hands or feet with missing digits is commonly referred to as "lobster-claw deformity." It typically results in the absence of the third distal ray with a deep triangular cleft extending to the level of the carpal bones. Fingers bordering the cleft may be fused or flexed, hypoplastic or missing entirely. The feet may also present a V-shaped deformity. The atypical form of this defect is an isolated finding, but others are associated with additional malformations.

Soft, midline chest defect possibly with visible palpitations

A cleft sternum is usually accompanied by a normally placed heart (congenital heart defects are rare). The midline sternal defect may be covered with skin, while the underlying internal tissue layers remain intact, or it may present as a discolored region or with a thinly covered, poorly epithelialized layer of skin that may move as the heart beats and through which the heart can be seen. There may be paradoxical movement of the chest during breathing. Sinus openings and lesions that look like sores have also been reported. Crying produces a dramatic increase in the apparent severity of the deformity. Transport is required; no special precautions are necessary other than ensuring that no pressure that may rupture the overlying skin or injure the heart is applied to the chest.

Atypical genitalia

It may be hard to determine if a baby really has atypical genitalia, as some cases are very subtle. Nevertheless, if atypical genitalia are even suspected, the baby should be transported for evaluation as soon as possible. These babies may suffer from salt-losing adrenal deficiency. If so, they are in grave danger of a systemic salt imbalance that can be fatal if not treated. You will not be able to rule this out at home; neonatal care and evaluation should take place without delay. The treatment for atypical genitalia is controversial. More details on this subject can be found in DIAGNOSTIC TESTS and HOLISTIC MIDWIFERY, Vol. III.

Tumors (swellings or any mass) in or Under the Skin

A number of different lesions may present with large lumps at birth. Most tumors will present as a visible or palpable mass. Those deep in the head or neck may be less obvious, although they may be large enough to produce respiratory distress from obstruction, compression or invasion. (Since the primary presenting symptom in these locations is respiratory distress, they are also covered in the subchapter entitled "Complicated Respiratory Distress" [item 1].) Hemangiomas, on rare occasions, may be present at birth; they are discussed more fully in the subchapter entitled "Examining the Skin." Most babies who have tumors but no symptoms do not require emergency transport, but should be evaluated shortly after birth. Those with large, obstructive tumors or teratomas should be transported per the protocols at the end of the discussion of teratomas.

Cystic hygroma

These tumors occur once in every 6000 term babies. They are a benign, localized cystic masses that are soft, ill defined, impressible, fluid filled and translucent on transillumination. They commonly appear on the neck and upper arm and rarely in the groin or behind the knee.

Dermoid cyst

These give a dramatic appearance as they often develop along the lines of fusion on the head, especially around the eyes and nose. There may be a sinus, often with a protruding hair. They may or may not be ruptured. Dermoid cysts contain ectodermal structures and may be attached to underlying structures; this should be excluded prior to removal.

Encephalocele

This variably sized fluctuant, sometimes pulsating mass may appear anywhere along the midline of the face or skull. It is discussed more fully in the subchapter entitled "Externalized Organs and Neural Tube Defects."

Lymphangioma

These masses of anomalous lymphatic vessels or channels vary in size, are usually greatly dilated, and are lined with normal endothelial cells. Lymphoid tissue is usually present in the peripheral portions of the lesions, which are present at birth or shortly thereafter and probably represent maldevelopment of lymphatic vessels (rather than true neoplasms). They occur most frequently in the neck and axilla but may also develop in the arm, mesentery, chest, retroperitoneum, and other sites. There are several types.

Lymphangioma simplex: These are singular, well defined, usually smooth, flesh colored, dermal and subcutaneous tumors that may occur anywhere on the skin or mucous membranes. They are most commonly found on the neck, upper trunk, inner surfaces of the arms and legs, and tongue.

Lymphangioma circumscriptum: The most common form of lymphangioma, this appears as clusters of deep-seated, thick-walled vesicles that have the appearance of frog eggs or grapes. These commonly appear on the inner surface of the limbs, shoulders, neck, axilla and adjacent chest wall, perineum, inguinal folds, tongue and mucous membranes.

Cavernous lymphangioma: These present as soft, diffuse masses of tissue. They consist of large cystic masses of dilated lymphatic vessels in the dermis and subcutaneous tissue and may involve the muscle layer. They are ill defined and often cover large areas of the face, trunk, limbs, and sometimes the tongue.

Nasal glioma

Very rarely, nasal gliomas present in newborns, affecting slightly more boys than girls. About 60% are extranasal, 30% are intranasal, and 10% are combined, passing through the nasal bones; rarely they may arise from the palate. Extranasal lesions are most common, presenting on the nasal bridge as a soft, skin-covered mass in the midline, or slightly to one side, resulting in widening of the nasal bones. As distinguished from an encephalocele, the glioma is a solid, nonpulsating mass that does not expand with crying.

Neurofibroma

These swellings may arise in any part of the body, especially in the subcutaneous tissues, either by themselves or in association with von Recklinghausen neurofibromatosis. They present as moderately firm, encapsulated tumors.

Tumor of the parotid or salivary glands

Several different varieties of tumors can arise from the parotid gland, including neurofibromas. These tumors present with swelling along one or both sides of the face, in front of the ear.

Tumor of the chest wall

A benign tumor of the chest wall presents a hard, fixed mass with marked rib deformation. It can produce respiratory distress if sufficiently large. Malignant chest tumors may also be visible at birth.

Hemangioma

Although uncommon, a hemangioma may present a visible lesion at birth. It can obstruct underlying tissues and organs if sufficiently large, giving rise to symptoms associated with impaired function of the organs involved.

Teratoma

Teratomas are tumors made up of tissues derived from all three germ layers. These tissues are arranged in a disorganized fashion, at varying degrees of maturation not normally found in the organs from which they arise. The tumor may contain all types of tissue, although neural tissue predominates. Malignancy may arise from any of its component tissues. Teratomas may be cystic, solid, or both. While the sites discussed in detail below are the most common, a teratoma can develop anywhere in the body; intracranial, orbital, intraoral (epignathus), cervical (including thyroid), mediastinal, intracardiac, gastric, renal, retroperitoneal, mesenteric, sacrococcygeal, ovarian and testicular varieties have all been noted in the literature. Most teratomas arise in the midline or para-axial position.

Sacrococcygeal teratoma is the most common teratoma and the most common tumor of the newborn, believed to occur in 1 out of every 40,000 live births, with a ratio of 4 affected girls for every boy. The tumor arises from the anterior portion of the coccyx. From here, it may extend into the pelvis (10%) with no external mass, as an external posterior mass (46%) or in both directions as a dumbbell-shaped mass (44%). Associated anomalies, including imperforate or stenotic anus and spina bifida, are found in about 10% of these babies. Musculoskeletal disorders are common, especially congenital hip dysplasia (7%) due to displacement by the tumor. Extrapelvic tumors are associated with spondylolysis of the lumbosacral spine, and intrapelvic tumors are seen with spina bifida occulta and other vertebral anomalies. The mother may suffer from "mirror syndrome" when she carries a baby with a sacrococcygeal teratoma, causing her to develop hypertension and a toxemic-like condition should her baby become hydropic.

While most babies are otherwise unaffected, some tumors may cause symptoms associated with their size or position or their physiological effects. Prior to birth, the fetus may develop hydrops, a large placenta and polyhydramnios, all of which are ominous and predict a fatal outcome. Rupture may lead to exsanguination. The size may approximate that of the head, resulting in dystocia during labor or at birth. The intrapelvic part may obstruct the urinary or intestinal tract, causing urinary retention, incontinence, constipation, or frequent stools (these symptoms appear later). Blood flow through the tumor may be such that high-output cardiac failure results. Respiratory insufficiency is a primary cause of early death from preterm birth, cardiac failure or both.

A sacrococcygeal teratoma appears as a large tumor, typically a mass that may approach half the baby's weight. It may be covered entirely with skin or have cystic, hemangioma-like or ulcerated areas. The anus faces forward, appearing as a large dimple beneath the genitalia. Smaller lesions are often far less obvious. The mass may be centered over the posterior sacrum, mimicking a lipoma or a meningocele. It may emerge from under the buttocks and present as a mass on a buttock or produce asymmetry of a gluteal muscle. Internal tumors can be detected during a rectal exam (do not try this at home). They usually extend between the posterior aspect of the rectum and the sacrum. The size may make it difficult to insert a finger during digital exam. The upper border of the tumor may be palpable in the lower abdomen. An internal sacrococcygeal teratoma may fill the pelvis, projecting anteroposteriorly to present as an abdominal mass with obstruction of urinary and gastrointestinal structures. Internal bleeding may be a serious problem.

Accompanying neurological problems suggest that malignant invasion from the teratoma into neural structures has taken place, that there is an associated meningocele, or that the mass is not a teratoma. Symptoms may be subtle; these include paralysis, pain or weakness of the lower limbs, and the same types of bowel and bladder symptoms that occur with simple obstruction. The perineum may appear swollen and full and the anus may pouch open. Benign tumors do not usually cause neurological symptoms.

A lateral mass in the lower abdomen may be an **ovarian teratoma**, although these rarely present prior to childhood. A **testicular teratoma** presents as a painless scrotal mass.

Differential diagnosis includes distinguishing a sacrococcygeal teratoma from a meningocele. Anteriorly placed meningoceles are rare and may be often confused with presacral teratomas, while posterior meningoceles are often confused with smaller posterior teratomas. A large anterior meningocele arising from the sacrum may appear as an abdominal mass. It can be associated with a neurogenic bladder and a patulous anal sphincter. Meningoceles have the following characteristics: they are totally cystic (fluid filled); the tension within the cyst increases with crying and reduces in size when the baby is quiet; there are often definite signs of neurologic compromise with weakness in the lower limbs; posterior bony defects may occur in association with a posterior meningocele. Small skin-covered sacral meningoceles may be more difficult to distinguish as leg movement is often normal. Also, a small teratoma emerging near the anus may be mistaken for a perirectal abscess or an anal fistula. A perirectal abscess has overlying redness and tenderness. A sacral lipomeningocele is seen as a round skin-covered mass directly over the sacrum.

Support and transport: Urgent transport is not necessary if the teratoma is skin-covered and the baby is stable. The parents can be allowed some time to bond with the baby. In the meantime, a pediatric consult should be obtained. An ulcerated area will require surgery before it becomes infected. The situation is emergent if the tumor has ruptured, as the baby could bleed to death. Bleeding within the tumor may be difficult to detect and quantify. Signs of hypovolemic shock will develop and vigorous resuscitation may be necessary. Direct pressure should be applied to the tumor if the source of bleeding can be determined.

The presence of hydrops indicates that the tumor has had adverse physiologic effects, with blood flow through the tumor significantly compromising the baby and often leading to fetal death, stillbirth or neonatal death. Hydropic babies have severe respiratory distress and impaired kidney function at birth. Surgery in uncomplicated cases can produce dramatic improvement.

Although a skin-covered defect with no open sinuses does not leave the baby immediately vulnerable to infection (as would an open defect), misplacement of organs by a tumor can involve the heart, abdominal organs or the spinal cord. Therefore, the baby should be transported for evaluation shortly after birth.

Signs and Symptoms in the Skin

Jaundice

Babies born yellow should be evaluated by a physician immediately. Collect cord blood samples at birth in both red- and purple-topped tubes. Jaundice at birth can be caused by blood incompatability with the mother, other forms of hemolytic disease, hepatic obstruction of the bile ducts or other problems. Jaundice caused by direct, unconjugated bilirubin is associated with severe hepatobiliary disorders; this is usually associated with dark urine and clay-colored stools and may be accompanied by liver enlargement. It can occur due to biliary atresia, choledochal cyst, spontaneous perforation of the bile ducts, biliary tumor, or gallbladder anomalies or disease; all can be treated surgically. Other causes of direct hyperbilirubinemia include intrauterine infection, certain metabolic disorders such as α_1-antitrypsin deficiency, or familial disease syndromes such as Dubin-Johnson or Rotor.

Blisters or fragile skin

Some babies are born with localized blisters that heal rapidly and do not spread. These can be a normal variation, but infection should be ruled out. Epidermolysis bullosa is an inherited skin disorder that causes localized tearing and separation of the skin with minimal friction (such as rubbing the skin) because of inadequate tissue bonding. It results in blistering with rupture, revealing red underlying tissue (Nikolsky's sign). It commonly affects the extensor surfaces of the limbs and the feet, as they are so active in utero. The wounds may resemble second-degree burns or a ruptured blister; one type of this disorder also produces atrophic changes in affected limbs. If the lesions are large, the baby is at risk for fluid and electrolyte loss as well as infection. A number of other, similar conditions may also be causative.

Severe peeling of the skin

Peeling, scaling and extreme dryness, which at times may be severe and may occur in large thin sheets of dead skin with underlying normal skin, may be seen in babies who are born postterm. Severe scaling is called **ichthyosis** because the baby's skin is like that of a fish. There are two main varieties of this disorder, with several exceedingly rare variations.

The skin appears shiny, shrink-wrapped (collodion baby): The baby is encased in a tight, glossy, cellophane-like membrane that distorts the face (especially the nose and ears) and the limbs. Occurring once in every 300,000 births, this condition may rarely accompany dysmaturity and postterm delivery, as well as a variety of inherited disorders of the skin. As soon as the skin begins to dry, which may begin within minutes of birth, the baby begins to appear to be wrapped in parchment. The underlying skin may appear bright red to almost normal in color. As the skin puckers, the eyelids or lips may be turned inside out, which makes sucking difficult. Peeling of this membrane begins shortly after birth and may leave bleeding fissures and raw areas. The infant becomes susceptible to dehydration, electrolyte imbalances, temperature instability and poor nursing. Blisters that appear in groups and vary from 0.5 to several centimeters in diameter are also present in bullous congenital ichthyosiform erythroderma. The baby may also aspirate dry skin flakes; the loss of skin integrity makes him susceptible to infections. Although this is not usually an isolated finding, at least 10% of these babies will have more or less normal skin after the initial shedding, which may take a few months. Babies with this disorder are typically born before term but experience few problems in the neonatal period.

Large thick, leathery scales and deep red cracks appear soon after birth (Harlequin fetus): The most severe congenital disorder of the skin, this condition also occurs once in every 300,000 births. As soon as the birth fluids start to dry, all of the baby's skin begins to harden into large, thick, leathery scales that resemble plates of armor. Cracks form between the scales, leaving deep red fissures. There are secondary deformities of the skeleton and soft tissues, with gangrene of the digits in some cases. The inflexibility of the skin restricts respiration and is often incompatible with life beyond the first few hours, although some of these babies do live somewhat longer.

Darkening bruises, enlarging hematoma, blood oozing from umbilicus or other signs of poor clotting

Scalp hemorrhaging that spreads over the vertex, down by the ear or to the bridge of the nose via the forehead is a subgaleal hemorrhage, which, when developing rapidly, can result in major blood loss, disseminated intravascular coagulation and collapse. Transport at once. (This type of scalp bleeding is further explained in the subchapter entitled "Examining the Head and Neck.")

Defects of primary hemostasis, such as thrombocytopenia, platelet function disorders and von Willebrand disease are usually associated with superficial bleeding in the skin and mucous membranes, classically presenting with petechiae, especially in exposed or dependent body surfaces subjected to minor trauma, pressure or increased venous pressure. Mucosal bleeding at sites of minor trauma can also occur, but spontaneous bleeding is unusual in any otherwise well baby with platelet counts over 20,000. Congenital or acquired infection is the most common cause of thrombocytopenia in the newborn. Clotting factor deficiencies cause deeper bleeding, typically resulting in the formation of large hematomas from relatively minor trauma; easy bruising and bleeding from the rectum or bladder is also seen. The breakdown of associated signs and their probable causes are summarized in the table below.

Transport considerations: Any baby who has signs of a bleeding problem should be given homeopathic Arnica 200C. Deep bleeding may respond better to bellis perennis 200C. Also consider administering vitamin K, apply pressure to external bleeding sites, and transport right away.

TYPE AND LOCATION OF BLEEDING	COAGULATION DISORDER
Intracranial hemorrhage	Severe hemophilia (A or B) Severe factor VII or XIII deficiency Vitamin K deficiency
Facial purpura (hemorrhage into the skin producing a red coloration that darkens to purple and fades to brownish-yellow)	Platelet dysfunction Severely low platelet levels Glanzmann thrombasthenia
Bleeding into the oral mucosa	Severely low platelet levels Severe von Willebrand disease
Cephalohematoma	Severe factor deficiencies Vitamin K deficiency
Intramuscular bleeding	
Blood-stained urine	Vitamin K def., renal vein thrombosis
Injury-related bleeding	Any coagulation defect
Umbilical stump oozing	Factor XIII deficiency Fibrinogen deficiency

Swelling Near the Umbilicus with Leakage of Urine or Meconium

Swelling without leakage

The most likely reason for swelling at the base of the cord is an umbilical hernia; this relatively common finding is discussed in the subchapter entitled "Examining the Abdomen and Groin." Next, an omphalocele, which is discussed in the subchapter entitled "Externalized Organs and Neural Tube Defects," should be ruled out.

Leakage of urine (patent urachus)

Persistence of the urachus occurs in 1 out of every 5000 births. It may take the form of a completely patent communication between the bladder and the urachus, a very tiny sinus opening to the umbilicus, a diverticulum of the bladder, a cyst along the otherwise obliterated path of the duct, or a peritonealized urachal chorda. The main symptom is urine discharging from the umbilicus, which may produce redness and swelling of the entire region surrounding the umbilicus. Careful inspection of the navel base usually reveals a small mucosal prolapse, which is the mouth of the fistula. Related cysts are sometimes mistaken for intra-abdominal cysts, but these cysts are far less mobile, as they are more superficial. A patent urachus must be distinguished from a patent omphalomesenteric duct, which exudes bilious fluid and gas. A urachal chorda produces a fibrous band where the duct once was; it can cause problems if bowel segments are caught inside it, leading to classic signs of bowel obstruction. When the base of the umbilicus appears abnormal, transport shortly after birth.

Rosette-like opening at the umbilicus (omphalomesenteric remnants)

A patent omphalomesenteric duct results in meconium and gas leaking from the umbilicus. This rare developmental defect, occurring in 1 out of every 15,000 live births, consists of a communication between the ileum (or, very rarely, the colon) and the umbilicus, resulting in bowel contents and gas extruding from a variably sized rosette-like opening at the umbilicus. There may be reddening and ulceration of the surrounding skin from constant contact with intestinal fluid.

Intra-abdominal pressure can cause the entire duct to prolapse; this will look like a small ileostomy or, in more extreme cases, like a little bright pink pair of horns with an intestinal opening at either end. It can lead to strangulation with infarction and symptoms of obstruction. It requires surgical correction. A tiny remnant of this duct, a vitelline duct cyst, can lie closed behind the umbilicus or be connected by a fine fistula containing whitish mucus. These cysts are prone to infection and are often not noticed at birth. The omphalomesenteric duct may also remain as a fibrous band that can cause small bowel obstruction or volvulus.

Mechel diverticulum occurs when the omphalomesenteric duct itself is obliterated but a small outpouching remains in the ileal wall. The primary symptom is blood in the stool, resulting from erosion of the mucosal walls, although there is no abdominal pain. Other complications, such as intussusception or volvulus, cause additional classic symptoms as described under those headings in the subchapter entitled "Abdominal Distension and Vomiting at Birth: Detecting Gastrointestinal Anomalies."

Floppy Baby (atonia)

Although muscle tone normally decreases when the baby is sleeping or dozing, no baby should be limp. Limpness at birth or shortly after strongly implies the need for resuscitative measures; however, if the baby is breathing well and the heart rate is normal, other causes must be investigated. Generally speaking, the floppy baby feels flabby. An increased range of passive joint movement with diminished resistance is possible, although care should be taken not to overextend the relaxed joint and cause injury. The head lags with poor control when the baby is pulled by her hands from a supine into a sitting position. The arms and legs dangle, the head droops and the trunk flexes when the baby is lifted by a hand under his chest. One of the most common causes of flaccidity is Down syndrome.

Is the infant weak as well as floppy? Check to see if strong movements can be induced reflexively (grasping, limb retraction, etc.), if the baby will pull away from a stimulus or both. If so, the baby is not weak and the cause of the floppiness is likely to be a central nervous system disease, metabolic disorder, connective tissue disorder or cerebral palsy. A baby who has normal motor activity in the upper body but diminished or absent movement from a certain point down is very likely to have a spinal defect or severe spinal injury. The baby who is uniformly weak as well as floppy is apt to have sluggish or absent reflexes from a disorder affecting the peripheral motor nerves or the muscle.

Whether the baby is just floppy or is weak and floppy, transport is called for shortly after birth for further evaluation. Evidence of spinal lesions should be sought by carefully examining the baby's back.

EXTERNALIZED ORGANS AND NEURAL TUBE DEFECTS

Babies may be born with one or more internal structures partially or fully outside the body. This most commonly occurs with the abdominal organs, the brain and the spinal cord and, more rarely, with the liver or heart. The risk of infection, drying and cracking, and torsion of the part are great whenever something that should be inside develops outside the body, especially if the part is not completely covered by normal skin. Gastrointestinal defects contraindicate normal feeding until obstruction and torsion can be ruled out or surgically corrected. In almost every case, the baby should be transported without delay to the nearest Level III or, if possible, a level IV neonatal intensive care unit.

Organs Exposed on the Anterior Surface of the Body

These types of defects most commonly involve the intestines and bladder region. Defects involving the major abdominal organs, such as hypogastric omphalocele or other abdominal wall defects, exstrophy complex, absence of hindgut, neural tube and vertebral defects, as well as heart defects, result when the caudal fold fails to develop.

Upper midline abdominal defects

Omphalocele [ohm-FAL-oh-seal]) (exomphalos): This defect occurs in 1 of every 3000 to 10,000 live births. It consists of an avascular, initially transparent sac consisting of peritoneum on the inside, amnion on the outside and a thin layer of Wharton's jelly between. The sac herniates through a defect in the midline of the abdominal wall. It contains abdominal contents and, occasionally, other organs. The sac that covers the defect may rupture during birth. The umbilical vessels are on the surface of the sac and join the umbilicus, which is broad and remains fluctuant after pulsations have stopped.

Associated defects: The defect may be small (< 4 cm in diameter) and contain only intestines. Large defects that exceed 4 cm in diameter allow the liver and other organs of the chest and genitourinary tract to protrude; these infants have a tendency to develop small narrow chests and downward-slanting ribs with associated pulmonary hypoplasia. There is a high incidence of other life-threatening congenital malformations associated with this defect, particularly thoracic, cardiac, other gastrointestinal defects, craniofacial defects such as cleft lip or palate and genitourinary anomalies. Extraintestinal defects will be found in 33 to 50% of these babies. A baby with an omphalocele positioned high near the chest will often have associated chest and cardiac defects, a sternal cleft and a diaphragmatic hernia. A narrow "dog" or bell-shaped chest suggests hypoplastic lungs, with the baby dying shortly after birth. In general, congenital heart defects and chromosomal anomalies (especially trisomies 13, 18, and 21), as well as neurological and renal defects, frequently accompany omphalocele and determine the ultimate outcome. Because this defect is enclosed, these babies are not in critically urgent need of surgery and can be fully evaluated after transport to ascertain whether any other defects are present before surgery is undertaken.

Gastroschisis (gas-trow-SKI-sis): This defect occurs once in every 4000 to 20,000 live births. A small, round, defect with a diameter of a few centimeters is located between the rectus muscles in the anterior abdominal wall, usually to the right of a normally situated umbilical cord. Fully exposed herniated intestines that are thickened, matted together, shortened, usually inflamed and edematous, with a leathery texture, protrude through this hole. Volvulus from malrotation occurs in a counterclockwise direction. A bridge of abdominal skin may separate the opening from the umbilical outlet. The herniated organs (usually intestines, with or without the stomach and bladder, and very rarely including the liver) are not covered by a membrane, although they may have a fibrous, peeling surface. The abdominal cavity appears small and empty. Few additional malformations are associated with this anomaly.

There is a tendency for the defect to partially close after birth, which can result in strangulation of the intestines, causing atresias. Prolonged exposure of the gut to amniotic fluid causes it to become thick and short. Babies with gastroschisis tend to be born preterm, are often of low birthweight and small for gestational age. The incidence of gastroschisis may be becoming more frequent.

These babies need surgery as soon as they are stable. They are at high risk for dehydration, heat loss and infection of the exposed organs, in addition to organ infarction from constriction of the blood supply as a result of twisting or inflammation.

FINDING	OMPHALOCELE	GASTROSCHISIS
Frequency	1 in 3000 to 10,000 live births	1 in 4000 to 20,000 live births
Gender association	3 males for every 2 females	Equal incidence in males and females
Gestational age & weight	Slightly preterm and underweight	More often more preterm and more underweight
Location	Within the umbilical ring	Separate opening to the right of the normal umbilicus
Size of defect	4 to 12 cm in diameter	Less than 4 cm in diameter
Sac	Present, may have ruptured	None
Location of umbilical cord	Enters on the surface of the sac	Normal
Liver involvement	Yes (may be damaged during yoni birth)	No
Bowel abnormalities:		
Malrotation	Yes	Yes
Appearance	Normal	Matted, thickened, shortened, edematous
Function	Normal	Dysmotile
Atresia	Rare	Common (11 to 23%)
Associated anomalies and syndromes	Found in up to two-thirds of babies with large omphaloceles	10 to 20% (16% intestinal atresia, midgut volvulus, intestinal stenosis). Rarely other defects are found, no associated syndromes.

Lower midline syndromes

Exstrophy (ECK-strow-fee) of the bladder: This exstrophy-epispadias defect occurs in 1 out of every 25,000 live births, three times more often in males than in females. It has a number of variants. Typically, the bladder protrudes through a fissure in the lower abdominal wall. The bladder, lying exposed in the suprapubic region, appears as a moist bundle of deep pink membranous tissue. The wall of the bladder is split and laid open, and the ureteric openings can be seen as two small, elevated tumor-like masses below the everted bladder. The size of the exstrophy varies and sometimes is as large as a normal bladder. The symphysis pubis is widely separated. There may be complete epispadias in both sexes, although this occurs much less commonly in girls. Rectal prolapse is also common. Seventy percent of these babies will be found to have other defects, and 30 to 40% of those will have associated genetic defects.

Cloacal exstrophy: This is the rarest and most extreme form of the exstrophy-epispadias complex, occurring only once in 200,000 to 400,000 live births. These babies are born with an exposed bladder and bowel complex that protrudes through an opening of variable size in the lower abdominal wall and perineal region. An omphalocele sits uppermost, below which is an open plate of mucosa. The bladder is usually split in half to either side of a central strip of intestinal epithelium, although it may also be above, below or joined with the externalized bowel. The bladder may or may not be covered by a thin skin. The surface of most of the defect will consist of moist, deep pink tissue. The ileocecal region of the small bowel often has three or four orifices. The lowermost orifice prolapses from a superior opening in the intestinal strip, resulting in an "elephant's trunk" appearance of this portion of the defect, which terminates in a minute stomal opening. A lower intestinal opening leads to a blind pouch in the colon. The anus is imperforate.

In boys, the penis is absent in 30% of these cases. When present, it may be a small, divided organ sitting on widely separated pubic bones; it may have an epispadias or be fully formed. Severely anomalous genitalia almost always accompany this condition.

Girls with a cloacal defect often have a single genital opening located beneath the clitoris, which is surrounded by a tiny vulva. This rare anomaly consists of a common cloacal channel, above which bladder, yoni and rectum all meet. This is not an intersex condition nor is it part of the adrenogenital syndrome. In girls, Mullerian structures may extrude below each half of the bladder, with blind-ended, duplicate yonis and a divided clitoris. Major associated anomalies may be found in up to 80% of these babies, including myelomeningocele and defects of the lower limbs, vertebral column and renal tract.

Upper midline syndromes involving the chest

Exposed heart (ectopia cordis): A cleft sternum may result in extrusion of the heart through the chest wall, the rarest of all exposed organ disorders. Occurring only 5.5 to 7.9 times in every million live births, there are three types:

Thoracic: The sternum may be intact superiorly or entirely split. The heart, with its apex orientated anteriorly, is uncovered and lies completely outside the chest wall (59% of cases).

Thoracoabdominal ectopia cordis (Cantrell pentalogy): The cephalic fold fails to develop properly, resulting in four, and sometimes five, associated defects, including a cleft in the lower sternum, anterior diaphragmatic hernia, exposed heart and heart defects. In addition, some babies have an adjacent or completely separate omphalocele (38% of cases).

Cervical: This is characterized by fusion between the apex of the heart and the mouth, with associated severe craniofacial anomalies. It is exceedingly rare (3% of cases) and uniformly fatal.

Ectopia cordis is a devastating anomaly that few babies survive because of associated heart defects and lack of room in the chest cavity in which to replace the heart. Surgical attempts to return the heart to the chest cavity often result in compressed blood vessels. The baby should be treated as for an exposed abdominal organ and transported without delay.

Care and transport considerations

Immediate care for babies with gastroschisis: With the baby lying supine, don sterile gloves and gently lift the bowel and arrange it on the top of the abdomen so that the surface of the mesentery is flat and untwisted from the bowel to its base, preventing traction on the mesentery. Inspect the bowel for color. Well-perfused bowel ranges from light pink to red orange. Compromised perfusion results in the bowel becoming cyanotic, with a blue or purple surface. Necrotic bowel is deep purple to black. Twisting of the mesentery can quickly lead to infarction of large portions of the bowel due to kinking or twisting of blood vessels. Alternatively, if the defect is too large to allow placement on the supine baby's abdomen (i.e., if the intestines slide off to the side when the baby is on his back), turn the baby on his right side and arrange the mesentery so that it is flat and untwisted.

Cord care for babies with exposed organs of the chest or abdomen: Cut the cord where it attaches to the placenta and clamp it. Explain to concerned ambulance attendants that a portion of the gastrointestinal tract may extend into a normal-looking cord on rare occasions and you'd rather be safe than sorry. This minimizes the chances that you will inadvertently cut through herniated intestines.

Transport protocols

Transport protocol for upper midline defects with exposed organs, gastroschisis or ruptured omphalocele: The two primary goals of transport are, first, preventing organs that are exposed or only covered with a thin membrane from drying out or becoming contaminated and, second, preventing the baby from becoming chilled. These babies are at great risk of heat loss. Be sure to take every precaution to maintain them in a thermoneutral state during transport. When drying is prevented by wet dressings, the baby can become chilled more easily.

Organs that are completely exposed or covered only by a thin membrane must be protected from dehydration. Your dressing, once it is in place, must be loose enough to prevent constriction. Position the baby to minimize friction and irritation, either on her back or side, depending upon the size of the defect. Generally, babies with a gastroschisis or upper midline defect can be positioned on their back.

1. Arrange a wide piece of clear, new plastic food wrap on a padded, portable surface.
2. Assess whether the baby should lie on her back or side, depending upon the size of the defect. The baby should be placed on her side if the defect is so large that it will fall to the side of the anterior torso when the baby is supine.
3. If the baby is to lie on her side, place dry gauze pads on the plastic wrap where the baby's defect will be positioned. Place sterile nonadherent dressings on top of these and soak them with warmed saline. This is to protect the underside of the defect from drying out and from abrasion. Place the baby on her side, on the transport surface with the defective tissues overlying the prepared moist surface.
4. Place the tip of a sterile feeding tube on the center of the defect. This will allow resaturation, if necessary, by attaching a syringe to the hub and injecting saline under the dressing.
5. Apply wet, nonadherent dressings over all membrane-covered or unencapsulated areas, then wrap everything loosely

with dry sterile gauze and soak with warmed saline.
6. Bring the ends of the plastic food wrap over the baby gently so as not to constrict the defect. Press the top and bottom edges against the baby above and below the defect to hold in heat and moisture.

Plain gauze will tend to stick, may leave lint on the defect and may abrade delicate membranes. Use only a nonadherent, lint-free dressing directly against the defect.

Once the defective area is covered:
1. Pass an orogastric or nasogastric tube and aspirate to prevent distension.
2. If the baby is on her back, place a small rolled towel between her legs to prevent rolling.
3. If the baby is on her side, place the rolled towel against her back to prevent rolling.
4. Be sure the defective parts are not compressed or twisted.
5. Loosely enclose the baby and transport surface with a space blanket to retain heat.
6. Use blow-by oxygen as needed. To avoid forcing air into the stomach, do not use positive pressure unless absolutely necessary. Use care with CPR to prevent trauma to the defective areas.

Transport protocol for an intact omphalocele: If the baby has an intact omphalocele, wet saline gauze pads need not be applied, which will help prevent chilling. Although not enclosed in normal skin, the covering of an omphalocele is sufficiently strong and resistant to drying to eliminate the need for moisture. The application of dressings is only recommended to keep the defect from sticking to the plastic wrap. If the defect is very large, the organs it contains must be protected from trauma due to jarring and tension on the surrounding membrane while the baby is being transported. To stabilize a large defect:
1. Place a wide piece of clear, new plastic food wrap on a padded, portable surface.
2. Place the baby supine on the cookie sheet.
3. Cover the omphalocele with dry nonadherent nonwicking dressings. Now wrap the plastic wrap up over and around the defect. Overlap the edges on the top to stabilize, but not strangle, the defect.
4. Carefully roll the baby onto his side to minimize jarring during transport and to prevent the omphalocele from pressing into the diaphragm, thereby producing respiratory distress.
5. Provide additional support for the defect by placing rolled towels around its edges.

Neural Tube Defects (involving brain or spinal tissue)

Babies with neural tube defects may display one or more of the following signs:
- Small indentation in the spine
- Membrane- or skin-covered sac along the spine
- Open lesion along the spine
- Membranous or skin-covered, fluid-filled sac that protrudes from the nape of the neck, the forehead or the back
- Enlarged head (only rarely very noticeable at birth when the birth has occurred normally, as a very enlarged head would have resulted in dystocia)
- Tufts of hair along the spine, midline dimples or sinus tracts
- Head tipped back with occiput fused to the cervical and thoracic spine; the defect is enclosed in skin (iniencephaly)
- Head tipped back with occiput fused to the cervical and thoracic spine, with an open spinal defect (craniorachischisis)
- Exposed cranium with missing cranial bones (anencephaly)
- The entire spinal cord is widely open (spinal rachischisis)

When a baby has a neural tube defect that contains nerve tissue, birth will be the first time this region is under the influence of gravity. Gravity may cause an extreme neurological response in the newly born baby, such as rapid breathing, accelerated heartbeat, etc. However, these babies typically stabilize quickly.

<u>**Care and transport issues**</u>

Membrane-covered or exposed defects: The primary aim of care should be to provide gentle support for defects enclosed in a membrane of fragile skin to distribute weight and minimize pressure and trauma. An exposed defect or one that is merely covered with a thin membrane is prone to injury. Both types also require constant moisture to prevent drying out. These babies should be transported right away.

Skin-covered defects: When a spinal defect is completely enclosed by normal skin, a little more time may be available for bonding at home prior to transport provided that the baby is stable, as the risk of infection is much less.

If the baby is anencephalic, consult a pediatrician by phone, if possible. If a house call is possible, immediate transport may not be necessary.

General transport procedures for spinal defects:

1. Keep baby warm and naked to avoid irritation of exposed organs.
2. Prepare the transport surface. Fold a towel or receiving blanket to the length of the baby's chest. The sides of the towel should extend beyond either side of the baby to provide a firm, stabilizing surface.
3. **If defect is small or not enclosed:** Place a long piece of plastic wrap centered across the towel. Lie the baby prone, with the head lower than the trunk. Bend the baby's legs in a frog position (spread apart at the hips and flat against the surface, knees flexed at a 90° angle). Place a rolled towel or diaper between the thighs to maintain this position, which stabilizes the baby and prevents him from rolling over. The primary goal is to avoid contamination or damage to the defect.

   If defect is very large and enclosed: Place the baby on her side on the towel. Place small rolled towels above and below the defect and lengthwise along her belly to prevent the baby from rolling backward onto the defect. A small rolled towel or washcloth can also be placed crosswise between the baby's legs for the same purpose.
4. Once baby is positioned correctly:

   If there are exposed or membranous surfaces: Apply saline-moistened nonadherent Telfa sponges. Cover these in sterile gauze, then soak with saline. Place a feeding tube carefully over or to the side of the defect so that more saline can be applied using a syringe attached to the coupler. Bring the ends of the plastic wrap up and over the defect, and carefully press the edges down above and below the defect to retain heat and moisture, taking care not to compress the defect

   Skin-covered defects: These need not be covered with gauze or plastic wrap.
5. Use full CPR if necessary: To do so place the baby on his side; be careful not to rupture or contaminate the defect. Another person should support the baby's head in a side-lying sniffing position. One hand can be placed against the baby's back to provide stabilization if chest compressions are required. This will be tricky to do.

<u>**Possible neural tube defects**</u>

Spina bifida refers to any condition arising from the abnormal or incomplete closure of the embryonic neural tube along the vertebral column. The overall incidence of all types of spina bifida (including occult forms that are never symptomatic) ranges from 1% to as high as 40% in the general population, depending on the study. The overall incidence of more severe spina bifida (meaning the spine is separated or cleft) is 1 in 2000 births. Cranium bifida refers to the range of defects that can occur in the skull and that involve the brain or meninges. An all-encompassing figure for the incidence of all types of cranium bifida is not available. The actual incidence of all these defects is influenced by many factors, including, to name a few, genetics, toxic exposures, and the folic acid level of the mother at the time of conception.

<u>**Anterior neural tube defects**</u>**:** These would more logically be called superior neural tube defects, as they have to do with brain development.

Anencephaly: Anencephaly is the most common major defect of the central nervous system, occurring in 1 out of every 1500 babies in North America, with a higher incidence in the United Kingdom. In the Western world, it is seen 37 times more often in girls than boys and the recurrence rate in families can be as high as 35%. The incidence is highest in Ireland, Scotland, Wales, Egypt and New Zealand, and lowest in Japan. This fatal defect occurs when the anterior neural tube does not close properly. The bones of the cranial vault are missing and the cerebral and cerebellar hemispheres, brainstem, and basal ganglia are either absent or very poorly formed. The defect begins at the vertex and may extend all the way down to the base of the neck at the foramen magnum. A soft, lumpy, bloody, exposed portion of the brain may be present in place of the normal skull vault, with no covering of either skin or membrane. Most commonly the forebrain and some amount of the upper brain stem is present and lying exposed. Anencephaly is frequently found in conjunction with adrenal hypoplasia and lung defects. This severe defect is incompatible with long-term survival, although the baby may live for several days or weeks.

Meroanencephaly: Meroanencephaly is a type of anencephaly in which both the brain and the bones of the cranial vault are present in rudimentary form.

Encephalocele (cephalocele): Encephaloceles are a class of defects involving the protrusion of part of the brain contents or meninges through a midline defect in the skull. The overall incidence is 1 in 5000 to 10,000 births. Incomplete closure of the neural tube results in a herniation of meninges, and sometimes brain tissue, into a sac filled with spinal fluid and possibly covered with skin or membrane only. The defect in the skull is referred to as a bifid cranium. Encephaloceles are classified according to location, as follows:

Occult cranium bifidum: A bifid cranium is present without anything protruding through it. This presents as a small tissue covered opening in the skull, similar to a fontanelle. Tufts of normal hair may surround the defect. It usually does not require surgery, and the skull frequently ossifies over the defect as the child grows.

Cranial meningocele: This bone defect involves an outpouching of spinal-fluid-filled meninges without any herniation of brain tissue.

Cranial encephalocele: These involve either the occipital, parietal or frontoethmoidal regions and are usually apparent at birth. They occur in the midline of the occipital bone in 75% of all cases; the second most common location is the glabella. However, less often they develop in the frontal, parietal, temporal or nasopharyngeal areas or as a protrusion from the eye socket.

Basal encephaloceles: These include transethmoidal, sphenoethmoidal and transsphenoidal defects and may not be evident at birth. Often the only hint of this lesion is a widening of the bridge of the nose or widely spaced eyes. They may produce symptoms of upper airway obstruction and may be mistaken for nasal polyps. Any intranasal mass in a newborn should be considered a basal encephalocele until this is ruled out.

The severity of the defect depends upon the size and contents of the sac, which may contain spinal fluid, meninges and brain tissue. The size of the sac gives no indication as to its contents. Defects vary in size from very small to huge masses the size of the skull or larger. The sac is usually completely covered with either normal or poorly developed skin. Some may leak fluid. These babies usually show no obvious neurological impairment, although subtle defects may develop later. Lower cranial nerves can be affected in low occipital lesions, giving rise to difficulties with sucking and swallowing as well as apnea and bradycardia. Hydrocephaly or microcephaly, spasticity, seizures and blindness are associated problems resulting from defects in the occipital lobe of the brain. An encephalocele can be transilluminated to reveal the amount of brain tissue it contains. However, since these structures are delicate and the baby must be transported in any event, do not risk rupturing the sac by attempting to transillumination at home. While skin-covered, nonleaking defects are not considered a surgical emergency, these babies should be transported soon after birth, as the complications from rupture of the sac are life threatening.

Both gender and ethnic distribution vary with the location of the defect. Frontoethmoidal defects are distributed equally among the sexes, while 70% of occipital defects occur in girls. Anterior defects are more common in South Asia (India, Sri Lanka, etc.) and Africa, while posterior defects represent 80% of those occurring in the Western Hemisphere and Europe. There is no known reason for this distribution. The reported overall frequency of these defects varies from 1 in 2400 to 1 in 12,500, but most estimates range between 1 in every 5000 to 9000 births.

Associated defects: Other defects are often found with encephalocele, with an overall incidence of 17 to 60%. These include microcephaly (up to 25%), hydrocephaly (12 to 24% in anterior defects and 16 to 51% in posterior defects), and anatomic defects of the brain (such as porencephaly, holoprosencephaly and lissencephaly). In addition, skeletal, maxillofacial, ocular, cardiac and renal defects are among many others that may occur. The frequency of these varies widely but is much less than those which involve the central nervous system.

Posterior neural tube defects: These defects are caused by incomplete closure of the posterior portion of the spinal vertebrae and can range from clinically insignificant to fatal.

Spina bifida occulta: The mildest of these defects, spina bifida occulta occurs most often in the lower lumbar or lumbosacral area when the spinous processes and lamina of one or two vertebrae fail to develop. This area is covered by skin and rarely involves the dura or any neurological tissues. The meninges and spinal cord are normally formed and placed. Tufts of hair, fatty tumors, areas of pigmentation, moles or openings may overlie such defects. While such bony defects are permanent, they rarely cause any problems and may exist in up to 20 to 40% of the general population.

Meningocele: Meningoceles account for 10% of all cases of spina bifida. This defect includes the same type of incomplete spinal closure found in the occulta form but with a herniation of the meninges filled with cerebrospinal fluid protruding through the vertebral defect. It is usually covered by a thin, hypoplastic layer of skin or a meningeal membrane. The spinal nerves are normally formed and placed, and neurological complications usually do not occur. An anterior meningocele arising from the inside of the sacrum may present an abdominal mass and may be associated with a neurogenic bladder and a patulous anal sphincter.

Lipomyelomeningocele: Here a mass composed of fat cells is included in the spinal defect. It may be associated with a true myelomeningocele or it may present as a simple benign fatty tumor (lipoma). Those associated with meningocele or simple spina bifida may be asymptomatic in newborns, but neurological problems may develop later from tethering of the spinal cord to the lesion as the child grows. This can result in progressive motor dysfunction of the legs, lower back and leg pain, bladder dysfunction and scoliosis. Surgery is required to prevent these complications.

Myelomeningocele: These lesions occur when spina bifida is severe. The defective vertebrae are widened on either side or may be absent entirely. The meninges, spinal cord and nerves protrude through the defect, covered only by the arachnoid layer, but not by dura or skin. The sac appears velvety red or yellow with fragile blood vessels embedded in the delicate membrane. The exposed portions of the spinal cord pass forward into the sac and the cord remains tethered to the bony defect. The neural tube is usually found on the outermost surface of the mass. Frequently the spinal cord ends in this sac and is splayed open, revealing the central core. Most of these lesions develop in the lumbar region. Abnormalities of neuromuscular function depend upon the specific nerve roots involved. (A chart outlining these correlations can be found in the subchapter entitled "Assessment of Cranial Nerve Function.") Ninety percent of these babies will have bowel or bladder dysfunction.

Associated anomalies: Arnold Chiari malformation (or simply Chiari malformation) is an anomaly of the hindbrain characterized by elongation and extension of the pons, medulla and cerebellar tonsils into the foramen magnum, a condition present in 90% of myelomeningocele cases and less frequently in milder forms of spina bifida. There may be no signs that this defect is present, although over half of affected babies will display swallowing difficulties, apneic spells and stridor. Other brain abnormalities may occur, as may other vertebral anomalies, although these usually will not present with clinical signs in the neonate.

Hydrocephalus is a frequently associated problem, found in 90% of these babies. Although external evidence of this is often absent at birth, the ventricles may still be enlarged. The higher up on the spine the defect occurs, the greater the degree of impairment of muscle use. Defects of the thoracic spine are also frequently associated with severe defects of spinal curvature, hips and legs. Extensive surgery and physical therapy will help these babies maximize their physical potentials.

In addition, babies with myelomeningoceles have a high incidence of associated anomalies, on average 2.2 additional defects are discovered in every baby. These include skeletal defects such as hip dislocation, clubfeet, extra digits, and craniofacial defects such as synostosis or cleft palate. About 7% of these infants have facial features similar to those found with Down syndrome, although they have normal chromosomal patterns. Genitourinary anomalies such as horseshoe kidney, exstrophy of the bladder, and hypospadias are more prevalent in these babies, as well as intestinal, cardiac, and esophageal defects.

Summary: The following table summarizes the range of neural tube defects that may occur.

Type of Defect	Anatomical Details and Incidence	Prognosis
Occult vertebral defects		
True occult spina bifida (spinal bifida aperta)	Failure of spinal bone fusion with no external evidence of lesions and rare tethering of the spinal cord. Rarely identified in infancy. (Up to 40% of general population.)	Excellent
Occult spina bifida with external evidence	Tumor-like lesion, sinus tract or atrophic skin overlying the bony defect; spinal tissue may be attached to the overlying skin.	Good
Spina bifida cystica		
Meningocele	Failure of spinal fusion with a protruding skin-covered sac of meninges anywhere along the neural tube but commonly in the lumbar region. No neurological deficit is evident, and the underlying cord is usually normal.	Excellent
Myelocystocele (Neuromeningocele)	Failure of spinal fusion; protruding skin-covered sac of meninges, often with some undifferentiated nerves attached, with associated neurological impairment. 99.5% are dorsal; ventral defects usually present as an anterior sacral meningocele. In females, this presents as a pelvic mass. Rare.	Good
Myelomeningocele (Meningomyelocele)	Failure of spinal fusion; an open cord defect over a limited length of spine presenting as a neural plaque, usually midline. Looks like dark pink smoked salmon, surrounded by a cystic lesion, thin skin and meninges. The lesion may be fairly flat or raised up in a cavity containing spinal fluid. Commonly located on the lower thoracic, lumbar and upper sacral regions, all of which are associated with significant neural compromise. Cervical and upper thoracic lesions have less severe neurological involvement (1 in 1000 births).	Variable
Lipomeningocele Lipomyelomeningocele	A fatty mass herniates through the bony spinal defect and attaches to the spinal cord and often the associated nerve roots. Can include both dorsal and ventral nerve roots, only the dorsal nerve roots or the filum terminale and conus medullaris. Not associated with hydrocephalus, but more severe than a simple meningocele.	Guarded, complex corrective surgery
Cranium bifidum		
Occultum	Persistently wide fontanelle, persistent parietal foramina or an extra fontanelle. Usually asymptomatic and only requires observation as it will eventually close.	Excellent
Encephalocele	10% of spina bifida cystica, more common in girls. Outpouching of brain and dura through midline defect in skull. Lesions pulse and become tense with straining or crying. In the US 80% are occipital; in Asia, most involve the frontal bone. In Pacific Rim countries, most are anterior lesions that present with hyper-telorism, obstructed nostrils, anterior skull masses, cleft palate and other defects.	Variable
Cranioschisis	Skull open and brain alone poorly developed	Fatal
Anencephaly (Meroanencephaly)	Brain and skull poorly developed, deformed forehead, large ears and eyes, with relatively normal lower facial features. (1 in 1000 to 8000 births.)	Fatal
Iniencephaly	Incompletely formed base of skull, resulting in extension of the head, no neck and extreme lordosis; scalp connects to the back, and the facial skin connects to chest.	Fatal
Exencephaly	The cranial vault is incomplete, with the brain herniated through the top.	Fatal
Craniorachischisis	Open brain-spinal defect; head extended, occiput fused to cervical and thoracic spine.	Fatal
Spinal rachischisis	The entire spine is widely open with an absence of varying amounts of spinal cord, nerve roots and meninges.	Fatal

BIRTH INJURIES (OTHER THAN CRANIAL AND INTRACRANIAL INJURIES)

Fortunately, birth injuries are rare when instrumental and surgical births are avoided, when physiologic birth is allowed to proceed unmanipulated, and when the fetal soft tissues are not unduly relaxed from the effect of maternal drugs. However, the term baby's bones are only partly ossified, and joints are very lax. Injuries can occur when the baby must be handled excessively to assist the birth, such as during a shoulder dystocia, a breech birth or an unusual cephalic presentation such as a face or brow, as well as when the head or another body part is forced into an unnatural position for many hours during a difficult labor or birth. The chances of injury are increased when the baby is either large or early (and more delicate). Suspect a birth injury if the baby presents with any of the following:

- Abnormal limb characteristics including rigidity, flaccidity, paralysis, distorted posture or irregular contours (lumps)
- Swelling, bruising, or both along the clavicular line
- Crying or otherwise exhibiting pain when a region of the body is moved or examined or when the baby is handled
- Localized bruising or a hematoma on the head, a limb or the torso
- A distorted, asymmetrical facial expression, especially when crying
- A distended abdomen, dark spots, signs of shock

The first three problems may be due to a broken bone, one of the most common birth injuries. A distorted posture or facial expression may be related to an accompanying nerve palsy or nerve damage from a traumatic birth, especially if the arms were manipulated, as might be the case with a baby who had a shoulder dystocia. Administer homeopathic arnica and hypericum and seek pediatric evaluation soon after birth.

Midwives do not usually take blood to check the newborn's hemoglobin at home (although this can be done with a portable testing device); however, increasing pallor, lethargy, sleepiness and localized regions of darkening or abdominal distension can all be signs of progressive internal bleeding.

Broken bones

The clavicle is the bone most frequently damaged by birth trauma in large, hypotonic babies who have shoulder dystocia, lateral neck traction or difficult arm extraction in a breech birth. It is often asymptomatic but can be discovered with palpation, which will detect movement of the broken ends. Associated injuries may include damage to the brachial plexus, spine and humerus. A limb that is broken without any evidence of accompanying neurological involvement should be stabilized until it can be evaluated by a pediatrician. A broken arm should be positioned straight along the side of the baby's body. An elastic support bandage should then be wrapped around the baby's trunk and arm to stabilize it. A broken leg should be wrapped with an elastic support bandage to keep the leg from bending. Care must be taken not to impede circulation whenever a binding is used. A broken clavicle usually does not require stabilization.

Fracture of the long bones usually occur in either the humerus or the femur. Injury to the humerus usually involves the upper epiphysis, presenting with a swollen, tender shoulder and pseudoparalysis. True dislocation rarely occurs, as the epiphysis will break before it dislocates. The shoulder should be immobilized in adduction and internal rotation with an elastic support bandage, and an orthopedic consult sought soon after birth (within 12 hours). Injury to the femur will result in pain during manipulation of the legs as well as the other general signs of bone injury. Injury to the proximal femoral epiphysis may mimic congenital hip dislocation, but simple hip dislocation is painless in the newborn.

Facial and mandibular fractures are significant traumatic injuries that are unlikely to occur at home. However, when they do, they present with bruising around the eye, facial asymmetry, an apparently small jaw and feeding difficulties. Their proximity to other structures such as the airway, eyes (and optic nerve) and subarachnoid space make them dangerous. Early alignment and immobilization are required to prevent damage and to achieve a good cosmetic result. Nasal fractures produce deviation of the septum. If severe, they may obstruct the airway. Give these babies Vitamin K and homeopathic arnica. Consult a pediatric orthopedist or osteopath as soon as possible.

Absence of bones: Note that the absence of a bone may cause the affected part to be held in an unusual, fixed posture without any injury having occurred. A typical location is the wrist when the radius is absent; this presents with a short forearm and bowing at the wrist that varies in severity according to how much of the radius is defective or absent. If any of the long bones of the leg are short or missing, the length of the leg will be obviously shorter than its mate.

Breakage of bones with normal birth and postpartum handling: Some congenital disorders involve extremely fragile bones. One of the most common is a hereditary disorder known as osteogenesis imperfecta which is often accompanied by blue sclera, deafness, a triangularly-shaped face, short stature, lateral curvature of the spine, high-pitched voice, excessive sweating, loose joints, easy bruising, respiratory problems and constipation as well as cardiac problems. There are four subtypes of this disorder with an overall incidence of 1 case per 20,000 live births. These babies may experience skull fracture during normal descent in labor and breakage of bones during normal handling after birth. They require extremely gentle care. If you suspect such a problem, transport for evaluation right away. There is no treatment for such disorders.

Nerve injuries

Peculiar facial expression or unusual posture (nerve damage): Always keep in mind that very peculiar postures can result from a baby's chosen position of comfort during gestation. At times, this involves dramatic alterations in other parts of the anatomy into which a limb was pressed, including chest depressions from knees, lopsided head contours, bent ears, and apparently malformed feet or legs. However, when the baby holds her face, arms or hands in an unusual posture with partial paralysis and cannot voluntarily move or be assisted to change from that posture, a palsy has occurred (rarely with a broken bone).

Asymmetrical facial features during crying may be the only clue to a facial palsy. Unilateral facial palsy results from peripheral nerve trauma. It presents with impaired movement, drooping mouth and flattened nasolabial fold (space above the upper lip), smooth forehead and a persistently open eye or elongated palpebral fissure on the affected side. Touching the face does not elicit normal muscular responses such as wrinkling the brow or grimacing. Normal facial expressions are absent or altered. Peripheral palsies can result from stress on the nerves due to prolonged pressure of the nerve against the mother's sacral promontory or traction on the nerves that traverse the neck during manipulation to resolve shoulder dystocia, although some 50% of these injuries occur without manipulation. The baby need not be transported immediately but should be evaluated in the first days after birth. Central nerve injury often results from contralateral nerve damage from trauma such as fracture of the temporal bone, posterior fossa bleeding or tissue destruction. It involves only the lower half to two-thirds of the face; the forehead and eyes are unaffected. It is more rare and more serious than peripheral palsy.

Nerve damage to the shoulders and arms: Brachial plexus injury occurs in 0.37 to 0.87 per 1000 live births. Erb or Duchenne palsy is confined to the upper spinal segment. Lesions affecting the 5th and 6th cervical segments make up 50 to 72% of all such injuries. A baby whose upper arm is paralyzed due to a stretching or tearing injury of the brachial plexus will hold the affected arm away from the body, rotate it posteriorly and flex the wrist, called the "waiter's tip position." The grasp reflex will be intact, but the Moro, biceps and radial reflexes will be absent on the affected side. Associated injuries include damage to the clavicle or humerus on the affected side (9%), diaphragmatic paralysis (5 to 9%), facial paralysis (5 to 14%) and injury to the parietal bone, scalp or face (rare).

Lower segment injury (Klumpke palsy), involving the 8th cervical segment and the first thoracic segment, is relatively rare. The intrinsic hand muscles and long flexor muscles of the fingers and wrist are affected, resulting in the loss of the grasp reflex. The eyelids may prolapse with contraction of the pupil, there may be a lack of sweat production, and inflammation of the tissues in the eye may develop if the sympathetic fibers from the first thoracic nerve root are involved. If the entire brachial plexus is involved, the arm will be fully paralyzed and all reflexes absent. Recovery depends upon the type and degree of damage. Brachial plexus palsy is further discussed in the chapter entitled "Shoulder Dystocia."

Radial nerve injury: Injury to the nerve of the wrist is often secondary to prolonged intrauterine compression due to a restricted fetal position, difficult birth and instrumental delivery. A hardened lesion with underlying fat necrosis often overlies the site of compression, which is frequently located over the lower portion of the nerve above the outer bony bump at the wrist. There is weakness of the extensors of the wrist, fingers and thumb; thus a typical wrist drop, which looks similar to a lower brachial plexus injury, presents. However, the grasp and other hand functions remain intact with a radial nerve injury.

Paralysis of the diaphragm: Unilateral paralysis occurs most often and is seen with injury to or congenital absence of the phrenic nerves at the 3rd, 4th, and 5th cervical nerve roots. It accompanies 5 to 7% of all brachial plexus injuries. There may be respiratory distress, lack of lung inflation and mediastinal shift. Bilateral paralysis will produce intractable respiratory distress since breathing is so dependent upon the excursion of the diaphragm.

Peroneal nerve injury: Compression of the peroneal nerve by amniotic bands may produce injury leading to "foot-drop," or flaccid limpness of the foot (the counterpart to wrist drop). Both ankle dorsiflexion and eversion are weakened. The injury is located along the superficial course of the nerve around the fibular head. The few cases on record show recovery by 3 to 6 months of age.

Spinal cord injury: Damage to the spinal cord is one of the most devastating of all birth injuries. Seventy percent of the most apparent injuries occur after a breech presentation (a third with spontaneous birth and two-thirds with forcible extraction), but subtle injuries occur much more frequently during manipulation of the baby's head in otherwise easy births. Breech presentations are commonly associated with injury between the 5th cervical and 1st thoracic segment. Cephalic presentations are more often associated with injury among the first 6 cervical segments. The primary cause is excessive traction, sometimes with torsion. Stretch injuries may be exaggerated by hyperflexion or hyperextension of the spine. However, injury to the spinal cord often occurs without any damage to the bones, but with laceration or severance, edema, congestion, bleeding, acute neurological injury and necrosis. Injury to the brainstem and spinal centers usually produces early death. Delayed death may occur when respiration is chronically insufficient. Some infants survive with residual paralysis; this last group is characterized by chronic respiratory depression with hypoxia and associated problems. Spinal cord injury should always be considered in any infant who has apnea, flaccidity and shock, especially if the birth was difficult.

Lumbosacral plexus injury is very rare. It involves both lumbar (L-2 to L-4) and sacral (S-1 to S-3) nerve roots and is associated with traction applied during frank breech births. It usually presents with total paralysis of the involved lower extremity, with reduced reflex response, especially in those babies with predominately lumbar involvement. This is a serious injury with incomplete recovery the rule.

Transporting babies with suspected spinal cord injury: Care should be taken not to move the baby's spine during transport. This can be accomplished by using prefabricated straps of cloth with Velcro fasteners.

1. Lay your straps down horizontally, spacing them so that the top one will be in line with the baby's forehead, the middle one will be level with the nipple line and the lower one will be level with the hips.
2. Place your padded transport surface over the center of the straps, with the long side perpendicular to the straps.
3. Carefully place the baby supine in the center of the transport surface, taking care to move the spine as little as possible.
4. Place two rolled washcloths lengthwise on either side of the baby's head.
5. Bring the end of the top strap across the baby's forehead. Position the closure to the side (not over the baby's head) and tighten it down to stabilize the head, but do not overtighten it.
6. Work the end of next strap up under the baby's arms to the nipple line, leaving the arms unrestrained. Position the closure to the side and tighten it down.
7. Bring the last strap up and over the baby's hips, position the closure to the side and tighten it down.
8. Make sure your strap closures are to the side, near the tray edge, to avoid pinching the baby.
9. Use four small cloth straps to make loops around each wrist and ankle and pin the loops to the towel to stabilize the limbs.
10. Cover the baby and the tray with a space blanket to retain heat.

If an airway must be established, use the jaw thrust maneuver, rather than cervical extension, to avoid further injury. The thermoregulatory ability of the baby may be compromised, so be sure to keep the baby warm.

Sciatic nerve injury: Sciatic nerve injury has been seen in babies after misplaced injection of drugs into the buttocks. Clinical features include deficits of abduction at the hip and of all movements at more distal joints. Necrosis of the buttock may also occur. This injury is distinguished from lumbosacral plexus injury by differing histories and intact hip flexion, adduction and external rotation in the babies with sciatic nerve injury. The prognosis varies, although many infants fail to recover.

Injuries to abdominal organs

A difficult birth may result in injury to the liver or spleen, usually in the form of a laceration or hematoma, and less commonly the adrenal glands. This is especially likely if the baby required manipulation during birth. Risk factors include a previously enlarged liver, breech presentation and the use of significant force. One of the most common abdominal injuries is a liver hematoma, which occurs when the peritoneal support ligaments are damaged by inappropriately applied traction. Alternatively, a hepatic hematoma can develop on the anterior surface of the liver when excessive pressure has been applied to the costal margin. This results in a baby who is poorly perfused because of internal bleeding and has abdominal distension, dullness on percussion and a falling hematocrit. The presence of free bleeding into the peritoneum may be suspected by scrotal discoloration or a dark bluish ring forming around the umbilicus (Cullen's sign). Bruising may also develop over the abdomen, although this does not always occur. Hematoma of the spleen is less common and is usually confined to the subcapsular locus, but has the same signs and symptoms. Both are serious emergencies requiring immediate transport.

Bowel injury leading to an intestinal hematoma forms only rarely. It presents with anemia, difficult feeding, and as the hematoma enlarges, intestinal obstruction, although it usually does not progress to shock.

A renal hemorrhage is confined to the retroperitoneal space. A distended bladder is easily injured if pressure is applied during pelvic manipulation. One of these should be suspected if you find a palpable flank mass with or without blood in the urine after a difficult breech birth.

Adrenal bleeding also collects retroperitoneally. It usually has a delayed onset of symptoms, including a palpable mass and persistent or late jaundice.

Eye injury

Traumatic eye injury occurs fairly often during instrumental births. It has been estimated that 20 to 25% of all babies have some minor eye injury, which is usually limited to bleeding into the sclera. The incidence is increased with difficult births, unusual presentations of the head and prolonged, strained pushing phases. All apparently significant eye injuries or surrounding bruising require immediate and often continued monitoring by a pediatric ophthalmologist. Different types of eye injury include:

Hyphema: Bleeding into the anterior chamber of the eye (highly associated with instrumental birth). Babies with hyphema are at increased risk for developing glaucoma as they mature.

Retinal hemorrhage: The incidence of bleeding into the retina varies from 2.6 to 50%, depending upon the amount of obstetrical intervention. Macular bleeding can increase the risk of subsequent amblyopia (poor vision resulting from inadequate stimulation of the brain).

Corneal injury: Rupture of Descemet's membrane occurs and may result in reduplication of the membrane and striae formation (similar to stretch marks) with resulting myopia, astigmatism, amblyopia, and severe impairment of vision. Corneal abscess can also develop, usually a result of staph infection.

Purtscher retinopathy: Usually the result of a midforceps birth, this consists of retinal edema, soft exudates and bleeding.

Hematic orbital cysts: Akin to blood blisters, these form in the orbit. They can lead to protrusion of the eyeball and may rupture, with resulting inflammation, pain and visual impairment.

Ear injury

Prolonged, difficult labor, cephalopelvic disproportion and unusual presentations may result in ear injuries. A large hematoma in the area of the ear may later produce lumpy thickening and firmness around the ear ("cauliflower ear") if not handled properly. Injury to the middle or inner ear results when the temporal bone is injured. It may lead to impairment of hearing or balance from damage to the ossicles or cochlea.

Soft-tissue injuries of the neck and shoulder girdle

The sternocleidomastoid muscle may be injured during hyperextension of the head. A hematoma develops and then undergoes fibrosis, resulting in a palpable mass after one week of age. This condition (known as **torticollis**) is covered in Volume III of this text.

Vocal cord injury may occur due to excessive head traction in a shoulder dystocia that damages the recurrent laryngeal nerve. Bilateral injury may also result from hypoxic ischemic central nervous system injury. Unilateral paralysis causes a hoarse cry and inspiratory stridor; it is treated with gentle handling and small frequent feedings. Bilateral injury presents with respiratory distress and absent vocalization; it may require surgical intervention. Both types, however, usually resolve on their own.

CRANIAL INJURIES

Cranial injuries can be divided into two broad categories: extracranial (outside the skull), which may include bleeding into the spinal tissues, and intracranial (within the skull). Here is a table giving an overview of these injuries.

SITE OF BLEEDING	RELATIVE FREQUENCY		COMMENTS
	PRETERM	TERM	
EXTRACRANIAL			
Subcutaneous (caput)	✓✓	✓✓✓	Edema in the skin layer with varying amount of bleeding*
Cephalohematoma	✓✓✓	✓✓	Bleeding bet. the periosteum and the skull, self-limited and usually not a problem
Subaponeurotic (subgaleal)	✓✓	✓✓✓	Usually associated with vacuum extraction and clotting disorders*
Retinal	✓	✓✓✓	Only associated with yoni birth, may cause serious eye damage*
Spinal (epidural space)	✓✓✓	✓	Found at autopsy, significance not fully established
INTRACRANIAL			
Extradural	✓	✓✓	Between the inner periosteal layer and the brain, rare and seldom problematic
Subdural			
Supratentorial	✓✓	✓✓✓	Usually from torn bridging veins of superior sagittal sinus, seldom direct cause of death*
Infratentorial	✓✓	✓✓✓	Usually from torn bridging veins of superior sagittal sinus, often fatal*
Subarachnoid			
Convexity	✓✓✓	✓✓✓	Associated with severe clotting disorders
Generalized, primary	✓✓✓	✓✓	Usually due to "anoxic" bleeding of leptomeninges
Generalized, secondary	✓✓✓	✓	Usually due to spread from intraventricular bleeding
Intracerebral			
Cortical	✓✓	✓✓✓	Usually related to infarction
White matter of brain	✓✓✓	✓✓	Venous infarction or spread from ependymal space
Subependymal	✓✓✓	✓	Usually germinal matrix bleeding in a preterm baby
Diffuse	✓✓✓	✓✓✓	Often bleeding from an infarction associated with infection
Cerebellar	✓✓✓	✓✓	Several types and causes; site varies with gestational age
Brain stem	✓✓✓	✓✓	Usually small, multiple bleeding sites; may be related to severe asphyxial gasping
Intraventricular extension			
From subependymal space	✓✓✓	✓	Site varies with gestational age
From another intracerebral site	✓✓✓	✓✓✓	May occur with all other types of intracerebral bleeding away from subependymal layer
From choroid plexus	✓	✓✓✓	Diagnosis by exclusion of other intracerebral sites

✓=Relative occurrence for gestation, but not if it is rare or common; one check in the preterm column and three in the term column show that the lesion is probably unrelated to gestation and is only more frequently seen at term because more babies are born at term.

*Typically associated with a traumatic birth (Table adapted from Pape & Wigglesworth, 1979)

Extracranial Injury

Extracranial injuries are by far the most common among babies born at home. For this reason, they are reviewed in detail in the subchapter entitled "Examining the Head and Neck." Fortunately, the two most common types, caput and cephalohematoma, are rarely serious. A cephalohematoma will require transport only on the rare occasion when the baby shows signs of compromise or when it continues to enlarge to massive proportions. However, a subgaleal hematoma, when severe, can be very serious, although it is exceedingly rare among homeborn babies. Be alert for a swelling that initially appears to be a cephalohematoma but spreads over the scalp, crosses suture lines and extends to the forehead and down to the ears and neck. Symptoms are the same as for any kind of hemorrhaging and may lead to hypovolemic shock. If you suspect a subgaleal hematoma, transport immediately.

PRIMARY FORMS OF TRAUMATIC EXTRACRANIAL HEMORRHAGE				
Lesion	**Characteristics**	**Enlarges after birth**	**Crosses sutures**	**Serious bleeding**
Caput succedaneum	Soft with pitting	No	Yes	No
Cephalohematoma	Firm but fluctuant	Yes	No	Rarely
Subgaleal hematoma	Firm and tense	Yes	Yes	Frequently

Intracranial Injury

Intracranial injury can cause a wide array of signs and symptoms that affect vital functions such as respiration, heart rate and muscle tone. Because of the multisystem nature of the impairment, you should be familiar with the early manifestations of such damage. While less extreme intracranial damage may take days before bleeding builds up enough to apply pressure to the brain and cause symptoms, severe hemorrhage results in obvious signs that something is wrong from birth onward. To minimize damage and restore systemic stability, any baby with suspected intracranial injury requires immediate transport for evaluation and possible decompression of the involved portions of the brain. If blood loss is extreme, the baby may also require transfusion. It is important to correlate the overall systemic disruption with the baby's history, although any baby displaying these abnormalities is in trouble and requires transport, regardless of the reason. The primary predisposing factors include a history of difficult birth, extreme moulding or a breech birth with difficult delivery of the head. Signs and symptoms of severe bleeding include:

- Lethargy or hyperirritability
- Regional, one-sided or complete hypotonia. Asymmetric popliteal angles in a baby born past 40 weeks gestation is seen in unilateral paralysis.
- Seizures
- Stupor (a state of impaired consciousness involving a markedly reduced response to environmental stimuli, with arousal only occurring with continual stimulation) leading to less and less arousability and culminating in coma (a state of profound unconsciousness from which the baby cannot be roused)
- Respiratory problems or apnea
- Rigid, extended or otherwise abnormal postures which may include but are not limited to:
  - Tight popliteal angles (excessive tone compared to that in the rest of the legs) is associated with intracranial bleeding.
  - Asymmetric popliteal angles in a baby born past 40 weeks gestation is found with hypertonia.
  - Isolated flexion of the index finger is associated with focal cerebral injury
- Pupils that are unequally dilated or one or both pupils partially or completely unresponsive to light
- Abnormal eye movements, deviated gaze or abnormal response to the doll's-eye maneuver
- Bulging fontanelle (seen only with massively increased intracranial build-up of blood)
- Slow heart rate
- Abnormal signs and symptoms, especially seizures, that are interspersed with periods of normal behavior and response

Presentation: The timing and onset of the preceding signs and symptoms are related to the location and size of the bleed. The faster the bleeding and the more pressure it applies to adjacent anatomy, the quicker the clinical picture will develop.

Transport: Do not use postural drainage to clear the airway. Lie the baby supine. Be prepared to provide CPR. Keep the baby warm and transport immediately.

Specific types of intracranial injury

Volpe (2001) lists five major categories of clinically important types of intracranial hemorrhage, which are shown in the table below.

LOCATION OF BLEEDING LESION	GESTATIONAL AGE	OVERALL FREQUENCY	GRAVITY
Subdural	> Full term < preterm	Uncommon	Variable
Primary subarachnoid	> Preterm < full term	Common	Variable
Intracerebellar	> Preterm < full term	Uncommon	Serious
Intraventricular	> Preterm < full term	Common	Serious
Miscellaneous intraparenchymal (other than cerebral)	> Full term < preterm	Uncommon	Variable

(How to read Gestational Age column: More common [>] in full term babies; less common [<] in preterm babies.)

Subdural hemorrhage: Minor subdural bleeding may occur in term babies and is usually asymptomatic. Serious subdural hemorrhage, rarely seen today, is the result of trauma and is also most often seen in term babies. The superior cerebral bridging veins are the most common site of hemorrhage. Stresses that rupture these vessels and that tear the tentorium are similar and coexist in many cases. Bleeding can occur from tears in the tentorium and straight sinus, rupture of the great vein of Galen or intratentorial veins, occipital diastasis with bleeding from the occipital sinuses, tears of the falx cerebelli with bleeding from the sagittal sinus, or rupture of the superficial cerebral veins. Signs of subdural bleeding include nonspecific lethargy or irritability. A subdural bleed within the posterior fossa usually results in the appearance of symptoms after a few hours or days of life, with decreased responsiveness, apnea, bradycardia, seizures and signs indicating a rise in intracranial pressure.

Tentorial tears: These tears usually occur just below the junction of the falx on one or both sides. Damage ranges from a separation of superficial fibers to a full-thickness tear that extends to the unattached edge of the tentorium. Tearing may lead to rupture of the lateral sinus, the great vein of Galen (resulting from rupture of the superficial cerebral veins) or the straight transverse sinus (involving laceration of the falx with rupture of the inferior sagittal sinus). Extensive tearing that involves the straight or transverse sinuses leads to subdural hemorrhage. Massive bleeding may also result from tentorial tears involving smaller fetal vessels that have persisted. Such trauma is rare in modern obstetric and midwifery practice because it usually occurs during difficult high forceps deliveries or forceful internal manipulations of the head.

Blood clots that extend into the posterior fossa may cause pressure on the brain, and large hemorrhages in this region result in neurological disturbances from birth, with signs of midbrain and upper pons compression, such as a sideways gaze that is not affected by the doll's-eye maneuver. The pupils will also respond unequally to light, eventually becoming fixed and dilated as the baby goes into a coma. Signs of building pressure in the lower brain stem are reflected in the abnormal eye movement and apnea. The baby may show varying degrees of opisthotonos, including a rigid posture with his head tilted back and arms held stiffly at his side and possibly extension of the trunk and legs. Bradycardia occurs with severe compression. As the clot increases in size, stupor turns into coma. Respiratory arrest may occur and can be fatal.

Laceration of the falx cerebri: Tears of the falx cerebri are also uncommon, but when they do occur, they tend to produce round or oval holes that usually do not extend to the free margin or the sagittal sinuses. As with most tentorial tears, they also arise from cranial trauma but do not lead to massive subdural hemorrhage. Bleeding occurs from the superior sagittal sinus. The development of a hematoma in the longitudinal cerebral fissure causes severe neurological signs as the clot extends infratentorially. Signs and symptoms match those for tentorial tearing.

Tearing of the superficial cerebral vein: This results in bleeding over the cerebral convexities. Three different symptom pictures may develop. The most common result of minor bleeding is either no evidence whatsoever or hyperirritability and a hyperalert state in the baby. The second presentation shows signs of localized impairment of cerebral function, commonly including seizures, weakness on one side of the body with deviation of the gaze toward the normally functioning side. The doll's-eye maneuver remains normal because the brain stem is uninvolved. Pressure on the oculomotor (third cranial) nerve results in impairment or unresponsiveness of the pupil to light on the side of the damage. In the third variety, there may be no evidence of bleeding during early infancy, manifesting only months later with enlargement of the head secondary to chronic subdural bleeding.

Primary subarachnoid hemorrhage: Bleeding results from damage to vessels within the subarachnoid space, located over the cerebral convexities. It is most often due to trauma or hypoxia. While this bleeding most commonly occurs in preterm babies, it can happen in term babies as well.

Small bleeds often go undetected because the baby displays no unusual signs or symptoms. A moderate amount of bleeding can cause seizure activity due to the build-up of pressure on the brain. The baby appears otherwise well and is stable between the seizures.

Massive subarachnoid hemorrhage is rare and is usually seen only after severe asphyxia and trauma. When it does occur, rapid deterioration and death are frequent sequelae. Those infants who survive may then develop hydrocephalus because of a decrease in spinal fluid absorption secondary to swelling and inflammation of the arachnoid villi in the subarachnoid space.

Intracerebellar hemorrhage: This occurs primarily among preterm infants, from a multiplicity of causes, usually circulatory problems of various sorts. In term infants, the pathogenesis is primarily associated with traumatic events such as a difficult breech birth or forceps delivery.

The clinical background is usually one of difficult breech birth or hypoxia at birth, although a few infants have no apparent associated factors. Onset is varied and ranges from the first day to two to three weeks of age. In term infants, onset within the first 24 hours is most common. Early onset in a preterm baby is ominous and usually occurs in those who die. Signs of brain stem compression (especially apnea, respiratory irregularities and sometimes bradycardia) and of obstructed cerebral spinal fluid circulation (such as bulging fontanelles and separated sutures), along with skew deviation of the eyes, facial paresis, intermittent tonic extension of the limbs, opisthotonic posture and a degree of quadriparesis, are often presenting evidence of this problem. Rapid progression and death is most often seen in small preterm babies. Slower deterioration or stabilization and improvement may also occur, especially in larger babies.

Periventricular and intraventricular hemorrhage: The spinal-fluid-filled space within the ventricles is called the **intraventricular space**. The area immediately outside the ventricles is called the **periventricular space**. After the 28th week, periventricular hemorrhage (PVH) occurs most often in the area of the caudate nucleus (a long, thick portion of gray matter that protrudes into each lateral ventricle) and the interventricular foramen (foramen of Monro), which is a short passageway centered under the inside border of each lateral ventricle and connecting them to the third ventricle of the diencephalon (Blackburn, 2003). The **choroid membrane** (tela choroidea) is a specialized portion of the pia mater that covers the ependyma, lining the roof and the medial wall of the lateral ventricles of the cerebral hemispheres. The portion of this structure that lines the third, fourth and lateral ventricles of the brain is called the **choroid plexus**. It is the predominant site of intraventricular hemorrhage (IVH) in term infants, with trauma being the most frequent cause (Blackburn, 2003).

Periventricular and intraventricular bleeding are the most common causes of intracranial hemorrhage in the region of the germinal matrix (described in the chapter entitled "Features of Fetal Anatomy Pertinent to the Birth Process") in preterm babies. Bleeding may begin in the fragile periventricular germinal matrix and be confined to this region, or it may burst into the adjacent ventricle; if bleeding is extensive enough, it may result in distension of the lateral ventricles. The surrounding cerebral tissue may also be damaged, leading to parenchymal clot or infarction.

The development of intraventricular hemorrhage in preterm infants may be related to abrupt increases in cerebral blood flow. The possibility of intraventricular damage is increased when the cord is clamped too quickly because the systemic pressure can suddenly rise to dangerous levels. This is most likely to be a problem in otherwise healthy preterm infants, who have more fragile cerebral vasculature. A similar problem arises for distressed infants in whom normal autoregulation of blood flow is impaired. Increased carbon dioxide levels and hypoxia are potent vasodilators. Faulty autoregulation following perinatal asphyxia may develop when maximal vasodilation has already occurred as a result of asphyxia. Maximally dilated arterioles and cerebral capillaries are more directly affected by arterial pressures. Therefore, if arterial pressures suddenly increase, the capillaries rupture because they are already stretched to their limit. This is less likely to occur when the umbilical cord is left intact until the baby has fully stabilized because the newborn system can then backwash blood via the umbilical vein, virtually eliminating the possibility of intolerable pressures building in these delicate cerebral capillaries. To further reduce the risk, ensure that the baby is not held with her head dependent and that the placenta is kept level with the baby.

A large intraventricular bleed often leads to hydrocephalus. Bleeding causes the arachnoid villi, which normally absorb spinal fluid, to become inflamed or scarred due to irritation from the blood and the particulate matter that accompanies it. This results in obstruction of fluid absorption. Less frequently, this may occur at the outlet of the third ventricle, when debris and swelling of the irritated tissues result in obstructed flow.

Two clinical presentations have been associated with this type of bleeding. Which one develops is thought to be related to the severity of the hemorrhage. The most severe and least common presentation involves focal or multifocal seizures (65% of cases), stupor that progresses to coma, shallow breathing that progresses to apnea and pupils that are fixed and unresponsive to light. The doll's-eye maneuver is abnormal. The eyes are fixed when the baby is lifted to an upright position, and there is a pronounced lack of muscle tone. As bleeding continues, the hematocrit falls, as do the blood pressure and heart rate. Other symptoms include fever and jitteriness. Metabolic acidosis and a bulging anterior fontanelle from the blood build-up are also noted on exam.

The baby with less severe bleeding displays signs of progressively decreasing alertness, hypotonia, lethargy, subtly abnormal eye movements and only a partially normal response to the doll's-eye maneuver. This decline in the baby's condition occurs over a number of hours, interspersed with periods of apparent stability and followed by a recurrence of these abnormal findings; this may go on for several days postpartum. In other cases, bleeding may be so minor as to only be detectable on ultrasound exam.

On rare occasions, intraventricular hemorrhage is also found in term babies, most commonly in the choroid plexus. Trauma and hypoxia are thought to be the primary causes. Bleeding is usually due to infiltration from major hemorrhagic infarctions, rupture of abnormal blood vessels, tumors or clotting disorders.

Miscellaneous causes of neonatal intracranial hemorrhage

Epidural bleeding: This rare injury results from detachment of the dura from the internal cranial periosteum with rupture of the dural emissary veins; 30 to 40% occur without associated skull fractures. Neonatal epidural bleeding is usually venous. This hemorrhage may be extremely difficult to diagnose, as it may have a prolonged asymptomatic period of up to several days postpartum. Early signs include a falling hematocrit, tense anterior fontanelle and increasing head circumference. Later, brainstem compression results in changes in pupillary response.

Hemorrhagic infarction: This lesion results when injured, although functional, capillaries within an ischemic infarct rupture due to an arterial obstruction from an embolus, an increase in venous pressure, or abnormal clotting.

Coagulation defect: Any type of coagulation defect may result in intracranial bleeding.

Vascular defect: Congenital arterial aneurysm and arteriovenous malformation are the two major forms of vascular defects that occur in the newborn. These commonly present with signs of increased intracranial pressure, focal motor seizures (simple, partial seizure with localized motor activity), congestive heart failure with cranial bruit, opisthotonic posture and paraplegia. Infants with coarctation of the aorta (a heart defect), are at particular risk for intracranial bleeding, although such a complication is rare.

Intracranial teratoma: This condition does not cause hemorrhage but must be considered when a baby presents with the signs and symptoms of intracranial trauma. This rare type of teratoma usually occurs as an isolated defect and is most frequently identified in childhood, rather than infancy. It most commonly arises from the pineal gland above the tentorium within the third ventricle or from within the subfrontal or subtemporal areas. The differential diagnosis includes intracranial hemorrhage, TORCH infections, ischemic brain necrosis or other intracranial tumors. These tumors are benign but can be locally invasive, with destruction of the base of the skull, the orbit and pharynx; they may also grow down the neck. The head is often enlarged, giving the impression of hydrocephalus. The prognosis is grim, as most babies with an intracranial teratoma do not survive.

Skull Fracture

Linear fractures

Normal babies can get skull fractures from extreme compression during birth, usually associated with instrumental delivery. Most are asymptomatic. They may be linear or depressed. A linear fracture exists when the edges are flush (not depressed) and are most commonly found on one of the parietal bones, followed by the occipital and frontal bones. Venous sinuses may be torn by the edge of a fractured or dislocated bone, leading to hemorrhaging that may produce a cephalohematoma, bleeding into the epidural or subdural space or a cerebral contusion. However, serious complications are rare. Osteogenesis imperfecta is a congenital disorder characterized by extremely brittle, fragile bones. These babies may experience fractures during a normal birth or even during gestation.

Depressed fractures

These occur when the skull becomes indented from external pressure, frequently over a parietal bone. Most are not associated with an actual fracture. While there are successful reports of a variety of low-tech remedies for elevating such depressions (including finger techniques and the application of suction with a breast pump or vacuum extractor as well as spontaneous resolution), the lesion should be evaluated with X-rays first to make sure no actual fracture is present. Some lesions may require surgical intervention and may also be associated with subdural, epidural, and even intracerebral bleeding. Fragments of fractured bone that are depressed more than 5 mm may result in focal encephalomalacia (abnormal softness of the cerebral parenchyma often due to ischemia or infarction), cerebral swelling, and the development of epilepsy. Skull fractures can also lead to leakage of spinal fluid from the nose, ear or mouth.

Occipital osteodiastasis

This the most common severe trauma in babies who die following forceful hyperextension of the head during extraction of the aftercoming head in a breech birth. It consists of a particularly dangerous disruption of the innominate synchondrodial joint that occurs when the edge of the squamous occipital bone is torn and pushed forward over the posterior edge of the condyle bone on one or both sides, leading to compression and sometimes tearing of the occipital venous sinus. The amount of bleeding that results varies widely because the occipital sinus varies in size and may be absent. Displacement of the bones narrows the foramen magnum and, depending upon the extent of the displacement, can compress the posterior spinal cord. The resultant bleeding escapes into the infratentorial posterior fossa areas, producing the same clinical signs that are noted with tentorial bleeding. In contrast, small bleeds into the posterior fossa will cause no symptoms initially. However, continued seepage and gradual build-up of blood with increasing intracranial pressure over the hours or days following birth leads to signs of impairment of brain stem function, causing respiratory depression, apnea, abnormal eye movements, partial paralysis of the face and, usually, seizures. Unless done with care, an autopsy may miss this lesion, as the bones of the skull vault are typically quite disrupted by the usual sequence of dissection by the time this part of the skull is revealed for examination (Pape & Wigglesworth, 1979).

Type of Fracture	Typical Location	Comments
Linear	Parietal bones, extending radially along the break line	Requires an extreme crushing force; seen with CPD difficult forceps deliveries. Any type of cranial bleeding may accompany this injury; may tear underlying dura with herniation of the brain or meninges (forming a leptomeningocele, which is a collection of blood in the pia mater layer). Most heal well.
Depressed	Parietal bones	Usually good outcome if corrected right away; may be associated with a small fracture.
Occipital osteodiastasis	Squamous and lateral parts of the occipital bone	Suboccipital pressure during breech extraction. Severe tearing leads to gross subdural bleeding; if severe, it is usually fatal.

DRUG WITHDRAWAL

Most drug withdrawal symptoms occur within 72 hours of birth, the range is from shortly after birth to as late as two weeks postpartum. Generally, the closer to birth the mother has used the drug, the greater the delay in the onset of symptoms in the baby.

Presentation

The mnemonic WITHDRAWAL can be used to help remember the symptoms of drug withdrawal in the neonate.

W–wakefulness
I–irritability
T–tremulousness, temperature instability, tachypnea
H–hyperactivity, high-pitched persistent cry, hyperacusis (abnormally sensitive hearing), hyperreflexia, hypertonus
D–diarrhea, diaphoresis (sweating), disorganized sucking
R–rub marks (from irritable fidgeting), respiratory distress, rhinorrhea (nasal discharge)
A–apneic attacks, autonomic nervous system dysfunction
W–an abnormal weight loss or failure to gain weight in the days and weeks following birth
A–alkalosis (respiratory)
L–lacrimation (excessive tearing)

The initial presentation of drug withdrawal can be very subtle in infants. However, it may become increasingly apparent over time. It is typical for symptoms to cycle, becoming worse and then subsiding for a time. Increased muscle tone and tremulousness are generally the earliest signs to appear. Hyperirritability or respiratory distress become more severe and withdrawal progresses. These reactions may mimic other problems such as infection, hypoglycemia or other metabolic disorders. The Moro and deep tendon reflexes will both be exaggerated and reflect an overall increased response to stimuli when the baby is awake. When the baby does sleep, he may experience longer periods of active sleep (rather than quiet sleep) because of the nervous system irritability, possibly reflecting decreased control of the nervous system. These babies may also have overvigorous sucking reflexes and fist sucking; however, other babies will exhibit decreased rates of sucking, nursing and percentage of time nursing during withdrawal. Not nursing, combined with the diarrhea and vomiting these babies also typically suffer, is a setup for dehydration and electrolyte imbalance.

Other signs and symptoms are less specific. These include autonomic dysfunction, respiratory distress, fever, flushing, yawning and mottled skin coloration. Nasal stuffiness is probably the number-one cause of tachypnea. Seizure activity tends to occur later in the withdrawal process.

Care and transport: If you suspect drug withdrawal in the infant, question the mother about possible drug use. Hopefully you will already know of a history of drug use from thorough prenatal care, but you may be in a position of caring for women whose care you have not provided during pregnancy. Depending upon the condition and stability of the baby as well as the drug in question, transport may be necessary. A neonatal consult should be sought. A meconium specimen will give the most accurate information about long-term exposure because it contains metabolites accumulated over a longer period of time, whereas urine will give more information about recent exposures (Ostrea et al., 1992). A sample of the first meconium passed should be collected in a clean specimen container. More about babies and drug withdrawal will be found in Volume III of this text.

RECOGNIZING BABIES WITH POSSIBLE GENETIC OR CHROMOSOMAL DISORDERS

One out of every 600 babies has some type of chromosomal syndrome. There are also hundreds of genetic defects, which no midwife is expected to be able to definitively diagnose. When three or more organ systems are malformed, the chance that there is a chromosomal abnormality is high. The following signs are common among many different defects. When several are present, it should raise your suspicions regarding the possibility of a chromosomal or genetically related condition. Whenever you have a question about a baby who has subtle differences, take a careful look at the parents' features and ask them again about family history. The following findings from your physical exam point to a syndrome, sequence, chromosomal or genetic disorder:

General impressions: Unusual visage, inappropriate size or structure of one or more external parts. Disparity of relationship of one part to another or of paired structures.

Skin color: Unusual overall color or unequal color distribution over the body (mottling, pallor)

Body proportion: Head, limbs and torso disproportionate

Size for dates: Small for gestational age

Arms and legs: Abnormal length or position; extreme bowing of limbs or digits; missing bones; extra, fused, webbed or missing digits; abnormal palmar or plantar creases; hyperflexion or limited flexion in the joints; webbing behind knees

Head: Cranial defects, premature closure of suture lines, micro- or macrocephaly, unusual hair texture or posterior hair line, continuous brow line across the orbital ridges, bald spots, abnormal hair whorl, raw scalp lesions (cutis aplasia), flat or bossed occiput

Face: Flat profile or midline elevation

Eyes: Droopy eyelids, abnormal pupils, cataracts, widely or narrowly set eyes, abnormal slant, small eye fissures

Nose: Flat nasal bridge, wide alae, choanal atresia

Mouth: Cleft lip or palate; smooth philtrum; high, arched palate; large tongue

Chin: Small or recessed

Ears: Low-set, rotated backward, poorly formed

Neck: Webbed, short, fusion of the cervical vertebrae

Chest: Small rib cage, abnormally placed nipples, missing pectoris muscle or clavicle

Abdomen: Two-vessel cord, failure of abdominal contents to reenter abdomen during development (especially with omphalocele, much less often with gastroschisis)

Genitourinary: Hypospadias, atypical genitalia, chordee (males)

Anus: Imperforate, misplaced, prolapsed

Spine: Curvature, neural tube defects

Trisomy 21 (Down syndrome)

This is the most common chromosomal defect, followed by trisomies 18, 13 and 15. A constellation of findings point to such syndromes, although all signs do not appear in the same infant. Most of the signs in the following table appear in over 70% of Down babies. Cardiac defects, especially atrioventricular canal and gastrointestinal defects, are more likely as well. Trisomies 13 and 18 display some of these signs, but these babies tend to have more major systemic defects than those with trisomy 21. The table on the next page outlines major findings for these common genetic defects.

Transport procedures for babies with suspected genetic or chromosomal abnormalities

Immediate transport is not necessary if the baby is stable and able to nurse, there are no exposed organs, no evidence of gastrointestinal or urogenital obstruction, the heart sounds good, color is normal and the sex of the baby can be clearly determined. Transport should take place soon after birth (within several hours, depending upon what other abnormalities appear to be involved). Even apparently stable babies can decompensate quickly because of unrecognized defects, such as major organ anomalies or associated metabolic imbalances. The baby should be evaluated within the first 12 hours of birth, regardless of how well the baby may appear.

Findings	Trisomy 21	Trisomy 18	Trisomy 13	Trisomy 15
Eponym	Down syndrome	Edward syndrome	Patau syndrome	Trisomy 15
Incidence per live births	1 in 800	1 in 8000	1 in 15,000	1 in 15,000
Prenatal associations				
Reduced fetal activity	Occasionally	Frequent	Occasionally	Occasionally
Preterm/term/postterm	Usually born at term	33% / 33% / 33%	Rarely an issue	Rarely an issue
Polyhydramnios	Occasionally	Frequent	Occasionally	Occasionally
Small placenta	Occasionally	Frequent	Occasionally	Occasionally
Low birthweight	May be symmetric SGA	Frequent	Occasionally	Occasionally
Single umbilical artery	Occasionally	Frequent	Frequent	Frequent
Neurologic disorders				
Tone	Hypotonia	Hypertonia	Hypo- or hypertonia	Hypo- or hypertonia
Seizures/apnea	Occasionally	Occasionally	Frequent	Frequent
Hearing impairment	Occasionally	Frequent	Frequent	Frequent
Cranial defects	Mild microcephaly, flat occiput, 3 fontanelles, abnormal palate	Microcephaly, prominent occiput	Microcephaly, sloping forehead, scalp defects over occiput, holoprosencephaly (single forebrain lobe)	Microcephaly; small, posteriorly displaced mandible; high, arched palate
Eye defects	Upslanting, epicanthal folds, Brushfield spots	Small palpebral fissures, corneal opacity	Small, close-set; iris coloboma; retinal dysplasia	
Outer ear defects	Small, low-set, folded upper helix	Low-set, malformed	Low-set, malformed	Malformed
Characteristic facial features	Protruding tongue; large cheeks; low, flat nasal bridge	Small mouth and tongue	Cleft lip and palate	Large nose; broad bridge; upturned nares; small mouth; narrow lips
Skeletal features and other identifying characteristics	Hands square and spade-like, 5th finger incurved with missing crease, Simian crease (50-60%), may have ulnar loops on all fingerprints; gap between toes 1 and 2. Excess nuchal skin, short stature.	Hands clenched, absent 5th finger distal crease, occasional Simian crease, hypoplastic nails, may have low arch fingerprints. Rocker-bottom feet. Short stature, thin ribs.	Hands clenched, Simian crease, flattish fingernails, extra digits placed behind usual location, occasionally hypoplastic toenails	Clenched hands; overriding fingers and toes; clubfeet; widely spaced nipples; short sternum; abnormal number of ribs; short, webbed neck; anteriorly displaced anus
Heart defects	40% (w/pallor or marbling)	60%	80%	Yes
Abdominal defects	Duodenal atresia (occasionally)	Omphalocele (occasionally)	Omphalocele (occasionally)	
Other defects		Polycystic kidneys	Other genetic anomalies, polycystic kidneys	Anteriorly displaced anus
Expected life span	Long-term survival (death usually due to heart defects)	90% die in first year of life	80% die in first year of life	Usually lethal prior to birth; survivors have mosaic form

References and Further Reading on Assessing, Supporting and Transporting the Baby in Need of Specialized Care

References Used in Multiple Chapters throughout This Section

Avery G, et al., eds. NEONATOLOGY: PATHOPHYSIOLOGY AND MANAGEMENT OF THE NEWBORN, 5th ed. Lippincott, Williams & Wilkins, Philadelphia PA, 1999.

Donn S, Faix R, eds. NEONATAL EMERGENCIES. Futura Pub, Mt. Kisco NY, 1991.

Duster M. "Pulmonary hypertension, high altitude," http://www.emedicine.com/ped/topic2783.htm, updated Sept 25, 2002. Accessed Apr 4, 2004.

Fletcher MA. PHYSICAL DIAGNOSIS IN NEONATOLOGY. Lippincott-Raven, Philadelphia PA, 1998.

Freeman N, et al., eds. SURGERY OF THE NEWBORN. Churchill Livingstone, Edinburgh UK, 1994.

Hatch D, et al. THE SURGICAL NEONATE: ANAESTHESIA AND INTENSIVE CARE, 3rd ed. Edward Arnold, London UK, 1995.

Illingworth R. THE DEVELOPMENT OF THE INFANT AND YOUNG CHILD: NORMAL AND ABNORMAL, 4th ed. E & S Livingstone, Ltd, Edinburgh UK, 1970.

Illingworth R. THE DEVELOPMENT OF THE INFANT AND YOUNG CHILD: NORMAL AND ABNORMAL, 6th ed. Churchill Livingstone, Edinburgh UK, 1975.

Illingworth R. THE DEVELOPMENT OF THE INFANT AND YOUNG CHILD: NORMAL AND ABNORMAL, 9th ed. Churchill Livingstone, Edinburgh UK, 1987.

Jaimovich D, Vidyasagar D, eds. HANDBOOK OF PEDIATRIC AND NEONATAL TRANSPORT MEDICINE. Hanley & Belfus, Inc, Philadelphia PA, 1996.

Marino B, Wernovsky G. Chapter 34: "Preoperative and postoperative care of the infant with critical congenital heart disease," Avery G, et al., eds. NEONATOLOGY: PATHOPHYSIOLOGY AND MANAGEMENT OF THE NEWBORN, 5th ed. Lippincott, Williams & Wilkins, Philadelphia PA, 1999.

Milner R, Herber S. A COLOUR ATLAS OF THE NEWBORN. Wolfe Medical Pub Ltd, London UK, 1984.

Morris R, Wood W, eds. OXFORD TEXTBOOK OF SURGERY, 2nd ed., VOL. 3. Oxford U, Oxford UK, 2000.

Nakayama D, et al., eds. CRITICAL CARE OF THE SURGICAL NEWBORN. Futura Pub Co, Armonk NY, 1997.

O'Doherty N. ATLAS OF THE NEWBORN, 2nd ed. MTP Press, Boston MA, 1985.

O'Doherty N. NEUROLOGICAL EXAMINATION OF THE NEWBORN: A ROUTINE FOR ALL. MTP Press, Lancaster UK, 1986.

Polin R, Spitzer A, eds. FETAL AND NEONATAL SECRETS. Hanley & Belfus, Inc, Philadelphia PA, 2001.

Rudolph A. ATLAS OF THE NEWBORN, VOLS. 1-5. BC Decker, Inc, Hamilton ONT, Canada, 1997.

Volpe J. NEUROLOGY OF THE NEWBORN, 4th ed. WB Saunders, Philadelphia PA, 2001.

Ziai M, et al., ASSESSMENT OF THE NEWBORN: A GUIDE FOR THE PRACTITIONER, 1st ed. Little, Brown and Co, Boston MA, 1984.

Neonatal Transport: An Overview

Donn SM, et al. "Neonatal transport," CURR PROBL PEDIATR, 15(4);1-65, Apr, 1985.

Vyas H, et al. "Efficacy of face mask resuscitation: does it lead to gastric distension?," ARCH DIS CHILD, 58(5); 373-375, May 1983.

Complicated Respiratory Distress

Beck W, Morsay D. "Eventration of the diaphragm," AMA ARCH SURG, 65(4);557-563, Oct, 1952.

Drew J, et al. "Neonatal whole blood hyperviscosity: the important factor influencing later neurologic function is the viscosity and not the polycythemia," CLIN HEMORHEOL MICROCIRC, 17(1);67-72, Jan-Feb, 1997.

Dunn P. "Perinatal factors influencing adaptation to extrauterine life," pp. 119-123, in Belfort P, et al., eds. ADVANCES IN GYNECOLOGY AND OBSTETRICS, VOL 5: PREGNANCY AND LABOR. Proceedings of the 12th World Congress of Gynecology and Obstetrics, Rio de Janeiro, Oct, 1988. Parthenon Pub, Carnforth Lancs UK, 1989.

Konner M, Worthman C. "Nursing frequency, gonadal function, and birth spacing among !Kung hunter gatherers," SCIENCE, 207(4432);788-791, Feb 15, 1980.

Morley G. "How the cord clamp injures your baby's brain," www.cordclamping.com, Feb 26, 2002a.

Morley G. "Respiratory Distress Syndrome," letter in response to an e-medicine article posted on www.emedicine.com, letter forwarded via e-mail, Aug 21, 2002b.

Cyanosis, Rapid Breathing, Congestive Heart Failure, Shock or Arrhythmia: Detecting Heart Defects in Newborns

Enning C. "Birth on demand," all day workshop on waterbirth, MIDWIFERY TODAY conf., Springfield OR, Mar, 2003.

Flanagan M, et al. Chapter 33: "Cardiac disease," in Avery G, et al., eds. NEONATOLOGY: PATHOPHYSIOLOGY AND MANAGEMENT OF THE NEWBORN, 5th ed. Lippincott, Williams & Wilkins, Philadelphia PA, 1999.

Litwin B. "Ectopia cordis," CHILDREN'S HOSPITAL OF WISCONSIN HEART MATTERS, 2(3), July, 1999, www.chw.org/Templates/PPF/ParentID/638/NID/638/PageID/1046/Mag.asp, accessed April 17, 2003.

Marino B, Wernovsky G. Chapter 34: "Preoperative and postoperative care of the infant with critical congenital heart disease," in Avery G, et al., eds. NEONATOLOGY: PATHOPHYSIOLOGY AND MANAGEMENT OF THE NEWBORN, 5th ed. Lippincott, Williams & Wilkins, Philadelphia PA, 1999.

DETECTING AND DIFFERENTIATING NEWBORN HYPOGLYCEMIA, SEPSIS AND HEART DEFECTS

Pati N, et al. "Transient neonatal hyperglycemia," INDIAN PEDIATR, 38(8), 898-901, Aug, 2001.

ABDOMINAL DISTENSION AND VOMITING: DETECTING GASTROINTESTINAL DEFECTS

Holgersen LO. "The etiology of spontaneous gastric perforation of the newborn: a reevaluation," J PEDIATR SURG, 16(4 S1);608-613, Aug, 1981.

Kamagata A, et al. "Peptic ulcer disease in neonates," J JAPANESE SOC PEDIATR SUR, 26;648-654, 1990.

VISIBLE DEFECTS AND ABNORMALITIES

Brenner B, et al., eds. WOMEN'S ISSUES IN THROMBOSIS AND HEMOSTASIS. Martin Dunitz, Ltd, London UK, 2002.

CRANIAL INJURIES

Blackburn S. MATERNAL, FETAL, AND NEONATAL PHYSIOLOGY: A CLINICAL PERSPECTIVE, 2nd ed. WB Saunders, Philadelphia PA, 2003.

Pape K, Wigglesworth J. HEMORRHAGE, ISCHAEMIA, AND THE PERINATAL BRAIN, Clinics in Dev Med (69/70). JB Lippincott Co, Philadelphia PA, 1979.

DRUG WITHDRAWAL

Ostrea E, et al. "Drug screening of newborns by meconium analysis: a large-scale, prospective, epidemiologic study," PEDIATR, 89(1);107-113, Jan, 1992.

PRODUCT AND EQUIPMENT SOURCES AND EDUCATIONAL RESOURCES

Birth Equipment and Remedies

Belly binder: Make your own from flannel, cotton, muslin or use a Rebozo.

Birth balls: Cutting Edge Press is a source for all sizes and shapes of birthing balls. Contact them at 287 Whiteface Mountain Dr., Johnson, VT, 05656, Phone: 802-635-2142. Web site: cuttingedgepress.net.

Birth Sling: Penny Simkin Productions, 1100 23rd Ave, E, Seattle, WA 98112, Phone: 206-325-1419. Web site: www.pennysimkin.com.

Birth tubs: Waterbirth International, PO Box 5578, Lighthouse Point, FL 33074. Phone: 954-821-9125, Web site: www.waterbirth.org. Yourwaterbirth.com also has waterbirth tubs and accessories for purchase on the web.

Burn box: Plain and decorated pine burn boxes for burning the cord in two can be gotten from www.cordburning.com.

Chart forms: Cascade Healthcare Products is the sole distributor of the MAWS chart forms that were developed by the midwives of Washington state. See contact information under supplies and equipment below.

deBy birth support stool: Seacoast Midwifery Services LLC, PO Box 381, Barrington, NH 03825. Web site: www.birthchair.com.

Laryngeal Mask Airway (LMA): Contact LMA North America, Inc., 4660 La Jolla Village Dr., Suite 900, San Diego CA 92122. Web site: www.lmana.com. Their classic model has the most sizes, including neonatal.

Mercury resuscitation equipment: Manufactured by Mercury Medical, 11300 49th St., Clearwater, FL 33762. Phone: 800-237-6418, Web site: www.mercurymed.com. Cascade HealthCare distributes this equipment.

Rebozo: To obtain a traditional rebozo shawl, contact Terra Experience, 2140 Regent St., Madison, WI 53726. Phone: 608-231-1247. Web site: www.terraexperience.org. To purchase a DVD and other materials about how to use a Rebozo in pregnancy and labor (available in both English and Spanish), contact Cutting Edge Press (see birth balls, above for contact information).

Second-stage enhancer (push and pull): NEEDS REVISION Diane Holmes, CPM, Gentle Childbirth, 832 N St., Rd. 15, Wabash, IN 46992. Phone: 260-563-9213. Admidwifecpm@comcast.net

Supplies and equipment: Cascade HealthCare Products is the largest specialty supplier to midwives in the United States. They have instruments, supplies and some textbooks. Contact them at 1826 NW 18th Ave, Portland, OR 97209. Phone orders: 800-443-9942. Customer service: 503-595-1720, Fax: 503-595-1726. Web site: www.cascade1.com. A number of smaller, cottage-industry suppliers operate in the US as well; check with your local midwifery community, for details regarding regional sources of supplies.

Sustainable healthcare products and practices: For information on this topic, there is still some information at www.sustainablehospitals.org but the site is no longer being updated.

TENS units: Available through several British suppliers as well as Cascade Healthcare Products in the US. See contact information under supplies and equipment, above.

Western Gas equipment: Western Gas produces a full line of fine-quality, innovative oxygen equipment. Contact them for a local distributor: 875 Bassett Rd., Westlake, OH, 44145-1142. Phone: 440-871-2160 or 800-783-7890. Fax: 440-871-2197.

Remedies

Aromatherapy: The American College of Healthcare Sciences, Portland, OR offers state-approved vocational training for herbology, aromatherapy and flower essences. Contact them at 800-487-8839 or visit their web site at www.achs.edu This is also an excellent source for the highest quality medicinal essential oils and other remedies.

Flower essences: Most but not all of the flower essences listed in this book can be purchased from Essencesonline. Web site: www.essencesonline.com. The ones they do not offer are listed below:

Flower essences of Fox Mountain: web site: www.foxmountain.net

Perelandra Flower Essences, Ltd., Jeffersonton, VA; US & Canada: **800-960-8806;** Overseas & Mexico: (540) 937-2153 web site: www.perelandra-ltd.com

Starmen of Kauài: Starmen Unlimited, HI, Telephone: 808-828-2166 Web site: www.starmen.com

www.flowervr.com also has a number of remedies from a variety of suppliers.

Herbal preparations: Frontier Natural Products Co-op is a great place to get reasonably priced, responsibly harvested herbs for making your own remedies and herbal bath packs. Website: www.frontiercoop.com.

To Enhance Your Study

Anatomical models

Anatomical Chart Company: This company has now been taken over by Lippincott Williams and Wilkins. They sell a finely featured fetal skull model. Website: www.lww.com. Enter the product code number 420r in the search bar.

Childbirth Graphics: This company sells an array of pelvises and dolls. They can be contacted at: www.childbirthgraphics.com

Denoyer-Gebbert: This company has the same fine quality fetal skull (product no. SK38). They also carry several nice looking female pelvic models but it is impossible to tell their actual size just from looking at a picture on the web, and most pelvic models are small in comparison to those of well-fed Western-European and American women because they are modeled after small Asian specimens. Web site: www.denoyer.com.

Educational and Scientific Products Ltd. manufactures the fine fetal skulls mentioned above in the UK. If you are in the UK or Europe, order directly from them at www.espmodels.co.uk; model no. ZJY-420-R.

Also, check the web with the search engine Google, using the search criteria such as "fetal doll model," "anatomical models," and "female pelvic model" to see what you can find.

Classes and seminars of interest

Emerson Training Seminars: This group offers training programs for parents and professionals that focus on specialized treatment procedures for prenatal and birth traumas. The group has been in existence for twenty-five years and has trained hundreds of people worldwide. The programs teach how prenatal and birth traumas can be healed during infancy, childhood, and adulthood. Trainings are offered in the US, Canada, and Europe. Phone: 707-763-7024. Web site: www.emersonbirthrx.com.

Resuscitation classes for homebirth midwives: Karen Strange, a CPM and homebirth midwife who is also a certified American Heart Association instructor in infant resuscitation, teaches classes far more thorough and relevant to the midwifery style and practice setting than classes taught by practitioners who have never attended a homebirth. Karen's enthusiasm for her topic is infectious. She includes controversial issues in her classes as well as protocols and techniques long considered standard practice in other industrialized countries, such as the initial inflation breaths discussed in this text. Karen travels around the country to teach Integrative Resuscitation of the Newborn. Website: www.newbornbreath.com.

Textbooks and periodicals

BREECH BIRTH: WOMAN-WISE by Maggie Banks: This wonderful book is available from www.midwiferytoday.com.

THE LABOR PROGRESS HANDBOOK by Penny Simkin and Ruth Ancheta: One of the most important childbirth assistance books ever written; the current edition is a must-have for your birth bag. It is small and slim, perfect for popping into your pocket for discrete reference when supporting women in the hospital post transport. Available at Penny Simkin Inc., 1100 23rd Ave. East, Seattle, WA, 98112. Phone: 206-325-1419. All of Penny's materials can be found on her web site at www.PennySimkin.com.

LET BIRTH BE BORN AGAIN! by Jean Sutton: This book contains the same content as the first book she co-authored with Pauline Scott entitled OPTIMAL FETAL POSITIONING, plus much more and is better edited. Find out about these and other titles by Jean Sutton at her website: optimal-foetal-positioning.co.nz.

MIDWIFERY TODAY: The best periodical for midwives working at home, chock-full of valuable information. They also sell a variety of books, including those by Maggie Banks and Jean Sutton. Web site: www.midwiferytoday.com.

TREATING BIRTH TRAUMA DURING INFANCY by William Emerson, PhD: Emerson Training Seminars offers a number of books and publications that describe prenatal and birth traumas, the psychological impact, and psychological and spiritual approaches to healing. A series of three videos show how birth trauma can be treated during infancy. Available through Emerson Training Seminars, 707 763-7024 or 763-4940, 3940 Bodega Ave., Petaluma, CA. 94952 Web site: www.emersonbirthrx.com. Also check their listing under "Classes and seminars of interest." (Mention my name for the possibility of a discount.)

PLACENTA: THE GIFT OF LIFE by Cornelia Enning. The placenta book is available through MidwiferyToday.com.

World Health Organization publications: These are informative from an international perspective. They may be ordered, and, in some cases downloaded from their website: www.who.int. It can be hard to tract down the books on pregnancy, try entering relevant keywords in their search bar.

Birth-related audio-visual presentations

RESOLVING SHOULDER DYSTOCIA by Gail Tully. Order this and other amazingly helpful materials from her website at www.spinningbabies.com.

SPIRITUAL MIDWIFERY DVD; produced by The Farm midwives. It is available at The Farm web site: www.farmcatalogue.com.

NORMALIZING THE BREECH DELIVERY by Valerie El Halta and Rahima Baldwin is available through Midwifery Today.

INDEX

NOTES: